ADAMS AND STASHAK'S LAMENESS IN HORSES

SIXTH EDITION

ADAMS AND STASHAK'S LAMENESS IN HORSES

SIXTH EDITION

GARY M. BAXTER, VMD, MS

DIPLOMATE ACVS

Department of Clinical Sciences, Veterinary Teaching Hospital
College of Veterinary Medicine and Biomedical Sciences
Colorado State University
Ft. Collins, Colorado

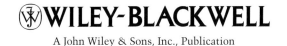

A John Wiley & Sons, Inc., Publication

This edition first published 2011 © 2011 by Blackwell Publishing, Ltd.
First through Fifth editions © 1962, 1966, 1974, 1987, 2002 Lippincott Williams & Wilkins

Blackwell Publishing was acquired by John Wiley & Sons in February 2007. Blackwell's publishing program has been merged with Wiley's global Scientific, Technical and Medical business to form Wiley-Blackwell.

Registered office: John Wiley & Sons Ltd, The Atrium, Southern Gate, Chichester, West Sussex, PO19 8SQ, UK

Editorial offices: 2121 State Avenue, Ames, Iowa 50014-8300, USA
The Atrium, Southern Gate, Chichester, West Sussex, PO19 8SQ, UK
9600 Garsington Road, Oxford, OX4 2DQ, UK

For details of our global editorial offices, for customer services and for information about how to apply for permission to reuse the copyright material in this book please see our website at www.wiley.com/wiley-blackwell.

Library of Congress Cataloging-in-Publication Data
Adams and Stashak's lameness in horses. – 6th ed. / [edited by] Gary M. Baxter.
   p. ; cm.
   Other title: Lameness in horses
   Rev. ed. of: Adams' lameness in horses. 5th ed. / [edited by] Ted S. Stashak. c2002.
   Includes bibliographical references and index.
   ISBN 978-0-8138-1549-7 (hardback : alk. paper) 1. Lameness in horses.   2. Horse shoeing.   I. Baxter, Gary M.   II. Adams, O. R. (Ora Roberts)   III. Adams' lameness in horses.   IV. Title: Lameness in horses.
   [DNLM: 1. Horse Diseases.   2. Lameness, Animal.   3. Horses–injuries. SF 959. L25 A2158 2011]
   SF959.L25A3 2011
   636.1'089758–dc22
                                    2010023258

A catalogue record for this book is available from the British Library.

Set in 10/10.5 pt Sabon by Toppan Best-set Premedia Limited
Printed and bound in Singapore by Fabulous Printers Pte Ltd

To my wife, Margaret, and daughters, Allison, Katherine, and Mary, for their encouragement, understanding, and support

And

To my parents, Arthur and Alice, for teaching me the importance of dedication and perseverance

TABLE OF CONTENTS

DVD included featuring additional anatomical images and video clips demonstrating key procedures and examples of conditions in motion.

LIST OF CONTRIBUTORS

GARY M. BAXTER, VMD, MS, DIPLOMATE ACVS
Department of Clinical Sciences
Veterinary Teaching Hospital
College of Veterinary Medicine and Biomedical
Sciences
Colorado State University
300 West Drake
Ft. Collins, CO 80523

JAMES K. BELKNAP, DVM, PhD, DIPLOMATE ACVS
Department of Veterinary Clinical Sciences
College of Veterinary Medicine
The Ohio State University
601 Vernon Tharp St.
Columbus, OH 43210

DWIGHT G. BENNETT, DVM, PhD, DIPLOMATE ACT
Professor Emeritus of Equine Medicine
Colorado State University
2307 Tanglewood Dr.
Ft. Collins, CO 80525

ALICIA L. BERTONE, DVM, PhD, DIPLOMATE ACVS
Trueman Family Endowed Chair and Professor
The Ohio State University
Veterinary Teaching Hospital
601 Vernon Tharp St.
Columbus, OH 43210

ROBIN M. DABAREINER, DVM, PhD, DIPLOMATE ACVS
7893 CR 246
Caldwell, TX 77836

NICOLAS S. ERNST, DVM, MS, DIPLOMATE ACVS
College of Veterinary Medicine
University of Minnesota
1365 Gortner Ave., 225 VMC
St. Paul, MN 55108

ANNA DEE FAILS, DVM, PhD
Department of Biomedical Sciences
Colorado State University
Ft. Collins, CO 80523

ELLIS G. FARSTVEDT, DVM, MS, DIPLOMATE ACVS
CSR Equine Medical Center and Sports Medicine
Team
Copper Spring Ranch
Bozeman, MT 59718

LUTZ S. GOEHRING, DVM, MS, PhD, DIPLOMATE ACVIM
Assistant Professor in Equine Medicine
Veterinary Teaching Hospital
Colorado State University
300 West Drake
Ft. Collins, CO 80523

NANCY L. GOODMAN, DVM
MG Equine Associates PC
6348 City Lights Lane
Loveland, CO 80537

LAURIE R. GOODRICH, DVM, PhD, DIPLOMATE ACVS
Assistant Professor in Equine Surgery and Lameness
College of Veterinary Medicine and Biomedical
Sciences
Colorado State University
Ft. Collins, CO 80523

KEVIN K. HAUSSLER, DVM, DC, PhD
Assistant Professor
Orthopaedic Research Center
College of Veterinary Medicine and Biomedical
Sciences
Colorado State University
300 West Drake
Ft. Collins, CO 80523

JAN F. HAWKINS, DVM, DIPLOMATE ACVS
Associate Professor of Large Animal Surgery
Purdue University
625 Harrison Street
West Lafayette, IN 47907-2026

CHERRY HILL, BS AN SCI
Livermore, CO 80536

TODD C. HOLBROOK, DVM, DIPLOMATE ACVIM
Associate Professor
Department of Veterinary Clinical Sciences
Center for Veterinary Health Sciences
Oklahoma State University
Stillwater, OK 74078

JEREMY HUBERT, BVSc, MRCVS, MS, DIPLOMATE ACVS
Veterinary Teaching Hospital
Colorado State University
300 West Drake
Ft. Collins, CO 80523

ROBERT J. HUNT, DVM, MS, DIPLOMATE ACVS
Hagyard-Davidson-McGee
4250 Iron Works Pike
Lexington, KY 40511

KIMBERLY JOHNSTON, VMD, DIPLOMATE ACVS
Veterinary Medicine and Surgery
Innovative BioTherapies
401 W. Morgan Road
Ann Arbor, MI 48108
*Affiliated with the College of Veterinary Medicine,
Michigan State University, during manuscript
preparation.*

ROBERT A. KAINER DVM, MS
Professor Emeritus Anatomy and Neurobiology
Colorado State University
Ft. Collins, CO 80523

CHRIS KAWCAK, DVM, PhD, DIPLOMATE ACVS
Iron Rose Ranch Chair
Equine Orthopaedic Research Center
Colorado State University
300 West Drake
Ft. Collins, CO 80523

KEVIN G. KEEGAN, DVM, MS, DIPLOMATE ACVS
Professor and Director, E. Paige Laurie Endowed
Program in Equine Lameness, Department of
Veterinary Medicine and Surgery
College of Veterinary Medicine
University of Missouri
Columbia, MO 65211

OMAR MAHER, DV, DACVS
New England Equine Medical and Surgical Center
15 Members Way
Dover, NH 03820

C. WAYNE MCILWRAITH, BVSc, PhD, DSc, FRCVS,
DIPLOMATE ACVS
University Distinguished Professor
Barbara Cox Anthony University Chair in
Orthopaedics
Director of Orthopedic Research
Colorado State University
Equine Orthopaedic Research Center
300 West Drake
Ft. Collins, CO 80523

FRANK A. NICKELS, DVM, MS, DIPLOMATE ACVS
Professor, Department of Large Animal Clinical
Science
College of Veterinary Medicine
Michigan State University
East Lansing, MI 48824

FOSTER NORTHROP, DVM
Louisville, KY

STEPHEN E. O'GRADY, DVM, MRCVS
Northern Virginia Equine
PO Box 746
Marshall, VA 20116

GENE OVNICEK, RMF
Equine Digit Support System, Inc.
506 Hwy 115
Penrose, CO 81240

RICHARD D. PARK, DVM, PhD, DIPLOMATE ACVR
Department of Environmental and Radiological
Health Sciences Colorado State University
300 West Drake
Ft. Collins, CO 80523

ANDREW PARKS, MA, VET MB, MRCVS, DIPLOMATE ACVS
Professor of Large Animal Surgery
Department of Large Animal Medicine
College of Veterinary Medicine
University of Georgia
Athens, GA 30622

ANTHONY P. PEASE, DVM, MS, DIPLOMATE ACVR
Michigan State University
College of Veterinary Medicine
Office G370
East Lansing, MI 48823

W. RICH REDDING, DVM, MS, DIPLOMATE ACVS
North Carolina State University
College of Veterinary Medicine
4700 Hillsborough St.
Raleigh, NC 27614

BONNIE R. RUSH, DVM, MS, DIPLOMATE ACVIM
Professor, Equine Internal Medicine
College of Veterinary Medicine
Kansas State University
1800 Denison Ave
Manhattan, KS 66506

MICHAEL SCHRAMME, DrMedVet, CertEO, PhD,
DIPLOMATE ECVS
Assistant Professor of Equine Surgery
North Carolina State University
College of Veterinary Medicine
4700 Hillsborough St.
Raleigh, NC 27606

JACK R. SNYDER, DVM, PhD, DIPLOMATE ACVS
Equine Surgery and Lameness Professor
Veterinary Medical Teaching Hospital
University of California
Davis, CA 95616

TED S. STASHAK DVM, MS DIPLOMATE ACVS
Professor Emeritus Surgery
Colorado State University
965 Los Alamos Road
Santa Rosa, CA 95409

PHILLIP F. STEYN, BVSc, MS, DIPLOMATE ACVR
Director of Professional Services and Chief
Radiologist
Antech Imaging Services

NARELLE C. STUBBS, B.APPSc(PT), M.ANIM
ST(ANIMAL PHYSIOTHERAPY)
Research Associate
McPhail Equine Performance Center
Large Animal Clinical Sciences
College of Veterinary Medicine
Michigan State University
East Lansing, MI 48824

KENNETH E. SULLINS, DVM, MS, DIPLOMATE ACVS
Professor of Surgery
Marion DuPont Scott Equine Medical Center
P.O. Box 1938
Leesburg, VA 20177

TERRY D. SWANSON, DVM
Littleton Equine Medical Center
8025 S. Santa Fe Dr.
Littleton, CO 80120

TROY N. TRUMBLE, DVM, PhD, DIPLOMATE ACVS
Assistant Professor
College of Veterinary Medicine
Veterinary Medical Center
University of Minnesota
1365 Gortner Ave., 225 VMC
St. Paul, MN 55108

TRACY A. TURNER, DVM, MS, DIPLOMATE ACVS,
DIPLOMATE ABT (AMERICAN BOARD OF THERMOLOGY)
Anoka Equine Veterinary Services
Elk River, MN 55330-6522

STEPHANIE J. VALBERG, DVM, PhD, DIPLOMATE ACVIM
Professor and Director
University of Minnesota Equine Center
Department of Veterinary Population Medicine
1365 Gortner Ave.
University of Minnesota
St. Paul, MN 55108

ALEJANDRO VALDÉS-MARTÍNEZ, MVZ, DIPLOMATE
ACVR
Assistant Professor, Department of Environmental and
Radiological Health Sciences
Veterinary Teaching Hospital
Colorado State University
300 West Drake
Ft. Collins, CO 80523

ROB VAN WESSUM, DVM, MS, CERT PRACT KNMvD (EQ)
1820 Darling Road
Mason, MI 48854
*Affiliated with the College of Veterinary Medicine,
Michigan State University during manuscript
preparation.*

PREFACE TO THE SIXTH EDITION

Welcome to the sixth edition of *Adams and Stashak's Lameness in Horses*. When Dr. Stashak approached me about being an editor for the new edition, I failed to realize the complexity of the endeavor. However, I have tried to modify the book with the specific goal of providing the most current information as concisely as possible. You will notice that Dr. Stashak's name has been added to the book title to reflect his numerous contributions to this text over the last few editions.

The primary objectives of the sixth edition were to update existing information and add new information without expanding the size of the book. This required re-organization, consolidation, and deletion of existing material in some cases. Expansive text on surgical procedures was condensed or eliminated in the sixth edition to focus on lameness and not surgery in horses.

You will notice that only chapters 1 through 5 and 12 are similar in content to previous chapters in the fifth edition. However, Chapter 4 (Diagnostic Procedures) has been expanded considerably to reflect the advances that have been made in this important area over the last several years. Chapters 6 through 11 are new, although much of the information from the fifth edition has been re-organized into a different format within these chapters. Chapter 6 was added because of the growing importance of the axial skeleton in lameness and poor performance, especially in certain occupations. Chapters 7 and 8 focus on the principles of musculoskeletal diseases and treatments, respectively, and hopefully permit the reader to better understand these basic disease processes as well as the multitude of treatment options that are available for the numerous disease conditions covered elsewhere in the text. Chapter 9 contains a wealth of information from experienced equine veterinarians regarding lameness conditions unique to a horse's specific sport. Knowing these specific occupation-related conditions can be extremely helpful in lameness diagnosis. Chapter 10 is a "catch all" for many conditions and situations that do not fit neatly within another chapter yet are important aspects of the musculoskeletal system in the horse. Examples include prepurchase examinations, saddle fit, headshaking, and assessment of the neurologic horse. Chapter 11 discusses the unique features of the musculoskeletal system in the growing horse and serves to remind us of the numerous differences between the immature and mature horse with respect to lameness.

A major effort was also made to include as many new color images and illustrations within the sixth edition as possible. Several older anatomical illustrations were converted to color but many of the black and white illustrations were retained because they remain excellent examples. Conventional radiographs were replaced with digital images whenever possible due to their improved quality and reproducibility. The goal was to have every image clearly illustrate what the author had intended.

An instructional DVD titled The "How to" Guide for Equine Lameness Evaluation complements the sixth edition. Its primary purpose is to demonstrate physical examination procedures, manipulative tests, and other diagnostic techniques that are somewhat unique to the horse. Perineural and intrasynovial anesthetic techniques are illustrated both with still images and live demonstrations. Examples of lameness cases were included so the observer could translate written text to the live horse regarding what to look for when evaluating a lame horse. Specific examples of uncommon musculoskeletal problems were also included with the idea that once you see one, you will never forget it. Finally, an example of how to evaluate lameness using objective data was included to make readers aware of the possible future of lameness diagnosis in the horse.

I wish to thank all who contributed to the text in any way, including the numerous horses, clients, and veterinarians who have provided me with the case material, knowledge, and experiences that have been included within this text. I hope that the sixth edition continues in the rich tradition of excellence that has been provided by previous editions of *Adams' Lameness in Horses*. However, as the specialty of equine lameness continues to evolve, ideas to further improve the text are always welcomed. Thank you.

PREFACE TO THE FIFTH EDITION

First and foremost, I want to extend my sincere thanks to the veterinary profession, veterinary students, students in related equine science programs, paraprofessionals in the equine industry, and horse owners throughout the world for their wide acceptance of the fourth edition of *Adams' Lameness in Horses*. The many favorable comments I received throughout the years have, to a large degree, provided me with the impetus to embark on the much-needed revision of the fourth edition. That being said, it pleases me to provide the veterinary profession and persons in equine-related fields with the extensively revised fifth edition of *Adams' Lameness in Horses*. As with the fourth edition, the changes are substantial, including the addition of new authors, the reorganization of material, and the reduction in the number of chapters from 14 to 9. As with the other editions, the fifth edition is designed to appeal to a wide audience in equine-related fields.

Chapter 1 has been revised to provide the reader with an updated version of the functional anatomy of the equine locomotor system. The latest information regarding the dermal microcirculation of the foot and the anatomy of various joint capsules and their distribution has been added with detailed illustrations to support the discussion. As usual, Dr. Kainer's attention to detail provides a complete reference for the various regions of the musculoskeletal system. I would like to thank Dr. Robert Bowker for his contributions to this chapter.

Chapter 2 has changed considerably and covers a discussion of conformation and locomotion. The part on conformation has been extensively revised and updated with as much reference material as possible in hopes of providing objective data from which to draw conclusions. Additionally, the discussion of normal movement, movement abnormalities, and factors that affect movement, which expands on the material from Chapter 13, "Natural and Artificial Gaits," from the fourth edition, has also been included. Cherry Hill's co-authorship has provided much needed insight from a certified (carded by the

U.S. breed associations) equine judge's standpoint. Cherry's background as a professional horse trainer and instructor has also added a practical perspective that I believe will appeal to veterinarians and horsemen alike.

Chapter 3 is presented in the same format as in the previous edition, with the addition of new material to make it as current as possible. Most of the anecdotal material has been removed except where personal experience was interjected to provide another perspective. Many new illustrations have been added to facilitate the discussion.

Chapter 4, the imaging chapter, has been completely updated and includes two new parts, one on ultrasound and one on nuclear medicine. The discussion of these two imaging modalities, used extensively for lameness diagnosis, has greatly increased the amount of material presented. Chapter 4 is divided into three parts. Part I, authored by Dr. Richard Park, provides an updated discussion of radiography in the diagnosis of equine lameness. This is followed by Part II, a comprehensive discussion by Dr. Robert Wrigley on the usefulness of ultrasound in lameness diagnosis. This part's many illustrations provide a useful and clear understanding of the anatomy being imaged. In Part III, Dr. Phillip Steyn provides a comprehensive discussion and presentation of illustrations on the value of nuclear medicine in the diagnosis of equine lameness. I would like to thank Dr. Richard Park for his leadership role in the development of this chapter.

Chapter 5 has also been completely updated with the addition of a new first author, Dr. Kate Savage, with Dr. Lewis acting as second author. This chapter provides the most current information regarding the role that nutrition plays in musculoskeletal development and disease.

Chapter 6 has also been completely revised and updated. With the departure of my colleague, Dr. Simon Turner, from the clinical arena to research, Dr. Gary Baxter has taken over as the first author of this chapter, with Dr. Turner serving as second author.

A significant addition to this chapter is a comprehensive and practical discussion of the emergency ("first aid") management of equine fracture patients for transport and/or treatment. Many illustrations have been added to support the discussion.

Chapter 7 has been extensively revised by Dr. Wayne McIlwraith. The addition of much research material to this chapter provides the reader with the most current information on the etiopathogenesis, diagnosis, and treatment of the various causes of joint disease and related structures. Many new illustrations have been added to augment the discussion of these various entities.

Chapter 8 has been extensively revised and greatly expanded, with the addition of new diseases. Dr. Alicia Bertone has updated discussion on the diseases associated with the fetlock region, including the metacarpus and carpus. Dr. Ken Sullins has updated discussion on the diseases of the hindlimb up to the coxofemoral joint. Dr. Dean Hendrickson has revised discussion on the diseases associated with the pelvis, back, and axial skeleton. The addition of these authors has greatly improved my ability to provide the reader with the most comprehensive and current discussion of the various diseases that cause lameness. As with the fourth edition, Chapter 8 concludes with discussion of "wobbler syndrome" and the various diseases of the spinal cord that can produce locomotor disorders that appear similar clinically. Dr. Alan Nixon has completely revised this section and, of note, has added a comprehensive discussion of the most current information on the diagnosis and treatment of equine protozoal myeloencephalitis (EPM).

Chapter 9 has been completely reorganized and updated and is presented in an entirely different format from that presented in the fourth edition. It incorporates information from Chapters 10 to 12 of the fourth edition. The addition of Cherry Hill, Richard Klimesh, and Gene Ovnicek as co-authors has greatly improved the presentation of this material, which should make this chapter most useful to all who read it. (Chapter 14, "Methods of Therapy," from the fourth edition has been eliminated, since most of this material is covered throughout the fifth edition for specific lesions or diseases and because many other texts cover the topic more completely than I possibly could in one chapter.)

With the expansion of the literature pertaining to lameness diagnosis and the recognition of new diseases, the reader will soon recognize that the reference lists have expanded in all portions of the text. In all cases the authors tried to include reference material from journals and text sources other than those of English-speaking countries. This was difficult at times, since frequently only summaries and abstracts were written in English.

I am grateful and indebted to Mark Goldstein for his untiring efforts and the many tasks he performed to make the fifth edition possible. Mark scanned the entire fourth edition onto computer. This unfortunately had to be done because the majority of the fourth edition text was lost in the archives of computer services. Following scanning, Mark proofread the material word for word, including checking superscripts and reference formatting. This had to be done, since the accuracy of the scanner at that time was only about 70%. Mark also did all the literature searches for the entire text and copied and organized the literature for distribution to contributing authors. Additionally, Mark combined new and old references for the fifth edition and added their numbered callouts in the text. Mark, thanks for your loyal and untiring effort; without you it would have been very difficult to complete the fifth edition.

The addition of numerous illustrations and photographs represents a tremendous time commitment and effort on behalf of the Computer-Assisted Teaching Service laboratory at Colorado State University. For the majority of the new illustrations I am deeply indebted to Jenger Smith for her skill and expertise in producing these fine illustrations for the fifth edition. Her desire to produce the best possible image and her untiring efforts are most appreciated. Additionally, I am grateful to Gale Mueller from Visible Productions for the excellent illustrations she made for Chapters 1, 3, and 7.

I am grateful to my colleagues, Drs. Baxter, Hendrickson, McIlwraith, and Trotter, including referring practitioners, for allowing me the courtesy of using some of their case material as examples. I also acknowledge the contribution of my colleagues and the surgical residents who have contributed to the care and treatment of some of the cases presented in this text. A special thanks is extended to the many practitioners who have referred cases that have been used in this text. Without their continued support, the accumulation of the case material would not have been possible. Additionally, I am grateful to the technicians who provided support in the care of these patients.

Dana Battaglia, Managing Editor, and the entire staff at Lippincott Williams & Wilkins have been most patient and helpful in the preparation of the fifth edition. I am grateful for their support and guidance. I also wish to thank Carroll Cann, former veterinary editor for Lippincott Williams & Wilkins, who provided early encouragement for this edition.

I hope the new fifth edition meets all the expectations and needs of those who read it. As always, I look forward to your cooperation in making corrections and suggested revisions for future editions.

Fort Collins, Colorado   TED S. STASHAK

PREFACE TO THE FOURTH EDITION

When I was contacted by Mr. George Mundorff, Executive Editor for Lea & Febiger, regarding the possibility of revising the third edition of "Lameness in Horses" by Dr. O. R. Adams, I was excited but naive to the task at hand. Dr. Adams had, in his previous three editions, established the state of the art of lameness diagnosis and treatment, presenting it in a unique manner that appealed to veterinarians, horse owners and trainers, and farriers. Without a doubt, he defined and directly influenced the course of this subject more than any other individual during this time. I was truly fortunate to train under him during my internship and surgical residency at Colorado State University. His never-ending thirst for knowledge, his humor, his friendship, and his love of the veterinary profession have inspired me throughout this endeavor. I only hope that I have served his memory well and that he would be proud of this fourth edition.

After considerable discussion with Lea & Febiger and the assurance of Mrs. Nancy Adams, Dr. Adams' widow, I embarked on the revision with some basic changes in format in mind. These included the addition of new authors, changes in chapter sequence and presentation, the addition of new chapters and deletion of some old ones, and the transition from a monograph to a reference text. Because I wanted the fourth edition to represent the school where Dr. Adams attended and taught, I selected mostly authors from our faculty on the basis of their expertise and their ability to provide a broad base of opinion for the reader.

With the idea of approaching the discussion of lameness as one would approach a lameness examination itself, I changed the sequence of presentation. Using the newest accepted nomenclature, Chapter 1 deals with the functional anatomy of the equine locomotor system and represents a complete revision of Chapter 2 in the previous edition. Dr. Kainer starts with the forelimb, advancing from the foot up the limb, describing the regional anatomy of each site. The hindlimb is covered in similar fashion. The nomenclature may be confusing initially to older graduates of American veterinary schools, but recent graduates as well as foreign veterinarians will be well versed in this terminology. We felt it was time to make this transition since the new nomenclature has been in use for at least 4 years. (Older terms are included parenthetically.)

Following a format similar to the previous edition, Chapter 2 deals with the relationship between conformation and lameness. I have eliminated "The Examination for Soundness," which was Chapter 3 in the previous edition, because it discussed many topics unrelated to lameness and, simply, because the subject of soundness is so comprehensive it could be covered in a separate text. The present Chapter 3 deals with the diagnosis of lameness. After defining lameness and establishing how to determine which limb is lame, the description of the physical examination begins at the foot of the forelimb and proceeds upward. Emphasis is placed on recognition of problems peculiar to the region examined. Following this is a description and illustration of perineural and intrasynovial anesthesia.

The next logical step in the diagnosis of lameness is radiology, which is discussed in Chapter 4. This chapter is comprehensive; nothing like it has been published elsewhere. The format of the text and illustrations should answer any question the reader may have regarding the techniques for taking radiographs and interpreting them. The artwork beautifully illustrates the different structures seen on various radiographic views, and the illustrations are labeled so that anatomic sites are easily identified.

Chapters 5 through 7 are new. Discussing the role of nutrition in musculoskeletal development and disease, Chapter 5 illustrates a unique approach not used elsewhere. Dr. Lewis provides a comprehensive review of specific nutritional disorders, their causes, and their treatment for all phases of growth and development in the foal, during pregnancy and lactation in the mare, and during maintenance of the working horse. This information will benefit both the horseman and the veterinarian. Chapter 6, by Dr. Turner, starts with a brief review of endochondral ossification and then discusses the diseases associated with bones and muscles and their treatment. In Chapter 7, Dr. McIlwraith describes the developmental anatomy of joints and related structures, disease processes, clinical signs, and treatments. Both of these chapters present in-depth reviews, with major emphasis on the pathogenesis and pathobiology of the diseases. They are heavily referenced, and will be of major interest to the veterinary profession.

Representing a complete revision of Chapter 8, "Lameness" updates the reader on new diseases as well as new findings and treatment for previously recognized entities. Unlike past editions, this material is heavily referenced. Information regarding the prevalence of the disease within various breeds according to sex and age introduces each subject. The format of the chapter has been changed to start with diseases relating to the foot region and then proceeding upward anatomically, consistent with the way most equine practitioners approach a systematic examination. Specific diseases of each region are discussed separately. This chapter, though referenced heavily and written technically, should be of interest to the horseman as well as the veterinary profession. I am particularly grateful to Dr. Alan Nixon for his thorough and comprehensive review of the diagnosis and treatment of the "wobbler's syndrome" in horses. His presentation is clear and well illustrated, giving the reader the confidence to differentiate among the diseases that cause this syndrome.

Chapters 9 through 12 were written primarily for the horseman and farrier, though they will also be of interest to the veterinarian, particularly the equine practitioner. I have updated these chapters with new information, as well as listing what the horseman should look for when the horse is properly trimmed and shod. Chapter 13, "Natural and Artificial Gaits," is essentially unchanged. Chapter 14, "Methods of Therapy," has been updated, and includes an extensive revision of different methods of external coaptation. This chapter is primarily directed toward the veterinary profession, though the horse owner will obtain insight into why different treatments are selected.

With the explosion of literature pertaining to musculoskeletal disease in the horse and the demands put on authors and editors alike, it became obvious that a transition from a monograph to a reference text was timely. To this end the authors have attempted to provide the latest information. As with any large text, however, authors and editors alike feel some-

what frustrated because at the time of publication some of this information will be out of date. With few exceptions, we stopped referencing material published in 1985. Occasionally publications in 1985 changed the presentation of the materials so much that it could not be denied and therefore was included.

I am grateful to Dr. Robert Kainer, Professor of Anatomy and author of the first chapter, for taking the time to review and advise me on the nomenclature used in this book. A special thanks is extended to Dr. A. S. Turner for his review and comments on Chapter 8. The fine contributions of all the authors is sincerely appreciated. I want to thank Dr. Robert Perce (California) and Mr. Richard Klimesh (farrier, Colorado) for their advice on the chapters dealing with trimming and shoeing horses.

The addition of many new illustrations and photographs represents a tremendous time commitment and effort on behalf of the Office of Biomedical Media at Colorado State University. For the illustrations, I am indebted to Mr. Tom McCracken and Mr. John Dougherty for their expertise and the cooperation they have given me. For the photographs I am grateful to Mr. Al Kilminster and Mr. David Clack, for their expertise, cooperation, and commitment to excellence. For the design of the book cover I thank Mr. Dave Carlson.

Most of the manuscript was typed by Mrs. Helen Acevedo. Her cooperation and patience with the many revisions necessary to complete this text are gratefully appreciated.

I am also grateful to my many colleagues who took the time to personally reveal their thoughts regarding certain topics. A special thanks is extended to the following: Dr. Joerg Auer (Texas), Dr. Peter Haynes (Louisiana), Dr. Larry Bramlage (Ohio), Dr. Joe Foerner (Illinois), Dr. Dallas Goble (Tennessee), Dr. Robert Baker (Southern California), Dr. Robert Copelan (Kentucky) and Dr. Scott Leith (deceased, Southern California).

Mr. Christian C. Febiger Spahr Jr., Veterinary Editor, Mr. George Mundorff, Executive Editor, Mr. Tom Colaiezzi, Production Manager, Ms. Constance Marino, and Mrs. Dorothy Di Rienzi, Manager of Copy Editors, and the entire staff at Lea & Febiger have been most helpful in the preparation of this book. I am grateful for their support and guidance.

I hope this book will be useful to all who read it. I hope to receive your cooperation in making corrections and suggested additions for further revisions.

Fort Collins, Colorado   Ted S. Stashak

ACKNOWLEDGEMENTS

The sixth edition of *Adams and Stashak's Lameness in Horses* has required considerable input from numerous people throughout its course. From the initial hallway talk with Dr. Stashak about being the next editor to the final publication, many people have contributed to its outcome and deserve recognition. These include Dr. Ted Stashak for asking me to become the new editor, Justin Jeffryes and the other staff at Wiley-Blackwell (Nancy Turner, Catriona Dixon, Elizabeth Bishop, and others) for helping with the publication, contributing authors for their excellent manuscripts, my colleagues at Colorado State University for providing images and case material, and Dave Carlson for creating all of the new color illustrations that have been included in the text and DVD. I would also like to thank Kathryn Visser and Ron Bend from Communications and Creative Services at Colorado State University for both filming and editing the DVD, and Shannon Nagasako who scanned images, proofed manuscripts, and critiqued the DVD. I am also indebted to Drs. Hendrickson, Hubert, Amend, and Keegan for the use of their video clips within the DVD. Lastly, I would also like to thank my wife and family and the equine faculty and staff at Colorado State University for their understanding and encouragement during this process.

GARY M. BAXTER

COMMON TERMINOLOGIES AND ABBREVIATIONS

Terminology	Abbreviations
Distal or third phalanx	P3; coffin bone
Middle or second phalanx	P2
Proximal or first phalanx	P1
Distal interphalangeal joint	DIP joint or coffin joint
Proximal interphalangeal joint	PIP joint or pastern joint
Metacarpo/metatarsophalangeal joint	MCP/MTP joint or fetlock joint
Distal sesamoidean ligaments	DSL
Distal sesamoidean impar ligament	DSIL
Collateral suspensory ligaments of navicular bone	CSL
Collateral ligaments of coffin joint	CLs of DIP joint
Deep digital flexor tendon	DDFT or DDF tendon
Superficial digital flexor tendon	SDFT or SDF tendon
Metacarpus/metatarsus	MC/MT or MC3/MT3 or MCIII/MTIII; cannon bone
Second and fourth metacarpal/metatarsal bones	MC2, MC4, MT2, MT4 or MCII, MCIV, MTII, MTIV; splint bones
Digital flexor tendon sheath	DFTS
Common digital extensor tendon	CDET
Long digital extensor tendon	LDET
Tarsometatarsal joint	TMT joint
Distal intertarsal joint	DIT joint
Proximal intertarsal joint	PIT joint
Tarsocrural joint	TC joint
Medial femorotibial joint	MFT joint
Lateral femorotibial joint	LFT joint
Femoropatellar joint	FP joint
Scapulohumeral joint	SHJ or shoulder joint
Sacroiliac joint	SI joint
Computed tomography	CT
Magnetic resonance imaging	MRI or MR
Ultrasonography	US
Osteochondrosis	OC/OCD
Osteochondritis dissecans	OCD
Subchondral cystic lesion	SCL
Angular limb deformity	ALD
Osteoarthritis	OA
Accessory ligament of deep digital flexor tendon	ALDDFT, ICL, or inferior check
Accessory ligament of superficial digital flexor tendon	ALSDFT, SCL, or superior check
Developmental orthopedic disease	DOD
Proximal suspensory desmitis	PSD
Suspensory ligament	SL
Nonsteroidal anti-inflammatory drug	NSAID
Hyaluronan or hyaluronic acid	HA

Polysulfated glycosaminoglycans	PSGAG; Adequan
Platelet-rich plasma	PRP
Interleukin receptor antagonist protein or conditioned serum	IRAP
Extracorporeal shockwave treatment	ESWT or shockwave
Intra-articular	IA
Dorsopalmar/plantar	DP
Mediolateral	ML
Triamcinolone	TA
Methyl prednisolone acetate	MPA or Depo-medrol
Dimethyl sulfoxide	DMSO
Diclofenac cream	Surpass
Mesenchymal stem cell	MSC
Proximal sesamoid bones	PSB

ADAMS AND STASHAK'S
LAMENESS IN HORSES

SIXTH EDITION

Functional Anatomy of the Equine Musculoskeletal System

ROBERT A. KAINER AND ANNA DEE FAILS

ANATOMIC NOMENCLATURE AND USAGE

Through the efforts of nomenclature committees, informative and logical names for parts of the horse's body, as well as positional and directional terms, have evolved (Nomina Anatomica Veterinaria).[32] Some older terminology is still in wide use. For example, navicular bone for distal sesamoid bone, coffin joint for distal interphalangeal joint, pastern joint for proximal interphalangeal joint, and fetlock joint for metacarpophalangeal joint, are acceptable synonyms. It behooves one to be familiar with many of the older terms. Acceptable synonyms are presented in this book, and the terms may be used interchangeably.

Figure 1.1 provides the appropriate directional terms for veterinary anatomy. With the exception of the eye, the terms anterior and posterior are not applicable to quadrupeds. Cranial and caudal apply to the limbs proximal to the antebrachiocarpal (radiocarpal) joint and the tarsocrural (tibiotarsal) joint. Distal to these joints, dorsal and palmar (on the forelimb) or plantar (on the hindlimb) are the correct terms. The adjective "solar" is used to designate structures on the palmar (plantar) surface of the distal phalanx and the ground surface of the hoof.

THORACIC LIMB

Digit and Fetlock

The foot and pastern comprise the equine digit, a region including distal (third), middle (second), and proximal (first) phalanges and associated structures (Figure 1.2). The fetlock consists of the metacarpophalangeal (fetlock) joint and the structures surrounding it. Because the digits and fetlocks of the thoracic limb and

Adams and Stashak's Lameness in Horses, 6e, edited by Gary M. Baxter
© 2011 Blackwell Publishing, Ltd.

the pelvic limb are similar in most respects, consider the following descriptions to pertain to both limbs unless otherwise indicated. When referring to structures of the forelimb, the term "palmar" is used; this will obviously be replaced with "plantar" when referring to the hindlimb. Likewise, such terms as metacarpophalangeal and metatarsophalangeal are counterparts in fore- and hindlimbs, respectively.

Foot

The foot consists of the epidermal hoof and all it encloses: the connective tissue corium (dermis), digital cushion, distal phalanx (coffin bone), most of the cartilages of the distal phalanx, distal interphalangeal (coffin) joint, distal extremity of the middle phalanx (short pastern bone), distal sesamoid (navicular) bone, podotrochlear bursa (navicular bursa), several ligaments, tendons of insertion of the common digital extensor and deep digital flexor muscles, blood vessels, and nerves. Skin between the heels is also part of the foot.

HOOF WALL, SOLE, AND FROG

The hoof is continuous with the epidermis at the coronet. Here the dermis of the skin is continuous with the dermis (corium) deep to the hoof. Regions of the corium correspond to the parts of the hoof under which they are located: perioplic corium, coronary corium, laminar (lamellar) corium, corium of the frog, and corium of the sole.

Examination of the ground surface of the hoof reveals the sole, frog, heels, bars, and ground surface of the wall (Figure 1.3). The ground surface of the forefoot is normally larger than that of the hind foot, reflecting the shape of the distal surface of the enclosed distal phalanx (coffin bone).

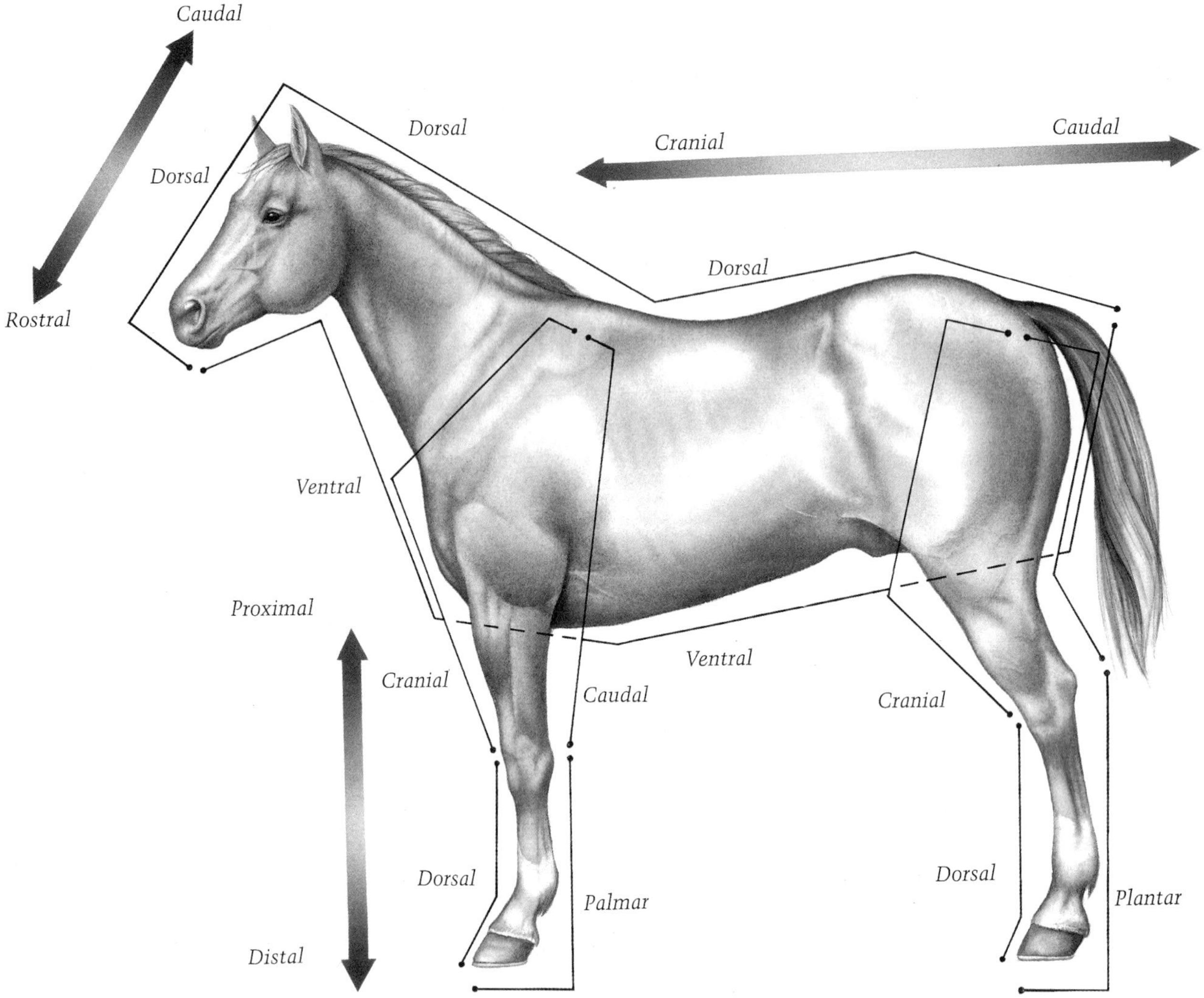

Figure 1.1. Positional and directional terms.

The hoof wall extends from the ground proximad to the coronary border where the soft white horn of the periople joins the epidermis of the skin at the coronet. Regions of the wall are the toe, the medial and lateral quarters, and the heels (Figures 1.3, 1.4). From the thick toe the wall becomes progressively thinner and more elastic toward the heels where it thickens again where it reflects dorsad as the bars. The wall usually curves more widely on the lateral side, and the lateral angle is less steep than the medial angle. Ranges for the angle of the toe between the dorsal surface of the hoof wall and the ground surface of the hoof vary widely.[1,17] In the ideal digit, the dorsal surface of the hoof wall and the dorsal surface of the pastern should be parallel, reflecting the axial alignment of the phalanges.

The highly vascular and densely innervated collagenous connective tissue of the coronary corium (dermis) gives rise to elongated, distally directed papillae. Laminar (lamellar) corium forms a series of laminae that interdigitate with epidermal laminae of the stratum internum of the hoof wall. Shorter papillae extend from the perioplic, solar and cuneate (frog) coria. The corium provides sensation as well as nourishment and attachment for the overlying stratified squamous epithelium comprising the ungual epidermis (L. *ungula*, hoof).

In the coronary region, the deepest layer (the stratum basale) of the ungual epidermis is a single layer of proliferating columnar keratinocytes lying upon and between long dermal papillae. This proliferation forces cells distad into the wide stratum medium of the hoof wall, forming tubular and intertubular epidermis that undergoes cornification.[2] A few layers of polyhedral cells joined by desmosomes make up a region corresponding to the stratum spinosum of cutaneous epidermis. The rest of the ungual epidermis is a stratum corneum of anucleate, squamous keratinocytes.

Most of the ungual epidermis, the horny stratum corneum, is devoid of nerve endings; it is the "insensitive" part of the foot. However, a few sensory nerve endings from nerves in the corium penetrate between cells of the stratum basale of the epidermis. In addition to many sensory nerve endings, the corium contains sympathetic motor endings to blood vessels.

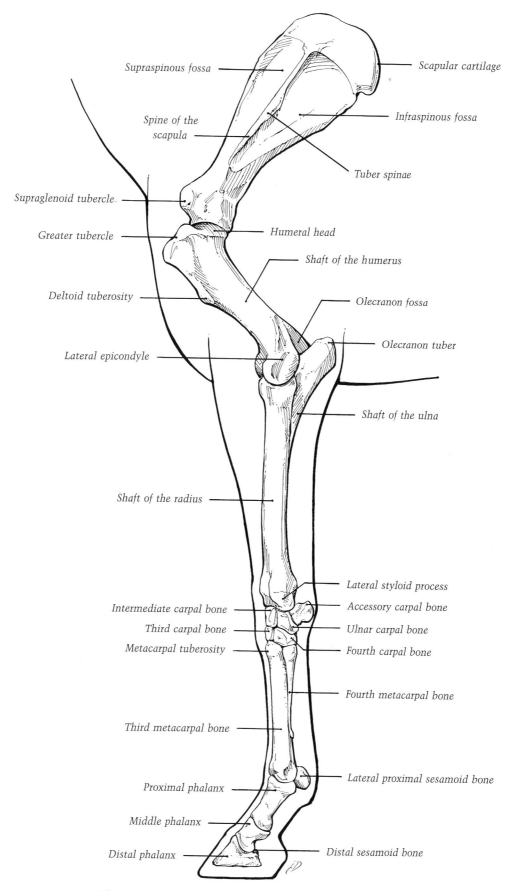

Supraspinous fossa

Scapular cartilage

Spine of the scapula

Infraspinous fossa

Tuber spinae

Supraglenoid tubercle

Humeral head

Greater tubercle

Shaft of the humerus

Deltoid tuberosity

Olecranon fossa

Lateral epicondyle

Olecranon tuber

Shaft of the ulna

Shaft of the radius

Lateral styloid process

Intermediate carpal bone

Accessory carpal bone

Third carpal bone

Ulnar carpal bone

Metacarpal tuberosity

Fourth carpal bone

Fourth metacarpal bone

Third metacarpal bone

Lateral proximal sesamoid bone

Proximal phalanx

Middle phalanx

Distal phalanx

Distal sesamoid bone

Figure 1.2. Bones of the left equine thoracic limb. Lateral view.

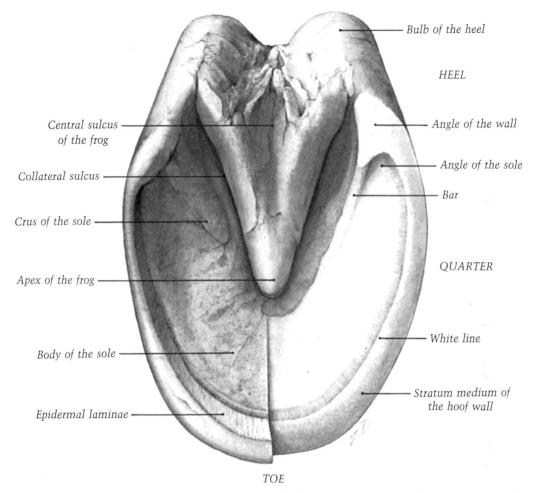

Central sulcus of the frog

Collateral sulcus

Crus of the sole

Apex of the frog

Body of the sole

Epidermal laminae

Bulb of the heel

HEEL

Angle of the wall

Angle of the sole

Bar

QUARTER

White line

Stratum medium of the hoof wall

TOE

Figure 1.3. Topography of the solar surface of the hoof. The right half has been trimmed to emphasize the region of the white line.

Three layers comprise the hoof wall: the stratum externum, stratum medium, and stratum internum (Figure 1.5). The superficial stratum externum is a thin layer of horn extending distad from the coronet a variable distance; this thin, soft layer, commonly called the periople, wears from the surface of the hoof wall so that it is present only on the bulbs of the heels and the proximal parts of the hoof wall. The bulk of the wall is a stratum medium consisting of horn tubules and intertubular horn. Horn tubules are generated by the stratum basale of the coronary epidermis covering the long papillae of the coronary corium.[2] Intertubular horn is formed in between the projections.

Distal to the coronary groove about 600 primary epidermal laminae of the stratum internum interleave with the primary dermal laminae of the laminar corium (Figures 1.6 and 1.7). Approximately 100 microscopic secondary laminae branch at an angle from each primary lamina, further binding the hoof and corium together (Figures 1.3 to 1.6). Some confusion exists concerning the terms "insensitive" and "sensitive" laminae. In the strictest sense the keratinized parts of the primary epidermal laminae are insensitive; the stratum basale, which includes all of the secondary epidermal laminae, and the laminar corium are "sensitive." The terms epi-

dermal and dermal (or corial) are more accurate adjectives.[49]

Growth of the hoof wall is primarily from the basal layer of the coronary epidermis toward the ground. Trauma or inflammation of the region stimulates greater keratinization, i.e., the production of horn. The laminar epidermis over terminal projections of the laminar corium keratinizes more heavily, forming pigmented horn and filling the spaces between the distal ends of the epidermal laminae. Ultrastructural studies indicate that progressive keratinization does not occur in cells of secondary epidermal laminae of the stratum internum and that during growth of the hoof, primary epidermal laminae move past the secondary epidermal laminae by breaking desmosomes between the two cell populations.[27] Submicroscopic, peg-like dermal projections increase the surface of attachment of the dermis (corium) and epidermis of the hoof.[49] This configuration and the blending of the laminar corium with the periosteum of the distal phalanx suspend and support the bone, aiding in the dissipation of concussion and the movement of blood.

The growth of the wall progresses at the rate of approximately 6 mm per month, taking from 9 to 12 months for the toe to grow out. The wall grows more

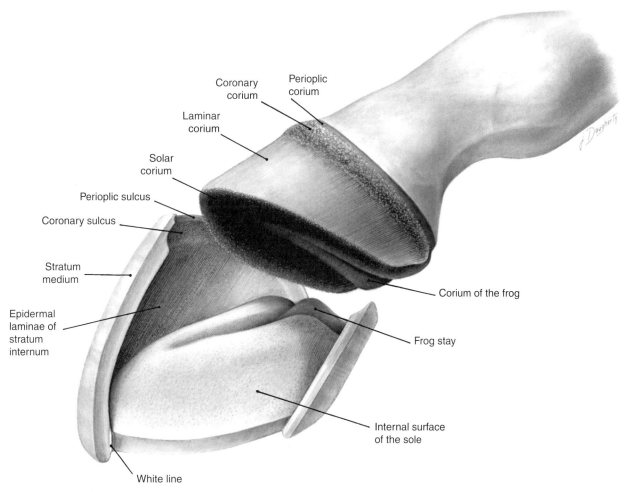

Coronary corium

Perioplic corium

Laminar corium

Solar corium

Perioplic sulcus

Coronary sulcus

Stratum medium

Epidermal laminae of stratum internum

Corium of the frog

Frog stay

Internal surface of the sole

White line

Figure 1.4. Dissected view of relationships of the hoof to underlying regions of the corium (dermis).

slowly in a cold environment. Growth is also slower in a dry environment when adequate moisture is not present in the wall. The hoof wall grows evenly distal to the coronary epidermis so that the youngest portion of the wall is at the heel (where it is shortest). Because this is the youngest part of the wall, it is also the most elastic, aiding in heel expansion during concussion.

Stratum medium may be pigmented or nonpigmented. Contrary to popular belief, pigmented hooves are not stronger than nonpigmented hooves. There is no difference in the stress-strain behavior of ultimate strength properties of pigmented and nonpigmented equine hooves.[25] It has also been demonstrated that pigmentation has no effect on fracture toughness of hoof keratin.[3] Water content of the hoof significantly affects its mechanical properties. In the natural hydration gradient in the hoof wall, the moisture content decreases from within outward, i.e., deep to superficial.[27] Very dry or extremely hydrated hoof wall is more likely to crack than normally hydrated hoof wall. A normally hydrated hoof is better able to absorb energy.[4]

The slightly concave sole does not normally bear weight on its ground surface except near its junction with the white line, but it bears internal weight transmitted from the solar surface of the distal phalanx through the solar corium. That portion of the sole at the angle formed by the wall and the bars is the angle of the sole. Two crura extend from the body of the sole to the angles. In the unworn, untrimmed hoof wall, insensitive laminae are seen on the internal surface as the wall extends distad to the plane of the sole (Figure 1.3). When the wall is trimmed, the white line (linea alba ungulae) of nonpigmented horn of the internal wall and pigmented horn over terminal papillae is evident where it blends with the horn of the sole. The sensitive corium is immediately internal to the white line that serves as a landmark for determining the proper position and angle for driving horseshoe nails.[14]

The frog (cuneus ungulae) is a wedge-shaped mass of keratinized stratified squamous epithelium rendered softer than other parts of the hoof by an increased water content.[49] Apocrine glands, spherical masses of tubules in the corium of the frog, extend ducts that deliver secretions to the surface of the frog.[50] The ground surface of the frog presents a pointed apex and central sulcus enclosed by two crura. Paracuneal (collateral) sulci separate the crura of the frog from the bars and the sole. The palmar aspect of the frog blends into the bulbs of the heels.

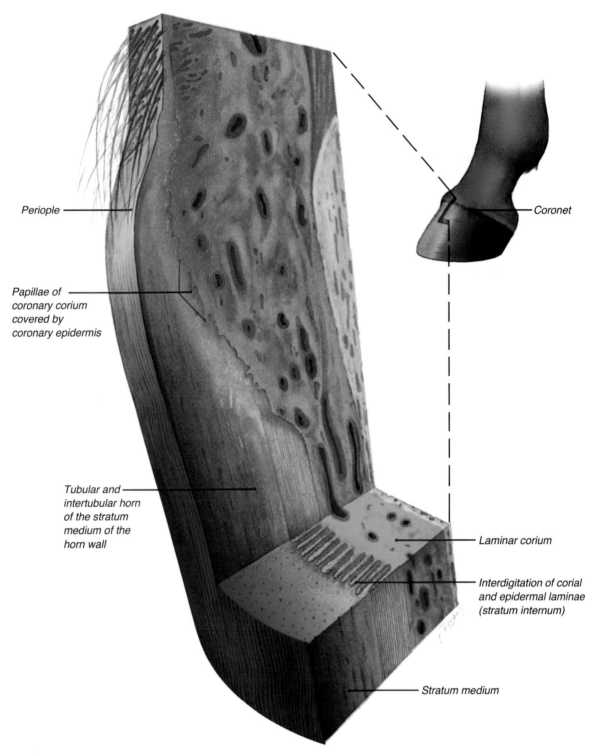

Periople

Papillae of coronary corium covered by coronary epidermis

Tubular and intertubular horn of the stratum medium of the horn wall

Coronet

Laminar corium

Interdigitation of corial and epidermal laminae (stratum internum)

Stratum medium

Figure 1.5. Three dimensional dissection of coronary region of the hoof wall.

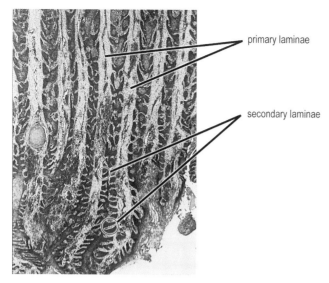

Figure 1.6. Photomicrograph of a cross section of the equine hoof. Interdigitations of primary epidermal laminae and dermal (corial) laminae can be appreciated. Notice the small secondary laminae.

primary laminae

secondary laminae

The dense white fibrous connective tissue of the hoof's corium is rich in elastic fibers, highly vascular, and well supplied with nerves. The arterial supply derives from numerous branches radiating outward from the terminal arch in small canals extending from the solar (semilunar) canal in the distal phalanx and from the dorsal and palmar branches of the distal phalanx from the digital arteries (Figure 1.8).

The coronary and perioplic coria and the stratum basale of the coronary and perioplic epidermis constitute the coronary band. Deep to the coronary band the subcutis is modified into the highly elastic coronary cushion. The coronary band and cushion form the bulging mass that fits into the coronary groove of the hoof. Part of the coronary venous plexus is within the coronary cushion. The plexus receives blood from the dorsal venous plexus in the laminar corium. Where the corium is adjacent to the distal phalanx, it blends with the bone's periosteum, serving (particularly in the laminar region) to connect the hoof to the bone.

INTERNAL STRUCTURES OF THE FOOT

The medial and lateral cartilages of the distal phalanx (ungual cartilages) lie under the corium of the hoof and the skin, covered on their abaxial surfaces by the coronary venous plexus. They extend from each palmar process of the bone proximal to the coronary border of the hoof where they may be palpated. The cartilages are concave on their axial surfaces, convex on their abaxial surfaces, and thicker distally where they attach to the bone. Toward the heels they curve toward one another. Each cartilage is perforated in its palmar half by several foramina for the passage of veins connecting the palmar venous plexus with the coronary venous plexus.

Five ligaments stabilize each cartilage of the distal phalanx (Figures 1.9 and 1.10):

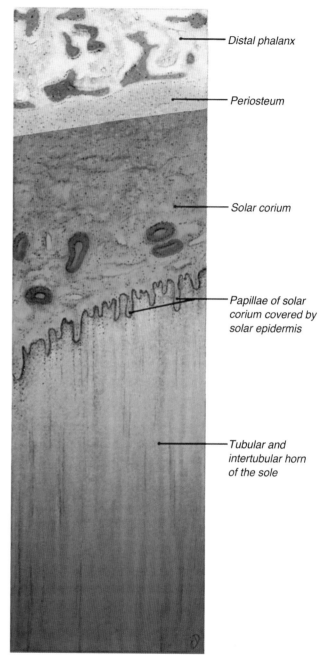

Distal phalanx

Periosteum

Solar corium

Papillae of solar corium covered by solar epidermis

Tubular and intertubular horn of the sole

Figure 1.7. Histological relationships of periosteum, corium, and horn of the sole.

1. A short, prominent ligament extends from the dorsal surface of the middle phalanx to the dorsal part of the cartilage.
2. A poorly defined elastic band extends from the side of the proximal phalanx to the proximal border of the cartilage and also detaches a branch to the digital cushion.
3. Several short fibers attach the distal part of the cartilage to the distal phalanx.
4. A ligament extends from the dorsal aspect of the cartilage to the termination of the tendon of insertion of the common digital extensor muscle. The dorsal part of each cartilage also serves as part of

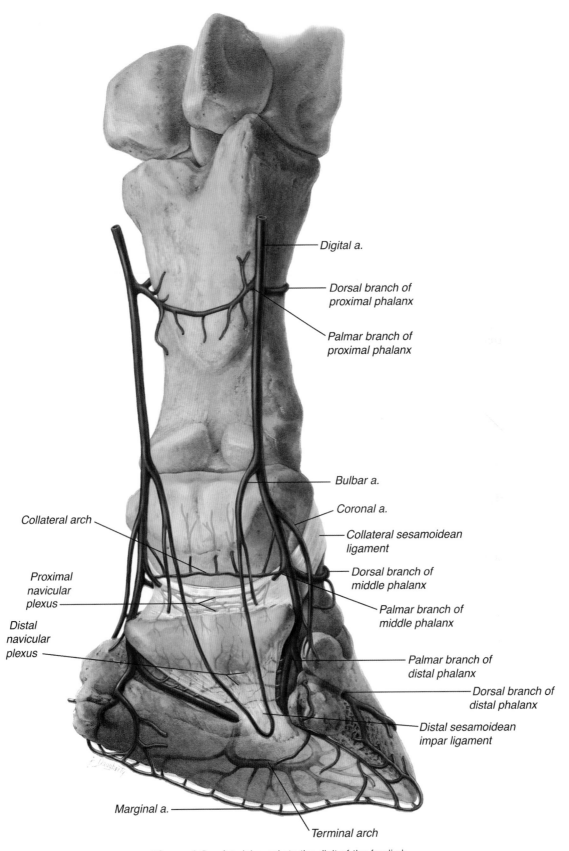

Digital a.

Dorsal branch of
proximal phalanx

Palmar branch of
proximal phalanx

Bulbar a.

Coronal a.

Collateral sesamoidean
ligament

Collateral arch

Dorsal branch of
middle phalanx

Proximal
navicular
plexus

Palmar branch of
middle phalanx

Distal
navicular
plexus

Palmar branch of
distal phalanx

Dorsal branch of
distal phalanx

Distal sesamoidean
impar ligament

Marginal a.

Terminal arch

Figure 1.8. Arterial supply to the digit of the forelimb.

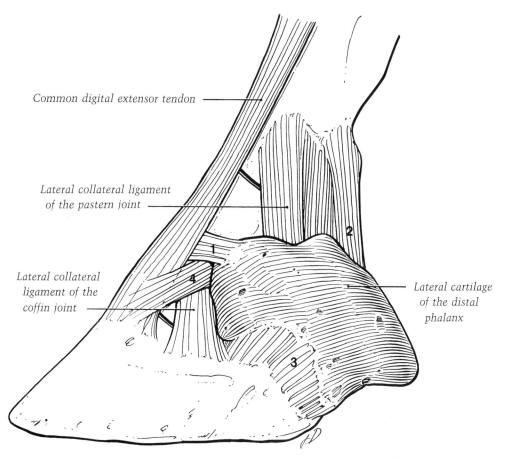

Figure 1.9. Four of the ligaments (1, 2, 3, and 4) that stabilize the cartilage of the distal phalanx.

Common digital extensor tendon

Lateral collateral ligament of the pastern joint

Lateral collateral ligament of the coffin joint

Lateral cartilage of the distal phalanx

the distal attachment for the respective collateral ligament of the coffin joint.

5. An extension of the collateral sesamoidean ligament attaches the end of the navicular bone to the cartilage of the distal phalanx.

Filling in between the cartilages is the digital cushion, a highly modified subcutis consisting of a meshwork of collagenous and elastic fibers, adipose tissue, and small masses of fibrocartilage (Figure 1.10). Only a few blood vessels ramify in the digital cushion. Dorsoproximally the digital cushion connects with the distal digital anular ligament. The apex of the wedge-shaped digital cushion is attached to the deep digital flexor tendon as the latter inserts on the solar surface of the distal phalanx. The base of the digital cushion bulges into the bulbs of the heels which are separated superficially by a central shallow groove. The structure and relationships of the digital cushion indicate its anticoncussive function.

As the deep digital flexor tendon courses to its insertion on the distal phalanx, it is bound down by the distal digital anular ligament, a sheet of deep fascia supporting the terminal part of the tendon and sweeping proximad to attach on each side of the proximal phalanx (Figure 1.11). The tendon passes over the complementary fibrocartilage, a fibrocartilaginous plate extending from the proximal extremity of the palmar surface of the middle phalanx. Then the tendon gives

off two secondary attachments to the distal aspect of the palmar surface of the bone (Figure 1.12). Continuing distad toward its primary attachment on the flexor surface of the distal phalanx, the deep digital flexor tendon passes over the navicular bursa (bursa podotrochlearis) interposed between the tendon and the fibrocartilaginous distal scutum covering the flexor surface of the navicular bone. From the exterior, the location of the navicular bursa may be approximated deep to the middle third of the frog on a plane parallel to the coronet over the quarters of the hoof wall.

The proximal border of the navicular bone (distal sesamoid bone) presents a groove containing foramina for the passage of small vessels and nerves. The distal border of the bone has a small, elongated facet that articulates with the distal phalanx. Several variously enlarged, foramina-containing fossae lie in an elongated depression palmar to that facet (Figure 1.13). Two concave areas on the main articular surface of the navicular bone contact the distal articular surface of the middle phalanx. The navicular bone is supported in its position by three ligaments comprising the navicular suspensory apparatus. A collateral sesamoidean (suspensory navicular) ligament arises from the distal end of the proximal phalanx (Figures 1.9 and 1.12). These collateral sesamoidean ligaments sweep obliquely distad, each ligament crossing the pastern joint, and then giving off a branch that joins the end of the

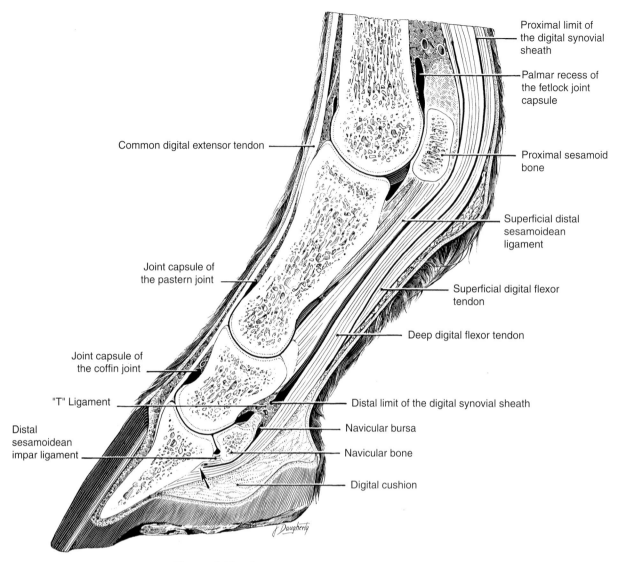

Figure 1.10. Sagittal section of equine fetlock and digit.

Proximal limit of the digital synovial sheath

Palmar recess of the fetlock joint capsule

Common digital extensor tendon

Proximal sesamoid bone

Superficial distal sesamoidean ligament

Joint capsule of the pastern joint

Superficial digital flexor tendon

Deep digital flexor tendon

Joint capsule of the coffin joint

"T" Ligament

Distal limit of the digital synovial sheath

Navicular bursa

Distal sesamoidean impar ligament

Navicular bone

Digital cushion

navicular bone to the cartilage of the distal phalanx and the angle of the bone. Each collateral sesamoidean ligament terminates by attaching to the proximal border of the navicular bone and joining with the contralateral ligament. Distally, the navicular bone is stabilized by the distal sesamoidean impar ligament, a fibrous sheet extending from the distal border of the bone to intersect with the deep digital flexor tendon (Figure 1.10).[8]

The distal articular surface of the middle phalanx, the articular surface of the distal phalanx, and the two articular surfaces of the navicular bone form the coffin joint, a ginglymus of limited range of motion. Short collateral ligaments arise from the distal end of the middle phalanx, pass distad deep to the cartilages of the distal phalanx, and terminate on either side of the extensor process and the dorsal part of each cartilage.

The synovial membrane of the distal interphalangeal (coffin) joint has a dorsal pouch that extends proximad on the dorsal surface of the middle phalanx under the common digital extensor tendon nearly to the pastern joint. The synovium has a complex relationship on its palmar side to the ligaments and tendons that are found

here. The proximal portions wrap around the distal ends of the collateral sesamoidean ligaments; the distal palmar pouch forms a thin extension between the articulation of the navicular bone and the distal phalanx. Distally, this pouch's synovial membrane surrounds the distal sesamoidean impar ligament on each side where the distal interphalangeal joint is closely associated with the neurovascular bundle that will enter the distal phalanx. Although a direct connection between the distal interphalangeal joint and the navicular bursa is rare, passive diffusion of injected dye and anesthetic occurs.[7]

The tendon of insertion of the common digital extensor muscle terminates on the extensor process of the distal phalanx, receiving a ligament from each cartilage of the distal phalanx as it inserts.

Pastern

Deep to the skin and superficial fascia on the palmar aspect of the pastern, the proximal digital anular ligament adheres to the superficial digital flexor tendon and

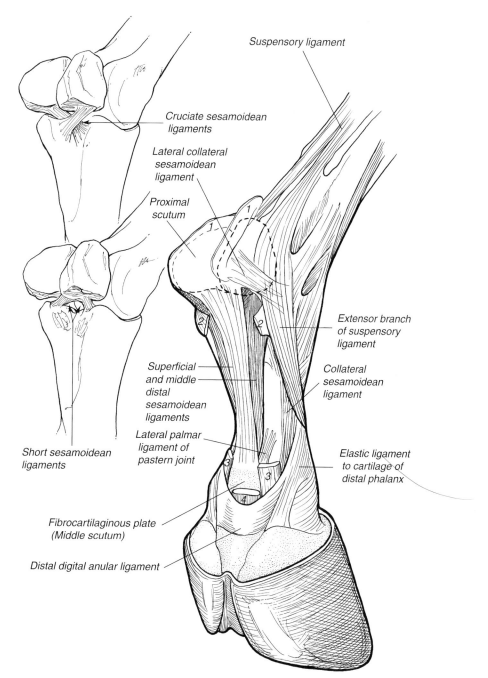

Figure 1.11. Sesamoidean ligaments. Dashed lines indicate positions of the proximal sesamoid bones embedded in the metacarpointersesamoidean ligament. Numbers indicate cut stumps of (1) palmar anular ligament, (2) proximal digital anular ligament, (3) superficial digital flexor, and (4) deep digital flexor tendon.

extends to the medial and lateral borders of the proximal phalanx (long pastern bone). This fibrous band of deep fascia covers the superficial digital flexor as it bifurcates and aids in binding down the deep digital flexor tendon as well.

Two distinct ligaments of the ergot diverge from beneath the horny ergot on the palmar skin of the fetlock. Each ligament descends obliquely just deep to the skin superficial to the proximal digital anular ligament, the terminal branch of the superficial digital flexor tendon, and the respective digital artery and palmar digital nerve, finally widening and connecting with the distal digital anular ligament. Its dense structure and glistening surface distinguish a ligament of the ergot from a digital nerve.

The tendon of insertion of the superficial digital flexor muscle terminates by bifurcating into two branches that insert on the proximal extremity of the middle phalanx just palmar to the collateral ligaments of the proximal interphalangeal (pastern) joint. Traditional parsing of the ligaments in this region has identified additional terminations of the superficial

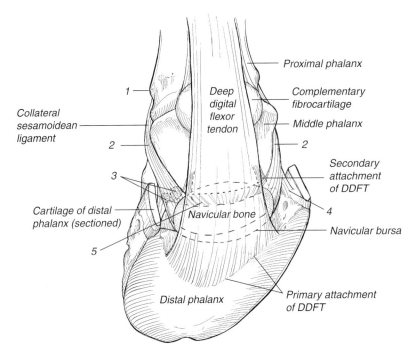

Figure 1.12. Attachments of deep digital flexor tendon and collateral sesamoidean ligaments (CSL). (1) Attachment of CSL to proximal phalanx, (2) attachment of CSL to middle phalanx, (3) abaxial outpocketings of palmar pouch of the synovial cavity of the distal interphalangeal joint, (4) attachment of CSL to cartilage of the distal phalanx, and (5) attachment of medial and lateral CSLs to navicular bone.

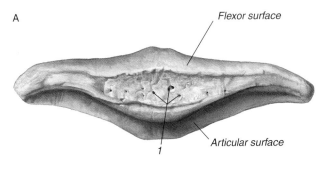

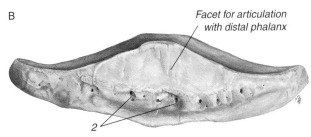

Figure 1.13. Distal sesamoid (navicular) bone. A. Proximal view. B. Distal view. (1) Foramina, (2) fossae.

digital flexor on the distal extremity of the proximal phalanx, although more recent studies have concluded that these attachments are not strictly part of the flexor tendon and instead represent associated palmar ligaments[51]. The tendon of insertion of the deep digital flexor muscle descends between the two branches of the superficial digital flexor tendon. A digital synovial sheath enfolds both tendons, including both branches of the superficial digital flexor tendon and continuing around the deep digital flexor tendon as far as the so-called "T ligament" (Figure 1.10). The latter is a fibrous partition attaching to the middle of the palmar surface of the middle phalanx.

Deep to the digital flexor tendons a series of ligaments (often collectively referred to as distal sesamoidean ligaments) extend distad from the bases of the two proximal sesamoid bones. The superficial straight sesamoidean ligament attaches distally to the fibrocartilaginous plate on the proximal extremity of the palmar surface of the middle phalanx, the triangular middle (oblique) sesamoidean ligament attaches distally to a rough area on the palmar surface of the proximal phalanx, and the deep pair of cruciate ligaments cross, each attaching distally to the contralateral eminence on the proximal extremity of the proximal phalanx (Figure 1.11).

A short sesamoidean ligament extends from the dorsal aspect of the base of each proximal sesamoid bone to the palmar edge of the articular surface of the proximal phalanx (see Figure 1.11).

An extensor branch of the suspensory ligament passes from the abaxial surface of the respective proximal sesamoid bone dorsodistad obliquely across each side of the proximal phalanx to the dorsal surface where each branch joins the tendon of insertion of the common digital extensor muscle near the distal extremity of the proximal phalanx. An elongated bursa under each extensor branch is extensive enough to be considered a synovial sheath.[17]

In the dorsal aspect of the pastern, the tendon of the common digital extensor muscle inserts partially on the middorsal aspect of the proximal extremities of the proximal and middle phalanges on its way to a definitive insertion on the extensor process of the distal phalanx. A bursa often occurs under the common digital extensor tendon near its union with the extensor branches of the suspensory ligament. The tendon of the lateral digital extensor muscle inserts lateral to the partial insertion of the common digital extensor tendon on the proximal middorsal surface of the proximal phalanx.

The proximal interphalangeal (pastern) joint is formed by two convex areas on the distal extremity of the proximal phalanx and two corresponding concave areas expanded by a palmar fibrocartilaginous plate on the proximal extremity of the middle phalanx.

Bones of the pastern joint are held together by two short collateral ligaments and four palmar ligaments. The collateral ligaments joining the distal extremity of the proximal phalanx with the proximal extremity of the middle phalanx are oriented vertically between the eminences on the bones rather than parallel to the axis of the digit. A central pair of palmar ligaments extends from the triangular rough surface on the proximal phalanx to the palmar margin of the proximal extremity of the middle phalanx; medial and lateral palmar ligaments pass from the proximal phalanx to the palmar surface of the proximal extremity of the middle phalanx. The central ligaments blend somewhat with the branches of the superficial digital flexor tendon and the straight sesamoidean ligament, and they may be difficult to discern as individual entities.

The joint capsule of the pastern joint blends with the deep surface of the common digital extensor tendon dorsally where it is accessible for arthrocentesis (Figure 1.10). It also blends with the collateral ligaments of the joint. The palmar aspect of the capsule extends slightly proximad, compressed between the middle phalanx and the terminal branches of the superficial digital flexor tendon and the straight sesamoidean ligament. These taut, overlying structures subdivide the capsule into medial and lateral pouches that are accessible for arthrocentesis.

Fetlock

The fetlock of the thoracic limb is the region around the metacarpophalangeal (fetlock) joint. On the palmar aspect of the fetlock, the horny ergot is a prominent cutaneous feature. Its dermal base gives origin to the two distally diverging ligaments of the ergot.

Deep to the skin and superficial fascia, the superficial transverse metacarpal ligament (palmar anular ligament of the fetlock) binds the digital flexor tendons and their enclosing digital synovial sheath in the sesamoid groove. The palmar anular ligament fuses lightly with the superficial digital flexor tendon and blends on the palmar border of each proximal sesamoid bone with the attachment of the collateral ligament of the proximal sesamoid bone. Distally, the palmar anular ligament of the fetlock blends with the proximal digital anular ligament.

The smooth depression between the proximal sesamoid bones through which the digital flexor tendons pass is formed by the fibrocartilage of the metacarpointersesamoidean ligament which covers the flexor surfaces of the proximal sesamoid bones. Immediately distal to the canal formed by the palmar anular ligament of the fetlock and the groove between the proximal sesamoids, the deep digital flexor tendon perforates through a circular opening in the superficial digital flexor tendon, the manaca flexoria.

The common and lateral digital extensor tendons pass over the dorsal aspect of the fetlock joint where a bursa is interposed between each tendon and the underlying joint. Small but common subcutaneous bursae may occur on the palmar surface of the fetlock joint and on the lateral aspect of the joint just proximal to the extensor branch of the suspensory ligament.[34]

The distal extremity of the third metacarpal bone (the cannon bone), the proximal extremity of the proximal phalanx, the two proximal sesamoid bones, and the extensive fibrocartilaginous metacarpointersesamoidean ligament in which the proximal sesamoids are embedded form the metacarpophalangeal (fetlock) joint. A somewhat cylindrical articular surface on the third metacarpal bone is divided by a sagittal ridge, and this surface fits into an accommodating depression formed by the proximal phalanx, the proximal sesamoid bones, and the metacarpointersesamoidean ligament.

Collateral ligaments of the fetlock joint extend distad from the eminence and depression on each side of the third metacarpal bone. The superficial part of each ligament attaches distally to the edge of the articular surface of the proximal phalanx; the shorter, stouter deep part of the ligament attaches to the abaxial surface of the adjacent proximal sesamoid and the proximal phalanx.

The palmar part of the fetlock joint capsule is thicker and more voluminous than the dorsal part. A consistent bursa deep to the digital flexor tendons at the distal extremity of the third metacarpal bone lies against the thickened capsule and may communicate with the joint cavity.[16] A palmar recess (pouch) of the fetlock joint capsule extends proximad between the third metacarpal bone and the suspensory ligament. This pouch is palpable and even visible when the joint is inflamed, distending the palmar recess with synovial fluid. The joint capsule is reinforced on each side by the collateral ligaments and dorsally by fascia attaching to the common digital extensor tendon.

Support for the fetlock and stabilization during locomotion is rendered by its suspensory apparatus, a part of the stay apparatus. The suspensory apparatus of the fetlock includes the suspensory ligament (interosseus medius muscle) and its extensor branches to the common digital extensor tendon and the distal sesamoidean ligaments extending from the bases of the proximal sesamoid bones distal to the proximal or middle phalanges. The proximal sesamoids embedded in the metacarpointersesamoidean ligament may be thought of as being intercalated in this ligamentous continuum.

Blood Vessels of the Digit and Fetlock

ARTERIAL SUPPLY

The arterial supply to the digit and fetlock of the thoracic limb is derived principally from the medial palmar artery which divides in the distal fourth of the metacarpus between the digital flexor tendons and the suspensory ligament into the medial and lateral digital arteries. An anastomotic branch from the distal deep palmar arch unites with the initial part of the lateral digital artery to form the superficial palmar arch. Branches from this arch supply the fetlock joint (Figure 1.8). Each digital artery becomes superficial on the proximal part of the fetlock covered by superficial fascia. The artery emerges palmar to its satellite vein between the ipsilateral palmar digital nerve and its dorsal branch (Figures 1.14 and 1.15). As each digital artery courses distad over the fetlock, it gives off branches to the fetlock joint, digital extensor and flexor tendons, digital synovial sheath, ligaments, fascia, and skin.

An anastomotic circle around the middle of the proximal phalanx is created as a short artery of the proximal phalanx arises from medial and lateral digital arteries; it divides immediately into dorsal and palmar branches of the proximal phalanx that encircle the proximal phalanx, thus providing an arterial supply to this bone and adjacent structures (Figure 1.8). The palmar branch extends between the proximal phalanx and the digital flexor tendons and joins the contralateral vessel between the straight and oblique sesamoidean ligaments. The dorsal branch anastomoses with the contralateral vessel deep to the common digital extensor tendon.

Near the level of the proximal interphalangeal joint, a prominent bulbar artery (artery of the digital cushion) arises from each digital artery. Its branches supply the frog, the digital cushion, palmar part of the cuneate corium, laminar corium of the heel and bar, and palmar parts of the perioplic and coronary coria. A small coronal artery detaches from the digital artery or the bulbar artery, and its branches supply the heel and perioplic corium, anastomosing with fine branches from the dorsal artery of the middle phalanx.

The dorsal branch of the middle phalanx is detached from each digital artery just below the middle of the middle phalanx and anastomoses with the contralateral branch deep to the common digital extensor tendon to form a coronary arterial circle. This vascular complex supplies branches to the distal interphalangeal joint, common digital extensor tendon, perioplic and coronary coria, fascia, and skin.

The palmar branches of the middle phalanx arise opposite the dorsal arteries. These vessels course inward parallel to the proximal border of the distal sesamoid bone, joining to complete an arterial circle around the middle phalanx. A collateral arch projects dorsad from the conjoined vessels supplemented by small branches from the digital arteries.[21] Branches from the conjoined palmar branches of the middle phalanx supply an anastomotic proximal navicular plexus providing several small arteries to foramina along the proximal border of the distal sesamoid bone.[10,21] The bone receives approximately one-third of its blood supply from this plexus.

Within the foot opposite each extremity of the navicular bone, an artery to the dermal laminae of the heel arising from the digital artery has been noted on radiographic angiograms.[9,18] At the level of the palmar process of the distal phalanx, the digital artery gives off the dorsal branch of the distal phalanx and then continues distad to the terminal arch. Before passing through a notch or foramen in the palmar process, the dorsal branch of the distal phalanx gives off a small artery supplying branches to the digital cushion and corium of the frog. Following passage through the notch or foramen in the palmar process, the dorsal branch of the distal phalanx bifurcates on the dorsal surface of the distal phalanx. One branch supplies the laminar corium of the heels and quarters; the other courses dorsad in the parietal sulcus of the distal phalanx to supply the laminar corium of the toe, eventually branching to join the palmar part of the marginal artery of the sole and branches of the coronal artery. The termination of the dorsal branch of the distal phalanx joins with a vessel coming through the distal phalanx from the terminal arch in the solar canal.

Immediately distal to each extremity of the distal sesamoid bone the ipsilateral digital artery gives off one to three small arteries that supply a total of three to six branches entering the distal border of the bone adjacent to the extremity (Figure 1.12). The lateral and medial digital arteries follow the solar grooves in the distal phalanx. Each artery detaches branches to the distal navicular plexus in the distal sesamoid impar ligament. Six to nine distal navicular arteries from the plexus enter the distal sesamoid bone through the distal border, anastomosing within the osseous foramina. Arterioles radiating from these supply the distal two-thirds of the distal sesamoid bone.[21]

Each digital artery enters a solar foramen and anastomoses with the contralateral artery to form the terminal arch within the solar (semilunar) canal of the distal phalanx (Figure 1.8). Branches from the terminal arch course through the bone, four or five of them emerging through mid-dorsal foramina on the parietal surface to supply the proximal part of the laminar corium; 8 to 10 vessels emerge through foramina near the solar border of the bone and anastomose to form the prominent marginal artery of the sole. The latter vessel supplies the solar and cuneate coria.

The arterial network of the corium has been divided into three regions with independent blood supplies: (1) the dorsal coronary corium, (2) the palmar part of the coronary corium and laminar corium, and (3) the dorsal laminar corium and solar corium.[17] Other regions are supplied by several arteries. Sequential angiographic studies indicate that blood flow within dermal laminae is from distal to proximal.[9]

Branches of the digital arteries in the hindfoot are essentially the same as in the forefoot except for the blood supply to the distal sesamoid bone. In 50% of hindfeet examined in a definitive study, the collateral arch from the plantar branches of the middle phalanx supplied the primary arteries to the proximal navicular network.[21]

DERMAL MICROCIRCULATION OF THE FOOT

A scanning electron microscopic study revealed the following vascular patterns in the dermal microcirculation of the foot with emphasis on the distribution of arteriovenous anastomoses.[36] Axial arteries branching from parietal arteries enter dermal laminae between pairs of axial veins. Interconnecting branches join adja-

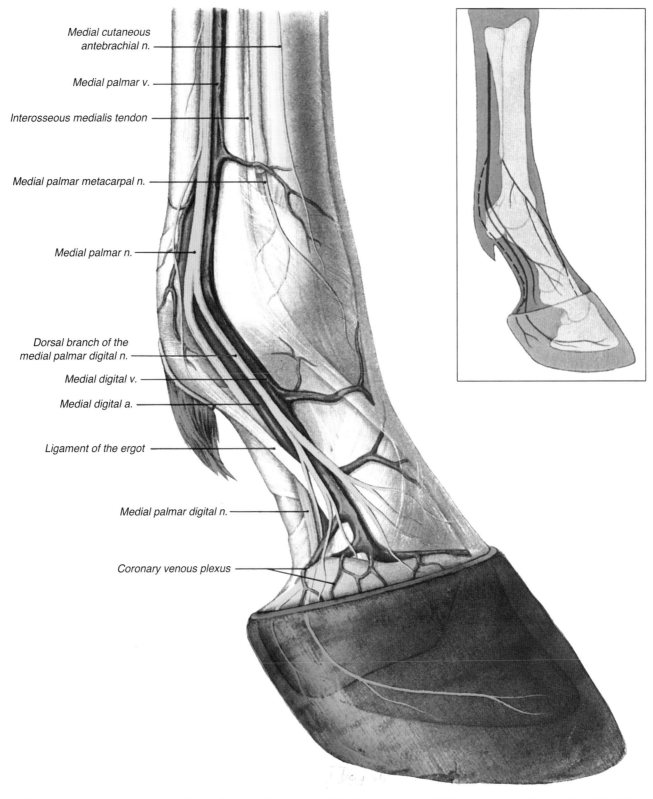

Medial cutaneous antebrachial n.

Medial palmar v.

Interosseous medialis tendon

Medial palmar metacarpal n.

Medial palmar n.

Dorsal branch of the medial palmar digital n.

Medial digital v.

Medial digital a.

Ligament of the ergot

Medial palmar digital n.

Coronary venous plexus

Figure 1.14. Medial aspect of distal metacarpus, fetlock, and digit with skin and superficial fascia removed. Inset: schematic of the distribution of major nerves; dashed lines indicate variant branches.

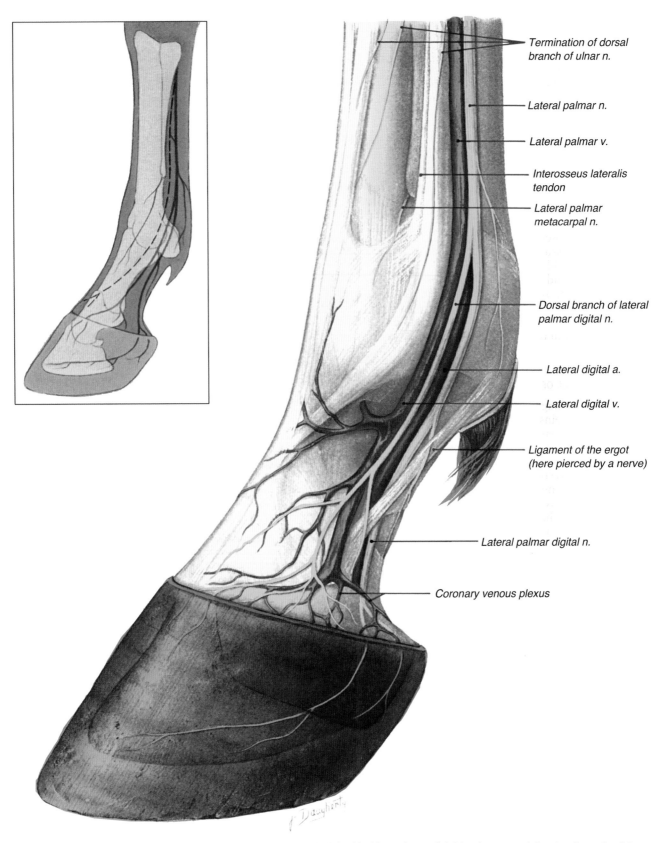

Termination of dorsal
branch of ulnar n.

Lateral palmar n.

Lateral palmar v.

Interosseus lateralis
tendon

Lateral palmar
metacarpal n.

Dorsal branch of lateral
palmar digital n.

Lateral digital a.

Lateral digital v.

Ligament of the ergot
(here pierced by a nerve)

Lateral palmar digital n.

Coronary venous plexus

Figure 1.15. Lateral aspect of distal metacarpus, fetlock, and digit with skin and superficial fascia removed. Inset: schematic of the distribution of major nerves; dashed lines indicate variant branches.

cent axial arteries and proximodistally oriented abaxial arteries. Anastomosing laminar veins drain the capillary network. In addition, numerous arteriovenous anastomoses occur in the laminar circulation with the largest and longest located near the origins of axial arteries. Dermal papillae of the periople, coronary band, distal laminae, frog, and sole each contain a central artery and vein ensheathed by a network of fine capillaries. Arteriovenous anastomoses occur at the base of each dermal papilla and between the central artery and vein.

Two functions have been suggested for these arteriovenous anastomoses.[36] The large number of arteriovenous anastomoses in dermal laminae may prevent cold-induced tissue damage by their periodic vasodilation. This would permit warm blood to bypass the capillary bed and enter the digits quickly to maintain temperatures above the freezing point. Another proposed function considers arteriovenous anastomoses as safety valves that help offset the large pressure changes that occur within the hoof capsule during galloping and jumping.

VENOUS DRAINAGE OF THE FOOT

Venous drainage from the laminar corium begins with parietal veins from the laminar circulation continuing into the parietal venous plexus and the coronary venous plexus (Figure 1.16). Veins from the periopic and coronary coria drain toward the coronary venous plexus, and those from the solar and cuneate coria drain into the solar venous plexus.

Two parallel veins in the solar canal come together at the level of the distal sesamoid bone to form the medial and lateral terminal veins. Each terminal vein

joins with branches of an inner venous plexus to form a digital vein. The digital vein receives branches from the distal sesamoid bone, coronary vein (draining the coronary region), inner venous plexus, and large bulbar vein carrying blood from the heel.

Most venous blood in the foot is drained by the veins located in the palmar aspect which are largely valveless. Some valves are present in the tributaries of the coronary and subcoronary veins and in the bulbar veins and their branches. Thus, the flow of blood may take different routes with the weightbearing force essential to its proximal flow[49].

Nerves of the Digit and Fetlock

As they descend to the proximal widening of the fetlock, the medial and lateral palmar nerves supply small branches to the fetlock and the flexor tendons, then continue as the medial and lateral palmar digital nerves. Each immediately gives off a dorsal branch (Figures 1.14 and 1.15). The corresponding digital artery lies between the dorsal branch and the continuation of the palmar digital nerve. The dorsal branch courses distad between the digital vein and artery. Midway down the pastern this nerve branches, the main part continuing dorsad superficial to the palmar digital vein. In approximately one-third of the cases, an intermediate branch arises from the dorsal aspect of the palmar digital nerve.[31] The dorsal and intermediate branches supply sensory and vasomotor innervation to the skin of the fetlock, dorsal part of the fetlock joint, dorsal parts of the interphalangeal joints, coronary corium and dorsal parts of the laminar and solar coria, and dorsal part of the cartilage of the distal phalanx.[6]

The main continuation of the palmar digital nerve descends palmar and parallel to the ipsilateral digital artery. The nerve and artery lie deep to the ligament of the ergot as it descends obliquely across the lateral aspect of the pastern. A branch may arise from the lateral palmar digital nerve and perforate the lateral ligament of the ergot (Figure 1.15).

The palmar continuations of the palmar digital nerves supply the fetlock joint capsule and then descend to supply the palmar structures of the digit: skin, pastern joint capsule, digital synovial sheath and flexor tendons, distal sesamoidean ligaments, coffin joint capsule, navicular bone and its ligaments, navicular bursa, palmar part of the cartilage of the distal phalanx, part of the laminar corium, coria of the sole and frog, and digital cushion.

A fine terminal branch of each palmar digital nerve and an accompanying small artery constitute a neurovascular bundle that descends adjacent to the synovial membrane of the distal interphalangeal joint to enter the distal phalanx.[5]

Further cutaneous innervation of the fetlock is supplied by terminal branches of the medial cutaneous antebrachial nerve dorsomedially and the dorsal branch of the ulnar nerve dorsolaterally. After supplying branches to the fetlock joint capsule, the medial and lateral palmar metacarpal nerves emerge immediately distal to the distal extremity of the respective small metacarpal bone and ramify in the superficial fascia of

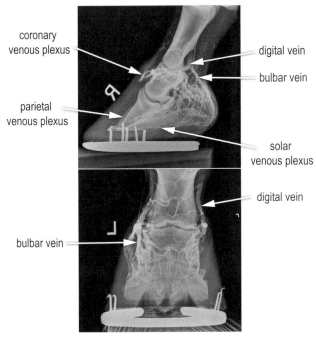

Figure 1.16. Venogram of equine foot. (Photo courtesy of Dr. Andrew Lewis.)

the pastern. It has been reported that in some instances, a terminal branch from the medial palmar metacarpal nerve descends to the coronary band (Figure 1.14).[23,34] An occasional variant, a palmarly directed branch from the medial palmar nerve in the distal metacarpus, courses palmar to the medial palmar digital nerve, reaching the digital cushion (Figure 1.14). Another variant branch may arise from the lateral palmar nerve in the proximal metacarpus, cross over the fetlock, and extend obliquely to the coronary band (Figure 1.15).

Electrophysiologic studies confirm that stimuli on the medial half of the digit and fetlock of a forelimb are mediated by the median nerve; stimuli on the lateral half are mediated by the median and ulnar nerves.[5]

Although direct communication between the distal interphalangeal joint and the navicular bursa is very rare, indirect communication via diffusion of molecules has been demonstrated.[6] Dye injected experimentally into the distal interphalangeal joint diffused into the navicular bursa and also stained the synovial coverings of the collateral sesamoidean ligaments and the distal sesamoidean impar ligament, and the medullary cavity of the navicular bone. Peptide immunocytochemistry and silver/gold axonal impregnation have identified sensory nerves superficially on the dorsal and palmar parts of the collateral sesamoidean ligaments and the distal sesamoidean impar ligament and in periarticular connective tissues.[6]

Functions of the Digit and Fetlock

In the standing position, the fetlock and digit are prevented from non-physiologic hyperextension by the suspensory apparatus of the fetlock (interosseus muscle, intersesamoidean ligament, and distal sesamoidean ligaments), digital flexor tendons, and collateral ligaments of the joints.

During flexion of the fetlock and digit, most of the movement is in the fetlock, the least amount of movement is in the pastern joint, and movement in the coffin joint is intermediate. Although the pastern joint is a hinge joint, providing only limited flexion and extension, manipulation can cause transverse flexion and some axial rotation when the joint is flexed.

Contraction of the common and lateral digital extensor muscles brings the bones and joints of the digit into alignment just before the hoof strikes the ground.

When the unshod hoof contacts the ground, the heels strike first, followed in sequence by the ground surfaces of the quarters and toe. Expansion of the heels is facilitated by the elasticity of the hoof wall which becomes thinner from toe to heels. Most of the impact is sustained by the hoof wall, and compression of the wall creates tension on the interlocking epidermal and dermal laminae and, hence, to the periosteum of the distal phalanx. Axial compressive force is transmitted through the phalanges. The concave sole does not support much force and it is depressed slightly by the pressure of the distal phalanx, causing expansion of the quarters. The position of the bars minimizes expansion of the sole. Descent of the coffin joint occurs as the navicular bone gives in a distopalmar direction, stretching its collateral (suspensory) and distal sesamoidean impar ligaments and pushing against the navicular bursa and tendon of

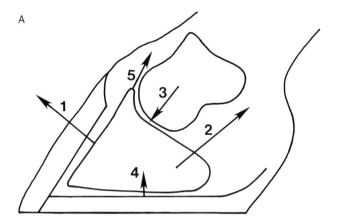

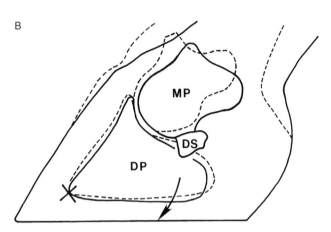

Figure 1.17. A. Diagram of forces acting on distal phalanx. (1) Forces from laminae of wall, (2) tensile force from deep digital flexor tendon, (3) compressive force from middle phalanx, (4) compressive force from sole, and (5) tensile forces from extensor branches of suspensory ligament and common (long, in pelvic limb) digital extensor tendon. B. Position changes in middle phalanx (MP), distal phalanx (DP), distal sesamoid (DS), and hoof wall resulting from weight-bearing. X = axis about which the distal phalanx rotates; arrow indicates rotation from unloaded (dotted line) to loaded (solid line) state. (Redrawn from Leach D. Biomechanical considerations in raising and lowering the heel. Proc Am Assoc Equine Pract 1983;33).

the deep digital flexor muscle. Forces acting on the distal phalanx are indicated in Figure 1.17. Magnitude and direction of the forces may change with limb position and loading state.[26] Concussion is further dissipated by pressure from the frog being transmitted to the digital cushion and the cartilages of the distal phalanx.

Lateral expansion of the hoof and cartilages of the distal phalanx compresses the venous plexuses of the foot, forcing blood proximad into the digital veins. The hydraulic shock absorption by the blood within the vessels augments the direct cushioning by the frog and digital cushion and the resiliency of the hoof wall.

During concussion, the palmar ligaments of the pastern joint, the straight sesamoidean ligament, and the tendon of the deep digital flexor provide the tension necessary to prevent overextension of the pastern joint. Contraction of the superficial digital flexor muscle tightens its tendon's insertions on the proximal end of the middle phalanx, preventing the pastern joint from buckling.

The suspensory apparatus of the fetlock and the digital flexor tendons ensure that overextension of the fetlock joint, i.e., decreasing the dorsal articular angle, is minimized when the hoof strikes the ground. Yet at a gallop, when all of the horse's weight is on one forelimb momentarily, the palmar aspect of the fetlock comes very close to the ground. During this descent of the fetlock, the coffin joint is flexed by the deep digital flexor tendon.

Metacarpus

The equine metacarpus consists of the large third metacarpal (cannon) bone, the second (medial) and fourth (lateral) small metacarpal bones (splint bones), and the structures associated with them. The shaft of each small metacarpal bone is united by an interosseous ligament to the large metacarpal bone. The cortex under the rounded dorsal surfaces of the metacarpal bones is thicker than the cortex under their concave palmar surfaces. Length and curvature of the shafts and the prominence of the free distal extremities ("buttons") of the small metacarpal bones are variable. The proximal extremities of the metacarpal bones articulate with the distal row of carpal bones; the second metacarpal articulating with the second and third carpals; the third metacarpal articulating with the second, third, and fourth carpals; and the fourth metacarpal with the fourth carpal bone.

Dorsal Aspect

The skin, fascia, and digital extensor tendons on the dorsal aspect of the metacarpus receive their blood supply from small medial and lateral dorsal metacarpal arteries originating from the dorsal carpal rete and descending between the large metacarpal bone and the respective medial or lateral metacarpal bone. Innervation to this region is furnished by the medial cutaneous antebrachial nerve (Figures 1.14 and 1.20) and the dorsal branch of the ulnar nerve (Figures 1.18 and 1.21). Deep to the skin the main tendon of the common digital extensor muscle inclines proximolaterad from its central position at the fetlock across the dorsal surface of the third metacarpal bone. Proximally the main tendon and the accompanying tendon of the radial head of the common digital extensor lie lateral to the insertional tendon of the extensor carpi radialis muscle on the prominent metacarpal tuberosity of the third metacarpal bone (Figure 1.20). The tendon of the lateral digital extensor muscle is lateral to the common extensor tendon, and the small radial tendon of the latter usually joins the lateral digital extensor tendon. Occasionally the radial tendon pursues an independent course to the fetlock. A strong fibrous band from the accessory carpal bone reinforces the lateral digital extensor tendon as it angles dorsad in its descent from the lateral aspect of the carpus.

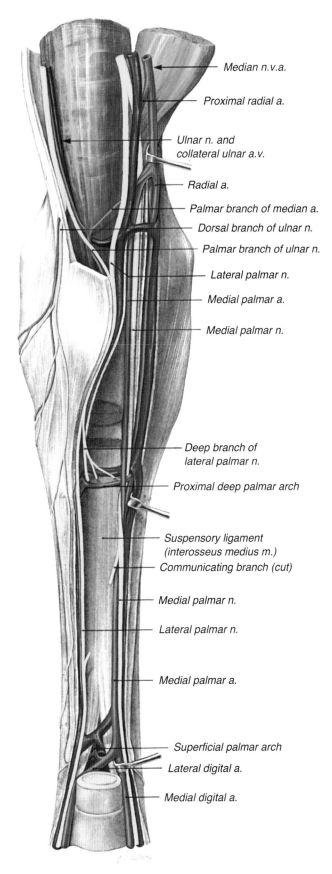

Figure 1.18. Caudal view of left carpus and metacarpus; most of the digital flexor tendons are removed.

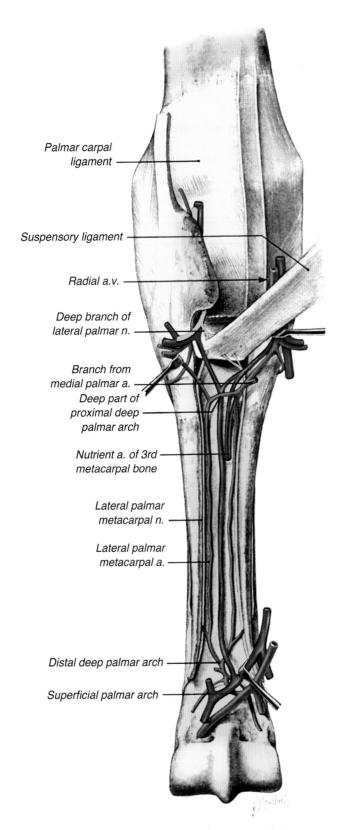

Palmar carpal ligament

Suspensory ligament

Radial a.v.

Deep branch of lateral palmar n.

Branch from medial palmar a.

Deep part of proximal deep palmar arch

Nutrient a. of 3rd metacarpal bone

Lateral palmar metacarpal n.

Lateral palmar metacarpal a.

Distal deep palmar arch

Superficial palmar arch

Figure 1.19. Deep dissection of caudal aspects of left carpus and metacarpus with medial palmar artery removed.

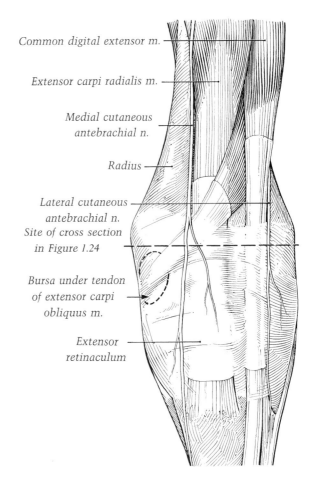

Common digital extensor m.

Extensor carpi radialis m.

Medial cutaneous antebrachial n.

Radius

Lateral cutaneous antebrachial n.
Site of cross section in Figure 1.24

Bursa under tendon of extensor carpi obliquus m.

Extensor retinaculum

Figure 1.20. Dorsal view of left carpus.

Medial and Lateral Aspects

From the medial digital vein at the fetlock, the medial palmar vein continues proximad on the medial aspect of the metacarpus. In the distal half of the metacarpus, the vein is related palmarly to the medial palmar nerve (Figure 1.14); in the proximal half, the large medial palmar artery is palmar to the vein (Figure 1.18). A similar relationship exists on the lateral side except that the very small lateral palmar artery does not intervene appreciably between the satellite vein and nerve. At the middle of the metacarpus, the medial palmar nerve detaches a communicating branch that angles distolaterad in the subcutaneous fascia across the digital flexor tendons to join the lateral palmar nerve distal to the middle of the metacarpus. The medial palmar nerve does not give off cutaneous branches proximal to the communicating branch.[12] The palmar nerves supply the digital flexor tendons and the skin over them. The palmar nerves are related to the dorsal border of the deep digital flexor tendon and edges of the suspensory ligament. Branches from the dorsal branch of the ulnar nerve ramify in the fascia and skin of the lateral aspect of the metacarpus. Branches from the medial cutaneous antebrachial nerve supply the medial and dorsal skin of the metacarpus with the large dorsal branch reaching the skin over the dorsomedial aspect of the fetlock.

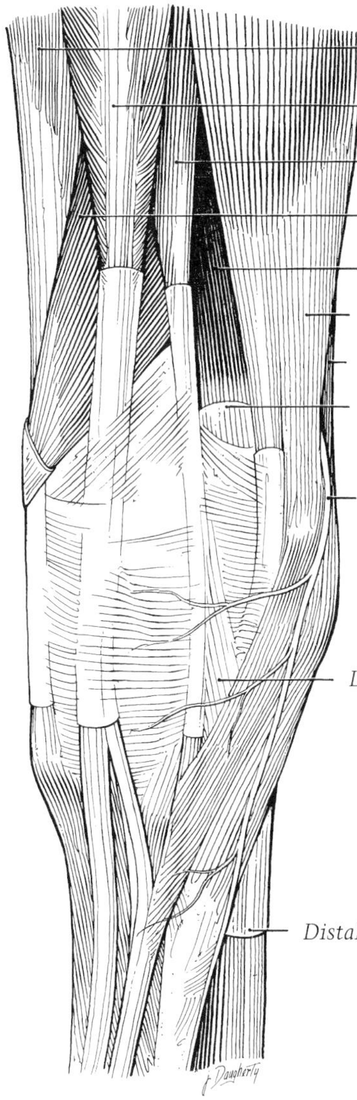

Extensor carpi radialis m.
Common digital extensor m.
Lateral digital extensor m.
Extensor carpi obliquus m.
Deep digital flexor m.
Ulnaris lateralis m.
Flexor carpi ulnaris m.
Proximal limit of carpal sheath
Dorsal branch of the ulnar n.
Lateral collateral ligament
Distal limit of carpal sheath

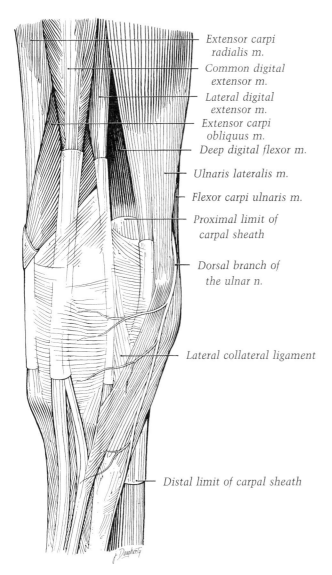

Figure 1.21. Lateral view of left distal forearm, carpus, and proximal metacarpus. Note that the ulnaris lateralis is now called extensor carpi ulnaris.

Palmar Aspect

The superficial digital flexor tendon is deep to the skin and subcutaneous fascia throughout the length of the metacarpus. Dorsally it is intimately related to the fascial covering of the deep digital flexor tendon. The latter, in turn, lies against the palmar surface of the suspensory ligament (m. interosseus medius, middle or third interosseous muscle). The carpal synovial sheath, enclosing both digital flexor tendons, extends distad as far as the middle of the metacarpus. At this level, the deep digital flexor tendon is joined by its accessory ligament (carpal check ligament or "inferior" check ligament), the distal continuation of the palmar carpal ligament (Figure 1.31, later in text). The medial and lateral lumbricales muscles, fleshy in other species, originate as fibrous slips from either side of the deep digital flexor tendon and insert under the ergot. The digital synovial sheath around the digital flexor tendons extends proximad into the distal fourth of the metacarpus (Figure 1.10).

The metacarpal groove, formed by the palmar surface of the third metacarpal bone and the axial surfaces of the second and fourth metacarpal bones, contains the suspensory ligament. The suspensory ligament arises from the distal row of carpal bones and the proximal end of the third metacarpal bone (Figures 1.18 and 1.19). It is broad, relatively flat, and shorter than the suspensory ligament of the hindlimb. Variable amounts of striated muscle fibers within the mainly collagenous suspensory ligament are organized into two longitudinal bundles within the proximal part and body of the ligament (hence, interosseus medius "muscle").[53] In the distal fourth of the metacarpus, the suspensory ligament bifurcates to become associated with the two proximal sesamoid bones (Figure 1.11). Each side crosses the abaxial surface of proximal sesamoid bone and extends across the abaxial aspect of the proximal phalanx where it contacts the origin of the ipsilateral collateral sesamoidean ligament. An extensor branch continues on to join the tendon of the common digital extensor muscle on the dorsal surface of the proximal phalanx (Figure 1.11). Two small interossei muscles originate on the respective small metacarpal bones with fine, strong tendons ending in the fascia of the fetlock.

Medial and lateral palmar metacarpal nerves and satellite vessels lie in the grooves formed by the third metacarpal bone with the respective small metacarpal bones (Figure 1.19). The two nerves originate from the deep branch of the lateral palmar nerve which supplies branches to the interosseus muscles, perforates the suspensory ligament, and then divides into the medial and lateral palmar metacarpal nerves. After sending branches to the fetlock joint capsule, each palmar metacarpal nerve emerges distal to the distal extremity (the "button") of the respective small metacarpal bone to ramify in the fascia and skin of the pastern (Figures 1.14 and 1.15).

The palmar metacarpal arteries originate from the proximal deep palmar arch, an anastomotic complex formed by the termination of the radial artery passing over the suspensory ligament to join the smaller palmar branch of the median artery (Figure 1.19). Part of the arch lies between the accessory ligament of the deep digital flexor tendon and the suspensory ligament; a smaller inconstant transverse branch lies deep to the suspensory ligament on the third metacarpal bone. Another contribution to this vascular complex may be provided by a prominent branch from the medial palmar artery which branches to anastomose with the radial artery and the medial palmar metacarpal artery (Figure 1.19). The medial palmar metacarpal artery supplies a nutrient artery to the third metacarpal bone and then often detaches a middle palmar metacarpal artery. Small branches from the medial and lateral palmar metacarpal arteries extend through interosseous spaces to join the medial and lateral dorsal metacarpal arteries. In the distal fourth of the metacarpus, the medial and lateral palmar metacarpal arteries join to form the distal deep palmar arch. A branch from this arch to the lateral digital artery is termed the superficial palmar arch.

A single, large palmar metacarpal vein courses proximad to join the venous deep palmar arch.

The vascular patterns described above are subject to variations, but the variations are of no clinical significance.

Carpus

The carpal region includes the carpal bones (radial, intermediate, ulnar, and accessory in the proximal row; first, second, third, and fourth in the distal row), the distal extremity of the radius, the proximal extremities of the three metacarpal bones, and the structures adjacent to these osseous components.

Dorsal Aspect

In the skin on the dorsal carpus a vascular network, the rete carpi dorsale, is formed by branches from the cranial interosseus, transverse cubital, and radial arteries. Medial and lateral cutaneous antebrachial nerves supply branches to the medial and dorsal aspects of the carpus. Tendon sheaths of the extensor carpi radialis, extensor carpi obliquus (abductor digiti I longus), and the common digital extensor muscles are enclosed in fibrous passages through the deep fascia and then through the extensor retinaculum. The tendon sheaths of the common digital and extensor carpi obliquus tendons extend from the carpometacarpal articulation proximad to 6 to 8 cm proximal to the carpus (Figure 1.20).

A subtendinous bursa lies between the ensheathed tendon of the extensor carpi obliquus and the medial collateral ligament of the carpus (Figure 1.20).[39] In most foals younger than 2 years, the bursa is a separate synovial structure; in older horses it communicates with the adjacent tendon sheath. A small tendon from the radial head of the common digital extensor muscle occupies the same synovial sheath as the main tendon; the small tendon may angle palmarad to join the tendon of the lateral digital extensor muscle, or it may pursue a course between the main extensor tendons to the fetlock. The tendon sheath of the extensor carpi radialis muscle terminates at the middle of the carpus, and then the tendon becomes adherent to the retinaculum as it extends to its insertion on the metacarpal tuberosity (Figure 1.20).

Deeply the extensor retinaculum serves as the dorsal part of the common fibrous joint capsule of the carpal joints—the antebrachiocarpal (radiocarpal), midcarpal, and carpometacarpal joints. The extensor retinaculum attaches to the radius, the dorsal intercarpal and dorsal carpometacarpal ligaments, the carpal bones, and the third metacarpal bone. Laterally and medially it blends with the collateral ligaments of the carpus.

Branches from the cranial interosseous artery supply the superficial structures of the lateral aspect of the carpal region. The proximal radial and lateral palmar arteries supply deeper structures. The dorsal branch of the ulnar nerve emerges between the tendon of insertion of the flexor carpi ulnaris muscle and the short tendon of the extensor carpi ulnaris or between the short and long tendons of the latter muscle (Figures 1.17 and 1.21). As it courses distad, the nerve supplies branches to the fascia and skin of the dorsal and lateral aspects of the carpus.

Lateral Aspect

The lateral collateral carpal ligament extends distad from its attachment on the styloid process of the radius (Figure 1.22). The superficial part of the ligament attaches distally on the fourth metacarpal bone and partly on the third metacarpal bone. A canal between the superficial part and the deep part of the ligament provides passage for the tendon of the lateral digital extensor muscle and its synovial sheath. The deep part of the ligament attaches on the ulnar carpal bone.

Palmar to the lateral collateral carpal ligament, four ligaments support the accessory carpal bone. These ligaments, named according to their attachments, are from proximal to distal, the accessorioulnar, accessoriocarpoulnar, accessorioquartal, and accessoriometacarpal ligaments (Figure 1.22). Tendons of two muscles are associated with the accessory carpal bone. The short tendon of the extensor carpi ulnaris muscle (formerly ulnaris lateralis m.) attaches to the proximal border and lateral surface of the bone; the muscle's long tendon, enclosed in a synovial sheath, passes through a groove on the bone's lateral surface and then continues distad to insert on the proximal extremity of the fourth metacarpal bone (Figure 1.21). Proximally, a palmarolateral pouch of the antebrachiocarpal joint capsule is interposed between the long tendon of the extensor carpi

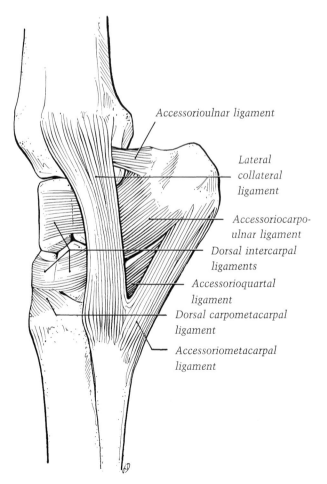

Accessorioulnar ligament

Lateral collateral ligament

Accessoriocarpo-ulnar ligament

Dorsal intercarpal ligaments

Accessorioquartal ligament

Dorsal carpometacarpal ligament

Accessoriometacarpal ligament

Figure 1.22.   Carpal ligaments, lateral view.

ulnaris and the lateral styloid process of the radius. The single tendon of the flexor carpi ulnaris muscle attaches to the proximal border of the accessory carpal bone, blending with the flexor retinaculum. A fibrous band from the accessory carpal bone attaches to the lateral digital extensor tendon.

Medial Aspect

On the medial side of the carpus the skin and fascia receive blood from branches of the radial artery. Innervation is supplied by the medial cutaneous antebrachial nerve.

The medial collateral carpal ligament extends from the medial styloid process of the radius and widens distally to attach to the proximal ends of the second and third metacarpal bones. Bundles of fibers also attach to the radial, second, and third carpal bones (Figure 1.23). Palmarly the ligament joins the flexor retinaculum. At this juncture a canal is formed that accommodates the passage of the tendon of the flexor carpi radialis and its synovial sheath as the tendon pursues its course to the proximal extremity of the second metacarpal bone. The inconstant first carpal bone may be embedded in the palmar part of the medial collateral carpal ligament adjacent to the second carpal bone.

Palmar Aspect

The flexor retinaculum is a fibrous band extending from the medial collateral ligament, distal end of the radius, radial and second carpal bones, and proximal

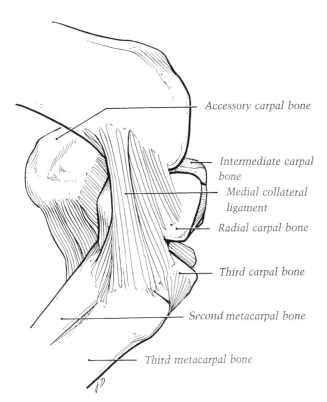

Figure 1.23. Carpal ligaments, medial view.

Accessory carpal bone

Intermediate carpal bone

Medial collateral ligament

Radial carpal bone

Third carpal bone

Second metacarpal bone

Third metacarpal bone

end of the second metacarpal bone laterad to the accessory carpal bone and the accessorioquartal and accessoriometacarpal ligaments. By bridging the carpal groove the flexor retinaculum forms the mediopalmar wall of the carpal canal. It blends proximally with the caudal antebrachial fascia, and distally with the palmar metacarpal fascia. Proximally, the fan-shaped accessory ligament of the superficial digital flexor tendon (radial check ligament) completes the medial wall of the carpal canal. The lateral wall is formed by the accessory carpal bone and its two distal ligaments. The palmar carpal ligament forms the smooth dorsal wall, its deep surface serving as the palmar part of the common fibrous capsule of the carpal joints. It attaches to the three palmar radiocarpal, three palmar intercarpal, and four carpometacarpal ligaments as well as the carpal bones. Distally, the palmar carpal ligament gives origin to the accessory ligament (carpal check) of the deep digital flexor tendon which joins the tendon at approximately the middle of the metacarpus.

The carpal canal (Figures 1.24 and 1.25) contains the following structures: the superficial and deep digital flexor tendons enclosed in the carpal synovial sheath; the medial palmar nerve and artery; and the lateral palmar nerve, artery, and vein. Medial to the carpal canal, the tendon of the flexor carpi radialis enclosed in its tendon sheath descends to its attachment on the proximal part of the second metacarpal bone. The radial artery and vein lie palmar to the tendon embedded in the flexor retinaculum.

The carpal synovial sheath enclosing the digital flexor tendons extends from a level 8 to 10 cm proximal to the antebrachiocarpal joint distad to near the middle of the metacarpus (Figure 1.25). Under the caudal antebrachial fascia, fibers from the accessory ligament of the superficial digital flexor tendon blend into the medial aspect of the wide proximal end of the carpal sheath. The distal end is covered by the palmar metacarpal fascia. Between the tendons, an intertendinous membrane attaches to the palmaromedial surface of the deep digital flexor tendon and the dorsomedial surface of the superficial digital flexor tendon, dividing the carpal synovial sheath into lateral and medial compartments.[47]

In the forearm proximal to the carpus, the palmar branches of the median and collateral ulnar arteries anastomose deep to the flexor carpi ulnaris muscle (Figure 1.18). The vascular network of the deep palmar carpal region, the rete carpi palmare, is supplied by small branches from the palmar branch of the median and proximal radial arteries (from the median artery). The lateral palmar artery continues distad to near the proximal end of the fourth metacarpal bone where it participates with the radial artery in forming the proximal deep palmar arch. Branches from the radial artery (also a terminal branch of the median artery) extend around the medial aspect of the carpus to contribute to the dorsal carpal rete.

Carpal Joints

The joints between the radius and proximal carpal bones (radiocarpal joint), ulna, and proximal carpal bones (ulnocarpal joint) together constitute the antebrachiocarpal joint. It and the midcarpal joint between

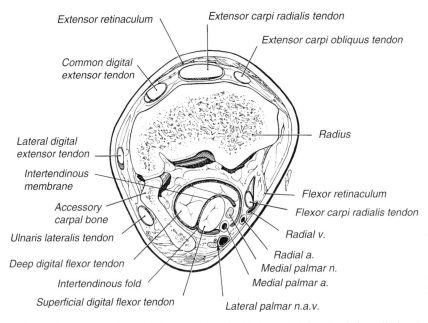

Figure 1.24. Cross section just proximal to the left antebrachiocarpal joint. Note that the ulnaris lateralis (tendon labeled here) is now called extensor carpi ulnaris.

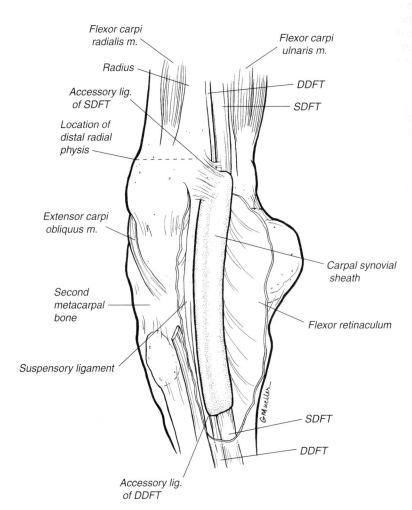

Figure 1.25. Palmaromedial view of carpus with flexor retinaculum cut and reflected. SDFT = superficial digital flexor tendon; DDFT = deep digital flexor tendon.

the proximal and distal rows of carpal bones act as hinge joints, whereas the carpometacarpal joint between the distal row of carpal bones and the three metacarpal bones is a plane joint with minimal movement. An extensive antebrachiocarpal synovial sac sends extensions between the carpal bones of the proximal row and also encompasses the joints formed by the accessory carpal bone. A palmarolateral pouch extends from the radiocarpal sac out between the long tendon of the extensor carpi ulnaris muscle and the lateral styloid process of the radius. The midcarpal synovial sac communicates with the small carpometacarpal sac between the third and fourth carpal bones.

The antebrachiocarpal and midcarpal joints are flexed by the combined action of the flexor carpi radialis, flexor carpi ulnaris, and probably the oddly-named extensor carpi ulnaris; the joints are extended by the extensor carpi radialis and extensor carpi obliquus (abductor digiti I longus) muscles. The palmar carpal ligament uniting the palmar aspect of the carpal bones serves to prevent overextension of the antebrachiocarpal and midcarpal joints.

Further stability is given to the extended carpus dorsally by the tendon of the extensor carpi radialis muscle and palmarly by the ligamentous support of the "check ligaments" and the digital flexor tendons. The accessory (radial check) ligament of the superficial digital flexor is a fan-shaped flat fibrous band originating on a ridge on the caudomedial aspect of the distal part of the radius and joining the tendon of the humeral head of the superficial digital flexor under the proximal part of the flexor retinaculum (Figure 1.32, later in text) and contributing to the medial wall of the carpal canal.

Antebrachium

The antebrachium (forearm) includes the radius and ulna and the muscles, vessels, nerves, and skin surrounding the bones. The prominent muscle belly of the extensor carpi radialis muscle bulges under the skin on the cranial aspect. A horny cutaneous structure, the chestnut, is present on the medial skin of the distal one-third of the forearm. The chestnut is considered to be a vestige of the first digit.

Superficial Nerves and Vessels

There is extensive overlapping among adjacent sensory cutaneous branches of the axillary, radial, musculocutaneous, and ulnar nerves in the forearm.[5] The axillary nerve detaches brachial cutaneous branches to the lateral aspect of the arm and terminates as the cranial cutaneous antebrachial nerve, crossing the insertion of the cleidobrachialis muscle and coursing distad in the fascia over the extensor carpi radialis muscle.

The lateral cutaneous antebrachial nerve is detached from the superficial branch of the radial nerve as the latter runs between the extensor carpi radialis and the lateral head of the triceps brachii (Figure 1.30, later in text). In its subcutaneous course the lateral cutaneous antebrachial nerve descends to supply the skin on the craniolateral distal part of the forearm. Terminal branches often course to the carpus and proximal metacarpus (Figure 1.20).

The medial cutaneous antebrachial nerve continues laterodistad from the musculocutaneous nerve, coursing in the subcutis over the biceps brachii muscle and then along the deep face of the lacertus fibrosus which blends with the antebrachial fascia and continues into the tendon of the extensor carpi radialis muscle. The nerve is readily palpable through the skin as it crosses the cranial edge and then the medial surface of the lacertus fibrosus where it divides into two main branches (Figure 1.26). The larger branch accompanies the accessory cephalic vein. The nerve continues distad on the dorsomedial aspect of the carpus and metacarpus to the fetlock. The smaller branch runs briefly with the cephalic vein and then courses obliquely across the medial surface of the radius where the bone is subcutaneous. This branch of the nerve is sensory to the skin as far as the medial aspect of the carpus. Whereas the medial cutaneous antebrachial nerve is primarily sensory, it also supplies motor fibers to the pectoralis transversus muscle.

Ascending over the cranial edge of the pectoralis transversus the cephalic vein lays in the groove between the pectoralis descendens and cleidobrachialis muscles. A small artery, the deltoid branch of the superficial cervical artery, accompanies the cephalic vein in the groove. Under cover of the cutaneous colli muscle, the cephalic vein empties into the jugular vein or occasionally into the subclavian vein. The accessory cephalic vein joins the cephalic vein after the latter detaches the median cubital vein (Figure 1.26). The median cubital vein courses proximocaudad over the short medial attachment of the biceps brachii to the radius and then passes over the median nerve and brachial artery to join the brachial vein in the distal fourth of the arm. Midway in its course the median cubital vein may receive a large branch emerging from between the radius and the flexor carpi radialis muscle.

The caudal cutaneous antebrachial nerve (from the ulnar nerve) emerges through the pectoralis transversus and ramifies in the superficial fascia on the caudal aspect of the forearm.

Fascia and Muscles

Beneath superficial antebrachial fascia the thick deep antebrachial fascia invests all of the muscles of the forearm and provides for insertion of the tensor fasciae antebrachii muscle medially, the cleidobrachialis muscle laterally, and the biceps brachii muscle cranially by means of the lacertus fibrosus. The deep fascia merges with the periosteum on the medial surface of the radius and attaches to the collateral ligaments and bony prominences at the elbow. Extensor muscles are invested more tightly than the flexor muscles. Intermuscular septa extend from the deep fascia between the common and lateral digital extensors, between the common digital extensor and extensor carpi radialis muscles, and between the radial and ulnar carpal flexors.

Extensor Muscles

The extensor carpi radialis is the largest of the extensor muscles of the antebrachium. It attaches proximally

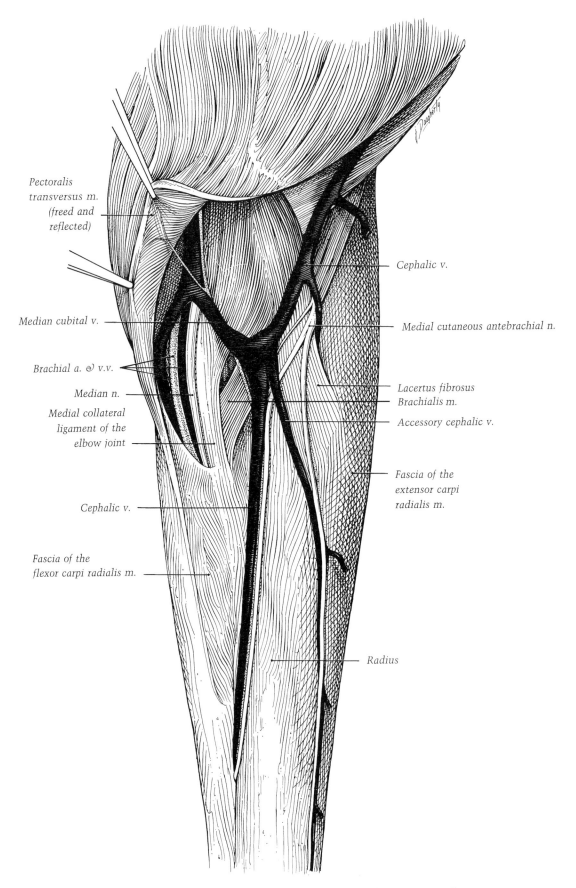

Pectoralis
transversus m.
(freed and
reflected)

Median cubital v.

Brachial a. & v.v.

Median n.

Medial collateral
ligament of the
elbow joint

Cephalic v.

Fascia of the
flexor carpi radialis m.

Cephalic v.

Medial cutaneous antebrachial n.

Lacertus fibrosus
Brachialis m.

Accessory cephalic v.

Fascia of the
extensor carpi
radialis m.

Radius

Figure 1.26. Caudomedial view of a superficial dissection of left elbow and forearm.

to the lateral epicondyle and radial fossa of the humerus (along with the tendon of origin of the common digital extensor) as well as attaching to the elbow joint capsule, the deep fascia, and the septum between the two muscles. The extensive tendon traversing the extensor carpi radialis blends with the deep fascia of the forearm after the fascia receives the lacertus fibrosus from the biceps brachii muscle. A tendon lying obliquely across the tendon of insertion of the extensor carpi radialis is that of the smallest muscle of the extensor group, the extensor carpi obliquus muscle (abductor digiti I longus) which originates on the lateral surface of the distal half of the radius. In its oblique course the muscle is at first deep to the common digital extensor, then its tendon crosses that of the extensor carpi radialis superficially. Its tendon sheath is adherent to the extensor retinaculum as the tendon angles over the carpus toward its insertion on the head of the second metacarpal bone. On the medial aspect of the carpus, the tendon and its sheath are related deeply to a bursa that usually communicates with the tendon sheath in older horses (Figure 1.20).[39]

The common digital extensor muscle (humeral head) takes common origin along with the extensor carpi radialis on the lateral epicondyle and radial fossa of the humerus, with additional attachments to the ulna, deep fascia, lateral aspect of the radius, and the lateral collateral ligament of the elbow. Its tendon of insertion, enclosed in its tendon sheath, occupies its respective groove on the distal extremity of the radius. A small tendon from the radial head of the muscle accompanies the main tendon as the two tendons enter the synovial sheath above the carpus. The lateral digital extensor muscle lies under the deep fascia against the radius and ulna between the extensor carpi ulnaris caudally and the larger common digital extensor muscle belly cranially (Figure 1.26). The lateral digital extensor originates from the radius, ulna, and lateral collateral ligament of the elbow joint, and the intermuscular septum from the deep fascia.

Flexor Muscles

The flexor carpi radialis muscle is related to the mediocaudal surface of the radius (Figure 1.26), extending distad from the medial epicondyle of the humerus to the proximal extremity of the second metacarpal bone. Caudal and partially deep to the preceding muscle, the flexor carpi ulnaris muscle is formed by an ulnar head from the olecranon and a humeral head from the medial epicondyle and extends to the accessory carpal bone. The next muscle belly caudal to the flexor carpi ulnaris is that of the extensor carpi ulnaris muscle (formerly ulnaris lateralis) that originates on the lateral epicondyle of the humerus caudal to the lateral collateral ligament of elbow joint. The muscle extends distad to insert on the proximal and lateral aspects of the accessory carpal bone and, by means of a longer, sheathed tendon, to the proximal end of the fourth metacarpal bone. Over the elbow joint a synovial sheath lies deep to the first part of the muscle. The synovial sheath opens into the elbow joint cavity. The preceding three muscles flex the carpal joint and extend the elbow joint, even though the extensor carpi ulnaris is morpho-

logically an extensor of the carpal joint and supplied by the radial nerve.

The humeral head of the superficial digital flexor muscle originates from the medial epicondyle of the humerus and then lies deep to the ulnar head of the deep digital flexor (which is quite superficial as it originates from the medial surface of the olecranon) and the flexor carpi ulnaris. The muscle belly of the superficial digital flexor lies flat against the large, partially subdivided head of the deep digital flexor muscle. Under the proximal part of the flexor retinaculum the tendon of the humeral head of the superficial digital flexor is joined by a flat, wide fibrous band, its accessory ligament (really a radial head of the muscle), which comes from its attachment on a ridge on the mediocaudal surface of the distal half of the radius (Figure 1.32, later in text).

The long, distinct tendon of the ulnar head of the deep digital flexor muscle joins the main tendon of the large humeral head proximal to the antebrachiocarpal joint just before the combined tendon becomes enclosed with the tendon of the superficial digital flexor in the carpal synovial sheath. When present, the tendon of the small radial head of the deep digital flexor also joins the main tendon at this level. The inconstant radial head takes origin from the middle half of the caudal surface of the radius and adjacent surface of the ulna deep to the humeral head. A synovial pouch from the elbow joint capsule protrudes distad beneath the humeral head's origin on the medial epicondyle of the humerus.

Nerves and Deep Vessels

The deep branch of the radial nerve descends over the flexor surface of the elbow and supplies branches to the extensor muscles of the forearm and the extensor carpi ulnaris.

Accompanied by the collateral ulnar artery and vein, the ulnar nerve crosses the medial epicondyle of the humerus, descends obliquely across the medial head of the triceps brachii muscle and the elbow, and then runs between the ulnar head of the flexor carpi ulnaris and the ulnar head of the deep digital flexor. The ulnar nerve gives branches to these two muscles and the superficial digital flexor. From this level the nerve pursues a distal course under the deep antebrachial fascia on the ulnar head of the deep digital flexor and then on the superficial surface of the superficial digital flexor muscle. The ulnar nerve continues distad between the superficial digital flexor and the extensor carpi ulnaris and finally between the latter and flexor carpi ulnaris muscles as they near their insertions. Here the ulnar nerve divides into its palmar and dorsal branches.

Distal to the elbow the median nerve lies along the caudal border of the medial collateral ligament of the elbow joint, lying against the cranial brachial vein cranial to the brachial artery (Figure 1.25). In the proximal part of the forearm, the median nerve supplies branches to the flexor carpi radialis muscle, the humeral and radial heads of the deep digital flexor muscle, and the periosteum of the radius and ulna. At about the middle of the forearm the median nerve divides into the medial and lateral palmar nerves which remain together in a common sheath before separating in the distal fourth of the forearm. The medial palmar nerve descends into the carpal canal; the lateral palmar nerve is joined by the palmar branch of the ulnar nerve and descends within the flexor retinaculum (Figure 1.18).

The common interosseous artery gives off a small caudal interosseous artery, then passes through the interosseous space, supplying nutrient arteries to the radius and ulna. The cranial interosseous artery is the main continuation of the common interosseous. Together with the transverse cubital artery the cranial interosseous provides branches to the cranial and medial aspects of the forearm.

Distal to the common interosseous artery, the brachial artery continues as the median artery between the flexor carpi radialis muscle and the caudomedial surface of the radius. In the distal part of the forearm, the median artery angles caudad and detaches the proximal radial artery, a small vessel that courses on the radius to the palmar aspect of the carpus. The median artery terminates at the distal end of the forearm by bifurcating into the large medial palmar artery, the much smaller lateral palmar artery, and, medially, the radial artery (1.18).

Two median veins accompany the median artery and nerve: a proximal continuation of the lateral palmar vein, which ascends caudal to the artery, and a vein formed by branches from the caudal antebrachial muscles, which ascends cranial to the artery.

Radioulnar Relationships

The interosseous ligament of the forearm attaches the shaft of a foal's ulna to the radius distal and proximal to the interosseous space. Ossification of the ligament distal to the space occurs in the young horse, but the proximal part of the ligament persists until it becomes ossified in very old horses.[17] Proximal to the interosseous space a radioulnar ligament extends from the borders of the ulna to the caudal aspect of the radius, stabilizing the proximal radioulnar joint.

Cubital (Elbow) Joint

Muscles adjacent to the equine cubital joint include two principal flexors, the biceps brachii and the brachialis (aided by the extensor carpi radialis and common digital extensor muscles), and three principal extensors, the tensor fasciae antebrachii, triceps brachii, and the anconeus (assisted by the flexors of the carpus and digit).

Cranially the terminal part of the biceps brachii muscle crosses the joint, its tendon of insertion branching into the lacertus fibrosus, which joins the deep fascia of the extensor carpi radialis, and a short tendon attaching to the radial tuberosity and medial collateral ligament of the cubital joint (Figure 1.27). The terminal part of the brachialis muscle, curving around from its location in the musculospiral groove of the humerus, passes between the biceps brachii and extensor carpi radialis muscles to attach to the medial border of the radius under the long part of the medial collateral ligament of the elbow joint (Figure 1.26). A bursa is situated between the tendon and the collateral ligament.[33] The medial collateral ligament represents the pronator teres muscle in the horse.

Over the medial aspect of the elbow joint deep to the cranial part of the pectoralis transversus muscle, the median nerve, cranial brachial vein, brachial artery, and caudal brachial vein lie caudal to the medial collateral ligament of the elbow joint (Figure 1.26). The short part of the collateral ligament is deep and attaches to the radial tuberosity. Proximocaudal to the joint the collateral ulnar artery and vein and the ulnar nerve and its cutaneous branch (caudal cutaneous antebrachial nerve) cross obliquely between the medial head of the triceps brachii and tensor fasciae antebrachii muscles.

All three principal extensors of the cubital joint insert on the olecranon tuberosity of the ulna. A subcutaneous bursa may cover the caudal aspect of the olecranon tuberosity; deeply a subtendinous bursa lies under the tendon of insertion of the long head of the massive triceps brachii muscle[33] (Figure 1.28). The medially located tensor fasciae antebrachii also inserts on and acts to tense the deep antebrachial fascia. Deep to the triceps brachii the small anconeus muscle originates from the caudal surface of the humerus, covers the olecranon fossa, and attaches to the elbow joint capsule, acting to elevate it when the joint is extended.

Laterally the cubital joint is covered by the distal part of the cutaneous omobrachialis muscle. A short, stout lateral collateral ligament extends from the lateral tuberosity of the radius to the lateral epicondyle of the humerus. Bands of fascia blend with the cranial part of the joint capsule. Caudally the joint capsule becomes thinner as it extends into the olecranon fossa deep to the anconeus muscle. The joint capsule is adherent to the anconeus muscle and tendons of surrounding muscles. Extensions of the synovial lining of the joint project under the origins of the extensor carpi ulnaris and the digital flexor muscles and into the radioulnar articulation. The cubital joint is supplied by branches from the transverse cubital artery cranially and a branch from the collateral ulnar artery caudally.

A fovea on the head and a ridge on the proximal extremity of the radius and the trochlear notch of the ulna articulate with the trochlea of the humerus, forming a ginglymus. The cranial articular angle is approximately 150° with a range of movement up to 60°. In flexion the forearm is carried laterad due to the slightly oblique axis of movement of the elbow joint.[16]

Arm and Shoulder

The arm is the region around the humerus. The shoulder includes the shoulder joint (scapulohumeral joint) and the region around the scapula that blends dorsally into the withers. The heavy deep fascia of the shoulder closely invests the underlying muscles and sends intermuscular septa in to attach to the spine and borders of the scapula. Within the superficial fascia over the lateral aspect of the shoulder and arm, the cutaneous omobrachialis muscle covers the deep fascia and extends as far distad as the cubital joint (Figure 1.28). The cutaneous muscle is innervated by the intercostobrachial nerve. Cutaneous sensation in this region is also mediated by brachial branches of the axillary and radial nerves. Superficial blood vessels are branches of the caudal circumflex humeral vessels.

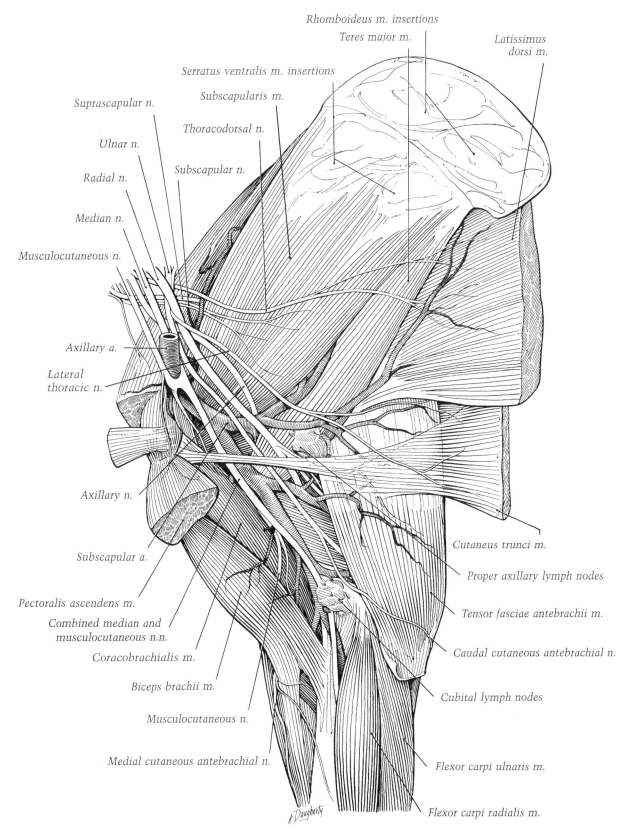

Suprascapular n.

Ulnar n.

Radial n.

Median n.

Musculocutaneous n.

Axillary a.

Lateral
thoracic n.

Axillary n.

Subscapular a.

Pectoralis ascendens m.

Combined median and
musculocutaneous n.n.

Coracobrachialis m.

Biceps brachii m.

Musculocutaneous n.

Medial cutaneous antebrachial n.

Serratus ventralis m. insertions

Subscapularis m.

Thoracodorsal n.

Subscapular n.

Rhomboideus m. insertions

Teres major m.

Latissimus
dorsi m.

Cutaneus trunci m.

Proper axillary lymph nodes

Tensor fasciae antebrachii m.

Caudal cutaneous antebrachial n.

Cubital lymph nodes

Flexor carpi ulnaris m.

Flexor carpi radialis m.

Figure 1.27. Medial view of left shoulder, arm, and proximal forearm. Veins are not depicted.

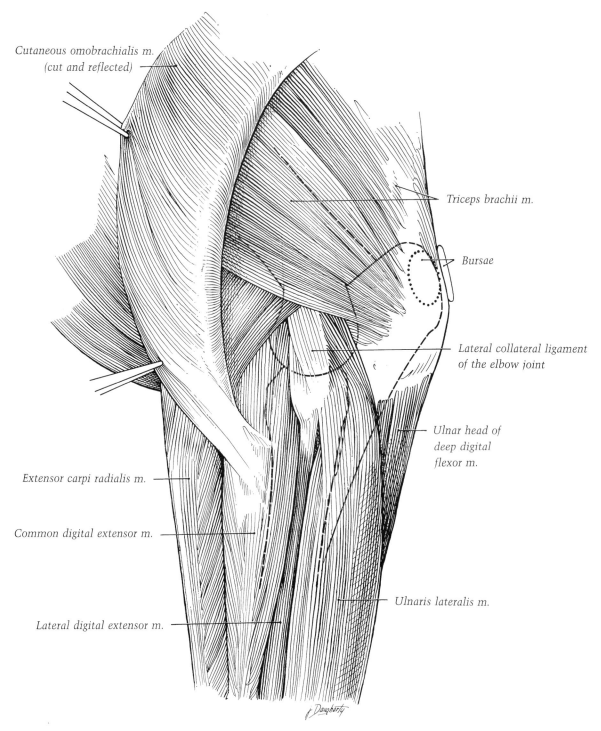

Cutaneous omobrachialis m.
(cut and reflected)

Triceps brachii m.

Bursae

Lateral collateral ligament
of the elbow joint

Ulnar head of
deep digital
flexor m.

Extensor carpi radialis m.

Common digital extensor m.

Ulnaris lateralis m.

Lateral digital extensor m.

Figure 1.28. Lateral view of left elbow. Dashed lines represent the locations of bony elements. Note that the ulnaris lateralis is now called extensor carpi ulnaris.

The cleidobrachialis muscle (of the brachiocephalicus) covers the craniolateral aspect of the shoulder joint and associated structures on the way to its insertion on the deltoid tuberosity, humeral crest, and the fascia of the arm (Figure 1.29). When the head and neck are fixed, this muscle acts as an extensor of the shoulder joint, drawing the forelimb craniad.

Muscles Substituting for Shoulder Joint Ligaments

Cranially the heavy, partly cartilaginous tendon of the biceps brachii muscle originates on the supraglenoid tubercle of the scapula and occupies the intertuberal groove of the humerus. A tendinous band from the pectoralis ascendens muscle extends from the lesser

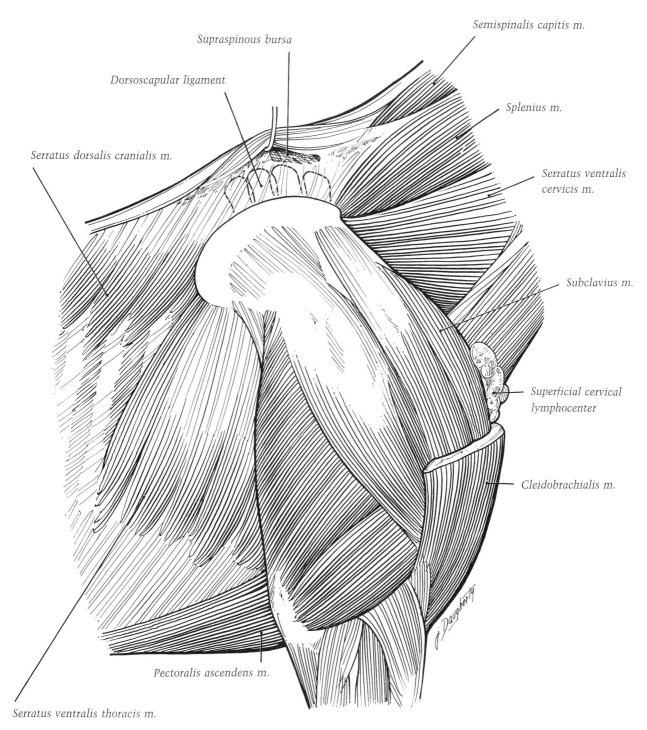

Semispinalis capitis m.

Supraspinous bursa

Dorsoscapular ligament

Splenius m.

Serratus dorsalis cranialis m.

Serratus ventralis cervicis m.

Subclavius m.

Superficial cervical lymphocenter

Cleidobrachialis m.

Pectoralis ascendens m.

Serratus ventralis thoracis m.

Figure 1.29. Right shoulder and dorsoscapular ligament. Spines of thoracic vertebrae 2 through 5 are outlined by dashed lines.

tubercle to the greater tubercle, serving to bind down the tendon of the biceps brachii. An intertuberal bursa lies under the tendon and extends around its sides. A tendinous intersection (an "internal tendon") extends distad through the muscle. In addition to flexing the elbow, the biceps brachii fixes the elbow and shoulder in the standing position. The musculocutaneous nerve supplies the biceps brachii. The supraspinatus muscle, which arises from the supraspinous fossa, the spine, and

cartilage of the scapula, divides distally to attach to the greater and lesser tubercles of the humerus, serving with the bicipital tendon to stabilize the shoulder joint cranially (Figure 1.30).

Laterally, the infraspinatus muscle extends from the scapular cartilage and infraspinous fossa to insert on the caudal eminence of the greater tubercle and a triangular area on the distal part of the tubercle distal to the insertion of the supraspinatus (Figure 1.30). The partly

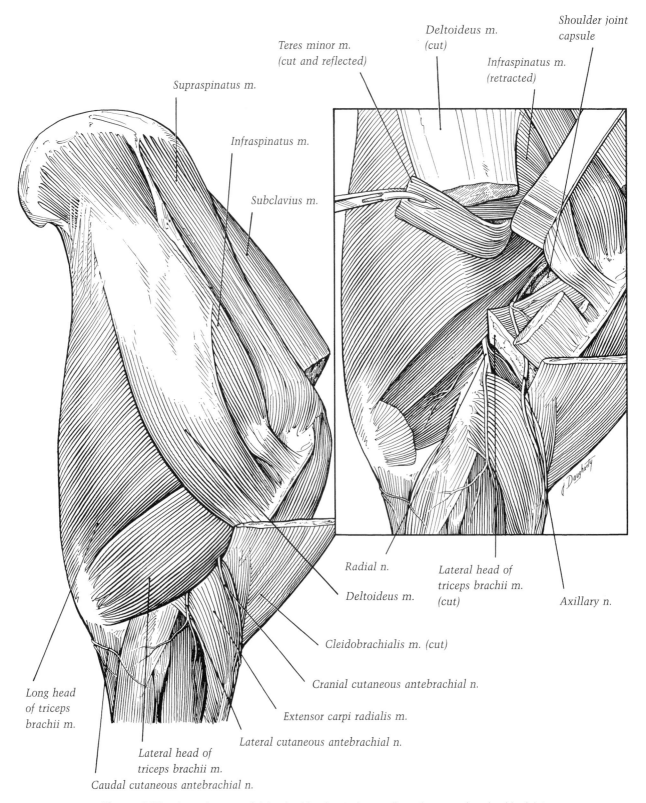

Figure 1.30. Lateral aspect of right shoulder. Inset: deeper dissection exposing shoulder joint.

cartilaginous tendon is protected from the underlying caudal eminence by adipose tissue and a constant synovial bursa that may communicate with the shoulder joint cavity. The tendon is the main lateral support of the shoulder joint assisted by the teres minor. This is a smaller, flat muscle arising from the infraspinous fossa, the caudal border, and a small tubercle on the distal extremity of the scapula and inserting proximal to and on the deltoid tuberosity. The lateral insertion of the supraspinatus muscle also lends some lateral support.

The supraspinatus muscle extends the shoulder joint; the teres minor muscle flexes the joint and, together with the infraspinatus, abducts the arm. The infraspinatus also rotates the arm laterad. The supraspinatus and infraspinatus muscles are supplied by the suprascapular nerve that reaches the supraspinous fossa by passing out between the subscapularis and supraspinatus muscles and then going around the distal fourth of the cranial border of the scapula.

The subscapularis muscle supports the shoulder joint medially. This adductor of the arm originates in the subscapular fossa of the scapula and inserts on the caudal eminence of the lesser tubercle of the humerus. Caudal support to the joint is rendered by the long head of the triceps brachii, the only head of this muscle originating from the scapula.

Flexor Muscles of the Shoulder Joint

In addition to the long head of the triceps brachii muscle, four muscles flex the shoulder joint: laterally, the deltoideus and teres minor (which also abduct the arm); medially, the teres major and coracobrachialis (which also adduct the arm); and the latissimus dorsi. The first three muscles are innervated by branches from the axillary nerve; the coracobrachialis, by the musculocutaneous nerve; and the latissimus dorsi, by the thoracodorsal nerve.

The deltoideus muscle originates from the proximal part of the caudal border of the scapula and the scapular spine via the aponeurosis investing the infraspinatus (Figure 1.30). The muscle lies in a groove on the lateral surface of the triceps brachii and partly on the infraspinatus and teres minor muscles as it extends distad to attach to the deltoid tuberosity of the humerus and the brachial fascia.

The teres major muscle extends from the caudal angle and border of the scapula across the medial surface of the triceps brachii to the teres major tuberosity of the humerus, where it inserts with the latissimus dorsi muscle (Figure 1.27).

The coracoid process of the scapula gives origin to the coracobrachialis muscle that crosses the medial aspect of the shoulder joint and proximal arm to attach to the humerus just proximal to the teres major tuberosity and on the middle of the cranial surface of the bone. A bursa is interposed between the tendon of origin of the coracobrachialis and the tendon of insertion of the subscapularis muscle[33].

Shoulder Joint

The fibrous part of the ample joint capsule of the shoulder joint attaches up to 2 cm from the margins of the articular surfaces. Two elastic glenohumeral ligaments reinforce the joint capsule as they diverge from the supraglenoid tubercle to the humeral tuberosities. A very small articularis humeri muscle lies on the flexion surface of the joint capsule. The muscle extends from the caudal part of the scapula proximal to the rim of the glenoid cavity passing through the origin of the brachialis muscle to terminate on the caudal surface of the humerus just distal to the head. Innervated by the axillary nerve, the articularis humeri tenses the joint capsule during flexion of the shoulder joint.

Within the shoulder joint the articular surface of the humeral head has approximately twice the area of the glenoid cavity of the scapula even with the small extension afforded by the glenoid lip around the rim. The articular configuration of this ball-and-socket joint and the support of the surrounding muscles give great stability to the joint. Major movements are flexion and extension. While standing, the caudal angle of the shoulder joint is 120° to 130°. The angle increases to approximately 145° in extension and decreases to 80° in flexion.[17] Muscles around the joint restrict abduction and adduction. Rotation is very limited.

MUSCLES

Beneath the skin over the scapular region the broad, triangular flat trapezius muscle covers parts of eight underlying muscles. The cervical part of the trapezius arises by a thin aponeurosis from most of the funicular part of the ligamentum nuchae and inserts on the scapular spine and fascia of the shoulder and arm. The aponeurosis of the thoracic part of the trapezius takes origin from the supraspinous ligament from the third to the tenth thoracic vertebrae, and the muscle inserts on the tuber of the spine of the scapula. An aponeurosis joins the two parts of the trapezius. Innervated by the accessory nerve and dorsal branches of adjacent thoracic nerves, the trapezius muscle elevates the shoulder and draws it either craniad or caudad, depending on the activity of the cervical or thoracic parts respectively.

Deep to the trapezius the rhomboideus cervicis originates from the funicular part of ligamentum nuchae, and the rhomboideus thoracis originates from the superficial surface of the dorsal part of the dorsoscapular ligament. Both parts of the rhomboideus muscle insert on the medial side of the scapular cartilage (Figure 1.27). This muscle is innervated by the sixth and seventh cervical nerves and dorsal branches of nerves adjacent to the rhomboideus thoracis. The rhomboideus draws the scapula dorsocraniad and, when the limb is stationary, the cervical part helps to raise the neck.

The widest muscle of the shoulder girdle, the latissimus dorsi, has roughly the shape of a right triangle with the origin arising through a broad aponeurosis from the thoracolumbar fascia. Thin at first, the muscle becomes thicker as it passes medial to the long head of the triceps brachii to converge on a flat, common tendon of insertion with the teres major muscle (Figure 1.27). As the tendon of insertion passes to its attachment on the teres major tuberosity of the humerus, it is attached lightly to the thin tendon of the cutaneus trunci muscle passing to that muscle's insertion on the lesser tubercle of the humerus.

From deep to superficial, the muscles contributing most substantially to the attachment of the thoracic limb to the trunk and neck are the serratus ventralis, pectoral muscles, subclavius, brachiocephalicus, and omotransversarius. The serratus ventralis cervicis extends from the transverse processes of the last four cervical vertebrae to the serrated face of the medial surface of the scapula and adjacent scapular cartilage; the serratus ventralis thoracis converges dorsad from the lateral surfaces of the first eight or nine ribs to the serrated face of the scapula and adjacent scapular cartilage. Elastic lamellae from the ventral part of the dorsoscapular ligament are interspersed through the attachments of the serratus ventralis on the scapula. The two parts of the muscle and the contralateral serratus ventralis form a support suspending the thorax between the thoracic limbs. When both muscles contract, they elevate the thorax; acting independently, each serratus ventralis shifts the trunk's weight to the ipsilateral limb. During locomotion the cervical part of the muscle draws the dorsal border of the scapula craniad; the thoracic part draws the scapula caudad. When the limb is fixed, the serratus cervicis extends the neck or pulls it laterad. The long thoracic nerve and branches from the fifth to the eighth cervical nerves supply this muscle.

Pectoral muscles attach to the sternum. There are two superficial pectoral muscles: (1) the pectoralis descendens muscle descending from the cartilage of the manubrium sterni to the deltoid tuberosity and the crest of the humerus and the brachial fascia and (2) the pectoralis transversus muscle extending from the ventral part of the sternum between the first and sixth sternebrae to the superficial fascia of the medial aspect of the antebrachium and to the humeral crest. The largest pectoral muscle, the deep pectoral (pectoralis ascendens) muscle (Figure 1.29), ascends from its attachments on the xyphoid cartilage, the ventral part of the sternum, the fourth to ninth costal cartilages, and the abdominal tunic to the cranial parts of the lesser and greater humeral tubercles and the tendon of origin of the coracobrachialis muscle. The subclavius has been traditionally grouped with the pectorales. It arises from the first four costal cartilages and the cranial half of the sternum and ends in an aponeurosis over the dorsal part of the supraspinatus muscle and the scapular fascia (Figure 1.29).

The superficial pectoral muscles adduct the thoracic limb and tense the antebrachial fascia. The deep pectoral and subclavius also adduct the limb and, if the limb is fixed in the advanced position, they pull the trunk craniad. Cranial and caudal pectoral nerves (with musculocutaneous and intercostal nerves contributing to the cranial pectoral nerves) supply these muscles.

As has been noted, the cleidobrachialis part of the brachiocephalicus muscle extends from the indistinct clavicular intersection to the arm. The mastoid part of the muscle (cleidomastoideus) lies between the intersection and its attachments to the mastoid process and nuchal crest, partly overlapping the omotransversius muscle dorsally. The omotransversarius originates from the wing of the atlas and the transverse processes of the second, third, and fourth cervical vertebrae and inserts on the humeral crest and fascia of the shoulder and arm. The dorsal branch of the accessory nerve passes through the cranial part of the omotransversius and then between that muscle and the trapezius.

DORSOSCAPULAR LIGAMENT

Further attachment of the shoulder to the trunk is afforded by a thickened, superficial lamina of the thoracolumbar fascia, the dorsoscapular ligament (Figure 1.31). It consists of two parts: a collagenous portion attaches to the third, fourth, and fifth thoracic spines under the flattened part of the nuchal ligament subjacent to the supraspinous bursa.[16] This part of the dorsoscapular ligament passes ventrad, ultimately attaching to the medial surface of the rhomboideus thoracis

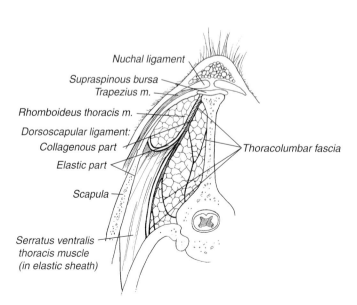

Figure 1.31. Cross section of right dorsoscapular ligament. (Reprinted with permission from Garrett PD. Anatomy of the dorsoscapular ligaments of horses. J Am Vet Med Assoc 1990;196:446.)

muscle. As it curves under the muscle, the collagenous part changes to an elastic part. A horizontal lamina of the elastic part forms the ventral sheath of the rhomboideus thoracis muscle. Several vertical laminae project from the ventral aspect of the horizontal lamina, surrounding bundles of the serratus ventralis muscle that insert on the scapula (Figure 1.31).

In this region, three other laminae detach from the thoracolumbar fascia. A superficial lamina gives origin to the splenius and serratus dorsalis cranialis muscles, an intermediate lamina passes between the iliocostalis thoracis and longissimus thoracis muscles, and a deep lamina passes between the longissimus thoracis and spinalis thoracis muscles to attach to the transverse processes of the first several thoracic vertebrae. The semispinalis capitis muscle attaches to the deep lamina.

Nerves and Vessels

The medial aspect of the arm and shoulder contains the large vessels and nerves supplying the thoracic limb (Figure 1.27). Suprascapular vessels accompany the suprascapular nerve, passing laterad between the cranial edges of the subscapularis and suprascapularis muscles. The median nerve descends with the axillary artery, forming an axillary loop distal to the artery by uniting with a large detachment from the musculocutaneous nerve. Proximal branches from the musculocutaneous nerve supply the coracobrachialis and biceps brachii muscles. Distal to the axillary loop, the median and musculocutaneous nerves are contained in a common sheath, coursing distad cranial to the brachial vein and medial to the brachial artery. In the middle of the arm the musculocutaneous nerve divides into a distal branch supplying the brachialis muscle and the medial cutaneous antebrachial nerve that spirals around the biceps brachii to that muscle's lacertus fibrosus. The median nerve crosses back over the brachial artery and descends caudal to it.

The axillary nerve traverses the medial surface of the subscapularis muscle and, together with the large subscapular vessels (from the axillary vessels), the nerve passes laterad between the subscapularis and teres major muscles. As the axillary nerve continues its course, it is accompanied by the caudal circumflex humeral artery, a branch of the subscapular artery.

The large radial nerve and smaller ulnar nerve descend close to each other medial to the subscapular artery, then caudal to the brachial vein. After supplying a branch to the tensor fasciae antebrachii muscle, the radial nerve plunges laterad between the teres major and medial and long heads of the triceps to the musculospiral groove of the humerus. In the groove it gives off lateral cutaneous branches to the caudodistal aspect of the arm and then supplies branches to the triceps brachii and anconeus muscles. Just proximal to the flexor surface of the elbow joint, the radial nerve divides into deep and superficial branches. The deep branch divides into branches supplying the craniolateral muscles of the antebrachium. The superficial branch courses laterad between the lateral head of the triceps brachii and the extensor carpi radialis muscles accompanied by the transverse cubital artery. The lateral cutaneous antebrachial nerve is detached and supplies sensory innerva-

tion to the fascia and skin of the lateral aspect of the forearm (Figure 1.30).

The ulnar nerve crosses the axillary vein and angles caudodistad to the middle of the arm. At the cranial edge of the tensor fasciae antebrachii muscle, the ulnar nerve detaches the caudal cutaneous antebrachial nerve that courses caudodistad across the medial surface of the muscle (Figure 1.27). The main trunk of the ulnar nerve continues its course by passing between the tensor fasciae antebrachii and the medial head of the triceps brachii accompanied by the collateral ulnar vessels. The nerve and vessels then cross the medial epicondyle of the humerus.

After giving off the cranial circumflex humeral vessels, the axillary vessels continue as the brachial artery and vein. As they descend the arm they give rise to the deep brachial vessels caudally and then the collateral ulnar vessels caudally and the bicipital vessels cranially. The transverse cubital vessels are given off cranially and pass distolaterad under the biceps brachii and brachialis muscles to the cranial aspect of the cubital joint. The nutrient artery of the humerus may come from the first part of the collateral ulnar artery or it may arise from the brachial artery.

Lymphatic Drainage

Lymphatic vessels from structures distal to the elbow are afferent to the cubital lymph nodes, a group of several small nodes found just proximal to the cubital joint (Figure 1.27). Efferent vessels from the cubital lymph nodes end in the proper axillary lymph nodes, an aggregate of lymph nodes on the medial surface of the teres major muscle (Figure 1.27). Lymph from the muscles of the arm and shoulder and from the adjacent skin and the ventrolateral trunk also drain to the proper axillary lymph nodes. Vessels from the proper axillary lymph nodes carry lymph to the several small axillary lymph nodes of the first rib. From these nodes efferents go to the nearby caudal deep cervical lymph nodes. Some efferents of the deep cervical nodes drain directly into the venous system; others pass to other regional nodes and therefore drain indirectly through these to the venous system[17].

Lymphatic vessels from the skin of the entire thoracic limb, neck, and dorsolateral trunk and more proximal parts of the limb are afferent to the superficial cervical lymphocenter on the cranial border of the subclavius muscle. Efferent lymphatic vessels from the superficial cervical lymph nodes terminate in the caudal deep cervical lymph nodes or by entering the common jugular vein.[17]

Stay Apparatus of the Thoracic Limb

In the standing position, interacting muscles, tendons, and ligaments constituting the stay apparatus of the thoracic limb fix the alignment of the bones of the manus, suspend the fetlock, lock the carpus, and stabilize the elbow and shoulder joints. This complex of structures functions almost entirely as a passive, force-resisting system.[38] It permits the horse to stand (and sleep) with a minimum of muscular activity (Figure 1.32).

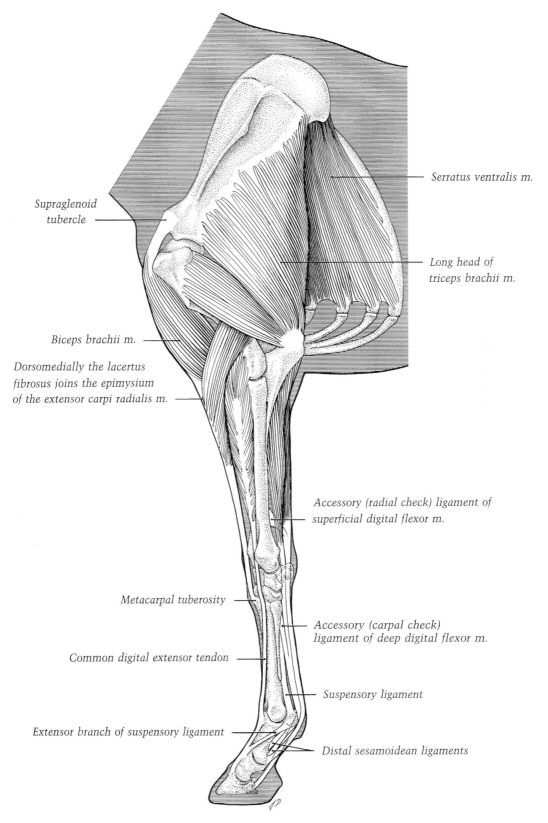

Supraglenoid
tubercle

Biceps brachii m.

Dorsomedially the lacertus
fibrosus joins the epimysium
of the extensor carpi radialis m.

Metacarpal tuberosity

Common digital extensor tendon

Extensor branch of suspensory ligament

Serratus ventralis m.

Long head of
triceps brachii m.

Accessory (radial check) ligament of
superficial digital flexor m.

Accessory (carpal check)
ligament of deep digital flexor m.

Suspensory ligament

Distal sesamoidean ligaments

Figure 1.32. Stay apparatus of the left thoracic limb.

The four palmar ligaments stretched tightly across the pastern joint, the straight distal sesamoidean ligament attached to the complementary cartilage of the middle phalanx, and the deep digital flexor tendon stabilize the pastern joint and prevent its overextension. Under tension in the standing position, the superficial digital flexor tendon prevents flexion by exerting palmar force on the joint.

The suspensory apparatus of the fetlock is a ligamentous continuum extending from the proximal end of the third metacarpal bone to the proximal and middle phalanges. It consists of the suspensory ligament, metacarpointersesamoidean ligament with its embedded proximal sesamoid bones, and the distal sesamoidean ligaments. The superficial and deep digital flexor tendons and their accessory (check) ligaments assist the suspensory apparatus of the fetlock in suspending the fetlock and preventing excessive overextension of the metacarpophalangeal joint and collapse of the fetlock during weight bearing, especially on striking the ground.[11] Disruption of the suspensory ligament alters its support of the fetlock, resulting in "sinking" or hyperextension of the fetlock.[53]

The normal carpus exhibits some stability in weight bearing; further stabilization is provided by the palmar carpal ligament and the collateral ligaments. Palmarly, the digital flexor tendons bridging the carpus in the carpal canal between their respective accessory ligaments and, dorsally, the extensor tendons, principally the extensor carpi radialis tendon attaching to the metacarpal tuberosity, lend further stability to the carpus.

A certain amount of muscle tone prevails in all "resting" muscles of the limb, even during most stages of sleep. Tension exerted by the long head of the triceps brachii muscle is essential to prevention of flexion of the elbow joint and collapse of the forelimb.[38] The elbow's eccentrically placed collateral ligaments allow it to exhibit considerable stability in the extended position, a stability enhanced by the triceps' tone. Flexion of the joint is further limited by the muscle belly and fibrous components of the superficial digital flexor muscle descending from its attachment of the medial epicondyle of the humerus.[11]

A tendinous continuum extending from the supraglenoid tubercle to the metacarpal tuberosity is formed by the main tendon of the biceps brachii muscle, its fibrous "internal tendon," and its superficial tendon (lacertus fibrosus) that blends into the fascia of extensor carpi radialis muscle and via it to the tendon of insertion of this muscle. This complex prevents flexion of the shoulder joint caused by the weight of the trunk via the scapular attachments of the serratus ventralis muscle and the dorsoscapular ligament. Additionally, the tendon of the extensor carpi radialis opposes flexion of the carpus.

HINDLIMB

Digit and Fetlock

The hindfoot is somewhat smaller and more elongate than the forefoot. It has been commonly reported that, compared to the forehoof, the angle of the toe of the hindhoof is slightly greater.[1] Within the hind pastern the middle phalanx is narrower and longer and the proximal phalanx somewhat shorter than their counterparts in the thoracic limb (Figure 1.33).

The long digital extensor muscle's tendon attaches to the dorsal surfaces of the proximal and middle phalanges and the extensor process of the distal phalanx, but the tendon of the lateral digital extensor usually does not attach to the proximal phalanx as it does in the thoracic limb. Digital flexor tendons, tendon sheaths, and bursae of the hind digit are not remarkably different. The suspensory apparatus of the fetlock and the configuration of the fetlock (metatarsophalangeal) joint are much the same as in the thoracic limb except that the dorsal articular angle of the fetlock is approximately 5° greater (i.e., is slightly more "upright").

Blood Vessels and Nerves of the Hind Digit and Fetlock

The principal blood supply to the fetlock and digit of the pelvic limb is derived from the continuation of dorsal metatarsal artery III, the distal perforating branch, which supplies branches to the distal deep plantar arch and then bifurcates into medial and lateral digital arteries in the distoplantar region of the metatarsus. A small secondary supply is contributed by the medial and lateral plantar arteries that join the digital arteries to form the superficial plantar arch just proximal to the enlargement of the fetlock (Figure 1.34). Branches of the digital arteries form a pattern similar to that in the thoracic limb except for the blood supply to the navicular bone. In contrast to all arteries of the proximal anastomotic network originating from palmar arterial branches of the middle phalanx, in the pelvic limb half of the primary arteries originate from the plantar arterial branches of the middle phalanx and half from the collateral arch. More significantly, a greater number of vessels enter the distal border of the navicular bone from the distal anastomotic network in the hindfoot than enter the same region in the forefoot.[21]

Venous drainage of the digit of the pelvic limb is similar to that of the forelimb. The medial digital vein carries blood to the plantar common digital vein II; the lateral digital vein carries blood to the plantar common digital vein III.

The pattern of distribution of the sensory plantar digital and plantar metatarsal nerves in the fetlock and digit of the pelvic limb is similar to the pattern of the counterpart nerves in the thoracic limb. Some differences exist, however. The dorsal branch of each plantar digital nerve is given off more distally than the corresponding branch in the pastern of the forelimb. Medial and lateral dorsal metatarsal nerves (from the deep fibular—formerly peroneal—nerve) course distad subcutaneously parallel and dorsal to the medial and lateral plantar metatarsal nerves (Figure l.34 and l.35). The lateral plantar metatarsal nerve extends distad over the fetlock to the lateral aspect of the pastern, while the medial plantar metatarsal nerve may reach the coronet; both dorsal metatarsal nerves continue into the laminar corium.[22] Terminal small branches of the saphenous nerve medially, the superficial fibular nerve dorsally and laterally, and the caudal cutaneous sural nerve (dorsolaterally) complete the sensory innervation to the skin of the fetlock.

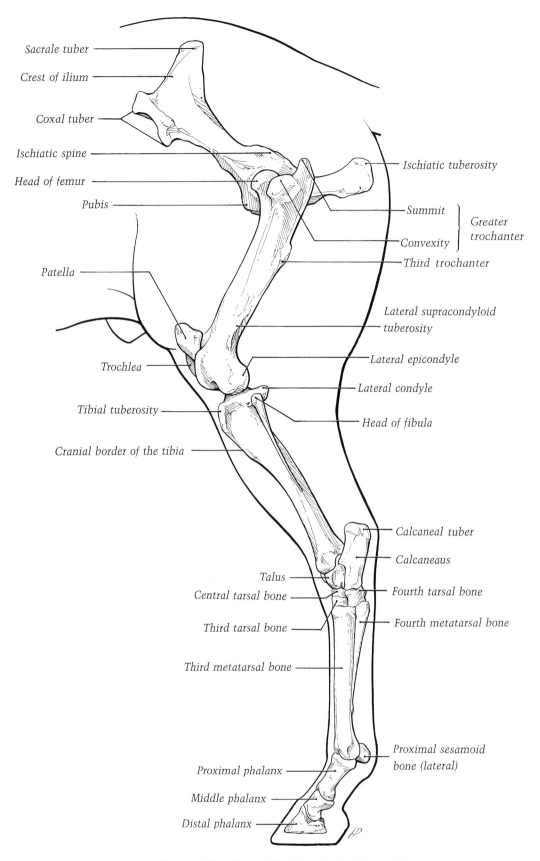

Figure 1.33. Bones of the left pelvic limb. Lateral view.

Sacrale tuber

Crest of ilium

Coxal tuber

Ischiatic spine

Head of femur

Pubis

Patella

Trochlea

Tibial tuberosity

Cranial border of the tibia

Talus

Central tarsal bone

Third tarsal bone

Third metatarsal bone

Proximal phalanx

Middle phalanx

Distal phalanx

Ischiatic tuberosity

Summit

Convexity

Greater trochanter

Third trochanter

Lateral supracondyloid tuberosity

Lateral epicondyle

Lateral condyle

Head of fibula

Calcaneal tuber

Calcaneaus

Fourth tarsal bone

Fourth metatarsal bone

Proximal sesamoid bone (lateral)

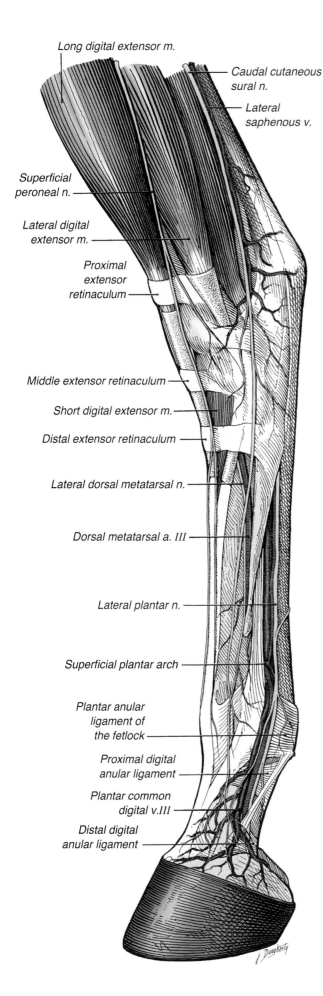

Long digital extensor m.

Caudal cutaneous sural n.

Lateral saphenous v.

Superficial peroneal n.

Lateral digital extensor m.

Proximal extensor retinaculum

Middle extensor retinaculum

Short digital extensor m.

Distal extensor retinaculum

Lateral dorsal metatarsal n.

Dorsal metatarsal a. III

Lateral plantar n.

Superficial plantar arch

Plantar anular ligament of the fetlock

Proximal digital anular ligament

Plantar common digital v.III

Distal digital anular ligament

Figure 1.34. Lateral view of left distal crus and pes. Please note that the term "fibularis" is currently preferred over "peroneus" (fibular rather than peroneal) although both are widely used.

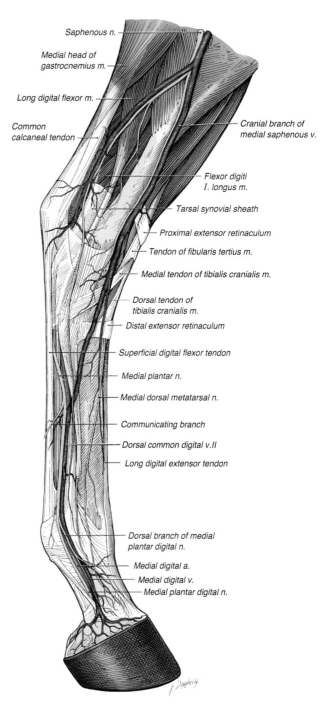

Saphenous n.

Medial head of gastrocnemius m.

Long digital flexor m.

Common calcaneal tendon

Cranial branch of medial saphenous v.

Flexor digiti I. longus m.

Tarsal synovial sheath

Proximal extensor retinaculum

Tendon of fibularis tertius m.

Medial tendon of tibialis cranialis m.

Dorsal tendon of tibialis cranialis m.

Distal extensor retinaculum

Superficial digital flexor tendon

Medial plantar n.

Medial dorsal metatarsal n.

Communicating branch

Dorsal common digital v.II

Long digital extensor tendon

Dorsal branch of medial plantar digital n.

Medial digital a.

Medial digital v.

Medial plantar digital n.

Figure 1.35. Medial view of left distal crus and pes. Please note that the term "fibularis" is currently preferred over "peroneus" (fibular rather than peroneal), although both are widely used.

41

Metatarsus

The equine metatarsus is about 16% longer than the corresponding metacarpus, and the third metatarsal bone is more rounded than the third metacarpal bone[17]. The fourth metatarsal bone, particularly its proximal extremity, is larger than the second metatarsal bone.

Dorsal Aspect

Three superficial nerves supply sensory innervation to the skin of the dorsal, lateral, and medial aspects of the metatarsus. Dorsally and laterally the two terminal branches of the superficial fibular nerve descend as far as the fetlock. The terminal branch of the caudal cutaneous sural nerve descends obliquely from the lateral aspect of the hock to course over the dorsolateral part of the third metatarsal bone, terminating in the skin of the fetlock, and the terminal branch of the saphenous nerve supplies medial skin of the metatarsus down to the fetlock.

The dorsal common digital vein II (great metatarsal vein) ascends from a venous arch proximal to the proximal sesamoid bones as the proximal continuation of the medial digital vein. At first, the dorsal common digital vein II lies along the medial border of the suspensory ligament, then in a groove on the proximal part of the dorsal surface of the third metatarsal bone to the hock where it continues into the cranial branch of the medial saphenous vein (Figure 1.35).

The tendon of the long digital extensor muscle extends the length of the metatarsus on the dorsal surface of the third metatarsal bone beneath the skin and fascia. At the proximal third of the metatarsus, the long digital extensor tendon is joined by the tendon of the lateral digital extensor muscle. Rarely, the tendon of the lateral digital extensor courses separately to the proximal phalanx. The angle formed by the conjoined long and lateral digital extensor tendons is occupied by the thin, triangular short digital extensor muscle. The short digital extensor originates on the lateral collateral ligament of the hock, the lateral tendon of the fibularis tertius muscle (most commonly called the peroneus tertius), and the middle extensor retinaculum, and inserts on the two large digital extensor tendons. All digital extensor muscles are bound down by the distal extensor retinaculum in the proximal third of the metatarsus (Figure 1.34).

Emerging under the distal edge of the distal extensor retinaculum, the large dorsal metatarsal artery III ("great metatarsal artery") pursues an oblique course distad to lie in the dorsolateral groove between the third and fourth metatarsal bones. The artery is accompanied by a very small satellite vein and the lateral dorsal metatarsal nerve that lies along the dorsal surface of the artery. The terminal branch of the caudal cutaneous sural nerve crosses superficial to the dorsal metatarsal artery III (Figure 1.34). Distally the artery passes between the third and fourth metatarsal bones, continuing deeply as the distal perforating branch that sends branches to the distal deep plantar arch and then divides into medial and lateral digital arteries adjacent to the plantar aspect of the third metatarsal bone in the distal fourth of the metatarsus. The lateral dorsal metatarsal nerve remains superficial, courses dorsodistad to the fetlock, and descends in the dorsal fascia of the pastern, eventually terminating in the laminar corium.

The slightly larger medial dorsal metatarsal nerve supplies sensory fibers to the hock joint capsule and a motor branch to the short digital extensor muscle. The nerve emerges under the medial edge of the long digital extensor tendon, and courses obliquely between the tendon and the second metatarsal bone to be distributed distally in the same manner as the lateral dorsal metatarsal nerve (Figure 1.35).

Lateral and Medial Aspects

The lateral and medial plantar nerves lie plantar to their satellite veins and arteries along the respective lateral or medial border of the deep digital flexor tendons (Figures 1.34 and 1.35). These nerves supply the lateral, medial, and plantar structures of the metatarsus. The lateral plantar nerve detaches a deep branch close to the tarsus; this is the parent trunk of the deeply located lateral and medial plantar metatarsal nerves that pursue courses homologous to the palmar metacarpal nerves in the forelimb. At about the mid-metatarsus the medial plantar nerve gives off the communicating branch that angles laterodistad across the superficial digital flexor tendon to join the lateral plantar nerve in the distal fourth of the metatarsus. The communicating branch is generally smaller than its counterpart in the metacarpus, and it may be absent.

On each side the small medial and lateral plantar arteries course down to the distal end of the metatarsus where they send branches to the respective digital arteries, forming the superficial plantar arch. The proximal deep plantar arch is supplied mainly by the proximal perforating branch from the dorsal pedal artery with minor contributing branches from the plantar arteries.

Plantar Aspect

The superficial digital flexor tendon is similar to the corresponding tendon in the metacarpus.[11] The deep digital flexor muscle's principal tendon is intimately related to the dorsomedial aspect of the superficial digital flexor tendon. In the proximal third of the metatarsus, the principal tendon is joined by the tendon of the medial digital flexor muscle (the medial head of the deep digital flexor muscle). A weakly developed, slender accessory ligament (tarsal or "inferior" check ligament) arises from the plantar aspect of the fibrous joint capsule of the hock. Longer than its counterpart in the forelimb, it joins the deep digital flexor tendon near the middle of the metatarsus. This slender accessory ligament may be absent in horses, and it is usually absent in mules and ponies.[17]

The suspensory ligament (middle or third interosseous muscle) takes origin from a large area on the proximal aspect of the third metatarsal bone and a smaller attachment on the distal row of tarsal bones. Lying within the metatarsal groove deep to the deep digital flexor tendon, the suspensory ligament of the hindlimb is relatively thinner, more rounded, and longer than the ligament of the forelimb. In some horses, e.g., Standardbreds, the suspensory ligament of the hindlimb contains more muscle than the suspensory ligament of the forelimb.[53] The two extensor branches pursue courses similar to those in the forelimb. Small medial (second) and lateral (fourth) interossei and lumbricales muscles are present in the metatarsus.

Distribution of the medial and lateral plantar metatarsal arteries coursing distad under the suspensory ligament to the distal deep plantar arch is similar to the distribution of the palmar metacarpal arteries. Satellite veins accompany the arteries. The dorsal common digital vein II lies along the deep digital flexor tendon in the distal half of the metatarsus, then deviates across the medial surface of the third metatarsal bone to ascend across the tarsus as the cranial branch of the saphenous vein.

Tarsus (Hock)

The bones of the tarsus include the talus; calcaneus; and central, first and second (fused), third, and fourth tarsal bones (Figure 1.33). Proximally, the trochlea of the talus articulates with the cochlear surface of the tibia in the tarsocrural joint; distally, the distal row of tarsal bones and the three metatarsal bones articulate in the tarsometatarsal joint. Extensive collateral ligaments span the latter two joints and the intertarsal joints. In the horse, nearly all the movement of the hock arises from the tarsocrural joint.

Dorsal Aspect

In the superficial fascia the large cranial branch of the medial saphenous vein continues proximad and crosses the mediodorsal aspect of the tarsus, lying upon the dorsomedial pouch of the tarsocrural joint capsule (Figure 1.36). An anastomotic branch joins the medial saphenous vein with the deeper cranial tibial vein just proximal to the tarsocrural joint. The cranial tibial vein is the proximal continuation of the dorsal pedal vein. The superficial fibular (peroneal) nerve lies in the fascia lateral and parallel to the tendon of the long digital extensor muscle. A fibrous loop, the middle extensor retinaculum, leaves the lateral tendon of insertion of the fibularis (peroneus) tertius muscle, wraps around the long digital extensor tendon and its sheath, and attaches to the calcaneus. The long digital extensor tendon's synovial sheath extends from the level of the lateral malleolus distad nearly to the junction of the tendon with the tendon of the lateral digital extensor muscle (Figure 1.34). The long digital extensor tendon is located just lateral to the palpable medial ridge of the trochlea of the talus. The proximal part of the short digital extensor muscle covers the tarsal joint capsule, the dorsal pedal artery continuing into the dorsal metatarsal artery III, and the termination of the deep fibular nerve as it bifurcates into the two dorsal metatarsal nerves (Figure 1.34).

As it crosses the dorsal surface of the tarsocrural joint, the tendon of the fibularis (peroneus) tertius muscle is superficial to the tendon of the tibialis cranialis muscle (Figures 1.35 and 1.36). Then the tendon of the fibularis tertius forms a sleeve-like cleft through which the tendon of the tibialis cranialis and its synovial sheath pass. The latter tendon then bifurcates into a dorsal tendon, which inserts on the large metatarsal bone, and a medial ("cunean") tendon, which angles mediodistad under the superficial layer of the long medial collateral ligament to insert on the first tarsal bone. A large bursa is interposed between the cunean tendon and the long medial collateral ligament (Figure 1.37).

After forming the cleft that admits passage of the tibialis cranialis tendon, the fibularis tertius divides into two tendons. The dorsal tendon passes under the cunean tendon and inserts on the third tarsal and third metatarsal bone, medial to the dorsal tendon of the cranial tibial muscle (Figure 1.37). The lateral tendon of the fibularis tertius extends distad deep to the long digital extensor tendon and continues laterad distal to the lateral ridge of the trochlea of the talus. The lateral tendon then bifurcates and inserts on the calcaneus and the fourth tarsal bone.

The main blood supply to the pes (tarsus, metatarsus, and digit), the cranial tibial artery, is continued as the dorsal pedal artery at the level of the tarsocrural joint (Figure 1.36). Small branches from the dorsal pedal artery form the dorsal tarsal rete in the tarsal fascia. Medial and lateral tarsal arteries are small vessels arising from the dorsal pedal artery and supplying their respective sides of the tarsus. Before continuing as the dorsal metatarsal artery III, the dorsal pedal artery gives off the proximal perforating branch which traverses the vascular canal formed by the central, third, and fourth tarsal bones. This branch supplies the proximal deep plantar arch. Satellite veins accompany the arteries.

Lateral Aspect

Innervation to the lateral aspect of the tarsus is provided by branches from the caudal cutaneous sural nerve as it courses superficial to the calcaneus and from the more dorsally located superficial fibular nerve (Figure 1.34).

Surrounded by its tendon sheath, the tendon of the lateral digital extensor muscle is bound by a fibrous band in a groove in the lateral malleolus of the tibia and then traverses a passage through the long lateral collateral ligament of the tarsus as the tendon angles dorsodistad (Figure 1.38). A synovial sheath enfolds the tendon from just proximal to the lateral malleolus to a point just proximal to the tendon's junction with the long digital extensor tendon. Plantar to the lateral extensor tendon, the lateroplantar pouch of the tarsocrural joint capsule protrudes between the lateral malleolus and the calcaneus.

Medial Aspect

A horny chestnut, the presumed vestige of the first digit, is located in the skin on the distomedial aspect of the tarsus. Branches from the cranial and caudal branches of the saphenous nerve and from the tibial nerve supply sensory innervation to the medial aspect of the tarsus. The large cranial branch of the medial saphenous vein courses subcutaneously, superficial to the dorsomedial pouch of the tarsocrural joint capsule. At the level of the medial malleolus of the tibia it sends an anastomotic branch to the cranial tibial vein. The

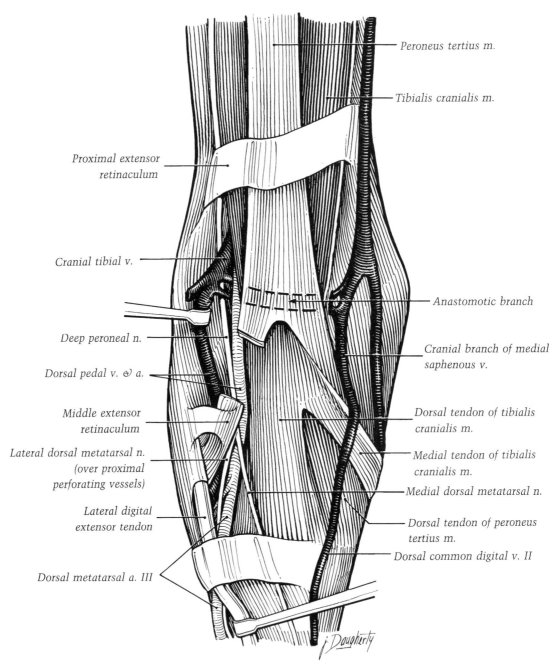

Peroneus tertius m.

Tibialis cranialis m.

Proximal extensor retinaculum

Cranial tibial v.

Anastomotic branch

Deep peroneal n.

Cranial branch of medial saphenous v.

Dorsal pedal v. & a.

Middle extensor retinaculum

Dorsal tendon of tibialis cranialis m.

Medial tendon of tibialis cranialis m.

Lateral dorsal metatarsal n. (over proximal perforating vessels)

Medial dorsal metatarsal n.

Lateral digital extensor tendon

Dorsal tendon of peroneus tertius m.

Dorsal common digital v. II

Dorsal metatarsal a. III

Figure 1.36. Dorsal dissection of right tarsus. The long digital extensor and short digital extensor muscles have been removed. The lateral tendon of the fibularis (peroneus) tertius is sectioned.

Please note that the term "fibularis" is currently preferred over "peroneus" (fibular rather than peroneal), although both are widely used.

caudal branch of the medial saphenous vein receives blood from branches in the medial and plantar regions of the hock.

A palpable feature of the medial aspect of the hock is the medial tendon of the tibialis cranialis muscle (colloquially called the "cunean tendon") as it inserts on the first tarsal bone. The bursa between the cunean tendon and the distal part of the long medial collateral ligament of the tarsus is not normally palpable (Figure 1.37). The tendon of the medial digital flexor (medial head of the deep digital flexor muscle, sometimes called

long digital flexor muscle) passes through a fascial tunnel plantar to the medial collateral ligament. A synovial sheath surrounds the tendon from the distal fourth of the tibia to the tendon's junction with the main tendon of the muscle (Figure 1.39). A compartment of the tarsocrural joint capsule, the medioplantar pouch, is located a short distance plantar to the medial digital flexor tendon and proximal to the sustentaculum tali of the calcaneus at the level of the medial malleolus.

The tarsal fascia thickens into a flexor retinaculum, bridging the groove on the sustentaculum tali of the

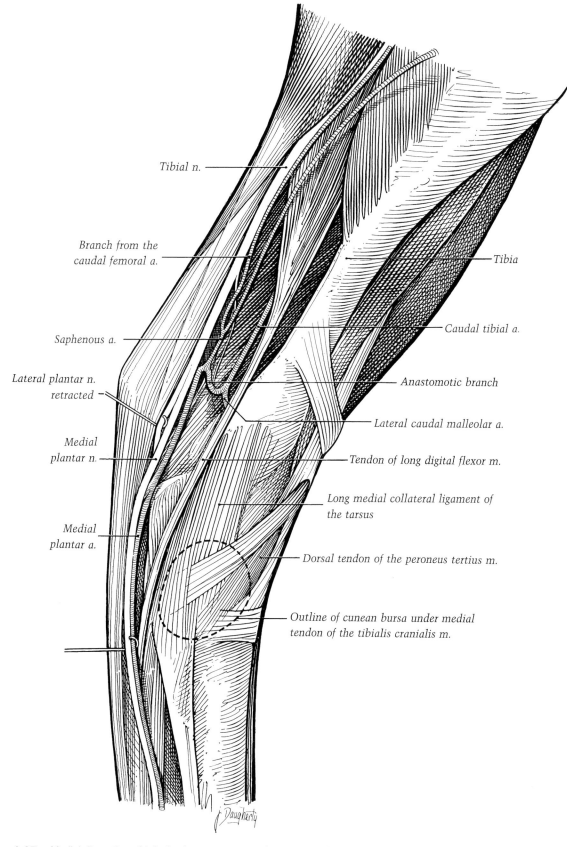

Tibial n.

Branch from the
caudal femoral a.

Saphenous a.

Lateral plantar n.
retracted

Medial
plantar n.

Medial
plantar a.

Tibia

Caudal tibial a.

Anastomotic branch

Lateral caudal malleolar a.

Tendon of long digital flexor m.

Long medial collateral ligament of
the tarsus

Dorsal tendon of the peroneus tertius m.

Outline of cunean bursa under medial
tendon of the tibialis cranialis m.

j. Daugherty

Figure 1.37. Medial dissection of left distal crus, tarsus, and metatarsus. Medial view. Please note that the term "fibularis" is currently preferred over "peroneus" (fibular rather than peroneal), although both are widely used.

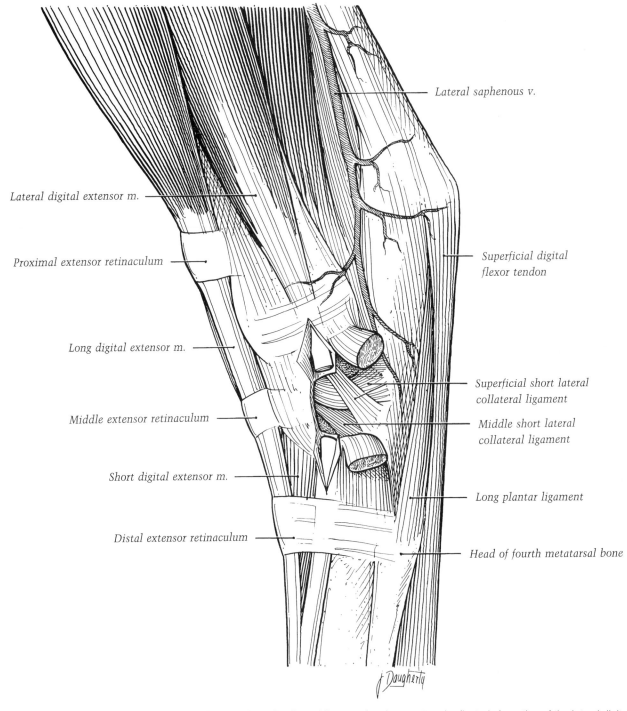

Lateral saphenous v.

Lateral digital extensor m.

Proximal extensor retinaculum

Superficial digital
flexor tendon

Long digital extensor m.

Superficial short lateral
collateral ligament

Middle short lateral
collateral ligament

Middle extensor retinaculum

Short digital extensor m.

Long plantar ligament

Distal extensor retinaculum

Head of fourth metatarsal bone

J Daugherty

Figure 1.38.   Lateral view of left tarsus. The long lateral collateral ligament has been cut and reflected. A section of the lateral digital extensor tendon has been removed.

calcaneus to form the tarsal canal containing the principal tendon of the deep digital flexor muscle. The tendon's synovial sheath, the tarsal sheath, extends from a level proximal to the medial malleolus to the proximal fourth of the metatarsus (Figure 1.35). After joining the anastomotic branch of the caudal tibial artery just proximal to the tarsus, the saphenous artery continues distad with the tendon (Figure 1.37). It bifurcates into small medial and lateral plantar arteries. Medial and lateral plantar nerves from the tibial nerve in the distal crural region also accompany the principal deep digital flexor tendon, lying lateral to the tendon in the tarsal canal (Figure 1.37). At the level of the tarsometatarsal joint, the medial plantar nerve and artery cross obliquely over the plantar surface of the deep digital flexor tendon to the medial side of the tendon.

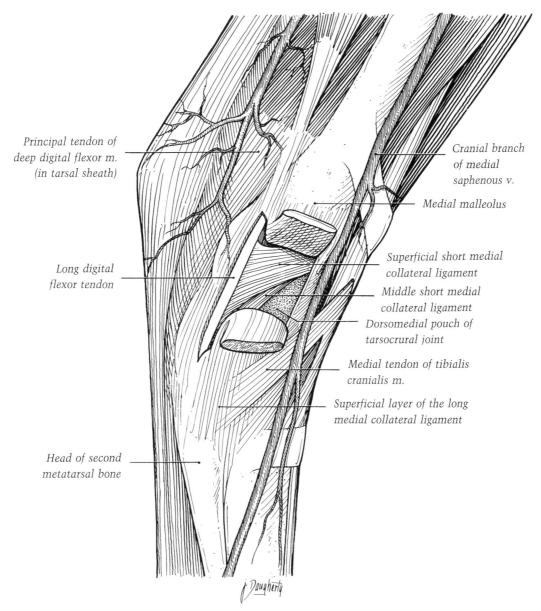

Principal tendon of
deep digital flexor m.
(in tarsal sheath)

Long digital
flexor tendon

Head of second
metatarsal bone

Cranial branch
of medial
saphenous v.

Medial malleolus

Superficial short medial
collateral ligament

Middle short medial
collateral ligament

Dorsomedial pouch of
tarsocrural joint

Medial tendon of tibialis
cranialis m.

Superficial layer of the long
medial collateral ligament

Figure 1.39. Medial view of left tarsus. The long medial collateral ligament has been cut and reflected. The tendon sheath of the long digital flexor tendon has been opened. Please note that "long digital flexor" is an older term for the medial head of the deep digital flexor muscle.

Plantar Aspect

In the distal third of the crus, the tendon of the superficial digital flexor muscle curls around the medial side of the tendon of the gastrocnemius muscle to become superficial as the tendons approach the calcaneal tuber. The superficial digital flexor tendon flattens and is joined by aponeurotic connections of the biceps femoris and semitendinosus muscles. This tendinous complex attaches to the point and sides of the calcaneal tuber. The tendon proper of the superficial digital flexor then narrows and continues distad superficial to the long plantar ligament. The calcaneal tendon of the gastrocnemius lies deep to the superficial digital flexor at the hock and inserts on the plantar surface of the calcaneal tuber. An elongated bursa is interposed between the two tendons just above the tarsus. A smaller bursa is present between the superficial digital flexor tendon and the calcaneal tuber. These two bursae usually communicate across the lateral surface of the gastrocnemius tendon.[33] An inconstant subcutaneous bursa may develop over the superficial digital flexor at the level of the calcaneal tuber.

Dorsolateral to the superficial digital flexor the long plantar ligament is attached to the plantar surface of the calcaneus, terminating distally on the fourth tarsal bone and the proximal extremity of the fourth metatarsal bone (Figure 1.38).

Tarsal Joint (Hock Joint)

The principal component of the composite tarsal joint is the tarsocrural joint. Deep grooves of the cochlear articular surface of the distal end of the tibia articulate with the surface of the trochlea of the talus at an angle of 12° to 15° dorsolateral to the limb's sagittal plane.[16] The interarticular and tarsometatarsal joints are plane joints capable of only a small amount of gliding movement. In the standing position, the dorsal articular angle of the hock is around 150°.[17] During flexion of the tarsocrural joint, the pes is directed slightly laterad due to the configuration of the joint.

A long collateral ligament and three short collateral ligaments bind each side of the equine hock (Figures 1.38, 1.39, and 1.40).[51] The long lateral collateral ligament extends from the lateral malleolus caudal to the groove for the tendon of the lateral digital extensor, attaching distally to the calcaneus, fourth tarsal bone, talus, and third and fourth metatarsal bones. The three short lateral collateral ligaments are fused proximally where they attach to the lateral malleolus cranial to the groove for the lateral digital extensor tendon. The superficial component, its fibers spiraling 180°, attaches distoplantarly to both the talus and calcaneus, whereas the middle and deep short lateral collateral ligaments attach solely on the lateral surface of the talus.

The long medial collateral ligament of the hock has less well-defined borders than its lateral counterpart. From its proximal attachment on the medial malleolus cranial to the groove for the long digital flexor muscle, the long medial collateral ligament extends distad and divides into two layers along its dorsal border. The superficial layer goes over the cunean tendon of the tibialis cranialis muscle and attaches to the fused first and second tarsal bones and the second and third

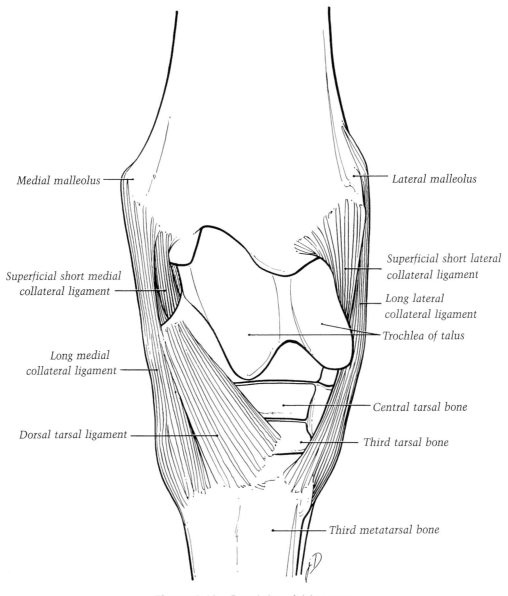

Figure 1.40.   Dorsal view of right tarsus.

metatarsal bones just distal to the distal edge of the cunean bursa. The deep layer attaches distally to the distal tuberosity of the talus and the central and third tarsal bones. The plantar edge of the ligament attaches to the deep fascia over the sustentaculum tali and the interosseous ligament between the second and third metatarsal bones.

The flat superficial short medial collateral ligament extends from the medial malleolus to the tuberosities of the talus and the ridge between them (Figure 1.39). The middle short medial collateral ligament extends obliquely from the medial tibial malleolus to the sustentaculum tali and central tarsal bone. It lies on the medial surface of the talus between the two tuberosities, varying in position during movement of the joints. The smallest component, the deep short medial collateral ligament, courses from the distal edge of the medial tibial malleolus obliquely to the ridge between the two tuberosities of the talus.

A dorsal tarsal ligament fans out distad from the distal tuberosity of the talus and attaches to the central and third tarsal bones and the proximal extremities of the second and third metatarsal bones (Figure 1.40). A plantar tarsal ligament attaches to the plantar surface of the calcaneus and fourth tarsal bone and the fourth metatarsal bone. Smaller, less distinct ligaments join contiguous tarsal bones.

The tarsal joint capsule is thinnest dorsally and thickest in its plantar and distal parts. Cartilage in the capsule covering the flexor groove of the sustentaculum tall provides a smooth surface for the deep digital flexor tendon. Distally the accessory (tarsal or "inferior" check) ligament of the deep digital flexor tendon takes origin from the fibrous joint capsule.

Three pouches can protrude (most notably with joint effusion) from the large tarsocrural synovial sac where it is not bound down by ligaments: the dorsomedial (largest), medioplantar, and lateroplantar pouches. This large synovial space consistently communicates with the synovial sac associated with the proximal intertarsal joint formed by the talus and calcaneus proximally and the central and fourth tarsal bones distally. The distal intertarsal sac, between the central tarsal and contiguous bones and the distal tarsal row, typically does not communicate with the proximal intertarsal sac, but may communicate with the synovial sac of the tarsometatarsal joint. Communications have been demonstrated in 8.3% to 23.8% of cases studied.[42]

Movements of the Tarsocrural Joint

The tarsocrural joint is flexed by contraction of the tibialis cranialis muscle and the passive pull of the tendinous fibularis (peroneus) tertius muscle. Contraction of the gastrocnemius, biceps femoris, and semitendinosus muscles and the passive pull of the tendinous superficial digital flexor muscle extends the joint. By virtue of its attachments in the extensor fossa of the femur proximally, and on the lateral aspect of the tarsus and dorsal surface of the third metatarsal bone distally, the fibularis tertius passively flexes the tarsocrural joint when the stifle joint is flexed. The superficial digital flexor muscle originates in the supracondyloid fossa of the femur and attaches to the calcaneal tuber. This part of the superficial digital flexor serves to passively extend the tarsocrural joint when the femorotibial joint is extended. The two tendinous, passively functioning muscles constitute the reciprocal apparatus (Figure 1.41).

Crus (Leg or Gaskin)

The crus or true leg is the region of the hindlimb containing the tibia and fibula. Thus, it extends from the tarsocrural joint to the femorotibial joint. The transversely flattened proximal end of the fibula articulates with the lateral condyle of the tibia. Distally the fibula narrows to a free end, terminating in the distal one-half to two-thirds of the crus as a thin ligament. An interosseous ligament occupies the space between the two bones. The cranial tibial vessels pass through the proximal part of the ligament. It should be noted that the current preference among anatomists is to replace the Greek word "peroneus" with its Latin equivalent "fibularis" in the naming of crural structures.

Beneath the skin and superficial fascia a heavy crural fascia invests the entire crural region. The superficial layer of the deep crural fascia is continuous with the femoral fascia; the middle layer is continuous with tendons descending from the thigh. In several places the two layers are inseparable. The crural fascia blends with the medial and lateral patellar ligaments and attaches to the medial tibia in the middle of the leg. Caudally, the crural fascia forms the combined aponeuroses of the biceps femoris and semitendinosus muscles that attach with the superficial digital flexor tendon to the calcaneal tuber. Under the two common fasciae a deeper layer covers the muscles of the leg.

Cranial Aspect

The belly of the long digital extensor muscle is prominent beneath the skin on the craniolateral aspect of the crus. It originates in common with the fibularis tertius from the extensor fossa of the femur, the common tendon descending through the extensor sulcus of the tibia (Figure 1.42). The long digital extensor muscle is related deeply to the tendinous fibularis tertius and the fleshy cranial tibial muscles and caudally to the lateral digital extensor muscle from which it is separated by a distinct intermuscular septum. The superficial fibular nerve courses distad in the groove between the digital extensor muscles and angles craniad toward the hock. The deep fibular nerve courses distad between the two muscles on the cranial surface of the intermuscular septum. At its origin this nerve sends branches to the digital extensor muscles and the fibularis tertius and tibialis cranialis muscles (Figure 1.38).

Deep to and intimately associated with the fibularis tertius, the cranial tibial muscle covers the craniolateral surface of the tibia, originating from the tibial tuberosity, lateral condyle, and lateral border, and from the crural fascia (Figure 1.42). After it passes through the interosseous space (between the tibia and fibula), the cranial tibial artery courses distad on the tibia deep to the cranial tibial muscle accompanied by two satellite veins.

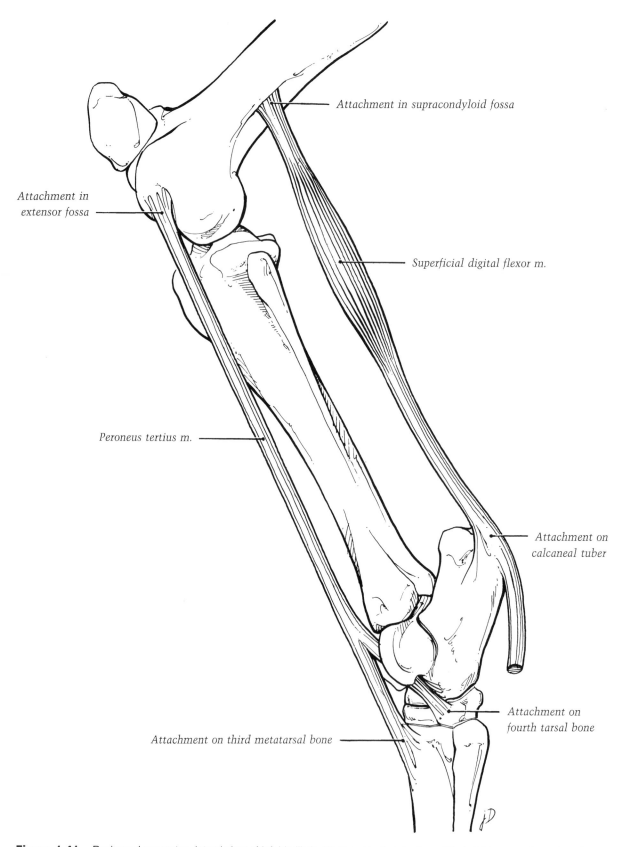

Attachment in supracondyloid fossa

Attachment in extensor fossa

Superficial digital flexor m.

Peroneus tertius m.

Attachment on calcaneal tuber

Attachment on fourth tarsal bone

Attachment on third metatarsal bone

Figure 1.41. Reciprocal apparatus, lateral view of left hindlimb. Please note that the term "fibularis" is currently preferred over "peroneus" (fibular rather than peroneal), although both are widely used.

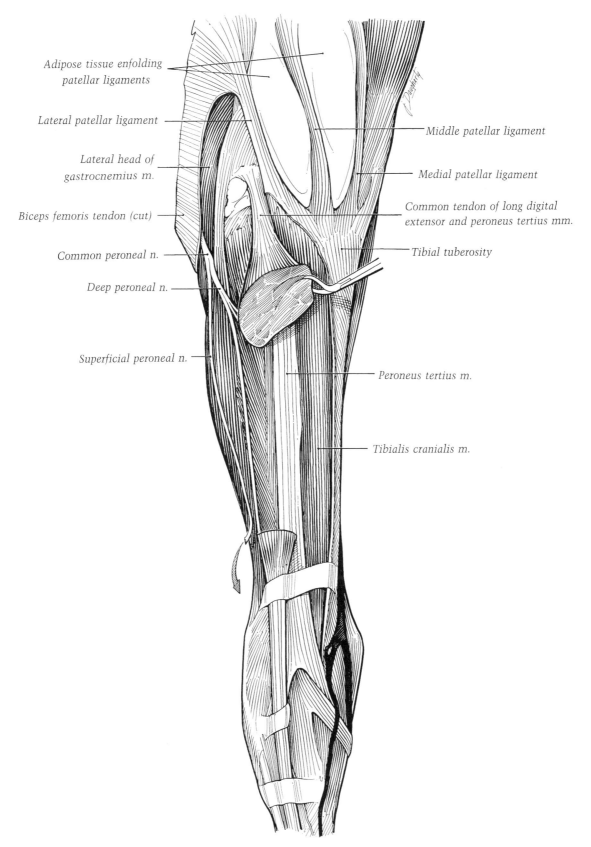

Adipose tissue enfolding patellar ligaments

Lateral patellar ligament

Lateral head of gastrocnemius m.

Biceps femoris tendon (cut)

Common peroneal n.

Deep peroneal n.

Superficial peroneal n.

Middle patellar ligament

Medial patellar ligament

Common tendon of long digital extensor and peroneus tertius mm.

Tibial tuberosity

Peroneus tertius m.

Tibialis cranialis m.

Figure 1.42. Dorsal view of right stifle, crus, and tarsus. The long digital extensor muscle belly has been removed, along with the terminal parts of the superficial fibular (peroneal) nerve (shown by arrow). Please note that the term "fibularis" is currently preferred over "peroneus" (fibular rather than peroneal), although both are widely used.

Lateral Aspect

The caudal cutaneous sural nerve is derived principally from the tibial nerve (Figure 1.43). In company with the lateral saphenous vein, the caudal cutaneous sural nerve courses laterad across both heads of the gastrocnemius muscle. The nerve and vein then descend under the crural fascia and tarsal attachment of the biceps femoris muscle to the distal third of the crus where the nerve penetrates the crural fascia and divides into several branches, one of which courses distad over the hock to the metatarsus (Figure 1.34). The tibial attachment of the biceps femoris muscle, a broad aponeurosis, sweeps across the proximal third of the lateral aspect of the crus to attach to the cranial border of the tibia. Deep to the belly of the biceps femoris, the common fibular nerve crosses the lateral surface of the lateral head of the gastrocnemius muscle and divides into superficial and deep fibular nerves (Figure 1.43). Caudal to these, the lateral digital extensor muscle extends distad from its origins on the fibula, interosseus ligament, lateral surface of the tibia, and the lateral collateral ligament of the femorotibial joint. The lateral head of the deep digital flexor muscle lies caudal to the belly of the lateral digital extensor.

The lateral head of the gastrocnemius originates on the lateral supracondyloid tuberosity of the femur. Under the crural fascia in the proximal half of the crus, the small soleus muscle extends from its origin on the fibula along the lateral aspect of the gastrocnemius muscle to join the gastrocnemius tendon (Figure 1.43).

Medial Aspect

Throughout most of its length, the medial surface of the tibia is subcutaneous (Figure 1.35). Sensation is provided to the medial and cranial aspects of the crus by numerous branches of the saphenous nerve ramifying in the superficial fascia. The distal continuation of the nerve follows the prominent cranial branch of the medial saphenous vein that angles across the medial surface of the tibia. Accompanied by the saphenous artery, the smaller caudal branch of the medial saphenous vein crosses medial to the medial head of the deep digital flexor muscle and joins the cranial branch of the vein superficial to the tibial attachment of the semitendinosus muscle.

Deep to the crural fascia and caudal to the caudal branch of the medial saphenous vein, the tibial nerve descends with branches of the caudal femoral vessels. The tibial nerve bifurcates about 8 to 10 cm proximal to the point of the calcaneal tuber into the medial and lateral plantar nerves. These nerves continue distad to the tarsus where they diverge to pursue their independent courses.

The caudal tibial vessels lie deep to the tendon of the medial head of the deep digital flexor as it passes distad. The anastomosis between the caudal tibial and saphenous vessels is located medial to the principal tendon of the deep digital flexor muscle (Figure 1.37).

Caudal Aspect

Descending from their origins on the supracondyloid tuberosities of the femur, the two heads of the gastroc-

nemius enclose the round, mostly tendinous superficial digital flexor. The tendon of the latter wraps medially from deep to superficial around the gastrocnemius tendon in the distal third of the crus.

The deep digital flexor muscle possesses three heads with a variety of names that appear in anatomical texts (Figure 1.43). In the horse, the tendons of all three heads unite with the main deep digital flexor tendon. In the distal third of the crus, the flat tendon of the caudal tibial (the superficial head) joins the larger tendon of the lateral head, whereas the tendon of the medial head (medial digital flexor m.) pursues its course over the medial aspect of the hock to join the principal tendon in the metatarsus.

Stifle (Genu)

The stifle is the region including the stifle joint (femorotibial joint plus the femoropatellar joint) and surrounding structures.

Cranial Aspect

Cutaneous innervation of the cranial aspect of the stifle is provided by terminal branches of the lateral cutaneous femoral nerve and lateral branch of the iliohypogastric nerve.

Deep to the skin three patellar ligaments descend from the patella, converging to their attachments on the tibial tuberosity. An extensive pad of adipose tissue is interposed between the ligaments and the joint capsule of the femoropatellar joint (Figure 1.42). The adipose tissue enfolds the ligaments, wrapping around their sides. The space between the medial and middle patellar ligaments is greater than the space between the middle and lateral ligaments. This difference reflects the origin of the medial patellar ligament from the parapatellar fibrocartilage. This is a large mass extending mediad from the patella in such a manner that its continuation, the medial patellar ligament, courses proximal and then medial to the medial ridge of the trochlea on the femur. The medial patellar ligament attaches to the medial side of the tibial tuberosity. As it descends from the patella to its insertion, two bursae lie under the middle patellar ligament, one between the proximal part of the ligament and the apex of the patella, and the other between the ligament and the proximal part of the groove. Inclining mediad from the lateral aspect of the cranial surface of the patella, the lateral patellar ligament serves as an attachment for a tendon from the biceps femoris muscle and then for the fascia lata just before the ligament attaches to the lateral aspect of the tibial tuberosity. The tendon from the biceps femoris continues on to the cranial surface of the patella.

The base, cranial surface, and medial border of the patella, and the parapatellar fibrocartilage and femoropatellar joint capsule, serve as attachments for the insertions of the quadriceps femoris muscle.

Lateral Aspect

The insertional parts of the biceps femoris muscle and, caudally, the semitendinosus muscle dominate the lateral aspect of the stifle region with the tendon from

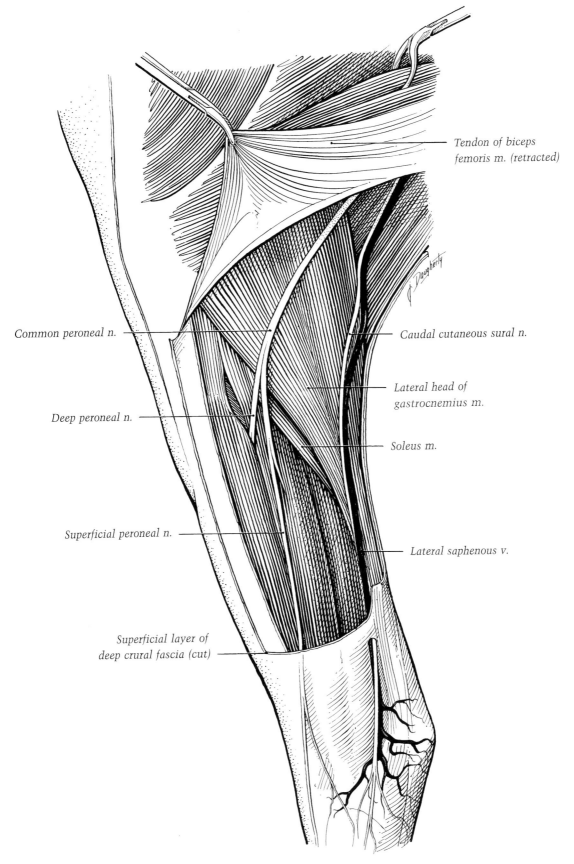

Labels on the figure:

Tendon of biceps femoris m. (retracted)

Common peroneal n.

Deep peroneal n.

Superficial peroneal n.

Superficial layer of deep crural fascia (cut)

Caudal cutaneous sural n.

Lateral head of gastrocnemius m.

Soleus m.

Lateral saphenous v.

Figure 1.43. Superficial dissection of lateral aspect of left stifle, crus, and tarsus. Please note that the term "fibularis" is currently preferred over "peroneus" (fibular rather than peroneal), although both are widely used.

the cranial division of the biceps femoris inserting on the lateral patellar ligament and the patella and the tendon from the middle division of the muscle sweeping craniodistad to the cranial border of the tibia.

Cutaneous innervation is supplied to this region by branches from several nerves: lateral branches of the iliohypogastric and ilioinguinal nerves, the lateral cutaneous sural nerve originating from the common fibular nerve and passing out between the middle and caudal divisions of the biceps femoris, the caudal cutaneous sural nerve (from the tibial nerve), and terminal branches of the caudal cutaneous femoral nerve (from the caudal gluteal nerve).

Reflection of the distal part of the biceps femoris muscle reveals the following (Figure 1.44): The lateral femoropatellar ligament extends obliquely from the lateral epicondyle of the femur to the lateral border of the patella. The lateral surface of the lateral head of the gastrocnemius muscle is crossed by the common fibular nerve and, further caudad, by the caudal cutaneous sural nerve and the lateral saphenous vein carrying blood to the caudal femoral vein. As it extends from the lateral epicondyle of the femur to the head of the fibula, the thick lateral collateral ligament of the femorotibial joint covers the tendon of origin of the popliteus muscle that also originates from the lateral epicondyle. A pouch from the lateral femorotibial joint capsule lies beneath

the tendon. A common tendon of the long digital extensor and fibularis (peroneus) tertius takes origin from the extensor fossa in the distal surface of the lateral epicondyle of the femur. The tendon is cushioned as it extends distad by an elongated pouch from the lateral femorotibial joint capsule.

Caudal Aspect

Under the skin and fascia on the caudal aspect of the stifle (supplied by branches of the caudal femoral nerve) the caudal part of the biceps femoris muscle covers the lateral head of the gastrocnemius, the tibial tendon of the biceps femoris going to the cranial border of the tibia, its tarsal tendon continuing distad. The semitendinosus muscle sweeps to its insertion on the cranial border of the tibia and distad toward its tarsal insertion, covering the medial head of the gastrocnemius. The tendons of the smaller medial head and larger lateral head of the gastrocnemius combine and, at first, the tendon lies superficial to the tendon of the superficial digital flexor muscle.

Separation of the two heads of the gastrocnemius muscle reveals the tendinous superficial digital flexor muscle that arises in the supracondyloid fossa of the femur between the two heads, its initial part embedded in the lateral head (Figure 1.45). After detaching the

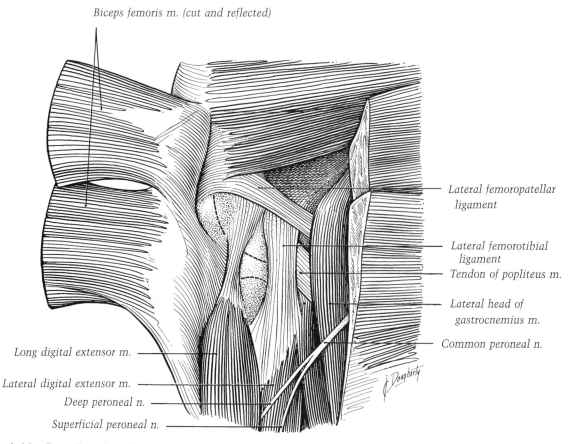

Biceps femoris m. (cut and reflected)

Lateral femoropatellar ligament

Lateral femorotibial ligament

Tendon of popliteus m.

Lateral head of gastrocnemius m.

Common peroneal n.

Long digital extensor m.

Lateral digital extensor m.

Deep peroneal n.

Superficial peroneal n.

Figure 1.44. Deep dissection of lateral aspect of left stifle with femoral and tibial condylar surfaces indicated by dashed lines. Please note that the term "fibularis" is currently preferred over "peroneus" (fibular rather than peroneal), although both are widely used.

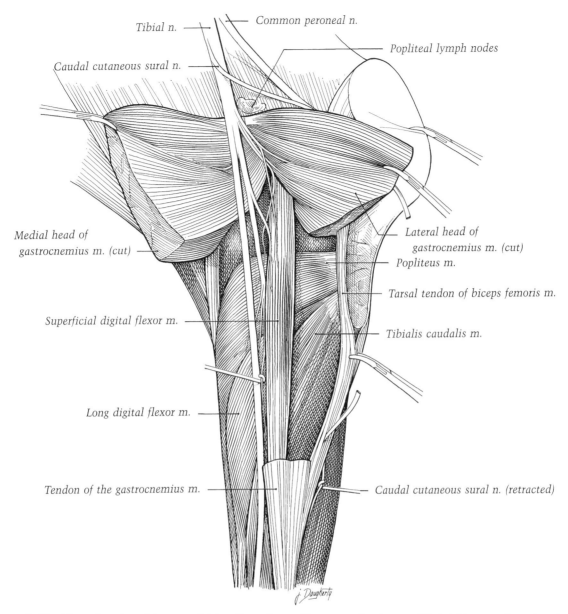

Figure 1.45. Dissection of caudal aspect of right stifle and crus. Please note that the term "fibularis" is currently preferred over "peroneus" (fibular rather than peroneal), although both are widely used.

caudal cutaneous sural nerve, the tibial nerve descends between the two heads of the gastrocnemius along the medial side of the superficial digital flexor. Branches from the tibial nerve supply the gastrocnemius, soleus, superficial digital flexor, deep digital flexor, and popliteus muscles. The femoral artery and vein terminate by giving off the distal caudal femoral vessels and continuing as the popliteal vessels that descend between the two heads of the gastrocnemius (Figure 1.46). Distal to the stifle joint, the popliteal vessels divide into cranial and caudal tibial vessels. The larger cranial vessels, the main blood supply to the pes, deviate laterad into the interosseous space between the tibia and fibula; the smaller caudal tibial vessels continue distad between the tibia and the popliteus muscle.

The triangular popliteus muscle extends mediodistad from its origin on the lateral epicondyle of the femur (Figure 1.44). The tendon of origin passes deep to the lateral collateral ligament of the stifle joint, cushioned by an extension of the lateral pouch of the femorotibial joint capsule. The popliteus spreads out and inserts on the medial part of the caudal surface of the tibia proximal to the popliteal line, contacting the medial head of the deep digital flexor (Figure 1.45).

Medial Aspect

Skin and fascia on the medial aspect of the stifle are supplied by the saphenous and lateral cutaneous femoral nerves. The region is crossed by the saphenous vein,

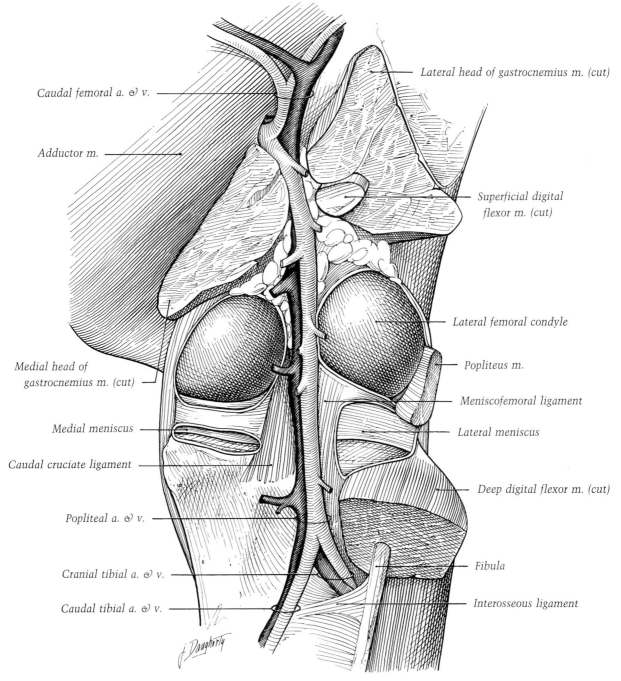

Figure 1.46. Deep dissection of caudal aspect of right stifle. The joint capsule of the femorotibial joint has been opened.

artery, and nerve. Cranially, the vastus medialis of the quadriceps femoris muscle attaches to the parapatellar fibrocartilage, medial border of the patella, and medial patellar ligament. The strap-like sartorius muscle attaches to the medial patellar ligament and the tibial tuberosity. Caudal to the sartorius, the gracilis muscle also attaches to the medial patellar ligament and to the medial collateral ligament of the femorotibial joint and the crural fascia (Figure 1.47).

A thinner medial collateral ligament of the femorotibial joint reaches from the medial epicondyle of the femur to just distal to the margin of the medial tibial condyle, detaching fibers to the medial meniscus (Figure 1.47). The adductor muscle inserts on the ligament and the medial epicondyle. The medial femoropatellar ligament is also thinner than its lateral counterpart, blending with the femoropatellar joint capsule as the ligament extends from the femur proximal to the medial epicondyle to the parapatellar fibrocartilage.

Stifle Joint

The stifle is the "true knee." It comprises two joints, the femoropatellar and femorotibial joints, which

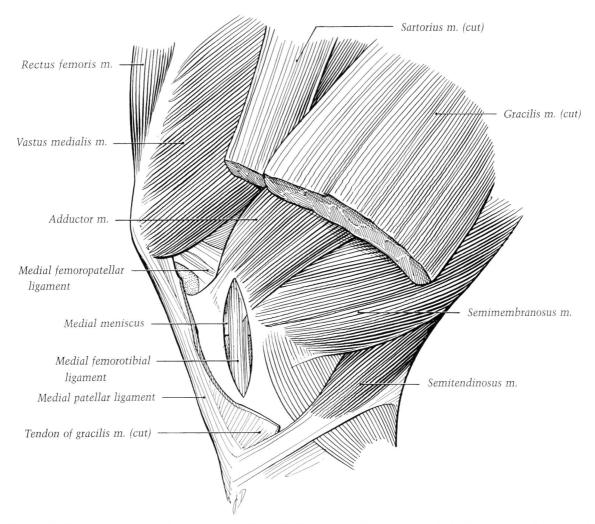

Figure 1.47. Deep dissection of medial aspect of left stifle. Tendon of adductor muscle is incised to reveal medial collateral ligament of the stifle.

together form a hinge joint. The synovial space of the stifle is significantly partitioned into three distinct sacs: the femoropatellar sac and right and left femorotibial joint sacs.[37]

Femoropatellar Joint

The patella is a sesamoid bone intercalated in the termination of the quadriceps femoris muscle with the three patellar ligaments constituting the tendon of insertion.

A thin, voluminous joint capsule attaches peripheral to the edge of the femoral trochlea, with its patellar attachment close to the edge of the patellar articular surface. A large pouch from the joint capsule protrudes proximad under a mass of adipose tissue and the distal part of the quadriceps femoris muscle. The distal extremity of the femoropatellar joint capsule contacts the femorotibial joint capsule. The vastus intermedius of the quadriceps femoris attaches, in part, to the femoropatellar joint capsule, acting to tense the capsule during extension of the femoropatellar joint.

The articular surface of the patella is much smaller than the trochlear surface of the femur; the larger gliding surface of the trochlea accommodates the proximal-distal movements of the patella. A wide groove separates the substantially larger medial ridge of the trochlea from the smaller, slightly more distal lateral ridge. Articular cartilage covers the entire large, rounded medial ridge; the cartilage covering the more regularly rounded lateral ridge extends only part way over the lateral surface. Contact between the patella and trochlea changes as the patella moves on its larger gliding surface during flexion of the stifle joint. The patella rolls on to its narrow distal articular surface (resting surface) as the parapatellar fibrocartilage maintains its tight relationship over the trochlea's medial ridge due to tension exerted by the medial patellar ligament. The narrow craniodorsal surface of the proximal part of the trochlea may be termed its resting surface.[41]

Femorotibial Joint

The fibrous part of the joint capsule is thick caudally, thin cranially. The cranial and caudal cruciate ligaments of the femorotibial joint lie between the joint capsule's medial and lateral synovial sacs. Two fibrocartilaginous menisci intervene between the femoral and tibial articular surfaces, thus partially subdividing each sac. An extension of the lateral synovial sac encloses the tendon of origin of the popliteus muscle and another protrudes distad under the common tendon of origin of the long digital extensor and fibularis tertius muscles.

The two fibrocartilaginous menisci are crescent-shaped, being thicker peripherally and thinner along the concave edge. Their proximal surfaces are concave to accommodate the convexity of the femoral condyles. Distally they conform to the peripheral parts of the articular surfaces of the tibial condyles. Cranial and caudal ligaments anchor each meniscus to the tibia, and a meniscofemoral ligament attaches the caudal aspect of the lateral meniscus to the caudal surface of the intercondyloid fossa of the femur.

In addition to the support rendered by medial and lateral collateral ligaments, the femur and tibia are joined by the two cruciate ligaments that cross one another in the intercondyloid space between the two synovial sacs of the femorotibial joint. The caudal cruciate ligament, the more substantial of the two, extends from the cranial surface of the intercondyloid fossa of the femur to the popliteal notch of the tibia, crossing the medial aspect of the cranial (or lateral) cruciate ligament. From its attachment on the lateral wall of the intercondyloid fossa, the cranial cruciate ligament attaches to a central fossa between the articular surfaces of the condyles.

The stifle is supplied principally by branches of the descending genicular artery that originates from the femoral artery and descends toward the medial aspect of the stifle joint deep to the sartorius and vastus medialis muscles.

Movements of the Stifle Joint

In the standing position, the caudal angle of the stifle joint is around 150°.[17] The quadriceps femoris muscle is relatively relaxed in this position. Extension of the stifle joint through action of the quadriceps femoris, tensor fasciae lata, and cranial division of the biceps femoris muscles plus passive traction exerted by the fibularis tertius is limited by tension from the collateral and cruciate ligaments. Flexion of the joint by the semitendinosus, middle division of the biceps femoris, popliteus, and gastrocnemius muscles, plus passive traction exerted by the superficial digital flexor, is limited only by the caudal muscle masses. During flexion the crus is rotated slightly mediad, and the femoral condyles and menisci move slightly caudad on the tibial condyles with somewhat more movement on the lateral surfaces.

When a horse shifts its weight to rest on one hindlimb, the supportive limb flexes slightly as the contralateral relaxed limb is brought to rest on the toe. The pelvis is tilted so that the hip of the supporting limb is higher. The stifle on the supporting limb is locked in position due to a slight medial rotation of the patella as the medial patellar ligament and parapatellar cartilage slip farther caudad on the proximal part of the medial trochlear ridge. The loop created by the parapatellar cartilage and medial patellar ligament is pulled proximad and mediad to engage the medial ridge of the femoral trochlea. The locked position achieved by this configuration together with the support rendered by the other components of the stay apparatus minimizes muscular activity in the supporting limb while the relaxed contralateral hindlimb is resting. A very small amount of muscle tone, confined to the vastus medialis, is necessary to stabilize the stifle in the locked position.[44]

Thigh and Hip
Lateral Aspect

Cutaneous innervation is supplied to the lateral aspect of the thigh and hip by the lateral branches of the iliohypogastric and ilioinguinal nerves, the caudal cutaneous femoral nerve, and the dorsal branches of the lumbar and sacral nerves.[19]

From caudal to cranial the superficial muscles of the lateral thigh and hip are the semitendinosus, biceps femoris, gluteus superficialis, gluteus medius, and tensor fasciae lata. Both the semitendinosus and biceps femoris have ischiatic and vertebral origins. The semitendinosus attaches to the first and second caudal vertebrae and fascia of the tail and the biceps femoris attaches to the dorsal sacroiliac ligament and the gluteal and tail fasciae. A prominent longitudinal groove marks the site of the intermuscular septum between the semitendinosus and the biceps femoris muscles.

The strong gluteal fascia gives origin to and unites the long caudal head and the cranial head of the gluteus superficialis (superficial gluteal) muscle. The two heads of the superficial gluteal muscle unite in a flat tendon that attaches to the trochanter tertius of the femur. Extending caudad from the aponeurosis of the longissimus lumborum muscle, the large gluteus medius (middle gluteal) muscle forms most of the mass of the rump. The middle gluteal muscle also takes origin from the gluteal surface of the ilium, the coxal tuber and sacral tuber, the sacrotuberal and dorsal sacroiliac ligaments, and the gluteal fascia. Distally the muscle attaches to greater trochanter, a crest distal to the greater trochanter and the lateral surface of the intertrochanteric crest.

The tensor fasciae latae muscle arises from the coxal tuber and fans out distally to insert into the fascia lata. An intermuscular septum attaches the caudal part of the muscle to the cranial head of the superficial gluteal. The fascia lata attaches to the patella and the lateral and middle patellar ligaments (Figure 1.48). The intermuscular septum between the biceps femoris and semitendinosus, the septa between the three divisions of the biceps femoris, and a septum between the biceps femoris and vastus lateralis all arise from the fascia lata (Figures 1.48 and 1.49).

Deeply on the lateral aspect of the hip the smaller deep part of the gluteus medius, the gluteus accessorius, has a distinct flat tendon that plays over the convexity of the greater trochanter on its way to attach on the crest distal to the trochanter. The large trochanteric bursa lies between the tendon and the cartilage covering the convexity (Figure 1.48). The small gluteus profundus muscle is deep to the caudal part of the gluteus medius, arising from the ischiatic spine and body of the

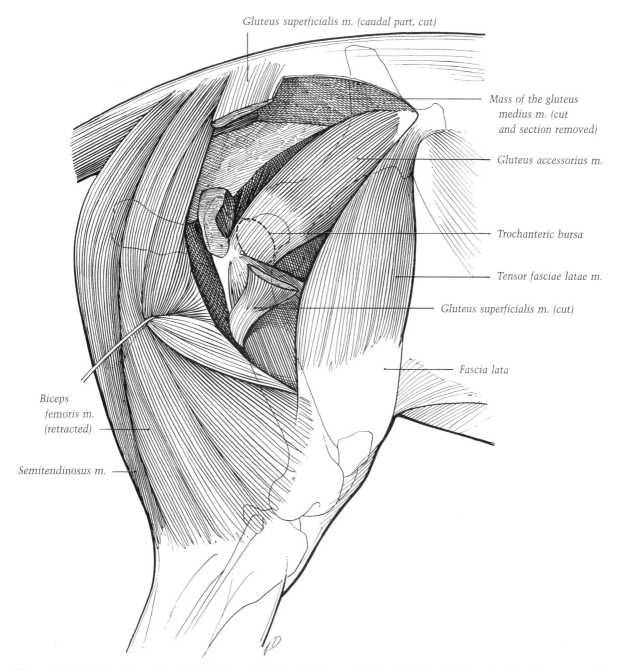

Gluteus superficialis m. (caudal part, cut)

Mass of the gluteus medius m. (cut and section removed)

Gluteus accessorius m.

Trochanteric bursa

Tensor fasciae latae m.

Gluteus superficialis m. (cut)

Fascia lata

Biceps femoris m. (retracted)

Semitendinosus m.

Figure 1.48. Lateral dissection of right thigh and hip. Most of the superficial and middle gluteal muscles have been removed.

ilium and attaching on the medial edge of the convexity of the greater trochanter (Figure 1.50). This muscle covers the hip joint and parts of the articularis coxae and rectus femoris muscles. A bursa is commonly present under the tendon of insertion of the gluteus profundus (Figure 1.49).[33]

On the caudal side of the proximal part of the femur the gemelli, external obturator, and internal obturator muscles come from their respective origins on the ischium, pubis, ilium, and wing of the sacrum to insert in the trochanteric fossa. The quadratus femoris muscle extends from the ventral aspect of the ischium to a line on the femur near the distal part of the lesser trochanter.

A broad sheet of dense white fibrous connective tissue, the sacrotuberous (sacrotuberal) ligament, forms most of the lateral wall of the pelvic cavity, attaching dorsally to the sacrum and first two caudal vertebrae and ventrally to the ischiatic spine and ischiatic tuber (Figure 1.50). The ventral edge of the sacrotuberal ligament completes two openings along the dorsal edge of the ischium: the lesser and greater ischiadic foramina which allow passage of neurovascular bundles from the lumbosacral region to the muscle of the rump.

Branches of the cranial gluteal vessels and the cranial gluteal nerve come through the greater ischiadic foremen to supply the gluteal muscles, the tensor fasciae latae, and the articularis coxae. The caudal gluteal vessels and

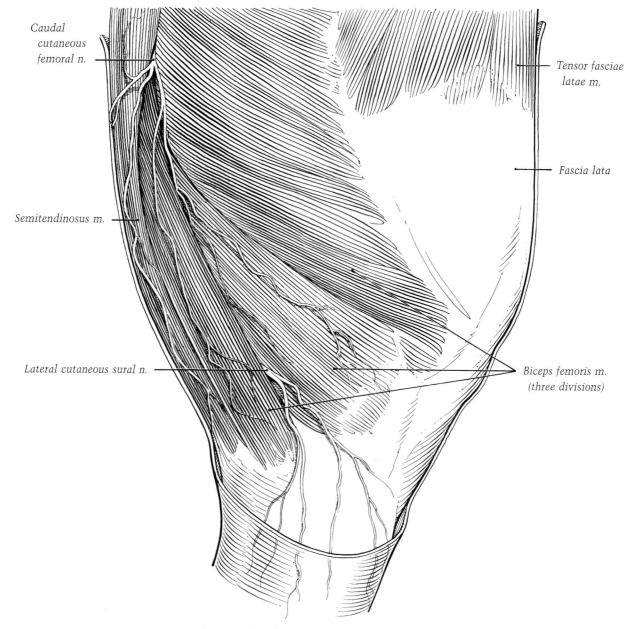

Caudal cutaneous femoral n.

Tensor fasciae latae m.

Fascia lata

Semitendinosus m.

Lateral cutaneous sural n.

Biceps femoris m. (three divisions)

Figure 1.49.   Lateral view of right stifle and thigh.

nerve perforate the sacrotuberal ligament dorsal to the ischiatic nerve. The caudal gluteal nerve divides into two trunks. The dorsal trunk supplies branches to the biceps femoris, middle gluteal, and long head of the superficial gluteal, and after supplying a branch to the semitendinosus, the ventral trunk continues as the caudal cutaneous femoral nerve. The latter nerve passes outward between the biceps femoris and semitendinosus to branch subcutaneously over the lateral and caudal surfaces of the thigh and hip. Muscles in this region are supplied by branches from the caudal gluteal vessels. In this region the internal pudendal artery courses on the deep face and within the sacrotuberous ligament. Iliolumbar vessels (from the cranial gluteal vessels) course laterad between the iliacus muscle and the ilium, supplying branches to the iliopsoas and longissimus

lumborum. The vessels then go around the lateral border of the ilium and supply branches to the middle gluteal and tensor fasciae latae.

The large, flat sciatic nerve passes through the greater ischiatic foremen and courses ventrocaudad on the sacrotuberale ligament and then on the origin of the gluteus profundus (deep gluteal). Turning distad, the ischiadic nerve passes over the gemelli, the tendon of the internal obturator, and the quadratus femoris, supplying branches to these muscles. A large branch is detached from the deep side of the nerve. This branch supplies branches to the semimembranosus, the biceps femoris and semitendinosus, and adductor medially and the biceps femoris laterally. The sciatic nerve terminates by dividing into common fibular and tibial nerves.

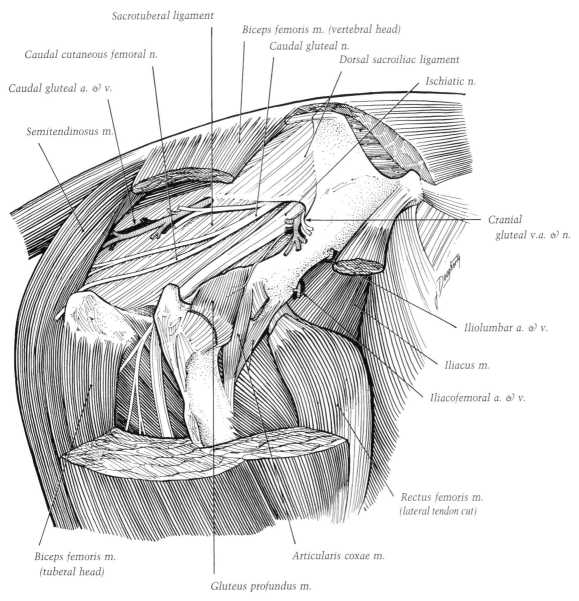

Caudal gluteal a. & v.

Caudal cutaneous femoral n.

Sacrotuberal ligament

Biceps femoris m. (vertebral head)

Caudal gluteal n.

Dorsal sacroiliac ligament

Ischiatic n.

Semitendinosus m.

Cranial gluteal v.a. & n.

Iliolumbar a. & v.

Iliacus m.

Iliacofemoral a. & v.

Rectus femoris m. (lateral tendon cut)

Biceps femoris m. (tuberal head)

Articularis coxae m.

Gluteus profundus m.

Figure 1.50. Deep dissection of right hip. Lateral view.

Medial Aspect

The lateral cutaneous femoral nerve; medial branches of the iliohypogastric, ilioinguinal, and genitofemoral nerves; and branches from the caudal cutaneous femoral and saphenous nerves supply cutaneous innervation to the medial aspect of the thigh.[19]

Accompanied by the small saphenous artery and the saphenous nerve, the large medial saphenous vein pursues a subcutaneous course proximad on the cranial part of the gracilis muscle, then between the gracilis and sartorius muscles to join the femoral vein. The broad gracilis muscle covers most of the medial aspect of the thigh, attaching proximally to the prepubic tendon, adjacent surface of the pubis, accessory femoral ligament, and middle of the pelvic symphysis. The muscle belly ends distally by joining a wide thin aponeurosis of insertion. The narrow sartorius muscle takes origin from the tendon of the psoas minor and ilial fascia and descends toward its insertion in the stifle which blends with the tendon of the gracilis.

Deep to the gracilis lies the pectineus muscle. It attaches proximally to the cranial border of the pubis, the prepubic tendon, and accessory femoral ligament. Distally the pectineus attaches to the medial border of the femur. The femoral canal, containing the neurovascular bundle supplying the pelvic limb, is delimited caudally by the pectineus, cranially by the sartorius, laterally by the vastus medialis and iliopsoas, and medially by the femoral fascia and cranial edge of the gracilis. The canal contains the femoral artery and vein, the saphenous nerve, and an elongated group of several lymph nodes of the deep inguinal lymphocenter embedded in adipose tissue. Within the canal the saphenous nerve detaches a motor branch to the sartorius muscle (Figure 1.51).

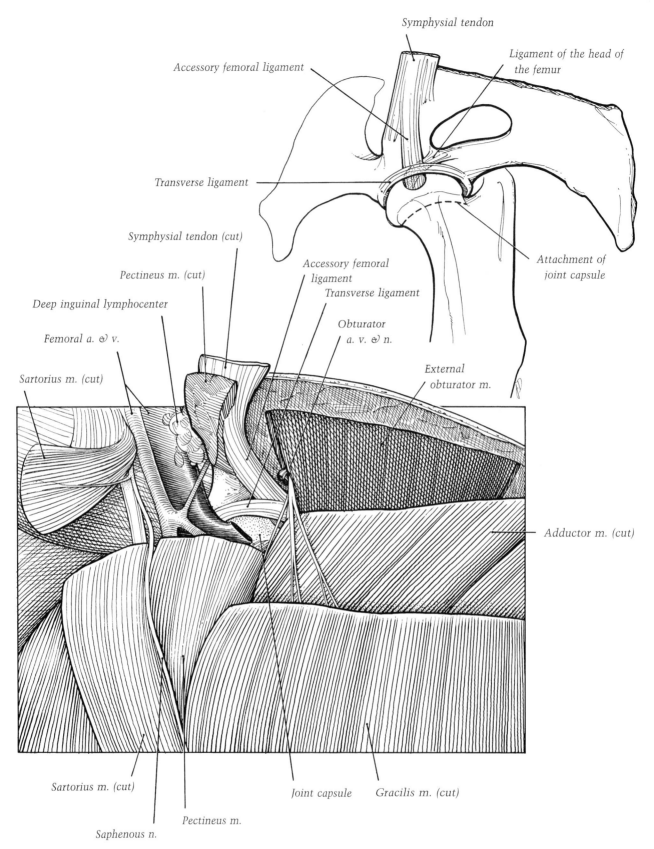

Figure 1.51. Deep dissection of right hip. Ventromedial view.

Symphysial tendon

Accessory femoral ligament

Ligament of the head of the femur

Transverse ligament

Symphysial tendon (cut)

Pectineus m. (cut)

Accessory femoral ligament

Deep inguinal lymphocenter

Transverse ligament

Femoral a. & v.

Obturator a. v. & n.

Attachment of joint capsule

Sartorius m. (cut)

External obturator m.

Adductor m. (cut)

Sartorius m. (cut)

Saphenous n.

Pectineus m.

Joint capsule

Gracilis m. (cut)

Caudal to the pectineus and vastus medialis the thick adductor muscle extends from the ventral surface of the ischium and pubis and the origin of the gracilis muscle to the caudal surface of the femur, the medial femoral epicondyle, and the medial collateral ligament of the femorotibial joint. The obturator nerve passes through the cranial part of the obturator foremen and external obturator muscle and branches to supply the external obturator, adductor, pectineus, and gracilis muscles (Figure 1.51). Branches from the obturator artery (from the cranial gluteal artery) supply the muscles in this region.

Cranial Aspect

The quadriceps femoris, articularis coxae, and sartorius muscles lie in the cranial part of the thigh and hip. In addition, the iliacus muscle crosses the cranial aspect of the hip where the muscle encloses the psoas major, creating the conjoined iliopsoas muscle. Their common tendon inserts on the lesser trochanter. The psoas major arises from the last two ribs and the lumbar transverse processes; the iliacus comes from the wing of the sacrum, ventral sacroiliac ligaments, sacropelvic surface of the ilium, and tendon of the psoas minor muscle.

Three heads of the quadriceps femoris muscles (the vastus lateralis, vastus intermedius, and vastus medialis) take origin from the shaft of the femur. The fourth head, the rectus femoris, originates from two tendons, one arising from a medial depression on the ilium craniodorsal to the acetabulum, and one from a lateral depression (Figure 1.50). A bursa is located under the lateral tendon.[33] All four heads of the quadriceps femoris attach to the patella. Bursae occur commonly under the insertions of the rectus femoris, vastus lateralis, and vastus medialis.

The femoral nerve passes between the psoas minor (a small muscle extending from the lumbar vertebral bodies to the ilium) and the psoas major, then between the iliopsoas and sartorius muscles. It supplies branches to the iliopsoas (which also receives innervation from lumbar nerves) and to all heads of the quadriceps femoris, and gives rise to the saphenous nerve.

Caudal Aspect

Innervation to the caudal skin of the thigh and hip is provided principally by the caudal cutaneous femoral nerve (Figure 1.49). The caudal rectal nerve supplies a small part dorsally. The main muscle mass is that of the semimembranosus with the semitendinosus with the caudal division of the biceps femoris related to it laterally and the gracilis medially. The long head of the semimembranosus attaches to the caudal border of the sacrotuberous ligament. The thicker short head attaches to the ventral part of the ischiatic tuber. The thick, roughly three-sided belly of the semimembranosus ends on a flat tendon that attaches to the medial femoral epicondyle.

Blood Supply to the Thigh

Before the external iliac artery passes through the femoral ring to continue as the femoral artery it gives off the deep femoral artery. This vessel courses between the sartorius and iliopsoas muscles and then between the latter muscle and the pectineus. After supplying small branches to the deep inguinal lymphocenter, the deep femoral artery gives off the large pudendoepigastric trunk. The trunk divides into the caudal epigastric artery and the external pudendal artery. The deep femoral artery continues caudad ventral to the pubis as the medial circumflex femoral artery that supplies the iliopsoas, pectineus, external obturator muscles, adductor (through which it passes), and semimembranosus (where its branches end). Branches are also supplied to the deep inguinal lymphocenter and the gracilis and quadratus femoris muscles. Satellite veins accompany the arteries.

The femoral artery courses distad through the femoral canal related caudally to the femoral vein and cranially to the saphenous nerve. Within the canal the femoral artery gives off the lateral circumflex femoral artery that passes craniodistad between the sartorius and iliopsoas muscles and then enters the quadriceps femoris, passing between the vastus medialis and rectus femoris.

The femoral artery directly supplies branches to muscles in this region. At the distal end of the femoral canal, the saphenous artery leaves the femoral artery and passes to the subcutaneous tissues between the gracilis and sartorius muscles. It courses caudodistad, related caudally to the much larger medial saphenous vein. The saphenous nerve accompanies the vessels as they course over the tendon of the gracilis. At the level of the tendon of insertion of the semitendinosus, the saphenous artery and medial saphenous vein each divide into cranial and caudal branches. In its course the saphenous artery supplies the sartorius, gracilis, and adductor muscles as well as fascia and skin.

The next branch of the femoral artery is the nutrient artery of the femur, and then the large descending genicular artery is detached from the cranial wall of the femoral artery. In the distal third of the thigh, the descending genicular artery courses distocraniad between the sartorius and vastus medialis and adductor, supplying these muscles and terminating in branches to the structures of the stifle.

The termination of the femoral artery gives off its last branch, the caudal femoral artery, and continues between the medial and lateral heads of the gastrocnemius as the popliteal artery (Figure 1.46). The caudal femoral artery pursues a short course caudad, giving off muscular branches to the superficial digital flexor and gastrocnemius. A branch runs distad to the crus where it joins a branch of the caudal tibial artery. Then the caudal femoral artery divides into an ascending branch and a descending branch. The ascending branch courses proximad between the semimembranosus and adductor, supplying these muscles and sending branches to the lateral head of the gastrocnemius, vastus lateralis, biceps femoris, and semitendinosus muscles. The descending branch of the caudal femoral artery runs distocaudad over the lateral head of the gastrocnemius in company with the lateral saphenous vein. Then the artery changes direction and passes proximad between the semitendinosus and the biceps femoris, supplying them and the small lymph nodes of the popliteal lymphocenter. A distally coursing branch supplies branches to both heads of the gastrocnemius and the superficial digital flexor and continues distad to join the saphenous artery.

Hip (Coxofemoral) Joint

The acetabulum of the os coxae is formed where the ilium, ischium, and pubis meet. The lunate surface of the acetabulum, a cup-shaped cavity arcing around a deep nonarticular fossa, articulates with the head of the femur. A fibrocartilaginous rim, the acetabular labrum, increases the articular surface of the acetabulum. The transverse acetabular ligament bridges the labrum across the medially located acetabular notch, binding two ligaments as they emerge from the fovea capitis of the femoral head (Figure 1.51). The shorter ligament of the head of the femur comes from the narrow apex of the fovea and attaches in the pubic groove. The thick accessory femoral ligament arises from the wider, peripheral part of the fovea and passes out through the acetabular notch to lie in the pubic groove. After giving partial origin to the gracilis and pectineus muscles, the accessory femoral ligament blends into the prepubic tendon.

The capacious joint capsule of the hip attaches to the acetabular labrum and on the neck of the femur a few millimeters from the margin of the femoral head (Figure 1.51). Within the joint the synovial membrane wraps around the ligaments. An outpocketing of the synovial membrane passes out through the acetabular notch to lie between the accessory femoral ligament and the pubic groove. A small pouch also lies under the ligament of the head of the femur. The fibrous joint capsule is intimately attached to the epimysium of the external obturator and deep gluteal muscles. Adipose tissue covers the capsule dorsally. The articularis coxae muscle is related to the lateral aspect of the hip joint, detaching some fibers to the joint capsule. During flexion of the hip joint, the articularis coxae can serve to tense the joint capsule.

Movements of the Hip Joint

While the hip joint is a ball-and-socket joint, capable only of very limited rotation, its principal movements are flexion and extension. Abduction of the thigh is restricted by the ligament of the head of the femur and the accessory femoral ligament. Adduction is checked by the attachments of the gluteal muscles on the femur. In the normal standing position, the caudolateral part of the head of the femur lies outside the acetabulum. The hip joint is slightly flexed in this position, the cranial angle being about 115°.[17] The range of motion between extreme flexion and extension is only 60°.[54]

Flexor muscles of the hip joint are the gluteus superficialis, tensor fasciae latae, rectus femoris, iliopsoas, sartorius, and pectineus. Extensor muscles of the hip joint are the gluteus medius, biceps femoris, semitendinosus, semimembranosus, adductor, and quadratus femoris. Muscles adducting the thigh include the gracilis, sartorius, adductor, pectineus, quadratus femoris, and obturatorius externus. Slight abduction is exerted on the thigh by all three gluteal muscles. The thigh is rotated laterad by the iliopsoas, external, and internal obturators and the gemelli. Medial rotation is accomplished through the combined action of the adductor and gluteus profundus muscles.

Pelvis

The equine pelvis, like that of other animals, comprises the ilium, ischium, and pubis; these bones are individually identifiable in the young but have fused by 10 to 12 months of age.[17]

The wing-shaped ilium presents two prominences, visible landmarks on the horse. The dorsally directed tuber sacrale inclines mediad toward its fellow, so that the two sacral tubers come within 2 to 3 cm over the first sacral spinous process. The ilial wing projects ventrolaterad in a bulky tuber coxae, creating the point of the hip.

Caudally, the ischial tuberosity presents as a laterally directed ridge to which muscles of the thigh attach. The acetabulum is formed through contributions from all three bones of the pelvis.

The pubis and ischium from each side meet ventrally at the symphysis pelvis. In the young animal fibrocartilage joins the bones. Later in life, a synostosis is formed as the cartilage ossifies in a cranial to caudal sequence.

Lymphatic Drainage

Two lymphocenters are involved in the lymphatic drainage of the pelvic limb. The popliteal lymphocenter consists of a few small deep popliteal lymph nodes embedded between the biceps femoris and semitendinosus muscles adjacent to the tibial nerve (Figure 1.44). They may be absent. The popliteal lymph nodes receive afferent lymphatic vessels from the distal pelvic limb. Its efferents drain to the deep inguinal lymphocenter in the femoral canal.

In addition to receiving lymphatic vessels from the popliteal lymphocenter, the lymph nodes of the deep inguinal lymphocenter (Figure 1.50) receive vessels from the caudal abdominal wall and superficial inguinal lymph nodes. Efferent vessels from the deep inguinal lymphocenter are afferent to the medial iliac lymph nodes[17].

Stay Apparatus of the Pelvic Limb (Figure 1.52)

The quadriceps femoris muscle and the tensor fasciae latae act to pull the patella, parapatellar cartilage, and medial patellar ligament proximad to the locked position over the medial trochlear ridge of the femur when the limb is positioned to bear weight at rest. Through the components of the reciprocal apparatus (cranially, the fibularis tertius from the femur to the lateral tarsus and proximal metatarsus and, caudally, the superficial digital flexor from the femur to the calcaneal tuber) the tarsus is correspondingly locked in extension. A small amount muscular activity in the quadriceps muscle assures continuation of this locked configuration, preventing flexion of the stifle and tarsocrural joints. Distal to the hock the digital flexor tendons support the plantar pes, the superficial digital flexor extending distad from its connection to the calcaneal tuber and the deep digital flexor usually receiving the

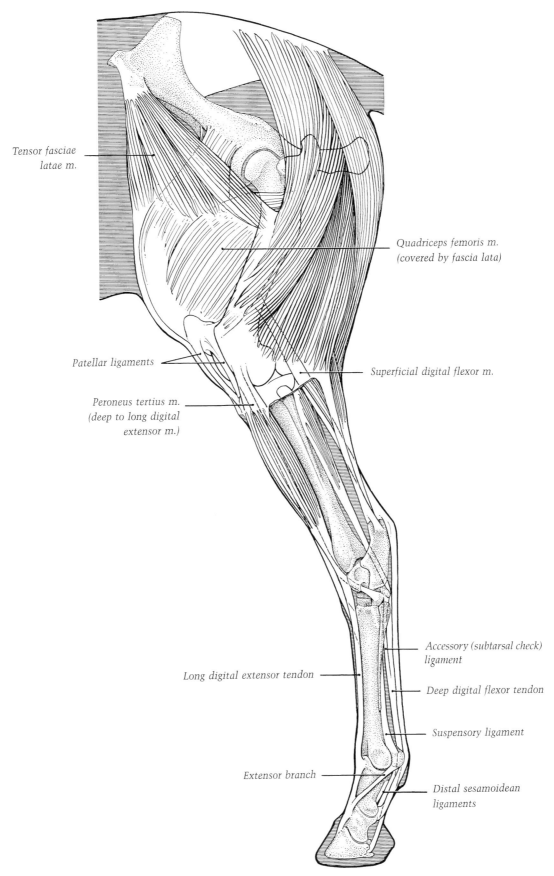

Tensor fasciae
latae m.

Quadriceps femoris m.
(covered by fascia lata)

Patellar ligaments

Superficial digital flexor m.

Peroneus tertius m.
(deep to long digital
extensor m.)

Accessory (subtarsal check)
ligament

Long digital extensor tendon

Deep digital flexor tendon

Suspensory ligament

Extensor branch

Distal sesamoidean
ligaments

Figure 1.52. Stay apparatus of the pelvic limb.

Table 1.1. Ranges of growth plate (physeal) closure times in equine thoracic limbs.[17]

Scapula	
Proximal	36+ months
Distal	9–18 months
Humerus	
Proximal	26–42 months
Distal	11–34 months
Radius	
Proximal	11–25 months
Distal	22–42 months
Ulna	
Proximal	27–42 months
Distal	2–12 months (some up to 4 years)
Third metacarpal bone	
Proximal	Before birth
Distal	6–18 months
Proximal phalanx	
Proximal	6–15 months
Distal	Before birth to 1 month
Middle phalanx	
Proximal	6–15 months
Distal	Before birth to 1 week
Distal phalanx	
Proximal	Before birth

Table 1.2. Ranges of growth plate (physeal) closure times in equine pelvic limbs.[17]

Ilium, ischium, pubis	10–12 months
Secondary centers for crest, tuber coxae, ischiatic tuber, and acetabular parts of pubis	4.5–5 years
Femur	
Proximal	36–42 months
Distal	22–42 months
Tibia	
Proximal	36–42 months
Distal	17–24 months
Fibula	
Proximal	3.5 years
Distal (lateral malleolus of tibia)	3–24 months (some up to 4 years)
Calcaneus	19–36 months

(Growth plate closure times for bones distal to tarsus are similar to those distal to carpus.)

accessory (tarsal check) ligament of the deep digital flexor tendon from the thick plantar part of the tarsal fibrous joint capsule. Prevention of overextension of the fetlock joint during the fixed, resting position is accomplished through the support rendered by the digital flexor tendons and the suspensory apparatus (suspensory ligament, proximal sesamoid bones, and their ligaments).

Growth Plate (Physeal) Closure

Several investigators have reported on closure times for the growth plates (physes or epiphyseal cartilages) of the bones in equine limbs.[16] Tables 1.1 and 1.2 summarize the ranges of reported closure times based on examination of radiographs and gross and microscopic specimens.

AXIAL COMPONENTS

Vertebral Column

The vertebral formula of the horse is 7 cervical, 18 thoracic, 6 lumbar, 5 sacral, and an inconsistent number of caudal vertebrae (ranging from 15 to 21). There is some individual variation in numbers of other vertebrae, most commonly in the number of lumbar vertebrae where 5 or 7 are sometimes seen (there is an increased incidence of 5 lumbar vertebrae in Arabian horses[48]). The typical vertebra possesses a ventrally placed, roughly cylindrical body whose cranial and caudal ends articulate with adjacent vertebrae at the intervertebral disc (Figure 1.53). A bony vertebral arch attaches to the body and surrounds the spinal cord. The aperture created within a given vertebrae by the dorsal aspect of the body and the medial and ventral parts of the arch is the vertebral foramen; where vertebral foramina of adjacent vertebrae are aligned to admit the spinal cord, the resulting passageway is called the vertebral canal. The vertebral canal is widest in the caudal cervical-cranial thoracic region, where it accommodates the cervical enlargement of the spinal cord. A second dilation of the canal occurs in the lumbar region where the lumbosacral enlargement of the cord resides.

The vertebral arch comprises the pedicles and laminae, which together create the "roof" over the spinal cord. The pedicles are the vertical bony attachments to the vertebral body. The dorsal part of the arch is created by the right and left laminae. The pedicles are characterized by vertebral notches, indentations on the cranial and caudal aspects of the pedicle. When individual vertebrae are articulated, the cranial vertebral notch of one vertebra abuts the caudal vertebral notch of another, creating an intervertebral foramen through which the spinal nerve emerges from the vertebral canal.

The vertebral arch features other bony processes that bear synovial joints between adjacent vertebrae and which serve as sites of attachment for epaxial muscles. Each vertebra has a single dorsal midline spinous process and two transverse processes that arise near the point at which the pedicle attaches to the body. The dorsal contour of the equine thorax and loin is largely determined by the relative size and prominence of the spinous processes of thoracic and lumbar vertebrae. Arising adjacent to the spinous process are a pair of cranial articular processes and a pair of caudal articular processes.

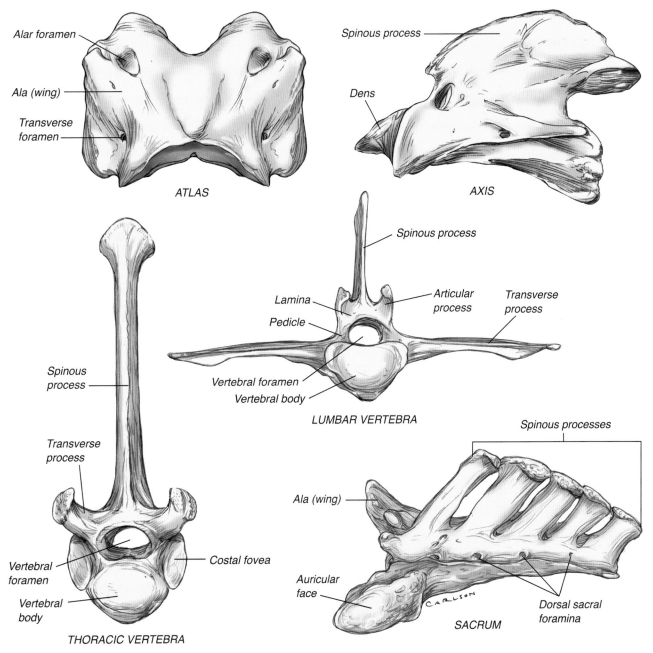

Figure 1.53. Vertebrae.

Cervical Vertebrae

The first 2 cervical vertebrae are highly modified to meet their specialized function in permitting movement of the head. The first vertebra is the atlas. It lacks the cylindrical body characteristic of other vertebrae, instead taking the form of a bony ring comprising dorsal and ventral arches. The spinous process is likewise absent. The transverse processes are modified into the wings of the atlas. These are robust, bent in a ventrolateral direction, and strongly concave ventrally. Their craniolateral edges form a prominent palpable ridge caudal to the ramus of the mandible. The dorsal

aspect of the wing of the atlas bears 3 foramina: the transverse foramen, the alar foramen, and the lateral vertebral foramen. The cranial aspect of the atlas possesses 2 deeply concave cranial articular foveae which form a synovial joint (the atlantooccipital joint) with the occipital condyles. The caudal articular foveae are also concave and participate in the synovial atlantoaxial joint.

The second cervical vertebra is the axis. The body of the axis is long. Its cranial extremity is modified into a scoop-like projection called the dens, which features a rounded ventral articular surface that articulates with the floor of the atlas. The caudal extremity of the axis' body is deeply concave where it articulates with the body of the third cervical vertebra. The spinous process of the axis is tall and long, modified into a thick midline sail. The transverse processes are small and caudally directed.

The third through seventh vertebrae are similar to one another and follow the basic pattern of most vertebrae. They are progressively shorter from cranial to caudal. Cervical vertebrae 3, 4, and 5 bear a distinct ventral crest on their bodies. This crest is diminished in size on the sixth and absent from the seventh cervical vertebra. Articular processes on these cervical vertebrae are large, with prominent oval fovea for articulation between vertebral arches. The cranial articular processes present their foveae in the dorsomedial direction; caudal articular processes have complementary foveae directed in the ventrolateral direction. Transverse processes are broad, each with 2 thick tubercles for muscular attachment. Transverse processes of the sixth cervical vertebra are especially robust, while those of the seventh are somewhat diminished relative to the other cervical vertebrae. The dorsocaudal aspect of the seventh cervical body features a costal fovea which participates in the synovial articulation of the head of the first rib with the seventh cervical and first thoracic vertebrae. The spinous process of the seventh cervical vertebra is tall compared to other cervical vertebrae.

Thoracic Vertebrae

There are usually 18 thoracic vertebrae in the horse, although on occasion there may be one more or one less than typical. The bodies of the thoracic vertebrae tend to be short with a small vertebral arch dorsally. The spinous processes are relatively tall, with the first 4 or 5 increasing in height and more caudal spinous processes gradually decreasing in height until at the level of the 12th thoracic vertebra, after which they are the same height as those of the lumbar vertebrae. The tall spinous processes of those first 12 vertebrae constitute the withers. The dorsal apex of the spines is somewhat expanded and in young horses surmounted by cartilage. The cartilage is replaced by bone as the horse ages, with the cartilages associated with the prominence of the withers persisting the longest at 10 years or more. The anticlinal vertebra is defined as the one whose spinous process is perpendicular to the long axis of the vertebral column. The spinous processes of more cranial vertebrae incline caudad, while those of more caudal vertebrae incline craniad. In the horse, the anticlinal vertebra is usually the 16th, and occasionally the 14th.

The vertebral bodies possess cranial and caudal costal foveae for articulation with the heads of ribs, excepting the last thoracic vertebra which features only cranial costal foveae. Transverse processes are irregular, largest in the cranial thoracic vertebrae and gradually decreasing in size toward the lumbar region. Mammillary processes appear in the caudal thoracic region. These are directed craniad and arise primarily from the transverse processes. In the most caudal of the thoracic vertebrae, they arise in common from the transverse and cranial articular processes and may for this reason be called mamilloarticular processes.

Lumbar Vertebrae

There are usually 6 lumbar vertebrae, although 5 and 7 have also been reported. The cylindrical bodies of the lumbar vertebrae are somewhat flattened dorsoventrally, especially the last 3; except for the seventh and sometimes the sixth lumbar vertebrae, a ventral crest is prominent. The spinous processes project slightly craniad. The vertebral arches tend to overlap dorsally, except at the L5-to-L6 and L6-to-S1 interspaces where the larger interarcuate spaces are much larger and clinically accessible. The cranial and caudal articular processes articulate in an approximation of the sagittal plane, an orientation which allows for a very slight degree of flexion and extension of the vertebral column but prevents lateral flexion. The transverse processes of the lumbar vertebrae are large and blade-like. They project laterad. The caudal aspect of the fifth transverse process articulates with the cranial aspect of the sixth. The caudal aspect of the sixth transverse process features a large concave facet through which it articulates with the sacrum.

Sacrum

The equine sacrum is a single bone formed through fusion of embryologically distinct sacral vertebrae, generally 5 of these, with 4, 6, and 7 sacral vertebrae also being reported.[48] Fusion is usually complete by 5 years of age. The sacrum is triangular and gently curving so as to present a slightly concave ventral aspect. Intervertebral foramina are transformed by the fusion of adjacent vertebrae into a row of 4 dorsal sacral foramina and 4 ventral sacral foramina, through which pass dorsal and ventral branches, respectively, of the sacral spinal nerves. The spinous processes remain individually distinct and incline slightly caudad, and the second through fifth end in slight enlargements that are not uncommonly bifid.

The first sacral vertebra gives rise to the wings of the sacrum. Their articular surfaces face dorsolateral to articulate with the auricular surface of the ilium. The ventral aspect of the first sacral vertebra is slightly rounded, forming the promontory of the sacrum, the point from which the conjugate diameter of the pelvis is measured.

Caudal Vertebrae

Although there is considerable individual variation, the average horse has 18 caudal vertebrae. Only the first 3 or so have vertebral arches, the remaining being represented by cylindrical bodies only. The first caudal vertebra is not uncommonly fused with the sacrum, especially in old horses.

Vertebral Articulations

Excluding the atlantoaxial joint (a pivot joint), the joints of the vertebral column all permit flexion, extension, lateral flexion, and limited rotation. These movements are fairly limited through thoracic and lumbar regions, but the cervical vertebral column is capable of extensive movement. Intervertebral discs of fibrocartilage are interposed between adjacent vertebral bodies. Further stabilization is provided to the vertebral column by (1) the continuous dorsal and ventral longitudinal ligaments on their respective surfaces of the vertebral bodies; (2) a supraspinous ligament that passes along the dorsal aspect of the spinous processes of thoracic, lumbar, and sacral vertebrae; and (3) interspinal ligaments that pass between adjacent spinous processes. In the thoracic region, intercapital ligaments pass transversely between the heads of contralateral ribs over the dorsal aspects of the intervertebral disks. Articulations between articular processes on vertebral arches are true synovial joints. In the cervical region, these constitute broad plates, oriented in a nearly horizontal plane to permit significant lateral bending. Articular facets on the cranial articular processes face dorsomediad while the complementary facets on the caudal articular processes face ventrolaterad. True joints also exist between the transverse processes of the fifth and sixth lumbar vertebrae and between the transverse processes of the sixth lumbar vertebra and the wings of the sacrum.

Sacroiliac Region

The axial skeleton and appendicular skeleton of the hindlimb are united at the sacroiliac joint (Figure 1.54).

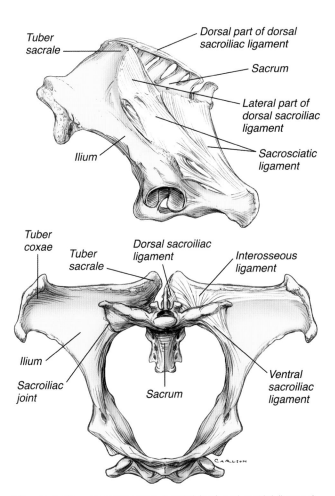

Figure 1.54. Sacroiliac joint. Lateral (top) and cranial (bottom) views.

This planar joint is created by the auricular face of the wings of the sacrum, which face dorsolaterad, and the auricular face of the wings of the ilia, which face ventromediad. This joint is histologically synovial, but is capable of only extremely limited gliding movement. Its principle purpose is probably therefore absorption of some of the concussive forces transmitted through the appendicular skeleton to the vertebral column. The joint capsule is close-fitting and is substantially reinforced by a series of sacroiliac ligaments that contribute markedly to the overall stability of the joint and probably act to transfer most of the weight of the trunk to the pelvic limbs. These ligaments can be summarized as comprising the ventral sacroiliac ligament, dorsal sacroiliac ligament, and interosseous ligament.

The ventral sacroiliac ligament surrounds the joint and fills the space between the ilium and the wing of the sacrum. The dorsal sacroiliac ligament presents two distinct portions. One arises from tuber sacrale and inserts on the spinous processes of the sacral vertebrae. The other, a more laterally placed sheet, arises from tuber sacrale and the caudal edge of the ilial wing and inserts along the lateral aspect of the sacrum. From here it blends ventrad into the broad sacrosciatic ligament that fills the space between the pelvis and sacrum. The interosseous ligament consists of strong, vertically oriented fibers between the ventral part of the wing of the ilium and the dorsal aspect of the wing of the sacrum.

Ligamentum Nuchae

The topline of the neck is in part determined by the presence of the ligamentum nuchae (nuchal ligament) which in horses extends from its cranial attachments on the external occipital protuberance to the spinous process of the third or fourth thoracic vertebra. Both parts of the nuchal ligament (funicular and laminar) are paired. The rope-like funicular part is connected to sheets which compose the laminar portions. These midline elastic sheets arise from the second through seventh cervical vertebrae and insert on the spines of the second and third thoracic vertebrae. Bursae are consistently found between the funicular part of the nuchal ligament and the atlas and between the nuchal ligament and the second thoracic spine. These are the bursa subligamentosa nuchalis cranialis and the bursa subligamentosa supraspinalis, respectively. A third bursa (bursa subligamentosa nuchalis caudalis) is inconsistently found between the nuchal ligament and the spine of the axis.[13,17]

Muscles of the Trunk and Neck

Muscles of the torso (neck, trunk, and tail) are roughly divided into those dorsal to the transverse processes (i.e., epaxial muscles) and those ventral to the transverse processes (i.e., hypaxial muscles). The epaxial muscles are innervated by dorsal branches of the spinal nerves while hypaxial muscles receive their innervation from ventral branches.

The epaxial muscles are extensors of the vertebral column and are roughly divided into 3 parallel bundles of fascicles: from lateral to medial these are the iliocostalis system, the longissimus system, and the

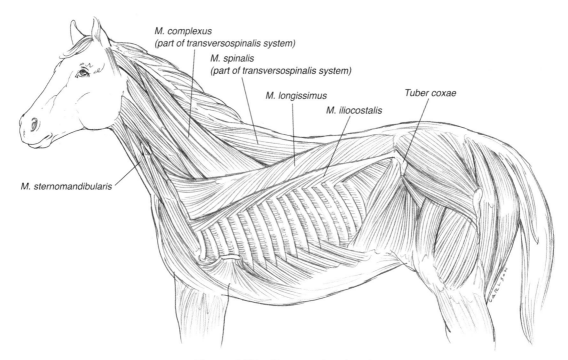

Figure 1.55. Deep muscles of trunk.

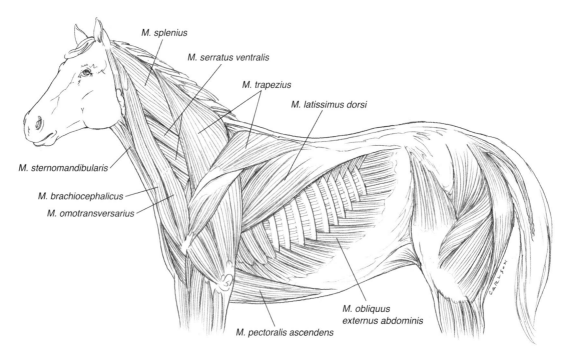

Figure 1.56. Superficial muscles of trunk. Cutaneous muscles have been removed.

transversospinalis system (Figure 1.55). The iliocostalis system (named for its attachments to the ilium and ribs) does not extend into the neck. The others continue into the cervical region and are associated with additional distinct muscles. Of these, the splenius muscle is most superficial (Figure 1.56). The splenius possesses capital and cervical parts. Both arise from the third, fourth, and fifth thoracic spines and from the funicular part of the nuchal ligament, and they insert on the nuchal crest of

the skull, the wing of the atlas, and the transverse processes of the third, fourth, and fifth cervical vertebrae. The splenius extends the neck and elevates the head, and it is largely the rhythmic contraction of this powerful muscle that creates the thrusting movements of the neck during the gallop.[30]

The longissimus group is described as having lumbar, thoracic, cervical, atlantal, and capital portions. It is most robust in the lumbar region, where it gives a well-conditioned horse's back its typical rounded appearance.

Hypaxial muscles of the trunk (the psoas minor, quadratus lumborum, and the 4 abdominal muscles on each side) act to flex the vertebral column during the gallop. Epaxial muscles extend the vertebral column. When they contract unilaterally, both hypaxial and epaxial muscles create lateral movement of the trunk and neck.

In the ventral neck, the equine m. longus colli is particularly well developed relative to other domestic species. The cervical portion of this muscle arises from the transverse processes and bodies of the third through sixth cervical vertebrae in paired bundles that converge to an insertion on the preceding vertebral bodies, sometimes bridging more than one intervertebral space. The most cranial attachment is on the ventral aspect of the atlas. The thoracic portion of the longus colli arises on the lateral vertebral bodies of thoracic vertebrae 1 through 6, passing craniad to insert on the transverse processes of cervical vertebrae 6 and 7.

The omohyoideus muscle is well-developed in the horse. It arises from an aponeurosis in the fascia near the shoulder joint. Its muscle belly is closely attached to the deep side of the brachiocephalicus until the neck's midpoint, where the omohyoideus becomes evident as a distinct muscle as it passes craniad deep to the sternocephalicus muscle. Near its insertion on the lingual process, it fuses with its partner from the contralateral side and with the sternohyoideus.

The right and left sternomandibularis muscles of the horse are fused on midline near their origin on the manubrium. Near mid-neck, the 2 halves separate, moving from their position ventral to the trachea to a more lateral location. As the muscle approaches its insertion on the sternomandibular tuberosity on the ramus of the mandible, it narrows to a distinct tendon that is visible in the cranial neck just caudal to the caudal border of the mandible. The tendon of insertion is classically considered one side of Viborg's triangle.

References

1. Balch O, White K, Butler D. Factors involved in the balancing of equine hooves. J Am Vet Med Assoc 1991;198:1980.
2. Banks WJ. Applied Veterinary Histology. 3rd ed. St. Louis, MO, Mosby-Yearbook, Inc. 1993.
3. Bertram JEM, Gosline JM. Fracture toughness design in horse hoof. J Exper Biol 1986;125:29.
4. Bertram JEA, Gosline JM. Functional design of horse hoof keratin: The modulation of mechanical properties through hydration effects. J Exper Biol 1987;130:121.
5. Blythe LL, Kitchell RL. Electrophysiologic studies of the thoracic limb of the horse. Am J Vet Res 1982;43:1511.
6. Bowker RM, Linder K, Van Wulfen KK, et al. An anatomical study of the distal interphalangeal joint in the horse: Its relationship to the navicular suspensory ligaments, sensory nerves and neurovascular bundle. Eq Vet J 1997;29:126.
7. Bowker RM, Rockershouser SJ, Vex KB, et al. Immunocytochemical and dye distribution studies of nerves potentially desensitized by injections into the distal interphalangeal joint or navicular bursa of horses. J Am Vet Med Assoc 1993;203:1708.
8. Bowker RM, Van Wulfen KK. Microanatomy of the intersection of the distal sesamoidean impar ligament and the deep digital flexor tendon: A preliminary report. Pferdheilkunde 1996;12:623.
9. Colles CM, Garner HE, Coffman JR. The blood supply of the horse's foot. Proc Am Assoc Equine Pract 1979;385.
10. Colles CM, Hickman J. The arterial supply of the navicular bone and its variation in navicular disease. Eq Vet J 1977;9:150.
11. Denoix JM. Functional anatomy of tendons and ligaments in the distal limbs (manus and pes). Vet Clinics of North Am 1994;10:273.
12. Derksen FG. Diagnostic local anesthesia of the equine front limb. Equine Pract 1980;2–41.
13. Dyce KM, Sack WO, Wensing CJG. Textbook of Veterinary Anatomy. Philadelphia, Elsevier Science. 2002.
14. Emery L, Miller J, Van Hoosen N. Horseshoeing Theory and Foot Care. Philadelphia, Lea and Febiger, 1977.
15. Ernst RR. Die Bedeutung der Wandepidermis (Hyponychium) des Pferdehufes fur die Hornbildung, Acta Anat 1954;22:15.
16. Garret PD. Anatomy of the dorsoscapular ligament of horses. J Am Vet Med Assoc 1990;196:446.
17. Getty R. Sisson and Grossman's The Anatomy of the Domestic Animals, 5th ed. Vol 1. Philadelphia, WB Saunders Co., 1975.
18. Goetz TE. Anatomic, hoof and shoeing considerations for the treatment of laminitis in horses. J Am Vet Med Assoc 1987;190:1323.
19. Grau H. Die Hautinnervation an den Gliedmassen des Pferdes. Arch Wschr Prakt Tierheilk 1935;69:96.
20. Grosenbaugh DA, Hood DM. Practical equine hoof wall biochemistry. Eq Pract 1993;15:8.
21. James PT, Kemler AG, Smallwood JE. The arterial supply to the distal sesamoid bones of the equine thoracic and pelvic limbs. J Vert Orthoped 1983;2:38.
22. Koch T. Die nervenversorgung der Hinterzehe des Pferdes Berl Munch Tierarztl Wsch 1939;28:440.
23. Koch T. Uber die Nervenversorgung der Gliedmassenspitzen des Pferdes. Tierraztl. Rundschau 1938;44:333.
24. Krolling O, Grau H. Lehrbuch der Histologie und vergleichenden mikroskopischen Anatomie der Haustiere, 10th ed., Berlin, P. Parey, 1960.
25. Landeau LJ, Barnett DJ, Batterman SC. Mechanical properties of equine hooves. Am J Vet Res 1983;44:100.
26. Leach D. Biomechanical considerations in raising and lowering the heel. Proc Am Assoc Equine Pract 1983;33.
27. Leach DH, Oliphant LW. Ultrastructure of equine hoof wall secondary epidermal lamellae. Am J Vet Res 1983;44:1561.
28. Mettam AE. On the development and histology of (1) the hoof wall and subjacent soft structures of the horse's foot, and (2) the structure of the frog, with a description of the sweat glands and some nerve-endings found therein. The Veterinarian 1896; 69:85.
29. Mishra PC, Leach DH. Extrinsic and intrinsic veins of the equine hoof wall. J Anat 1983;136:543.
30. Nickel R, Schummer A, Seiferle E, et al. The locomotor system of the domestic mammals. In: The anatomy of the domestic animals. New York, Springer-Verlag. 1986.
31. Nilsson SA. Bidrag till kannedomen om fotens innervation hos hast. (Engl. summary), Skandinavisk Veterinar-Tidskrift 1948; 38:401.
32. Nomina Anatomica Veterinaria: World Association of Vet Anatomists. 5th ed., 2005.
33. Ottaway CA, Worden AN. Bursae and tendon sheaths of the horse. Vet Rec 1940;52:477.
34. Pohlmeyer K, Redecker R. Die fur die Klinik bedeutsamen Nerven an dem Gliedemassen des Pferdes einschliesslich moglicher Varianten. Deutsche Tieraztl. Wschr 1974;81:5001.
35. Pollitt CC, Molyneux GS. A scanning electron microscopical study of the dermal microcirculation of the equine foot. Equine Vet J 1990;22:79.
36. Preuss F, Eggers H. Zur Radialislhahmung des Pferdes. Tierarztliche Umschau 1951;6:435.
37. Reeves MJ, Trotter GW, Kainer RA. Anatomical and functional communications between synovial sacs of the equine stifle joint. Eq Vet J 1991;23:215.
38. Rooney JR, Quddus MA, Kingsbury HB. A laboratory investigation of the function of the stay apparatus of the equine foreleg. J Em Med Surg 1978;2:173.
39. Sack WO. Subtendinous bursa on the medial aspect of the equine carpus. J Am Vet Med Assoc 1976;165:315.
40. Sack WO. Nerve distribution in the metacarpus and front digit of the horse. J Am Vet Med Assoc 1975;167:298.
41. Sack WO, Habel RE. Rooney's Guide to the Dissection of the Horse. Ithaca, NY. Veterinary Textbooks, 1977.
42. Sack WO, Orsini PG. Distal intertarsal and tarsometatarsal joints in the horse: Communication and injection sites. J Am Vet Med Assoc 1981;179:3555.

43. Schummer A, Wilkens H, Vollmerhaus B, et al. Schummer and Seiferle's The Anatomy of the Domestic Animals. Vol 3, New York, Heidelberg, Berlin, Springer-Verlag, 1981.

44. Schuurman SO, Kersten W, Weijs WA. The equine hind limb is actively stabilized during standing. J Anat 2003;202:355–62.

45. Smallwood JE. A Guided Tour of Veterinary Anatomy. Philadelphia, WB Saunders Co, 1992.

46. Smith F. A Manual of Veterinary Physiology. 4th ed., London, Bailliere, Tindall and Cox, 1912.

47. Southwood LL, Stashak TS, Kainer RA. Tenoscopic anatomy of the equine carpal flexor synovial sheath. Vet Surg 1997;27:150–7.

48. Stecher RM. Anatomical variations of the spine in the horse. J Mam 1962;43:205.

49. Stump JE. Anatomy of the normal equine foot, including microscopic features of the laminar region. J Am Vet Med Assoc 1967;151:1588.

50. Talukdar AJ, Calhoun ML, Stinson AW. Sweat glands of the horse: A histologic study. Am J Vet Res 1970;31:2179.

51. Updike SJ. Functional anatomy of the equine tarsocrural collateral ligaments. Am J Vet Res 1984;45:867.

52. Weaver JC, Stover SM, O'Brien TR. Radiographic anatomy of soft tissue attachments in the equine metacarpophalangeal and proximal phalangeal region. Equine Vet J 1992;24:310.

53. Wilson DA, Baker GJ, Pijanowski GJ, et al. Composition and morphologic features of the interosseous muscle in Standardbreds and Thoroughbreds. Am J Vet Res 1991;52:133.

54. Wright C. Unpublished data, 1983.

Conformation and Movement

GARY M. BAXTER, TED S. STASHAK, AND CHERRY HILL

To develop an appreciation of lameness and gait defects, it is important to have an understanding of conformation and movement. While many lameness problems occur in the lower limbs, the causative factors may be located in the upper limbs or body; therefore, overall conformation should be considered. Certain conformation traits can predispose to lameness and these should be eliminated through responsible breeding. Understanding the relationship between conformation, movement, and lameness is essential for making wise breeding decisions and devising sound management and training programs. However, breed conformational traits can differ and many conformational traits are not always related to performance and soundness.[24,30] Furthermore, conformation is often a subjective assessment based on what a particular breed may consider to be "ideal." Objective techniques to quantify conformation have been developed and are currently being used especially in Europe.[24,29,30] Although a list of quantified conformational features of horses for sale or stallions at stud may be desirable, it seems unlikely to completely replace subjective conformational assessment and the art of selection.[10]

CONFORMATION

Conformation refers to the physical appearance and outline of a horse as dictated primarily by bone and muscle structures.[24,29] It is impractical to set a single standard of perfection or to specifically define *ideal* or *normal* conformation because the guidelines depend on the classification, type, breed, and intended use of the horse.[29,30] Therefore, conformation evaluation should relate to function,[8,9] but objective studies relating conformational traits to performance or lameness problems can be difficult to perform.[24]

When conformational discrepancies are identified, it is important to differentiate between "blemishes" and "unsoundnesses." Blemishes are scars and irregularities

that do not affect the serviceability of the horse. Unsoundnesses cause a horse to be lame, limit performance, or be otherwise unserviceable.[36] Superficial scars from old wire cuts, non-painful swellings or enlargements, and white spots from old injuries are considered blemishes if they do not affect the horse's soundness.

TYPES AND BREEDS

Horses are classified as draft horses, light horses, or ponies. Classifications are further divided by type according to overall body style and conformation and the work for which the horse is best suited. Light (riding and driving) horses can be described as one of six types: pleasure horse, hunter, stock horse, sport horse, animated (show) horse, and race horse.

Pleasure horses have comfortable gaits, are conformed (designed) for ease of riding, and are typified by smooth movement in any breed. Hunters move with a long, low (horizontal) stride, are suited to cross-country riding and negotiating hunter fences, and are typified by the American Thoroughbred. Stock horses are well muscled, agile, and quick; are suited to working cattle; and are typified by the American Quarter horse. The sport horse can be one of two types: a large, athletic horse suited for one or all of the disciplines of eventing (dressage, cross-country, and jumping) and typified by the European Warmbloods, or a small, lean, tough horse suited for endurance events and typified by the Arabian. The animated or gaited horse is one with highly cadenced, flashy gaits (usually with a high degree of flexion), often suited for the show ring, and is typified by the American Saddlebred and Tennessee Walking horse. The race horse is lean in relation to height with a deep but not round barrel and is typified by the racing Thoroughbred.

A "breed" is a group of horses with common ancestry and usually strong conformational similarities. In most cases, a horse must come from approved breeding stock to be registered with a particular breed. If a horse is not eligible for registration, it is considered to be a "grade" or "crossbred" horse. Several breeds can have similar makeup and be of the same type. For example,

Adams and Stashak's Lameness in Horses, 6e, edited by Gary M. Baxter
© 2011 Blackwell Publishing, Ltd.

most Quarter horses, Paint horses, and Appaloosas are considered to be stock horse types. In addition, racing Quarter horses often have considerable Thoroughbred background. Some breeds contain individuals of different types within the breed; Thoroughbreds can be of the race, hunter, or sport horse type.

METHOD OF EVALUATION

Although breed characteristics may vary, the process of evaluating any horse should be similar. A general systematic assessment of the horse's four functional sections is made (head and neck, forelimbs, trunk, and hindlimbs), giving each area approximately equal importance (Figure 2.1).[36] The horse's specific conformational components or traits are then evaluated in detail.

Systematic Evaluation of Conformation

The evaluation begins by viewing the horse from the near (left) side in profile and assessing balance by comparing the forehand (head, neck, and forelimbs) to the hindquarters (hindlimbs and croup). Attention should be paid to the curvature and proportions of the top line, and observations made from poll to tail and down to the gaskin. The attachment of the appendicular skeleton (limbs) to the axial skeleton (head and trunk) should be observed with emphasis placed on limb angles. There is a strong relationship between long bone lengths and wither heights at differing ages, suggesting that horses should be proportional regardless of their size.[1]

From the front of the horse, the limbs and hooves are evaluated for straightness and symmetry. The depth and length of the muscles in the forearm and chest are observed. The head, eyes, nostrils, ears, and teeth are

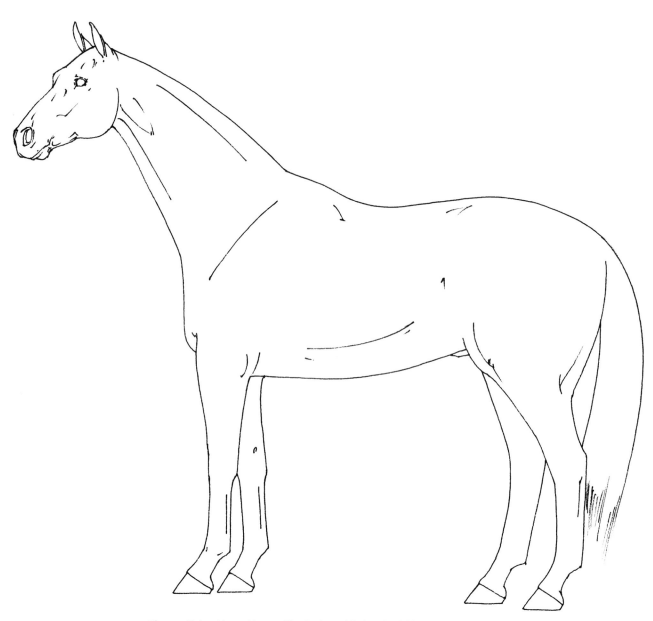

Figure 2.1. Normal horse. The body and limbs should be well proportioned.

also evaluated. Evaluation of balance, top line, and limb angles is confirmed by viewing the off (right) side of the horse.

From directly behind the tail, the hindquarters; the straightness and symmetry of the back, croup, point of the hip, and buttock; and the limbs are evaluated. Observation should be made slowly from the poll to the tail because this is the best vantage point for evaluating back muscling, alignment of the vertebral column, and (provided the horse is standing square) left-to-right symmetry. The spring (width and curve) of rib is also best observed from the rear.

The observer should then make another entire circle around the horse, this time stopping at each quadrant to look diagonally across the center of the horse. From the rear of the horse, the observer should look from the left hindlimb toward the right forelimb, and from the right hindlimb toward the left forelimb. This angle will often reveal abnormalities in the limbs and hooves that were missed during the side, front, and rear examinations. The horse is then viewed from the front in a similar diagonal approach. While observing the horse, it is helpful to obtain an overall sense of correctness of each of the four functional sections: head/neck, forelimbs, trunk (barrel), and hindlimbs.

Head and Neck

The vital senses are located in the head, so it should be correct and functional. The size or shape of the head is often breed-specific, but does not appear to influence performance or lameness. The neck acts as a lever to help regulate the horse's balance while moving; therefore, it should be long and flexible with a slight convex curve to its top line.[8,9,24] Jumping horses have been found to benefit from longer necks, probably because they make it easier to maintain balance over the fence.[24]

Forelimbs

Kinematic studies have confirmed that at the beginning of the stance phase, the distal portion of the forelimb is subjected to more stress from weight-bearing forces than the distal portion of the hindlimb.[6] The forelimbs tend to "bounce," whereas the hindlimbs "slide".[24] The forelimbs are considered to support approximately 60% to 65% of the horse's body weight, so they should be well muscled and conformed normally.[9,36]

Trunk (Barrel)

The horse should have adequate heart girth and width (spring) to the ribs to house the vital organs. The back should be well muscled and strong so that the horse is able to carry the weight of its internal organs, and the rider and saddle.

Hindlimbs

The hindlimbs are the source of power for propulsion and stopping.[36] The hindlimb muscling should be appropriate for the type, breed, and use of the horse. The croup and points of the hip and buttock should be symmetrical, and the limbs should be straight and sound.

CONFORMATION COMPONENTS AND TRAITS

Balance

Balance refers to the relationship between the forehand and hindquarters, between the limbs and the body, and between the right and the left sides of the body (Figures 2.1 to 2.3). It is a subjective assessment based on the overall conformation of the horse. A well-balanced horse is thought to move more efficiently, thereby experiencing less stress on the musculoskeletal system.

The center of gravity is a theoretical point in the horse's body around which the mass of the horse is equally distributed. It is located at a point of intersection of a vertical line dropped from the highest point of the withers and a line from the point of the shoulder to the point of the buttock. The center of gravity is usually just behind the xyphoid and two-thirds the distance down from the top line of the back.[36] (Figure 2.3).

Although the center of gravity remains relatively constant when a well-balanced horse moves, most horses must learn to rebalance their weight (and that of the rider and tack) when ridden. To pick up a front foot to step forward, the horse must shift its weight toward the rear. The amount of this weight shift depends on the horse's conformation, the position of the rider, the gait, the degree of collection, and the style of the performance. The higher the degree of collection, the more the horse must step under the center of gravity with the hindlimbs.

If the forehand is proportionately larger than the hindquarters, particularly if it is associated with a downhill top line, the center of gravity tends to shift forward. This causes the horse to travel heavy on his front end, setting the stage for increased concussion, stress, and lameness. When the forehand and hindquarters are balanced and the withers are level with or higher than the level of the croup, the horse's center of gravity is located more toward the rear. Such a horse can carry more weight with his hindquarters, thus moving in balance and exhibiting a lighter, freer motion with the forehand than the horse with withers lower than the croup. However, hip height was consistently 2 to 3 cm greater than wither height in young growing thoroughbreds suggesting that level top lines may only develop with maturity, if at all.[37] Even with a level top line, if the forehand is heavily muscled in comparison to the hindquarters, the horse may travel heavy on the forehand.

A balanced horse has approximately equal lower limb length and depth of body. The lower limb length (chest floor to the ground) should be equal to the distance from the chest floor to the top of the withers (Figure 2.3). Proportionately shorter lower limbs are associated with a choppy stride. The horse's height or overall limb length (point of the withers to the ground) should approximate the length of the horse's body (the point of the shoulder to the point of the buttock) (Figure 2.3). A horse with a longer body than its height often experiences difficulty in synchronization

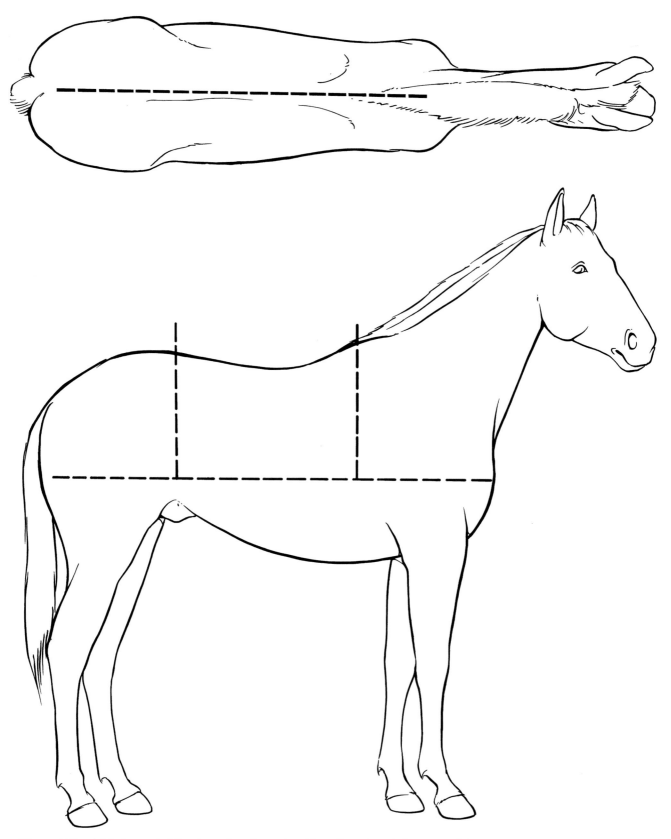

Figure 2.2. Axial alignment. A line drawn from the center of the withers through the center of the back should roughly divide the body into two equal halves. Bottom. Balance is evaluated by dividing the body into three equal parts.

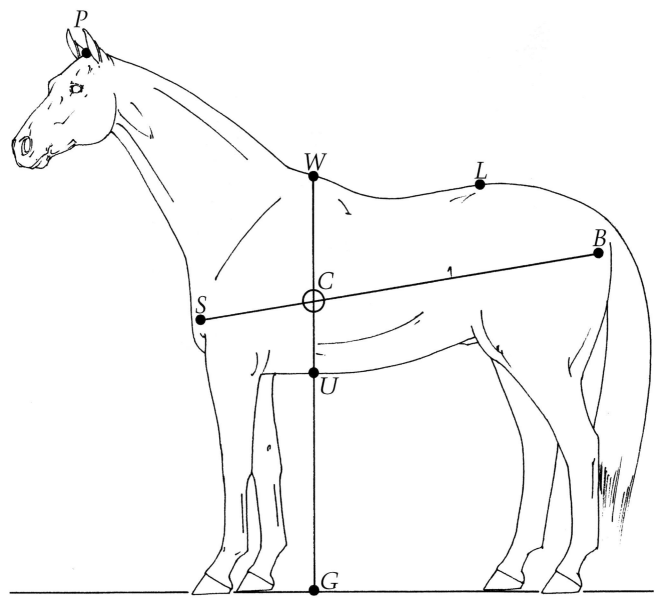

Figure 2.3. Proportions. P = poll, W = highest point of withers, L = caudal loin, B = point of buttock, S = point of shoulder, C = center of gravity, U = underline, G = ground, WU = depth of body, UG = lower limb length, WG = height and overall limb length, SB = length of body, PW = length of neck, WL = length of back, LB = length of hip. (Reprinted with permission from Hill, C., Klimesh R. Horse Hoof Care. Storey Publishing. North Adams, MA, 2009.)

and coordination of movement. A horse with limbs proportionately longer than the body may be predisposed to forging, over-reaching, and other gait defects. Overall, the right side of the horse should be symmetrical with the left side.

Proportions and Curvature of the Top Line

The ratio of the top line's components, curvature of the top line, strength of loin (longissimus dorsi muscles in the lumbar region), sharpness of withers, slope to the croup, and length of the underline in relation to the length of back all affect a horse's movement (Figures 2.2 and 2.3).[36]

The neck is measured from the poll to the highest point of the withers (Figure 2.3). The back measure-

ment is taken from the withers to the caudal extent of the loin located in front of the pelvis. The hip length is measured from the caudal loin to the point of the buttock (Figure 2.3).

A neck that is shorter than the back tends to decrease a horse's overall flexibility and balance. A back that is much longer than the neck tends to hollow (flex down or is more concave). A very short hip, in relation to the neck or back, is associated with lack of propulsion and often a downhill configuration. A general rule of thumb is that the neck length should be greater than or equal to the back length, and that the hip should be at least two-thirds the length of the back (Figure 2.3).

The shape of the neck is determined by the "S" shape formed by the seven cervical vertebrae. The neck should have a graceful shape that rises up out of the withers,

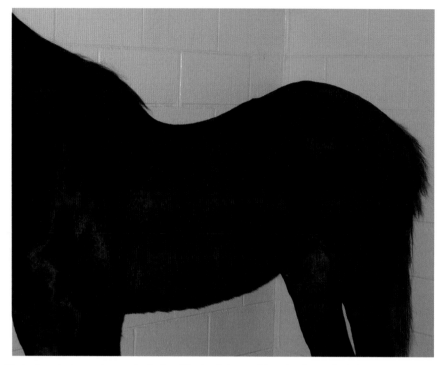

Figure 2.4. Marked ventral curvature or lordosis of the back is considered to be undesirable because it may predispose to back problems.

not dipping ventral (downward) in front of the withers. A longer, flatter (more horizontal) attachment of the upper cervical vertebrae (C1 to C2) at the poll is thought to result in a cleaner, more flexible throat latch. The attachment of the lower neck (caudal cervical region) should be short and shallow and should attach relatively high on the horse's chest. The thickest point in the neck should be at the ventral limits. Ewe-necked horses often have a long, ventral curve to the neck that appears to attach low on the chest. The attachment of the neck muscles to the shoulders should be smooth. Prominent depressions in the muscles in front of the shoulders are undesirable.

The dorsal (upper) neck length (poll to withers) should be twice the ventral (lower) neck length (throat latch to chest). This is dictated to a large degree by the slope of the shoulder. A horse with a steep shoulder has an undesirable ratio (approaching 1:1) between the dorsal and ventral neck lengths.[36]

The withers should blend gradually into the back, ending ideally at about the midpoint of the back. The back behind the withers should resemble a natural place for a saddle, beginning with prominent withers located above or behind the heart girth. The neck and forearm muscles and the ligamentum nuchae should attach at the highest point of the withers. There should not be a prominent dip in the muscles in front of or behind the withers (Figure 2.4). Low (mutton) withers limit a horse's ability to raise its back as it lowers and extends its neck. A horse with a well-sloped shoulder usually has correctly placed withers.

The longissimus muscles that run along the spine should be flat and appear strong rather than sloped and weak. The back muscles aid to counteract the gravitational pull from the weight of the horse's internal organs and to support the rider's weight.

The loin is located along the lumbar vertebrae from the last thoracic vertebrae to the lumbosacral junction (Figures 2.2 to 2.4). The loin should be well muscled and relatively short. Horses termed "long-backed" often have an acceptable back length but a long, weak loin. A horse with a weak and/or long loin and loose coupling (flanks) tends to have a hollow back. (The coupling is the area behind the ribs and in front of a vertical line dropped from the point of the hip). A horse that has a chronic hollow back may be predisposed to focal lumbar pain, pinched nerves, or vertebral damage.[36] In addition, kinematic studies have documented that even subtle hindlimb lameness can alter movement of the thoracolumbar region, potentially contributing to secondary musculoskeletal pain in the region.[19]

The loin and coupling transfer the motion of the hindquarters up through the back and forward to the forehand; therefore, they should be strong and well connected. A short, heavily muscled loin may have great strength, power, and durability but may lack the flexibility of a more moderately muscled loin. A lumpy appearance in the loin may indicate abnormal alignment (subluxations) of the vertebrae or damage to the supraspinous ligament.[36]

The croup is measured from the lumbosacral junction to the tail head. The croup should be fairly long, because this is associated with a good length to the hip and a desirable forward-placement of the lumbosacral articulation. The top line (the back) should be short in relation to the underline. Such a combination indicates strength plus desirable length of stride.

Head

The head should appear symmetrical and functional (Figure 2.1). The length from the ear to the eye should be at least one-third the distance from the ear to the nostril. The width between the eyes should be similar to that from the ear to the eye. A wide-open throat latch allows for an adequate airway during flexion; a narrow throat latch is often associated with a ewe-neck attachment. Large eyes located at the edge of the forehead enhance the arc of vision.[9] The eye should have a prominent bony orbit and the expression of the eye should indicate a quiet, tractable temperament.

The muzzle should be trim, but if too small, the nostrils may be pinched and there may be inadequate space for the incisor teeth, resulting in dental malalignments. The width of the cheek bones indicates the space for molar teeth; adequate room is required for sideways grinding of food. The shape of the nasal bone and forehead is largely a matter of breed preferences.

Quality

Quality is depicted by "flat" cannon (third metacarpal/metatarsal) bones, clean (lack of swelling) joints, sharply defined (refined) features, smooth muscling, overall blending of parts, and a fine, smooth hair coat. "Flat" bone is a misnomer because "flat" refers to well-defined tendons that stand out cleanly behind the cannon bone and give the impression, when viewed from the side, that the cannon bone is flat.

Substance

Thickness, depth, and breadth of bone, muscle, and other tissues are described as "substance." Muscle substance is described by the type, thickness, and length of the muscle, and the position of attachment. Other substance factors include weight of the horse, height of the horse, size of the hoofs, depth of the heart girth and flank, and spring of rib.

"Spring of rib," which is best viewed from the rear, refers to the curvature of the ribs. In addition to providing room for the heart, lungs, and digestive tract, a well-sprung rib cage provides a natural, comfortable place for a rider's legs. A slab-sided horse with a shallow heart girth is difficult to sit upon properly; an extremely wide-barreled horse can be stressful to the rider's legs.

"Substance of bone" refers to adequacy of the bone to the horse's weight ratio. Traditionally, the circumference around the cannon bone just below the carpus serves as the measurement for substance of bone. For riding horses, an adequate ratio is approximately 0.7 inches of bone for every 100 lbs. of body weight.[36] Using this rule, a 1,200-lb. horse should have an 8.4-inch cannon bone circumference.

Correctness of Angles and Structures

The correct alignment of the skeletal components provides the framework for muscular attachments. The length and slope to the shoulder, arm, forearm, croup, hip, stifle, and pasterns should be appropriate and work well together. There should be a straight alignment of bones when viewed from the front and rear, large clean joints, high-quality hoof horn, adequate height and width of heel, concave sole, and adequate hoof size.

Forelimbs

CRANIAL VIEW

Both forelimbs should be of equal length and size and should appear to bear equal weight when the horse is standing squarely. A line dropped from the point of the shoulder (middle of the scapulohumeral joint) to the ground should bisect the limb. The manner in which the shoulder blade and arm (humerus) are conformed and attach to the chest often dictates the alignment of the lower limb. Whether the toes point in or out is often related to upper limb structures, which is why it may be counterproductive to alter a limb's alignment through radical hoof adjustments. The toes should point forward and the width of the feet on the ground should be the same as the width at the origin of the limbs in the chest (Figure 2.5). The shoulder should be well muscled without being heavy and coarse.

The medial-lateral slope of the humerus is evaluated by finding the point of the shoulder and a spot in front of the point of the elbow on each side. The four points are then connected visually. If the resulting box is square, the humerus lies in an ideal position for straight lower limbs. If the bottom of the box is wider, the horse may toe-in and travel with loose elbows and paddle. If the bottom of the box is narrower, the horse will probably toe-out, have tight elbows, and wing in.

The muscles of the forearm (antebrachium) should extend to the knee, tapering gradually rather than ending abruptly a few inches above the knee. This is believed to allow the horse to use its front limbs in a

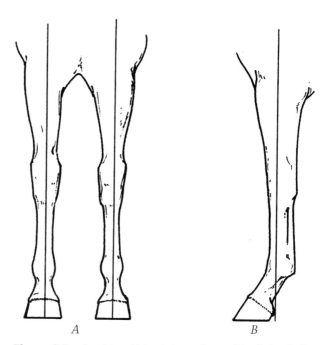

Figure 2.5. Cranial and lateral views of normal forelimbs. A. A line dropped from the point of the shoulder joint should bisect the limb. B. A line dropped from the tuber spinae of the scapula should bisect the limb down to the fetlock and end at the heel bulbs.

smooth, sweeping, forward motion. The pectoral muscles should also extend far down onto the limb. The pectoral and the forearm muscles help a horse to move its limbs laterally and medially, and to elevate the forelimb. It is believed by some horseman that long forearms and short cannon bones are conducive to speed[26] but this has not been documented.[29]

The carpal joints should be balanced and should not deviate toward, or away from, one another. The cannon bone should be centered under the carpus and not to the lateral side (bench knees). Deviations from a straight limb may cause strain on the collateral support structures and asymmetrical loading (compression) of the hinge joints in the forelimb.

LATERAL VIEW

When viewed from the side, limbs should exhibit a composite of moderate angles so that shock absorption is efficient (Figure 2.6). The shoulder angle is measured along the spine of the scapula, from the point of the shoulder to the point of the withers. The angle of the scapula and shoulder tend to increase (become more upright) as horses mature from foals to adults.[1] The shorter and straighter the shoulder, the shorter and quicker the stride, and the more stress and concussion that is transmitted to the limb.[22,24] Studies in dressage horses and show jumpers have found that a more horizontal scapula was related to a higher level of performance.[21,27] Also important is the angle the shoulder makes with the arm, which should be at least 90°. Horses with a more horizontally positioned scapula or a more flexed shoulder joint show more maximal extension of the elbow joint relative to the angle at initial ground contact.[5] This prolongs the stance phase.[5] It is also known that good gait and collection in performance horses is associated with longer stance duration in the forelimbs.[23,24] A long sloping scapula is ergonomically efficient and may place the rider more to the rear of the horse, resulting in improved balance.[24] The scapulohumeral (shoulder) joint is supported entirely by the muscles and tendons surrounding it. Because this muscle support is so important to proper movement, a horse should have well developed muscles in this region.

The length of the humerus (from the point of the shoulder to the point of the elbow) also affects stride length (Figure 2.6). A long humerus is associated with a long, reaching stride and good lateral ability; a short humerus is related to a short, choppy stride and poor lateral ability. A long humerus corresponds to a long triceps muscle that facilitates a larger range of elbow movements.[24] In general, the steeper the angle of the humerus, the higher the action; the closer the angle is to horizontal, the lower the action.

The angle formed by the humerus and radius and ulna at the elbow joint should be between 120° and 150°.[36] A more flexed elbow together with a horizontal scapula results in a longer stance duration, which is thought to improve gait quality with more collection in the forelimbs.[23] Straighter conformation (lesser angulation) at this joint may result in a short, choppy gait and increased concussion on the distal limb. The radius and ulna should be of sufficient length to provide good muscular function.

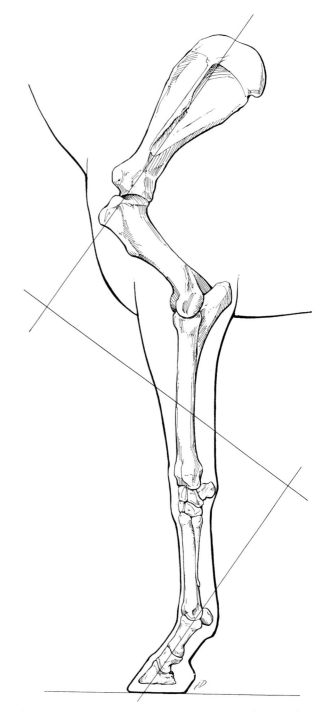

Figure 2.6. The angle of the shoulder usually influences the angle of the pastern.

Ideally the limb should form a straight column from the elbow joint to the fetlock. This conformation will disseminate the axial compression forces to all bony surfaces equally. With malalignment, axial compressive forces become focused on one side and tensional forces are created opposite to it, increasing the stress and strain on musculoskeletal structures.[36]

The carpus (knee) is a complex joint and functions in flexion, absorption of concussion, and extension. Flexion primarily occurs at the radiocarpal and middle

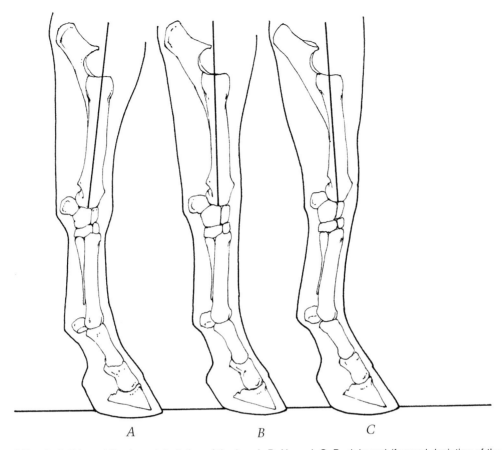

Figure 2.7. A. Calf-kneed (backward deviation of the knee). B. Normal. C. Buck-kneed (forward deviation of the knee).

carpal joints. Concussion is absorbed by all three carpal joints and extension occurs by a locking mechanism while the horse is weight-bearing during the extension phase of the stride. The carpal bones should be in good axial alignment with the radius and third metacarpal bone, and of sufficient size to support this downward force. The muscles of the forearm should be well developed to support the flexion and extension functions of the carpus. The carpus should appear straight and not deviate forward or backward (Figure 2.7).

Fetlock joints should be large enough and angled to permit free movement. A more extended fetlock joint resulted in more maximal extension, which correlated with a good gait in the forelimbs in one study.[5] It has also been found that a straighter hindlimb fetlock joint angle results in a longer stride and swing duration.[5] A study on Swedish Warmblood horses found the mean front fetlock angle to between 146° and 155° and the mean hind fetlock angle between 153° and 161°.[21]

This is considerable variation in the literature regarding what the "normal" hoof-pastern axis of the forefoot should be. Previous reports of angles less than 50° are currently considered to be too low and normal angles are thought to be approximately 54°.[7,11,12,29,36] However, these angles may vary considerably but the angle of the dorsal hoof wall should be similar to the angle of the pastern.[9] Exceptionally long, sloping pasterns or a broken back hoof-pastern axis are thought to increase strain to flexor support structures of the fetlock and

phalanges (Figure 2.8). Short, upright pasterns or a broken forward hoof-pastern axis are thought to cause greater concussive stresses to the fetlock, phalangeal joints, and foot.[7,9,29] They may also be associated with suspensory and tendon injuries in racehorses.[29]

The hoof should be appropriately sized for the size for the horse, well shaped (more round than egg-shaped) and symmetric. It should have high-quality hoof horn, adequate height and width of heel, a concave sole, and a robust frog. The bulbs of the heel should lie vertically below the central axis of the cannon bone in the sagittal plane (Figure 2.5B). Normally trimmed hooves usually impact the ground heel first or flat footed.[7,12,36] Studies have documented that lower hoof angles predispose racehorses to musculoskeletal injuries and contribute to a multitude of lameness problems in the palmar aspect of the foot.[26,29,31]

Faults in Conformation of the Forelimbs

BASE-NARROW (Figure 2.9)

In base-narrow conformation, the distance between the center of the feet on the ground is less than the distance between the center of the limbs at their origin in the chest when viewed from the front. This is often seen in horses with large chests and well-developed pectoral muscles, such as the Quarter horse. This conformation may be accompanied by a toe-in

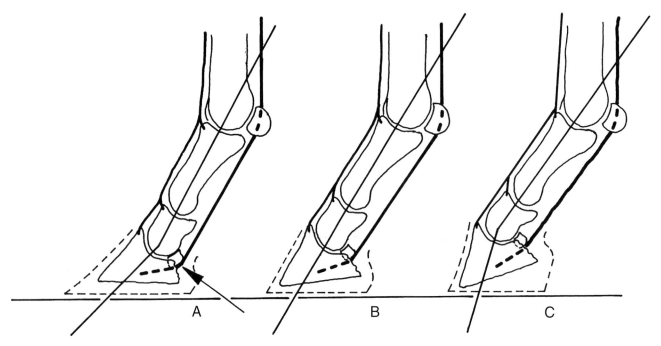

Figure 2.8. A. broken back pastern axis contributes to increased pressure in the navicular region (arrow). B. Normal or straight pastern axis. It is considered normal for the coffin bone to be 3° to 5° above the horizontal. C. Broken forward pastern axis. (Reprinted with permission from Hill, C., Klimesh R. Horse Hoof Care. Storey Publishing. North Adams, MA, 2009.)

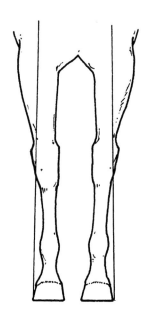

Figure 2.9. Base-narrow conformation. The distance between the center lines of the limbs is greater than the distance between the center lines of the feet on the ground.

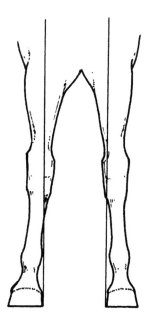

Figure 2.10. Base-wide conformation. The distance between the center lines of the feet is greater than the distance between the center lines of the limbs at the chest.

(pigeon-toed) or toe-out (splay-footed) conformation. Base-narrow conformation inherently causes the horse to bear more weight on the outside of the foot than on the inside.

BASE-WIDE (Figure 2.10)

In base-wide conformation, the distance between the center of the feet on the ground is greater than the distance between the center of the limbs at their origin in the chest when viewed from the front. This condition is found most commonly in narrow-chested horses and may be accompanied by toe-out (splay-footed) position of the feet. Base-wide, toe-out conformation usually causes winging of the limb to the inside (Figures 2.11 and 2.12). Base-wide conformation forces the horse to land on the inside of the foot, increasing weight-bearing forces on the inside of the foot and entire limb.

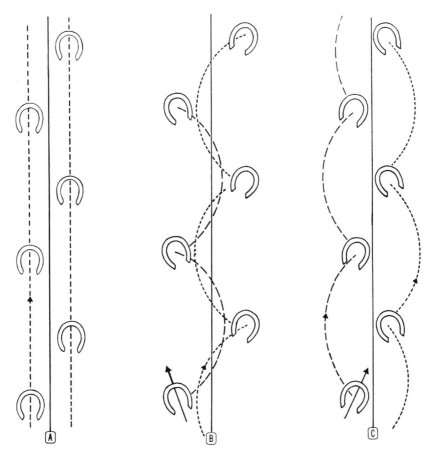

Figure 2.11. Examples of how toe-in and toe-out conformation affect foot path. A. Normal foot path. B. A horse with toe-out conformation. C. A horse with toe-in conformation.

TOE-IN OR PIGEON-TOED (Figure 2.13)

Toe-in is the position of the feet in which the toes point toward one another when viewed from the front (Figure 2.14). Its point of origin can be as high as the chest or as low as the fetlock down. It is often accompanied by a base-narrow conformation but rarely is present when the horse is base-wide. In the young foal, the condition may be seen as the result of an angular limb deformity. Proper trimming and corrective shoeing of the feet may prevent worsening of the condition, especially in growing horses. Toed-in horses tend to paddle with their feet (Figures 2.11C and 2.15) and have an outward deviation of the foot during flight. The foot breaks over the outside toe and lands on the outside wall. Base-narrow, toe-in conformation can cause interference, especially at the fetlock region. One study documenting variations in conformation in Swedish Warmblood horses found a 50% frequency of mild toe-in conformation in elite sport horses, indicating minor deviations do not impair soundness or performance.[21]

TOE-OUT OR SPLAY-FOOTED (Figures 2.16 and 2.17)

In a toe-out or splay-footed conformation, the toes point away from one another when viewed from the front. The point of origin is usually at the chest but the condition can be associated with outward rotation of the fetlock. It may be accompanied by either base-wide or base-narrow conformation. As with a toe-in conformation, it may be controlled or partially corrected by corrective trimming or shoeing. The flight of the foot goes through an inner arc when advancing, contributing to interference with the opposite forelimb (Figures 2.11B and 2.12). A toe-out, base-narrow conformation is thought to increase the likelihood of limb interference and plaiting.

BASE-NARROW, TOE-IN CONFORMATION (Figure 2.13)

Base-narrow, toe-in conformation causes excessive strain on the lateral collateral support structures of carpus, fetlock, and phalangeal joints. It often causes paddling (Figure 2.11C) and appears to be a common conformational abnormality (Figure 2.14).

BASE-NARROW, TOE-OUT CONFORMATION (Figure 2.16)

Base-narrow, toe-out conformation is one of the worst types of conformation in the forelimb. Horses having this conformation can seldom handle heavy work. The closely placed feet, combined with a tendency to wing inwardly from the toe-out position, commonly cause limb interference or plaiting. The hoof breaks over the inside toe, swings inward, and lands on

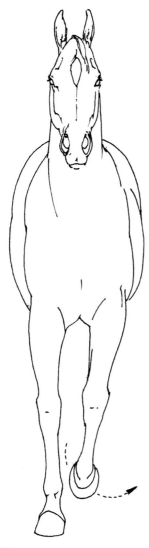

Figure 2.12. Winging, which may cause interference, is caused by a toe-out position of the foot.

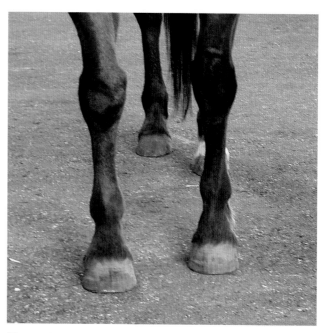

Figure 2.14. Horse with a slight varus deviation of the distal limb. Slight toe-in or pigeon-toe conformation is relatively common and does not appear to contribute to lameness in many cases.

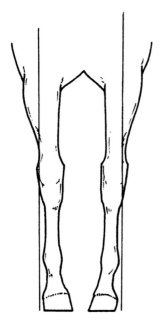

Figure 2.13. Base-narrow, toe-in conformation.

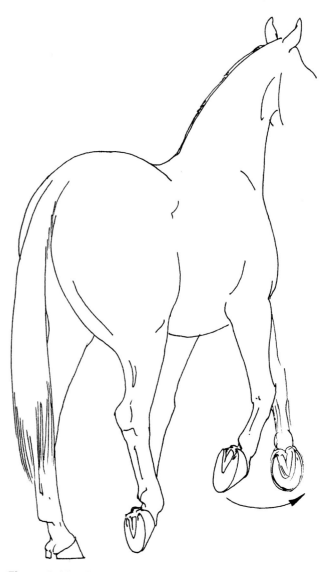

Figure 2.15. Paddling often accompanies toe-in conformation.

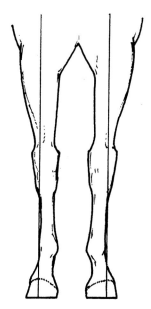

Figure 2.16. Base-narrow, toe-out conformation.

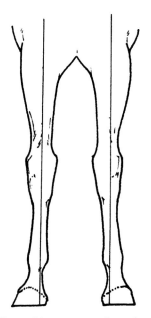

Figure 2.17. Base-wide, toe-out conformation.

the outside wall, contributing to increased strain on the limb below the fetlock. The base-narrow limb position places the weight on the outside wall, as with base-narrow, toe-in conformation.

BASE-WIDE, TOE-OUT CONFORMATION (Figure 2.17)

When a horse is base-wide, the feet usually toe-out. The base-wide conformation places the greatest stress on the inside of the limb. The foot usually breaks over the inside toe, wings to the inside, and lands on the inside hoof wall. Interference is common, similar to any type of toe-out conformation.

BASE-WIDE, TOE-IN CONFORMATION

This type of conformation is unusual. The base-wide position of the limbs places the greatest stress on the inside of the limb. In most cases, a horse affected with base-wide, toe-in conformation will paddle to the outside even though it breaks over the inside toe and lands on the inside wall.

PLAITING

Some horses, especially those with base-narrow, toe-out conformation, tend to place one foot directly in front of the other. This is an undesirable characteristic, because it can produce interference and stumbling when the advancing limb contacts the one placed in front of it. Plaiting tends to be seen more commonly in the hindlimbs than the forelimbs.

PALMAR (BACKWARD) DEVIATION OF THE CARPUS (HYPEREXTENDED KNEES, CALF KNEES, OR SHEEP KNEES) (Figure 2.7)

Backward deviation of the carpus (back at the knee) is thought to place increased stress on the palmar soft tissue structures and increase compression on the dorsal aspect of the carpus. Backward knee conformation is thought to make horses working at speed more susceptible to carpal injuries but this is not widely accepted, especially in Europe.[29] Hyperextension of the carpus is not the only reason for carpal injuries; long toes were associated with carpal problems in Thoroughbred racehorses in one study.[31] Additionally, injury to the palmar soft tissue structures of the carpus may contribute to this conformation, suggesting that it may not be a strictly genetic influence.

DORSAL (FORWARD) DEVIATION OF THE CARPUS (BUCKED KNEES OR KNEE SPRUNG) (Figure 2.7)

This condition may also be called "goat knees" or "over in the knees." It is generally believed that "bucked knees" is a less serious problem than the calf-knee condition and may protect against carpal disease in racehorses.[29] However, severe dorsal deviation may be more dangerous for the rider because the horse's knees are on the verge of buckling forward. Forward deviation of the carpus may be caused by contraction of the carpal flexors (i.e., ulnaris lateralis, flexor carpi ulnaris, and flexor carpi radialis) in young horses and may place increased strain on the extensor carpi radialis and the suspensory ligament.[36] Congenital forms are nearly always bilateral and may be accompanied by a forward knuckling of the fetlocks. The condition is often present at birth and usually disappears by 3 months of age if it is not severe. One study documenting the variations in conformation in Swedish Warmblood horses found considerably more elite sport horses were "buck kneed" than "calf kneed," while the reverse was true in riding school horses.[21]

MEDIAL DEVIATION OF THE CARPUS (KNOCK KNEES, CARPUS VALGUS, OR KNEE-NARROW CONFORMATION) (Figure 2.18B)

Medial angular deviation of the carpus (or lateral deviation of the distal limb) can result from

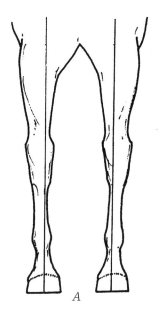 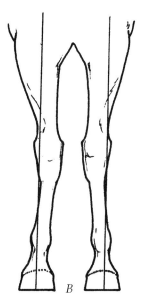

Figure 2.18. Examples of abnormal carpal conformation as compared to Figure 2.5. A. carpal varus or bowlegs. B. carpal valgus or knock-knees. Some degree (<5° to 7°) of carpal valgus is considered to be within normal limits in most horses.

abnormalities of the distal metaphysis, physis, and epiphysis of the radius; from abnormal development and alignment of the carpal bones; or from carpal joint laxity. This deviation contributes to increased tensional strain on the medial collateral ligaments of the carpus and compression forces on the lateral (concave) surface of the carpus. Varying degrees of stresses are also transmitted to the joints proximal and distal to the carpus. Varying degrees of outward rotation of the cannon bone, fetlock, and foot may accompany this entity. Mild carpal valgus (5° to 7°) may have a protective mechanism against carpal injuries, and is preferred over completely straight front limbs. The odds for carpal fracture and effusion decreased with an increase in carpal angle in Thoroughbred racehorses.[3] In general, carpal valgus appears to be less problematic in performance horses than carpal varus.

LATERAL DEVIATION OF THE CARPUS (BOWLEGS, CARPAL VARUS, OR BANDY-LEGGED CONFORMATION) (Figure 2.18A)

Carpal varus is an outward deviation of the carpus (or inward deviation of the distal limb) when viewed from the front of the horse. It may be accompanied by a base-narrow, toe-in conformation. This condition increases tension on the lateral surface of the carpus and compression on the medial surface of the carpus and carpal bones (Figure 2.19). This deviation may be correctable in young horses but growth of the knee reached a plateau at approximately 140 days of age in Thoroughbreds, suggesting that carpal deviations (lateral or medial) should be corrected before this age.[37]

BENCH KNEES (OFFSET KNEES) (Figure 2.20)

Bench knee is a conformation in which the cannon bone is offset to the lateral side and does not follow a straight line down from the radius when viewed from the front. Increased weight bearing on the medial splint

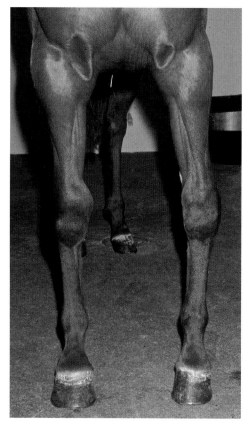

Figure 2.19. A Quarter horse yearling with varus deformity of the carpus associated with physitis of the distal radial physis. This type of deviation of the carpus is likely to contribute to lameness problems.

bone is thought to occur in benched kneed horses. This is thought to contribute to increased stress on the interosseous ligament predisposing to "splints." In a study documenting the conformational abnormalities in 356

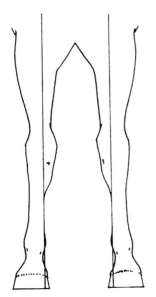

Figure 2.20. Offset knees (bench knees), which are characterized by the cannon bones being set too far laterally.

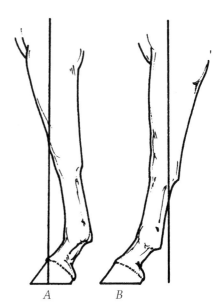

Figure 2.21. A. Standing under in front. B. Camped out in front.

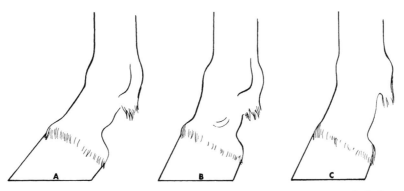

Figure 2.22. Examples of pastern conformation. A. A normal angulation of hoof wall and pastern. B. A short upright pastern. C. A long upright pastern.

Warmblood horses, more than 50% were bench kneed.[21] The combination of bench knees and carpal valgus is common, and offset knees has been associated with fetlock problems in racing Thoroughbreds.[2]

STANDING UNDER IN FRONT (Figure 2.21A)

With this deviation the entire forelimb from the elbow down is placed too far under the body when the horse is viewed from the side. This stance may occur in certain diseases and may not be a conformational fault. With this conformation, the base of support is shortened, the forelimbs become overloaded, the cranial phase of the stride is shortened, and the arc of foot flight may be low. This may predispose the horse to stumbling but is not problematic in many horses.

CAMPED IN FRONT (Figure 2.21B)

This is a condition opposite that described above. The entire forelimb, from the body to the ground, is too far forward when viewed from the side. This limb position may be present with certain lameness conditions, such as bilateral navicular syndrome and laminitis.

SHORT UPRIGHT PASTERN (Figure 2.22)

A short upright pastern is believed to increase concussion and injuries to the fetlock and phalangeal joints, the navicular bone region, and soft tissue structures within the metacarpus.[29,36] If the angle of the hoof is more upright than that of the pastern, it is referred to as a broken forward hoof-pastern axis.[24] This type of conformation is often associated with a base-narrow, toe-in conformation and is often seen in horses with short limbs and a powerful body and limb musculature.[36] Additionally, a straight shoulder (more vertical) usually accompanies a short upright pastern.

LONG SLOPING PASTERN (Figure 2.23)

A long sloping pastern is characterized by a normal or subnormal angulation of the forefoot (less than 50° to 54°) with a pastern that is too long for the length of the limb. If the angle of the hoof is more acute (lower) than that of the pastern, it is referred to as a broken backward hoof-pastern axis.[24] It is often seen in horses with long toes and/or low heels and may predispose a horse to injury of the navicular region, flexor tendons, sesamoid bones, and suspensory ligament (Figure 2.24).[36] Long pasterns were also found to increase the odds of Thoroughbred racehorses fracturing a front limb.[2]

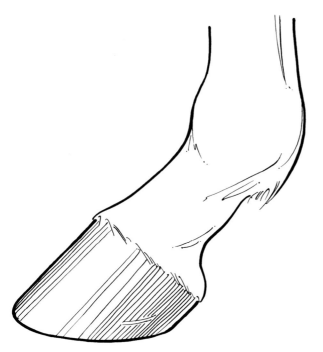

Figure 2.23. Example of a long sloping pastern that is often associated with a broken-back hoof pastern axis. A long toe and a low heel often contribute to this conformation. The weight-bearing surface of the foot is well forward of the metacarpus/metatarsus.

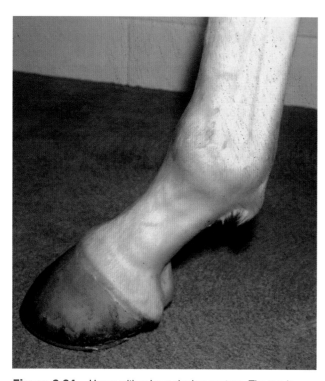

Figure 2.24. Horse with a long sloping pastern. The toe is long and the heels are low.

The Hindlimbs

The hindlimbs constitute the "engine" of the horse regardless of its intended use. Endurance horses are characterized by longer, flatter muscles, stock horses are characterized by shorter, thicker muscles, and all-around horses have moderate muscling. Lack of hindlimb musculature or a disparity between the amount of forelimb vs. hindlimb muscle development may suggest chronic hindlimb lameness problems.

LATERAL VIEW

When viewed from the side, the hindlimbs should exhibit a composite of moderate angles so that shock absorption will be efficient (Figure 2.25). A line from the point of buttock to the ground should touch the hock and end slightly behind the bulbs of the heels. A hindlimb in front of this line is often standing under (Figure 2.26) or sickle-hocked (Figure 2.27); a hindlimb behind this line is often post-legged (Figure 2.28) or camped out (Figure 2.29). The hindquarter should be symmetric and well connected to the barrel and the lower limb. The gluteal muscles should tie well forward into the back and the hamstrings should extend down low into the Achilles tendon of the hock.

The relationship of the length of the bones, the angles of the joints, and the overall height of the hindlimb

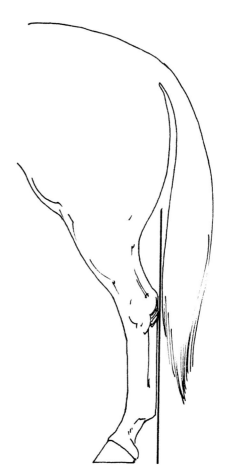

Figure 2.25. Normal hindlimb conformation as viewed from the side. A line dropped from the point of the buttock (tuber ischii) should follow the cannon bone.

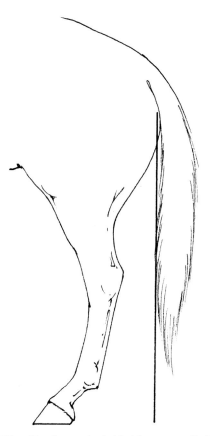

Figure 2.26. Standing under behind (compare with Figure 2.25).

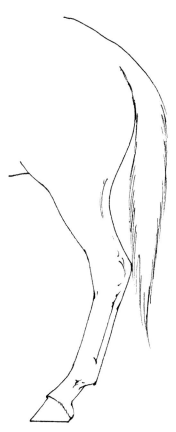

Figure 2.27. Sickle hocks. The angle of the hock looks excessive but is actually less than normal. Hocks with an angle of less than 150° to 153° are considered to be sickle.

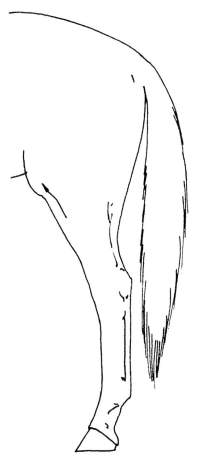

Figure 2.28. Post-legged refers to too little angulation of the hock and stifle joints. The hock is very straight and angles of more than 165° to 170° are considered to be abnormal.

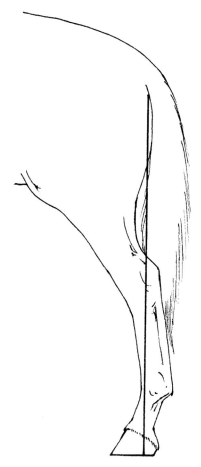

Figure 2.29. Camped out behind (compare with Figure 2.25).

often dictate the type of action and amount of power produced. The length and slope to the pelvis (croup) are measured from the point of the hip to the point of the buttock. A flat, level croup is associated with hindlimb action that occurs behind the hindquarters rather than underneath it. A "goose rump" is a very steep croup that places the hindlimbs so far under the horse's belly that structural problems may occur due to the over-angulation. Somewhere between these two extremes is ideal. In general, a more flexed hip causes a more pro-tracted position of the hindlimb at the stance phase and a more horizontal femur during the swing phase. This causes the horse to keep its hindlimbs more under its body, which is important for collection in dressage horses and lift-off in show jumpers.[23]

Probably the most important individual conforma-tional detail in sport horses is the femur. A long and forwardly sloping femur places the hindlimbs more under the horse, which allows the horse to keep its balance more easily because the limb is closer to the center of gravity.[24] A forwardly sloping femur has also been shown to have a positive effect on soundness. A long femur is thought to result in a longer stride with more reach. A short femur is associated with the short, rapid stride characteristic of a sprinter. The gaskin length (stifle to hock) should be shorter than the femur length (buttock to stifle). A gaskin length longer than the femur length tends to be associated with cow hocks and sickle hocks.

Hindlimbs with less angulation (open angles, straighter hindlimbs when viewed from the side) usually have a shorter overall limb length and produce efficient movement suitable for hunters or racehorses. Generally, hindlimbs with more angulation (closed joints) have a longer overall limb length and produce a more vertical, folding action necessary for collection characteristic of dressage horses.[36] An overall limb length that is too long may contribute to either a camped-out or sickle-hocked conformation. Elite Warmblood horses were found to have larger hock angles (straighter) than other groups of horses.[21] A positive relationship between large hock angles and soundness in Standardbred trotters has also been found.[28] Horses with lameness and back problems usually have significantly smaller hock angles than sound horses.[24]

Caudal View

From the rear, both hindlimbs should be symmetri-cal, the same length, and bear equal weight (Figure 2.30). A left-to-right symmetry should be evident between the peaks of the croup (tuber sacrale), the points of the hip, the points of the buttock, and the midline position of the tail. A study in Standardbred trotters found that hindquarter asymmetry (tuber sacrale at unequal heights) and associated factors had a negative effect on performance(Figure 2.31).[15] In addi-tion, poor development of the epaxial muscles in the thoracolumbar region and asymmetry of the hindquar-ter musculature but not asymmetry of the tuber sacrale were common findings in sport horses with documented sacroiliac disease.[16] The widest point of the hindquar-ters should be the width between the stifles. A line dropped from the point of the buttock to the ground should essentially bisect the limb; however, the hindlimbs

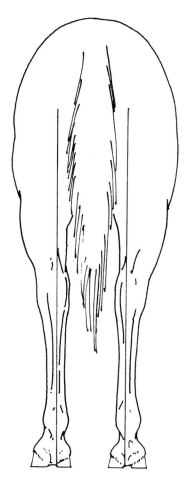

Figure 2.30. Normal hindlimbs as viewed from the rear. A line dropped from the point of the buttock (tuber ischii) should bisect the limb.

are not designed to point absolutely straight forward.[29] About 80% of all Warmblood riding horses and Standardbred trotters have outwardly rotated hindlimbs.[24] It is also normal for the stifles to point slightly outward, which in turn causes the points of the hocks to face slightly inward and the toes to point slightly outward. The rounder the belly and/or the shorter the loin and coupling, the more the stifles must point outward and the points of the hocks appear to point inward. When the cannon bone faces outward, the horse is considered to be cow-hocked (Figure 2.32); when the cannon bones face inward, the horse is bow-legged (Figure 2.33).

Faults in Conformation of the Hindlimbs

Standing Under Behind (Figure 2.26)

Viewed from the side, the entire limb is placed too far forward or sickle hocks are present. A perpendicular line drawn from the point of the buttock (tuber ischii) would strike the ground well behind the limb.

Excessive Angulation of the Hock (Sickle Hocks, Small Hock Angles) (Figure 2.27)

Mean hock angles in normal horses are thought to be approximately 155° to 165°.[18,24] Hock angles less

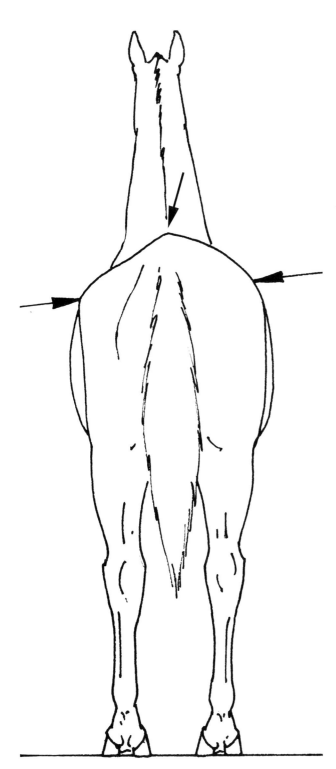

Figure 2.31. Asymmetry between the peaks of the croup, points of the hip, and points of the buttock (arrows).

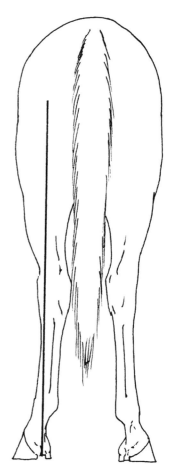

Figure 2.32. Cow hocks accompanied by base-wide conformation (compare with Figure 2.25). Such horses are often base-narrow at the hocks and base-wide from the hocks down.

of Icelandic horses.[3] Small hock angles may also impair a horse's ability to attain the level of collection required for good performance in advanced classes. One study on elite Swedish Warmblood sport horses found that none of the show jumpers and only one of the dressage horses were "sickle hocked."[21] In general, sickle-hocked horses or horses with small hock angles should be avoided,[24] although others state that many of these horses can be effectively managed.[29]

EXCESSIVELY STRAIGHT LIMBS, "STRAIGHT BEHIND" (Figure 2.28)

When viewed from the side, there is very little angle between the tibia and femur, and the hock is excessively straight (large hock joint angle of more than 165° to 170°).[18,29] This is believed to predispose the horse to bog spavin, thoroughpin, upward fixation of the patella, and high suspensory disease.[29,36] Horses with large tarsal angles showed less tarsal flexion and less energy absorption at the tarsus during the impact phase, potentially contributing to the development of OA.[18] Generally, the pastern conformation is also too straight when the tarsus is too straight.

CAMPED BEHIND (Figure 2.29)

"Camped behind" means that the entire limb is placed too far caudally when viewed from the side. A

than 150° to 153° are considered sickle.[22,24,29] When viewed from the side, the angle of the hock is decreased so that the horse is standing under from the hock down. This places the hock under greater stress and may predispose to synovial distention in the stifle and hock joints, and bone spavin.[24,29] A small tarsal angle was significantly associated with radiographic signs of osteoarthritis (OA) in the distal tarsus in a large number

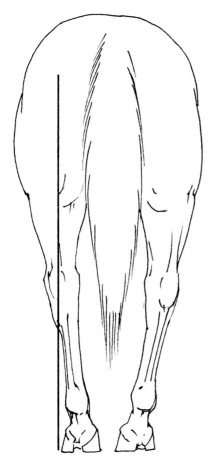

Figure 2.33. Base-narrow behind (compare with Figure 2.25). This is often accompanied by "bowlegs," as shown.

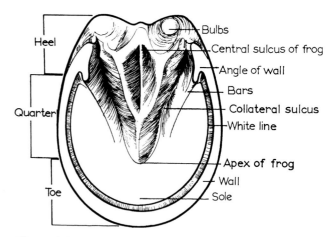

Figure 2.34. Normal forefoot with structures labeled.

perpendicular line dropped from the point of the buttock would hit the toe, or halfway between the toe and heel. Upright pasterns often accompany this condition.

BASE-WIDE (Figure 2.32)

Base-wide means that when viewed from behind, the distance between the center of the feet on the ground is greater than the distance between the center of the limbs in the thigh region. Base-wide conformation is not as frequent in the hindlimbs as in the forelimbs and is often associated with cow hocks.

MEDIAL DEVIATION OF THE HOCK (COW HOCKS OR TARSAL VALGUS) (Figure 2.32)

"Cow-hocked" means that the limbs are base-narrow down to the hock and then base-wide from the hock to the feet. The hocks are too close together and point toward one another, and the feet are widely separated. Cow-hocked conformation is a common defect and some believe that it is a serious hindlimb conformation flaw.[36] However, others feels that a slight valgus deformity of the hindlimbs, provided that the metatarsal bones remain vertical, is not a cause for concern.[29] Sickle hocks and cow hocks can occur concurrently and may have a compounding effect on hindlimb lameness problems.

BASE-NARROW (Figure 2.33)

Base-narrow conformation of the hindlimbs means that the distance between the center of the feet is less than the distance between the center of the limbs in the thigh region, when viewed from behind. This is observed most commonly in heavily muscled horses. It causes excessive strain on the lateral aspect of the limb and most of the horse's weight is placed on the outside of the hooves. Base-narrow conformation is often accompanied by "bowlegs" or a condition in which the hocks are too far apart. The limbs may appear fairly straight to the hock and then deviate inward, and the hocks may bow outward during movement. When a horse has good conformation in front and is base-narrow behind, many types of interference can occur between the forelimbs and hindlimbs.[36]

Conformation of the Foot

Hoof anatomy and conformation are also discussed in Chapters 1 and 12.

THE FOREFOOT (Figure 2.34)

Ideally, the forefoot should be round and wide in the heels, and the size and shape of the heels should correspond to the size and shape of the toe. The bars should be well developed. The wall should be thickest at the toe and should thin gradually toward the heels; the inside wall should be slightly straighter than the outside wall. The sole should be slightly concave medial to lateral and front to back, but excessive concavity may suggest a chronic foot problem. There should be minimal contact between the ground and the sole, because it is not a weight-bearing structure. Toe lengths of greater than 1 1/2 inches cranial to the apex of the frog when viewed from the bottom of the foot often suggest excessive toe length.

The mean hoof angle of the forefoot is usually 50° to 55° and the angle of the heel should be approximately the same as the angle of the toe.[7,9,11,12] However, the angle of the hoof is less important than the hoof pastern axis when evaluating foot conformation. Toe wall length relative to heel wall length should be approximately 2 : 1 in the forefoot and 2 : 1.5 in the

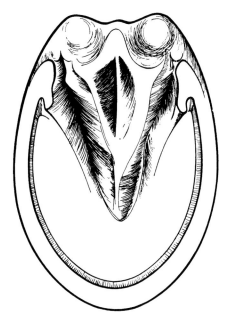

Figure 2.35. Normal hindfoot (compare with Figure 2.34). The toe of the hindfoot is more pointed than that of the forefoot.

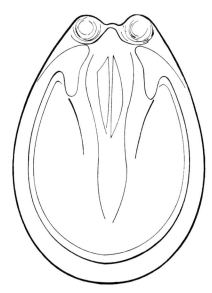

Figure 2.36. Contracted foot illustrating narrowing of the heels and quarters (compare with Figure 2.34).

hindfoot.[7] Break-over should occur squarely over the center of the toe and not over the medial or lateral portions of the toe. The wall should show even wear throughout.

The frog should be large and well developed with a good cleft, have normal consistency and elasticity, and be dry and soft. It should divide the sole into two nearly equal halves, and the apex should point to the center of the toe. In most horses, the apex of the frog should end approximately 1 to 1 1/2 inches behind the toe. Unequal size of the two halves of the frog may indicate a base-wide or base-narrow conformation.

THE HINDFOOT (Figure 2.35)

The hindfoot is usually narrower, has a larger hoof angle, and has a more pointed appearance at the toe than does the forefoot.[6,7] Break-over should be evident straight over the toe, and the frog should divide the sole into equal halves. The mean hoof angle in the hindfoot is usually 55° or greater, and there should be no defects in the wall.[7,11,36] The walls should show normal wear on the medial and lateral sides, and the sole should be slightly concave medial to lateral and front to back. The sole of the hindfoot is normally more concave than that of the forefoot.

Abnormal Conformation of the Foot

FLAT FEET

A flat foot lacks the natural concavity in the sole; it is not a normal condition in light horses but is present in some draft breeds. Flat feet may be heritable and are observed more commonly in the forefeet than in the hind. The horse may land on the heels to avoid sole pressure with this condition. Sole bruising is a common sequelae of flat feet. There is no known cure for flat foot, but corrective shoeing may help prevent resultant lameness.

CONTRACTED FOOT OR CONTRACTED HEELS (Figure 2.36)

A contracted foot is a condition in which the foot is narrower than normal, especially the back half of the foot. This condition is much more common in the front feet than in the hindfeet, and it may be unilateral or bilateral. Hoof contraction can occur rapidly in the heels with a long-toe, low-heel conformation resulting in a low hoof.[17] Heel contraction also occurs with disuse of the foot as is seen with chronic lameness conditions. Heel contraction can be quantified using several techniques (Figure 2.37).

Certain breeds of horses normally have a foot that more closely approaches an oval than a circle in shape. A narrow foot is not necessarily a contracted foot; donkeys and mules normally have a foot shape that would be called contracted in a horse. Foot contraction may be present in the Tennessee Walking horse and American Saddlebred when these horses are used for show because the hoof wall is allowed to grow excessively long.

A unilateral contraction of one forefoot may be present in some horses. This may be congenital or developmental, but it is not known whether it is a heritable abnormality. The contracted foot may or may not eventually show lameness, but it should be regarded as an undesirable feature. A small foot on one side may also indicate a chronic lameness and can be associated with a club foot. This is often referred to as "mismatched" feet.

BUTTRESS FOOT (Figure 2.38)

"Buttress foot" is a swelling above the dorsal surface of the hoof wall at the coronary band. This swelling may be from low ringbone or a fracture of the extensor process of the distal phalanx (coffin bone). A conical deformity of the toe from the coronary band to the ground surface occurs due to the deformed hoof growth associated with chronic swelling at the coronary band. This often results in a triangular or pyramidal shape to the foot (Figure 2.39).

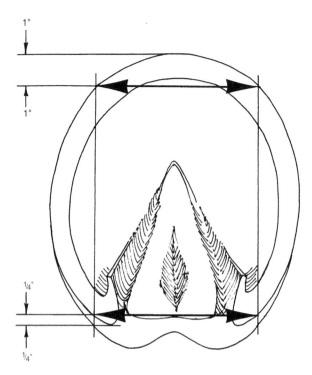

Figure 2.37. One method to quantify heel contraction. The width of the heels 1/4 inch from the heel buttresses should equal or exceed the width of the trimmed foot 1 inch behind the toe.

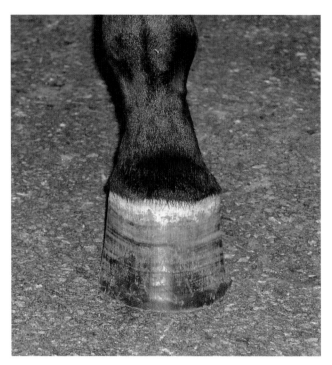

Figure 2.39. Front view of a horse with a buttress foot associated with a large extensor process fracture of the distal phalanx. The foot has assumed a triangular or pyramidal shape.

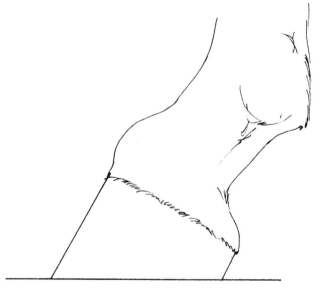

Figure 2.38. Buttress foot.

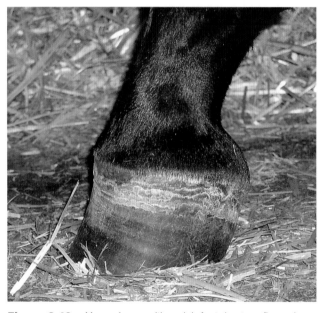

Figure 2.40. Young horse with a club foot due to a flexural deformity of the deep digital flexor tendon. There can be many causes of a club foot and not all contribute to lameness.

CLUB FOOT (Figure 2.40)

A "club foot" usually refers to a foot with a foot axis greater than or equal to 60°. A unilateral club foot may be due to an injury that has prevented proper use of the foot (disuse due to chronic lameness) or from a flexural deformity involving the deep digital flexor tendon, seen primarily in foals. It may be developmental or acquired, and may or may not contribute to a lameness problem.[29]

COON-FOOTED (Figure 2.41)

The pastern alignment of the coon-footed horse slopes more than the dorsal surface of the hoof wall. In other words, the hoof-pastern axis is broken forward at the coronary band. It may occur in the front or hind-

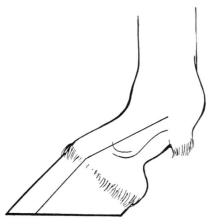

Figure 2.41. Broken angle between the hoof and pastern axis where the foot axis is steeper than the pastern axis (coon-footed).

feet and causes strain on the flexor support structures and the common/long digital extensor tendon.[36]

THIN WALL AND SOLE

Thin walls and soles accompany one another and are thought to be heritable. The conformation of the foot may appear to be normal, but the hoof wall either wears away too rapidly or does not grow fast enough to avoid sole pressure. This condition is especially noticeable at the heels, where the hoof-pastern axis may be broken backward by the tendency of the heels to be low.

MOVEMENT

Movement comprises a horse's travel and action. Although the lower limbs are the focal point of evaluation, movement is a combined effort of the horse's entire body (Box 2.1). "Travel" refers to the flight of

---

Box 2.1. Terms Associated with Movement.

1. **Action:** The style of the movement, including joint flexion, stride length, and suspension; usually viewed from the side.
2. **Asymmetry:** A difference between two body parts or an alteration in the synchronization of a gait; when a horse is performing asymmetrically, he is often said to be "off."
3. **Balance:** The harmonious, precise, coordinated form of a horse's movement as reflected by equal distribution of weight from left to right and an appropriate amount of weight carried by the hindquarters.
4. **Breakover:** The moment between the stance and swing phases as the heel lifts and the hoof pivots over the toe.
5. **Cadence:** See "Rhythm."
6. **Collection:** A shortening of stride within a gait, without a decrease in tempo; brought about by a shift of the center of gravity rearward; usually accompanied by an overall body elevation and an increase in joint flexion.
7. **Directness:** Trueness of travel, the straightness of the line in which the hoof (limb) is carried forward.
8. **Evenness:** Balance, symmetry, and synchronization of the steps within a gait in terms of weight bearing and timing.
9. **Extension:** A lengthening of stride within a gait, without an increase in tempo; brought about by a driving force from behind and a reaching in front; usually accompanied by a horizontal floating called "suspension."
10. **Gait:** An orderly footfall pattern such as the walk, trot, or canter.
11. **Height:** The degree of elevation of the arc of the stride, viewed from the side.
12. **Impulsion:** Thrust, the manner in which the horse's weight is settled and released from the supporting structures of the limb in the act of carrying the horse forward.
13. **Overtrack "tracking up":** The horse's hind feet step on or ahead of the front prints.
14. **Pace:** The variations within the gaits such as working trot, extended trot, collected trot; a goal (in dressage) is that the tempos should remain the same for the various paces within a gait. Pace also refers to a specific two-beat lateral gait exhibited by some Standardbreds and other gaited horses.
15. **Power:** Propelling, balancing, and sometimes pulling forces.
16. **Rapidity:** Promptness, quickness; the time consumed in taking a single stride.
17. **Regularity:** The cadence, the rhythmical precision with which each stride is taken in turn.
18. **Relaxation:** Absence of excess muscular tension.
19. **Rhythm:** The cadence of the footfall within a gait, taking into account timing (number of beats) and accent.
20. **Step:** A single beat of a gait; a step may involve one or more limbs. In the walk, there are four individual steps. In the trot, there are two steps, and each involves two limbs.
21. **Stiffness:** Inability (pain or lack of condition) or unwillingness (bad attitude) to flex and extend the muscles or joints.
22. **Stride, length of:** The distance from the point of breaking over to the point of next contact with the ground of the same hoof; a full sequence of steps in a particular gait.
23. **Suppleness:** Flexibility.
24. **Suspension:** The horizontal floating that occurs when a limb is extended and the body continues moving forward; also refers to the moment at the canter and gallop when all limbs are flexed or curled up, reorganizing for the next stride.
25. **Tempo:** The rate of movement, the rate of stride repetition; a faster tempo results in more strides per minute.
26. **Travel:** The path of the hoof (limb) flight in relation to the midline of the horse and the other limbs; usually viewed from the front or rear.

the hoof in relation to the other limbs and is often viewed from the front or rear (Box 2.2). "Action" takes into account joint flexion, stride length, suspension, and other qualities and is usually assessed from a side view.

The Natural Gaits

The "walk" is a four-beat gait (Figure 2.42) that should have a very even rhythm as the feet land and take off in the following sequence: left hind, left fore, right hind, right fore. A horse that is rushing at the walk might either jig or prance (impure gaits composed of half walking, half trotting) or might develop a pacey walk. The "pace" (Figure 2.43) is a two-beat lateral gait in which the two right limbs rise and land alternately with the two left limbs. Although the pace is a viable gait for a Standardbred racehorse, a pacey walk is considered an impure gait for most riding horses because the even four-beat pattern of the walk is broken.[36]

The "trot" is a two-beat diagonal gait (Figure 2.44). The right fore and left hind rise and fall together alternately with the diagonal pair left fore and right hind. Often, the trot is a horse's steadiest and most rhythmic gait. Traditionally, the trot referred to an English gait with a moderate to great degree of impulsion. The (western) jog is a shorter-strided trot with less impulsion. If a horse is jogged too slowly, the gait becomes

---

Box 2.2. Defects in Travel.

1. **Paddling:** The foot is thrown *outward* in flight, but the foot often lands *inside* the normal track; often associated with wide and/or toed-in conformation.
2. **Winging:** The foot swings *inward* in flight but often lands *outside* the normal track; often associated with narrow and/or toed-out conformation; dangerous because it can result in interfering.
3. **Plaiting:** Also called rope-walking. The horse places one foot directly in front of the other; dangerous due to stumbling and tripping; associated with narrow, toed-out conformation.
4. **Interfering:** Striking a limb with the opposite limb; associated with toed-out, base-narrow conformation; results in tripping, wounds.
5. **Forging:** Hitting the sole or the shoe of the forefoot with the toe of the hindfoot on the same side; associated with sickle-hocked or short-backed/long-limbed conformation, a tired, young, or unconditioned horse, one that needs its shoes reset, or one with long toes.
6. **Over-reaching:** Hitting the heel of the forefoot with the hindfoot on the same side before the forefoot has left the ground; also called "grabbing"; often results in lost shoes.

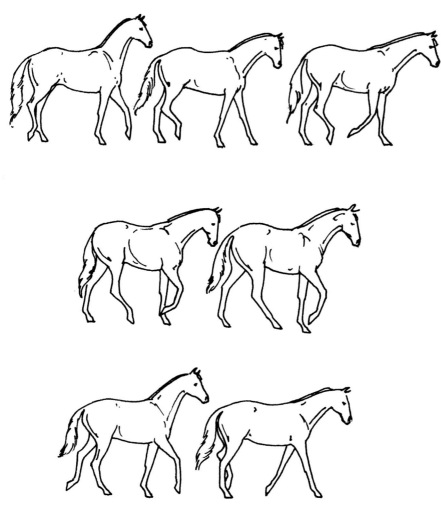

Figure 2.42. The walk.

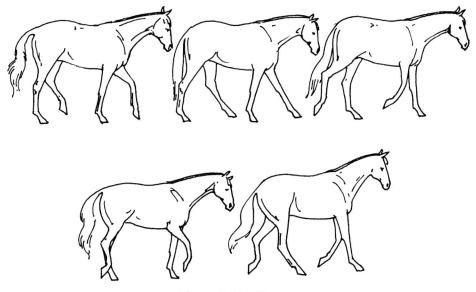

Figure 2.43. The pace.

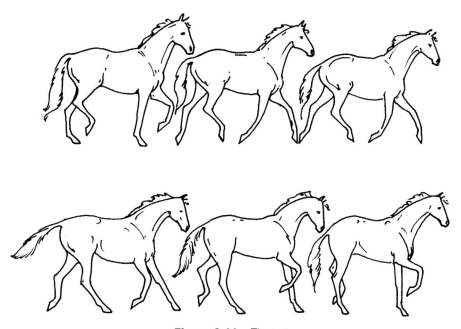

Figure 2.44. The trot.

impure as the diagonal pairs break and the horse essentially walks behind and trots in front.

The "canter" or "lope" (Figure 2.45) is a three-beat gait with the following sequence: one hindlimb, then the other hindlimb simultaneously with its diagonal forelimb, and finally the remaining forelimb. If a horse is on the right lead, the initiating hind will be the left hind, the diagonal pair will be the right hind (sometimes referred to as the supporting hind) and the left fore, and the final beat will occur when the leading forelimb (the right fore) lands. Then there is a moment of suspension as the horse gathers its limbs underneath itself to get

organized for the next cycle. When observing a horse on the right lead from the side, it is evident that the right limbs will reach farther forward than the left limbs. A change of lead (Figure 2.46) can occur during the moment of suspension so that the horse can change both front and hind simultaneously.

The "gallop" or run is a four-beat variation of the canter (Figure 2.47). With increased impulsion and length of stride, the diagonal pair breaks, resulting in four beats. The footfall sequence of a right lead gallop is left hind, right hind, left fore, and right fore. As in the canter, the right limbs reach farther forward than

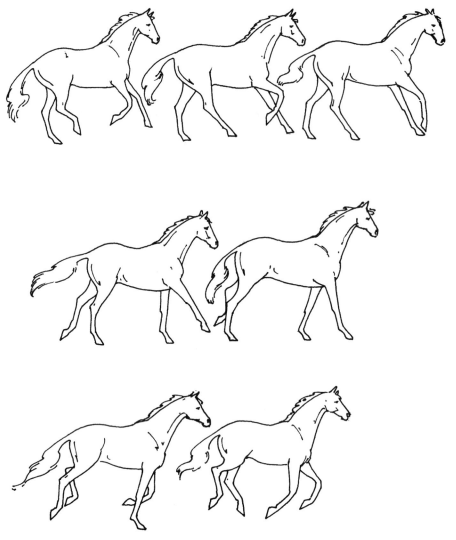

Figure 2.45. The canter, right lead.

the left limbs when the horse is in the right lead. There is more suspension at the gallop than at the canter.

The Phases of a Stride

The five phases of a horse's stride are landing, loading, stance, break-over, and swing (Figures 2.48 to 2.50).

LANDING (Figure 2.48)

The hoof touches the ground, and the limb begins to receive the impact of the body's weight.

LOADING (Figure 2.48)

The body moves forward, and the horse's center of gravity passes over the hoof. Usually, this is when the fetlock descends (extends) to its lowest point, sometimes resulting in an almost horizontal pastern. The geometry of the foot also changes when loaded; the heels expand and sink caudally, and the toe retracts.

STANCE (Figure 2.49)

The fetlock rises to a configuration comparable to the horse's stance at rest. The transition between the loading phase and the stance phase can be stressful to the internal structures of the hoof and lower limb. The horse's center of gravity moves ahead of the hoof. The flexor apparatus lifts the weight of the horse and rider, and the fetlock begins to move upward. The pastern straightens and the limb begins to push off the ground.

BREAK-OVER (Figure 2.49)

"Break-over" is the phase when the hoof leaves the ground. It starts when the heels lift and the hoof begins to pivot at the toe. The knee (or hock) relaxes and begins to flex. Break-over is measured from the time the heels leave the ground to the time the toe leaves the ground. The onset and duration of break-over are sensitive to changes in hoof balance, especially hoof angle and toe length.[7] The deep digital flexor tendon (assisted by the suspensory ligament) is stretched just prior to the

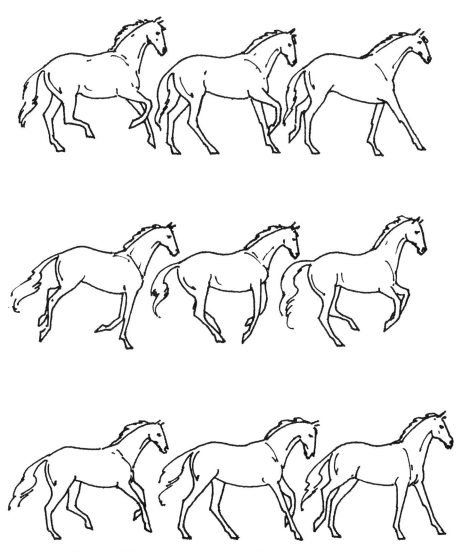

Figure 2.46. Canter with flying lead change, right lead to left lead.

beginning of break-over to counteract the downward pressure of the weight of the horse's body.

SWING (Figure 2.50)

The limb moves through the air and straightens out in preparation for landing.

Stride Length

Leaving the toe of a hoof long has been thought to increase a horse's stride length, thereby contributing to a smooth and efficient stride and fewer strides over a given distance. However, it has been shown that horses with long toes and an acute hoof angle do not take longer strides.[13,14] Long toes (often accompanied by low, run-under heels) move the pivot point of the hoof farther forward than normal. The long toe acts as a lever arm during break-over, making it more difficult for the heels to rotate around the toe; consequently, tension in the deep digital flexor tendon and navicular bone ligaments may be prolonged and/or

exaggerated.[29,36] The delayed break-over permits the mass of the horse's body to move farther forward over the horse's limbs before the limbs leave the ground. To support this further, rolled toe shoes have been shown to improve the ease of movement and to lower peak loading of the distal limb during break-over.[38]

The arc of hoof flight is also not significantly changed by trimming.[7,10] However, the approach to the loading phase and the landing phase can be affected. With a normally trimmed hoof, the toe of the hoof is elevated slightly prior to landing as the hoof prepares for a heel-first or flat-foot impact. The hoof with an acute angle approaches the ground toe first, often landing with the toe impacting first.[13,29] Such stabbing into the ground with the toes often results in a broken, jarring motion rather than smooth action. Additionally, when the front feet are trimmed normally and the hind toes are long, the hind feet leave the ground significantly later than their diagonal forefeet.[13] However, the hindlimbs compensate for the delay in break-over by moving through the air more rapidly so that they can catch up and land at the same time as their corresponding diagonal

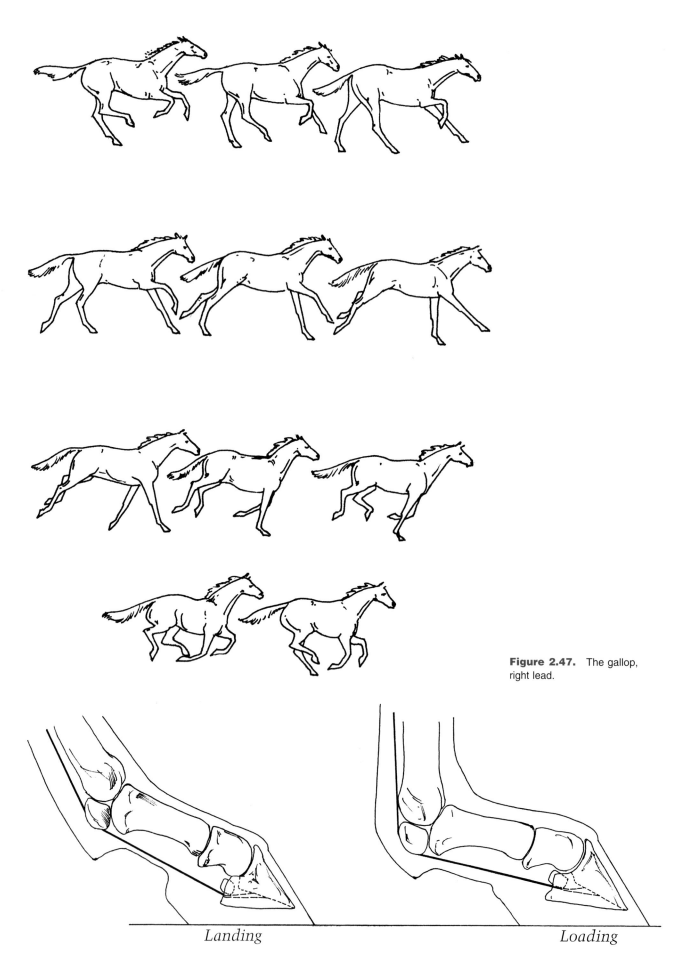

Figure 2.47. The gallop, right lead.

Landing

Loading

Figure 2.48. Phases of the stride: landing and loading (Reprinted with permission from Hill, C., Klimesh R. Horse Hoof Care. Storey Publishing. North Adams, MA, 2009.)

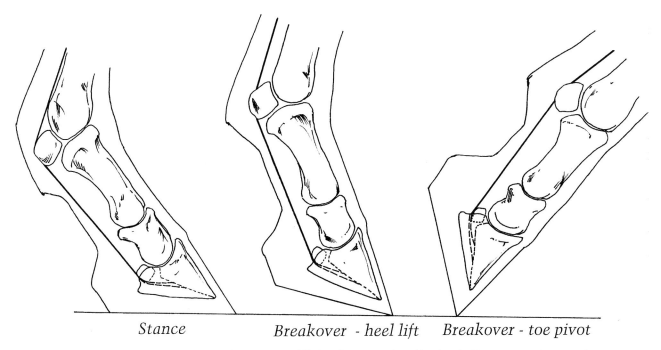

Stance   *Breakover - heel lift*   *Breakover - toe pivot*

Figure 2.49. Phases of the stride: stance, breakover-heel lift, breakover-toe pivot. (Reprinted with permission from Hill, C., Klimesh R. Horse Hoof Care. Storey Publishing. North Adams, MA, 2009.)

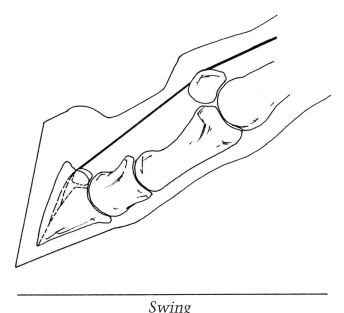

Swing

Figure 2.50. Phases of the stride: swing. (Reprinted with permission from Hill, C., Klimesh R. Horse Hoof Care. Storey Publishing. North Adams, MA, 2009.)

forefeet. This results in an uneven gait; the horse is first delayed behind and then hurries the movement of the hindlimbs.

The popular theory that long toes in the hind may make a horse reach farther forward has been discarded.[13] Rather than the hindlimbs reaching farther forward, the horse's mass moves farther ahead of the weight-bearing limbs before they leave the ground. This tends to put the cycle of the forelimb movement farther under the horse, thereby lessening the potential for (hindquarter) engagement.

Normal Movement

The straight foot flight pattern that is used as the basis when referring to deviations has often been termed "ideal." Such a foot flight is ideal only for a horse with ideal body and limb conformation. Horses with structural imperfections, which include virtually all horses, have individual ideal foot flight patterns that compensate for imperfections; such an individual pattern may not be "textbook pretty," but it may be functional. Instead of thinking of the straight foot flight as ideal, think of it as "standard," so that rather than representing a goal to strive for, the term indicates a baseline for comparison.

The standard for forelimb movement starts with a straight bony column and a series of hinge joints all symmetrically conformed and working in a true forward-backward plane. Add to this a balanced hoof, and the result should be a straight foot flight.

Because hindlimbs nearly always turn out to some degree, the standard for hindlimb foot flight is different than the front. Depending on the conformation of the hindquarters, this turning out of the limb facilitates a freer working of the stifle. The bone structure of a heavily muscled horse may, by genetic design, turn out to permit more drive and reach with the hindlimbs as well as to counteract the inward pull characteristic of a horse with heavy inside gaskin muscles.

Movement Abnormalities

"Gait defects" are movement abnormalities that consistently occur during regular work (Box 2.2).

FORGING (Figure 2.51)

Forging is a gait defect that is commonly heard when a horse is trotting. Forging occurs when a hindfoot contacts a front foot on the same side. Frequently, contact is made when the hindfoot is gliding in for a landing and the front foot is beginning its swing phase.

If the front foot is delayed in its break-over, the hindfoot may arrive before the foot has a chance to get out of the way. As the front fetlock begins flexing, the toe of the front shoe may swing back and slap the toe of the landing hind shoe. This creates a characteristic "clicking" sound as the shod horse trots and a dull "thwacking" sound if the horse is barefoot.

Forging customarily refers to the contact made between shoes or hoofs but is related to over-reaching. Over-reaching (Figure 2.52) usually indicates that a front shoe has been pulled off by a hind or that the

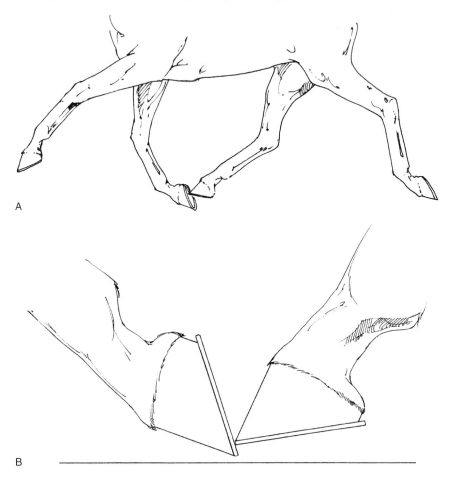

A

B

Figure 2.51. A. Forging at the trot; hindfoot and front foot on the same side make contact. B. Close-up of foot contact. (Reprinted with permission from Hill, C., Klimesh R. Horse Hoof Care. Storey Publishing. North Adams, MA, 2009.)

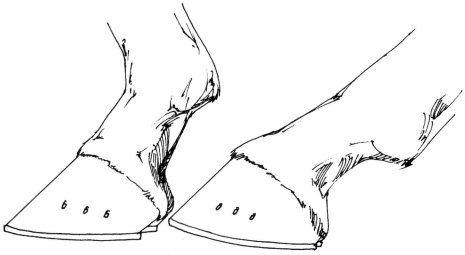

Figure 2.52. Overreaching or grabbing can occur when the front feet are delayed in breakover. (Reprinted with permission from Hill, C., Klimesh R. Horse Hoof Care. Storey Publishing. North Adams, MA, 2009.)

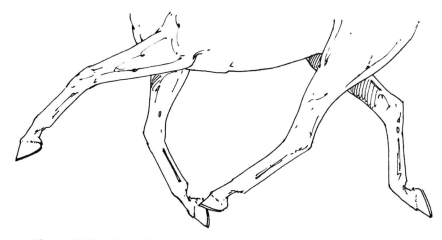

Figure 2.53. Cross firing at the pace; the hindlimb strikes the opposite forelimb.

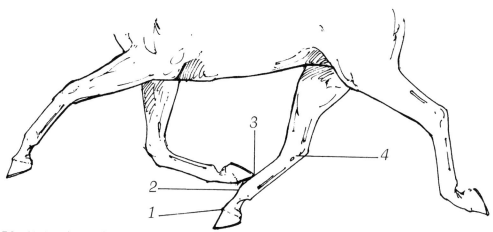

Figure 2.54. Various forms of hindlimb contact that can occur at the trot. (1) Scalping, (2) speedy cutting, (3) shin hitting, and (4) hock hitting.

hindfoot has injured some part of the forelimb such as the heel bulb or coronary band. A horse that forges or over-reaches may also be prone to stumbling or falling, especially at the moment when the shoe is stepped on or pulled off. If the conditions that cause a horse to forge are ignored or inadvertently perpetuated, the stride imbalances may progress to over-reaching. Other movement abnormalities include cross firing (Figure 2.53) and scalping (Figure 2.54).

Forging and over-reaching are indications that the horse's movement is out of balance. Balance is customarily discussed in terms of dorsal-palmar (DP) balance, left-right (LR) balance, and medial-lateral (ML) balance. DP balance can refer to the relationship between the front and rear of the horse's entire body as well as to the relationship between the toe and heel of the hoof. LR balance refers to the relationship between the left and right sides of the horse's body. There are inherent discrepancies in LR balance in most horses. ML balance is often used to describe the relationship between the two halves of a limb or hoof when viewed from the front or rear (Figure 2.55). The most graphic examples of ML imbalance are seen in the knees, hocks, fetlocks, and hoofs. These imbalances are implicated as causes

of gait defects such as winging in and paddling. Although LR and ML imbalances can be associated with forging and over-reaching, they are mainly attributed to DP imbalances.

A horse's balance during movement is affected by many factors: conformation, conditioning, energy level, mental attitude, footing, level of training, gait or maneuver being performed, proficiency of the rider, and shoeing. All of these factors can affect break-over, but the theoretical discussion of break-over usually deals with the function of one limb at a time. To correct forging, the timing and direction of break-over of all of the hooves must be coordinated so that the limbs work in harmony and avoid collision.

LATERAL GAIT DEFECTS

A lateral gait defect is one that involves a regularly occurring, abnormal sideways swing of a limb. Some lateral gait defects cause physical contact with an opposite limb; others do not. Paddling or dishing, often seen with bow-legged, toed-in, or wide-chested and base-narrow horses, is a swinging out of the limb from the midline so that contact rarely results. In contrast,

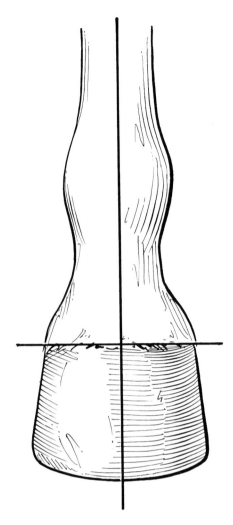

Figure 2.55. A hoof is considered to be in ML balance when an imaginary line through the coronet is parallel to the ground surface and perpendicular to a line that bisects the limb axis when viewed from the front.

interfering is frequently associated with narrow and/or toed-out horses. Such chest conformation places the limbs closer together and the toed-out hoof predisposes the horse to winging, i.e., swinging the limb toward the midline during flight. As one limb swings inward, it passes the opposite weight-bearing limb, and contact can potentially occur. The higher up the limb the turned-out deviation is located, the greater the torque that is imparted to the limb and the worse the winging-in will be. Swinging in of the limb, often called "brushing," is commonly referred to as "interfering" when contact between the two limbs is made.

Interfering occurs most commonly at the trot or any other type of two-beat diagonal gait. The speed and energy level of limb movement affects its tendency to interfere. One horse may interfere at a jog but not at the extended trot; another horse may move with adequate clearance at the jog but not at an energetic trot. Similarly, one horse performing a quiet rein back might place its limbs carefully, but if asked to speed up the limbs might swing from side to side and collide. Another

horse may work its limbs with piston-like precision while backing quickly and straight but might exhibit an altered foot flight if asked to slow down.

Interference can occur from the knee distally in the forelimbs and usually from the fetlock distally in the hindlimbs. Often the first signs of interference may be pain, heat, or swelling in the area of contact. The problem may escalate to include missing hair, bruises, cuts, chronic sores, and perhaps underlying bone damage. Additionally, a horse may sometimes show reluctance to perform certain maneuvers that have caused it to hit itself in the past. The horse may try to avoid circular or lateral work by stiffening the back and working with short hopping strides with the hindlimbs. With a reining horse, interference problems in the forelimbs may make it reluctant to add speed to its turnaround.

Factors that Affect Movement

There are many elements that affect a horse's movement. When lameness is a concern, the factors that are traditionally considered are lower limb conformation, pain, and shoeing. However, other factors should be considered because, in many cases, understanding the whole picture will result in a better treatment program and ultimately a more effective plan for lameness prevention.

CONFORMATION

There are no absolutes when it comes to predicting whether a horse will paddle, wing-in, or travel straight. Generalizations related to stance, breed, or type are frequently proven incorrect. Lateral gait defects can affect a pair of limbs or a single limb. Conformational components that should be evaluated in the front limb include shoulder to rib cage attachment, width of chest, width at knees, fetlock, and hoof, and straightness of forearm, cannon, and pastern regions. Normally, the fetlock and carpal joints work in a hinge-like fashion, backward and forward in a straight line, parallel with the horse's midline. An abnormally developed joint tends to hinge in a swivel-like motion at an angle to the horse's midline. This arc causes the limb to deviate in flight.

Many factors influence how close a horse's front and hind feet come together when it is moving: the relationship between the height at the wither and the height at the hip; the amount of muscling and the width of the chest and hips; the length, proportion, and shape of the top line components; the relationship between the length of the top line to the length of the underline; and, perhaps, most commonly, the length of underline to the length of the limbs. Horses with short backs and long limbs, and especially those with short forelimbs and long hindlimbs, are the most likely to have contact between the fore and hindlimbs.

PAIN

A horse with conformational traits that theoretically add up to straight travel may break all of the conformation rules if it experiences pain during movement. Horses usually attempt to use their limbs in a manner that creates the least stress and pain in any given area. An injury or soreness in a limb or an associated structure can cause a horse to protect one portion of the limb when landing, subsequently altering the arc of the foot's flight. For example, if the horse is sore in the navicular region of the front feet, instead of landing heel first and rolling forward, it may land toe first, which will shorten the stride.

When a horse is painful in a part of the body other than the hooves or limbs, its balance during movement may be negatively altered as it compensates for the soreness. For example, back soreness can mimic lower limb lameness problems and alter foot flight. A variety of other factors can cause the horse to carry its body in a stiff or crooked fashion (e.g., muscle cramping or poor fitting tack). Sometimes, the stiffness or pain is subtle but just enough to prevent the horse from tracking straight.

IMBALANCE

There are three forces at work when a horse moves: the vertical force of the weight of the horse and rider, the horizontal force of the horse moving forward, and the swinging or side-to-side motion of the horse at various gaits. Limb placement under its body is determined in a large part by the interaction of these three forces and the direction of their composite. Gait defects often occur simply because the horse is trying to keep its balance. The horse is attempting to keep its limbs under its center of mass. A barefoot horse moving free in a pasture rarely interferes. It is when a horse carries a rider and is asked to perform in collected and extended frames at both faster and slower speeds that interfering occurs most commonly.

A rider can make a horse move well or poorly. Rider proficiency determines how the horse distributes its weight (from front to rear and from side to side), how the horse changes the speed of the stride or the length of a stride within a gait, and how the horse adapts the stride when turning, stopping, and performing such maneuvers as lead changes. Inadequate riding skills can exaggerate the deficiencies in a horse's conformation and way of going. Because no horse moves perfectly at all times, it takes a knowledgeable and competent rider to compensate for a horse's shortcomings. A rider's balance and condition, as well as talent, coordination, and skill at choosing and applying the aids, greatly affect a horse's coordination. Morales performed kinematic analysis of elite riding horses and concluded that rider-effect must be taken into consideration when well-gaited horses are selected for dressage purposes.[33]

Inexperienced riders often ask a cold or poorly conditioned horse to do multiple things at once, such as come to a hard stop from a thundering gallop, make a sharp turn, and lope off in the opposite direction, without properly preparing the horse or helping him perform in a balanced fashion. When a horse is asked to do something he is not physically ready to do, such as a flying lead change, a deep stop, a fast burst out of the roping box, or a sharp turn, he can easily over-reach or interfere.

An unskilled rider can also throw off a horse's balance. Inexperienced riders often commit one or more of these imbalance errors: sit off to one side of the saddle, ride with one stirrup longer, ride with a twisted pelvis, lean one shoulder lower than the other, hold one shoulder farther back than the other, or sit with a tilted head. All of these postures can alter the horse's composite center of mass and cause the horse to make adjustments to stay balanced. Riders that let their horses ramble on in long, unbalanced frames, heavy on the forehand, also seem to have more forging problems. Some horses are able to compensate for an imbalanced rider without forging or interfering and others are not.

Some horses simply have an imbalanced way of going. Certain horses are uncoordinated, inattentive, and sloppy, whereas others move precisely, gracefully, and balanced. Training, conditioning, and conscientious shoeing can improve a poor mover's tendencies, but some horses, no matter how talented the rider and farrier, will consistently move in an imbalanced fashion.

SHOEING

Recent but improper shoeing can be responsible for gait defects. A long-toe, low-heel shoeing style predisposes a horse to forge and possibly interfere. When a horse is overdue for shoeing, the hooves have potentially grown out of balance enough to contribute to gait abnormalities and lameness. When a horse is shod the hoof wears mainly in the heel region, contributing to a lower hoof angle and increased extension of the coffin joint as the hoof grows.[7] Sound Warmblood horses were found to compensate for hoof conformation change during an 8-week shoeing interval, which led to increased extension of the distal interphalangeal joint and increased loading of the deep digital flexor tendon.[32] Sometimes, just going a week past the horse's needs can adversely alter gait synchronization and lameness originating in the foot.

FOOTING

The surface the horse is worked on directly affects its movement. Traction on dirt occurs when the horse's weight descends through the bony columns of the limbs, causing the hoofs to drop 0.5 inch or more into the ground. Simultaneously, the soil is cupped upward toward the sole. This occurs whether a horse is barefoot or shod. Shoes basically extend the hoof wall, creating a potentially deeper cup to the bottom of the hoof, therefore increasing traction in dirt or soft footing.

Ideal arena footing is light and does not stay compressed, so some dirt falls out of the hoof with every stride. Hard surfaces absorb little energy, shorten the impact time, and potentially contribute to a higher incidence of lameness.[7] In dry arenas, the moderate amount of dirt the shoe comes in contact with results in good traction. However, if conditions are damp to wet and the footing is heavy, the hooves may pack and mound, thereby decreasing stability and traction. Packed dirt left in for prolonged periods of time creates constant pressure on the sole and can cause sole and frog bruises. Therefore, for work in soft, wet, and/or deep footing, it is important for shoes to be self-cleaning. They should permit mud, manure, or snow to move out at the base of the frog. This will ensure that the horse has an open sole and maximum traction potential for each stride.

Heavy footing (sand, mud, snow, long grass) generally delays front foot break-over. If a horse must be worked on footing he is unaccustomed to, protective boots may be helpful. Bell boots and scalping boots may prevent injury to the heels and coronary bands. Over-reaching boots provide protection to the tendons.

TRACTION

In some instances, a horse requires greater traction than would be provided by a standard shoe. Generally, the wider the web of the shoe, the less traction the shoe provides. The extreme is the sliding plate, which can be more than 1 inch wide and allows the horse to "float" over the ground surface. Optimum traction can increase horse and rider safety, increase a horse's feeling of security so it will stride normally, and help a horse to maintain its balance in unstable footing such as mud, ice, snow, or rock.

Permanent calks, those driven into the shoe, forged into the shoe, or brazed or welded onto the shoe, provide good traction. However, such calks cannot be changed between shoeing and may lose their effectiveness as they wear down. Removable screw-in calks (studs) may be the best answer when performance requirements or footing are constantly changing. Event riders can use large studs for the cross country phase of competition and take them out or replace them with smaller studs for dressage and stadium jumping.

Jar calks (either rectangular or triangular pieces of steel) can be brazed on the shoes to prevent sideways slipping while allowing the hoof to slide forward on landing. They are usually applied at the heels and set in the direction of travel, not parallel to the sides of the shoe. However, if the goal is to decrease both sideways and forward/backward slipping, the jar calks can be placed parallel to the sides of the shoe.

Toe grabs, as the name implies, are placed on the front of the shoe. They are commonly used in racehorses to improve traction. Studies have documented that toe grabs are associated with increased odds of both non-fatal and fatal musculoskeletal injuries and specifically suspensory ligament problems in Thoroughbred racehorses.[20,25] Increasing the height of the toe grabs also was associated with increased odds of injury.[20,25] Conversely, horses shod with rim shoes appeared to have a decreased risk of injury.[25] The use of toe-grabs in racehorses has been banned in some states due to their potential to increase musculoskeletal injuries.

CONDITIONING AND LEVEL OF FITNESS

A horse's level of fitness and energy level affect its movement. In general, a horse has 15 minutes of peak performance whether in a daily work session or at a competition. The horse may be either approaching that peak period or coming away from it. A rider must know how to properly warm up a horse to establish the most

natural and efficient way of going for that horse; then the rider must assist (and not hinder) the horse in working in a balanced frame during the peak period. Finally, a rider must know how to gradually let the horse come down from its peak. A horse predisposed to forging or over-reaching may likely do so if:

1. It is permitted to dawdle around on the forehand during the warm-up
2. The bridle reins are pulled up suddenly and the horse is put to work when it is "cold"
3. Contact is "thrown away" all at once
4. Engagement is allowed to slip away during work
5. The horse is allowed to fall on its forehand immediately following the completion of its peak performance.

If a rider asks too much in relation to a horse's current physical capabilities or fitness level, many horses will attempt to adapt while complying. If overworked, many horses will continue to move forward but will modify their stride to minimize fatigue and discomfort to flexor muscles and tendons. One kinematic study done on unmounted and mounted horses at a walk before and after treadmill exercise concluded that strenuous workload significantly influenced kinematics, even at a walk, although each horse kept its characteristic gait pattern.[35] Gait defects can occur when a tired horse adjusts the timing of the various phases of its stride. If the hindquarters have not been properly conditioned and strengthened, a horse will rely heavily on the forehand for both propulsion and support. This makes it even harder for the already heavily weighted forehand to get out of the way of the incoming hindfeet.

Poor condition or fatigue may also cause a horse to fling its limbs aimlessly; the horse does not have the muscle strength or energy necessary to project its limbs in a controlled fashion. In some cases, when a lazy horse moves slowly at a trot, it may move sloppily and carelessly, causing him to occasionally interfere. Requiring such a horse to move out with more energy may smooth out gait defects. This situation can be interpreted as an exception to the general rule that an increase in speed usually brings an increase in the potential to interfere. The amount of weight that a horse is carrying can also exaggerate its lateral limb movements. An overweight horse or heavy rider may cause more side-to-side sway, which will alter the net force of forward movement.

AGE AND STAGE OF DEVELOPMENT

A study that evaluated longitudinal development of equine locomotion from foal to adult concluded that there is a high similarity and a good correlation between foal and adult locomotor variables.[4] Certain characteristics of jumping observed in 4-year-olds were already detectable when these same horses were foals.[34] These studies suggest that there may be a reasonably accurate prediction of adult kinematics from those recorded in foals.[4,34] However, young horses that do not have fully developed muscles may lack the width of chest, stifle, or hip that will prevent them from interfering once they are adults. The relationship between the inside (axial) and outside (abaxial) muscles also can affect how the limb swings. A horse with heavy outside gaskin muscling, especially if the hindlimbs toe-out, may have difficulty keeping its limbs under its body during a stop. This can be a major problem for a stock horse. There simply is not enough inside gaskin muscle power to counteract the outward rotation of the limb during the stop. To complicate things, this type of limb tends to wing inward during forward movement so interference might occur.

TRAINING

One of the main causes of intermittent gait defects is asking a horse to perform something beyond its level of training. One of the first goals of training is to teach a horse to track straight. Until a horse learns to decisively step up underneath itself, its travel is often wobbly and inconsistent. Working on circles and lateral maneuvers before a horse is balanced and supple can cause it to make missteps and interfere. Asking a horse to perform advanced movements such as the passage, canter pirouette, or turnaround before the horse is physically developed and trained can increase the possibility of interference. These movements are characterized by either higher action, greater speed, or a greater degree of joint flexion, all of which tend to increase rotational forces of the limb and the possibility of interference. Gait defects tend to surface with an increase in speed within a gait as well as the extension of a stride within a gait.

TACK

Poor-fitting saddles can be a cause of back pain and subsequently poor movement. If the tree is too narrow, it may compress the withers, contributing to muscle and ligament pain at the sites of their attachments. If the tree is too wide, it may cause the weight of the saddle and rider to be borne directly by the vertebrae (see Chapter 10 for more information). Additionally, bit-related problems may contribute to head shaking and other types of performance issues that may contribute to alteration in movement.

References

1. Anderson TA, McIlwraith CW. Longitudinal developmental of equine conformation from weanling to 3 years of age in the Thoroughbred. Equine Vet J 2004;36:571–575.
2. Anderson TA, McIlwraith CW, Douay P. The role of conformation in musculoskeletal problems in racing Thoroughbreds. Equine Vet J 2004;36:571–575.
3. Axelsson M, Bjornsdottir S, Eksell P, et al. Risk factors associated with hindlimb lameness and degenerative joint disease in the distal tarsus of Icelandic horses. Equine Vet J 2001;33:84–90.
4. Back W, Schamhardt HC, Hartman W, et al. Predictive value of foal kinematics for locomotor performance in adult horses. Res Vet Sci 1995;59:64–69.
5. Back W, Schamhardt HC, Barnveld A. The influence of conformation on fore and hind limb kinematics of trotting Dutch Warmblood horses. Pferdeheilkunde 1996;12:647–650.
6. Back W, Schamhardt HC, Hartman W, et al. Kinematic differences between the distal portions of the forelimbs and hind limbs of horses at the trot. Am J Vet Res 1995;56:1522–1528.
7. Back W. The role of the hoof and shoeing. In Equine Locomotion, Back W, Clayton HM, eds. WB Saunders, Philadelphia, 2001;135–166.
8. Beeman GM. Correlation of defects in conformation to pathology in the horse. Proceedings Am Assoc Eq Pract 1973; 19:177–197.
9. Beeman GM. Conformation of the horse; Relationship of form to function. Proceedings Am Assoc Eq Pract 2008;54;1–5.
10. Belloy E, Bathe AP. The importance of standardizing the evaluation of conformation in the horse. Equine Vet J 1996; 28:429–30.
11. Bushe T, Turner TA, Poulos PW, et al. The effects of hoof angle on coffin, pastern and fetlock joint angles. Proceedings Am Assoc Eq Pract 1987;33:729–738.
12. Clayton HM. Comparison of stride of trotting horses trimmed with a normal and a broken-back hoof axis. Proceedings Am Assoc Eq Pract 1988;33:289–298.
13. Clayton HM. The effect of an acute hoof wall angulation on the stride kinematics of trotting horses. Equine Vet J (Suppl) 1990; 9:86–90.
14. Clayton HM. Comparison of the stride kinematics of the collected, working, medium, and extended trot in the horses. Equine Vet J 1994;26:230–234.
15. Dalin G, Magnuson LE, Thafvelin BC. Retrospective study of hind quarter asymmetry in standardbred trotter and its correlation with performance. Equine Vet J 1985;17:292–296.
16. Dyson S, Murray R. Pain associated with the sacroiliac joint region: a clinical study of 74 horses. Equine Vet J 2003; 35:240–5.
17. Glade MJ, Salzman RA. Effects of hoof angle on hoof growth and contraction in the horse. J Eq Vet Sci 1985;5:45.
18. Gnagey L, Clayton HM, Lanovaz JL. Effect of standing tarsal angle on joint kinematics and kinetics. Equine Vet J 2006; 38:628–33.
19. Gomez Alvarez CB, Bobbert MF, Lamers L, et al. The effect of induced hindlimb lameness on thoracolumbar kinematics during treadmill locomotion. Equine Vet J 2008;40:147–152.
20. Hill AE, Stover SM, Gardner IA, et al. Risk factors for and outcome of noncatastrophic suspensory apparatus injury in Thoroughbred racehorses. Am J Vet Res 2001;218:1136–1144.
21. Holmstrom M, Magnusson LE, Phillipsson J. Variation in conformation of Swedish Warmblood horses and conformational characteristics of elite sport horses. Equine Vet J 1990; 22:186–193.
22. Holmstrom M, Phillipsson J. Relationship between conformation, performance and health in 4-year old Swedish Warmblood riding horses. Livestock Prod Sci 1993;33:293–312.
23. Holmstrom M, Fredricson I, Drevemo S. Biokinematic effects of collection on trotting gaits in the dressage horse. Equine Vet J 1995;27:281–287.
24. Holmstrom M. The Effects of Conformation. In Equine Locomotion, Back W, Clayton HM eds. WB Saunders, Philadelphia 2001;281–296.
25. Kane AJ, Stover MS, Gardner IA, et al. Horseshoe characteristics as possible risk factors for fatal musculoskeletal injury of thoroughbred racehorses. Am J Vet Res 1996;57:1147–52.
26. Kobluk CN, Robinson A, Gordon BG, et al. The effect of conformation and shoeing: A cohort study of 95 Thoroughbred racehorses. Proceedings Am Assoc Eq Pract 1990; 36:259–274.
27. Konen EPC, Velduizen AE, Brascamp EW. Genetic parameters of linear scored conformation traits and their relation to dressage and show jumping performance in the Dutch Warmblood riding horse population. Livestock Production Science 1995; 43:85.
28. Magusson LE, Thafvelin B. Studies on the conformation and related traits of Standardbred trotters in Sweden. IV: Relationship between conformation and soundness of Standard trotters. Thesis SLU Skara ISBN91-576-2315-5.
29. Marks D. Conformation and soundness. Proceedings Am Assoc Eq Pract 2000;46:39–45.
30. Mawdsley A, Kelly EP, Smith FH, et al. Linear assessment of the Thoroughbred horse: An approach to conformation evaluation. Equine Vet J 1996;28:461–467.
31. McIlwraith CW, Anderson TA, Douay P, et al. Role of conformation in musculoskeletal problems in the racing Thoroughbred and racing Quarter Horse. Proceedings Am Assoc Eq Pract 2003;49:59–61
32. Moleman M, van Heel MC, van Weeran PR, et al. Hoof growth between two shoeing sessions leads to a substantial increase of the moment about the distal, but not the proximal, interphalangeal joint. Equine Vet J 2006;38:170–174
33. Morales JL, Manchado M, Vivo J, et al. Angular kinematic patterns of limbs in elite and riding horses at trot. Equine Vet J 1998;30:528–533.

34. Santamaria S, Bobbet ME, Back W, et al. Evaluation of consistency of jumping technique in horses between the ages of 6 months and 4 years. Am J Vet Res 2004;65:945–950.

35. Sloet van Oldruitenborgh-Oosterban MM, Barnveld A, Schamhardt HC. Kinematics of unmounted and mounted horses at a walk before and after treadmill exercise Pferdeheilkunde 1996;12:651–655.

36. Stashak TS, Hill C. Conformation and movement. In: Adams' Lameness in Horses. Stashak TS ed. 5th ed. Lippincott Williams and Wilkins, Philadelphia. 2002;73–111.

37. Thompson KN. Skeletal growth-rates of weanling and yearling thoroughbred horses. J Anim Sci 1995;73:2513–2517.

38. Van Hell MC, van Weeren PR, Back W. Shoeing sound Warmblood horses with a rolled toe optimizes hoof-unrollment and lowers peak loading during break-over. Equine Vet J 2006;38:258–262.

Examination for Lameness

HISTORY, VISUAL EXAM, PALPATION, AND MANIPULATION

GARY M. BAXTER AND TED S. STASHAK

INTRODUCTION

Lameness is an indication of a structural or functional disorder in one or more limbs or the back that is evident while the horse is standing or at movement.[28] Lameness can be caused by trauma (single event or repetitive work), congenital or acquired anomalies, developmental defects, infection, metabolic disturbances, circulatory and nervous disorders, or any combination of these. The diagnosis of lameness requires a detailed knowledge of anatomy, an understanding of kinematics, and an appreciation for geometric design and resultant forces. It is important to differentiate between lameness resulting from pain and nonpainful alterations in gait, often referred to as "mechanical lameness," and lameness resulting from neurologic (nervous system) dysfunction.[1,28] Lameness due to pain is most common in the horse.

A complete lameness examination helps to differentiate among the many types of lameness problems in the horse. The objectives of a lameness examination are to determine:

1. Whether the horse is lame
2. Which limb or limbs are involved
3. The site or sites of the problem
4. The specific cause of the problem
5. The appropriate treatment
6. The prognosis for recovery

The steps to perform a routine or traditional lameness examination include:

1. Complete history including signalment and use
2. Visual exam of the horse at rest
3. Palpation of the musculoskeletal system including hoof tester examination of the feet
4. Observation of the horse in motion (usually at a straight walk and trot/lope followed by circling)
5. Manipulative tests such as flexion tests
6. Diagnostic anesthesia if necessary
7. Diagnostic imaging

Please refer to the accompanying DVD for further information about how to perform a lameness evaluation.

Palpation of the limbs and axial skeleton and hoof tester examination of the feet are usually performed prior to exercising the horse. However, some clinicians prefer to observe the horse at exercise prior to palpation of the musculoskeletal system. Diagnostic anesthesia and imaging often follow to document the location of the pain, specific cause of the problem, extent of injury, and prognosis for recovery.

ADAPTIVE STRATEGIES OF LAME HORSES

Horses adapt to lameness with compensatory movements of specific body parts.[5,6,33] With most lameness conditions, the horse attempts to "unload" the lame limb during weight-bearing or the stance phase of the stride. In a kinetic study of forelimb lameness, the vertical force peak had the highest sensitivity and specificity for lameness classification.[13] Horses accomplish this by abnormal movement of a body part (head nod or pelvic hike), weight shifting (to the contralateral or diagonal limb or torso), change in joint angles (lack of fetlock extension), and alterations in foot flight.[33] For example, hyperextension of the fetlock has been shown to be an indirect measure for the vertical ground reaction force

Adams and Stashak's Lameness in Horses, 6e, edited by Gary M. Baxter
© 2011 Blackwell Publishing, Ltd.

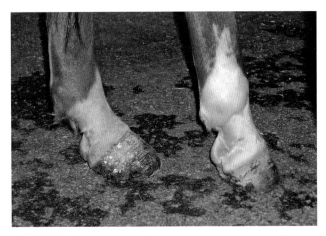

Figure 3.1. Chronic hindlimb lameness that has resulted in a wide flat foot on the sound left hindlimb and a narrow, upright hoof on the lame right hindlimb.

and is reduced in the lame limb at the stance phase proportionally to the degree of lameness.[4,23,33] In addition, in horses with chronic lameness, the limb with the flatter hoof exhibits higher vertical loads because it is the non-lame limb (Figure 3.1).[33] Detecting these compensatory movements is an integral part of diagnosing lameness in the horse. The most consistent compensatory movements that are observed are the vertical displacement and acceleration of the head in forelimb lameness and of the sacrum and tuber coxae in hindlimb lameness.[3,33] Although overlap of these movements can occur (head movement with hindlimb lameness and pelvic movement with forelimb lameness), they tend to occur primarily in moderate to severe lameness. In addition, more subtle lameness causes fewer compensatory changes, making lameness diagnosis more difficult, and problems within the axial skeleton (back) may also alter the movement of the limbs.[12,33]

Four compensatory mechanisms determined by quantitative gait analysis have been reported to reduce structural stress (peak vertical force) on the lame limb at a trot:[33]

1. With increasing lameness, horses reduce total vertical impulse/stride by increasing stride frequency.
2. The diagonal vertical impulse decreases selectively in the lame diagonal, causing a faster transition time from the lame to the sound diagonal. The vertical trunk movement is reduced on the lame limb.
3. The limb impulse shifts to the lame diagonal with forelimb lameness and to the contralateral hindlimb with hindlimb lameness. This corresponds to changes in the body center of mass movement.
4. The rate of loading and the peak forces are reduced by prolonging the stance duration. This occurs in the lame limb and in the contralateral limb to neutralize the extra force it will receive from unloading the lame limb.

Although some of these gait changes may be difficult to appreciate during visual examination of a lame horse, it should be remembered that the primary adaptive strategy of the horse is to redistribute load to compensate for pain in a limb without causing an overload situation in other limbs.[33]

CLASSIFICATION OF LAMENESS

There are a variety of ways to classify lameness in the horse. In most cases there is a primary or baseline lameness that contributes to the most obvious gait abnormalities. Compensatory, secondary, or complementary lameness results from overloading of the other limbs as a result of the primary lameness.[24] Lameness may also be classified according to when it occurs (or is best observed) within the stride. The different classifications of lameness are defined below.

1. Supporting limb lameness: Apparent when the foot first contacts the ground or when the limb is supporting weight (stance phase). Injury to bones, joints, soft tissue support structures (e.g., ligaments and flexor tendons), and the foot are considered causes of this type of lameness. This is by far the most common type of lameness identified in the horse.
2. Swinging limb lameness: Evident when the limb is in motion. A variety of pathologic changes may be the cause, and the majority of these problems are thought to involve the upper limbs or axial skeleton.[28]
3. Mixed lameness: Evident both when the limb is moving (swing phase) and when it is supporting weight (stance phase). Mixed lameness can involve any combination of structures affected in swinging or supporting-limb lameness.
4. Primary or baseline lameness: Most obvious lameness or gait abnormality that is observed before flexion or manipulative tests.[24] This can be complicated by lameness in multiple limbs, but in most cases the lameness that is the worst is considered the primary lameness. Evaluation of the primary lameness should be performed initially before scrutinizing complementary lameness problems.
5. Compensatory or complementary lameness: Pain in a limb can cause uneven distribution of weight on another limb or limbs, which can produce lameness in a previously sound limb. It is common to have complementary lameness produced in a forelimb as a result of lameness in the opposite forelimb.[28] Also, a lameness in a hindlimb can result in lameness in the opposite forelimb (e.g., left hind and right fore) or can mimic a forelimb lameness on the ipsilateral side (right hind and right fore). Quantitative lameness evaluations suggest that an apparent lameness in the forelimb and hindlimb on the same side often suggests a primary hindlimb lameness and a false compensatory forelimb lameness.[18] Additionally, lameness in one hindlimb may contribute to lameness in the opposite hind.

Even minor changes in weight-bearing can produce complementary lameness at high speeds, especially over long distances. The feet, suspensory ligament, sesamoid bones, hocks, and flexor tendons seem to be affected most commonly.[28] Complementary lameness in the same limb usually results when excess stress occurs to an otherwise healthy structure in an attempt to protect a painful region in that limb. For example, a horse with navicular syndrome often lands toe first, potentially contributing to toe bruising and/or pedal osteitis.

By observing the gait from a distance, one can usually determine whether the lameness is supporting-limb,

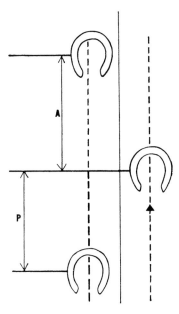

Figure 3.2. Phases of the stride. A. The cranial phase of the stride is the half of the stride in front of the print of the opposite foot. P. The caudal phase of the stride is the half of the stride in back of the print of the opposite foot.

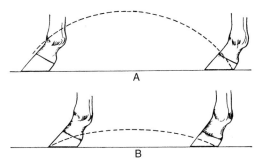

Figure 3.3. A. Normal arc of the foot flight. B. Low arc of foot flight caused by lack of flexion in either the forelimbs or hindlimbs.

swinging-limb, or mixed. Some conditions that cause supporting-limb lameness may cause the horse to alter the movement of the limb to protect the foot when it lands. This can be mistaken for swinging-limb lameness. Because of this and other adaptive strategies that occur in lame horses, some clinicians feel that mixed lameness occurs most commonly in horses.[24]

Character of the Stride

The character of the stride of a limb is important to the diagnosis of lameness. When observing the stride, the following characteristics should be observed:

The Phases of the Stride: The stride consists of a cranial phase and a caudal phase. The cranial phase of the stride is in front of the footprint of the opposite limb, and the caudal phase is behind it (Figure 3.2). With lameness, the cranial or caudal phases may be shortened. If the cranial phase is shortened, there may be a compensatory lengthening of the caudal phase, and vice versa.

Alterations in phase of the stride are best viewed from the side of the horse. Potential causes for a short-ened cranial phase of the stride include navicular syn-drome, joint problems such as osteoarthritis (OA), trauma to the extensor tendons, shoulder problems, gonitis, and bone spavin. Causes of shortened caudal phase of the stride include digital anular ligament des-mitis and tendonitis or tenosynovitis involving the flexor tendons.[28]

The Arc of Foot Flight: The arc of foot flight (Figure 3.3) is changed when there is pain anywhere in the limb. The arc of one foot is compared to that of the opposite member when viewed from the side. In some cases, the arc is changed in both forefeet (bilateral navicular syn-drome, laminitis) or in both hindfeet (bilateral bone

spavin). In the hindlimb, the arc may be changed enough to cause the toe to drag when the limb is advanced because of reduced flexion of the hock or stifle joints. In some lameness, the horse will overflex the lame limb while leaving the sound limb as close to the ground as possible; thus, the sound limb has a decreased height of the foot flight arc.

Most horses exhibiting a decrease in height of the foot flight arc also show alteration in their phase of stride. For subtle alterations in the hoof flight arc of the hindlimb, it is sometimes helpful to observe the horse from the rear to compare the extent and duration that the horse presents the solar surfaces of both feet to the observer. In general, the less sole that can be seen, the lower the arc of foot flight in the limb.[28]

The Path of the Foot in Flight: If the foot travels inward, it may cause an interference problem (e.g., trauma to the medial aspect of the limb). When the foot travels in an outward path (paddling), no special problem usually results. However, if paddling does develop, it may be a sign of bilateral carpal pain.

How the Foot Lands: When a painful condition is present in the foot, the horse usually indicates the pain by placing its weight opposite to the pain. For example, with pain in the heel region, the horse may only toe-touch. If the lesion is in the lateral portion of the sole, the weight is carried on the medial side of the foot, and vice versa.

Joint Extension: The degree of extension of the fetlock (how close the back of the fetlock approaches the ground) during weight-bearing is a sensitive indica-tor of how much weight the horse is willing to bear on that limb. Reduction in fetlock extension during weight-bearing usually indicates the lame limb (Figure 3.1). This sign can be observed at a walk and/or a trot.

Joint Flexion Angles: Joint flexion angles are best viewed from the side and may or may not be associated with alterations in the hoof flight arc and phase of stride. One limb is compared to the other and the degree of flexion is assessed. In some cases, horses compensate with an increased flexion of the unaffected limb.

Symmetry and Duration of Gluteal Use: To identify hindlimb lameness, it is helpful to observe the horse from the rear to compare the symmetry and duration of gluteal use and to correlate these findings with altera-tions in the character of the stride viewed from the side.

Head and Pelvic Movement: Horses use their pelvis or hemi-pelvis with hindlimb lameness similar to how they use their head and neck with forelimb lameness. Both are used as a method to "unweight" the lame limb and the amount of movement of each is often proportional to the degree of lameness. Movement of the head and pelvis (or hemi-pelvis) are best observed from the side and should be correlated with gait changes.

Other Lameness Factors

It is generally considered that the majority of lameness problems in horses occur in the forelimb due to the increased weight-bearing on the forelimbs (60% to 65%) and the shock of landing that the forelimbs absorb during movement.[28] The hindlimbs propel the horse during movement and carry less of the overall weight. This results in greater concussion to the structures of the forelimbs. However, breed and use can alter this typical relationship. For instance, horses that pull carts or perform events such as dressage, cutting, and reining, which place greater stress on the hindquarters, often have a higher percentage of hindlimb lameness. Many hindlimb lameness problems involve the hock and/or stifle. Horses within a discipline that do different activities may also have different limbs that are affected most commonly. For instance, horses used for heading in team roping have more problems in the right forelimb and horses used for heeling have more bilateral hindlimb lameness problems.[8] Although there is considerable overlap, common lameness conditions that are associated with the specific type of work should be suspected first (Table 3.1). See Chapter 9 for further information on occupation-related lameness conditions.

It is also believed that approximately 95% of lameness in the forelimb occurs distal to the carpus.[28] Close evaluation of the distal limb should be performed in any horse with forelimb lameness before considering an upper limb problem, unless a more proximal condition is obvious. In the hindlimb, approximately 80% of lameness problems are thought to involve the hock or stifle.[28] Therefore, after preliminary examination of the foot and distal limb, the hock and stifle should be closely evaluated until conditions of those two regions can be eliminated. In many cases, diagnostic anesthesia can be very helpful to rule in or rule out problems in these commonly affected sites.

Multiple other factors that may contribute to lameness should also be considered. Horses that are improperly or irregularly shod may become lame. Surfaces that are too soft, too hard, slippery, or rocky may aggravate conformational imperfections or may be the outright cause of lameness. Improper conditioning resulting in muscle fatigue is considered to be a common cause of performance-related injuries. Young horses in work may develop lameness problems more easily than older horses due to the immaturity of their musculoskeletal system. With the emphasis on racing and showing 2-year-olds, many lameness problems may be produced that would not occur in older, more mature horses.

SIGNALMENT AND USE

Patient age and use are important considerations when determining potential lameness conditions. For example, an aged crossbred horse used for ranch work, occasional rodeo performance, and trail riding will have a higher incidence of problems associated with the forefeet, low motion joints (e.g., pastern and distal tarsal joints), and ligaments. In contrast, a young racehorse will often have lameness problems associated with high motion joints (e.g., carpus and fetlock), sprain/strain of flexor support structures, and stress-related fractures. Horses used for competitive trail or endurance riding often sustain a higher incidence of sprain/strain injuries, tendonitis, and stress-related fractures to the phalanges. Young cutting horses appear to be prone to stifle issues and any young horse just beginning training may become lame from developmental orthopedic-related problems.

HISTORY (ANAMNESIS)

A detailed medical history should be obtained on every horse. Records should include specific information regarding the duration and intensity of the lameness, the symptoms, the activity immediately preceding the lameness, and any previous treatments or therapies employed. The following questions should be answered:

1. How long has the horse been lame? (Acute vs. chronic injury.)
2. Has the horse been rested or exercised during the lameness period? (The horse may not exhibit the same lameness if it has been rested.)
3. Has the lameness worsened, stayed the same, or improved? (May indicate severity of the problem.)
4. Was the cause of the lameness observed? (This should include the character of the lameness at the onset.)
5. Does the horse warm out of the lameness?
6. What treatment has been given, and was it helpful? (Response to treatment may help predict the prognosis of the case but may also mask the severity of lameness and give a false impression of recovery.)
7. When was the horse last shod or trimmed? (Lameness directly after shoeing may suggest that the feet were trimmed too short or a nail was driven into or near sensitive tissue.)

LAMENESS EXAMINATION

Visual Examination at Rest

A careful visual examination is made with the horse standing squarely on a flat surface at rest.[1,28] This should be done at a distance and then up close, viewing the horse from all directions. From a distance, the body type is characterized (stocky vs. slender); conformation is noted; and body condition and alterations in posture, weight shifting, and pointing are also noted. It is important to look for changes in contour of the limbs and asymmetry between limbs.

Under normal circumstances, the forelimbs bear equal weight and are opposite each other. With bilateral forelimb involvement the weight may be shifted from one foot to the other, or both limbs may be placed too far out in front of the horse. In the hindlimbs, it is normal for the horse to shift its weight from one limb to the other. If the horse consistently rests one hindlimb and refuses to bear weight on it for a length of time or

Table 3.1. Occupation-related lameness problems (See Chapter 9 for further information.)

Occupation	Lameness Conditions
TB and QH racehorse (Fatigue-associated repetitive overuse)	Foot bruising, quarter cracks, heel pain Forelimb fetlock synovitis and fractures Carpal synovitis and fractures Bucked shins in young horses Fatigue/stress fractures—MC/MT, P1, humerus, tibia, pelvis SDFT tendonitis Suspensory injuries Coffin joint arthrosis—QH Proximal suspensory desmitis—QH Catastrophic fractures—sesamoids, P1, MC/MT, and humerus Distal tarsitis/OA
STD racehorse (hindlimb > forelimb)	Front feet bruising and corns Hindlimb fetlock synovitis and fractures Carpal synovitis and fractures (C3) Fatigue/stress fractures—similar to TB and QH but tibia most common SDFT tendonitis Suspensory injuries, especially PSD Hock, stifle, and sacroiliac problems
Endurance horse	Muscle disorders including tying-up and muscle spasm, cramps, and strains Forelimb and hindlimb suspensory desmitis Foot bruising, pedal osteitis, and laminitis Fetlock synovitis/OA SDFT tendonitis
Show/pleasure horse	Navicular syndrome/disease Coffin joint synovitis/OA Forelimb and hindlimb PSD Distal tarsitis or bone spavin Reverse angle of P3 in hind feet Lumbar and sacroiliac problems
Western performance horses (Cutting, reining, roping, barrel racing, rodeo, gymkhana, and ranch horses)	Navicular syndrome/disease Phalangeal fractures (primarily P2) Pastern ringbone Fetlock and carpal synovitis/OA Distal tarsitis or bone spavin Stifle synovitis/OA Forelimb and hindlimb PSD Thoracolumbar myositis Hindlimb muscle strains
Jumping/dressage/eventing	Navicular syndrome/disease including DDFT injuries Suspensory branch injuries Forelimb and hindlimb PSD Fetlock synovitis/OA SDFT tendonitis Distal tarsitis or bone spavin Stifle injuries Thoracolumbar myositis—back problems Sacroiliac problems
Draft horses	Hoof cracks and laminitis Subsolar abscesses, canker, and thrush Ringbone Sweeny Bone and bog spavin Stifle synovitis/OA Shivers and PSSM

TB, Thoroughbred; QH, Quarter horse; STD, Standardbred.
P1, first phalanx; P2, second phalanx; P3, third phalanx; MC/MT, metacarpus/metatarsus; C3, third carpal bone; PSD, proximal suspensory desmitis; SDFT, superficial digital flexor tendon; OA, osteoarthritis; PSSM, polysaccharide storage myopathy.

cannot be forced to bear weight on it at all, lameness in that hindlimb should be considered.

At close observation, each limb and muscle group should be observed and compared to its opposing member for symmetry. Feet are observed for abnormal wear, hoof cracks, imbalance, size, and heel bulb contraction (Figure 3.4). All joints and tendons and their sheaths are visually inspected for swelling and the muscles of the limbs, back, and rump are observed for swelling and atrophy. Comparing one side to the other is most important. Each abnormal finding should be ruled out as a cause of lameness during exercise and palpation examination. For the forelimbs, the limb with the narrowest (smallest) foot and highest heel with varying degrees of extensor muscle atrophy is usually

the lame or lamest (if the problem is bilateral) limb. The foot is smaller due to chronic alteration in weight-bearing and the muscle atrophy results from a reluctance to extend that limb. For the hindlimb, atrophy of the middle gluteal and/or gracilis muscles usually indicates the lame limb (Figures 3.5 and 3.6). Generally, if one tuber sacrale is higher than the other and/or the pelvis appears tilted, the horse will usually have an asymmetrical gait (Figure 3.7).

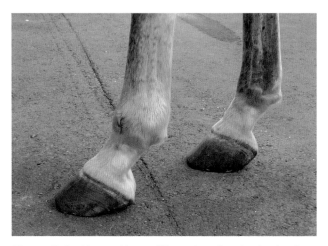

Figure 3.4. Horse with two different front feet: low heel and long toe on the left fore and a more upright hoof conformation on the right front. Unlike many horses with this hoof conformation, this horse was lame on the left forelimb.

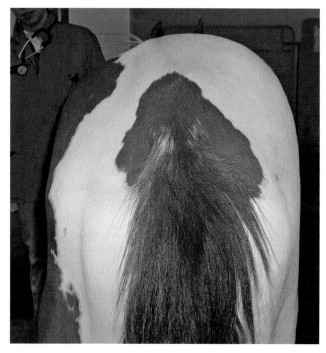

Figure 3.6. Example of atrophy of the gluteal muscles (left hindlimb) that often accompanies pelvic fractures in horses.

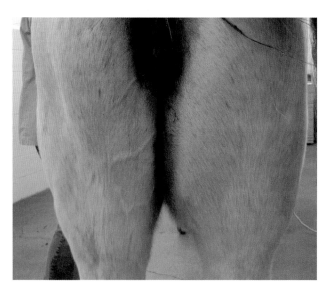

Figure 3.5. Example of atrophy of the inner and outer thigh muscles of the left hindlimb that occurred secondary to an upper hindlimb lameness.

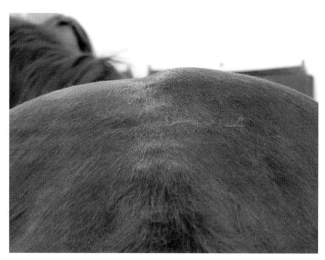

Figure 3.7. Rear view of the pelvis of a horse with a history of an acute onset of right hind lameness. There is asymmetry to the sacroiliac region visible and pain on firm palpation of the right tuber sacrale.

Visual Exam at Exercise

Visual examination of the horse at exercise focuses on the gait characteristics of all limbs and is usually performed from a distance. In most cases, it is best to observe the forelimbs first, and then the hindlimbs. Once a person is able to accommodate his eyes to observe all limbs at once, then each limb individually, the diagnosis of lameness is simplified. In most cases, the horse is observed at exercise without removing the shoes, although the shoes can be removed if necessary.

The main objective in exercising the horse is to identify the limb or limbs involved and the degree of lameness and/or incoordination in movement. The horse should be observed at a walk and trot in a straight line, then while lunging in circles. Foot placement is usually best observed from the side with the horse at a walk, and from the front or rear with the horse walked toward or away from the observer, respectively. In general, forelimb lameness is best viewed from the front and side, and hindlimb lameness is best observed from the side and rear. The examiner is looking for head nodding, gait asymmetry, alterations in height of the foot flight arc, alterations in foot flight, length of stride, joint flexion angle, foot placement, degree of fetlock extension with weight-bearing, action of the shoulder musculature, symmetry in gluteal rise and use, and movement of the pelvis, hemi-pelvis, and croup. The two most important concepts in lameness detection in the horse are the "head nod" for forelimb lameness and the "pelvic hike or rise" for hindlimb lameness.[3,24,33] Kinematic gait analysis indicates that maximal vertical acceleration of the head and displacement amplitude of the tuber sacrale are the best indicators to quantify a forelimb and hindlimb lameness, respectively.[3] In both scenarios the horse tries to unweight the lame limb by elevating the head and neck for a forelimb problem and elevating the pelvis or hemi-pelvis and croup for a hindlimb problem. However, objective analysis of lame horses suggests that elevation of the head and neck and pelvic hike may only occur in horses with substantial forelimb and hindlimb lameness.[14-16]

Abnormal movement of the head and pelvis and other gait abnormalities are best viewed at a distance from the front, side, or rear of the horse. An overall impression of how the horse moves should be obtained initially by paying close attention to movement of the head and neck and pelvis and croup. The action of all four limbs should then be observed followed by the limb in question. It is important to observe the opposite limb for a comparison. For subtle gait changes, it may require visual shifting from one limb to the other and back again. In some cases, it is helpful to observe the horse while being ridden or driven, or at speed on a treadmill. Because of the logistics of training a horse to use the treadmill, most horses are evaluated further while in work instead of on a treadmill. Videography of the horse at work, especially if it can be viewed in slow motion, may also be used to detect subtle abnormalities that are not present on a routine lameness examination.[6] Gait analysis is also possible but is not commonly performed because of the special equipment that is needed.[6,15-17] Methods to objectively measure lameness in the horse are covered later in this chapter.

How to Handle the Horse

The handler or "jogger" plays a very important role in lameness evaluation. In general, horses should be held loosely with their heads centered in line with their bodies, and exercised at a constant speed in a straight line as slowly as practical. Movement of the head and neck from side to side often results in an asymmetric gait. If the handler holds the horse too tightly, subtle head nodding is difficult to observe. Fast trotting or cantering makes it more difficult to focus on limb movement, but in some cases, it maybe helpful in identifying a neurologic deficit because more coordination is required for movement at speed. Additionally, the handler should not look at the horse and should be far enough in front of the forelimbs so as not to obscure the examiner's view.

Circling a horse at a trot usually accentuates low-grade lameness on the inside limb. This can be done by the handler jogging in a circle or preferably by lunging the horse in a circle. The horse should be relaxed at a trot, starting with a large circle that gradually gets smaller. The smaller circle will sometimes reveal lameness not seen in a larger circle. Horses with bilateral forelimb lameness not seen at a trot in a straight line will often show lameness on the inside limb. This is manifested when the lame limb contacts the ground by head and neck lifting, splinting the shoulder muscles in anticipation of weight-bearing and by placing the head and neck to the outside of the circle to unweight the lame limb. In some cases horses will attempt to make a square out of the circle or act up or stop periodically when circled to the lame side. If the lameness persists or is exaggerated when the limb is on the outside of the circle one should consider high suspensory ligament desmitis, collateral ligament injury, medial carpal problems, medial splint bone problems, or medial sesamoid bone problems.[28] Circling usually accentuates the lameness on the inside limb with many hindlimb lameness problems as well. However, this generalization is less consistent in the hindlimb compared to the forelimb. A more delayed protraction of the limb, a shorter cranial phase of the stride, and a greater degree of unweighting of the limb (pelvic hike and lack of extension of the fetlock) are often seen. A toe drag may also become more apparent in a circle than at a straight trot.

If the horse is flighty or apprehensive, the examination can be facilitated by the administration of 10 to 20 mg of acepromazine IV or IM to a 450-kg horse.[1,28] The tranquilization allows the horse to relax, making the lameness more apparent, and should not alter the severity of the lameness. This is particularly true for painful conditions that alter the gait. Alternatively, the horse may be sedated with romifidine to perform nerve blocks, and then reversed with yohimbine to permit re-evaluation of the lameness. If the horse is unbroken it can be encouraged to move in a round pen without the assistance of a handler. When dealing with a foal, the dam can be exercised and the foal examined as it follows the mare.

Selection of Surfaces

In most cases, the evaluation of lameness is best carried out on a hard level surface. A hard surface provides more concussion than a softer surface, and it affords the examiner the opportunity to listen to as well as visualize foot placement. There is usually an obvious difference in the horse's landing between the unsound and sound foot. The unsound foot makes less noise because less weight is taken on that foot and often results in a "clip-clop" sound. This is true for both the forelimbs and hindlimbs. Because hard surfaces typically do not apply sole and frog pressure, horses with suspected foot problems can be exercised on dirt, turf, or gravel (short distance) surfaces to accentuate the lameness. This is particularly true of horses with chronic symmetric conditions involving the feet. When exercised on asphalt, they may travel with a stilted, shuffling-like gait but appear comfortable. When placed on gravel, a bilateral lameness may become quite evident. Foot placement is also best observed on hard surfaces because softer surfaces tend to envelop the foot, making placement more difficult to see. This is especially true when evaluating medial-to-lateral foot balance.

The Forelimbs

Observations that may be used to detect forelimb lameness include:

1. Head and neck movement or "head nod"; head up on the lame limb or head down on the sound limb
2. Tensing of the shoulder musculature: shoulder of lame limb fixes or "props" just before it hits the ground
3. Alterations in height of the foot flight arc
4. Alterations in foot flight (paddling, winging-in, etc.)
5. Length of stride (cranial or caudal)
6. Joint flexion angles
7. Degree of fetlock extension or "drop" with weight-bearing
8. Front-to-back rocking of torso
9. Gait asymmetry—asymmetric side-to-side motion
10. Sound differences between lame and sound limb

Most forelimb lameness is best viewed from the side, paying close attention to head and neck movement, the shoulder musculature, and length of the stride. With an obvious lameness in a forelimb, the head will drop when the sound foot lands and rise when weight is placed on the unsound foot or limb. However, the severity of head and neck movement may be greatly attenuated in horses with bilateral forelimb lameness (such as those with navicular disease). If trotted on a hard surface, the sound foot will produce a louder sound when it contacts the ground. Additionally, splinting of the caudal neck and shoulder muscles in anticipation of weight-bearing on that limb may be seen. The cranial phase of the stride is often reduced with bilateral forelimb lameness and with problems in the upper limb (shoulder).

In the normal gait, the heel is lifted first when the limb is advanced. When the foot lands, the hoof should land flat or the heel should hit just before the toe. Selective weight-bearing and alteration in the phases of stride may be observed when pain involves one region of the foot. If pain is present in the lateral portion of the foot, the weight may be taken medially. In general, pain in the toe region causes a shortened caudal phase of the stride, whereas involvement of the heel region of the foot causes a shortened cranial phase of the stride.[28]

The arc that the foot makes in flight may suggest the site of pain in the limb (Figure 3.3). If the foot flight is too low in the forelimb, there may be interference with flexion of the shoulder, knee, or fetlock due to pain or mechanical injury. Fixation of these joints reduces the arc of the foot flight, limits the cranial phase of the stride, and lengthens the caudal phase. With shoulder problems, the scapulohumeral joint usually remains semi-fixed when the limb is advanced (swing phase of stride), and the head may show marked lifting and may be pulled toward the unaffected side. With bilateral forelimb involvement, the gait often appears unanimated (stilted or stiff), giving the false impression of shoulder involvement.

Multiple factors such as conformation, shoeing, and lameness may contribute to contact problems in the limbs of horses. However, contact problems can occur in well-shod horses with good conformation as a result of the type of work they are performing. For instance, in barrel racing, cutting, pole bending, and reining, the horse's weight is suddenly shifted and the horse may be off balance, resulting in uncoordinated movement and contact. Various forms of limb contact are defined as follows: (See Chapter 2 for more information.)

1. Brushing: General term for light striking, especially as in interfering.
2. Cross-firing: Usually consists of the inside of the hindfoot hitting the inside quarter of the diagonal forefoot.
3. Elbow hitting: When the elbow is hit with the shoe of the same limb, and may be seen in horses with weighted shoes.
4. Forging: The toe of the hind foot hits the sole or shoe of the forefoot on the same side. It can also be described as the front sole or shoe slapping the toe of the hind foot as it comes gliding in for a landing.
5. Knee hitting: A case of high interference, generally seen in gaited horses.
6. Interfering: Can occur in both the fore- and hindfeet. It is a striking, anywhere between the coronary band and the cannon bone, by the opposite foot that is in motion.
7. Over-reaching: The toe of the hindfoot catches the forefoot on the same side, usually on the heel. The hindfoot advances more quickly than in forging, stepping on the heel of the forefoot, and may cause shoe pulling.
8. Scalping: Here the toe of the forefoot hits the hairline at the coronary band or above on the hindfoot of the same side. It may hit the dorsal (front) face of the pastern or cannon bone.
9. Speedy cutting: Speedy cutting is difficult to determine and can literally be defined as any type of limb interference at fast gaits. It may be the same as cross-firing or it may mean that the outside wall of the hindfoot comes up and strikes the medial aspect of the forelimb on the same side.

The Hindlimbs

Observations that may be used to detect hindlimb lameness include:

1. "Pelvic hike or rise"—Upward movement of the pelvis or hemi-pelvis and croup on lame limb; unweighting of lame limb and shifting of weight to sound limb.
2. Excess vertical displacement of tuber coxae or croup—More movement on one side than the other.
3. Alterations in height or arc of foot flight.
4. Head and neck movement; head down on the lame limb; only in substantial hindlimb lameness and often accompanied by a pelvic hike resulting in a rocking horse motion.
5. Length of stride (cranial or caudal phase).
6. Gluteal rise and gluteal use.
7. Hip hike or hip roll.
8. Reduced flexion of lame leg (joint angles).
9. Degree of fetlock extension or "drop" with weight-bearing.
10. Drifting away from lame limb.

There is much confusion as to what to observe for in horses with hindlimb lameness. In addition, there is more subjectivity in evaluating hindlimb lameness than forelimb lameness. Many clinicians most likely observe the same thing but refer to it as something different. For instance, the rapid elevation of the hip and gluteals recognized as a "hip hike" or "upward flick" on the affected side is most likely the same thing as the "pelvic hike" that others refer to. One set of clinicians prefers to focus on what happens on the lame limb (one side of the pelvis)[28] while others prefer to look at the entire pelvis or hemi-pelvis.[24] In both scenarios, the horse is attempting to get off the lame hindlimb more quickly, shift weight to the opposite hindlimb, and unweight the limb. This usually causes upward movement of the pelvis and croup, gluteal muscles, and tuber coxae, resulting in a "pelvic hike," "hip hike," "gluteal rise," "upward flick," and more movement of the tuber coxae.

All of these terms most likely describe the same observation that is similar to what we do when we are lame. However, it is important to remember that the upward movement of the pelvis, hemi-pelvis, hip, or tuber coxae in hindlimb lameness is the clinical impression of the change in height and not necessarily the absolute or measured height. In addition, most horses that are trying to unweight a hindlimb will have reduced gluteal muscle contraction, which may lead to a shortened duration of gluteal use and a subsequent "hip roll" or hip "drop off."[28] The stance phase is shortened giving the impression that the hip drops more on the lame limb. In a study of hindlimb lameness by May, the lame hip was often not elevated above the hip on the sound side (6 cases were elevated, 7 cases were not elevated).[20] In fact, the midpoint of the vertical displacement for each hip marker was lower in the lame limb in all 13 cases. However, the croup (gluteal rise) was always higher when the lame limb started to bear weight.[20] This may explain the confusion as to whether the hip hikes up or drops off in the lame hindlimb.

Some clinicians prefer to place markers (usually tape) on the tuber coxae or gluteal muscles and observe for asymmetrical movement between the hindlimbs. The limb with more total movement as viewed from behind is usually the lame limb. The asymmetry of the gluteal rise and duration of gluteal use (movement of the croup)

are also best evaluated from the rear. The rise is evident during the swing phase of the stride; the use is evident during the support (stance) phase of the stride.[28] A symmetric gluteal rise as the hindlimbs are brought forward indicates that both limbs are swinging symmetrically and subsequently are elevated to the same height. On the other hand, the duration of gluteal use is a function of weight-bearing with subsequent contraction of the gluteal muscles as the limb moves from cranial to caudal during weight-bearing (support/stance phase of the stride). Stashak has described 3 different scenarios between gluteal rise and gluteal use in horses with hindlimb lameness:[28]

1. A depressed gluteal rise and a decreased use. This is usually seen in horses that are in pain during the swing phase of the stride. Often structures above the stifle are involved. Along with muscle atrophy, this gait is commonly seen with problems involving the hip and/or sacroiliac regions.
2. A symmetric gluteal rise but a decreased gluteal use. This is usually seen in cases with subtle hindlimb lameness. Head nodding is usually not seen and only subtle changes in the height of the foot flight arc, phase of stride, and flexion angles may be observed.
3. A rapid and increased gluteal rise ("hip hike" or "upward flick") in which the affected limb gluteal is brought up rapidly, and the duration of gluteal use is shortened. This situation is usually seen in horses that are in considerable pain during the support phase of the stride. Varying degrees of head nodding will be seen, and the height of the foot flight arc, phase of stride, and flexion angles are usually altered.

Observation of pelvic hike or movement of the hemi-pelvis is often best performed from the side in a similar manner to observing head and neck movement. A line or marker at a constant height in the background can be a useful reference point to view upward and downward movement of the head and pelvis. The severity of pelvic hike is usually proportional to the severity of the lameness; therefore, pelvic hike may be difficult to observe in horses with subtle lameness. The severity of pelvic hike may also be attenuated in horses with bilateral hindlimb lameness. Observation of subtle pelvic hike can sometimes be facilitated by observing the horse from the front using the horse's topline as a frame of reference.[24] However, objective lameness evaluations of lame horses suggests that pelvic hike may only occur in horses with severe hindlimb lameness.[14,18] Because of the difficulties of "seeing" subtle lameness, more objective methods to evaluate lameness, especially hindlimb lameness, are being developed.[17,18] (These methods are discussed in the section on objective assessment of lameness.)

The arc of the foot flight in the hindlimb is best viewed from the side (Figure 3.3). Problems with the hock and stifle generally reduce the arc of the foot flight and thereby shorten the cranial phase of the stride with a compensating lengthening of the caudal phase. Because of the reciprocal apparatus of the hock and stifle, incomplete limb flexion is characteristic of involvement of both joints. The toe may also be worn excessively with involvement of the hock or stifle.

Although head and neck movements can be observed from the rear, they are best viewed from the side at the trot. With mild hindlimb lameness, abnormal movements of the head and neck are usually not evident. In moderate to severe lameness, the head and neck will rise as the unaffected hindlimb contacts the ground and lower when the affected hindlimb contacts the ground. In severe cases, horses will not only lower their head and neck but will also extend their head. The lowering of the head and neck reduces the weight placed on the affected hindlimb when it contacts the ground. Movement of the head and neck in horses with severe hindlimb lameness is nearly always accompanied by a pelvic rise producing a "rocking horse" type motion.

Forelimb vs. Hindlimb Lameness

When observing head and neck movement at the trot one must be cautious not to confuse a left hind lameness with a left fore lameness, or a right hind lameness with a right fore lameness. In most cases a hindlimb lameness will mimic a forelimb lameness on the ipsilateral side, not the diagonal forelimb.[18,24,28] This could occur when a hindlimb is lame at the trot because the horse will often land more solidly on the sound opposite forelimb. For example, if a left hindlimb is lame at the trot, the horse will lower its head when the left hind and right fore land, taking more weight on the right fore. On a hard surface, this gives the impression that the horse is yielding or has upward head movement on the left fore, suggesting lameness in that limb. Keegan suggests that an ipsilateral fore- and hindlimb lameness suggests a primary hindlimb lameness, whereas contralateral fore and hind lameness suggests primary forelimb lameness or lameness in both limbs.[18] Careful attention to the pelvis and croup can help differentiate between primary forelimb and primary hindlimb lameness. There should be minimal to no movement of the pelvis (no pelvic hike, hip hike, or gluteal asymmetry) in horses with a forelimb lameness at a straight trot or when circled.

Occasionally, left hindlimb lameness may be confused with right forelimb lameness. This usually occurs in cases in which there is little or no head movement at the trot. The non-lame diagonals (right hind and left fore) contact the ground with such force that it appears that the horse is protecting the right forelimb. Most confusion occurs when watching the horse from the side view. Observing it from behind usually reveals the hip and pelvic asymmetry typical of hindlimb lameness. Head movement may also be absent with bilateral involvement of the limbs, especially forelimb lameness, or with mild lameness.

GRADING/SCORING THE LAMENESS

The degree of lameness should be recorded as part of a complete medical record. Although using mild, moderate, and severe may suffice, a more objective approach using a grading system is recommended. A lameness grading system is not only beneficial because it defines the degree of lameness, but it also makes record keeping easier and it provides the examiner with an objective reference to assess improvement at reevaluation. However, just as the determination of lameness

Table 3.2. AAEP grading system.[29]

Grade	Description of Lameness
0	Lameness is not perceptible under any circumstances.
1	Lameness is difficult to observe; not consistently apparent regardless of circumstances (i.e., weight carrying, circling, inclines, hard surface, etc.).
2	Lameness is difficult to observe at a walk or in trotting a straight line; consistently apparent under certain circumstances (i.e., weight carrying, circling, inclines, hard surface, etc.).
3	Lameness is consistently observable at a trot under all circumstances.
4	Obvious lameness: marked nodding, hitching, or shortened stride.
5	Minimal weight–bearing in motion and/or at rest; inability to move.

is somewhat subjective, so is grading or scoring the lameness. This subjectivity increases with milder lameness. In a study that evaluated lameness on a treadmill, scoring of lameness was more repeatable by experienced clinicians than residents and interns.[15] However, scoring of mild lameness as detected by kinematic gait analysis was not reliable even by experienced clinicians. Another study indicated that the reliability of lameness scoring was good intra-assessor, but not as good inter-assessor.[11] However, scoring of a change in lameness was reliable throughout the study.[11]

Many grading systems exist but there is no universally accepted approach. A 5-point scale and a 10-point scale are used most commonly. The lameness grading system recommended by the American Association of Equine Practitioners (AAEP) is used by the author and is outlined in table 3.2.[29] Although this system is useful, it has limitations because it grades lameness at both a walk and a trot.[24] In addition there are inconsistencies with the different grades. For example, horses that are not lame at the trot but are consistently lame in the circle, by definition should be considered a grade 2. However, many clinicians would consider them as a grade 1 because of the lack of lameness at a straight trot. As long as the same veterinarian is interpreting the scale the same way, then accurate re-assessment of a lame horse is possible. However, multiple clinicians with multiple interpretations of the same grading scale make accurate comparisons difficult.

Palpation and Manipulation

Palpation of the musculoskeletal system is a very important aspect of the lameness evaluation. With experience, subtle abnormalities can be detected that are often indicative of the site of the problem. The authors usually perform a thorough palpation of the patient prior to observing it at exercise. Most manipulative tests

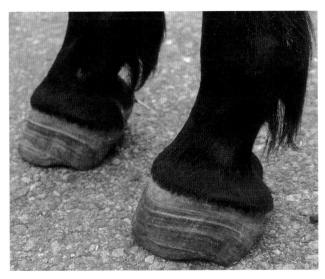

Figure 3.8. Bilaterally symmetrical hoof wall rings that were not associated with lameness or any other known problem within the hoof wall.

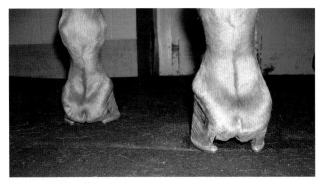

Figure 3.9. View of both front feet in a horse with forelimb lameness. The front feet of the same horse as viewed from the side is illustrated in Figure 3.10. The medial wall of the right foot is concave with the coronary band pushed proximally suggesting excessive concussion. In addition the heels are contracted and overgrown.

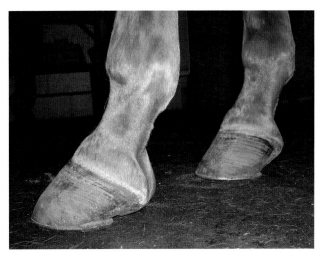

Figure 3.10. Front feet of the horse in Figure 3.9 as viewed from the side. The front feet have markedly different hoof angles. The right foot has contracted heels resulting in a very upright conformation compared to a low under-run heel with a long toe on the left foot resulting in a low hoof conformation. In addition, the coronary band on the right has an abnormal contour suggesting foot imbalance.

are performed after exercise. A systematic approach of palpation is recommended to avoid missing abnormalities. The first author palpates the forelimb proximally to distally with it weight-bearing, and then distally to proximally with the limb picked up or unweighted. Palpation of the hindlimbs is performed in the same manner, paying close attention to the medial aspects of the stifle and tarsus. The back and axial skeleton are palpated last because some horses become agitated with manipulation of the back. Hoof tester examination of the feet is usually performed after the entire musculoskeletal system has been palpated. The following discussion briefly describes how to visually examine and palpate the different anatomic regions of the equine musculoskeletal system.

Foot

The size and shape of the foot on the lame limb should be compared to its opposite member. The examiner is looking for asymmetry in foot size, abnormal hoof wear, ring formation and heel bulb contraction, shearing of the heels and quarters, hoof wall cracks, swellings that are primarily associated with the coronet, and foot imbalances.[28,31] Asymmetry in foot size may be a result of trauma, lack of weight-bearing leading to contraction, and congenital or developmental defects. In general, the limb with the smallest foot is usually the lame limb. Hoof wall ring formation can be unilateral (trauma) or bilateral (selenium toxicosis, laminitis, or systemic disease) and is not always associated with lameness (Figure 3.8). Heel contraction often results from decreased weight-bearing of the affected limb and is usually a symptom rather than the cause of the lameness (Figures 3.9 and 3.10). Visual examination of heel bulb contraction is best performed with the examiner standing or squatting near the flank and looking at both right and left heel bulbs at once (Figure 3.9). Asymmetry in heel bulb height (sheared heels) is most frequently associated with improper trimming and shoeing. Hoof wall cracks may or may not be associated with lameness but should be ruled out with hoof tester examination and in some cases nerve blocks. Swellings at the coronary band can result from superficial scar formation from wire cuts, constant bruising during exercise, or from deeper involvement (e.g., gravel, keratoma, or quittor). Foot imbalances can either be dorsopalmar/plantar (D-P), lateral medial (LM), or a combination of the two (Figures 3.9 and 3.10). These imbalances often alter the shape of the hoof wall and can result in abnormal stresses applied to the foot and other support structures.

After superficial cleaning of the sole, abnormal wear of the shoe and/or sole, collapsed heels, heel bulb contraction, and frog atrophy should be noted (Figure 3.11). Secondary frog atrophy may accompany heel

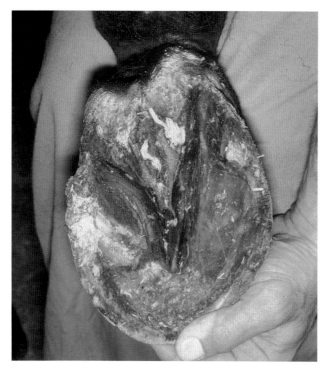

Figure 3.11. A hindfoot with overgrown bars and heels that have resulted in atrophy of the frog. The frog should be prominent and approximately level with the widest part of the heels.

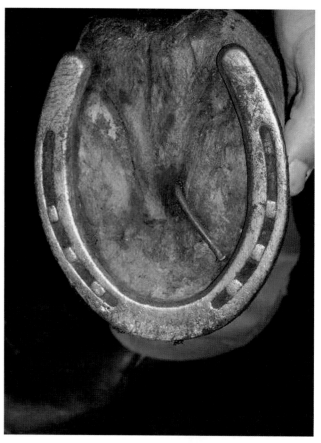

Figure 3.12. This horse presented for an acute onset hindlimb lameness. A nail was found protruding from the apex of the frog. Based on the location, entry into the navicular bursa would be unlikely.

contraction in chronic cases. The shape of the sole should be observed. A slightly concave shape is normal. Some horses are flatfooted and therefore predisposed to sole bruising. Convexity dorsal to the apex of the frog ("dropped soles" in front of the frog) is considered abnormal and is often associated with rotation of the distal phalanx. In some cases, the offending cause of lameness may be identified immediately, such as a nail wedged in the frog (Figure 3.12). However, the clefts of the frog may need to be opened with a knife to properly evaluate the depths of the sulci for evidence of thrush or canker.

A hoof tester is an instrument that permits deep palpation of the sole, frog, and wall of the hoof (Figure 3.13). When applied properly, the examiner tries to identify and localize hoof sensitivity. Most normal horses should be able to withstand a fair bit of hoof tester pressure without showing signs of discomfort. The arm of the hoof tester that is applied to the hoof wall is continually checked so pressure is not being applied to the coronary band.

The order of hoof tester application is less important than being systematic and complete. One method is to begin at the lateral or medial angle of the sole and continue hoof tester pressure at 2- to 3-cm intervals until the entire surface of the sole is checked. This is followed by pressure applied to the frog (caudal, central, and cranial) from both the medial and lateral heel. Lastly, the hoof tester is applied to the hoof wall across the heels, and then it can be applied diagonally from the medial heel to the dorsolateral hoof and then from the lateral heel to the dorsolateral hoof. If sensitivity is encountered, it is necessary to confirm whether the response is from pain and not just a whimsical reaction

by the horse. Repeatability is the key to being confident with your findings. True sensitivity is identified by repeated intermittent hoof tester pressure that results in persistent reflexive withdrawal (flexing the shoulder) with hoof tester pressure. Obviously varying amounts of hoof tester pressure are applied to elicit a response, and this is dependent on sole thickness and the painfulness of the condition. Hoof tester responses should be compared to those obtained from the opposite foot.

In general, diffuse sole sensitivity may suggest a sagittal fracture of the distal phalanx, diffuse pedal osteitis, and in some cases laminitis. More localized hoof tester sensitivity is usually obtained with corns, sole bruising, puncture wounds, close or hot nail, and localized subsolar abscesses or gravel. Hoof tester sensitivity over the central third of the frog usually suggests navicular syndrome and/or sheared heels and quarters (Figure 3.14). Pain across the most cranial portion of the frog may indicate a problem at the attachment of the deep digital flexor tendon to the distal phalanx.[28] Pain across the heels without pain over the frog suggests bruised heels, sheared heels, contracted heels, or other problems related to shoeing. Any other region of sensitivity associated with cracks or abnormal discoloration of the sole may need to be explored with a hoof knife.

A hoof tester or a hammer can also be used to strike (percuss) the hoof wall. If this is painful, laminitis or

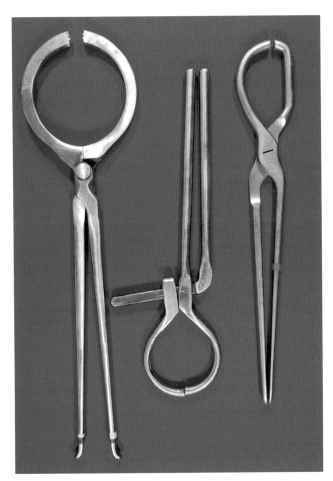

Figure 3.13. Examples of several types of hoof testers. Left, GE Forge and Tool Works, 959 Highland Way, Grover Beach, CA, 93433. Middle, Ryding Hoof Tester, Jorgenson Labs, 2198 W 15th St., Loveland, CO, 80537. Right, Kane Enterprises, AG-TEK Division, P.O. Box 1043, Sioux Falls, SD, 57101.

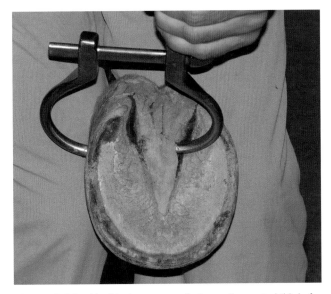

Figure 3.14. Hoof testers are applied over the central third of the frog of the forefoot to produce direct pressure over the navicular region. The authors prefers the Ryding Hoof Tester.

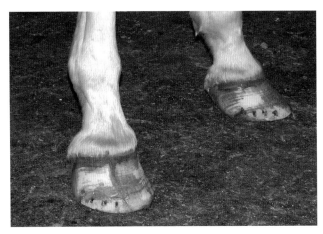

Figure 3.15. Partial-thickness dorsal hoof crack associated with a long toe and a concavity of the dorsal hoof wall. Both factors most likely contributed to the development of the crack in this horse.

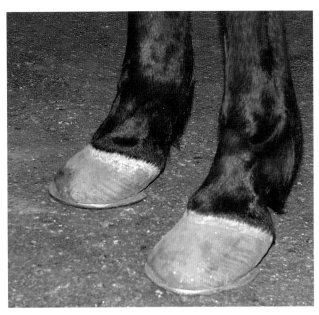

Figure 3.16. Concavity of the left front foot in a horse with chronic laminitis. This horse was most lame in the left forelimb.

gravel may be the problem. If a hollow sound is heard over the dorsal hoof wall, there is probably a separation between the sensitive and insensitive laminae (e.g., white line disease or incomplete avulsion of hoof wall). The hoof wall is checked for cracks that may extend into the sensitive laminae (they are most common in the toe and quarter), uneven wear, and excessive dryness (Figure 3.15). Dishing (concavity) of the dorsal aspect of the hoof wall is often indicative of chronic rotation of the distal phalanx or a flexural deformity involving the deep digital flexor tendon (Figure 3.16).

The coronary band should be palpated for heat, swelling, and pain on pressure. A generalized increase in the temperature of the coronary band of both limbs is consistent with laminitis, whereas selective swelling with or without pain on deep palpation just dorsal and

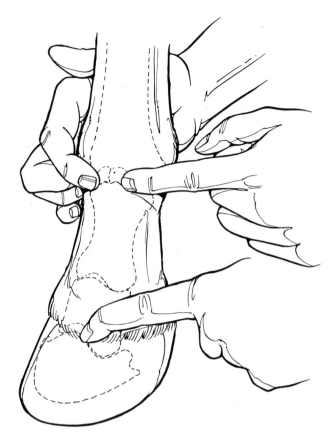

Figure 3.17. Lower finger marks the site of swelling and pain associated with fracture of the extensor process. Upper fingers are applied over the dorsal aspect of the fetlock to identify synovial distention and thickening of the joint capsule.

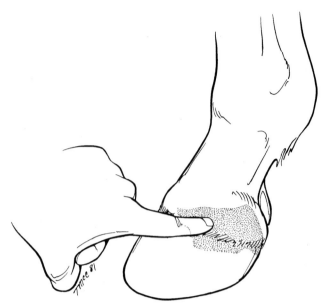

Figure 3.18. Finger marks area in which gravel and/or quittor occurs. Signs of inflammation and drainage are common in affected animals.

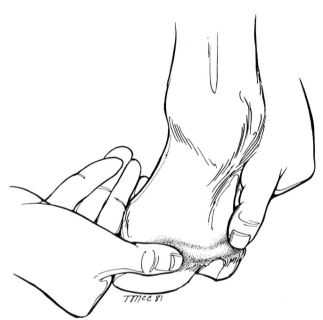

Figure 3.19. Palpation of the heel bulbs to identify heat, pain, and swelling that may be associated with subsolar abscesses.

proximal to the coronary band may suggest effusion of the distal interphalangeal joint (Figure 3.17).[9] Firm, often nonpainful swelling in this region may also be evidence of low ringbone. Point swelling and pain with or without drainage at the coronet in the mid-quarter region may indicate an abscess along the white line or infection of the collateral cartilage of the distal phalanx if the swelling is more diffuse (Figure 3.18). Heat, pain, and swelling with or without drainage of one of the heel bulbs are often found in horses with subsolar abscesses (Figure 3.19). Most penetrating wounds not involving the white line or navicular bursa that develop into an abscess eventually break out in the heel bulb region. In situations in which a small puncture hole in the sole has been identified, hoof tester pressure adjacent to the hole may force pus out of the hole, confirming the presence of a subsolar abscess.

Pastern

The dorsal, medial, and lateral surfaces of the proximal interphalangeal (PIP) joint should be palpated for enlargement and heat, which may indicate ringbone (Figure 3.20). Comparison to the opposite pastern is always recommended. However, it is not uncommon to have the lateral to medial dimensions of one pastern to be slightly larger than its opposite member. With the limb off the ground, the distal sesamoidean ligaments and flexor tendons (superficial and deep digital flexors) are palpated deeply for pain, heat, and swelling (Figure 3.21). Particular attention is paid to the lateral and medial branches of the superficial digital flexor tendon (SDFT) as they attach to the middle phalanx. Tendonitis of the deep digital flexor tendon (DDFT) and/or tenosynovitis of digital flexor tendon sheath (DFTS) are often identified by swelling, effusion, and sometimes pain in this region (Figure 3.22). Deep palpation of the lateral and medial eminences (wings) of the middle

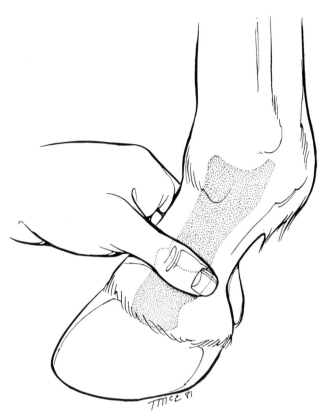

Figure 3.20. Palpation of the pastern. Thickening in this region may suggest the presence of ringbone.

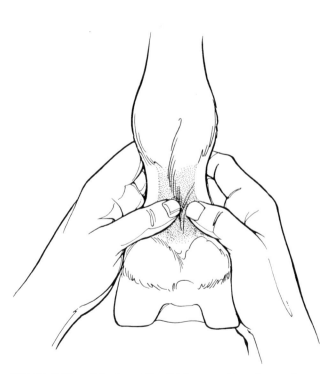

Figure 3.21. Palpation of the distal sesamoidean ligaments, branches of the superficial digital flexor tendon, and the deep digital flexor tendon in the palmar/plantar aspect of the pastern.

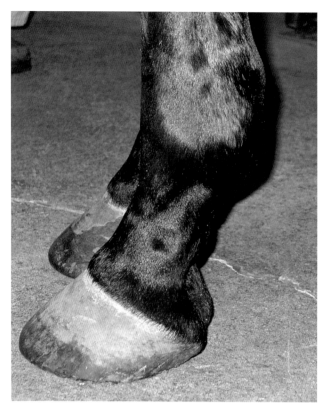

Figure 3.22. Horse with effusion of the digital flexor tendon sheath that had a prominent outpouching of fluid in the palmar pastern region.

phalanx may elicit pain if a fracture is present. With the hands placed on the hoof wall, the phalangeal joints should be rotated medially and laterally. Pain can often be elicited with OA or with proximal and middle phalangeal fractures. The collateral ligaments can be stressed, laterally and medially, by placing one hand lateral or medial over the pastern joint while the other hand is used to pull the foot toward that side (Figure 3.23). This bending force creates increased tension on the collateral ligaments of the phalangeal joints.

Fetlock

The dorsal and palmar/plantar joint pouches of the metacarpophalangeal/metatarsophalangeal joint should be palpated for swelling, effusion, or thickening of the joint capsule. These abnormalities may indicate idiopathic synovitis, chronic synovitis/capsulitis secondary to osteoarthritis, or any type of articular fracture (Figures 3.17 and 3.24). Pressure should be applied to the lateral and medial branches of the suspensory ligament just above their attachments to the proximal sesamoid bones. Pain and swelling may indicate desmitis, sesamoiditis, or apical/abaxial fractures of the sesamoid bone. The superficial and deep digital flexor tendon and digital sheath should be palpated for heat, pain, swelling, or effusion (Figure 3.25). Some distention of the digital flexor tendon sheath of all four limbs is not uncommon in performance horses. This often is referred to as "wind puffs." The annular ligament should be palpated for evidence of constriction.

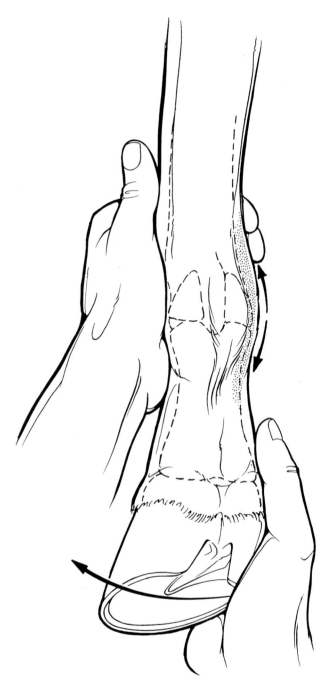

Figure 3.23. Tension is applied to the collateral ligaments supporting the fetlock and interphalangeal joints (pastern and coffin) to identify pain.

With the limb off the ground, thumb or finger pressure is applied to the basilar, body, and apical portions of the proximal sesamoid bones (Figure 3.26). Sensitivity and pain may indicate a sesamoid fracture or desmitis of the suspensory ligament. The fetlock is rotated and the collateral ligaments are checked in a similar manner to that of the pastern joint (Figure 3.23). Additionally, the fetlock joint should be passively flexed to identify pain and assess the range of motion. This is done by extending the carpus as much as possible and flexing the fetlock by placing one hand on the pastern (Figure

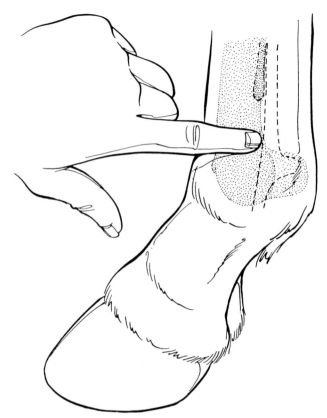

Figure 3.24. Finger marks the palmar recesses of the fetlock joint capsule. Distention at the site results from synovial effusion.

3.27). This technique flexes the fetlock joint separate from the phalangeal joints in contrast to all of the joints of the distal limb (Figure 3.28).

Metacarpus/Metatarsus (MC/MT)

Palpation of the dorsal aspect of the metacarpus should be performed, especially in racehorses. Firm pressure applied with the fingertips often elicits a painful response in horses with dorsal metacarpal disease (buck shins). Heat and swelling over the dorsal middle third of the metacarpus may also be present (Figure 3.29). The extensor tendons on the dorsal surface of the MC/MT should be palpated for swelling, thickness, and pain, especially in horses with a history of trauma/laceration to this region. Scarring of the extensor tendon is more common in the MT than the MC and is often an incidental finding.

The entire length of each small metacarpal/metatarsal bone (splint bone) should be palpated for heat, pain, and swelling with the limb weighted and unweighted. With the limb elevated the palmar/plantar and axial surfaces of the splint bones can be palpated by pushing the suspensory ligament toward the opposite side (Figure 3.30). The splint bone can be palpated with the thumb applying pressure as needed. Heat, pain, and swelling may indicate a fracture or a condition referred to as "splints" if located in the proximal aspect of MCII. Splint fractures most commonly involve the medial splint bone in the forelimb and the lateral splint

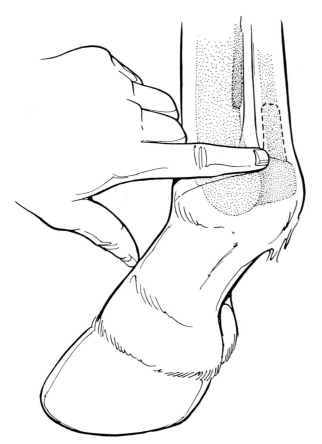

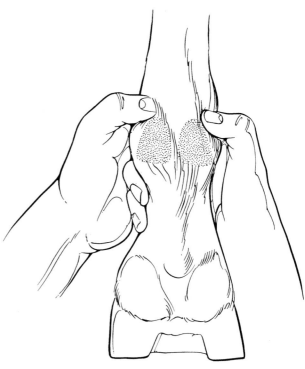

Figure 3.26. Digital pressure applied to the apical sesamoid region to detect pain, heat, and asymmetry. Palpation of the midbody and basilar aspects of the bones should also be performed.

Figure 3.25. Palpation of the digital flexor synovial sheath around the superficial and deep digital flexor tendons is performed behind the branch of the suspensory ligament. Synovial distention of the sheath is often referred to as wind puffs.

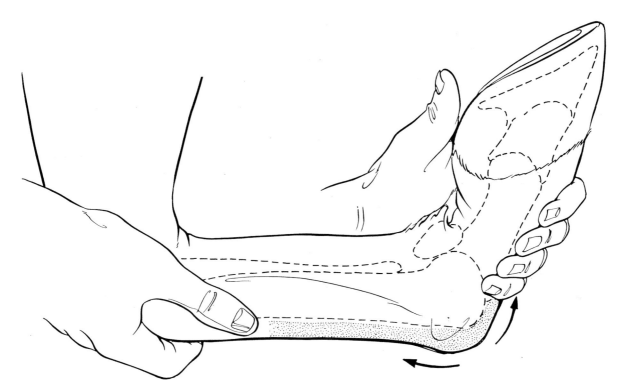

Figure 3.27. Fetlock flexion test is performed by extending the carpus and flexing the fetlock joint. One hand is placed on the dorsal aspect of the pastern to create fetlock flexion without flexion of the interphalangeal joints.

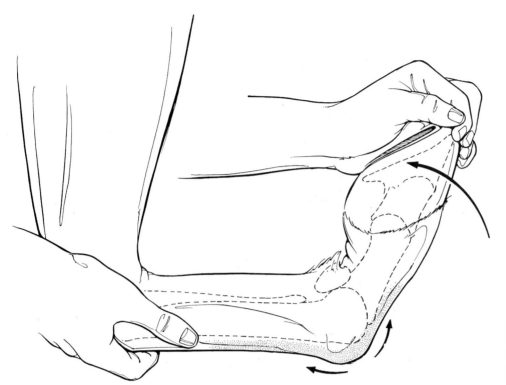

Figure 3.28. Distal limb flexion test in which the interphalangeal (pastern and coffin) and fetlock joints are flexed simultaneously.

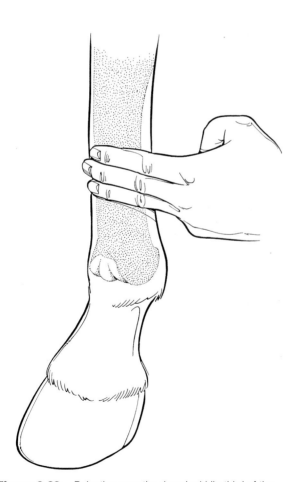

Figure 3.29. Palpation over the dorsal middle third of the metacarpus to identify heat, pain, and swelling associated with dorsal metacarpal disease.

bone of the hindlimb. A chronic splint bone fracture associated with excessive swelling and pain presenting with a history of recurrent drainage usually indicates infection/sequestration. It is not uncommon to palpate nonpainful enlargements of the splint bones which are often incidental findings. However, many middle and proximal splint bone fractures heal with excessive callus that may contribute to lameness.

Suspensory Ligament

The suspensory ligament (interosseus medius muscle) lies just palmar/plantar to the splint bones in the metacarpal/metatarsal groove. It should be palpated with the limb weight-bearing and with the limb flexed. Deep palpation is often needed to identify swelling and pain, and comparison between the lateral and medial branches may be helpful.[10] Damage to the suspensory tends to occur distally within the branches of the suspensory ligament or at its proximal attachment to the MC/MT. However, secondary suspensory desmitis may be associated with a healing splint fracture anywhere along its length. With the limb held in a flexed position, the proximal attachment of the suspensory ligament to the MC/MT can be palpated by pushing the flexor tendons to the side and applying pressure with the thumb (Figure 3.31). Alternatively, pressure can be applied to this region by placing the palm of the hand on the dorsal MC and wrapping the fingers around the medial side of the MC. The fingertips are used to "squeeze" the limb and apply pressure to the proximal palmar MC region (Figure 3.32). Many horses may react initially by withdrawing (flexing) the limb. However, with constant pressure this response often fatigues. A painful withdrawal that persists (does not fatigue) may indicate a

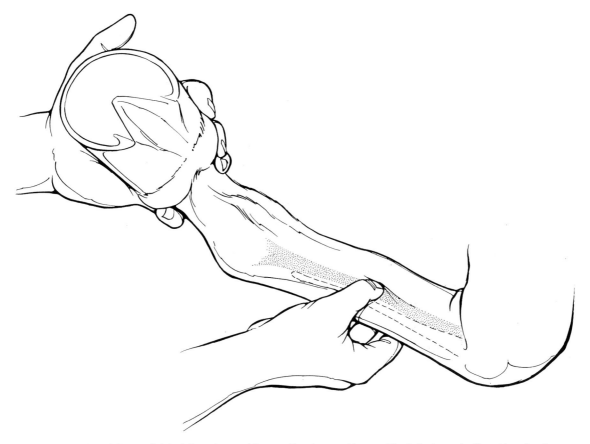

Figure 3.30. Palpation of the medial (axial) surfaces of the small metacarpal bones. The fetlock can be flexed to relax the suspensory ligament to permit easier palpation.

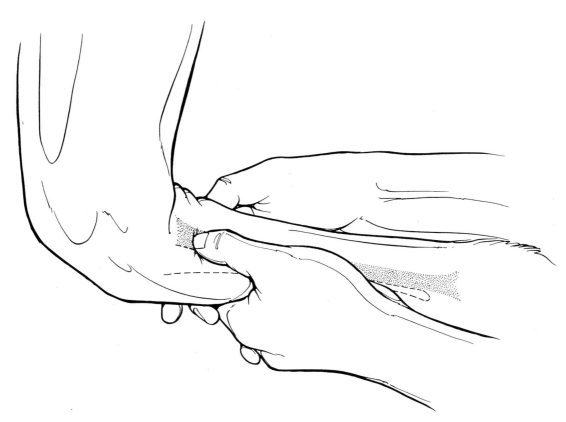

Figure 3.31. Palpation of the origin of the suspensory ligament in the proximal aspect of the metacarpal region. A repeatable painful response may suggest proximal suspensory desmitis.

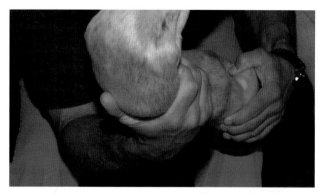

Figure 3.32. Method used to apply digital pressure to the suspensory ligament in the proximal palmar metacarpal region.

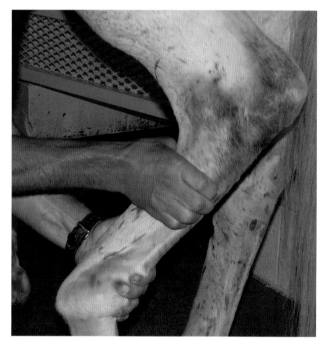

Figure 3.33. Method used to apply digital pressure to the suspensory ligament in the proximal plantar metatarsal region.

problem at the origin of the suspensory ligament, inferior check ligament desmitis, or a fissure fracture of the proximal palmar metacarpus.[10,21,26] Palpation of the proximal suspensory is more difficult in the hindlimbs than the forelimbs because it is more closely surrounded by the small metatarsal bones and the superficial digital flexor tendon is less easily pushed to the side (Figure 3.33).

Inferior (Carpal) Check Ligament

The inferior check ligament (accessory ligament of the deep digital flexor tendon) originates from the palmar carpal ligaments and attaches in a cup-like manner to the deep digital flexor tendon at about the middle of the metacarpus. It lies directly palmar to the suspensory ligament and can be palpated by holding the ligament between the index finger and the thumb or by applying pressure from the palmar aspect with the thumb.

Flexor Tendons

The superficial and deep digital flexor tendons are located palmar to the suspensory ligament and are intimately associated with each other. The proximal one-third of the flexors (associated with the carpus) and distal one-third (associated with the fetlock) are encased in tendon sheaths, whereas the central one-third is covered by a paratendon only. Each region should be palpated carefully for heat, pain, and swelling with the tendons weighted and relaxed. With the limb held in one hand an attempt should be made to roll or separate the superficial flexor tendon from the deep digital flexor tendon with the thumb and forefinger (Figure 3.34). If normal, they can be easily separated and differentiated. With pathology such as tendonitis, varying degrees of adhesions between the two as well as thickening will result in an inability to separate them. Most horses respond slightly to "pinching" the superficial digital flexor tendon between the thumb and index finger. Pain will be elicited easily with palpation in most horses with tendonitis.

Carpus

The carpus is visualized for swelling/effusion on the dorsal and palmar surfaces. Point swelling associated with the radiocarpal and middle carpal joints that occurs medial to the extensor carpi radialis tendon is often present in horses with osteochondral chip fractures and/or OA (Figure 3.35). More diffuse swelling of these joints may indicate more severe articular pathology such as slab fractures, advanced OA, and proliferative exostosis (carpitis). Distention of the tendon sheaths of the extensor tendons overlying the carpus (common digital and extensor carpi radialis) may indicate tenosynovitis and/or rupture, particularly of the common digital extensor tendon in foals (Figure 3.36). A diffuse fluctuant, subcutaneous swelling over the dorsal surface of the carpus is consistent with acute hematoma/seroma or chronic hygroma (Figure 3.37). Swelling/effusion of the palmar carpal canal may be found with accessory carpal bone fractures, tenosynovitis (carpal tunnel syndrome), or osteochondroma formation of the caudal distal aspect of the radius (Figure 3.38).[28]

Palpation of the carpal joints and bones including the accessory carpal bone are best done with the carpus flexed. The degree of carpal flexion or range of motion should also be evaluated. In the normal horse the flexor surface of the metacarpal region can approximate that of the forearm when the carpus is flexed (Figure 3.39). Carpal flexion should be performed slowly in horses with severe lameness with suspected carpal pathology to avoid a severely painful response. Reduced degrees of flexion with a painful response are consistent with most intra-articular carpal problem and possibly desmitis of the proximal attachment of the suspensory ligament.[28] After flexion, the carpus should be rotated by swinging the metacarpus laterally and medially (Figure 3.40). With the carpus held in flexion, the individual carpal bones are evaluated by deep digital pressure along the dorsal articular surfaces (Figure 3.41). With the carpus flexed, and the tension of the ulnaris lateralis and flexor carpi ulnaris reduced, the accessory carpal bone can be manipulated, potentially identifying a fracture (Figure 3.42). In some cases, an osteochondroma

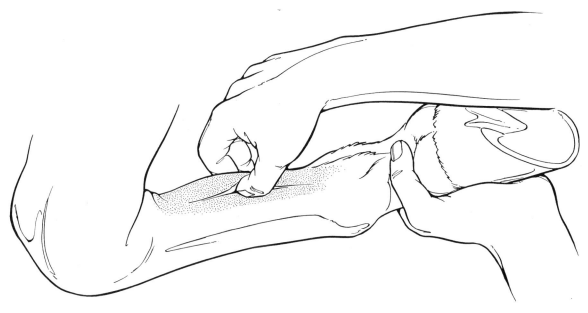

Figure 3.34. Palpation of the flexor tendons with the fetlock flexed to permit separation of the superficial and deep digital flexor tendons. Inability to separate the tendons usually suggests tendonitis.

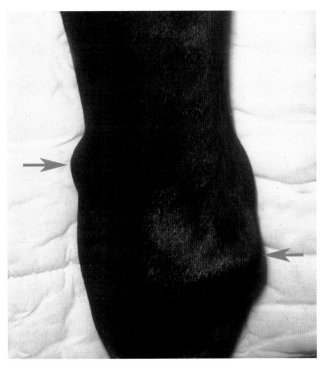

Figure 3.35. Effusion of radiocarpal joint was visible and easily palpable on the dorsomedial and palmarolateral joint pouches (arrows) in this horse.

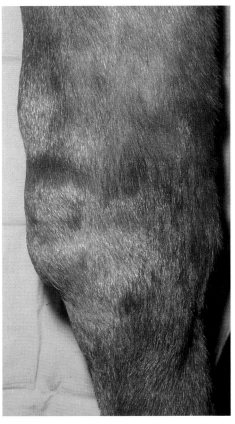

Figure 3.36. Effusion of the extensor carpi radialis tendon sheath is usually characterized by swelling that courses up and down the cranial aspect of the carpus.

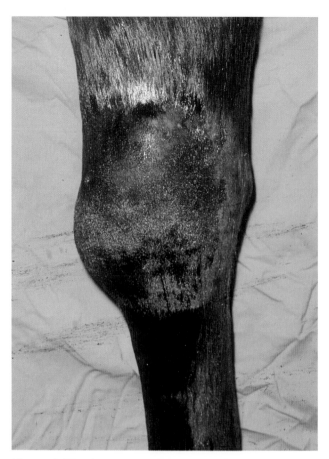

Figure 3.37. A hygroma of the carpus is a fluid-filled swelling located under the skin on the cranial aspect of the carpus. It is usually confined to the cranial aspect of the carpus and does not course up the limb.

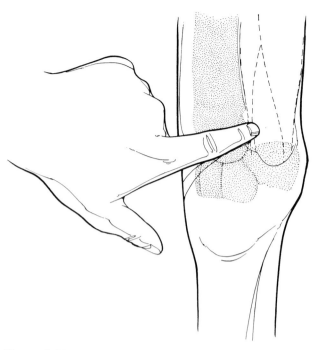

Figure 3.38. Finger marks the carpal canal. Effusion within the carpal sheath usually courses longitudinally up the medial aspect of the carpus but may also be present laterally.

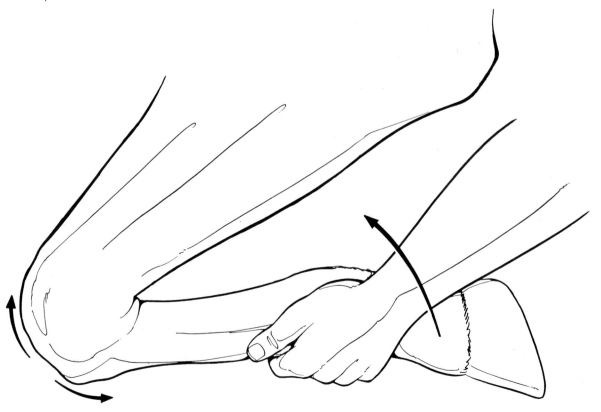

Figure 3.39. Flexion of the carpus to identify a painful response. In the normal horse, the flexor surface of the metacarpus approximates that of the forearm.

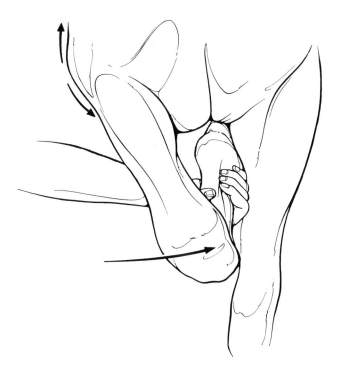

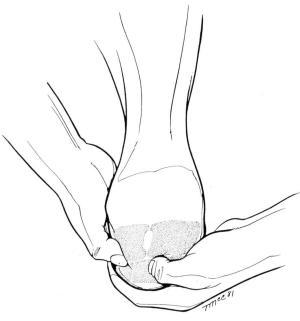

Figure 3.40. Adduction of the elbow and carpus places stress on the lateral support structures and may be used to identify a painful area.

Figure 3.41. The dorsal articular margins of the carpal bones can be palpated after the carpus is flexed to identify pain within the individual carpal bones and/or capsulitis.

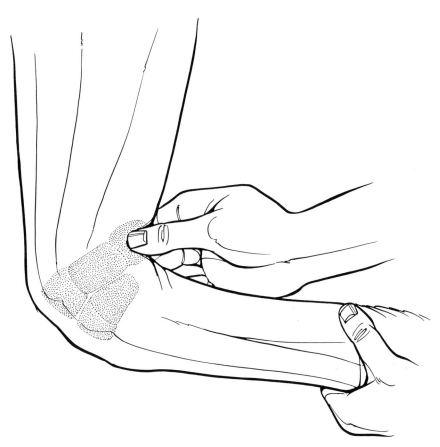

Figure 3.42. Palpation of the accessory carpal bone to identify a possible fracture. This is best done with the carpus flexed to decrease the tensional influence of the tendinous insertions of the ulnaris lateralis and flexor carpi ulnaris muscles.

on the caudodistal aspect of the radius may be palpable if effusion of the carpal canal is present.

Forearm (Antebrachium) and Elbow

The soft tissues of the forearm and elbow joint (cubital joint) should be palpated for signs of inflammation, particularly swelling. A firm swelling associated with the flexor muscles may be consistent with a myositis or a fibrotic or ossifying myopathy of these structures. The distal aspect of the radius should be palpated for swelling, heat, and pain. A firm, usually nonpainful but fluctuant swelling at the point of the elbow is consistent with an elbow hygroma, also known as olecranon bursitis (Figure 3.43). Severe swelling and an inability to extend the limb (dropped elbow) are consistent with a fracture of the olecranon. In cases of non-displaced or chronic olecranon fractures, palpation of the caudal aspect of the olecranon may reveal variable degrees of swelling and pain with digital pressure. Elevation of the limb into extension will also often cause pain (Figure 3.44). The collateral ligaments of the elbow joint can be evaluated by abducting and adducting the elbow (Figure 3.40). This, however, is not selective because the carpal and shoulder joints are manipulated as well. Severe swelling, crepitation, and pain may be observed in horses with humeral fractures and can be confused with fractures of the olecranon.

Shoulder and Scapula

The soft tissues around the shoulder joint (scapulohumeral joint) are observed and palpated for swelling or atrophy (Fig 3.45). Particular attention is paid to the bicipital bursa region (cranial aspect of shoulder), and deep digital palpation is applied in an attempt to elicit pain. The muscle and tendon should be grasped with the fingers and thumb and pulled laterad. Young horses

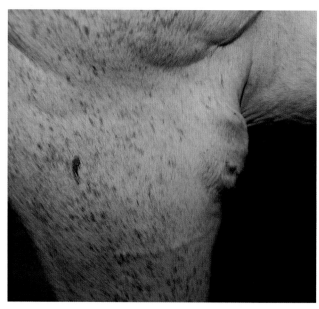

Figure 3.43.   A small fluid-filled swelling was present on the point of the elbow in this horse, consistent with olecranon bursitis. The skin was also thickened in the region but no lameness was present.

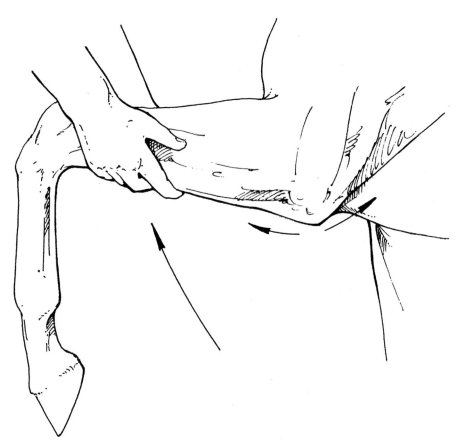

Figure 3.44.   Elevating the limb into extension to flex the elbow joint extends the shoulder and increases the tension on the triceps brachii tendon at its insertion on the olecranon process.

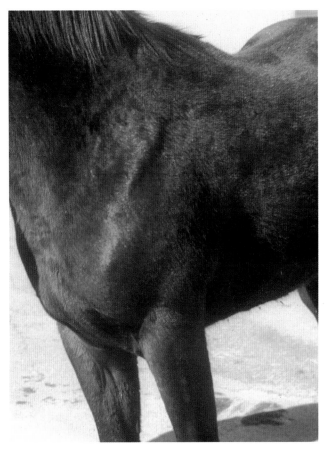

Figure 3.45. Atrophy of the shoulder muscles in young horses is often seen with osteochondrosis of the shoulder joint.

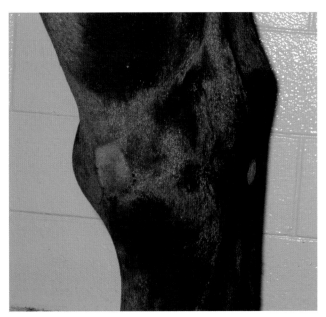

Figure 3.46. Young horse with effusion of the tarsocrural joint that is easily compressible and nonpainful.

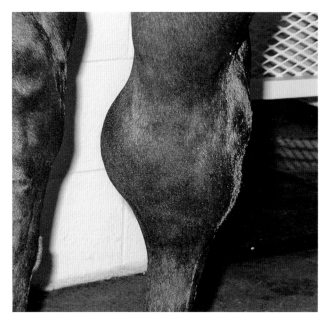

Figure 3.47. This young horse had a history of previous trauma to the tarsus. Part of the swelling was firm and painful to palpation but there was also effusion within the tarsocrural joint.

exhibiting obvious shoulder lameness at exercise and variable degrees of pain on manipulation often have osteochondrosis of the shoulder joint.[2,28] Degenerative change within the shoulder joint as well as fractures of the scapula and proximal humerus are also painful on manipulation. Elevation of the limb as described for the elbow joint may also result in a painful response, particularly if a fracture or a lesion within the joint is present (Figure 3.44). Another test to evaluate the shoulder region is to place one arm over the midline at the withers and the other hand over the distal one third of the scapula. The hand overlying the distal scapula is forced axially rapidly then released.

The infraspinatus and supraspinatus muscles should be observed for atrophy, which is found with suprascapular nerve paralysis or osteochondrosis (Figure 3.45), and swelling, which is consistent with external trauma. Deep palpation and manipulation in conjunction with a stethoscopic examination at the swollen site may define a fracture. Horses with mid-body scapular fractures may have an external swelling located above the shoulder joint. Extension or flexion and abduction or adduction of the shoulder joint may elicit pain in these horses.

Tarsus (Hock)

The tarsus is visualized and should be palpated for:

1. Tarsocrural joint effusion (synovitis, bog spavin, osteochondrosis)
2. Thickening of the fibrous joint capsule (capsulitis, chronic OA, previous trauma)
3. Bone proliferation of the distal tarsal joints (bone spavin)
4. Distension of the tarsal sheath (thoroughpin)

5. Inflammation of the long plantar ligament or superficial digital flexor tendon (curb)
6. Luxation of the superficial digital flexor tendon over the calcaneus
7. Capped hock
8. Subtendinous bursal effusion (calcaneal bursitis)

In general, there are three different types of soft tissue swelling that may be seen within the tarsus.[28] The first is a fluctuant fluid distension of the tarsocrural joint, often referred to as "bog spavin." The synovial effusion can be easily compressed from the dorsal medial pouch to distend the plantar pouches of the joint capsule and vice versa (Figure 3.46). The second type of swelling is a firm distension of the tarsocrural joint capsule, and the synovial fluid is difficult to compress from one pouch to the other. This "firmness" is due to synovial inflammation of the fibrous layer of the joint capsule (capsulitis) and often suggests a chronic problem such as OA or trauma to the fibrous joint capsule. The third type of swelling is a firm, diffuse swelling of the entire tarsal joint region (Figure 3.47). It is usually due to a severe sprain to the fibrous joint capsule and surrounding ligamentous support structures associated with trauma.

The medial aspect of the distal tarsal joint region (distal intertarsal and tarsometatarsal joints) should be closely examined visually and with palpation (Figure 3.48). In the normal horse there is a smooth contour that tapers to the distal tarsal bones as they join the proximal metatarsus. This is easily visualized from the rear and palpated from the side. If this region appears boxy with obvious enlargement, OA of the distal intertarsal and/or the tarsometatarsal joints (bone spavin) should be suspected. These medial enlargements have also been referred to as "tarsal shelves" (Figure 3.49). Applying pressure over the medial aspect of the distal tarsus has been referred to as the Churchill pressure test. Using the index and middle fingers, firm pressure is applied to the plantar aspect of the proximal end (head) of the second metatarsal (splint) bone (Figure 3.50). The test is considered positive if the horse flexes and abducts the limb away from the pressure.[7] A positive Churchill test may indicate distal tarsal OA or cunean bursitis, especially if there is a marked difference in the response between the two tarsi.

Effusion/swelling of the tarsal sheath is often referred to as "thoroughpin" and can usually be observed and palpated on the medial aspect of the tarsus. Unlike effusion of the tarsocrural joint, the effusion is asymmetrical on the limb (medially) and runs in a distal to proximal direction (Figure 3.51). Tarsocrural joint effusion is symmetrical and courses circumferentially around the tarsus. Tarsal sheath effusion may be a cosmetic blemish but can be indicative of problems of the deep digital flexor tendon or the sustentaculum tali of the talus (Figure 3.51). The plantar aspect of the tuber calcis should be palpated for inflammation of the plantar ligament ("curb") (Figure 3.52), tendonitis of the superficial flexor tendon (Figure 3.53), displacement of the superficial digital flexor tendon (Figure 3.54), and a fluid swelling at its proximal limits, referred to as "capped" hock. Swelling associated with a capped hock is subcutaneous, whereas effusion within the calcaneal

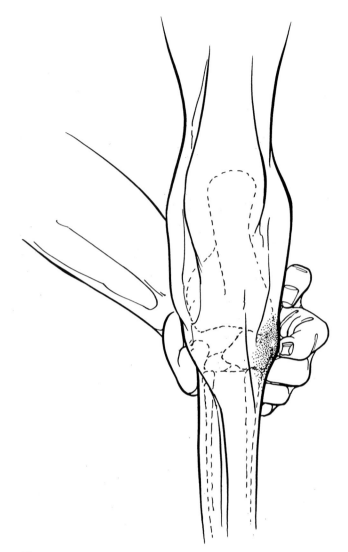

Figure 3.48. Palpation over the distal tarsal joints on the medial aspect of the tarsus, often referred to as the "Churchill test."

bursa is beneath the superficial digital flexor tendon (Figure 3.55). Effusion of the calcaneal bursa is often characterized by small pockets of fluid on each side of the tendon above and below the point of the hock (Figure 3.56).

Tibia

The tibial region can be difficult to detect abnormalities both visually and with palpation. Swelling in the caudal tibial region may indicate myositis of the semimembranosus and semitendinosus muscles or gastrocnemius tendonitis. Focal swelling of the distal medial epicondyle of the tibia could be associated with a fracture or sprain to the medial collateral ligament of the tarsus. Severe pain with deep digital palpation of the distal third of the tibia, together with a severe lameness and a positive spavin test, may suggest the possibility of an incomplete tibial fracture. A complete fracture of the tibia is associated with non-weight-bearing lameness, severe swelling, limb deviation, and crepitation on palpation and manipulation.

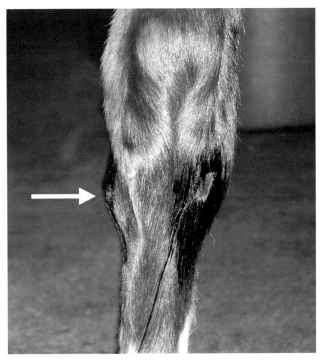

Figure 3.49. Enlargement of the medial aspect of the distal tarsus (arrow) consistent with distal tarsal OA (bone spavin).

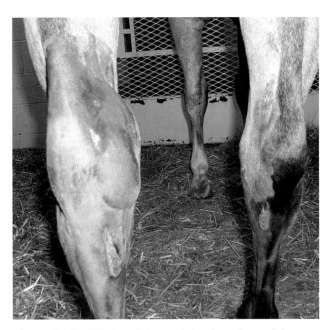

Figure 3.51. Effusion of the tarsal sheath on the medial aspect of the tarsus that was associated with fragmentation of the sustentaculum tali.

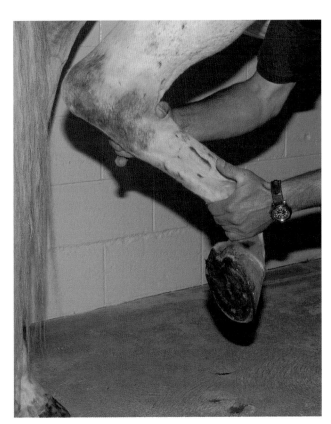

Figure 3.50. Limb and hand positioning to perform the "Churchill" test to detect pain on the medial aspect of the distal tarsal joints.

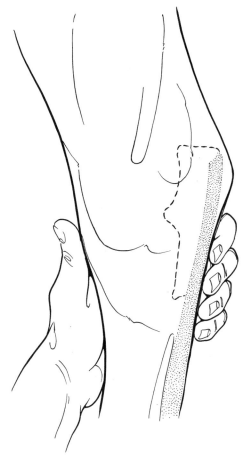

Figure 3.52. Palpation of the long plantar ligament over the plantar aspect of the calcaneus. Swelling in this region is often referred to as a curb but may represent tendonitis of the superficial digital flexor tendon instead. Foals with a "curby" appearance may also have incomplete ossification of the tarsal bones.

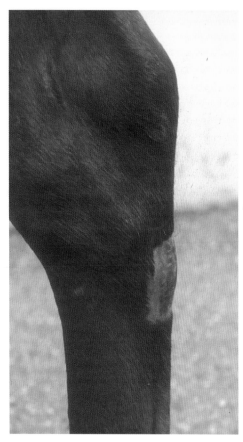

Figure 3.53. Tendonitis of the superficial digital flexor tendon in the proximal metatarsal region, which can be misdiagnosed as a curb in some horses.

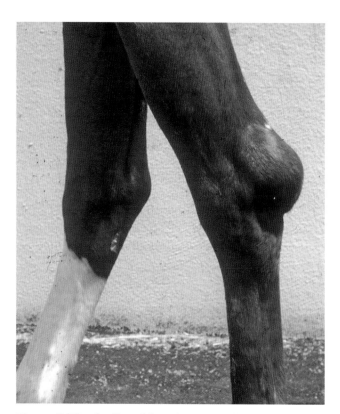

Figure 3.55. Swelling of the subcutaneous bursa at the point of calcaneus, often referred to as a "capped hock."

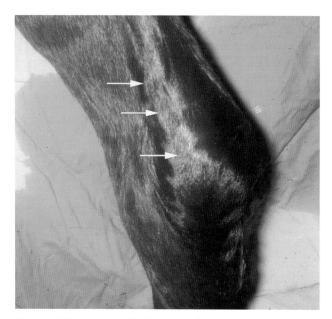

Figure 3.54. Lateral displacement of the superficial digital flexor tendon from the point of the calcaneus (arrows). Effusion of the calcaneal bursa is also usually present in these horses.

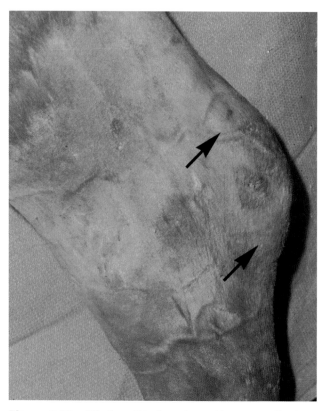

Figure 3.56. Effusion within the calcaneal bursa can often be palpated as fluid outpouchings above and below the retinaculum of the superficial digital flexor tendon (arrows).

The semimembranosus and semitendinosus muscles should be palpated for any evidence of pain and swelling indicative of myositis (hamstring pull) and for firm scarring/fibrosis that is often present with fibrotic myopathy (Figure 3.57). Although an uncommon site for problems, the gastrocnemius tendon should be palpated for swelling and pain. An attempt should also be made to extend the hock joint if clinical signs consistent with rupture of the peroneus tertius muscle are present during exercise. With the stifle flexed, the hock can be extended and a characteristic dimpling of the gastrocnemius tendon occurs (Figure 3.58).

Stifle

The stifle should be observed and palpated for swelling and/or atrophy of the associated muscle groups and for fluid distention of the joints. Distension of the femoropatellar joint is best seen from the lateral view (Figure 3.59) and distention of the medial femorotibial (MFT) is best observed from the cranial aspect (Figure 3.60). However, palpation is the preferred method to detect effusion within the stifle joints. The femoropatellar joint pouch is located on the cranial aspect of the stifle beneath the patella ligaments. In general, effusion of the femoropatellar joint makes palpation of the three distal patellar ligaments more difficult. These ligaments should be easily palpable across the dorsal aspect of the stifle and are the landmarks to locate the three synovial

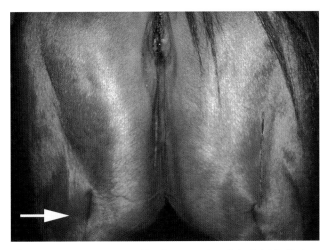

Figure 3.57. Horse with fibrotic myopathy of the left hindlimb. There is atrophy of the semitendinosus muscle and firm scar tissue palpable in the caudal tibial region (arrow).

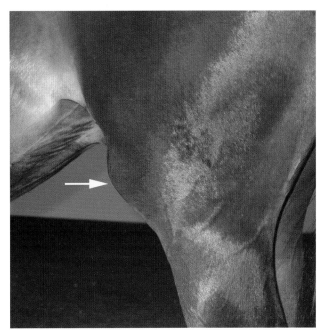

Figure 3.59. Effusion can be seen and palpated within the femoropatellar joint cranial to the patella ligaments (arrow).

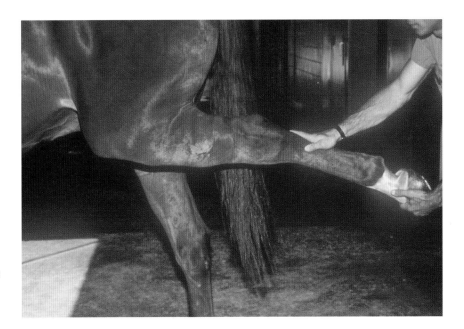

Figure 3.58. Horse with rupture of the peroneus tertius as suggested by the ability to simultaneously extend the hock and flex the stifle.

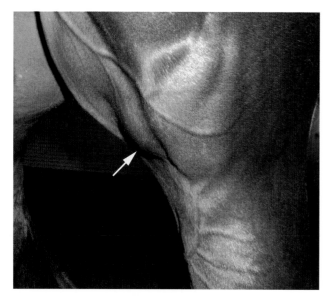

Figure 3.60. Visible and palpable effusion within the medial femorotibial joint is present just behind the medial patella ligament (arrow).

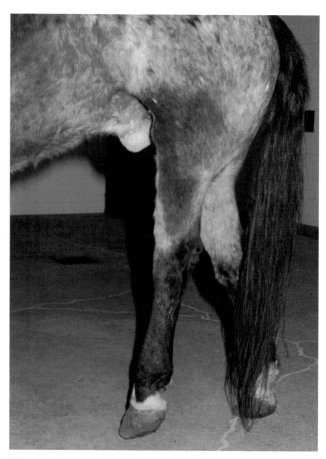

Figure 3.61. The stifle and hock are locked in extension as is seen with upward fixation of the patella.

pouches of the stifle. The patella ligaments should be palpated for evidence of desmitis, and the medial patellar ligament should be evaluated for scarring that may suggest previous surgery for upward fixation of the patella. Fluid distension of the femoropatellar pouch may indicate pathology within the femoropatellar joint or within the MFT joint because they communicate with each other. The MFT joint pouch is located medial to the medial patella ligament directly above the tibial plateau. The lateral femorotibial joint is located lateral to the lateral patella ligament and effusion within this joint is rarely detected. Palpation of the stifle joints for effusion should always be compared to the opposite limb. In general, abnormalities within the stifle joint are usually accompanied with synovial effusion. Effusion of the femoropatellar and MFT joints can be associated with a variety of problems (see the stifle section in Chapter 5 for details).

The patella should be palpated for parapatellar inflammation and pain, crepitation, and displacement. The patellar displacement test can be performed by placing the base of the patella between the thumb and forefinger. The patella is then displaced proximally (upward) and laterally (outward) in an attempt to engage the medial patellar ligament over the medial trochlea. Most horses object to this manipulation and will attempt to flex the stifle to prevent the forced upward displacement of the patella. If the patella is easily displaced upward with apparent locking, the horse is walked off and its reaction observed. With complete upward fixation the horse will be unable to flex its stifle or hock and may drag its limb behind in extension (Figure 3.61).

Manipulative tests may also be performed on the stifle to assess the cruciate ligaments and medial collateral ligament.[28] These tests are very subjective and only used in those horses when other clinical signs suggest injury to these structures. The cruciate test can

be performed from either the caudal or cranial aspect of the limb. With the caudal approach, the examiner stands behind the horse with his/her arms brought around the limb and the hands clasped together at the proximal end of the tibia (Figure 3.62). The examiner's knees or knee should be in close contact with the plantar aspect of the calcaneus, and the examiner's toe is placed between the bulbs of the heels. This positioning helps to stabilize the limb. In this position the examiner pulls the tibia sharply caudally and releases it to go cranially, feeling for looseness and crepitation which may suggest cruciate ligament damage. With a cranial cruciate ligament rupture, the looseness is felt as a sliding movement in a cranial direction (cranial drawer sign). However, a generalized looseness within the stifle is often the only definitive finding because it is difficult to identify the phase (caudal or cranial) in which the movement occurs.

With the cranial approach, the examiner stands in front of the affected limb with one hand placed on the proximal tibial tuberosity. The other hand is used to pull the tail to that side to force the horse into weight-bearing. The tibia is pushed caudally as quickly and forcibly as possible, which is thought to stress the cranial and caudal cruciate ligaments (Figure 3.63). This may be repeated multiple times, after which the horse may be trotted off and the degree of lameness observed. An increase in lameness may indicate a

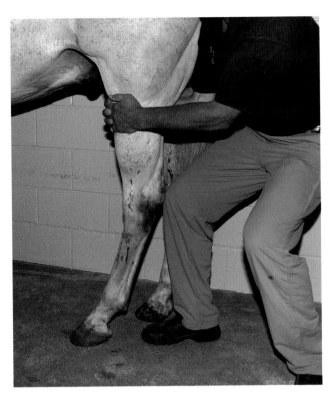

Figure 3.62. The caudal cruciate test is performed by grasping the tibia from behind and quickly pulling the tibia caudally. Increased movement of the tibia or a painful response may suggest damage to one of the cruciate ligaments.

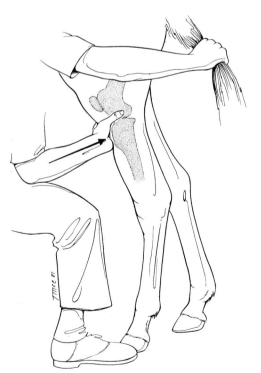

Figure 3.63. Positioning to check for problems with the cranial cruciate ligament. The examiner places one hand on the proximal tibia and forces it caudally (arrow) to check for increased movement (cranial drawer) of the tibia in relation to the femur. The examiner may also repeatedly push the tibia caudally several times and then trot the horse off to see if this manipulation worsens the lameness.

sprained or ruptured cruciate ligament, but is not specific for this injury.[28]

The medial collateral ligament test is performed by placing the shoulder or outside hand over the lateral aspect of the stifle and abducting the distal limb with the other hand (Figure 3.64). Increased lateral movement of the distal limb indicates complete rupture of the medial collateral ligament. The opposite approach may be performed to test the integrity of the lateral collateral ligament but injuries to this ligament are uncommon. If a sprain to the ligament is suspected, the limb may be abducted 5 to 10 times, after which the horse is trotted off and the degree of lameness assessed.

Femur

The muscles surrounding the femur are primarily examined for swelling and/or atrophy (Figure 3.65). The femoral artery should be palpated for the quality of pulsations on the medial side of the thigh in the groove between the sartorius muscle cranially and the pectineus muscle caudally. If the pulse is weak or nonexistent, thrombosis of the iliac artery may be contributing to the lameness. Pressure can be applied to the greater trochanter, and if painful, middle gluteal muscle strain or trochanteric bursitis (whirlbone disease) should be suspected.[7] Complete fractures of the femur usually result in non-weight-bearing lameness with severe swelling and limb shortening due to overriding of the fracture (Figure 3.65). Femoral neck fractures are more difficult to diagnose because they typically cause less swelling and lameness than diaphyseal femoral fractures. With time the swelling may migrate distally on the medial side of the thigh, giving the impression that the distal femoral region is involved.

Hip

The hip should be examined for asymmetry, swelling, and atrophy of associated muscle groups. With hip problems, swelling over the coxofemoral joint may be visually apparent and pain can often be elicited with deep palpation directly over the joint using the palm of the hand. At a walk, a stifle-out, hock-in, toe-out gait (external rotation) is frequently observed, with an apparent shortening of the limb length (Figure 3.66). From the side, the affected limb may appear to be straighter than the contralateral limb. With the metatarsus held in-hand, the coxofemoral joint can be manipulated into extension, flexion, and abduction to check for evidence of pain and crepitation. Additionally, the hip can be intermittently flexed and auscultated with a stethoscope at the same time to identify crepitation. Limb abduction is often painful to horses with hip conditions, and repeated limb abduction will often exacerbate the lameness.

Pelvis

Visual identification of asymmetry of the bones and musculature of the pelvis is an important aspect of examination of the pelvis. This includes the tuber coxae, the tuber ischium, the tuber sacrale, and the gluteal muscles on each side. Asymmetry of the bony pelvis

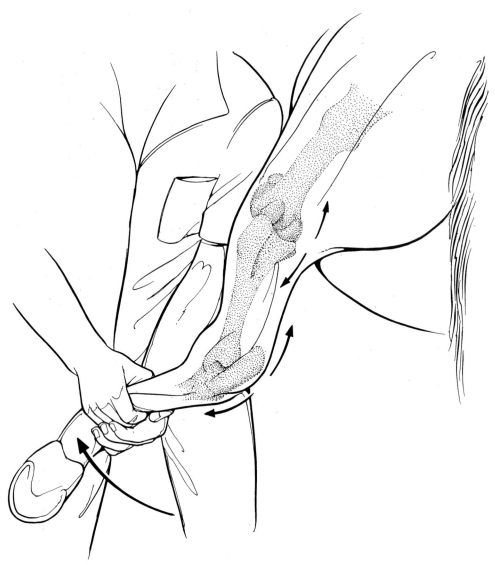

Figure 3.64. Test to stress the medial collateral ligaments of the hock and stifle. Alternatively, one hand can be placed on the medial aspect of the distal tibia to selectively stress the medial collateral ligament of the femorotibial joint. The examiner's shoulder can be placed over the middle of the tibia and both hands on the distal metatarsus to selectively stress the medial aspect of the hock.

often suggests a pelvic fracture, subluxation of the sacroiliac region, or fracture of the specific bony prominence. Gluteal muscle atrophy often accompanies chronic pelvic fractures but can be seen with any chronic hindlimb lameness (Figure 3.67). Crepitus associated with pelvic fractures can usually be elicited by swaying the horse from side to side or can sometimes be picked up by rectal examination.

Back

Visual assessment of the horse's back includes observing the muscle contour from the side and axial alignment from the rear (Figure 3.68). The dorsal spinous processes should be palpated for axial alignment, protrusion or depression, and interspinous distance (Figure 3.69). Malalignment of these processes may indicate fracture, luxation or subluxation, or overlapping of the dorsal spinous processes. Any muscle swelling, atrophy, or asymmetry in the epaxial musculature should also be noted.

Palpation is usually best performed with firm fingertip pressure using both hands simultaneously (Figure 3.70). Alternatively, the palm of the hand can be used to apply downward pressure to the epaxial muscles. Palpation of the epaxial muscles lateral to the dorsal spinous processes along the entire length of the back should be performed. Many horses may respond to downward pressure in the lumbar region by ventroflexing their backs but this response often fatigues and withdrawal is less prominent. In horses that have clinically significant back pain, ventroflexion of the back is often severe and any increase in finger or palm-applied pressure greatly increases this response. The horse attempts to "drop down" to get away from hand pressure. Palpation may also cause the horse to vocalize,

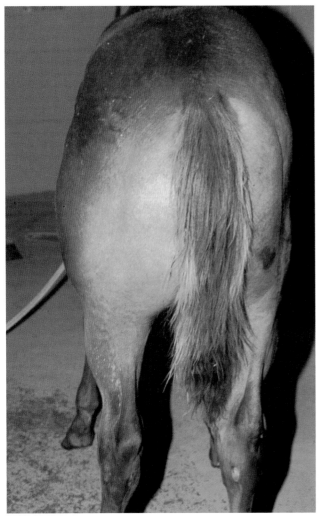

Figure 3.65. Swelling of the femoral region associated with a fracture of the distal femur in a yearling Quarter horse.

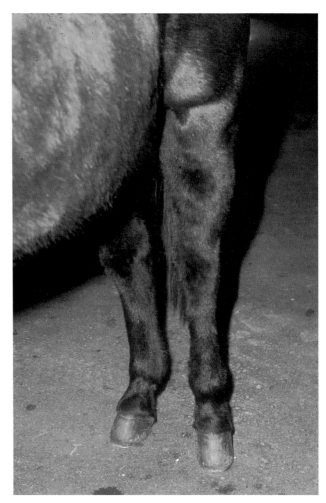

Figure 3.66. Typical toe-out, hock-in stance that often accompanies problems within the hip and pelvic region.

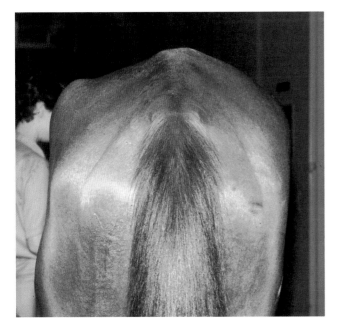

Figure 3.67. Severe atrophy of the left gluteal muscles secondary to a pelvic fracture. Disuse gluteal atrophy tends to occur more quickly and more profoundly with pelvic fractures than other lameness problems more distal in the limb.

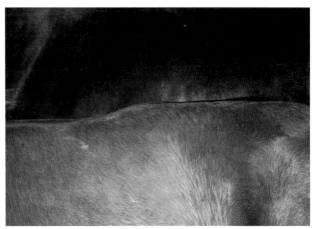

Figure 3.68. Kyphosis of the thoracolumbar region was present in this foal and was due to a developmental malformation of the vertebral column in this location.

141

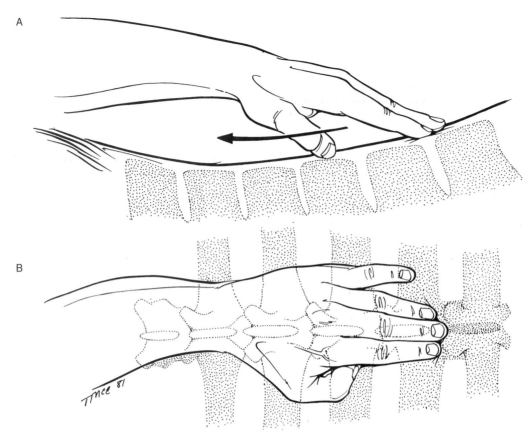

Figure 3.69. A. Palpation of the summits of the dorsal spinous processes to identify depressions or protrusions that may indicate subluxation or fracture. B. Palpation of the axial alignment of the dorsal spinous processes.

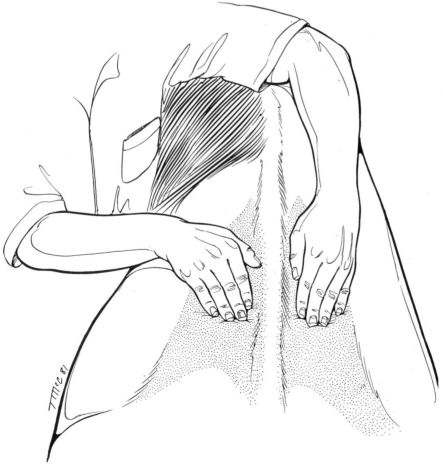

Figure 3.70. Firm pressure applied to the back musculature from the withers to the tuber sacrale to identify a painful response. The fingers should be held flat to prevent "digging in" with the fingertips.

swish its tail, or actually kick out behind. Back palpation is somewhat subjective and, therefore, the assessment requires clinical experience. In some cases, tightening of the longissimus dorsi muscle may be felt with palpation rather than a painful withdrawal response. This usually signifies that the horse is attempting to fix the vertebral column because ventroflexion is painful.

The examiner may also wish to assess the horse's willingness to ventroflex, dorsiflex, and lateroflex its thoracic and lumbar vertebrae.[88] Assessment of the horse's ability to ventroflex the back is obtained by exerting downward pressure to the muscles in the thoracolumbar region. A blunted instrument (needle cap) run over the croup usually causes dorsiflexion or arching of the back. Lateral flexion can usually be assessed by firmly stroking either side of the thoracolumbar region with a blunted instrument. Reluctance to flex the back in any of these directions may suggest muscle tightening and back rigidity within the thoracolumbar region (see Chapter 6 for further information on examination of the back and axial skeleton).

Neck

The neck should be examined for contour from the side and axial alignment from the front and rear. Excessive ventral arching of the neck in the mid-cervical region may be seen in some cases of cervical vertebral malformation. A straight (extended) poll can be seen with atlanto-occipital and atlanto-axial malformations. Axial deviations of the neck are most commonly due to developmental problems (e.g., hemivertebrae) or trauma. Splinting and spastic contraction of the neck muscles with or without signs of spinal ataxia is often consistent with vertebral fracture. Generally these horses are very painful.

Palpation should be done to identify muscle atrophy or swelling and to document the alignment of the vertebrae. The transverse processes should be palpated for alignment and symmetry. Muscle atrophy is most often observed in the caudal neck region dorsal to the cervical vertebrae and may be symmetric or asymmetric. Potential causes for muscle atrophy include cervical vertebral malformation, articular facet joint osteoarthritis, and neurologic problems such as equine protozoal myelopathy. Swelling of the neck either lateral or ventral is generally a sign of trauma and or infection.

The neck should be flexed laterally and ventrally and extended to assess flexibility, range of motion, and pain. Lateral flexing can be done by pulling the horse's head by the halter to one side and then to the other. Alternatively, lateral neck flexion can be encouraged by holding a treat at the horse's shoulder. Most horses should be able to flex their neck laterally enough that the muzzle almost contacts the craniolateral shoulder region. Ventroflexion is assessed by feeding the horse from the ground level and extension is evaluated by elevating the head and neck. Resistance to neck movement in any direction is usually due to pain and can be from many potential causes.

Flexion Tests/Manipulation

Most flexion tests, regardless of the location, are usually performed for 30 to 60 seconds and are a sub-jective method to further isolate the site of the lameness. However, the response to flexion tests must be interpreted in light of clinical findings because many otherwise normal horses may demonstrate positive responses.[22,32] These positive responses were thought to be directly related to the force applied to the limb since 20 of 50 horses responded to a "normal" distal limb flexion and 49 of 50 horses responded to a "firm" distal limb flexion.[22] Another study revealed that more than 60% of 100 sound horses had a positive response to distal limb flexion and that the positive outcome increased significantly with age.[5] Both of these studies question the validity of distal limb flexion tests to predict future joint-related problems.[5,22] In addition, false-positive responses to flexion seem to occur more commonly in horses in active work than in horses that have been rested or turned out to pasture.[25] In general, there are more false positive results to flexion at any location than false negative results but both can occur. False-positive responses are most common in the front fetlock.

Because both the amount of force and the duration for which it is applied affect the response to flexion[19,32], the procedure should be standardized as much as possible to minimize variability. For instance, the same person should flex the right and left limbs at any location for the same period of time so they can be accurately compared. Different people may have slight differences in the way they hold the limb or apply pressure to the limb, which can alter the responses. Despite this potential for variability, the flexion techniques performed by experienced veterinarians are usually sufficient to objectively assess responses to flexion.[19]

Passive flexion usually refers to manipulation of a joint during routine palpation of the horse and pain detected with passive flexion often predicts a significant response to a 30- to 60-second flexion test. However, flexion tests can also be used to subjectively assess the severity of damage within an affected joint(s). In general, the severity of damage is often proportional to the severity of the response to the flexion test. For instance, horses with severe responses to carpal, fetlock, or stifle flexion typically have significant intra-articular or extra-articular pathology. However, flexion tests are not specific for the joint because it is nearly impossible to flex a single joint without affecting other nearby joints and soft tissues. Flexion of a joint not only increases the intra-articular and subchondral bone intra-osseous pressures within the joint, but also compresses and stretches the joint capsule and surrounding soft tissues.[25,27] The numerous other "structures" that are being manipulated with any flexion test should always be considered when interpreting the clinical significance of flexion tests.

The responses to flexion should be graded in some manner and included in the records. This is most important when re-evaluating the lameness to more accurately determine whether improvement is being made. The author uses a grading scale of negative, mild response, moderate response, and severe response to assess the flexion tests. Alternatively, a plus-minus system may be used with "−" being no response, 1+ equating to mild, 2+ to moderate, and 3+ to severe. Regardless of the system used, the responses to flexion are a very

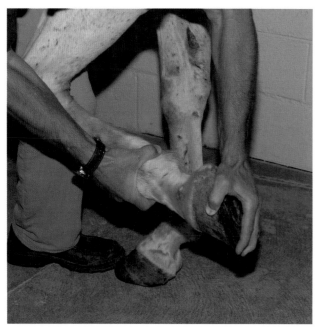

Figure 3.71. Hand and limb positioning to perform flexion of the phalangeal joints without flexing the fetlock.

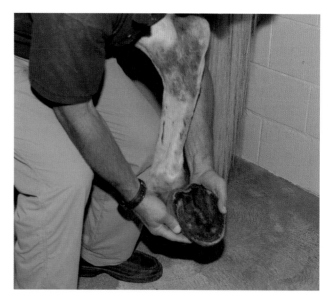

Figure 3.72. Hand and limb positioning to perform distal limb flexion (phalangeal and fetlock joints) of the hindlimb.

important aspect of the lameness examination, and should be recorded. Additionally, changes in lameness in the limb not being flexed (weight-bearing limb) should also be recorded because this is often an important clinical finding. This contralateral response to flexion tends to occur most commonly in horses with bilateral hock and carpal problems.[25]

Distal Limb/Phalangeal/Fetlock Flexion

Attempts can be made to isolate the fetlock joint from the pastern and coffin joints during flexion of the distal limb. However, it is nearly impossible to only flex the fetlock or only flex the pastern or coffin joints. Flexion of the fetlock joint is performed by placing one hand on the dorsal metacarpus/metatarsus and pulling up on the pastern with the opposite hand (Figure 3.27).[25] Flexion of just the phalangeal joints is performed by maintaining fetlock extension by placing one hand on the fetlock while flexing the phalanges by pulling up on the toe with the opposite hand (Figure 3.71). All three joints can be flexed together (distal limb flexion) by pulling up on the toe and phalanges with both hands while facing toward the back of the horse (Figure 3.28). In general, it is much more difficult to isolate the phalanges from the fetlock region in the hindlimb; therefore, most distal limb flexion tests performed in the hindlimb include all 3 joints (distal limb flexion test; Figure 3.72).

Regardless of how the flexion test is performed, the fetlock/phalanges are held in position for 30 seconds, after which the horse is trotted off and lameness is observed. Differences in the severity of the responses may be used to suggest whether there may be a problem in the fetlock vs. the pastern or coffin joints. A painful response to phalangeal flexion and a negative response to fetlock flexion may suggest a problem in the coffin

or pastern joint or any soft tissue structure in the area. A negative response to phalangeal flexion together with positive responses to both the fetlock and distal limb flexion suggest a fetlock problem. Any positive signs should be checked with the opposite limb because a marked asymmetry in responses to distal limb flexion tests is an important clinical finding, and further indicates a potential problem in the area. However, false positive fetlock flexion tests do occur, especially in horses in work, and many horses may show a positive response if a large amount of force is applied to the fetlock/distal limb. One study in normal horses evaluating the force applied for the fetlock and phalangeal flexion test by different examiners found that the force varied considerably and was frequently too high.[32] Methods to standardize the fetlock flexion test have been recommended (calibrated measuring device) but are not being used clinically by most clinicians.[32]

Carpal Flexion

The carpal flexion test is very useful to help isolate a problem to the carpus. A negative response does not rule out a problem in the carpus (many horses with osteochondral fragmentation are not positive to carpal flexion) but a positive response is highly suggestive of a carpal problem (few false positive responses). This is in contrast to the fetlock, where false positive responses are much more common. Carpal flexion is performed by grasping the metacarpus with the outside hand while facing the horse, pulling up on the distal limb (Figure 3.39). The foot should be able to contact the caudal aspect of the olecranon in normal horses. The carpus is held in this position for 60 seconds, after which the horse is jogged away and observed for increased lameness.

Elbow Flexion

It is difficult to completely separate the elbow from the shoulder when performing upper limb flexion tests

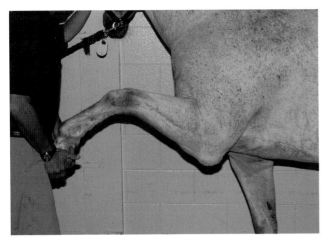

Figure 3.73. Upper limb flexion test in which the limb is pulled cranially and upward to "stress" the shoulder region.

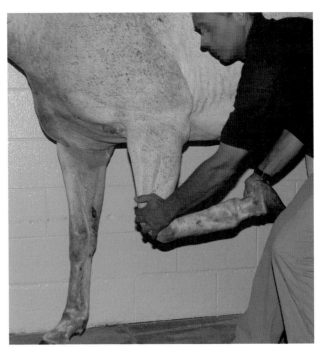

Figure 3.74. Flexion of the upper forelimb can be performed by grasping the antebrachium and foot and pulling the limb caudally.

in the forelimb. This is analogous to the tarsus and stifle in the hindlimb because flexion of one area often affects the other. However, flexion of the elbow can be performed by lifting the antebrachium (forearm) so that it is parallel to the ground and not pulled forward (Figure 3.44). This flexes the elbow and causes the carpus and distal limb to hang freely. The limb is held in this position for 60 seconds and the horse is jogged off. Elbow flexion is not part of a routine lameness evaluation and is usually performed when an abnormality in the elbow region is found on physical examination.

Shoulder/Upper Forelimb Flexion

Manipulation of the upper forelimb can be performed either by pulling the limb cranially and upward or by pulling the limb caudally. The cranial approach is similar to flexing the elbow, only the limb is pulled forward and will flex the elbow and extend the shoulder. This is usually performed by standing in front of the limb, grasping the antebrachium, and lifting the limb up and forward (Figure 3.73). This exacerbates lameness problems in the caudal aspect of the elbow (olecranon, triceps brachii) and the cranial aspect of the shoulder (bicipital bursa, biceps brachii). The more the limb is elevated, the more pressure is applied to the cranial aspect of the shoulder. The position is maintained for 60 seconds (or as long as the horse tolerates it) and the horse is trotted. Horses with supraglenoid tubercle fractures of the scapula and horses with bicipital bursitis often respond to this type of shoulder manipulation.

The caudal approach to flex the shoulder joint can be performed by placing one hand on the olecranon process and pulling the limb caudally. Alternatively, the cranial antebrachium may be grasped and pulled caudally together with the distal limb instead of applying pressure to the olecranon (Figure 3.74). The position is maintained for 60 seconds (or as long as the horse tolerates it), after which the horse is trotted and the degree of lameness is evaluated.

Tarsal/Hock Flexion

The tarsal flexion test or spavin test is somewhat of a misnomer because it flexes the fetlock, stifle, and hip in addition to the hock. A positive response to hock flexion is not synonymous with a tarsal problem but can be used together with other physical examination findings to suggest a problem in the tarsus. Hock flexion is performed by placing the outside hand when facing the rear of the horse on the plantar surface of the distal third of the metatarsus and elevating the limb to flex the hock (Figure 3.75). The opposite hand is then placed around the metatarsus and the limb is held with both hands while facing the back of the horse. The grip should avoid the sesamoid bones and be loose enough to avoid excessive pressure to the flexor tendons and suspensory ligament. The fetlock and phalanges should not be forcibly flexed.

Alternatively, the tip of the toe can be held so the pastern and fetlock joints are extended and the hock is flexed (Figure 3.76). It may also be beneficial to gradually flex the tarsus to its fullest extent over a 15-second period to avoid resentment by the horse. In some cases in which the horse tends to lean away from the examiner it may be helpful to place the horse adjacent to a solid support (i.e., wall or fence) or have an assistant provide counterbalance to the tuber coxae of the opposite hip. Once the tarsus is in full flexion, it is held in this position for 60 seconds, the limb is released gradually, and the horse is trotted off.

A positive hock flexion test is indicated by an increase in lameness of the flexed limb. However, increased lameness of the opposite limb (standing limb) is thought to occur with some upper limb lameness problems (sacroiliac problems). The first few steps the horse takes after this test are often the most important. If there is

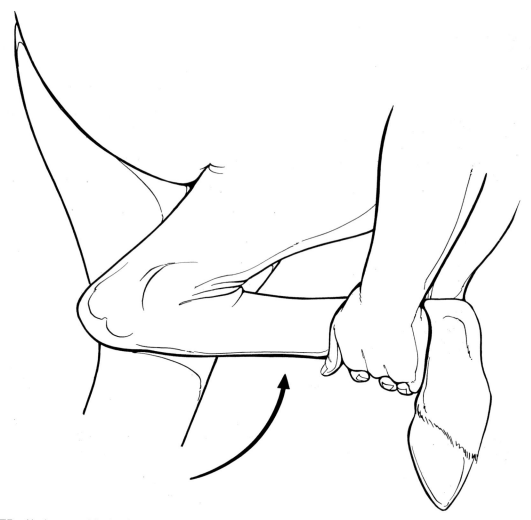

Figure 3.75. Hock or tarsal flexion (spavin) test. The hindlimb is flexed so that the metatarsus is approximately parallel to the ground. This test is not specific for the tarsus because it flexes both the stifle and the fetlock to some degree.

any question regarding the validity of the flexion test, it should be repeated. Two of the most common errors in performing this test are not obtaining full tarsal flexion and spooking the horse so that it balks at the onset of the test rather than jogging off at a smooth pace. The response to tarsal flexion should nearly always be compared to the opposite limb because an asymmetrical response is often an important clinical finding.

Stifle Flexion

The stifle flexion test is often used in an attempt to separate stifle pain from tarsal pain in horses that respond to a tarsal flexion test. In most cases the stifle flexion test will flex the hock less than the tarsal flexion test will flex the stifle. In many cases it can be more specific for stifle problems but this is debatable. It is performed by grasping the distal tibia and pulling the limb backward and upward until maximal stifle flexion is achieved (Figure 3.77). It is best to face toward the back of the horse with the limb in front of you when performing this test. The limb is held in this position for 60 seconds and the horse is trotted off. Some clinicians prefer to perform the stifle flexion test before the

hock flexion test, while others do it afterwards. A positive tarsal flexion together with a more positive stifle flexion may suggest that the lameness is due to a stifle problem and vice versa.

Full Limb Forelimb and Hindlimb Flexion

Full limb forelimb and hindlimb flexion tests can be used as quick screening tests to determine whether more isolated flexion tests may be necessary. If there is no response to flexing all of the joints at one time, the potential for getting positive responses to individual flexion tests is thought to be unlikely. Full-limb forelimb flexion is performed by grasping the foot and lifting the leg to flex the fetlock, carpus, and elbow. The opposite hand is placed on the metacarpus and the limb elevated and pulled forward to extend the shoulder (Figure 3.78). Full-limb hindlimb flexion is performed by grasping the foot and flexing the fetlock, hock, and stifle simultaneously. The hindlimb is pulled out behind the horse to help flex the stifle (Figure 3.79). The limb is usually held in position for 60 seconds. A negative response is thought to suggest that individual flexion responses will also be negative, but this has not been determined definitively for either the forelimb or hindlimb.

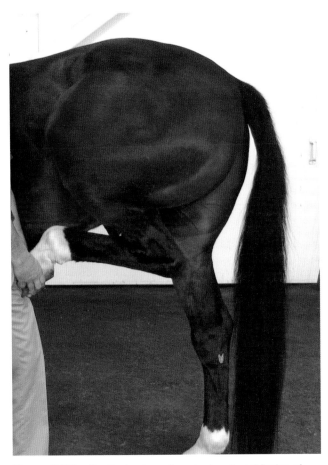

Figure 3.76. Positioning to perform hock or tarsal flexion of the hindlimb where the limb is held by the hoof.

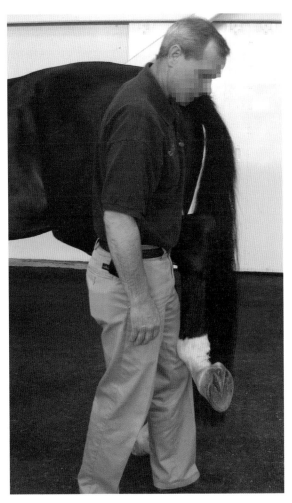

Figure 3.77. Flexion of the stifle is performed by pulling the hindlimb caudally and lifting up on the distal tibia.

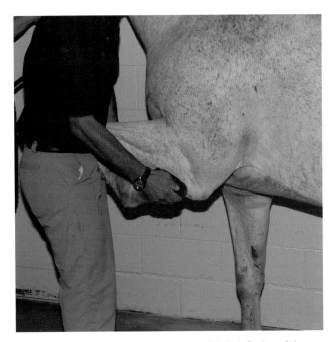

Figure 3.78. Positioning to perform a full limb flexion of the forelimb. All of the joints in the limb are flexed simultaneously.

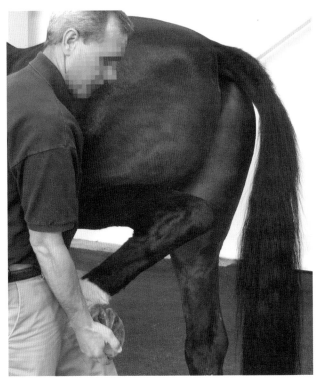

Figure 3.79. Positioning to perform a full limb flexion of the hindlimb.

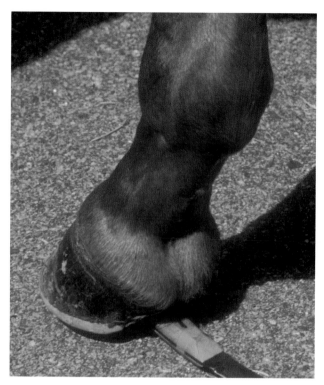

Figure 3.80. One method to apply pressure to the navicular region is to place a wooden object beneath the frog and have the horse stand on the limb for a few seconds.

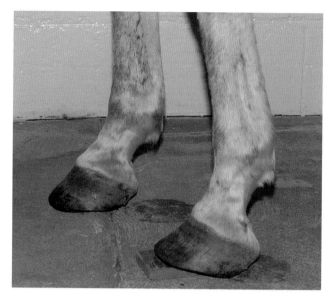

Figure 3.81. The navicular wedge test is performed by elevating the toe with a wooden block to increase the tension on the deep digital flexor tendon in the navicular region.

Navicular Wedge Test

The navicular wedge test can be performed in two different ways.[30] A wedge (usually a block of wood) may be placed beneath the frog of the affected foot while the opposite limb is held up (Figure 3.80). It is thought to apply direct pressure to the frog area, similar to hoof testers, and is usually performed for one minute, after which the horse is trotted off.[30] Alternatively, the toe is forced into an elevated position in relation to the heel by placing a wooden wedge under the toe (Figure 3.81). This serves to increase the tension on the deep digital flexor tendon and increase pressure over the navicular bone. The wedge may also be applied to the medial or lateral aspects of the foot to manipulate the soft tissues of the digit.[25] The opposite limb is elevated for one minute, and the horse is trotted off. Although these tests are often used for horses with navicular syndrome, any cause of heel/foot pain may be exacerbated with these tests.

Direct or Local Pressure Plus Movement

The premise for applying direct pressure to a specific site and watching the horse trot is to confirm the significance of palpation findings. A positive response to static palpation does not necessarily indicate the site of the problem. However, increasing the baseline lameness by deep palpation of a suspicious area or anatomic structure will often confirm the potential of a problem in the area. Direct pressure is usually applied manually, but hoof testers can be used to apply pressure to the sole of the foot. The limb is usually elevated, the site is compressed for 15 to 30 seconds, and the horse is trotted off. Exacerbation of the lameness by one or more grades is considered a positive response.[25] The direct pressure test is most commonly performed over swellings of the splint bones, dorsal metacarpus, flexor tendons, suspensory body and branches, and medial aspect of the tarsus. It also may be used to assess pain in the proximal suspensory region of both the forelimb and hindlimb and several areas of the axial skeleton.

Rectal Examination

A rectal examination may be indicated in some horses with upper hindlimb lameness. It is most commonly performed in horses with suspected pelvic fractures or problems in the sacral region. Information also may be obtained rectally in horses with iliopsoas myositis, fractured vertebrae, or thrombosis of the iliac arteries.[28] Rectal examination is usually performed with the horse standing still but it may be beneficial to walk the horse while performing the rectal exam (so called "walking rectal"). The examination is often performed in a cranial to caudal direction. Pressure should be applied to the iliopsoas muscle located cranial to the pelvic brim (Figure 3.82). Swelling or pain in the muscle may suggest a local myopathy or fracture of the lumbar vertebrae. The aorta and iliac arteries should be checked for normal pulsation. The symmetry of the pelvis is palpated by comparing one side to the other (Figure 3.83). With displaced ilial fractures an obvious asymmetry may be present, and rocking the horse from side to side may reveal crepitus or movement of the bones. Rocking the pelvis by pushing down on the tuber coxae may also cause separation of the fracture. The ventral aspect of the sacral vertebral bodies should be checked for alignment and any depression or protrusion into the

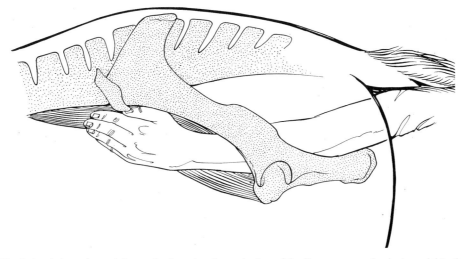

Figure 3.82. Lateral view of a rectal examination showing palpation of the iliopsoas muscles just cranial to the pelvic brim.

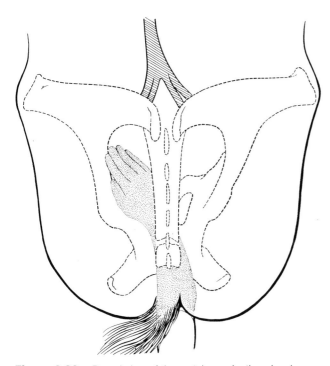

Figure 3.83. Dorsal view of the rectal examination showing evaluation of the symmetry of the pelvis. One side of the pelvis should be compared with the other. The pelvis can also be palpated for crepitation while the horse is swayed from the side to side while standing or during movement.

pelvic canal, which may indicate fracture or subluxation. Rectal ultrasound of the pelvis may be performed at the same time as palpation to further document abnormalities.

Neurological Examination

Any horse with a suspected neurological problem should have a complete neurological examination performed (see Chapter 10 for this description). However, determining the presence of hindlimb weakness and correct limb placement can be performed quickly and may help suggest neurological problems. Hindlimb weakness can be assessed by either pushing the horse from one side to the other or more commonly be pulling its tail to each side. This has been referred to as the sway test or tail pull test.[28] Normal horses resist pulling the tail, while many ataxic horses appear relatively weak and do very little to resist being pulled from one side to the other. However, this test is very subjective and many young Warmblood horses with underdeveloped hindlimb musculature often appear to be very weak but are not neurological.

Limb placement can be assessed by walking the horse over a curb, circling, positioning the limb across midline while standing, and trotting in a serpentine pattern. Repeated stumbling, hitting the curb, circumduction of the hindlimbs, and a general sense of not knowing where the hind feet are suggest a neurologic problem. Some horses that have bilateral hindlimb ataxia may also appear very "bouncy" when trotted, and when stopped suddenly from a trot may stumble in the hindlimbs. The most common neurological problems that may be confused with lameness problems are cervical vertebral malformation and equine protozoal myelopathy (see Chapter 10 for more information on neurologic examination).

References

1. Beeman GM. The clinical diagnosis of lameness. Compend Contin Educ Pract Vet 1988;10:172–179.
2. Bertone AL, McIlwraith CW, Powers BE, et al. Arthroscopic surgery for the treatment of osteochondrosis in the equine shoulder joint. Vet Surg 1987;16:303–311.
3. Buchner HH, Savelberg HH, Schamhardt HC, et al. Head and trunk movement adaptations in horses with experimentally induced fore- or hindlimb lameness. Equine Vet J 1996;28:71–76.
4. Buchner HH, Savelberg HH, Schamhardt HC, et al. Limb movement adaptations in horses with experimentally induced fore- or hindlimb lameness. Equine Vet J 1996;28:63–70.
5. Busschers E, van Weeren PR. Use of the flexion test of the distal forelimb in the sound horse: repeatability and effect of age, gender, weight, height and fetlock joint range of motion. J Vet Med A Physiol Pathol Clin Med 2001;48:413–427.

6. Caron JP. Objective and subjective gait analysis techniques. In Current Techniques in Equine Surgery and Lameness, White NA, Moore JN, eds. WB Saunders, Philadelphia 1998;501–504.

7. Churchill EA. The methodology of diagnosis of hind leg lameness. Proceedings Am Assoc Equine Pract 1979;25:297–304.

8. Dabareiner RM, Cohen ND, Carter GK, et al. Lameness and poor performance in horses used for team roping: 118 cases (2000–2003). J Am Vet Med Assoc 2005;226:1694–1699.

9. Dyson SJ. Lameness due to pain associated with the distal interphalangeal joint: 45 cases. Equine Vet J 1991;23:128–135.

10. Dyson SJ, Arthur RM, Palmer SE, et al. Suspensory ligament desmitis. Vet Clin North Am Equine Pract 1995;11:177–215.

11. Fuller CJ, Bladon BM, Driver AJ, et al. The intra- and inter-assessor reliability of measurement of functional outcome by lameness scoring in horses. Vet J 2006;171:281–286.

12. Gomez Alvarez CB, Bobbert MF, Lamers L, et al. The effect of induced hindlimb lameness on thoracolumbar kinematics during treadmill locomotion. Equine Vet J 2008;40:147–152.

13. Ishihara A, Bertone AL, Rajala-Schultz PJ. Association between subjective lameness grade and kinetic gait parameters in horses with experimentally induced forelimb lameness. Am J Vet Res 2005;66:1805–1815.

14. Keegan KG, Wilson DA, Kramer J. How to evaluate head and pelvic movement to determine lameness. Proceedings Am Assoc Equine Pract 2004;50:206–211.

15. Keegan KG, Wilson DA, Wilson DJ, et al. Evaluation of mild lameness in horses trotting on a treadmill by clinicians and interns or residents and correlation of their assessments with kinematic gait analysis. Am J Vet Res 1998;59:1370–1377.

16. Keegan KG, Pai PF, Wilson DA, et al. Signal decomposition method of evaluating head movement to measure induced forelimb lameness in horses trotting on a treadmill. Equine Vet J 2001;33:446–451.

17. Keegan KG, Yonezawa Y, Pai PF, et al. Evaluation of a sensor-based system of motion analysis for detection and quantification of forelimb and hindlimb lameness in horses. Am J Vet Res 2004;65:665–670.

18. Keegan KG. Evidence-based lameness detection and quantification. Vet Clin North Am Equine Pract 2007;23:403–423.

19. Keg PR, van Weeren PR, Back W, et al. Influence of the force applied and its period of application on the outcome of the flexion test of the distal forelimb of the horse. Vet Rec 1997;141:463–466.

20. May SA, Wyn-Jones G. Identification of hindleg lameness. Equine Vet J 1987;19:185–188.

21. Pleasant RS, Baker JB, Muhlbauer MC, et al. Stress reaction and stress fractures of the proximal palmar aspect of the third metacarpal bone in horses: 58 cases (1980–1990) J Am Vet Med Assoc 1992;201:1918–1923

22. Ramey DW. Prospective evaluation of forelimb flexion tests in practice: clinical response, radiographic correlation, and predictive value for future lameness. Proceedings Am Assoc Equine Pract 1997;43:116–120.

23. Riemersma DJ, Schamhardt HC, Hartman W, et al. Kinetics and kinematics of the equine hindlimb: in vivo tendon loads and force plate measurements in ponies. Am J Vet Res 1988;49:1344–1352.

24. Ross MW. Movement. In Diagnosis and Management of Lameness in the Horse, Ross MW, Dyson SJ, eds. Saunders, St. Louis, MO 2003;60–73

25. Ross MW. Manipulation. In Diagnosis and Management of Lameness in the Horse, Ross MW, Dyson SJ, eds. Saunders, St. Louis, MO 2003;74–81.

26. Ross MW, Ford TS, Orsini PG. Incomplete longitudinal fracture of the proximal palmar cortex of the metacarpal bone in horses. Vet Surg 1988;17:82–86.

27. Strand E, Martin GS, Crawford MP, et al. Intra-articular pressure, elastance and range of motion in healthy and injured racehorse metacarpophalangeal joints. Equine Vet J 1998;30:520–527.

28. Stashak TS. Examination for Lameness. In Adams' Lameness in Horses, Stashak TS, ed., 5th ed. Lippincott Williams and Wilkins, Philadelphia. 2002;113–183.

29. Swanson TD. Guide for Veterinary Service and Judging of Equestrian Events. 3rd ed. Golden, CO. Am Assoc Equine Pract, 1984;24.

30. Turner T. Diagnosis and treatment of navicular disease in horses. Vet Clin N Am Equine Pract. 1989;5:131–143.

31. Turner TA. How to subjectively and objectively examine the equine foot. Proceedings Am Assoc Equine Pract 2006;52:531–537.

32. Verschooten F, Verbeeck J. Flexion test of the metacarpophalangeal and interphalangeal joints and flexion angle of the metacarpophalangeal joint in sound horses. Equine Vet J. 1997;29:50–54.

33. Weishaupt MA. Adaptation strategies of horses with lameness. Vet Clin North Am Equine Pract 2008;24:79–100.

EVALUATION OF HORSES AT WORK

Terry D. Swanson

Some lameness is best demonstrated while the horse is at work because neither the weight of the rider nor the characteristics of specific movements can be duplicated in-hand or discovered by palpation of the horse. In addition, the evaluation of a horse in work can validate the findings of the in-hand examination. Due to attitude or disposition, some horses do not lend themselves to detailed in-hand evaluation, and working under saddle can be the best presentation. It is important to remember that the concerns found by palpation and in-hand movement will not always represent the root of the lameness, and can be distractions from the underlying problem. Also, the working of a horse during the diagnostic procedures could be the only way to demonstrate improvement from diagnostic blocks. In these circumstances one must acknowledge that not all cases are safe to ride while under the influence of a diagnostic block.

REASONS TO EVALUATE HORSES AT WORK

In most instances, work means under saddle with a rider, but this must also consider horses that pull carts, wagons, or sulkies or perform without riders, such as exhibition horses. Fortunately, most horses with lameness that need to be worked to observe the lameness and make a diagnosis are the exceptions. With most equine lameness, in-hand evaluations are sufficient.

Even if the horse is going to be worked, the horse is first evaluated in-hand, which allows the examining veterinarian to become familiar with the horse. This physical exam includes visual evaluation and palpation, moving the horse in-hand and on the lunge line, and performing flexion or stress tests. For most lameness the cause or etiology will be identified during this exercise; for other lameness or performance problems it is not possible to demonstrate or identify the etiology with the physical exam. Instead, as mentioned before, it takes the weight of the rider and tack or the rider asking the horse for specific maneuvers. Also, identifying the areas that are abnormal or suspicious before the work session can suggest more specific observations during the work. In most cases the working examination is for horses with subtle lameness (grade 1 or grade 2), cases that have more than 1 leg with a lameness problem, or horses that are simply resistant to training without an observable lameness.

Dressage horses that are having difficulties with their side passes, reining horses that have trouble with their spins, and any horse that is having trouble with collection and head set are examples of cases that can be better evaluated under saddle. In some cases, however, it may be determined by the physical exam that the horse does not need to be worked or that it would be unsafe for the rider or the horse to be put to work.

PROCEDURE TO EVALUATE HORSES AT WORK

The procedure to examine horses at work is based on the availability of the appropriate facilities, tack, and rider or driver. Limitations of facilities, tack, and personnel can cause a compromise in how the horse is worked. Nevertheless, the effort may still demonstrate the problems being considered and should be performed unless there are safety issues. Often a small turf area or round pen can be sufficient to demonstrate the problem. In some cases the horse must perform a specific task or maneuver to demonstrate the problem. The horse's particular discipline can compromise a specific working examination. In a clinic or hospital setting it is often impossible to observe the horse at work; speed horses or cattle-working horses are good examples. Special arrangements often must be made in these circumstances.

When examining a horse at work, if possible the veterinarian should observe the horse being tacked and observe the rider mounting the horse. There are several things to consider when examining a horse under saddle or in work. First, the veterinarian should have a good understanding of the type of work the horse performs. Once the horse begins to work it is important to evaluate the general attitude the horse displays. This information is noted for later interpretation. Most horses enjoy the work they perform and it shows in their attitude while working. If they develop a significant veterinary problem, their performance attitude can change. However, not all sound horses work as if they enjoy their job and the owner or trainer should be consulted regarding the horse's behavior if this is a concern. When a horse displays an attitude problem it is important to verify with the rider that there are no known physical reasons for the observed changes.

The whole horse and its performance are observed. The evaluation of the horse's movements must be tempered by the individual's athletic ability. Watch for subtle changes in the fluid motions, flexions, extensions, normal swaying, or swinging of the gaits. The movements a horse makes are determined by the discipline that it is performing. The level of training adds another factor to consider when evaluating a horse's movements or maneuvers.

Symmetry in movement is important. This includes leg movement, with the left and right leg strides being equal in length, and the specific gaits being equal to the left and to the right. Head and neck flexions and extensions should be supple and symmetrical. The body from the neck to the croup should be arched lateral to the extent of the circle in which the horse is traveling. The rear quarters should not shift into the circle or drift to the outside. Likewise, the shoulders should not drop to the inside of the circle and the head should not turn to the outside of the circle unless the rider is asking for these specific movements. The rear quarters should be able to move up under the horse when asked. The transitions from one gait to another should be smooth and balanced. This includes when the horse gains speed to another gait and as it slows to a slower gait. As mentioned previously, the level of training and/or the response to training must be considered when evaluating a horse at work. Remember that the discipline in which the horse is working may also affect body positioning and movement. An example is a team-roping horse that some trainers and riders only move in the left lead and they are not asked for the right lead because all of the work flows to the left.

All situations require that the veterinarian work in concert with the trainer or rider to determine whether the horse is exhibiting a training/resistance problem or a lameness problem. In some situations the trainer cannot or will not recognize the lack of proper training as the root of the performance problem. An example is a horse having lead change problems. It may be improperly prepared for the task, rather than having a veterinary problem.[1] To successfully manage this circumstance requires a tactful approach by the veterinarian.

If the veterinarian does not have a good knowledge of a horse's job, she can obtain a reasonable understanding of the performance requirements from an observant and communicative owner or trainer. This makes the working session more productive and can greatly aid in interpreting the observations. Occasionally circumstances prevent working the horse. In that case, video imaging can be a very useful tool for lameness evaluation. In most instances lameness is well demonstrated by a quality video recording.

Specific Observations of Performance Horses at Work

The equine practitioner should always remember that if the client's concern about their horse's performance cannot be demonstrated by palpation or in-hand evaluation, he should take advantage of the luxury of evaluating the horse at work. An example is the dressage horse that has problems with a particular lateral movement but does not exhibit a specific lameness. Under saddle the gait abnormality is observed only going one direction while the horse is performing the specific lateral movement. Observing the movement and the limb structures involved along with previous experiences can give valuable clues to the etiology of the performance deficit. There may or may not be palpable changes to support the diagnosis.

Reluctance to enter the arena or show ring may be due to training resistance or it could be a response to anticipated pain during the upcoming performance. An example is a roping horse that is unruly in the scoring box while waiting for the steer or calf. This could be related to the anticipated pain it will feel while performing in the area, and the pain could result from veterinary issues or how the horse is ridden or trained. It also may be possible that the horse has not been properly prepared to handle the pressure of the job.

Note the horse's head position. Watching how the horse controls or sets its head can be helpful; this becomes more important if there is a recent change

reported by the rider. Neck or back pain can cause the horse to resist bit contact. Extending the head and neck may also be an effort to reduce impact on the front legs or feet. Furthermore, ruling out dental or temporomandibular joint pain is important. Observe the horse's neck flexions or extension, and watch for the horse to flex the neck equally to the left and right as well as its willingness to flex and extend the neck, depending upon body position. Resistance in any of these motions can be an indication of a neck problem.

It is important to observe how the horse uses its back. Watch the lateral flexion, ventral flexion, and dorsal extension as it moves. Rider position and tack adjustments can also affect these motions; therefore, experience in seeing the whole picture is important. A horse with dorsal spinous process "kissing" lesions will be reluctant to extend the back and there will be reduced bounce to the back and torso as the horse moves forward. Observing the horse's inability to arch or bend its body to the same curve as it turns could indicate back issues, which can be muscular or vertebral. The rider may comment that the hindquarters shift to the inside of the circle in this situation. Another cause for this posturing could be a lameness associated with the outside rear leg, often the medial femorotibial joint.

Reluctance of the tie-down roping horse or team roping horse to take the jerk could indicate a back, hock, or even front foot problem. An improper saddle fit at the withers or the loin could also account for signs of back pain. A team roping horse that is reluctant to pull or log the steer could also have hock or saddle fit problems. Again, improper training of the horse to position for the jerk may be a factor.

Lumbosacral or sacroiliac soreness may cause a decrease in performance without a specific lameness being observed. There are many different gait changes with pain in this area. English discipline horses often kick up or give a small buck as they round a corner. Dressage horses have trouble with their lateral work with pain in this area. The horse's movement may make it difficult for the rider to sit in the saddle. The barrel racing horse can have trouble making a tight turn and the team roping horse often shifts its rear quarters one way or the other to log or pull the steer due to pain in the sacroiliac area. Some horses with sacroiliac pain may or may not demonstrate a specific lameness.

Poor stifle function can cause a loss in performance. With delayed patella release problems there may not be specific lameness noted but only changes in performance. Stumbling on the rear leg at the canter or lope is common. Somewhat exaggerated elevation of the rear quarters occurs as the horse makes the transition up from a trot to a canter or down from a canter to a trot or a trot to a walk. Another example of delayed patellar release syndrome is a western horse moving at a slow jog, which involves a dramatically shortened step with one or both hindlimbs looking very lame, but exhibiting no lameness when extended to a faster trot.[2] A horse with delayed patellar release is also more reluctant to go straight down steeper slopes and prefers to zig-zag. Front feet soreness also may cause reluctance to going downhill. It is important to remember that horses with delayed patella release syndrome can also have other concurrent hindlimb lameness problems.

Lower grade stifle lameness or soreness will often affect the horse going in the opposite direction of the affected rear leg. Lead changes to the opposite direction can be difficult, that is, if the left stifle is sore, the change from the left to the right lead will be more difficult. This condition ranges from a slight problem to a significant problem depending upon the magnitude of the lameness.

Front lead changes to the respective direction can often be the result of lower leg soreness of the respective front leg. That is, if the left front foot or lower leg is sore, the horse is reluctant to extend that leg for the respective lead change.

If the horse shows lameness of the outside front leg while traveling in a circle, there are several areas of potential soreness to consider. First, the suspensory ligament of the outside leg could be sore, especially if the lameness is more pronounced in soft footing. In some cases a carpal injury would account for the outside leg lameness, and a reduced ability to move the outside leg forward can be due to a shoulder or upper limb muscular injury.

Horses with sore front feet can buck or crow hop when asked to move out. When jumping horses are sore-footed they stay flat over the jumps to limit the impact when they land. They also may refuse jumps or they may hurry or rush over the jumps. Rodeo horses with sore front feet are reluctant to accelerate to their top speed.

A horse jumping over fences that is sore on a rear leg will often move toward the sore leg as he goes over the jump because he pushes off most with the sound rear leg and therefore shifts toward the sore leg. In most situations horses in other disciplines drift away from the sore leg.

Horses with sore hocks can have trouble with their rear lead changes. Their movement is labored when pushing up hill or pushing off to go over a jump. They can lack the impulse to go forward. Rodeo horses are reluctant to work deep into their stop or turns. Cutting horses have difficulty making their turns back to the opposite direction with the cow.

It is helpful to further observe the horse with subtle hindlimb lameness by observing the horse's response to the rider's posting at the trot. Subtle rear leg lameness is enhanced when the rider's weight comes down or sits when the affected leg is weight-bearing. Ask the rider to post the trot on the correct diagonal and then the opposite diagonal while trotting, both to the left and to the right. This could be helpful to determine which leg

is lame or which leg is the most lame. It is also helpful to ask the rider to set the trot, because this can enhance the lameness signs.[3]

The way in which most horses exhibit lameness differently depends on how collected they are with the bridle when ridden. It is important to see the horse with little collection and again with relatively full collection. In addition, some horses with lower cervical or upper thoracic vertebral injuries will only show their lameness when tacked, girthed, and carrying a rider.

A significant variable for performance horses is their ability to perform with discomfort. For any specific disease process diagnosed, there is a predicted level of pain or discomfort. Some horses with above average athletic ability can cope with problems that would cause other horses to struggle. The horse's individual tolerance of pain, attitude in general, or willingness to work, and the specific lameness problem with which they are dealing, all influence what the veterinarian will observe.

Another variable is the ability of the trainer to manage the horse's performance. Techniques include not asking the horse for a higher level of performance than it can physically achieve, not over training the horse between events, and a riding style that can be supportive for the horse with physical problems. Trainers who use these techniques can successfully exhibit a horse with certain veterinary problems.

Experienced and observant riders or trainers are extremely helpful to the veterinarian when assessing a horse at work. At the same time, the veterinarian must keep an open mind about the remarks from the trainer in relation to his observations. Questioning the trainer should be done in a respectful manner, remembering that the best outcome for the horse will be achieved when all of the professionals work together as a team.

The information from this section is to be used with discretion with each individual case and in conjunction with the history and physical exam. These ideas are presented as helpful guides to unraveling the complications of lower grade lameness affecting a horse's performance. They are not "rules" for lameness diagnosis.

References

1. Anderson GF. 2009. Personal communication.
2. Beeman, GM. 1973. Personal communication.
3. Ross MW. Movement. In Diagnosis and Management of Lameness in the Horse, Ross MW and Dyson SJ, eds. Saunders, St. Louis, MO 2003;73.

OBJECTIVE ASSESSMENT OF LAMENESS

Kevin G. Keegan

The standard of practice to detect and assess severity of lameness in horses is observing the horse in motion with the naked eye and then scoring using a discrete scale, for example the AAEP lameness grades. This is sufficient for the majority of cases. However, there is anecdotal and experimental evidence that detection and evaluation of lameness in horses using the naked eye is insufficient in some cases, especially when the severity of lameness is mild.[9,10,13] Multiple limb involvement and compensatory movement in the opposite half of the body contribute to variability in assessment. Agreement, even between experts, for the detection of mild lameness between AAEP grades 1 and 2 or for picking the most affected limb is only slightly above chance.[16] The most likely explanation for this is limited temporal resolution of the human eye to detect fast events in the movement of the horse. Furthermore, un-blinded subjective assessment is predisposed to bias.[1] Objective assessments of lameness by precise and accurate measurement of ground reaction force or asymmetry of movement at high sampling rates can be used to mitigate these limitations.

MEASUREMENT OF GROUND REACTION FORCES (KINETICS)

Most lameness causes pain during weight-bearing. A horse will bear less weight on an affected limb to decrease pain, resulting in decreased ground reaction force, which can be objectively measured. The stationary force plate, force measuring treadmill, force-measuring devices attached to the bottom of the hoof, and pressure-sensitive mats have been used to measure ground reaction forces in moving horses. The stationary force plate is the most commonly used and cited method.

During an evaluation for lameness with the stationary force plate the horse is moved over the force plate so that at least one, and preferably just one, hoof strikes the force plate completely within the confines of the surface of the force plate (Figure 3.84). Ground reaction forces can be measured in all 3 directions—vertical, horizontal, and transverse (Figure 3.85). Decreased vertical ground reaction force and to some extent, altered horizontal ground reaction forces, are most often associated with lameness in the horse. Peak forces and impulse (area under the force vs. time curve) decrease with severity of lameness. It is also likely that the shape of the vertical and horizontal ground reaction force curves contains information relevant to determining timing of lameness and differentiating whether pain is maximum during limb impact, in the first half of stance or during pushoff, in the last part of stance. Some work has been done in this area[8] but more is needed before the force plate is reliable for aiding in localizing lameness within the limb.

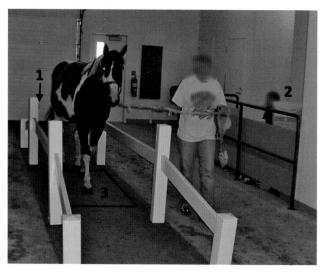

Figure 3.84. Stationary force plate set for evaluation of lameness in horses. (1) Electric eye to detect subject velocity. (2) Workstation with software. (3) Approximate outline of size of force plate embedded into the ground and covered to prevent shying. (Courtesy of Dr. Charles MacAllister.)

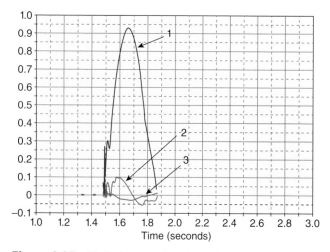

Figure 3.85. Typical output of stationary force plate. Ground reaction force curves reported in all directions: (1) vertical, (2) horizontal, (3) transverse. Y-axis units are proportionate of ground reaction force to body weight, with 1.0 = 100% body weight. (Data courtesy of Dr. Charles MacAllister.)

The stationary force plate is a precise and accurate instrument. Variability between trials is low (coefficients of variation below 10%) and sensitivity is high enough to detect subclinical lameness.[11,12,19] However, acquiring data requires controlled conditions. The hoof must strike completely within a relatively small area, often requiring multiple attempts. Speed of movement is also controlled, both to increase the chance of successful hoof strike and to decrease variability between hoof strikes. The stationary force plate is a gold standard for objective lameness evaluation in horses, but the controlled conditions required for acquiring consistent results make it unlikely to be adopted for routine use in clinical practice. Although it has been shown to vary with breed, the forelimb of sound horses trotting across the force plate at moderate speed will strike the force plate with force approximately equal in magnitude to 100% of its body weight.[2] Horses with AAEP grade 4 lameness will strike the forelimb with a force as low as 50% of their body weight. At this time the same estimates are not available for hindlimb lameness.

MEASUREMENT OF MOVEMENT (KINEMATICS)

Kinematics is the measurement and study of movement. Limb and torso pain alter the normal movement of the horse. If pain predominates in one side of the body, the normal, symmetric movement between right and left parts of the stride will become asymmetric. Kinematics, like kinetics, can be used to quantify absolute movement measures that may correlate well with lameness. However, most applications quantify lameness by measuring the asymmetry of movement between left and right sides of the body. Many different motion

parameters have been studied and used to detect and evaluate forelimb and hindlimb lameness in horses, including vertical movement of the torso (head bob, pelvic fall and rise),[4] stride and step length and timing,[7] pelvic rotation (hip hike and dip),[17] limb and hoof flight pattern,[5] and joint angle extremes and range of motion.[7] Asymmetric vertical movement of the torso, because it is more directly associated with vertical ground reaction force, is most likely the most sensitive kinematic measure of asymmetry of movement due to lameness.[6,14] More detailed descriptions of the kinematic parameters useful for detection and evaluation of lameness in horses are covered in the next section of this chapter.

Body motion changes due to lameness are more variable than changes in ground reaction force. Variability can be decreased by either strictly controlling conditions of evaluation or collecting multiple contiguous strides or both. The most common kinematic technique is camera-based. The horse is filmed while moving and body motion is quantified by analyzing trajectories of markers attached to the body of the horse (Figure 3.86). The camera-based kinematic technique is more sensitive than subjective evaluation for detecting asymmetry of motion because the sampling rate of the camera can exceed the temporal resolution of the unaided human eye. In order to collect multiple contiguous strides at maximum spatial resolution, kinematic evaluation of lameness in horses is usually performed on the equine treadmill. Because of this it is unlikely that camera-based kinematic evaluation of lameness will be adopted for routine use in clinical practice.

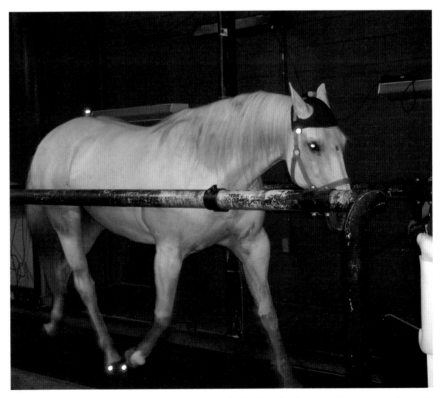

Figure 3.86. Marking of the horse with reflective spheres (head, right hoof walls, pelvis) for camera-based kinematic evaluation of lameness.

Asymmetry of motion can also be measured using inertial sensors attached to the horse's body.[3,15,18] Sensor data can then either be stored or wirelessly transmitted to the evaluator. Motion data from multiple contiguous strides in an over-ground setting can be collected and evaluated. Wireless transmission of body-mounted inertial sensor data offers a possibility of using kinematics to objectively evaluate lameness in horses in a natural clinical environment. The remainder of this section describes some of the technology being developed or available today for this purpose. Because the author is more familiar with the output of Lameness Locator® by Equinosis™, this system is discussed in more depth. Further information can be obtained by contacting the developers directly (www.equusys.com; www.equinosis.com; www.centaure-metrix.com).

EquuSense by Equusys Inc.

Equusys, Inc. of Sudbury, Massachusetts, has developed and is marketing EquuSense Equine motion capture and analysis systems to equine professionals for analysis of equine performance and lameness. EquuSense Equine systems are composed of 8 to 18 inertial sensor nodes that use accelerometers, gyroscopes, and magnetometers to sense motion; a wireless telemetry system that transmits the data from the nodes; a small hub fixed on or near the horse; and a workstation with software. Each sensor provides objective and accurate information on its position, velocity, acceleration, orientation, and rotation (±2 mm, ±2 degrees). They are sampled and transmitted at up to 2,000 samples per second in real time. The sensors weigh 75 grams and can be attached to the horse with specially-designed boots and pouches (Figure 3.87). Data is analyzed to give the user objective output and presented to the user as animated flight paths of body parts or as an animated moving "stick figure" horse. This system can be considered a field-ready, and therefore more practical, replacement for the more familiar camera and marker kinematic systems.

The software, which comes in 2 versions (one primarily for the researcher and one for practicing veterinarians) enables the user to visualize parameters that may be of interest for analysis of lameness, such as the relative height of the horse during each stance phase of each of the forelimbs, maximal vertical acceleration of the head, relative height and shape of the hoof flight arc, fetlock extension during the stance phase, and displacement amplitude of the tuber sacrale. Users can make comparisons among the limbs of a particular horse, between different sessions of a particular trial such as before and after a flexion test or pre- and postblocking, against a baseline from an earlier session, or against a typical population of horses. Samples of data corresponding to a particular set of parameters can be saved as "snapshots" on a remote server for archiving and sharing with other professionals.

Lameness Locator® by Equinosis™

Lameness Locator® was specifically designed as an aid to the practicing equine veterinarian for detection and evaluation of difficult lameness in horses. It was developed by equine veterinarians and engineers at the

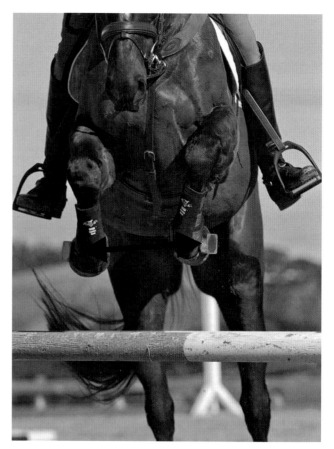

Figure 3.87. EquuSense motion capture and analysis system by Equusys Inc. Inertial sensors attached to both forelimbs (double-headed arrow) wirelessly report to the user in real time position, velocity, acceleration, and orientation of sensors. Other sensors attached to other body parts give additional trajectory information. (Courtesy of Michael Davies, Equusys Inc.)

University of Missouri in collaboration with the Hiroshima Institute of Technology in Japan. It is licensed to Equinosis™ in Columbia, Missouri, for further development and commercialization.

Lameness Locator® consists of 3 inertial sensors (2 accelerometers and 1 gyroscope), a tablet PC for data analysis, a sensor battery charger, and accessories for attaching the sensors to the horse's body (Figure 3.88). The inertial sensors are attached to the head, right forelimb pastern or hoof wall, and pelvis. Each sensor is 1.5 inches by 1.25 inches by 0.75 inches and weighs 28 grams. Vertical accelerations of the head and pelvis and angular velocity of the right distal forelimb are measured and wirelessly transmitted in real time to a handheld tablet computer. Range of transmission is up to 150 meters. Custom-designed algorithms are used to detect and quantify forelimb and hindlimb lameness when the horse is trotting. Trotting strides are automatically detected by the software when the horse is moving.

Lameness Locator® algorithms were developed from previous kinematic research. Best sensor type and locations were determined by data mining of accumulated motion data from groups of sound horses, horses

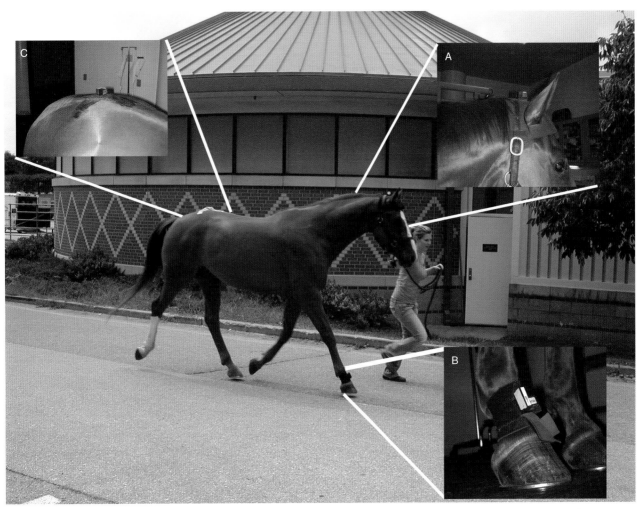

Figure 3.88. Lameness Locator® inertial sensor-based lameness evaluation system. A. Head accelerometer attached to head bumper. B. Right forelimb gyroscope attached to pastern pouch. C. Pelvic accelerometer attached with strip of 3M dual lock tape.

with naturally occurring lameness, and horses with various models of induced lameness. Vertical head and pelvic acceleration are converted to distance and separated into components by custom error-correction algorithms. Random movement is discarded. Remaining periodic movement is separated into movement due to lameness at stride frequency and natural vertical motion at twice stride frequency. Lameness is detected and quantified by reporting (1) the ratio of vertical movement due to lameness to natural vertical movement, and (2) the means and standard deviations of maximum and minimum height differences of the head (for forelimb lameness evaluation) and pelvis (for hindlimb lameness evaluation) position. Location of lameness to limb and timing of peak lameness within the stride phase of a limb are determined by the association of head and pelvic movement to angular velocity of the right forelimb.

Lameness evaluation results are reported in a graphical display that depicts amplitude of impact and propulsion asymmetry in each stride. Compensatory or multiple limb lameness patterns can be determined by studying the distribution of impact and pushoff asym-

metry in all 4 limbs. Improvement in the severity of lameness after block or treatment can be quantified. Response to flexion tests can be quantified. The developers of Lameness Locator® claim that it will be most useful to experienced equine veterinarians evaluating horses with mild, subtle, or multiple limb lameness and in objectively evaluating partial improvements after blocking. At the time of this writing Lameness Locator® is being used in 35 private practice and university veterinary teaching hospital sites in the United States, Canada, and Europe. It became commercially available in December 2009. Lameness Locator® is marketed only to veterinarians.

Detecting Forelimb Lameness with Lameness Locator®

Forelimb lameness is reported in a graphical display of a ray diagram and by calculating 4 lameness values (Figure 3.89). The forelimb lameness ray diagram plot is a qualitative description of the forelimb lameness. Each ray on the plot is a stride. The length of the ray is representative of the amplitude of asymmetric head motion for that stride. The location of the ray on the

Forelimb Evaluation

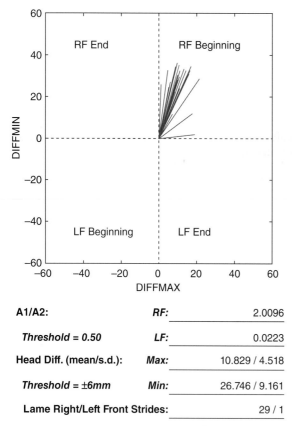

A1/A2:	*RF:*	2.0096
Threshold = 0.50	*LF:*	0.0223
Head Diff. (mean/s.d.):	*Max:*	10.829 / 4.518
Threshold = ±6mm	*Min:*	26.746 / 9.161
Lame Right/Left Front Strides:		29 / 1

Figure 3.89. Output of Lameness Locator® indicating right forelimb impact lameness. All rays pointing in quadrant 1. A1/A2 RF value >0.50. Head diff max and head diff min > threshold of ±6 mm. Standard deviations of head diff max and head diff min less than mean head diff max and head diff min, indicating consistent lameness.

plot represents the side and timing of lameness for that stride. Rays in quadrant 1 represent lameness in the right forelimb maximum during the first half of stance, from impact to midstance; rays in quadrant 2 represent lameness in the right forelimb maximum during second half of stance, midstance to pushoff; rays in quadrant 3 represent lameness in the left forelimb during the first half of stance; and rays in quadrant 4 represent lameness in the left forelimb during the second half of stance.

The 4 lameness values give a more quantitative description of the forelimb lameness. The RF and LF A1/A2 values are the ratios of vertical head movement from lameness to expected, normal vertical head movement distributed to the right and left forelimbs, respectively. These values represent an overall measure of forelimb lameness distributed to each limb. The approximate threshold value between sound and lame states for both RF and LF A1/A2 values is 0.50. This threshold value was determined by an independent study comparing Lameness Locator® results to simultaneous subjective evaluation of sound and lame horses by at least 2 experienced equine veterinarians. Values of RF or LF A1/A2 above 0.50 are supportive of lameness in that limb. Values of RF or LF A1/A2 below 0.50 are sup-

portive of soundness in that limb. Because the RF and LF values represent a quality of the entire collected signal, these values are considered gross measures of the severity of forelimb lameness. The 95% confidence interval for a single measure is approximately 30% of the RF or LF A1/A2 values.

Forelimb lameness is also quantified by calculation of the difference in maximum head position between left and right forelimb strides (diff max head) and the difference in minimum head position between left and right forelimb strides (diff min head). Diff max head and diff min head are calculated for every stride collected and the mean and standard deviation over all strides are reported. The signs of diff max head and diff min head determine side and timing of lameness. Because the diff max head and diff min head values are calculated for every stride, these measures are considered more specific indicators of lameness in a particular forelimb. The approximate threshold between sound and lame for these values is ±6 mm. The 95% confidence interval for a single measure for these values is ±6 mm.

Detecting Hindlimb Lameness with Lameness Locator®

Hindlimb lameness is reported in a graphical display that depicts deficiency of right and left hindlimb impact (first half of stance) or pushoff (second half of stance) and by calculating 4 lameness values (Figure 3.90).

The hindlimb lameness display is a qualitative description of the hindlimb lameness. The left side of the display represents qualities of the left hindlimb function. The right side of the display represents qualities of the right hindlimb function. Each vertical line on the display moving from left to right is a measure of either the deficiency of impact or the deficiency of pushoff for that limb. The length of the line is representative of the amplitude of asymmetric pelvic motion for that stride.

The 4 lameness values give a more quantitative description of the hindlimb lameness. The RH and LH A1/A2 values are the ratios of vertical pelvic movement from lameness to expected, normal vertical pelvic movement distributed to the right and left hindlimbs, respectively. These values represent an overall measure of hindlimb lameness distributed to each limb. The approximate threshold value between both RH and LH A1/A2 values is 0.17. This threshold value was determined by an independent study comparing Lameness Locator® results to simultaneous subjective evaluation of sound and lame horses by at least 2 experienced equine veterinarians. Values of RH or LH A1/A2 above 0.17 are supportive of lameness in that limb. Values of RH or LH A1/A2 below 0.17 are supportive of soundness in that limb. Because the RH and LH A1/A2 values represent a quality of the entire collected signal, these values are considered gross measures of the severity of hindlimb lameness. The 95% confidence interval for a single measure is approximately 25% of the RH or LH A1/A2 values.

Hindlimb lameness is also quantified by calculation of the difference in maximum pelvic position between left and right hindlimb strides (diff max pelvis) and the difference in minimum pelvic position between left and right hindlimb strides (diff min pelvis). Diff max pelvis

Strides Evaluated (front/hind): 48 / 47

Hindlimb Evaluation

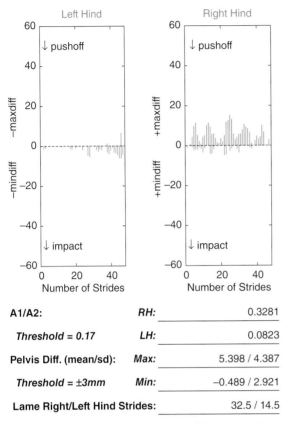

A1/A2:	*RH:*	0.3281
Threshold = 0.17	*LH:*	0.0823
Pelvis Diff. (mean/sd):	*Max:*	5.398 / 4.387
Threshold = ±3mm	*Min:*	−0.489 / 2.921
Lame Right/Left Hind Strides:		32.5 / 14.5

Figure 3.90. Output of Lameness Locator® indicating right hindlimb pushoff lameness. Most red rays (pelvic diff max) are on right side. This indicates most pelvic diff max of strides are + in sign, i.e., the pelvis is thrust up less after pushoff of right hindlimb compared to left hindlimb. A1/A2 RH value >0.17. Pelvic diff max > threshold of ±3 mm. Standard deviation of pelvic diff max less than mean of pelvic diff max, indicating consistent lameness.

and diff min pelvis are calculated for every stride collected and the mean and standard deviation over all strides are reported. The signs of diff max pelvis and diff min pelvis determine side and timing of lameness. Positive values indicate right hindlimb lameness and negative values indicate left hindlimb lameness. High diff max pelvis absolute values indicate pushoff type hindlimb lameness. High diff min pelvis absolute values indicate impact type hindlimb lameness. Because the diff max pelvis and diff min pelvis values are calculated for every stride, these measures are considered more specific indicators of lameness in a particular hindlimb. The approximate threshold between sound and lame for this value is ±3 mm. The 95% confidence interval for a single measure is ±3 mm.

Detecting Compensatory Lameness with Lameness Locator™

In trotting quadrupeds a primary lameness in the front half of the body will cause compensatory move-

ments in the back half of the body and vice versa, such that an apparent multiple limb lameness is present. Interpretation of these compensatory movements is sometimes referred to as the "law of sides." The first part of the law of sides states that an apparent ipsilateral lameness, i.e., forelimb and hindlimb lameness on the same side of the body, is likely primary hindlimb lameness and a compensatory but false forelimb lameness. The second part of the law of sides states that an apparent contralateral lameness, i.e., forelimb and hindlimb lameness on opposite sides of the body, is likely primary forelimb lameness and a compensatory but false hindlimb lameness.

Experimental studies have determined that the first part of the law of sides is, for the most part, true. Although there is significant variability from horse to horse that is likely dependent on the type of primary hindlimb lameness, even slight primary hindlimb lameness may cause compensatory movement in the head that mimics significant forelimb lameness. This suggests the possibility, depending on the sensitivity of detection, of missing the primary hindlimb lameness because of the more apparent compensatory but false forelimb lameness. The increased sampling frequency of the inertial sensors compared to the unaided human eye decreases the chance of this confusion (Figure 3.91).

The second part of the law of sides is slightly misleading. Primary forelimb lameness frequently causes compensatory movements in the vertical movement of the pelvis attributable to both hindlimbs such that false hindlimb lameness could be measured in both sides. Primary forelimb lameness causes the horse to shift its center of gravity slightly toward the back half of the body during the stance phase of the affected forelimb. This causes the pelvis to fall more in the contralateral hindlimb compared to the ipsilateral hindlimb, mimicking impact type lameness in the ipsilateral hindlimb. However, in a horse that is forced to progress forward, the opposite sound diagonal hindlimb (ipsilateral to the forelimb with primary lameness) will push off greater than the hindlimb in the lame diagonal, causing the pelvis to rise more and giving the appearance of a contralateral pushoff type hindlimb lameness. Thus, primary forelimb lameness may cause compensatory movements that mimic ipsilateral hindlimb impact type hindlimb lameness but contralateral pushoff type hindlimb lameness. These compensatory pelvic movements are small compared to the asymmetric head movements of primary forelimb lameness and not usually visible to the naked eye unless the primary forelimb lameness is considerable. However, compensatory pelvic movement patterns with primary forelimb lameness are regularly measured with the increased sensitivity of the inertial sensors and these patterns are useful for helping to detect and evaluate forelimb lameness (Figure 3.92).

Using Lameness Locator™ to Quantify Response to Flexion Tests

Lameness Locator™ can be used to objectively quantify the effect of flexion tests. Thresholds and confidence intervals established for trotting in a straight line and collecting at least 25 contiguous strides, however, are not

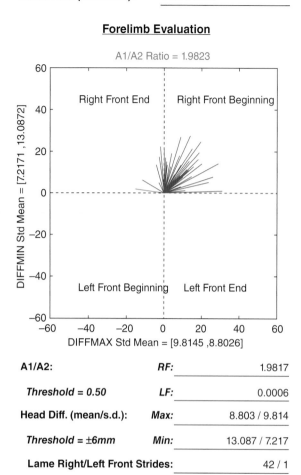

Stride Rate (front/hind):   1.461 / 1.461   **Strides Evaluated (front/hind):**   43 / 43

Forelimb Evaluation

A1/A2 Ratio = 1.9823

A1/A2:	RF:	1.9817
Threshold = 0.50	LF:	0.0006
Head Diff. (mean/s.d.):	*Max:*	8.803 / 9.814
Threshold = ±6mm	*Min:*	13.087 / 7.217
Lame Right/Left Front Strides:		42 / 1

Hindlimb Evaluation

A1/A2:	RH:	0.4058
Threshold = 0.17	LH:	0.0009
Pelvis Diff. (mean/sd):	*Max:*	3.713 / 2.14
Threshold = ±3mm	*Min:*	5.163 / 1.984
Lame Right/Left Hind Strides:		41.5 / 1.5

Figure 3.91. Output of Lameness Locator® indicating primary right hindlimb lameness and compensatory (false) right forelimb lameness, according to the first "law of sides." Pelvis diff max and pelvis diff min are both positive (right hindlimb lameness) and outside threshold (±3 mm). A1/A2 RH = 0.41, which is greater than threshold of 0.17. This is the primary right hindlimb lameness. In forelimb plot all rays are in the first quadrant, and A1/A2 RF, head diff max, and head diff min are all above thresholds, and head diff max and head diff min are positive, all indicating RF early stance lameness. Because lameness is ipsilateral (right hind and right fore), primary lameness is most likely hindlimb, and forelimb is likely compensatory.

applicable. The effect of flexion tests is usually dissipated after fewer numbers of strides and the veterinarian usually evaluates the effects of flexion tests by trotting the horse off in one direction only. Therefore, a baseline trot off in one direction without flexion must be collected for comparison. A positive response to flexion is then ascertained by simply comparing the amplitude of the lameness values for that limb before and after flexion (Figure 3.93).

Using Lameness Locator® to Evaluate Lameness During the Lunge

Lameness Locator® can be used to objectively quantify lameness while the horse is trotting in a circle. Some lameness conditions in horses are more apparent when the horse is moving in a circle. Thresholds and confidence intervals established for trotting in a straight line and collecting at least 25 contiguous strides, however,

are not applicable. When the horse is trotting in a circle the torso is tilted slightly toward the center of the circle. Depending on the horse and the radius of the circle this tilt can be significant. Torso tilt is measured by the inertial sensors as asymmetric vertical motion. However, the effect of tilt can be predicted and in sound horses the tilt and asymmetric motion are equal in amplitude but opposite in direction. For example, in some horses downward motion of the pelvis during the stance phase of the inside limb is less, resulting in an increase in the diff min pelvis absolute value and upward motion of the pelvis on the outside limb is less, resulting in an increase in the diff max pelvis absolute value. Horses trotting to the right can be expected to have negative max diff pelvis values and positive diff min pelvis values. Horses trotting to the left can be expected to have positive diff max pelvis values and negative diff min pelvis values. However, if the amplitude of asymmetry is opposite in direction but equal in amplitude, this should be considered normal (Figure 3.94).

Forelimb Evaluation

Hindlimb Evaluation

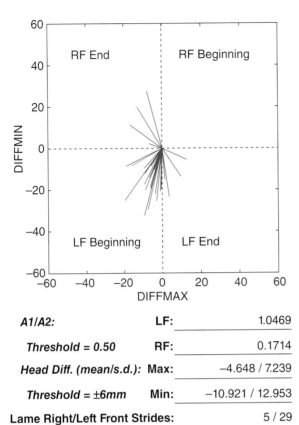

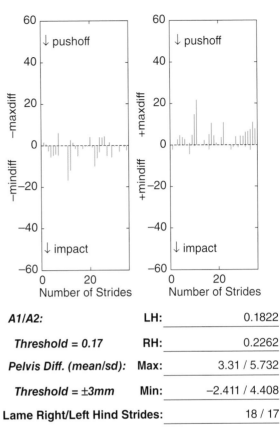

A1/A2:	LF:	1.0469
Threshold = 0.50	RF:	0.1714
Head Diff. (mean/s.d.):	Max:	−4.648 / 7.239
Threshold = ±6mm	Min:	−10.921 / 12.953
Lame Right/Left Front Strides:		5 / 29

A1/A2:	LH:	0.1822
Threshold = 0.17	RH:	0.2262
Pelvis Diff. (mean/sd):	Max:	3.31 / 5.732
Threshold = ±3mm	Min:	−2.411 / 4.408
Lame Right/Left Hind Strides:		18 / 17

Figure 3.92. Output of Lameness Locator® indicating primary left forelimb lameness and compensatory (false) movement in pelvis in both hindlimbs; less upward movement of the pelvis after pushoff of the contralateral (right) hindlimb and less downward movement of the pelvis during landing of the ipsilateral (left) hindlimb.

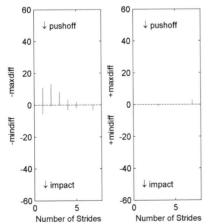

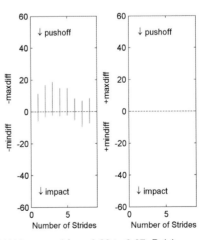

Hindlimb Evaluation

A1/A2; Threshold = 0.17

0.0299	RH	0.00
0.3622	LH	0.6732

Pelvis Diff. (mean/sd)
Threshold = ±3mm

−4.949 / 5.789	Max	−12.348 / 4.448
−1.872 / 2.392	Min	−4.878 / 2.717

Lame Right/Left Hind Strides

1.5 / 5.5	~	0 / 8

Figure 3.93. Output of Lameness Locator® indicating positive response to left hindlimb flexion test. Red and green rays on right side of report (after flexion) are longer than on left side of report (before flexion). A1/A2 LH increased from 0.36 to 0.67. Pelvic max diff becomes more negative (−4.9 mm to −12.3 mm).

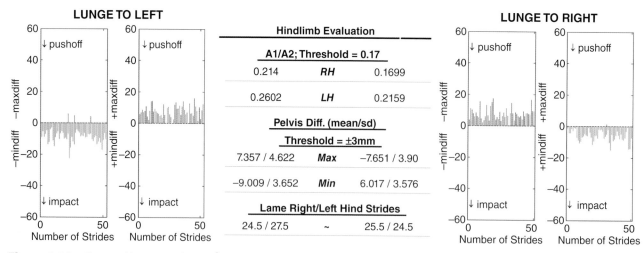

Figure 3.94. Output of Lameness Locator® indicating a normal profile of vertical pelvic movement during the lunge, first to the left (left side of report) and then to the right (right side of report). Pelvic fall is less on inside hindlimb with a negative pelvic min diff lunging to the left and a positive pelvic min diff lunging to the right. Pelvic rise is less on the outside hindlimb with a positive pelvic max diff lunging to the left and a negative pelvic max diff lunging to the right.

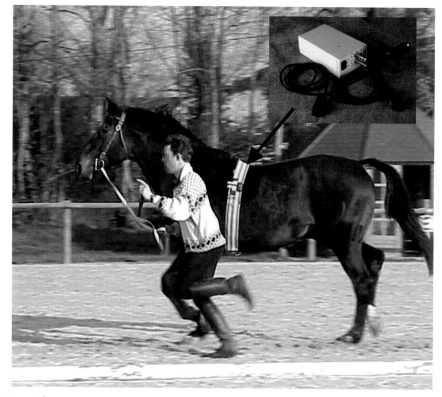

Figure 3.95. Equimetrix® system for lameness evaluation. Accelerometers and data logger attached to the girth strap worn by the horse. (Courtesy of Dr. Eric Barrey, Centaure-Métrix, Evry, France.)

One advantage of using Lameness Locator® to evaluate lameness during the lunge is the ability to collect many contiguous strides in a small area at small effort to the handler. Collection of data from large numbers of contiguous strides decreases variability. However, some horses do not lunge well and many horses misbehave more during the lunge by tossing and shaking the head. This increases variability of vertical torso movement and renders measurement of lameness by Lameness Locator® less reliable. Evaluation of hindlimb lameness by Lameness Locator™ during the lunge is more consistent than evaluation of forelimb lameness.

Equimetrix® by Centaure-Métrix™

Equimetrix® is a 3-dimensional, accelerometer system attached to girth of an exercising horse (Figure 3.95). It is marketed by Centaure-Metrix™ in Evry, France.

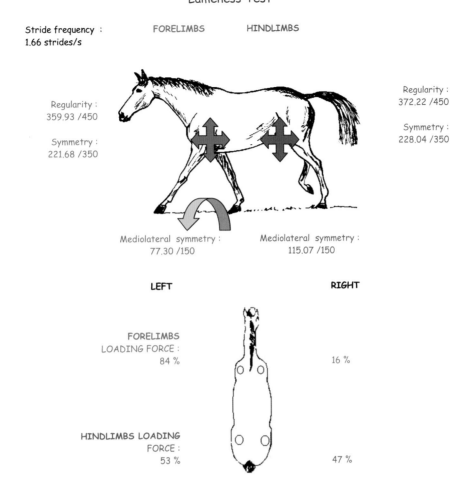

Figure 3.96. Output of the Equimetrix® system for lameness evaluation. Loading force of left forelimb significantly higher than right forelimb, indicating right forelimb lameness. (Courtesy of Dr. Eric Barrey, Centaure-Métrix, Evry, France.)

Three-dimensional torso acceleration is collected and logged as the horse is exercising. The data is then analyzed and output is used to measure stride characteristics such as regularity, frequency, length, and propulsion power. Although the output of Equimetrix® is directed primarily toward assessing performance in exercising horses (race, endurance, jumping, dressage), existing algorithms calculate regularity and symmetry indexes, which are specifically used for lameness evaluation in horses (Figure 3.96). The Equimetrix® process is also validated for the dog, cat, and human (Locometrix®) locomotion evaluation and used for routine examination and clinical trials.

References

1. Arkell M, Archer RM, Guitian FJ, May SA. Evidence of bias affecting the interpretation of the results of local anesthetic nerve blocks when assessing lameness in horses. Vet Rec 2006;159:346–349.
2. Back W, MacAllister CG, van Heel MCV, et al. Vertical frontlimb ground reaction forces of sound and lame Warmbloods differ from those in Quarter horses. J Equine Vet Sci 2007;27:123–129.
3. Barrey E, Hermelin M, Vaudelin JL, et al. Utilisation of an accelerometric device in equine gait analysis. Equine Vet J Suppl 1994;17:7–12.
4. Buchner HHF, Savelberg HCCM, Schamhardt HC, et al. Head and trunk movement adaptations in horses with experimentally induced fore or hindlimb lameness. Equine Vet J 1996;28:71–76.
5. Buchner HHF, Salvelberg HHCM, Schamhardt HC, Barneveld A. Limb movement adaptations in horses with experimentally induced fore- or hindlimb lameness. Equine Vet J 1996;28:63–70.
6. Buchner HHF, Obermüller S, Scheidl M. Body centre of mass movement in the sound horse. Vet J 2000;160:225–234.
7. Buchner HHF. Limb movement pattern in forelimb and hindlimb lameness. Proceedings Am Assoc Equine Pract 2005;51:128–133.
8. Eliashar E, McGuigan MP, Wilson AM. Relationship of foot conformation and force applied to the navicular bone of sound horses at the trot. Equine Vet J 2004;36:431–435.
9. Fuller CJ, Bladon BM, Driver AJ, Barr ARS. The intra- and inter-assessor reliability of measurement of functional outcome by lameness scoring in horses. Vet J 2006;171:281–286.
10. Hewetson M, Christley RM, Hunt ID, Voute LC. Investigations of the reliability of observational gait analysis for the assessment of lameness in horses. Vet Rec 2006;158:852–857.
11. Hu HH, MacAllister CG, Payton ME, Erkert RS. Evaluation of the analgesic effects of phenylbutazone administered at a high and low dosage in horses with chronic lameness. Am J Vet Res 2005;226:414–417.
12. Ishihara A, Bertone AL, Rajaala-Schultz PJ. Association between subjective lameness grade and kinetic gait parameters in horses with experimentally induced forelimb lameness. Am J Vet Res 2005;66:1805–1815.

13. Keegan KG, Wilson DA, Wilson DJ, et al. Evaluation of mild lameness in horses trotting on a treadmill by clinicians and interns or residents and correlation of their assessments with kinematic gait analysis. Am J Vet Res 1998;59:1370–1377.

14. Keegan KG, Arafat S, Skubic M, et al. Detection of lameness and determination of the affected forelimb in horses by use of continuous wavelet transformation and neural network classification of kinematic data. Am J Vet Res 2003;64:1376–1381.

15. Keegan KG, Yonezawa Y, Pai PF, et al. Evaluation of a sensor based system of equine motion analysis for the detection and quantification of forelimb and hindlimb lameness in horses. Am J Vet Res 2004;65:665–670.

16. Keegan KG, Dent EV, Wilson DA, et al. Agreement Among Veterinarians for Subjective Evaluation of Lameness in Horses. Proceedings Am Assoc Equine Pract 2008;54:260.

17. Kramer J, Keegan KG, Wilson DA, et al. Kinematics of the equine hindlimb in trotting horses after induced distal tarsal lameness and distal tarsal anesthesia. Am J Vet Res 2000;61:1031–1036.

18. Pfau T, Robilliard JJ, Weller R, et al. Assessment of mild hindlimb lameness during over ground locomotion using linear discriminant analysis of inertial sensor data. Equine Vet J 2007; 39:407–413.

19. Symonds KD, MacAllister CG, Erkert RS, Payton MC. Use of force plate analysis to assess the analgesic effects of etodolac in horses with navicular syndrome. Am J Vet Res 2006;67: 557–561.

KINEMATICS/KINETICS

Kevin G. Keegan

KINEMATICS

Kinematics is the measurement and study of movement. Kinematics can be used as an objective assessment of lameness in horses. Compared to the force plate, kinematics should be considered a less direct method of detecting and quantifying lameness in horses. A lame horse will bear less weight on the affected limb and this can be measured directly as decreased ground reaction force. Lameness also alters normal motion of the torso, head, neck, and limbs during weight-bearing or while the limb is in the swing phase of the stride. Unless the horse is equally lame in both right and left limbs, the change in movement usually manifests as an increasing asymmetry of movement between the right and left strides. However, asymmetric motion of the torso, head, neck, and limbs may be seen for many reasons other than lameness; for example, conformational disparity between right and left limbs and "leggedness" or preference to use one limb over the other. Motion asymmetry is more variable than change in ground reaction force due to lameness. Higher variability of kinematic data compared to the force plate means that it is potentially less precise than the force plate for measurement of lameness. However, data from multiple contiguous strides can be easily collected kinematically, thereby mitigating the effect of potentially lower precision on sensitivity to detect lameness or small change in lameness.

Despite the higher variability compared to the force plate, results of kinematic evaluation of lameness are generally more intuitive and easy to understand for the veterinary practitioner. Significant findings in kinematic studies of lameness can be more easily applied by the practicing veterinarian for use in a standard lameness evaluation technique.

Until only very recently the most commonly used kinematic technique for evaluation of lameness in horses was camera- and body-marker-based. Body parts are "marked" in some way and the horse is filmed (Figure 3.97). Computer assistance is then used to quantify and record the trajectories of the marked body parts. Analysis of the trajectories, most likely the asymmetry of trajectory motion between right and left parts of the stride, can then be used to detect and measure lameness. Although there are many different commercially-available, camera-based systems, they all depend on unobstructed, line-of-site light transmission. Because of the desirability to collect multiple contiguous strides, most kinematic studies of lameness in horses are performed when the horse is moving on a treadmill. Recent developments in wireless inertial sensor system design, however, have made it possible to conduct kinematic studies of lameness in horses over ground. Information on inertial sensor systems for kinematic study of lame-

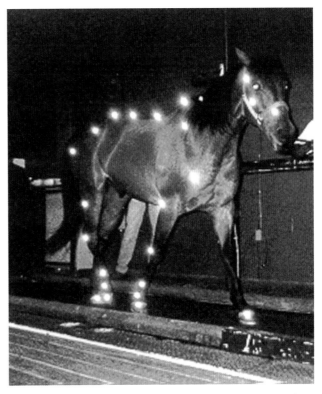

Figure 3.97. Horse on treadmill marked at head, back, and limb joint centers on right side of body in preparation for camera-based kinematic analysis of movement.

ness in horses can be found in the previous section of this chapter on objective assessment of lameness.

Many motion parameters have been measured and studied as lameness indicators in horses. It is not unusual to find in the literature reports of kinematic studies in which many different motion parameters were measured but few were found to be significantly associated with lameness. Although there is considerable overlap, there is also considerable contradiction between studies as to which motion parameters are sensitive indicators of lameness in horses. Some difference can be explained by differences in the models of lameness being studied. Despite these qualifications, some motion parameters can be considered sensitive indicators of lameness in horses.

Joint Angle Measurements Associated with Lameness

Decreased weight-bearing due to lameness in the forelimbs or hindlimbs will decrease maximum fetlock extension and maximum coffin joint flexion during the stance phase of the lame limb compared to the stance phase of the contralateral sound limb (Figure 3.98).[6] Maximum fetlock extension and coffin joint flexion during stance are sensitive indicators of both forelimb and hindlimb lameness in the horse. Fetlock extension during lame limb stance was 8° less than sound limb stance in a sole pressure-induced lameness model of a grade 2 (out of 5) lameness.[7] Carpal extension during stance is reduced but only with moderate to severe lameness.[12] Proximal limb joints become more flexed during weight-bearing of the lame limb, resulting in an overall limb shortening during stance.[10]

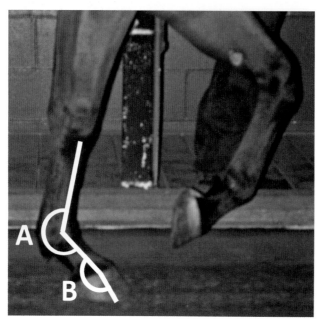

Figure 3.98. (A) Fetlock extension and (B) coffin flexion angles during full weight-bearing. With lameness (A) decreases and (B) decreases.

Stride Timing Variables Associated with Lameness

Except when weight-bearing lameness is severe, stance duration (Figure 3.99) for the lame limb is greater than for the sound limb.[15] Stance duration is increased to spread total vertical ground reaction force out over time so that peak amplitude of vertical ground reaction force is decreased. Step duration, or the time between pushoff of one limb and impact on the contralateral limb (Figure 3.100), on the other hand, is shorter between pushoff of the lame and impact of the sound limb than between pushoff of the sound limb and impact of the lame limb.[4]

Limb Flight Arc Variables Associated with Lameness

The length and shape of the forelimb and hindlimb hoof flight arc during the swing phase of the stride is commonly perceived to be associated with lameness. Forelimb protraction, the cranial phase of the hoof flight arc, will either decrease or increase with lameness, depending upon type of lameness.[12] For example, in the foot, heel lameness generally decreases but toe lameness generally increases forelimb retraction. However, hindlimb protraction is usually decreased in most cases of hindlimb lameness.[13] Unilateral decreased hindlimb protraction is easy to recognize in the lame limb at the trot by visualizing the distance between the affected hindlimb at full protraction and the ipsilateral forelimb at full retraction (Figure 3.101). This distance is longer on the lame side.

The reliability of other swing phase measures to detect lameness has not been objectively studied to sufficient extent. Stride length of the lame limb is decreased compared to the sound limb but significant difference may not be appreciated or detected until lameness is of moderate severity.[2] Step length, or the distance between placements of opposite limbs, such as step duration, is less between placements of the lame and then sound

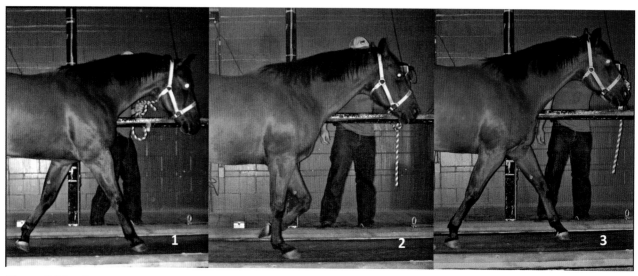

Figure 3.99. Stance duration continues from (1) impact, through (2) midstance, to (3) end of break-over. Stance duration is increased in horses with mild to moderate lameness.

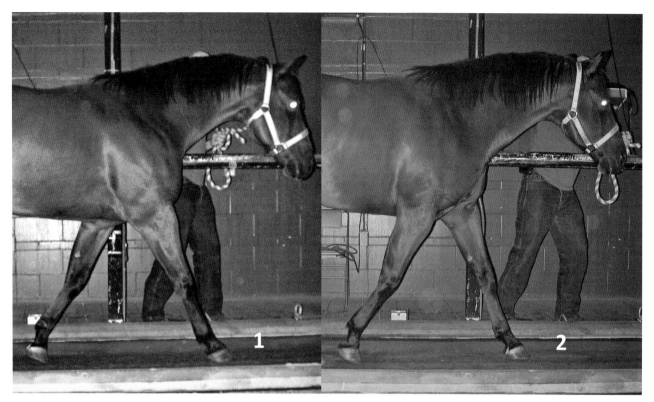

Figure 3.100. Step duration is the duration between (1) impact of one limb and (2) impact of the contralateral limb. Step duration is longer from the sound to the lame limb compared to step duration from the lame to the sound limb. Because stance duration is increased in the lame limb in horses with mild to moderate lameness the largest percent change between sound and lame limbs is a decrease in duration of the swing phase of the sound limb.

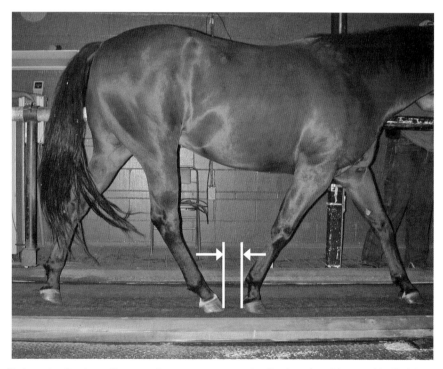

Figure 3.101. Hindlimb protraction is easily seen when viewing from the side of the horse. The hoof of the retracted ipsilateral forelimb acts as a point of reference. Hindlimb protraction is reduced in most hindlimb lameness; thus, the space between the retracted forelimb and protracted hindlimb is greater (arrows) on the lame hindlimb side.

limbs than between placement of the sound and then lame limb.[4] Height of foot flight arc may be increased or decreased in the lame forelimb compared to the sound forelimb, and the shape may be different, depending on the cause of lameness.[6] Dragging the hindlimb toe is commonly thought to be a sign of subtle hindlimb lameness but this may not always be true. In the hindlimb, the height of hoof flight arc is determined by 2 competing factors with the strongest determining the overall effect. Decreased propulsion during pushoff of the lame hindlimb causes the rear torso to rise less. In order to bring the affected limb forward during the swing phase of the stride without dragging it on the ground, the proximal limb joints will flex more. The comparative extents of the decreased torso rise and increased limb flexion determine the height of the hoof flight arc.

The extent of limb abduction or adduction during the swing phase of the stride is thought to be helpful for determination of forelimb and hindlimb lameness in horses. For example, horses with carpal lameness are subjectively thought to abduct the forelimb during the swing phase of the stride. Distal tarsal arthritis is thought to induce adduction and stifle pain is thought to induce abduction of the hindlimb during the swing phase of the stride. However, the phenomenon of altered limb flight arc in the frontal plane due to lameness has not been sufficiently proven by objective kinematic studies.

Vertical Movement of the Torso Associated with Lameness

Most of the evidence suggests that asymmetric vertical movement of the torso is the most sensitive kinematic measure for detection and evaluation of lameness in horses.[5] Stride-to-stride variability in the movement of head and pelvis is less than that of the limbs. Asymmetry of movement of the torso and proximal limb parts is lower than distal limb parts in sound horses.[8] In horses with weight-bearing lameness, asymmetry of trunk and proximal limb movement is greater than that of the distal limb.[1] Thus, if using asymmetry between right and left as the determinant of lameness, the most likely good indicator will be movement of the

torso. Significant load redistribution due to the pain of lameness is most effectively accomplished by altering the vertical movement of the trunk. In the front part of the torso these alterations are magnified by vertical movement of the head and neck.

When a horse trots in a straight line its head and pelvis follow the vertical movement of the torso and move down and then up twice during a single complete stride (Figure 3.102).[5] The head and pelvis move down during the first half of stance and then, depending on the speed of movement, begin moving up at about midstance. In the sound horse this downward and then upward movement is nearly symmetrical in time in a pattern that is regular and of unchanging amplitude. With lameness this constant, regular vertical amplitude is perturbed; the greater the lameness, the greater the perturbation.

With forelimb lameness the normal, expected vertical head movement at the trot is perturbed by vertical movement in the opposite direction, away from the vertical movement of the torso. If the lameness is in the first half of stance, when the head is normally moving down, it moves down but ends its downward progression early to a higher absolute height to the ground than during sound limb stance (Figure 3.103). If the lameness is in the second half of stance, when the head is normally moving up, it moves up more, to a higher absolute height to the ground than after sound limb stance (Figure 3.104). If the forelimb lameness is predominant

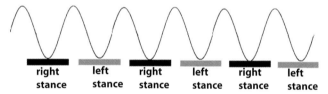

Figure 3.102. Graphic of normal vertical head and pelvic movement in a sound horse. Both head and pelvis move down during the first part of stance and then up in the second part of stance. Amplitude of downward and upward movement are the same in each half-cycle of a complete stride. Also, local maximum and minimum height positions of head and pelvis during each half-cycle of the stride are equivalent.

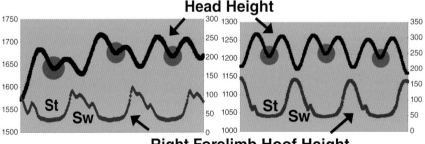

Head Height

Right Forelimb Hoof Height

Figure 3.103. Graphic of impact type forelimb lameness. Primary perturbation of normal vertical head movement is less than expected downward movement of the head during the first part of the stance phase of the lame forelimb. Red circles indicate approximate vertical position of head during midstance of the lame (right) forelimb. St = stance phase of right forelimb (swing phase of the left forelimb). Sw = swing phase of right forelimb (stance phase of the left forelimb). Head height during stance phase of lame right forelimb is higher than during stance phase of sound left forelimb.

Head Height

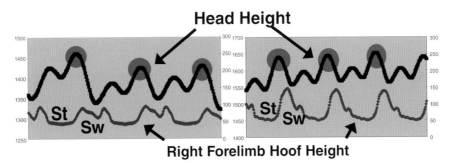

Right Forelimb Hoof Height

Figure 3.104. Graphic of pushoff type forelimb lameness. Primary perturbation of normal vertical head movements is greater than expected upward movement of the head during the second part and after the stance phase of the lame right forelimb. Red circles indicate approximate vertical position of head after the end of the stance of the lame right forelimb. St = stance phase of right forelimb (swing phase of the left forelimb). Sw = swing phase of right forelimb (stance phase of the left forelimb). Head height during second part of and after stance phase of the lame right forelimb is higher than during the second part of and after the stance phase of the sound left forelimb.

in one side, then this perturbation of normal movement occurs once per stride or at one-half the frequency of the normal up-and-down motion of the head.

This perturbation of vertical movement is what many equine practitioners "see" when they evaluate horses for forelimb lameness and it is routinely expressed as a "head bob" or "nod." "Down on sound" and "up on bad" are both used to describe the vertical asymmetric motion of the head in horses with forelimb lameness. However, neither of these simple explanations is correct in every case. "Down on sound" will be correct for most forelimb lameness conditions because most forelimb lameness conditions manifest primarily during the first half of stance (an impact-type lameness). "Down on sound," however, may pick the wrong side if the lameness is predominantly a pushoff-type lameness. "Up on bad" will be correct for some forelimb lameness conditions but is most appropriate for detecting the odd forelimb lameness that primarily manifests during the acceleratory phase of the stride (a pushoff-type lameness). Although this interpretation of forelimb lameness is most likely highly dependent upon speed of movement, knowledge of whether the lameness is manifested primarily during the first or second half of stance is valuable to the practitioner in helping to localize lameness within the affected forelimb.

There are 2 good indicators of asymmetric torso movement for determination of hindlimb lameness in the horse: (1) differential vertical movements of the right and left tuber coxae, and (2) asymmetric vertical movement of the entire pelvis (Figure 3.105).[5,13] The first method, which is easiest to see because the motion is greater, relies on pelvic anatomy symmetry and pelvic rotation around the lumbosacral joint. It is frequently referred to as the pelvic rotation or hip hike technique. The second method, which is more difficult to see in some horses because the amplitude of vertical displacement can be small, depends directly on the force of impact and pushoff of the hindlimbs. This method is referred to as the "vertical pelvic movement" method.

The pelvic rotation or hip hike technique takes advantage of the fact that vertical displacement of the lame-side hemipelvis is greater than that of the sound-side hemipelvis (Figures 3.105 and 3.106). If the lame-

ness is primarily in the first half of hindlimb stance the pelvis will not fall as hard on the affected side and the tuber coxae on the lame side will appear to reach higher relative to the tuber coxae on the sound side hemipelvis immediately before the beginning of stance. If the lameness is primarily in the second half of hindlimb stance the pelvis will not be pushed up as high as the opposite sound side after stance. Lower pelvic height requires the affected limb to flex more for the limb to be brought forward without hitting the ground. The pelvis appears to rotate toward the side of lameness and the tuber coxae on the lame side will reach a lower height than on the sound side. Because it is likely that many hindlimb lameness conditions cause decreased pushoff strength (the hindlimb is the primary propulsive power generator for moving the horse forward), the second observation, or dipping of the tuber coxae on the affected side, is probably the most correct method to use most of the time.

The best position for the evaluator using the pelvic rotation method is behind the horse with the horse moving away from the evaluator. This method has been criticized as being sometimes misleading in horses with pre-existing pelvic asymmetry because the pelvis appears to rotate toward the down side pelvis independent of whether or not force of impact or pushoff are asymmetric. The pelvic rotation method, in some form, is used by most practitioners today for detection and evaluation of hindlimb lameness.

The second, or vertical pelvic movement, method detects the whole pelvis moving down to a lower height during the stance phase of the sound hindlimb or the pelvis moving up to a greater height after pushoff of the sound limb (Figure 3.105). An easily visible marker fixed to the most dorsal aspect of the pelvis between the tuber sacrale may help to detect this asymmetric movement. Horses with impact-type hindlimb lameness display a down-on-sound pattern, with the whole pelvis falling to a lower height during the stance phase of the sound hindlimb.

Horses with a pushoff-type of lameness or lack of impulsion display a less-up-on-bad pattern, with the whole pelvis rising to a lower height just after the stance phase of the lame hindlimb. Using this method the

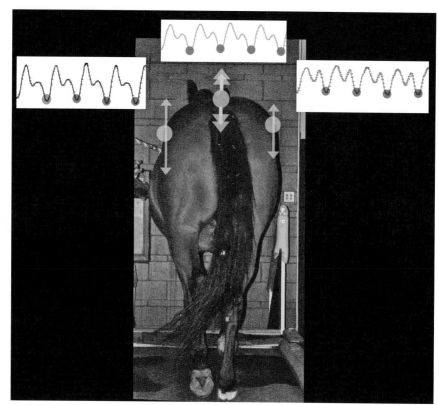

Figure 3.105. Two methods of hindlimb lameness detection and evaluation. Vertical pelvic movement method evaluates imaginary "ball" on midline of pelvis, between the tuber sacrale. Pelvic rotation method evaluates imaginary "balls" located at left and right tuber coxae. Vertical pelvic movement method relies on temporal asymmetry of movement of entire pelvis, with less downward movement of the pelvis (pelvis stops downward movement at higher height) during stance phase of lame limb and/or less upward movement of the pelvis (pelvis stops upward movement at lower height) after pushoff of the lame limb, depending on whether the lameness is impact or pushoff or both.

Top curve (green) indicates dorsal pelvic movement through 4 strides of horse with left hindlimb lameness with black circle at time of sound (right) hindlimb stance (synchronous with picture). Pelvic rotation method relies on greater total vertical movement of the tuber coxae on the lame hindlimb side. Curve on left (black) indicates left tuber coxae vertical movement through 4 strides in horse with left hindlimb lameness with black circles at time of sound (right) hindlimb stance (synchronous with picture). Curve on right (red) indicated right tuber coxae vertical movement through 4 strides in horse with left hindlimb lameness with black circles at time of sound (right) hindlimb stance (synchronous with picture).

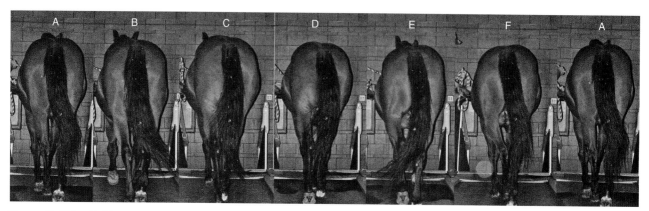

Figure 3.106. Pelvic rotation method of hindlimb lameness detection. Horse has impact and pushoff left hindlimb lameness. A. Left hindlimb impact. B. Left hindlimb midstance. C. Left hindlimb pushoff. D. Right hindlimb impact. E. Right hindlimb midstance. F. Right hindlimb pushoff. Left tuber coxae is higher relative to right tuber coxae during left hindlimb impact (A) than right tuber coxae relative to left tuber coxae during right hindlimb impact (D). This is the impact part of the hindlimb lameness. Also,

left tuber coxae is lower relative to right tuber coxae during right hindlimb midstance (E) than right tuber coxae relative to left tuber coxae during left hindlimb midstance (B). This is the pushoff part of the hindlimb lameness. "Hip hike" is the greater vertical movement of the left tuber coxae from right hindlimb midstance (E) to left hindlimb impact (A) than right tuber coxae movement from left hindlimb midstance (B) to right hindlimb impact (D).

evaluator can be either behind the horse as it moves away or beside the horse as it passes by. This method is more difficult to see (compared to the pelvic rotation method) because vertical movement of the pelvis at the midline is relatively small, especially in some breeds such as Missouri Foxtrotters. Furthermore, the tail head in other breeds, such as American Saddlebreds, frequently projects upward and effectively obscures the dorsum of the pelvis, making asymmetric vertical movement of this area difficult to see. Nevertheless, this method is less sensitive to pre-existing pelvic asymmetry, and can be mastered with practice. This method is also more robust because it can be employed by the evaluator from any direction around the horse. Both impact- and pushoff-type hindlimb lameness are suspected to occur in horses.

Knowledge of and ability to detect the different types of pelvic asymmetry (i.e., down on sound or less up on bad) is helpful to veterinary practitioners isolating lameness within the affected limb.

KINETICS

In physics, kinetics can be considered a branch of dynamics or classical mechanics, concerned with the motion of bodies and the forces acting upon them. In human and veterinary medicine, kinetics usually refers to measurement of ground reaction forces acting on a body for the purpose of measuring locomotion. In equine medicine ground reaction forces are measured primarily with the stationary force plate to evaluate hoof-surface interaction; for example, to evaluate trimming or shoeing manipulations, and, of interest to this section, to measure and evaluate musculoskeletal or neurological abnormalities. Although force-measuring treadmills for horses exist and force-measuring horse shoes have been described, this section only concerns the stationary force plate to evaluate lameness in horses.

The stationary force plate has been used for many years to evaluate lameness in horses. Compared to using cameras or inertial sensors (kinematics), the stationary force plate should rightly be considered a more direct method of identifying and quantifying lameness in horses. The stationary force plate has the requisite qualities for it to be considered a gold standard for lameness quantification in horses. The general principal of using the force plate to measure lameness is that a horse with lameness will bear less weight on the affected limb resulting in decreased ground reaction force against the affected limb. Most stationary force plates use highly sensitive load transducers (strain or capacitance gauges, or piezoelectric or piezoresistive sensors) distributed around and under a flat surface structure. The simplest force plate measures only the vertical component of ground reaction force at the geometric center of the force plate surface, but more advanced force plates measure vertical, horizontal, and transverse ground reaction forces at the net center of the point of application of force, center of pressure, or ground reaction force center. The installation and proper maintenance of a force plate facility requires considerable planning, expertise, and oversight.

When evaluating a horse for lameness using the stationary force plate, the horse is led, usually either at the walk or trot, over the force plate until one of the limbs strikes the surface of the force plate completely within the confines of the borders of the plate surface. Successful hoof strikes do not usually occur on every trip over the force plate area. Controlled conditions, such as starting the horse the same distance from the force plate on each trial, keeping the speed of the horse approximately the same on each trial, and camouflaging the force plate, help to increase the percentage of successful hoof strikes. For complete evaluation of bilateral or multiple limb lameness, each limb needs to be evaluated individually. To account for stride-to-stride variability, even under strictly controlled conditions, most investigators suggest collecting at least 5 to 6 valid hoof strikes from each limb being evaluated. Ground reaction forces correlate strongly with speed of movement. For this reason most force plate facilities additionally incorporate some method of measuring speed of movement, such as electronic switches activated by interrupting the transmission of laser light path, or using high speed cameras to track markers attached to the approximate center of mass of the horse.

Stationary force plates are capable of measuring ground reaction forces in all 3 orthogonal directions: vertical, horizontal (caudocranial), and transverse (side to side). Peak (highest) force within the signal and force impulse (area under the force signal curve) are specific measures usually reported in force plate investigations of lameness. Peak force measures can be reported in units of Newtons (kg × m/sec^2), normalized between horses by reporting in Newtons/kg of body weight, or as percentage of body weight (9.8 N/kg = 100% body weight). Event duration, such as stance phase duration or braking phase duration (see below), and time variables, such as time of peak vertical force or time of transition between negative horizontal (braking) and positive horizontal (propulsion) forces, can be collected and have also been investigated for their relation to lameness. Duration and time variables are reported either in raw units (i.e., seconds) or they are normalized between horses and strides by calculating and reporting in units of percent stance or stride duration.

The vertical ground reaction force signal is most strongly associated with lameness and, therefore, most frequently used by equine lameness investigators as the signal of interest. Also, the trial-to-trial variability of vertical ground reaction force measures is generally lower than measures in the horizontal and transverse directions, with coefficients of variation below 10%.[11] Thus, measurement of vertical ground reaction forces with the stationary force plate should be considered a sensitive and specific objective lameness measurement tool in clinical investigations of equine lameness. Using lameness measures with low trial-to-trial variability increases the likelihood of finding small differences between treatment groups with fewer numbers of control and treated subjects. There is objective evidence that supports the belief that the stationary force plate is more sensitive than the human eye at detecting lameness in horses.[11]

Amplitude of vertical ground reaction forces in a sound horse at a moderate speed trot (3 to 4 m/s) varies between breeds. In sound Quarter horses, peak vertical ground reaction force in the forelimbs is about 95% to

103% of body weight in the forelimbs and 92% of body weight in the hindlimbs.[3] This is about 5,000 Newtons for the average 1,000-pound horse or about 9 to 10 Newtons/kg of body weight. By comparison, peak vertical ground reaction force in sound Warmbloods is higher, with normal reported values ranging from 118% to 126% for the forelimbs and 96% for the hindlimbs.[3] For each grade of lameness on the AAEP scale, peak vertical ground reaction force decreases by about 12% in Quarter horses and about 20% in Warmbloods.[3] Presumably similar amplitude decreases would be seen in other breeds of horses.

Although more work needs to be completed in this area, there is some evidence for disease-specific changes in the shape of the vertical ground reaction force signal.[9] Thus, it may be possible in the future to use the force plate to help further localize lameness within an affected limb. For example, differentiating between lameness with peak pain occurring during impact, as would be expected with a hoof or distal limb cause, and lameness with peak pain occurring later in the stance phase, as would be expected with some flexor tendon, suspensory apparatus, or upper limb soft tissue injury.

References

1. Audigié F, Pourcelot P, Degueurce C, et al. Kinematic analysis of the symmetry of limb movements in lame trotting horses. Equine Vet J Suppl 2001;33:128–134.
2. Back W, Barneveld A, van Weeren PR, van den Bogert AJ. Kinematic gait analysis in equine carpal lameness. Acta Anat 1993;146:86–89.
3. Back W, MacAllister CG, van Heel MCV, et al. Vertical frontlimb ground reaction forces of sound and lame Warmbloods differ from those in Quarter horses. J Equine Vet Sci 2007;27:123–129.
4. Buchner HHF, Savelberg HHCM, Schamhardt HC, et al. Temporal stride patterns in horses with experimentally induced fore and hindlimb lameness. Equine Vet J Suppl 1995;18:161–165.
5. Buchner HHF, Savelberg HHCM, Schamhardt HC, et al. Head and trunk movement adaptations in horses with experimentally induced fore- and hindlimb lameness. Equine Vet J 1996;28:71–76.
6. Buchner HHF, Savelberg HHCM, Schamhardt HC, et al. Limb movement adaptations in horses with experimentally induced fore or hindlimb lameness. Equine Vet J 1996;28:63–70.
7. Buchner HHF. Limb movement pattern in forelimb and hindlimb lameness. Proceedings Am Assoc Equine Pract 2005;51:128–133.
8. Degueurce C, Pourcelot P, Audigié F, et al. Variability of the limb joint patterns of sound horses at trot. Equine Vet J Suppl 1997;23:89–92.
9. Eliashar E, McGuigan MP, Wilson AM. Relationship of foot conformation and force applied to the navicular bone of sound horses at the trot. Equine Vet J 2004;36:431–435.
10. Hjertén G, Drevemo S. Shortening of the forelimb in the horse during the stance phase. Acta Anat 1993;146:193–195.
11. Ishihara A, Bertone AL, Rajaala-Schultz PJ. Association between subjective lameness grade and kinetic gait parameters in horses with experimentally induced forelimb lameness. Am J Vet Res 2005;66:1805–1815.
12. Keegan KG, Wilson DA, Smith BK, et al. Changes in kinematic variables seen with lameness induced by applying pressure to the frog and to the toe in adult horses trotting on the treadmill. Am J Vet Res 2000;61:612–619.
13. Kramer J, Keegan KG, Wilson DA, et al. Kinematics of the hindlimb in trotting horses after induced lameness of the distal intertarsal and tarsometatarsal joints and intra-articular administration of anesthetic. Am J Vet Res 2000;61:1031–1036.
15. Weishaupt MA. Compensatory load redistribution in forelimb and hindlimb lameness. Proceedings Am Assoc Equine Pract 2005;51:141–148.

PERINEURAL AND INTRASYNOVIAL ANESTHESIA

Gary M. Baxter and Ted S. Stashak

Local anesthesia is commonly used during a lameness examination to confirm or identify the site or sites of pain where obvious pathology may not exist.[7,15,23,54,55] It can also be useful to prove the location of a lameness to a client who may be suspicious of another site. Local anesthesia may be accomplished by perineural infiltration (local nerve block), ring block, direct infiltration of a painful region, or intrasynovial injection (joints, tendon sheaths, and bursae). The reader is referred to the accompanying DVD for further information and demonstration of these techniques.

Perineural infiltration and ring blocks are used to localize the source of pain to a specific region and, therefore, should be performed in a systematic manner starting with the distal extremity and progressing proximally. Direct infiltration and intrasynovial anesthesia are used to identify the involvement of a specific structure and do not have to be performed in a systematic manner.[7] It is not uncommon to perform several different types of local anesthesia in the same horse (perineural together with intrasynovial), depending on the specific clinical signs and problem. With lameness, local anesthesia is important to document the specific site of the problem so that diagnostic imaging (radiography, ultrasonography, or magnetic resonance imaging) can be used to determine the cause of the problem. Other uses of local anesthesia include providing analgesia during and after surgery and pain control for other painful conditions.

TYPES OF LOCAL ANESTHETICS

The local anesthetics most frequently used are 2% lidocaine hydrochloride (Xylocaine hydrochloride) and 2% mepivacaine hydrochloride (Carbocaine). These solutions are potent and rapidly effective, but can be locally irritating. Because mepivacaine is longer lasting and less irritating than lidocaine, it is used most frequently.[3,42,55] Lidocaine is thought to last only 60 minutes with the maximum effect at 15 minutes.[61] However, a recent study using force plate evaluations indicated that mepivacaine was also only fully effective for 15 to 60 minutes after a palmar digital (PD) nerve block was performed.[3] The effect of the block began to subside between 1 and 2 hours, but gait characteristics persisted beyond 2 hours. This is very important to remember when performing multiple nerve blocks on any given horse over a prolonged period of time. Bupivacaine hydrochloride (marcaine) may be used if the goal is to provide a longer duration of analgesia (4 to 6 hours), such as following surgery.[42] The duration of anesthesia may also be prolonged by combining the local anesthetic with epinephrine. Combining epinephrine with lidocaine can provide up to 6 hours of total anesthesia.[61] However, swelling is usually more severe and the potential to cause skin necrosis over the site of injection is a serious concern.[61,62]

SKIN PREPARATION AND RESTRAINT

The only skin preparation necessary for most sites of regional anesthesia is scrubbing/wiping the area with gauze soaked in alcohol until clean. However, there are a few sites for perineural anesthesia that are very close to synovial structures where during injection the needle may inadvertently enter a synovial cavity. These exceptions include the low four-point block (digital tendon sheath or fetlock joint), the high palmar/plantar blocks (carpometacarpal or tarsometatarsal joints), and the lateral palmar block (middle carpal joint or carpal sheath). A more thorough skin preparation of these sites is recommended to avoid potential complications. A minimum 5-minute scrubbing of the skin and hair with an antiseptic and alcohol is recommended for intrasynovial injections.[26] The horse may be clipped if the hair is unusually long or soiled, but this is not necessary.[26] In all cases, the least amount of local anesthetic should be used to reduce tissue irritation and local diffusion of anesthetic that may complicate the interpretation of the block.

When performing local anesthesia, the horse should be haltered and restrained by an attendant who is standing on the same side of the horse. For intrasynovial anesthesia, a twitch is usually applied so that there is minimal limb movement during the insertion of the needle and injection of the anesthetic. When using local anesthesia in the hindlimb, the practitioner should always be in a position so that minimal bodily harm will result if rapid movement occurs. In most cases the needle is inserted rapidly and the syringe applied just tight enough to prevent loss of local anesthetic solution during injection.

PERINEURAL ANESTHESIA

Perineural anesthesia is used when the lame limb has been identified but the exact region affected cannot be determined by other methods. Even if a suspicious region is identified, it is often useful to anesthetize the region to confirm that the lameness is emanating from a single location. It is not uncommon to find several regions on one limb or find that other limbs may be contributing to the overall lameness problem. In these cases local anesthesia allows one to interpret the percentage that each region is contributing to the lameness. In addition, the degree of improvement with perineural blocks may aid in the interpretation of the findings on imaging. This is especially true for conditions that may be contributing to palmar heel pain.

Perineural anesthesia is typically performed in a stepwise manner starting from the distal limb and progressing proximally. In general, the accuracy of desensitizing a nerve is greater in the distal limb (distal to the carpus and tarsus) than more proximally where the nerves are deeper and covered with soft tissue. Also, the more distal the nerve, the more specific or smaller the region is that is anesthetized. In most cases perineural anesthesia is thought to desensitize the skin and all deep structures distal to the site of injection. However, aberrant nerves exist and should be remembered when interpreting the response to a block. Some feel that ring blocks are more reliable to completely desensitize the skin than local perineural blocks.[62] However, ring blocks are not commonly performed when attempting to accurately locate the site of lameness. Guidelines for performing perineural anesthesia are given in Table 3.3.

A thorough knowledge of the neuroanatomy of the involved region and a good understanding of the limitations of perineural anesthesia are necessary to properly apply and interpret perineural anesthesia. Accurately determining whether the nerve has been completely desensitized by the block is often the first step in interpreting the result. Complete desensitization of the nerve is often evaluated by checking the skin sensation distal to the point of injection. This can be performed with a blunt object such as a pen, hemostat, or needle cap. These objects should not be jabbed into the skin, but applied gently at first with a gradual increase in pressure. Most horses are receptive to this technique, and will quietly respond if the nerves are not totally desensitized. However, some horses are difficult to read and skin sensation may persist even with an effective block. This is especially true for blocks performed more proxi-

Table 3.3. Guidelines for perineural local anesthesia.

Specific block	Needle size	Volume of anesthetic	Skin prep recommended (Yes or No)	Location
Palmar/plantar digital (PD)	25 g, 5/8″	1–1.5 mL	No	Just above collateral cartilages
Basisesamoid (High PD)	25 g, 5/8″	1.5–2 mL	No	At the base of the proximal sesamoid bone
Pastern ring block	22 g, 1.5″	2–3 mL	No	Above collateral cartilages and directed dorsally
Abaxial sesamoid	25 g, 5/8″	1.5–2 mL	No	Abaxial surface of proximal sesamoid bone
Low palmar or 4-point	22–25 g, 5/8–1″	2–3 mL/site	Yes	Distal metacarpus (above buttons of splint bones)
High palmar or 4-point	25 g 5/8″ and 20–22 g 1.5″	3–5 mL/site	Yes	Proximal metacarpus
Lateral palmar (lateral approach)	20–22 g 1″	5–8 mL	Yes	Distal to accessory carpal bone
Lateral palmar (medial approach)	25 g, 5/8″ or 22 g 1″	2–4 mL	No	Medial aspect of accessory carpal bone
Ulnar	20 g 1.5″	10 mL	No	4″ above accessory carpal bone
Median	20–22 g 1.5–2.5″	10 mL	No	Caudal to radius below pectoralis muscle
Medial cutaneous antebrachial	22–25 g 1–1.5″	5–10 mL	No	Mid-radius near cephalic and accessory cephalic veins
Low plantar or 6-point	25 g, 5/8″ or 22 g 1″	2–3 mL/site	Yes	Distal metatarsus and each side of long digital extensor tendon
High plantar, high 4-point or subtarsal	25 g 5/8″ and 20–22 g 1.5″	3–5 mL/site	Yes	Proximal metatarsus
Deep branch of lateral plantar	20–22 g 1.5″	5–7 mL/site	Yes	Lateral aspect of proximal metatarsus
Tibial/peroneal	20–22 g 1.5″	10–20 mL/site	No	4″ above point of hock on lateral and medial aspects of limb

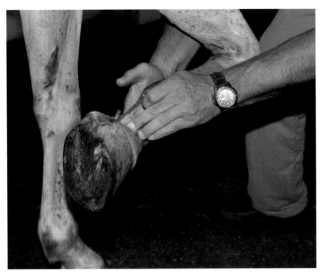

Figure 3.107. This image illustrates the positioning to perform a PD nerve block when facing the back of the horse and holding the limb with one hand. The needle is directed toward the hoof and is inserted at or below the level of the collateral cartilages.

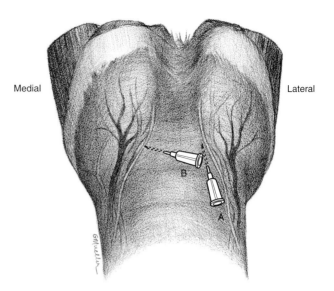

Medial   Lateral

Figure 3.108. Injection sites for a PD nerve block. In (A), the needle is inserted parallel to the lateral PD nerve, while in (B), the needle enters just off midline and is inserted in the subcutaneous tissues to approximate the medial PD nerve.

mally in the limb (above the fetlock). Other manipulative tests that previously caused pain (such as hoof tester examination, deep palpation, and flexion) may need to be repeated to accurately determine if the block worked. The ultimate test is whether lameness is no longer present, but for those horses that have not improved accurate interpretation of complete nerve desensitization is important. Therefore, it is recommended that multiple approaches be used before deciding whether perineural anesthesia has or has not been successful.

The Forelimb

Palmar Digital (PD) Block

The medial and lateral palmar digital nerves are located just palmar to their respective artery and vein and lie along the dorsal border of the SDFT proximal to the pastern joint and along the DDFT distal to the pastern joint. The injection is done with the foot elevated in most cases. Some prefer to stand with their backs toward the animal's rear end while holding the hoof between their knees. Others prefer holding the pastern with one hand while injecting with the other and assume either a lateral or frontal position in relation to the limb (Figure 3.107). The PD nerves should be anesthetized just distal to or at the proximal border of the collateral cartilages (Figure 3.107 and 3.108). Blocking the nerves at this location reduces the risk of anesthetizing the dorsal branches of the PD nerve.[54,55] If the PD block is performed 2 to 3 cm above the collateral cartilages, the PIP joint is often desensitized in addition to the foot.[51] The PD nerve and neurovascular bundle are easily palpable at the level of the collateral cartilage just behind the DDFT. A 25-gauge, 5/8-inch (1.5-cm) needle is inserted into the subcutaneous tissue in a proximal to distal direction over the nerve, and 1

to 1.5 ml of local anesthetic solution is injected perineurally.[55,62] The needle is retracted slightly and redirected if excessive pressure is needed to inject. Since there are several tissue planes, it is advisable to inject a small amount of local anesthetic as the needle is being withdrawn. Each nerve can be injected individually (preferred by the author) or the needle can be directed across midline under the skin to inject the contralateral nerve (Figure 3.108).

Loss of skin sensation at the coronary band in the heel region and loss of deep sensation between the heel bulbs after 5 to 10 minutes is a reliable indication that the block was successful.[42] Previous hoof tester pain should also be gone following the block. Once the block has been assessed to be successful, the horse is exercised in a manner similar to that which led to the original signs of lameness. In cases of navicular syndrome, the lameness will often shift to the opposite forelimb. In general, other conditions affecting this region, such as wing fractures of the distal phalanx, subsolar abscess, and pedal osteitis, are often unilateral, and the lameness should be greatly reduced or eliminated. Structures that are desensitized with a biaxial PD nerve block include the entire sole, the navicular apparatus and soft tissues of the heel, the entire DIP joint of the forelimb, the distal portion of the DDFT, and some of the distal sesamoidean ligaments.[18,42,54,55] Partial desensitization of the PIP joint is also thought to occur in some horses.[51]

Pastern Ring or Semi-ring Block

A pastern ring block is performed just above the collateral cartilages of the distal phalanx at the same site as the PD block (Figure 3.109). A 20- to 22-gauge needle is used to inject 3 to 4 mL of anesthetic subcutaneously laterally and medially from the site of the respective PD block. The needle is directed dorsally

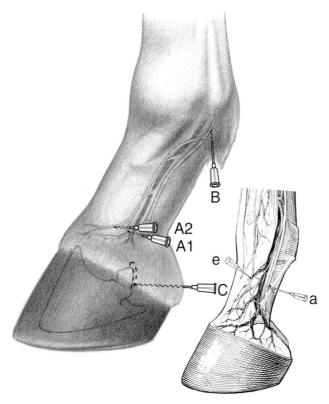

Figure 3.109. Injection sites for local anesthesia. A1 and A2. Sites for the pastern ring block. B. Site for the digital nerve block at the base of the sesamoid bones (basisesamoid block). C. Site for the navicular bursa block. Inset: a. Plantar digital nerve. e. Lateral and medial dorsal metatarsal nerves from the deep peroneal.

perpendicular to the long axis of the pastern to about the level of the medial and lateral collateral ligaments. This will anesthetize the dorsal branches of the PD nerve and will desensitize all the deep structures distal to the block. However, because the dorsal branches of the digital nerves are thought to contribute little to sensation within the foot, the pastern ring block is unlikely to improve lameness that has not been ameliorated with a PD nerve block.[18,42] The pastern ring block can be performed with the limb in a full weight-bearing position but is easier to perform with the foot off the ground. Horses tend to resent this block more than the PD or basisesamoid nerve blocks.

Basisesamoid or High PD Block

An alternative to the pastern ring block is the basisesamoid block. This block is performed similarly to the PD block, only it is more proximal on the limb at the base of the proximal sesamoid bones (often referred to as a high PD block). The PD nerves can be palpated at this location and 1.5 to 2 mL of anesthetic is deposited directly over the nerves using a 25-gauge, 5/8-inch (1.5-cm) needle (Figure 3.109). The basisesamoid block will desensitize the dorsal branch and the PD nerve at a more proximal location in the pastern. This block desensitizes the palmar/plantar soft tissue structures of

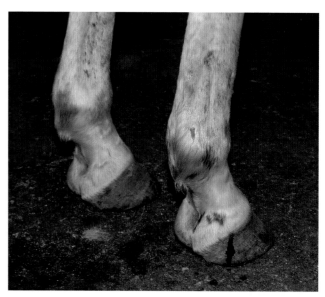

Figure 3.110. Needle location to perform an abaxial sesamoid nerve block in the forelimb.

the pastern, PIP joint, and all structures of the foot. Because it is performed at the base of the sesamoid bones, it is unlikely to desensitize any of the fetlock joint.

Abaxial Sesamoid Block

The neurovascular bundle is easily palpable at the abaxial surface of the proximal sesamoid bone. With the limb elevated by holding the fetlock in the palm of the hand, the palmar nerve can be isolated by rolling it away from the artery and vein with the thumb or forefinger. A 5/8-inch (1.5-cm), 25-gauge needle is used to inject 2 mL of anesthetic perineurally (Figure 3.110). It is best to use a small volume of anesthetic and direct the needle distally to avoid partial desensitization of the fetlock joint.[55] The biaxial block desensitizes the foot, middle phalanx, PIP joint, distopalmar aspects of proximal phalanx, distal portions of the SDFT and DDFT, distal sesamoidean ligaments, and digital annular ligament.[13,42,55] Loss of skin sensation at the coronary band in the toe region together with loss of skin sensation on the palmar pastern is used to determine the success of the block.[42] While it is common to find that skin sensation still exists over the dorsal surface of the phalanges, this does not mean that the phalanges and all the deep structures are not desensitized.

Low Palmar Block (Low 4-Point Block)

The low palmar block is often referred to as the low 4-point block because both palmar and palmar metacarpal nerves are anesthetized at the distal aspect of the metacarpus/metatarsus (Figure 3.111). The lateral and medial palmar nerves lie between the suspensory ligament and the DDFT. Since they assume a vein-artery-nerve relationship, these nerves are located closer to the DDFT and lie on its dorsal edge.[43] These nerves are relatively deep but can be reached in most cases with

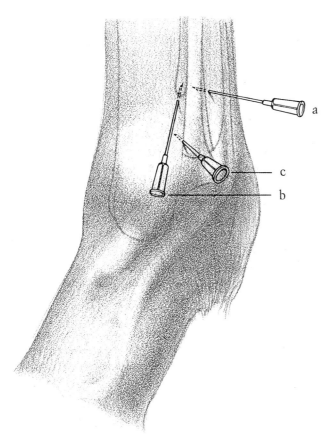

Figure 3.111. Low palmar or 4-point block. a. Site for palmar nerve block, but it is recommended to go 1 cm proximal to the distal end of the small metacarpal bones. b. Site for palmar metacarpal nerve block at the distal end of the splint bones. c. Site for intrasynovial anesthesia of the palmar/plantar pouch of the fetlock joint.

a 5/8-inch (1.5-cm) 25-gauge needle (a 1-inch, 22-gauge needle may also be used), after which 2 to 3 mL of local anesthetic is deposited. It is best to perform these blocks 1 cm proximal to the distal ends of the splint bones to avoid injection into the digital flexor tendon sheath.[30,42]

Blocking the palmar nerves alone will not completely desensitize the fetlock joint. Two additional nerves, the medial and lateral palmar metacarpal nerves, innervate the deep structures of the fetlock.[47,62] These nerves course parallel and axial to the second and fourth metacarpal bones. A 5/8-inch (1.5-cm) 25-gauge needle or a 1-inch (2.5-cm), 22-gauge needle is used to inject 2 to 3 mL of anesthetic around these nerves as they emerge distal to the ends of the second and fourth metacarpal bones (Figure 3.111b). However, because the palmar pouches of the fetlock joint can be inadvertently entered at this location, these nerves can also be anesthetized more proximally.[42]

Both the palmar and palmar metacarpal nerve blocks can be performed while the horse is bearing full weight or the limb can be held with the opposite hand. It is usually easier to perform in the standing position. Anesthesia of these four nerves effectively desensitizes the deep structures of the fetlock region and all structures distally.[42] Anesthesia of the skin over the dorsal aspect of the pastern and fetlock indicates that the block was successful. Some skin sensation may be present over the dorsal surface of the fetlock joint as a result of the sensory supply from the medial cutaneous antebrachial distribution.[47]

High Palmar (High 4-Point Block)

The high 4-point or high palmar block is analogous to the low 4-point block because the same 4 nerves are anesthetized in the proximal aspect of the metacarpus just below the carpometacarpal joint. However, the high palmar block is more difficult to perform because the soft tissue structures are more closely confined to the metacarpus and the palmar metacarpal nerves are located deeper within the axial borders of the second and fourth metacarpal bones. In addition, the distal outpouchings of the carpometacarpal joint extend approximately 2.5 cm distal to the joint in close proximity to the nerves, and can be entered when blocking the palmar metacarpal nerves.[20,30] Therefore, aseptic preparation of the injection sites is recommended when blocking the palmar metacarpal nerves.

The proximal palmar nerves are anesthetized in the groove between the suspensory ligament and the DDFT. The nerves lie under heavy fascia, palmar to the vein and artery, and rest against the dorsal, lateral, and medial aspects of the deep digital flexor tendon. A 5/8-inch (1.5 cm), 25-gauge needle is inserted through the heavy fascia and 3 to 5 mL of anesthetic is deposited (Figure 3.112 a and b).[42] Blocking just the palmar nerves will not completely desensitize the deep structures of the metacarpus.[62] The palmar metacarpal nerves run parallel and axial to the second and fourth metacarpal bones and each can be desensitized by infiltration of 3 to 5 mL of local anesthetic along the axial surfaces of the metacarpal bones. (Figure 3.113 b_1 and b_2). A 20- to 22-gauge, 1.5-inch needle is directed toward the palmar metacarpus along the axial borders of the splint bones until bone is contacted. The needle is withdrawn slightly and aspirated to be certain that the needle is not within the carpometacarpal joint before the anesthetic is deposited. Blocking the palmar metacarpal nerves is usually performed with the limb held, whereas anesthesia of the palmar nerves is often easier with the limb weight-bearing.[42]

These four nerve blocks will effectively desensitize the deep structures of the metacarpus with the exception of the origin of the suspensory ligament.[30] The medial and lateral palmar metacarpal nerves innervate the interosseous ligaments of the second and fourth metacarpal bones, the interosseous lateralis and medialis muscles, and the suspensory ligament (interosseus muscle).[47] The palmar nerves innervate the flexor tendons and the inferior check ligament.[42] Horses that become sound after this block warrant diagnostic imaging of the metacarpal region. Lack of improvement with a high palmar block does not necessarily rule out a problem at the origin of the suspensory.

Lateral Palmar Block (Lateral Approach)

The lateral palmar nerve originates at a variable distance proximal to the carpus and represents a

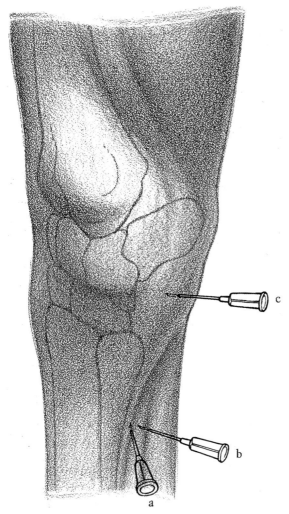

Figure 3.112. High 4-point block. a and b. Needle positioned lateral and medial to block the palmar nerves. c. Needle positioning to perform the lateral approach to block the lateral palmar nerve. Needle positioning to block the palmar metacarpal nerves is not shown but is located axial to the heads of the splint bones.

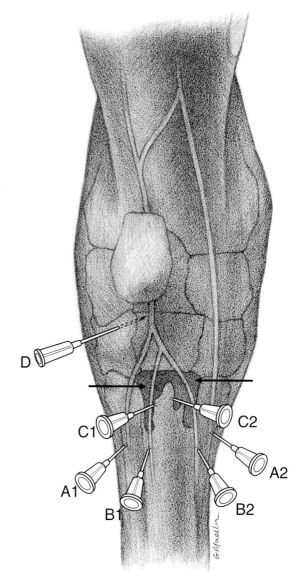

Figure 3.113. Palmar view of the carpometacarpal region of the left forelimb showing the synovial outpouchings of the carpometacarpal joint (arrows). A1 and A2. Sites for injection of the palmar nerves. B1 and B2. Sites for injection of the palmar metacarpal nerves. C1 and C2. Sites for direct infiltration of the origin of the suspensory ligament. D. Site for injection of the lateral palmar nerve using the lateral approach.

continuation of the median nerve plus the palmar branch of the ulnar nerve. The lateral palmar nerve courses in a dorsolateral direction distal to the accessory carpal bone and runs along the palmar-distal aspect of the accessoriometacarpal ligament (Figure 3.113d). At the proximal end of the fourth metacarpal bone, the lateral palmar nerve gives off its deep branch that detaches branches to the origin of the suspensory ligament and divides into the lateral and medial palmar metacarpal nerves (Figure 3.113 b_1 and b_2).[62] The lateral palmar nerve can be anesthetized just below the accessory carpal bone (lateral approach) or axial to the accessory carpal bone in a more proximal location (medial approach). This block desensitizes the origin of the suspensory and ligament and other deep structures of the palmar metacarpus. Performing this block avoids the necessity of direct infiltration of the suspensory ligament and anesthesia of the palmar and palmar metacarpal nerves independently.[21,30]

The lateral palmar nerve is anesthetized with 5 to 8 mL of anesthetic administered through a 1-inch (2.5-cm), 20-gauge needle midway between the distal border of the accessory carpal bone and the proximal end of the fourth metacarpal bone on the palmar border of the accessoriometacarpal ligament (Figures 3.112c and 3.113d). The needle is directed in a palmarolateral-to-dorsomedial direction and must penetrate the 2- to 3-mm thickness of the flexor retinaculum of the carpus.[30] This block may be performed with the horse standing or with the carpus slightly flexed.[30] Skin sensation is not useful to evaluate the effect of the block. Instead, lack of any response to deep palpation of the proximal suspensory ligament often suggests an effective block.

Lateral Palmar Block (Medial Approach)

The lateral palmar nerve may also be blocked medial to the accessory carpal bone.[8] This medial technique is thought to reduce the risk of inadvertent injection into the carpal canal which may occur with the lateral approach to the lateral palmar nerve.[21,42] The site of injection is a longitudinal groove in the fascia palpable over the medial aspect of the accessory carpal bone, palmar to the insertion of the flexor retinaculum that forms the palmaromedial aspect of the carpal canal.[8,42] With the limb weight-bearing, a 25-gauge, 5/8-inch needle is inserted into the distal third of the groove in a mediolateral direction perpendicular to the limb. The needle should contact the bone and 2 mL of anesthetic is injected (Figure 3.114). In the first author's experience with this technique, injection may be difficult until the needle is withdrawn slightly or redirected. The author uses a 22-gauge, 1-inch (2.5 cm) needle and 2 to 4 mL of anesthetic for this technique. Skin sensation is not useful to evaluate the effect of the block and palpation of the suspensory ligament is necessary.

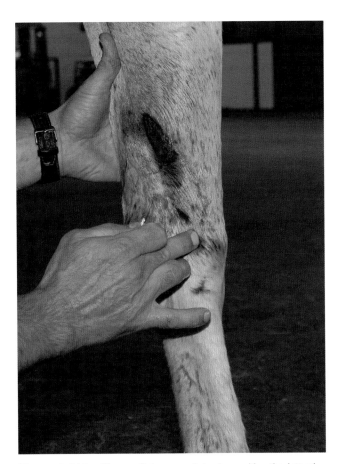

Figure 3.114. The medial approach to desensitize the lateral palmar nerve is located on the axial border of the accessory carpal bone.

High 2-Point Block

The high 2-point block is a combination of the lateral palmar block and the high medial palmar block (1 nerve of the high 4-point block). When performed, all deep and superficial structures on the palmar aspect of the metacarpus distal to the block will be desensitized. This includes the proximal aspects of the second and fourth metacarpal bones and the origin of the suspensory ligament.

This block can be used instead of the high 4-point and is easier to perform with less risk of complications. However, some clinicians have found it unnecessary to block the medial palmar nerve in conjunction with blocking the lateral palmar nerve.[62]

Ulnar, Median, and Medial Cutaneous Antebrachial Blocks

Perineural anesthesia is used most frequently up to the level of the carpus because the nerves lie superficial and the injection techniques are relatively easy to perform. Above this region intrasynovial anesthesia is often used to identify the site of lameness. However, the carpus and distal aspect of the limb can be desensitized by blocking the ulnar, median, and medial cutaneous antebrachial nerves. The medial cutaneous antebrachial nerve innervates only the skin so it is primarily used to anesthetize the limb for a surgical procedure.[42] The median and ulnar nerve blocks may be used to locate a painful condition in the distal limb during a lameness examination. For instance, this procedure could be used to rule out lameness of the distal limb if an upper forelimb lameness was suspected.

The ulnar nerve is anesthetized approximately 4 inches (10 cm) proximal to the accessory carpal bone on the caudal aspect of the forearm (Figure 3.115c). Careful palpation reveals a groove between the flexor carpi ulnaris and ulnaris lateralis muscles. A 20-gauge, 1-inch (3.8-cm) needle is inserted through the skin and fascia perpendicular to the limb. Although the depth of this nerve varies, it is usually about 0.25 to 0.5 inches (1 to 1.5 cm) below the skin surface. The local anesthetic (10 mL) is infused both superficially and deeply in this region. Because the palmar branch of the ulnar nerve gives rise to the lateral palmar and palmar metacarpal nerves, anesthesia desensitizes the lateral skin of the forelimb distal to the injection site down to the fetlock.[42] Also, the accessory carpal bone and surrounding structures, palmar carpal region, carpal canal, proximal metacarpus, SDFT, and suspensory ligament are partially blocked by this technique. Lame horses with lesions in the very proximal aspect of the SDFT may only improve after an ulnar block.[9]

The median nerve is anesthetized on the caudomedial aspect of the radius, cranial to the origin of the flexor carpi radialis muscle (Figure 3.115A). The injection site is located just below the elbow joint where the ventral edge of the posterior superficial pectoral muscle inserts in the radius.[42] At this point the nerve is superficial and lies directly on the caudal surface of the radius. A 2- to 2.5-inch (5- to 6.2-cm), 20-gauge needle is inserted obliquely through the skin and fascia to a depth of 1 to 2 inches (2.5 to 5 cm). The needle should be kept as

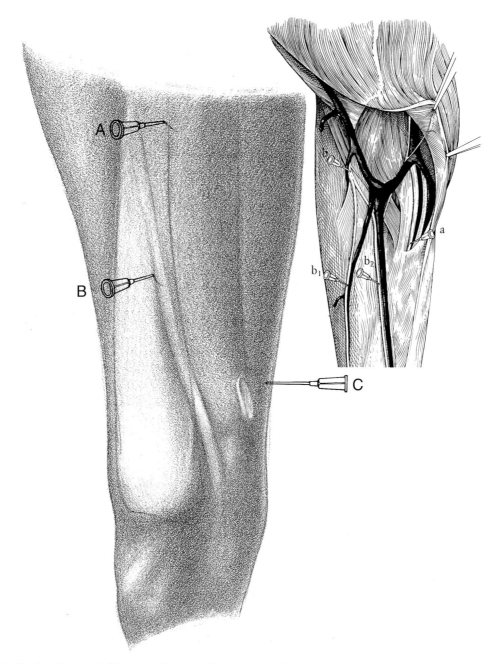

Figure 3.115. Forelimb blocks. A. Site for median nerve block. B. Site for medial cutaneous antebrachial nerve block. C. Site for ulnar nerve block. Inset: a. Site for median nerve block. b. Site for medial cutaneous antebrachial nerve block as nerve crosses the lacertus fibrosus, which blocks both the cranial (b1) and the caudal (b2) branches.

close to the radius as possible to avoid the median artery and vein which lie caudal to the nerve.[62] At least 10 mL of anesthetic is usually injected. Blocking this nerve alone accomplishes little more than a medial and lateral palmar nerve block. However, blocking the median nerve in conjunction with the ulnar nerve effectively anesthetizes most important areas of lameness distal to the blocks.

The two branches of the medial cutaneous antebrachial nerve are blocked on the medial aspect of the forearm halfway between the elbow and the carpus, just cranial to the cephalic vein and just cranial to the accessory cephalic vein (Figure 3.115b$_1$ and b$_2$).[62] The nerve

is usually just below the skin; however, its location can vary. It is best to block the subcutaneous tissues both cranial and caudal to the cephalic vein.[62] A 22-gauge, 1-inch (2.5-cm) needle is used to deposit 5 ml of anesthetic solution. Alternatively, the medial cutaneous antebrachial nerve may be blocked as it crosses the lacertus fibrosus before it branches (Figure 3.115b).[42,62]

The Hindlimb

The neuroanatomy of the distal hindlimb below the tarsus is somewhat similar to that of the forelimb below the carpus. The majority of perineural techniques described previously for the forelimb are similar in the hindlimb. However, limb positioning, restraint, and the technique may vary slightly. One difference in the neuroanatomy is that lateral and medial dorsal metatarsal nerves from the deep peroneal (fibular) nerve course over the dorsolateral and dorsomedial surfaces of the third metatarsal bone and digits (Figure 3.109 inset).[62] Therefore, it is recommended that additional anesthetic solution be injected dorsally when performing plantar digital nerve blocks at the pastern and proximal (abaxial) sesamoid bones and low and high 4-point plantar nerve blocks. Anesthesia of the dorsal metatarsal nerves is accomplished by injecting 2 to 3 mL of local anesthetic subcutaneously, lateral and medial to the long digital extensor tendon using a 5/8-inch (1.5-cm), 25-gauge needle. Blocking the dorsal metatarsal nerves effectively anesthetizes all structures innervated by the nerves distal to block.

Intrasynovial anesthesia is performed most frequently proximal to (above) the metatarsus in the hindlimb. However, perineural anesthesia of the tibial and peroneal nerves can be used to desensitize the tarsal region. The tibial and peroneal nerve blocks can also be used to determine whether the pain from a severe lameness without clinical findings is located proximal or distal to the hock region. Horses exhibiting subtle lameness are generally not good candidates for tibial and peroneal anesthesia because blocking the peroneal nerve may affect the horse's ability to extend the digit, thus making interpretation of the results difficult.[7]

When dealing with the hindlimb, proper restraint and body positioning are important to prevent bodily harm. In most cases a twitch is applied and the handler should stand on the same side as the veterinarian. All blocks should be performed with the veterinarian facing toward the back of the horse. The authors routinely begin diagnostic nerve blocks at the level of the proximal sesamoid bones unless there is uncertainty regarding foot involvement. If the foot is suspected, a high PD nerve block in the pastern is usually performed because often there is less concern about anesthetizing more proximal structures. In addition, a low PD block is difficult to perform in the hindfeet because the fetlock flexes when the limb is picked up.

The PD and abaxial sesamoid blocks are best performed with the limb extended behind the horse in a position similar to that when performing a fetlock flexion test or applying a horseshoe. The point of the hock is held fast by cradling it with the inside of the arm and axilla. This position reduces the ability of the horse to withdraw the limb to kick. Perineural blocks performed proximal to the abaxial sesamoid block are usually performed while standing close to the horse and with the limb on the ground. If the horse is prone to kicking, the limb can be held fast by grasping the foot, after which the limb is brought forward (similar to that done with a spavin test) to perform the block.[7]

High Plantar Block

The high plantar block anesthetizes the medial and lateral plantar and plantar metatarsal nerves just below the tarsus analogous to the high palmar block of the forelimb. Anesthesia of the dorsal metatarsal nerves just

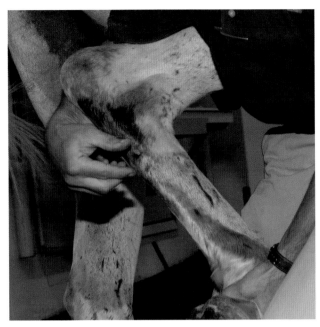

Figure 3.116. The high plantar or subtarsal nerve block can be performed in the proximal metatarsal region in a similar manner as the high palmar block.

below the tarsometatarsal joint may be included in this block to provide complete analgesia to structures in the metatarsal region and below.[42] The plantar metatarsal nerves can be blocked using a 1.5-inch (3.8-cm), 20-gauge needle inserted axial to the second and fourth metatarsal bones and directed dorsally toward the plantar aspect of the metatarsus (Figure 3.116). Three to 5 mL of local anesthetic is injected into the region of the origin of the suspensory ligament. Inadvertent administration of anesthetic into the tarsal sheath or the tarsometatarsal joint can occur when performing anesthesia of the plantar metatarsal nerves.[7,14,30,42] Because of the potential for intrasynovial injection, careful skin preparation prior to performing this block is recommended.[14,30]

The medial and lateral plantar nerves can be anesthetized by placing 3 to 5 mL of anesthetic through the heavy fascia adjacent to the dorsal surface of the DDFT in the proximal metatarsal region using a 25-gauge, 5/8-inch needle. If a large volume of anesthetic (7 to 10 mL) is used at the site of the lateral plantar nerve block, the deep branch of the lateral plantar nerve can also be anesthetized.[42] This will block both the medial and lateral plantar metatarsal nerves, negating the need to block these nerves individually. The high plantar block effectively desensitizes the second and fourth metatarsal bones, the suspensory ligament and its origin, and the flexor tendons in the metatarsal region. One study concluded that the high plantar nerve block cannot be used to differentiate between flexor tendon and suspensory ligament lesions because horses with both conditions improved after the block.[35] In addition, the high plantar block is difficult to perform, can inadvertently block the tarsal sheath or tarsometatarsal joint, and is not commonly performed by the first author.

Deep Branch of the Lateral Plantar Nerve (DBLPN) Block

The deep branch of the lateral plantar nerve (DBLPN) innervates the proximal suspensory in the hindlimb and is removed to treat some horses with hindlimb proximal suspensory desmitis. This nerve can be selectively desensitized to aid more accurate diagnosis of this condition. Two different techniques have been described. With the first approach, a 23-gauge, 1-inch (2.5-cm) needle is inserted 15 mm distal to the head of the fourth metatarsus and directed perpendicular to skin between the axial border of the fourth metatarsus and the SDFT to a depth of approximately 25 mm.[31] This single-injection technique was considered to be 95% accurate to block the DBLPN in a cadaver and live horse study. Alternatively, an 18- to 20-gauge, 1.5-inch (3.8-cm) needle is inserted 20 mm distal and plantar to the head of the fourth metatarsus and directed proximodorsally and axial to the bone (Figure 3.117). The needle is advanced to a depth of 1 to 2 cm and 5 to 7 mL of anesthetic is deposited.[22] It is usually best to hold the limb to perform either of these techniques. The single-injection technique for the DBLPN is thought to provide a reliable method for perineural analgesia of the deep branch of the lateral plantar nerve for diagnosis of proximal suspensory desmitis of the pelvic limb with a minimal risk of inadvertently desensitizing structures within the tarsal sheath and the tarsometatarsal joint.[22,31]

Tibial and Peroneal Block

Anesthetizing the tibial and deep and superficial peroneal nerves above the point of the hock desensitizes the entire distal limb.[42] These blocks can be helpful to diagnose some horses with hock lameness, or they can be used to rule out whether the pain causing the lameness is located within the hock or distal limb. However, blocking the peroneal nerve, particularly the common trunk, can affect the ability of the horse to extend the limb and may cause dragging of the toe or knuckling of the fetlock.[7,62] This may complicate the ability to assess improvement in the lameness and injure the horse during the lameness evaluation.

The site for injection of the tibial nerve is approximately 4 inches (10 cm) above the point of the hock on the medial aspect of the limb, between the Achilles tendon and the deep digital flexor muscle (Figure 3.118). When the horse is weight-bearing, the nerve lies close to the caudal edge of the deep digital flexor muscle. The nerve (6 mm in diameter) can be palpated caudal to the deep flexor muscle by unweighting the limb and grasping firmly cranial to the Achilles tendon with the thumb and forefinger.[62] The block may be performed by either standing on the lateral side of the limb to be blocked or by reaching across from the opposite limb to access the medial aspect of the limb. A small amount of anesthetic placed in the skin and subcutaneous tissues may minimize the horse's reaction to the block. A 20- to 22-gauge, 1.5-inch (3.8-cm) needle is used to deposit 15 to 20 mL of anesthetic in several tissue planes in the fascia that overlies the deep digital flexor muscle. Blocking the tibial nerve provides anesthesia to the plantar tarsus, metatarsus, distal Achilles tendon, calcaneus, suspensory ligament, and most of the foot.[7,62]

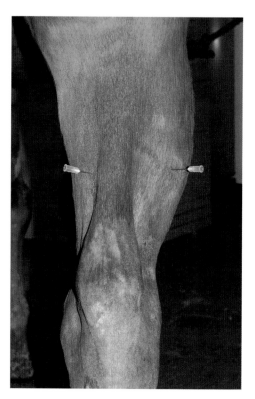

Figure 3.118. Image illustrating the locations to block the tibial and peroneal nerves. The site for injection of the tibial nerve is approximately 4 inches (10 cm) above the point of the hock on the medial aspect of the limb, between the Achilles tendon and the deep digital flexor muscle. The location to block the peroneal nerves is approximately 4 inches (10 cm) above the point of the hock on the lateral aspect of the limb in the groove formed by the muscle bellies of the lateral and long digital extensor muscles.

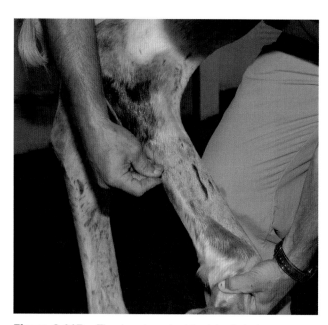

Figure 3.117. The deep branch of the lateral plantar nerve (DBLPN) can be desensitized by inserting a needle 20 mm below the head of the lateral splint and directing it proximodorsally and axial to the bone.

To completely desensitize the hock and limb distal to the hock, the deep and superficial peroneal (fibular) nerves must be anesthetized.[42,62] The deep peroneal nerve lies near the lateral edge of the cranial tibial muscle close to the tibia. The superficial peroneal nerve lies slightly caudal to the septum of the two extensor muscles and more superficial. The location of injection is approximately 4 inches (10 cm) above the point of the hock on the lateral aspect of the limb in the groove formed by the muscle bellies of the lateral and long digital extensor muscle (Figure 3.118). To block the deep peroneal nerve, a 1.5- to 2-inch (3.8- to 5-cm), 20-gauge needle is inserted in a slightly caudal direction until the needle contacts the caudal edge of the tibia. Ten to 15 ml of anesthetic is injected on the lateral border of the cranial tibial muscle close to the tibia. The needle is then retracted and another 10 to 15 mL of local anesthetic is injected more superficially in several planes to be sure that the superficial peroneal nerve is blocked. The depth of the superficial peroneal nerve can vary, so the more superficial injection should include a region from 0.6-cm to 2.5-cm deep.[62]

An alternative to blocking the superficial and deep peroneal nerves individually is to block the common peroneal nerve proximal to its division.[7] This can be accomplished by blocking the nerve near the origin of the long digital extensor tendon. The nerve can be palpated at this point and it is anesthetized using a 1.5-inch (3.8-cm), 20-gauge needle to inject 20 mL of anesthetic.

Direct Infiltration of Anesthetic

Direct infiltration of anesthesia can be used anywhere a sensitive area is identified. However, it is used most often at sites of insertions of ligaments and tendons (e.g., the proximal interosseous muscle), or at bony prominences (i.e., splints or swellings). The region is infused directly with local anesthetic instead of performing perineural anesthesia. This approach often permits the clinician to be more definitive regarding whether a painful region is contributing to the lameness. The amount of local anesthetic administered depends on the location and dimensions of the area involved.

The origin of the suspensory ligament can be desensitized by direct infiltration (Figure 3.113c$_1$ and c$_2$) but perineural anesthesia using the lateral palmar nerve block in the forelimb and the DBLPN block in the hindlimb is preferred. Direct infiltration of the proximal suspensory is best performed with the limb held with the opposite hand. A 1-inch (2.5-cm), 20- to 22-gauge needle is inserted between the attachments of the suspensory ligament and the inferior check ligament in the forelimb or between the fourth metatarsus and the SDFT in the hindlimb.[62] The needle is directed toward the origin of the suspensory ligament and 5 to 8 mL of anesthetic is injected. Both the lateral and medial sides can be blocked in the same manner, but this usually is unnecessary, especially in the hindlimb. Inadvertent injection into the carpometacarpal joint in the forelimb and the tarsometatarsal and tarsal sheath in the hindlimb can occur with these techniques.[62]

INTRASYNOVIAL ANESTHESIA

The use of intrasynovial anesthesia plays an important role in the diagnosis of equine lameness.[25,30,38,43,64] In most cases, it is more specific and efficient to anesthetize the specific synovial structure (joint capsule, tendon sheath, or bursa) that is thought to be the cause of the lameness than performing local perineural anesthesia. This is especially true in horses that tend to have joint problems (racehorses) or if the clinical findings suggest involvement of a synovial structure. In addition, intrasynovial anesthesia is commonly performed above the carpus and tarsus where perineural anesthesia becomes more difficult. If intrasynovial anesthesia needs to be performed after perineural anesthesia, it is best to wait at least 2 hours for sensation to return.[3,62] However, gait changes may persist beyond 2 hours and it is probably safest to perform intrasynovial anesthesia on a different day.[3]

Intrasynovial anesthesia is thought to be more specific than perineural anesthesia because if the lameness improves, the synovial cavity is considered the site of the problem. The three major exceptions to the specificity of intrasynovial blocks are the distal interphalangeal (DIP) joint, middle carpal joint, and the tarsometatarsal (TMT) joint. These exceptions are usually related to regional nerves being close to synovial outpouchings of the synovial cavities or passive diffusion of local anesthetic from the synovial cavity.[22,52–56] Intrasynovial anesthesia of the DIP joint can anesthetize the nerves innervating the foot,[4–6,15,16] and intrasynovial anesthesia of the middle carpal joint or TMT joint can provide analgesia of the proximal palmar metacarpal/plantar metatarsal regions, respectively.[14,20,21] In general, the more anesthetic that is used, the greater the likelihood of inadvertent analgesia of surrounding structures.[52,55] Less commonly, nerves that lie close to the site of intrasynovial injection also may be inadvertently desensitized. For example, the lateral plantar nerve may be desensitized when injecting local anesthetic into the TMT joint[14] and the lateral palmar/plantar nerve at the level of the fetlock may be desensitized when injecting anesthesia into the digital tendon sheath using the palmar axial sesamoidean approach.

General Technique: Site Preparation, Restraint, Interpretation

There are several different anatomic approaches that can be used for intrasynovial injections in most synovial cavities. Knowledge of the anatomic landmarks for intrasynovial injections is imperative to be able to competently perform these injections. Practice on cadaver limbs can be very beneficial to improve the proficiency in performing the injection techniques because repeated attempts to locate the synovial cavity are not well tolerated by most horses.

Proper preparation of the site for injection is necessary to prevent subsequent infection within the synovial cavity. Iatrogenic infection appears very rare following anesthesia of a synovial cavity but is prone to occur when synovial cavities are treated with medications, especially corticosteroids. Clipping the hair is unnecessary because there is no appreciable difference in bacteria-forming units in clipped and haired skin after 5 minutes of preparation with povidone iodine scrub followed by an alcohol rinse.[26] However, if the hair is very long and soiled, it is best to clip the hair overlying the injection site. In general, the authors tend to clip a very small area (1 to 2 cm square) over the site unless the owners/trainers request otherwise. Clipping the hair also has the advantage of marking the site of injection so that a helper knows exactly where to prep the skin. A 5-minute sterile skin preparation is recommended using either povidone iodine or chlorhexidine and alcohol.

An experienced helper makes performing intrasynovial injections much easier and safer. Proper restraint of the horse is also required to prevent injury to personnel and damage to the articular cartilage, and to reduce the risk of needle breakage. Be sure to always keep in mind that the handler and any person observing becomes your assumed responsibility.[43] Twitch restraint is recommended by the authors for all intrasynovial injections unless it is not tolerated by the horse. Horses being treated by intrasynovial injections are often routinely tranquilized but this is not usually possible for injections used for diagnostic purposes. Local anesthetic (1 to 2 mL) at the site of injection also may aid in the injection process, especially for synovial cavities in the proximal aspect of the limbs. In addition, the smallest possible gauge needle (usually 20-gauge or smaller) should be used to minimize objection by the horse.

Sterile gloves are recommended to permit careful palpation of the anatomic landmarks and to be able to handle the shaft of the needle without contamination. The injection should be done carefully but also as rapidly as possible. Once the needle has penetrated the synovial space, synovial fluid may be observed draining from the needle hub. The synovial fluid is allowed to run freely until its ejection pressure is reduced to a slow drip. The syringe is then inserted on the finger-stabilized needle hub, and the anesthetic is injected as rapidly as possible. If synovial fluid is not observed, a small syringe can be attached to the needle to withdraw fluid. However, lack of synovial fluid does not necessarily mean that the needle is not within the synovial cavity. To confirm correct needle placement, one can inject a small amount of sterile solution; if there is little or no plunger pressure, it is reasonable to assume that the needle is within the synovial space. However, the only definitive method to confirm that the needle is in the correct location is to obtain synovial fluid. Mepivacaine is usually the anesthetic of choice for intrasynovial anesthesia because there is some evidence that it is less irritating than lidocaine after intra-articular injection.[6,42] Guidelines for performing diagnostic intrasynovial anesthesia, including suggested volumes of anesthetic to use, are given in Table 3.4.

Assessment of intrasynovial blocks is usually performed 5 to 30 minutes after completion of the injection. If there is no improvement after 30 minutes it is unlikely that waiting longer will change the response. In a study documenting the onset and duration of intra-articular mepivacaine in the horse, lameness induced by injection of *Escherichia coli* endotoxin into the middle carpal joint was not apparent after 5 minutes and the improvement lasted for 55 minutes.[1] In addition,

improvement in lameness within 5 to 8 minutes of injection is often seen after intra-articular injection of the DIP joint in horses with navicular disease or experimentally induced navicular bursal pain.[16,44,54] Evaluation of the effectiveness of the block should include repeating the exercise that resulted in the most significant signs of lameness and possibly re-performing the manipulative/flexion test that made the examiner suspicious that this region was involved. It is important to remember that structures superficial to the synovial cavity may retain their sensitivity.[62] In addition, false negative intrasynovial blocks have been reported but tend to be uncommon. One report identified a failure of intra-articular anesthesia of the radiocarpal joint to abolish lameness associated with chip fracture of the distal radius.[59] Diffusion of anesthetic to local structures, inadvertent anesthesia of peripheral nerves closely associated with the synovial cavity outpouchings, and the possibility that the injection was not in the synovial cavity should all be considered when assessing the response to intrasynovial injections.

Distal Interphalangeal (DIP) Joint

The DIP joint can be entered using three dorsal approaches (perpendicular, parallel, or dorsolateral) and one lateral approach. These approaches are usually best performed in the standing patient and a maximum of 4 to 6 mL of anesthesia is recommended.[55] The dorsolateral and dorsal parallel approaches are used most commonly by the first author. The site of injection for the dorsolateral approach is 0.5 inch (1 cm) above the coronary band and .75 to 1 inch (2 to 3 cm) lateral (or medial) to midline. A 1.5-inch (3.8-cm), 20-gauge needle is inserted from a vertical position and directed distally and medially toward the center of the foot at approximately a 45° angle. The needle should enter the DIP joint capsule at the edge of the extensor process (Figure 3.119). If entry into the joint is uncertain the needle can be directed at a more acute angle (more horizontal) to the skin and inserted until the needle contacts the distal end of P2. It then is "walked" distally until the joint is penetrated.[64]

Some prefer to enter the joint on the dorsal midline using the proximal outpouching of the DIP joint above the extensor process (Figures 3.119B and 3.120A).[42,54,55] The injection site is just above the coronary band 0.25 to 0.5 inches (8 to 12 mm) above the edge of the hoof wall on the dorsal midline of the foot. With the dorsal perpendicular approach the needle is directed downward perpendicular to the bearing surface of the foot.[42] With the dorsal parallel approach, the needle is directed parallel or slightly downward (hub of the needle is moved proximally) to the ground to a depth of approximately 0.5 inches (12 to 15 mm). The dorsal parallel approach is usually easier to perform and is recommended by many clinicians.[42,54,55]

The site for injection for the lateral approach is bounded distally by a depression along the proximal border of the collateral cartilage approximately midway between the dorsal and palmar/plantar border of P2 (Figure 3.120B). A 1-inch (2.5-cm), 20-gauge needle is directed downward at a 45° angle toward the medial weight-bearing hoof surface.[66] Most horses appear to

Table 3.4. Guidelines for intrasynovial anesthesia.

Synovial cavity	Needle size	Volume of anesthetic	Approaches and limb position (standing or held
Coffin joint	20–22 g, 1–1.5″	4–6 mL	Dorsal approaches: standing Lateral approach: standing or held
Pastern joint	20–22 g, 1.5″	4–6 mL	Dorsal and dorsolateral approaches: standing Palmar/plantar approach: held
Fetlock joint	20–22 g, 1–1.5″	8–12 mL	Proximal palmar/plantar approaches: standing or held Collateral sesamoidean approach: held Distal palmar/plantar approach: standing Dorsal approach: standing
Carpal joints	20–22 g, 1–1.5″	8–10 mL	Doral approaches: held Palmar approaches: standing
Elbow	20 g, 1.5″ or 20 g, 3.5″	20–30 mL	All approaches: standing
Shoulder	18–20 g, 3.5″	20–40 mL	All approaches: standing
Tarsometatarsal joint	20 g, 1–1.5″	4–6 mL	All approaches: standing
Distal intertarsal joint	25 g, 5/8″ or 22 g, 1″	3–5 mL	All approaches: standing
Tarsocrural joint	20–22 g, 1.5″	15–20 mL	All approaches: standing
Femoropatellar joint	20 g, 1.5–3.5″	30–40 mL	All approaches: standing
Medial femorotibial joint	20 g, 1.5″	20–30 mL	All approaches: standing
Lateral femorotibial joint	20 g, 1.5″	20–30 mL	All approaches: standing
Coxofemoral joint	16–18 g, 6–8″ spinal	30–60 mL	All approaches: standing
Sacroiliac joint	15–16 g, 10″ spinal	7–10 mL	All approaches: standing
Digital flexor tendon sheath	20–22 g, 1–1.5″	8–15 mL	Proximal approach: standing All other approaches: held
Carpal sheath	20 g, 1.5–3.5″	15–30 mL	Medial approach: standing Lateral approach: held
Tarsal sheath	20 g, 1.5″	15–20 mL	Medial approach: standing
Extensor carpi radialis sheath	20 g, 1.5″	10–20 mL	All approaches: standing or held
Calcaneal bursa	20 g, 1.5″	10–15 mL	Distal approach: standing Proximal approach: standing or held
Bicipital bursa	18–20 g, 3.5–5″ or 20 g, 1.5″	20–30 mL	All approaches: standing
Trochanteric bursa	18–20 g, 1.5–3.5″	7–10 mL	All approaches: standing
Cunean bursa	20–22 g, 1″	2–3 mL	Medial approach: standing

tolerate this technique very well. However, the specificity of the lateral approach is thought to be less than the dorsolateral approach. In one study using cadavers and live horses, contrast material entered the DIP joint in 100% of the cases injected using the dorsolateral approach and 85% of the cases in which the palmar/plantar lateral approach was used.[66] Importantly, with the lateral approach, only 65% of the limbs had contrast exclusively in the DIP joint, 20% had contrast in the digital sheath, and 5% had contrast in the subcutaneous tissues.[66] Because of this and the ease of performing any of the dorsal approaches to the DIP joint, the lateral approach is rarely used by the authors.

Several studies have documented that injection of the DIP joint with a local anesthetic is not selective for the joint and it will cause analgesia of the podotrochlear apparatus, navicular bone, and navicular

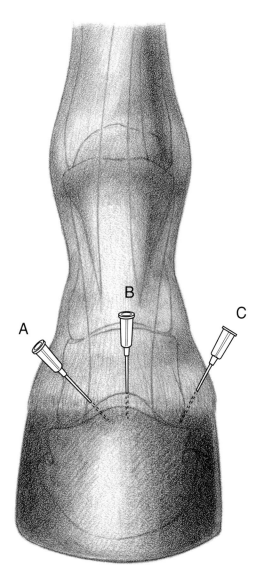

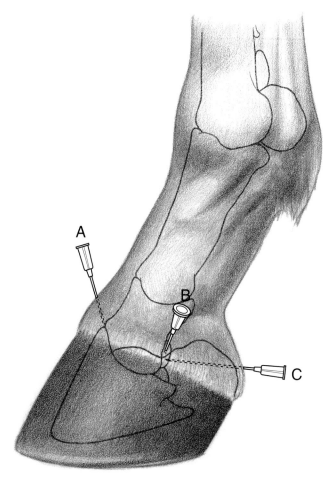

Figure 3.120.   Lateral view of the injection sites for the coffin joint. A. Dorsal approach. B. Lateral approach. C. Palmer approach.

Figure 3.119.   Dorsal view of the injection sites for the coffin joint. A. Dorsal lateral approach. B. Dorsal perpendicular approach. C. Lateral approach.

bursa.[5–6,15,34,44,53,56] In addition, injection of the DIP joint may cause partial, and often complete, analgesia of the sole, toe, and heel regions of the foot.[52,53] The analgesic effect increased with time and 10 mL of anesthetic was more effective than 6 mL in alleviating pain in the foot.[52] To improve the selectivity of DIP joint anesthesia, a maximum of 5 to 6 mL of anesthesia is recommended and assessment of the block should be performed within 10 minutes of injection.[54,55]

Podotrochlear (Navicular) Bursa

There are various techniques for needle entry into the navicular bursa but the technique through the heel bulbs is thought to be most accurate.[45,55] With this approach, a 20-gauge, 3.5-inch (8.9-cm) spinal needle is inserted between the heel bulbs just above the coronary band. Local anesthesia at the site of the injection

or perineural anesthesia above the heel bulbs may be used to provide skin analgesia prior to the injection. The needle is advanced along a sagittal plane aiming for a point 1 cm below the coronary band, midway between the toe and the heel (Figure 3.121). The needle is advanced until bone is contacted. Only 2 to 4 mL or anesthetic or medication can usually be injected and flexing the lower limb will decrease the resistance to injection. A special wooden block for foot placement that unweights the heel and flexes the distal limb is used by some clinicians. Radiographic or fluoroscopic documentation of the needle's location is recommended in most cases because it is easy to pass the needle over to the proximal border of the navicular bone into the DIP joint (Figure 3.122).[25,42] Including radiographic contrast medium into the injection solution and taking a radiograph immediately after the injection can also be used to document a successful injection.

Another approach to the navicular bursa is through the lowest part of the depression between the heel bulbs. A 1.5-inch (3.8-cm), 20-gauge needle is directed dorsally toward the coronary band and inserted to a depth of approximately 1 cm before the navicular bone is contacted.[25,62] The advantages to this approach are that a spinal needle is not needed and the injection site is

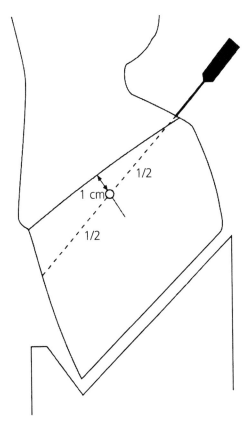

Figure 3.121. Lateral view of the foot demonstrating the approximate location of the navicular bone (circle) and the correct angulation of the spinal needle to enter the navicular bursa using the palmar approach between the heel bulbs. (Reprinted with permission from Schumacher J, Schumacher J, Schramme MC. Diagnostic analgesia of the equine forefoot. Equine Vet Educ 2004;16(3):159–165.)

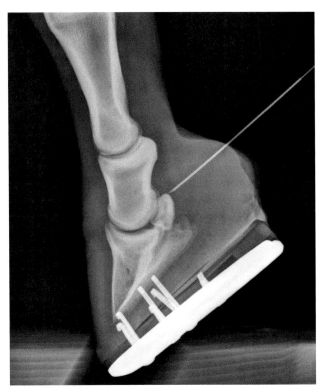

Figure 3.122. Lateral radiograph of the foot after needle placement to confirm the correct location of the needle palmar to the navicular bone. The authors prefer to locate the needle at the proximal edge of the navicular bone so injected material can accumulate within the proximal outpouching of the bursa.

further from the ground, potentially lessening the risk of contamination. The disadvantage is that the needle is more likely to enter the palmar/plantar aspect of the DIP joint.

The navicular bursa can also be entered from the lateral or medial sides (abaxial position) just proximal to the collateral cartilage of the distal phalanx. This is the same location that is used to insert the arthroscope into the navicular bursa for endoscopy.[67] A 3.5-inch (8.9-cm), 20-gauge needle is directed distally toward the opposite heel between the middle phalanx and the DDFT.[25,67] The needle is directed beneath the deep digital flexor tendon and digital tendon sheath to enter the bursa. The primary advantage of this technique is that the needle does not penetrate the DDFT which may decrease the morbidity associated with the injection. The disadvantages include possible entry into the tendon sheath and the difficulty of placing the needle at the correct angulation. As with all navicular bursal injections, confirmation of correct needle placement is recommended with some type of imaging either before or after the injection.

A positive response to administration of local anesthesia into the navicular bursa may indicate problems of the navicular bursa, navicular bone and/or its sup-

porting ligaments, sole and/or toe, or distal aspect of the DDFT.[15,42,54,55] Even though diffusion of local anesthetic into the navicular bursa occurs following DIP joint injection[4–6,34,44] the converse does not occur, and analgesia of the navicular bursa does not result in analgesia of the DIP joint.[55] Pain from the DIP joint can likely be excluded as a cause of lameness if analgesia of the navicular bursa improves the lameness within 10 minutes.[55] In addition, a positive response to intra-articular analgesia of the DIP joint together with a negative response to navicular bursa analgesia incriminates pain within the DIP joint as the cause of lameness.[16,55]

Proximal Interphalangeal (PIP) Joint

There are two dorsal and one palmar/plantar approach for arthrocentesis of the PIP joint. One dorsal site of injection is on the midline approximately 0.5 cm dorsal to an imaginary line drawn from the medial and lateral eminences of the proximal end of P2. A 20-gauge, 1.5-inch (3.8-cm) needle is directed slightly distally and medially to enter the joint capsule underneath the extensor tendon (Figures 3.123A and 3.124A). The dorsolateral approach can be done while the horse is standing or with the limb extended and the sole supported on the knee. The condylar eminences of the distolateral aspect of P1 are identified and a 1.5-inch (3.8-cm), 20-gauge needle is inserted parallel to the ground

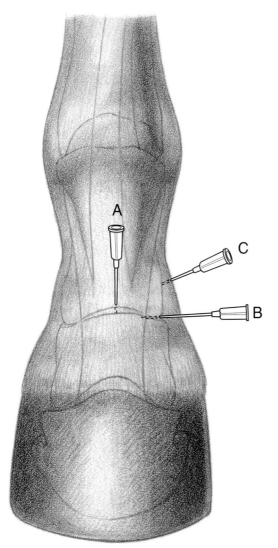

Figure 3.123. Dorsal view of the injection sites for the pastern joint. A. Dorsal approach. B. Dorsolateral approach. C. Palmar/plantar approach.

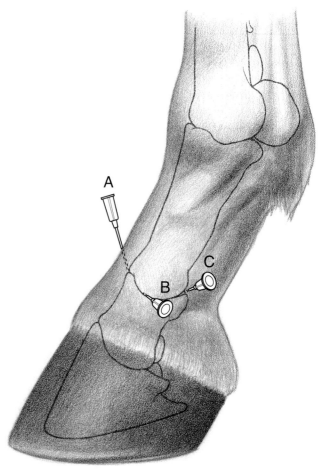

Figure 3.124. Lateral view of injection sites for the pastern joint. A. Dorsal approach. B. Dorsolateral approach. C. Palmar/plantar approach.

surface 0.5 inches (1.2 cm) distal to the palpable eminence.[42,62] The needle is directed underneath the edge of the extensor tendon to enter the joint at a depth of 0.5 inches(Figures 3.123B and 3.124B).

The palmaro/plantaroproximal approach is best performed with the distal limb in a flexed position. A 1.5-inch (3.8cm), 20-gauge needle is inserted perpendicular to the limb into the palpable V-depression formed by the palmar aspect of P1 dorsally, the distal eminence of P1 distally, and the lateral branch of the SDFT as it inserts on the eminence of P2 palmarodistally[40] (Figures 3.123C and 3.124C). This corresponds to the transverse bony prominence on the proximopalmar/plantar border of P2 that is usually easily palpable. The first author prefers to angle the needle slightly dorsally to contact P1, and then direct the needle along the palmar/plantar aspect of the bone. This ensures that the needle is just behind P1 where it will enter the PIP joint capsule at a depth of approximately 1 inch (2.5 cm).

Metacarpophalangeal/Metatarsophalangeal (Fetlock) Joints

Three palmar/plantar approaches and one dorsal approach can be used for arthrocentesis of the fetlock joint. The proximal palmar/plantar approach can be performed with the limb weight-bearing or held, the approach through the collateral sesamoidean ligament must be performed with the fetlock joint flexed, and the distal palmar/plantar and dorsal approaches are usually performed in the standing limb. The dorsal and proximal palmar/plantar approaches are usually reserved for horses with significant effusion to avoid damage to the articular cartilage and inadvertent hemorrhage, respectively. Which technique to use is often based on personal preference, although some are easier to perform in the forelimb than the hindlimb. Approximately 8 to 12 mL of anesthetic is usually used for diagnostic anesthesia.[42]

Proximal Palmar/Plantar Pouch

The boundaries of the palmar/plantar pouches of the fetlock joint are the apical border of the proximal sesamoid bones distally, the distal ends of the splint bones

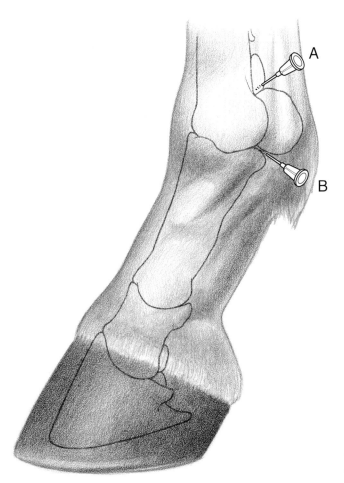

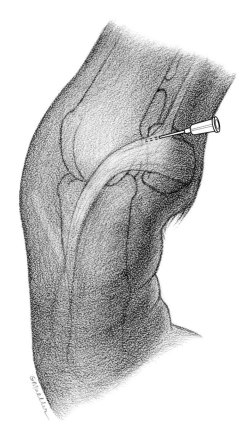

Figure 3.125. Lateral view of injection sites for the fetlock joint. A. Proximal palmar/plantar approach. B. Distal palmar/plantar approach at the base of the sesamoid bone.

Figure 3.126. Lateral view of the injection site for the flexed fetlock joint. The site illustrated is through the collateral sesamoidean ligament. The needle also may be inserted just above the ligament in a depression made by the collateral sesamoidean ligament and the branch of the suspensory ligament.

proximally, the third metacarpal/metatarsal bone dorsally, and the branch of the suspensory ligament palmar/plantarly (Figure 3.125A). In the normal horse, these pouches appear as a depression, and attempts to retrieve synovial fluid or inject substances may be difficult. However, they are usually easily identified in horses with fetlock effusion. When performing this approach in the standing patient, a 1-inch (2.5-cm), 20-gauge needle is inserted from lateral to medial and directed distally at a 45° angle to the long axis of the limb. The disadvantages of this approach are the possibility of contaminating the synovial fluid sample with blood because of the highly vascular synovial membrane and the inability to aspirate synovial fluid because the synovial villi plug the needle.[30,41]

Performing the palmar/plantar approach with the fetlock flexed can potentially minimize these complications. With the fetlock flexed there is a very palpable depression at the very distal aspect of the pouch just above the branch of the suspensory ligament. A 1-inch (2.5-cm), 20-gauge needle is inserted at this location and directed distally at a 45° angle. The more distal location in the palmar/plantar pouch reduces the risk of iatrogenic hemorrhage.

Collateral Sesamoidean Approach

Arthrocentesis of the fetlock through the lateral collateral sesamoidean ligament is probably the best approach to obtain a hemorrhage-free synovial fluid sample. The fetlock is flexed to increase the space between the articular surfaces of the proximal sesamoid bones and the metacarpus/metatarsus. The depression between the bones is palpated and a 1-inch, 20-gauge needle inserted through the collateral sesamoidean ligament perpendicular to the limb (Figure 3.126).[41] If the needle fails to advance, it is most likely contacting bone and will need to be redirected to enter the joint space.

Distal Palmar/Plantar Approach

The distal palmar/plantar approach is performed in the palpable depression formed by the distal aspect of the proximal sesamoid bone and the proximopalmar/plantar eminence of P1. The landmarks are the distal aspect of the proximal sesamoid bone and collateral sesamoidean ligament proximally, the proximal palmar/plantar eminence of P1 distally; and the digital vein, artery, and nerve palmar/plantarly.[60] A 1.5-inch (3.8-cm), 20-gauge needle is inserted in the depression and directed slightly dorsally (10° to 20°) and proximally

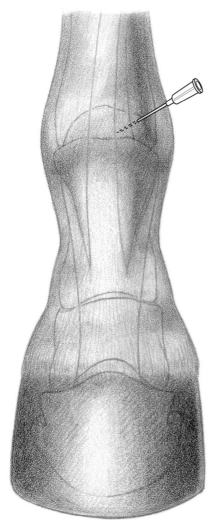

Figure 3.127. Dorsal view of the injection site for the dorsal approach to the fetlock joint in the standing horse.

(10°) until the joint is entered (Figure 3.125B). To avoid penetration of the digital sheath it is important that the needle be inserted dorsal to the palmar digital artery, vein, and nerve. The advantages to this approach are that the landmarks are easily palpable, synovial fluid is often obtained, it can be performed in the standing horse, and horses tolerate the procedure well.[60]

Dorsal Approach

The dorsal approach is usually performed with the limb weight-bearing. The needle is inserted proximal to the proximodorsal limits of P1 in the palpable joint space in a slightly oblique manner, either lateral or medial to the extensor tendon (Figure 3.127). The fetlock joint capsule is thicker in this location than in the palmar/plantar pouch and appears to cause greater discomfort to the horse than the other techniques.

Digital Flexor Tendon Sheath (DFTS)

There are several outpouchings of the DFTS that may be used for synoviocentesis. In general, the proximal

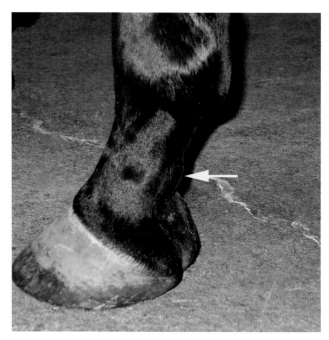

Figure 3.128. The distal outpouching of the digital flexor tendon sheath (arrow) can be used for synoviocentesis when distended.

pouch palmar/plantar to the suspensory and the distal recess in the pastern superficial to the DDFT are difficult to penetrate without sheath effusion. However, they can often be the easiest approaches to perform if effusion is present. The site for injection of the proximal pouch of the DFTS is 1 cm proximal to the palmar/plantar annular ligament and 1 cm palmar/plantar to the lateral branch of the suspensory ligament. A 1- to 1.5-inch, 20-gauge needle is directed slightly distally until the sheath is penetrated. The distal outpouching of the pastern is often palpable as a distinct "bubble" when effusion is present (Figure 3.128). It is located between the proximal and distal digital annular ligaments and between the diverging branches of the SDFT where the DDFT lies close to the skin.[42] A 20-gauge, 1-inch needle is directed in a lateral to medial direction just beneath the skin so as not to penetrate the DDFT.

The axial sesamoidean approach at the level of the fetlock and the medial or lateral approach between the annular ligament and proximal digital annular ligament can be performed in the distended and non-distended DFTS. Both approaches are best performed with the limb held with the fetlock slightly flexed. The axial sesamoidean approach is performed 3 mm axial to the palpable border of the midbody of the lateral proximal sesamoid bone using a 1-inch (2.5-cm), 20-gauge needle.[28] The needle is directed at a 45° angle to the saggital plane to a depth of approximately 1.5 to 2 cm. Alternatively, the needle can be inserted into the outpouching of the DFTS abaxial and distal to the sesamoid bones between the annular and proximal digital annular ligaments. The needle is inserted in a distal to proximal direction at approximately a 45° angle to the sagittal plane. Ten to 15 mL of anesthetic is recommended for diagnostic purposes. Improvement of lameness in horses after intrasynovial analgesia of the DFTS is usually due to attenuation of pain within the structures contained in the DFTS. Analgesia of the DFTS has little effect on lameness caused by pain originating in the sole, DIP joint, or the navicular bone.[27]

Carpal Joints

Arthrocentesis of the radiocarpal and middle carpal joints can be performed using either a dorsal or palmar approach. The dorsal approach is performed with the carpus flexed and the palmar approach is performed in the weight-bearing limb and can be somewhat difficult in the nondistended joint. Approximately 10 mL of anesthetic is recommended. Because the carpometacarpal joint and the middle carpal joint communicate, anesthetics injected into the middle carpal joint also desensitize the carpometacarpal joint. Additionally, the carpometacarpal joint has palmar pouches that extend palmarodistally adjacent to the origin of the suspensory ligament. Anesthetic injected into the middle carpal joint may also desensitize the proximal suspensory ligament and proximal palmar metacarpal region.[20,21]

The sites of injection for the radiocarpal and middle carpal joints are located in palpable depressions lateral or medial to the extensor carpi radialis tendon on the dorsal aspect of each joint (Figure 3.129). The injection is made with a 1-inch (2.5-cm), 20-gauge needle midway between the distal radius and proximal row of carpal bones (for the radiocarpal joint) or the proximal and distal rows of carpal bones (for the middle carpal joint). Because the surfaces of the carpal bones are at an angle, the needle should be directed slightly proximally to avoid hitting the articular cartilage.[62]

The landmarks for the palmarolateral approach to the radiocarpal joint are the palmarolateral aspect of the radius, proximolateral aspect of the accessory carpal bone, and palmarolateral aspect of the ulnar carpal bone (Figure 3.130A).[43,64] A 1-inch (2.5-cm), 20-gauge needle is inserted in this palpable depression at 90° to the long axis of the limb and the needle is directed dorsomedially. Another palmarolateral approach is at the midaccessory carpal bone level in a palpable "V" between the tendons of the ulnaris lateralis and the lateral digital extensor.[42] The needle is inserted perpendicular to the skin in a small depression 0.5 to 1 inch (8 to 12 mm) distal to the "V" in the space between the distal lateral aspect of the radius (vestigial ulna) and the proximal lateral aspect of the ulnar carpal bone.[42,43]

The palmarolateral approach to the middle carpal joint is best used if the joint is distended (Figure 3.130B). With distension the joint capsule is superficial and protrudes palmar and lateral to the ulnar and fourth carpal bones distal to the accessory carpal bone. The injection site is approximately 1 inch (2.5 cm) distal to the site of injection of the radiocarpal joint.[62] A 1-inch, 20-gauge needle is inserted perpendicular to the skin to a depth of about 0.5 inches (1.2 cm).

Elbow Joint

There are three major approaches to the elbow joint: lateral, caudolateral, and caudal. The lateral approach

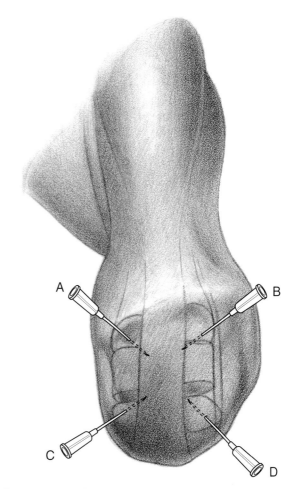

Figure 3.129. Cranial view of the injection sites for the carpus. Needles can enter the radiocarpal joint (A and B) or middle carpal joint (C and D), either lateral or medial to the extensor carpi radialis tendon. When the lateral site is chosen, the lateral digital extensor tendon must be avoided.

is within the radiohumeral articulation, whereas the caudolateral and caudal approaches are within the humeroulnar articulation. All three techniques are best performed while the horse is standing, but can be done with the limb flexed.[62] Injection of the elbow is more difficult than many other joints in the horse and approximately 20 to 30 mL of anesthetic is needed for diagnostic purposes.[42]

Lateral Approach

The landmark for the lateral approach is the lateral collateral ligament that extends across the joint from the lateral epicondyle of the humerus to the lateral tuberosity of the radius. Both of these bony landmarks are easily palpated. The elbow joint can be entered either cranial or caudal to the collateral ligament. The site for injection is two-thirds the distance distally measured from the lateral epicondyle of the humerus to the lateral tuberosity of the radius (Figure 3.131A and B).[30,62] A 1.5-inch (3.8-cm), 20-gauge needle is inserted at a 90° angle to the skin just cranial or caudal to the lateral collateral ligament to a depth of 1 inch.[30,42] If

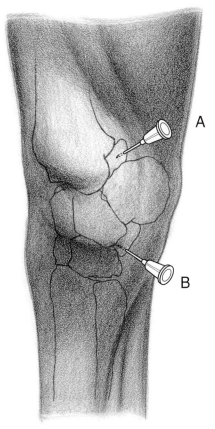

Figure 3.130. Lateral view of the palmarolateral injection sites for the carpal joints. A. Site for the radiocarpal joint. B. Site for injection of the middle carpal joint.

injected cranially, it is important to verify that the needle is within the joint because periarticular anesthetic may desensitize the distal branches of the radial nerve, causing temporary paralysis of the extensor carpi radialis and common digital extensor muscles. This will cause the horse to be unable to lock its carpus in extension. If injected caudally, the needle may enter the bursa of the ulnaris lateralis muscle which is thought to communicate with the elbow joint.[49] However, communication between the bursa and the elbow joint occurred in only 9 of 24 (37.5%) of the joints examined.[49] To avoid the ulnaris lateralis bursa, the needle may be inserted more caudally in the elbow in a palpable depression formed by the caudal epicondyle of the humerus, the caudal proximal tuberosity of the radius, and the anconeal process (Figure 3.131C).[62]

Caudolateral Approach

The caudolateral approach is an alternative to placing the needle directly caudal to the collateral ligament using the lateral approach. The injection site is caudal to the palpable humeral epicondyle in the aconeal notch within the humero-ulna joint. This palpable V-shaped depression is usually just below the triceps muscles and 6 to 8 cm cranio-distal from the point of the olecranon process.[62] A 1.5- to 3.5-inch (3.8- to 8.8-cm), 20-gauge needle is inserted at a 45° angle to the skin and directed craniomedially (Figure 3.131C).

Caudal Approach

The large caudal joint pouch of the elbow can be entered from a more proximal location. The landmarks

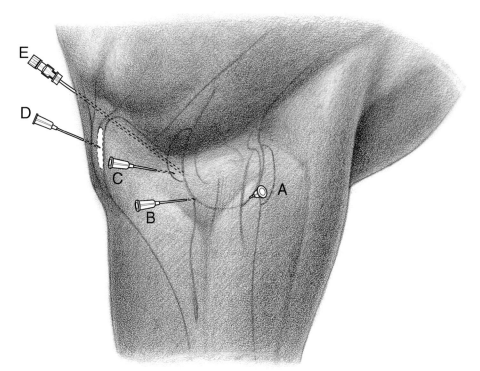

Figure 3.131. Lateral view of injection sites for the elbow joint and bursa. A and B. Lateral approaches cranial (A) or caudal (B) to the collateral ligament. C. Caudolateral approach with a 1.5-inch, 20-gauge needle. D. Site for olecranon bursa. E. Approach to caudal joint pouch along the shaft of the olecranon.

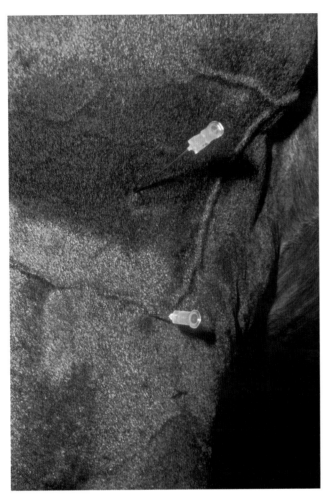

Figure 3.132. The approach to the large caudal outpouching of the elbow joint is 0.5 inches (1 cm) proximal to and one-third of the distance measured caudally from the supracondylar eminence to the point of the olecranon. A 3.5-inch (8.9-cm), 18- to 20-gauge spinal needle is directed distomedially through the triceps musculature at a 45° angle to the long axis of the limb into the olecranon fossa (top needle).

are the lateral supracondylar crest of the distal humerus and the most proximal point of the olecranon process.[30,42,49] The injection site is 0.5 inches (1 cm) proximal to and one-third of the distance measured caudally from the supracondylar eminence to the point of the olecranon. A 3.5-inch (8.9-cm), 18- to 20-gauge spinal needle is directed distomedially through the triceps musculature at a 45° angle to the long axis of the limb into the olecranon fossa (Figure 3.132). Alternatively, the spinal needle can be directed downward along the lateral shaft of the olecranon process (Figure 3.131E).[62] The injection site is 3 cm distal and 2 cm cranial to the point of the olecranon, and the needle is directed distally and cranially to enter the caudal joint pouch just proximal to the anconeal process.

Scapulohumeral (Shoulder) Joint

Arthrocentesis of the shoulder can be difficult due to the depth of the joint. It is a large joint and 20 to 40 mL

of anesthetic is usually used for diagnostic purposes. It is always performed with the horse standing on the limb. The shoulder joint may communicate with bicipital bursa in a small percentage of horses and temporary anesthesia of the suprascapular nerve and paralysis of the infraspinatus and supraspinatus muscles may occur with periarticular injection of anesthetic.[42,62] Some clinicians prefer to use only 10 mL of anesthetic to block the joint in hopes that this volume will be less likely to involve the suprascapular nerve.[38]

Craniolateral Approach

The site for the craniolateral approach to the shoulder joint is located in the notch formed between the cranial and caudal prominences of the lateral tuberosity of the humerus. The caudal prominence (point of the shoulder) is easiest to palpate and by exerting deep finger pressure the depression for needle insertion can be palpated 3.5 to 4 cm cranial to the caudal prominence. This notch is not as readily palpable in heavily muscled horses. A 3.5-inch (8.8-cm), 18- to 20-gauge spinal needle is inserted into this notch and directed parallel to the ground in a caudomedial direction toward the opposite elbow (Figure 3.133A).[42,62] The depth of penetration depends on the size of the horse, but the joint capsule is usually entered at a depth of 2 to 3 inches (5 to 7 cm). Synovial fluid can usually be aspirated and is the only definitive method to document correct needle placement. Alternatively, the spinal needle may be inserted slightly more proximal on the limb in a distinct depression located 1 to 1.5 cm cranial to the infraspinatus tendon and slightly proximal and cranial to the point of the shoulder. The needle is placed parallel to the ground or slightly downward and directed caudomedially at a 45° angle until bone is contacted.

Lateral Approach

The landmarks for the lateral approach to the shoulder are the lateral humeral tuberosity and the infraspinatus tendon. A 3.5-inch (8.9-cm), 18- to 20-gauge spinal needle is inserted 1 to 2 cm caudal and distal to the infraspinatus tendon in line with the lateral humeral tuberosity.[62] The needle is directed slightly caudally and upward toward the lateral aspect of the humeral head. In general, this approach is more difficult than the craniolateral approach.

Bicipital Bursa

The bicipital bursa lies cranial to the shoulder and humerus under the biceps brachii muscle. It is a relatively large synovial structure (20 to 30 mL of anesthetic) but can be difficult to enter because of its depth and the landmarks for injection are not easily palpable. In a recent study that compared two different injection techniques (distal and proximal) to enter the bicipital bursa, the accuracy of injecting the bursa was only 28% and 39%, respectively.[57] The authors concluded that clinicians without previous experience of injecting the bicipital bursa were unlikely to be successful with either approach. This study confirmed the difficulty of injecting the bicipital bursa and suggested that radiographic

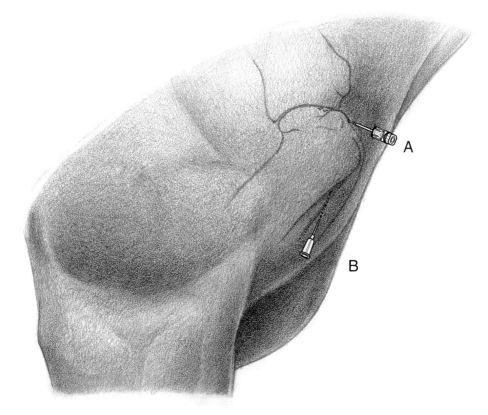

Figure 3.133. Lateral view of the injection sites for the shoulder region. A. Site for the shoulder joint. B. Site for the distal approach to the bicipital bursa.

examination after injecting radiopaque contrast medium may be necessary to assess the success of centesis if synovial fluid is not obtained. The proximal and distal approaches to the bursa are usually performed with the limb weight-bearing, but the proximal approach may be done with the limb held.

Distal Approach

The cranial prominence of the lateral tuberosity of the humerus is used as the landmark, as was done for the shoulder joint. The site of injection is 2.5 inches (5 to 6 cm) distal and 3 inches (7 to 8 cm) caudal to this prominence. A 3.5-inch (8.9-cm), 18- to 20-gauge spinal needle is directed proximomedially toward the intertubercal groove until it contacts the humerus (Figure 3.133B). The depth of the needle depends on the size of the horse, but a 3.5-inch (8.9-cm) spinal needle is usually inserted to the hub in most mature horses.[42] Alternatively, the deltoid tuberosity of the humerus can be palpated and used as a landmark. A 3.5-inch (8.9-cm), 18- to 20-gauge spinal needle is inserted 1.5 inches (3 to 4 cm) proximal to the distal aspect of the deltoid tuberosity and directed proximomedially (toward to opposite ear) to a depth of 2 to 3 inches (5 to 7 cm).[42,62]

Proximal Approach

The proximal approach is performed in the intertubercal groove which can be palpated medial to the edge of the cranial prominence of the lateral tuberosity of the humerus.[42,57] A 1.5-inch (3.8-cm), 20-gauge needle is inserted into the intertubercal groove in a plane parallel to the bearing surface of the foot at about a 45° angle to the sagittal axis of the horse until the needle strikes cartilage. The primary advantages of the proximal approach compared to the distal approach are a slightly improved accuracy of entering the bursa and not needing a 3.5-inch (8.9-cm) spinal needle.

Tarsal (Hock) Joints

There are four joint spaces associated with the tarsus: tarsocrural, proximal intertarsal (PIT), distal intertarsal (DIT), and tarsometatarsal (TMT). The tarsocrural joint is considered a high-motion joint, whereas the PIT, DIT, and TMT joints are low-motion joints. Numerous studies have been done to determine the consistency of communication between these joints. The tarsocrural and PIT joints communicate consistently and are usually considered as one joint as far as intra-articular injection. Reports of communication between the DIT and TMT joints vary from 8% to 38%.[2,14,37] To complicate things further, the PIT and DIT, and the PIT and the TMT joints may also communicate occasionally.[37] Because of these findings, the interpretation of intra-articular anesthesia in the tarsus is not always straightforward. In addition, the communication patterns may differ in the diseased tarsus compared to a normal tarsus, and diffusion of medication may occur between the TMT and

DIT joints regardless of the communication pattern. Corticosteroids injected into the TMT joint were consistently found within the DIT joint in all horses sampled.[58]

Tarsocrural Joint

The tarsocrural joint is the largest joint pouch in the tarsus and is easy to enter, especially if synovial effusion is present. The joint may be entered dorsally (dorsomedial) or plantarly depending on the clinical situation. For the dorsomedial approach, a 1-inch (2.5-cm), 20-gauge needle is inserted 1 to 1.5 inches (2 to 3 cm) distal to the medial malleolus of the tibia, medial or lateral to the cranial branch of the medial saphenous vein (Figure 3.134A). The needle is advanced in a plantarolateral direction at approximately a 45° until synovial fluid flows from the needle. The dorsomedial approach is usually performed in the weight-bearing limb from the opposite side of the horse, but can be performed from the same side of the horse. Fifteen to 20 mL of local anesthetic is recommended.

The medial or lateral plantar outpouchings of the tarsocrural joint may be used for arthrocentesis, especially if significant synovial effusion is present. The palpable landmarks of the lateral plantar pouch are bordered by the tuber calcis caudally, the caudal aspect of the distal tibia cranially, and the proximal aspect of the lateral trochlear ridge of the talus distally.[30] Confirmation that fluid swellings in this location are part of the tarsocrural joint can be determined by applying finger pressure to the swellings and feeling the dorsal pouches of the tarsocrural joint distend. A 1-inch (2.5-cm), 20-gauge needle is inserted perpendicular to the skin at the site of the effusion with the limb weight-bearing.

Distal Intertarsal (DIT) or Centrodistal Joint

The site for injection of the DIT joint is on the distomedial surface of the tarsus. The injection is performed from the opposite side of the horse with the limb weight-bearing. One technique is to draw an imaginary line between the palpable distal tubercle of the talus and the space between the second and third metatarsal bones (MT II and III) at their proximal limits.[48,62] A small depression can often be felt with a fingernail just distal to the cunean tendon along this imaginary line. Another approach is to identify the medial eminence of the talus and medial eminence of the central tarsal bone. The site for injection is halfway between these landmarks and 0.5 inch (1 cm) distal to the eminence of the central tarsal bone.[42] A 1-inch (2.5-cm), 22- to 25-gauge needle is directed perpendicular to the long axis of the limb (or slightly caudally) to enter the joint space between the combined first and second tarsal bones, the third, and the central tarsal bones. The needle is advanced to about 0.5 inches (1 cm) and 3 to 5 mL of local anesthetic is injected (Figure 3.134B). The needle is determined to be within the DIT joint by low resistance to injection without developing a subcutaneous swelling and the ability to aspirate the injected contents of the syringe.[42] The DIT joint is thought to communicate frequently with the cunean bursa.[24]

The DIT or centrodistal joint can also be entered using a dorsolateral approach.[33] The injection site is 2 to 3 mm lateral to the long digital extensor tendon and 6 to 8 mm proximal to a line drawn perpendicular to the axis of the third metatarsal bone through the head of the fourth metatarsal bone. This is usually distal to the palpable lateral trochlear ridge of the talus. The needle is directed plantaromedially at an angle of approximately 70° from the sagittal plane until bone is contacted (Figure 3.135). This approach is safer for the clinician because it is performed on the lateral aspect of the tarsus but is technically more difficult in the author's hands.

Tarsometatarsal (TMT) Joint

The TMT joint is best approached from the plantarolateral aspect of the tarsus with the limb weight-bearing. The landmarks for injection are the proximal head of the fourth metatarsal (MT IV) bone and the lateral edge of the SDFT. A 1- to 1.5 inch (2.5- to 3.8-cm), 20- to 22-gauge needle is inserted in the small palpable depression 0.25 inch (0.5 to 1 cm) proximal to the head of MT IV (Figure 3.136). The needle is directed toward the dorsomedial aspect of the tarsus in a slightly

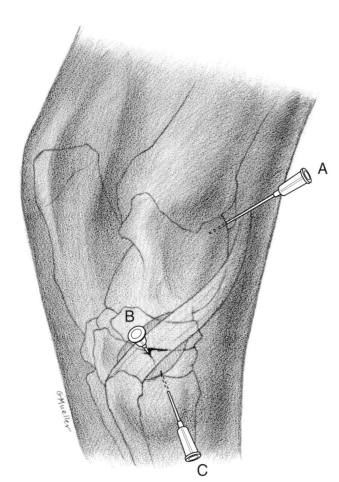

Figure 3.134. Medial view of the injection sites for the tarsal joints. A. Sites for the tarsocrural joint. B. Site for the distal intertarsal joint. C. Site for the cunean bursa.

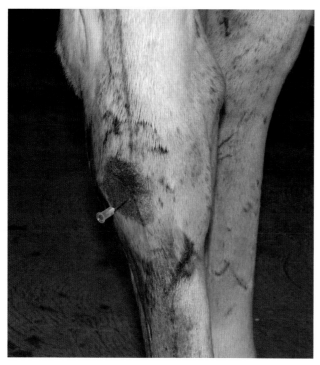

Figure 3.135. The craniolateral approach to the DIT joint is 2 to 3 mm lateral to the long digital extensor tendon and approximately 6 to 8 mm proximal to a line drawn perpendicular to the axis of the third metatarsal bone through the head of the fourth metatarsal bone. This is usually distal to the palpable lateral trochlear ridge of the talus. The needle is directed plantaromedially at an angle of approximately 70° from the sagittal plane until bone is contacted.

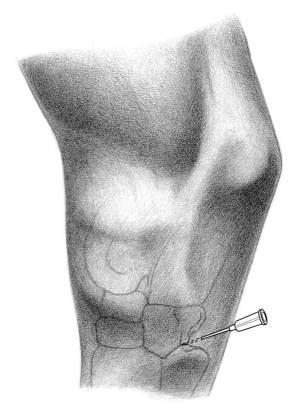

Figure 3.136. Lateral view of the injection site for the tarsometatarsal joint.

downward direction to a depth of 0.5 to 1 inch (1 to 3 cm).[42,43] Synovial fluid is often observed in the needle hub and 3 to 5 mL of anesthetic is used for diagnostic purposes. Injecting the anesthetic under pressure was thought to force anesthetic into the DIT joint but instead it causes it to accumulate in the subcutaneous tissues.[42] In addition, the anesthetic may enter the tarsal sheath and extend around the tendons of the tibialis cranialis and fibularis tertius when using this approach.[14] A more difficult alternative approach to the TMT joint is from the distomedial aspect of the tarsus. The site for injection is approximately 0.5 inches (1 to 2 cm) distal to the site used for the medial approach to the DIT joint.[62]

Cunean Bursa

The cunean bursa is located on the medial surface of the distal tarsus between the medial collateral ligament of the tarsus and the medial branch of the tibialis cranialis (cunean) tendon. The bursa is relatively small and is not routinely anesthetized or treated alone because it often communicates with the DIT joint.[24] A 1-inch (2.54-cm), 22-gauge needle is inserted under the distal border of the cunean tendon and directed proximally to enter the bursa (Figure 3.134C). Some clinicians treat the cunean bursa concurrently when medicating the DIT joint in horses with distal tarsal OA.

Calcaneal Bursa

The calcaneal bursa is located between the SDFT and the caudal aspect of the calcaneus. When distended, the bursa has synovial outpouchings medial and lateral to the tendon both proximal and distal to the SDFT retinaculum. These can often be seen as 4 distinct pockets of fluid surrounding the point of the hock in horses with bursal distention. Synovial aspiration is best performed using the lateral synovial outpouchings either above or below the SDFT retinaculum with the horse weight-bearing. A 1-inch (2.5-cm), 20-gauge needle is angled proximally within these outpouchings to avoid the SDFT. The sites for needle placement are the same as those described for insertion of the arthroscope into the calcaneal bursa: 1 cm dorsal to the SDFT and 1 cm distal to the medial or lateral aspect of the SDFT retinaculum (Figure 3.137).[32] Approximately 8 to 12 mL of anesthetic is used to block the bursa.

Stifle Joint

The stifle joint is comprised of three synovial compartments: the femoropatellar and the lateral and medial femorotibial joints. Contrast studies have shown that the frequency of communication between the femoropatellar and the medial femorotibial (MFT) joint is approximately 60% to 65%.[46,65] The communication, however, is variable, and appears to depend on the direction of flow of the injectable agent, the amount of joint inflammation, and anatomic variation. Communication between the femoropatellar and the MFT joint is observed more frequently when the MFT joint is injected than when the femoropatellar joint is injected. Communication between the femoropatellar joint and the lateral femorotibial (LFT) joint occurs rarely, and communication between the MFT and LFT joints does not occur under normal situations. Some clinicians feel that each synovial compartment of the stifle should be injected separately to ensure accurate distribution of local anesthetic.[62] However, greater diffusion of local anesthetic between compartments of the stifle probably occurs than what has previously been assumed based on anatomic, latex-injection, and contrast arthrography

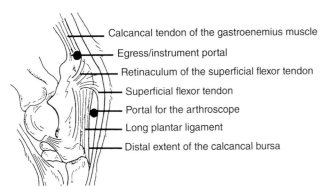

Figure 3.137. Injection sites for the calcaneal bursa are located either above or below the retinaculum of the superficial digital flexor tendon (black dots). These injection sites can be difficult to find without effusion.

studies.[24,42] The majority of the injection approaches to all compartments of the stifle are performed in the weight-bearing limb and approximately 20 to 30 mL of anesthetic is usually recommended in each joint.

Femoropatellar Joint

The femoropatellar joint is the largest of the compartments and it can be entered from the cranial (on either side of the middle patella ligament) or lateral (caudal to the lateral patella ligament) aspects. In one cranial approach, a 3.5-inch (3.8- or 8.9-cm), 18- to 20-gauge needle is inserted approximately 1 to 1.5 inches (3 to 4 cm) proximal to the tibial crest between the middle and medial patella ligaments, and is directed proximally under the patella (Figure 3.138A). This approach is best performed with the limb in a partial weight-bearing (slightly flexed) position.[62] Alternatively, the needle can be directed parallel to the ground with the limb fully weight-bearing.[42] The femoropatellar joint can also be entered just distal to the apex of the patella on either side of the middle patellar ligament with the limb weight-bearing (Figure 3.139a).[64] The joint capsule is superficial at this location and a 1.5-inch (3.8-cm), 18- to 20-gauge needle is directed at right angles to the skin.

The lateral approach to the femoropatellar joint is performed with the horse weight-bearing (Figure 3.138B).[29] The lateral cul-de-sac of the joint is located caudal to the lateral patellar ligament and approximately 2 inches (5 to 6 cm) proximal to the lateral tibial condyle. A 1.5-inch (3.8-cm), 18- to 20-gauge needle is

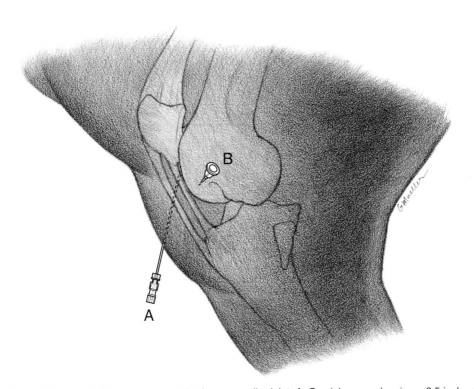

Figure 3.138. Lateral view of the injection sites for the femoropatellar joint. A. Cranial approach using a 3.5-inch spinal needle. B. Lateral approach behind the lateral patellar ligament.

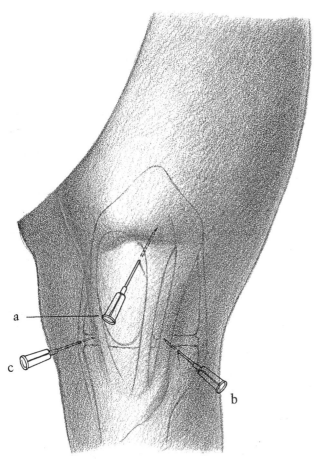

Figure 3.139. Cranial view of the injection sites for the stifle joints. (a) Needle inserted medial to the middle patellar ligament to enter the femoropatellar joint. (b) Needle inserted caudal to the lateral patellar ligament to enter the lateral femorotibial joint. (c) Needle positioned medial to the medial patellar ligament to enter the medial femorotibial joint.

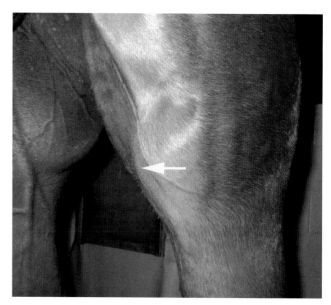

Figure 3.140. With the cranial approach to the MFT joint, the needle is directed in a cranial-to-caudal direction in the depression between the medial patella ligament and the tendon of insertion of the sartorius muscle to enter the proximal outpouching of the joint (arrow).

inserted into the recess perpendicular to the long axis of the femur until the nonarticular portion of the lateral trochlea is contacted. Synovial fluid can be retrieved in most cases and this approach is usually well tolerated by the horse.

Medial Femorotibial (MFT) Joint

The site for injection of the MFT joint is located in the space between the medial patellar and medial collateral ligaments just above the palpable proximomedial edge of the tibia in the weight-bearing limb (Figure 3.139c).[42] A 1.5-inch (3.8-cm), 18- to 20-gauge needle is inserted just caudal to the medial patellar ligament, 1 cm proximal to the tibia and directed perpendicular to the long axis of the limb. The needle may need to be repositioned slightly cranially or caudally to help obtain synovial fluid. The medial meniscus will be contacted (penetrated) if the needle is inserted too far caudally or too close to the proximal tibia.[30,64] This approach may be performed from the same side (facing the stifle) or from the opposite side, reaching under the horse's belly.

Another approach to the MFT joint is located 0.5 to 1 inch (1 to 2 cm) proximal to the medial tibial plateau in the depression between the medial patella ligament and the tendon of insertion of the sartorius muscle.[63] A 1.5-inch (3.8-cm), 20-gauge needle is directed in a cranial to caudal direction parallel to the ground and parallel to a plane the bisects the limb (Figure 3.140). The needle enters a medial outpouching of the MFT joint and avoids inadvertent penetration of the medial meniscus and the medial femoral condyle. In addition, synovial fluid is often obtained.

Lateral Femorotibial (LFT) Joint

The site for injection of the LFT joint is slightly caudal to the palpable edge of the lateral patellar ligament just above the proximolateral edge of the tibia with the limb weight-bearing (Figure 3.139b). A 1.5-inch (3.8-cm), 18- to 20-gauge needle is inserted at right angles to the long axis of the femur and directed from lateral to medial to a depth of 1 inch (2 to 3 cm). An alternative approach is to insert the needle just proximal to the tibia in the space between the lateral collateral ligament of the LFT joint and the tendon of origin of the long digital extensor tendon (Figure 3.141).[30,42] The palpable head of the fibula helps to identify these structures. The needle is inserted slowly to a depth of approximately 1 inch (2 to 3 cm) until the joint capsule is entered.[42] Deeper insertion may result in penetration of the lateral meniscus and a painful response.[62]

Single Approach for All Three Joints

All three joints in the stifle can be injected from one cranial site 1.5 cm proximal to the tibia between the

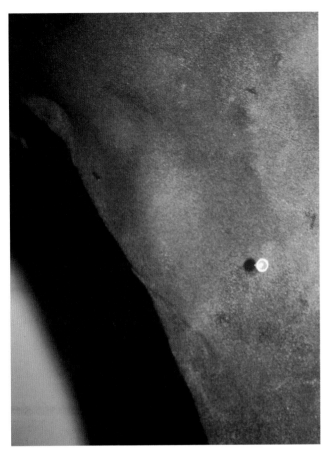

Figure 3.141.   Injection site for the lateral femorotibial joint just proximal to the tibia in the space between the lateral collateral ligament of the joint and the tendon of origin of the long digital extensor tendon. The palpable head of the fibula helps to identify these structures.

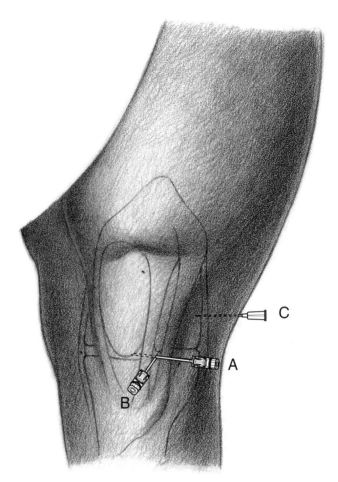

Figure 3.142.   Cranial view of using a single cranial injection site for both femorotibial joints. A. Site for the medial femorotibial joint using a spinal needle. B. Site for the lateral femorotibial joint using a spinal needle. C. Lateral approach to the femoropatellar joint.

lateral and middle patellar ligaments with the stifle slightly flexed.[62] Local skin and subcutaneous anesthesia at the injection site is helpful for this technique. A 3.5-inch (8.9-cm), 18- to 20-gauge spinal needle is inserted and directed caudomedially parallel to the tibial crest toward the MFT joint (Figure 3.142A). The needle is then withdrawn to the subcutaneous tissue and redirected caudolaterally parallel to the tibial crest toward the LFT joint and anesthetic is deposited (Figure 3.142B). The needle is again withdrawn to the subcutaneous tissue and redirected proximally under the patella into the femoropatellar joint.

Trochanteric Bursa

The trochanteric bursa is located beneath the tendon of insertion of the middle gluteal muscle on the cranial aspect of the greater trochanter of the femur (Figure 1.48 in Chapter 1). The site for injection is between the tendon and the lateral surface of the greater trochanter at the most cranial aspect of the palpable greater trochanter. A 1.5-inch (3.8-cm), 18-gauge needle is usually all that is needed, although larger Warmblood horses may require a longer needle in some cases.[25] The needle is inserted and directed horizontally at right angles to

the sagittal plane until bone is encountered. Seven to 10 ml of anesthetic is injected. An alternate method is to direct the needle medially through the middle gluteal muscle directly over the bursa toward the trochanter.[62]

Coxofemoral (Hip) Joint

The coxofemoral joint is one of the most difficult joints to enter.[38,42] This is particularly true in mature, heavily muscled horses. The joint is well away from the proximal end of the femur and the landmarks for injection are often difficult to palpate. The procedure is best performed with the horse standing squarely and restrained within stocks. Mild sedation is often advised because movement during the injection procedure may cause the needle to bend or break.

The most important landmarks to palpate are the paired summits of the greater trochanter of the femur. The trochanter is located about two-thirds of the distance between the tuber coxae and the tuber ischii.[42] The greater trochanter is approximately 4 inches (10 cm) wide with a notch between the cranial and

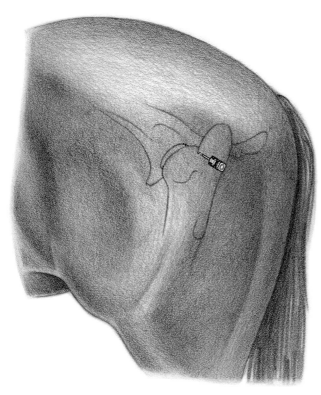

Figure 3.143. Lateral view of the injection site for the coxofemoral joint. The needle is inserted in the trochanteric notch and directed at a 45° angle with the long axis until the joint is entered.

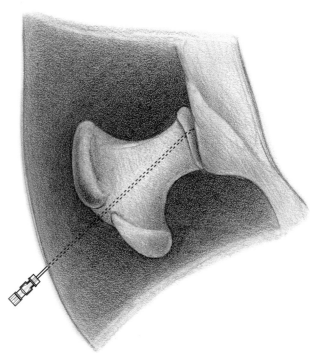

Figure 3.144. Overhead view of the injection site for the coxofemoral joint. The needle is inserted just caudal to the greater trochanter and directed at a 45° angle to enter the joint.

caudal protuberances that can be difficult to palpate. The site for injection is about 0.5 inches (1 to 2 cm) above the middle of the proximal summit of the trochanter (Figure 3.143).[42] A small bleb of local anesthetic is injected subcutaneously over the injection site and a small stab incision may aid needle insertion. A 6- to 8-inch (15- to 20-cm), 16- to 18-gauge spinal needle is directed in a horizontal plane perpendicular to the vertebral column (Figure 3.144). The needle should be directed slightly downward to stay close to the femoral neck so that it is approximately 0.5 inches (1 to 2 cm) lower than the insertion site after it has been advanced 3 to 4 inches (8 to 10 cm). Firm fibrous tissue is often felt just before the needle penetrates the joint capsule at approximately 4 to 6 inches (10 to 15 cm). Synovial fluid is often aspirated and 30 to 60 mL of anesthetic is recommended.[30,42] If unsuccessful, the needle should be withdrawn to just under the skin and then re-directed. Ultrasound may also be used to help direct needle insertion into the coxofemoral joint.[10]

Sacroiliac (SI) Joint

The SI joint is not a true synovial joint, but treatment of this region has become more common in the last several years. Anesthesia of the SI joint may cause partial paralysis of the sciatic nerve, making horses recumbent for variable periods of time. Therefore, anesthesia of this region is not performed commonly by the first author.

The described technique by Engeli and Haussler is used by the first author and is described here.[19] The horse is usually sedated, restrained in stocks, and the injection site anesthetized with local anesthesia. The landmark for injection is the cranial aspect of the tuber sacrale. A 10-inch (25-cm), 15- to 16-gauge spinal needle is bent to an angle of about 40° in the direction of the needle's bevel. The needle is inserted through a stab incision in the skin 1 inch (2 cm) cranial to the contralateral tuber sacrale, and directed at a 60° angle to the vertical plane. The needle is advanced across midline aiming for a point midway between the ipsilateral tuber coxae and the greater trochanter of the femur until it contacts the medial aspect of the tuber sacrale (Figure 3.145). The needle hub is lifted and the needle is advanced at a steeper angle along the medial aspect of the ilial wing until it contacts the dorsal surface of the sacrum at a depth of approximately 6 to 8 inches (15 to 20 cm).[42] Approximately 8 to 10 mL of anesthetic can be used for diagnostic purposes or when medication is injected. An alternative technique is to insert a 6-inch (15-cm), 18-gauge needle near the cranial aspect of the tuber sacrale. The needle is directed ventrocaudolateral toward the SI joint of the opposite side at a 20° to 40° angle to the vertical plane.[17] The latter technique is thought to be a less precise technique for both anesthesia and treatment of the SI region.[42] Ultrasound guided SI injections may also be performed and both cranial and caudal approaches have been described.[12]

See Chapter 6 for additional information on SI injection techniques.

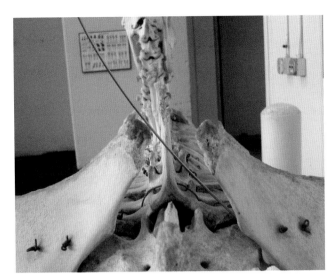

Figure 3.145. Needle location and angulation of the spinal needle used to inject the contralateral sacroiliac joint from the cranial aspect of the tuber sacrale. A 10-inch (25-cm), 15- to 16-gauge spinal needle is bent to an angle of about 40° in the direction of the needle's bevel. The needle is inserted through a stab incision in the skin 1 inch (2 cm) cranial to the contralateral tuber sacrale, and directed at a 60° angle to the vertical plane.

Cervical Facets

Centesis of a cervical facet joint is usually performed to administer a corticosteroid into the joint of a horse that has clinical signs suggestive of disease within the cervical articulation. Lesions of the cervical facets tend to occur most commonly in vertebrae C5 to C6 and C6 to C7.[39] The procedure is performed in the standing, sedated horse with the help of ultrasound, and is usually performed bilaterally unless a specific side of the lesion has been documented. The approximate location of the injection can be made by using one width of the hand to represent the length of one cervical vertebra.[42] The facet joint is imaged with the ultrasound probe, and a 3.5-inch (8.9-cm), 18- to 20-gauge spinal needle is advanced toward the joint at an angle so the tip of the needle can be seen. Ultrasound is used to direct the needle into the joint and the medication or anesthetic is deposited.

References

1. Andreen DS, Trumble TN, Caron JP, et al. Onset and duration of intra-articular mepivacaine in the horse. Proceedings Am Assoc Equine Pract 1994;40:151.
2. Bell BTL, Baker GJ, Foreman JH, et al. *In vivo* investigation of communication between the distal intertarsal and tarsometatarsal joints in horses and ponies. Vet Surg 1993;22:289–292.
3. Bidwell LA, Brown KE, Cordier A, et al. Mepivacaine local anaesthetic duration in equine palmar digital nerve blocks. Equine Vet J 2004;36:723–726.
4. Bowker RM, Rockershouser SJ, Vex KB, et al. Immunohistochemical and dye distribution studies of nerves potentially desensitized by injections into the distal interphalangeal joint or the navicular bursa of horses. J Am Vet Med Assoc 1993;203:1708–1714.
5. Bowker RM, Van Wulfen KK, Grentz DJ. Nonselectivity of local anesthetics injected into the distal interphalangeal joint and navicular bursa. Proceedings Am Assoc Equine Pract 1995;41:240–242.
6. Bowker RM, Linder K, Van Wulfen KK, et al. Distribution of local anesthetics injected into the distal interphalangeal joint and podotrochlear bursa: An experimental study. Pferdehilkunde. 1996;12:609–612.
7. Carter GK, Hogan PM. Use of diagnostic nerve blocks in lameness evaluation. Proceedings Am Assoc Equine Pract 1996;42:26–32.
8. Castro FA, Schumacher JS, Pauwels F, et al. A new approach for perineural injection of the lateral palmar nerve in the horse. *Vet Surg* 2005;34:539–542.
9. Chesen AB, Dabareiner RM, Chaffin MK, et al. Tendonitis of the proximal aspect of the superficial digital flexor tendon in horses: 12 cases(2000–2006) J Am Vet Med Assoc 2009;234:1432–1436.
10. David F, Rougier M, Alexander K, et al. Ultrasound-guided coxofemoral arthrocentesis in horses. Equine Vet J 2007;39:79–83.
11. Day TK, Skarda RT. The pharmacology of local anesthetics. Vet Clin North Am Equine Pract 1991;7:489–500.
12. Denoix JM, Jacquet S. Ultrasound-guided injections of the sacroiliac area in horses. Equine Vet Educ 2008;April:203–207.
13. Denoix JM. Diagnostic techniques for identification and documentation of tendon and ligament injuries. Vet Clin North Am Equine Pract 1994;10:365–407.
14. Dyson SJ, Romero JM. An investigation of injection techniques for local analgesia of the equine distal tarsus and proximal metatarsus. Equine Vet J 1993;25:30–35.
15. Dyson SJ. Comparison of responses to analgesia of the navicular bursa and intra-articular analgesia of the distal interphalangeal joint in 102 horses. Proceedings, Am Assoc Equine Pract 1995;41:234–239.
16. Dyson SJ. The puzzle of distal interphalangeal joint pain. Equine Vet Edu 1998;10:119–125.
17. Dyson SJ, Murray R. Pain associated with the sacroiliac joint region: a clinical study of 74 horses. Equine Vet J 2003;35:240–245.
18. Easter JL, Watkins JP, Stephens SL, et al. Effects of regional anesthesia on experimentally induced coffin joint synovitis. Proceedings, Am Assoc Equine Pract 2000;46:214–216.
19. Engeli E, Haussler KK, Erb HN. Development and validation of a periarticular injection technique of the sacroiliac joint in horses. Equine Vet J 2004;36:324–330.
20. Ford TS, Ross MW, Orsini PG. Communication and boundaries of the middle carpal and carpometacarpal joints in horses. Am J Vet Res 1988;49:2161–2164.
21. Ford TS, Ross MW, Orsini PG. A comparison of methods for proximal palmar metacarpal analgesia in horses. *Vet Surg* 1989;18:146–150.
22. Gayle JM, Redding WR. Comparison of diagnostic anaesthetic techniques of the proximal metatarsus in the horse. Equine Vet Education 2007;May:222–224.
23. Goodman NL, Baker BK. Lameness diagnosis and treatment in the Quarter Horse racehorse. Vet Clin North Am Equine Pract 1990;6:85–108.
24. Gough MR, Munroe GA, Mayhew G. Diffusion of mepivacaine between adjacent synovial structures in the horse. Part 2: tarsus and stifle. Equine Vet J 2002;34:85–90.
25. Grant BD. Bursal Injections. Proceedings, Am Assoc Equine Pract 1996;42:64–68.
26. Hague BA, Honnas CM, Simpson RB, et al. Evaluation of skin bacterial flora before and after aseptic preparation of clipped and nonclipped arthrocentesis sites in horses. Vet Surg 1997;26:121–125.
27. Harper J, Schumacher J, Degraves F, et al. Effects of analgesia of the digital flexor tendon sheath on pain originating in the sole, distal interphalangeal joint or navicular bursa of horses. Equine Vet J 2007;39:535–539.
28. Hassel DM, Stover SM, Yarbrough TB, et al. Palmar-plantar axial sesamoidean approach to the digital flexor sheath in horses. J Am Vet Med Assoc 2000;217:1343–1347.
29. Hendrickson DA, Nixon AJ. A lateral approach for synovial fluid aspiration and joint injection of the femoropatellar joint of the horse. Equine Vet J, 1992;24:397–398.
30. Hogan PH, Honnas CM. Diagnostic Neural and Articular Anesthesia. In Current Techniques in Equine Surgery and Lameness, White NA, Moore JN, eds. WB Saunders, Philadelphia 1998;490–500.
31. Hughes TK, Eliashar E, Smith RK. *In vitro* evaluation of a single injection technique for diagnostic analgesia of the proximal suspensory ligament of the equine pelvic limb. Vet Surg 2007;36:760–764.

32. Ingle-Fehr JE, Baxter GM. Endoscopy of the calcaneal bursa in horses. Vet Surg 1998;27:561–567.

33. Just EM, Patan B, Licka TF. Dorsolateral approach for arthrocentesis of the centrodistal joint in horses. *Am J Vet Res* 2007;68:946–952.

34. Keegan KG, Wilson DA, Kreeger JM, et al. Local distribution of mepivacaine after distal interphalangeal joint injection in horses. Am J Vet Res 1996;57:422–426.

35. Keg PR, Barneveld A, Schamhardt HC, et al. Clinical and force plate evaluation of the effect of a high plantar nerve block in lameness caused by induced mid-metatarsal tendonitis. Vet Q 1994;16 Suppl 2:S70–75.

36. Kiely RG, McMullan W. Lateral arthrocentesis of the equine carpus. Eq Pract 1987;9:22–24.

37. Kraus-Hansen AE, Jann HW, Kerr DV, et al. Arthrographic analysis of communication between the tarsometatarsal and distal intertarsal joints of the horse. Vet Surg 1992;21:139–144.

38. Lewis RD. Techniques for arthrocentesis of equine shoulder, elbow, stifle and hip joints. Proceedings, Am Assoc Equine Pract 1996;42:55–63.

39. Mattoon JS, Drost WT, Grguric MR, et al. Technique for equine cervical articular process joint injection. Vet Radiol Ultrasound 2004;45:238–240.

40. Miller SM, Stover SM. Palmaroproximal approach for arthrocentesis of the proximal interphalangeal joint in the horse. Equine Vet J. 1996;28:376–380.

41. Misheff MM, Stover SM. A comparison of two techniques for arthrocentesis of the metacarpophalangeal joint. Equine Vet J, 1991;23:273–276.

42. Moyer W, Schumacher J, Schumacher J. A Guide to Equine Joint Injection and Regional Anesthesia. Veterinary Learning Systems, Yardley, Pa. 2007;6–65.

43. Moyer W, Carter GK. Techniques to facilitate intra–articular injection of equine joints. Proceedings, Am Assoc Equine Pract 1996;42:48–54.

44. Pleasant RS, Moll HD, Leg WB, et al. Intra-articular anesthesia of the distal interphalangeal joint alleviates lameness associated with the navicular bursa in horses. Vet Surg 1997;26:137–140.

45. Piccot-Crezollet C, Cauvin ER, Lepage OM. Comparison of two techniques for injection of the podotrochlear bursa in horses. J Am Vet Med Assoc 2005;226:1524–1527.

46. Reeves M, Trotter GW, Kainer R. Anatomic and functional communications between the synovial sacs of the equine stifle joint. Equine Vet J 1991;23:215–218.

47. Sack WO. Nerve distribution in the metacarpus and front digit of the horse. J Am Vet Med Assoc 1975;167:298–335.

48. Sack WO, Orsini PG. Distal intertarsal and tarsometatarsal joints in the horse: Communication and injection sites. J Am Vet Med Assoc 1981;179:355–359.

49. Sams AE, Honnas CM, Sack WO, et al. Communication of the ulnaris lateralis bursa with the equine elbow joint and evaluation of caudal arthrocentesis. Equine Vet J. 1993;25:130–133.

50. Schramme MC, Boswell JC, Hamhougias K, et al. An *in vitro* study to compare 5 different techniques for injection of the navicular bursa in the horse. Equine Vet J 2000;32:263–267.

51. Schumacher J, Livesey L, DeGraves FJ, et al. Effect of anaesthesia of the palmar digital nerves on proximal interphalangeal joint pain in the horse. Equine Vet J 2004;36:409–414.

52. Schumacher J, de Graves F, Steiger R, et al. A comparison of the effects of two volumes of local analgesic solution in the distal interphalangeal joint of horses with lameness caused by solar toe or solar heel pain. *Equine Vet J* 2001;33:265–268.

53. Schumacher J, Steiger R, de Graves F, et al. Effects of analgesia of the distal interphalangeal joint or palmar digital nerves on lameness caused by solar pain in horses. Vet Surg 2000;29:54–58.

54. Schumacher J, Schramme MC, Schumacher J, et al. A review of recent studies concerning diagnostic analgesia of the equine forefoot. Proceedings, Am Assoc Equine Pract 2003;49:312–316.

55. Schumacher J, Schumacher J, Schramme MC. Diagnostic analgesia of the equine forefoot. Equine Vet Educ 2004;June:199–204.

56. Schumacher J, Gillette R, DeGraves F, et al. The effects of local anesthetic solution in the navicular bursa of horses with lameness caused by distal interphalangeal joint pain. Equine Vet J 2003;35:502–505.

57. Schumacher J, Livesey L, Brawner W, et al. Comparison of 2 methods of centesis of the bursa of the biceps brachii tendon of horses. Equine Vet J 2007;39:356–359.

58. Serena A, Schumacher J, Schramme MC, et al. Concentration of methylprednisolone in the centrodistal joint after administration of methylprednisolone acetate in the tarsometatarsal joint. Equine Vet J 2005;37:172–174.

59. Shepherd MC, Pilsworth RC. Failure of intra-articular anaesthesia of the antebrachiocarpal joint to abolish lameness associated with chip fracture of the distal radius. Equine Vet J. 1993;25:458–461.

60. Southwood LL, Baxter GM, Fehr JE. How to perform arthrocentesis of the fetlock joint by using a distal palmar (plantar) approach. Proceedings, Am Assoc Equine Pract 1997;43:151–153.

61. Spoormakers TJ, Donker SH, Ensink JM. Diagnostic anaesthesia of the equine lower limb: a comparison of lidocaine and lidocaine with epinephrine. Tijdschr Diergeneeskd 2004;129:548–551.

62. Stashak TS. Examination for Lameness. In Adams' Lameness in Horses. Stashak TS, ed., 5th ed. Lippincott Williams and Wilkins, Philadelphia. 2002;113–183.

63. Swiderski CE, Linford R. How to inject the medial femorotibial joint: an alternate approach. Proceedings, Am Assoc Equine Pract 2005;51:476–480.

64. Trotter GW, McIlwraith CW. Clinical features and diagnosis of equine joint disease. In Joint Disease in the Horse McIlwraith CW and Trotter GW, eds. WB Saunders, Philadelphia. 1996;125–134.

65. Vacek JR, Ford TS, Honnas CM. Communication between the femoropatellar and medial and lateral femorotibial joints in horses. Am J Vet Res 1992;53:1431–1434.

66. Vazquez de Mercado R, Stover SM, Taylor KT, et al. Lateral approach for arthrocentesis of the distal interphalangeal joint in horses. J Am Vet Med Assoc 1998;212:1413–1418.

67. Wright IM, Phillips TJ, Walmsley JP. Endoscopy of the navicular bursa: a new technique for the treatment of contaminated and septic bursae. Equine Vet J 1999;31:5–11.

EQUINE DIAGNOSTIC ACUPUNCTURE EXAMINATION (DAPE)

Kevin K. Haussler and Gary M. Baxter

Palpation along acupuncture channels/meridians and at specific acupoints can be used for diagnostic purposes in both animals and people.[4,21] This is termed the diagnostic acupuncture examination (DAPE), and can be used to complement the Western approach to examine horses with musculoskeletal abnormalities. (The reader is referred to the DVD for a demonstration of performing a DAPE.) The primary difference between the two approaches lies in the emphasis given to the information that is obtained.[4] The DAPE detects trigger points or painful sites along the acupuncture channels/meridians that may indicate focal myofascial pain or "referred pain" from problems at other locations of the musculoskeletal system. For example, trigger points found along the bladder (BL) channel in the thoracolumbar region of the horse may represent local pain in the back musculature or suggest problems in the tarsus or stifle.[4] However, it is very difficult to prove referred zones of pain in animals such that a trigger point found in the back indicates a potential problem in the tarsus.[8,10]

TRIGGER POINTS

Trigger points or myofascial trigger points are known to exist in humans and are defined as hyperirritable spots, usually within a taut band of skeletal muscle, which is painful on compression and can give rise to characteristic referred pain, motor dysfunction, and autonomic phenomena.[9] Others have termed trigger points as objectively demonstrable foci within muscles[8] or as localized tender spots in a taut band of skeletal muscle.[10] These foci are usually identified subjectively by a local twitch response using a strumming palpation technique.[10] Objectively, they can be demonstrated with algometry, pressure threshold measurements, magnetic resonance thermography, and histology.[8]

Increased electromyographic (EMG) activity has been demonstrated at trigger point sites compared to normal muscle in both humans and horses.[7,10] The study in horses concluded that equine myofascial trigger points can be identified and have similar objective signs and EMG properties to those documented in human and rabbit skeletal muscle.[10] However, the important differences from findings in human studies are that referred pain patterns and the reproduction of pain profile cannot be determined in animals.[10] To date, there is no scientific evidence to suggest that myofascial trigger points found in the horse can be used as an indicator of disease elsewhere in the musculoskeletal system. However, veterinarians familiar with acupuncture and the DAPE use this information routinely as evidence of referred pain.[4]

HOW TO PERFORM A DAPE

The DAPE is another approach to evaluate the musculoskeletal system other than traditional palpation and manipulation. The goal is to obtain further information that may help localize the site(s) of the problem. It is not necessarily helpful in all lameness cases and in general is more beneficial for hindlimb problems than forelimb problems. The authors primarily use the DAPE for horses with subtle hindlimb lameness, performance-limiting lameness, and other nebulous musculoskeletal problems. In addition, a DAPE is often performed if no abnormalities are found with traditional palpation and manipulation, and minimal lameness is observed.

The information obtained by the DAPE is directly related to the skill and experience of the person performing the exam.[4] Consistency of pressure applied during the exam is critical and an unbiased approach to each horse must be taken. The examination can be performed with the fingers, or a blunt object such as a needle cap can be used.[4] Devices that apply consistent pressure, such as an algometer, may also be used to improve the overall accuracy of the exam. The authors usually perform the DAPE with a 16-gauge needle case and attempt to apply consistent pressure using a smooth, uninterrupted stroke instead of inserting pressure at individual points.

The examination is divided into specific regions of the body, beginning with the head and neck, and progressing to the chest and forelimb, back and abdomen, sacral region, and ending with the hindlimbs.[4] The exam is then continued on the opposite side of the horse in the same manner. The goal is to detect focal areas of myofascial pain that may represent local pain but may also suggest problems elsewhere in the musculoskeletal system. However, most trigger points found over the back along the BL channel/meridian in horses most likely represent local soft tissue pain and do not represent referred pain. Finding several trigger points during a DAPE that all suggest a problem at another specific location usually warrants further investigation.[4] In addition, the findings of the Western examination must be taken into account when interpreting the DAPE.

DETAILED DIAGNOSTIC ACUPUNCTURE EVALUATION

The traditional Chinese medicine (TCM) examination is based on pattern recognition and includes four components: looking (inspection), hearing and smelling (auscultation and olfaction), asking (history taking), and feeling (palpation).[22] Practitioners collect general and seemingly unrelated information about temperament; behavior; activity; and detailed history of the onset, provocation, and improvement of the chief complaint to formulate a tentative diagnosis.[13]

For evaluation of lameness or back pain, palpation of reactive acupuncture points along each meridian using either finger pressure or a needle cap often provides the most useful information. Reactivity to palpation of acupuncture points along the dorsal epaxial musculature of the neck, back, and croup is graded on a 1-to-4 scale.[13,14] Grade 1 corresponds to a normal, supple, and non-painful response to deep palpation. Grade 2 is a mild pain response and transient muscle contraction that quickly disappears with repeated stimulation. Grade 3 is consistent pain or avoidance to deep palpation with repeated stimulation. Grade 4 reactivity is characterized by a strong avoidance response, which may include an attempt to kick or bite. Horses with Grade 1 or 2 responses are characterized as having balanced acupuncture meridians or normal responses to applied pressure. The presence of Grade 3 and 4 reactivity is characterized as unbalanced acupuncture meridians and is considered an indication for acupuncture treatment.[14] From a TCM perspective, reactivity to light pressure indicates an excess, acute, or superficial (*Yang*) condition, whereas, a positive response to deep pressure is thought to indicate a chronic or deficiency (*Yin*) condition.[6]

Palpation usually focuses on body regions and proceeds from the head to the tail in a systematic manner. Based on TCM principles, any pathology along the course of a meridian should produce palpable reactive diagnostic points.[5,19] However, in a study of 189 horses with thoracic limb lameness, only 41% (78) of horses had reactive diagnostic acupuncture points.[15] Reactivity at 5 diagnostic acupuncture points for the thoracic limb was significantly more prevalent in cases of laminitis (83%) and acute or chronic heel pain (69%), compared to subsolar abscesses (0%).[15]

Reactivity at certain acupuncture points has been empirically associated with specific disease conditions; however, there is little scientific evidence to support these claims.[4] The presence of diagnostic acupuncture points may also have different interpretations based on reactivity of other local or regional acupuncture points.[18] For example, reactivity at large intestine 16 (LI-16), which is located at the intersection of the cranial border of the scapula and the dorsal border of the brachiocephalicus muscle, may be reactive due to thoracic limb lameness, cervical hyperesthesia, or contralateral pelvic limb lameness. Neurologic diseases, such as equine herpes (EHV-1) and equine protozoal myelitis (EPM), have also been postulated to activate specific diagnostic acupuncture points; however, controlled studies have refuted these hypotheses.[2,3]

A more appropriate use of acupuncture point reactivity is to identify local pain and tissue inflammation or regional musculoskeletal dysfunction. Acute back pain is often diagnosed based on identifying sites of pain or muscle spasms. The diagnosis of chronic back pain is often based on a thorough history, physical examination, change in performance, and radiographic findings.[11] However, radiographic examination alone is considered one of the least effective methods of diagnosing back pain in horses. Acupuncture evaluation and treatment must be used in conjunction with a thorough physical examination and complete lameness examination to provide a definitive diagnosis of the source of lameness or back pain.

Superficial palpation of the DAPE begins on the lateral face to identify pain or sensitivity within the masseter muscles and around the temporo-mandibular joint region, which may be indicative of temporo-mandibular or dental disorders. The examination continues into the poll region and lateral cervical spine to identify localized regions of pain or cervical dysfunction.[6] The chest and proximal forelimb musculature is assessed for hypertonic muscles or trigger or *Ah shi* points that may suggest the presence of a forelimb lameness.[10] No direct relationship exists between lameness and the severity or distribution of reactive acupuncture points.[13] Based on several large case series, it has been hypothesized that intra-articular pathologies activate acupuncture meridians and extra-articular pathologies (e.g., foot abscess, splints, tendonitis, and subchondral bone disease) do not; little scientific evidence exists to support this theory.[13]

The Back *shu* (association) points are considered the most important diagnostic points and are located along the bladder meridian traveling in two parallel lines over the longissimus and iliocostalis muscles.[4,21] These points correspond to segmental distribution of the thoraco-lumbar spinal nerves. The governing vessel is palpated along the dorsal midline from the withers to the base of the tail. *Hua Tou Jia Jia* points are located lateral to the dorsal spinous process and may be reactive with impinged spinous processes. Back pain associated with myopathies, poor saddle fit, rider-induced injuries, inappropriate training programs, or possible pelvic limb lameness may also produce sensitivity along the BL meridian.[18] Additional reactions along the BL meridian have been reported with visceral disease due to the presence of somatovisceral reflexes associated with colic or urogenital pain. Intercostal spaces along the lateral thorax are also assessed for reactivity.

The croup and proximal pelvic limb musculature are examined along the bladder meridian for trigger points or reactive acupuncture points indicative of pelvic limb lameness.[12] Regions around the bony pelvic prominences (e.g., tuber coxae) are evaluated for sensitivity within muscular attachments. Meridian reactivity within the pelvic limb has been associated with intra-articular pathology of the distal tarsus and metatarso-phalangeal and distal interphalangeal joints.[12] *Ting* points are diagnostic acupuncture points located around the periphery of the coronary band of all 4 limbs. The presence of depressions, edema, or focal pain are indicative of meridian imbalances and are considered diagnostically important.[4]

HOW TO INTERPRET A DAPE

Interpreting the results of the DAPE is often the most difficult aspect of this diagnostic test. Horses are individuals and may react differently to the same amount of pressure.[4] Occasionally, the legitimacy of the results may be questioned depending on the demeanor of the horse. However, consistency and repeatability of the resultant trigger points are often very helpful to document the accuracy of the findings. In addition, asymmetry in responses from cranial to caudal and the left to the right sides of the horse often suggest that the findings are real.

Consistency between the Western exam and the DAPE also further supports the validity of the findings. Negative findings on the DAPE are just as important as positive findings in the authors' opinion, because many horses without back and hindlimb issues will not respond to the DAPE in these locations. A negative DAPE exam together with negative palpation/manipulation can often rule out the back and hindlimbs as the source of a performance-limiting problem. However, a definitive diagnosis can never be made based strictly on the DAPE.

WHEN TO PERFORM THE DAPE

Most reports of the use of acupuncture for lameness problems in horses have focused on horses with back pain.[1,17] When the DAPE is performed during the lameness examination is less important than how it is performed. However, in the second author's opinion it is best to perform the DAPE after palpation but before observing the horse for lameness to ensure that the DAPE is not biased in any way. In general, the DAPE appears to be most useful to help detect problems in the upper fore- and hindlimbs and those along the neck, back, and sacrum. The DAPE is primarily used for horses with subtle hindlimb lameness, performance-limiting lameness, and other nebulous musculoskeletal problems. The second author has also found it beneficial in some cases to help differentiate between a musculoskeletal or neurological problem. The DAPE and a Western examination are both used to obtain as much information as possible in these horses. The DAPE complements the Western examination and does not replace it.

VALIDITY OF DIAGNOSTIC ACUPUNCTURE

Findings of the palpation phase of the acupuncture examination must be combined with history, inspection, physical examination, and results of orthopedic tests and diagnostic imaging to establish a definitive diagnosis. However, acupuncture is considered useful for evaluation of poor performance and vague back or lameness complaints that defy traditional veterinary diagnostics.[16] Patterns of reactive acupuncture points are considered useful to localize pain and lameness and help to identify the presence of concurrent limb or axial skeletal pain.[18,20] In the prepurchase examination of 235 sport horses, 66% (156) were sound at their working gaits and 34% (79) had observable lameness.[14] Lame horses had a significantly higher proportion (66%; 52) of palpable meridian imbalances, compared to sound horses (29%; 46). Significantly more sound horses with no meridian imbalances were sold, compared to sound horses with unbalanced meridians or lame horses. The presence of reactive meridians in sound horses suggests the possibility of muscle soreness or subclinical lameness and a need for changes in the training program,

management, shoeing, or other contributing factors.[14] However, several authors have questioned whether referred pain can be determined in animals,[8,10] suggesting that trigger point pain at specific locations along an acupuncture channel/meridian may not indicate a problem elsewhere in the limb. More objective assessments of the DAPE are needed before concrete associations can be made between it and the Western examination.

References

1. Chan WW, Chen KY, Liu H, et al. Acupuncture for general veterinary practice. J Vet Med Sci 2001;63:1057–1062.
2. Chvala S, Nowotny N, Kotzab E, et al. Use of the meridian test for the detection of equine herpesvirus type 1 infection in horses with decreased performance. J Am Vet Med Assoc 2004;225:554–559.
3. Fenger CK, Granstrom DE, Langemeier JL, et al. Equine protozoal myeloencephalitis: Acupuncture diagnosis. Proc Amer Assoc Equine Practitioners 1997;43:327–329.
4. Fleming P. Diagnostic Acupuncture Palpation Examination in the Horse. In Veterinary Acupuncture. 2nd ed. Schoen AM. ed. Mosby Inc. St. Louis, MO. 2001:433–442.
5. Flemming P. Acupuncture for musculoskeletal and neurologic conditions in horses. Vet Acupunct 1994;28:513–521.
6. Fleming P. Equine acupuncture. In Complementary and alternative veterinary medicine: principles and practice. Schoen AM, Wynn SG, eds. Mosby, St. Louis. 1998;169–184.
7. Fricton JR, Auvinen MD, Dykstra D, et al. Myofascial pain syndrome: electromyographic changes associated with local twitch response. Arch Phys Med Rehabil 1985;66:314–317.
8. Janssens LA. Trigger point therapy. Probl Vet Med 1992;4:117–124.
9. Lavelle ED, Lavelle W, Smith HS. Myofascial trigger points Med Clin North Am 2007;91:229–239.
10. Macgregor J, Graf von Schweinitz D. Needle electromyographic activity of myofascial trigger points and control sites in equine cleidobrachialis muscle—an observational study. Acupunct Med 2006;24:61–70.
11. Martin BB Jr., Klide AM. Diagnosis and treatment of chronic back pain in horses. Proc Amer Assoc Equine Practitioners 1997;43:310–311.
12. McCormick WH. The origins of acupuncture channel imbalance in pain of the equine hindlimb. J Equine Vet Sci 1998;18:528–534.
13. McCormick WH. Understanding the use of acupuncture in treating equine lameness and musculoskeletal pain. In Diagnosis and management of lameness in the horse. Ross MW, Dyson SJ, eds. Saunders, St. Louis, MO. 2003;798–803.
14. McCormick WH. The incidence and significance of excess acupuncture channel imbalance in the equine sport horse purchase examination, 1999–2004. J Equine Vet Sci 2006;26:322–325.
15. McCormick WH. Oriental channel diagnosis in foot lameness of the equine forelimb. J Equine Vet Sci 1997;17:315–321.
16. Merriam JG. Acupuncture in the treatment of back pain and hind leg pain in sport horses. Proc Amer Assoc Equine Practitioners 1997;43:325–326.
17. Ridgway K. Acupuncture as a treatment modality for back problems. Vet Clin North Am Equine Pract 1999;15:211–221.
18. Schoen AM. Equine acupuncture: incorporation into lameness diagnosis and treatment. Proc Amer Assoc Equine Practitioners 2000;46:80–83.
19. Snader M. Diagnostic acupuncture in horses. Vet Acupunct 1994;27:466–468.
20. Sutherland EC. Integration of acupuncture and manipulation into a standard lameness examination and treatment approach. Proc Amer Assoc Equine Practitioners 1997;43:319–321.
21. Xie H, Colahan P, Ott EA. Evaluation of electroacupuncture treatment of horses with signs of chronic thoracolumbar pain. J Am Vet Med Assoc 2005;227:281–286.
22. Xie H, Liu H. Equine traditional Chinese medical diagnosis. In Veterinary acupuncture: Ancient art to modern medicine. Schoen AM, ed. Mosby Publications, St. Louis, MO. 2001;503–513.

Diagnostic Procedures

RADIOLOGY

Alejandro Valdés-Martínez and Richard D. Park

Digital radiography has replaced screen-film systems in most university veterinary teaching hospitals during the past decade. This technology has also become more popular in the private sector, from large referral hospitals to ambulatory practice. However, the conversion from conventional to digital radiography is currently in transition and the use of film-based radiography remains widely acceptable worldwide.

Regardless of the radiographic system used, the X-ray machine and radiation safety practice remain exactly the same for either conventional or digital radiography. The veterinarian must be familiar with the basic instrumentation of an X-ray machine and the radiation safety techniques commonly practiced in radiography. An understanding of the normal equine radiographic anatomy, basic radiographic interpretation principles, examination techniques, and post-capture image processing or darkroom equipment and procedures is essential to perform diagnostic radiographic studies. Too often, knowledge of these basic concepts is overlooked, resulting in inferior radiographic examinations. Poor-quality radiographs may result in erroneous diagnoses and conclusions. The axiom "No radiograph is better than a poor quality radiograph" is true in equine radiology.

This section is not intended to comprehensively cover the physics behind the different radiographic systems (conventional and digital); however, a review of the various technologies available in veterinary medicine including dark room equipment, post-capture digital image processing, and image display and storage are included. More detailed information is available elsewhere.[21,24,42–44,54,55,57] The normal equine radiographic anatomy with standard projections used in the diagnosis of lameness in addition to the common radiographic signs of bone and soft tissue response to different pathologic processes are also discussed.

EQUIPMENT

Knowledge of radiography equipment including X-rays machines, detector systems, film processing, image viewing devices, and accessory equipment is necessary for obtaining good quality diagnostic radiographs safely. The reader should also be aware of the advantages and disadvantages of the different equipment options that are available for veterinary practice, especially when deciding to upgrade from conventional to digital radiography.

X-Ray Machines

The basic control settings of an X-ray machine, the milliamperage (mA), exposure time, and kilovoltage potential (kVp), are located on the control panel and may be changed to vary the exposure (Figure 4.1). Milliamperage is the tube current and refers to the quantity of electrons flowing per second in the X-ray tube. Ultimately, it determines the quantity of X-rays emitted from the X-ray tube.

Exposure time is an important variable in equine radiology. Because of problems related to patient and detector movement, exposure time should be 0.1 second or less, if possible, for equine limb examinations. The use of electronic timers is recommended for accurate timing when the exposure is less than 0.1 second. For equine radiology, an electronic timer with 2-step exposure button is desirable.[39] The first step warms the X-ray tube filament; the exposure is made in the second step. The 2-step exposure button prolongs the X-ray tube life. Because exposure time (in seconds) multiplied by

Adams and Stashak's Lameness in Horses, 6e, edited by Gary M. Baxter
© 2011 Blackwell Publishing, Ltd.

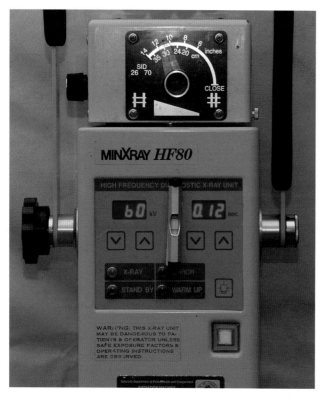

Figure 4.1. Control panel for a 30-mA portable X-ray machine.

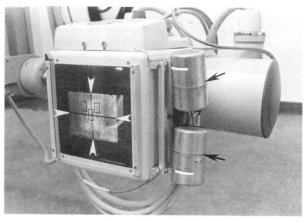

Figure 4.2. Adjustable light-beam collimator. The primary beam is limited by adjustable leaves in the collimator. A light source within the collimator defines the limits of the primary beam (white arrows). A double light source within the canisters on the side of the collimator provides a converging double line on the cassette to position the X-ray tube at the correct FFD (black arrows).

the milliamperage equals milliamperage-seconds (mAs), radiation exposure is directly related to milliamperage-seconds:

$$0.1 \text{ second} \times 10 \text{ mA} = 1 \text{ mAs}$$
$$0.1 \text{ second} \times 15 \text{ mA} = 1.5 \text{ mAs}$$
$$0.2 \text{ second} \times 10 \text{ mA} = 2 \text{ mAs}$$

Kilovoltage determines the energy of X-rays being produced. Kilovoltage potential should range from 70 to 90 for equine limb radiographs on mature horses when a portable X-ray machine is used. A 10% increase or decrease in kilovoltage potential effectively doubles or halves the radiation exposure.

The focal spot-film distance (FFD) is the distance from the X-ray tube focal spot to the detector. The focal spot location is usually marked on the outside tube housing; if it is not, the approximate center of the tube housing can be used for its location. A constant FFD is necessary to minimize improper exposures because the intensity of X-rays that expose the film is inversely proportional to the square of the FFD. Therefore, a small difference in the FFD can dramatically change the exposure on the X-ray film. For example, if the FFD were changed from 36 to 40 inches, the exposure from the X-ray machine would have to be increased by 23% to maintain a constant film exposure. In other words, if 10 mAs provided a good exposure at an FFD of 36 inches, 12.3 mAs would be required at 40 inches.

Some method of measuring the FFD before each exposure should be employed (Figures 4.2 and 4.3). Such things as a lightweight metal bar or a small rope can be used for fast FFD measurement. More elaborate

measuring devices with converging light beams at the correctly set FFD may also be used. The FFD for equine limb radiography should be between 36 and 40 inches (85 and 100 cm) and no less than 24 inches (60 cm). When the FFD is less than 24 inches, the object is magnified and spatial resolution is reduced. FFDs greater than 40 inches can be used if exposure times are not excessively long.

Collimation is the process of limiting or restricting the primary X-ray beam to the appropriate size to cover the anatomical region of interest within the X-ray detector being used. Collimating the primary beam is a safety practice that must be monitored for each exposure and must be reset if the cassette size changes. Limiting the size of the primary X-ray beam is a major factor in reducing scatter radiation, which keeps radiation exposure to personnel as low as possible. Fixed cylinders or cones and adjustable light-beam collimators are available (Figure 4.2). The disadvantage of fixed primary beam restrictors is that they do not conform to different cassette sizes. Adjustable light-beam collimation is recommended for equine radiography. Adjustable collimators can be affixed to most X-ray machines. They come with an internal light source, preferably 40 W or greater,[39] so the limits of the primary X-ray beam are projected on the X-ray cassette/detector as visible light.

The type of X-ray machines best suited for equine practice depends on the type of practice: out-of-hospital vs. in-hospital. The features of the X-ray machines must be matched to fit different practice situations. Some compromises or trade-offs must be made, e.g., less milliamperage or kilovoltage potential for more portability. An ideal X-ray machine for equine radiography has the following features:

1. Easily and quietly movable, with a tube head that can extend to the floor or ground surface
2. Adjustable milliamperage and kilovoltage potential setting

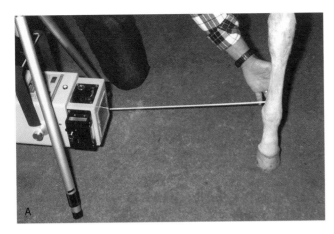

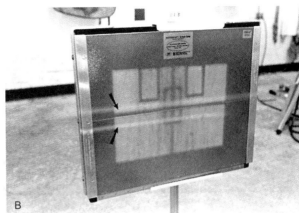

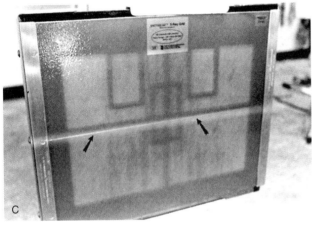

Figure 4.3. Methods of measuring FFD. A. Some portable X-ray machines come with a built-in measuring tape. B and C. Other machines use a converging light-bar system. When the cassette is not at the preset FFD, a double light bar, projected from the canisters (see Figure 4.2), is present (B, arrows). When the cassette is at the preset FFD, a single light bar is seen (C, arrows).

3. Electronic, 2-step timer capable of accurate exposure times of 0.1 second or faster
4. Some form of tube head support so that handholding the X-ray tube during the exposure is not necessary
5. Line voltage compensator and compensation meter
6. Primary X-ray beam restrictor (the preferred system is an adjustable light-beam collimator)
7. Absence of radiation or electrical hazards

Types of X-ray machines available for equine radiography are portable, mobile, and fixed (ceiling suspended) (Figure 4.4). These machines differ in size and capacity, from small, portable 15-mA machines to large, fixed 800-mA machines. Portable X-ray machines are best suited for out-of-hospital locations. They are lightweight (30 to 55 lbs) and can be easily stored for transport.

Even though portable machines are lightweight and easily moved, for radiation safety purposes they should be used with a stand or other mechanical support system. Impediments for using X-ray tube stands include cost, incompatibility with the machines, and lack of field versatility. A two-legged stand system is the most adaptable to the variety of conditions encountered in the field.[20] The maximum milliamperage on portable X-ray machines is between 10 and 40 mA, and the kilovoltage potential varies between 50 and 100 kVp. Milliamperage and kilovoltage potential settings on portable X-ray machines are usually interdependent, e.g., 10 mA at 80 kVp and 20 mA at 60 kVp. Desirable control settings on a portable X-ray machine are multiple kilovoltage potential settings and multiple time settings. Time setting increments should be 50% or less below 0.5 second.

High-frequency transformers that reduce the exposure time are available for portable X-ray machines. They are equivalent to a 3-phase, 12-pulse X-ray generator and provide a 40% to 50% increase in exposure compared with a full-wave rectified machine. The practical application is to reduce the exposure time and still obtain an adequate exposure for a diagnostic radiograph. A line voltage compensator is also desirable for portable X-ray machines. It is especially important in field situations, where the line voltage may fluctuate with the simultaneous use of the electrical equipment, and it can compensate for a line voltage drop when a long electrical extension cord is used.

Mobile X-ray machines are best suited for in-hospital radiography. They can be moved easily and quietly,

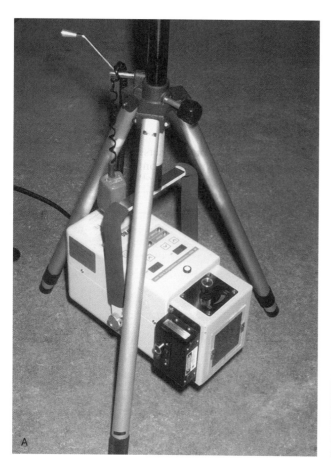

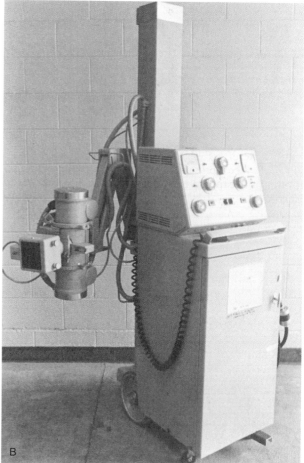

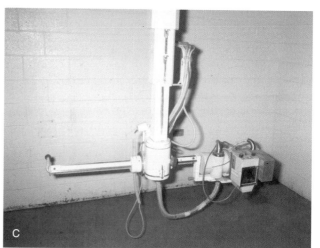

Figure 4.4. Types of X-ray machines used in equine radiography. A. Portable 30-mA, 90-kVp machine on a tripod stand. B. Mobile 200-mA machine. C. Fixed or ceiling-suspended 800-mA machine with a 3-m telescoping crane that extends to the floor. The exposure capabilities and mobility of each type of X-ray machine determine how and where they may be most effectively used.

although they are not as easily moved as portable machines. Mobile X-ray machines generally have a milliamperage range between 100 and 200 mA. The X-ray tube should be movable in the vertical plane to extend to the floor. Sometimes, mechanical modifications must be made to provide the necessary degree of X-ray tube travel. Timers on mobile X-ray machines usually have exposure times as fast as 1/60th or 1/120th of a second.

Fixed X-ray machines are usually suspended from the ceiling. They are limited to use within a single room. These machines can be coupled with large transformer systems that are capable of providing high milliamperage (800 to 1,000 mA). Ceiling-suspended tubes are easily movable and can be locked into position by magnetic locks while the X-ray exposure is made. The tube should be capable of extending to the floor. X-ray machines with high milliamperage capability have fast exposure times, eliminating most motion artifacts when radiographing equine limbs.

Detectors, Film Processing, and Viewing Devices

The differences between digital and conventional radiography equipment is the detector used for image capture, post-capture image processing, and the image viewing devices. Conventional radiography uses screen-film technology in which the film, after being exposed to radiation, is processed in a dark room, and then the radiograph evaluated on a viewbox. Digital radiography can be divided into computed radiography (CR) or direct digital radiography (DDR).

CR uses a detector panel that stores the image and then uses a separate image read-out unit. In DDR, the detector panel converts the X-rays into electrical charges by means of a direct read-out process. DDR systems can be further divided into direct or indirect conversion technologies depending on the type of X-ray conversion used. Both CR and DDR systems convert the electronic signal to digital data and send it to an acquisition device. At this point, the digital data is considered "raw" and it can be further processed.

The term "image processing" is ample and incorporates multiple steps in the acquisition of a digital image before the study is completed. During the image processing, the raw image can be manipulated with the purpose of having the best image possibly available for interpretation at the viewing station. One of the key factors that can be manipulated is the lookup table (LUT), which allows the operator to change the gray-scale of the image by altering the actual pixel values. Once the study is completed, the images are sent to the viewing station where Digital Imaging and Communication in Medicine (DICOM) viewing software is used for image display on a computer monitor. A complete discussion of image processing is beyond the scope of this chapter. More in-depth information is available in textbooks of diagnostic radiology physics and radiology journal articles.[7,21,24]

Screen-film System for Conventional Radiography

Conventional radiography most commonly uses cassettes equipped with intensifying screens and loaded with radiographic film. An alternative is the use of non-screen film protected with a cardboard holder. The basic function of intensifying screens is to convert X-ray photons into a visible light pattern when the photons strike the phosphor layer within the screen. This visible light pattern contains the same information as the original X-ray beam. In the conversion process, the latent image is intensified, which makes possible a properly exposed film with approximately 50× less X-ray exposure than would be necessary if intensifying screens were not used. On the other hand, the spatial resolution is decreased when using intensifying screens due to the diffusion of light emitted by the phosphor layer. This diffusion is greater for thicker (fast speed) screens than for thinner (slow speed) screens; therefore, screen speed and spatial resolution have an inverse relationship. Fast screens require less exposure from the X-ray machines for a properly exposed film, but fine anatomic detail within the film will be decreased.

Non-screen film systems are not recommended in equine radiography due to the high exposure settings required to obtain a diagnostic radiograph, the unnecessary radiation exposure to personnel, and the increased probability of motion artifacts.

Rare earth screens are recommended for equine conventional radiography. The following are some advantages of rare earth intensifying screens:[19]

- Exposure to personnel can be decreased 40% to 60%, depending on the screen speed used.
- Diagnostic capabilities of low-milliamperage X-ray machines can be increased (e.g., a 30-mA machine may have the potential of a 60- to 80-mA machine). This is particularly important in equine radiography, because low-milliamperage, portable X-ray machines are used extensively.
- Workload on X-ray generators and tubes can be reduced, which prolongs the life of the X-ray tube and machine and thus reduces costs.
- Exposure time can be decreased, thereby reducing motion artifacts.
- A smaller focal spot, which increases spatial resolution, may be used with machines that have more than one focal spot.
- Different speed screens are available, providing examination flexibility.

The combination of different films and screens determines the relative system speed, i.e., the film-screen speed. When matched correctly, rare earth screen and film combinations provide tremendous advantages for the examination of equine extremities (Table 4.1). With portable X-ray machines, a medium-speed combination (400 to 600) is recommended for routine examination of the extremities distal to the antebrachial carpal and the tarsocrural joints. A slow-speed combination (100) may be used for the occasional view that requires higher spatial resolution, e.g., navicular bone or distal phalanx. A high-speed combination (800) may be used for examinations proximal to the antebrachial carpal and the tarsocrural joints. With mobile or fixed X-ray machines, a slow-speed combination (100 may be used for examination of the extremities distal to the antebrachial carpal and tarsocrural joints) and medium-speed combinations (400 to 600) may be used proximal to these joints.

Radiographic Film Processing

Basic darkroom equipment and developing, fixing, and final wash solution properties have been covered elsewhere and are not discussed in this section.[33] However, the practitioner should be aware that many of the mistakes made in the process of obtaining a radiograph occur while processing the film in the darkroom, regardless of whether an automatic processor or hand techniques are used. Therefore, strict rules should

Table 4.1. Rare earth intensifying screen and film combinations.

Screen (manufacturer)	Film	Relative speed
Trimax (3M)		
2	XDA	100–125
6/12	XDA	400
6/12	XM	800
12	XDA	600
12	XM	1,200
Lanex (Kodak)		
Fine	T-Mat L	75–100
Regular	Ortho L	400
Regular	Ortho H	800
Fast	T-Mat L	600
Quanta (DuPont)		
Detail	Cornex 4L	100
Fast detail	Cornex 4L	400
III	Cornex 4L	800

be followed to have a clean, dry, and lightproof darkroom and maintain good quality chemical control.

Radiographic Film Viewing Devices

The entire X-ray examination will have been done in vain if the X-ray film cannot be adequately viewed or is read with poor illumination. A good quality X-ray viewer and a bright light are necessary equipment. They should be placed in an area where external light can be subdued. Each properly exposed film should be inspected with a bright light where it may reveal soft tissue structures and subtle bone changes not apparent with regular X-ray viewers.

DIGITAL RADIOGRAPHY SYSTEMS

Computed Radiography

CR systems are similar to screen-film systems, in which a cassette stores the latent image until processing. The difference is the way the latent image is stored. As explained above, screen-film systems store the latent image in the radiographic film after the light from the intensifying screen strikes the silver crystals on the film. CR detectors eliminate the intensifying screens and replace the radiographic film with an imaging plate that is also protected in a cassette. This imaging plate has photostimulable phosphors (PSP) made of a mix of europium activated bromide, chlorine, or iodide (e.g., $BaFBr:Eu^{2+}$).[21]

After the imaging plate is exposed to X-ray photons, the PSP change to a higher energy state and store the latent image. The PSP can store the latent image while remaining in that higher energy state for several hours, depending on the phosphor crystals used.[45] The information stored in a CR imaging plate contains analog data.

CR Reading Process

The data stored in the imaging plate phosphor (PSP) must be released to create a visible image. This process occurs when the cassette is placed in the reader unit (Figure 4.5). Once the cassette is inserted in the reader unit, the imaging plate is automatically removed from the cassette and scanned by a laser beam. The laser light stimulates the energy trapped in the PSP and visible light is released from the plate. The released light strikes a photomultiplier tube and is converted into an electronic signal. The magnitude of the electronic signal represents the degree of X-ray attenuation of the structure that was imaged and is also assigned a corresponding shade of gray after conversion from analog to digital format.[55] The data is then stored temporarily in a local hard disk. Subsequently, the imaging plate is exposed to bright white light to erase any residual trapped energy before it is returned to the cassette for reuse.[7] The whole readout process for a 14×17 inch image plate takes approximately 30 to 40 seconds.[21]

Direct Digital Radiography

As mentioned above, direct digital radiography systems can be further divided into direct and indirect conversion. The main difference is that indirect technology converts the X-rays to light, which is then converted into an electrical charge, as opposed to direct technology, which immediately converts X-rays to an electrical charge with no light conversion during the process. Both the direct and indirect conversion systems have a direct readout, meaning that the detector sends the signal straight to the computer instead of using a reading unit such as the CR system. The time lapse between exposure to image display takes less than 10 seconds,[21] which increases the patient through-put and becomes an important factor to consider, especially in high patient load hospitals.

Direct Conversion

A direct flat panel detector (Figure 4.6) is formed by different layers consisting of photoconductors, and thin film transistors that contain rows and columns of individual detector elements with storage capacitors and readout electronics.[7,8,36] The photoconductors can be made of amorphous selenium (most common used), lead iodide, lead oxide, thallium bromide, and gadolinium compounds.[21] The photoconductors are the first layer in contact with the X-ray photons that exit the patient and are responsible for converting them into electrical charges. The electrical charges are stored in capacitors and then read row by row and the informa-

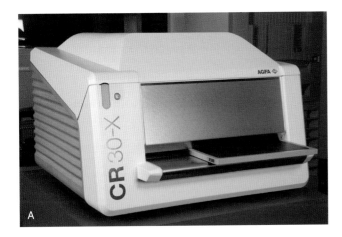

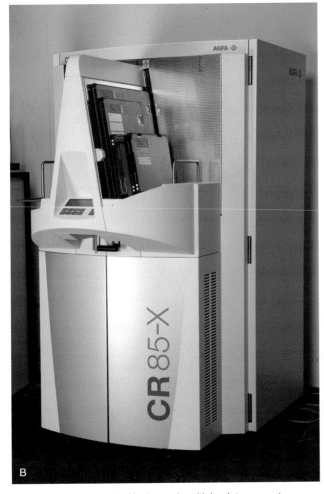

Figure 4.5. A and B. Single- and multiple-plate computer radiography reading units. (Used with permission from Agfa HealthCare Corporation, Copyright 2009. All rights reserved.)

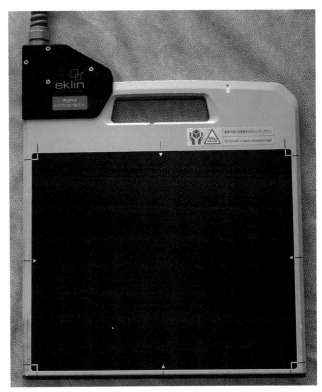

Figure 4.6. Direct flat panel detector (9 × 11 inch imaging area).

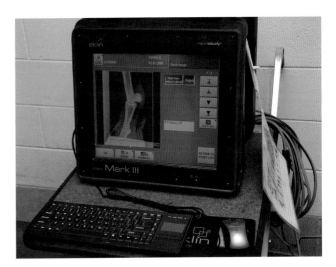

Figure 4.7. Mark III portable digital radiography system.

tion sent to the computer after analog-to-digital conversion (Figure 4.7). More detailed information is available in radiology journal articles.[21,55]

Indirect Conversion

Indirect conversion can be done with two technologies: indirect flat panel detector or charged coupled device (CCD). An indirect flat panel detector consists of a scintillator layer (usually made of cesium iodide crystals), an amorphous silicon photodiode circuit layer, and a thin film transistor array. Light is produced by the scintillator after being irradiated by the X-rays exiting the patient. The light is absorbed and converted to electrical charges by the photodiodes. The readout of the electrical charges is accomplished with the thin film transistor array in a similar way as in the direct digital radiography systems.[21]

A charged coupled device is also a light-sensitive unit for recording images. The X-rays from the patient are converted to light after striking the scintillator in a similar way as an intensifying screen in conventional screen-film systems. The light is then usually minified with a lens to fit in the small CCD where it is recorded and converted into electrical charges. In the process of light minification, some of the light photons are lost and do not reach the CCD unit. This results in increased image noise compared with the flat panel detectors in which minification is not applied.[55]

Other materials used in the scintillator layer include gadolinium based crystals. The advantage of cesium iodide scintillators is that the crystals can be structured into 5 to 10 um wide parallel needles, which reduce the spreading of light within the scintillator. Hence, the spatial resolution is increased.

Digital Image Display

A computer used in a digital image viewing station consists of two basic parts: 1 or more monitors (hardware) and a DICOM viewer (software) (Figure 4.8). A monitor used for digital radiography should have excellent resolution, high brightness (luminance), and wide dynamic range. The resolution of a monitor is dictated by the pixel and matrix size. As the pixel size decreases and the matrix size increases, the monitor's resolution improves. Due to the high spatial resolution (ability to distinguish or separate two objects that are close to each other) required for evaluating digital radiographs, medical grade monitors with at least 2 to 3 megapixels are recommended. Monitor brightness or luminance is calculated in foot-lamberts (ft-L) or nit (candela/m^2) and should be at least 50 ft-L.[42] The dynamic range of a monitor is the luminance ratio between the darkest (black) shade and the brightest (white) shade that the monitor can display. The dynamic range of a monitor is usually correlated to the luminance; thus, the

higher the monitor brightness, the higher the dynamic range.

A wide variety of Windows or Macintosh based DICOM software programs are available and include free Internet downloadable versions to more sophisticated software that requires purchase or leasing contracts. The different DICOM viewing software provides the user with the ability to further manipulate and improve the image displayed on the monitor. Features such as modifying contrast (window and level), image sharpening, edge enhancement, zoom, measurement tools, etc. are included in most DICOM viewers, but differ among vendors depending on the quality of the software.

Conventional Radiography vs. CR vs. DDR

Several aspects need to be evaluated and the practitioner must be aware of the advantages and limitations among the different technologies when making a decision to purchase radiographic equipment.

Exposure latitude or dynamic range is the degree of over- or underexposure tolerable in a correctly processed film to maintain an acceptable radiographic image. As the exposure latitude becomes wider, the degree of over- or underexposure tolerance increases. One of the main limitations of the conventional screen-film systems is a narrow exposure latitude when compared to digital systems. It is not uncommon to have to retake radiographic projections, especially in ambulatory practice where the power outlets may have subtle changes in voltage. Other disadvantages of the screen-film systems include the need to maintain good quality control of dark room and processing chemical solutions, the need to constantly purchase radiographic film, film storage concerns, lack of image processing/manipulation, and the need to digitize radiographs or use mail/shipping services for second opinions. Advantages of screen-film systems over digital radiography systems include reduced equipment cost, portability, and higher spatial resolution.

In general, digital radiography systems are more expensive than screen-film systems. The slight decrease in spatial resolution of digital radiography systems, when compared to screen-film systems, is usually more than compensated for by the increased contrast resolution provided by digital radiography. This is supported by the fact that digital radiography has shown advantages over conventional screen-film systems, even in studies in which spatial resolution is critical, such as in breast cancer detection in humans.[23,40]

The portability of digital radiography equipment is improving as the technology advances. Now it is not uncommon to see ambulatory practitioners using direct digital radiography systems in the field. An advantage of this is the opportunity to almost immediately repeat a projection if it was not of diagnostic quality, instead of having to process it in a darkroom. Improved image contrast, increased patient through-put, the ability to do image processing/manipulation, and teleradiology are also advantages of digital radiography over conventional radiography.

In summary, the advantages of digital radiography over conventional radiography have, in many instances,

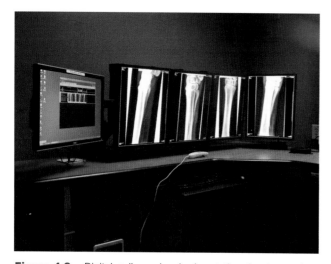

Figure 4.8. Digital radiography viewing station. A color monitor (far left) is used to access the Picture Archive and Communication System (PACS). Four black-and-white, 3MP medical grade monitors are used for display and evaluation of the radiographs.

overcome its higher monetary value so that the replacement of conventional systems by digital systems is imminent in the near future.

Digital Image Storage, HIS/RIS, PACS, and DICOM

An advantage of replacing films with digital radiographic images includes a smaller physical storing area (magnetic tape, CD, DVD, hard drives, USB flash drives, etc.), which consequently eases the organization and provides quick retrieval of previous exams. The digital image quality does not degrade with time, as occurs with conventional radiographs. In addition, the capability of referring a study for a second opinion is literally only an e-mail away. The practice of teleradiology is becoming more popular among veterinary radiologists, both in private practice and academia, as a service to referring veterinarians.

Most university-based veterinary teaching hospitals and some large private referral hospitals have a Hospital or Radiology Information System (HIS or RIS), a Picture Archive and Communication System (PACS), and DICOM viewing software. The combination of these three technologies tremendously improves the daily work flow of busy operations. Every step in the process of obtaining a diagnostic imaging study, from the time the patient enters the hospital to the time that it exits, is directed using a HIS or RIS, PACS, and a DICOM image viewer. This improves the efficiency of a radiology unit, increasing patient through-put, having immediate access to digital images, retrieving imaging reports electronically, and practically eliminating errors such as having the wrong patient information and losing/mixing studies.

Detailed information regarding digital image storage, HIS/RIS, PACS, and DICOM is beyond the scope of this chapter and is available elsewhere.[43,44,54]

Accessory X-Ray Equipment

Accessory X-ray equipment for equine musculoskeletal examinations has special requirements. Good-quality, well-maintained accessory equipment is necessary to ensure that quality radiographic examinations are performed safely. Accessory equipment consists of grids, markers, and film-marking systems, detector holders, padded tables for radiographic projections under general anesthesia, and positioning aids. These pieces of equipment are used with conventional or digital radiography. Most accessory equipment is available commercially, but because of the unique requirement of equine radiology, some equipment, such as cassette holders, padded tables, and positioning aids, may have to be custom-built locally.

Grids

A radiographic grid is a thin wafer consisting of lead foil strips separated by X-ray-transparent spacers. Grids differ by grid ratio, lines per inch, and pattern. Grid ratio is the height of the lead foil strings relative to the width between the strips and may vary from 5 : 1 to 16 : 1. Lines per inch are the number of lead foil stripes per inch. The more lines per inch, the less apparent the lines are on the exposed X-ray film. Grid patterns differ depending on the longitudinal orientation of the lead strips, and can be linear, linear focus, and cross-hatched. The clinician must consider these variables when purchasing a grid for use in equine radiography.

Grids are generally used to decrease the amount of scattered radiation that exposes the X-ray film. Because scattered radiation exposes film from several directions, it has the effect of decreasing details and "fogging" the film. A fogged film has a gray or flat appearance and decreased contrast.

Stationary grids are the most common grids used in equine radiography. The grid may be placed over the front of the detector or may be fixed permanently in the detector holder. Examination of areas more than 12 cm thick is best performed with a grid; this usually includes the limbs proximal to the carpus and tarsus. A grid is desirable for the caudocranial view of the stifle but may not be necessary for the lateromedial view. A grid may also be helpful for foot examinations when the X-ray cassette is positioned under the foot and in a cassette tunnel that has a thick protecting cover between the horse's foot and X-ray cassette.

A nonfocused linear grid with 6 : 1 ratio and more than 100 lines per inch is adequate for equine limb examinations. A smaller ratio and/or fewer lines per inch may be used with less powerful X-ray machines to facilitate a decrease in exposure time.

The advantages of using a grid are increased film detail and contrast, which improve the diagnostic quality of the film. The disadvantages of a gird are cost, increased radiation exposure to personnel, and the need for more precise centering of the X-ray beam and positioning of the grid to prevent grid cutoff artifact. Increased radiation exposure is particularly important in equine radiography, for which low-output X-ray machines are extensively used. The grid must be perpendicular to the X-ray beam, and if a focused grid is used, the center of the X-ray beam must be aligned with the center of the gird. Improper positioning results in grid cutoff and a non-diagnostic radiograph.

Film Markers and Marking Systems

Adequate, legible film marking is necessary but often overlooked in equine radiography. Proper identification procedures are necessary for follow-up comparative examinations and for accurately documenting when, where, what, and by whom the examination was performed. Such documentation on the film in a proper permanent fashion may also be needed for medical-legal purposes.

Radiographs should be identified with the veterinarian's name and/or hospital or the place where the radiograph was made, the date, and the animal's name or number. The view and anatomic part examined should also be recorded at the time the film is exposed. Acceptable methods of film labeling include lead impregnated tape, lead letters and/or numbers, and a photo-flash marking system. Adhesive tape and coins are not acceptable methods of marking radiographs.

A permanent aluminum plate containing the veterinarian's name and other information can be used with lead-impregnated tape and lead letters. These plates are placed on the front of the cassette before the radiograph is made and provide legible figures on the radiograph.

The photofinish marking system requires a permanent lead blocker impregnated in the corner of the X-ray cassette. This area is exposed with identification information that is written or typed on a card placed in the photoflash machine.

The part examined and the X-ray view used should also be labeled with lead letters or other available lead markers. The part examined should be labeled left (L) or right (R) for the examinations and labeled fore or hind distal to the carpus and tarsus. Regardless of the system used, the essential information must be on the radiograph in clear legible form.

Most digital radiography systems allow selecting the site within the radiograph (usually the corners) where the appropriate information such as hospital, practice or veterinarian's name, patient's demographics, date of examination, technique, and projection label will appear at the time of image display. Because the "left" or "right" label must be set in a predetermined area, it will not always be helpful in indicating which side is medial or lateral, especially in examinations of the distal limb. Therefore, current metallic labels are still used with digital radiography.

Detector Holding and Positioning Aids

Detector holders and positioning blocks are necessary for radiation safety purposes and to facilitate consistent views or projections of an examined part. Detector holders and blocks enable personnel who hold the cassette to position their hands away from the primary X-ray beam, even though they are wearing lead-impregnated gloves. For equine limb examinations, a handled detector holder, a detector holder (tunnel) for weight-bearing foot studies, and a positioning block are necessary. More sophisticated equipment, such as padded tables for radiographic projections with the horse under general anesthesia, are available at university teaching hospitals and most large referral clinics (Figure 4.9). A radiography table usually has multiple adjustable spaces for placing the detector and grid in a

tunnel underneath the horse, in a way that it can be properly adjusted once the horse is positioned on the table. The table should be conditioned with enough padding to prevent pressure injuries from the horse's body weight, but should be thin enough for the detector to be properly exposed. Radiographic examination such as pelvic projections and cervical myelography are studies normally performed with a table.

There are many types of detector holders made of aluminum or wood for conventional radiography cassettes (Figure 4.10). Digital radiography detectors usually have a handle for secure holding that, in conjunction with good collimation techniques, keeps the personnel's lead-protected hand from being directly exposed to the primary beam. However, some vendors provide an extension that attaches to the handle to further minimize radiation exposure (Figure 4.11). One wood block with two grooves in the top can be used

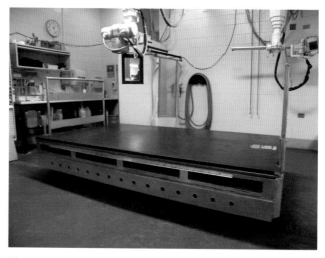

Figure 4.9. Padded table used for equine radiographic studies under general anesthesia. Four channels along the side allow multi-level positioning of the X-ray detector to radiograph different anatomical areas.

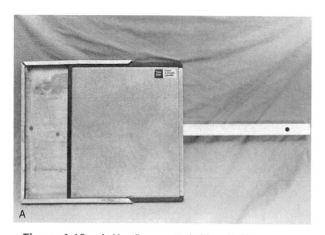

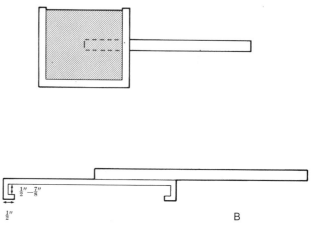

Figure 4.10. A. Handle cassette holder with X-ray cassette partially inserted into it. B. Line diagram and dimensions of a handle cassette holder.

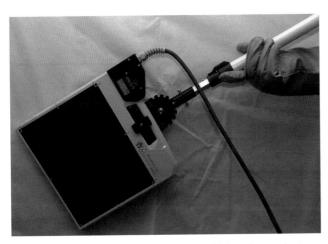

Figure 4.11. Direct flat panel detector with handle attached.

for phalangeal and navicular examinations (Figure 4.12). A 55° wedge may be added to an end of the block to accommodate an upright foot examination, and a metal strip may be recessed into the flat surface to mark the plane of the sole. A detector holder (tunnel) can be used for weight-bearing studies of the feet and navicular bone (Figure 4.13). The detector holder protects the detector from damage caused by direct weight-bearing by the horse. Lead may be added to the underside of the holder to prevent back-scattered radiation from fogging the film. Detector holders that have thick (more than 0.25-inch) plexiglass trays may produce excess scatter radiation, and therefore require a grid to obtain an acceptable radiograph of the navicular bone. These positioning aids allow routine examinations of the limb to be performed in a safe, consistent manner.

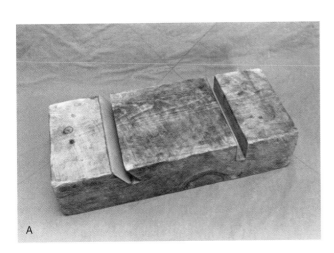

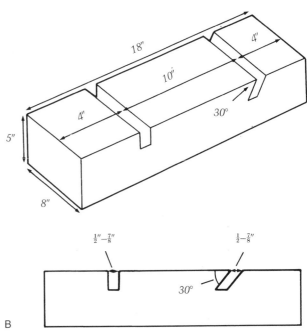

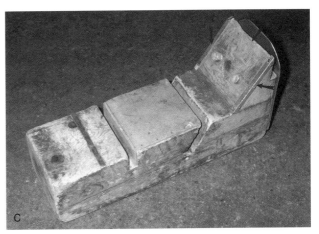

Figure 4.12. A. Wood positioning block. B. Line diagram and dimensions of a wood positioning block. C. Modified wood positioning block with 55° angled wedge at one end (arrow) to facilitate the dorsal 60° proximal-palmarodistal oblique projection of the distal phalanx and navicular bone.

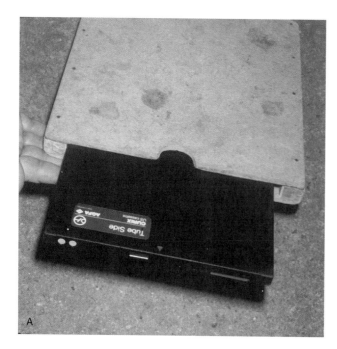

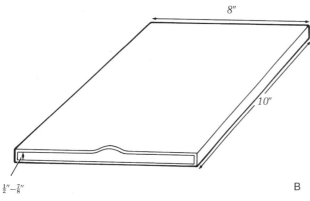

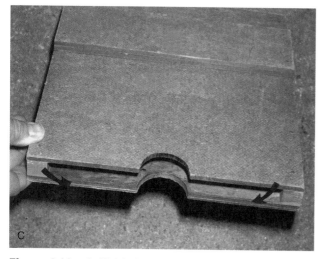

Figure 4.13. A. Weight-bearing cassette holder with the cassette partially inserted into the holder. B. Line diagram and dimensions of a weight-bearing cassette holder. C. A 1-mm-thick piece of lead can be added to the bottom of the cassette holder (arrows) to stop radiation backscatter from the ground to the X-ray detector. Radiation backscatter produces background film fog and decreases the image quality.

RADIATION SAFETY

Radiation safety becomes even more important as the use of radiology increases in equine practice. Safe radiation procedures are often not followed because of insufficient knowledge of biologic radiation effects, lack of awareness of radiation safety principles, inadequate radiation safety equipment, and/or neglect of radiation safety practices because these practices require too much time and effort. None of these reasons justifies the unsafe use of radiation.

Veterinarians in equine practice may receive low doses of radiation over long periods of time. Because the clinician's extremities (hands, eyes, and feet) are the most common body parts to be exposed to radiation, they are subject to chronic radiation injury. Chronic radiation injury may manifest as skin ridge flattening on fingertips, ridging of fingernails, or, in severe cases, skin carcinomas. Such changes may result from not routinely following safe radiation procedures.

The general principles of radiation safety are:

1. Keeping personnel as far away from the radiation source (X-ray tube) as possible
2. Using protective barriers
3. Reducing X-ray exposure factors
4. Using a radiation monitoring system

Keeping personnel as far away from the X-ray source as possible can be accomplished by having nonessential personnel leave the immediate area, using cassette holders and positioning blocks, providing tranquilization or general anesthesia when needed,[3] using an X-ray tube stand or support, and having a 1- to 2-meter-long cord connected to the exposure button. No part of the body should be exposed to the primary X-ray beam.

Protective barriers should always be used. Walls and lead screens are good protective barriers to use when practical. Adequate wall thickness in a new or remodeled facility should be determined by consulting with a health physicist. The personnel subject to the greatest exposure when performing equine examinations are those holding the horse's limb, the detector holder, and those holding the halter.[3] Therefore, if personnel must be near the animal when the X-ray examination is performed, they should wear lead aprons and gloves. Periodically aprons and gloves should be radiographed to check for cracks and holes in the lead-impregnated lining (Figure 4.14).

Fast film-screen combinations and a decreased FFD can be used to reduce X-ray exposure factors. As mentioned, for good-quality films, the FFD should not be less than 24 inches and preferably not more than 36 inches.

A radiation-monitoring system should be used by all radiology personnel. These systems not only provide safety guidance but also protect against possible legal implications. Film-badge monitoring systems and service can be purchased from commercial sources.

Equipment necessary for safely operating an X-ray machine includes detector holders, lead aprons and gloves, aluminum filters, and an adjustable light-beam collimator. Detector holders eliminate the need to hand-hold detectors, increasing the distance between hands and the X-ray beam. They should be durable and light-

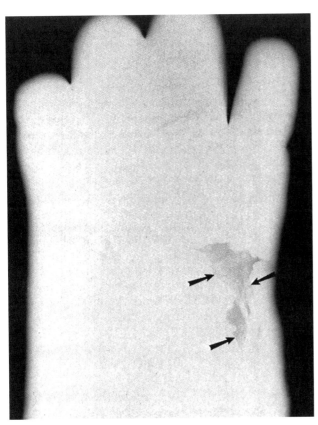

Figure 4.14. Radiograph of a lead glove, showing a lucent area (arrows) that represents a defect or hole in the lead lining.

weight. As discussed previously, several designs for detector holders are available (Figures 4.10 and 4.11).

Lead aprons and gloves should be worn by everyone assisting with the X-ray examination. Protective gear should have at least 0.5-mm lead equivalent. Lead aprons and gloves provide adequate protection from secondary and scattered radiation but not from primary radiation. The life of lead aprons and gloves can be prolonged by hanging them up when they are not in use. This prevents cracks or holes forming from improper care (Figure 4.14).

Primary beam filtration should be at least 2.5-mm aluminum. The filtration should be added at the X-ray tube port. Filtration makes the X-ray beam more energetic (hardens) and reduces the amount of less energetic (soft) radiation. This has the effect of decreasing the amount of scattered radiation to surrounding personnel.

An X-ray beam-limiting device or collimator (Figure 4.2) is one of the important, yet overlooked, pieces of radiation safety equipment. The size of the primary X-ray beam is a major factor in determining radiation dose to the hands. Several beam-limiting devices are available. Fixed-size cones and cylinders and adjustable light-beam collimators limit the primary X-ray beam. Adjustable light-beam collimators have the advantage of limiting the primary X-ray beam to the exact cassette size, regardless of the FFD. The light also assists alignment of the primary X-ray beam with the cassette. Every X-ray machine should have a primary beam-

limiting device. An adjustable light-beam collimator is highly recommended.

Recent studies in human radiography have shown that some digital radiography systems may be capable of reducing the exposure settings while minimally compromising the diagnostic value of the radiograph.[5,22,49,53] However, the reduction of the exposure is limited to some extent and depends on the area of examination and the clinical indication.[38,53] Radiation exposure reduction to both the patient and personnel can be simply achieved by minimizing the number of non-diagnostic radiographs due to technique factors. This is most feasible in digital radiography as a result of the wider dynamic range of these systems.

In summary, the following safety measures should be observed:

- Never handhold the X-ray detector during an exposure. Detector holders or general anesthesia should be used.
- All personnel not needed for assistance with the X-ray examination should leave the immediate area.
- Lead gloves and aprons should be worn by all individuals assisting with the X-ray examination.
- A primary X-ray beam-restricting device should be used, preferably an adjustable light-beam collimator.
- Primary beam filtration equivalent to 2.5-mm aluminum should be used.
- If possible, rotate personnel responsible for holding the detector; avoid routinely using the same person for this job.
- Do not allow anyone under 18 years of age or anyone who is pregnant to assist with an X-ray examination.
- Use consistent X-ray exposures and darkroom techniques. Repeat exposures require unnecessary radiation exposure to personnel.
- Use a radiation-monitoring system.

The veterinarian in charge is responsible for the radiation safety practices used by his/her employees. Providing necessary radiation safety equipment and following these rules should keep exposure levels below the limits recommended by the National Council on Radiation Protection.[2]

TECHNIQUE CHARTS

A technique chart should be formulated for each X-ray machine, because no two machines have exactly the same exposure characteristics (Figure 4.15). A technique chart ensures consistent exposure factors from the X-ray machine settings, decreasing the number of repeat radiographs and thus reducing radiation exposure to personnel and the wasting of X-ray film.

Several variables should be kept constant when a technique chart is being formulated: FFD, film-processing conditions, line voltage, type of intensifying screen, type of X-ray film, type of collimation, and amount of primary beam filtration. If these variable are changed, the indicated setting from the chart may no longer be valid.

The following general rules and principles should be observed when a technique chart for equine limb examinations is being formulated: (1) the exposure times

HF100 EQUINE TECHNIQUE CHART*

X-ray Unit: MinXray, Inc. **Model *HF100***
Screen/Film Combination: Sterling Ultravision Rapid Screens/Ultravision L Film/**400** Speed Combination
Focal Film Distance (FFD): As Specified (Adjust Exposure Time If Using Different FFD)

	Thk, cm	FFD, in	kV	mA	Time, sec	mAs
P3						
Lateral	16	40	68	20.0	0.05	1.0
D65P-PD view	11	40	62	20.0	0.05	1.0
DP	11	40	70	20.0	0.05	1.0
Navicular						
Lateral	11	40	68	20.0	0.05	1.0
D65P-PD (cone)	11	40	68	20.0	0.07	1.4
Flexor	N/A	16	65	20.0	0.04	0.8
Fetlock						
Lateral	11	40	68	20.0	0.05	1.0
Oblique	8	40	70	20.0	0.05	1.0
D15P-PD	9	40	72	20.0	0.05	1.0
Carpus						
Lateral	10	40	72	20.0	0.05	1.0
Oblique	9	40	74	20.0	0.05	1.0
DP	12	40	78	20.0	0.04	0.8
Skyline	N/A	31	74	20.0	0.05	1.0
Tarsus						
Lateral	10	40	72	20.0	0.05	1.0
Oblique	10	40	72	20.0	0.05	1.0
DP	13	40	92	20.0	0.04	0.8
Stifle						
Lateral	24	40	78	20.0	0.08	1.6
CC	26	40	96	20.0	0.10	2.0
Skull						
Lateral (Nasal)	16	40	80	20.0	0.08	1.6
Lateral (Teeth)	16	40	80	20.0	0.12	2.4
Lateral (Guttural Pouch)	16	40	88	20.0	0.13	2.6

These are recommended starting techniques. Final results depend upon many factors. Please note examples of adjustments that follow.

Adjustments in kV for Variations in Thickness:

<u>40-80 kV</u> - Add or subtract 2kV for each 1cm increase or decrease in thickness
<u>80-100kV</u> - Add or subtract 3kV for each 1cm increase or decrease in thickness

Adjustments in Time for Variations in Film Density:

If films are too dark (overexposed), decrease time.
If films are too light (underexposed), increase time.

Developed At:

THE UNIVERSITY OF TENNESSEE
COLLEGE OF VETERINARY MEDICINE
KNOXVILLE, TN

ur

Radiology Section

Figure 4.15. Technique chart for equine examinations. (Reprinted with permission from the University of Tennessee College of Veterinary Medicine, Knoxville, TN.)

should be as fast as possible to limit motion artifacts on the radiograph and (2) the kilovoltage potential range should be between 70 and 90 kVp for most examinations but may be higher when mobile or fixed X-ray machines are used.

Manipulation of exposure factors on the X-ray machine is often necessary when a technique chart is being formulated and used. To double or halve the X-ray exposure by changing the milliamperage-seconds, simply double or halve either the milliamperage or time. To double or halve the X-ray exposure by changing the kilovoltage potential, simply add or subtract approximately 10% from the original kilovoltage potential (Table 4.2).

A technique chart may be formulated with or without a grid. A grid is usually not used and is not necessary

Table 4.2. Equivalent exposures.

80 kVp	15 mA	0.1 second	1.5 mAs
90 kVp	15 mA	0.05 second	0.75 mAs
70 kVp	30 mA	0.1 second	3.0 mAs
70 kVp	15 mA	0.2 second	3.0 mAs

for most extremity examinations because of insufficient part thickness. If a grid is used, exposure factors must be increased. The amount of increase depends on the grid type, grid ratio, and lines per inch.

Table 4.3. Example technique chart for carpus.

Trial exposures

    Good trial exposure: 70 kVp, 1.5 mAs

    More film contrast (black and white): 60 kVp, 3.0 mAs

    Less film contrast (more gray shades): 80 kVp, 0.75 mAs

Refinements per view[a]

    Dorsopalmar (DPa): 70 kVp, 1.5 mAs

    Dorsolateral-palmaromedial oblique (D45L-PaMO): 70 kVp, 1.5 mAs

    Dorsomedial-palmarolateral oblique (D45M-PaLO): 70 kVp, 1.5 mAs

    Lateromedial (LM): 75 kVp, 1.5 mAs

    Flexed lateromedial (flexed LM): 75 kVp, 1.5 mAs

[a]If more or less film contrast is desired, adjust the kilovoltage potential and milliamperage-seconds.

A trial exposure should be made on each part to find the most suitable exposure. For example, for the fetlock (metacarpophalangeal joint), foot (distal phalanges), metacarpus, and metatarsus, a baseline exposure with FFD of 30 inches (75 cm) and exposure setting of 2.0 mAs and 70 kVp with a 400-speed rare earth film-screen combination and no grid may be used. The baseline exposure should be slightly higher for tarsal and carpal studies and decreased by half for dorsopalmar-plantar studies of the distal phalanx.

These trial exposures should be made on each part: the baseline exposure, an exposure half the baseline, and an exposure twice the baseline. If all three exposures are too light (underexposed) or too dark (overexposed), the baseline exposure should be adjusted to compensate and the three exposures should be repeated. A good-quality film should eventually be made with one trial film darker and one trial film lighter. A good-quality film should show soft tissue as well as bone without the use of a bright light, and bone trabeculae should be identifiable. Once a good exposure is made for a given part, it should be recorded on the technique chart. With additional work, the chart can be refined to include more specific exposure information for each view (Table 4.3).

The technique charts should be established for an average-sized horse. For smaller and larger horses, the exposure factors must be adjusted to produce acceptable radiographs.

CONTRAST EXAMINATIONS

A contrast radiographic examination consists of using contrast material to better define suspicious lesions detected clinically or radiographically but not distinctly seen on survey radiographs. Triiodinated contrast material is most useful for contrast examinations

Table 4.4. Organic iodide contrast material.

Brand name	Generic name	Manufacturer
Hypaque sodium 20%	20% Diatrizoate Na	Nycomed[a]
Hypaque sodium 25%	25% Diatrizoate Na	Nycomed
Hypaque sodium 50%	50% Diatrizoate Na	Nycomed
Hypaque meglumine 60%	60% Diatrizoate meglumine	Nycomed
Omnipaque[b]	Iohexol	Nycomed
Reno-DIP	30% Diatrizoate meglumine	Bracco[c]
Renocal-76	66% Diatrizoate meglumine and 10% Diatrizoate Na	Bracco
Reno-30 and 60	30% and 60% Diatrizoate meglumine	Bracco
Renovist	35% Diatrizoate Na and 10% Diatrizoate meglumine	Bracco
Isovue[b] 200, 250, 300, and 370	41%, 51%, 61%, and 76% Iopamidol	Bracco

[a]Nycomed Inc, 90 Park Avenue, New York, NY.
[b]Nonionic contrast medium.
[c]Bracco Diagnostics, Princeton, NJ, 08543.

in lame horses. Positive-contrast agents are commercially available in an injectable form (Table 4.4). The use of negative-contrast agents (gas) has been reported[4] but has not found widespread, routine acceptance. Procedures most commonly performed are injection of a draining tract (sinography or fistulography) and myelography. Other contrast examinations such as arthrography and tendonography have become unpopular, and in the majority of cases replaced by ultrasound, computed tomography, magnetic resonance imaging, or arthroscopy.

Fistulography or Sinography

Fistulograms provide valuable diagnostic information when chronic draining tracts or recent traumatic puncture wounds are present. Survey radiographs of the area should be made first. If the source or cause of the draining tract or puncture wound is not clearly identified on the survey radiographs, a fistulogram can be performed to obtain additional diagnostic data.[9,11,25,27]

The technique consists of injecting undiluted water soluble triiodinated contrast material into the draining tract as aseptically as possible. Water-soluble contrast material is used because it is less viscous and penetrates chronic draining tracts more easily than oil-based contrast material. To avoid contrast material draining from the tract after injection, an inflatable, cuffed

(Foley) catheter or a small polyethylene tube inserted some distance into the tract can be used before injecting the material. Filling is best accomplished if the contrast material is injected under pressure; thus, some form of occlusion of the tract opening is necessary.

When the distal extremity is being examined, it is important to flex and extend the region slowly. This allows a tract that may be closed while the horse is standing to open up, permitting the contrast to enter the tract. The volume needed for injection is not consistent, and when fistulograms are performed, the injection of an insufficient volume is a common error.[25] Contrast material should be injected until back pressure is felt on the syringe plunger or external leakage is observed. A single radiograph can also be made to determine if an adequate volume of contrast material was injected. After contrast material has been injected to delineate the entire tract, orthogonal radiographic views should be made for complete evaluation. Any contrast material that leaks onto the skin surface should be removed before radiographs are made.

A fistulogram may demonstrate (1) the extent and direction of the tract to aid in surgical exploration, (2) communication with underlying soft tissue structures (e.g., tendon sheaths or synovial joints) (Figure 4.16A), (3) osseous involvement (e.g., sequestra or osteomyelitis associated with surgical implants), and (4) filling defects (which appear radiolucent because of displacement of contrast material) (Figure 4.16B).[11] Filling defects may be caused by fibrous reaction within the tract or by foreign bodies. Fibrous tissues generally have irregular borders, whereas foreign bodies such as wood splinters have sharp, straight borders. Small foreign bodies may not be identifiable on a fistulogram because of the overlying opacity of the contrast material. In such cases, ultrasound imaging may provide additional diagnostic information.[9]

Myelography

Myelography in the horse is used to substantiate cervical spinal cord compression suspected from a neurologic and/or radiographic examination. It also serves to identify the location, extent, and type of compressive lesion present, which is necessary for determining the prognosis and indication for surgical intervention.

A survey radiographic examination is performed by making neutral lateral radiographs centered on the cranial, mid, and caudal cervical regions. In addition to ruling out fractures/fissures, discospondylosis, osteochondrosis, and malformations, survey radiographs should be evaluated for 5 important parameters, including: (1) encroachment of the caudal physis dorsally into the vertebral canal ("ski jumps"), (2) caudal extension of the dorsal aspect of the arch of the vertebral canal, (3) intervertebral malalignment (Figure 4.17), (4) abnormal ossification of the articular facets, and (5) degenerative joint disease of the articular facets (Figure 4.18).[31] The accuracy of the subjective evaluation of survey radiographs for predicting a compressive lesion has been reported to be 70% at C3 to C4 and only 40% in all other levels of the cervical spine.[37]

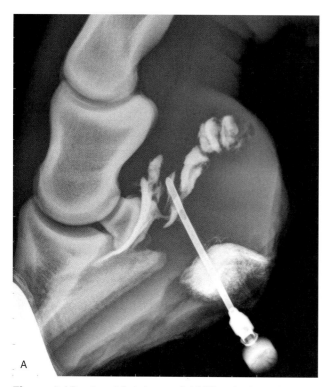

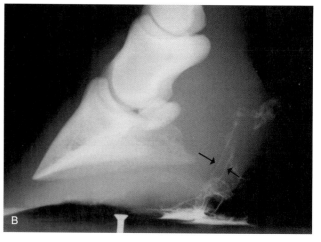

Figure 4.16. A and B. Lateromedial (LM) projections of the distal limb after injection of iodinated contrast material into an externally draining tract. Image A shows filling of the navicular bursa with contrast material consistent with a communication between the draining tract and the bursa. Image B shows a well-defined filling defect outlined by contrast material representing a wood foreign body (arrows).

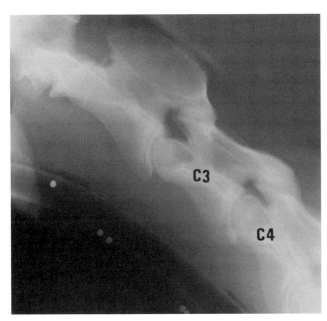

Figure 4.17. Lateral survey radiograph of the cranial cervical spine, showing a possible dynamic cervical stenosis. A mild kyphotic malalignment is present between C3 and C4.

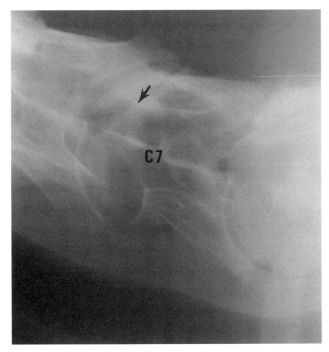

Figure 4.18. Lateral survey radiograph of the caudal cervical spine, showing bony proliferation around the articular facets, sclerosis of the rostral dorsal lamina of C7 (arrow), and narrowing of the spinal canal at the rostral aspect of C7.

There are different methods for quantitatively assessing cervical spine survey radiographs to try to predict a possible compressive spinal cord lesion. Mayhew et al., in 1993, introduced a semi-quantitative method used in Thoroughbred yearlings that consisted of scoring survey radiographs and giving values according to the presence

of any of the 5 radiographic abnormalities mentioned above and the presence of vertebral canal stenosis based on measuring the minimum sagittal diameter. Scores of or equal to 12 were consistent with cervical vertebral malformation.[29] Moore et al., in 1994, suggested the intra-vertebral sagittal ratio which represents the ratio of the minimum sagittal diameter of the vertebral canal to the maximum sagittal diameter of the corresponding vertebral body, obtained at the cranial aspect of the vertebra and perpendicular to the vertebral canal. A sagittal ratio of less than or equal to 50% from C4 to C6 or less than or equal to 52% at C7 is a strong predictor (26.1 to 41.5 likelihood ratio) of vertebral canal narrowing. The sensitivity and specificity of this method for detecting cervical stenotic myelopathy is greater than or equal to 89% at each vertebral site from C4 through C7.[32] Mayhew and Green, in 2000, suggested the inter-vertebral sagittal ratio as a way to evaluate survey radiographs for cervical vertebral malformation. This technique represents the ratio of the minimal distance taken from the most cranial aspect of the vertebral body to the most caudal aspect of the vertebral arch of the vertebra located cranially and the maximal sagittal diameter of the vertebral body.[30] A recent study by Hahn et al. in 2008 compared the utility of the intra- and inter-vertebral sagittal ratio methods for diagnosing cervical vertebral malformations. It was concluded that a sagittal diameter ratio of less than or equal to 48% at any intra- or inter-vertebral site from C2 to C7 represents cervical vertebral malformation.[15] Considering the above discussion, the practitioner should be aware of the inevitable false positive results because some horses may have a narrow vertebral site and not necessarily represent a spinal cord compressive lesion.

Myelography with nonionic, water-soluble contrast material has proven to be an acceptable and safe diagnostic procedure in the horse.[6,26,28,35] Iohexol and iopamidol are nonionic contrast agents that have relatively few side effects.[26,28,56] With the horse under general anesthesia and in the lateral recumbent position, its head is elevated, and approximately 40 to 50 mL iopamidol 300, or 370 mg iodine/mL or iohexol 300, or 350 mg iodine/mL is injected into the subarachnoid space at the cisterna magna.[6,28] Iohexol may produce slightly less of an inflammatory reaction than iopamidol,[6] but both contrast agents are relatively safe for myelography in the horse. The higher concentration contrast material provides better contrast in large horses.

Lateral cervical radiographs centered over the cranial, mid cervical, and caudal cervical regions are made with the spine in a neutral position. A flexed lateral projection is made in the mid cervical region, and an extended lateral one is made in the caudal cervical region. Additional flexed and extended projections at different sites may be necessary. The contrast material can be visualized via ventro-dorsal radiographs over the cranial and mid cervical regions, but because of the thickness of the body area, it is usually not possible to visualize the contrast material in the caudal cervical region of the adult horse.

On a normal myelogram study, several variations need to be noted and not confused with false positive lesions. On neutral lateral radiographs, there are areas of some degree of elevation of the ventral contrast column at each intervertebral disk. On flexed lateral radiographs, there is also narrowing of the dorsal subarachnoid space, most frequently at C3 to C4 and C4 to C5, and the ventral column at these locations appears as a thin line. On extended lateral views, the dorsal column does not narrow and the ventral column is increased in width.

Most lesions detected via cervical myelograms in the horse are compressive lesions from cervical stenosis, either bony or ligamentous, or the result of vertebral instability (Figure 4.19). These lesions may cause substantial narrowing, obliteration, or displacement of the contrast column. The most common sites of compression, in order of decreasing frequency, are C3 to C4,

C6 to C7, C5 to C6, and C4 to C5.[37] Suggested methods for assessment of a spinal cord compressive lesions include: the reduction of 50% or more of the dorsal contrast column compared with the thickness of the subarachnoid space cranial to the narrowing,[35] narrowing of the dorsal and ventral contrast columns by more than 50% in diametrically opposed sites,[37] and 40% reduction of the entire dural diameter.[50]

The results obtained from these methods should be interpreted with caution due to the risk of false positive results. It has been suggested that a reduction of 70% of the dorsal contrast column is needed to avoid false positive diagnosis.[51] A study by van Biervliet et al. in 2004 showed a high sensitivity and specificity of the reduction of 20% of the entire dural diameter at C6 to

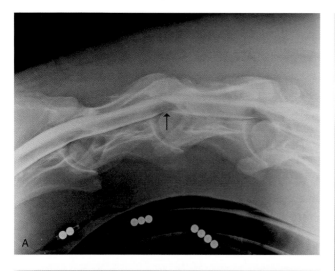
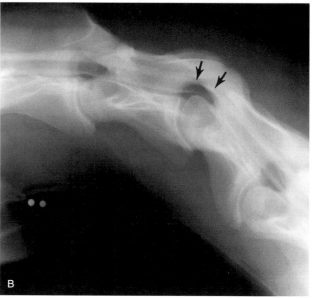
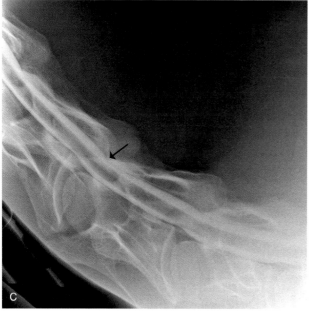

Figure 4.19. A. Normal flexed lateral myelogram of the cranial cervical region, showing contrast material in the subarachnoid space and narrowing of the ventral column at C3 to C4 (arrow). No narrowing of the dorsal column or significant spinal cord compression is present. B. Flexed lateral myelogram of the cranial cervical region, showing ventral and dorsal (arrows) contrast columns narrowed by more than 50% and a narrowed spinal cord, suggesting dynamic cervical stenosis. C. Extended lateral myelogram of the mid cervical region at the level of C4 to C5, showing stenosis of the spinal canal on the cranial aspect of C5 with narrowing of the dorsal contrast column by at least 50% (arrow).

C7 in neutral or flexed myelographic projections for diagnosing cervical stenotic myelopathy. Using this parameter at any other site, the test had only low sensitivity and high specificity.[52] One should be aware that besides obtaining false positive results, misinterpretation of myelograms can occur with suboptimal technique or when the lesion is lateralized and only lateral radiographic views are made.

Arthrography

Although arthrography in most cases has been replaced by more advanced imaging modalities and arthroscopy, positive and double contrast examinations may provide diagnostic information when evaluating possible open joints, dissecting cartilage flaps, or synovial defects (fistulae or hernias), especially in joints in which some advanced imaging studies are difficult to obtain, such as the shoulder.[34]

Tendonography

During the last two decades many practitioners have become familiar with the basic use and interpretation of equine ultrasonography, making it the modality of choice for the evaluation of equine limb soft tissue structures. The fact that ultrasound equipment is now more available and affordable for most practitioners, a diagnostic technique such as tendonography is now considered unpopular and almost obsolete. However, in rare cases such as synovial herniations and intrasynovial communications that could represent a greater diagnostic challenge when using ultrasonography, contrast examinations may be more effective and easier to interpret.[10]

Other modalities such as computed tomography and magnetic resonance imaging have proved to add substantial diagnostic information in the diagnosis of soft tissue and bone injuries and will be discussed further in this chapter.

PRINCIPLES OF RADIOGRAPHIC INTERPRETATION

There are three basic steps to radiographic interpretation: (1) evaluating the film and quality of the examination, (2) reading the radiograph, and (3) formulating a radiographic impression, diagnosis, and/or prognosis. Film quality should be evaluated by checking film exposure, labeling, collimation, and positioning. This is an important step because poor-quality radiographs result in missed or improperly diagnosed conditions. A properly exposed radiograph should have enough film contrast latitude to allow observation of bone and soft tissue outlines, and the film detail should be sufficient to demonstrate bone trabeculae. Exposure becomes a less critical factor when using digital radiography systems due to the greater contrast latitude. The person evaluating the study should be familiar with artifacts that may originate from the patient or be associated with the system used.

Positioning should be evaluated by inspecting joint space and bone alignment. Poorly positioned studies may result from the horse standing with the limb not perpendicular to the ground, the cassette not parallel with the limb, or the X-ray tube not perpendicular to the X-ray cassette or the part being examined.

A thorough radiographic examination should be done on each part for which pathology is expected from the physical examination. The routine examination may consist of 2 to 8 views, depending on the part examined. Sometimes, additional views are needed to better define and demonstrate suspected lesions.

The second step in radiographic interpretation is reading the radiograph. If the clinician is in a hurry to make a diagnosis, this step may be overlooked or cut short, resulting in interpretational errors. A systematic thorough inspection of the entire film should be done so that nothing is missed. Identifying radiographic abnormalities requires knowledge of both radiographic anatomy and radiographic signs of disease. Without knowledge of either, a correct radiographic interpretation is usually not made.

The third step is formulating a radiographic impression, diagnosis, or differential diagnosis. Knowledge of disease pathophysiology and its relationship to radiographic signs is necessary for this step. Finally, the radiographic diagnosis should be integrated with other diagnostic information, such as history, physical examinations, and perineural anesthesia results, to arrive at a final diagnosis.

If these basic steps of radiographic interpretation are not followed, the clinician may reach erroneous conclusions, leading to a faulty impression, diagnosis, and/or prognosis.

Radiology of Soft Tissue Structures

Soft tissue changes may be primary pathologic changes, secondary to more serious bone changes, or incidental findings of no clinical significance. A bright light is helpful for evaluating soft tissue structures when using conventional (screen-film) radiographic systems. Fascial planes, tendons, ligaments, and some portion of joint capsules may be seen because of adipose tissue (fat) within and around these structures. Fat is less opaque and appears slightly darker than muscle, skin, tendons, or ligaments on a radiograph (Figure 4.20). Soft tissue structures should be evaluated for thickening, mineralization, and free gas (radiolucencies).

Soft Tissue Thickening

Soft tissue thickening in the equine extremity is usually caused by swelling secondary to inflammation from infection or trauma. However, non-clinically significant soft tissue thickening can also be identified radiographically such as in cases of elbow or carpal hygroma where the thickening originates from chronic trauma but is simply a cosmetic blemish. The soft tissue thickening may be localized or diffuse. Localized thickening may be identified radiographically within or around joints, tendons, or muscles (Figure 4.21). Radiographic signs of soft tissue thickening include an increased soft tissue prominence, displacement of fat bodies (adipose tissue) around the joint capsule or tendon sheaths, and mottling or obliteration of adipose tissue in fascial planes around muscles, joint capsules, or tendons.

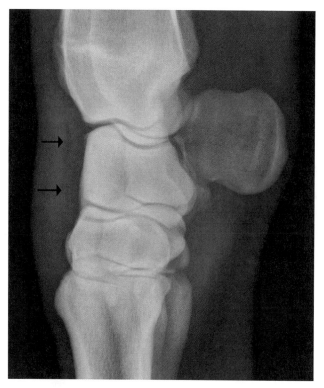

Figure 4.20. Lateromedial (LM) projection of a normal carpus showing the fat pads (adipose tissue bodies) as lucent structures within the dorsal soft tissues (arrows).

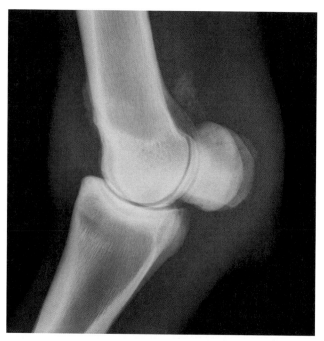

Figure 4.22. Lateromedial (LM) projection of the metacarpophalangeal joint. Amorphous soft tissue mineralization is present just palmar to the distal MCIII and proximal to the sesamoid bones, consistent with dystrophic mineralization of the palmar joint capsule. Note also the irregular periosteal reaction on the distal dorsal cortex of MCIII, consistent with enthesopathy of the origin of the joint capsule. An irregular palmar border of one of the sesamoid bones is likely secondary to chronic desmitis of the corresponding suspensory ligament branch. (Courtesy of New Bolton Center, University of Pennsylvania.)

Mineralization

Soft tissue mineralization in equine limbs may be dystrophic or metastatic. Dystrophic mineralization is most frequent and is present in damaged tissues after physical, chemical, or thermal trauma (Figure 4.22). Hematomas and necrotic and post-inflammatory foci and cartilaginous areas are frequent sites of dystrophic mineralization. Calcinosis circumscripta is a form of dystrophic mineralization and is most frequently seen periarticular in the horse. Metastatic mineralization primarily occurs in normal soft tissue from a disturbance in calcium and phosphorus metabolism but is seldom observed in the horse.

Radiographic signs of soft tissue mineralization include an amorphous radiopacity within soft tissue structures, absence of trabecular or cortical bone within the radiopacity, indistinct borders with dystrophic mineralization, and well-defined and distinct borders. A round "cauliflower-shaped" appearance is usually present with calcinosis circumpscripta.

Gas

Gas may be present in the soft tissue structures of equine limbs as a result of traumatic lacerations, puncture wounds, needle centesis, or gas-producing bacterial

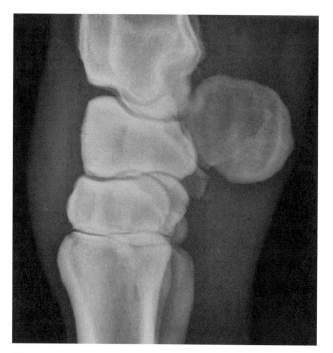

Figure 4.21. Lateromedial (LM) projection of carpal effusion. Note the soft tissue thickening on the dorsal aspect of the carpus obliterating the normal fat pads (see Figure 4.20). There are multiple, small, irregular osseous bodies on the palmar and dorsal aspects of the carpus consistent with osteochondral fragments.

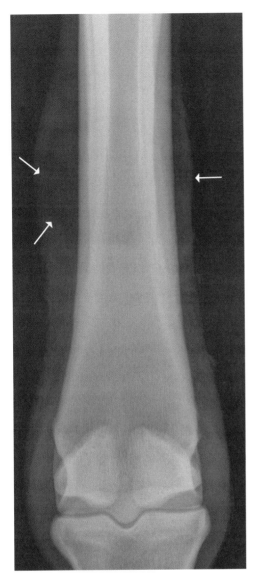

Figure 4.23. Dorsopalmar (DP) projection of the metacarpus. Surrounding the mid third metacarpal bone, the skin margins are irregular and there is gas within the thickened soft tissue secondary to a skin laceration (arrows).

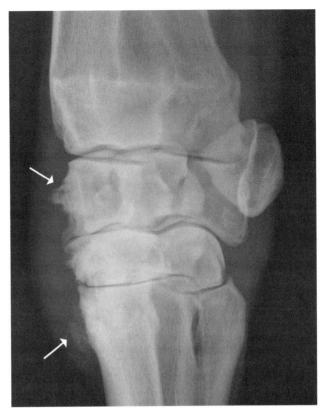

Figure 4.24. Dorsolateral-palmaromedial oblique (D45L-PMO) projection of the carpus with periarticular osteophytosis and lysis at the middle carpal and carpo-metacarpal joints secondary to osteoarthritis. Note the rounded, bone proliferation on the dorsal surface of the radial and third carpal bones and proximal aspect of the third metacarpal bone, consistent with enthesopathy of the insertion of the joint capsule and extensor carpi radialis, respectively (arrows).

organisms (Figure 4.23). Radiographic signs of soft tissue emphysema include radiolucent regions within soft tissue structures (the radiolucencies should be differentiated from fat) and a focal accumulation of gas with an air-fluid level that occurs with abscesses. The radiographic evidence of gas within the soft tissues in addition to an irregular skin surface should prompt the diagnosis of skin laceration.

Gas lucencies can be identified radiographically in subcutaneous tissue, muscle fascial planes, intramuscular tissue, and within the joint. Localization of soft tissue gas is important diagnostically and prognostically. Gas within muscle tissue occurs with a gas phlegmon, intra-articular gas may be associated with the "vacuum phenomenon" (non-clinically significant) when a joint is flexed,[14,47] or an air-fluid level within soft tissue may be diagnostic of an abscess.

Entheses

An enthesis is a point in the bone at which a soft tissue structure attaches. The soft tissues involved can include tendons, ligaments, or joint capsule. A pathologic change at these sites is known as enthesopathy and can be secondary to many disorders, but most commonly includes trauma or degenerative or inflammatory conditions, and may be intra- or extra-articular (Figure 4.24). In cases of an acute traumatic event, an avulsion fracture at the enthesis may occur (Figure 4.25). Radiographic changes associated with enthesopathy include bone erosion, bone proliferation or hyperostosis (thickening of cortical bone), sclerosis, fragmentation, and adjacent soft tissue mineralization.

Radiology of Bone

Knowledge of normal radiographic anatomy and basic bone response patterns is essential for evaluating bone structures radiographically in equine limbs. If the veterinarian is not familiar with physeal closure and ossification times of both epiphyses and apophyses in immature animals, he/she can easily look them up in anatomy textbooks (see Chapter 1 for information on growth plate closure times). The clinician should be

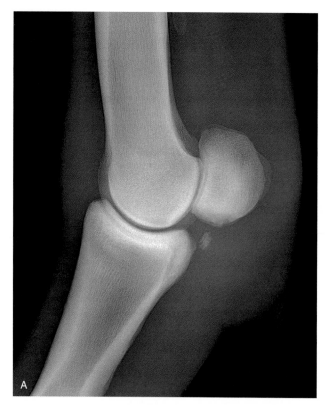

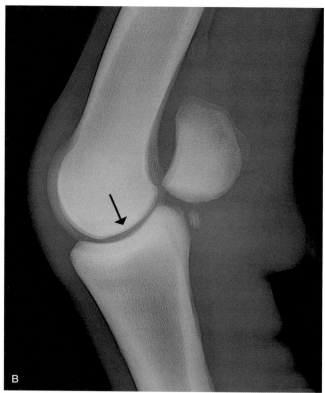

Figure 4.25. (A) Lateromedial (LM) and (B) flexed lateromedial (flexed LM) projections of the metacarpophalangeal joint. An irregular osseous body is seen just distal to the proximal sesamoid bones, consistent with an avulsion fracture of the base of one of the sesamoid bones. Note the origin of the avulsion fracture as an irregular concavity on the basal surface of the sesamoid bones. Also, mild flattening of the articular surface of the MCIII condyles is present (arrow). (Courtesy of Dr. Katherine Garrett.)

familiar with the normal shape of bones and the location and appearance of protuberances and fossae in mature animals; this information is available in standard references.

Fundamental Patterns of Bone Response

The response of bone to different pathologic processes is limited and consists in one or a combination of the following processes: new bone production/formation, bone resorption/destruction, or shape alteration. Bone remodeling and bone modeling are two terms commonly used interchangeably when referring to musculoskeletal radiology. Physiologically, osteoclastic and osteoblastic activities occur in both processes.

During the bone remodeling process, the osteoblasts and osteoclasts are coupled and act together; therefore, bone resorption and formation occur at the same time and at the same site on a bone surface.[13] On the other hand, during the bone modeling process, the bone alterations result from independent actions from osteoclasts and osteoblasts. This means that the bone resorption and formation may occur on different sites. In addition, modeling may cause large changes in bone structure, whereas remodeling will replace bone, maintaining the current amount of bone structure.[12] Therefore, the correct term for describing visible bone structural changes is modeling rather than remodeling.

Radiographically, new bone production commonly is manifested as a periosteal or endosteal reaction (adjacent to the cortex), new bone at periarticular margins or entheses, or increased bone opacity (sclerosis). Areas of bone destruction are seen as bone lysis (aggressive bone lesions or osteoarthritis) or decreased bone opacity (osteopenia). Pathologic shape alteration is commonly seen radiographically in, but not limited to, skeletally immature horses, usually secondary to physeal problems or abnormal weight-bearing. To formulate a correct diagnosis, the clinician should note fundamental bone response patterns and distribution within bones and any associated soft tissue changes on equine limb radiographs. The clinician also should be able to differentiate whether these changes are a response to pathologic processes or secondary to normal bone modeling as adaptation to a particular athletic activity.

Periosteal Reactions

The periosteum is stimulated when elevated by hemorrhage, pus, edema, or infiltrating neoplastic cells. In the horse, direct trauma; extension of soft tissue infections; and avulsion of ligaments, tendons, and/or joint capsules are most frequently associated with periosteal new bone production. Periosteal bone production may be acute or chronic (Figure 4.26). Acute periosteal bone production has an irregular, indistinct border and may

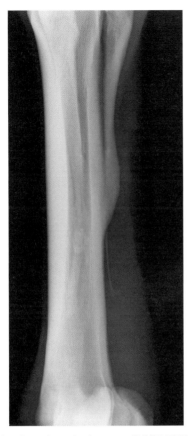

Figure 4.26. Dorsolateral-palmaromedial (DLPMO) oblique projection of the metacarpus. Note the smooth periosteal reaction and cortical thickening of the mid-distal diaphysis of MCIV, consistent with a chronic exostosis. (Courtesy of New Bolton Center, University of Pennsylvania.)

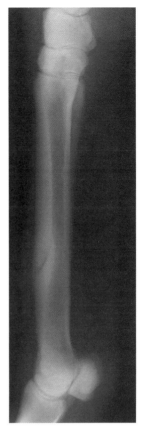

Figure 4.27. Lateromedial (LM) projection of the metacarpus. A radiolucent line is seen through the dorsal cortex of the mid MCIII, consistent with a stress fracture. There is also associated cortical and soft tissue thickening.

be continuous or interrupted, laminated or speculated. Acute periosteal reaction is usually active. Chronic periosteal bone production has a smooth, well-defined border, is solid, and often blends with the adjacent cortex. This type of periosteal reaction is usually inactive and often indicates a healed process such as a healed fracture or previous active periosteal bone production that has changed to a chronic, probably inactive stage.

Cortical Changes

Cortical changes that can be identified radiographically consist of defects, erosions, lysis, and changes in thickness. Cortical defects seen most frequently in equine extremities are caused by fractures. Fractures must be differentiated from nutrient foramina, physeal lines, and edge enhancement shadows caused by superimposed bones (Figure 4.27). Long bone cortical stress fractures may not be evident in all cases as a distinct fracture line (Figure 4.28); a periosteal and/or endosteal reaction may be the only visible radiographic change (Figure 4.29). Cortical lysis is usually caused by infection and typically has a permeative and/or moth-eaten pattern. A sequestrum also may be associated with a

focal area of cortical lysis (Figure 4.30). In such cases, a dense sequestered piece of bone can be identified surrounded by a lytic zone (cloaca), which in turn is surrounded by bone sclerosis, producing an involucrum.

Cortical erosion changes can extend from either the endosteal or the periosteal surface. In the horse, they are most frequently encountered adjacent to the periosteal surface. Erosive changes with an irregular border usually result from infiltration into the bone and are most often caused by infectious processes. Cortical erosive areas with a smooth border are the result of pressure erosion (Figure 4.31), such as that seen with proliferative synovitis in the metacarpophalangeal or metatarsophalangeal joints.

Cortical erosions seen on the flexor surface of the navicular bone are secondary to a degenerative disorder initiated and promoted by excessive and sustained forces of compression against the flexor surface (most of them on the distal half), mainly from a faulty conformation (Figure 4.32).[41] Similar microscopic changes, consisting of focal cartilage degeneration and lysis, thickened subchondral bone, and fibrous ankylosis to the opposing surface at the sites of subchondral bone destruction, are also seen in the periarticular margins and articular surfaces of high-load, low-motion joints;

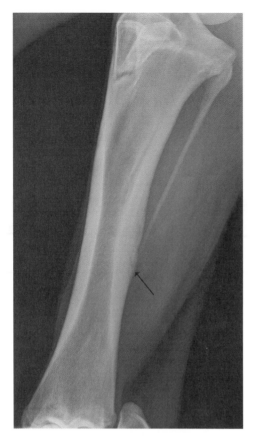

Figure 4.28. Craniolateral-caudomedial oblique projection of the tibia. A stress fracture of the tibia is present on the latero-caudal cortex of the mid diaphysis. Note the smooth, thickened periosteal reaction with a faint radiolucent cortical fracture line (arrow). A subtle endosteal reaction is also present at that level. (Courtesy of New Bolton Center, University of Pennsylvania.)

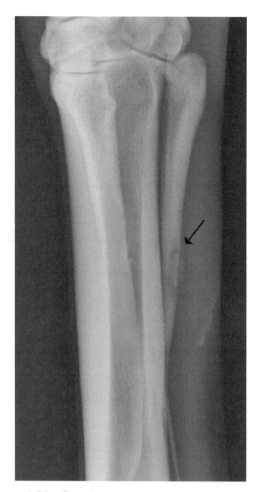

Figure 4.30. Dorsolateral-palmaromedial oblique (DL-PMO) projection of the metacarpus showing a well defined osseous body (sequestrum) surrounded by a radiolucent rim (cloaca) on the mid diaphysis of MCIV. There is mild surrounding sclerosis and a small periosteal reaction just proximal to the cloaca, representing the involucrum (arrow).

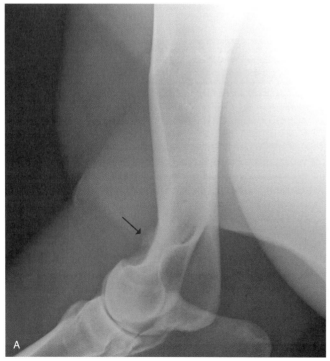

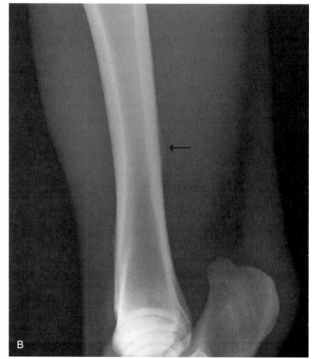

Figure 4.29. Examples of humeral (A) and tibial (B) stress fractures with only radiographic evidence of a periosteal reaction (arrows). (Courtesy of New Bolton Center, University of Pennsylvania.)

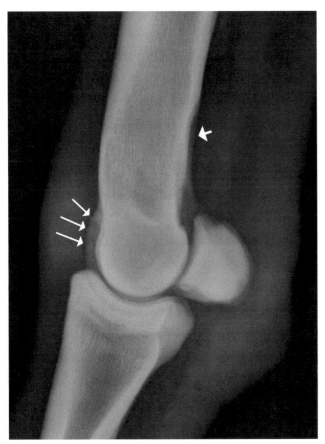

Figure 4.31. Lateromedial (LM) projection of the metacarpophalangeal joint with osteochondritis dessicans, evident by the osseous bodies seen on the dorsal aspect of the joint (long arrows). Note the soft tissue thickening, consistent with joint effusion, and the marked supracondylar bone loss on the palmar cortex of distal MCIII (short arrow), secondary to chronic inflammation.

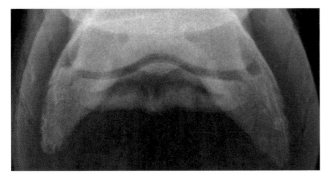

Figure 4.32. Palmaroproximal-palmarodistal oblique (Pa45Pr-PaDiO) projection of the navicular bone. On the flexor aspect of the navicular bone, note the poor corticomedullary definition, irregular medullary sclerosis, and cortical erosions consistent with degenerative changes.

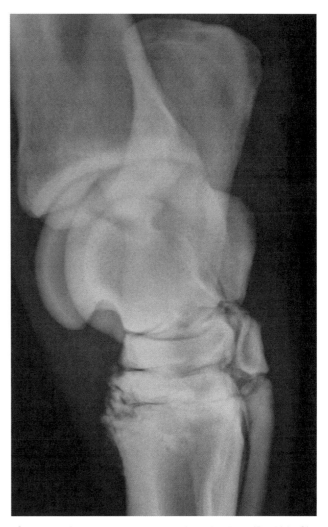

Figure 4.33. Dorsomedial-plantarolateral oblique (D55M-PLO) projection of the tarsus. Sclerosis of the dorsal aspect of the central and third tarsal bones and irregular periarticular osteophytosis and subchondral bone erosions are present at the dorsolateral aspect of the distal intertarsal and tarsometatarsal joints, consistent with severe osteoarthritis. Irregular periosteal reaction is also seen on the proximal dorsolateral aspect of MTIII secondary to enthesopathy at the insertion of the peroneus tertius and tibialis cranialis muscles.

for example, the proximal interphalangeal joint and the distal intertarsal and tarsometatarsal joints (Figure 4.33).[16]

Increased cortical width is usually produced by increased weight-bearing. Such changes in cortical width are frequently present with valgus or varus limb abnormalities.

Generalized bone opacity may be decreased or increased. Decreased bone density is seen secondary to disuse of the limb or distal to a fracture. The osteopenia that develops in these limbs can be recognized radiographically as a coarse primary trabecular pattern with or without thin cortices (Figure 4.34). Increased bone opacity is identified radiographically with loss of the trabecular pattern secondary to bone deposition within the medullary cavity (Figure 4.35). Sclerosis is common on the third carpal bone and the proximal MCIII or MTIII at the origin of the suspensory ligament (Figures 4.36 and 4.37).[17,48]

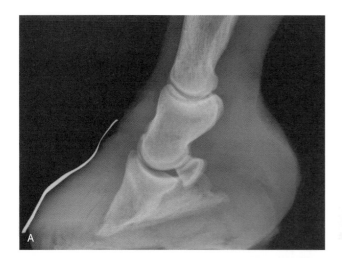
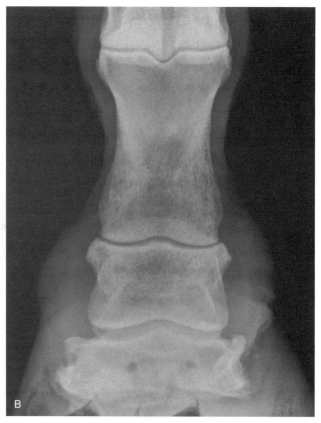

Figure 4.34. (A) Lateromedial (LM) and (B) dorsopalmar (DP) projections of a distal limb with rotating laminitis. Note the coarse trabecular pattern (more noticeable on distal P1 and proximal P2) secondary to disuse osteopenia from chronic non-weight-bearing.

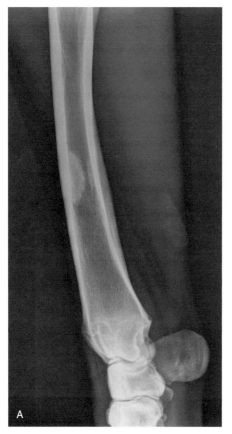
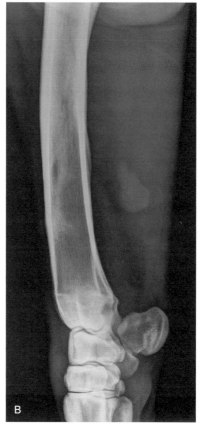

Figure 4.35. Lateromedial (LM) projections of the radius. (A) shows a well defined, oval medullary sclerosis adjacent to the endosteal surface of the cranial mid diaphysis and a similar elongated opacity adjacent to the caudal endosteal surface at the same level. (B) shows a diffused, irregular medullary sclerosis affecting mostly the proximal and mid thirds of the diaphysis. Nuclear medicine exams showed increased radiopharmaceutical uptake in both cases, which is consistent with enostosis-like lesions. (Courtesy of Dr. Jeremy D. Hubert.)

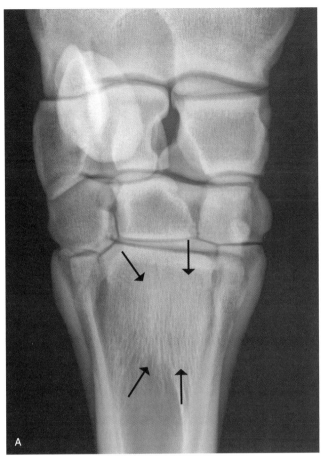

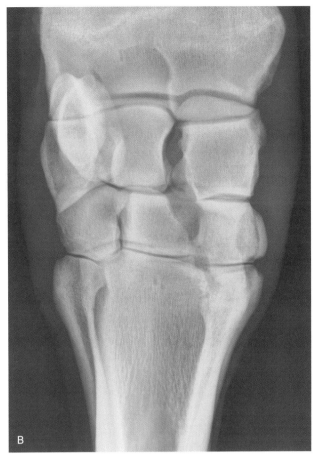

Figure 4.36. Dorsopalmar (DP) projections of the carpus. A. Sclerosis of the proximal aspect of MCIII with partial loss of the trabecular pattern, suggesting desmitis at the origin of the

suspensory ligament (arrows). Compare with normal image (B), where a well defined trabecular pattern is present.

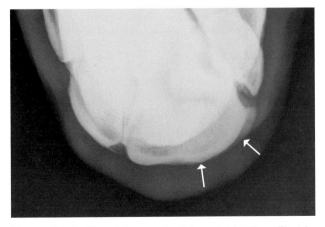

Figure 4.37. Flexed dorsoproximal-dorsodistal oblique (flexed D30Pr-DDiO) projection of the distal row of carpal bones. Note the sclerosis of the radial facet of the articular surface of the third carpal bone with partial loss of the corticomedullary definition (arrows).

Radiographic Signs (Bone Response Patterns) with Osteomyelitis

Osteomyelitis in equine limbs may be hematogenous in origin or result from penetrating wounds or open fractures. The region affected depends on the source and route of infection. Both acute and chronic osteomyelitis can be identified radiographically (Figures 4.38 and 4.39). It generally takes 7 to 10 days after clinical signs of acute osteomyelitis are observed before the earliest detectable radiographic bone changes occur because at least 50% of mineral content must be depleted from the bone to be radiographically visible.

Because osteomyelitis can affect any bone in an equine limb and must be differentiated from other focal bone lesions, it will be used to illustrate the use of radiographic signs or bone response patterns to arrive at a radiographic diagnosis. Identifying radiographic signs requires close inspection of the radiograph and is an important step in accurately establishing a specific or differential diagnosis.

The following are radiographic signs manifested by acute osteomyelitis:

- Soft tissue thickening adjacent to the bone. This thickening is manifested by increased opacity, mottling, and obliteration of adipose tissue in fascial planes.

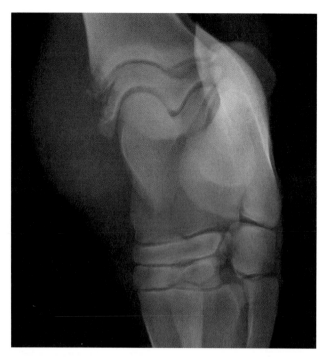

Figure 4.38. Dorsolateral-plantaromedial oblique (D35L-PIMO) projection of the tarsus, showing focal widening of the medial aspect of distal tibial physis with adjacent subchondral bone lysis and marked soft tissue thickening consistent with septic physitis. (Courtesy of Dr. Jeremy D. Hubert.)

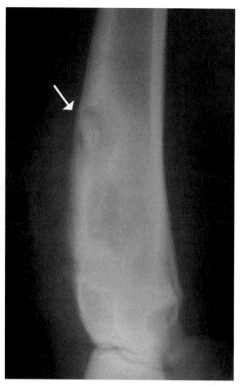

Figure 4.39. Lateromedial (LM) projection of the distal radius with radiographic changes, consistent with osteomyelitis. Note the irregular and discontinued periosteal reaction with lysis of the craniodistal cortex of the distal radius and adjacent ill defined increased medullary opacity and soft tissue thickening. On the most proximal aspect of the lesion, the cranial cortex is wider and presents a circular mineral opacity with a surrounding radiolucent rim and sclerosis, suggesting the presence of a sequestrum (arrow). (Courtesy of Dr. Gary Baxter.)

- Periosteal new bone production. This new bone has an irregular, indistinct border and parallels the bone cortices. Subtle areas of subperiosteal bone lysis may be seen in association with the acute periosteal bone reaction. These changes are not usually seen until 7 to 10 days after clinical signs of the disease have been observed. As the disease progresses, the periosteal bone production parallels the cortex and spreads proximal and distal from the original infection site.
- Permeative lysis is observed as small round lucent areas, 2 to 3 mm in size, within cortical bone and may extend into the medullary cavity. A moth-eaten pattern of lysis with larger lucent areas can also be seen in acute and active aggressive lesions. These changes are usually seen in association with acute periosteal bone production.
- Areas of bone lysis within the physis, metaphysis, or epiphysis secondary to septic osteomyelitis in young animals is very aggressive and mostly destructive, giving little or no opportunity to the body to produce bone in the attempt to ward off the infection.

Chronic osteomyelitis may have the following radiographic changes:

- Large cortical defects, some of which may be as large as 1 cm in size and can also involve the medullary cavity. Although rare, bone abscesses may appear as a geographic pattern of lysis represented by a single well-defined medullary lytic area with surrounding sclerosis.[18,58]
- Localized increased bone densities (sclerosis), which are produced within the host bone, e.g., thick cortices, and in which a sequestrum sometimes may be

identified within the sclerotic and lytic bone patterns
- Periosteal bone production, which is usually abundant with a well-defined irregular or smooth border.

It is often impossible to determine radiographically whether the chronic osteomyelitis is active or inactive. This diagnosis is probably best determined by physical examination, clinical signs, or other imaging techniques, such as nuclear scintigraphy.

Radiology of Synovial Joints

Radiographic evaluation of joints in the equine limb is an important part of the diagnostic workup for lameness and encompasses evaluation of several joint structures or areas, including soft tissue structures (both intracapsular and extracapsular); joint margins; subchondral bone; the "joint space"; ligament, tendon, and joint capsule attachment areas; and joint alignment (Figure 4.40).

Normal Joint Structures

The joint capsule and periarticular soft tissue structures should not be distended. Fat bodies and adipose

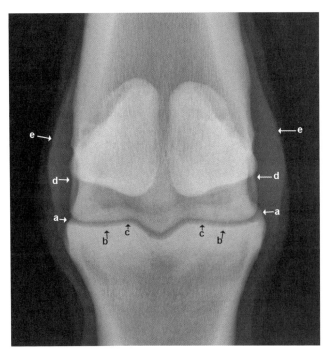

Figure 4.40. Dorsoproximal-distopalmar oblique (D30Pr-DiPaO) projection of a normal metacarpophalangeal joint, showing the structures that should be evaluated around a joint. (a) Joint margins. (b) Subchondral bone. (c)"Joint space" (articular cartilage). (d) Areas for collateral ligament attachment. (e) Joint capsule and general joint alignment.

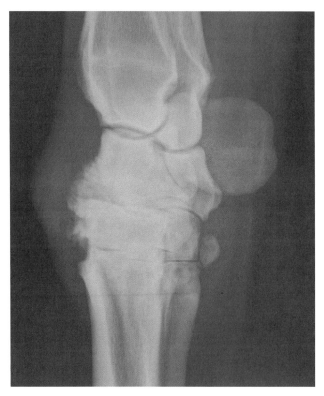

Figure 4.41. Dorsomedial-palmarolateral oblique (D30M-PLO) projection of the carpus. Severe periarticular osteophytosis is present at the middle carpal and the carpo-metacarpal joints with sclerosis of the cuboidal bones involved and focal soft tissue thickening consistent with osteoarthritis.

tissue within muscle fascial planes can be identified around some normal joints. Visibility and location of adipose tissue may change with inflammation or joint capsule distension or thickening. The normal location and the presence of fat bodies vary, depending on the joint and animal being examined.

Joint margins are bony regions at the edge of articular cartilage that also coincide with the edge of the subchondral bone. Articular cartilage, the periosteum, and the joint capsule meet in this region. In the normal joint, the margins are smooth and blend with the surrounding bone structures. Subchondral bone is a dense, compact bony zone 1 to 3 mm in width and adjacent to the articular cartilage. The subchondral bone surface adjacent to the articular cartilage is smooth and even.

The so-called "joint space" as seen on a radiograph is not an actual space but is composed of articular cartilage with a thin layer of synovial fluid between the opposing cartilaginous surfaces. It appears radiolucent on a radiograph, compared with the adjacent radiopaque subchondral bone. The joint space should be of even thickness throughout a specific joint, but thickness differs from joint to joint, e.g., the distal interphalangeal joint space is wider than the proximal interphalangeal joint space, which is wider than the metacarpophalangeal joint space.

Ligaments, tendons, and the joint capsule, which attach periarticularly, add stability to the joint. The attachment areas vary with the joint and may be located at different distances both proximal and distal to the joint margins. It is important to know regions of insertion for ligaments and tendons around specific joints.

The normal subchondral bone surfaces should align evenly. Positional changes of the horse or of the X-ray tube when the radiograph is made may make a normal joint appear slightly malaligned.

Radiographic Changes Associated with Joint Disease

The radiographic examination is helpful for evaluating the type and extent of joint disease. The radiographic manifestations of joint disease occur in the soft tissue and bone structures and may develop before or after clinical signs of the disease develop. The bone changes follow clinical signs in septic arthritis and may precede or follow clinical manifestations with osteoarthritis (OA).

Soft tissue changes that may be observed radiographically are periarticular soft tissue thickening, joint capsule distension, and mineralization. The location of fat bodies (adipose tissue masses) and adipose tissue in fascial planes can be used to evaluate periarticular swelling and joint capsule distension. Periarticular mineralization may be associated with numerous causes, but in the horse is predominantly dystrophic or secondary to blunt soft tissue trauma.

Marginal joint changes consist of periarticular osteophyte formation and bone lysis. Marginal periarticular

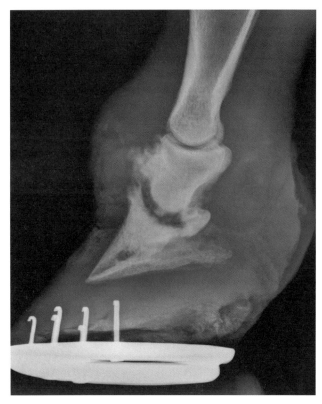

Figure 4.42. Lateromedial (LM) projection of the distal limb showing radiographic changes consistent with septic arthritis. Note the severe irregular subchondral bone lysis on the adjacent articular surfaces of the distal interphalangeal joint (DIPJ) with marked articular cartilage loss, the irregular periosteal proliferation on the dorsal and palmar surfaces of P2 and dorsal P3, and the severe soft tissue thickening with irregular skin surface centered over the dorsal aspect of the DIPJ. In addition, there is a coarse trabecular pattern on P1 consistent with disuse osteopenia.

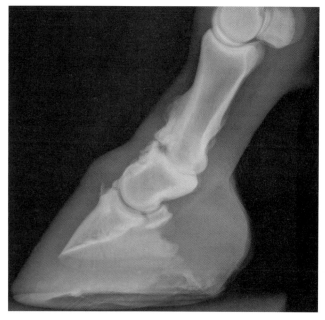

Figure 4.43. Lateromedial (LM) projection of the distal limb. Severe chronic degenerative changes are present on the proximal and to a lesser degree the distal interphalangeal joints consistent with osteoarthritis (high and low "ringbone"). Note the marked bone proliferation (osteophytes and enthesophytes) with rounded borders on the dorsal aspect of distal P1, P2, and the extensor process of P3; loss of the "joint space" is present at the proximal interphalangeal joint with adjacent subchondral bone sclerosis. Enthesophytes are also seen on the palmar aspect of distal P1 and proximal P2. (Courtesy of Dr. Gary Baxter.)

osteophytes are usually associated with OA (Figure 4.41), whereas marginal bone lysis is most often seen with septic arthritis (Figure 4.42). In early stages, marginal changes may be subtle, but with advanced or more severe disease, the changes are easily identified.

Subchondral bone changes consist of sclerosis, lysis, and fragmentation (Figure 4.43). Subchondral bone sclerosis may be present with OA, although it seems to be recognized radiographically in only the more pronounced or longstanding cases. Subchondral bone lysis can have a local or general distribution within the joint and may be seen in association with subchondral bone fragments. Subchondral bone lysis may be present with septic arthritis, OA, osteochondrosis, or "traumatic arthritis". Localized or general subchondral lytic patterns with irregular, indistinct margins are associated with septic arthritis. Localized, well-defined lytic lesions are seen with osteochondrosis, which may develop into subchondral cyst-like lesions. Focal subchondral lytic areas associated with bone fragments are seen with osteochronditis dissecans and traumatic arthritis lesions from chronic mircofractures in the subchondral bone. Traumatic arthritis lesions are usually seen on the dorsal

surfaces of joints and are caused by hyperextension trauma.

The joint space width may be increased or decreased. An increased width may be associated with joint effusion, although in weight-bearing studies, this is seldom apparent. An increased joint space associated with subchondral bone lysis can be seen with extensive septic arthritis. A decreased joint space, either general or localized within the joint, is associated with cartilaginous lesions and degeneration and occurs predominately with OA (Figure 4.43).

Periarticular enthesiophytes are usually associated with joint capsule, ligament, or tendon damage or avulsion from their bony attachments (Figure 4.24). The enthesiophytes (periosteal new bone production) are irregular in the acute stages, which distinguishes them from marginal periarticular osteophytes, and occur at tendinous and ligamentous attachment areas.

Alignment abnormalities may consist of subluxation or luxation of a joint or may simply result in an abnormal degree of flexion or extension of a joint in a resting position. Abnormal joint alignment may be associated with ligament laxity and/or injury (Figure 4.44), tendon injury or contracture, abnormal bone growth, i.e., angular limb deformities in foals, and healed, malaligned fractures. Chronic alignment abnormalities predispose the joint to degenerative joint disease from abnormal weight-bearing and stress distribution through the joint.

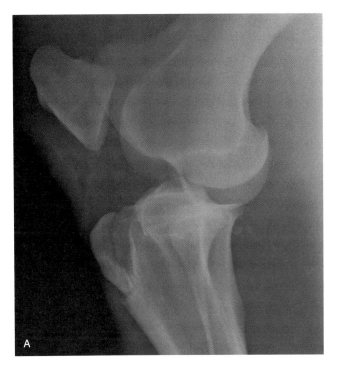

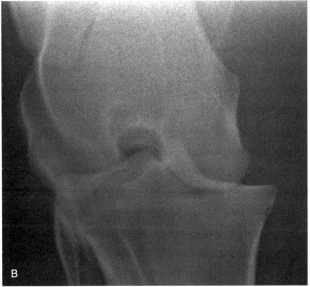

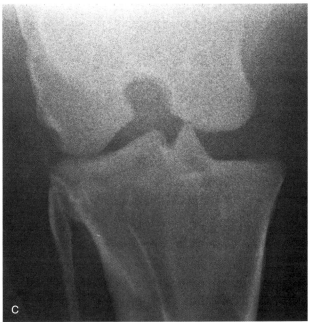

Figure 4.44. (A) Lateromedial (LM) and (B and C) caudo-cranial (Ca-Cr) projections of the stifle. Image A shows cranial displacement of the tibia with partial loss of the cranial fat pad, consistent with cranial subluxation and stifle joint effusion, likely secondary to cranial cruciate ligament injury. (B and C) Show a marked variation on the medial and lateral joint space width and medial displacement of the tibia, consistent with lateral to medial instability secondary to collateral ligament injury.

Radiographic Changes with Specific Joint Conditions

Degenerative joint disease, osteoarthrosis, or osteo-arthritis (OA) is a secondary condition in the horse (Figures 4.33, 4.41, and 4.45). The severity of radiographic changes usually correlates with the severity and/or duration of the disease process. The following are radiographic changes seen in the horse, listed in order from most common to least common:

• Marginal periarticular osteophytes
• Narrowed joint space, which may involve all or only part of the joint; distinct, smooth borders remain on the subchondral bone adjacent to the articular cartilage
• Well-defined subchondral bone lucencies, as seen in chronic OA of the tarsus and carpus
• Subchondral bone sclerosis
• Subchondral bone cystic degeneration, which occurs infrequently as sequelae to degenerative joint disease

Septic arthritis may be hematogenous in origin or result from extension of an adjacent osteomyelitis, cellulitis, or penetrating injury (Figures 4.42 and 4.46). The following are radiographic signs of septic arthritis:

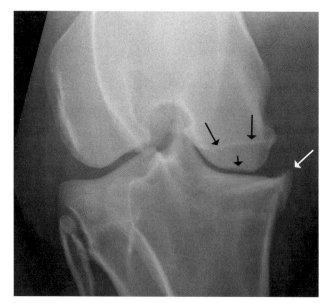

Figure 4.45. Caudo-cranial (Ca-Cr) projection of the stifle. A rounded periarticular osteophyte is present on the medial periarticular margin of the medial tibial condyle, consistent with osteoarthritis (white arrow). Also note the mild flattening of the articular surface of the medial femoral condyle, likely representing an osteochondrosis lesion (short black arrow) and the faint radiopaque line corresponding to the cranial margin of the medial femoral condyle (long black arrows), likely representing enthesophytosis at the insertion of the medial femorotibial and , medial aspect of the femoropatellar joint capsules.

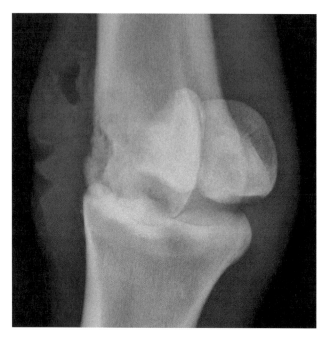

Figure 4.46. Dorsomedial-palmarolateral oblique (DMPLO) projection of the metacarpophalangeal joint. An area of permeative lysis is present on the dorsal aspect of the lateral condyle of MCIII. Marked narrowing of the joint space, mild irregular periosteal reaction on the dorolateral aspect of proximal P1, and associated soft tissue thickening with subcutaneous gas is also present. These findings are consistent with septic arthritis.

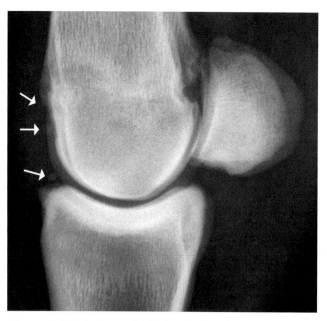

Figure 4.47. Lateromedial (LM) projection of the metacarpophalangeal joint. Three small, well defined, circular osseous bodies are seen on the dorsal aspect of the joint (arrows), consistent with osteochondritis dessicans.

- Periarticular soft tissue thickening and joint capsule distension
- Marginal bone lysis, which may occur early in the disease
- Subchondral bone destruction, which may be an extension from or occur without the marginal lysis
- Periosteal reactions, which may be adjacent to the joint but are generally distributed around the joint; when septic arthritis has occurred from extension of an adjacent osteomyelitis or cellulitis, the periosteal reaction may precede the intra-articular changes

Osteochondrosis is associated with regions of high predilection in specific joints, which should be observed when diagnosing the condition. It is caused by defective osteochrondral development, which usually involves subchondral bone (Figures 4.47 to 4.50). The following are radiographic changes present with osteochondrosis:

- Flattening of the subchondral bone surface
- Localized subchondral bone defect (lysis)
- Osteochondral bone fragments, which are seen radiographically as osseous bodies representing osteochondritis dessicans
- Secondary degenerative joint disease changes that may also be present
- Subchondral cyst-like lesions that may develop secondary to osteochondrosis

Traumatic osteochondrosis or traumatic joint disease also manifests with subchondral bone lysis. These lesions must be differentiated from true osteochondrosis lesions. Areas of predilection for traumatic joint disease

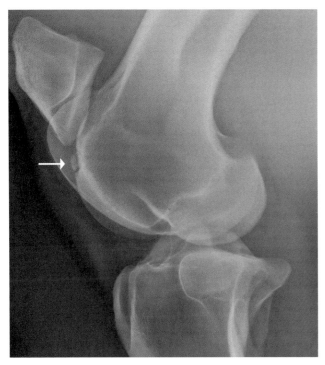

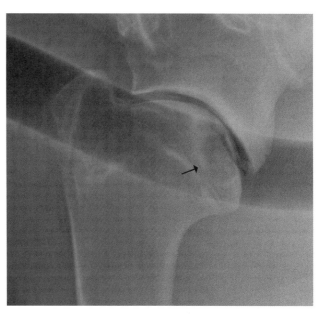

Figure 4.48. Lateromedial (LM) projection of the stifle. Note the well defined, oval, osseous body associated with a concave subchondral bone defect on the lateral trochlea ridge (arrow), consistent with osteochondritis dessicans.

Figure 4.49. Mediolateral (ML) projection of the shoulder. A large radiolucent subchondral bone defect (cyst) surrounded by a rim of sclerosis is seen on the caudal aspect of the humeral head (arrow), consistent with osteochondrosis.

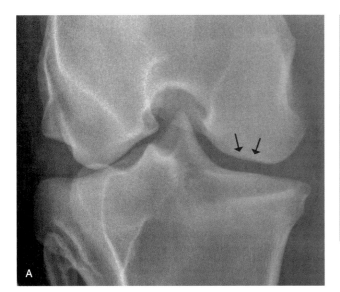

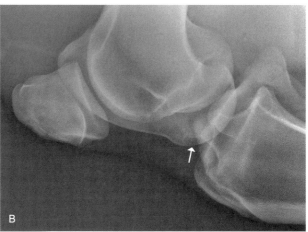

Figure 4.50. (A) Caudo-cranial (Ca-Cr) and (B) flexed lateromedial (flexed LM) projections of the same stifle. (A) shows a mild flattening and sclerotic region on the articular surface of the medial femoral condyle (arrows). (B) shows the cranial aspect of the medial femoral condyle free of superimposition, which allows the identification of a well defined, subchondral bone defect (cyst) surrounded by sclerosis (arrow), consistent with an osteochondrosis lesion that may be congenital or acquired secondary to trauma.

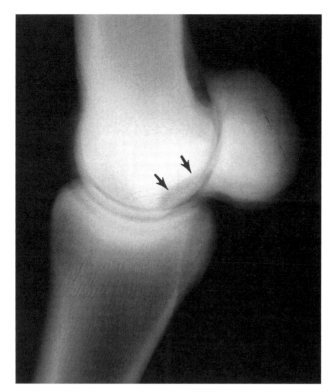

Figure 4.51. Lateromedial (LM) projection of the metacarpophalangeal joint showing a traumatic osteochondrosis lesion on the distal palmar surface of MCIII (arrows).

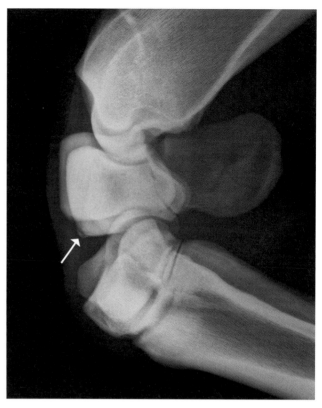

Figure 4.52. Flexed lateromedial (flexed LM) projection of the carpus. An area of lysis with a well defined associated osseous body (chip fracture) is present on the dorsodistal periarticular margin of the radial carpal bone secondary to traumatic hyperextension injury (arrow). (Courtesy of New Bolton Center, University of Pennsylvania.)

are the metacarpophalangeal joints (Figure 4.51) and carpus (Figure 4.52).

Traumatic osteochondrosis develops from increased weight-bearing and stress on a joint surface, resulting in bone sclerosis and eventual microfractures, which leads to subchondral bone lysis. Traumatic joint disease may also develop after hyperextension injury in joints such as the carpus, producing microfractures, subchondral bone lysis, and small subchondral bone fragments. The following are radiographic signs of traumatic joint disease:

- Focal subchondral bone lysis with indistinct borders
- Subchondral bone sclerosis
- Bone fragments, which may be adjacent to the subchondral bone lysis
- Incomplete articular fractures (stress fractures)
- Changes in contour of the bones, such as flattening of the medial femoral condyle or condyles of MCIII/MTIII

Systematic use of the radiographic signs of bone and joint disease discussed in this chapter provide the basis for correct, consistent radiographic diagnosis. Without close observation of the radiograph for these changes, missed or incorrect diagnoses will be made. History, signalment, and physical exam findings should always be taken into consideration at the time of interpreting the radiographic findings to give the correct diagnosis or most accurate list of differential diagnosis.

LIMITATIONS OF RADIOGRAPHY

Radiography is the most common imaging modality that has been widely used for the diagnosis of musculoskeletal injuries. However, it is well known that with the lack of detailed soft tissue visualization, radiography has a limited role in the evaluation of areas surrounding the bone. In the majority of cases, soft tissue thickening can be identified in plain radiographs and in combination with the history, clinical signs, and location; the practitioner will be able to differentiate whether the soft tissue thickening is secondary to active inflammation or a chronic condition. However, in order to have the most accurate diagnosis and subsequently be able to provide the best care to the patient, visualization of architectural changes within the soft tissues is essential. Ideally, in these cases, other imaging modalities (i.e., ultrasound or MRI) should be considered to complement the radiographic findings.

Skeletal abnormalities are identified radiographically based on changes in bone density/opacity (reduced or increased) and shape. Because skeletal lesions may only be detected with radiographs after approximately 50% change in bone mineralization is present, some conditions such as acute osteomyelitis, early synovitis, early cartilage loss/erosive arthritis, and minimally or nondisplaced fractures may not be recognized on the initial radiographic exam. It may take up to 2 weeks before the bone changes are detected with plain radiographs.

In cases of comminuted fractures, radiography may be unable to define the lesion clearly. In these cases, computed tomography with multiplanar and 3D reconstructions should be considered for surgical planning.

In summary, the practitioner should be aware of the above-mentioned limitations of radiography and that the combined results of different imaging modalities may be necessary to obtain a diagnosis. More important, it should always be remembered that radiographic changes do not necessarily represent lameness; therefore, a complete history and a thorough physical and lameness examinations are imperative in every clinical situation.

NORMAL RADIOGRAPHIC ANATOMY

Recognition of normal radiographic anatomy and variations of normal in the mature and immature horse is essential in equine radiology. Erroneous diagnoses or misdiagnoses may result if normal anatomy is not known. The normal radiographic anatomy of horse extremities is presented for reference in the following pages (Figures 4.54 to 4.101). A diagram accompanies each of the radiographic projections, demonstrating the position of the X-ray machine and detector in relation to the anatomical site of interest, as well as the angle orientation of the X-ray beam. In addition, radiographic projections commonly not included in a standard examination are described. A brief explanation of the advantage of obtaining these projections is also included.

The nomenclature system used in this chapter is that proposed by the Nomenclature Committee of the American College of Veterinary Radiology,[46] which uses proper veterinary anatomic directional terms[1] and describes the direction in which the central X-ray beam penetrates the body part of interest, from the point of entrance to the point of exit (Figure 4.53). The standard abbreviation for the view is given in parentheses in the figure legends.

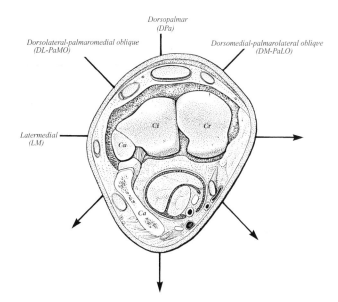

Figure 4.53. Cross-sectional diagram at the level of the proximal row of carpal bones demonstrating the nomenclature and method for labeling radiographic projections. Cr = radial carpal bone, Ci = intermediate carpal bone, Cu = ulnar carpal bone, Ca = accessory carpal bone.

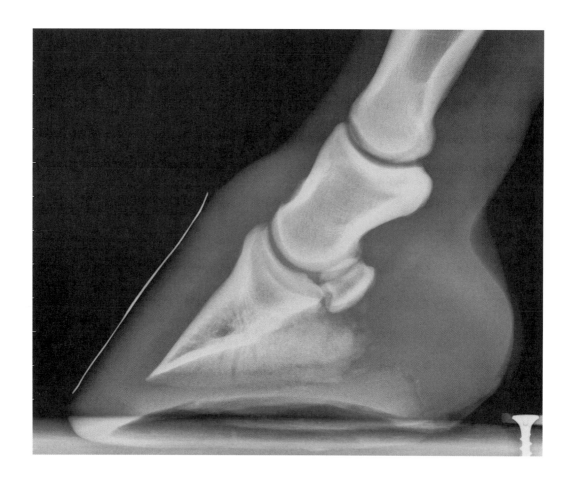

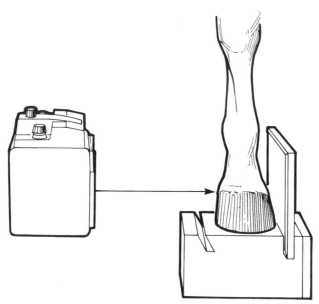

Figure 4.54.

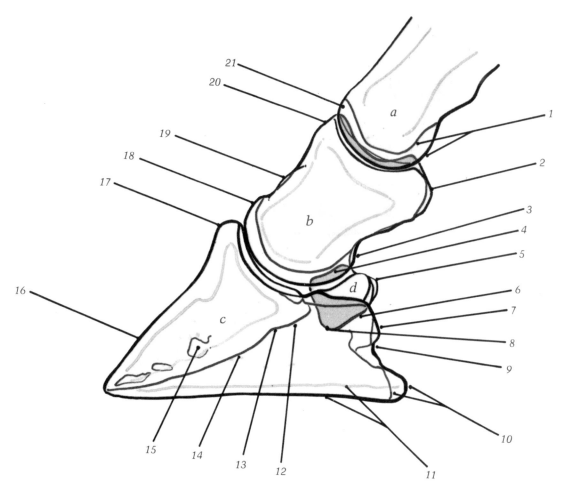

Figure 4.54. (*Continued*) Lateromedial (LM) projection of the distal phalanges and navicular bone. (a) Proximal phalanx, (b) middle phalanx, (c) distal phalanx, (d) navicular bone.

1. Palmar aspect of the medial and lateral condyles on the distal extremity of the proximal phalanx.
2. Transverse bony prominence on the proximopalmar aspect of the middle phalanx.
3. Superimposed medial and lateral condyles on the distopalmar aspect of the middle phalanx.
4. Articular surface of the navicular bone.
5. Proximal border of the navicular bone.
6. Flexor cortex and surface of the navicular bone; the medullary cavity (spongiosa) is the less opaque area in the center of the navicular bone.
7. Superimposed medial and lateral proximal parts of the palmar process on the distal phalanx. The size of this palmar process varies depending on the mineralization and ossification of the collateral cartilages. The palmar process also superimposes over the navicular bone, sometimes creating confusing opacities.
8. Distal border of the navicular bone, the border of which may appear as a distinct ridge or may blend with the contour of the navicular bone. Slight obliquity on the lateromedial projection alters the navicular bone's apparent shape.
9. Palmar process incisure.
10. Superimposed distal parts of the medial and lateral palmar processes on the distal phalanx.
11. Medial and lateral distal (solar) borders of the distal phalanx. On oblique projections, these borders may be separated farther.
12. Flexor surface of the distal phalanx, where the deep digital flexor attaches.
13. Semilunar line on the solar surface of the distal phalanx.
14. Opaque line representing the bone cortex on the concave solar surface of the distal phalanx.
15. Solar canal of the distal phalanx on end. This canal makes a semicircular loop in the distal phalanx, and its visibility depends on its size and the X-ray beam angle.
16. Dorsal surface of the distal phalanx.
17. Extensor process of the distal phalanx, which may have a single, double-humped, or pointed appearance. The surface should always be smooth.
18. Dorsal extent of the distal articular surface on the middle phalanx. The slight projection on the articular margin should not be mistaken for an osteophyte.
19. Eminences for collateral ligament attachments from the distal interphalangeal joint. They may be prominent or small, but their surface should be smooth; they should not be mistaken for periosteal bone production.
20. Extensor process of the middle phalanx.
21. Distal dorsal articular surface of the proximal phalanx.

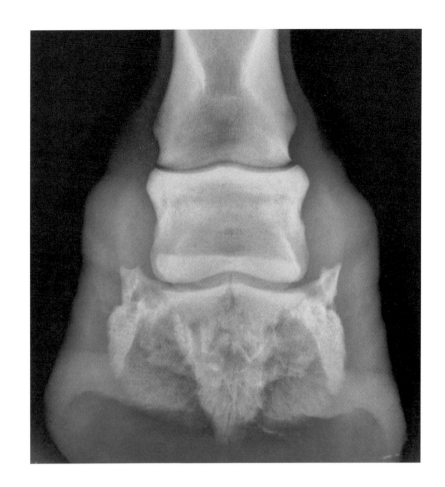

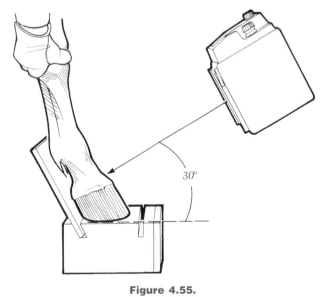

Figure 4.55.

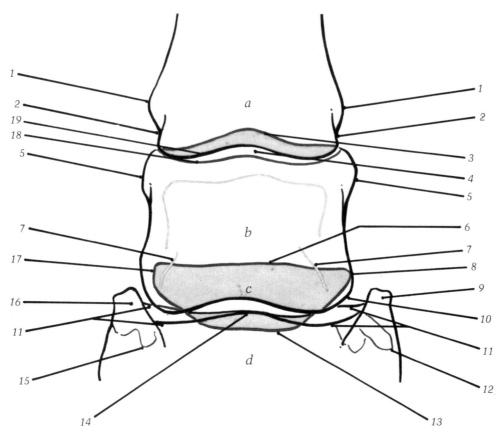

Figure 4.55. (*Continued*) Dorsoproximal-palmarodistal oblique (D30Pr-PaDiO) projection of the distal phalanges and navicular bone (foot). (a) Proximal phalanx, (b) middle phalanx, (c) navicular bone (distal sesamoid bone), (d) distal phalanx.

1. Medial and lateral eminences on the distal extremity of the middle phalanx for attachment of collateral ligaments.
2. Medial and lateral depressions for attachment of collateral ligaments.
3. Proximal palmar border of the middle phalanx.
4. Articular cartilage thickness in the proximal interphalangeal joint space, which is approximately half the thickness of the articular cartilage in the distal interphalangeal joint.
5. Medial and lateral eminences for ligamentous and tendinous attachments on the proximal palmar aspect of the middle phalanx.
6. Proximal border of the navicular bone, which is seen with the least amount of distortion on this projection. It should be straight, smooth, and distinct.
7. Dorsal eminences on the medial and lateral aspects of the middle phalanx for attachment of the collateral ligaments of the distal interphalangeal joint.
8. Medial extremity of the navicular bone, which is slightly more rounded in appearance than the lateral extremity.

9. Proximal part of the medial palmar process on the distal phalanx.
10. Medial aspect of the distal articular surface on the middle phalanx.
11. Proximal articular surface of the distal phalanx; palmar and dorsal borders.
12. Fossa on the palmar medial surface of the distal phalanx.
13. Distal palmar border of the navicular bone, which cannot be adequately evaluated on this projection because of superimposition over the distal interphalangeal joint.
14. Extensor process for the distal phalanx.
15. Fossa on palmar lateral surface of the distal phalanx.
16. Proximal part of the lateral palmar process, the size of which depends on the extent of ossification in the cartilages of the distal phalanx. Separate ossification centers may occur in this region and should not be mistaken for fracture fragments.
17. Lateral extremity of the navicular bone, which has a sharper angled appearance than the medial extremity.
18. Proximal articular surface (articular fovea) of the middle phalanx.
19. Distal articular surface of the proximal phalanx.

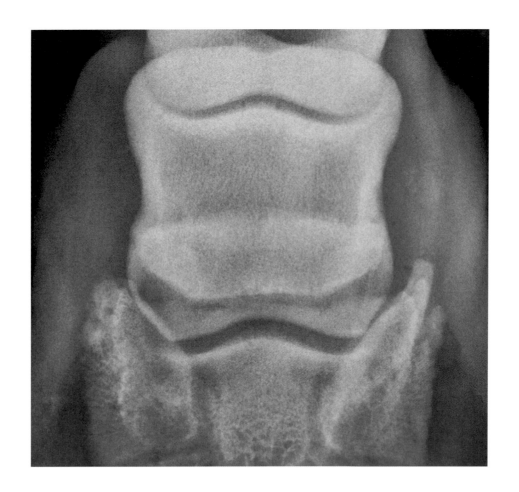

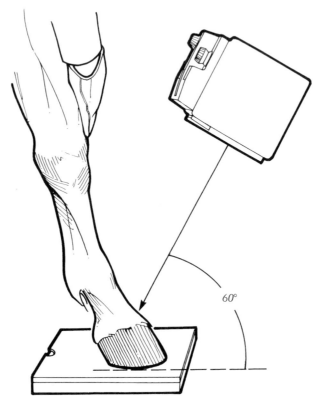

Figure 4.56.

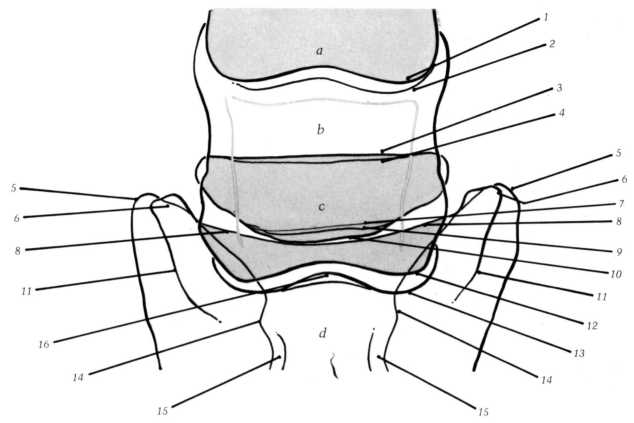

Figure 4.56. (*Continued*) Dorsoproximal-palmarodistal oblique (D60Pr-PaDiO) projection of the distal phalanx and navicular bone (foot). This projection is used extensively for evaluating the navicular bone. Position and exposure are critical for optimal visualization. (a) Proximal phalanx, (b) middle phalanx, (c) navicular bone (distal sesamoid bone), (d) distal phalanx.

1. Distal articular surface of the proximal phalanx.
2. Proximal articular surface of the middle phalanx.
3. Proximal border of the flexor surface on the navicular bone.
4. Proximal border of the articular surface on the navicular bone, which often looks indistinct and slightly irregular on this projection because of the projection angle of the X-ray beam.
5. Distal part of the medial and lateral palmar processes.
6. Proximal part of the medial and lateral palmar processes.
7. Groove on the distal navicular bone between the flexor and articular margins. Vascular foramina are in this groove.
8. Palmar articular margin of the distal phalanx.
9. Distal margin on the navicular bone.
10. Distal margin of the flexor surface on the navicular bone.
11. Medial and lateral parietal sulci on the distal phalanx.
12. Distal articular surface of the middle phalanx.
13. Articular border of the distal phalanx.
14. Medial and lateral solar grooves on the solar surface of the distal phalanx.
15. Solar canal.
16. Extensor process of the distal phalanx.

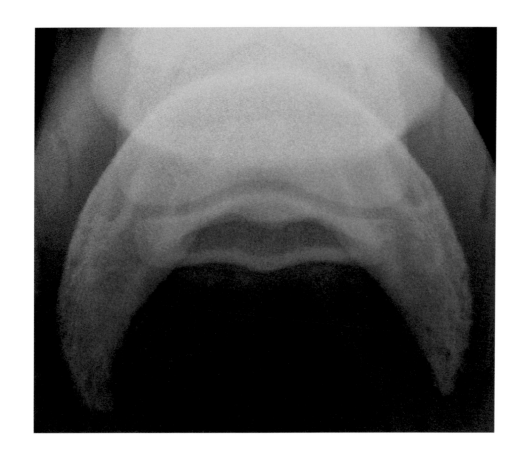

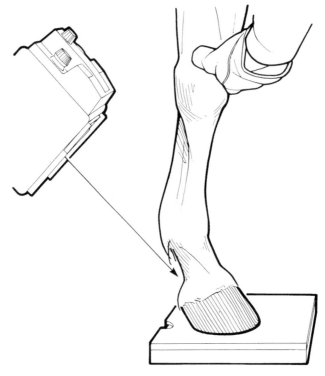

Figure 4.57.

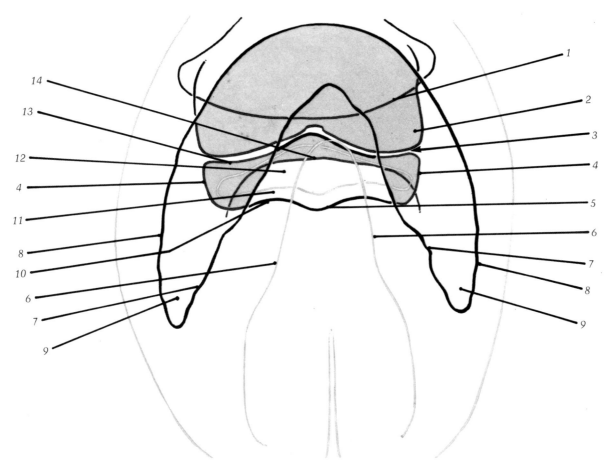

Figure 4.57. (*Continued*) Palmaroproximal-palmarodistal oblique (Pa45Pr-PaDiO) projection of the distal phalanx and navicular bone (foot). This projection shows the navicular bone with minimal superimposition over other bones. The angle of the X-ray beam and exposures are critical for eliminating projection artifacts, e.g., lack of good cortical and medullary cavity definition of superimposition of the distal phalanx over the navicular bone.

1. Palmar border of the middle phalanx.
2. Distal medial condyle of the middle phalanx.
3. Articulation between the navicular bone and the middle phalanx.
4. Medial and lateral extremities of the navicular bone.
5. Central eminence on the flexor surface of the navicular bone.
6. Collateral (paracureal) sulci of the frog.
7. Semilunar line on the solar surface of the distal phalanx.
8. Medial and lateral aspects of the solar border of the distal phalanx.
9. Distal part of the medial and lateral palmar processes.
10. Flexor surface of the navicular bone.
12. Medullary (spongiosa) cavity of the navicular bone.
13. Articular surface of the navicular bone.
14. Palmar articular border of the distal phalanx.

249

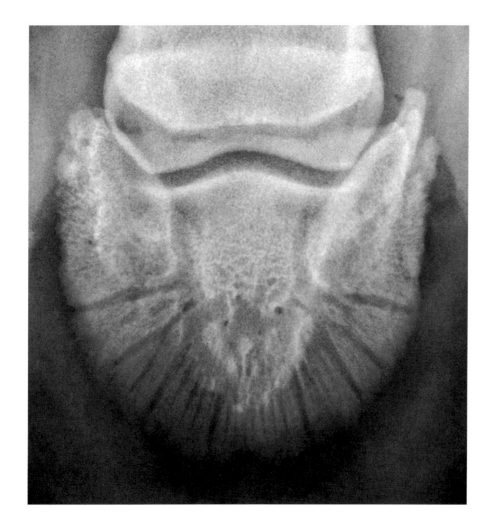

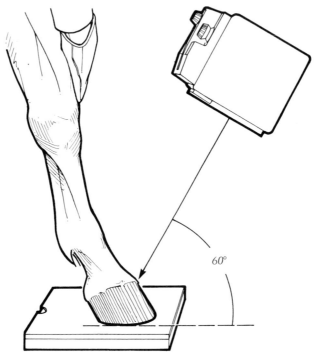

Figure 4.58.

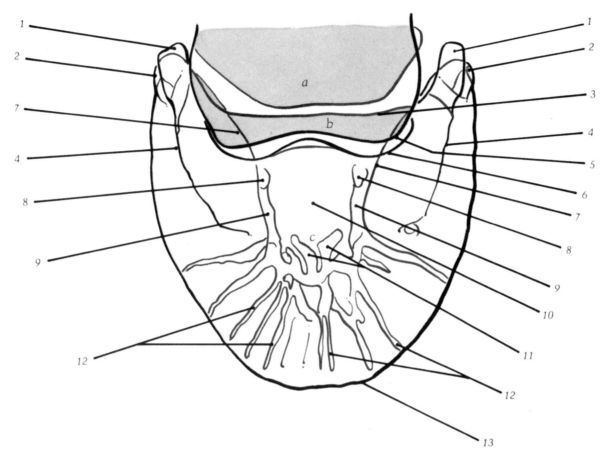

Figure 4.58. (*Continued*) Dorsoproximal-palmarodistal oblique (D60Pr-PaDiO) projection of the distal phalanx (foot). The X-ray beam for this projection is centered at the coronet, and the exposure is half that necessary for visualizing the navicular bone. (a) Navicular bone (distal sesamoidean bone), (b) middle phalanx, (c) distal phalanx.

1. Proximal part of the medial and lateral palmar processes.
2. Distal part of the medial and lateral palmar processes.
3. Palmar articular margin of the distal phalanx.
4. Medial and lateral parietal sulci on the distal phalanx.
5. Distal articular surface of the middle phalanx.
6. Proximal dorsal margin of the articular surface of the distal phalanx.
7. Borders of the medial and lateral solar grooves.
8. Medial and lateral solar foramina.
9. Solar canal, the width and distinctness of which are variable in normal distal phalanges.
10. Flexor surface of the distal phalanx, where the deep digital flexor tendon attaches.
11. Vascular canals in the region of the solar canal.
12. Peripheral vascular canals. The vascular canals may be of variable width in normal distal phalanges. The peripheral solar border of the distal phalanx should be relatively smooth and symmetrical, although a slight irregular peripheral border may be considered normal in older animals.
13. Distal solar margin of the distal phalanx. The normal distal border of the distal phalanx may be convex or have some degree of concavity. A middistal notch, when present, is the crena marginis solaris.

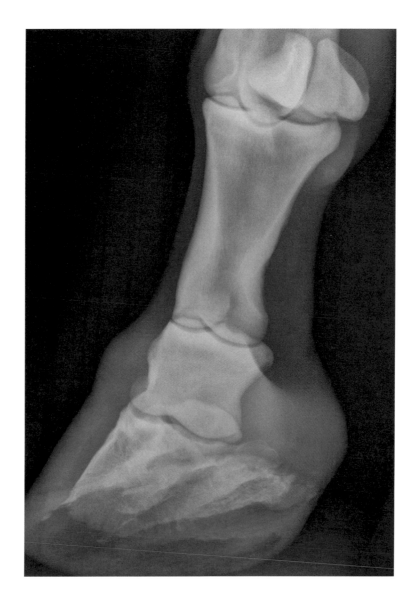

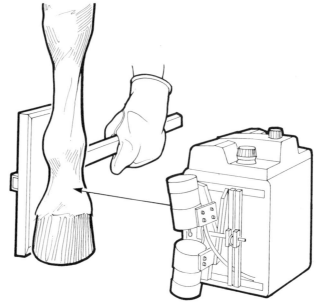

Figure 4.59.

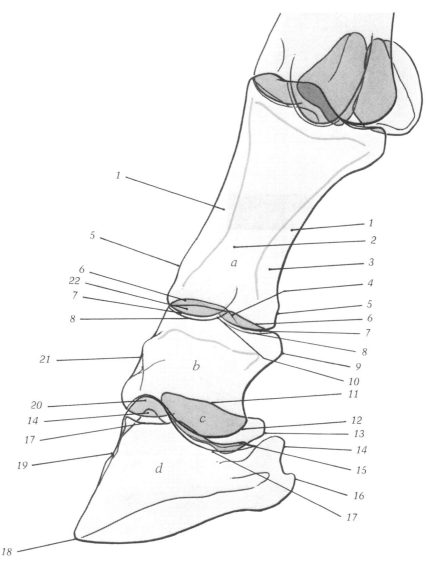

Figure 4.59. (*Continued*) Dorsomedial-palmarolateral oblique (D35M-PaLO) projection of the phalanges. (a) Proximal phalanx, (b) middle phalanx, (c) navicular bone, (d) distal phalanx.

1. Mediopalmar and dorsolateral cortices of the proximal phalanx.
2. Medullary cavity of the proximal phalanx, which can sometimes be distinctly seen as a 2- to 3-cm lucency in the center of the proximal phalanx.
3. Surface for attachment of the middle (oblique) distal sesamoidean ligament.
4. Sagittal ridge on the proximal articular surface of the middle phalanx.
5. Eminences for attachment of the medial and lateral collateral ligaments of the proximal interphalangeal joint on the distal aspect of the proximal phalanx.
6. Palmar border of the articular fovea on the base of the middle phalanx.
7. Medial and lateral condyles of the distal aspect of the proximal phalanx.
8. Articular fovea on the base of the middle phalanx.
9. Medial proximal eminence for attachment of the medial collateral ligament and the medial branch of the tendon of the superficial digital flexor on the middle phalanx.

10. Sagittal ridge between the fovea on the base of the middle phalanx.
11. Proximal border of the navicular bone.
12. Distal medial condyle of the middle phalanx.
13. Medial extremity of navicular bone.
14. Proximal part of the medial palmar process of the distal phalanx.
15. Palmar part of the medial palmar process of the distal phalanx.
16. Distal part of the medial palmar process of the distal phalanx.
17. Medial and lateral aspects of the coronary border of the articular surface on the distal phalanx.
18. Solar border of the distal phalanx.
19. Depression and bony prominence on the lateral parietal surface of the distal phalanx for lateral collateral ligament attachment. The bony prominence has a smooth surface and should not be mistaken for bone production.
20. Extensor process of the distal phalanx.
21. Eminence on the dorsal surface of the middle phalanx for collateral ligament attachment, which has a smooth surface and should not be mistaken for periosteal bone production.
22. Dorsolateral articular border on the middle phalanx.

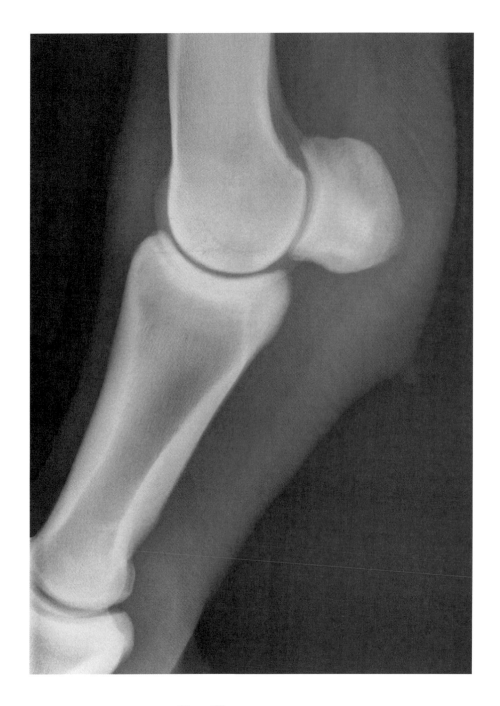

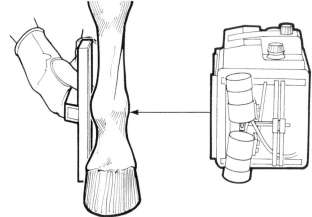

Figure 4.60.

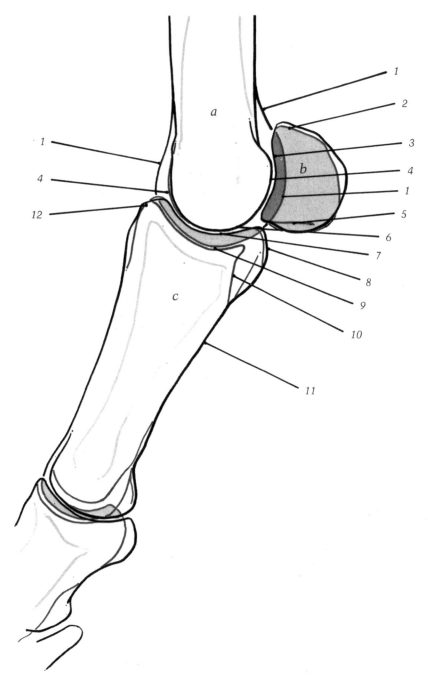

Figure 4.60. (*Continued*) Lateromedial (LM) projection of the metacarpophalangeal joint. (a) Third metacarpophalangeal bone, (b) proximal sesamoid bone, (c) proximal phalanx.

1. Sagittal ridge on the distal extremity of the third metacarpal bone.
2. Apex of the superimposed proximal sesamoid bones.
3. Articular surface of the proximal sesamoid bones.
4. Articular surface of the superimposed medial and lateral condyles of the third metacarpal bone.
5. Superimposed base of the proximal sesamoid bones.
6. Transverse ridge on the distal articular surface of the third metacarpal bone, which divides the distal metacarpal articular surface into dorsal and palmar areas. It varies in size and visibility.
7. Superimposed medial and lateral articular fovea of the proximal phalanx.
8. Superimposed medial and lateral tuberosities on the proximal caudal aspect of the proximal phalanx for ligamentous attachment.
9. Sagittal groove on the proximal articular surface of the proximal phalanx, which articulates with the sagittal ridge of the third metacarpal bone.
10. Midpalmar surface of the proximal phalanx located between the lateral and medial tuberosities.
11. Palmar surface of the proximal phalanx, where the middle (oblique) distal sesamoidean ligament attaches.
12. Superimposed medial and lateral bony eminences for attachment of the extensor tendon on the proximal phalanx.

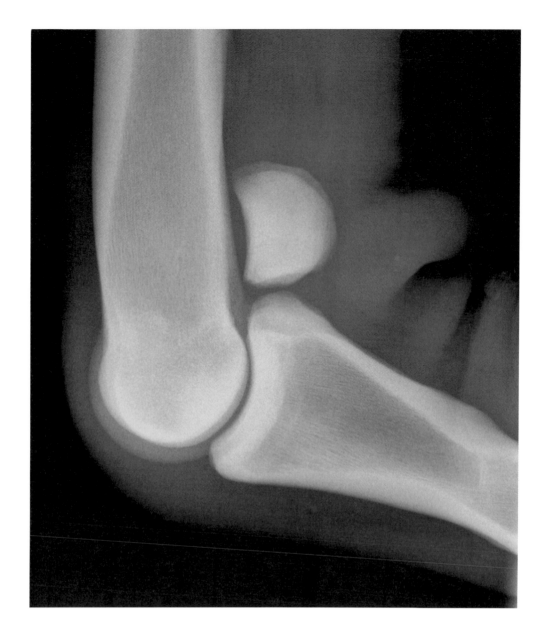

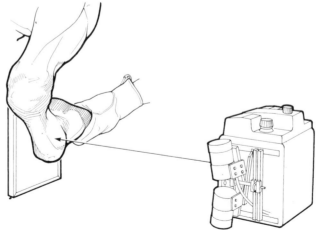

Figure 4.61.

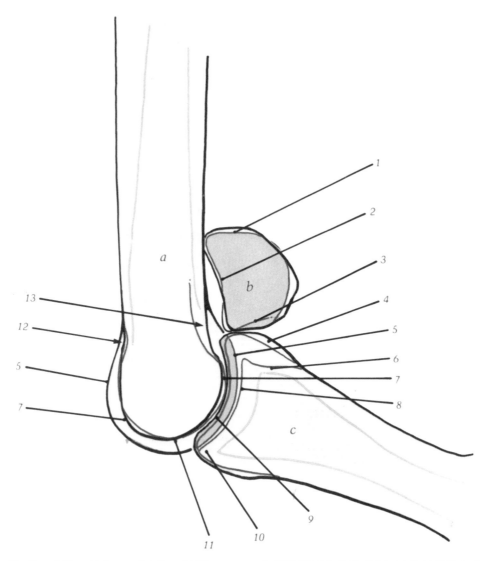

Figure 4.61. (*Continued*) Flexed lateromedial (flexed LM) projection of the metacarpophalangeal joint. This projection allows the most effective evaluation of the articular surface of the sesamoid bones, offers good visualization of small articular basilar sesamoid fractures and changes, and provides a distinct projection of the proximal tuberosities. Furthermore, the dorsal articular surface of the third metacarpal bone can be evaluated without superimposition of the proximal phalanx. (a) Third metacarpal bone, (b) proximal sesamoid bones, (c) proximal phalanx.

1. Apex of the superimposed proximal sesamoid bones.
2. Superimposed articular surfaces of the proximal sesamoid bones.
3. Bases of the superimposed proximal sesamoid bones.
4. Superimposed medial and lateral tuberosities on the proximal caudal aspect of the proximal phalanx, where ligamentous attachments occur.
5. Sagittal ridge on the distal articular surface of the third metacarpal bone; the dorsal and palmar aspects are labeled.
6. Midpalmar surface of the proximal phalanx, located between the medial and lateral tuberosities.
7. Palmar and dorsal aspects of the superimposed medial and lateral condyles of the third metacarpal bone.
8. Sagittal groove on the proximal articular surface of the proximal phalanx, which articulates with the sagittal ridge on the distal third metacarpal bone.
9. Superimposed fovea (articular surface) of the proximal extremity of the proximal phalanx.
10. Superimposed medial and lateral parts of the extensor eminence of the proximal phalanx.
11. Transverse ridge on the distal articular surface of the third metacarpal bone, which separates the distal articular surface of the third metacarpal bone into dorsal and palmar parts.
12. Bony depression where the proximal dorsal recess from the metacarpophalangeal joint is located.
13. Bony depression where the proximal palmar recess from the metacarpophalangeal joint is located.

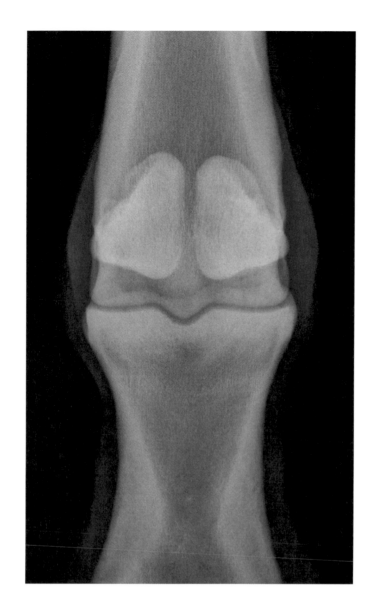

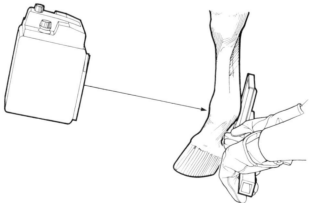

Figure 4.62.

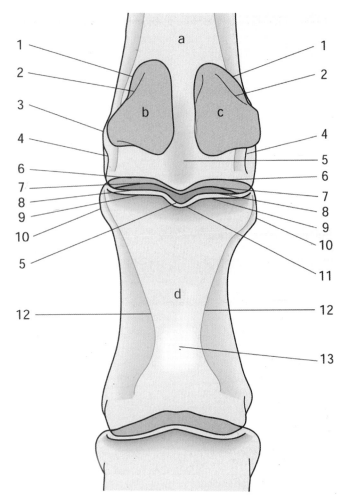

Figure 4.62. (*Continued*) Dorsoproximal-palmarodistal (D30Pr-PaDi) projection of the metacarpophalangeal joint. (a) Third metacarpal bone, (b) lateral proximal sesamoid bone, (c) medial proximal sesamoid bone, (d) proximal phalanx.

1. Peripheral abaxial margins of the proximal sesamoid bones. The peripheral margin of the medial proximal sesamoid bone is more convex than that of the lateral proximal sesamoid bone.
2. Abaxial margin of the surfaces of the medial and lateral proximal sesamoid bone.
3. Eminence for attachment of the lateral collateral ligament.
4. Depression on the medial and lateral aspects of the third metacarpal bone where collateral ligaments attach.
5. Sagittal ridge on the distal articular surface of the third metacarpal bone.

6. Medial and lateral palmar margins of the articular fovea on the proximal extremity of the proximal phalanx.
7. Medial and lateral dorsal margins of the articular fovea on the proximal extremity of the proximal phalanx.
8. Medial and lateral condyles (articular surface) of the third metacarpal bone.
9. Articular fovea on the proximal extremity of the proximal phalanx.
10. Medial and lateral palmar tuberosities on the proximal extremity of the proximal phalanx for ligament attachment.
11. Sagittal groove on the proximal articular surface of the proximal phalanx.
12. Bony ridges on the palmar surface of the proximal phalanx for attachment of the middle (oblique) distal sesamoidean ligament.
13. Medullary cavity in the proximal phalanx.

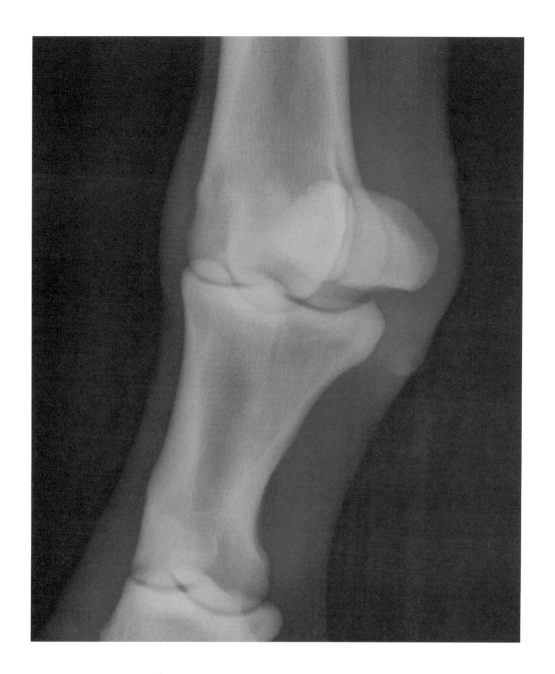

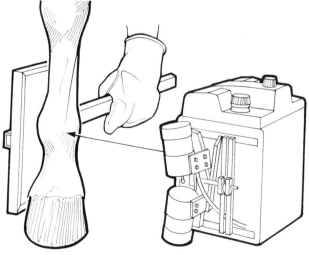

Figure 4.63.

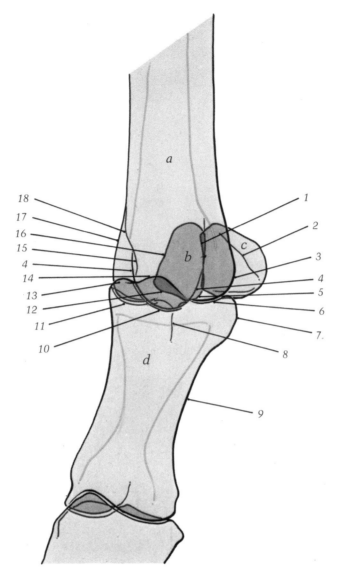

Figure 4.63. (*Continued*) Dorsolateral-palmaromedial oblique (D45L-PaMO) projection of the metacarpophalangeal joint.
(a) Third metacarpal bone, (b) medial proximal sesamoid bone, (c) lateral proximal sesamoid bone, (d) proximal phalanx.

1. Articular surface of the lateral proximal sesamoid bone.
2. The difference in radiographic opacity is caused by a difference in bone thickness on the lateral proximal sesamoid bone. The base and body are more opaque than the apex and peripheral border. The convex shape on the abaxial surface produces the distinct line between the two opacities.
3. Palmar surface of the lateral condyle distal aspect of the third metacarpal bone.
4. Palmar and dorsal aspects of the sagittal ridge on the distal third metacarpal bone.
5. Junction of the peripheral and basilar margins of the medial proximal sesamoid bone.
6. Lateral articular fovea of the proximal extremity of the proximal sesamoid bone.
7. Lateral tuberosity on the proximal palmar aspect of the proximal phalanx.
8. Medial tuberosity on the proximal palmar aspect of the proximal phalanx.
9. Lateral bony ridge for attachment of the middle (oblique) distal sesamoidean ligament.

10. Sagittal groove on the proximal articular surface of the proximal phalanx.
11. Medial articular fovea of the proximal extremity of the proximal phalanx.
12. Basilar margin of the medial proximal sesamoid bone.
13. Medial dorsal margin of the articular fovea on the proximal phalanx.
14. Lateral dorsal margin of the articular fovea on the proximal phalanx. Both margins (13, 14) are visible on correctly exposed and positioned oblique projections of the metacarpophalangeal joint.
15. Depression (concave surface) for attachment of the medial collateral ligament on the distal third metacarpal bone. The visibility and distinctness of the concave line change on different projections. It may be more prominent on some examinations and not visible on others.
16. Abaxial articular margin of the medial proximal sesamoid bone.
17. Dorsal aspect of the medial condyle on the third metacarpal bone.
18. Eminence on the third metacarpal bone for attachment of the medial collateral ligament.

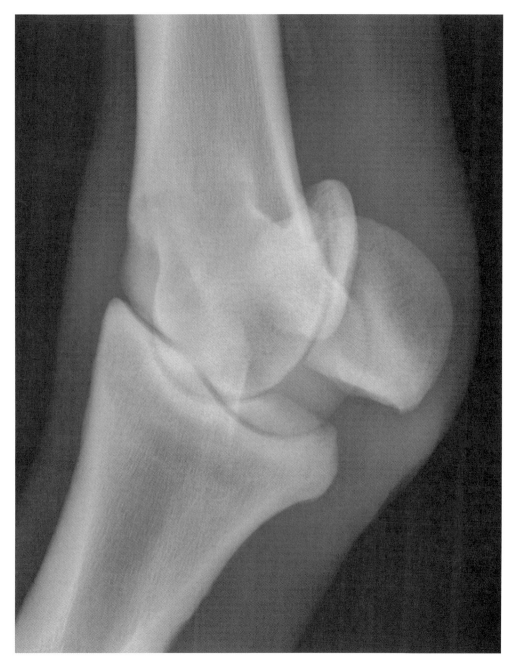

Figure 4.64.

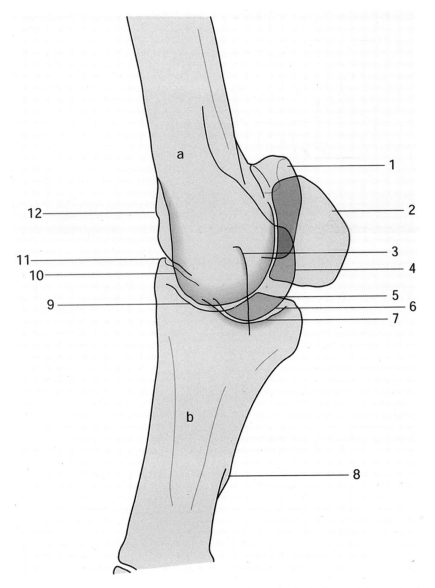

Figure 4.64. (*Continued*) Lateroproximodorsal-mediodistopalmar oblique (L20Pr20D-MDiPaO) projection of the metacarpophalangeal joint. (a) Third metacarpal bone, (b) proximal phalanx.

1. Medial proximal sesamoid bone.
2. Peripheral margin of the lateral proximal sesamoid bone.
3. Medial proximal palmar border of the proximal phalanx.
4. Lateral condyle of the third metacarpal bone.
5. Lateral palmar eminence of the proximal phalanx.
6. Lateral condyle (articular surface) of the third metacarpal bone.
7. Lateral articular fovea of the proximal phalanx.
8. Bony ridge for attachment of the middle (oblique) distal sesamoidean ligament.
9. Sagittal groove on the proximal articular surface of the proximal phalanx.
10. Distal surface of the sagittal ridge of the third metacarpal bone.
11. Medial articular margin of the articular fovea on the proximal phalanx.
12. Dorsal border of the medial condyle of the third metacarpal bone.

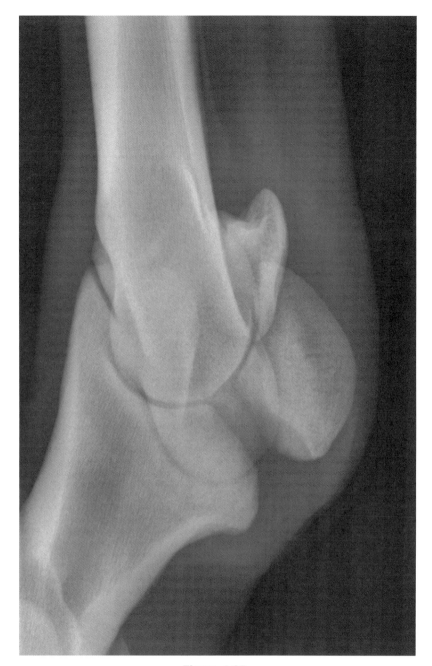

Figure 4.65.

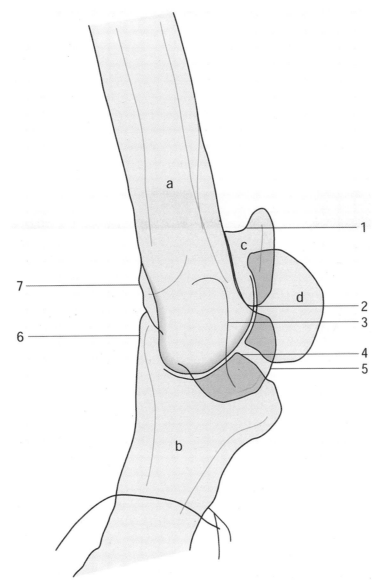

Figure 4.65. (*Continued*) Lateroproximal-distomedial oblique (L45P-DiMO) projection of the metacarpophalangeal joint. (a) Third metacarpal bone, (b) proximal phalanx, (c) medial proximal sesamoid bone, (d) lateral proximal sesamoid bone.

1. Abaxial surface of the medial proximal sesamoid bone.
2. Palmar surface of the sagittal ridge of the third metacarpal bone.
3. Medial proximal border of the proximal phalanx.
4. Lateral palmar eminence of the proximal phalanx.
5. Lateral condyle of the third metacarpal bone.
6. Proximal medial surface of the proximal phalanx.
7. Dorsal border of the medial condyle of the third metacarpal bone.

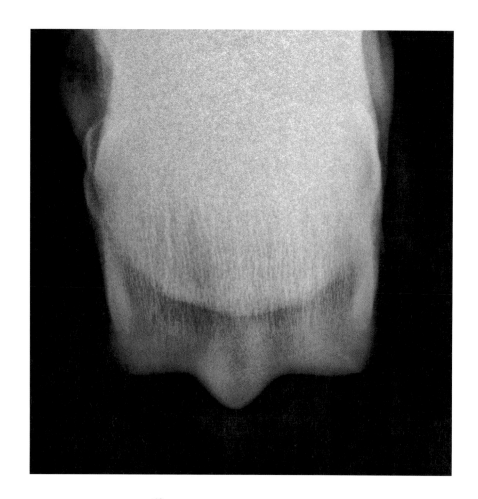

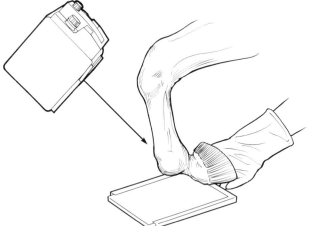

Figure 4.66.

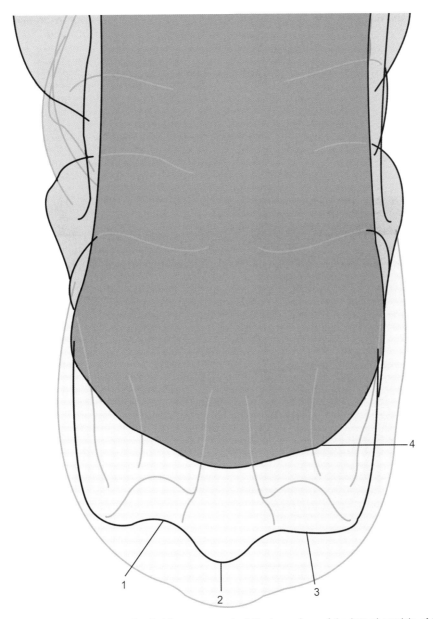

Figure 4.66. (*Continued*) Dorsoproximal-dorsodistal oblique (D45–70Pr-DDiO) projection of the metacarpophalangeal joint. In this projection, the flexed fetlock joint is held on top of the detector. The primary X-ray beam is directed distally in a 45° to 70° dorso-proximal dorso-distal direction and is centered on the dorsal aspect of the mid sagittal ridge of metacarpus/metatarsus for evaluation of the dorsal articular surface of the condyle of MCIII/MTIII.

1. Articular surface of the lateral condyle of the third metacarpal bone.
2. Sagittal ridge on the distal articular surface of the third metacarpal bone.
3. Articular surface of the medial condyle of the third metacarpal bone.
4. Proximal dorsal aspect of the proximal phalanx.

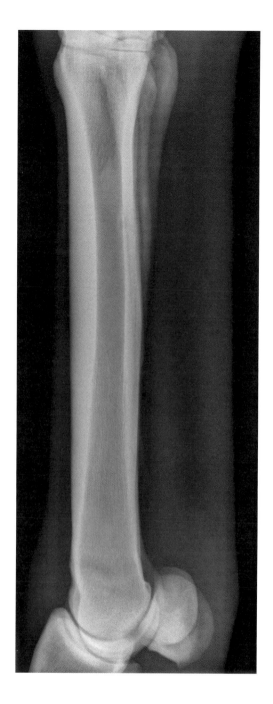

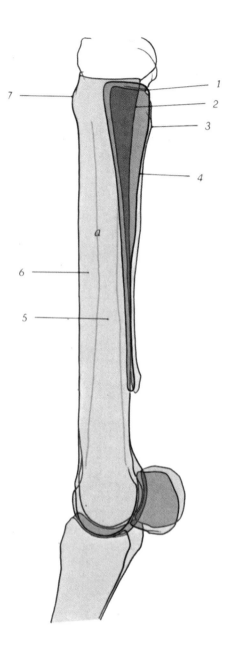

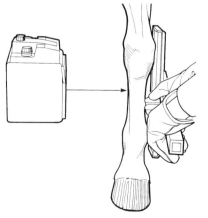

Figure 4.67. Lateromedial (LM) projection of the metacarpus. (a) Third metacarpal bone.

1. Articulation between the second carpal and the second metacarpal bone.
2. Proximal palmar surface of the third metacarpal bone, where the suspensory ligament (interosseus muscle) attaches. The nutrient foramen is frequently present on the palmar surface of the third metacarpal bone at approximately the junction of the proximal and middle thirds; it may be mistaken for a nondisplaced cortical fracture.
3. Palmar surface of the second metacarpal bone.
4. Palmar aspect of the fourth metacarpal bone. The superimposition of the cortices on the metacarpal bones produces longitudinal lucent lines that may be mistaken for longitudinal fractures.
5. Medullary cavity of the third metacarpal bone.
6. Dorsal cortex of the third metacarpal bone, which is fusiform in shape, i.e., thick in the center and thin toward both extremities.
7. Metacarpal tuberosity.

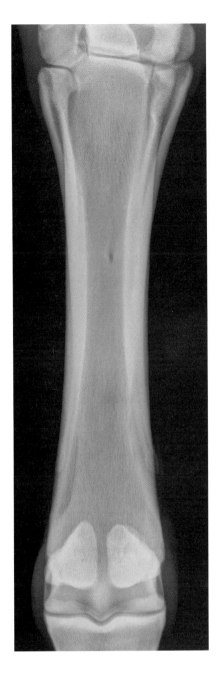

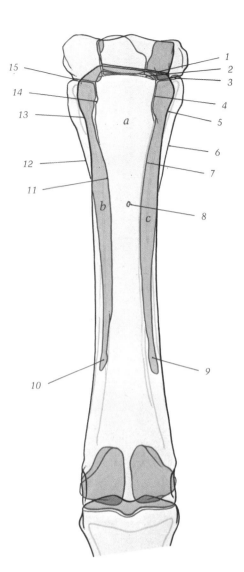

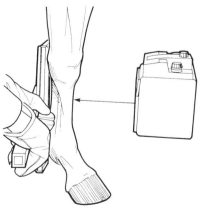

Figure 4.68. Dorsopalmar (DPa) projection of the metacarpus. (a) Third metacarpal bone, (b) fourth metacarpal bone, (c) second metacarpal bone.

1. Dorsal aspect of the articulation between the third carpal and the third metacarpal bone.
2. Palmar aspect of the articulation between the third carpal and the third metacarpal bone.
3. Articulation between the second carpal and the second metacarpal bone.
4. Articulation between the second and third metacarpal bones.
5. Medioproximal border of the third metacarpal bone.
6. Abaxial border of the second metacarpal bone.
7. Axial border of the second metacarpal bone.
8. End-on projection of the nutrient foramen on the palmar surface of the third metacarpal bone.
9. Distal extent of the second metacarpal bone. The normal shape and position of this bone may be variable. The position may vary in axial and abaxial direction and in proximal or distal direction.
10. Distal extent of the fourth metacarpal bone. The normal shape and position of this bone may be variable. The position may vary in axial and abaxial direction and in proximal or distal direction.
11. Axial border of the fourth metacarpal bone.
12. Abaxial border of the fourth metacarpal bone.
13. Lateral border of the third metacarpal bone.
14. Articulation between the third and fourth metacarpal bones.
15. Articulation between the fourth carpal and the fourth metacarpal bone.

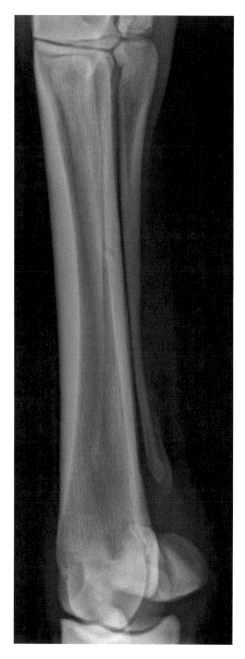

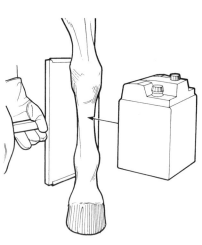

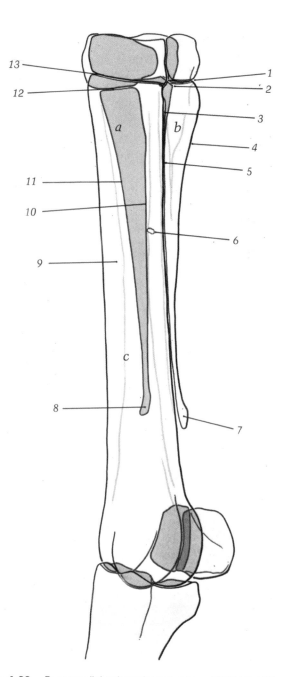

Figure 4.69. Dorsomedial-palmarolateral oblique (D55M-PaLO) projection of the metacarpus. (a) Fourth metacarpal bone, (b) second metacarpal bone, (c) third metacarpal bone.

1. Articulation between the second carpal and the second metacarpal bone.
2. Proximal palmar medial angle of the third metacarpal bone.
3. Junction between the second and third metacarpal bones.
4. Palmar border of the second metacarpal bone.
5. Dorsal border of the second metacarpal bone.
6. Nutrient foramen on the palmar surface of the third metacarpal bone.
7. Distal end of the second metacarpal bone.
8. Distal end of the fourth metacarpal bone.
9. Dorsolateral cortex of the third metacarpal bone.
10. Palmar surface of the fourth metacarpal bone.
11. Dorsal surface of the fourth metacarpal bone.
12. Articulation between the fourth carpal and the fourth metacarpal bone.
13. Articulation between the third carpal and the third metacarpal bone.

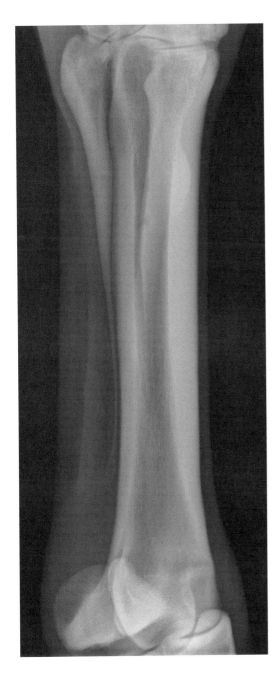

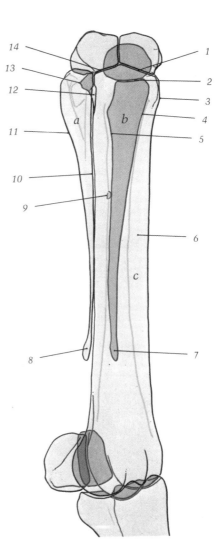

Figure 4.70. Dorsolateral-palmaromedial oblique (D55L-PaMO) projection of the metacarpus. (a) Fourth metacarpal bone, (b) second metacarpal bone, (c) third metacarpal bone.

1. Articulation between the third carpal and the third metacarpal bone.
2. Articulation between the second carpal and the second metacarpal bone.
3. Metacarpal tuberosity on the dorsomedial surface of the proximal extremity of the third metacarpal bone.
4. Dorsal border of the second metacarpal bone.
5. Palmar border of the second metacarpal bone.
6. Dorsomedial cortex of the third metacarpal bone. The dorsal cortex is normally thick, and the periosteal surface of the cortex should be straight and smooth.
7. Distal end of the second metacarpal bone which may vary in size, shape, and position.
8. Distal ends of the fourth metacarpal bone which may vary in size, shape, and position.
9. Nutrient foramen on the palmar surface of the third metacarpal bone, which may be prominent or not visualized, depending on its size and the projection.
10. Dorsal border of the fourth metacarpal bone.
11. Palmar border of the fourth metacarpal bone.
12. Articulation between the third and fourth metacarpal bones, the visualization of which depends on the incident angle of the primary X-ray beam.
13. Proximal-palmar-lateral angle of the third metacarpal bone.
14. Articulation between the fourth carpal and the third metacarpal bone.

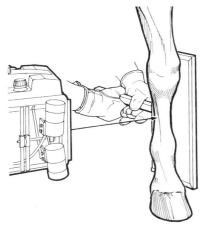

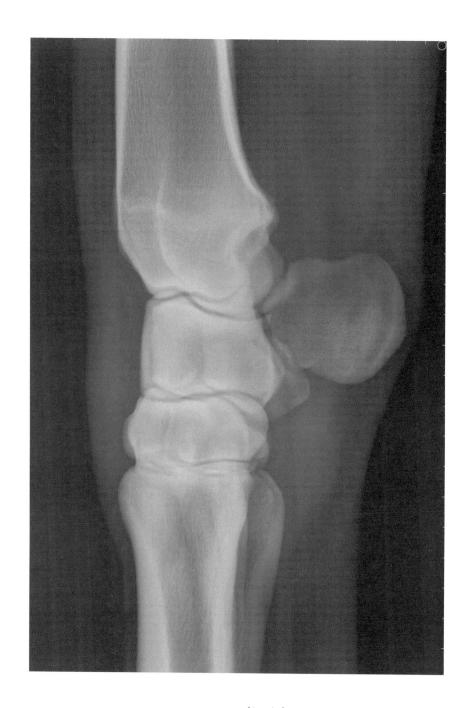

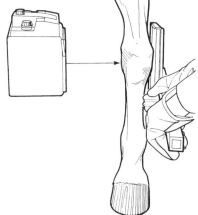

Figure 4.71.

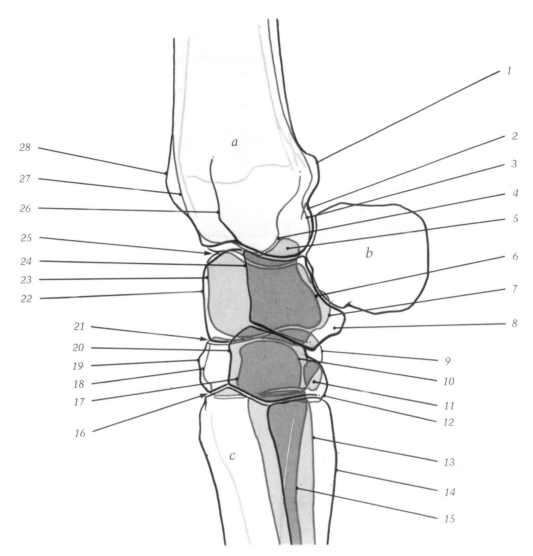

Figure 4.71. (*Continued*) Lateromedial (LM) projection of the carpus. The relative positions of the bony ridges of the distal cranial radius depend on the X-ray beam projection angle. (a) Radius, (b) accessory carpal bone, (c) third metacarpal bone.

1. Transverse crest, which projects caudad from the closed distal radial physis.
2. Lateral facet of the radial trochlea (lateral styloid process), which articulates with the ulnar carpal bone.
3. Medial facet of the radial trochlea (medial styloid process), which articulates with the radial carpal bone.
4. Intermediate facet of the radial trochlea, which articulates with the intermediate carpal bone.
5. Tuberosity from the proximal palmar aspect of the intermediate carpal bone.
6. Palmar border of the intermediate carpal bone.
7. Palmar border of the radial carpal bone.
8. Palmar border of the ulnar carpal bone. The position of 6, 7, and 8 may change with slight changes in angulation of the X-ray tube or the horse's limb.
9. Palmar border of the third carpal bone.
10. Palmar border of the second carpal bone.
11. First carpal bone, which sometimes is not present.

12. Palmar border of the fourth carpal bone.
13. Proximal palmar border of the second metacarpal bone.
14. Proximal palmar border fourth metacarpal bone.
15. Proximal palmar border of the third metacarpal bone.
16. Carpometacarpal joint.
17. Dorsal border of the second carpal bone.
18. Dorsal border of the third carpal bone.
19. Transverse ridge on the dorsal border of the third carpal bone, which projects with varying degrees of prominence in each horse.
20. Dorsal border of the fourth carpal bone.
21. Midcarpal joint.
22. Dorsal border of the radial carpal bone.
23. Dorsal border of the intermediate carpal bone.
24. Dorsal border of the ulnar carpal bone.
25. Antebrachiocarpal (radiocarpal) joint.
26. Lateral bony ridge of the distal cranial radius, adjacent to the common digital extensor tendon.
27. Bony ridge of the distal cranial radius, adjacent to the medial border of the extensor carpi radialis tendon.
28. Bony ridge of the distal cranial radius between the common digital extensor tendon and the extensor carpi radialis tendon.

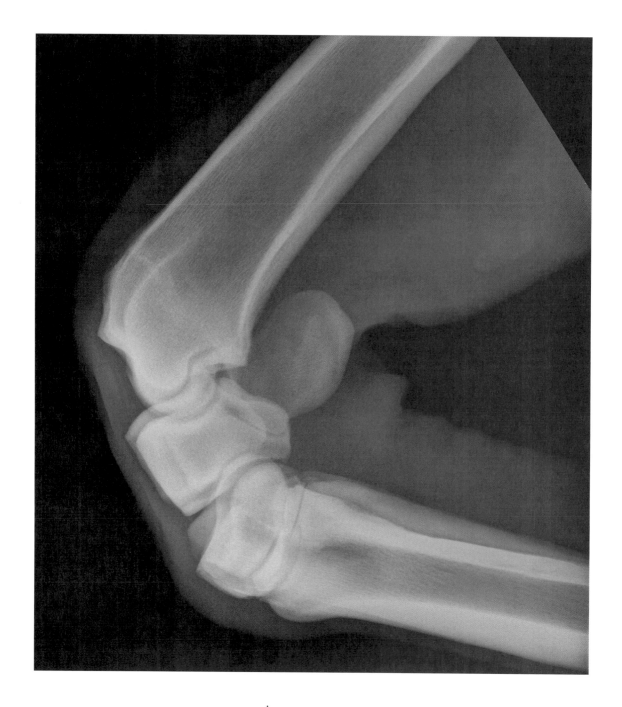

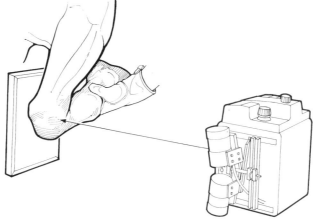

Figure 4.72.

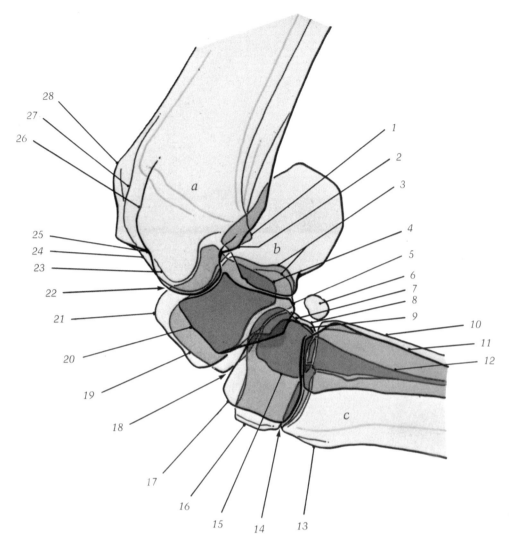

Figure 4.72. (*Continued*) Flexed lateromedial (flexed LM) projection of the carpus. The size and shape of the first and fifth carpal bones may vary, and sometimes the bones are absent. The palmar borders of the carpal and metacarpal bones are closely superimposed in this projection, and the positions may vary slightly with X-ray tube angulation and/or the horse's limb positions. Projection of the bony ridges and facets of the radial trochlea may vary with the positions of the limb and the angle of the X-ray beam. (a) Radius, (b) accessory carpal bone, (c) third metacarpal bone.

1. Transverse crest, which projects from the caudal aspect of the closed distal radial physis.
2. Ridges produced by the caudal aspect of the medial (medial styloid process) and lateral (lateral styloid process) parts of the radial trochlea.
3. Palmar border of the radial carpal bone.
4. Palmar border of the intermediate carpal bone.
5. Palmar border of the ulnar carpal bone.
6. First carpal bone.
7. Palmar border of the fourth carpal bone.
8. Palmar border of the third carpal bone.
9. Palmar border of the second carpal bone.
10. Proximal palmar border of the second metacarpal bone.
11. Proximal palmar border of the fourth metacarpal bone.
12. Proximal palmar border of the third metacarpal bone.
13. Metacarpal tuberosity which may vary in prominence.

14. Carpometacarpal joint. Numerous joint space lines are produced by the irregular contour of the bones forming this joint.
15. Dorsal border of the second carpal bone.
16. Dorsal border of the third carpal bone.
17. Dorsal border of the fourth carpal bone. The proximal dorsal aspect of the fourth carpal bone (17) projects proximal to the third carpal bone (16) on the flexed lateral projection.
18. Middle carpal joint.
19. Dorsal border of the radial carpal bone.
20. Dorsal borders of the ulnar carpal bone.
21. Dorsal borders of the intermediate carpal bone. The dorsal borders of the radial (19) and intermediate (21) carpal bones are closely superimposed and may vary slightly. The intermediate carpal bone usually projects proximal to the radial carpal bone on the flexed lateral projection.
22. Antebrachiocarpal (radiocarpal) joint.
23. Intermediate facet of the radial trochlea, which articulates with the intermediate carpal bone (21).
24. Medial border of the radial trochlea.
25. Lateral border of the radial trochlea.
26. Lateral bony ridge adjacent to the lateral border of the common digital extensor tendon.
27. Bony ridge adjacent to the medial border of the extensor carpi radialis.
28. Bony ridge between the lateral digital extensor tendon and the extensor carpi radialis tendon.

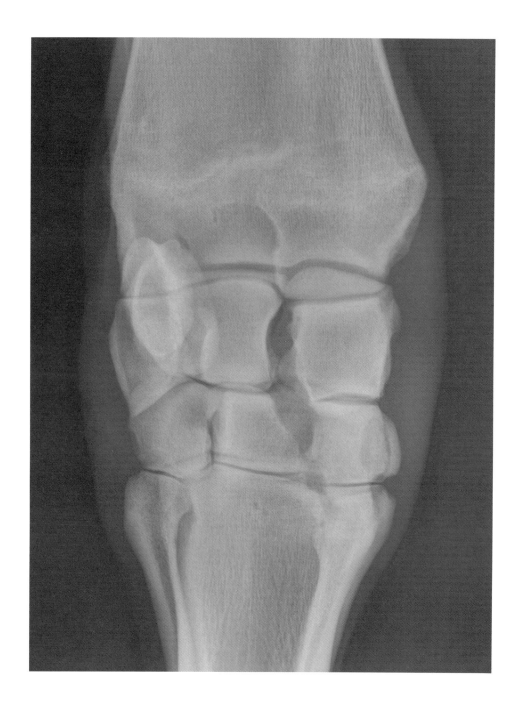

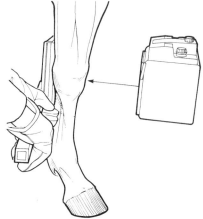

Figure 4.73.

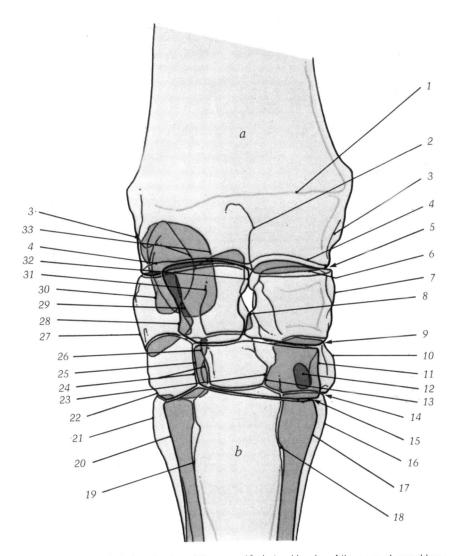

Figure 4.73. (*Continued*) Dorsopalmar (DPa) projection of the carpus. (a) Radius, (b) third metacarpal bone.

1. Physeal scar in the distal extremity of the radius after physeal closure.
2. Caudolateral border of the medial facet (medial styloid process) on the radial trochlea.
3. Depression in the medial and lateral styloid processes for attachment of medial and lateral collateral ligaments. Their appearances and apparent depths can changes with a slight obliqueness of the limb.
4. Cranial articular margin on the distal radius.
5. Antebrachiocarpal (radiocarpal) joint.
6. Medial facet (medial styloid process) on the distal radial trochlea, which articulates with the radial carpal bone (7 and 8).
7. Medial border of the radial carpal bone.
8. Lateral border of the radial carpal bone.
9. Midcarpal joint. The different levels of the joint space are the result of many bones forming the articular surfaces and of slight angulation of the X-ray tube or positions of the horse's limb.
10. Medial border of the second carpal bone.
11. Dorsomedial border of the third carpal bone.
12. First carpal bone superimposed over the second and third carpal bone.
13. Lateral border of the second carpal bone.
14. Palmar aspect of the carpometacarpal joint space.
15. Dorsal aspect of the carpometacarpal joint space.
16. Proximomedial border of the second metacarpal bone.
17. Proximomedial border of the third metacarpal bone.
18. Articulation between the second and third metacarpal bones.
19. Articulation between the third and fourth metacarpal bones.
20. Lateral border of the third metacarpal bone.
21. Lateral border of the fourth metacarpal bone.
22. Lateral border of the fourth carpal bone.
23. Medial border of the palmar process on the third carpal bone.
24. Medial border of the fourth carpal bone.
25. Dorsolateral border of the third carpal bone.
26. Lateral border of the palmar process on the third carpal bone.
27. Lateral border of the ulnar carpal bone.
28. Lateral border of the intermediate carpal bone.
29. Medial border of the ulnar carpal bone.
30. Lateral border of the accessory carpal bone.
31. Lateral border of the palmar tuberosity on the intermediate carpal bone.
32. Medial border of the intermediate carpal bone.
33. Concave medial surface of the accessory carpal bone.

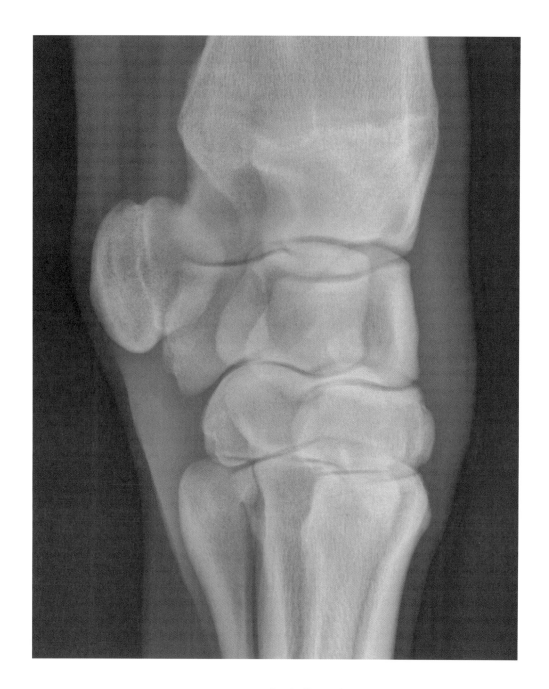

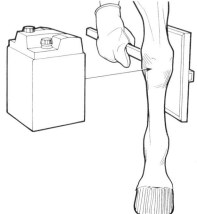

Figure 4.74.

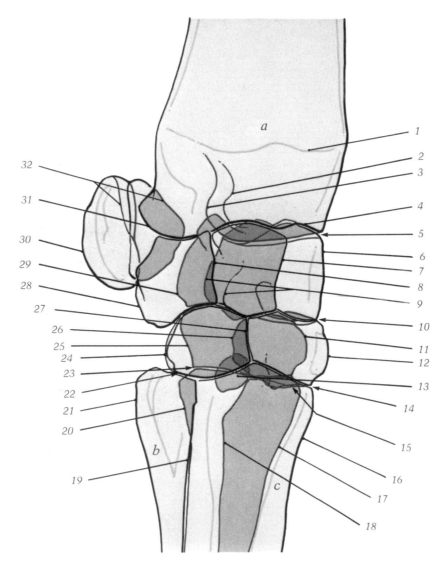

Figure 4.74. (*Continued*) Dorsolateral-palmaromedial oblique (D45L-PaMO) projection of the carpus. (a) Radius, (b) fourth metacarpal bone, (c) third metacarpal bone.

1. Physeal scar remaining after distal radial physeal closure.
2. Caudal aspect of the intermediate facet on the radial trochlea.
3. Caudal aspect of the medial facet (medial styloid process) on the radial trochlea.
4. Cranial articular margin on the radial trochlea.
5. Dorsomedial aspect of the antebrachiocarpal (radiocarpal) joint.
6. Dorsomedial border of the radial carpal bone.
7. Dorsomedial border of the intermediate carpal bone.
8. Dorsomedial border of the ulnar carpal bone.
9. Tubercles on the palmar surface of the radiocarpal bone.
10. Dorsomedial aspect of the midcarpal joint.
11. Dorsomedial border of the second carpal bone.
12. Transverse ridge on the dorsomedial border of the third carpal bone.
13. First carpal bone, which is difficult to see on this projection because of superimposition.
14. Medial aspect of the carpometacarpal joint.
15. Dorsal aspect of the carpometacarpal joint. The multiple joint spaces are associated with the carpometacarpal joint and vary in appearance on different projection angles.
16. Dorsomedial border of the third metacarpal bone.
17. Dorsomedial border of the second metacarpal bone.
18. Palmarolateral border of the second metacarpal bones.
19. Dorsomedial border of the fourth metacarpal bone.
20. Palmarolateral border of the third metacarpal bone.
21. Palmarolateral border of the fourth metacarpal bone.
22. Palmarolateral aspect of the carpometacarpal joint between the fourth carpal bone and the third and fourth metacarpal bones.
23. Palmar aspect of the carpometacarpal joint between the third carpal and the third metacarpal bone.
24. Tubercle on the palmarolateral border of the fourth carpal bones.
25. Palmarolateral border of the third carpal bone.
26. Palmarolateral border of the second carpal bone.
27. Dorsomedial border of the fourth carpal bone.
28. Palmarolateral border of the ulnar carpal bone.
29. Palmarolateral border of the intermediate carpal bone.
30. Palmarolateral border of the accessory carpal bone.
31. Lateral facet (lateral styloid process) on the radial trochlea.
32. Medial, concave surface of the accessory carpal bone.

279

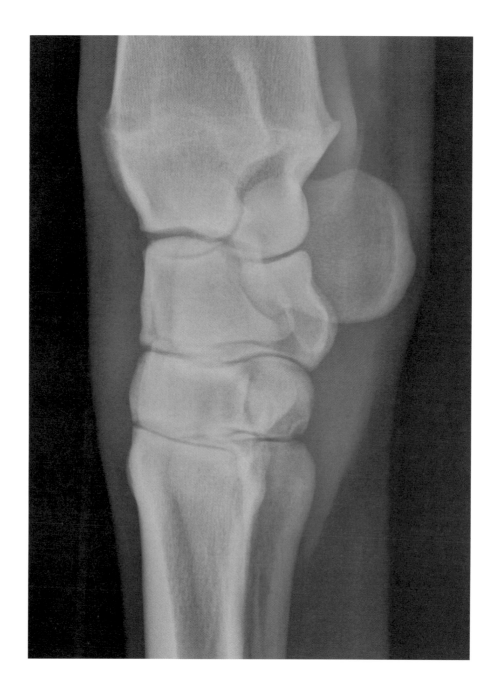

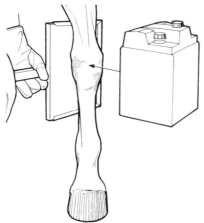

Figure 4.75.

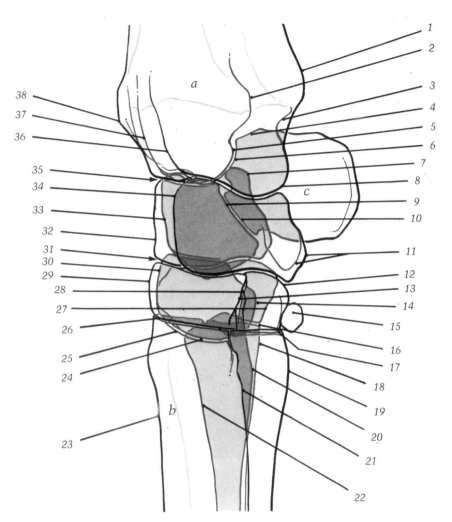

Figure 4.75. (*Continued*) Dorsomedial-palmarolateral oblique (D60M-PaLO) projection of the carpus. The relative positions of the bony ridges on the distocranial aspect of the radius change slightly with different X-ray beam projections. (a) Radius, (b) third metacarpal bone, (c) accessory carpal bone.

1. Bony projection from the mediocaudal surface of the radius.
2. Transverse crest proximal to the lateral facet (lateral styloid process) of the radial trochlea.
3. Indentation proximal to the medial facet (medial styloid process) of the radial trochlea.
4. Proximal border of the accessory carpal bone.
5. Caudal border of the lateral and intermediate facets of the radial trochlea superimposed.
6. Proximal articular surface of the accessory carpal bone.
7. Palmaromedial border of the intermediate carpal bone.
8. Medial facet (medial styloid process) of the radial trochlea.
9. Palmaromedial border of the ulnar carpal bone.
10. Distal articular surface of the accessory carpal bone.
11. Palmaromedial border of the radial carpal bone.
12. Palmaromedial border of the second carpal bone.
13. Palmaromedial border of the third carpal bone.
14. Palmaromedial border of the fourth carpal bone.
15. First carpal bone.
16. Carpometacarpal articulation between the third carpal and the third metacarpal bone.
17. Carpometacarpal articulation between the second carpal and the second metacarpal bone.
18. Palmaromedial border of the third metacarpal bone.
19. Palmaromedial border of the second metacarpal bone.
20. Palmaromedial border of the fourth metacarpal bone.
21. Dorsolateral border of the second metacarpal bone.
22. Dorsolateral border of the fourth metacarpal bone.
23. Dorsolateral border of the third metacarpal bone.
24. Carpometacarpal articulation between the fourth carpal and the fourth metacarpal bone.
25. Carpometacarpal articulation between the fourth carpal and the third metacarpal bone.
26. Carpometacarpal articulation between the third carpal and the third metacarpal bone.
27. Palmaromedial border of the third carpal bone.
28. Dorsal border of the second metacarpal bone.
29. Dorsal border of the third metacarpal bone.
30. Dorsal border of the fourth metacarpal bone.
31. Dorsolateral aspect of the midcarpal joint.
32. Dorsal border of the intermediate carpal bone.
33. Dorsal border of the ulnar carpal bone.
34. Dorsal border of the radial carpal bone. The relative position and appearance of the dorsal borders of 32, 33, and 34 may change with slight projection differences of the X-ray beam.
35. Antebrachiocarpal (radiocarpal) joint.
36. Bony ridge forming the medial border of the groove for the common digital extensor tendon.
37. Bony ridge along the lateral border of the extensor carpi radialis tendon.
38. Bony ridge between the grooves for the common digital extensor and the extensor carpi radialis tendons.

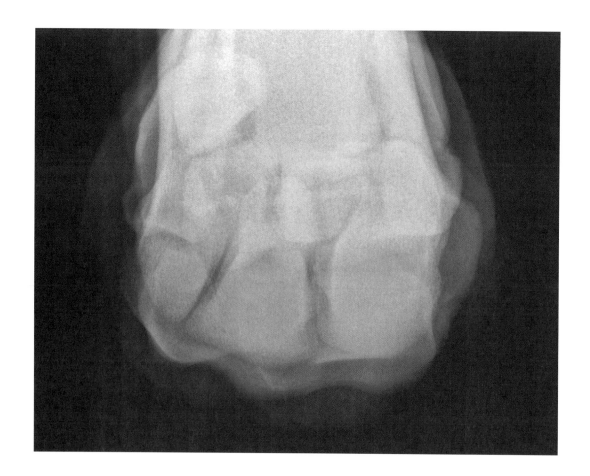

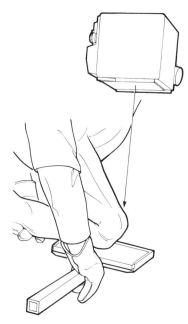

Figure 4.76.

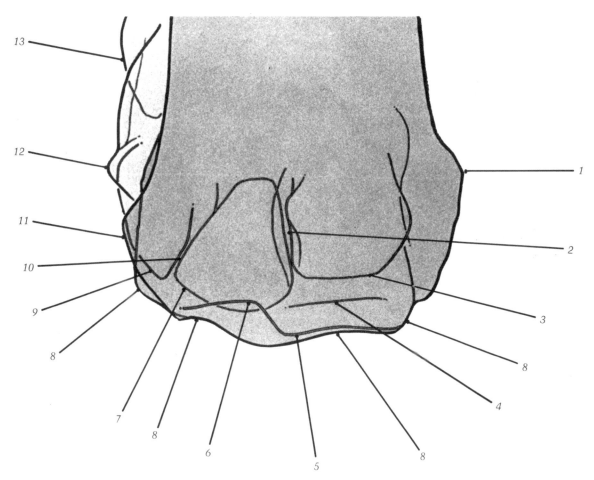

Figure 4.76. (*Continued*) Flexed dorsoproximal-dorsodistal oblique (flexed D80Pr-DDiO) projection of the distal radius.

1. Tuberosity on the distomedial aspect of the radius for attachment of the medial collateral ligament.
2. Junction between the radial and intermediate carpal bones.
3. Dorsal border of the radial carpal bone.
4. Dorsoproximal border of the radial carpal bone.
5. Medial facet (medial styloid process) of the radial trochlea.
6. Intermediate facet of the radial trochlea.
7. Dorsal border of the intermediate carpal bone.
8. Dorsal articular margin of the radial trochlea.
9. Dorsal border of the ulnar carpal bone.
10. Junction between the ulnar and intermediate carpal bones.
11. Tuberosity on the distal lateral radius for attachment of the lateral collateral ligament.
12. Lateral border of the accessory carpal bone.
13. Proximolateral border of the fourth metacarpal bone.

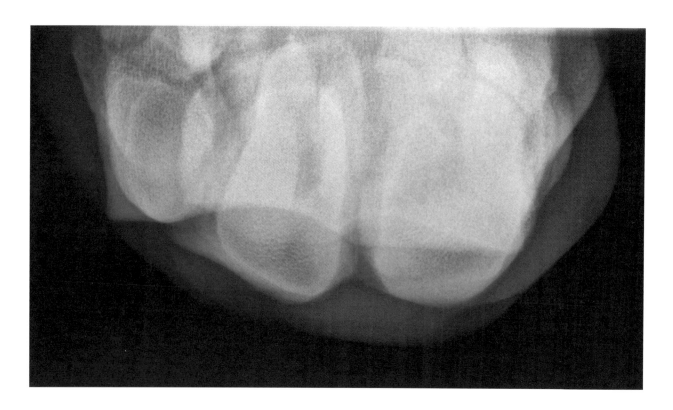

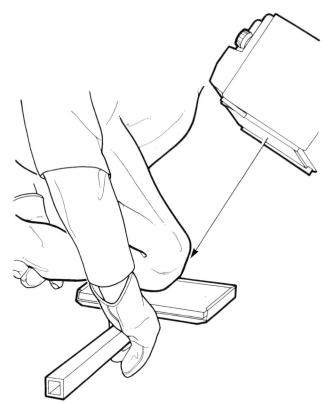

Figure 4.77.

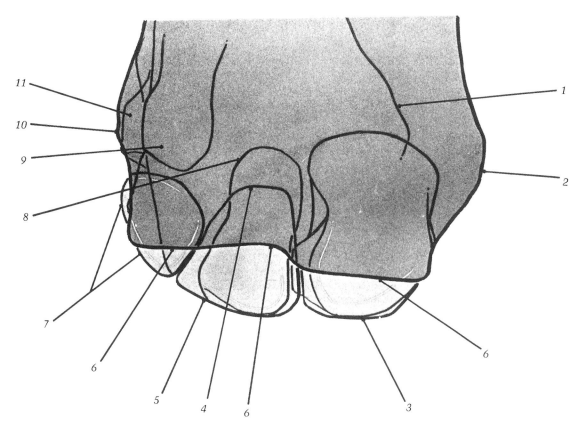

Figure 4.77. (*Continued*) Flexed dorsoproximal-dorsodistal oblique (flexed D55Pr-DDiO) projection of the proximal row of carpal bones. The position of the distal extremity of the radius relative to the proximal carpal bones varies with position of the horse's limb and the angulation of the primary X-ray beam. Slight changes in either may cause different degrees of superimposition of the radius and carpal bones.

1. Medial border of the second metacarpal bone.
2. Tuberosity on the distomedial aspect of the radius for attachment of the medial collateral ligament.
3. Dorsal border of the radial carpal bone.
4. Proximopalmar border of the intermediate carpal bone.
5. Dorsal border of the intermediate carpal bone.
6. Radial trochlea.
7. Dorsolateral border of the ulnar carpal bone.
8. Palmarodistal border of the intermediate carpal bone.
9. Proximal aspect of the fourth metacarpal bone.
10. Lateral tuberosity on the distal extremity of the radius for attachment of the lateral collateral ligament.
11. Accessory carpal bone.

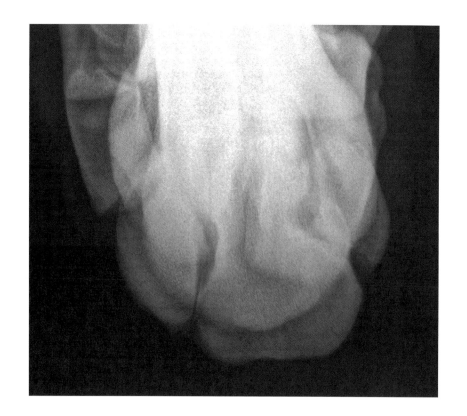

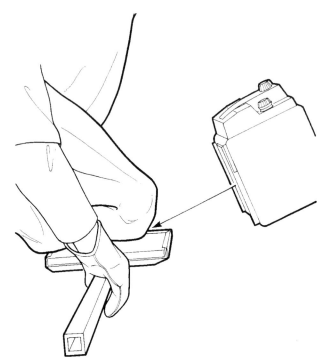

Figure 4.78.

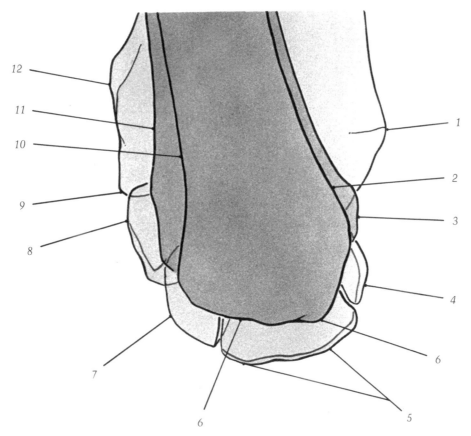

Figure 4.78. (*Continued*) Flexed dorsoproximal-dorsodistal oblique (flexed D30Pr-DDiO) projection of the distal row of carpal bones. The apparent shape of the third carpal bone may be changed by X-ray tube angulation and the position of the horse's limb, and may appear more elongated than shown here. The dorsal cortex and medullary cavity should be evident on the medial aspect of the normal third carpal bone if properly positioned.

1. Medial tuberosity on the distal radius for attachment of the medial collateral ligament.
2. Medial border of the third metacarpal bone.
3. Medial border of the second metacarpal bone.
4. Second carpal bone.
5. Dorsal border of the third carpal bone.
6. Superimposed dorsal border of the proximal carpal bones and the third metacarpal bone.
7. Fourth carpal bone.
8. Lateral border of the accessory carpal bone.
9. Lateral aspect (lateral styloid process) of the radial trochlea.
10. Lateral border of the third metacarpal bone.
11. Lateral border of the fourth metacarpal bone.
12. Lateral tuberosity on the distal extremity of the radius for attachment of the lateral collateral ligament.

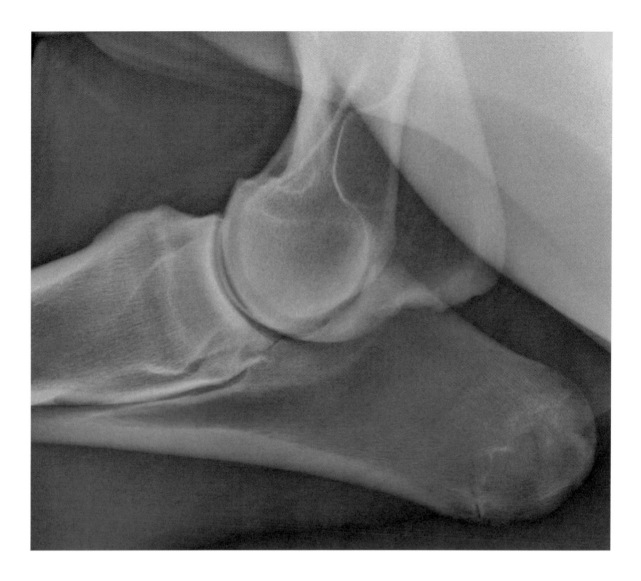

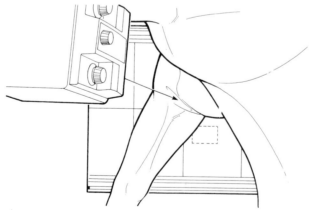

Figure 4.79.

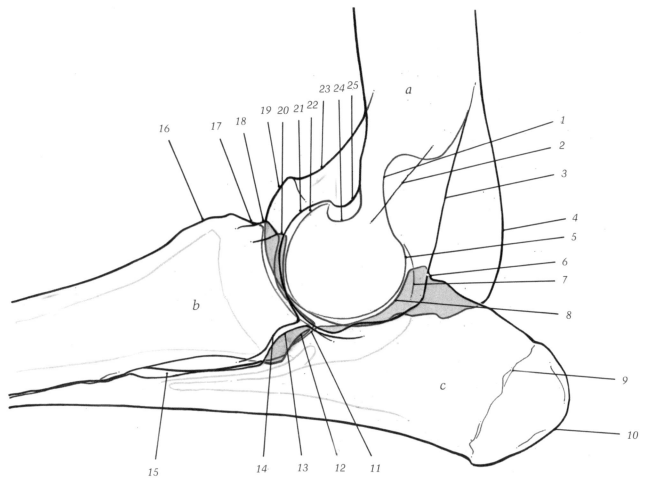

Figure 4.79. (*Continued*) Mediolateral (ML) projection of the humeroulnar and humeroradial joint (elbow). (a) Humerus, (b) radius, (c) ulna.

1. Floor of the olecranon fossa.
2. Lateral supracondylar crest on the distal extremity of the humerus.
3. Lateral epicondyle of the distal humerus.
4. Medial epicondyle of the distal humerus.
5. Sagittal trochlear groove on the medial humeral condyle.
6. Anconeal process of the ulna.
7. Articular surface of the trochlea (medial condyle) on the humerus.
8. Trochlear notch (ulnar articular surface).
9. Growth plate (physis) in the proximal ulna.
10. Olecranon tuberosity.
11. Medial aspect of the coronoid process of the ulna.

12. Middle caudal border of the radial head.
13. Lateral aspect of the coronoid process of the ulna.
14. Laterocaudal border of the radial head.
15. Interosseous space between the radius and ulna.
16. Radial tuberosity.
17. Craniomedial border of the radial head.
18. Midcranial border of the radial head.
19. Trochlea (medial condyle) of the humerus.
20. Cranial lateral border of the radial head.
21. Capitulum of the humerus.
22. Cranial surface (floor) of the sagittal groove on the trochlea of the humerus.
23. Medial border of the radial fossa.
24. Floor of the radial fossa.
25. Lateral border of the radial fossa.

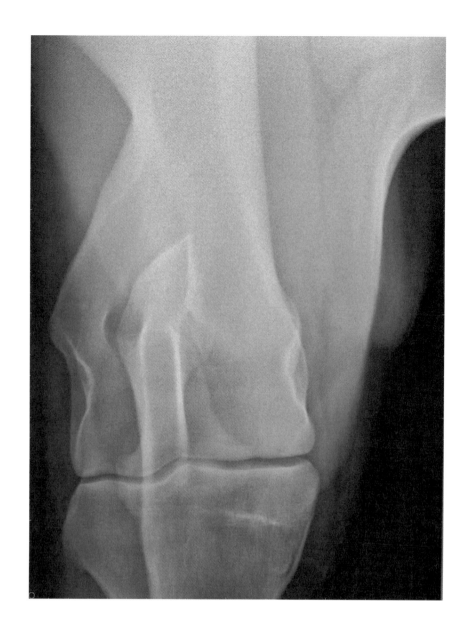

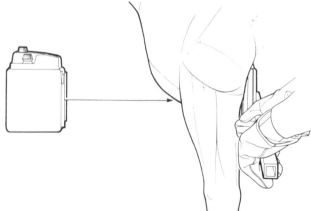

Figure 4.80.

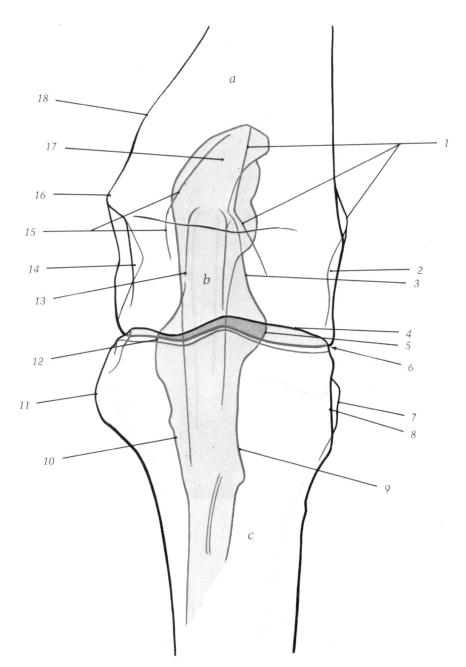

Figure 4.80. (*Continued*) Craniocaudal (CrCa) projection of the humeroulnar and humeroradial joint (elbow). (a) Humerus, (b) ulna, (c) radius.

1. Medial epicondyle of the humerus, which is large and superimposed over the distal extremity of the humerus except for a slight convex projection on the distal medial humerus where the medial collateral ligament attaches.
2. Depression on the distomedial aspect of the humerus.
3. Medial border of the trochlear notch on the ulna.
4. Caudal margin of the capitular fovea (proximal radial articulation).
5. Medial aspect of the coronoid process of the ulna.
6. Humeroradial articulations.
7. Radial tuberosity.
8. Medial tuberosity of the radius for collateral ligament attachment.
9. Medial border of the ulna.
10. Lateral border of the ulna.
11. Lateral tuberosity of the radius for collateral ligament attachment.
12. Lateral aspect of the coronoid process of the ulna.
13. Lateral border of the trochlear notch on the ulna.
14. Depression for attachment of the lateral collateral ligament.
15. Lateral border of the olecranon fossa.
16. Lateral epicondyle of the humerus.
17. Olecranon tuberosity of the ulna.
18. Lateral supracondylar crest.

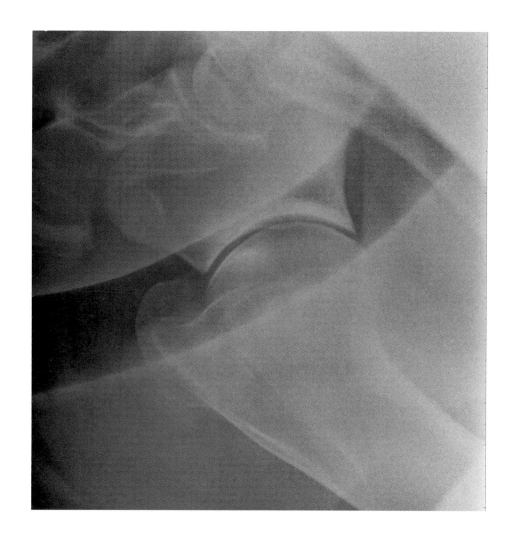

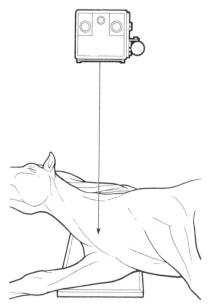

Figure 4.81.

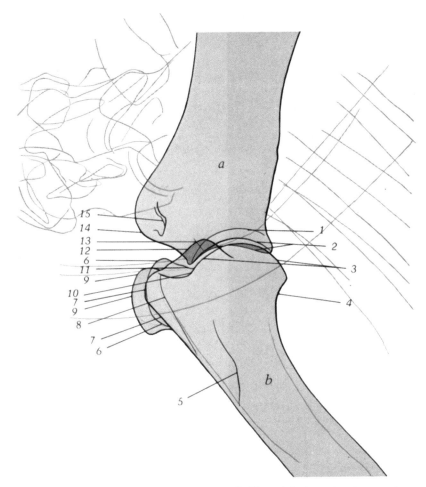

Figure 4.81. (*Continued*) Mediolateral (ML) projection of the scapulohumeral joint (shoulder). (a) Scapula, (b) humerus.

1. Subchondral bone on the concave surface of the glenoid cavity.
2. Medial and lateral borders of the glenoid cavity.
3. Cranial and caudal borders of the humeral head.
4. Caudal border of the humeral neck.
5. Deltoid tuberosity superimposed on the humerus.
6. Proximal and distocranial borders of the lesser (medial) tubercle.
7. Cranial border of the greater (lateral) tubercle.

8. Floor of the intertuberal groove between the lateral and intermediate tubercles.
9. Intermediate tubercle.
10. Fossa between the tubercles and the humeral head.
11. Caudal part of the lesser (medial) tubercle.
12. Caudal part of the greater (lateral) tubercle.
13. Glenoid notch, which is more or less apparent, depending on the X-ray beam projection angle and development in the horse.
14. Supraglenoid tubercle.
15. Coracoid process.

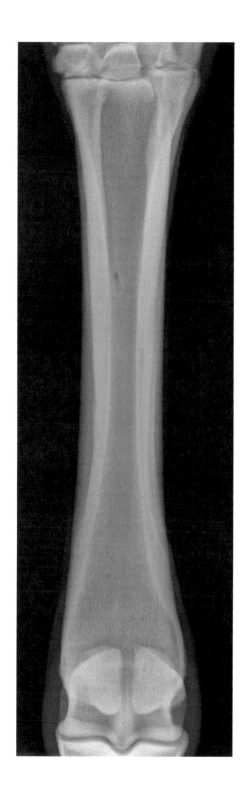

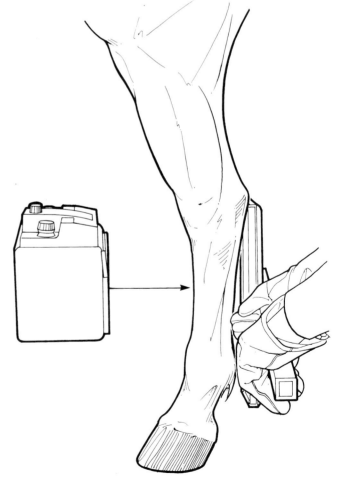

Figure 4.82.

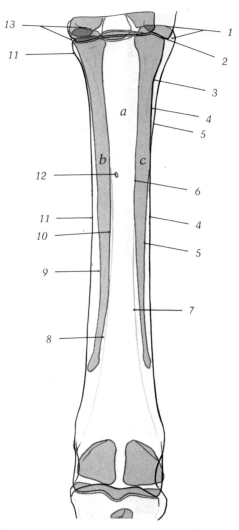

Figure 4.82. (*Continued*) Dorsoplantar (DPI) projection of the metatarsus. (a) Third metatarsal bone, (b) second metatarsal bone, (c) fourth metatarsal bone.

1. Proximal extremity (base) of the fourth metatarsal bone, which is larger than the second metatarsal bone and is superimposed over the third and fourth tarsal bones.
2. Articulation between the fourth tarsal and the third metatarsal bone.
3. Lateral surface of the third metatarsal bone.
4. Abaxial surface of the fourth metatarsal bone.
5. Axial surface of the fourth metatarsal bone.
6. Axial surface of the fourth metatarsal bone.
7. Endosteal surface on the lateral cortex of the third metatarsal bone.
8. Endosteal surface on the medial cortex of the third metatarsal bone.
9. Abaxial surface of the second metatarsal bone.
10. Axial surface of the second metatarsal bone.
11. Medial surface of the third metatarsal bone.
12. Nutrient foramen on the plantar surface of the third metatarsal bone.
13. Proximal extremity (base) of the second metatarsal bone, which is superimposed over the fused first and second tarsal bones and the third tarsal bone.

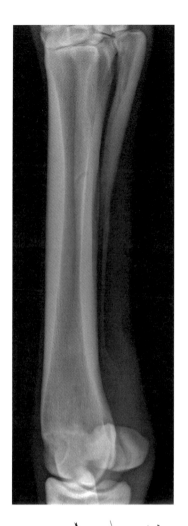

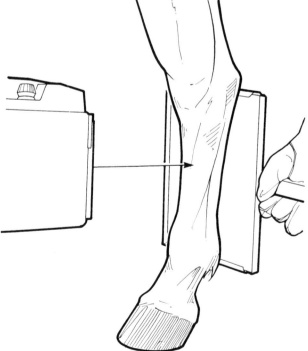

Figure 4.83.

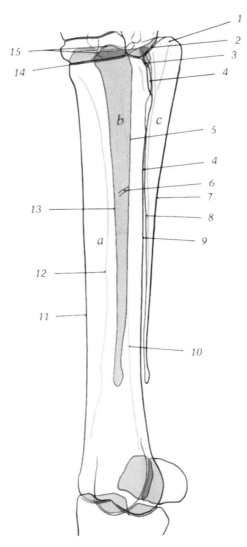

Figure 4.83. (*Continued*) Dorsolateral-plantaromedial oblique (D45L-PIMO) projection of the metatarsus. (a) Third metatarsal bone, (b) second metatarsal bone, (c) fourth metatarsal bone.

1. Proximal extremity (base) of fourth metatarsal bone.
2. Articulation between the fourth metatarsal and the fourth tarsal bone.
3. Articulation between the fourth and third metatarsal bones.
4. Interosseous space between the third and fourth metatarsal bones.
5. Plantarolateral border of second metatarsal bone.
6. Nutrient foramen on the plantar surface of the third metatarsal bone.
7. Plantarolateral border of fourth metatarsal bone.
8. Dorsomedial border of fourth metatarsal bone.
9. Plantarolateral border of third metatarsal bone.
10. Endosteal surface on the plantarolateral cortex of third metatarsal bone.
11. Dorsomedial surface of third metatarsal bone.
12. Endosteal surface on the dorsomedial cortex of third metatarsal bone.
13. Dorsomedial surface of second metatarsal bone.
14. Articulation between the third tarsal and the third metatarsal bone.
15. Proximal extremity (base) of the second metatarsal bone superimposed over the distal tarsal bones.

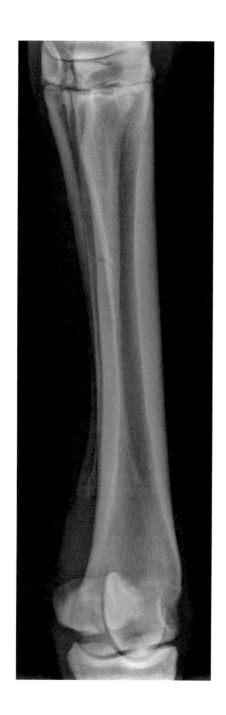

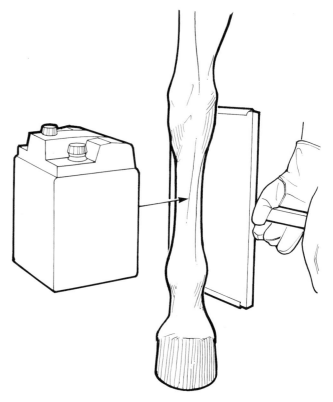

Figure 4.84

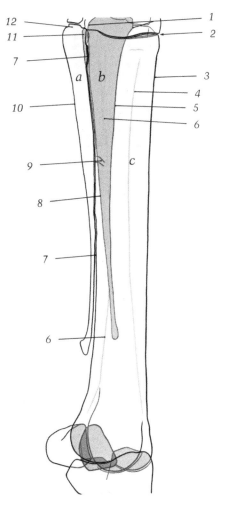

Figure 4.84. (*Continued*) Dorsomedial-plantarolateral oblique (D45M-PILO) projection of the metatarsus. (a) Second metatarsal bone, (b) fourth metatarsal bone, (c) third metatarsal bone.

1. Proximal extremity (base) of the fourth metatarsal bone.
2. Articulation between the third tarsal and the third metatarsal bone.
3. Dorsolateral surface of the third metatarsal bone.
4. Endosteal surface on the dorsolateral cortex of the third metatarsal bone.
5. Dorsolateral surface of the fourth metatarsal bone.

6. Endosteal surface on the plantar medial cortex of the third metatarsal bone.
7. Interosseous space between the second and third metatarsal bones.
8. Plantaromedial surface of the fourth metatarsal bone.
9. Nutrient foramen on the plantar surface of the third metatarsal bone.
10. Plantaromedial surface of the second metatarsal bone.
11. Articulation between second and third metatarsal bones.
12. Proximal extremity (base) of the second metatarsal bone.

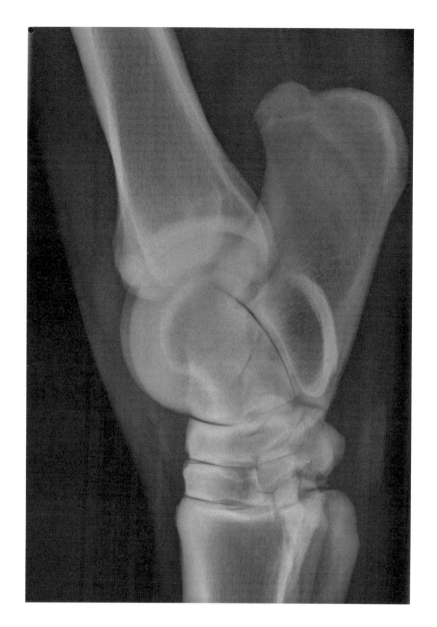

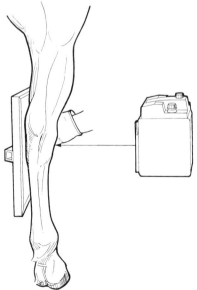

Figure 4.85.

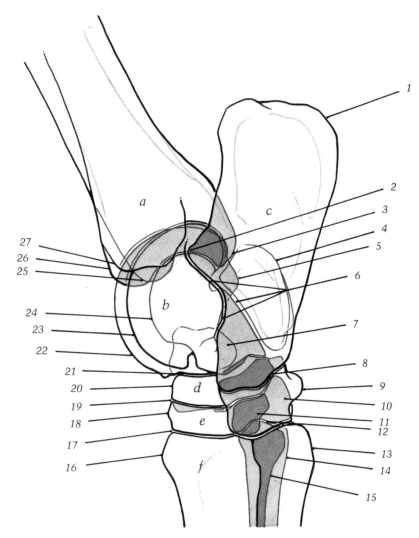

Figure 4.85. (*Continued*) Lateromedial (LM) projection of the tarsus. Depending on obliquity of the radiographic projection, the cranial borders of the malleoli and trochlear ridges may be in different relative positions. (a) Tibia, (b) talus, (c) calcaneus, (d) central tarsal bone, (e) third tarsal bone, (f) third metatarsal bone.

1. Calcaneal tuber.
2. Coracoid process of the calcaneus.
3. Caudal intermediate part of the tibial cochlea.
4. Sustentaculum tali of the calcaneus.
5. Proximomedial tuberosity of the talus for ligamentous attachments (superficial short medial collateral ligament).
6. Articulation between the talus and the calcaneus. All of these joint surfaces may not be distinguishable on any one radiograph; they should not be mistaken for fractures.
7. Distomedial tuberosity of the talus for ligamentous attachment (dorsal tarsal ligament).
8. Articulation between the calcaneus and the fourth tarsal bone.
9. Plantar surface of the fourth tarsal bone.
10. Second tarsal bone. The first and second tarsal bones are fused and project as different densities because of superimposition.
11. First tarsal bone.
12. Plantar aspect of the tarsometatarsal articulations.
13. Plantar border of the fourth metatarsal bone. The fourth metatarsal bone is larger than the second metatarsal bone and projects on the plantar surface.
14. Plantar border of the second metatarsal bone.
15. Plantar border of the third metatarsal bone.
16. Dorsoproximal ridge on the third metatarsal bone for attachment of the tibialis cranialis.
17. Articulation between the third tarsal and the third metatarsal bone.
18. Dorsal border of the third tarsal bone.
19. Articulation between the third and central tarsal bones.
20. Dorsal border of the central tarsal bone.
21. Articulation between the central tarsal bone and the talus.
22. Medial trochlear ridge of the talus. The small bony projection on the distal part of the medial trochlear ridge is variable in size and shape and should not be mistaken for a periarticular osteophyte or any other bony abnormality.
23. Lateral trochlear ridge of the talus.
24. Depth of the trochlear groove between the trochlear ridges on the talus.
25. Distocranial border of the medial tibial malleoli.
26. Cranial intermediate part of the tibial cochlea.
27. Distocranial border of the lateral tibial malleoli.

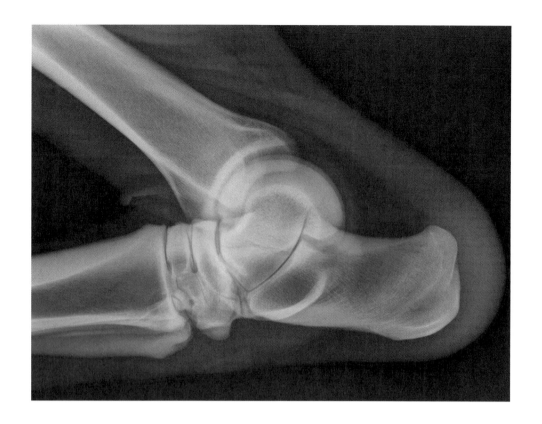

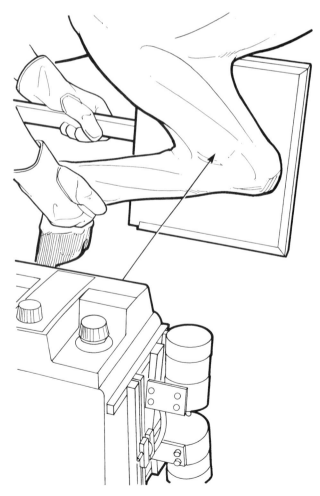

Figure 4.86.

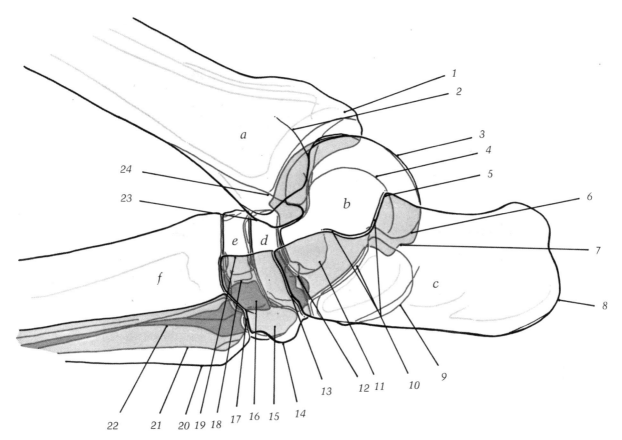

Figure 4.86. (*Continued*) Flexed lateromedial (flexed LM) projection of the tarsus. (a) Tibia, (b) talus, (c) calcaneus, (d) central tarsal bone, (e) third tarsal bone, (f) third metatarsal bone.

1. Caudal intermediate part of the tibial cochlea.
2. Distocaudal border of the lateral tibial malleolus.
3. Superimposed medial and lateral trochlear ridges of the talus.
4. Depth of the trochlear groove between the trochlear ridges of the talus.
5. Coracoid process of the calcaneus.
6. Plantar border of the lateral trochlear ridge on the talus.
7. Plantar border of the medial trochlear ridge on the talus.
8. Calcaneal tuber.
9. Sustentaculum tali.
10. Articulations between the talus and calcaneus, the visualization of which depends on the projection angle.
11. Distomedial tuberosity of the talus for ligamentous attachment (dorsal tarsal ligament).
12. Articulation between the talus and the central tarsal bone.
13. Articulation between the calcaneus and the fourth tarsal bone.
14. Plantar border of the fourth tarsal bone.
15. Second tarsal bone. The first and second tarsal bones are fused.
16. First tarsal bone.
17. Tarsometatarsal articulation.
18. Junction between the first and third tarsal bones, which is not always distinctly visible. Do not mistake the junction, when present, for a slab fracture.
19. Dorsal border of the fourth tarsal bone.
20. Plantar border of the fourth metatarsal bone.
21. Plantar border of the second metatarsal bone.
22. Plantar border of the third metatarsal bone. The superimposed plantar border of the third metatarsal bone and the dorsal borders of the second and fourth metatarsal bones may produce pseudolongitudinal fracture lines.
23. Cranial intermediate part of the tibial cochlea.
24. Cranial border of the medial tibial malleolus.

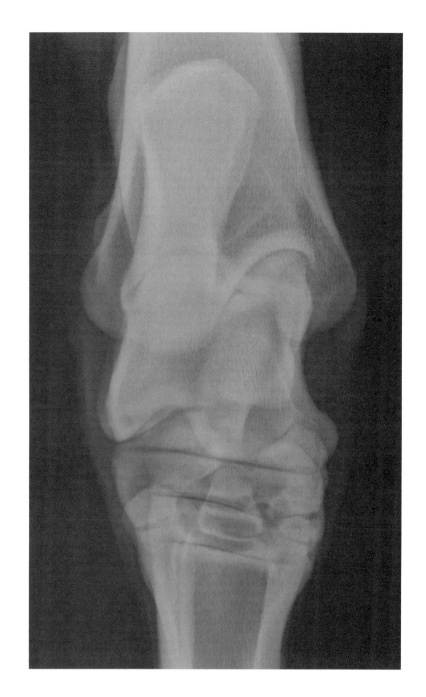

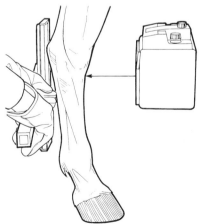

Figure 4.87.

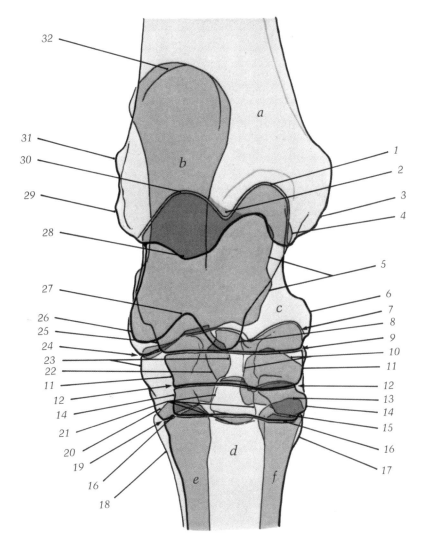

Figure 4.87. (*Continued*) Dorsoplantar (DPI) projection of the tarsus. The bones and joints of the tarsus are irregular and have complex shapes; thus, their appearance can vary with little change in projection angle. Therefore, careful observation is necessary when the tarsus is being evaluated radiographically. (a) Tibia, (b) calcaneus, (c) talus, (d) third metatarsal bone, (e) fourth metatarsal bone, (f) second metatarsal bone.

1. Articulation between the medial trochlear ridge of the talus and the medial cochlear groove of the tibia (tarsocrural joint).
2. Intermediate ridge of the tibial cochlea.
3. Medial malleolus on the distal tibia, where the medial collateral ligaments attach.
4. Proximal medial tuberosity on the talus, where the superficial short medial collateral ligament attaches.
5. Sustentaculum tali.
6. Distal medial tuberosity on talus for ligamentous attachment.
7. Plantar medial aspect of the talocalcaneocentral (proximal intertarsal) joint.
8. Distomedial border of the medial trochlear ridge on the talus.
9. Dorsomedial aspect of the talocalcaneal central (proximal intertarsal) joint. The difference in position of the plantar and dorsal aspects of this joint is caused by the curved contour of the articular surfaces in the proximal intertarsal joint.
10. Medial and lateral borders of the second tarsal bone.
11. Medial and lateral borders of the central tarsal bone.
12. Articulation between the third and central tarsal bones (tarsodistal or distal intertarsal joint).
13. Proximal border of the second metatarsal bone superimposed on the first and third tarsal bones.

14. Medial and lateral borders of the third tarsal bone.
15. Articulation between the second metatarsal and the fused first and second tarsal bones.
16. Medial and lateral aspects of the articulation between the third tarsal and the third metatarsal bone.
17. Proximomedial border of the second metatarsal bones.
18. Proximolateral border of the fourth metatarsal bone.
19. Articulation between the fourth tarsal and the fourth metatarsal bone (tarsometatarsal joint).
20. Proximal border of the fourth metatarsal bone superimposed over the fourth tarsal bone.
21. Bony prominence on the plantar surface of the third tarsal bone.
22. Prominence on the plantar surface of the central tarsal bone.
23. Lateral and medial borders of the fourth tarsal bone.
24. Articulation of the fourth tarsal bone and the calcaneus (calceneoquartal or proximal intertarsal joint).
25. Distal lateral border of the talus.
26. Lateral trochlear ridge of the talus.
27. Groove between medial and lateral trochlear ridges on the talus.
28. Caudal aspect of the intermediate ridge on the tibial cochlea.
29. Cranial part of the lateral malleolus.
30. Articulation between the lateral trochlear ridge on the talus and the lateral tibial cochlear groove in the tarsocrural (tibiotarsal) joint.
31. Caudal part of the lateral malleolus.
32. Calcaneal tuber.

305

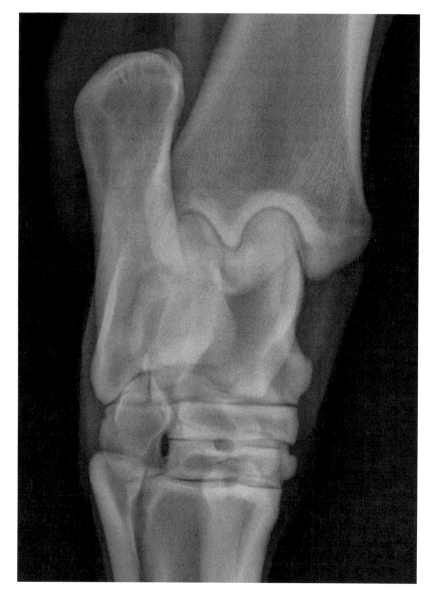
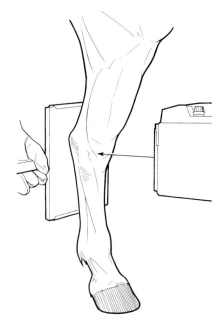

Figure 4.88. Dorsolateral-plantaromedial oblique (D35L-PlMO) projection of the tarsus. (a) Tibia, (b) calcaneus, (c) talus, (d) third metatarsus, (e) fourth metatarsal bone, (f) second metatarsal bone.

1. Articulation between the medial trochlear ridge of the talus and the medial tibial cochlear groove in the tarsocrural (tibiotarsal) joint.
2. Medial malleolus.
3. Articulation between the intermediate ridge of the tibial cochlea and the groove in the trochlea tali in the tarsocrural joint.
4. Cranial aspect of the intermediate ridge on the tibial cochlea.
5. Caudal aspect of the intermediate ridge on the tibial cochlea.
6. Medial trochlear ridge of the talus.
7. Lateral trochlear ridge of the talus.
8. Dorsomedial border of the sustentaculum tali.
9. Distomedial tuberosity of the talus for ligamentous attachment.
10. Plantaromedial aspect of the talocalcaneocentral (proximal intertarsal) joint.
11. Dorsomedial aspect of the talocalcaneocentral (proximal intertarsal) joint.
12. Dorsomedial aspect of the articulations between the central and third tarsal bone (centrodistal or distal intertarsal joint).
13. Medial and lateral borders of the fused first and second tarsal bones.
14. Prominent ridge for ligamentous attachment on the dorsomedial surface of the third tarsal bone.
15. Articulation between the fused first and second tarsal bones and the second metatarsal bone.
16. Dorsomedial aspect of the articulation between the metatarsal bone and the third metatarsal bone (tarsometatarsal joint).
17. Dorsomedial border of the third metatarsal bone.

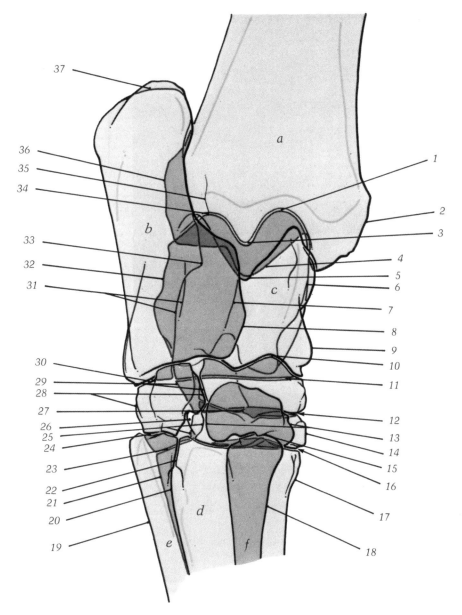

Figure 4.88. *(Continued)*
18. Dorsomedial border of the fourth metatarsal bone.
19. Plantarolateral border of the fourth metatarsal bone.
20. Interosseous space between the third and fourth metatarsal bone.
21. Lateral border of the third metatarsal bone dorsal to the fourth metatarsal bone.
22. Articulation between the third and fourth metatarsal bone.
23. Articulation between the fourth tarsal and the third metatarsal bone.
24. Articulation between the fourth tarsal and the fourth metatarsal bone.
25. Plantarolateral and plantaromedial borders of the third tarsal bone.
26. Vascular tarsal canal, which encloses the perforating tarsal artery and vein and a deep perineal nerve branch. It may be more or less apparent on this projection, depending on the projection angle.
27. Nonvascular area between the central and the third tarsal bones. These nonarticular areas may simulate subchondral

bone lysis and must be differentiated from erosion by their location.
28. Plantarolateral and dorsomedial borders of the fourth tarsal bone.
29. Plantarolateral and plantaromedial borders of the central tarsal bone.
30. Articulation between the calcaneus and the fourth tarsal bone (calcaneoquarteral or proximal intertarsal joint).
31. Borders of the sinus tarsi, which is a space between the calcaneus and talus that appears as a more or less lucent region.
32. Plantarolateral border of the sustentaculum tali.
33. Coracoid process of the calcaneus.
34. Articulation between the lateral trochlear ridge of the talus and the lateral tibial cochlear groove in the tarsocrural joint (tibiotarsal joint).
35. Cranial part of the lateral malleolus.
36. Caudal part of the lateral malleolus.
37. Calcaneal tuber.

307

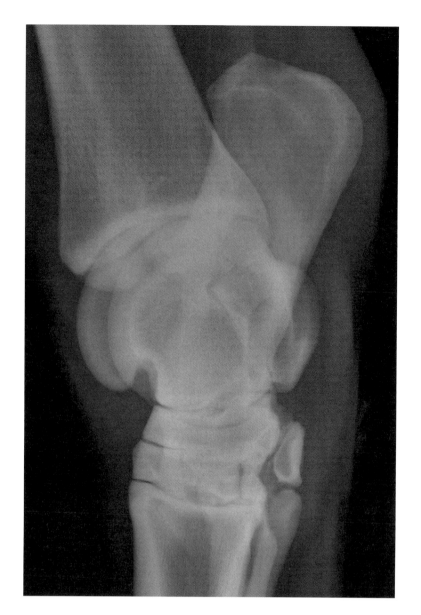

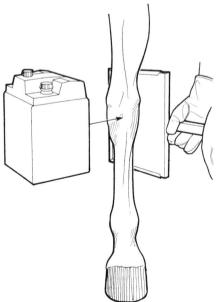

Figure 4.89.

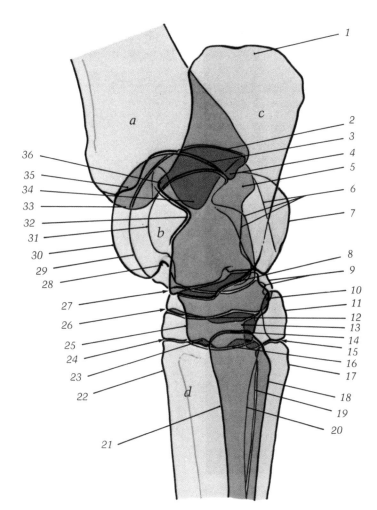

Figure 4.89. (*Continued*) Dorsomedial-plantarolateral (D55M-PILO) projection of the tarsus. (a) Tibia, (b) talus, (c) calcaneus, (d) third metatarsal bone.

1. Calcaneal tuber
2. Articulation between the medial trochlear ridge of the talus and the medial tibial cochlear groove of the tarsocrural joint.
3. Articulation between the lateral trochlea of the talus and the lateral tibial cochlear groove of the tarsocrural joint.
4. Caudal aspect of the intermediate ridge of the tibial cochlea.
5. Proximomedial tuberosity of the talus.
6. Plantar borders of the talus superimposed on the calcaneus.
7. Plantar border of the sustentaculum tali.
8. Nonarticular depression between the talus and the central tarsal bone. These nonarticular depressions, which appear more of less distinct depending on the angle of the X-ray beam projection, may simulate subchondral bone lysis.
9. Medial and lateral plantar borders of the central tarsal bone.
10. Plantar border of the fourth tarsal bone.
11. Plantar border of the fused first and second tarsal bone.
12. Area of nonarticular depression between the central and third tarsal bones.
13. Junction between the fused first and second tarsal bones and the medial plantar border of the third tarsal bone.
14. Articulation between the fourth tarsal and the fourth metatarsal bone.
15. Articulation between the fused first and second tarsal bone and the second metatarsal bone.
16. Articulation between the fourth tarsal bone and the third metatarsal bone.
17. Plantar border of the second metatarsal bone.

18. Plantar border of the fourth metatarsal bone.
19. Interosseous space between the second and third metatarsal bones.
20. Plantar border of the third metatarsal bone.
21. Dorsolateral border of the fourth metatarsal bone.
22. Dorsolateral border of the third metatarsal bone.
23. Nonarticular depressions in the adjacent surface of the third tarsal and the third metatarsal bone.
24. Dorsolateral aspect of the articulation between the third tarsal and the third metatarsal bone (tarsometatarsal joint).
25. Dorsolateral border of the fourth tarsal bone.
26. Dorsolateral aspect of the articulation between the central and the third tarsal bone (centrodistal or distal intertarsal bone).
27. Dorsolateral aspect of the talocalcaneal central (proximal intertarsal joint).
28. Notch at the distal aspect of the lateral trochlear ridge on the talus.
29. Medial trochlear ridge of the talus.
30. Lateral trochlear ridge of the talus.
31. Depth of the groove between the medial and lateral trochlear ridges on the talus.
32. Articulation between the talus and the calcaneus (talocalcaneal articulation), the visibility of which depends on the X-ray beam projection.
33. Cranial aspect of the intermediate ridge on the tibial cochlea.
34. Medial malleolus superimposed over the talus and calcaneus.
35. Lateral malleolus superimposed over the intermediate tibial cochlear ridge and the lateral trochlear ridge of the talus.
36. Coracoid process of the calcaneus.

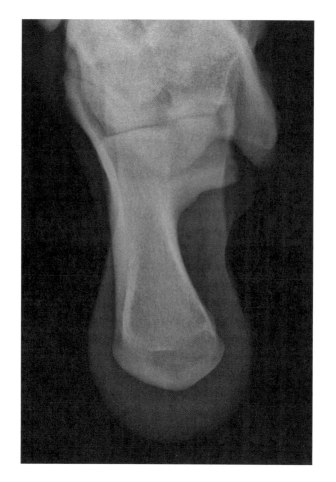

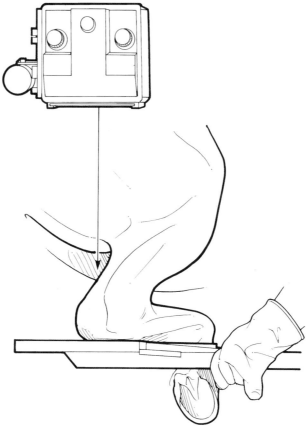

Figure 4.90.

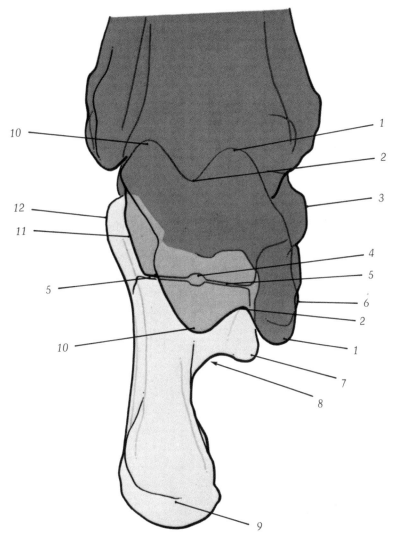

Figure 4.90. (*Continued*) Flexed dorsoplantar (flexed DP) projection of the tarsus.

1. Medial trochlear ridge on the talus.
2. Groove between the medial and lateral trochlear ridges of the talus.
3. Distomedial tuberosity of the talus.
4. Nonarticular depressions between the talus and calcaneus. This opening communicates with the sinus tarsi.
5. Medial and lateral aspects of the articulation between the talus and calcaneus.
6. Proximomedial tuberosity of the talus.
7. Sustentaculum tali
8. Tarsal groove for the deep digital flexor principal tendon.
9. Calcaneal tuber.
10. Lateral trochlear ridge on the talus.
11. Areas of attachment of the lateral collateral ligament on the talus.
12. Areas of attachment of the lateral collateral ligament on the calcaneus.

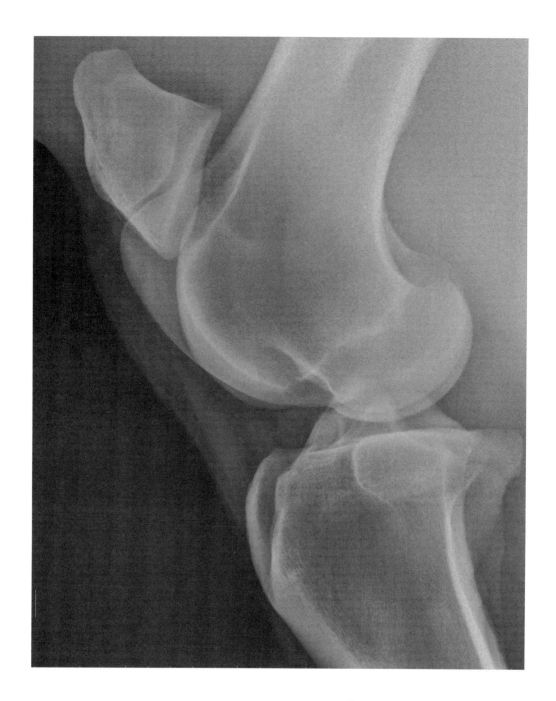

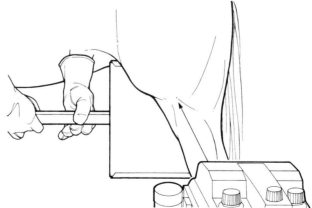

Figure 4.91.

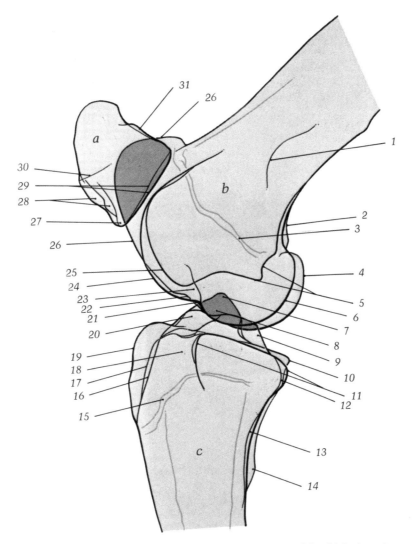

Figure 4.91. (*Continued*) Lateromedial (LM) projection of the femorotibial and femoropatellar joints (stifle joint). (a) Patella, (b) femur, (c) tibia.

1. Supracondyloid fossa.
2. Medial supracondyloid tuberosity.
3. Distal femoral growth plate.
4. Medial femoral condyle.
5. Intercondyloid fossa.
6. Lateral femoral condyle.
7. Medial tubercle on the intercondyloid eminence of the tibia.
8. Central intercondylar area.
9. Medial part of the articular surface on the lateral tibial condyle.
10. Medial tibial condyle.
11. Lateral tibial condyle.
12. Popliteal notch.
13. Concavity of the popliteal incisure.
14. Tubercle on the caudal medial surface of the tibia.
15. Growth plate on the proximal tibia.
16. Groove for the medial patellar ligament.

17. Medial part of the tibial tuberosity.
18. Extensor sulcus.
19. Lateral part of the tibial tuberosity.
20. Lateral tubercle on the intercondyloid eminence of the tibia.
21. Ridge connecting the lateral trochlear ridge and the lateral condyle on the femur.
22. Ridge connecting the medial trochlear ridge and the medial condyle on the femur.
23. Extensor fossa.
24. Lateral femoral trochlear ridge.
25. Compact bone in the femoral trochlear between the lateral and medial trochlear ridge.
26. Medial femoral trochlear ridge.
27. Apex of the patella.
28. Areas of ligamentous attachment on the cranial surface of the patella.
29. Articular surfaces of the patella.
30. Edge of the medial articular surface and medial border of the patella.
31. Base of the patella.

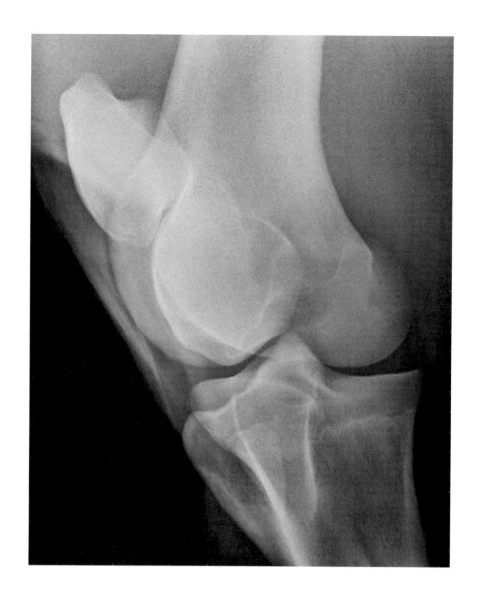

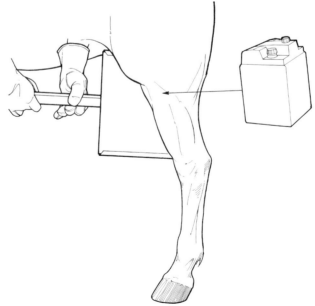

Figure 4.92.

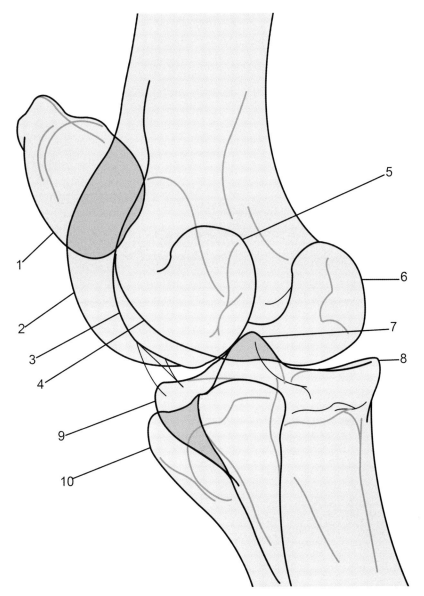

Figure 4.92. (*Continued*) Laterocaudal-craniomedial oblique (L45Ca-CrMO) projection of the stifle joint. From a straight latero-medial position, the primary X-ray beam is directed parallel to the ground with a 45° caudal angle and is centered on the caudal aspect of the stifle joint for a different approach in the evaluation of the medial femoral condyle. This projection also shows a large area of the weight-bearing articular surface of the medial femoral condyle free of superimposition with the lateral condyle, and can be an alternative to the flexed projection. However, in both projections, the medial femoral condyle is projected differently and one lesion may be seen in one and not the other.

1. Patella.
2. Lateral femoral trochlear ridge.
3. Intercondylar groove.
4. Medial femoral trochlear ridge.
5. Lateral femoral condyle.
6. Medial femoral condyle.
7. Medial tubercle on the intercondyloid eminence of the tibia.
8. Medial tibial condyle.
9. Lateral tibial condyle.
10. Tibial tuberosity.

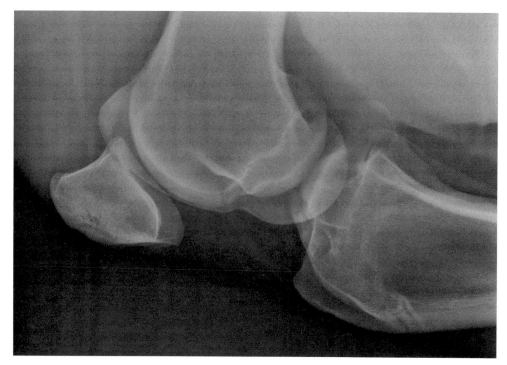

Figure 4.93.

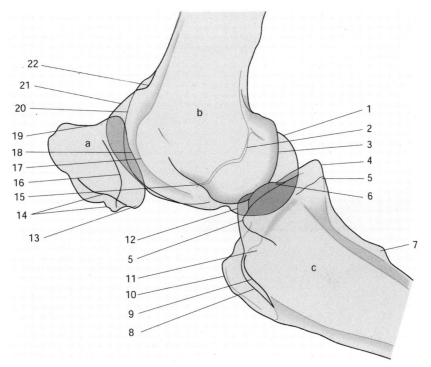

Figure 4.93. (*Continued*) Flexed lateromedial (flexed L0-20Cr-CaMO) projection of the femorotibial and femoropatellar joints (stifle). (a) Patella, (b) femur, (c) tibia. This projection shows the articular surface of the medial femoral condyle free of superimposition with other osseous structures. This projection can be performed in two different ways. The limb can be flexed and abducted and the X-ray beam directed parallel to the ground with a 0°- to 20°-laterocranial obliquity; if the limb can not be abducted, an approximately 10° distal obliquity (L0-20Cr10Di-PrMO) should be added to the X-ray beam direction.

1. Medial femoral condyle.
2. Intercondyloid fossa.
3. Lateral femoral condyle.
4. Lateral tibial condyle.
5. Medial tibial condyle.
6. Medial tubercle on the intercondyloid eminence of the tibia.
7. Tubercle on the caudal medial surface of the tibia.
8. Medial part of the tibial tuberosity.
9. Groove for the medial patellar ligament.
10. Lateral part of the tibial tuberosity.
11. Extensor sulcus.
12. Lateral tubercle on the intercondyloid eminence of the tibia.
13. Apex of the patella.
14. Areas for ligament attachment on the cranial surface of the patella.
15. Extensor fossa.
16. Medial aspect of the articular surface of the patella.
17. Subchondral bone in the femoral trochlea between the lateral and medial trochlear ridges.
18. Lateral aspect of the articular surface of the patella.
19. Base of the patella.
20. Lateral femoral trochlear ridge.
21. Medial femoral trochlear ridge.
22. Nonarticular fossa between the femoral trochlear ridges.

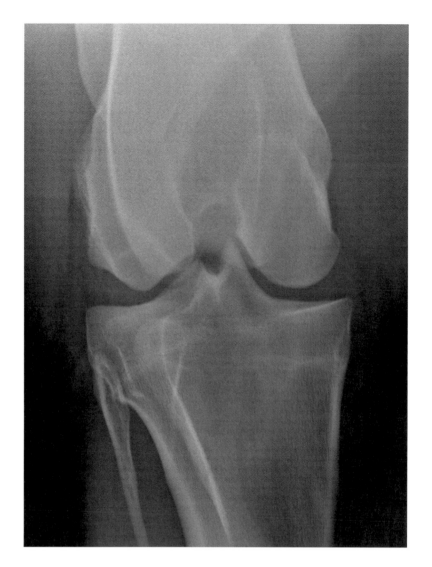

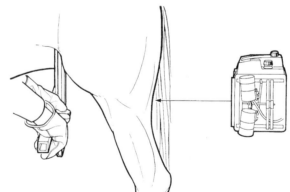

Figure 4.94.

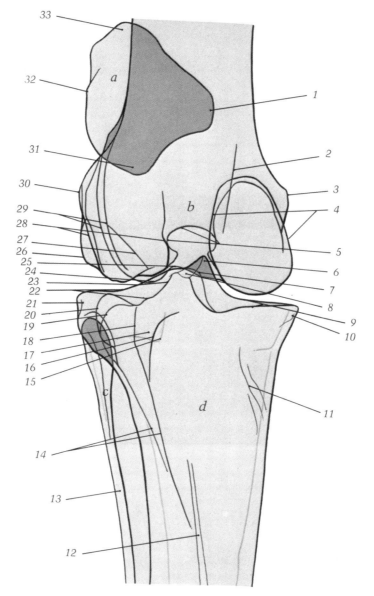

Figure 4.94. (*Continued*) Caudocranial (CaCr) projection of the femorotibial and femoropatellar joints (stifle). The entire patella may or may not be seen depending on the X-ray exposure. The patella is normally located to the lateral side of the distal aspect of the femur. The fibula may be a complete bone (as here), but it is usually rudimentary with only the proximal part present or with one or two transverse lines that give the mistaken appearance of fractures. (a) Patella, (b) femur, (c) fibula, (d) tibia.

1. Medial angle of the patella. A large cartilaginous process extends from the medial angle of the patella and is not visible radiographically.
2. Lateral border of the medial trochlear ridge on the distal femur, the visibility of which depends on the X-ray exposure.
3. Medial epicondyle for ligamentous attachment.
4. Medial and lateral borders of the medial femoral condyle.
5. Intercondyloid fossa on the caudal aspect of the distal femur.
6. Medial tubercle on the intercondylar eminence on the proximal tibia.
7. Lateral tubercle on the intercondylar eminence of the proximal tibia.
8. Central intercondylar area.
9. Cranial and caudal borders of the articular surface of the medial tibial condyle.
10. Medial tibial condyle.
11. Tubercle on the caudal medial tibial surface.
12. Muscular lines on the caudal tibial surface.

13. Fibula.
14. Tibial crest.
15. Bony margin of the extensor sulcus.
16. Medial part of the tibial tuberosity.
17. Groove between the medial and lateral parts of the tibial tuberosity for the medial patellar ligament.
18. Medial border of the lateral part of the tibial tuberosity.
19. Cranial aspect of the lateral tibial condyle.
20. Lateral proximal border of the lateral part of the tibial tuberosity.
21. Caudal aspect of the lateral tibial condyle.
22. Cranial and caudal articular surfaces on the lateral tibial condyle.
23. Articular surface on the medial part of the lateral tibial condyle.
24. Distal aspect of the lateral trochlear ridge on the femur.
25. Distal aspect of the groove between the distal femoral trochlear ridges.
26. Lateral femoral epicondyle for ligamentous attachment.
27. Bony borders of the extensor fossa on the distal femur.
28. Lateral and medial borders of the lateral femoral condyle.
29. Lateral trochlear ridge on the distal extremity of the femur.
30. Proximolateral border of the lateral femoral condyle.
31. Apex of the patella
32. Lateral angle and the patella.
33. Base of the patella.

319

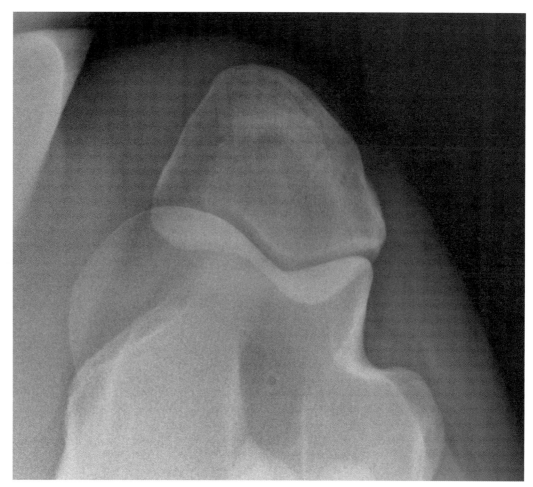

Figure 4.95.

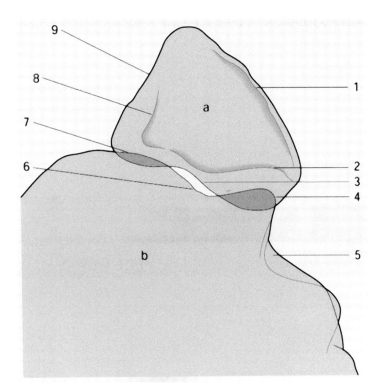

Figure 4.95. (*Continued*) Cranioproximal-craniodistal oblique (CrPR-DiCrO) projection of the patella. (a) Patella, (b) femur.
1. Dorsal surface and area of ligament attachment on the patella.
2. Distal articular surface on the patella.
3. Proximal articular surface on the patella.
4. Lateral femoral trochlear ridge.
5. Extensor fossa.
6. Trochlear groove between the medial and lateral trochlear ridges.
7. Medial femoral trochlear ridge.
8. Distal medial border of the patella.
9. Proximal medial border of the patella.

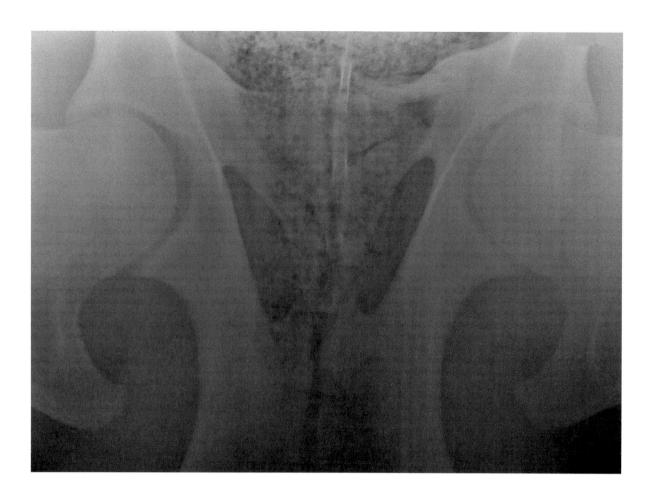

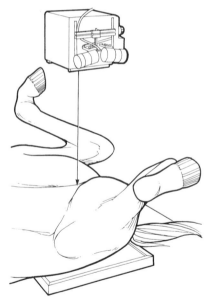

Figure 4.96.

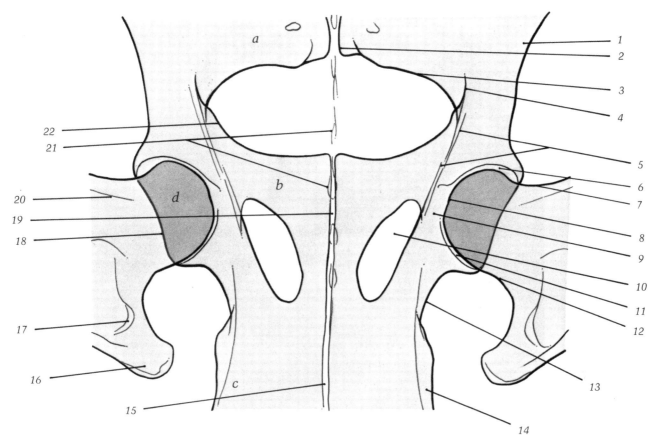

Figure 4.96. (*Continued*) Ventrodorsal (VD) projection of the pelvis. (a) Right ilium, (b) right pubis, (c) right ischium, (d) right femoral head.

1. Body of the ilium
2. Tuber sacrale. Fecal material in the large colon may be superimposed over the tuber sacrale and the sacrum, compromising good radiographic evaluation of these structures.
3. Great ischiatic notch on the dorsal border of the ilium.
4. Ventral border of the ilium.
5. Ischiatic spine.
6. Articulation between the cranial border of the acetabulum and the femoral head.
7. Medial border of the femoral neck.
8. Fovea capitis femoris, which is a flattened region on the femoral head, the visibility of which depends on the angulation and position during radiography.
9. Acetabular fossa. Because there is no articular cartilage or subchondral bone in the region of the acetabular fossa, it

appears as a break or defect in the articular surface of the acetabulum, but it is normal.
10. Obturator foramen.
11. Articulation between the caudal border of the acetabulum and the femoral head.
12. Lateral border of the femoral neck.
13. Lateral border of the ischium.
14. Ischiatic tuberosity.
15. Ischiatic symphysis.
16. Caudal part of the greater trochanter.
17. Cranial part of the greater trochanter.
18. Dorsal rim of the acetabulum.
19. Pubic symphysis.
20. Lesser trochanter superimposed over the femur.
21. Dorsal spinous processes of the sacrum.
22. Cranial border of the pubis.

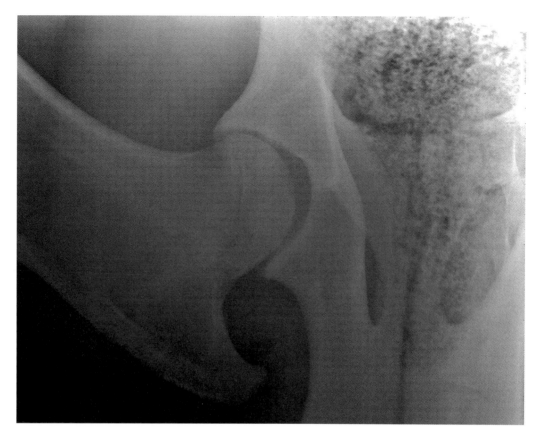

Figure 4.97.

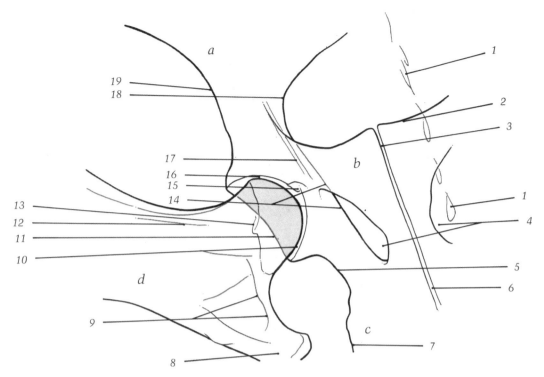

Figure 4.97. (*Continued*) Ventromedial-dorsolateral oblique (V25M-DLO) projection of the pelvis. (a) Ilium, (b) pubis, (c) ischium, (d) femur.

1. Dorsal spinous process of the sacrum.
2. Cranial border of the pubis.
3. Pubic symphysis.
4. Obturator foramina.
5. Lateral border of the ischium.
6. Ischiatic symphysis.
7. Ischiatic tuberosity.
8. Caudal part of the greater trochanter.
9. Cranial part of the greater trochanter.
10. Articulation between the caudal aspect of the acetabulum and the femoral head.
11. Dorsal acetabular rim.
12. Lesser trochanter superimposed over the femur.
13. Growth plate (physis) between the femoral head and the neck.
14. Medial dorsal border of the ischium.
15. Acetabular fossa.
16. Articulation between the cranial acetabulum and the femoral head.
17. Ischiatic spine on the dorsal border of the ischium.
18. Medial dorsal border of the ilium.
19. Lateral border of the ilium.

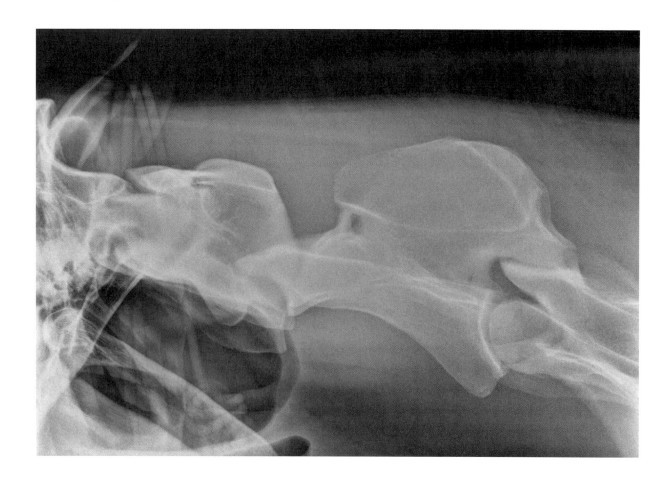

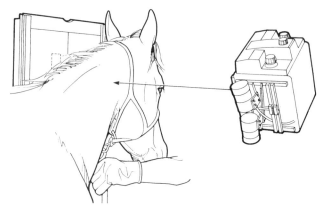

Figure 4.98.

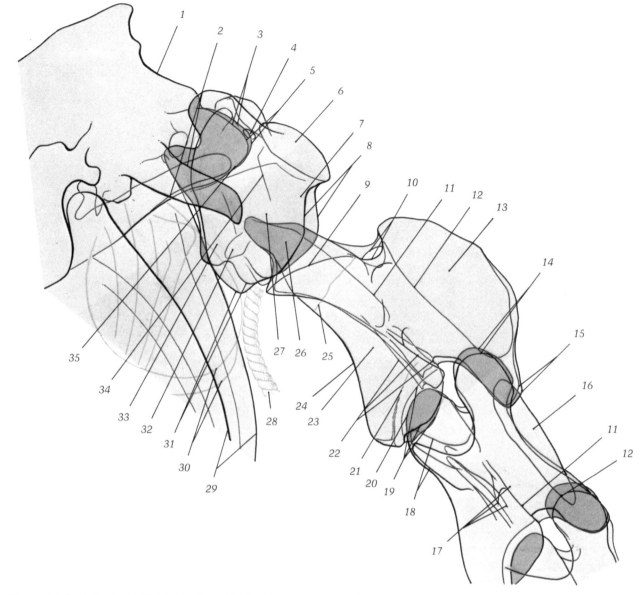

Figure 4.98. (*Continued*) Right-to-left lateral (Rt-LeL) projection of the cranial cervical vertebral column (C1 to C3).

1. Occipital bone.
2. Jugular process.
3. Dorsal surface of the right and left occipital condyles.
4. Right and left margins of the lateral foramen of the atlas.
5. Caudal borders of the occipital condyle (atlantooccipital articulation).
6. Dorsal tubercle of the atlas.
7. Atlas.
8. Caudal margins of the articular fovea.
9. Cranial articular process of the axis.
10. Margins of the lateral vertebral foramen.
11. Ventral margin of the vertebral column.
12. Dorsal margin of the vertebral column.
13. Dorsal spinous process of the axis.
14. Right and left cranial articular fovea of C3.
15. Caudal articular fovea of the atlas.
16. Dorsal spinous process of C3.
17. Base of the transverse processes of C3.
18. Transverse process of C3.
19. Concave margins of the caudal extremity of the axis.
20. Convex cranial extremity of C3.
21. Caudal growth plate of the axis.
22. Multiple linear opacities produced by the wide bases on the right and left transverse processes of the axis.
23. Axis.
24. Ventral border of the axis.
25. Cranial growth plate of the axis.
26. Dens of the axis.
27. Atlas.
28. Shadow produced by braided rope used for alter.
29. Right and left rami of the mandible.
30. Right and left ventral margins of the guttural pouches.
31. Right and left ventrocaudal margins of the axis.
32. Shadow caused by margins of the transverse foramen.
33. Base of the wings of the atlas.
34. Shadow formed by the concavity of the atlantal fossa.
35. Right and left caudal margins of the occipital condyles.

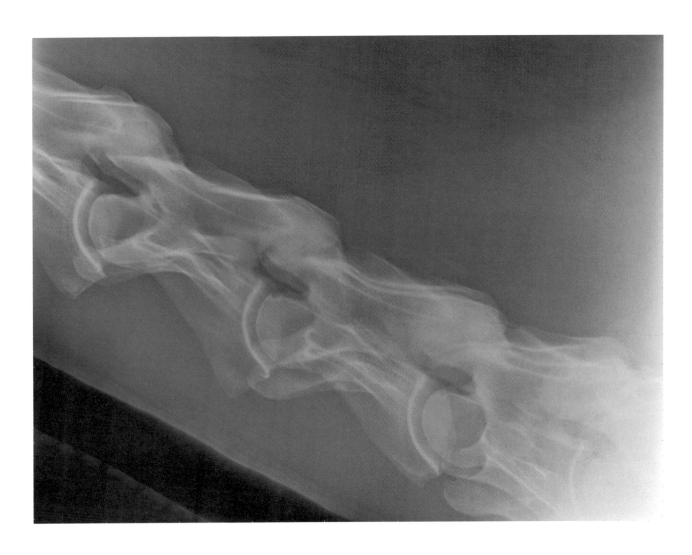

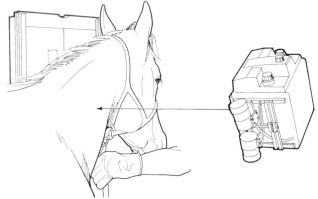

Figure 4.99.

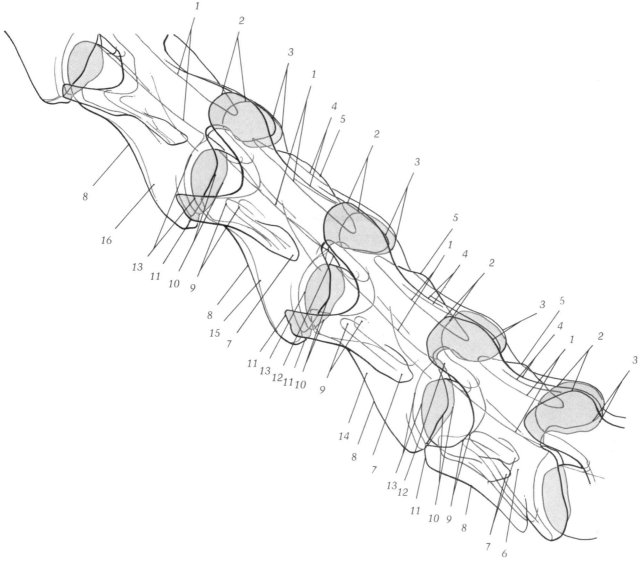

Figure 4.99. (*Continued*) Right-to-left lateral (Rt-LeL) projection of the midcervical spine (C3-C6).

1. Dorsal and ventral borders of the vertebral canal.
2. Right and left cranial articular processes.
3. Right and left caudal articular processes.
4. Shadows formed by vertebral arches on either side of the spinous processes.
5. Dorsal spinous processes of C4, C5, and C6.
6. C6.
7. Bases of lateral transverse vertebral processes.
8. Ventral borders of the vertebrae.
9. Bases of the transverse processes, which also form the ventral and dorsal margins of transverse foramina.
10. Caudal extremities of the vertebrae.
11. Transverse processes.
12. Dorsal tuberculums.
13. Concave borders of the caudal extremities.
14. C5.
15. C4.
16. C3.

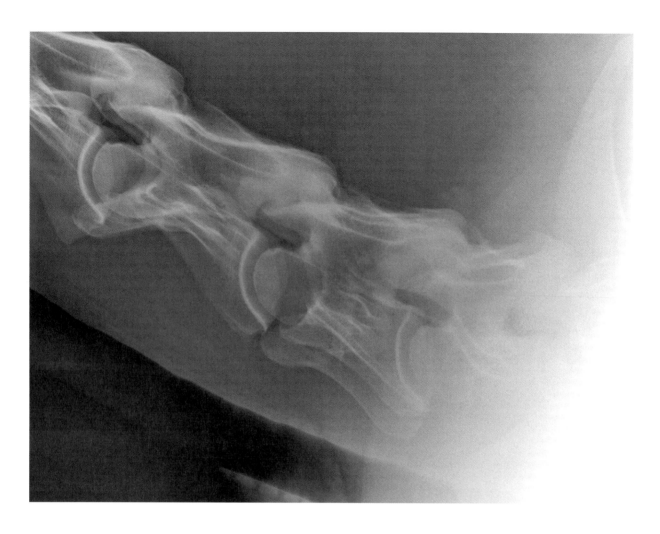

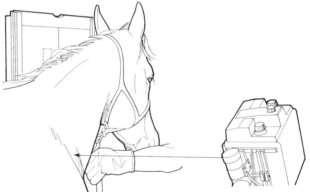

Figure 4.100.

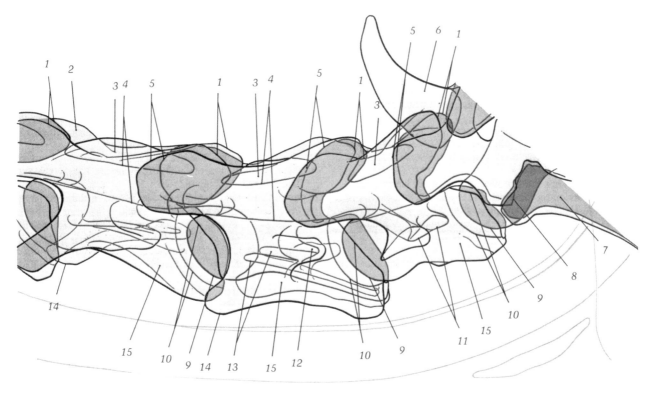

Figure 4.100. (*Continued*) Right-to-left lateral (Rt-LeL) projection of the caudal cervical spine (C5 to C7).

1. Caudal articular processes.
2. Vertebral lamina on either side of the spinous process.
3. Dorsal spinous processes and dorsal laminae.
4. Dorsal and ventral borders of the vertebral canal.
5. Cranial articular border.
6. Dorsal spinous process of T1.
7. First rib.
8. Tubercle of the first rib.
9. Cranial extremities of the vertebrae.
10. Caudal extremities of the vertebrae.
11. Bases of the transverse processes.
12. Shadow of the transverse foramen.
13. Bases of the transverse processes.
14. Cranial part of the transverse processes of C6 and C7.
15. C5, C6, and C7.

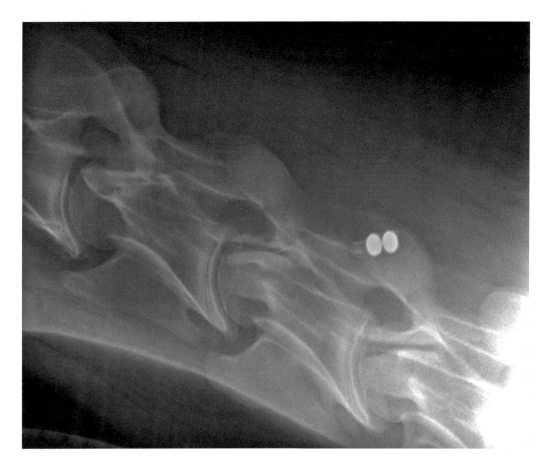

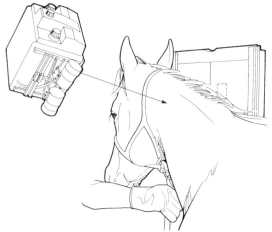

Figure 4.101A.

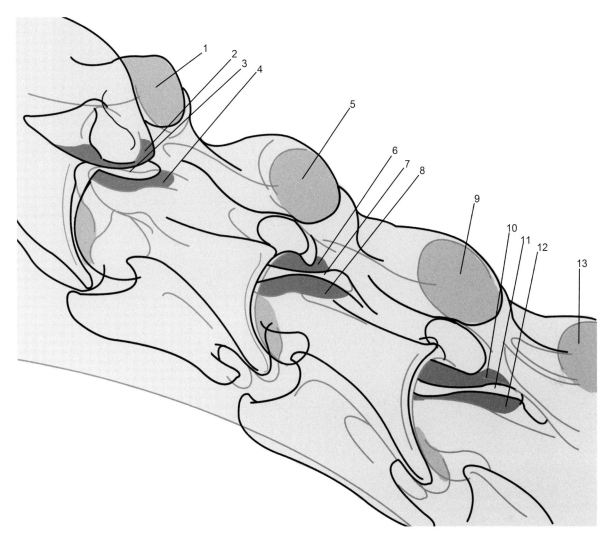

Figure 4.101A. (*Continued*) Laterodorsal-lateroventral oblique (La45D-LaVO) projections of the cervical vertebral facets. A. Cranial-mid cervical spine. B. Mid-caudal cervical spine. These projections are used to free the articular facets from superimposition with each other with the goal of having more discernible facet borders and detecting unilateral or bilateral changes.

A. Cranial-mid cervical spine.
1. Superimposed articular facets of C2 and C3.
2. Caudal articular facet of C2.
3. Joint space between articular facets of caudal C2 and cranial C3.
4. Cranial articular facet of C3.
5. Superimposed articular facets of C3 to C4.
6. Caudal articular facet of C3.
7. Joint space between articular facets of caudal C3 and cranial C4.
8. Cranial articular facet of C4.
9. Superimposed articular facets of C4 and C5.
10. Caudal articular facet of C4.
11. Joint space between articular facets of caudal C4 and cranial C5.
12. Cranial articular facet of C5.
13. Superimposed articular facets of C5 and C6.

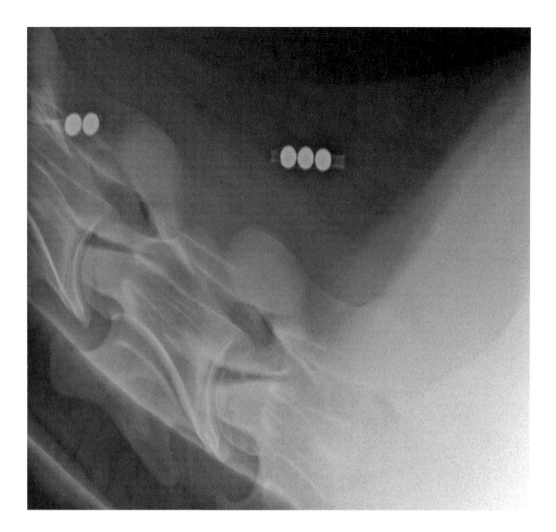

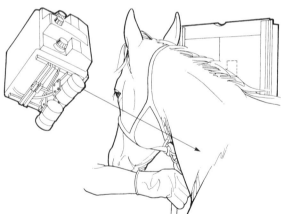

Figure 4.101B. (*Continued*)

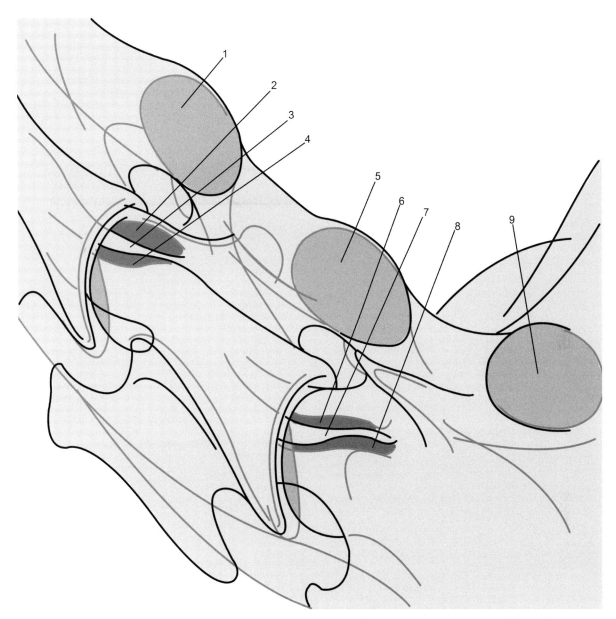

Figure 4.101B. (*Continued*)
B. Caudal cervical spine.
   1. Superimposed articular facets of C5 and C6.
   2. Caudal articular facet of C5.
   3. Joint space between articular facets of caudal C5 and cranial C6.
   4. Caudal articular facet of C6.
   5. Superimposed articular facets of C6 and C7.
   6. Caudal articular facet of C6.
   7. Joint space between articular facets of caudal C6 and cranial C7.
   8. Cranial articular facet of C7.
   9. Superimposed articular facets of C7 and T1.

References

1. International Committee on Veterinary Anatomical Nomenclature. Distributed by Dept. of Anatomy, New York State Veterinary College, Vienna, 1973.
2. National Council on Radiation Protection and Measurements. Radiation Protection in Veterinary Medicine. National Council on Radiation Protection and Measurements. Washington, DC 1970.
3. Ackerman N, Spencer CP, Hager DA, et al. Radiation exposure during equine radiography. Vet Radiol Ultrasound 1988; 29:198–201.
4. Arnbjerg J. Contrast radiography of joints and tendon sheaths in the horse. Nord Vet Med 1969;21:318.
5. Bacher K, Smeets P, Bonnarens K, et al. Dose reduction in patients undergoing chest imaging: digital amorphous silicon flat-panel detector radiography versus conventional film-screen radiography and phosphor-based computed radiography. AJR Am J Roentgenol 2003;181:923–929.
6. Burbidge HM, Kannegieter N, Dickson LR, et al. Iohexol myelography in the horse. Equine Vet J 1989;21:347–350.
7. Bushberg JT, Seibert JA, Leidholdt Jr. EM, et al. Digital Radiography. In The Essential Physics of Medical Imaging, Bushberg JT, Seibert JA, Leidholdt Jr EM, Boone JM, eds. Second ed., 2002. Lippincott Williams and Wilkins, Philadelphia, 293–316.
8. Chotas HG, Dobbins JT 3rd, Ravin CE. Principles of digital radiography with large-area, electronically readable detectors: a review of the basics. Radiology 1999;210:595–599.
9. Dik KJ. Fistulographie beim Pferd—retrospecktive Auswertung. Pferdeheilkunde 1987;3:255–261.
10. Dik KJ, Keg PR. The efficacy of contrast radiography to demonstrate 'false thoroughpins' in five horses. Equine Vet J 1990;22:223–225.
11. Farrow C. Sinography in the horse. Proceedings Am Assoc Equine Pract 1987;505–521.
12. Frost HM. Skeletal structural adaptations to mechanical usage (SATMU): 1. Redefining Wolff's law: the bone modeling problem. Anat Rec 1990;226:403–413.
13. Frost HM. Skeletal structural adaptations to mechanical usage (SATMU): 2. Redefining Wolff's law: the remodeling problem. Anat Rec 1990;226:414–422.
14. Gottschalk RD, Kirberger RM, Fourie SL. Vacuum phenomenon in equine carpal, metacarpophalangeal and metatarsophalangeal joints. J S Afr Vet Assoc 1999;70:5–8.
15. Hahn CN, Handel I, Green SL, et al. Assessment of the utility of using intra- and intervertebral minimum sagittal diameter ratios in the diagnosis of cervical vertebral malformation in horses. Vet Radiol Ultrasound 2008;49:1–6.
16. Hoffman KD, Pool RR, Pascoe JR. Degenerative joint disease of the proximal interphalangeal joints of the forelimbs of two young horses. Equine Vet J 1984;16:138–140.
17. Hopper BJ, Steel C, Richardson JL, et al. Radiographic evaluation of sclerosis of the third carpal bone associated with exercise and the development of lameness in Standardbred racehorses. Equine Vet J 2004;36:441–446.
18. Huber MJ, Grisel GR. Abscess on the lateral epicondyle of the humerus as a cause of lameness in a horse. J Am Vet Med Assoc 1997;211:1558–1561.
19. Koblik PD, Hornof WJ, O'Brien TR. Rare earth intensifying screens for veterinary radiography: An evaluation of two systems. Vet Radiol Ultrasound 1980;21:224–232.
20. Koblik PD, Toal R. Portable veterinary X-ray support systems for field use. J Am Vet Med Assoc 1991;199:186–188.
21. Korner M, Weber CH, Wirth S, et al. Advances in digital radiography: physical principles and system overview. Radiographics 2007;27:675–686.
22. Kroft LJ, Geleijns J, Mertens BJ, et al. Digital slot-scan charge-coupled device radiography versus AMBER and Bucky screen-film radiography for detection of simulated nodules and interstitial disease in a chest phantom. Radiology 2004;231:156–163.
23. Lewin JM, Hendrick RE, D'Orsi CJ, et al. Comparison of full-field digital mammography with screen-film mammography for cancer detection: results of 4,945 paired examinations. Radiology 2001;218:873–880.
24. Lo WY, Puchalski SM. Digital image processing. Vet Radiol Ultrasound 2008;49: S42–47.
25. Lundin CS, Clem MF, Debowes RM, et al. Diagnostic fistulography in horses. Comp Cont Educ Equine Pract 1988;10:639–645.
26. Maclean AA, Jeffcott LB, Lavelle RB, et al. Use of iohexol for myelography in the horse. Equine Vet J 1988;20:286–290.
27. May SA, Wyn-Jones G. Contrast radiography in the investigation of sinus tracts and abscess cavities in the horse. Equine Vet J 1987;19:218–222.
28. May SA, Wyn-Jones G, Church S, et al. Iopamidol myelography in the horse. Equine Vet J 1986;18:199–202.
29. Mayhew IG, Donawick WJ, Green SL, et al. Diagnosis and prediction of cervical vertebral malformation in thoroughbred foals based on semi-quantitative radiographic indicators. Equine Vet J 1993;25:435–440.
30. Mayhew IG, Green SL. Accuracy of diagnosing CVM from radiographs. 39th British Equine Veterinary Association Annual Congress 2000;74–75.
31. Mayhew IG, Whitlock RH, DeLahunta A. Spinal cord disease in the horse. Cornell Vet 1978;68:44.
32. Moore BR, Reed SM, Biller DS, et al. Assessment of vertebral canal diameter and bony malformations of the cervical part of the spine in horses with cervical stenotic myelopathy. Am J Vet Res 1994;55:5–13.
33. Morgan JP, Silverman S. Techniques of Veterinary Radiography. Iowa State University Press, 1989.
34. Nixon AJ, Spencer CP. Arthrography of the equine shoulder joint. Equine Vet J 1990;22:107–113.
35. Nyland TG, Blythe LL, Pool RR, et al. Metrizamide myelography in the horse: clinical, radiographic, and pathologic changes. Am J Vet Res 1980;41:204–211.
36. Okamura T, Tanaka S, Koyama K, et al. Clinical evaluation of digital radiography based on a large-area cesium iodide-amorphous silicon flat-panel detector compared with screen-film radiography for skeletal system and abdomen. Eur Radiol 2002; 12:1741–1747.
37. Papageorges M, Gavin PR, Sande RD, et al. Radiographic and myelographic examination of the cervical vertebral column in 306 ataxic horses. Vet Radiol Ultrasound 1987;28:53–59.
38. Peer R, Lanser A, Giacomuzzi SM, et al. Storage phosphor radiography of wrist fractures: a subjective comparison of image quality at varying exposure levels. Eur Radiol 2002;12: 1354–1359.
39. Phillips D. Radiology in your practice: Choosing the right equipment. Vet Med 1987;6:587–598.
40. Pisano ED, Gatsonis C, Hendrick E, et al. Diagnostic performance of digital versus film mammography for breast-cancer screening. N Engl J Med 2005;353:1773–1783.
41. Pool RR, Meagher DM, Stover SM. Pathophysiology of navicular syndrome. Vet Clin North Am Equine Pract 1989;5:109–129.
42. Puchalski SM. Image display. Vet Radiol Ultrasound 2008;49: S9–13.
43. Robertson I. Image dissemination and archiving. Clin Tech Small Anim Pract 2007;22:138–144.
44. Robertson ID, Saveraid T. Hospital, radiology, and picture archiving and communication systems. Vet Radiol Ultrasound 2008;49: S19–28.
45. Rowlands JA. The physics of computed radiography. Phys Med Biol 2002;47: R123–166.
46. Smallwood JE, Shively MJ, Rendano VT, et al. A standardized nomenclature for radiographic projections used in veterinary medicine. Vet Radiol Ultrasound 1985;26:2–9.
47. Specht TE, Poulos PW, Metcalf MR, et al. Vacuum phenomenon in the metatarsophalangeal joint of a horse. J Am Vet Med Assoc 1990;197:749–750.
48. Stickle R, Tetens J, Stick J, et al. Radiographic diagnosis: Proximal suspensory desmitis. Vet Radiol Ultrasound 1996;37: 105–107.
49. Strotzer M, Volk M, Reiser M, et al. Chest radiography with a large-area detector based on cesium-iodide/amorphous-silicon technology: image quality and dose requirement in comparison with an asymmetric screen-film system. J Thorac Imaging 2000;15:157–161.
50. Tomizawa N, Nishimura R, Sasaki N, et al. Efficacy of the new radiographic measurement method for cervical vertebral instability in wobbling foals. J Vet Med Sci 1994;56:1119–1122.
51. van Biervliet J, Mayhew J, de Lahunta A. Cervical Vertebral Compressive Myelopathy: Diagnosis. Clinical Techniques in Equine Practice 2006;5:54–59.
52. van Biervliet J, Scrivani PV, Divers TJ, et al. Evaluation of decision criteria for detection of spinal cord compression based on cervical myelography in horses: 38 cases (1981–2001). Equine Veterinary Journal 2004;36:14–20.

53. Volk M, Strotzer M, Holzknecht N, et al. Digital radiography of the skeleton using a large-area detector based on amorphous silicon technology: image quality and potential for dose reduction in comparison with screen-film radiography. Clin Radiol 2000;55:615–621.
54. Wallack S. Digital image storage. Vet Radiol Ultrasound 2008;49:S37–41.
55. Widmer WR. Acquisition hardware for digital imaging. Vet Radiol Ultrasound 2008;49:S2–8.
56. Widmer WR. Iohexol and iopamidol: new contrast media for veterinary myelography. J Am Vet Med Assoc 1989;194: 1714–1716.
57. Wright MA, Ballance D, Robertson ID, et al. Introduction to DICOM for the practicing veterinarian. Vet Radiol Ultrasound 2008;49: S14–18.
58. Young BD, Hendrickson DA, Park RD. What is your diagnosis? Mixed lytic-proliferative lesion in the left tibia. J Am Vet Med Assoc 2002;221:1251–1252.

ULTRASOUND

W. Rich Redding

INTRODUCTION

Diagnostic ultrasound was introduced to equine veterinarians in the early 1980s. At that time veterinary ultrasound systems were predominantly designed and used for reproductive examinations with large 5-MHz rectal probes. While these probes were less than ideal for examining the superficial structures of the musculoskeletal system, a few innovative equine veterinarians embraced this new technology and started to evaluate the flexor tendons of the metacarpus. Shortly thereafter, higher frequency mechanical sector scanners with multiple frequency transducers (3.5 to 7.5 MHz) became available and allowed detailed examination and classification of soft tissue injuries of the palmar/plantar metacarpus/metatarsus and pastern.[33,35,53,54,55,61] This was the first time soft tissue structures of the distal limb could be seen as a tomographic or body slice image. It was now possible to evaluate the flexor tendons and suspensory ligament for morphological change.

Over the last couple of decades, ultrasound technology has dramatically improved and linear array ultrasound systems have been developed that are better suited for musculoskeletal examinations. Many of these high end systems have 14- to 18-MHz linear tendon probes and 8- to 10-MHz microconvex probes with variable focusing capabilities and multiple frequencies. In addition, mainframe ultrasound platforms have been reduced to the size of notebook-sized computers and the miniaturization of electronics has reduced the quality differences between portable and stationary technologies. Ultrasonography is now considered the imaging modality of choice to evaluate soft tissue injuries in the horse.

SCIENCE OF ULTRASOUND

Ultrasonography is a 2-dimensional real-time imaging technique that uses the transfer and propagation of sound waves into soft tissue.[3,40,45,49,54,55,61] Ultrasound is defined as sound above the audible range. Ultrasound waves behave as classic sound waves that operate at frequencies spanning 1 to 20 MHz. These sound waves are mechanical waves that require some sort of medium to allow the waves to form and travel. The propagating medium determines how fast the sound waves travel, how easily they can be formed, and how well the traveling waves can remain together.

Ultrasound machines produce a sound wave of longitudinal orientation in which the elements of the medium are compressed and rarefied. The distance between the start of one cycle of compression and rarefaction and the next is considered the wavelength, and most wavelengths are 1 mm or less. Propagation speed of the ultrasound wave is determined by the density and stiffness of a given tissue, with bone propagating at higher speeds, while fluid-filled structures propagate at medium speeds and air propagates at the lowest speeds. Average propagation velocity of the sound wave in soft tissues is around 1,540 meters/second.

Ultrasound waves lose energy to the medium in the form of heat through a process termed absorption. Absorption increases directly with distance and frequency. A transducer produces short bursts of specific frequency sound waves which are transmitted into the patient and reflected back at different tissues and tissue interfaces. The transducer then detects the reflected sound waves and these waves are converted to electrical energy. A computer plots the time the sound waves traveled along with the amplitude of the reflected sound waves. Echoes are produced at tissue interfaces of different acoustic impedance, which is a measure of how easily waves can be formed and depends on sound velocity and tissue density. The greater the differences in acoustic impedance of the reflecting interfaces the greater the intensity of the returning echo.

Ultrasound waves constantly encounter changes in soft tissue that can affect propagation of the sound wave which cause scatter and a weakening of the return echoes. The brightness of the dot on the monitor screen correlates to the amplitude of the returning echo. Terms to describe the appearance of an image relate to the tissue's echo intensity or echogenicity. The echogenicity of a structure or the degree to which the structure reflects sound waves determines the brightness of objects on ultrasound. All of this information is displayed as a cross sectional image developed by an entirely different set of physical parameters of structures (objects) than those measured by other imaging modalities.

The frequency of the sound wave is determined by the piezoelectric crystals in the scan head. These crystals are man-made and designed to vibrate at high frequencies and produce a specific wavelength sound beam. The crystals receive sound waves coming back from the tissues and convert them to electrical energy. The wavelength dictates the resolution and the energy contained by this sound beam. High-frequency transducers have smaller crystals and the sound pulses are close together and the wavelengths are shorter. The shorter the wavelength, the better the axial resolution, which is a measure of the ability to show two interfaces as separate along the axis of the beam.

Axial resolution is determined by the wavelength (pulse length), and the wavelength is determined by the frequency. Lateral resolution is the minimum distance that two dots can be distinguished from one another in a plane perpendicular to the sound wave. Lateral resolution is best in the focal zone and depends on the width of the sound beam. Improving lateral resolution requires focusing the beam to the narrowest width possible. Axial resolution is usually superior to lateral resolution. Images should be obtained with the highest frequency probe possible to obtain the best resolution of the structure of interest. However, sound is attenuated at 1 dB/cm depth per megahertz (MHz). Higher frequencies are therefore attenuated at higher rates, which reduces the penetration of the sound wave. Lower frequencies are attenuated at lower rates, which allow them to penetrate deeper into tissue.

Most current musculoskeletal ultrasound systems use variable focus linear and convex array transducers. Flat-face linear and microconvex probes are the most popular probes for musculoskeletal imaging. Linear probes give superior images at tissue depths of 2 cm or less due to decreased distortion and artifact creation in the near field. Linear probes have stand-off pads available that improve contact with the skin, increasing the footprint and moving the superficial structures into the near field focal zone and away from the near field artifact. A stand-off also increases the footprint or image field of the scan head, and linear probes also provide excellent evaluation of longitudinal fiber alignment.

Convex array transducers are used when the skin is contoured and it is difficult to seat the flat-face transducer. The divergent beam allows the examiner to image from a smaller skin contact point. These convex probes can be more difficult to use because it is easier to inadvertently change the beam angle, especially when doing longitudinal assessments of fiber alignment. In addition to the superior imaging, these transducers have lower purchase prices and lower maintenance costs when compared to sector technology. Many of these probes have multiple frequencies available, which allows the examiner to easily change the frequency without needing to change the probe. Structures within 5 to 7 cm of the skin should be evaluated with transducers of a minimum of 7.5 to 10 MHz or higher. Structures within 7 to 14 cm should be evaluated with 5-MHz transducers. Anything deeper than 14 cm requires lower frequencies such as 2.5 to 3.5 MHz.

DIAGNOSTIC ULTRASOUND TO EVALUATE TENDONS AND LIGAMENTS

Ultrasonography has significantly advanced the diagnosis and management of a variety of musculoskeletal injuries in performance horses.[13,18,28,33,34,35,53,54,55,61] A working knowledge of the normal anatomy is critical for tendon and ligament ultrasonographic examinations as well as those involving joints, sheaths, and bursae.[24,38,66,70,79] Ultrasonography is routinely used to define morphological change in the superficial digital flexor tendon (SDFT), deep digital flexor tendon (DDFT), suspensory ligament (SL), accessory ligament of the DDFT (ICL) and distal sesamoidean ligaments (DSL) of the pastern region. The subcutaneous tissue, peritendinous tissue, vessels, and contour of the cortical bone in the region should be assessed as well. Most importantly, diagnostic ultrasound is the most useful and practical tool to monitor the repair of these structures and guide the rehabilitation of tendinous and ligamentous structures. Many other soft tissue structures can be evaluated, including muscle, musculotendinous junctions, tendon sheaths, and bursae associated with the tendons and ligaments.

Joint injury (which is discussed later in the chapter) is very effectively examined with radiography and ultrasonography. These imaging tools are considered complementary and provide more information about a joint than either tool used alone. Joint examination should include evaluation of the periarticular structures such as the collateral ligaments and extensor/flexor tendons, joint capsule, and joint fluid accumulations.

Real-time imaging capability of ultrasonography allows the use of interventional techniques (such as needle insertion for injection or aspiration/biopsy), which can provide additional clinical information.[6,11,41,44,72] Ultrasonography is also used to evaluate a variety of other problems such as fractures of long bones, osteitis/osteomyelitis, foreign body penetration, and implant infection, as well as being used intra-operatively to assist with some surgical procedures.[7,62,84]

Patient Preparation and Scan Protocol

Confirmation that lameness is associated with a specific structure or area is critical. Localization of lameness should include a clinical examination and the use of diagnostic nerve blocks when necessary. In most instances injection of diagnostic anesthesia into an area will not interfere with the ultrasonographic examination. Occasionally gas bubbles in the injectate may inhibit sound transmission and necessitate performing the exam on a subsequent day. Tranquilization may be necessary and can assist the examination.

Patient preparation is very important and should include clipping with a #40 blade. Both limbs should be clipped and prepped because strain-induced tendon and ligament injury can occur bilaterally, with one limb being more severely affected than the other. Shaving is frequently required to give a higher resolution image. A scrub with a detergent is generally necessary to remove dirt and debris. Many clinicians do a 5-minute sterile prep with antiseptic solution/detergent followed by an alcohol rinse. Liberally coat the prepped area with ultrasound gel and let stand on the limb for 5 minutes. Excessive gel can cause a lateral image artifact which may compromise image quality. When clipping and shaving is not possible, the limb should be thoroughly washed with warm water and detergent. Application of alcohol to the hair coat may enhance the sound transmission. To acquire the best image, a scan head with a frequency of at least 7.5 MHz should be used, but frequencies of 10 to 18 MHz are preferable. Low frame rates should be used to give higher line density and improved resolution. Most superficial structures can be visualized at a scan depth of 2 to 4 cm, often with the use of a stand-off pad.

The ultrasonographic examination should be performed in a systematic manner with each structure evaluated from proximal to distal to ensure a complete and thorough tendon/ligament evaluation. The examiner should develop a systematic approach to screening the limb, such as the technique described by Genovese and Rantanen.[33,35,54,55] This approach provides a survey of all structures, including veins, arteries, subcutaneous tissue, paratendinous tissue, and bone contour at specific levels in the metacarpus/metatarsus. A standardized scanning protocol has numerous advantages, but most importantly it provides a means for clinicians to effectively screen the limb as well as provide a method for veterinarians to accurately communicate their findings.

This imaging protocol is based on the metacarpus being approximately 24 cm in length or roughly 3 hand-widths of a person's hand (8 cm/hand breadth). The metatarsus is longer that the metacarpus and measures approximately 32 cm or roughly 4 hand-widths in length. Theses zones are numbered 1 through 3 in the forelimb and 1 through 4 in the hindlimb. Each of these zones is further subdivided into 2 equal zones named A and B (each being 4 cm) such that the forelimb has zones 1A, 1B, 2A, 2B, 3A, 3B.

The area associated with the proximal sesamoids of the fetlock is considered zone 3C (or 4C in the hindlimb). Some authors use a simple numerical scheme with the forelimb having levels 1 through 7 and the hindlimb having levels 1 through 9. These levels are the same zones mentioned above but without the letter designations (Figures 4.102 to 4.110) To more completely assess the architecture of the SL branches it is necessary to incline the transducer more medial to lateral or lateral to medial as the examiner progresses distally until they attach to the proximal aspect of their respective proximal sesamoid bone (Figure 4.111).

The imaging protocol for the pastern is based on zones related to the proximal and middle pastern bones.

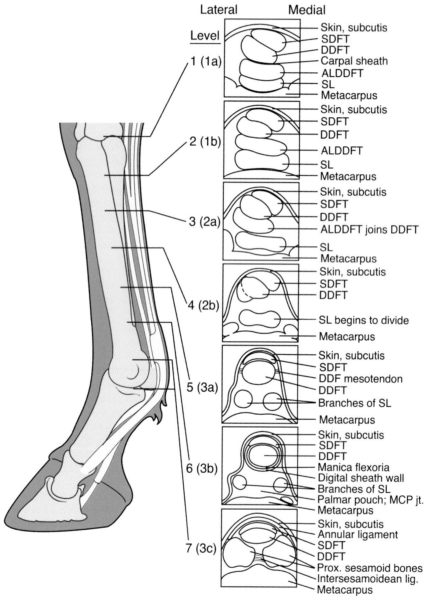

Figure 4.102. Ultrasonographic imaging of the metacarpus is based on the length being approximately 24 cm in length or roughly 3 hand-widths of a person's hand (8 cm/hand breadth). Theses zones are numbered 1 through 3 in the forelimb. These zones are further subdivided into two equal zones named A and B (each being approximately 4 cm) such that the forelimb has zones 1A, 1B, 2A, 2B, 3A, 3B. The area associated with the proximal sesamoid bones (PSB) of the fetlock is considered zone 3C. Some authors use a simple numerical scheme, with the forelimb having levels 1 through 7. The structures identified from the transducer to the palmar metacarpus are the SDFT, DDFT, ICL, and SL.

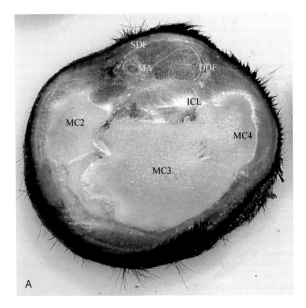

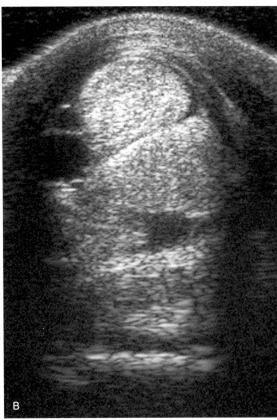

Figure 4.103. A. In Z1A the SDFT is round but with a flat border dorsally where it is adjacent to the DDFT. The DDFT is rounded in shape. The ICL is located dorsal to the DDFT with the carpal sheath visualized as an anechoic triangular structure between these two structures. The SL is located dorsal to the ICL but may only have a few fibers apparent in proximal Z1A. The SL

becomes more apparent, progressing distally in this zone. B. This ultrasound image is taken at the proximal aspect of Z1A to correspond to the gross section slice plane that is close to the carpometacarpal joint. At this level the ICL is the only structure apparent dorsal to the DDFT. The median artery and large metacarpal vein are prominent on the medial aspect of the DDFT.

Figure 4.104. In Z1B the palmar metacarpal structures appear much as they did in zone 1A. The SDFT appears to flatten palmar to dorsal and the DDFT becomes more rounded. The ICL becomes more inclined toward the DDFT. Fibers of the SL become more pronounced and this structure widens medial to lateral (A). However, ultrasound imaging of this area has inherent problems with edge artifacts and acoustic enhancement artifacts which can make evaluation of the SL difficult (B).

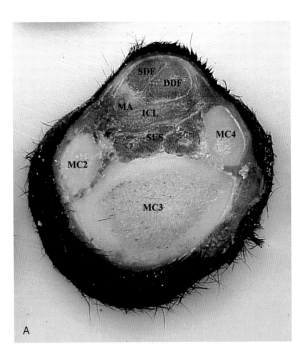

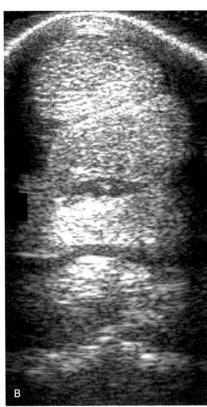

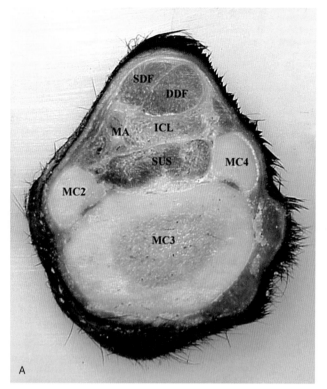

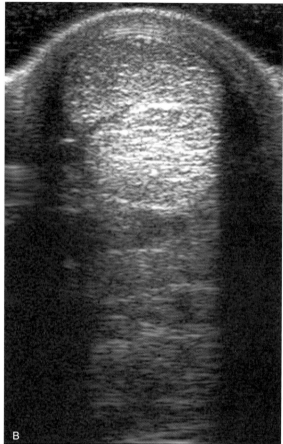

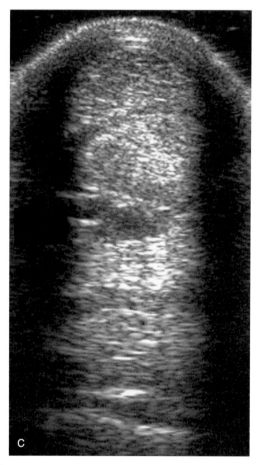

Figure 4.105. In Z2A the ICL narrows palmar to dorsal and the SL increases in area, becoming more discreet and separated from the palmar cortex of MC3 (cannon bone). The large metacarpal vessels can be seen medially and laterally (A). These vessels also create edge and acoustic enhancement artifacts, compromising interpretation of the SL architecture. B and C.

These ultrasound images demonstrate these artifacts and also highlight the importance of focal zone placement. The focal zone in (B) is placed on the SDFT/DDFT junction with the deeper structures out of focus and poorly imaged, and the focal zone in (C) is placed at the level of the SL.

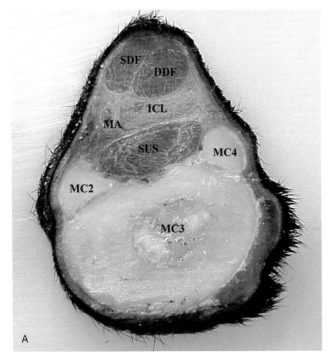

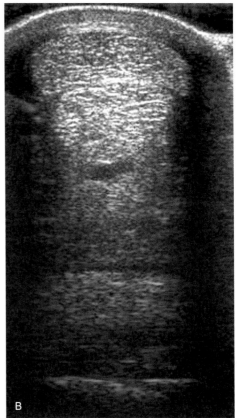

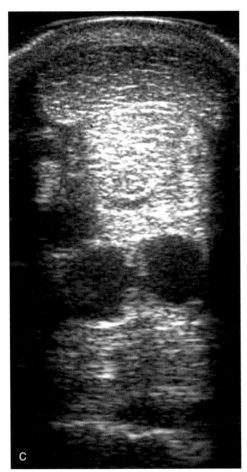

Figure 4.106. A. In Z2B the SDFT becomes flatter and the ICL remains distinct from but closely associated with the DDFT. The metacarpal vessels converge to midline between the ICL and the SL. B. This ultrasound image with the focal zone placed superficially demonstrates the fibers of the SDFT/DDFT interface, while (C) shows focal zone at the level of the SL and the convergence of the large metacarpal vessels palmar to the SL.

343

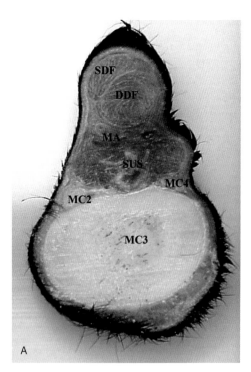

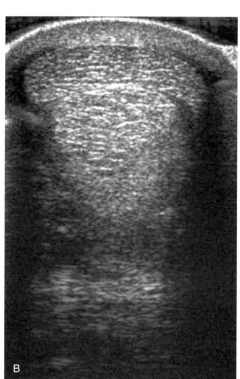

Figure 4.107. A. In the proximal aspect of zone 3A the SDFT thins and begins to expand medial to lateral and appears crescent shaped. The DDFT and ICL are beginning to blend together and can appear as one structure. In the proximal aspect of this zone the SL has not divided and continues to appear as one structure. B. There may appear to be a hypoechoic area within the central aspect of the SL just prior to the formation of the branches but this should not be confused with a lesion.

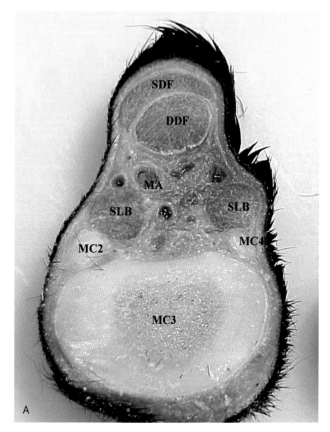

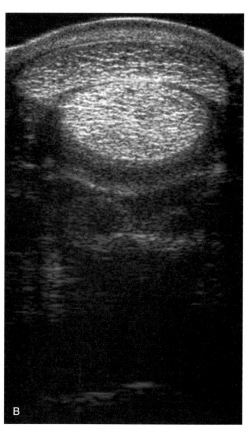

Figure 4.108. A. The distal aspect of Z3A demonstrates the SDFT as elongated in a medial-to-lateral direction and the division (splitting) of the SL into branches (SLBs). B. This ultrasound image with the focal zone at the junction of the SDFT and DDFT demonstrates the widening of the SDFT and blending of the fibers of the DDFT and the ICL.

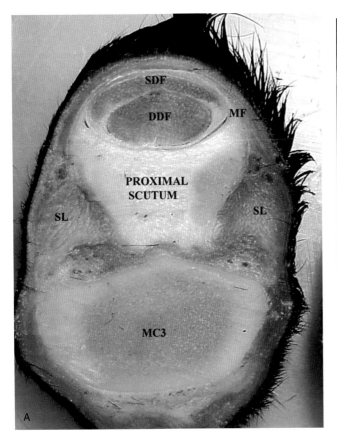

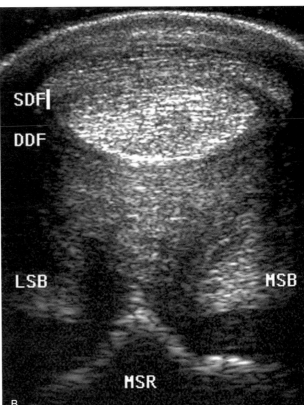

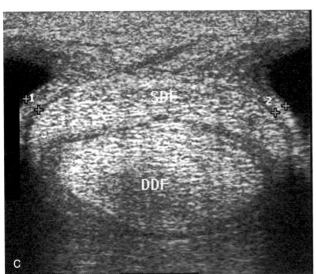

Figure 4.109. A and B. Zone 3B is somewhat longer than the other zones and several important landmarks can be seen in this area. The SDFT and DDFT widen in a medial to lateral direction. These structures can be difficult to image together so each must be examined independently. At the junction of Z3A and 3B after the SL divides into medial and lateral branches, the proximal scutum and palmar aspect of the fetlock joint just proximal to the PSBs can be seen. The proximal aspect of the midsagittal ridge of the palmar metacarpus can be seen. C. This ultrasound image demonstrates a moderate amount of effusion within the DFTS and allows the natural axial connection of the DFTS to the palmar border of the SDFT proximal to the MCP joint to be visualized. This should not be considered abnormal.

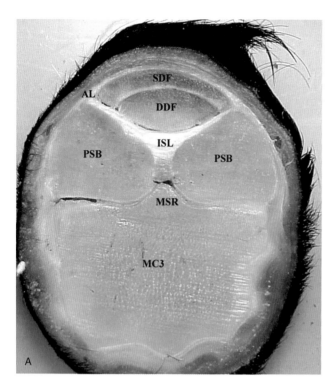

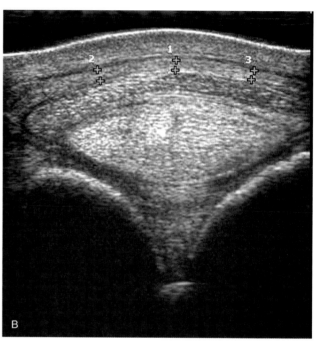

Figure 4.110. A. Zone 3C begins at the level of the PSBs and extends through the fetlock canal. The primary anular ligament (PAL) extends from the palmarolateral to palmaromedial border of the PSBs (abaxial border of each PSB). B. This ultrasound image demonstrates the PAL wrapping around the SDFT and DDFT. It may be necessary to rotate the transducer in the medial to lateral plane to evaluate the fibers of the PAL. A more abaxial orientation of the transducer may also be necessary to image the attachment to the PSBs.

The proximal pastern (P1) has 3 2-cm zones associated with it and named P1A, P1B, and P1C. The middle pastern bone (P2) is shorter and has just 2 2-cm zones associated with it: P2A and P2B (Figures 4.112 to 4.119).[42]

The overall length of the pastern and height of the collateral cartilages of the distal phalanx can significantly affect the ability to image the deep digital flexor tendon (DDFT) in zone P2A. To evaluate the origin of the oblique sesamoidean ligaments (OSLs) on the distal aspect of the proximal sesamoid bone it is necessary to incline the transducer more dorsally such that a medial-to-lateral or lateral-to-medial orientation is obtained. The pastern is more difficult to examine than the metacarpus because positioning the probe between the distal aspect of the sesamoid bones (and the ergot) and the proximal aspect of the collateral cartilages can be difficult. Placing the foot on a block of wood with the limb more caudal than the opposite limb increases the extension of the fetlock joint and positions the axis of the pastern in a more upright position (Figure 4.120). In general the distal sesamoidean ligaments (DSLs) and branches of the superficial digital flexor tendon (SDFT) are smaller and inclined at different angles as they course to their insertions, which requires that different scan planes be used to evaluate each of these structures.

Each structure should be examined on cross section and on longitudinal orientation with appropriate placement of the focal zone(s) on the structure of interest at each location. In the metacarpus each level should have 2 transverse scans performed. The first should have a stand-off placed on the transducer with the focal zone(s) and transducer angle directed initially at the SDFT and DDFT. The second scan should be acquired with or without a stand-off with focal zone(s) and transducer angle directed at the inferior check ligament (ICL) and suspensory ligament (SL) (Figure 4.121). In some instances it may be helpful to use a microconvex transducer for this scan because the divergent beam can improve assessment of the medial and lateral borders of the SL. The transverse scan plane should be positioned such that the structures on the left side of the horse are placed to the left side of the screen. Some clinicians like to place the medial side of the limb on the left side of the screen and the lateral side of the limb on the right side of the screen.[61] In addition, the sagittal scan plane should position structures of the proximal aspect of the limb to the left of the screen and structures of the distal aspect of the limb to the right side of the screen. Some clinicians place these structures opposite with the proximal aspect of the limb to the right of the screen.[61] Whatever protocol is used, it should be done consistently with appropriate labeling on the recorded image.

Careful attention should be paid to all tendinous/ligamentous structures because multiple structures are often involved. The examiner should also be aware that an injury can extend proximally into the carpal sheath or distally into the digital sheath/pastern area. If an abnormality exists the lesion should be mapped and

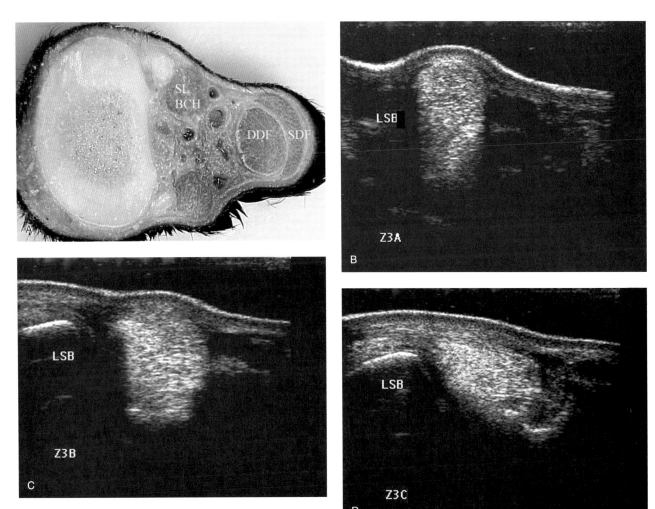

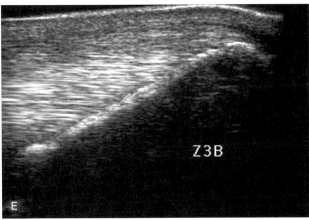

Figure 4.111. A to E. The branches of the suspensory ligament (SLBs) are best imaged from a medial-to-lateral and/or lateral-to-medial orientation. These structures should be evaluated at the level where they begin to divide in distal 3A until their attachments to the PSBs. B. Initially the SLBs have an oval shape. C. Further distally the branch becomes somewhat D-shaped. D. The branch appears to rotate in a dorsal-to-palmar direction, becoming oval-shaped just prior to their attachment onto the PSBs. E. The SLBs should also be evaluated in the longitudinal plane from their beginning to their attachments to the PSBs.

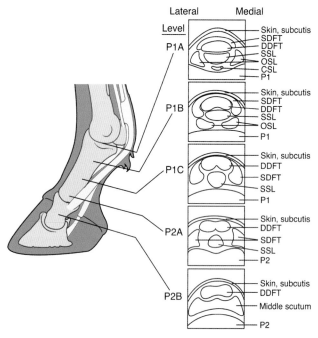

Lateral   Medial

Level

P1A — Skin, subcutis / SDFT / DDFT / SSL / OSL / CSL / P1

P1B — Skin, subcutis / SDFT / DDFT / SSL / OSL / P1

P1C — Skin, subcutis / DDFT / SDFT / SSL / P1

P2A — Skin, subcutis / DDFT / SDFT / SSL / P2

P2B — Skin, subcutis / DDFT / Middle scutum / P2

Figure 4.112. The SDFT and DDFT continue into the pastern. The DSLs (SSL, paired OSLs, and paired CSLs) originate on the PSBs and course distally onto insert on the distal aspects of P1 and P2. The SSL originates from the axial region of the PSBs and crosses the pastern joint onto insert on the palmaroproximal aspect of P2. The OSLs originate from the abaxial region of the PSBs and insert on the roughened triangular area of P1. The cruciate sesamoidean ligaments cross from the PSB to the contralateral aspect of palmaroproximal P1. The SDFT encircles the DDFT as they course out of the fetlock canal. The fibers of the SDFT incline abaxially, moving distally in the pastern to form teardrop-shaped branches that insert on the abaxial area of palmaroproximal P2. The DDFT continues distally and becomes bi-lobed in the midpastern area. The DDFT widens in a medial-to-lateral direction as it courses into the foot to insert on the distal phalanx (P3).

measured in centimeters from a reference point such as the accessory carpal bone in the forelimb and the point of the hock or tarsometatarsal joint (head of the lateral splint) in the hindlimb. The extent and severity of the lesion should be documented and mapped by measuring the proximal most extent of the lesion from the appropriate anatomical reference point to the distal most extent of the lesion. The lesion should be evaluated on both cross section and longitudinal scan planes. The lesion's maximum size should be determined and mapped. Echogenicity and fiber alignment should be subjectively evaluated throughout the abnormal tissue.

Each image should be labeled with the date, owner's name, patient's name, limb being examined, and location of the lesion(s). A description of the scan plane should be included in every image and every image recorded as part of the medical record. Documentation of the lesion location, lesion echogenicity, and extent or degree of change with appropriate labeling should be included on the image before being stored and maintained as part of the permanent medical record. Images can be stored as thermal prints (which degrade over time), video recordings, or digital images (DICOMs) for

comparison at later examinations. Most current machines provide software that allows the image to be traced, which provides a cross sectional area of the tendon/ligament and lesion. As mentioned earlier, this is critical for the rehabilitation process so healing can be accurately assessed.

Tendons and ligaments appear similarly as moderately echogenic structures with relatively well-defined margins due to their parallel fascicular arrangement. It is this arrangement of fibers, aligned to resist tensile forces, that creates the intense specular reflections (echoes) seen when the sound beam is perpendicular to the direction of the fascicles. The examiner must pay particular attention to the course of the tendon or ligament being imaged, and maintain the transducer at 90° to the structure. The structures of the metacarpus/metatarsus and the pastern change orientation as they incline distally toward their insertion sites.

To perform a complete examination, each structure should be evaluated independently with careful attention being paid to correct beam angle and focal zone placement. The horse should be weight-bearing on the limb and the tendons and ligaments loaded during the ultrasound examination. Imaging while the horse is not bearing weight or only partially bearing weight can create changes in shape and size of these structures, referred to as relaxation artifacts.

Relaxation artifacts appear as hypoechoic areas within the normally bright specular reflections seen during routine examination of tendons and ligaments, which can compromise the accuracy of the study. Relaxation artifacts can also occur in some abnormal conditions. For example, complete disruption of the suspensory apparatus relieves the tension in the straight sesamoidean ligament (SSL), resulting in relaxation artifacts in the SSL. This is also apparent when evaluating lacerations or rupture of a tendon/ligament, which relaxes the tensile forces in the affected structures and can create relaxation artifacts most often proximal but also distal to the site of injury.

There are some indications for off-weighted examination of some structures. Proximal anular ligament syndrome of the digital flexor tendon sheath frequently has a proliferative tenosynovitis which can obscure the borders of the SDFT and DDFT, diminishing the ability of ultrasonography to define these structures as separate. Off-weighted scanning of this area is indicated to determine whether adhesions may have developed between the flexor tendons within the digital flexor tendon sheath. Lifting the limb off the ground and flexing the fetlock joint through a full range of motion while performing an ultrasonographic examination in longitudinal scan plane may be necessary to demonstrate a lack of independent movement of the tendons. A lack of independent movement suggests the formation of adhesions between these two structures.

In addition, horses with proximal anular ligament syndrome may have a compartmentalization syndrome, which can compress the tendons, obscuring significant pathology in the standing animal. Lifting the limb off the ground and placing it through a range of motion while imaging in transverse scan plane may allow the architecture of the SDFT and DDFT to be assessed more completely.

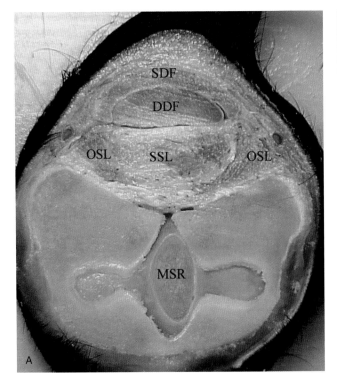

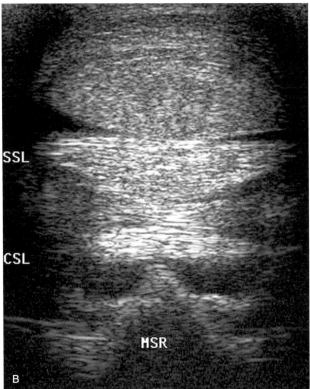

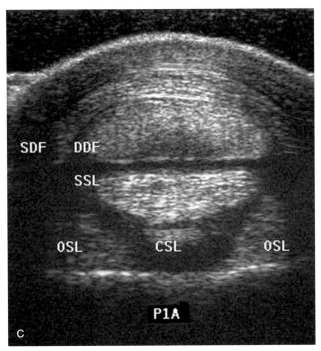

Figure 4.113. A. In ZP1A the contour of the palmar border of the proximal P1 is a V-shaped hyperechoic line. From the midline position the OSLs are positioned on the abaxial surfaces of P1 (palmar tuberosities). The SDFT encircles the oval DDFT with a uniform palmar-to-dorsal dimension. The SSL is triangular in shape at its origin from the intersesamoidean ligament (ISL) and

PSBs. B. Angling the transducer proximad allows the distal aspect of the midsagittal ridge to be seen. The DDFT is oval at this level, while the SSL is triangular at its origin; the cruciate sesamoidean ligament (CSL) can be seen dorsal to the SSL. C. At the level proximal of P1 the DDFT and the SSL are easily imaged but the OSL will require a more abaxial position of the transducer.

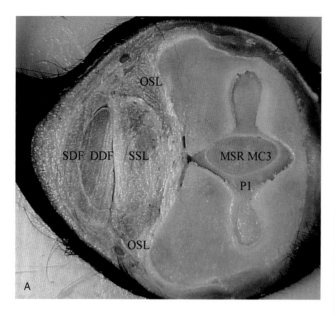

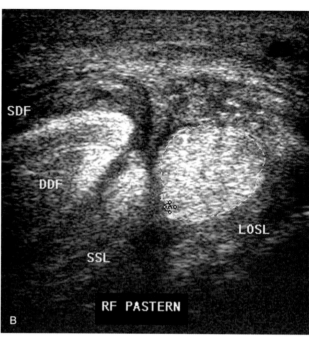

Figure 4.114. A. To best image the origin of the OSLs, the transducer should be placed more abaxially and directed toward the base of the PSBs. B. In transverse section the OSLs appear somewhat rounded at this level. The transducer should also be placed longitudinally to image the origin of the OSLs to their respective PSBs.

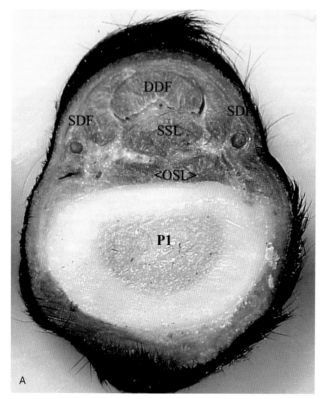

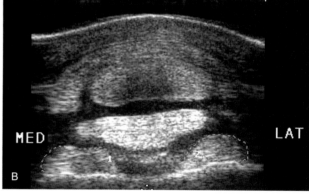

Figure 4.115. A. Zone P1B is considered the middle of the proximal phalanx (P1). The bone contour of P1 is flat at this level. The fibers of the SDFT incline abaxially to the medial and lateral aspect of the DDFT as they begin to divide into branches. The DDFT develops a central depression on its dorsal surface and becomes bilobed in appearance. The SSL becomes more rounded in appearance. The OSLs incline more axially on P1, blending together to form a rectangular structure. B. The ultrasound image shows that the SSL appears hyperechoic relative to other structures. When the SSL is in focus the DDFT is hypoechoic, necessitating that each structure be imaged independently. The SDFT cannot be adequately imaged with this transducer orientation.

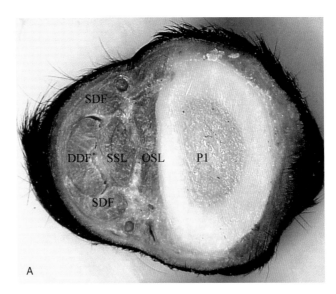

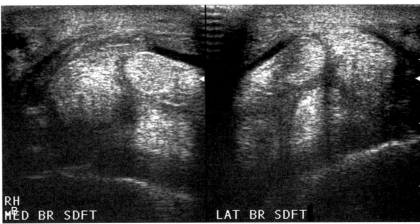

Figure 4.116. A and B. To examine the SDFT branches the transducer must be placed more abaxially, which allows the individual SDFT branches to be imaged as they incline to their insertion onto the medial and lateral aspects of proximal P2.

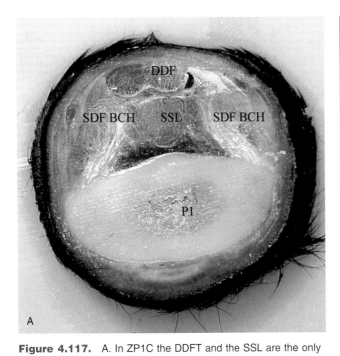

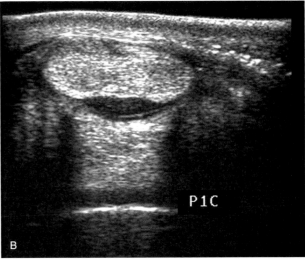

Figure 4.117. A. In ZP1C the DDFT and the SSL are the only structures easily imaged when the transducer is on midline in a palmar position. The DDFT is bilobed and now expands in a medial-to-lateral direction. The SSL is rounded just prior to insertion onto palmar P2 and the middle scutum. B. The SDFT branches are more abaxial and difficult to image with this transducer orientation (see Figure 4.116).

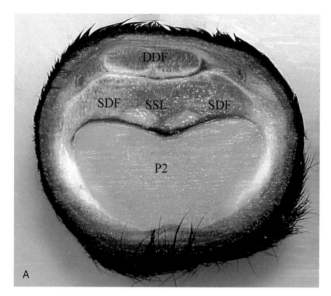

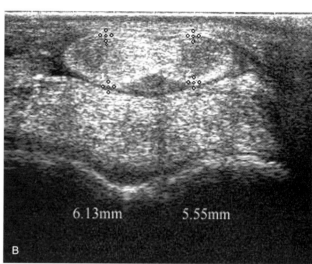

Figure 4.118. A. Zones P2A and P2B are associated with the middle phalanx (P2). Zone P2A begins when the ultrasound examination visualizes the structures of the pastern crossing the proximal interphalangeal joint. The SSL, medial, and lateral SDFT branches and the axial and abaxial ligaments of the pastern joint blend together to form the cartilaginous attachment onto P2, called the middle scutum. B. There is a normal hypoechoic area within the SSL just prior to insertion onto P2.

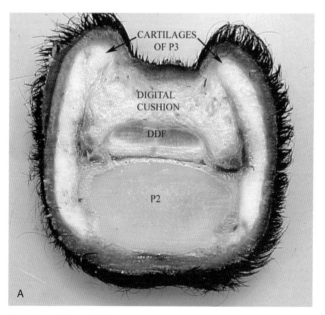

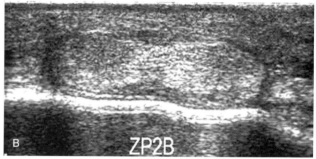

Figure 4.119. A. Ultrasound imaging of Z2PB in the distopalmar aspect of P2 can be difficult due to the presence of the collateral cartilages of the distal phalanx. B. The collateral cartilages interfere with proper placement of the transducer distal enough to assess the DDFT with a perpendicular orientation of the sound beam to the fiber pattern of the tendon.

Another indication for off-weighted but also off-incidence beam angle is when trying to perform a complete examination of the proximal suspensory ligament.[18] Relaxation of the flexor tendons allows them to become hypoechoic and brings the suspensory ligament closer to the transducer and within the focal zones of the transducer.

Ultrasonographic Assessment of Tendon/Ligament Pathology

Tendon and ligament injury is recognized ultrasonographically by changes in size, shape, architecture, position (with respect to surrounding anatomy), and fiber alignment. Cross sectional area (CSA) measurements are considered a very sensitive indicator of inflammation and the best way to assess increases in size from the transverse images (Figure 4.122). Subtle enlargements of a structure may require comparison to the opposite limb. Any enlargement suggests structural thickening and the rest of the examination should attempt to determine whether the change is a result of acute, subacute, or chronic injury.

Most current ultrasound machines have the capability to trace the CSA of the frozen image on the screen. Some machines have software that allows stored images

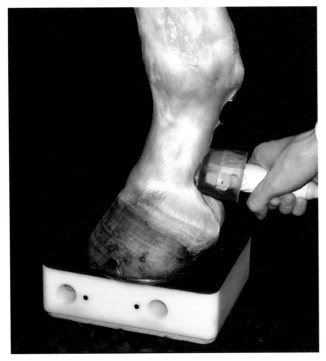

Figure 4.120. Placing the limb on a small block with the leg more caudal allows a more comfortable examination of the structures of the pastern region. Notice the stand-off pad placed over the probe to move the near field artifact away from the superficial structures.

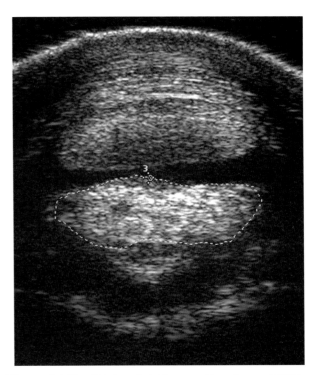

Figure 4.122. This is a straight sesamoidean ligament (SSL) injury. There is enlargement with an irregular outline associated with the heterogeneous appearance of the ligament. Tracing of the cross sectional area is helpful to follow the rehabilitation process. Tendon and ligament damage is represented by changes in size, shape, architecture, position (with respect to surrounding anatomy), and fiber alignment.

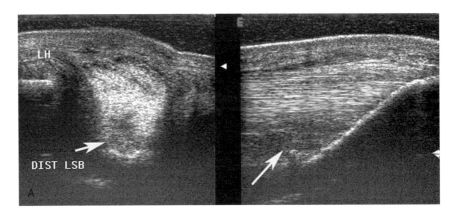

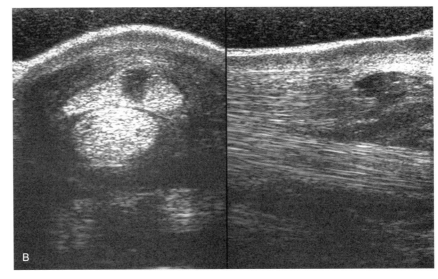

Figure 4.121. A. Longitudinal and cross sectional ultrasound image of a suspensory ligament attachment injury. Notice the loss of fiber pattern and the calcification at the attachment to the proximal sesamoid bone on transverse and longitudinal sections. B. Longitudinal and cross sectional ultrasound image of the SDFT with a core type defect of the central aspect of the tendon.

to be processed after recovery and storage. Post processing of the image to determine a CSA can be accomplished with digitizing software, provided the images are stored as DICOMs; however, this can be quite time consuming (Dicom Works). Lesion CSA can be compared to the tendon/ligament CSA measurement to calculate the proportion of tendon involved. An accurate CSA must be obtained because this measurement will be used as a baseline in the rehabilitation of tendon and ligaments. CSA may increase for 2 to 3 weeks after an injury due to persistent inflammation. A repeat scan at 2 weeks will provide a more accurate maximum lesion and tendon CSA to compare back to during rehabilitation.

Normal values for Standardbred and Thoroughbred horses have been published.[61] If normal values for CSA for a structure are not available they can be obtained from the opposite limb at the same level. As the tendon/ligament remodels, the CSA will progressively diminish during the rehabilitation process. Increases in CSA during the rehabilitation period must be carefully assessed and often indicate that a reduction in the level of activity is warranted.

The tendons and ligaments of the distal limb (and to certain extent proximal limb as well) have been found to have consistent but unique shapes at each level of the examination.[12,24,33,35,38,42,53–56,63,66,70,79] It is normal for these structures to change shape as they course distally in the limb. Therefore, if the examiner perceives a structure to have an abnormal shape it should be compared to the same structure in the opposite limb at the exact same level. It is also helpful in those horses with a change in shape to assess their position with respect to the surrounding anatomy.

Architecture (or texture) is a subjective assessment of the ultrasound image that attempts to describe morphological change or damage. Terms used to describe the architecture of an image relate to the tissue's ultrasonographic intensity. Architectural change is described as a change in echogenicity or the whiteness/brightness of a structure. Echogenicity is a function of each structure's particular density based on several things including cellular composition, fiber alignment, and blood supply. Alterations in echogenicity are subjective interpretations and have been described with the terms isoechoic, anechoic, hypoechoic, and hyperechoic. Isoechoic implies a normal echogenicity, whereas hypoechoic and hyperechoic imply less than and more than isoechoic, respectively. Anechoic implies the structure (or lesion) is mostly black. Fluid is often considered anechoic. In general, the denser the structure, the more echoes it returns and the whiter the structure appears. Alterations in echogenicity reflect changes in cellular and extracellular composition of the tissue. Changes in echogenicity can range from barely perceptible with a mild loss of fiber pattern to complete disruption of fiber pattern from fiber rupture with focal anechoic hemorrhage and/or serous fluid accumulation.

Fibers have a parallel alignment in most normal tendon and ligamentous structures. This parallel fiber bundle alignment is best assessed on longitudinal images. Injury to and inflammation of tendons and ligaments can disrupt fiber bundle alignment. Subtle changes in fiber alignment are best seen on the longitudinal plane images. More severe fiber bundle alignment changes can begin to be appreciated on transverse images. Damage seen on cross section should be confirmed on longitudinal orientation with the longitudinal plane obtained through the affected tissue. Fiber disruption seen as echolucent areas surrounding the fibers is compatible with hemorrhage and edema seen with acute injuries. Nonparallel or random fiber alignment without echolucent fluid content is compatible with chronic injury. Tendon injury can be focal or generalized such that the distribution of fiber damage can be quite variable. Tendon fiber damage is seen as a continuum of changes, ranging from fiber slippage to fiber rupture. Early mild fiber slippage may not be appreciated ultrasonographically; however, mild increases in CSA may indirectly indicate tendinitis. Loss of echogenicity usually indicates fiber disruption but may also reflect edema of the tendon or paratendinous tissue with fluid accumulation. Acute tendinitis can have a variable appearance based on the severity of conditions. Typically these changes are manifested as decreased echogenicity with increased tendon volume frequently represented as a rounding of the structure in cross section. Fibroblasts migrate into the damaged area and begin to deposit collagen and form granulation tissue. This collagen is laid down randomly and cross links are produced between the fibers. This random disorganized tissue appears hypoechoic on ultrasound and can persist for some time post injury. Rehabilitation with increasing levels of exercise precipitates remodeling of the collagen and a return of the echogenicity and alignment to normal (Figure 4.123).

LIMITATIONS OF ULTRASONOGRAPHY

Ultrasonography has many limitations that must be recognized. The quality of the image is directly related to the operator, the equipment, and the anatomical area being examined. This imaging tool is influenced by the skill of the operator more than any other imaging technique. The operator is responsible for positioning and steering the sound beam as well as determining the equipment settings during image acquisition. Artifacts are easily produced and can create inaccuracies in the image, which can significantly compromise interpretation. Artifacts most often involve operator error and an assortment of sound-tissue interactions that may or may not be controllable.

One common but easily corrected artifact is created by inadequate skin preparation, which leads to poor transmission of sound and a corresponding dark image. The limb should be clipped and prepped to maximize skin contact and sound transmission. High-frequency transducers produce better images but often require using a razor to shave the area to be examined. Improving skin-transducer contact is critical to obtain the best images possible.

Another common artifact due to operator error occurs when the ultrasound beam is off incidence to tissue interfaces and tendinous structures. Off incidence artifact occurs when the ultrasound beam is not at 90° to the fibers of the target structure which reflect the returning echoes away from the transducer. This creates a hypoechoic area that mimics a lesion(s) within the

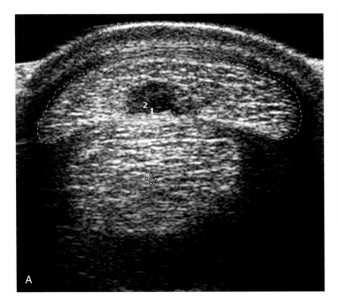

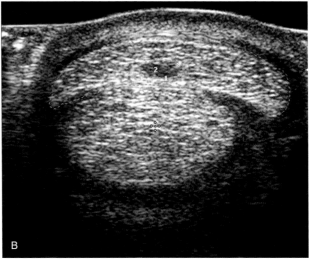

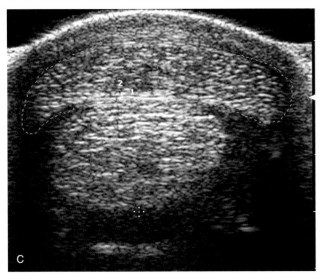

Figure 4.123. A, B, C. These are sequential scans acquired over 12 weeks (4, 8, and 12 weeks) of an iatrogenic tendon lesion created in the central aspect of the SDFT. Acute tendonitis initially appears as a decrease in echogenicity with corresponding increased tendon volume (cross sectional area) which is frequently represented as a rounding of the structure. Early in the repair process cellular infiltration with fibroblasts and vascular cells fills the damaged area and begins to deposit collagen and form granulation tissue which can increase the echogenicity of the lesion. Collagen is laid down randomly and cross links are produced between the fibers. Random disorganized tissue may appear hypoechoic on ultrasound and can persist for some time post injury (into the remodeling phase of healing). Rehabilitation with increasing levels of exercise precipitates remodeling of the collagen and a return of the echogenicity and alignment to normal. The lesion size and cross sectional area tend to progressively decrease over time.

targeted structure. Improper gain and power settings and inappropriate focal zone position can also lead to suboptimal images. Near gain and power settings that are set too high reduce the ability to differentiate the tissues. Gain settings should be adjusted to produce a uniform gray scale across the entire image. Focal zones are variable in number and position and should be adjusted to the level of the specific structure(s) to optimize image quality.

Artifacts created by sound-tissue interactions include acoustic enhancement, refractive scattering (edge artifacts), reverberation, and acoustic shadowing. Acoustic enhancement occurs when sound passes through a fluid structure. Fluid attenuates sound less than soft tissue. Enhancement results from relatively increased amplitude of deeper echoes by an overlying structure of low attenuation. This creates the appearance of increased echogenicity of the tissue deep to the fluid-filled structure (far field enhancement). The most common structure(s) that can cause enhancement artifacts in the musculoskeletal examinations are veins and arteries.

Refractive artifacts are generated from the edge of a curved surface and are created because part of the sound beam is refracted off the curved structure and does not return to the transducer. Shadow artifacts are displayed distal to the lateral margins of curved or cystic

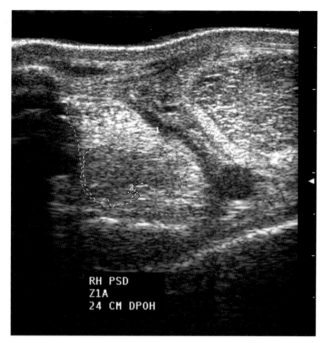

Figure 4.124. Transverse scan of the proximal plantar metatarsal area with the inherent artifacts that occur in this area due to edge shadowing, acoustic enhancement, and acoustic shadowing that occur because of the bony anatomy and overlying SDF and DDF and vessels. This lesion was found to be a false positive when the horse had a normal MRI examination of this area. The operator must find an acoustic window that minimizes the interference of the splint bones as well as prevents or limits the development of refraction and enhancement artifacts from the overlying tendons and vessels.

structures. Edge artifacts are consistent and particularly troublesome when examining specific anatomical locations. The SDFT, DDFT, and ICL are superimposed over the SL in the metacarpus and metatarsus and the size differential (the SL is wider than the SDFT/DDFT/ICL) between these structures allows refractive or edge artifacts to occur in the SL. In addition, the presence of vessels over the SL creates enhancement artifacts in the image.

The proximal plantar metatarsal region is another good example of how these artifacts can affect the quality of the ultrasonographic examination of the origin of the SL (Figure 4.124). At this location there are large oval/rounded structures of different echogenicity (SDFT, DDFT, ICL, and origin of the SL), all with a slightly different fiber orientation and acoustic impedances. The operator must find an acoustic window that minimizes the interference of the splint bones as well as prevents or limits the development of refraction and enhancement artifacts from the overlying tendons and vessels. Dilatation of the vessels in this area due to the inflammatory response of the damaged SL makes scanning this area even more problematic and significantly compromises interpretation of the SL morphology. Scanning at a more plantaromedial to dorsolateral oblique orientation may be necessary to improve image quality. However, the experience of the operator scanning areas such as the proximal plantar metatarsus will

improve the diagnostic accuracy of the ultrasound exam even though the image may still be suboptimal.

Ultrasound remains a practical, inexpensive, and readily accessible imaging technique for soft tissue injuries of the horse. However, with the recent introduction of magnetic resonance imaging (MR) to equine musculoskeletal imaging, soft tissue and bone injuries can be evaluated in detail not possible with any other imaging technique. MR is now considered the gold standard to assess lameness originating from the carpus and tarsus distally (especially of the foot within the horny hoof capsule) but it is not always practical or necessary to make a diagnosis. Lesion(s) seen with standard ultrasonographic imaging are not typically candidates for MR examination.

While ultrasonography and MR remain the optimal choices for soft tissue imaging, the most effective imaging tool in all cases remains unclear. Many studies in humans compare the diagnostic accuracy and utility of ultrasound compared to MR for a variety of orthopedic problems. These studies are lacking in horses and need to be performed. A limited number of studies have been performed and have looked at the collateral ligaments of the distal interphalangeal joint and the proximal plantar metatarsal region.[4,26,27] In those studies a negative ultrasound exam did not rule out an abnormality and positive ultrasonographic findings should be regarded with caution. It is hoped that further experience comparing ultrasound with MR along with the completion of more comparative studies between MR and ultrasound will identify specific indications for each imaging modality. It is hoped that MR will improve the capabilities of ultrasonographers.

USE OF DIAGNOSTIC ULTRASOUND TO EVALUATE JOINT INJURY

Radiology, ultrasonography, thermography, nuclear imaging, CT, and MRI all have a place in lameness diagnostics and each may be warranted in selected cases.[39,46,78] An accurate diagnosis of the cause of joint pain is critical to select the most appropriate treatment plan and rehabilitation regimen. Good quality baseline radiographic and ultrasonographic images are important for an accurate diagnosis but are also helpful in the re-evaluation of the joint during the rehabilitation process.

Joint injury, osteochondrosis, and degenerative joint disease are significant causes of lameness.[50,51] Many of these problems can be accurately assessed with a combination of radiographs and ultrasound. Radiographic examination has proven to be very effective at imaging the bony structures of the joints of the equine limb, but there can be poor correlation between clinical and radiographic findings.[40,46] Often, intra-articular anesthesia significantly improves the lameness and localizes it to a particular joint, but the radiographic study may be inconclusive. In such a case, the cause of lameness is presumed to be soft tissue injury, and often empirical treatment is instituted. Ultrasonography has recently become incorporated in the evaluation of a variety of joint conditions and can provide valuable information about the cartilage, subchondral bone surface, and the ligaments and tendons associated with the joint.[1,14–16,19,43,59,60] Ultrasonography has the added advantage of providing immediate, detailed information, but generates a relatively limited field of view when compared to other imaging techniques. Global survey of a joint can be potentially time-consuming. When used in combination, radiography and ultrasonography can supply more information about an orthopedic problem than when each modality is used alone.

Successful management of lameness requires the clinician to incorporate all of the information at his disposal to develop an accurate diagnosis and choose the most appropriate treatment. However, to best utilize all of the imaging modalities available requires a good working knowledge of the anatomy of the area. The clinician must also understand the advantages and limitations of each imaging modality as well as the appearance of the normal anatomy and pathology characteristic with each technique. When using diagnostic ultrasound to evaluate joints it is necessary to become familiar with the appearance of many of these structures in transverse, longitudinal (sagittal), and frontal planes. Normal anatomical variations exist and it is important that the clinician recognize these variations as normal to prevent an inaccurate diagnosis. The opposite limb can and should be used for comparison when possible, recognizing that disease can occur at the same location in the opposite limb.

In general the stability of a joint is provided by the congruent contours of the joint surfaces of the bony column, collateral (and in some joints the intra-articular) ligaments, integrity of the joint capsule, and surrounding tendons and ligaments. In the proximal limb, additional stability is provided by various muscle groups and tendons that cross the joint. Most joints of the appendicular skeleton in the horse are designed to work in the sagittal plane, with flexion and extension the predominant motion. This necessitates that a joint have a redundant joint capsule at the dorsal and palmar/plantar surfaces. In addition, tendons and ligaments that pass over joints with a wide range of motion typically have sheaths or bursae to allow these structures to effectively glide across the joint surface throughout their full range of motion. Development of fluid or effusion in any of these structures must be accurately defined to effectively manage the cause of the effusion.

Indications for Ultrasonography of Joints

A complete set of radiographs should be acquired to assess the bony structures of the joint when the clinical examination has localized the source of pain to a joint. Ultrasonography should be considered as complementary to radiography in joint examinations and should be used to assess the soft tissues of the joint. The radiographic study should be acquired and evaluated before the ultrasound study. Ultrasonography is indicated when:

1. The radiographic study is inconclusive, especially when the joint is enlarged with synovial effusion, or there is joint capsule thickening or focal swelling associated with any of the soft tissue structures of the joint
2. The radiographic study of the joint demonstrates an abnormality but further evaluation of the soft tissues

is necessary (i.e., an apical sesamoid fracture should be assessed for the degree of SL involvement to provide a more accurate prognosis)
3. Diagnostic radiographs are difficult to obtain, such as the pelvis and coxofemoral joint. Ultrasonography has proven very helpful to assess both the soft tissues and bony contours of this joint.
4. Diagnostic ultrasound can be used as an interventional procedure to help obtain clinical information about the joint or to aid appropriate treatment. Ultrasound has been very helpful to confirm that either local anesthetic or medication has been deposited into the appropriate joints or sheaths, particularly in areas where it can be difficult to confirm accurate placement of the needle (articular facets of the cervical spine, shoulder joint, coxofemoral joint, bicipital bursa, navicular bursa, etc).[6,11,41,44,72] Visually documenting needle placement and injection into the synovial space of joints, sheaths, or bursae is important to prevent confusing results (false positive and false negative results). In addition, collection of fluid samples can be directed by ultrasonography, improving the recovery rate in situations such as septic arthritis.
5. Information about a joint can sometimes be acquired before radiographic survey is available. This is only pertinent when using radiographic equipment that is not digital and requires additional time to develop the radiographic image, particularly in septic joints and wounds or punctures that are close to a joint and are suspected to have contaminated the joint.
6. To assist with preoperative planning of candidates for joint surgery. The joint should be thoroughly evaluated for coexisting problems which might alter the prognosis. Evaluation of some bone fragments may be necessary to determine the extent of soft tissue attachments and document the position of the fragment as intra- or extra-articular, fixed, or mobile (e.g., an apical and abaxial proximal sesamoid fracture).
7. To assist intraoperatively by guiding the surgical approach or retrieval of bony fragments (i.e., lateral malleolar fractures of the distal tibia).

Equipment and Technique

The same equipment used for tendon and ligament examinations is ideal for joint evaluations. The joint should be prepared as for a tendon or ligament examination with the joint being clipped (and possibly shaved, depending on the operator's preference); cleansed to remove dirt, hair, and other surface debris; and liberally coated with a conducting gel. Most joint examinations require clipping and prepping the entirety of the joint surface.

The majority of the structures evaluated during joint ultrasonography are superficial in location well within the focal zones of most high-frequency transducer. Flat-face linear transducers of 10 to 18 MHz are often used because of superior near-field resolution and broad field of view. It is helpful to evaluate most of the structures of the joint at a scan depth of 2 to 4 cm. Stand-off pads move the superficial structures out of the near field artifact and into the near focal zone of the probe.

Stand-off pads also improve the footprint by conforming to the skin surface. Lower frequency transducers (5 or 7.5 MHz) may be necessary to image deeper aspects of the joint such as the caudal aspect of the stifle. In the proximal limb the joints are farther from the skin due to muscle coverage. The overlying muscle mass provides a good window for the sound transmission to the deeper aspects of the joint. However, lower frequency probes, which have poorer resolution and somewhat compromised image quality, may need to be used. Microconvex or macroconvex probes have the added advantage of a divergent beam which allows image acquisition from a smaller skin contact point.

Unlike the palmar/plantar metacarpal exam in which the transverse images are typically acquired, it is helpful to begin the examination of a joint with the longitudinal scan plane. This allows the examiner to easily identify the articular surfaces of a joint and provides orientation for the rest of the examination. Global evaluation of a joint can be time-consuming because multiple scan planes are required. The articular surface of the weight-bearing and nonweight-bearing areas, the extensor and flexor surfaces (and the soft tissues such as the flexor tendons that cross these areas), and the collateral ligaments of the joint all should be examined. For example, examination of the fetlock, which is considered a simple joint, is divided into quadrants. The quadrants of the fetlock are dorsal, palmar/plantar, medial/lateral, and dorsomedial/dorsolateral scan planes.[17,22] In more complex joints, additional scan planes may be indicated due to additional structures associated with the joint (i.e., the stifle has the patellar ligaments, long digital extensor tendon, popliteal tendon, etc.). Numerous reference materials report the anatomy and techniques required to examine joints in the horse.[2,5,6,8–11,20,21,23,29,36,37,47,48,52,64–69,72,74–77,80,83]

All tendinous or ligamentous structures should be evaluated in both transverse and longitudinal scan planes. A description of the scan plane used to acquire the image should be documented on the stored image. Scan planes should be labeled similar to the nomenclature used for radiographic projections. These oblique projections are described by the direction that the central ray of the primary beam penetrates the body part of interest, from the point of entrance to the point of exit. Soft tissue structures should be examined first, followed by the cartilage and subchondral bone surfaces. Much of the cartilage and subchondral bone surface in the nonweight-bearing areas can be imaged in the standing horse. However, dynamic examination of the cartilage and subchondral bone surfaces of the weight-bearing areas of the joint requires lifting the limb and placing the probe on the dorsal joint surface, all while attempting to place the probe 90° to the subchondral surface while flexing and extending the joint. This maneuver requires considerable practice, but it can be expedited by having someone hold the limb (or placing the limb in a stand) while the examiner positions the transducer while manipulating the limb. Maximally flexing the leg is necessary to access the major weight-bearing areas of a joint. Unfortunately, flexion of an inflamed joint will likely be resented, making it more difficult to evaluate the weight-bearing surface.

The joint examined and the area of interest within the joint is, in many cases, directed by the signalment (and by any prior radiographic findings). For example, racehorses have a high incidence of problems involving the dorsal articular surfaces of the high-motion joints, particularly the fetlock and carpus; younger horses may have developmental orthopedic disease which, when involving a joint, frequently involves the trochlear ridges of the stifle, the distal intermediate ridge of the tibia, or the trochlear ridges of the talus; Warmbloods often have a similar distribution of osteochondrosis lesions and they also tend to develop periarticular changes in the coffin, pastern, and fetlock joints. In each case, it is important to perform as complete an examination of the joint as possible because many joint conditions involve multiple structures and/or multiple areas of the joint. For example, OA tends to cause cartilage degeneration and thinning in the loaded areas of the articular surface. Along with these cartilage changes, periarticular remodeling occurs in the form of osteophyte and/or enthesiophyte formation. Joint capsule thickening, with or without metaplasia, is also a common feature of OA. Many of the osteochondral fractures that occur in the joints of performance horses occur on the dorsal surface due to hyperextension of the joint. However, hyperextension may also cause damage to the palmar/plantar soft tissues (flexor tendons, suspensory ligament, and distal sesamoidean ligaments), which can significantly alter the prognosis.

Dynamic examination of the joint as described for the examination of the weight-bearing cartilage allows the evaluation of redundant parts of the joint capsule in high-motion joints. For example, the dorsal surface of the fetlock joint has redundancy of the joint capsule that is relaxed when the horse is bearing weight on the limb. Flexion of the fetlock tenses the dorsal aspect of the joint capsule, allowing better evaluation of this part of the joint. Tearing of the dorsal joint capsule is more accurately imaged if the structure is under tension while the joint is in flexion. Flexion and extension of the joint during ultrasonographic examination can also be helpful in demonstrating mobility of an osteochondral fragment and in evaluating fluid movement within the joint.

The same joint on the contralateral limb should serve as a comparison when evaluating articular and periarticular structures. However, there are two precautions: (1) the examiner must make certain to use the same orientation of the transducer and image the contralateral joint at exactly the same location when making comparisons, and (2) it is important to bear in mind that some joint conditions, in particular osteochondrosis in young horses and osteochondral fragmentation in racehorses, can be present bilaterally.

The major obstacle to the effective use of diagnostic ultrasound in the examination of joints is the need to understand the unique anatomy of each joint and appreciate how the various tissue types are influenced by sound-tissue interactions. It is also important to understand the information and misinformation (artifacts) created during any ultrasound evaluation (see the section on limitations of ultrasound, earlier in this chapter). Many texts describe the anatomy of specific joints in the horse[24,38,66,70] as well as the use of diagnostic ultrasound in the examination of joints.[1,14–16,19,31,32,43,50,51,59,60,81,82] It is recommended that these textbooks be available as reference materials to assist with the examination. Descriptions of the ultrasonographic examination of the specific joints are beyond the scope of this chapter. However, a discussion of some general features unique to the use of ultrasound in the examination of joints follows.

Periarticular Structures

Appearance of Periarticular Structures

The joints of the appendicular skeleton in the horse are designed to work predominantly in the sagittal plane with flexion and extension as the primary range of motion. A major component of the stability of a joint is provided by the periarticular soft tissues, particularly the collateral ligaments. The collateral ligaments are designed to impart stability to the joint throughout its entire range of motion. This unique task is accomplished either with paired structures (i.e., multiple bundles of the fetlock, tarsal joints) or by unpaired structures (i.e., single bundle of coffin joint).

Knowing the anatomic arrangement of the collateral ligaments of each specific joint becomes extremely important because the ultrasonographic appearance of these ligaments is determined by the fiber orientation. Most of the collateral ligaments have a uniform fascicular orientation, and therefore a homogeneous ultrasonographic appearance. Some have a mixed fascicular arrangement which gives them a heterogeneous appearance. The lateral collateral ligaments of the stifle, hock, and elbow, and the collateral ligaments of the fetlock and carpus, have spiral or crossed fibers.[14] This mixed arrangement of fascicles within the CLs is one of the arrangements that allow the collateral ligaments to function in both extension and flexion (Figure 4.125). In the tarsocrural joint, the superficial collateral ligaments are under tension while the limb is extended, and relaxed while the limb is flexed, whereas the short collateral ligaments are tensed only when the tarsus is flexed.[79] Therefore, the short collateral ligaments should be examined while the leg is flexed.

As discussed in the previous section of this chapter, tendons and ligaments appear as moderately echogenic structures with relatively well-defined margins, and injury is recognized ultrasonographically by changes in size, shape, architecture, position, and fiber alignment. Ultrasonographic examination of the tendons at the level of the joint is no different except from a couple of perspectives. First, the examiner must pay particular attention to how the tendon or ligament courses over a joint because there can be quite remarkable changes in direction. This is important because the transducer must constantly be adjusted to maintain a perpendicular orientation to the structure to prevent beam angle artifact. Second, the periarticular portions of tendons have

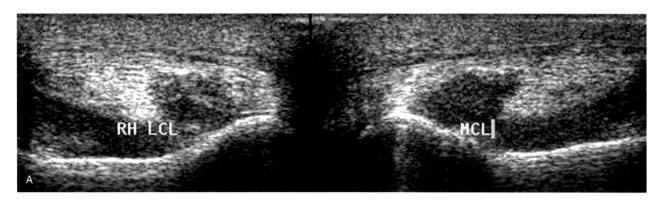
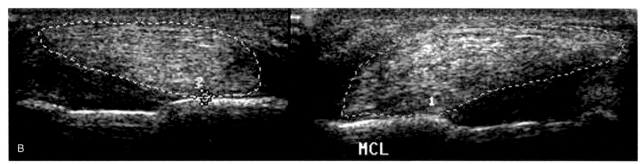

Figure 4.125. A mixed arrangement of fascicles within the CLs of many joints is one of the unique arrangements of ligaments that allow a collateral ligament to function in both extension and flexion. This mixed arrangement of fibers can produce a heterogeneous appearance of the collateral ligament on ultrasound examination. A. This is a transverse ultrasound image of the CLs of the fetlock joint that appears to have a hypoechoic lesion within the dorsal aspect of the medial CL. However, the lateral CL has the same appearance and similar cross sectional area, suggesting that this is a variation of normal in this horse. B. This transverse image of an MCP CL demonstrates a thickened CSA with a heterogeneous fiber pattern, consistent with chronic desmitis.

sheaths (and occasionally bursae) associated with them. Injury to these tendons/ligaments may also manifest as the development of fluid or effusion within the sheaths or bursae. To further confuse the matter, the effusion may occur without structural damage to the tendon or ligament. Therefore, effusion of the sheaths and bursae associated with these structures requires careful evaluation to define the cause and to differentiate the fluid accumulation as separate from joint effusion.

Joint Capsule

The joint capsule is primarily connective tissue with low cell density. The joint capsule is continuous with the periosteum or perichondrium, but it does not insert directly at the perimeter of the articular cartilage (Figure 4.126). There tends to be redundancy of the joint capsule in the high-motion joints, such as the fetlock, carpus, tarsus, and stifle. In fact, this redundancy can cause relaxation artifacts if the redundant aspect of the joint is examined in the weight-bearing position rather than during flexion. Inflammatory conditions within the joint can cause capsular changes that include thickening (initially due to hemorrhage and edema, and later, fibrosis), calcification, and insertional capsulopathies (enthesiophytes). Osteoarthritis in high-motion joints typically involves periarticular changes which begin with congestion and thickening of the joint capsule. The synovial membrane becomes hyperplastic and, in more chronic cases, synoviocyte metaplasia may lead to the formation of synovial chondromas, which are seen as nodules of cartilage. These nodules may undergo endochondral ossification, resulting in ovoid radiodense bodies within the joint capsule.

Synovium

Synovitis usually accompanies capsulitis and joint injury; however, thickening of the thin synovial membrane is difficult to appreciate ultrasonographically. Synovial effusion is helpful in assessing synovial mem-

brane proliferation and thickening. In cases of severe synovitis, synovial fluid that is fibrinous, cellular, or hemorrhagic can cloud evaluation of the joint capsule and synovium.

Synovial Fluid

There is usually minimal synovial fluid in a normal joint, so the joint capsule and synovium are normally in close apposition with the articular cartilage. Synovial fluid accumulation occurs with many abnormal joint conditions, so thorough evaluation of the various articular structures is indicated when synovial effusion is present. The ultrasonographic properties of the synovial fluid can help assess the nature of the fluid (Figure 4.127). Effusion associated with acute synovitis typically is anechoic, with occasional fibrinous accumulations. Hemorrhage or sepsis increases the cellularity and fibrin deposition within the joint, and appears as echogenic fluid. Ultrasonography can aid in aspiration of synovial fluid by identifying areas of fluid accumulation. Utilization of this technique, particularly in the deeper joints such as the hip and the shoulder, can minimize trauma to the joint and reduce the potential for blood contamination of the fluid sample.

Sonographic Features of the Articular Surface

With ultrasonography, reflections of the sound beam occur at interfaces between tissues of different material densities. Articular cartilage is primarily water, so it produces a sonolucent (anechoic to hypoechoic) image between the echogenic joint capsule/synovium and subchondral bone. However, the distinction between joint fluid and cartilage cannot always be appreciated. The ultrasound beam cannot pass through bone, so the subchondral bone interface is seen as a dense, hyperechoic line that follows the normal contour of the joint surface. Normally, there are distinct soft tissue-cartilage and cartilage-bone interfaces. When synovial fluid is seen between the synovial membrane and the cartilage

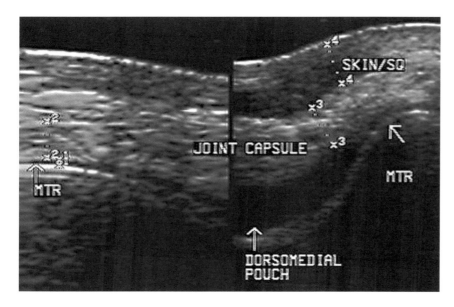

Figure 4.126. Ultrasound image of the dorsomedial aspect of the tarsocrural joint. There is mild edema of the subcutaneous tissues and synovial effusion within the joint, allowing visualization of the joint capsule. Fluid accumulation within the joint can allow delineation of the synovium.

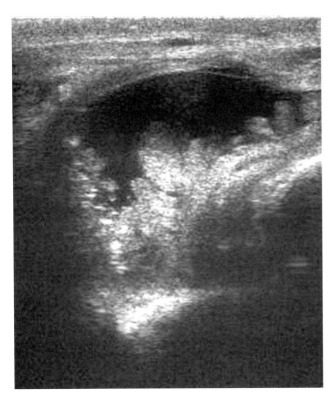

Figure 4.127. Synovial fluid accumulation occurs with many joint, sheath, or bursal conditions. A thorough evaluation of the various structures of the joint or synovial sheath is indicated when effusion is present. This image demonstrates a proliferative synovial membrane from a chronic synovial effusion that was due to a previously undiagnosed osteochondrosis lesion of the medial malleolus of the tibia.

surface, the interface between the fluid and the cartilage may create a thin, echogenic line.[14] Accurate definition of the thickness and detection of changes in the surface and internal characteristics of articular cartilage requires that the sound beam be perpendicular to the cartilage surface.

Normal Cartilage Thickness

To accurately define the thickness and to detect changes in surface and internal characteristics of cartilage, the sound beam must be perpendicular to the cartilage surface. Normal articular cartilage thickness in horses remains to be well defined in all but a few joints. A recent study in healthy adult horses showed that the mean cartilage thickness on the lateral and medial trochlear ridges of the talus and on the distal intermediate ridge of the tibia was 0.57, 0.58, and 0.70 mm, respectively.[76] The trochlear ridges of the talus were chosen in that study because of the high incidence of osteochondrosis and the potential for cartilage thickening at these sites. Fetlock cartilage thickness was found to be thicker proximally (0.8 mm) than distally (0.4 mm).[17]

In humans, cartilage thickness varies somewhat between joints, and even within a particular joint. For example, in the human knee the cartilage thickness on the femoral condyles normally ranges from 1.2 to 1.9 mm, with cartilage thickness on the medial condyle being less than that on the intercondylar notch and the lateral condyle.[1]

From the limited number of equine studies and based on clinical impression, there is also variation in cartilage thickness both between and within joints in horses. Compare, for example, the difference in articular cartilage thickness between the lateral and medial trochlear ridges of the femur in the normal femoropatellar joint. The cartilage is thinner on the medial trochlear ridge; this is normal and should not be mistaken for a pathologic process.

Normal Variations

Articular cartilage has a fairly uniform thickness and a smooth contour. There are, however, a couple of areas where cartilage thickness and contour vary normally. Synovial fossae occur in some joints that are bilaterally symmetrical and most often located in a nonweight-bearing part of the articular surface (e.g., humeroradial, tarsocrural, and coxofemoral joints). If an area is found that is of concern, the same site in the opposite limb should be evaluated for comparison (bearing in mind that some developmental lesions often occur bilaterally). The articular cartilage at the perimeter of a concave epiphysis and the cartilage at the center of a convex epiphysis is thickest.[40]

Immature Cartilage and Bone

Epiphyseal cartilage ossifies from a secondary ossification center, and the carpal and tarsal bones ossify by endochondral ossification. Ossification radiates out toward the articular surface so that articular cartilage of immature joints can appear thickened and the interface with the subchondral bone irregular. A more distinct cartilage-subchondral bone interface develops with maturity. Thus, measurements of articular/epiphyseal cartilage thickness in foals may vary greatly with age, and possibly with the joint involved. In neonates, articular/epiphyseal cartilage thickness on the medial trochlear ridge of the femur can be as much as 25 mm; the articular cartilage is about 1 mm thick, and the remaining thickness is unossified epiphyseal cartilage, although the differentiation between the two types of cartilage is not appreciable ultrasonographically.[31] The thickness of articular cartilage can be quite variable depending on the stage of development and the amount of calcification that exists. As epiphyseal ossification continues, the thickness of cartilage covering the epiphyseal bone decreases.[31,32]

Osteochondral Lesions

Ultrasonography complements radiography in the early diagnosis of cartilage osteochondrosis in growing animals. In young horses, articular cartilage lesions associated with osteochondrosis can cause significant joint effusion, and in many cases there are cartilage or osteochondral fragments either *in situ* or free-floating within the joint. Areas of thickened cartilage or osteochondral fragment(s) are often apparent over an

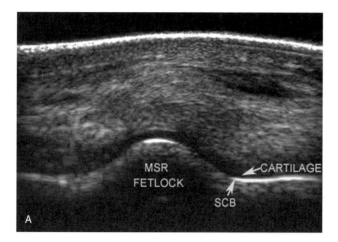

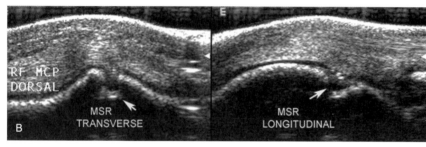

Figure 4.128. Osteochondrosis in the developing animal manifests articular cartilage lesions that are often associated with significant joint effusion, and in many cases there are cartilage or osteochondral fragments either *in situ* or free-floating within the joint. A. This is a transverse ultrasound image of the dorsal aspect of a normal MCP joint. The anechoic cartilage is seen overlying the hyperechoic subchondral bone surface. Notice the smooth subchondral surface of the normal joint. B. This transverse and longitudinal ultrasound image demonstrates an irregular subchondral surface of the sagittal ridge of this MCP joint, consistent with osteochondrosis.

irregular subchondral bone surface (Figure 4.128). This irregular surface is thought to be associated with a continuum of changes that occur in the development of osteochondrosis lesions, starting with a linear fissure or fold formation in the thickened articular cartilage which can progress to an undermined cartilage flap with lysis of the underlying bone.[50,51] Developmental abnormalities in the articular cartilage and subchondral bone can occur bilaterally, so use of the contralateral limb for comparison may be misleading.

Clinical signs often precede radiographic evidence of osteochondrosis in young horses. Radiographic assessment of osteochondrosis lesions commonly underestimates the extent of the articular lesion when compared with what is seen arthroscopically. Ultrasonography has proven to be a very useful imaging technique to evaluate the cartilage/subchondral surface and is indicated in any young horse with joint effusion that is suspected of having osteochondrosis. Serial examination of affected joints can be particularly useful when deciding whether surgery is necessary. Progression of an osteochondrosis lesion is a good indicator for surgical debridement. When serial examination demonstrates a static osteochondrosis lesion or even progression to a normal cartilage-subchondral bone surface, surgery is not indicated.

Osteoarthritis

Osteoarthritis manifests as thinning and erosion of the articular cartilage and progresses to osteophyte formation and periarticular soft tissue changes such as enthesis new bone at the joint capsule attachments. In the horse, early cartilage thinning has been difficult to identify ultrasonographically. More advanced stages of

the disease may be easier to demonstrate in high-motion joints, particularly when the joint capsule is seen to be in close contact with the subchondral bone surface when pressure is applied with the transducer. The advanced stages of the disease often manifest significant soft tissue changes such as enthesis new bone and periarticular lipping. In the low-motion joints, such as the distal hock joints and the pastern, ultrasonographic evidence of OA generally is limited to periarticular changes because access to the cartilage surface is limited.

A study in humans showed that ultrasound was useful in identifying early OA of the knee.[43] Changes included a decrease in cartilage thickness and blurring of cartilage margins which made cartilage measurements less precise. In general, ratings of clarity and sharpness correlated better with clinical status than absolute thickness of the articular cartilage in that study. Further experience with ultrasonographic examination with higher frequency transducers will hopefully allow similar criteria to be established for horses.

Subchondral bone sclerosis is also a feature of OA, but cannot be detected with ultrasonography because the sound beam does not penetrate the subchondral bone surface. Except in foals, the subchondral bone surface should be uniform.

Lesions on the Medial Femoral Condyle

Horses with hindlimb lameness that improves after intra-articular anesthesia of the medial femorotibial joint should have a radiographic and ultrasonographic examination performed.[81] Ultrasonography should be used to evaluate the medial meniscus, medial collateral

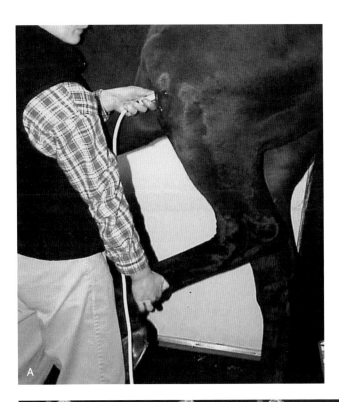

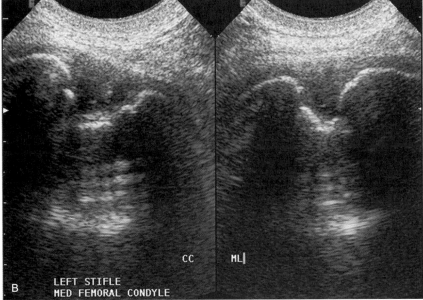

Figure 4.129. A. The weight-bearing area of the medial condyle is evaluated by flexing the stifle and placing the probe between the medial and middle patellar ligament just above the tibial crest. B. The ultrasound image demonstrates a large subchondral defect in the medial femoral condyle of the femur, consistent with a subchondral cystic lesion.

ligament, cranial ligament of the medial meniscus, and cartilage/subchondral bone of the medial condyle. The weight-bearing area of the medial condyle is evaluated by flexing the stifle and placing the probe between the medial and middle patellar ligament just above the tibial crest (Figure 4.129). Cartilage lesions with underlying subchondral bone defects are readily identified and their size and position documented with ultrasonography. Subchondral cystic lesions are also readily identified and ultrasound can help characterize the size of the cyst opening and depth of the cyst.

Interestingly, some medial meniscal injuries are easier to demonstrate with ultrasound when performing dynamic assessment of the joint. Some clinicians have reported using ultrasound to guide the placement of a needle percutaneously into the cyst cavity. Treatment is directed at placing various medications directly in the cystic cavity (corticosteroids, bone marrow, stem cells, etc.).[82] As in other joint injuries, radiographic and ultrasonographic examination is complementary and should be performed together to more accurately assess lesions within the femoropatellar, medial femorotibial, and lateral femorotibial joints. Identifying a specific injury within these joints may preclude the use of intraarticular medications and direct the clinician to explore the joint arthroscopically.

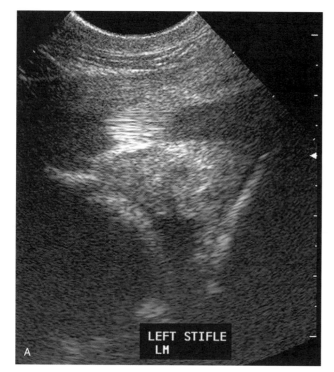

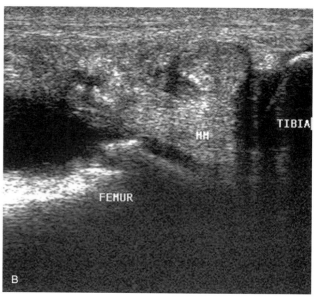

Figure 4.130. Damage to the medial meniscus is manifested ultrasonographically by a change in size, shape, echogenicity, or position relative to the femoral condyles and proximal tibia. A. This ultrasound image of a damaged meniscus demonstrates an axial injury of the meniscus. B. This image represents a more severe injury of the meniscus with prolapse of the meniscus.

Menisci

The equine stifle has two menisci that are composed of specialized fibrocartilage. A frontal scan (lateral-to-medial or medial-to-lateral longitudinal orientation) of the femorotibial joints produces the best images of the menisci and collateral ligaments of the stifle. The menisci have a triangular shape and a homogeneous appearance when the transducer is perpendicular to their abaxial border. A complete description of the ultrasonographic examination of the stifle is presented in various texts and should be studied before the examiner attempts to evaluate the stifle.[14,15]

Meniscal evaluation is enhanced by fluid accumulation within the joint. A complete assessment of the entire meniscus is essential and should include the cranial and caudal horns. The cranial horns of the lateral and medial menisci (MM) are visible between the lateral and middle patellar ligaments and the medial and middle patellar ligaments in the standing horse, respectively. The cranial and caudal horns of the meniscus have a similar ultrasonographic appearance when imaged from the cranial and caudal aspects of the joint and with the stifle flexed. Documentation of caudal horn involvement with ultrasonography indicates exploratory arthroscopy should also involve a caudal approach because damage to the caudal horn of the meniscus often is not appreciated via the normal cranial arthroscopic approach to the femorotibial joint. Damage to the meniscus is manifested ultrasonographically by a change in size, shape, echogenicity, or position relative to the femoral condyles and proximal tibia. (Figure 4.130)

Hyperechoic areas casting shadows are indicative of calcification and point toward chronic damage. Loss of the normal triangular shape is indicative of tearing. Linear hypoechoic images indicative of tears are seen crossing horizontally through the MM, and are best identified with the stifle in slight flexion. Large hypoechoic areas in cross-section can be associated with chronic lameness, and compatible with edema, fiber disruption, and degenerative processes. Extrusion of part of the meniscus from its normal position can occur if the tearing is severe. Collapse of the joint space and joint effusion may also be appreciated when both the collaterals and menisci are involved. When synovial distention is extensive and the synovial membrane is thickened, a hypoechoic space can be identified between the MM and the superficial structures (fascia and MCL). This gap between the MM and the MCL is abnormal, because these two structures normally are adhered to each other.

Identifying Incomplete Ossification

Ultrasonography can be useful to determine the stage of endochondral ossification in young foals. It is particularly useful for identifying incomplete ossification of the cuboidal bones in the carpus or tarsus of neonates. Unlike radiography, ultrasonography provides the information immediately in a field situation, allowing appropriate treatment or management changes to be instituted without delay.

Conclusions

Ultrasonography is vastly underutilized in the clinical assessment of joint problems in horses. A complete radiographic study of a joint can demonstrate osseous lesions, but it gives little information about the articular cartilage and soft tissue structures of the joint which are important sites of pathology in most types of joint disease. These tissues are readily imaged using ultrasonography (within the anatomical limitations of the particular joint being imaged). Arthroscopy allows direct visualization of lesions found on radiography and assessment of the articular cartilage surfaces and other intra-articular structures. The major restrictions to its use are that arthroscopy requires general anesthesia and it is invasive and expensive. Ultrasonography is noninvasive, rapidly performed, widely available, well tolerated by the patient, and inexpensive.

Ultrasonography offers many advantages in the clinical assessment and management of joint problems in horses. Ultrasonography can potentially detect lesions not evident radiographically, allowing treatment to be instituted and/or management changes made to slow or arrest lesion progression and prolong the useful life of the horse. In particular, ultrasonography may identify soft tissue and cartilage defects over radiographically normal bone which can cause lameness but that otherwise may be identified only at surgery or postmortem examination.

As an isolated study of a joint, ultrasonography may not always provide a specific diagnosis. But even though the initial examination may be negative or inconclusive, repeat ultrasound examination may reveal early changes indicative of a potentially serious joint problem. In humans, ultrasonography is purported to be a more sensitive indicator of early OA than radiography.[43] It allows monitoring of lesion progression or resolution over time, which can aid surgical decision-making, direct management and rehabilitation strategies, and increase the understanding of joint disease in horses. This approach not only aids the surgeon in deciding which cases warrant surgical intervention, it also enables a more accurate prognosis to be made before the client commits to surgery.

Ultrasonography can enhance the equine practitioner's ability to accurately diagnose and manage joint-related problems in performance horses. However, it is only one tool at the clinician's disposal; clinical acumen and selective use of other imaging modalities are needed to accurately diagnose many types of joint disease. Currently, the gold standard for assessing soft tissue injuries in humans is magnetic resonance imaging (MRI). However, in human medicine ultrasonography remains a very useful imaging modality for evaluating the popliteal space, knee, patellar tendon, shoulder (especially the rotator cuff), and neonatal hip. Extensive use of ultrasonography in the examination of equine joints has already demonstrated the sensitivity of this modality in defining articular lesions not apparent radiographically. In time, there will undoubtedly be certain joint conditions in horses that will most readily be identified with ultrasonography.

ULTRASONOGRAPHY OF SYNOVIAL STRUCTURES OTHER THAN JOINTS

Swellings of the synovial sheaths and bursae of the equine limb are common. The clinical significance of some of these disorders can be difficult to ascertain. Acute effusions of these synovial structures may be due to a primary inflammatory response, or they may be secondary to an injury of one or more of the associated tendons or ligaments. Effective management of these disorders therefore requires an accurate diagnosis that identifies the structure involved and the specific damage incurred.

General Synovial Sheath Anatomy

Tendons are bound to the limb by annular ligaments or retinacula. An annular ligament or retinaculum is a bandlike thickening of the deep fascia that crosses over one or more tendons and begins and ends on a close bony prominence. Where there is increased motion or a severe change in direction of the tendon, such as at a joint, it is surrounded by a synovial sheath (vagina synovialis tendinis). A synovial sheath is composed of inner visceral (pars tendinae) and outer parietal (pars parietalis) layers. Closely surrounding and included in the parietal layer is the fibrous portion of the sheath. Both layers are lined with synovial cells that produce a synovial-like fluid medium that facilitates movement of the tendon by minimizing friction and thereby aiding the gliding action of the tendon. The visceral and parietal layers of a sheath are continuous through the mesotendon, which carries the extrinsic blood supply to the tendon. In areas of increased motion, the mesotendon disappears or is replaced by threads of tissue called vincula.

The proximal aspect of a synovial sheath has a redundant sickle-shaped fold of the parietal and fibrous layer that allows the tendon to travel freely within the sheath. The distal aspect of most sheaths does not have a large range of movement and therefore inserts directly on a distal aspect of the tendon. For simplicity, some anatomists have classified sheaths as bursae that are folded over the tendon. This characterization may be seen more clearly when viewing some tendon sheaths that do not surround the tendon fully at all levels, particularly the sheaths of the extensor surface of the carpus.

The tendons that cross a joint are bound to the limb by retinacula or anular ligaments. For instance in the digit the SDFT and DDFT are surrounded by the digital flexor tendon sheath (DTFS). The primary anular ligament (PAL) crosses between the proximal sesamoid bones (PSBs) to hold the tendons tightly in the fetlock canal. As the tendons course out of the fetlock canal they are held in place initially by the proximal digital anular ligament (PDAL), and further distally the DDFT is encircled by the distal digital anular ligament (DDAL) just prior to going into the hoof. Injury of either the SDFT or DDFT anywhere in the digit can cause effusion in the sheath that prolapses around the restricting anular ligaments. Chronic injury to any of these structures may manifest as thickening of the mesotendon which is the vascular supply to the tendon within a sheath. In the case of the DFTS the medial mesotendinous attachment contains the primary vascular supply to the DDFT within the sheath.

The most commonly affected sheaths, in order of occurrence, are the DFTS (all 4 limbs), tarsal sheath, carpal sheath (covers the DDF and SDF tendons), sheaths of the digital extensor tendons as they cross the dorsal aspect of the carpus and tarsus. A description of the DFTS follows.

Digital Flexor Tendon Sheath

Ultrasonographic examination of the structures of the fetlock canal and palmar pastern has been frequently reported, probably due to the complex anatomy of the structures in this area as well as the frequency with which this area is involved in lameness of the distal limb.[12,15,22,25,33,42,55–58,63,71] Most of the literature emphasizes examination of the SDFT and DDFT, the SL, and the DSLs. The anatomy of the structures of the DFTS is unique (Figure 4.131). The SDFT has a natural axial connection of the sheath wall and anular ligament, whereas the DDFT has mesotendinous attachments to the medial and lateral borders. The SDFT also forms the proximal and distal rings around the DDFT called the manica flexoria. The SDFT and DDFT are maintained in the fetlock canal by the primary anular ligament attaching to the PSBs. Injury to the DSLs may manifest as a DFTS problem. Acute tenosynovitis of the DFTS of a performance horse necessitates close evaluation of all these structures. In addition, injury to the DSLs (particularly the OSL and SSL), which are outside the DFTS in the digit, may also cause acute tenosynovitis because of the proximity of the inflammatory response.

Traumatic injuries to this area are more likely to involve multiple structures or severe injuries to a single structure that instigate an intense and prolonged inflammatory response and are more likely to lead to chronic tenosynovitis of the DFTS. Clinical and ultrasonographic examinations frequently reveal an inflammatory response characterized by fibrous thickening of the DFTS. Chronic tenosynovitis of the DFTS may cause type 2 anular ligament constriction syndrome within the palmar or plantar fetlock canal.[22] Lameness is more likely to be present in horses with chronic tenosynovitis due to injuries to either of the tendons inside the DFTS. Type 3 anular ligament constriction syndrome is characterized by thickening of the annular ligament and a loss of echogenicity of the SDFT. Both of these conditions may appear to have a notched appearance along the palmar or plantar border of the fetlock when viewed from the side. In both syndromes, horses may have a history of chronic lameness that does not improve with rest and worsens with exercise.

Intrasynovial corticosteroid injection may provide temporary relief in the case of chronic tenosynovitis. The need for repeated injections indicates a more severe problem that usually requires tenoscopy. The use of tenoscopy or endoscopy to explore the sheaths and

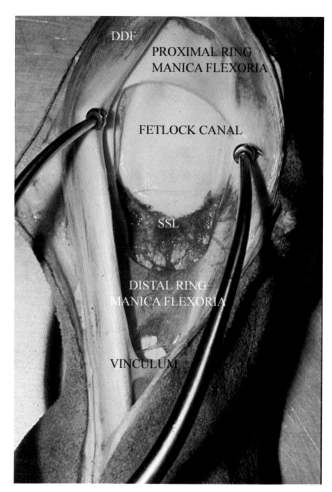

Figure 4.131. The structures within the digital flexor tendon sheath (DFTS) are exposed via a longitudinal incision through the SDFT at the level of the fetlock joint. The unique anatomy at this level begins with the mesotendinous attachments (not seen in this section) to the DDFT at the medial and lateral borders in the proximal sheath. Progressing distally the SDFT produces the proximal ring of the manica flexoria encircling the DDFT. Just distal to the manica flexoria the SDFT and DDFT are bound within the fetlock canal by the primary anular ligament (PAL) which has been incised in this section. Just distal to the fetlock canal the SDFT makes another ring (smaller) around the DDFT called the distal ring of the manica flexoria. Just distal to this ring the vincula attaches to the midline of the DDFT on its dorsal border.

bursae of the equine limb have allowed comparison of ultrasonography and tenoscopy in identifying tendon/ligament injury.[30,57,58,71,85] Tenosynovitis of the DFTS may result from tears in the DDFT or SDFT, manica flexoria, or other structures that communicate with the synovial fluid and thus can generate an intense synovial response in the DFTS. However, some of these lesions can be identified confidently only by tenoscopy, which also permits appropriate lesion management.[71] Longitudinal tears of the DDFT should also be suspected if ultrasonographic changes are present lateral or medial to the border of the DDFT, but tenoscopic examination of the tendon sheath is essential to establish an accurate diagnosis and an effective treatment.[85]

The DFTS is also commonly involved in lacerations and puncture wounds. Close inspection of wounds or punctures to the area of the palmar/plantar fetlock and pastern region is essential to rule out involvement of the DFTS. Lacerations that involve the sheath should be examined ultrasonographically to ascertain tendon involvement. Meticulous debridement of wound edges with copious lavage should allow the sheath to be sutured primarily. Horses with wounds to the DFTS should have a repeat ultrasonographic exam to determine whether adhesions have formed.

Villonodular synovitis has been reported to occur in the DFTS and the calcaneal bursa. Isolated masses may be found, or the condition may be part of a chronic proliferative tenosynovitis.

Carpal Sheath

The carpal sheath in the proximal palmar metacarpus is seen on routine ultrasonographic examinations as an anechoic space between the DDFT and the ICL. Mild effusions of the carpal sheath may be seen primarily as an enlargement of this anechoic space in the proximal palmar metacarpus. Some effusions may extend to the midmetacarpus or as far as the proximal DFTS. Larger effusions may extend proximal to the carpus with pronounced swellings laterally between the ulnaris lateralis and lateral digital extensor muscles and medially between the flexor carpi ulnaris and flexor carpi radialis muscles.

Although idiopathic tenosynovitis occasionally occurs in the carpal sheath, acute tenosynovitis is more common. Acute tenosynovitis of the carpal sheath may be due to injuries to the DDF or SDF tendon in the proximal metacarpus. Tendinitis of the DDF and/or SDF tendons should therefore be ruled out before therapy for primary tenosynovitis is instituted. Acute tenosynovitis of the carpal sheath accompanied by severe lameness on flexion of the carpus may be due to fractures within the carpus, particularly fracture of the accessory carpal bone. A complete set of radiographs should routinely be included in evaluations of horses with acute tenosynovitis with mild to moderate lameness of the forelimb.

Various conditions may create chronic tenosynovitis of the carpal sheath. Direct trauma to the soft tissues of the carpal canal and fractures of the palmar aspect of the carpus (accessory carpal bone) may cause acute synovitis of the carpal sheath. Continued trauma to the soft tissues of the palmar carpus and callus formation resultant from fracture repair may lead to chronic tenosynovitis of the carpal sheath.

Osteochondroma or slow-growing exostosis of the distal caudal radius may create chronic tenosynovitis. Ultrasonography can aid in determining the presence of DDF tendinitis within the carpal canal; however, the absence of ultrasonographic changes does not preclude the presence of injury to the tendon.[64]

Proliferative fibrous thickening of the carpal sheath characteristic of chronic tenosynovitis of the carpal sheath can result in carpal canal syndrome from compression of the neurovascular structures that course through the carpal canal. Intrasynovial corticosteroid may provide temporary relief, but carpal canal syndrome frequently requires sectioning of the flexor retinaculum for return to soundness. Osteochondromas should be removed, and if this is not successful, sectioning of the flexor retinaculum may be required.

Tarsal Sheath

The normal tarsal sheath is not routinely visualized on ultrasonographic examinations of the plantar tarsus. A moderate amount of effusion is typically present and is apparent as two swellings cranial to the calcaneal tendon on both medial and lateral aspects of the distal crus. In more pronounced effusions of the tarsal sheath, a distal swelling may be seen distal to the hock on the medial aspect of the tarsometatarsal joint.

Swellings of the tarsal sheath are called thoroughpin. Thoroughpin is a morphologic description and can exist with varying degrees of inflammation. Most cases of thoroughpin, however, are classified as idiopathic tenosynovitis, which can occur bilaterally and in some instances is probably due to conformation.

Acute tenosynovitis of the tarsal sheath, however, can manifest with varying degrees of inflammation and lameness. This necessitates a more accurate definition of the underlying cause of acute tenosynovitis of the tarsal sheath.

Acute tarsal sheath effusion usually occurs unilaterally, with sudden onset of moderate to severe lameness. Acute tenosynovitis of the tarsal sheath is thought in most instances to be traumatically induced. Frequently, the horse has a history of a known trauma to the medial aspect of the tarsus. Fractures of the bones of the tarsus, avulsion fracture of the sustentaculum tali (around the attachment of the middle short medial tarsocrural ligament, which attaches to the distomedial aspect of the sustentaculum tali), or overstretching of the sheath may cause aseptic tenosynovitis of the tarsal sheath. Radiographs of the tarsus including the dorsomedial-plantarolateral and dorsopalmar (flexed) projections should be included in the diagnostic work-up. Chronic unilateral tarsal sheath effusion with lameness frequently reveals new bone production on the sustentaculum tali and fibrillation of the DDFT. Contrast radiography may assist in further defining both acute and chronic tarsal sheath abnormalities.

Wounds to the tarsus should be evaluated for the possibility of penetration into the tarsal sheath and the closely positioned tarsocrural joint. Chronic septic tenosynovitis may progress to osteomyelitis of the sustentaculum tali and adhesions of the DDFT, and carries an unfavorable prognosis.

Idiopathic Tenosynovitis

Idiopathic tenosynovitis is present when there is synovial effusion within a tendon sheath without obvious signs of inflammation, pain, or lameness. Clinical examination reveals a nonpainful synovial distention of the tendon sheath and, if a synovial sample is collected, a normal synovial fluid analysis. Effusion without inflammation is thought to occur insidiously from low-grade chronic trauma. Poor conformation is thought to predispose animals to some forms of tenosynovitis, such as that seen in tarsal sheath effusion (thoroughpin). Tendon sheath effusion may occur because of stretching of the sheath resulting from an increasing workload, obesity, or pregnancy. The most common sites for idiopathic effusion are the digital sheath, tarsal sheath, and extensor tendon sheaths of the carpus. Most cases of idiopathic tenosynovitis are considered cosmetic blemishes but ultrasonography is necessary to document normal architecture of the sheath and associated structures.

Acute Tenosynovitis

Acute tenosynovitis is present when effusion, inflammation, pain, or lameness rapidly develops within a tendon sheath. (Figure 4.132) Acute tenosynovitis is usually associated with some form of traumatic injury. A known incident such as hitting a jump or a fall during a work or turnout may indicate the origin of the injury. Structural damage to one or more of the tendons or ligaments associated with the tendon sheath may be the underlying cause of the effusion present in the sheath.

Ultrasonographic examination is indicated to preclude further damage to injured structures. Documentation of the specific structures involved and classification of the injury are necessary to institute appropriate therapy and to monitor the reparative process. Those horses without ultrasonographic evidence of structural damage to the soft tissues associated with the sheath should have a complete set of high-

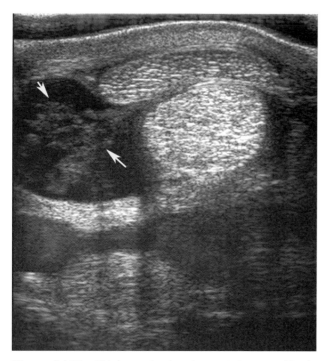

Figure 4.132. This horse developed an acute tenosynovitis of the DFTS following a traumatic injury to the distal limb. Ultrasound examination is indicated in acute tenosynovitis cases due to the potential for several structures to be affected, all of which can instigate an intense and prolonged inflammatory response. In this case there is a large clot within the DFTS adjacent to the DDFT (arrows) but little evidence of structural damage to the flexor tendons or DSLs.

detail radiographs taken to rule out osseous abnormalities such as fractures. Those horses with tendinitis or desmitis should have therapy aimed at reducing inflammation of the appropriate structure (see discussion on treatment of tendon and ligament injuries).

Chronic Tenosynovitis

Chronic tenosynovitis typically is unresolved acute tenosynovitis. Persistent effusion and inflammation present in chronic tenosynovitis frequently leads to a thickening of the fibrous portion of the sheath. Typically, the function of the sheath must be compromised to be classified as chronic. Fibrous adhesions of the parietal and visceral layers of the sheath may form and may restrict the gliding motion of the tendon through the sheath. Structural damage to the sheath, tendon, or related structures without appropriate rest or therapy is frequently the cause of the persistent inflammation.

An attempt to define the inciting cause of the inflammation should be made before treatment is instituted. Ultrasonographic examination frequently reveals a diffuse proliferative response of the sheath that complicates accurate identification of underlying structural damage. Proliferative nodular masses occur within synovial sheaths. Care should be taken to define the location of these nodular masses as intraluminal or extraluminal and to determine that no other masses exist. Adhesions between a tendon and the sheath and between a tendon and another tendon or between any of these structures and a mass(es) may be found on ultrasonographic examination.

Off-weighted ultrasonographic examination while placing the joint through a range of motion may help demonstrate adhesions between structures within the sheath. It may become necessary to inject a contrast or fluid medium to define the synovial membrane and the structures within the sheath. Persistence of lameness after medical therapy indicates that surgical exploration is necessary to define the specific problem. Endoscopy with an arthroscope allows good access to the structures of the digital sheath. Resection of the retinaculum or the annular ligament may be warranted to relieve compression on soft tissue structures within a carpal or fetlock canal, respectively.

Septic Tenosynovitis

Horses with infection of any synovial sheath or closed space usually present with a severe, nonweight-bearing lameness with heat, pain, and diffuse swelling. Punctures, lacerations, and iatrogenic infections are the most common causes of septic tenosynovitis, although infections of hematogenous origin occur. The nonspecific action of many of the enzymes of inflammation can destroy the fibrils and matrix of the tendon within the synovial sheath. Fibrin deposition within the synovial sheath may lead to fibrous adhesion formation. Therapy should be aggressive and should follow the same principles as for septic arthritis.

Ultrasonographic examination is not necessary to make a diagnosis of septic tenosynovitis, but it is a very useful adjunct to help find a pocket of fluid for collection of a synovial fluid sample for culture and sensitivity testing and synovial fluid analysis. The ultrasonographic appearance of the synovial fluid can vary depending on the cellular content and the formation of fibrin. The prognosis can be modified based on the extent of degenerative changes of the tendon or tendons. Placement of a closed-suction drain at the distal-most extent of the sheath may be assisted by the use of ultrasound. Sequential ultrasonographic examinations should be used to assess the response to therapy. This is particularly important to evaluate the effectiveness of a closed-suction apparatus in collecting the accumulating fluid formed within the sheath.

General Bursal Anatomy

A bursa (bursa synovialis) is a closed sac lined with a membrane closely resembling a synovial membrane. A bursa is present on a limb or at specific areas of the body that generally have limited movement but untoward pressure against a portion of bone, tendon, or ligament. A bursa can also be found in areas to facilitate the gliding action of a tendon, particularly in an area of stress such at a sesamoid bone but also in the vicinity of the tendon's attachment. The surface of the bone or the portions of the tendon or ligament contacting the bone may become cartilaginous.

Bursae have been classified based on anatomic position (subcutaneous, subfascial, subligamentous, submuscular, and subtendinous) or by the method of formation (congenital and acquired). Congenital bursae are located in a predictable position and are termed true or constant bursae. Acquired bursae typically develop subcutaneously in response to pressure and friction and are called inconstant bursae. Skin movement causes tearing of the subcutaneous tissue, allowing fluid to accumulate that later becomes encapsulated by fibrous tissue. In the later stages of development, bursae develop a synovial-like membrane that has a similar structural appearance to congenital bursae. In general, bursae beneath the deep fascia or among tendon, muscle, and bone are constant, whereas those between the skin and other structures (subcutaneous bursae) are inconstant. Occasionally a bursa may communicate with a joint or tendon sheath that is in close proximity (e.g., bursa beneath the long digital extensor tendon and the lateral femorotibial joint of the stifle, subtendinous bursa with the tendon sheath of the abductor pollicis longus in older horses, and bicipital bursa and the scapulohumeral joint). These may become clinically apparent because of effusions from the respective joint or sheath that cause filling of the bursa.

The constant bursae found to be of most clinical significance are the navicular bursa, bicipital bursa, subtendinous bursae of the common calcaneal tendon, and occasionally the cunean bursa. The acquired bursae most commonly found to be of clinical significance are the olecranon bursa, subcutaneous calcaneal bursa, and carpal hygroma.

Navicular Bursa (Bursa Podotrochlearis)

The navicular bursa is interposed between the DDFT and the navicular bone (NB) before insertion of the tendon onto P3. The bursa is lined by a synovial membrane, except along the fibrocartilage of the NB and along the surface of the DDFT, which apposes the fibrocartilage.

Evaluation of the navicular area requires two approaches. The palmar approach through the skin of the pastern area allows the inspection of the DDFT, suspensory ligament of the navicular apparatus, palmar proximal pouch of the navicular bursa, proximal border of the navicular bone, and palmar aspect of the DIP joint. The transcuneal approach is used to inspect the digital cushion, DDFT, distal sesamoidean impar ligament, navicular bone, and navicular bursa. However, diagnostic quality images of the navicular area and specifically the DDFT require that the sound beam be perpendicular to the fiber orientation of the tendon. Unfortunately, the course of the DDFT within the foot is not perpendicular to the windows (frog and bulbs of the heel) normally used to image structures within the foot, making it impossible to obtain the pertinent architectural information about the fibers of the DDFT.

The examination of many of the soft tissue structures within the foot is limited to the proximal aspect of the structure present above the horny hoof capsule or through the frog. In addition, access through the frog can be influenced by environmental conditions that influence the water content of the frog. Dry conditions may require soaking the foot to increase sound transmission and the quality of the image. In addition, the horse with chronic lameness associated with the foot will frequently have an atrophied frog, further limiting the window available to evaluate the internal structures of the foot. MR studies of the foot have demonstrated that many of the DDFT lesions are more abaxial, either in the medial or lateral lobes, and probably not apparent during the ultrasonographic examination. The transcuneal ultrasonographic approach provides good demonstration of needle insertion into the navicular bursa.

Bicipital Bursa (Bursa Intertubercularis)

The bicipital bursa lies deep to the biceps tendon as it courses through the intertubercular groove. The bursa is interposed between the biceps brachii tendon and the proximal humerus. The bursa extends around the medial and lateral lobes of the biceps brachii tendon, assuming a more sheath-like function. The bicipital bursa does not routinely communicate with the scapulohumeral joint, but occasionally a communication does exist.[25,70] There is also a bursa located between the infraspinatus tendon and the caudal part of the greater tubercle. Occasionally, a bursa can be found at the supraglenoid tubercle[70] that protects the supraspinatus muscle as it divides into the lateral and medial lobes. The tendon of origin of the biceps brachii is the supraglenoid tubercle of the scapula. The tendon appears tri-lobed and is heterogeneous due to adipose tissue within the tendon and interposed between the tendon and the humerus in the region between the supraglenoid tubercle and the tubercles of the humerus. The tendon then becomes bi-lobed in shape and more homogenous in echogenicity and is partly cartilaginous at the level of the humeral tubercles as it is closely molded around the intermediate tubercle of the humerus.

A complete ultrasonographic examination of the shoulder area should include the biceps tendon, bicipital bursa, humeral tubercles, infraspinatus bursa and tendons of attachment of the supraspinatus muscle, and infraspinatus muscle as well as the shoulder joint. When evaluating the biceps brachii tendon, the zoning system and reference measurements previously described should be used.[10,75]

Ultrasonography of the shoulder area should be considered when the lameness is eliminated with intra-articular analgesia of the scapulohumeral joint or intra-bursal analgesia of the bicipital bursa, or when there is a history of trauma or any swelling associated with the shoulder area (Figure 4.133). Ultrasonographic exam is often indicated even when there is a radiographic apparent abnormality because the soft tissues of the shoulder should be carefully evaluated. Careful radiographic and ultrasonographic exam of the shoulder is usually indicated when nuclear scintigraphy demonstrates active uptake of the radiopharmaceutical, even though this is more indicative of a bony problem of the shoulder.

Ultrasonography has proven very helpful in assessing soft tissue injuries as well as some bony injuries that are poorly defined by radiographs. In general, ultrasonographic and radiographic examination should be considered complementary imaging modalities, and it is essential to combine the 2 modalities in heavily muscled areas such as the shoulder. Radiography allows good evaluation of the bony structures of the shoulder but is limited in the number of projections that can be obtained to accurately image the joint. Ultrasonography, on the other hand, provides information about the surrounding soft tissues as well as the shoulder joint itself. Injections of medications can be more effectively deposited into the intrasynovial space by using ultrasonographically guided needle placement.[6] When used in the field, ultrasonography can effectively aid in diagnosing a fracture of the supraglenoid tubercle and greater tubercle.

Acquired Bursitis

OLECRANON BURSITIS

Olecranon bursitis (shoe boil, capped elbow) is an acquired bursitis typically due to trauma from contact of the ipsilateral horseshoe with the elbow. The injury may occur when the animal lies down or, in the gaited horse, during work. Repeated trauma is prevented by wrapping the foot in a boot or cotton bandage. In the acute stages, fluid is usually present within the bursa. Lameness is typically not present unless the bursitis has become septic. Draining tracts suggest infection, which may be iatrogenic or due to a foreign body. As the condition becomes chronic, the fluid is often replaced by fibrous tissue.

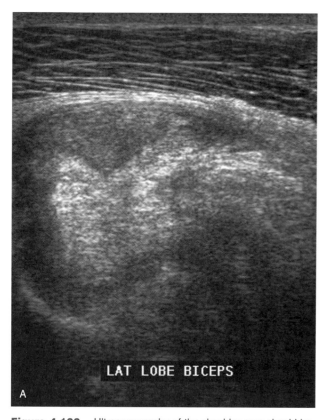
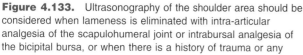
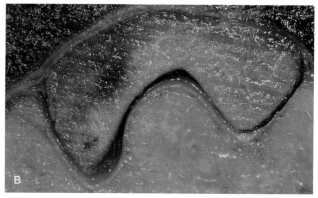

Figure 4.133. Ultrasonography of the shoulder area should be considered when lameness is eliminated with intra-articular analgesia of the scapulohumeral joint or intrabursal analgesia of the bicipital bursa, or when there is a history of trauma or any swelling associated with the shoulder area. This ultrasound image (A) and cross section (B) demonstrate a chronic active tendonitis of the lateral lobe of the bicipital tendon.

Ultrasonographic exam typically reveals a subcutaneous position of the bursa and may be helpful to characterize the bursitis as acute or chronic (fluid filled or fibrous). The presence of a foreign body or bone involvement may be seen ultrasonographically. Once infection can be ruled out, then drainage and injection with a corticosteroid may be necessary, provided conservative therapy has not been effective. Strict aseptic technique is necessary to prevent infection of the acquired bursa. Once the bursa wall thickens with fibrous tissue, treatment becomes more problematic. Surgical drainage and the placement of drains may become necessary. More extreme measures may be necessary if there is no response. Repeated ultrasonographic examination can assist the clinician in determining the response to each stage of treatment.

Calcaneal Bursitis

Acquired calcaneal bursitis (capped hock) is thought to be due to trauma, usually from a horse kicking the wall or trailer. Ultrasonographic exam typically reveals a subcutaneous position of the bursa and, in the early stages, a primarily fluid-filled pocket. The fluid may have fibrin or the appearance of a large clot within the cavity. A capped hock appearance has been reported in cases of gastrocnemius tendinitis and in some bony abnormalities of the tuber calcis. Plantar ligament desmitis, or curb, manifests as a swelling along the plantar aspect of the calcaneus. Curb occurs commonly and may be related to conformation. Lameness is typically minimal and of short duration. Horses with persistent lameness with swelling more distal to the plantar ligament should be evaluated more carefully. Superficial digital flexor tendinitis of the proximal metatarsus may have a similar appearance, with swelling distal to the calcaneus. Occasionally, similar swelling exists without lameness. This swelling has a fluid consistency and appears ultrasonographically as a fluid pocket surrounding the SDFT. Drainage may alleviate the problem, but persistence of the fluid may warrant corticosteroid injection.

The constant bursa of the calcaneus can develop effusion in luxation of the SDFT. The constant bursa can be involved in septic processes, particularly punctures and lacerations around the tarsus. Appropriate treatment includes systemic antibiotics, surgical debridement as necessary, and possibly placement of drains. Radiographs may provide evidence of osteomyelitis or sequestrum formation or osteomyelitis, which may be the primary problem, with the bursa secondarily infected.

Carpal Hygroma

A carpal hygroma is a subcutaneous swelling that develops after repeated trauma to the dorsal carpus. In the acute stage, a carpal hygroma contains fluid that appears consistent with a hematoma. Ultrasonographically, this fluid can have a range of cellular and inflammatory debris, frequently with an organized clot. Fluid aspiration and pressure bandaging may be sufficient to resolve the problem initially. In the chronic state,

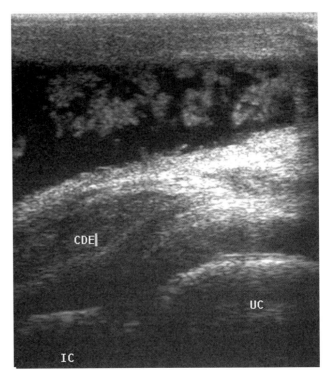

Figure 4.134. This ultrasound image is of an acquired bursa on the face of the carpus (hygroma). A carpal hygroma is a subcutaneous swelling that develops after trauma to the dorsal carpus. This ultrasound image demonstrates multiple irregularly sized flocculent particles within anechoic fluid, suggestive of fibrin.

loculation of fluid by fibrous bands can occur, but more commonly, a distinct bursal cavity develops. Ultrasonographic evaluation is useful in differentiating swellings of the dorsal aspect of the carpus (Figure 4.134). Synovitis of the extensor carpi radialis tendon sheath, subcutaneous herniation of a carpal joint capsule, ganglion, synovial fistula of the extensor sheaths and carpal joints, and synovitis of the carpal joints all may cause swellings of the dorsal carpus, each with a unique treatment. Once the formation of a carpal hygroma has been confirmed, it may be necessary to surgically drain the bursa and place a Penrose drain in the cavity, and to maintain a pressure wrap on the limb.

OTHER INDICATIONS FOR ULTRASONOGRAPHY OF THE MUSCULOSKELETAL SYSTEM

Evaluation of Bone

Bone appears as a bright hyperechoic line with a strong acoustic shadow. This is due to the high acoustic impedance when compared to the soft tissues. The bone surface appears to be of uniform thickness. Ultrasonography has proven especially useful in the diagnosis of fractures in areas that are not readily accessible to radiographic examination such as the pelvis, femur, scapula, humerus, and spine. Ultrasonography is often used in conjunction with nuclear scintigraphy to focus on areas of bone injury not apparent on radiographs. Fractures can be seen as anechoic to hypoechoic lines that are visible in the cortical bone. Often there is displacement (distraction) of the bone edges, evident as a step in the cortical margin.

Osteitis and osteomyelitis can also be evaluated with diagnostic ultrasound and appear as a fluid interface at the bone surface.[62] Acute trauma may have hemorrhage at the bone surface, which can appear similar to osteitis and may indicate more detailed radiographs to rule out a fracture. A repeat scan should be performed in 4 to 5 days to document resolution or resorption of the hemorrhage of the fluid interface.

Progression to osteitis is demonstrated by the persistence of fluid, which can vary from hypoechoic to anechoic and may contain hyperechoic echoes consistent with gas in the fluid. Hypoechoic tracts that begin at or just under the skin surface can occasionally be seen tracking to the bone surface. The bone surface may begin to demonstrate a raised area of periosteal new bone production, consistent with involucrum formation at the margins of the sequestrum or bone fragment(s). These periosteal changes can be seen earlier with ultrasound than radiographs. Sequestra appear as hyperechoic structures that cast acoustic shadows (Figure 4.135). Sequestra typically remain adjacent to parent bone and are surrounded by hypoechoic to anechoic fluid. Occasionally the sequestra can be seen displaced from the involucrum and lying in the tract leading to the skin surface. Areas with a predisposition to form

sequestra include the metacarpal/metatarsal bone, spine of the scapula, and medial aspect of the radius, but any area with cortical bone that is close to the skin surface may develop a sequestrum.

Ultrasonography is also helpful to assess fractures that have been repaired with internal fixation. In the early postoperative period the repair appears much like acute trauma cases, with hemorrhage and edema surrounding the implants. However, 5 to 7 days postoperatively this fluid interface should begin to become more organized unless there is increased motion or infection of the repair. If this fluid interface persists and the animal manifests systemic signs such as pain, heat, and swelling at the incision site; fever; and/or lameness, then infection of the implants should be suspected.

Evaluation of Punctures and Lacerations

Ultrasonography has proven particularly helpful in defining the extent of damage incurred during wounding, either from a puncture or a laceration. Lacerations over the extensor or flexor tendons in the distal extremities require careful examination of the tendons to document involvement and then determine the extent of damage incurred at wounding (Figure 4.136). Also, because these tendinous structures are frequently associated with sheaths and bursae, it is important to determine if these synovial structures are involved.

The wound should have a sterile prep applied to the wound margins and the wound bed flushed with a balanced electrolyte solution to clean dirt and debris from the wound. Sterile lubricant can be applied to the wound bed and a sterile glove or sheath placed over the probe. The probe can then be placed into the wound to examine the structures deep within the wound bed.

Air introduced into the wound may block sound transmission and compromise the study, which can be performed on another day after keeping the wound under a bandage. Documentation of tendon or sheath involvement significantly changes the management of these types of wounds. Diagnostic ultrasound can be useful to identify synovial distention and assess the character of the synovial fluid. An increase in cellularity and fibrin content in the synovial fluid increases its echogenicity. The presence of gas shadows suggests either an open joint space or the presence of gas-producing organisms in the joint fluid. Treatment must be directed at eliminating any foreign material, reducing bacterial numbers, removing contaminated and devitalized material, and neutralizing and eliminating inflammatory enzymes and other inflammatory products. Puncture wounds involving the tendons and ligaments around the joint can significantly affect the prognosis.

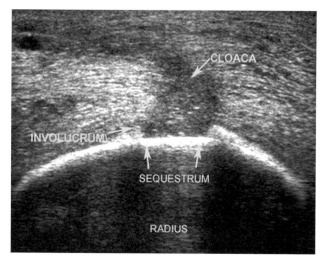

Figure 4.135. This horse had a draining tract of the medial radius. Radiographs were suggestive but not conclusive for a sequestrum, but ultrasonography proved to be diagnostic. There are small gas shadows within the middle of the tract (cloaca) which courses from surface of the radius to the skin. New bone is being deposited at the periphery of the sequestrum. The margins of the sequestrum have raised periosteal new bone production consistent with involucrum formation. Sequestra appear as hyperechoic structures that cast acoustic shadows. These periosteal changes can be seen earlier with ultrasound than radiographs.

Evaluation of Muscle

Acute muscle injury occurs due to blunt trauma, violent contraction against resistance, and myositis. Muscle has a heterogeneous appearance with hypoechogenic muscle fibers laced with and surrounded by fascia, connective tissue, and fat. On transverse images normal muscle has a marbled or speckled appearance.[62] Each muscle has a fairly unique appearance that can change between weight-bearing and nonweight-bearing.

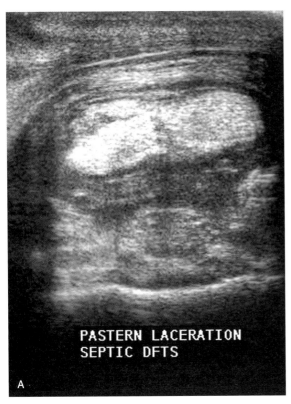

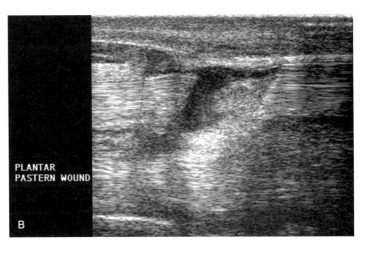

Figure 4.136. Lacerations over the extensor or flexor tendons of the distal extremities require careful examination of the tendons and any associated sheaths/bursas to determine the extent of damage incurred at wounding. A. Transverse ultrasound image of a DDFT injury in the pastern. There is a proliferative response within the DFTS that suggests an active inflammatory process. Due to the penetrating injury sepsis is likely. B. Longitudinal ultrasound image of a laceration which demonstrates a severe DDFT injury. There is complete transaction of the DDFT with retraction of the proximal stump of the tendon.

More severe muscle injuries may have fluid-filled areas with loculation seen on ultrasonographic examination, which is suggestive of significant muscle fiber tearing and hemorrhage. It can be more difficult to define minor injuries because ultrasonographic changes are less obvious. Minor injuries may simply manifest as an enlargement of the muscle belly with very little loss of the normal striated muscle pattern and a decrease in echogenicity. The paired structure on the opposite limb should be used for comparison (Figure 4.137). Ultrasonography can be used to monitor the repair process. The hematoma is slowly resorbed and the area gradually filled in with granulation tissue. The infiltration of fibrocytes and capillaries create a more heterogenous appearance to the muscle injury over time.

Fibrotic myopathy is a chronic muscle condition that is probably the result of some acute muscle damage that heals with exuberant scar. This scar creates a restricted gait in which the limb is rapidly slapped to the ground at the end of swing phase (described as goose stepping). Palpable muscle scarring can usually be found within the semimembranosus, semitendinosus, and occasionally the gracilis muscles. The ultrasound appearance of this mass is consistent with excessive fibrosis, seen as hyperechogenic areas within the body of the muscle. There may be hyperechogenic areas suggestive of mineralization or dystrophic calcification that cast acoustic shadows within or adjacent to the affected tissue.

Evaluation of Foreign Bodies

A number of different materials, when introduced into the soft tissues, can create a significant foreign body reaction in the horse. The most common foreign bodies include wood, lead (bullets or buckshot), metallic objects (such as wire or fencing materials), glass, plant material, hair, and suture material (Figure 4.138).

Wood appears as a linear hyperechoic structure that casts a strong acoustic shadow. The most common wood foreign bodies are associated with fencing materials that splinter after penetrating the skin. It is important to carefully evaluate the wounded area for multiple wood splinters before initiating retrieval because air introduced into the wound either at wounding or during surgery can block ultrasound transmission, further limiting the evaluation of tissues deep to it.

Bullets and metallic structures can appear to have variable shapes and contours, but like wood, these objects can cast strong acoustic shadows. However, plant material and hair appear to have small hyperechoic shadows that may or may not cast acoustic shadows. This hyperechoic material is usually seen within a hypoechoic tract. Metal such as surgical instruments appear similarly and cast strong acoustic shadows that can be used to the clinician's advantage when ultrasonographically guided retrieval is used. Placement of an instrument such as a mosquito forceps around the

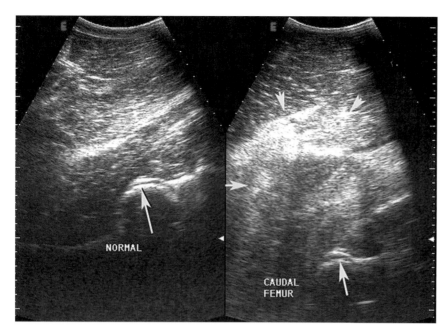

Figure 4.137. This is a longitudinal ultrasound image of the caudal femur of the stifle. The cartilage covering the caudal condyle is apparent (lower arrows). Proximal is to the left and distal is to the right. This horse incurred a caudal reciprocal apparatus breakdown and the gastrocnemius muscle can be seen to have significant damage (smaller arrows surrounding the damaged area).

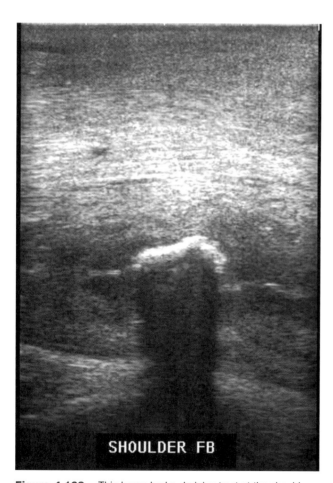

Figure 4.138. This horse had a draining tract at the shoulder region. There appears to be a dense foreign body several centimeters deep, consistent with a bullet. The surgical approach to the foreign body was mapped out with ultrasonography intraoperatively.

foreign body can be easily seen. If retrieval of the foreign body is more complicated, then the area should be mapped out with ultrasonography before retrieval.

References

1. Aisen AM, McCune WJ, MacQuire A. Ultrasonographic evaluation of the cartilage of the knee. Radiology 1984;153:781–784.
2. Almanza A, Whitcomb MB. Ultrasonographic diagnosis of pelvic fractures in 28 horses. Proc Am Assoc Eq Pract 2003; 49:50–54.
3. Benson CB. Ultrasonography of the musculoskeletal system. In. Musculoskeletal Imaging—MRI, CT, Nuclear Medicine, and Ultrasound in Clinical Practice. Markisz JA, ed. Little Brown and Company, Boston. 1991 201–210.
4. Bischofberger AS, Konar M, Ohlerth S, et al. Magnetic resonance imaging, ultrasonography and histology of the origin of the suspensory ligament—a comparative study of the normal equine anatomy. Eq Vet J 2006;38:508–516.
5. Brenner S, Whitcomb MB. How to Diagnose Equine Coxofemoral Subluxation with Dynamic Ultrasonography. Proc Am Assoc Eq Pract 2007;53:433–437.
6. Carnicer D, Coudry T, Denoix JM. Ultrasonographic guided injection of the scapulohumeral joint in horses. Eq Vet Educ 2008;20(2):103–106.
7. Cartee RE, Rumph PF. Ultrasonographic detection of fistulous tracts and foreign objects in the muscles of horses. J Am Vet Med Assoc 1984;184:1127.
8. Cauvin EJ. Soft tissue injuries in the shoulder region: systematic approach to differential diagnosis. Eq Vet Educ 1998;10: 70–74.
9. Cauvin ER, Munroe GA, Boyd JS, et al. Ultrasonographic examination of the femorotibial articulation in horses: imaging of the cranial and caudal aspects. Equine Vet J 1996;4:285–96.
10. Crabill, MR, Chaffin, KM, Schmitz, DG. Ultrasonographic morphology of the bicipital tendon and bursa in clinically normal Quarter horses. Am J Vet Res 1995;56:5–10.
11. David F, Rougier M, Alexande K, et al. Ultrasound-guided coxofemoral arthrocentesis in horses. Eq Vet J 2007;39(1):79–83.
12. Denoix JM, Crevier N, Azevedo C. Ultrasound examination of the pastern in horses. Proc Am Assoc Eq Pract 1991;33: 363–380.
13. Denoix JM, Farres D. Ultrasonographic imaging of the proximal third interosseous muscle in the pelvic limb using a plantaromedial approach. J Eq Vet Sci 1995:15:346–350.

14. Denoix JM. Ultrasonographic examination in the diagnosis of joint disease. In Joint Disease in the Horse. McIlwraith CW, Trotter G, eds. W.B. Saunders Co., Philadelphia. 1996; 165–202.

15. Denoix JM. Joints and miscellaneous tendons. In Equine Diagnostic Ultrasonography. Rantanen NW, McKinnon AO, eds. Williams and Wilkins, Philadelphia. 1998;475–514.

16. Denoix JM, Busoni V. Ultrasonography of joints and synovia. In Current Techniques in Equine Surgery and Lameness. 2nd ed. White NA, Moore JN, eds. W.B. Saunders, Philadelphia. 1998;643–654.

17. Denoix JM, Jacot S, Perrot P. Ultrasonographic anatomy of the dorsal and abaxial aspect of the equine fetlock, Eq Vet J 1996 28:54–62.

18. Denoix JM, Coudry V, Jacquet S. Ultrasonographic procedure for a complete examination of the proximal third interosseous muscle (proximal suspensory ligament) in the equine forelimbs. Eq Vet Educ 2008;20(3):148–153.

19. Denoix JM. Ultrasonographic evaluation of joints. In Diagnosis and Management of Lameness in the Horse. Ross MW, Dyson SJ, eds. WB Saunders, Philadelphia. 2003;189–194.

20. Dik KJ. Radiographic and ultrasonographic imaging of soft tissue disorders of the equine carpus. Tijdschr Diergeneeskd 1990; 115:1168–1174.

21. Dik KJ. Ultrasound of the equine tarsus. Vet Rad and Ultrasound 1993;34:36–43.

22. Dik KJ, Van Den Belt JM, Keg PR. Ultrasonographic evaluation of fetlock annular ligament constriction in the horse. Equine Vet J 1991;23:285–288.

23. Dik KJ. Ultrasonography of the equine shoulder. Eq Pract 1996;18:13–18.

24. Dyce KM, Sack WO, Wensing CJ. Textbook of Veterinary Anatomy. W.B. Saunders Co., Philadelphia, 1987;542–595.

25. Dyson S, Dik, KJ. Miscellaneous conditions of tendons, tendon sheaths, and ligaments. Vet Clin N Am 1995;11:315–338.

26. Dyson S, Murray R, Schramme M. Collateral desmitis of the distal interphalangeal joint in 18 horses (2001–2002). Eq Vet J 2004;36:160–166.

27. Dyson S, Murray R. Collateral desmitis of the distal interphalangeal joint in 62 horses (January 2001–December 2003), in 50th Proc Am Assoc Eq Pract 2004;248–256.

28. Dyson SJ, Genovese R. The suspensory apparatus. In Diagnosis and Management of Lameness in the Horse. Ross MW, Dyson SJ, eds. W.B. Saunders, Philadelphia, 2003;654–672.

29. Dyson SJ. Normal ultrasonographic anatomy and injury of the patellar ligaments in the horse. Eq Vet J 2002;34;258–64.

30. Edinger J, Mobius G, Ferguson J. Comparison of tenoscopic and ultrasonographic methods of examination of the digital flexor tendon sheath in horses. Vet Comp Orthop Traumatol 2005; 1:84:209–14.

31. Firth EC. Functional joint anatomy and its development. In Joint Disease in the Horse. McIlwraith CW, Trotter G, eds. WB Saunders Co, Philadelphia, 1996;80–86.

32. Firth EC, Greydanus Y. Cartilage thickness measurements in foals. Res Vet Sci 1987;42:35–46.

33. Genovese RL, Rantanen NW, Simpson BS. The use of ultrasound in the diagnosis and management of injuries to the equine limb. Comp Cont Educ Pract Vet 1987;9:945–955.

34. Genovese RL. The suspensory apparatus. In Diagnosis and Management of Lameness in the Horse, Ross MW, Dyson SJ, eds. W.B. Saunders, Philadelphia, 2003;654–672.

35. Genovese RL, Rantanen N, Hauser M, Simpson BS. Diagnostic ultrasonography of equine limbs. Vet Clin N Am Equine Pract 1986;2:145.

36. Goodrich LR, Werpy NM, Armentrout A. How to ultrasound the normal pelvis for aiding diagnosis of pelvic fractures using rectal and transcutaneous ultrasound examination. Proc Am Assoc Eq Pract 2006;52:609–612.

37. Grewel J, McClure S, Booth L, et al. Assessment of the ultrasonographic characteristics of the podotrochlear apparatus in clinically normal horses and horses with navicular syndrome. J Am Vet Med Assoc 2004;225:1881–1888.

38. Kainer RA. Functional anatomy of the equine locomotor organs. In Adams' Lameness in Horses, 4th ed. Stashak TS, ed. Lea and Febiger, Philadelphia, 1987;1–70.

39. Lamb CR. Contrast radiography of equine joints, tendon sheaths, and draining tracts. Vet Clin N Am Aug 1991;241–258.

40. Mack LA, Scheible W. Diagnostic ultrasound, radiography, and related diagnostic techniques in the evaluation of bone, joint, and soft tissue diseases. In Diagnosis of Bone and Joint Disorders, 3rd ed. Resnik D, ed. W.B. Saunders Co., Philadelphia, 1995; 219–236.

41. Mattoon JS, Drost WT, Grguric MR. Technique for equine cervical articular process joint injection. Vet Rad and Ultrasound 2004;45:238–240.

42. McClellan PD, Colby J. Ultrasonic structure of the pastern. J Eq Vet Sci 1986;6:99.

43. McCune WJ, Dedrick DK, Aisen AM. Sonographic evaluation of osteoarthritic femoral condylar cartilage—correlation with operative findings. Clin Orthop 1990;254:230.

44. Nielsen JV, Berg LC, Thoefner MB, et al. Accuracy of ultrasound-guided intra-articular injection of cervical facet joints in horses: a cadaveric study. Eq Vet J 2003;35;657–661.

45. Nyland TG, Matoon JS. Small Animal Diagnostic Ultrasound, WB Saunders, Philadelphia, 2002;1–28.

46. O'Callaghan MW. The integration of radiography and alternative imaging in the diagnosis of equine orthopedic disease. Vet Clin N Am Aug 1991;339–364.

47. Olivier-Carstens A. Ultrasonography of the solar aspect of the distal phalanx in the horse. Vet Rad and Ultrasound 2004; 45(5):449–57.

48. Penninck D, Nyland T, O'Brien T, et al. Ultrasonography of the equine stifle. Vet Rad and Ultrasound 1990;31:293–298.

49. Powis RL. Ultrasound Science for the Veterinarian. Equine Diagnostic Ultrasonography. Rantanen NW, McKimmon AO, eds. Williams and Wilkins, Baltimore, 1998;1–18.

50. Pool RR. Traumatic injury and osteoarthritis. In Joint Disease in the Horse. McIlwraith CW, Trotter G, eds. W.B. Saunders Co., Philadelphia, 1996;87–104.

51. Pool RR, Meagher DM. Pathological findings and pathogenesis of racetrack injuries. Vet Clin N Am 1990;6:1–30.

52. Pugh CR, Johnson PJ, Crawle G, et al. Ultrasonography of the equine bicipital tendon region: a case history and review of anatomy. Vet Radiol and Ultrasound 1994;35:183–188.

53. Rantanen NW. The use of diagnostic ultrasound to detect structural damage to the soft tissues of the extremities of horses. J Eq Vet Sci 1985;3:134–135.

54. Rantanen NW. Examination procedures and normal anatomy. In Rantanen NW, McKinnon AO, eds. Equine diagnostic ultrasonography. The Williams and Wilkins Co., Baltimore. 1998; 114–117.

55. Rantanen NW, Jorgensen JS, Genovese RL. Ultrasonographic evaluation of the equine limb. In Diagnosis and Management of Lameness in the Horse. Ross MW, Dyson SJ, eds. WB Saunders, Philadelphia. 2003;166–188.

56. Redding WR. Distal sesamoidean ligament injuries and desmitis of the accessory ligament of the deep digital flexor tendon. Proc Dubai International Eq Symp, 1996;227–240.

57. Redding WR. Sonographic exam of the digital flexor tendon sheath, distal flexor tendons, and soft tissues of the palmar pastern region. Proc Am Assoc Eq Pract 1993:39:11–16.

58. Redding WR. Ultrasonic imaging of the structures of the digital sheath. Comp Cont Educ Pract Vet 1991 13:1824–1832.

59. Redding WR. Sonographic examination of the joints of horses; Part 1: Indications, techniques and equipment. Eq Vet Educ Aug 2001;3(4):250–259.

60. Redding WR. Sonographic examination of the joints of horses; Part 2: Examination of articular structures. Eq Vet Educ 2001 Oct, 13(5):275–279.

61. Reef VB. Musculoskeletal ultrasonography. In Equine Diagnostic Ultrasound. WB Saunders Co., Philadelphia. 1998;43–100.

62. Reef VB. Ultrasonography and Orthopedic (nonarticular) Disease. In Diagnosis and Management of Lameness in the Horse. Ross MW, Dyson SJ, eds. Saunders, Philadelphia. 2003; 194–197.

63. Reimer JM. Ultrasonography of the pastern: 1. anatomy and pathology; 2. outcome of selected injuries in race horses. Proc Am Assoc Eq Pract 1996;42:123–125.

64. Ruggles AJ. The carpus. In Diagnosis and Management of Lameness in the Horse. Ross MW, Dyson SJ, eds. WB Saunders, Philadelphia. 2003; p. 1253–1266.

65. Ruohoniemi M. Monitoring the Progression of Tarsal Ossification with Ultrasound and Radiography in Three Immature Foals. Vet Rad and Ultrasound. 1995;36(5):402–410.

66. Sack W, Habel R. Rooney's Guide to the Dissection of the Horse, Rooney J. ed. Veterinary Textbooks, Ithaca. 1977;542–595.

67. Sage AM, Turner TA. Ultrasonography of the soft tissue structures of the equine foot, Eq Vet Educ 2002;14(4):221–224.

68. Schneider RK, Jenson P, Moore RM. Evaluation of cartilage lesions on the medial femoral condyle as a cause of lameness in horses: 11 cases (1988–1994). J Am Vet Med Assoc 1997; 210:1649–1652.

69. Shepherd MC, Pilsworth RC. The use of ultrasound in the diagnosis of pelvic fractures. Eq Vet Educ 1994;6:223–227.

70. Sisson S. Equine Osteology, Syndesmology, and Myology. In Sisson and Grossman's The Anatomy of the Domestic Animals, 5th ed. Getty R, ed. W.B. Saunders Co, Philadelphia. 1975;255–453.

71. Smith MR, Wright IM. Noninfected tenosynovitis of the digital flexor tendon sheath: a retrospective analysis of 76 cases. Eq Vet J 2006;38 (2):134–41.

72. Spriet M, David F, Rossier Y. Ultrasonographic control of navicular bursa injection. Eq Vet J 2004;36:637–639.

73. Stashak TS. Diagnosis of Lameness. In Adams' Lameness in Horses, 4th ed. Stashak TS, ed. Lea and Febiger, Philadelphia, 1987;100–156.

74. Tnibar M, Kaser-Hotz B, Auer JA. Ultrasonography of the dorsal and lateral aspects of the equine carpus: technique and normal appearance. Vet Rad and Ultrasound 1993;34:413–425.

75. Tnibar MA, Auer JA, Bakkali S. Ultrasonography of the equine shoulder: technique and normal appearance. Vet Rad and Ultrasound 1999;40:44–57.

76. Tomlinson J, Redding WR, Sage A. Ultrasonographic evaluation of tarsocrural joint cartilage in normal adult horses. Vet Rad and Ultrasound 2000;41(5):457–460.

77. Tomlinson JE, Sage AM, Turner TA. Detailed ultrasonographic mapping of the pelvis in clinically normal horses and ponies. Am J Vet Res 2001;62:1768–1775.

78. Turner TA. Thermography as an aid to the clinical lameness evaluation. Vet Clin N Am 1991;311–338.

79. Updike, SJ. Functional anatomy of the equine tarsocrural collateral ligaments. Am J Vet Res 1984;45:867–874.

80. Vanderperren K, Raes E, Hoegaerts M, et al. Diagnostic imaging of the equine tarsal region using radiography and ultrasonography. Part 1: the soft tissues Eq Vet J 2009;179(2):179–87.

81. Von Rechenberg B, McIlwraith CW, Auer JA. Cystic bone lesions in horses and humans: a comparative review. Vet Comp Orthop Traumatol 1998;11:8–18.

82. Wallis TW, Goodrich L, McIlwraith W, et al. Arthroscopic Injection of Corticosteroids Into Subchondral Cystic Lesions of the Medial Femoral Condyle in Horses. Proc Am Assoc Eq Pract 2007;53:414–415.

83. Walmsley J. Vertical tears of the cranial horn of the meniscus and its cranial ligament in the equine femorotibial joint: 7 cases and their treatment by arthroscopic surgery. Eq Vet J 1995; 27:20–25.

84. White NA. Ultrasound-guided transection of the accessory ligament of the deep digital flexor muscle in horses. Vet Surg 1995;24:373–378.

85. Wilderjans H, Boussauw B, Madder K, et al. Tenosynovitis of the digital flexor tendon sheath and annular ligament constriction syndrome caused by longitudinal tears in the deep digital flexor tendon: a clinical and surgical report of 17 cases in Warmblood horses. Eq Vet J 2003;35(3):270–5.

NUCLEAR MEDICINE

Alejandro Valdés-Martínez and Philip F. Steyn

Nuclear medicine techniques image the blood flow to bone as well as the function or the physiological activity of bone, whereas radiography, ultrasound, computerized tomography (CT), and magnetic resonance imaging (MRI) produce images that reveal anatomic detail. Nuclear medicine imaging is a very sensitive tool that augments but does not replace the basic lameness examination.[10,57,59,71,77,78,93,96] Most academic institutions and several private clinics have nuclear medicine imaging facilities, making this modality within the reach of many equine practitioners worldwide. This chapter discusses the principles, techniques, indications for, and interpretations of nuclear medicine imaging in the evaluation of the musculoskeletal system of horses.

PRINCIPLES OF NUCLEAR MEDICINE

Nuclear medicine imaging, also known as scintigraphy, is based on the functional distribution of a radio-pharmaceutical in the body. The radio-pharmaceutical is made of a radionuclide, most commonly Technetium-99m (^{99m}Tc), and is labeled to a pharmaceutical, which determines the target tissue of the radio-pharmaceutical in the body. Technetium-99m decays by emitting a 140-kEv γ-ray. A γ-ray is identical to an X-ray, except that it originates from the nucleus of an unstable atom (^{99m}Tc in this case) as the atom strives toward a more stable state. Nuclear medicine imaging can also be described as an emission imaging technique because the image is made by γ-rays that are emitted by the ^{99m}Tc inside the horse. Radiography is considered a transmission imaging technique because the X-rays that produce the image are transmitted through the patient.

Technetium-99m can be produced on site using a molybdenum-99m generator, or it can be ordered from a nuclear pharmacy when needed. Technetium-99m has a relatively short natural half-life ($T_{1/2}$) of 6 hours, which means that, e.g., 100 mCi of ^{99m}Tc will decay to 50 mCi in 6 hours, or an exposure rate of e.g., 4 mrem/hour (0.04 Millisievert [mSv]) will decrease to 2 mrem/hour (0.02 mSv) in 6 hours. However, the effective $T_{1/2}$ of a radiopharmaceutical is generally shorter than the natural $T_{1/2}$ due to biological excretion of the tracer.

The pharmaceutical part of the radiopharmaceutical determines the distribution of the tracer radionuclide in the body. There are various molecules or cells that can be labeled. Red blood cells can be labeled for the evaluation of the circulating blood compartment, most commonly to study cardiac function. Intravenous administration of ^{99m}Tc-pertechnetate (^{99m}TcO$_4$) or ^{99m}Tc-labeled red blood cells (^{99m}TcRBCs) are scintigraphic techniques for looking at the perfusion (blood flow) of soft tissue structures such as the joints of the distal limbs. White blood cells can be selectively labeled with ^{99m}Tc-HMPAO to look for areas of active inflammation/infection.[9,48,61] ^{99m}Tc-labeled biotin (^{99m}TcEB1)

has also been used to detect soft tissue inflammation in horses.[44] Renal function can be studied using ^{99m}Tc-DTPA, and quantitative hepato-billiary studies can be performed with ^{99m}Tc-Disophenin. Functional lung ventilation studies have been described using aerosolized ^{99m}Tc-DTPA[59] and lung perfusion with ^{99m}Tc macro aggregates of albumin (MAA).[8] Although each of these techniques uses ^{99m}Tc, the distribution of the radiopharmaceutical varies, based on the biokinetics of the pharmaceutical or cell to which the ^{99m}Tc has been labeled.

Bone scans are conducted using radiolabeled polyphosphanates, which have a high affinity for the Ca-hydroxy-apatite molecules in bone. Images made at 2 to 4 hours post injection are a representation of the uptake pattern in the bones. A very predictable uptake pattern is seen in normal animals and increased radiopharmaceutical uptake (IRU) is seen with increased blood flow or increased osteoblastic activity. Either ^{99m}Tc-oxidronate (HDP) or ^{99m}Tc-methylene diphosphanate (MDP) is administered intravenously at a dose of about 0.35 mCi/kg body weight. ^{99m}Tc-HDP has the advantage of faster soft tissue clearance, thus allowing image acquisition to begin sooner after injection.[4] A second advantage of ^{99m}Tc-HDP is improved visualization of bones surrounded by large amounts of muscle, e.g., spine, pelvis, and hips. An average 450-kg horse receives about 160 mCi (5.92 GBq) of the radiolabel. The dose rate can be adjusted for age, i.e., increased by about 10% in older patients and decreased by about 10% in juveniles because of the difference in metabolic activity of bone tissue. Approximately 50% of the injected radiolabel is excreted in the urine, which results in the effective $T_{1/2}$ being shorter than the natural $T_{1/2}$.[66]

A nuclear medicine evaluation of the musculoskeletal system may consist of 3 phases. Phase 1, known as the blood flow or vascular phase, represents the radio-pharmaceutical in the blood vessels before diffusion into the extracellular fluid. It lasts for 1 or 2 minutes after injection. The body region to be evaluated must be positioned in front of the γ camera at the time of injection, and dynamic rapid frame acquisition is made as the radiolabel perfuses the vasculature. Multiple images are acquired over the first few minutes while the radiolabel is within the vascular system, before diffusion into the extravascular space occurs. The vascular phase is used to compare the blood flow, especially to the distal limbs, e.g., in cases of degloving injuries, but it can also be used to document perfusion deficits in different anatomical regions.

Phase 2, known as the pool or soft tissue phase, represents the radio-pharmaceutical distribution in the extracellular fluid and is visualized from 3 to approximately 10 minutes post injection. This phase is used to evaluate blood flow to soft tissues. An increased signal is observed with hyperemia due to edema, inflammation, etc. Increased radioactivity during the pool or soft tissue phase is best used in the distal limbs and has been associated with navicular syndrome as well as inflamed joints and tendinitis or desmitis.

Early intense bone uptake of the radio-pharmaceutical (^{99m}Tc-HDP or ^{99m}Tc-MDP) can sometimes be seen as soon as 5 minutes after injection, especially in cases of intense delayed phase bone uptake, e.g., fractures or infectious processes. This can sometimes make the evaluation of soft tissues challenging at best, if not impossible. A scintigraphic technique for looking at soft tissues only, without any possibility of bone uptake, is to use ^{99m}Tc-O$_4$ (pertechnetate, unlabeled to a pharmaceutical) administered intravenously and images made as soon as radiopharmaceutical equilibrium in the extracellular space is achieved. A similar dose to that of the bone-scanning agents is recommended. ^{99m}Tc-RBC is another alternative for evaluating blood perfusion to soft tissues without the risk of bone uptake overlap.[79]

Phase 3, known as the delayed or bone phase, occurs several hours later when approximately 50% of the injected radiopharmaceutical has attached to bone. The remainder of the tracer is excreted by the kidneys in the first 1 or 2 urine voids post injection. The uptake pattern of normal bone is quite predictable and is described later in this chapter. The diaphysis of long bones has the least uptake, and greatest uptake of the tracer occurs in the juxtaphyseal and subchondral bone in normal subjects. Increased uptake by or near the joints during the delayed (bone) phase has been related to osteoarthritis (OA), various enthesopathies, periarticular bone sclerosis, and septic arthritis, etc. These changes from the normal uptake pattern are discussed later in this chapter.

RADIATION SAFETY AND PROTECTION

The ALARA procedures and protocols as described by the local radiation safety officer should always be followed. ALARA means that the radiation dose to which one is exposed will be kept *"As Low As Reasonably Achievable."* These procedures and protocols are intended to protect the clinician, others, and the environment from unnecessary risks due to radiation exposures.

Radiation detection equipment is used to find ^{99m}Tc traces that may have accidentally spilled, or to detect the levels of radiation in a patient before releasing the patient back to the public. Geiger Muller survey instruments and wipe tests are used to survey areas and surfaces for spills (Figure 4.139) and ion chambers are used to record the levels of radioactivity in patients (Figure 4.140). Film badges (personal dosimeters) should always be worn to monitor the total cumulative radiation dose. Finger (ring) thermoluminescent dosimetry (TLD) film badges should be worn by personnel preparing and injecting the radiopharmaceutical (Figure 4.141).

Eating, drinking, or smoking while handling a radioactive patient or radioactive materials is not permitted.[95] Lead or tungsten syringe shields are designed to help reduce the radiation dose to the fingers (Figure 4.142). An indwelling jugular catheter with a short extension tube should be placed prior to the study to

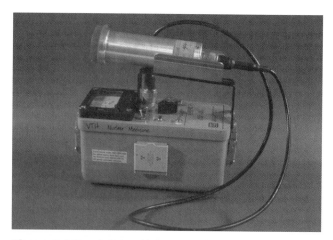

Figure 4.139. A Geiger Muller survey instrument is used to scan for radioactive spills and possible contamination.

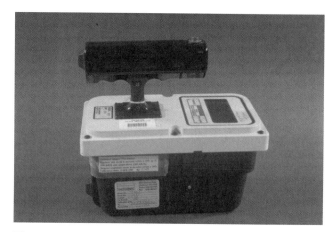

Figure 4.140. An ion chamber records the levels of radioactivity in patients, e.g., to determine whether they can be released. Acceptable radioactivity levels depend on state law but should be defined in the license description for each nuclear medicine clinic.

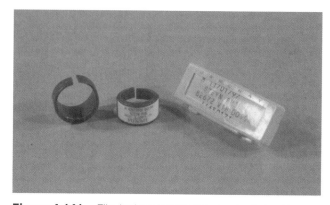

Figure 4.141. Film badges (personal dosimeters) should always be worn to monitor the total cumulative radiation dose. Finger (ring) thermoluminescent dosimeter film badges should be worn by personnel who prepare and inject the radiopharmaceutical.

help reduce the radiation exposure to the fingers of the injector.

The nuclear medicine clinician should be conscious of two basic methods of exposure to ionizing radiation: internal contamination and external radiation. Care must be taken to avoid internal contamination through the accidental ingestion of the radionuclide. This most commonly occurs by contamination of the hands and subsequent accidental ingestion, although absorption by the mucus membranes of the eyes and nose or inhalation can also occur if the dose is accidentally sprayed (for example, during injection). Direct injection per accidental hypodermic needle stick is less likely though possible route of internal contamination. Latex gloves should always be worn when working with radiophar-

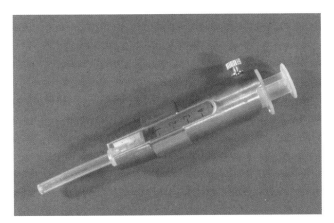

Figure 4.142. Lead syringe shields are designed to help reduce the radiation dose to the fingers.

maceuticals or radioactive patients. These gloves and other items used to treat the horse should be disposed of appropriately, as described by the local radiation safety officer.

External radiation occurs when one is in the immediate vicinity of the horse, for example, when scanning. The three basic rules of radiation safety are "time, distance, and shielding". Therefore, the time spent with the horse should be only that necessary for performing the study. Doubling the distance between the horse and the personnel reduces the radiation exposure by one-fourth. Similarly, the exposure is quadrupled by halving the distance from the horse. Standing 1 meter away from the horse significantly reduces the radiation exposure to personnel. For example, the exposure rate at the surface of a horse of 6.6 mrem/hour decreases to 1.3 mrem/hour at 1 meter.

Syringe shields should be used to reduce the radiation dose to the fingers (Figure 4.142). Personnel who scan horses on a frequent basis should consider wearing a lead apron and a lead thyroid shield (Figure 4.143). Protective lead clothing reduces the radiation exposure dose by 3 to 4-fold. For example, if the exposure at the surface of the horse is 6.6 mrem/hour, the exposure to a person wearing a lead apron (at skin surface) is only 1.5 mrem/hour.[80] Thus, in this example, standing 1 meter away from the horse and wearing a lead apron reduces the exposure to about 0.5 mrem/hour.

Appropriate radiation warning signs and patient handling procedures, as determined by the radiation safety officer, should be posted on the stall in which a radioactive horse has been housed. The horse is hospitalized until the radiation exposure levels at skin level are below a certain level. This level is determined by

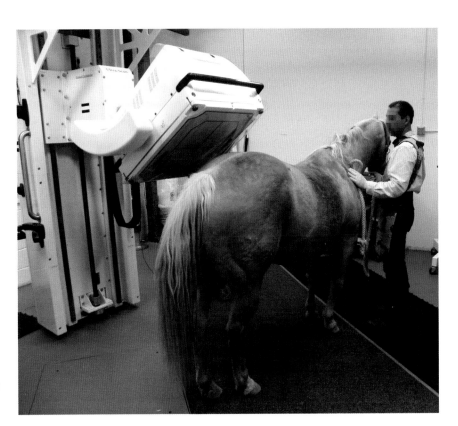

Figure 4.143. A lead apron and thyroid shield reduce the radiation dose to the personnel. Latex gloves prevent skin contamination, e.g., by radioactive urine.

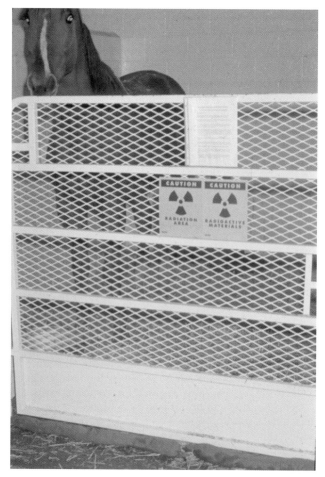

Figure 4.144. Horses should be housed in stalls approved by the radiation safety officer until skin levels reach the standards set by the state. Radioactive warning signs and patient handling procedures should be posted on the stall, and absorbent material such as socks can be used on the floor in front of the stall to absorb potentially radioactive urine.

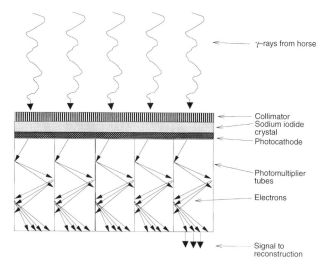

Figure 4.145. In the gamma camera, the γ-photons from the ^{99m}Tc in the horse are changed to light photons by the sodium iodide crystal and then to electrons by the photocathode. The electrons are amplified by the photomultiplier tubes, and the signal is used for image reconstruction by the computer.

each state, and varies from 1 to 5 mrem/hour at skin level. Survey meters such as Geiger counters (Figure 4.139) and ion chambers (Figure 4.140) are used to monitor the work area for possible contamination and to monitor the patient for release purposes. After the horse has been released the stall is closed off for an additional 24 hours before it is cleaned. This allows 4 more half-lives of natural decay of the ^{99m}Tc that was excreted via the urine, reducing the exposure to the personnel even further (ALARA). Radiation safety rules may vary from state to state; therefore, the practitioner should consult the local radiation safety officer and comply with the specific state regulations. Other precautionary steps, for example placing absorbent material (socks) in front of stalls to prevent radioactive urine from leaking into the walkway, should be considered when indicated (Figure 4.144).

IMAGING EQUIPMENT

The gamma camera contains a collimator made of small holes in a lead plate that allows only perpendicu-

lar γ-rays through (Figure 4.145). This reduces scatter, thereby improving image resolution. The γ-rays interact with a fluorescent crystal (a thallium-activated sodium iodide crystal is commonly used), changing the γ-energy to light photons. The light photons interact with a photocathode, generating electrons that are amplified by an array of photomultiplier tubes. The x-y co-ordinates of the electrons are then recorded and the image is reconstructed. Therefore, the image represents the geographic distribution of the radiopharmaceutical in the horse. Images are acquired in a 256×256 matrix to optimize image resolution without requiring excessive computer storage capabilities.

Various techniques have been devised to suspend the gamma camera, including stationary systems such as forklifts, hydraulic systems, or systems that are available to move anywhere around the nuclear medicine suite such as track-and-hoist or track-and-column mounted detectors (Figure 4.146).[67] The advantage of the track system is that the horse can be positioned anywhere in the room and the detector moved around the horse to obtain different views. The gamma camera and collimator weigh approximately 1,500 lbs (680 kg) and must be kept very still for the acquisition time (about 30 to 90 seconds).

The gamma camera computer acquires the data and reconstructs the images and sends the digitized images to the processing computer. That computer is usually dedicated to the nuclear medicine facility and is used to perform post processing of the images and maintain image storage (Figure 4.147). Hard copies of nuclear medicine images can be made to X-ray type film, but have become less popular. With recent advances in technology, DICOM (Digital Imaging and Communications in Medicine) images can be produced with most software products and sent to a computer station with PACS (Picture Archiving and Communication Systems) for reviewing and storage.

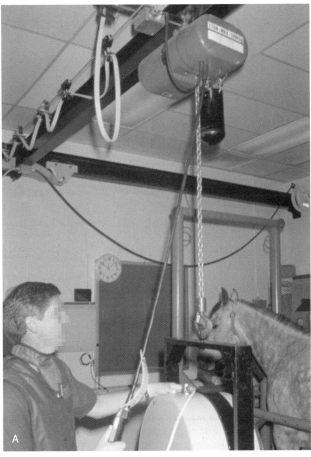
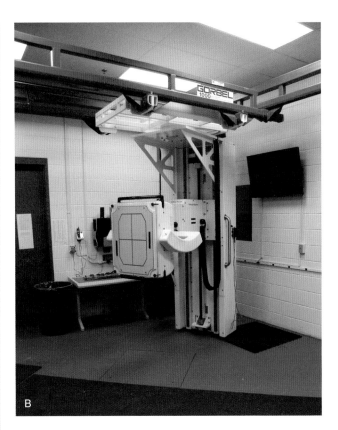

Figure 4.146. A. The gamma camera suspended by a chain hoist. B. The gamma camera mounted on a lift system with a yoke to move the camera in different directions. Both cameras can be positioned anywhere around the horse using a track system.

The equipment needed for a nuclear medicine imaging service consists of relatively high technology electronic instrumentation and must be maintained appropriately under controlled temperature to ensure that optimal diagnostic images are acquired. Although the maintenance of the equipment is beyond the scope of this text, it should be noted that image quality and resolution can be affected by, among others, one or more of the following factors:

1. Insufficient counts, e.g., too short acquisition time, too low ^{99m}Tc dose, extravascular injection of radio-pharmaceutical, inadequately peaked camera
2. Incorrect collimator
3. Inadequate correction floods
4. Motion of patient, camera, or both
5. Excessive distance between gamma camera and patient.

Image acquisition is determined either by the number of counts or the acquisition time. The number of counts/image is the most critical factor in terms of image quality. A certain minimum number of counts is needed for a diagnostic image, and more counts result in a superior image. Table 4.5 offers suggestions for minimum counts/image. A longer image acquisition time is needed for more counts/image, although at some stage a long image acquisition time becomes impracti-

cal. Most horses will stand still for about 60 seconds when sedated with IV butorphanol and detomidine, so an image is rarely acquired for less than 60 seconds. For example, if a 60-second image of the foot results in 250,000 counts (minimum 100,000 to 150,000 counts needed), the image is acquired for 60 seconds rather than 30 seconds, which would still have given a diagnostic image albeit with less resolution.

The risk with limiting the acquisition to a certain number of counts (as opposed to time) is that if there is urine contamination under a foot or another limb or the urinary bladder is in the field of view, then the counts recorded by the acquisition computer will include these aberrant γ-rays which do not contribute to image quality. In fact, they reduce image quality by diminishing the number of γ-rays used for image reconstruction. It is therefore better to use acquisition time than counts/image when scanning, given the premise that the number of counts is the more critical factor in image quality.

METHOD FOR A SCINTIGRAPHIC EXAM OF THE MUSCULOSKELETAL SYSTEM

The radiolabeled pharmaceutical, either ^{99m}Tc-MDP (methylene diphosphanate) or ^{99m}Tc-HDP (oxidronate), is generally used at a dose of 0.35 mCi/kg (0.16 mCi/

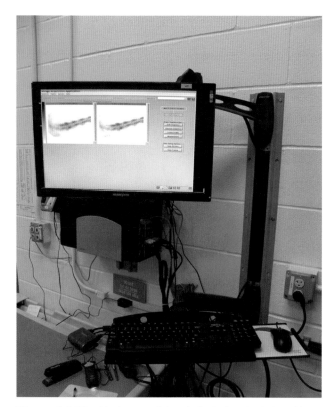

Figure 4.147. Nuclear medicine dedicated work station with the software for image acquisition and processing. Digital images may also be stored in the work station.

Table 4.5. Minimum image acquisition counts.

Body region	Number of counts (×1,000)
Foot	100–150
Carpus	100–150
Elbow	150–200
Shoulder	200–300
Tarsus	150–200
Stifle	150–200
Sacroiliac area	200–300
Spine	200–300
Soft tissue (pool) phase image	75–100

lb). The radiolabel must be given intravenously; otherwise, slow release of the ^{99m}Tc will result in sub-optimal images due to continuous release and thus high levels of circulating radioactivity. Patient control is very important because images generally take about 60 seconds to acquire. Chemical restraint is useful in preventing patient motion; a combination of IV detomidine

and butorphanol has shown to be useful at the authors' institution. The use of general anesthesia has also been used at some institutions with the objective of obtaining greater numbers of counts and subsequently improved image resolution. However, a disadvantage of general anesthesia is that the patient is at risk of exacerbating a lesion during recovery. Newer image viewing and processing software packages have integrated motion correction tools that allow some degree of motion with minimal or no image deterioration.

Imaging Technique

The tracer is given IV and the blood flow (phase 1) images are acquired immediately if required. Pool phase images are acquired within the next 10 minutes if desired. Pool phase images must be limited to about 3 or 4 anatomical regions to ensure that they are completed before significant bone uptake occurs. Delayed phase images are acquired from 2 to 4 hours after injection to allow an optimal bone-to-soft-tissue ratio. Furosemide is given IV 60 to 90 minutes before the delayed phase starts if lumbar spine, pelvis, and stifle images are being acquired. This increases the chances of an empty bladder because the ^{99m}Tc-HDP is excreted by the kidneys and urine in the bladder obscures visualization of the stifles, lumbosacral junction, sacroiliac (SI) joints, and the coxofemoral joints (Figure 4.148).

Lateral images of the limbs are made, being careful to position the camera lateral to the region being imaged (which is not necessarily lateral to the horse). Dorsal views of the carpi are generally performed. Orthogonal views of a lesion should always be attempted to help document the third dimension. Lead sheets are used to shield scatter radiation from the other limbs (Figure 4.149). Lead also should be placed medial to the olecranon and the stifle to shield the sternum and the penis/urinary bladder, respectively. Slightly overlapping the views will ensure that no area is left unscanned. Be aware that increased soft tissue uptake during the soft tissue (pool) phase can be detected for up to at least 14 or 17 days after intra-articular or perineural anesthesia, respectively.[87,88] Local nerve blocks (intra-articular or perineural) do not, however, affect bone uptake in the delayed phase.[35]

The following views are recommended for the full evaluation of the thoracic and pelvic limbs and spine using a detector with a 20-inch (50-cm) field of view.

Thoracic Limb

Lateral and dorsal views of the foot (these views include distal metacarpus, metacarpophalangeal joint and phalanges), solar distal phalanx, lateral and dorsal carpus, lateral and cranial humerus (Figure 4.150), and lateral scapula. The metacarpus is included in the views of the foot and the carpus, the radius and elbows are included in the views of the carpus and humerus, and the shoulder is included in the views of the humerus and scapula. If an area of abnormal uptake is seen in the metacarpus, radius, or elbow, or in an area where only lateral views were obtained, additional images including orthogonal views centered over the areas of interest should be acquired.

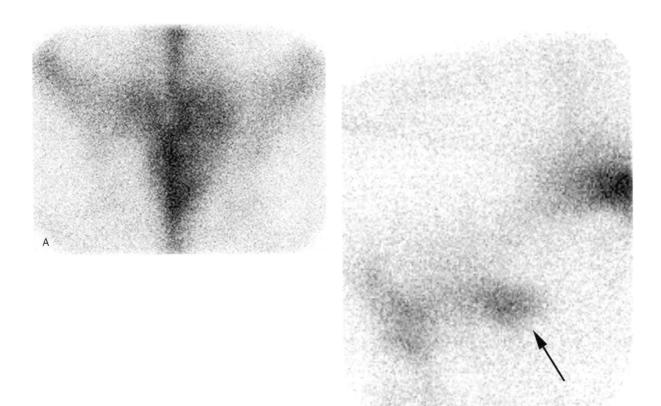

Figure 4.148. Delayed phase dorsal (A) and lateral (B) views of the pelvis of a normal horse. Note the diffuse IRU seen in the region of the sacrum on the dorsal view that corresponds to radioactive urine in the urinary bladder, as seen on the lateral image (arrow).

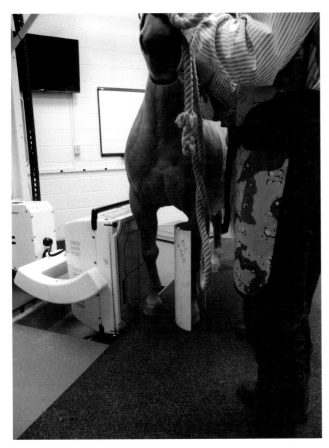

Figure 4.149. Gamma camera positioned in a pit below floor level for the lateral view of the right fore distal limb. Lead shielding is used to block out the contralateral limb.

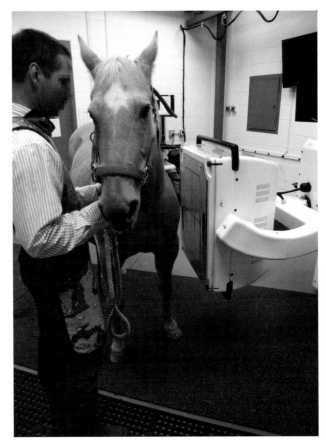

Figure 4.150. Gamma camera positioned for the lateral view of the left shoulder joint.

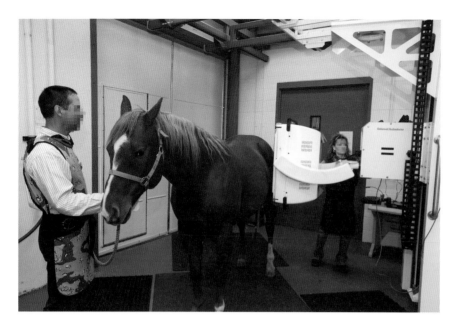

Figure 4.151. Gamma camera positioned for the lateral view of the left hip joint.

Pelvic Limb

Lateral and plantar foot (these views include distal metatarsus, metatarsophalangeal joint and phalanges), lateral and plantar tarsus, lateral and caudal stifle, lateral femur, right and left lateral hip (Figure 4.151), right and left dorsal oblique (RDO/LDO) hip, dorsal pelvis, caudal pelvis, and (RDO/LDO) sacrum. The metacarpus is included in the views of the foot and the tarsus, and the tibia is included in the views of the tarsus and stifle. As on the thoracic limb, if an area of IRU is seen on the metatarsus, tibia, or femur, additional images including plantar/caudal views centered over the area of interest should be obtained.

Spine

Right and left lateral views of the cervical spine (cranial, mid, and caudal), RDO/LDO cranial thoracic spine, RDO/LDO caudal thoracic spine, RDO/LDO lumbar spine, RDO/LDO lumbosacral junction (Figure 4.152), dorsal pelvis (Figure 4.153), caudal pelvis (tail on detector, TOD), and RDO/LDO sacrum. Lateral and dorsal views of the spine are less effective due to the great distance that the camera is from the vertebra. They can, however, be included as orthogonal views when a lesion is found. A point source, also known as fiducial marker, (e.g., cobalt marker or the syringe and needle that was used for the ^{99m}Tc-HDP injection, sealed in a latex glove) can be placed along the dorsum of the back to localize the exact position of a lesion, which is then marked with a permanent marker.

Foot

Different options exist for obtaining lateral, dorsal, and palmar views of the feet. In some institutions, the nuclear medicine suite has a pit in the floor into which the gamma camera is lowered to have it centered over the distal limb (Figure 4.154). In these cases, the horse is positioned to obtain lateral, dorsal, and palmar views.

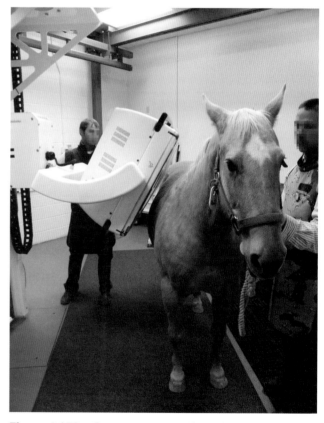

Figure 4.152. Gamma camera positioned for the right dorsal oblique (RDO) view of the thoracolumbar spine.

These views can also be made by placing both forefeet (or both hindfeet) on a wooden box about 25 cm high (Figure 4.155). The top of the box should be strong enough (3.75 cm or 1.5 inches, plywood) to support a large horse. The gamma camera can then be lowered to acquire the views. Some clinics have constructed a platform for the horse to stand on during the entire exam.

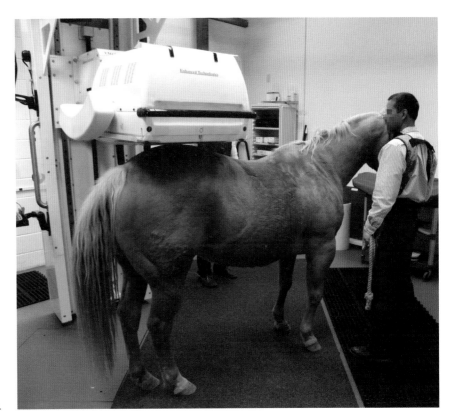

Figure 4.153. Gamma camera positioned for the dorsal view of the pelvis.

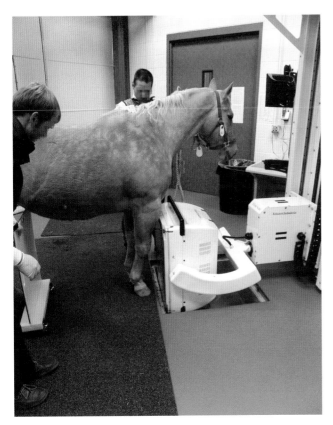

Figure 4.154. Gamma camera positioned in a pit below floor level for the dorsal view of both fore distal limbs. Lead shielding is used to block out the hindlimbs.

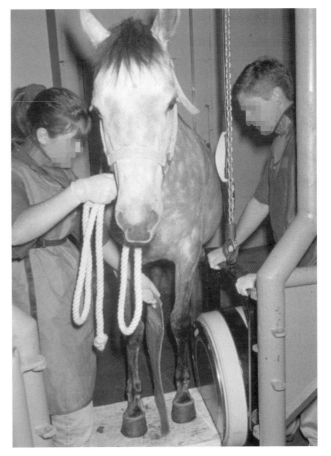

Figure 4.155. Camera positioned for the lateral view of the left fore distal limb. The horse is standing on a wooden box to allow the gamma camera to be located distal enough to be centered over the foot. Lead shielding is used to block out the contralateral limb.

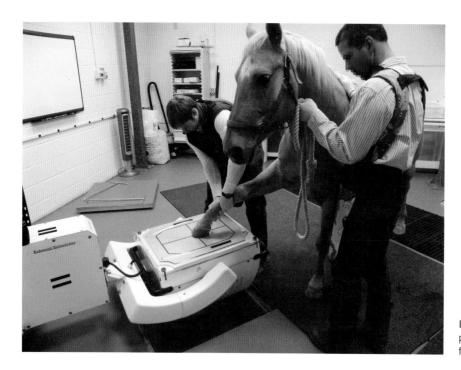

Figure 4.156. Gamma camera positioned for the solar view of the right forefoot.

At these facilities the camera moves around the horse and is placed where needed, including below foot level for lateral, dorsal, and palmar views of the foot. An alternative option is to have a ramp on which the horse can place the front- or hindfeet. Both the platform and ramp take up more space, and in most cases the horse cannot remain still on it for the entire examination.

Solar views of the feet (for the navicular bone) are best made by stretching the forefoot out cranially and placing it on the camera face which has a plexiglass covering to protect the collimator (Figure 4.156). The solar view of the feet has been shown to be more sensitive for the evaluation of the navicular bone than the lateral view.[43] The camera is positioned face-up in front of the horse, with the surface of the camera at or just below the level of the carpus. A solar view of the hindfoot is done less frequently and can be made by stretching the limb caudally, placing the foot on a wooden box and positioning the camera behind it. An alternative method is to have a pit in the floor into which the camera is placed face-up. The pit is covered with appropriate material and the horse stands over the camera. While it is easier to position the horse over the pit than to stretch the foot out forward and hold it on the camera, the downside is superimposition of the pastern and fetlock over the navicular bone region.

INDICATIONS FOR NUCLEAR SCINTIGRAPHY OF THE MUSCULOSKELETAL SYSTEM IN HORSES

Vascular Phase (Phase 1)

The vascular phase is an excellent technique for the evaluation of blood flow to specific areas, and is of particular importance in the evaluation of trauma to the distal extremities or to areas where inadequate blood perfusion is suspected. Decreased blood flow in the foot region may be seen in cases of laminitis. The vascular phase can also be helpful in documenting aortoiliac thromboembolism. Increased blood flow to a particular region may be associated with acute inflammatory conditions or infectious processes. In most institutions, the vascular phase is not included as part of a routine scintigraphic exam of the musculoskeletal system.

Soft Tissue Phase (Phase 2)

Soft tissue phase (pool phase) images provide more useful information in cases of acute lameness, particularly in the distal limb, because of the ability to identify changes (especially increases) in blood flow to local areas. For example, hyperemia of the synovium or joint capsule secondary to acute synovitis/capsulitis, or at the proximal attachment of the suspensory ligament due to acute desmitis, may be detected during the soft tissue phase.[28] Focal areas of trauma can also be evaluated for altered soft tissue perfusion. It can sometimes be difficult to differentiate between early bone uptake by a lesion and increased blood flow to an area. Therefore, the more accurate soft tissue phase images are those done with pertechnetate ($^{99m}TcO_4$) or labeled RBCs (^{99m}Tc-RBC), and not with a bone-seeking radiolabel.

The practitioner should be aware that detection of increased blood flow to a specific region is more common in acute conditions and a negative result on a soft tissue phase does not rule out a subtle or more chronic injury.

Delayed Phase (Phase 3)

Delayed phase images provide information for evaluation of the skeleton. The high sensitivity of this phase to detect early changes in bone metabolism before these changes are radiographically evident make this part of the study most useful for evaluation of acute lameness; e.g., incomplete or stress fractures in racehorses or high performance horses. The delayed phase may also help

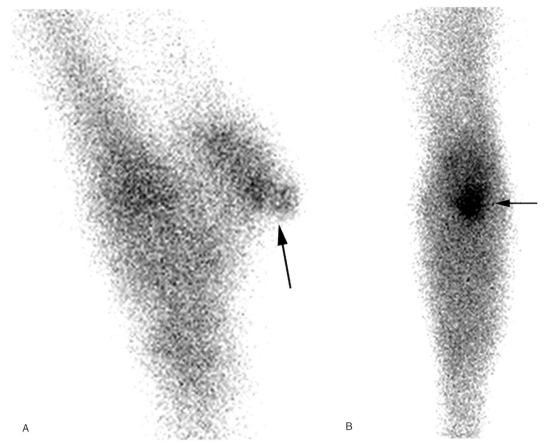

A

B

Figure 4.157. Delayed phase lateral (A) and plantar (B) views of the left tarsus, showing an IRU area within the soft tissues just plantar and distal to the calcaneal tuberosity (arrows), corresponding to dystrophic mineralization of the superficial digital flexor tendon. (Courtesy of Dr. Erik Bergman.)

in the diagnostic work-up of horses presenting for other reasons such as ill-defined lameness or lameness that is difficult to diagnose with regional anesthesia; multiple causes of lameness in the same limb or different regions of the body; acute lameness of unknown origin; recheck of known lesion (to follow progress of healing); evaluation of the physiologic activity of radiographic lesions; and evaluation of areas that are difficult to radiograph such as the proximal thoracic and pelvic limb, spine, and pelvis including the SI and coxofemoral joints. Delayed phase imaging is also useful for the assessment of bone viability and as a general survey in pre-purchase examinations. Soft tissue uptake in the muscles, seen during the delayed phase, can be seen in cases of rhabdomyolysis[13,56] or dystrophic mineralization of soft tissues (Figure 4.157).

A scintigraphic examination should not replace a complete physical and lameness examination. False negative scintigraphic results do not rule out a possible source of lameness suspected during clinical evaluation of the patient.

NORMAL BONE SCAN

Vascular phase images are best viewed as a cine loop on the acquisition computer (a computer software application that allows the images to be viewed sequen-tially in rapid order). A composite of vascular phase images also can be generated, and it should show good perfusion. When looking at the distal limbs, try to have both limbs in a dorsal or palmar/plantar view and look for perfusion symmetry. Composite images of the distal aorta should show the bifurcation of the aorta into the internal and external iliac arteries (Figure 4.158).

Soft tissue (pool) phase images of the foot show some vascular activity, but the fetlock and pastern regions should have homogeneously smooth uptake (Figure 4.159). The palmar/plantar blood vessels are seen as a distinct linear activity, and the coronet also has increased activity due to a vascular plexus. Additionally, the distal phalanx has a generous blood supply to the sensitive laminae and increased activity is seen. Soft tissue images proximal to the carpus or tarsus are usually unrewarding due to the normal IRU of overlying musculature.[26]

Normal delayed phase uptake patterns vary among horses, depending on the patient's age, breed, and occupation.[92] For example, in athletic horses, most of these normal variations represent an exercise-induced bone remodeling secondary to an ongoing bone response to stress, and do not necessarily produce clinical signs of lameness. Skeletally immature animals normally have bilaterally symmetric increased areas of uptake at growth plates and secondary centers of ossification (Figure 4.160).

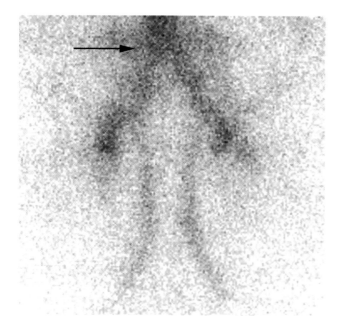

Figure 4.158. Composite image of blood flow in the region of the caudal aorta, showing normal bifurcation of the aorta (arrow) into internal and external iliac arteries.

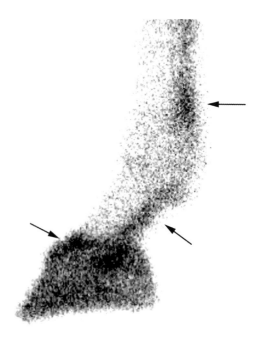

Figure 4.159. Soft tissue (pool) phase view of a normal left forefoot, showing vascular activity on the palmar aspects proximal and distal to the fetlock and in the area of the coronary band (arrows). Note that the fetlock and pastern regions have homogeneously smooth uptake.

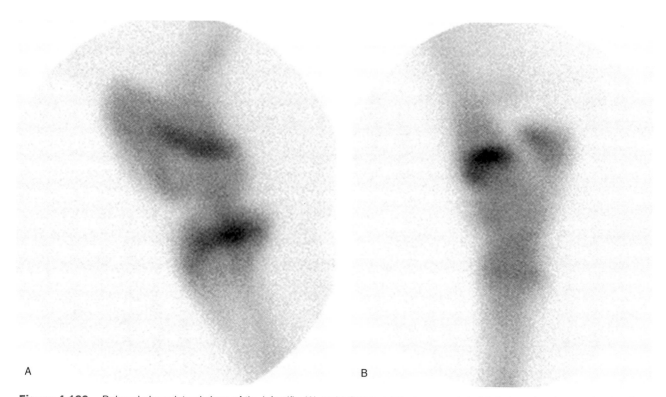

A

B

Figure 4.160. Delayed phase lateral views of the left stifle (A) and left tarsus (B) of a normal skeletally immature horse, showing IRU in the region of the physes. (Courtesy of Dr. Erik Bergman.)

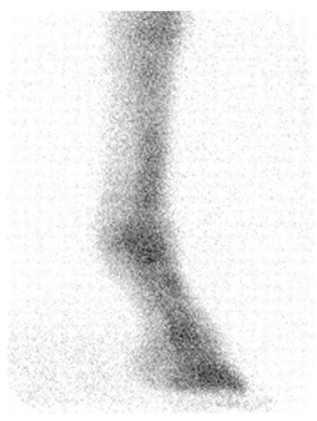

Figure 4.161. Delayed phase lateral view of the distal limb of a normal horse. Note the similar uptake between the fetlock, pastern, and coffin joints. (Courtesy of Dr. Erik Bergman.)

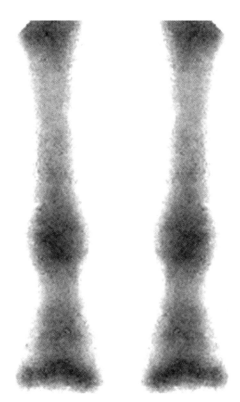

Figure 4.162. Delayed phase dorsal view of both fore distal limbs of a normal horse. The uptake should be uniformly similar between both limbs.

The diaphyses of long bones have less uptake than other parts of the bones, due to relatively low metabolism in the diaphyses of normal subjects. The uptake should, however, be smoothly homogenous with no focal areas of increased uptake. Contralateral imaging can be useful when evaluating borderline lesions. Physes, epiphyses, and apophyses demonstrate increased uptake due to increased metabolic rates of bone tissue in these regions.

Distal Limb (Foot, Pastern, and Fetlock)

On the lateral view, a normal horse has similar uptake in the coffin, pastern, and fetlock joints. The navicular bone should not be seen as a distinct entity due to a homogeneous uptake with the rest of the distal phalanx (Figure 4.161). Normal mild decreased uptake in the metacarpal condyles, when compared to the proximal phalanx and sesamoid bones, has also been reported.[97] The dorsal view (plantar view if evaluating the pelvic limbs) is useful for comparison of ipsilateral structures in the same image (Figure 4.162).

The solar view of a normal horse has a very uniform pattern of uptake with less than 10% change between the regions of the navicular bone, deep digital flexor tendon (DDFT) insertion, toe, and medial and lateral aspects of P3 (Figure 4.163).[24] Mild increases in radiopharmaceutical uptake can be seen at the insertion of

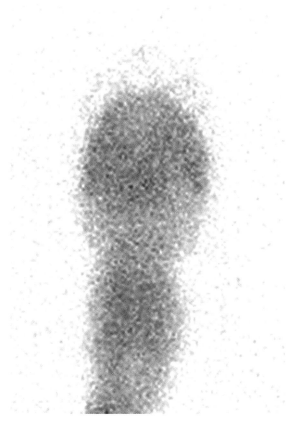

Figure 4.163. Delayed phase solar view of a normal horse. Note the homogenous uptake throughout the entire image without distinction of any particular area.

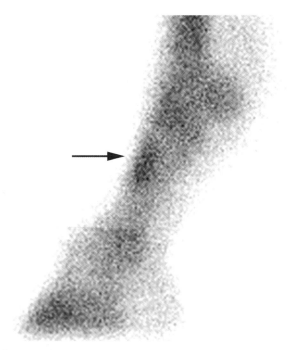

Figure 4.164. Delayed phase lateral view of the left distal limb of a normal horse. The focal IRU on the dorsoproximal diaphysis of P1 (arrow) is a normal finding as a response to the athletic activity usually seen bilaterally in performance horses. (Courtesy of Dr. Erik Bergman.)

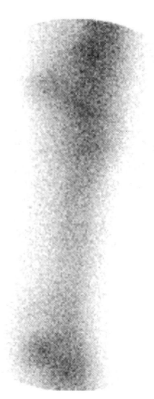

Figure 4.165. Delayed phase lateral view of the right metacarpus of a normal horse. Note the uniform uptake along the diaphysis. (Courtesy of Dr. Erik Bergman.)

the DDFT or the lateral or medial aspects of P3 secondary to low heel conformation or lateral-medial hoof imbalances.

A focal increase uptake, usually bilateral and not associated with lameness, can be seen on the dorso-proximal diaphysis of the proximal phalanx, especially on dressage, show jumping, or eventing horses (Figure 4.164).[6] The palmar or plantar cortices may also show focal IRU. The etiology of this uptake is uncertain but it is believed to be secondary to adaptive remodeling from a normal response to training.

Metacarpus and Metatarsus

There should be a uniform uptake along the diaphysis of the metacarpus and metatarsus with no distinction between the second, third, and fourth metacarpal bones (Figure 4.165).

Carpus and Tarsus

Radiopharmaceutical uptake is normally uniformly greater in the carpal and tarsal bones when compared with the diaphysis of the metacarpus and radius or metatarsus and tibia, respectively (Figure 4.166). Focal areas of IRU associated with the cuboidal bones are considered abnormal.

Upper Limb Long Bones

The distal physis of the radius and tibia can be seen with an increased uptake for a few years, even after evidence of radiographic closure. Growth is no longer

occurring at these sites, but there is still sufficient osteoblastic activity to differentiate the physis from the adjacent metaphysis and the epiphysis. The increased uptake in those areas is the result of different histologic architecture after closure, which exposes more bone crystal to diphosphonate binding.[92] A uniform pattern of uptake should be seen along the diaphysis of the normal tibia[94] (Figure 4.167) and radius. The deltoid tuberosity is easily visualized as an area of IRU on the cranio-proximal cortex of the humerus (Figure 4.168). The third trochanter is an important landmark and should be seen as an area of IRU in all horses. The cranial and caudal parts of the greater trochanter should be identified as separate structures. (Figure 4.169)

Elbow, Shoulder, and Stifle Joints

Increased uptake is often seen in the radioulnar joint of normal elbows (Figure 4.170). The normal shoulder joint demonstrates increased uptake in the areas of the greater and lesser tubercles and the humeral head (Figure 4.171). The glenoid cavity, however, should have less activity than the humeral head.

A similar uptake between the patella, trochlea, and condyles should be seen in the stifle joint (Figure 4.172). However, in adult horses it is also normal to see a mild IRU on the patella secondary to adaptive bone remodeling.[21] In immature horses, a normal bi-lobed appearance of the proximal tibia is commonly seen, formed by areas of IRU corresponding to the center of ossification of the tibial tuberosity and the superimposition of the

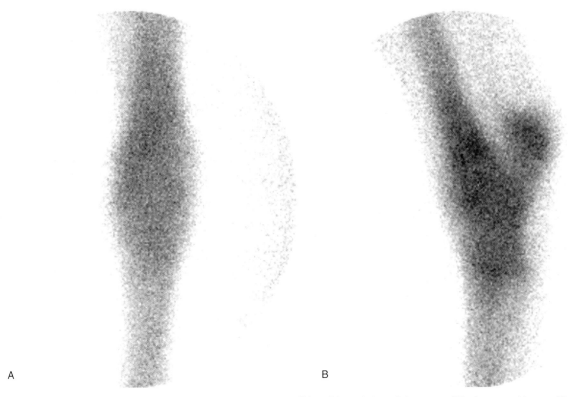

A   B

Figure 4.166. Delayed phase dorsal view of the carpus (A) and lateral view of the tarsus (B) of a normal horse. (Courtesy of Dr. Erik Bergman.)

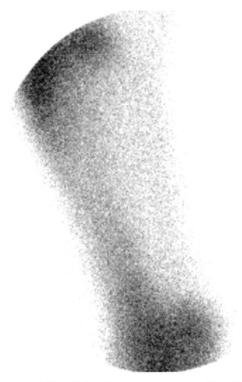

Figure 4.167. Delayed phase lateral view of the tibia. Note the uniform uptake along the diaphysis. (Courtesy of Dr. Erik Bergman.)

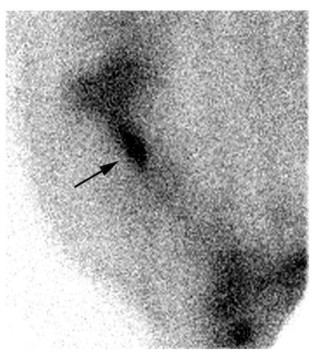

Figure 4.168. Delayed phase lateral view of the shoulder of a normal horse. A focal area of IRU on the cranial aspect of the proximal diaphysis represents the deltoid tuberosity (arrow).

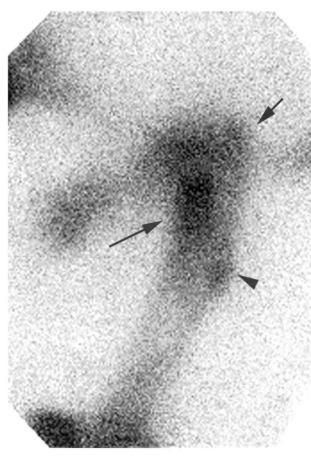

Figure 4.169. Delayed phase lateral view of the femur of a normal horse. Note the cranial (large arrow) and caudal (small arrow) parts of the greater trochanter, and the third trochanter (arrowhead) as separate structures.

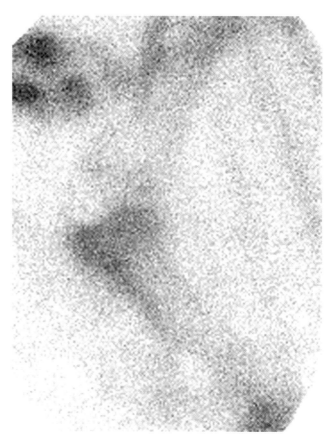

Figure 4.171. Delayed phase lateral view of the shoulder joint of a normal horse.

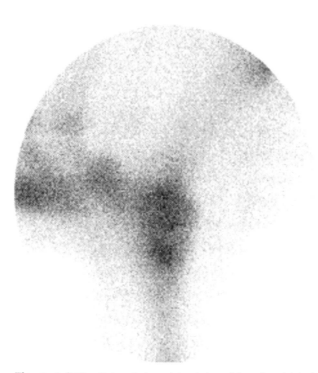

Figure 4.170. Delayed phase lateral view of the elbow joint of a normal horse. (Courtesy of Dr. Erik Bergman.)

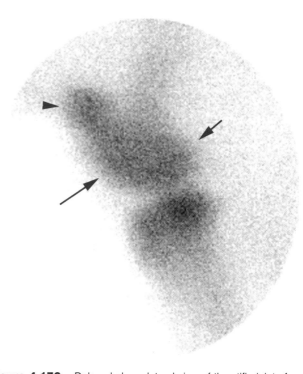

Figure 4.172. Delayed phase lateral view of the stifle joint of a normal horse. Note the uniform uptake between the patella (arrowhead), trochlea (large arrow), and condyles (small arrow). (Courtesy of Dr. Erik Bergman.)

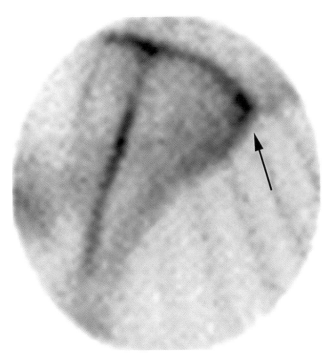

Figure 4.173. Delayed phase lateral view of the scapula of a normal horse. Note the spine of the scapula and a superimposition artifact (arrow) created by overlap between the caudodorsal angle of the scapula and the thoracic vertebral bodies. (Courtesy of Dr. Erik Bergman.)

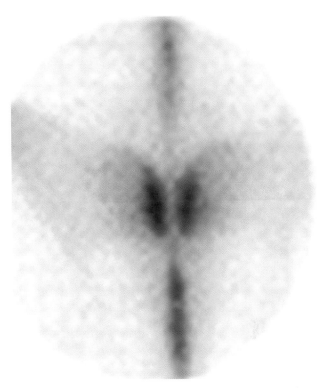

Figure 4.174. Delayed phase dorsal view of the sacrum of a normal horse. The two oval and symmetric focal areas of IRU correspond to the sacral tuberosities. (Courtesy of Dr. Erik Bergman.)

caudal tibial plateau and the head of the fibula.[21,69] Adult horses show less uptake at the tibial tuberosity than the caudal tibial plateau/fibular head region. In addition to the superimposition of the head of the fibula and the caudal aspect of the tibial plateau, IRU in this region also has been attributed to the weight-bearing distribution and greater load transmission in this area.[21]

Scapula

The scapula should be easy to visualize and in some cases the withers can be evaluated at the same time (Figure 4.173). Superimposition artifact from the withers and thoracic spine often occurs on images of the scapula, creating an area of perceived increased uptake. The caudal border and the spine of the scapula have normally greater uptake than the supra- and infra-spinatus fossae.

Pelvis, SI, and Coxofemoral Joints

The dorsal view of the pelvis is the best view for the evaluation of the tuber sacrale. The uptake is normally increased due to the close distance and minimal soft tissue attenuation between the sacral tuberosities and the γ-ray detector (Figure 4.174). The SI joints can be evaluated on a dorsal view or a dorsal 45° oblique view. Asymmetric uptake can be better visualized on the dorsal oblique view and the entire extent of the joint can be better seen on the oblique view with less superimposition of pelvic canal structures (Figure 4.175). Although the dorsum of the sixth and seventh lumbar

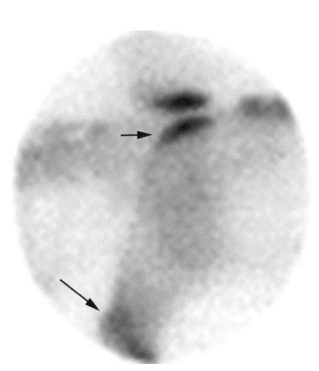

Figure 4.175. Delayed phase oblique view of the sacroiliac joint of a normal horse. Note the sacral (small arrow) and iliac (large arrow) tuberosities. (Courtesy of Dr. Erik Bergman.)

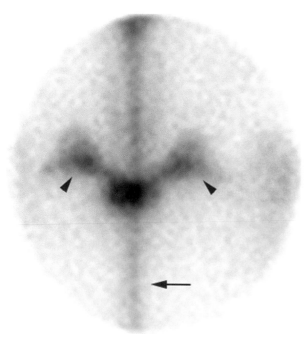

Figure 4.176. Delayed phase tail on detector (TOD) view of a normal horse. Note the good visualization of the floor of the pelvis, especially the symmetric ischiatic tuberosities (arrowheads). The tail is seen as a midline structure (arrow). (Courtesy of Dr. Erik Bergman.)

vertebrae and the sacrum can also be seen on the dorsal view, the dorsal spinous processes are best evaluated on the dorsal oblique views.

The caudal view of the pelvis (tail-on detector view, TOD) is essential for the evaluation of the floor of the pelvis and the tuber ischii (Figure 4.176). The camera is positioned directly behind the pelvis of the horse for the TOD view. It is important to make sure that the gamma camera is equidistant from the left and right tuber ischii during the acquisition of this view because if not, then the closer tuber ischiadicum will appear to have more uptake and vice versa. Asymmetric uptake by the tuber ischiadicum is considered abnormal. Angling the camera dorsally (slope of the rump) should be done if the urinary bladder interferes with the image. This projects the bladder above the tuber ischiadicum.

Lateral images of the coxofemoral joint should identify the cranial and caudal portions of the greater trochanter and third trochanter of the femur (Figure 4.177). Commonly, IRU is seen in the coxofemoral joint region on the lateral view because the cranial part of the greater trochanter (convexity) is partially superimposed over the joint region. Dorsal oblique views (approximately 45°) of the coxofemoral joint allow improved visualization of the femoral head and neck and acetabular region without superimposition of other structures (Figure 4.178). The normal acetabulum should not be seen as a separate entity (i.e., the acetabulum should not have a signal greater that of the ilium). Urine in the urinary bladder sometimes obscures visualization of the hip joint and can be mistaken for disease. Dorsal or caudal views of the hip region should be made to differentiate the urinary bladder (a midline structure) from the coxofemoral joints.

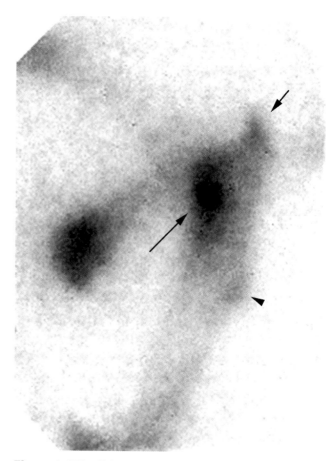

Figure 4.177. Delayed phase lateral view of the left coxofemoral joint of a normal horse. Note the cranial (large arrow) and caudal (small arrow) parts of the greater trochanter and the third trochanter (arrowhead) as separate structures.

Spine

Lateral images of the cervical spine should show similar uptake between articular facets and their corresponding vertebral bodies with the exception of the C6-C7 articular facets where, usually, a relatively higher uptake is seen in the body of C6 due to the shorter and thicker transverse processes. Similar uptake should be seen between cervical articular facets at adjacent levels (Figure 4.179). The region of the dens usually has a higher radiopharmaceutical uptake than the surrounding bony structures (Figure 4.180).

The thoracic and lumbar spine can be evaluated with lateral images; however, the large rib cage and epaxial musculature maintain a great distance between the vertebrae and the γ-ray detector, making subtle areas of increased uptake difficult to detect. Therefore, left and right dorsal oblique images are invaluable for the evaluation of the spine (Figure 4.181). When obtaining the dorsal oblique view, care should be taken when evaluating the caudal thoracic vertebrae for superimposition of the vertebral bodies and the normal increased uptake in the right kidney. Overlap should exist between views to include all anatomical regions. Resolution of the dorsal spinous and transverse processes should be possible in all horses; however, patients greater than 1,500 lbs. can be so bulky that the γ-rays may be reduced or

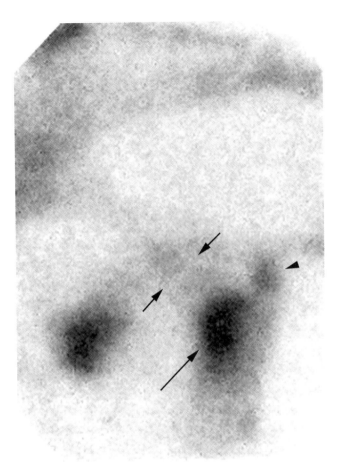

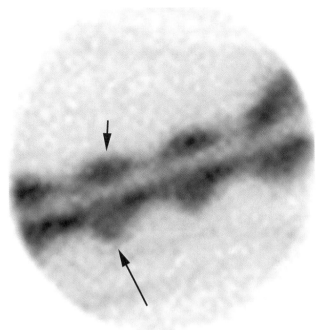

Figure 4.178. Delayed phase oblique view of the left coxofemoral joint of a normal horse. The coxofemoral joint is located between the two small arrows and is not superimposed over the greater trochanter. The cranial and caudal parts of the greater trochanter (large arrow and arrowhead, respectively) are still visualized as separate structures.

Figure 4.179. Delayed phase right lateral view of the mid cervical region of a normal horse. Note the similar uptake between the articular facets (short arrow) and the vertebral body (large arrow). (Courtesy of Dr. Erik Bergman.)

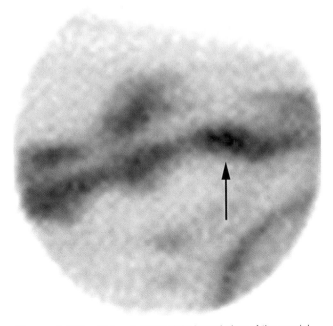

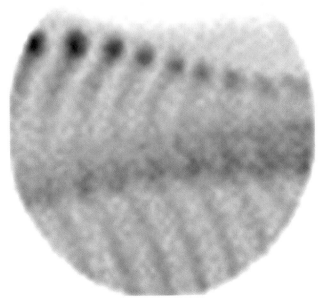

Figure 4.180. Delayed phase right lateral view of the cranial cervical region of a normal horse. Note the normal IRU in the region of the dens (arrow). (Courtesy of Dr. Erik Bergman.)

Figure 4.181. Delayed phase dorsal oblique view of the thoracic spine of a normal horse. Note the good resolution of the dorsal spinous processes and the ribs. (Courtesy of Dr. Erik Bergman.)

attenuated significantly enough to reduce dorsal spine and transverse process resolution. The most dorsal aspect of the dorsal spinous processes of the withers usually have normal focal areas of IRU (Figure 4.182). Adjacent spinal units should have similar amounts of uptake to each other. Be sure to evaluate the dorsal spines, articular facets, and transverse processes of the entire spine, including the sacrum and tail head (sacro-coccygeal region).

The dorsal view provides limited information in most clinical cases. However, soft tissue and delay phase dorsal views should be obtained when a lesion is suspected after clinical evaluation.

Although the distribution of the radiopharmaceutical in the normal horse, young and old, is predictable, experience is necessary for interpreting bone scans. Comparing the relative uptake in opposite limbs, or comparing images from horses of a similar age, can assist in arriving at significant conclusions.

It is important to look at relative uptake between structures on the same image, and then compare it with the ratio between the same structures on the contralateral image. This is important because of the phenomenon that occurs when an entire leg might have less uptake than the opposite limb. In these cases it is inappropriate to compare the uptake of, for example, the fetlock of one limb with the uptake of the fetlock of the other. It is more accurate to evaluate the uptake ratio between the fetlock and the pastern region in one limb and compare it with the same ratio in the other limb. This reduces the over-reading of radiopharmaceutical uptake disparities that occur as natural phenomena or as image acquisition artifacts (for example, camera-body-distance inequalities, collimator decentering, etc).

The same interpretation philosophy of comparing relative uptake ratios should be used in other body regions. Generally speaking, the more intense the uptake, the more severe the condition.

SCINTIGRAPHIC SIGNS OF DISEASE

Vascular Phase

Increased blood flow can be seen as a sub-acute or chronic response to trauma during the healing phase. Vascular imaging is useful to determine the amount of perfusion to the distal extremity and can therefore help determine the best therapy as well as prognosis. It generally takes about one minute for the leading edge of the tracer to reach the distal limb. The radiopharmaceutical can reach the distal limb quicker if the horse is sedated with acepromazine.[75]

The images can be viewed either individually or as a composite image, or the data from the individual images can be displayed in the form of a graph. Figure 4.183 illustrates the composite image of the vascular phase of a horse that suffered from a near de-gloving injury to the distal left metacarpus 1 week prior. Ninety images of 2 seconds each were acquired after the intravenous administration of about 150 mCi ^{99m}Tc-O$_4$. The study was performed to evaluate whether there was blood flow to the pastern region.

The composite image shows increased blood flow to the distal metacarpus, where granulation tissue had already started to form. The pastern, however, showed

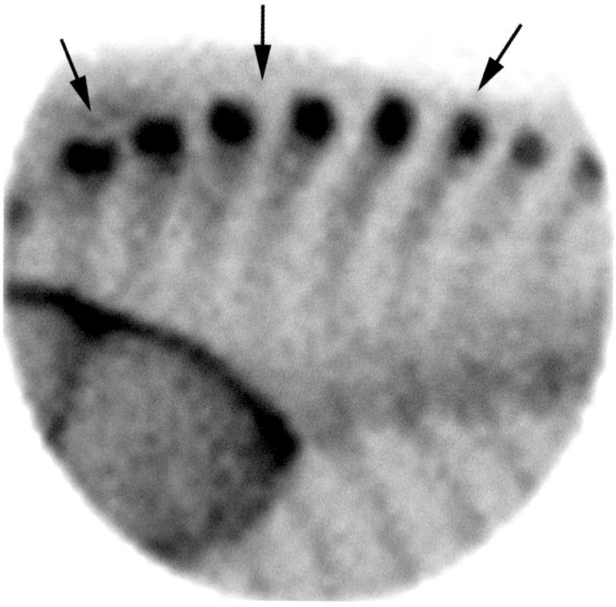

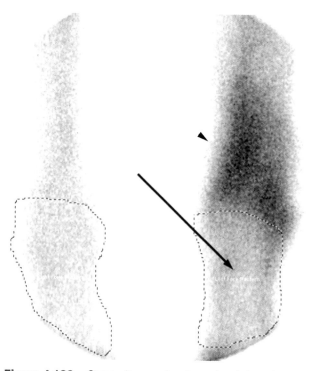

Figure 4.182. Delayed phase left dorsal oblique (LDO) view of the cranial thoracic spine of a normal horse. Note the normal IRU on the most proximal aspect of the dorsal spinous processes of the withers (arrows). (Courtesy of Dr. Erik Bergman.)

Figure 4.183. Composite vascular phase dorsal view of the pastern area of a horse 1 week after a near-degloving injury to the distal left fore cannon bone region, showing moderately increased blood flow to the left pastern region (arrow) and markedly increased blood flow to the distal left cannon bone region (arrowhead).

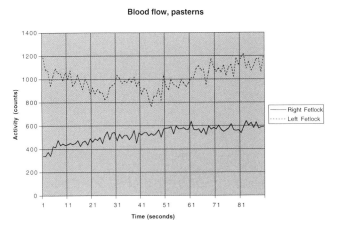

Blood flow, pasterns

Figure 4.184. Graph of the data from the composite image shown in Figure 4.183, confirming that the left pastern had more blood flow than the right one.

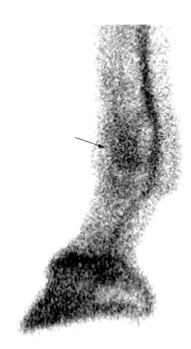

Figure 4.185. Soft tissue (pool) phase image of the left forefoot, showing increased blood flow to the fetlock region (arrow), which is suggestive of hyperemia associated with joint synovitis and/or capsulitis. Figure 4.159 provides the normal comparison.

more blood flow than the (normal) contralateral pastern region. This was thought to be due to reflex hyperemia secondary to the healing process, and was considered a positive sign, indicating that there was good blood flow to the foot. Figure 4.184 is a graphical representation of the vascular phase. The curve represents the amount of radioactivity in the left and right pastern regions, determined by the region of interest that was drawn around them. Each data point on the curve is 1 of the 90 images. Quantitation of the respective blood flow can be done by determining the area under the curve of each pastern and calculating the percentage of total flow. Empirical evaluation of the images is generally sufficient in most clinical cases.

Decreased blood flow to a region is often associated with nonviable bone or other tissue. Although rare, this can be used to evaluate large sequestra, cases of severe blood flow compromise from a traumatic/degloving injury (especially distal limb), or different conditions such as aortoiliac thrombosis.[18]

Soft Tissue Phase

Increased activity in soft tissues is a good method to document increased blood flow to specific regions, for example joints with synovitis/capsulitis. In these cases, nuclear scintigraphy is very sensitive at detecting increased periarticular blood flow around inflamed joints before radiographic changes of OA are evident. A fetlock joint capsulitis has a region of IRU over the joint when compared with the distal metacarpal region and proximal phalanx (Figure 4.185; compare with normal, Figure 4.159). Increased soft tissue phase uptake with a normal delayed phase image is compatible with a more acute degenerative condition, whereas if it is accompanied by increased uptake in the delayed phase, the condition is probably more chronic in nature.

Soft tissue phase imaging is helpful in diagnosing desmitis or avulsion type injuries of the proximal attachment of the suspensory ligament. These injuries are not necessarily evident on ultrasound or radiographic studies. Deep lying regions, for example the coxofemo-

ral and SI joints, are difficult if not impossible to evaluate during the soft tissue phase because of the meager nature of the signal and the large amount of other tissues between the hip and the camera. These tissues make up several half-value layers (a layer of tissue resulting in the reduction of the signal by one-half) which attenuate the beam significantly before reaching the gamma camera.

Care must be taken to not overinterpret soft tissue phase images when severe increased uptake is also seen in the delayed phase images. Soft tissue phase "hot spots" in these cases often represent early bone uptake. For example, the soft tissue image in Figure 4.186A probably represents early bone uptake of the radiopharmaceutical by the proximal phalanx because of the intense uptake seen in the proximal phalanx in the delayed phase (Figure 4.186B). This horse had a fissure fracture of P1 which was also seen radiographically (Figure 4.186C).

Delayed Phase

Regions with increased blood flow and osteoblastic activity demonstrate increased uptake of the radiopharmaceutical. The severity or intensity of the increased uptake can vary, and is often associated with conditions such as fractures, stress fractures, osteoarthritis, enthesopathy, osteomyelitis, and neoplasia. Fractures and infectious processes have similar scintigraphic behavior in most bones and in some cases it is difficult to differentiate between the two conditions. Therefore, correlation with clinical signs and other imaging findings is extremely important for making the diagnosis.

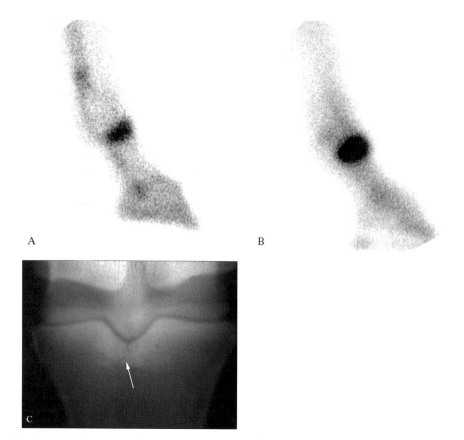

Figure 4.186. Right forefoot of a horse suffering from a chronic proximal first phalanx fracture. A. Soft tissue (pool) phase image showing marked increased blood flow to the proximal portion of the first phalanx. B. Delayed phase image showing marked IRU by the proximal portion of the first phalanx. C.

Radiograph showing a proximal first phalanx fracture (arrow). The IRU seen in the soft tissue image likely represents early radiopharmaceutical uptake by the bone, not just increased blood flow, because of the marked IRU seen in the delayed phase image.

The amount of tracer uptake that a fracture demonstrates may help determine the time of onset (acute vs. chronic) or the nature (pathologic vs. traumatic) of the fracture. Chronic and sub-acute fractures (older than 48 hours) have intense increased uptake due to the considerable osteoblastic activity (Figure 4.187). Acute fractures have less radiopharmaceutical uptake because it takes approximately 24 hours for the osteoblastic activity to be greater than surrounding bone. In fact, acute traumatic fractures less than 24 hours duration fail to show increased tracer uptake when compared with adjacent bone. Figure 4.188 is a delayed phase image of a comminuted middle phalangeal fracture 48 hours post injury. Although mild increased uptake is seen, the fracture is best diagnosed due to anatomic abnormality and not its physiologic peculiarity. Compare this with Figure 4.186, a chronic proximal phalangeal fracture with intense uptake but minimal anatomic displacement. Fracture uptake in humans is expected at about 24 hours post injury (although it takes longer in older patients) and is expected to last for 6 to 12 months or longer in older patients.[85] The uptake by a fracture should decrease over time as fracture healing occurs.

Multifocal areas of IRU have been described with different diseases such as enostosis-like lesions,[7,63] hypertrophic osteopathy,[49] neoplasia,[27,41] and horses with a bone fragility disorder,[2] a recently reported condition of unknown etiology that affects the axial and proximal appendicular skeleton. Figure 4.189 shows intestinal adenocarcinoma metastases to the ribs and distal left humerus. The same horse also had metastatic disease to several cervical, thoracic, and lumbar vertebrae; multiple ribs; and the sternum.

Localized delayed phase uptake of the radiopharmaceutical by soft tissues is not commonly seen, and can occur with various conditions, e.g., dystrophic mineralization of ligament and tendon injuries, regional anesthesia,[1] rhabdomyolysis,[13,39,56] and repeated intramuscular injection of butorphanol[47](Figures 4.157, 4.190, 4.191). Rhabdomyolysis (tying up) is seen as linear or diffuse uptake patterns in the muscles, such as the gluteals, semimembranosus, and semitendinosus.

ABNORMAL CONDITIONS FOR SPECIFIC ANATOMICAL REGIONS

Distal Limb (Foot, Pastern, and Fetlock)

The distal phalanx and navicular bone can experience different pathologic conditions involving the osseous anatomy or the multiple soft tissue structures related to them. Radiographic changes of the navicular bone can be difficult to interpret because many different architectural variations have been seen in both lame and

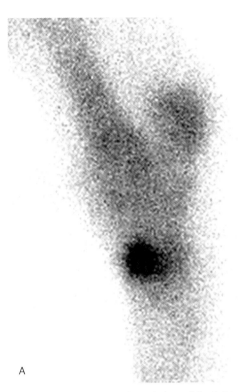

A

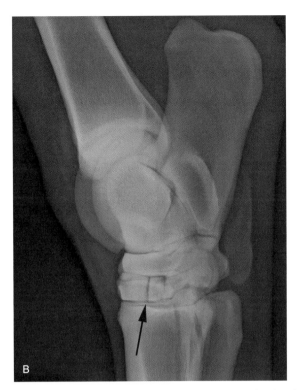

B

Figure 4.187. A. Delayed phase lateral view of the left tarsus of a horse with focal and intense IRU in the region of the distal tarsus corresponding to a third tarsal bone fracture.

B. Lateromedial radiograph of the same tarsus showing the well-defined radiolucent fracture line extending from the proximal to the distal articular surfaces of the third tarsal bone, consistent with a slab fracture (arrow). (Courtesy of Dr. Erik Bergman.)

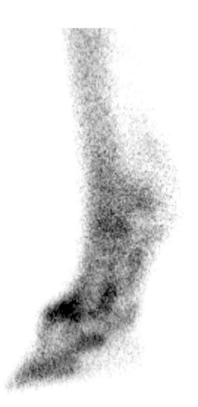

Figure 4.188. Delayed phase image of a comminuted left fore middle phalangeal fracture 48 hours postinjury. Anatomic displacement is apparent, although radiopharmaceutical uptake is only mildly increased.

sound horses.[42] The presence of IRU in the navicular bone region in the delayed phase is highly sensitive for the diagnosis of active navicular disease,[89] especially when solar views are obtained.[43] Remember that the navicular bone should not be seen as a separate entity on the normal foot; therefore, IRU in that region is indicative of active disease (Figure 4.192). Laminitis results in moderate to severe radiopharmaceutical uptake in the distal aspect of the distal phalanx, seen on both the lateral but especially the solar view (Figure 4.193). Other conditions, such as P3 osteitis, P3 fractures, and subsolar bruising, can also appear as areas of IRU (Figures 4.194 and 4.195).

A normal scintigraphic image does not show a discrete insertion of the DDFT on P3 and collateral ligaments of the DIP joint. However, the anatomical location of these structures can be identified, especially on solar views (Figure 4.196). If possible, abnormal uptake at these sites should also be documented on the lateral and dorsal/palmar views. Areas of IRU in these regions in combination with a positive response to local anesthesia help to identify active pathologic changes (Figure 4.197). These changes could be further characterized with MRI.

Osteoarthritis of the DIP or PIP joints, also known as low and high ringbone, respectively, and fetlock joint can be identified when IRU is seen at these regions when compared to the adjacent joints and relative radiopharmaceutical uptake ratios in the opposite limb (Figure 4.198).

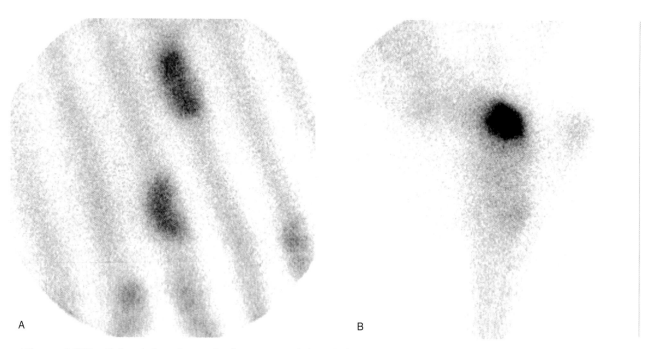

Figure 4.189. Delayed phase image showing a metastatic intestinal adenocarcinoma, which resulted in focal and intense IRU in (among others) the ribs (A) and distal left humerus (B).

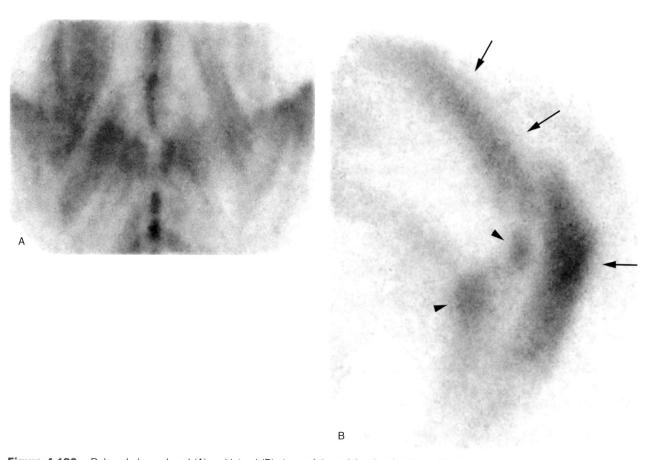

Figure 4.190. Delayed phase dorsal (A) and lateral (B) views of the pelvis, showing linear IRU (arrows) in the muscles of a horse with rhabdomyolysis (tying-up syndrome). (Courtesy of Dr. Kent Allen.)

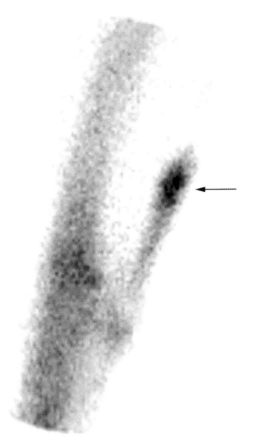

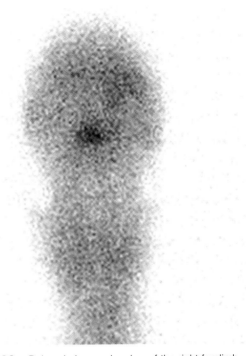

Figure 4.192. Delayed phase solar view of the right forelimb, showing a focal and intense IRU in the region of the navicular bone, consistent with navicular disease. (Courtesy of Dr. Erik Bergman.)

Figure 4.191. Lateral delayed phase view of the left carpus obtained 3 weeks after an ulnar nerve block. Note the soft tissue IRU at the injection site proximal to the accessory carpal bone (arrow).

The proximal articular surface of the first phalanx is a common location for IRU that represents active injuries to the subchondral bone that in many instances are not detected radiographically and would benefit from additional studies such as computed tomography and magnetic resonance imaging.[25,51,70] The proximal sesamoid bones are also susceptible to inflammatory changes that may appear as areas of IRU, which likely are related to stress from the different ligamentous attachments (Figure 4.199). Injuries to the axial border of the proximal sesamoid bones are usually, but not necessarily, traumatically induced, involving the inter-sesamoidean ligament, and can be the result of septic or nonseptic inflammation.[12,25,48,98]

Metacarpus and Metatarsus

Areas of IRU are often seen in the distal cannon bone of racing Thoroughbreds and Standardbreds. Both front- and hindlimbs can be affected, but Thoroughbreds more frequently show IRU in the distal metacarpus and Standardbreds in the distal metatarsus.[5,53] Stress remodeling and incomplete condylar fractures are common attributable pathologic changes for this increase uptake.[53,68,72]

Diffuse dorsal metacarpal IRU is common in racing horses and represents reactive periostitis or stress remodeling[45] (Figure 4.200). Focal and intense areas of IRU on the dorsal cortex of the cannon bone are likely indicative of a stress fracture (Figure 4.201).

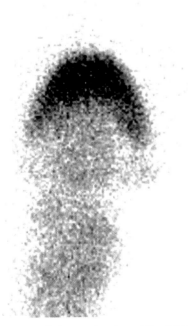

Figure 4.193. Delayed phase solar view of the right hindlimb, showing intense IRU along the distal portion of P3, compatible with laminitis.

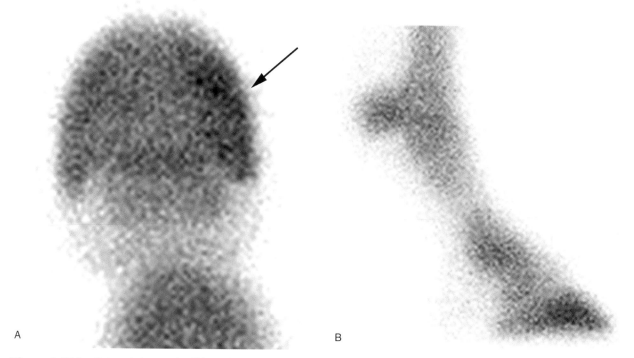

Figure 4.194. Delayed phase solar (A) and lateral (B) views of the distal limb of a horse with diffuse IRU along the medial aspect of the solar margin of P3 (arrow), compatible with pedal osteitis. (Courtesy of Dr. Erik Bergman.)

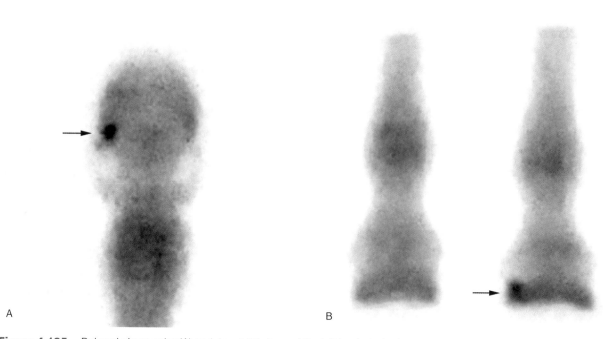

Figure 4.195. Delayed phase solar (A) and dorsal (B) views of the left forefoot of a horse with a focal and intense IRU on the medial aspect of P3 (arrows) representing a palmar process fracture. (Courtesy of Dr. Kent Allen.)

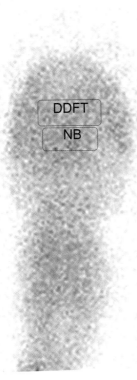

Figure 4.196. Delayed phase solar view of a normal horse. Note the uniform uptake along the entire image. NB = navicular bone area, DDFT = deep digital flexor tendon area.

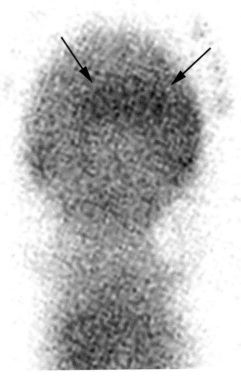

Figure 4.197. Delayed phase solar view of a horse with moderate diffused uptake in the region of insertion of the DDFT (arrows), suggesting tendinitis and enthesopathy. (Courtesy of Dr. Erik Bergman.)

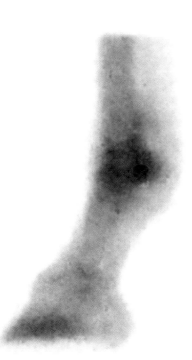

Figure 4.198. Delayed phase lateral view of the left fore distal limb of a horse showing diffuse IRU in the fetlock joint region, consistent with osteoarthritis. Note the difference in uptake between the abnormal fetlock and the normal proximal and distal interphalangeal joints. (Courtesy of Dr. Kent Allen.)

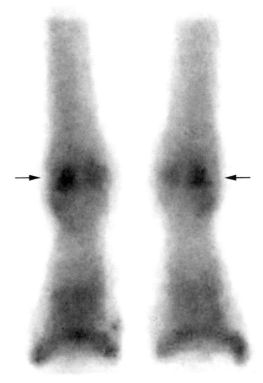

Figure 4.199. Delayed phase dorsal view of both front distal limbs of a horse with focal and intense IRU in the region of the lateral sesamoid bones (arrows), consistent with sesamoiditis. (Courtesy of Dr. Kent Allen.)

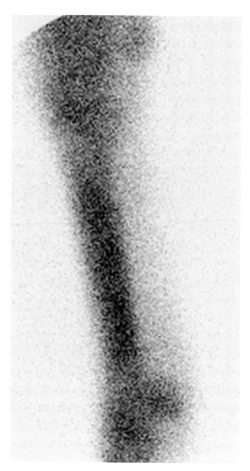

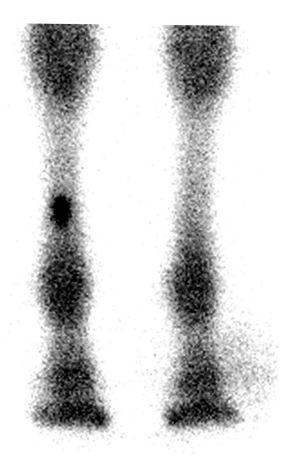

Figure 4.200. Delayed phase lateral view of the left metacarpus of a horse showing diffuse IRU along the diaphysis of MCIII, compatible with dorsal metacarpal disease ("buckshins"). (Courtesy of Dr. Erik Bergman.)

Figure 4.201. Delayed phase dorsal view of the distal forelimbs of a horse with a focal and intense IRU on the mid-distal diaphysis of the right MCIII, consistent with a stress fracture.

Increased radiopharmaceutical uptake on the palmar or plantar proximal cannon bone is a common finding in cases of desmitis at the origin of the suspensory ligament that produces stress reaction or avulsion fracture on the bony attachment[28] (Figure 4.202).

Carpus

Exercise-induced bone remodeling is seen frequently on the third carpal bone, especially in Standardbreds,[29] but it may be seen in other racing breeds and Warmbloods. The IRU on the third carpal bone corresponds to sclerosis or fractures seen in radiographs (Figure 4.203).

Upper Limb Long Bones

Stress fractures are common injuries seen on the tibial and humeral diaphyses in racing horses[60] that appear as a focal and intense areas of IRU located near a cortical margin. Humeral stress fractures are more common in Thoroughbreds than Standardbreds.[46] Common sites of tibial stress fractures in Thoroughbreds include the lateral cortex of the mid diaphysis, caudal cortex of the proximal diaphysis, and less commonly the medial cortex of the distal diaphysis (Figure 4.204).[52,60] Stress fractures in the humerus occur at the cranio- and caudo-distal, caudo-proximal, and less commonly cranio-proximal cortices (Figure 4.205).[60] Stress fractures of the radius are less common and have been reported to have a mid diaphyseal occurrence.[50]

Focal increase radiopharmaceutical uptake in the medullary cavity of long bones was first described as "bone infarcts"[65] and subsequently as enostosis-like lesions (Figure 4.206).[7,63] These lesions are frequently seen in the tibia, radius, humerus, and third metacarpal/metatarsal bones. Radiographically, the lesions appear as well-defined areas of increased opacity in the medullary cavities. It appears to be a transient condition with the lesions resolving in follow-up radiographic and scintigraphic examinations. The pathophysiology of these lesions is not well understood and it has been reported that not all of the lesions are associated with lameness.[7,63]

Increased radiopharmaceutical uptake on the caudal aspect of the distal femoral diaphysis just proximal to the stifle joint on a lateral view and localized laterally on the caudal view has been seen in cases of injury to the origin of the gastrocnemius muscle.[84]

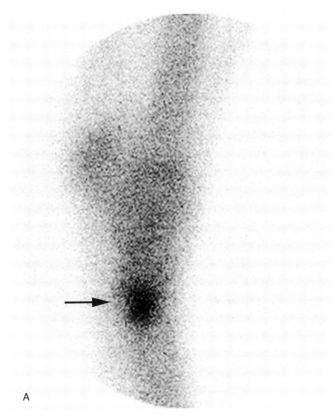

A

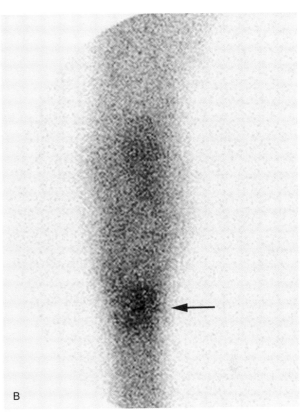

B

Figure 4.202. Delayed phase lateral (A) and plantar (B) views of the right tarsus of a horse, showing focal and intense IRU at the origin of the suspensory ligament on the proximal and plantar aspects of MTIII (arrows), compatible with an origin of the suspensory desmitis and enthesopathy. (Courtesy of Dr. Erik Bergman.)

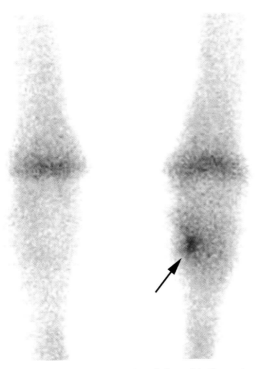

Figure 4.203. Delayed phase dorsal view of both carpi, showing a focal and intense IRU in the medial aspect of the left third carpal bone region (arrow), suggestive of sclerosis, chip fracture, or slab fracture. (Courtesy of Dr. Ryan Carpenter.)

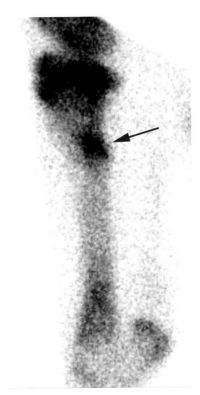

Figure 4.204. Delayed phase lateral view of the left tibia of a horse, showing a focal and intense IRU on the caudoproximal cortex of the tibia (arrow), consistent with a stress fracture.

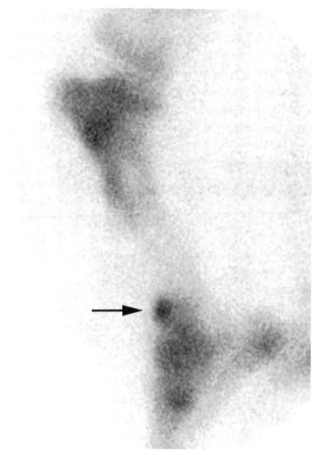

Figure 4.205. Delayed phase lateral view of the left humerus, showing a focal and intense IRU on the craniodistal humeral diaphysis (arrow), consistent with a stress fracture. (Courtesy of Dr. Ryan Carpenter.)

Elbow

Ulnar fractures are relatively common, especially in young horses.[14] Other traumatic injuries such as Salter-Harris fractures and subluxations can also occur. These injuries are usually diagnosed clinically and radiographically. However, fractures can sometimes be very small or minimally displaced; in such cases scintigraphy may add useful information in the diagnosis. Osteomyelitis secondary to trauma to the proximal radius with possible progression to septic elbow arthritis has been documented as a large and intense area of IRU in that region.[83] Radiographically, these lesions may be subtle or not apparent if the infection has not advanced enough to cause substantial bone lysis.

Subchondral bone cysts and cartilage lesions may not show scintigraphic abnormalities unless the underlying subchondral bone is affected.

Shoulder and Scapula

Injuries to the shoulder and scapula in the horse are uncommon. Fractures of the greater tubercle may occur, but frequently the diagnosis is based on clinical evaluation in combination with radiography or ultrasonog-

raphy.[55,91] An area of IRU in the cranio-proximal humerus may represent a fracture of the tubercle(s) or extension of an infectious/inflammatory process related to the bicipital bursa (Figure 4.207). An unusual case of IRU in the cranio-proximal humerus corresponding to a cyst-like lesion of the intermediate tubercle in absence of bicipital bursitis was reported.[64] In general, subchondral bone cysts and small cartilage defects are lesions that are not detected scintigraphically unless there are inflammatory changes extending to the adjacent subchondral bone.

The supraglenoid tubercle is the most frequent location for a traumatic fracture of the scapula.[19,20] Complete fractures of the neck and body of the scapula have also been reported sporadically.[19,20] The scintigraphic diagnosis of stress fractures of the scapula has been documented in a report of two cases in which the location of the focal and intense IRU corresponding to the fractures was located in the caudal mid body and the ventral aspect of the neck, respectively.[15]

Tarsus

Distal tarsal IRU is usually seen in jumping horses, followed by racing Standardbreds and less commonly Thoroughbreds.[5,29,30] The IRU can be unilateral or bilateral; a distribution along the entire area of the distal tarsal region of the dorsal aspect is the most common pattern.[58] Increased radiopharmaceutical uptake in the distal tarsal region corresponds to OA or degenerative changes that may or may not be radiographically apparent (Figure 4.208). Talocalcaneal OA is rare but has also been documented as focal and intense IRU predominantly medially and more plantar and proximal than distal tarsal IRU (Figure 4.209).[74]

Scintigraphy is very useful in localizing fractures of the central and third tarsal bones, especially when the fracture is not displaced, hence radiographically occult.[81] These horses have a history of acute onset of lameness, usually following exercise. The fracture will appear as a focal and intense region of IRU in the mid to distal tarsal region. Incomplete sagittal fracture of the talus is a rare condition in horses and can be a diagnostic challenge because the patient can present without evidence of soft tissue swelling or tarsocrural joint effusion.[16]

A focal and moderate-to-intense area of IRU at the level of the proximal talus should lend suspicion to a sagittal fracture, which is not always evident on radiographs.[16] A similar pattern of IRU was also reported on a 2-year-old Thoroughbred with unusual osteochondral lesions at the proximal articular margin of the medial trochlear ridge of the talus.[73] Osseous cyst-like lesions in the tarsus have been described as focal areas of IRU in the distal tibia (medial or lateral malleoli or intermediate sagittal ridge) or talus.[34] Adding a flexed lateral view to the routine scintigraphic exam protocol of the tarsus can help to differentiate whether the IRU is located in the distal tibia or the talus.

Stifle

Medial femoral condyle subchondral bone cysts are one of the most common pathologic changes seen in the stifle joint of horses. However, as previously mentioned,

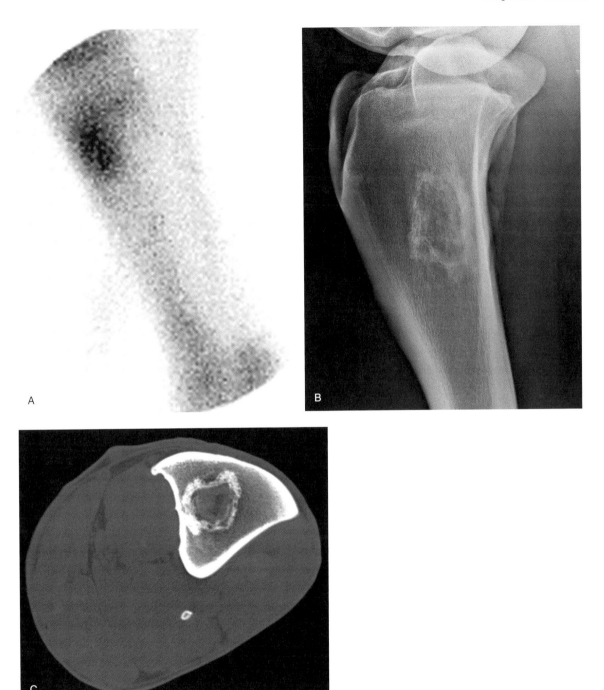

Figure 4.206. A. Delayed phase lateral view of the left tibia of a horse, showing a focal and intense IRU in the medullary cavity of the proximal diaphysis, suggestive of enostosis-like lesion. Radiographic (B) and computed tomographic (C) images showing the presence of ill defined, irregular medullary sclerosis, compatible with an enostosis-like lesion. (Courtesy of Dr. Erik Bergman.)

these lesions do not appear as areas of IRU unless an osteoblastic response or juxta-cyst osteosclerosis occurs in the adjacent subchondral bone (Figure 4.210). A case of a yearling horse with radiographically evident bilateral enlarging subchondral bone cysts after surgical debridement was reported to have normal postoperative follow-up scintigraphic examinations, despite the persistence of lameness localized to the stifle joints.[76] It was proposed that the lesions were mostly osteoclastic, hence no IRU was observed. Subchondral cystic lesions can also appear in the proximal tibia secondary to osteochondrosis or as a manifestation of OA, which scintigraphically may exhibit focal IRU.[86]

Ligamentous/tendinous avulsions may be suspected when a localized area of IRU is seen at an enthesis during the delayed phase. In these cases, other approaches such as ultrasound, MRI, or arthroscopy should be considered for better evaluation of the soft tissues.

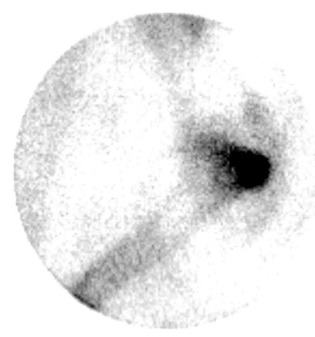

Figure 4.207. Delayed phase lateral view of the right humerus, showing focal and intense IRU in the greater tubercle, caused by a suppurative process.

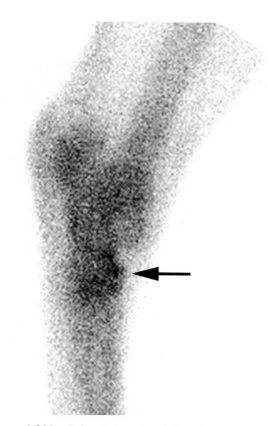

Figure 4.208. Delayed phase lateral view of the right tarsus of a horse, showing focal areas of IRU on the dorsal aspect of the distal intertarsal and tarsometatarsal joints (arrow), consistent with osteoarthritis. (Courtesy of Dr. Erik Bergman.)

Pelvis, SI, and Coxofemoral Joints

Complete, stress, and avulsion fractures at different anatomical locations in the pelvic region have been documented as areas of IRU in delayed phase scintigraphy.[11-13,36,62] Injuries to superficial structures such as the tuber coxae, ischial tuberosity, dorsal sacrum/tail head, greater trochanter, and third trochanter can be the result of direct trauma, often blunt in nature, from a kick, trailer accident, or self-inflicted as can occur from rapid movement or falling accidents. Fractures of the tuber coxae and tuber ischium can be detected by the intense IRU (Figure 4.211) and the possible asymmetric location of the IRU between affected and unaffected sides in cases of displaced fractures. Decreased uptake of a fractured tuber coxae has been associated with a ventrally displaced fracture fragment.[13] Oblique views of the pelvis are very useful for evaluating the iliac wing in suspected cases of stress fractures.[40] Trochanteric bursitis is more common in Standardbred racehorses, usually as a result of trauma, either direct or related to stress from racing.[54] Most of the time the lesion involves soft tissue structures, but in some cases the subchondral bone and cartilage overlying the greater trochanter are injured and a focal IRU is seen over the greater trochanter (Figure 4.212).

Coxofemoral joint pathology is very difficult to assess with dorsal views due to the great γ-ray attenuation from the superimposed musculature. Forty-five degree oblique views are very useful in cases of suspected hip pathology (Figure 4.213).[13]

The SI region is also susceptible to pathology commonly attributed to SI desmitis or OA. Injuries to the sacral tuberosity at the origin of the SI ligaments have been described as IRU at the affected enthesis[23] possibly with the tuberosity being displaced cranially.[13] The SI joint can be evaluated on the dorsal oblique view and the straight dorsal view.[31] The straight dorsal view is better to compare left and right on the same image; however, the oblique view gives a better evaluation of the extent of joint surface because it appears wider and in some cases helps to avoid superimposition of the urinary bladder. Areas of IRU at the SI joint region are often correlated with SI joint pain/injury (Figure 4.214).[22,90] However, IRU in the SI region has also been found in normal horses and those in which the lameness was attributed to a different anatomical region.[13,23] Variations on the anatomical conformation of the sacral wings and the cranial sacral borders may also play a role in the pattern of radiopharmaceutical uptake.[37] Areas of IRU in the SI region should be interpreted with caution and the diagnosis of pathology should not be based on the scintigraphic findings alone because of the lack of a "gold standard" and the possibility of false-positive results.[3,23]

In general, the results of pelvic scintigraphic evaluations should be strongly correlated with clinical and physical exam findings and supported, as frequently as possible, with ultrasound or radiography and/or local anesthesia.

Spine

Degenerative changes in the spine are most commonly associated with impingement of the dorsal

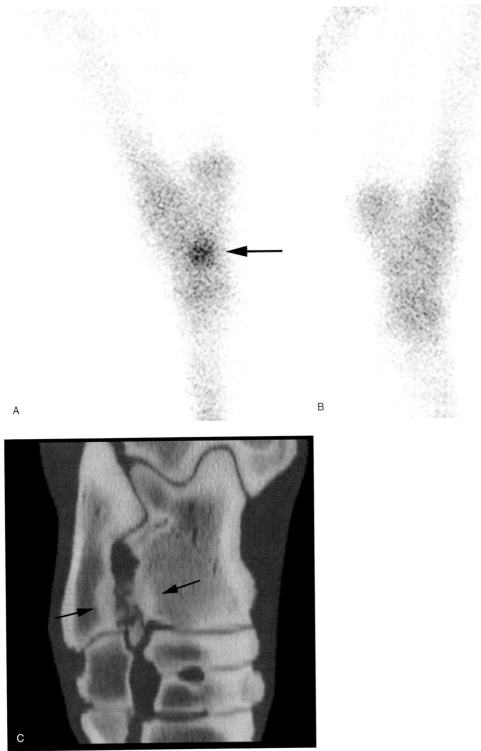

A

B

C

Figure 4.209. Delayed phase lateral views of the left (A) and right (B) tarsi. Note the focal and intense IRU seen in the region of the talocalcaneal joint on the left tarsus (arrow), compatible with osteoarthritis. Compare with the uniform uptake of the normal right tarsus. Computed tomographic image (C) of the left tarsus confirms the osteoarthritis with evidence of irregular bone margins with adjacent sclerosis and soft tissue mineralization of the intertarsal region (arrows). (Courtesy of Dr. Sarah M. Puchalski.)

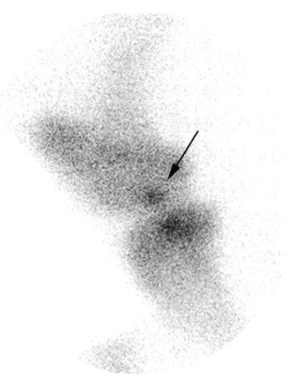

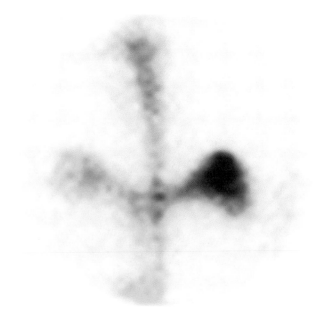

Figure 4.211. Delayed phase tail on detector (TOD) view of the pelvis of a horse, showing focal and intense IRU on the right ischial tuberosity, compatible with a fracture. (Courtesy of Dr. Erik Bergman.)

Figure 4.210. Delayed phase lateral view of the left stifle joint of a horse, showing a focal IRU at the articular surface of the condyles (arrow), suggestive of a bone cyst with reactive adjacent subchondral bone. (Courtesy of Dr. Erik Bergman.)

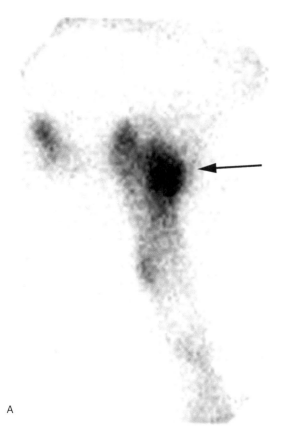

A

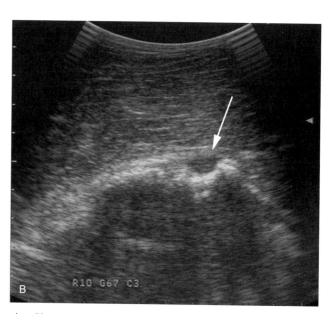

B

Figure 4.212. A. Delayed phase lateral view of the right hip joint of a horse, showing focal and intense IRU in the region of the right greater trochanter (arrow), compatible with trauma and gluteal muscle (medial or deep) enthesopathy, aseptic trochanteric bursitis, or a suppurative process. B. Transverse ultrasound image of the greater trochanter seen in (A), showing a mildly distended trochanteric bursa (arrow). Ultrasound-guided local anesthetic injection resulted in significant lameness improvement.

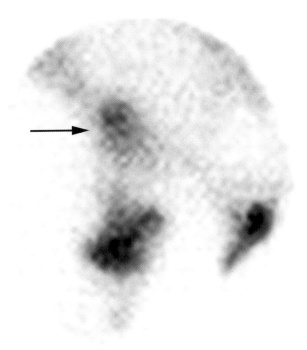

Figure 4.213. Delayed phase left dorsal oblique (LDO) view of the left hip joint showing a mild IRU in the region of the joint (arrow), suggestive of osteoarthritis. (Courtesy of Dr. Erik Bergman.)

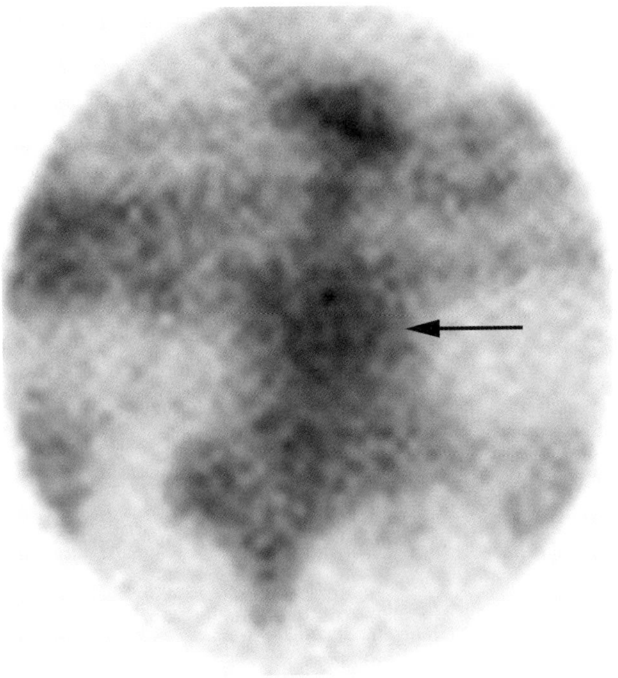

Figure 4.214. Delayed phase LDO of the left sacroiliac region of a horse, showing marked and diffuse IRU in the sacroiliac joint (arrow), compatible with osteoarthritis. (Courtesy of Dr. Erik Bergman.)

spinous processes (kissing spines), as well as OA of the articular facets. Impingement of the dorsal spinous process is common on the thoracic and lumbar spine. Good quality radiographs of these regions, especially the lumbar spine, can be very difficult to obtain because of the large amount of musculature causing considerable scatter radiation and because if the technique is increased, the most dorsal aspect of the dorsal spinous processes can be overexposed. This makes the scintigraphic evaluation of the spine an invaluable tool for evaluation of the back (Figure 4.215). Left and right dorsal oblique views of the spine are the best, although straight lateral and dorsal views are made if a lesion is found. Areas of mild IRU in the region of the dorsal spinous processes can be seen in horses with no clinical signs of back problems; therefore, these findings should be interpreted with caution.[32,33] Focal and intense areas of IRU can be seen with fractures, severe impingement with or without ligamentous damage, osteomyelitis, or neoplasia (Figures 4.216 and 4.217). Diagnostic differentials should be made, taking into consideration history, physical/clinical exam, and blood analysis.

Increased radiopharmaceutical uptake in the cervical articular facets is most commonly seen in cases of OA. The IRU can be identified when the bone activity in the region of the articular facets is greater than in the corresponding vertebral body or adjacent joints. Affected cervical vertebral facets may be unilateral or bilateral and more than one joint may be affected (Figures 4.218 and 4.219) Therefore, left and right views should be obtained and the practitioner should be aware of the possibility of multiple adjacent sites affected and not

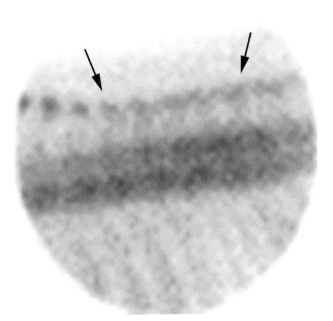

Figure 4.215. Delayed phase LDO view of the mid thoracic vertebrae of a normal horse. Note the relative increased uptake of the vertebral bodies when compared with the corresponding dorsal spinous processes (arrows). (Courtesy of Dr. Erik Bergman.)

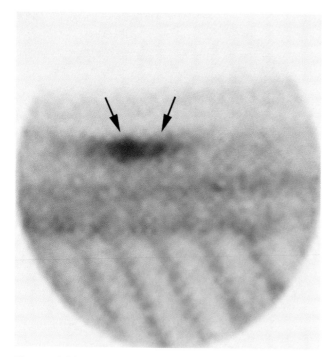

Figure 4.216. Delayed phase LDO view of the mid thoracic vertebrae of a horse, showing focal and intense IRU at at least two adjacent dorsal spinous processes (arrows), suggestive of impingement. (Courtesy of Dr. Erik Bergman.)

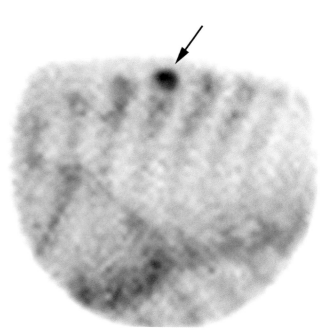

Figure 4.217. Delayed phase LDO view of the withers of a horse, showing a focal and intense IRU involving only the most proximal aspect of one of the dorsal spinous processes (arrow), suggestive of a fracture. (Courtesy of Dr. Erik Bergman.)

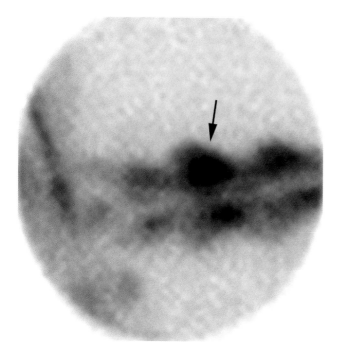

Figure 4.218. Delayed phase right lateral view of the caudal cervical region of a horse, showing marked, focal, and intense IRU at the articular facets of C6 to C7 (arrow), compatible with osteoarthritis. (Courtesy of Dr. Erik Bergman.)

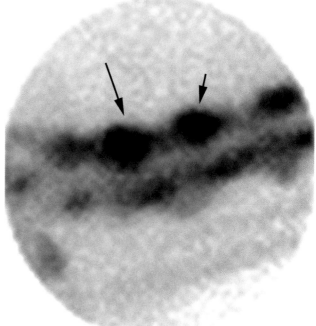

Figure 4.219. Delayed phase right lateral view of the caudal cervical region of a horse, showing marked, focal, and intense IRU at the articular facets of C5 to C6 (short arrow) and C6 to C7 (long arrow), compatible with osteoarthritis. (Courtesy of Dr. Erik Bergman.)

rely only on the comparison of adjacent joints for increased uptake evaluation.

Increased radiopharmaceutical uptake in the vertebral bodies is uncommon and has been reported with spondylosis deformans[17] and cases of discospondylitis.[38,82]

LIMITATIONS OF NUCLEAR MEDICINE

As mentioned previously, nuclear medicine traces physiologic processes in the different body systems and therefore has a high sensitivity in detecting early changes in the metabolism. This is the main reason why nuclear scintigraphy of the musculoskeletal system is an invaluable diagnostic tool in equine lameness. However, the specificity of bone scintigraphy is very low in the majority of cases. During the evaluation of the bone scintigraphy results, the practitioner should be aware that an area of IRU only means that there is an area of increased osteoblastic activity in a particular region. If the IRU is considered pathologic, in most situations a list of differential diagnoses should be made and further imaging performed to gain a better idea of the anatomical changes of the affected region.

In general, bone scintigraphy is used to localize an area of abnormal bone metabolism that may explain the source of lameness and not necessarily the specific pathologic change. There are some cases in which the diagnosis can be made from the bone scintigraphy results. For example, one can diagnose a stress fracture in a sound racehorse that becomes lame immediately after a training session or a race and has a focal IRU area in the diaphysis of the tibia. On the other hand, if a similar IRU area is found in a retired older horse that spends most of the time in the pasture, other differential diagnoses should be considered, such as blunt trauma with or without a fracture, enostosis-like lesion, osteomyelitis, or neoplasia.

False negative results occur secondary to many different reasons and can be considered as a limitation of bone scintigraphy. For example, a bone lesion with minimum uptake in the proximal region of a limb may not be apparent due to the significant γ-ray attenuation produced by the surrounding musculature. As in cases of subchondral bone cysts, cartilage or meniscal injuries will likely give a false negative result if the adjacent bone is not affected.

In summary, the practitioner should be aware of the potential limitations when interpreting the results of a nuclear medicine examination, correlate them with the signalment, history, clinical signs, and physical/lameness exam findings, and consider further diagnostics when appropriate.

References

1. Allhands RV, Twardock AR, Boero MJ. Uptake of ^{99m}Tc-MDP in muscle associated with peripheral nerve block. Vet Radiol Ultrasound 1987;28:181–184.
2. Anderson JD, Galuppo LD, Barr BC, et al. Clinical and scintigraphic findings in horses with a bone fragility disorder: 16 cases (1980–2006). J Am Vet Med Assoc 2008;232:1694–1699.
3. Archer DC, Boswell JC, Voute LC, et al. Skeletal scintigraphy in the horse: current indications and validity as a diagnostic test. Vet J 2007;173:31–44.
4. Arndt J, Pauwels E, Camps J, et al. Clinical differences between bone-seeking agents. Eur J Nucl Med 1985;11:330.
5. Arthur RM, Constantinide D. Results of 428 nuclear scintigraphic examinations of the musculoskeletal system at a Thoroughbred racetrack. Proceedings Am Assoc Equine Pract 1995;84.
6. Bailey RE, Dyson SJ, Parkin TD. Focal increased radiopharmaceutical uptake in the dorsoproximal diaphyseal region of the equine proximal phalanx. Vet Radiol Ultrasound 2007; 48:460–466.
7. Bassage LH, Ross MW. Enostosis-like lesions in the long bones of 10 horses: scintigraphic and radiographic features. Equine Vet J 1998;30:35–42.
8. Berry CR, Daniel GB. Pulmonary and mucociliary scintigraphy. In Textbook of Veterinary Nuclear Medicine, 2nd ed. Daniel GB, Berry CR, eds. North Carolina State University Press, Raleigh, NC, 2006;303–327.
9. Butson RJ, Webbon PM, Fairbairn SM. ^{99m}Tc-HMPAO labeled leucocytes and their biodistribution in the horse: a preliminary investigation. Equine Vet J 1995;27:313–315.
10. Chambers MD, Martinelli MJ, Baker GJ, et al. Nuclear medicine for diagnosis of lameness in horses. J Am Vet Med Assoc 1995;206:792–796.
11. Dabareiner RM, Cole RC. Fractures of the tuber coxae of the ilium in horses: 29 cases (1996–2007). J Am Vet Med Assoc 2009;234:1303–1307.
12. Dabareiner RM, Watkins JP, Carter GK, et al. Osteitis of the axial border of the proximal sesamoid bones in horses: eight cases (1993–1999). J Am Vet Med Assoc 2001;219:82–86.
13. Davenport-Goodall CLM, Ross MW. Scintigraphic abnormalities of the pelvic region in horses examined because of lameness or poor performance: 128 cases (1993–2000). J Am Vet Med Assoc 2004;224:88–95.
14. David GW, Elizabeth R. Nonsurgical Management of Ulnar Fractures in the Horse: A Retrospective Study of 43 Cases. Vet Surg 1985;14:283–286.
15. Davidson EJ, Martin BB, Jr. Stress fracture of the scapula in two horses. Vet Radiol Ultrasound 2004;45:407–410.
16. Davidson EJ, Ross MW, Parente EJ. Incomplete sagittal fracture of the talus in 11 racehorses: outcome. Equine Vet J 2005;37:457–461.
17. Denoix JM. Discovertebral pathology in horses. Equine Veterinary Education 2007;19:72–73.
18. Duggan VE, Holbrook TC, Dechant JE, et al. Diagnosis of aorto-iliac thrombosis in a Quarter horse foal using Doppler ultrasound and nuclear scintigraphy. J Vet Intern Med 2004;18 753–756.
19. Dyson S. Shoulder lameness in horses: an analysis of 58 suspected cases. Equine Vet J 1986;18:29–36.
20. Dyson S. Sixteen fractures of the shoulder region in the horse. Equine Vet J 1985;17:104–110.
21. Dyson S, McNie K, Weekes J, et al. Scintigraphic evaluation of the stifle in normal horses and horses with forelimb lameness. Vet Radiol Ultrasound 2007;48:378–382.
22. Dyson S, Murray R. Pain associated with the sacroiliac joint region: a clinical study of 74 horses. Equine Vet J 2003; 35:240–245.
23. Dyson S, Murray R, Branch M, et al. The sacroiliac joints: evaluation using nuclear scintigraphy. Part 2: Lame horses. Equine Vet J 2003;35:233–239.
24. Dyson SJ. Subjective and quantitative scintigraphic assessment of the equine foot and its relationship with foot pain. Equine Vet J 2002;34:164–170.
25. Dyson SJ, Murray R. Osseous trauma in the fetlock region of mature sport horses. Proceedings Am Assoc Equine Pract 2006;443–456.
26. Dyson SJ, Weekes J. Orthopedic imaging. In Equine Scintigraphy. Dyson SJ, Pilsworth RC, Twardock AR, Martinelli MJ, eds. Equine Veterinary Journal, LTD, Suffolk, UK, 2003;85.
27. East LM, Steyn PF, Dickinson CE, et al. Occult osseous metastasis of a colonic adenocarcinoma visualized with technetium ^{99m}Tc hydroxymethylene diphosphate scintigraphy in a horse. J Am Vet Med Assoc 1998;213:1132–1133, 1167–1170.
28. Edwards RB, Ducharme NG, Fubini SL, et al. Scintigraphy for diagnosis of avulsions of the origin of the suspensory ligament in horses: 51 cases (1980–1993). J Am Vet Med Assoc 1995; 207:608–611.
29. Ehrlich PJ, Dohoo IR, O'Callaghan MW. Results of bone scintigraphy in racing standardbred horses: 64 cases (1992–1994). J Am Vet Med Assoc 1999;215:982–991.

30. Ehrlich PJ, Seeherman HJ, O'Callaghan MW, et al. Results of bone scintigraphy in horses used for show jumping, hunting, or eventing: 141 cases (1988–1994). J Am Vet Med Assoc 1998;213:1460–1467.

31. Erichsen C, Berger M, Eksell P. The scintigraphic anatomy of the equine sacroiliac joint. Vet Radiol Ultrasound 2002; 43:287–292.

32. Erichsen C, Eksell P, Holm KR, et al. Relationship between scintigraphic and radiographic evaluations of spinous processes in the thoracolumbar spine in riding horses without clinical signs of back problems. Equine Vet J 2004;36:458–465.

33. Erichsen C, Eksell P, Widstrom C, et al. Scintigraphic evaluation of the thoracic spine in the asymptomatic riding horse. Vet Radiol Ultrasound 2003;44:330–338.

34. Garcia-Lopez JM, Kirker-Head CA. Occult subchondral osseous cyst-like lesions of the equine tarsocrural joint. Vet Surg 2004;33:557–564.

35. Gaughan EM, Wallace RJ, Kallfelz FA. Local anesthetics and nuclear medical bone images of the equine fore limb. Vet Surg 1990;19:131–135.

36. Geissbuhler U, Busato A, Ueltschi G. Abnormal bone scan findings of the equine ischial tuberosity and third trochanter. Vet Radiol Ultrasound 1998;39:572–577.

37. Gorgas D, Luder P, Lang J, et al. Scintigraphic and radiographic appearance of the sacroiliac region in horses with gait abnormalities or poor performance. Vet Radiol Ultrasound 2009; 50:208–214.

38. Hillyer MH, Innes JF, Patteson MW, et al. Discospondylitis in an adult horse. Vet Rec 1996;139:519–521.

39. Hornof WJ, Koblik PD. The scintigraphic detection of muscle damage. Equine Vet J 1991;23:327–328.

40. Hornof WJ, Stover SM, Koblik PD, et al. Oblique views of the ilium and the scintigraphic appearance of stress fractures of the ilium. Equine Vet J 1996;28:355–358.

41. Jorgensen JS, Geoly FJ, Berry CR, et al. Lameness and pleural effusion associated with an aggressive fibrosarcoma in a horse. J Am Vet Med Assoc 1997;210:1328–1331.

42. Kaser-Hotz B, Ueltschi G. Radiographic appearance of the navicular bone in sound horses. Vet Radiol Ultrasound 1992; 33:9–17.

43. Keegan KG, Wilson DA, Lattimer JC, et al.: Scintigraphic evaluation of ^{99m}Tc-methylene diphosphonate uptake in the navicular area of horses with lameness isolated to the foot by anesthesia of the palmar digital nerves. Am J Vet Res 1996;57:415–421.

44. Kleine LG, Solano M, Rusckowski M, et al. Evaluation of technetium ^{Tc}99m-labeled biotin for scintigraphic detection of soft tissue inflammation in horses. Am J Vet Res 2008;69:639–646.

45. Koblik PD, Hornof WJ, Seeherman HJ. Scintigraphic appearance of stress-induced trauma of the dorsal cortex of the third metacarpal bone in racing Thoroughbred horses: 121 cases (1978–1986). J Am Vet Med Assoc 1988;192:390–395.

46. Kraus BM, Ross MW, Boswell RP. Stress remodeling and stress fracture of the humerus in four Standardbred racehorses. Vet Radiol Ultrasound 2005;46:524–528.

47. Lamb CR. Non-skeletal distribution of bone-seeking radiopharmaceuticals. Vet Radiol Ultrasound 1990;31:246–253.

48. Long CD, Galuppo LD, Waters NK, et al. Scintigraphic detection of equine orthopedic infection using Tc-HMPAO labeled leukocytes in 14 horses. Vet Radiol Ultrasound 2000;41:354–359.

49. Long MT, Foreman JH, Wallig MA, et al. Hypertrophic osteopathy characterized by nuclear scintigraphy in a horse. Vet Radiol Ultrasound 1993;34:289–294.

50. Mackey VS, Trout DR, Meagher DM, et al. Stress fractures of the humerus, radius, and tibia in horses. Vet Radiol Ultrasound 1987;28:26–31.

51. Martinelli MJ. Subchondral bone and injury. Equine Veterinary Education 2009;21:253–256.

52. Martinelli MJ, Arthur RM. The American Thoroughbred. In Equine Scintigraphy. Dyson S, Pilsworth RC, Twardock AR, Martinelli MJ, eds. Equine Veterinary Journal LTD, Suffolk, UK, 2003;151.

53. Martinelli MJ, Chambers MD, Baker GJ, et al. A retrospective study of increased bone scintigraphy uptake in the palmar-plantar fetlock and its relationship to performance: 50 cases (1989–1993). Proceedings Am Assoc Equine Pract 1994;53.

54. McIlwraith CW. Diseases of joints, tendons, ligaments, and related structures. In Adam's Lameness in Horses, 5th ed. Stashak TS, ed. Lippincott Williams and Wilkins, Philadelphia, 2002;642.

55. Mez JC, Dabareiner RM, Cole RC, et al. Fractures of the greater tubercle of the humerus in horses: 15 cases (1986–2004). J Am Vet Med Assoc 2007;230:1350–1355.

56. Morris E, Seeherman HJ, O'Callaghan MW, et al. Scintigraphic identification of skeletal muscle damage in horses 24 hours after strenuous exercise. Equine Vet J 1991;23:347–352.

57. Morris EA, Seeherman HJ. Clinical evaluation of poor performance in the racehorse: the results of 275 evaluations. Equine Vet J 1991;23:169–174.

58. Murray RC, Dyson SJ, Weekes JS, et al. Scintigraphic evaluation of the distal tarsal region in horses with distal tarsal pain. Vet Radiol Ultrasound 2005;46:171–178.

59. O'Callaghan MW. The integration of radiography and alternative imaging methods in the diagnosis of equine orthopedic disease. Vet Clin North Am Equine Pract 1991;7:339–364.

60. O'Sullivan CB, Lumsden JM. Stress fractures of the tibia and humerus in Thoroughbred racehorses: 99 cases (1992–2000). J Am Vet Med Assoc 2003;222:491–498.

61. Peters AM. Imaging infection and inflammation in veterinary practice. Equine Vet J 1995;27:242–244.

62. Pilsworth RC, Shepherd MC, Herinckx BM, et al. Fracture of the wing of the ilium, adjacent to the sacroiliac joint, in thoroughbred racehorses. Equine Vet J 1994;26:94–99.

63. Ramzan PH. Equine enostosis-like lesions: 12 cases. Equine Vet Educ 2002;14:143–148.

64. Ramzan PH. Osseous cyst-like lesion of the intermediate humeral tubercle of a horse. Vet Rec 2004;154:534–536.

65. Rantanen NW, Rose J, Grisel GT, et al. Apparent bone marrow infarcts in Thoroughbred racehorses. J Eq Vet Sci 1994; 14:126–127.

66. Riddolls LJ, Byford GG, McKee SL. Biological and imaging characteristics and radiation dose rates associated with the use of technetium-99m-labelled imidodiphosphate in the horse. Can J Vet Res 1996;60:81–88.

67. Riddolls LJ, Willoughby RA, Dobson H. A method of mounting a gamma detector and yoke assembly for equine nuclear imaging. Vet Radiol Ultrasound 1991;32:78–81.

68. Ross MW. Scintigraphic and clinical findings in the Standardbred metatarsophalangeal joint: 114 cases (1993–1995). Equine Vet J 1998;30:131–138.

69. Ross MW. The Standardbred. In Equine Scintigraphy. Dyson S, Pilsworth RC, Twardock AR, Martinelli MJ, eds. Equine Veterinary Journal, LTD, Suffolk, UK, 2003;153.

70. Schoenborn WC, Rick MC, Hornof WJ. Computed tomographic appearance of osteochondritis dessicans-like lesions of the proximal articular surface of the proximal phalanx in a horse. Vet Radiol Ultrasound 2002;43:541–544.

71. Seeherman HJ, Morris E, O'Callaghan MW. The use of sports medicine techniques in evaluating the problem equine athlete. Vet Clin North Am Equine Pract 1990;6:239–274.

72. Shepherd MC, Pilsworth RC. Stress reactions to the plantarolateral condyles of MTIII in UK Thoroughbreds: 26 cases. Proceedings Am Assoc Equine Pract 1997;128–131.

73. Simpson CM, Lumsden JM. Unusual osteochondral lesions of the talus in a horse. Aust Vet J 2001;79:752–755.

74. Smith RK, Dyson SJ, Schramme MC, et al. Osteoarthritis of the talocalcaneal joint in 18 horses. Equine Vet J 2005; 37:166–171.

75. Solano M, Welcome J, Johnson K. Effects of acepromazine on three-phase ^{99m}Tc-MDP bone imaging in 11 horses. Vet Radiol Ultrasound 2005;46:437–442.

76. Squire KRE, Fessler JF, Cantwell HD, et al. Enlarging bilateral femoral condylar bone cysts without scintigraphic uptake in a yearling foal. Vet Radiol Ultrasound 1992;33:109–113.

77. Steckel RR. The role of scintigraphy in the lameness evaluation. Vet Clin North Am Equine Pract 1991;7:207–239.

78. Stewart M. Clinical applications of musculoskeletal scintigraphy in the horse. Aust Equine Vet 1994;12:71–75.

79. Steyn PF, Ramey DW, Kirschvink J, et al. Effect of a static magnetic field on blood flow to the metacarpus in horses. J Am Vet Med Assoc 2000;217:874–877.

80. Steyn PF, Uhrig J. The role of protective lead clothing in reducing radiation exposure rates to personnel during equine bone scintigraphy. Vet Radiol Ultrasound 2005;46:529–532.

81. Stover SM, Hornof WJ, Richardson GL, et al. Bone scintigraphy as an aid in the diagnosis of occult distal tarsal bone trauma in three horses. J Am Vet Med Assoc 1986;188:624–628.

82. Sweers L, Carstens A. Imaging features of discospondylitis in two horses. Vet Radiol Ultrasound 2006;47:159–164.

83. Swinebroad EL, Dabareiner RM, Swor TM, et al. Osteomyelitis secondary to trauma involving the proximal end of the radius in horses: five cases (1987–2001). J Am Vet Med Assoc 2003;223:486–491.

84. Swor TM, Schneider RK, Ross MW, et al. Injury to the origin of the gastrocnemius muscle as a possible cause of lameness in four horses. J Am Vet Med Assoc 2001;219:215–219.

85. Taylor AJ, Datz FL. Clinical practice of nuclear medicine. Churchill Livingstone Inc., 1991;397.

86. Textor JA, Nixon AJ, Lumsden J, et al. Subchondral cystic lesions of the proximal extremity of the tibia in horses: 12 cases (1983–2000). J Am Vet Med Assoc 2001;218:408–413.

87. Trout DR, Hornof WJ, Fisher PE. The effects of intra-articular anesthesia on soft tissue and bone phase scintigraphy in the horse. Vet Radiol Ultrasound 1991;32:251–255.

88. Trout DR, Hornof WJ, Liskey CC, et al. The effects of regional perineural anesthesia on soft tissue and bone phase scintigraphy in the horse. Vet Radiol Ultrasound 1991;32:140–144.

89. Trout DR, Hornof WJ, O'Brien TR. Soft tissue- and bone-phase scintigraphy for diagnosis of navicular disease in horses. J Am Vet Med Assoc 1991;198:73–77.

90. Tucker RL, Schneider RK, Sondhof AH, et al. Bone scintigraphy in the diagnosis of sacroiliac injury in twelve horses. Equine Vet J 1998;30:390–395.

91. Tudor R, Crosier M, Love NE, et al. Radiographic diagnosis: Fracture of the caudal aspect of the greater tubercle of the humerus in a horse. Vet Radiol Ultrasound 2001;42:244–245.

92. Twardock AR. Equine bone scintigraphic uptake patterns related to age, breed, and occupation. Vet Clin North Am Equine Pract 2001;17:75–94.

93. Twardock AR. Scintigraphy. Nuclear medicine scans complement X-rays as equine diagnostic tool. Large Animal Veterinarian 1995;50:30–31.

94. Valdes-Martinez A, Seiler G, Mai W, et al. Quantitative analysis of scintigraphic findings in tibial stress fractures in Thoroughbred racehorses. Am J Vet Res 2008;69:886–890.

95. Voute LC, Webbon PM, Whitelock R. Rules, regulations and safety aspects of scintigraphy. Equine Vet Educ 1995;7:169–172.

96. Weaver MP. Twenty years of equine scintigraphy—a coming of age? Equine Vet J 1995;27:163–165.

97. Weekes JS, Murray RC, Dyson SJ. Scintigraphic evaluation of metacarpophalangeal and metatarsophalangeal joints in clinically sound horses. Vet Radiol Ultrasound 2004;45:85–90.

98. Wisner ER, O'Brien TR, Pool RR, et al. Osteomyelitis of the axial border of the proximal sesamoid bones in seven horses. Equine Vet J 1991;23:383–389.

MAGNETIC RESONANCE IMAGING

Michael Schramme and W. Rich Redding

INTRODUCTION

Magnetic resonance imaging (MRI) is a relatively new multiplanar cross–sectional imaging modality in horses that is fast becoming the gold standard for diagnosis of musculoskeletal injury of the distal limbs in the equine patient. MRI allows soft tissue and bone structures to be evaluated in ways not previously possible. It provides superior contrast and detail, especially of soft tissue structures, and some physiological information on both soft tissue and osseous injuries.

As with any new imaging modality, it is essential to understand the factors that influence the signal characteristics that produce the diagnostic images and to learn the strengths and weaknesses of the technique. The clinician must understand the basic physics of MRI and the MRI sequences used for acquisition in order to comprehend the relationship between signal abnormalities and pathological abnormalities and between signal and normal anatomical variations. As more and different MRI systems, both high- and low-field, become available for imaging equine patients, it is also important to remain constantly critical of image quality.

The increasing use of MRI in equine sports medicine requires every equine practitioner to have a basic knowledge of MRI interpretation concepts. Accurate knowledge of the pros and cons of MRI help clinicians make a careful selection of horses that undergo MRI. MRI is not a substitute for in-depth clinical investigation and more conventional imaging techniques, and many diagnoses can and will continue to be made without MRI. Nonetheless, the use of MRI has highlighted the potential shortfalls of both radiography for imaging bone and ultrasonography for imaging soft tissue lesions.

GENERAL PRINCIPLES AND PHYSICS OF MRI

MRI produces a gray-scale image of tissue hydrogen protons by placing tissues in a large magnetic field, exposing them to a radio-frequency pulse, and measuring the magnetic resonance caused by this pulse. A computer interprets the data and creates images that display the different resonance characteristics of different tissue types.

The resonance that is measured originates from the magnetic properties of the positively charged proton in the nuclei of hydrogen atoms in biological tissues. The positively charged proton spins, resulting in a magnetic moment, which allows it to interact with the external magnetic field. Normally, hydrogen atoms are randomly oriented in tissues. However, when tissues are placed in the bore of a large magnet (Figure 4.220) and exposed to an external magnetic field, all hydrogen atoms align parallel with this field. Subsequently, a radio-frequency coil (Figure 4.221) is applied to the anatomical area of interest within the large magnet. Radio-frequency coils are made for human shoulders, knees, and other body parts. The coil is a large inductor with a defined wavelength that can transmit the short radio-frequency pulse

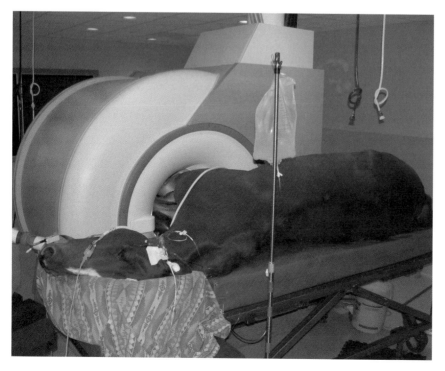

Figure 4.220. The 1.5 Tesla Siemens Symphony high field magnet (Siemens, Malvern, PA) used for MRI of horses under general anesthesia at the Veterinary Teaching Hospital of North Carolina State University. The horse is positioned in lateral recumbency with the lame(r) limb lowermost. The region of interest in the limb, in this case the foot, is positioned in the isocenter of the magnet.

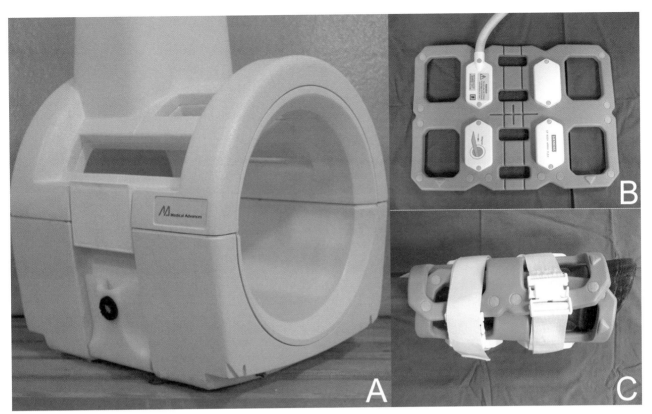

Figure 4.221. Radiofrequency coils manufactured for human MRI are used in equine MRI. A knee coil is a transmit-receive quadrature coil (volume coil) that surrounds the entire body part and has good field homogeneity (A). A human torso array coil is a receive-only flexible phased array coil (B) that can be wrapped around the horse's limb and secured with Velcro straps (C).

that makes MRI possible. The coil may also function to detect (receive) the magnetic resonance from the tissues. Radio-frequency coils can be differentiated by their function into transmit-receive coils, transmit-only coils, or receive-only coils.

When exposed to a short radio-frequency pulse specific for hydrogen by the radio-frequency coil, hydrogen nuclei absorb this pulse and change their alignment within the main magnetic field according to the direction of the radio-frequency pulse. Following discontinuation of the radio-frequency pulse, the hydrogen nuclei resume their previous orientation of parallel alignment with the main magnetic field, thereby making the transition from a high-energy to a low-energy state. This transition results in energy release that is used to generate a signal. The exchange of energy between spin states is called the resonance, and thus the name magnetic resonance imaging.

The time required for the hydrogen nuclei to resume equilibrium within the main magnetic field is the relaxation time, measured in milliseconds. The relaxation of hydrogen nuclei can be divided into two separate components, the longitudinal and transverse relaxations. Longitudinal relaxation is influenced by interaction of spinning protons with the tissue lattice. The transverse relaxation refers to the interaction of adjacent spinning protons with each other. Spin-lattice or longitudinal relaxation time is called T1. Spin-spin or transverse relaxation time is called T2 and is much shorter than T1. Most tissues can be characterized by their T1 and

T2 signal properties. Images are constructed with the different signals obtained from the various tissue parts. The collected signal is called an echo and it is detected by the radio-frequency receiver coil placed around the area of interest in the limb. Because fat and water both contain a high concentration of hydrogen atoms, the strength of the resonance signal depends on the amount of fat and water in the tissue. High-signal areas are white and low-signal areas are black.

Field gradients can be created within the main magnetic field by three additional gradient coils that surround the bore of the large magnet and change the intensity of the static magnetic field in transverse, dorsal, and sagittal directions. As a result, the intensity of signal produced by a given hydrogen proton can be used to position it precisely in space and create a 3-dimensional (3D) image. Hence, the magnetic field gradients allow tissue sampling as a slice in any chosen orientation or as 3D data sets. Three-dimensional signal acquisition allows thinner slice thickness and improves signal-to-noise ratio.

EQUIPMENT AND PRACTICALITIES OF MRI OF HORSES

Magnetic field strength is expressed in tesla units. One tesla (T) is approximately 20,000× the strength of the earth's magnetic field. High-strength magnetic fields measure in excess of 1 T, low-strength fields less than 0.5 T, and mid-strength fields between 0.5 and 1 T.

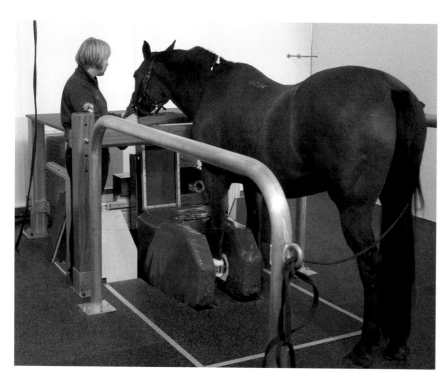

Figure 4.222. The Hallmarq Equine Limbscanner® (Hallmarq Veterinary Imaging, Guilford, UK) is an open, low-field magnet, mounted vertically at floor level, that allows MRI to be performed on standing, sedated horses.

Superconducting, closed, cylindrical bore magnets (Figure 4.220) generate high-strength magnetic fields, while resistive or permanent, open magnets (Figure 4.222) produce low-strength fields. Signal strength is proportional to the strength of the magnetic field. Consequently, lower field systems generate less tissue signal, require longer acquisition times, and produce lower resolution images. The uniformity or homogeneity of the main magnetic field is also higher in closed than in open magnets. Image quality and resolution increase with increasing magnetic field strength. Both high-field and low-field MRI units are currently in clinical use for horses.

Though a clinical 3-T magnet has been introduced recently, 1.5 T is considered the gold standard for high-field imaging of horses (Figure 4.220). The area of the limb to be imaged must be positioned in or near the isocenter of the cylindrical bore of the magnet, which lies at the intersection of all 3 gradient coils and in the optimal position for imaging. This requires the horse to be recumbent and therefore under general anesthesia, which increases the cost and, to some extent, the risk of the procedure. Although high-field magnets are generally capable of imaging limbs of horses from the carpus and tarsus distally, this capability is limited by how far the horse can be pulled into the bore of the magnet. Therefore, not all high-field magnets are equal in this respect. Positioning in isocenter is more difficult in longer and narrower cylindrical bores than in some newer short-bore magnets with flared ends. In addition, some high-field magnets have a much tighter imaging window around the isocenter than others, which makes it harder to pull areas of interest further proximal than the fetlock region into the imaging window.

Low-field MRI of horses is currently performed with 1 of 2 permanent, open magnets with a field strength ranging from 0.20 to 0.26 tesla. One open low-field MRI scanner designed specifically for imaging distal limbs of horses (Hallmarq Equine Limbscanner®, Hallmarq Veterinary Imaging, Guilford, UK) is mounted vertically at floor level and allows imaging to be performed on standing, sedated horses (Figure 4.222). However, imaging of areas proximal to the foot is susceptible to motion artifact in these units. Other low-field magnets (Vet MR® and Vet MR Grande®, Universal Medical Systems, Inc. Solon, OH) are oriented horizontally on a pedestal and require horses to be placed under general anesthesia. Low-field magnets produce a lower signal-to-noise ratio resulting in reduced image resolution and detail. Even so, low-field magnets are capable of producing diagnostic-quality images of the distal limb, and many examples of pathology visible with these magnets are available.[7,31,43–45,72–74,82]

Radio-frequency coils designed for human imaging are used in equine MRI. The choice of coil is dictated by manufacturer availability. Most distal limb studies are performed with human knee coils or torso array coils. Knee coils are transmit-receive quadrature coils (volume coils) that surround the entire body part and have good field homogeneity over a large area. A human torso array coil is a surface or flexible phased array coil that can be wrapped around the limb and secured with Velcro straps (Figure 4.221). Surface array coils are receive-only coils that have a good signal-to-noise ratio with an additional 20% signal gain over volume coils. They allow faster scanning with finer detail and have greatest sensitivity nearest to the coil surface.

Horses undergoing MRI must have all metal and ferrous material removed to avoid interference with the magnetic field and generation of susceptibility artifacts. This includes shoes, nails, metallic debris in the nail holes and sole, and the occasional metallic implant. Other ferromagnetic materials such as horse transport tables and anesthetic equipment may interfere with the homogeneity of the magnetic field and should be avoided in the radio-frequency-shielded MRI room. Customized nonferrous tables and MRI-compatible anesthetic machines, ventilators, and monitoring equipment are available.

INDICATIONS, CASE SELECTION, ADVANTAGES, AND DISADVANTAGES OF MRI

Magnetic resonance imaging is indicated when a lameness problem has been localized to an anatomical area and other imaging modalities have failed to provide an unequivocal diagnosis. Lameness should first be localized to an anatomical area because unlike nuclear scintigraphy, MRI is not a screening technique. The examination is costly and time-consuming and should be focused and completed within a fixed time period sufficient to scan 1 area of interest in the lame limb and the contralateral limb for comparison. Such protocol avoids problems associated with prolonged anesthesia in high-field magnets or motion during prolonged standing examination in a low-field magnet. Moreover, the overwhelming detail seen with MRI can make it difficult to decide which signal abnormalities are clinically significant. Therefore, accurate knowledge of the localization of the cause of lameness with diagnostic analgesia is indispensable when interpreting MR images.

MRI is particularly useful in anatomical areas where conventional imaging modalities have limitations, such as the foot, palmar/plantar soft tissues, and joints of the distal limbs. Ultrasonography is limited by the hoof capsule in lameness of the foot. Ultrasonographic findings may be equivocal in lameness associated with the palmar/plantar soft tissues of the distal limb. Radiography is incapable of detecting subtle or early cartilage or subchondral bone abnormalities in joint lameness. Radiographic abnormalities also may not be present in some cases of lameness associated with scintigraphic abnormalities.

Although MRI is the only imaging modality that can assess all tissues in a single examination, the availability of MRI should not result in the omission of radiographic and ultrasonographic examinations. MRI should not replace but rather complement radiographic and ultrasonographic findings. Information obtained from radiographic, ultrasonographic, and scintigraphic examinations helps in the interpretation of MRI findings and a full set of diagnostic images always provides a better basis for an accurate diagnosis. Radiography in particular has better bone vs. soft tissue contrast when compared to MRI and may therefore be more sensitive to subtle bone contour changes such as osteophytes and enthesiophytes.

MRI has numerous advantages over other imaging modalities. It does not use ionizing radiation. It has high intrinsic contrast and resolution, particularly for soft tissues, resulting in good anatomic separation between different tissues. Next to anatomic information, MRI also displays information that is pathophysiological. As a 3-D cross-sectional imaging modality, MRI is able to scan an object in any image plane.

The main disadvantages of MRI are its cost (installation and running costs), still limited availability, limited accessibility restricted to examination of the distal limbs and head only, need for general anesthesia with high-field magnets, relatively lower tissue signal and interference of patient movement with low-field magnets, and need for specialist training. MR image acquisition involves some complicated physics and a bewildering choice of pulse sequences, of which the nomenclature varies between manufacturers. A lack of uniformity or consensus exists regarding the most appropriate sequences to use. Image quality can be influenced by many different parameters, including time, signal-to-noise ratio, size of the object of interest, slice thickness, field of view, and other imaging specifications. In addition MRI, gives rise to a number of unfamiliar imaging artifacts that may mimic the presence of lesions or render a scan nondiagnostic. It is important to know how signal characteristics are influenced by all of the above mentioned parameters so that the clinician can assure image quality. The large number of images generated with each study also makes interpretation time consuming. For all of the above mentioned reasons, interpretation of images requires dedicated training.

SEQUENCES AND PROTOCOLS FOR EQUINE MRI

MRI examinations rely on the use of several different acquisition sequences. Each sequence name describes the radio-frequency pulse applied, the weighting of that pulse, and the associated magnetic field gradients. Different sequences used in conjunction to image a given anatomical area define the imaging protocol. It is necessary to use several sequences in multiple image planes within a protocol to identify pathological conditions accurately.

The common categories of conventional MRI sequences are spin echo (SE), turbo spin echo (TSE), gradient echo (GE), and inversion recovery (IR). The difference between these MR sequences relies on the method and timing of how the radio-frequency signals are pulsed into the tissues and how the resonance is collected to generate an image. Two parameters that define the sequence type are the repetition time (TR) and the echo time (TE). TR defines the time interval between radio-frequency pulses, and TE the time interval between the introduction of a radio-frequency pulse and the collection of resonance signal. These time intervals determine the tissue contrast of spin echo and fast spin echo images.

Spin echo sequences have long acquisition times and are impractical for live horse imaging. Fast or turbo spin echo sequences are used as a more practical alternative to reduce acquisition times while maintaining signal-to-noise ratio. The purpose of gradient echoes is to further decrease acquisition times and allow 3-D acquisitions. However, these advantages of gradient echoes are accompanied by disadvantages such as decreased soft tissue contrast and increased susceptibility to magnetic field inhomogeneities and susceptibility artifacts. Gradient echoes can be T1-weighted or T2-weighted. While some clinicians routinely use a clinical imaging protocol based on dual echo fast spin echo sequences,[80] others prefer 3-D gradient echo sequences because of the faster scanning times, thinner slices, higher detail, and increased sensitivity to hemorrhage in 3-D acquisitions.[21]

Inversion recovery sequences are produced using a similar method to spin echo sequences. However, the first radio-frequency pulse applied causes rotation of protons over 180° with a selected time of inversion. The selected time of inversion is used to suppress the returning signal from a specific tissue, usually fat. During this acquisition, it is useful to adjust the location of the digital fat suppression process manually to exactly 220 MHz away from the water peak.

Fat suppression can also be achieved by a high-detail spectral presaturation technique, although results of this technique are less consistent than those of inversion recovery. As a result of fat suppression, adipose tissue appears black, making fluid the only remaining source of hyperintense signal on an inversion recovery image, amid dark bone, soft tissues, and fat. The short tau inversion recovery (STIR) sequence is commonly used in orthopedics for the detection of abnormal fluid in bone. However, STIR sequences have an increased acquisition time, decreased signal-to-noise ratio, and decreased resolution. Fat suppression techniques require good homogeneity of the system's main magnetic field and are therefore more easily obtained with high-field systems.

Depending on whether T1 or T2 relaxation is measured during acquisition, sequences are called T1-weighted, T2-weighted, or intermediate between both T1 and T2, which is referred to as a proton density sequence (PD). PD images display any change in the density of protons as a change in signal intensity. T1 and T2 have characteristic values for each type of tissue and can be used to describe the magnetic properties of all tissues (Table 4.6, Figure 4.223). On T1-weighted images, adipose tissue has high signal (white), muscle has low to intermediate signal (dark to medium gray),

Table 4.6. The signal intensity of different tissues in different contrast weightings.

Sequence	T2	T1	Proton density	Inversion recovery
Cortical bone	Black	Black	Black	Black
Cancellous bone	Light gray	Light gray	Light gray	Light gray
Cartilage	Dark gray	Light gray	Gray	Gray
Tendon	Black	Black	Black	Black
Ligament	Black	Gray to black	Black	Black
Fat	Light gray	White	White	Black
Fluid	White	Dark gray	Light gray	White

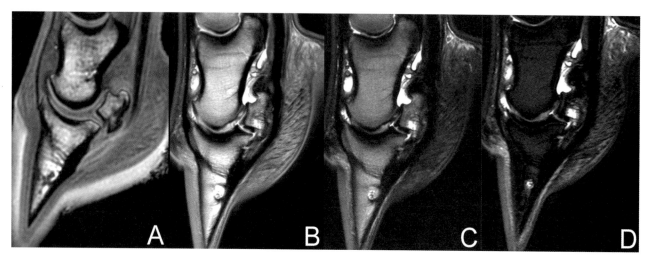

Figure 4.223. T1-weighted (A), proton density (B), T2-weighted (C), and short tau inversion recovery (STIR) sagittal images of the foot of a horse with navicular bone disease. Cortical bone, tendons, and ligaments are black on all sequences. On the T1-weighted image (A), fat is white and fluid is dark gray. On the proton density image (B), fat is white and fluid is light gray. On the T2-weighted image (C), fat and fluid are white. On the STIR image (D), fat is black and fluid is white. In general, T1-weighted and PD images show anatomical detail well, while T2-weighted and inversion recovery images show less detail but have higher fluid contrast.

and fluid has low signal (dark gray). On T2-weighted images, fat signal intensity is lower than in T1 and is bright to medium gray, muscle is still medium gray, and fluid has high signal (white). On PD images, fat is white or light gray, muscle is medium gray, and fluid has intermediate signal and is medium to lighter gray. In general, T1-weighted and PD images show anatomical detail well, whereas T2-weighted and inversion recovery images show less detail but have higher fluid contrast and are thus more likely to demonstrate pathology characterized by accumulation of fluid.

A range of time intervals is used to produce PD, T1, or T2 weighting of sequences. T1-weighted images are produced using short TR and TE values. T2-weighted images have long TR and TE values. PD images have long TR and short TE values. Manipulation of TR and TE values can produce more or less T1 or T2 weighting of any sequence and thereby result in different signal intensities for the same tissue within the same sequence definition. This feature may result in identical sequences with a different appearance between different MRI systems.

Standard protocols consist of proton density fast spin echo, T2-weighted fast spin echo, short tau inversion recovery (STIR) fast spin echo, and 3-D gradient echo (3-D GE) sequences. T2-weighted scans can take a long time to acquire; therefore, T2 and PD echoes can be collected concurrently as dual echoes with identical TR but different TE to minimize scanning times. PD images are easiest to evaluate ligament and tendon margins and symmetry. T2-weighted images have high fluid contrast, making them useful for looking at fluid in soft tissues. However, they have minimal shades of gray, resulting in poor definition of soft tissue margins. STIR images show inflammatory fluid in bone and soft tissues most easily but have a low resolution. T2-weighted or spoiled T1-weighted gradient echo sequences are used in 3-D acquisitions for evaluation of the fine anatomical detail in thin tissue slices.

The choice of protocol is determined by the type of scanner, the region under scrutiny, and the preference of the attending clinician. Consequently, protocols may differ between hospitals. With an endless number of combinations of sequences, weightings, and image planes available, it is tempting to continue scanning every patient until the clinician feels all questions have been answered. However, this approach lacks consistency and may cause problems. Sequences and image planes should be standardized to allow for consistent comparison between limbs and between horses. Deviation from the standardized protocol complicates interpretation and may lead to misdiagnosis. Moreover, excessive scanning times and prolonged recumbency within a confined magnet space with limited padding can result in postanesthetic complications.

Table 4.7 shows the routine protocols that have proven useful at North Carolina State University, with a typical MRI examination taking approximately 1 hour to complete. For optimal assessment of an anatomical region, images are generally obtained in three planes: sagittal, dorsal, and transverse. As part of the protocol, the authors routinely image the area of interest in the lame(r) limb as well as the contralateral limb for comparison. This allows recognition of the presence of normal anatomical variations and bilateral pathology, and is essential for determining the significance of signal abnormalities (Table 4.7).

ARTIFACTS OF MRI

MRI produces a wide range of artifacts and variations that can confuse the interpreter. In addition, MRI is susceptible to artifacts that are created by acquisition of images at oblique angles. Even slightly asymmetric positioning of image slices can create significant problems of image interpretation. Consequently, MRI is an imaging technique that can easily lead the examiner to over interpret images as well as miss lesions. Knowledge of the regional anatomy and familiarity with the image acquisition process are necessary to understand the origin of MRI artifacts. More than with other imaging modalities, practice and experience are essential to become proficient at evaluating MRI studies.

Artifacts can be classified as motion artifacts, magnetic field heterogeneity artifacts, and digital imaging artifacts. Motion artifacts generally result in ghosting, which results from displaced reduplications of the image in the phase encoding direction, or in marked blurring of the image. Respiration and blood flow can cause multiple motion ghosting (Figure 4.224). Respiratory motion is most often manifested in the upper limbs of anesthetized horses and can be reduced with sandbags or by interrupting mechanical ventilation for the duration of the more sensitive sequences. Ghost images of blood flow in vessels occur in the phase-encoding direction and it is important to select a phase encoding direction in which motion artifacts are not superimposed on areas of particular interest (e.g., the proximal part of the suspensory ligament).

Artifacts from magnetic field heterogeneity lead to image distortion or alterations in signal intensity and are more common in low-field than high-field magnets. Magnetic susceptibility artifacts are caused by the presence of ferrous material in metal or blood breakdown products from hemorrhage in tissues. Susceptibility artifacts result in an area of zero signal around the ferrous object and create distortion of the rest of the image (Figure 4.225). Gradient echoes are particularly susceptible to these artifacts. Feet should be radiographed routinely prior to MRI to ensure that all metal fragments and debris have been removed. Chemical shift artifacts are caused by the presence of fat and water adjacent to each other. This causes the position of fat signal to shift in the frequency-encoding direction of the image. A specific fat-water cancellation artifact occurs in T2 images with TE around 13 obtained with the Hallmarq Equine Limb Scanner® (Hallmarq Veterinary Imaging, Ltd. Guilford, UK)[84]. In areas of medullary bone (e.g., in the navicular bone) with an equal amount of water and fat, signals from both fat and water cancel each other out and are replaced with an area of zero signal (black) in the medullary cavity of the affected bone. This can lead to an erroneous diagnosis of medullary sclerosis.

Magic angle artifact causes a sudden increase in signal in tendons and ligaments where collagen is orientated at an angle of around 55° to the main magnetic field (Figure 4.226). This is most obvious at the inser-

Table 4.7. Siemens Symphony 1.5-tesla magnetic resonance imaging protocols for horses.

Slice plane	Sequence	TR msec	TE msec	FA°	Matrix size pixels	NEX #	FOV mm	Slice #	Slice width mm	Gap mm	Scan time min
Foot											
Sagittal	STIR	5840	26	180	256 × 192	1	140	23	3.5	0.5	2:51
Sagittal	PD TSE	3800	14	180	320 × 224	2	140	23	3.5	0.5	5.47
Sagittal	T2 TSE	3800	95	180	320 × 224	2	140	23	3.5	0.5	***
Transverse	PD TSE	3940	14	180	320 × 203	2	150	30	4.0	0.5	3:07
Transverse	T2 TSE	4750	81	180	320 × 203	2	150	30	4.0	0.5	3:07
Transverse	STIR	7610	26	180	256 × 192	1	150	30	4.0	0.5	3.19
Transverse	3-D FLASH* FS #	36	10	40	256 × 256 IP	1	120	40	2.0	−2.0	4.09
Dorsal	3-D FLASH* #	18	10	40	256 × 256 IP	1	140	32	2.0	−2.0	2:30
Oblique transverse	PD TSE FS	2760	30	180	320 × 224	1	150	26	3.0	0.6	2.08
Fetlock											
Sagittal	STIR	5490	28	180	256 × 256	1	170	21	3.0	0.5	2.30
Sagittal	PD TSE	4370	14	180	384 × 189	2	170	21	3.0	0.5	4.02
Sagittal	T2 TSE	4370	112	180	384 × 189	2	170	21	3.0	0.5	***
Transverse	PD TSE	5740	12	180	320 × 224	2	144	30	4.0	0.5	6.26
Transverse	T2 TSE	5740	124	180	320 × 224	2	144	30	4.0	0.5	***
Transverse	STIR	7610	26	180	256 × 192 IP	1	144	30	4.0	0.5	3.42
Dorsal	3-D FLASH #	18	10	40	256 × 218	1	160	36	2.0	−2.0	2.31
Sagittal	3-D FLASH FS #	37	10	40	256 × 256	1	120	40	2.0	−2.0	4.14
MC/MT											
Sagittal	STIR	5490	28	180	256 × 256	1	170	21	3.0	0.5	2.30
Sagittal	PD TSE	3800	14	180	384 × 189	1	170	21	3.0	0.5	2.30
Sagittal	T2 TSE	3800	112	180	384 × 189	1	170	21	3.0	0.5	***
Transverse	PD TSE^	3020^	12	180	384 × 269	1	144	30	4.0	0.5	3:39
Transverse	T2 TSE^	3020^	117	180	384 × 269	1	144	30	4.0	0.5	***
Transverse	STIR*	7900	29	180	256 × 192 IP	1	144	30	4.0	0.5	3.51
Transverse	3-D FLASH FS #	36	10	40	256 × 256 IP	1	120	30	2.0	−2.0	4.09
Dorsal	3-D FLASH #	18	10	40	256 × 256	2	140	36	2.0	−2.0	3.45
Carpus/tarsus											
Sagittal	STIR	5490	28	180	256 × 256	1	170	21	3	0.5	2:30
Sagittal	PD TSE	3800	14	180	384 × 189	1	170	21	3	0.5	2:30
Sagittal	T2 TSE	3800	112	180	384 × 189	1	170	21	3	0.5	**
Transverse	PD TSE	3060^	13	180	384 × 269	1	144	30	4	0.5	4:06
Transverse	T2 TSE	3060^	119	180	384 × 269	1	144	30	4	0.5	**
Transverse	STIR	7900	29	180	256 × 192	1	144	30	4	0.5	3:51
Dorsal	3-D FLASH #	36	10	40	256 × 256 IP	1	120	30	2.0	−2.0	4.09
Sagittal	3-D FLASH # FS	18	10	40	256 × 256	2	140	36	2.0	−2.0	3.45

TR = repetition time, TE = echo time, FA = flip angle, FOV = field of view, NEX = number of excitations, PD = proton density, TSE = turbo spin echo sequence, 3-D = three-dimensional, FLASH = fast low angle shot sequence, FS = fat saturated, STIR = short tau inversion recovery sequence, IP = interpolated, # = RF spoiling, ∧ = 2 concatenations.

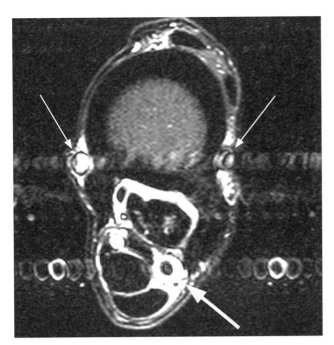

Figure 4.224. Transverse STIR image of the right hind proximal metatarsal region. Multiple motion ghosting caused by blood flow results in displaced reduplications of the images of the lateral and medial dorsal metatarsal arteries (narrow arrows) and the medial metatarsal artery (broad arrow) in the phase encoding direction.

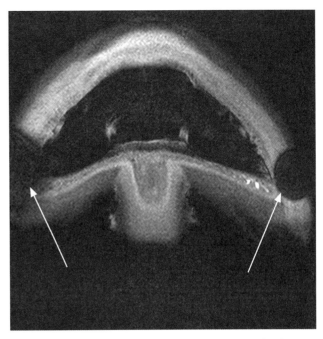

Figure 4.225. Transverse T1-weighted fast low angle shot (FLASH) image with fat saturation of a foot at the level of the insertion of the deep digital flexor tendon to the distal phalanx. The presence of small amounts of metallic debris in nail holes has resulted in areas of zero signal and image distortion around the ferrous material (arrows).

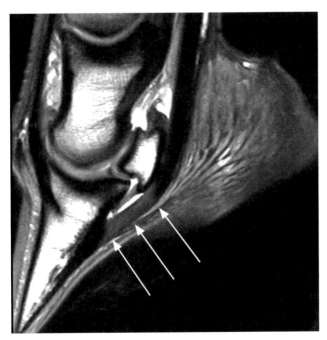

Figure 4.226. Sagittal proton density image of the central part of the foot of a forelimb. The magic angle effect causes an abrupt increase in signal intensity of the deep digital flexor tendon from the distal border of the navicular bone distally to its insertion onto the distal phalanx (arrows).

tion of the DDFT to the distal phalanx[10,78] but can also appear in the oblique distal sesamoidean ligaments (DSL) and collateral ligaments of the joints of the distal limb.[76,77] Magic angle artifact is particularly noticeable

in sequences with a short TE and is less evident on T2-weighted images.

Partial volume averaging artifacts occur when the different signal intensities of more than 1 tissue type within the same voxel are digitally averaged, resulting in a misleading shade of gray. This artifact results in blurring of the margins of structures and image inaccuracies. Curved and thin structures are most susceptible to the volume averaging effect. For example, it may be impossible to distinguish the margin of articular cartilage when imaging the articular surfaces of the equine metacarpophalangeal joints (Figure 4.227). The volume averaging effect can be reduced by using thinner slices.

Phase wrap artifacts occur when a portion of the object that lies outside the field of view is represented out of position in the image. Gibbs truncation artifacts or Gibbs ringing artifacts are seen when lines of bright signal are repeated parallel with an interface of abrupt signal change between 2 objects of markedly different signal intensity in the image. This is an effect of under sampling and disappears with use of a higher acquisition matrix. The acquisition matrix represents the number of pixels in the frequency-encoding and phase-encoding directions.

INTERPRETATION OF MR IMAGES

Signal intensity describes the shade of gray of a specific tissue on an MR image. Bright or white signal is described as hyperintense or as having high signal intensity. Dark or black tissues are hypointense or have low

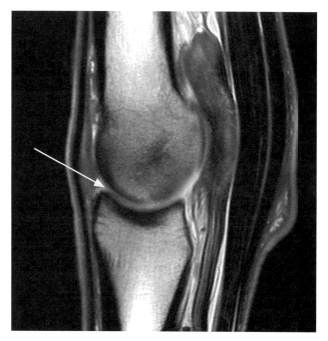

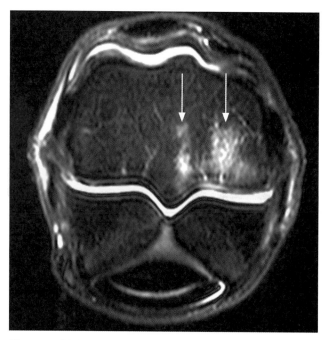

Figure 4.227. Sagittal proton density image of the central part of the fetlock of a forelimb. The slice is positioned immediately adjacent to the sagittal ridge of the distal aspect of the third metacarpal bone. The articular cartilage layers of the third metacarpal bone and the proximal phalanx are poorly distinguishable from each other and from adjacent subchondral bone (arrow). The margins are blurred due to volume averaging effect of slices across the curved articular surfaces.

Figure 4.228. Transverse STIR image of the distal aspect of the right third metacarpal bone at the level of the proximal sesamoid bones. There are hyperintense areas of abnormal intra-osseous fluid in the palmar aspect of the lateral condyle and sagittal ridge of the third metacarpal bone (arrows).

signal intensity. Isointense is used as a comparative term for two tissues that have similar signal intensity. Unlike other diagnostic imaging modalities, MRI is unique in that it produces images in which the same tissue may have a different appearance (signal intensity) depending on the sequence used for image acquisition.

Injury results in changes in biochemical composition and fluid content, and therefore signal intensity of tissues. Bone sclerosis, increased tissue fluid, and presence of fibrous tissue can be readily detected because of alterations in signal intensity. For a complete assessment of injury, images must be analyzed in all pulse sequences and planes. A protocol that combines information from T1-weighted, T2-weighted, and fat-suppressed images is most useful for a complete evaluation. Some clinicians prefer to substitute the T1-weighted with PD sequences within such protocols because they contain more contrast. In general, fluid is hypointense on T1-weighted and hyperintense on T2-weighted and PD images. Increased protein or cellular content in fluid can lead to increased signal intensity of fluid on T1-weighted images. On T2-weighted images, the presence of blood leads to a relative decrease in signal intensity compared with fluid. Immature granulation tissue has high signal intensity on T2-weighted and T1-weighted images, whereas mature fibrotic tissue has low signal intensity on T2-weighted images but can retain higher signal intensity on T1-weighted images[85].

Normal cortical bone is black on all sequences and has clearly defined margins. Cancellous bone is more heterogeneous because of the presence of adipose and

connective tissues in addition to mineralized bone. Bone remodeling can result in changes in bone contour and the presence of cancellous bone fluid and cancellous bone mineralization.

Bone contour changes may be observed as osteophytes or enthesiophytes typically seen on individual image slices. Bone contour changes may also be manifested as periosteal and endosteal new bone formation, cortical bone lysis, and irregularities in the outline of subchondral bone. Changes in trabecular architecture are visible as loss in signal homogeneity and thickening or loss of trabeculae.

The presence of abnormal fluid in bone is recognized as a combination of high signal on fat-suppressed and T2-weighted images and low signal on T1-weighted images (Figure 4.228). Although this combination of signal changes is commonly referred to as bone edema or bone bruising, it has been shown to reflect a wider range of possible pathologic changes including bone necrosis, hemorrhage, inflammation, trabecular microdamage, fibrosis, fat necrosis, and bone edema.[51,59,88] Even so, the ability to detect the presence of fluid in bone makes MRI extremely sensitive in the diagnosis of subtle bone injuries.

Areas of increased density or mineralization of cancellous bone (sclerosis) are characterized by low signal on both T2- and T1-weighted images (Figure 4.229). Sclerosis is visible on MR images before it becomes visible radiographically. Damage to bone can also occur at the origin or insertion of ligaments and tendons and may consist of localized signal increase on fat suppressed images, signs of sclerosis, enthesiophyte formation, or endosteal reaction. Occasionally an osseous

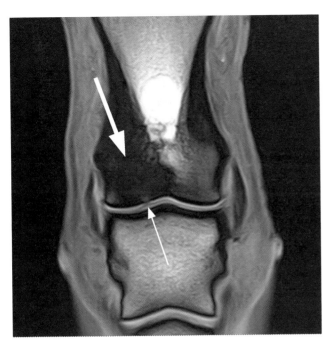

Figure 4.229. Dorsal T1-weighted spoiled gradient echo image of the proximal interphalangeal joint of the right forelimb of a horse with septic arthritis of 5 weeks duration. There is a small, focal, hyperintense subchondral bone lesion (narrow arrow) surrounded by a wide area of extensive loss of signal from the cancellous bone of the laterodistal aspect of the proximal phalanx (broad arrow). When accompanied by a similar loss of signal in paired T2-weighted images, this indicates increased density or mineralization of cancellous bone (osteosclerosis).

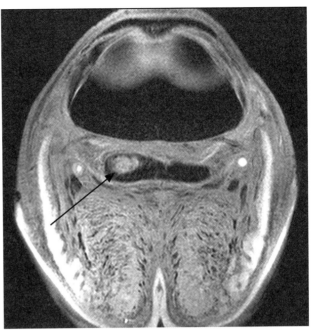

Figure 4.230. Transverse T1-weighted fast low angle shot (FLASH) image with fat saturation of the right front foot at the level of the middle phalanx of a horse with acute onset foot lameness. There is abnormal signal hyperintensity in a large core lesion of the medial lobe of the deep digital flexor tendon (arrow).

cyst-like lesion can be observed at the attachment site of a ligament or tendon. Fractures are seen as defects in the bone contour and structure and as lines of high signal on T2-weighted and fat-suppressed images.

Normal tendons emit zero signal on T1- and T2-weighted images. Normal ligaments produce more signal variation than tendons and vary from light gray to black. Not only do some ligaments contain muscle fibers and surrounding connective tissue that produce signals of mixed intensity (e.g., suspensory ligament), but ligaments also are often composed of fiber bundles with different orientations which makes them more susceptible to magic angle effects than tendons. The degree of signal variability depends on the specific ligament, the density of collagen bundles, and the sequence used for imaging.

Gradient echo sequences inherently produce less soft tissue contrast which may result in difficulty detecting ligament margins as they tend to blend into a gray background of the surrounding soft tissues. This lack of soft tissue contrast in gradient echo sequences is more apparent on low-field images. Therefore, T2-weighted fast spin echo sequences should always be included when evaluating possible ligament abnormalities.

Mild signal increase also may be seen in normal areas of cartilaginous tissue in tendons and ligaments, such as at the insertion of the straight DSL, the insertion of the collateral sesamoidean ligaments (CSLs), and the dorsal aspect of the deep digital flexor tendon (DDFT)

in the fetlock region. In general, increased signal intensity in tendons or ligaments indicates tissue damage. Mild damage may be detected by the presence of periligamentous signal increase on T2-weighted images. More severe damage is characterized by either focal or diffuse intratendinous or intraligamentous increase in signal intensity (Figure 4.230). This may be accompanied by enlargement and shape changes.

A partial tear may result in thinning, elongation, or a wavy or partially interrupted contour of a ligament or tendon. With complete tears, the contour is interrupted by a visible defect and stumps may be present at the ligament or tendon ends. In the acute and subacute stages of tendon or ligament injury, signal increase is present in both T1- and T2-weighted images, the latter due to the presence of fluid signal associated with acute necrosis and inflammation. At later stages of fibrosis and healing, T2 signal progressively returns to normal while T1 signal hyperintensity persists, sometimes indefinitely.[5,11,21,37,67] MRI may therefore not be able to establish when a patient with a previous tendon or ligament injury can safely resume sporting activities.

Some authors make a distinction between tendinitis and tendonosis.[81] Tendinitis has been characterized by the presence of inflammation and increased fluid signal in T2-weighted images in the early stages of injury and healing. Tendonosis, on the other hand, has been described as a degenerative process in tendons due to cumulative overload microtrauma without evidence of inflammation.[81] It has been suggested that tendonosis results in intratendinous signal hyperintensity in T1-weighted and PD images but not in T2-weighted and fat-suppressed images.[81] However, with severe intratendonous necrosis and myxoid degeneration, even in the absence of inflammation, fluid signal intensity may still be present in fat-suppressed images.

In one study of clinical core lesions in the digital part of the DDFT, tendons with fascicular necrosis had signal increase on fat-suppressed images and T1-weighted images, whereas signal intensity in fat-suppressed images was normal in core lesions with core fibroplasia rather than necrosis[5]. Similarly, the presence of increased signal on fat-suppressed images was associated with the most severe histological grades of collagen fiber disruption in one study of human Achilles tendonosis[36].

Normal articular cartilage has medium signal intensity on PD images, medium to high signal intensity on T1-weighted images, and medium to low signal intensity on T2-weighted images. It can be clearly defined from hypointense subchondral bone and from synovial fluid, which is hypointense on T1-weighted and hyperintense on T2-weighted images. Spoiled gradient echo sequences with fat suppression have been found to be most useful for defining margins and thickness of equine articular cartilage in the carpal joints[50].

Cartilage damage can be visualized directly as a change in signal, thickness, and/or surface contour of cartilage. Surface irregularities may indicate the presence of superficial fibrillation but more substantial lesions (erosions and wear lines) can be visualized as defects in the cartilage surface contour. These cartilage defects allow pooling of synovial fluid, which results in focal T2 and STIR signal hyperintensity and T1 signal hypointensity (Figure 4.231). Full-thickness defects are

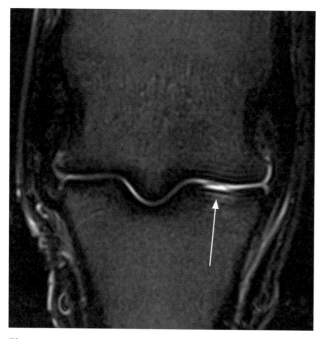

Figure 4.231. Dorsal STIR image of the right fore fetlock of a horse with acute right fore fetlock lameness. There is abnormal signal hyperintensity at the level of the articular cartilage proximal to a small subchondral bone irregularity in the proximomedial articular surface of the proximal phalanx (arrow). There is mild signal hyperintensity in the subchondral bone adjacent to the articular cartilage hyperintensity. Necropsy confirmed the presence of a full-thickness cartilage injury at this site.

usually accompanied by changes of the subchondral bone, including thickening and irregularity of the borders of the subchondral bone plate and focal bone edema that may draw attention to the less obvious cartilage signal changes.

Although MRI has been reported as a good imaging modality for evaluation of articular cartilage, accurate MRI evaluation of degenerative and traumatic cartilage lesions in distal limb joints remains difficult.[33,65] This is true not only in the distal limbs of horses but also in the human knee. Comparisons between MRI and arthroscopic evaluation of the human knee have indicated a better correlation between the prediction and finding of meniscal lesions than of articular cartilage defects.[30,38,47] Imaging difficulties arise mainly from the thickness (lack thereof) of equine distal limb cartilage that is frequently too thin for the spatial resolution of clinical MRI. In addition, the articular surfaces of equine distal limb joints are markedly curved. Both factors promote partial volume-averaging across image slices resulting in blurring of cartilage margins.[14]

Normal synovial fluid has high signal intensity on T2-weighted and low signal intensity on T1-weighted images. Joint capsule has medium to low signal intensity on all sequences. Joint effusion results in displacement of the joint capsule margins. Increased protein or hemorrhage in the synovial fluid may cause an increase in T1 signal and a decrease in T2 signal intensity of the fluid. Chronic hemarthrosis may result in the presence of small susceptibility artifacts on gradient echoes due to the presence of hemosiderin in the synovial membrane.

Blood in the lumen of a normal artery or vein may appear as low intensity, high intensity, or mixed intensity signal depending on the imaging parameters and blood flow characteristics. Hemorrhage can be differentiated into acute and chronic stages on MR images.[53] In the acute stage, hemorrhage is like other fluids, hypointense on T1-weighted images and hyperintense on T2-weighted images. After approximately 1 week, methemaglobin release leads to increased T1 signal intensity. In the chronic stage, hemosiderin causes zero signal areas to appear due to susceptibility artifacts, especially on gradient echoes.[6] The center of old hemorrhage may remain hyperintense on T1-weighted and T2-weighted images due to persistence of methemaglobin.

EVALUATION OF EQUINE MRI STUDIES

A standard high-field MRI protocol produces hundreds of high-detail images, each of which may contain important information. In order to turn this information into a useful diagnosis, a methodical and consistent approach should be used to reading the MRI study. All of the imaging sequences and planes should be checked in a repeatable order and each structure evaluated in a standard order for each sequence. One such methodical approach is to start the evaluation of images with the anatomical sequences first (sagittal, transverse, and dorsal T1-weighted gradient echo or PD fast spin echo sequences).

Next the fat-suppressed fast spin echo sequences could be evaluated for the presence of bone abnormalities. Subsequently the fast spin echo T2-weigthed sequences should be assessed for the presence of soft tissue abnormalities. Finally, specialized selected 3-D spoiled gradient echo sequences might be evaluated for the finer detail of a specific anatomical structure (e.g., the distal border of the navicular bone or the DDFT). Alternatively, the fat-suppressed sequences can be evaluated first to screen the bony structures, followed by the fast spin echo T2-weighted sequences to screen the soft tissue structures, while the anatomical sequences are used as reference images.

The interpreter should select 1 area of interest in 1 image plane of the anatomical sequence (e.g., the insertion of the DDFT in the sagittal PD or T1-weighted images) and scroll through all of the images of that particular image plane while continuing to focus on that same area of interest. Attention can then be shifted to another area of interest and the same process repeated in that same image plane. When the entire image has been covered with overlapping areas of interest, the next image plane of the anatomical sequence (transverse or dorsal PD or T1-weighted images) can be evaluated in a similar fashion. This process can be repeated until all sequences have been evaluated.

Any suspect abnormality should be defined by signal intensity, size, shape, and contour in comparison with normal. Throughout the evaluation process the clinician should cross reference any suspected signal abnormality in two ways, i.e., by anatomical cross referencing and by contrast cross referencing. Anatomical cross referencing is performed by comparing the appearance of a suspected lesion with its appearance in other image planes of the same sequence. In other words, any suspected abnormality visible on a sagittal PD (or T1-weighted) image should also be visible on corresponding images of the transverse and dorsal PD (or T1-weighted) sequences. Contrast cross referencing refers to the process of comparing the signal intensity of a suspected lesion in a PD or T1-weighted image with its signal intensity in the corresponding T2-weighted and fat-suppressed images.

As a general rule, an abnormality should be identifiable in at least 2 different imaging planes and 2 different contrast weightings for it to be considered a true lesion. Frequently more than one true lesion is identified during an MRI examination, causing a diagnostic dilemma. The clinician must decide on the likely hierarchy of clinical significance of lesions encountered in light of the physical examination, the results of diagnostic analgesia, and the current knowledge of which MRI lesions are most common in any given anatomical region of the limb.

SPECIALIZED MRI TECHNIQUES

New sequences aimed at improving articular cartilage contrast are constantly evolving and under investigation. These include volumetric interpolated breath-hold examination (VIBE), double echo in the steady state (DESS), true fast imaging with steady-state free precession (true-FISP), fast imaging employing steady-state acquisition (FIESTA), multiple-echo data image combination (MEDIC), fluctuating equilibrium MRI (FEMR), driven equilibrium Fourier transform (DEFT), and delayed gadolinium-enhanced MRI of cartilage (dGEMRIC).[41]

T2-mapping has been successfully performed in equine stifles and allowed good distinction between normal and abnormal cartilage[86].

Contrast enhanced orthopedic MRI has been used to help define and follow the healing of soft tissue injuries. Post contrast fat-saturated T1-weighted sequences are obtained following intravenous administration of gadolinium diethlyentriaminepentaacetic acid (0.02 mmol/kg IV)[28] or gadopentetate dimeglumine (0.1 mL/kg IV),[34] as the conspicuity of these paramagnetic contrast agents is increased on T1-weighted images. Gadopentetate dimeglumine is considered an extracellular fluid agent and leaks into the extracellular compartment to become detectable on MR images following tissue injury with inflammation and capillary breakdown.[27] Contrast enhanced imaging has helped to define the dynamic state of injury and healing in the Achilles tendon[69–71] and the tendon sheaths of wrists.[79] The technique was found to be particularly useful in the detection of subtle MRI lesions in the feet of horses. Significant contrast enhancement was observed in lesions of the DDFT, desmitis of the distal sesamoidean impar ligament (DSIL), desmitis of the CSLs, and palmar erosions of the flexor cortex of the navicular bone (Figure 4.232).[34]

Direct MRI arthrography with a saline-gadopentate dimeglumine mixture (1.0 mL gadopentate dimeglumine/250 mL saline) has been used in the assessment of complex intra-articular soft tissue structures in human patients.[58] With respect to cartilage imaging, MRI arthrography has reportedly resulted in 10% improvement in chondral lesion detection relative to conventional MRI studies.[40] Better cartilage contrast may be achieved following direct MRI arthrography with saline than with gadolinium.[12,66]

Indirect MRI arthrography is performed following intravenous injection of paramagnetic MRI contrast media. Similar sensitivities and specificities have been reported for indirect MRI arthrography when compared to direct MRI arthrography in the diagnosis of rotator cuff, glenoid labrum, and meniscal injuries.[89]

MAGNETIC RESONANCE IMAGING OF THE FOOT

Introduction

The true causes of pain in horses with foot lameness have often remained elusive. This has led to debate about the relevance or lack thereof of radiographic findings in the navicular bones.[18] It has become apparent that in addition to degeneration of the navicular bone and the distal interphalangeal joint, soft tissue injuries make an important contribution to pain in the foot.[21,87] MRI has become the gold standard of diagnosis in these patients, because of its ability to show superior soft tissue contrast and detail. Many of the causes of foot lameness we know today can not be conclusively identified without the use of MRI.

MRI Protocol

An effective high-field foot protocol is shown in Table 4.7. This protocol consists of sagittal and transverse PD, T2-weighted and inversion recovery fast spin echo sequences. Image planes span from the level

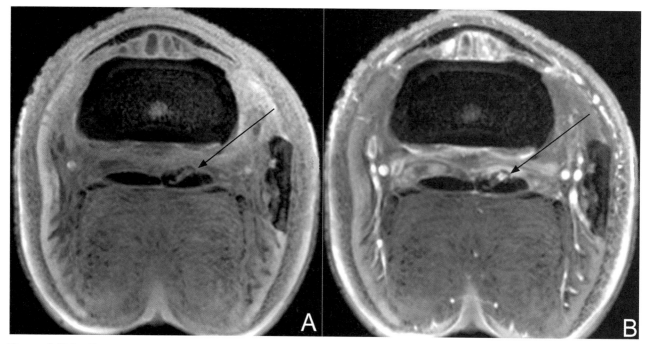

Figure 4.232. Transverse volumetric interpolated breath-hold examination (VIBE) images at the level of the middle phalanx of the right front foot of a horse with chronic foot lameness, before (A) and after (B) intravenous administration of gadolinium contrast material. There is an area of abnormal signal hyperintensity in the lateral lobe of the deep digital flexor tendon at the level of the proximal border of the navicular bursa (arrows). This lesion is enhanced by the administration of intravenous contrast as the relative signal intensity of the core lesion is increased in Figure B (arrow). (Courtesy of Dr. Carter Judy.)

of the insertion of the straight DSL to the middle scutum proximally through the tip of the distal phalanx distally. Transverse sequences are oriented perpendicular to the flexor surface of the navicular bone. Three other sequences supplement the basic dual echo and fat-suppressed sequences, including the 3-D transverse and dorsal T1-weighted spoiled gradient fast low angle shot sequences (FLASH) and an oblique transverse, fat-saturated PD echo.

The transverse FLASH sequence is oriented perpendicular to the flexor surface of the navicular bone and is intended to provide high detail information on the DDFT at this level (Figure 4.233). The dorsal FLASH sequence is oriented parallel with the flexor surface of the navicular bone and highlights the contour of the navicular bone in detail. It is particularly useful for the recognition of synovial invaginations and osseous fragments of the distal border of the navicular bone (Figure 4.234).

The oblique transverse, fat-saturated PD sequence is oriented perpendicular to the long axis of the collateral ligaments of the distal interphalangeal joint and aligned parallel with the solar surface of the foot. It is most suitable for detection of signal change and size variation in these ligaments. An additional, optional, fat-saturated PD sequence suitable for evaluation of the collateral ligaments can be oriented in the dorsal plane, parallel with the long axis of the collateral ligaments of the distal interphalangeal joint and at the same time perpendicular to the solar surface of the foot. An alternative protocol has been proposed using 3-D T2 gradient and T1-weighted spoiled gradient echoes in all 3 imaging planes supplemented with 1 or 2 fat-suppressed sequences.[16]

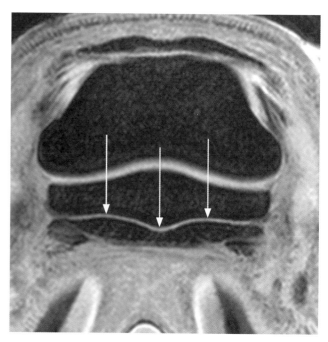

Figure 4.233. Transverse T1-weighted FLASH image with fat saturation at the level of the navicular bone, oriented perpendicular to its flexor surface. The thin slices of this sequence are ideal for detailed evaluation of the dorsal surface of the DDFT at the level of the navicular bone (arrows).

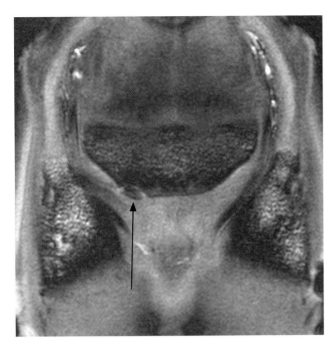

Figure 4.234. Dorsal T1-weighted FLASH image at the level of the navicular bone, oriented parallel with its flexor surface. The narrow slice thickness of this sequence allows for detailed evaluation of the distal border of the navicular bone for the presence of osseous fragments (arrow).

Lesion Incidence

There have been several reports on the incidence of injuries diagnosed with both low- and high-field MRI in horses with foot lameness that could not be elucidated with conventional imaging modalities. Some of these[7,21,24,43,46,68] are summarized in Table 4.8. Overall, injury of the DDFT was the most commonly observed lesion with MRI with a total incidence ranging from 30% to 64%. Navicular bone lesions were the next most common diagnosis (8% to 77%), followed by injuries of the collateral ligaments of the distal interphalangeal joint (6% to 43%). These numbers reflect the total incidence of each injury and do not imply that each lesion encountered was considered the primary cause of lameness. Abnormalities in the distal interphalangeal joint and navicular bursa were diagnosed frequently in 2 low-field studies[43,46] but less commonly in high-field studies. Injuries to all other structures occurred with markedly lower frequency, generally in less than 10% of horses. The absence of significant abnormalities was mentioned in 4 studies and a diagnosis was not made in up to 14% of horses in these studies. Although MRI is the most sensitive and specific diagnostic modality for the diagnosis of injuries of all tissues in the horse's foot,[51] not all causes of foot lameness can be readily identified (Table 4.8).

Table 4.8. Incidence of MRI findings in 7 retrospective MRI studies of foot lameness. The total incidence of each lesion is represented, rather than only the incidence of lesions considered as the primary cause of lameness. Several horses had simultaneous incidence of more than one lesion.

MRI lesions % total incidence	Mair et al. 2003[43] N = 35	Sherlock et al. 2007[72] N = 41	Dyson et al. 2005[21] N = 199*	Dyson et al. 2007[23] N = 347*	Boswell et al. 2006[7] N = 170	Mitchell et al. 2006[46] N = 98	Schramme and Redding 2009[68] N = 172*
DDFT tendinitis	49	29	60	48	52	64	30
Navicular disease	31	32	19	29	8	77	50
CL desmitis DIP joint	6	7	31	43	23	21	16
Navicular bursitis	—	17	—	—	—	49	1
Collateral sesamoidean desmitis	14	10	—	10	—	13	8
Distal sesamoidean impar desmitis	9	—	10	15	1	4	6
DIP joint synovitis/OA	23	37	3	2	9	68	9
Bone bruising middle or distal phalanx	—	5	7	4	6	2	3
Distal sesamoidean desmitis	6	—	1	2	1	—	2
Distal annular desmitis	—	—	—	—	—	—	4
Multiple injuries	NS	15	17	33	4	NS	24
No abnormalities detected	14	12	NS	NS	6	NS	10

* = high-field MRI system, DDFT = deep digital flexor tendon, CL = collateral ligament, DIP = distal interphalangeal, OA = osteoarthritis, NS = not specified.

MRI Abnormalities in the Foot

Tendinitis of the DDFT

The normal DDFT can clearly be seen as a well delineated, bi-lobed, elliptical structure of homogeneous low signal (black) on all transverse and sagittal MR images. A generalized signal increase at the insertion of the DDFT can be caused by the magic angle effect distal to the distal border of the navicular bone, where the tendon changes its orientation and comes to lie close to 55° relative to the main magnetic field (Figure 4.226).[10,78]

The MRI appearance of the normal DDFT has a strong left-to-right-limb as well as medial-to-lateral-lobe symmetry of both signal intensity and cross-sectional area measurements.[49] The cross sectional area of the distal portion of the DDFT increases with the body weight and height of the horse.[49] The DDFT is characterized by the presence of a dorsal zone of T1 and PD signal hyperintensity, both at the level of the navicular bone and proximal to the navicular bone.[66] At the level of the navicular bone, the layer of T1 signal hyperintensity is very thin and cannot be differentiated on T1-weighted images from the hyperintense palmar fibrocartilage of the navicular bone, except when saline contrast bursography is used.[66] Proximal to the navicular bone the dorsal zone of T1 and PD signal hyperintensity occupies up to 30% of the dorsopalmar dimension of the tendon. This zone coincides with the presence of a dorsal layer of fibrocartilage rich in elastic fibers.[3]

Tendon damage is seen as focal or diffuse, marginal or central, intratendinous signal increase on both T1- and T2-weighted sequences, that is variably accompanied by swelling of the affected lobe in the acute stage of injury.[17] Lesions may occur at the insertion to the distal phalanx, at the level of the flexor surface of the navicular bone, proximal to the navicular bone, or in any combination of these 3 levels at the same time. Lesions are frequently restricted to 1 lobe.

There is a good correlation between the MRI appearance of DDFT lesions and their pathological classification into core lesions, sagittal plane splits, insertional lesions, and dorsal surface lesions.[4,11,51,65] Core lesions (Figure 4.235) result in focal, circular areas of signal increase in the center of or near the dorsal border of the affected lobe, and are completely surrounded by normal, low-intensity tendon signal. Core lesions mostly occur proximal to the proximal border of the navicular bone.

Sagittal plane splits (Figure 4.236) form linear hyperintensities of variable depth arising from the dorsal surface of the tendon and progressing palmarly in the sagittal plane of the limb. Splits are mostly seen at the level of the flexor surface and proximal to the proximal border of the navicular bone. The presence of a core lesion or a parasagittal split at the insertion constitutes an insertional injury (Figure 4.237). In addition, insertional enthesopathy can result in cortical irregularity, caused by focal bone loss or enthesiophyte formation at the insertion of the DDFT to the flexor surface of the distal phalanx, and in diffuse signal loss in the cancellous bone, caused by localized palmar sclerosis of the distal phalanx.

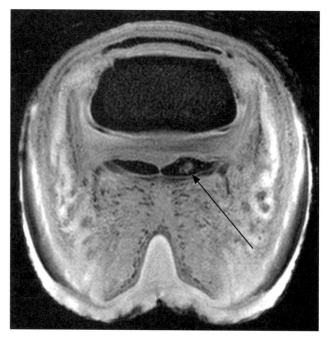

Figure 4.235. Transverse T1-weighted FLASH image with fat saturation of the right front foot at the level of the middle phalanx of a horse with acute onset foot lameness. The lateral lobe of the DDFT is enlarged and contains a core lesion characterized by a central, circular area of signal hyperintensity (arrow) surrounded by normal, low intensity, tendon signal.

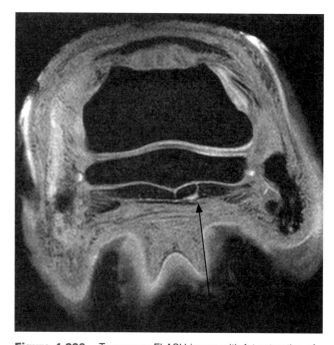

Figure 4.236. Transverse FLASH image with fat saturation of the right foot at the level of the navicular bone of a horse with acute onset foot lameness. A linear signal hyperintensity arises from a defect in the dorsal surface of the deep digital flexor tendon and progresses in a dorsopalmar direction, resulting in a full-thickness parasagittal split of the lateral lobe (arrow).

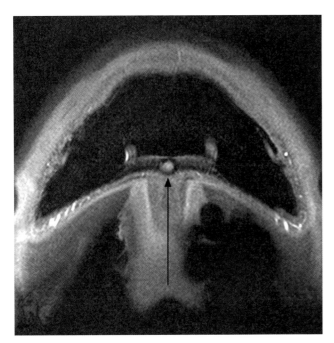

Figure 4.237. Transverse FLASH image with fat saturation of a foot at the level of the insertion of the deep digital flexor tendon onto the distal phalanx of a horse with foot lameness. A hyperintense core lesion is present in the central part of the tendon (arrow) and extends distally to the bone-tendon interface.

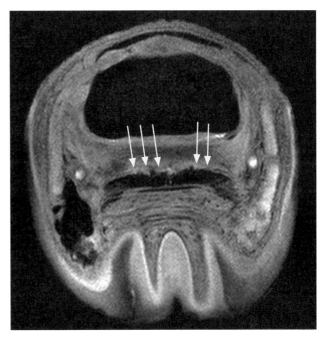

Figure 4.238. Transverse FLASH image with fat saturation of the foot at the level of the middle phalanx of a horse with foot lameness. The dorsal surface of the deep digital flexor tendon is irregular due to the presence of fibrillations and short, incomplete sagittal splits disrupting the smooth dorsal contour of the tendon (arrows).

Superficial fibrillations of the dorsal border of the DDFT (Figure 4.238) are characterized by irregularity of the dorsal margin of the tendon where it apposes the flexor surface of the navicular bone, consisting of small sagittal plane splits or punctate focal hyperintensities at the flexor surface-tendon interface. More severe erosive lesions cause signal increase extending from the dorsal border toward the center of the affected lobe. Dorsal fibrillations of the DDFT may be accompanied by adhesions between the dorsal surface of the tendon and the palmar surface of the CSLs and the DSIL within the navicular bursa. Other signs of navicular bursitis accompanying damage to the dorsal surface of the DDFT include fluid increase in the proximolateral and proximomedial pouches of the bursa and thickening and proliferation of the bursal synovium in the proximal recess of the navicular bursa. Thickening of the CSLs and the DSIL may also be seen. Lesions of the flexor cortex of the navicular bone are frequently accompanied by adhesions between the navicular bone and the dorsal surface of the DDFT (Figure 4.241).

In the chronic stages of healing by fibrosis, signal intensity in core lesions generally decreases in T2-weighted sequences, but remains hyperintense in T1-weighted sequences. In some cases of DDFT injury in the foot, focal intralesional signal hyperintensity remained present on T1-weighted sequences for more than 12 months, in spite of histological evidence of mature scar tissue.[65] Therefore, a focal area of abnormally high signal in the DDFT on a T1-weighted sequence that is not accompanied by high signal on the corresponding T2 and fat-suppressed images may reflect a previous chronic or healed injury without current inflammation or myxoid degeneration.

Lesions of the Navicular Bone

MR images of the navicular bone in horses with navicular bone disease may show 1 or more of 3 main abnormalities: remodeling changes in the medulla, degenerative changes of the flexor border, and osteochondral fragments of the distal border. The most common type of abnormality seen in the navicular bones of horses with recent onset navicular syndrome is STIR signal hyperintensity in the medullary cavity of the navicular bone with or without additional areas of T2 and PD signal hypointensity (Figure 4.239).[64]

Medullary STIR hyperintensity is best seen on fat-suppressed images and has been referred to as fluid signal or bone edema.[11,64] It has been speculated that bone edema may be an acute inflammatory or post traumatic finding in horses with recent onset navicular syndrome.[64] However, in pathological studies, MRI evidence of bone edema in navicular bones was usually not associated with acute inflammation but with evidence of chronic osteonecrosis, medullary fibrosis, loss of trabecular structure, thickening of trabeculae, prominent capillary infiltration, and, in some horses, adipose tissue necrosis.[3,11]

In one pathological study, all but 1 horse with medullary STIR hyperintensity had concurrent degenerative changes of the flexor surface of the navicular bone.[65] However, these pathological studies did not include horses with recent onset lameness and it therefore remains possible that medullary STIR hyperintensity can represent acute inflammatory fluid in the medullary cavity of the navicular bone.[64]

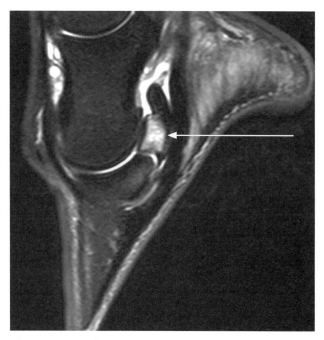

Figure 4.239. Sagittal STIR image of the foot of a horse with lameness that is abolished by anesthesia of the palmar digital nerves. There is marked STIR hyperintensity of cancellous bone in the medullary cavity of the navicular bone (arrow), indicating the presence of abnormal medullary fluid, medullary fibrosis, or medullary fat necrosis.

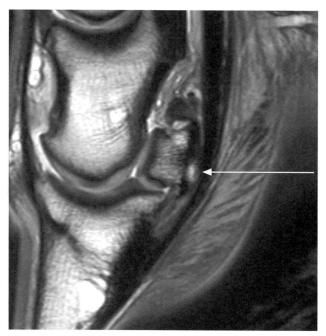

Figure 4.240. Sagittal proton density image of the foot of a horse with chronic navicular bone degeneration. There is localized signal hyperintensity in the distal third of the flexor border of the navicular bone due to loss of cortical bone and the presence of fibrous tissue and bursal synovial fluid in the defect (arrow). There is diffuse loss of signal in the medullary cavity of the navicular bone due to osteosclerosis. There is loss of separation between the palmar surfaces of the thickened collateral sesamoidean and distal sesamoidean impar ligaments on the one hand, and the dorsal surface of the deep digital flexor tendon on the other, suggestive of abnormal adherence between these structures.

Medullary STIR hyperintensity may be focal near the distal border of the navicular bone, or extend from the distal border in a vertical band along the palmar cortex to the proximal border of the bone, or spread diffusely throughout the medullary cavity. Based on the extent and intensity of intra-osseous STIR hyperintensity, medullary bone edema can be graded from mild to severe. Lower grades of medullary STIR hyperintensity have been encountered in nonlame control limbs, but severe medullary edema pattern was strongly associated with the presence of lameness.[51,64] Areas of signal hypointensity may also be seen in the medullary cavity of the navicular bone and may be focal or diffuse. Loss of T1 signal represents replacement of medullary fat by fluid, whereas loss of T2 and PD signal indicates the presence of medullary mineralization and sclerosis, usually in response to degenerative changes of the flexor surface of the navicular bone.

In horses with chronic navicular syndrome, the most common MRI abnormality is the presence of abnormal signal hyperintensities at the level of the flexor border of the navicular bone (Figure 4.240).[65] This can be a subtle, focal increase caused by synovial fluid pooling at a site of early fibrocartilage loss and thinning, best seen on PD or T2-weighted images. MRI bursography with saline has been shown to improve the conspicuity of fibrocartilage lesions.[66] Signal increase at the flexor surface can also be more extensive and extend deeper within the cortical bone of the flexor cortex when cortical bone erosion is present (Figure 4.240). Focal bone loss from the flexor surface is best seen on fat-suppressed images. These flexor cortex lesions may not be easily detected radiographically.[73] In affected horses, there is usually concurrent irregularity of the normally smooth endosteal surface of the flexor cortex, especially opposite the site of focal signal increase of the palmar surface. Fibrocartilage loss at the palmar aspect of the flexor surface of the navicular bone is also frequently accompanied by fibrillation of the dorsal aspect of the DDFT. Areas of advanced fibrocartilage and cortical bone loss from the flexor surface of the navicular bone are prone to adhesion formation to the dorsal surface of the DDFT (Figure 4.241).

Another form of navicular bone disease may be caused by the presence of osseous fragments at the distal border of the navicular bone (Figure 4.234).[65] Motion between the fragment and parent bone can cause a remodeling response in the adjacent distal margin of the navicular bone that may be reflected by the presence of localized STIR hyperintensity, T2 and PD hypointensity, and an irregular cortical and endosteal outline, especially when these fragments are large. A distal border fragment accompanied by focal medullary bone edema and sclerosis of the navicular bone is likely to be associated with lameness.

Smaller distal border fragments may be asymptomatic, especially if there is no MRI evidence of remodeling of the distal border of the navicular bone adjacent to the fragment. In horses with a complete navicular

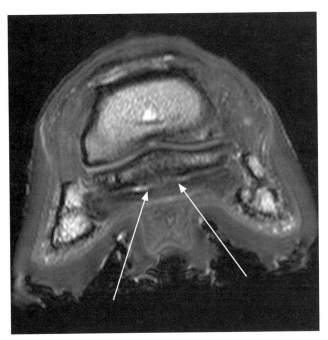

Figure 4.241. Transverse T2 gradient echo image of the foot of a horse with chronic navicular bone disease. The palmar border of the navicular bone is irregular due to degenerative erosion of the flexor cortex. There is sclerosis of the medullary cavity of the navicular bone. The normal hyperintense synovial fluid layer separating the palmar border of the navicular bone from the dorsal surface of the deep digital flexor tendon is interrupted by hypointense fibrous adhesions between both surfaces (arrows).

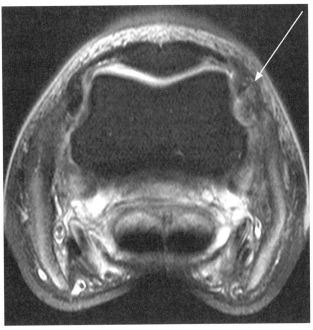

Figure 4.242. Transverse proton density image with fat saturation oriented parallel with the solar surface of the foot of a horse with collateral desmitis of the distal interphalangeal joint. The affected collateral ligament is enlarged and its margins are irregular (arrow). There is loss of architecture, and irregular areas of signal hyperintensity are dispersed throughout the cross section of the ligament (arrow).

bone fracture, MRI can demonstrate the fracture configuration on 3-D images and elucidate whether any associated damage to the DDFT is present, prior to possible attempts at surgical repair.

Lesions of the Collateral Ligaments of the Distal Interphalangeal Joint

Normal collateral ligaments can be seen as well delineated elliptical structures of homogeneous low signal with smooth endosteal margins at the origin and insertion on most transverse MR images. They also appear as curved banana-shaped bands on dorsal images that are obtained in an image plane parallel with the direction of the collateral ligaments and perpendicular to the solar surface of the foot. Symmetry between the lateral and medial collateral ligaments is used as a normal baseline reference, although lateromedial differences are possible due to anatomical variation. In order for lateromedial symmetry to form an accurate basis for assessment, it is critical that transverse image planes transect both collateral ligaments at the same level. Any deviation from accurate symmetrical positioning results in asymmetry in signal intensity and shape, especially at the proximal extent of the ligaments, and may lead to an inaccurate diagnosis of collateral desmitis. Signal asymmetry at the proximal aspect of the collateral ligament may occur even with perfect slice positioning, because the collateral ligaments may be of different thickness and length.[19,20,53]

Desmitis is characterized by increased cross-sectional area, irregular contour, and increased signal intensity of the collateral ligament (Figure 4.242).[19,31,92] Because there may be normal adaptive asymmetry in size between both collateral ligaments,[20] altered signal intensity and contour are more selective criteria for desmitis than size changes. The medial collateral ligament is more frequently affected than the lateral[19,20]. Signal hyperintensity can be diffuse or focal.

Enlargement and signal increase of a collateral ligament are best recognized on transverse T1-weighted or PD images in a high-field magnet. However, enlargement and signal increase of a collateral ligament must also be evaluated in transverse T2-weighted spin echo images and fat-suppressed images to verify whether signal increase is truly caused by tissue damage.

High signal on a T1-weighted gradient echo sequence that is not accompanied by high signal on the corresponding T2-weighted and STIR images is not a reliable indicator of injury. High intraligamentous signal on a T1-weighted gradient sequence can be caused by the variable orientation of collagen fibers in the collateral ligament that results in a variation in signal intensity. Intraligamentous signal hyperintensity on T1-weighted gradient sequences only may also reflect the presence of scar tissue from a previous, old injury. High signal on both T1 and T2 images represents injury that may be acute or chronic. STIR hyperintensity indicates the presence of acute injury.

Damage at the origin or insertion of a collateral ligament causes signal alteration in the adjacent bone. In approximately 40% of cases of collateral ligament disease, osseous abnormalities are identified on MRI. These osseous abnormalities can consist of cortical and endosteal irregularities or defects, osseous cyst-like lesions, abnormal mineralization, or fluid-like signal in cancellous bone adjacent to the origin or insertion of the collateral ligament. Avulsion of a collateral ligament from its insertion on the distal phalanx results in pooling of hyperintense synovial fluid from the distal interphalangeal joint in the defect, outlining the distal stump of the collateral ligament (Figure 4.243). Collateral desmitis of the distal interphalangeal joint may occur in conjunction with severe ossification of the collateral cartilages.[45] Signs of osteoarthritis or misalignment of the distal interphalangeal joint caused by subluxation associated with collateral ligament injury may occur but are rare.

Since the first report of MRI diagnosis of collateral desmitis of the distal interphalangeal joint,[19] several authors have identified the high incidence of normal signal variation in this anatomical structure. This variation is due to the heterogeneous fiber orientation in ligaments[81] and the prevalence of magic angle effect in this structure.[75,77] Unless MRI signs of both osseous and ligamentous abnormalities are evident, it may be difficult to establish the clinical significance of mild signal changes in collateral ligaments. Corroborating scintigraphic evidence of bone remodeling at the attachment sites of the collateral ligament can be a helpful finding to strengthen the diagnosis.

Lesions of the Distal Sesamoidean Impar Ligament (DSIL)

The anatomy of the DSIL renders it difficult to interpret accurately on MR images, especially low-field images. It is composed of individual fiber bundles with interdigitations of the synovial membrane and fluid of the distal interphalangeal joint, and small branches of the palmar digital arteries. The presence of multiple fluid-fiber interfaces in this small ligament results in a high susceptibility to partial volume averaging. Therefore, increased signal intensity within the DSIL is not necessarily synonymous with a lesion, unlike in other ligaments. In addition, the ligament is thicker and more intimately apposed to the dorsal border of the DDFT axially than abaxially, which may confound identification of ligament thickening and adhesion formation. Although one study identified abnormalities in the DSIL of 36% of horses examined,[64] desmitis of this ligament is rarely considered the primary cause of lameness.

Clear signs of pathology of the DSIL include marked thickening, extensive adhesion of the palmar surface of the ligament to the dorsal surface of the DDFT, and osseous signal irregularities at the insertion of this ligament to the distal phalanx. These osseous irregularities include increased fluid signal, sclerosis, new bone production, or bone lysis (Figure 4.244). Occasionally there may be focal fluid signal or mineralization in the navicular bone adjacent to the origin of the DSIL. Generalized thickening of the DSIL and adhesions between the DSIL and the DDFT occur most commonly in association with marked pathology of the DDFT and may be

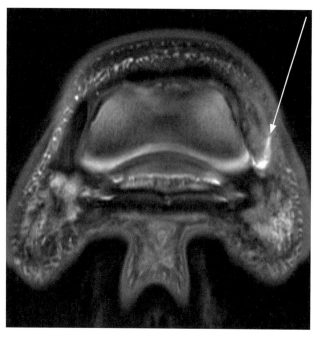

Figure 4.243. Oblique transverse proton density image of the foot of a horse with collateral desmitis of the distal interphalangeal joint. Slice direction is perpendicular to the flexor surface of the navicular bone. There is pooling of hyperintense synovial fluid in a defect resulting from avulsion of collateral ligament fibers from their insertion on the distal phalanx (arrow). There is enlargement, loss of architecture, increased signal intensity, and loss of margination of the affected ligament. The hyperintense fluid outlines the distal stump of the torn collateral ligament (arrow).

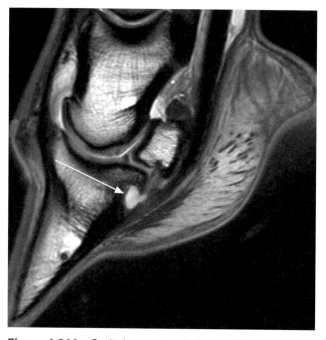

Figure 4.244. Sagittal proton density image of the central part of the foot of a horse with chronic foot lameness. There is localized signal hyperintensity in an osseous cyst-like lesion at the insertion of the distal sesamoidean impar ligament to the distal phalanx, indicating chronic enthesopathy of this ligament (arrow).

an integral part of secondary generalized bursal inflammation.

Lesions of the Collateral Sesamoidean Ligaments (CSLs)

It has been reported that the paired CSLs have uniform low intensity signal in all image sequences and are symmetrical in thickness medially and laterally.[61] However, the presence of signal hyperintensity is a common, normal variation on all sequences, especially near the insertion to the proximal border of the navicular bone. Signal heterogeneity in the CSLs may be due to magic angle effect because of variable fiber orientation or fibrocartilaginous metaplasia within the ligament.[3,78] The dorsal and palmar borders of the ligaments are clearly demarcated by the adjacent high signal of fluid in the palmar recess of the distal interphalangeal joint and the navicular bursa in PD, T2-weighted, and fat-suppressed sequences.

CSL injury may be evident as an altered shape with signal heterogeneity in the body of the ligament. Uniaxial thickening of a CSL is most easily identified when the paired ligament is normal (Figure 4.245). Generalized thickening of the CSL and loss of separation due to adhesions between the palmar surface of the ligament and dorsal surface of the DDFT occur most commonly in association with pathology of the dorsal surface of the DDFT and/or pathology of the navicular bone, and may be an integral part of secondary generalized inflammation of the navicular bursa with resulting periligamentous swelling.

Primary injury to the CSL is rare and seems to occur mainly as an enthesopathy characterized by new bone formation or focal STIR hyperintensity of the proximal border of the navicular bone. The prevalence of CSL desmitis has been reported as 75%, though it was only considered the primary cause of lameness in 15% of horses.[64]

Navicular Bursitis

Fluid in the navicular bursa produces high-intensity signal on all sequences except T1-weighted images. Some mild pooling of fluid can normally be observed in the proximolateral and proximomedial pouches of the navicular bursa. There is visible separation between the dorsal surface of the DDFT and the palmar surfaces of the collateral and distal impar sesamoidean ligaments in normal navicular bursae.

Navicular bursitis results in effusion with enlargement of the proximolateral and proximomedial pouches and sometimes in dorsal deviation of the central part of the CSLs. Fibrous scar tissue formation can be present in the distended synovial outpouchings and may indicate the presence of chronic bursitis. Lack of separation between the dorsal surface of the DDFT and the palmar surface of the CSLs is suggestive of bursitis with adhesion formation in the proximal recess of the navicular bursa. MRI bursography improves the conspicuity of adhesions in the navicular bursa by separating the DDFT from the palmar surfaces of the navicular bone and its associated ligaments.[42,66] The presence of

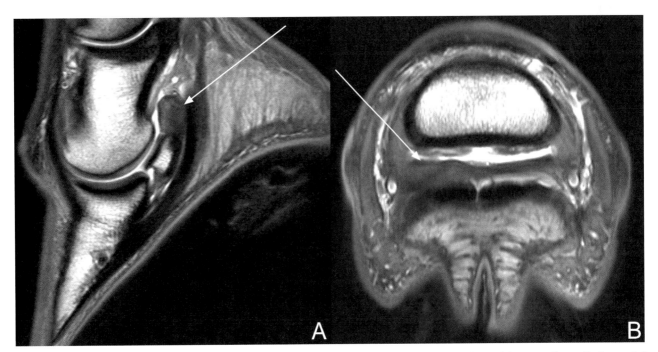

Figure 4.245. Sagittal proton density image lateral to the sagittal midline (A) and transverse proton density image at the level of the proximal aspect of the navicular bursa (B) of the left foot of a horse with chronic lameness that can be eliminated by anesthesia of the palmar digital nerves. The lateral collateral sesamoidean ligament contains areas of increased signal intensity and is markedly thickened (arrows) in comparison with the medial ligament. Swelling has resulted in loss of separation between the palmar surface of the lateral collateral sesamoidean ligament and the dorsal surface of the lateral lobe of the deep digital flexor tendon. The presence of adherence between both structures cannot be ruled out.

adhesions in the proximal and distal recesses of the navicular bursa is usually associated with pathology of the dorsal surface of the DDFT and/or the palmar surface of the navicular bone and is frequently accompanied by thickening of the CSLs and the DSIL. Simple distension of the navicular bursa is a frequent nonspecific finding in many horses irrespective of the primary injury site.[21] It is rarely considered the primary cause of lameness.[64]

Lesions of the Distal Interphalangeal Joint

The presence of joint distension can be readily deduced from enlargement of the dorsal and palmaroproximal outpouchings of the distal interphalangeal joint with fluid. Distension may cause palmar deviation of the axial part of the CSLs. Distension of the dorsal joint pouch is generally more prominent in standing horses than in recumbent horses. Distension of the distal interphalangeal joint is a frequent nonspecific finding in many horses irrespective of the primary injury site.[21,64]

The distal interphalangeal joint usually has smoothly curved articular surfaces. These curved articular surfaces make it difficult to assess the articular cartilage accurately due to partial volume averaging, so that focal cartilage defects may be missed. Cartilage lesions may be observed as cartilage surface irregularity, cartilage thickness change, or focal increase in signal intensity caused by pooling of synovial fluid in a cartilage defect (Figure 4.246).

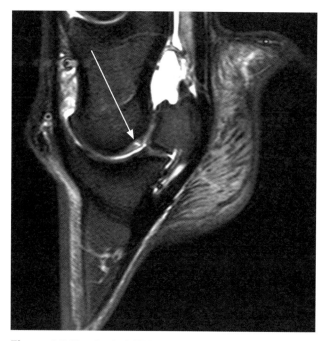

Figure 4.246. Sagittal STIR image of the central part of the right foot of a horse with lameness that can be abolished with intra-articular anesthesia of the distal interphalangeal joint. There is a focal signal hyperintensity within the hyaline cartilage layer of the distal articular surface of the middle phalanx (arrow). This focal signal increase is caused by pooling of synovial fluid within an articular cartilage defect. An oblique full-thickness cartilage cleft was identified at necropsy.

Altered surface contour of cartilage can only be assessed accurately in areas where the articular surface is relatively flat and not affected by partial volume averaging across the width of the MRI slice. Signal changes in small cartilage lesions can be subtle and are best seen on PD and T2-weighted images. Careful slice-per-slice comparison with the contralateral limb is necessary. Altered thickness of the subchondral bone plate, bone signal increase on fat-suppressed images, and endosteal irregularity may be useful indicators for the presence of an adjacent area of cartilage damage. Small osseous cyst-like lesions with STIR hyperintensity can be present in the central weight-bearing part of the distal phalanx. Osteophytes may be visible as small spur formations on the extensor process of the distal phalanx, palmar margin of the middle phalanx, and dorsoproximal border of the navicular bone.

Lesions of the Distal and Middle Phalanges

Osseous trauma to the phalanges is most often seen on MR images as focal or diffuse STIR hyperintensity on fat-suppressed images and hypointensity on T1-weighted images. It is commonly referred to as bone bruising. Signal intensity may initially also be high on T2-weighted sequences and gradually diminishes as reactive mineralization occurs in the area of the bone bruise. There is usually associated increase in radiopharmaceutical uptake on scintigraphic images.

Bone bruises of the phalanges occur mostly in the region of the palmar process of the distal phalanx[21] and the dorsodistal aspect of the middle phalanx.[57] Bone bruises of the palmar processes of the distal phalanx can be associated with irregularity of the cortical margin and disruption of the adjacent laminar architecture. Mineralization of a palmar process of the distal phalanx is usually seen in conjunction with other MRI abnormalities. Bone bruising of the dorsodistal aspect of the middle phalanx is becoming more commonly diagnosed as a cause of foot lameness (Figure 4.247).[84] The bruise usually involves a well circumscribed area of cancellous bone adjacent to the dorsal half of the distal interphalangeal joint and can be located axially or abaxially in the middle phalanx.

MRI may identify incomplete or complete fractures of the phalanges that are not visible radiographically because the fracture plane does not coincide with the direction of the standard radiographic projections.

Osseous cyst-like lesions are seen as well demarcated, hyperintense subchondral bone defects surrounded by a diffuse region of bone with hypointense signal.[44] The content of the osseous cyst-like lesions is usually hyperintense on all sequences consistent with proteinaceous fluid. Recently, osseous cyst-like lesions of the distal phalanx have been described in the subchondral bone, at the insertion of the collateral ligaments of the distal interphalangeal joint, and at the insertion of the DSIL.[44] The clinical significance of osseous cyst-like lesions in the phalanges may not always be clear but their presence is frequently associated with lameness.[44]

Other Abnormalities

The straight DSL has a thickened appearance distally and frequently contains a focal triangular area of

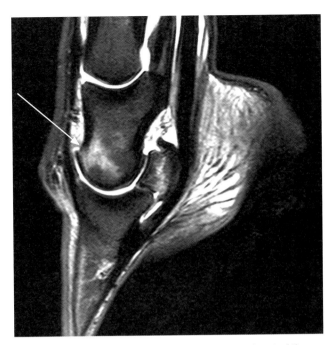

Figure 4.247. Sagittal STIR image of the central part of the foot of a horse with acute onset foot lameness. There is an area of marked signal hyperintensity at the dorsodistal aspect of the middle phalanx adjoining the articular surface of the distal interphalangeal joint (arrow). This appearance is suggestive for the presence of bone edema or a localized bone bruise of the middle phalanx.

increased signal intensity close to its insertion in normal horses, which may be difficult to distinguish from desmitis. Isolated cases of desmitis of the distal and proximal digital annular ligaments,[13] proximal ligament of the digital cushion, chondrocompedal ligament, and chondrosesamoidean ligament have also been observed.[68] MRI characteristics of desmitis consist of focal or diffuse thickening, focal or diffuse areas of signal hyperintensity, and occasionally adhesion formation.

MRI can accurately evaluate which structures have been damaged following a puncture wound to the solar surface of the foot. Damage to the DDFT from a puncture wound may result in long-term pain even after resolution of infection and healing of the solar defect. MRI evidence of a previous puncture wound may consist of focal areas of hypointense signal in the solar soft tissues typical of hemosiderin deposition, with severe focal lesions penetrating the DDFT and DSIL.[6]

MRI may also improve visualization of pathology associated with chronic laminitis. Signs that were consistently observed with MRI but not radiography included evidence of laminar disruption, circumscribed areas of laminar gas, laminar fluid, bone medullary fluid, increased size and number of vascular channels, and alterations in the coronary corium.[49]

Lesions that Are Poorly Detectable with MRI

Some tissue abnormalities in the foot do not show up well on MR images. Abnormalities of the hoof and sensitive laminae of the solar and heel regions of the foot may not result in obvious signal abnormalities. Although some marked subsolar abscesses or bruises may result in laminar and osseous signal increase in the solar region of the foot, many horses with solar pain responsive to application of hoof testers may have unremarkable foot MR images. Similarly, horses with poor dorsopalmar foot balance resulting in palmar heel pain may produce unremarkable MRI scans. Early hyaline or fibrocartilage degeneration in the distal interphalangeal joint or navicular flexor surface as well as mild fibrillation of the dorsal surface of the DDFT in the navicular bursa may also be difficult to identify.[65]

Pathological Validation of MRI of the Foot

The accuracy of MRI in depicting pathological lesions in the horse's foot has been reported in several studies as good to excellent.[3–5,11,21,51,54,65] Although differences exist due to system and operator variations, MRI was highly sensitive and specific for all abnormalities of the navicular bone and the DDFT, with exception of partial thickness fibrocartilage degeneration on the palmar surface of the bone and mild to moderate fibrillation of the dorsal surface of the DDFT within the navicular bursa, for which the sensitivity was low.[65] Cartilage degeneration in the distal interphalangeal joint proved difficult to diagnose, while abnormalities of the DSIL were easily overinterpreted.[65] MRI was also reasonably reliable for the diagnosis of collateral ligament damage, but some false negative results were reported.[26]

Comparison of High-field and Low-field MRI for the Foot

Pathological validation studies showing a high diagnostic accuracy for MRI in the equine distal limb have all been performed with 1.5-T high-field magnets.[3,4,11,54] The substantial investment required for purchase and maintenance of high-field systems makes them prohibitively expensive for widespread use in equine practice. Low-field MRI systems are cost-effective and, when correctly acquired, produce diagnostic studies.[7,31,43–45,72–74,82] A good agreement has been reported between the incidence of MRI lesions in the feet of lame horses with high- and low-field systems.[7] Nevertheless, high-field systems produce higher signal and therefore higher resolution and allow shorter acquisition times. Higher resolution of high-field images yields greater confidence in the diagnosis of lesions.[82] High-field systems have been calculated to improve contrast-to-noise ratio by 20% for T1-weighted images and up to 40% for T2-weighted images.[60]

Low-field MRI is less prone to susceptibility artifacts and magic angle effects at the insertion of the DDFT because the tendon is never oriented at 55° degrees to the main magnetic field in a standing foot. On the other hand, high-field MRI is less susceptible to magnetic field heterogeneity and partial volume averaging. The ability to reduce the effects of partial volume averaging by using thinner slices with high-field systems results in improved delineation of articular cartilage, flexor surface of the navicular bone, and the DSIL[82]. Low-field scans performed on standing horses are also particularly susceptible to motion artifacts, especially for regions proximal to the foot, in spite of the development of motion correction software.

Few studies are available to define the difference in diagnostic accuracy between high-field and low-field MRI systems for use in equine distal limbs.[55,83] One study of surgically created chondral and osteochondral defects in metacarpophalangeal joints concluded that cartilage defects could not be detected and that motion prevented accurate identification of small subchondral bone defects with low-field MRI.[83] Another study, using cadaver limbs of horses with distal limb lameness, found that anatomical structures appeared similar in both high- and low-field systems but that the margins of some structures were less clearly defined with low-field MRI, likely due to partial volume effect.[55] It was concluded that the level of detection of moderate to severe lesions in the foot was similar between high- and low-field systems. However, small tendon, articular cartilage, and ligament and bone lesions were better detected using a high-field system.[55]

MAGNETIC RESONANCE IMAGING OF THE FETLOCK REGION

Introduction

Conventional imaging techniques have limitations in the fetlock region. Radiography and scintigraphy are not capable of detecting early cartilage loss and subchondral bone injury without marked structural bone damage or demineralization,[23,74,90] and ultrasonographic evaluation lacks sensitivity for injuries of the straight and oblique DSLs.[63,76] Hence, MRI is being used increasingly to diagnose the causes of lameness in the fetlock region of horses.[23,29,63,74,76,90]

The primary indication for MRI of the fetlock region is pain localized to the fetlock region with diagnostic analgesia but without radiological or ultrasonographic abnormalities sufficient to explain the degree of lameness.[25] Some authors consider the presence of synovial effusion of the joint or digital flexor tendon sheath a stronger indication for endoscopic exploration than for MRI.[25] The normal MRI anatomy of the fetlock joint has been described.[25]

Imaging Protocol

An effective high-field fetlock protocol is shown in Table 4.7. This protocol consists of sagittal and transverse PD, T2-weighted, and inversion recovery fast spin echo sequences. Image planes extend from the proximal aspect of the suspensory ligament branches to a level just distal to the insertion of the oblique DSLs to the proximal phalanx. Limbs are placed in a neutral position with a dorsal fetlock angle of 180°. Transverse sequences are oriented perpendicular to the long axis of the third metacarpal/metatarsal bone (MC3/MT3) and parallel with the distal articular surface of the MC3/MT3. Additional transverse, sagittal, and dorsal 3-D T1-weighted spoiled gradient FLASH sequences can be used to provide high detail information on the flexor tendons and articular cartilage.

Table 4.9. Lesions identified with MR imaging in 40 horses with metacarpo(tarso)phalangeal region lameness in the order of incidence. Twenty-five horses had simultaneous occurrence of 2 or more injuries.

MRI Diagnosis (n = 40)	Incidence %
Subchondral bone injury	47.5
Distal sesamoidean desmitis	32
OA and cartilage injury	20
Suspensory branch desmitis	20
Osteochondral fragmentation	18
Proximal sesamoid bone injury	18
Intersesamoidean desmitis	10
DDFT tendinitis within DFTS	10
Collateral desmitis	7.5
SDFT tendinitis	5
Enostosis-like lesion	5
Palmar annular desmitis	2
Proximal digital annular desmitis	2
Dystrophic mineralization of LDET	2

OA = osteoarthritis, DDFT = deep digital flexor tendon, SDFT = superficial digital flexor tendon, DFTS = digital flexor tendon sheath, LDET = lateral digital extensor tendon.

Lesion Incidence

Studies on the incidence of MRI diagnoses in the fetlock region are scarce. The results of one study[29] are summarized in Table 4.9. The most common MRI diagnoses in the fetlock region were subchondral bone abnormalities of the distal metacarpus and lesions of the DSLs. Cartilage or osteochondral lesions in the fetlock joint and injuries of the suspensory ligament branches and proximal sesamoid bones were less common but also occurred with regular frequency. Abnormalities of subchondral bone and lesions of the DSLs were also frequently diagnosed in other reports.[23,63,76] Subchondral bone injuries can be diagnosed with low-field MRI[74] but there are currently no reports on low-field MRI studies of DSL injuries. Combinations of injuries are common in the fetlock region, with 63% of horses being identified with multiple MRI abnormalities. Concurrent soft tissue injuries were present in 65% of horses with subchondral bone injury, most commonly involving components of the suspensory apparatus.[29]

MRI Abnormalities in the Fetlock Region

Subchondral Bone Abnormalities

The subchondral bone thickness of the distal aspect of the MC3/MT3 varies from dorsal to palmar and

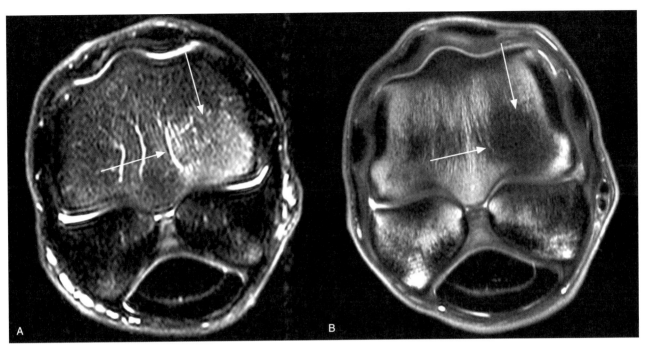

Figure 4.248. Transverse STIR image (A) and transverse proton density image (B) at the level of the proximal sesamoid bones of the right fore metacarpophalangeal joint of 2 different 3-year-old racehorses with fetlock lameness and abnormal MR signal in the palmar aspect of the lateral condyle of the third metacarpal bone. STIR signal hyperintensity suggestive of abnormal bone fluid is present in A (arrows), while an area of signal hypointensity indicates the presence of palmar osteosclerosis in B (arrows).

from abaxial to axial, being thinnest axially and thickest in the middle of each condyle, especially toward the palmar aspect.[25] Subchondral bone thickness of the distal aspect of the MC3/MT3 is likely to change with the type of exercise the horse performs. The subchondral bone thickness of the proximal phalanx increases slightly toward the palmar aspect of each condyle. There is reasonable symmetry in subchondral bone thickness of both the MC3/MT3 and proximal phalanx.

Abnormal MRI signal in subchondral bone is manifested as diffuse or focal signal increase in fat-suppressed images consistent with bone edema or bruising, and diffuse T1, PD, and T2 signal decrease consistent with trabecular thickening and osteosclerosis (Figure 4.248). Focal T1, PD, and T2 signal increase is observed in the presence of trabecular necrosis in osseous cyst-like lesions. Fluid-like signal in bone appears more commonly in the acute stage of injury, while sclerosis reflects more chronic bone damage with reactive remodeling. Focal osteonecrosis may be visible in the center of an area of sclerosis. When located close to the articular surface, osteonecrosis may lead to secondary articular cartilage loss from the palmar surface of the affected condyle of the MC3/MT3. Subchondral bone damage may or may not be associated with primary or secondary cartilage loss. Some authors consider the presence of post traumatic subchondral bone edema a risk factor for the development of degenerative articular cartilage lesions in human patients.[15,56]

Lesions are predominantly located in the medial condyle of the distal part of the MC3/MT3[29] with a preference for the palmar/plantar aspect of the condyle.[23,74,90] The dorsal aspect of the condyles may also be affected, especially in non racehorses.[29]

Distal Sesamoidean Ligament Injuries

The straight DSL has a heterogeneous appearance with multiple high and low signal areas spread throughout most of its length.[76] A normal small, homogeneous, triangular signal hyperintensity exists at the insertion of the straight DSL onto the middle phalanx. The oblique DSLs have heterogeneous signal intensity throughout their entire length to the insertion. The lateral oblique DSL is frequently larger and more hyperintense than the medial ligament.[76] In a standing horse, images of the proximal third of the oblique DSLs are susceptible to magic angle effect, especially medially. This effect results from the divergence of fibers within the proximal third of each oblique DSL, and the tendency for the medial oblique DSL to be at a more oblique angle to the vertical than the lateral oblique DSL. Magic angle effect results in increased signal intensity in the ligaments, thereby confounding image interpretation.[75]

The heterogeneity of the DSLs varies between individual horses.[76] Normal signal heterogeneity should not be confused with the presence of abnormal signal hyperintensity. Abnormal signal intensity in a lesion commonly covers a larger cross-sectional area than the focal signal hyperintensities caused by normal signal variation in the DSLs.[76] In contrast to anatomical focal signal hyperintensities, abnormal signal intensity in lesions can typically also be observed in more than 1 slice. Lesions within the oblique and straight DSLs can result in discrete or diffuse areas of signal hyperintensity within the

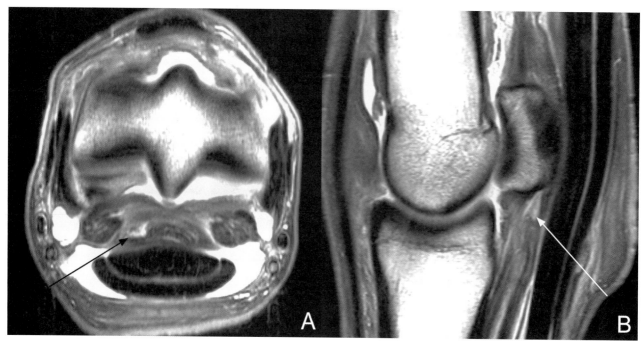

Figure 4.249. Transverse (A) and sagittal (B) proton density images of the metacarpophalangeal joint of a horse with chronic fetlock lameness. There is abnormal focal signal hyperintensity within the proximolateral aspect of the straight distal sesamoidean ligament (black arrow), indicative of local fiber disruption. The lesion originates at the distal border of the lateral proximal sesamoid bone (white arrow) and extends 11 mm distally.

body or along the edge of the affected ligament. One or multiple small core lesions with focal signal increase may be observed in affected ligaments, extending from 5 to 30 mm in a proximodistal direction (Figure 4.249). Enlargement of a ligament may also occur with or without abnormal signal increase, but this finding is less consistent. In 1 study, 30% of DSLs affected with desmitis were not enlarged.[29] Lesions may occur biaxially or bilaterally.

The location of lesions within ligaments and the distribution of lesions varies between studies.[29,63,76] Straight sesamoidean desmitis occurs more commonly in the distal part of the ligament, proximal to its insertion on the middle phalanx,[63,76] although proximal lesions near the origin were most common in 1 study (Figure 4.249).[29] Oblique distal sesamoidean desmitis can occur proximally or throughout the entire length of the ligament.[29,63,76] Cruciate distal sesamoidean desmitis is very rare.[76]

Reports suggest that distal sesamoidean desmitis is frequently regarded as the primary cause of lameness,[29,63] although 1 author considered lesions to be the sole cause of lameness in only 2 of 58 horses with evidence of desmitis.[76] The majority of horses with oblique or straight distal sesamoidean desmitis diagnosed with MRI do not have a palpable enlargement nor ultrasonographic abnormalities.[29,63,76]

Suspensory Ligament Branch Injuries

The suspensory ligament branches are paired triangular structures of low signal intensity that flatten in a dorsopalmar direction and widen lateromedially as they move distally toward their insertion on the proximal sesamoid bones. The margins of the branches are sharply delineated. Close to the insertion, the branches become D-shaped on cross section and faint, linear, high-intensity, dorsopalmar striations appear near the ligament-bone interface, possibly associated with the presence of adaptive fibrocartilaginous metaplasia at the insertion. A small hyperintense indentation may be present in the palmar border of the normal suspensory branch immediately proximal to its insertion. Suspensory branch lesions are characterized by an intraligamentous focus of signal hyperintensity in PD, T2, and STIR images, usually near the palmar/plantar border of the affected branch, with or without enlargement of the branch (Figure 4.250).

Injuries of the Proximal Sesamoid Bones

Abnormal MRI signal in the proximal sesamoid bones includes osteosclerosis, STIR hyperintensity consistent with bone edema or contusion, and focal trabecular bone loss associated with osseous cyst-like lesions at the attachment site of ligaments (Figure 4.251). Hyperintense lesions associated with osteolysis may be found at the axial margin of the proximal sesamoid bones in association with intersesamoidean desmitis. Osteophyte formation at the proximal and distal margins of the sesamoid bones may be present in association with osteoarthritis of the fetlock joint.

Articular Cartilage Abnormalities

The distal surface of the MC3/MT3 in the fetlock joint is the most difficult to image with MRI because of its curvature and the thin articular cartilage layer. This

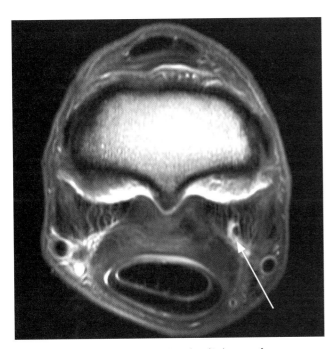

Figure 4.250. Transverse proton density image of a metatarsophalangeal joint of a horse with lameness localized to the fetlock region. There is a small, linear hyperintensity reflecting the presence of a tear in the plantar border of the lateral branch of the suspensory ligament (arrow).

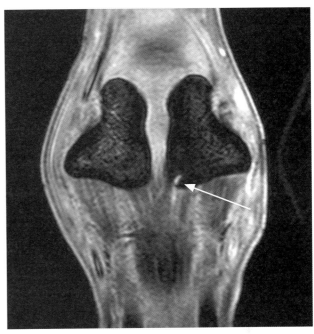

Figure 4.251. Dorsal FLASH image with fat saturation of the proximal sesamoid bones of a horse with lameness localized to the metacarpophalangeal joint. There is focal and intense signal hyperintensity at the base of the medial proximal sesamoid bone (arrow), indicative of a small osseous cyst-like lesion associated with a small vertical tear of the straight distal sesamoidean ligament.

Figure 4.252. Sagittal (A) and transverse (B) proton density images of the fetlock of a horse with chronic metacarpophalangeal joint lameness. There is an elliptical area of full-thickness cartilage loss on the dorsodistal aspect of the medial condyle of the third metacarpal bone (arrows). This is characterized by replacement of the normal hypointense cartilage layer with pooling of hyperintense synovial fluid in the cartilage defect (arrows). A wavy, thin, hypointense line overlying the cartilage defect may indicate the presence of pannus tissue along with synovial fluid (A).

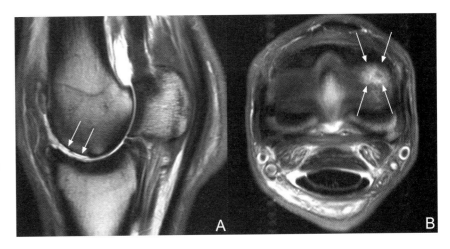

joint tests the limits of MRI systems and the capability to resolve fine detail.[83]

Cartilage lesions may occur as isolated focal injuries with localized cartilage loss and little evidence of osteoarthritis or as part of the disease complex of an osteoarthritic joint. Cartilage injury or degeneration resulting in wear lines or erosions is usually identified by the focal accumulation of hyperintense joint fluid in the cartilage defects on PD and STIR images. A focal, irregular island of fluid hyperintensity associated with pooling of synovial fluid in a chondral defect can sometimes be recognized on transverse PD, T2, or STIR images that are located exactly parallel with and through the affected articular surface (Figure 4.252B). Cartilage defects have been identified on all articular surfaces in the fetlock joint.[29] MRI tends to underestimate the size and extent of cartilage loss in the fetlock joint compared to arthroscopic findings.[29]

Osteophytes may be seen as contour changes of the proximal and distal articular margins of the proximal sesamoid bones and the dorsoproximal, lateral, and medial margins of the proximal phalanx. However, osteophytes may be more easily recognized on radiographs due to the radiographic summation effect and the better radiographic contrast between cortical bone and soft tissue attachments at the joint margins.

Osteochondral Fragmentation

Some osteochondral fragments from the dorsoproximal margin of the proximal phalanx and the basilar margin of the proximal sesamoid bones that are not visible radiographically may be recognized as focal, osseous hypointensities separated from parent bone on all sequences. Osseous fragments may be difficult to distinguish from end-on blood vessels near joint margins because both may appear hypointense on MR images. Avulsion fragments are always difficult to differentiate from the tendon or ligament in which they are embedded, due to the similarities in signal intensity between bone, tendon, and ligaments. Sagittal FLASH and PD images are most helpful in identifying osseous fragments.

Abnormalities of the Digital Flexor Tendon Sheath

Injuries to the superficial digital flexor tendon (SDFT) or DDFT in the digital flexor tendon sheath may be recognized as dispersed small, focal areas of signal hyperintensity, distinct hyperintense core lesions, thickening of the affected lobe(s), and/or longitudinal parasagittal splits of the lateral or medial border of the tendon with partial separation of the tendon margin (Figure 4.253). Lesions of the DDFT within the digital

flexor tendon sheath may continue distally into the navicular bursa and the insertion to the distal phalanx. Lesions of the SDFT within the digital flexor tendon sheath may extend into one of the branches of the tendon and its insertion on the middle scutum. Hyperintensities and contour changes of the flexor tendons within the digital sheath are most obvious in transverse FLASH images and frequently not visible ultrasonographically. Increased fluid distension and intrathecal soft tissue proliferation of the digital flexor tendon sheath and thickening and signal change in the palmar annular ligament of the fetlock have also been recognized.[29]

Other Abnormalities

Other injuries have been reported in the fetlock region with a lower incidence than those listed above, including desmitis of the intersesamoidean and collateral ligaments.[29] Intersesamoidean desmitis results in a large or small, focal, central area of hyperintensity within the intersesamoidean ligament in T2, PD, and STIR images (Figure 4.254). Loss of normal contour of the axial margin of the proximal sesamoid bones due to osteolysis can usually be seen as an area of intraosseous hyperintensity confluent with the area of signal increase in the intersesamoidean ligament.

Collateral desmitis is characterized by enlargement of the superficial or deep part of the collateral ligament relative to the contralateral limb and by the presence of hyperintensity in T2 and PD images in the affected part of the ligament. Signal increase may be difficult to recognize in the deep part of the collateral ligament because

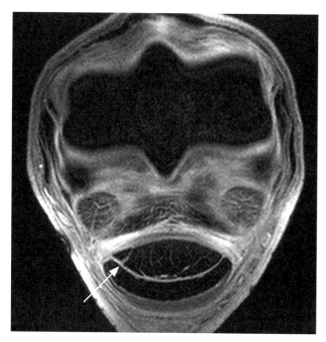

Figure 4.253. Transverse FLASH image with fat saturation immediately distal to the base of the proximal sesamoid bones of a horse with chronic lameness localized to the digital flexor tendon sheath. There is a small linear hyperintensity (arrow) compatible with the presence of a longitudinal tear of the lateral margin of the deep digital flexor tendon. The detached lateral margin of the tendon is slightly displaced. This lesion was confirmed and treated tenoscopically.

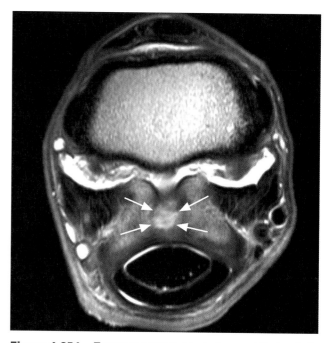

Figure 4.254. Transverse proton density image at the level of the apices of the proximal sesamoid bones of a horse with acute severe metacarpophalangeal joint lameness. There is a circular area of signal hyperintensity indicative of fiber disruption and desmitis in the intersesamoidean ligament (arrows).

this structure frequently appears hyperintense on PD and T1-weighted MR images. This phenomenon is most likely due to the presence of magic angle effect caused by the oblique fiber orientation in the deep part of the collateral ligament relative to the main magnetic field. Evidence of endosteal irregularity may be present at the origin of a collateral ligament. A small avulsion fragment at the base of the epicondylar fossa in association with collateral desmitis has been described.[29]

MAGNETIC RESONANCE IMAGING OF THE METACARPAL AND METATARSAL REGIONS

Introduction

Lameness from pain associated with the proximal palmar metacarpal and plantar metatarsal regions has been increasingly recognized in equine athletes. There are a number of differential diagnoses for proximal metacarpal/metatarsal pain, including avulsion fractures of the origin of the suspensory ligament, palmar or plantar proximal cortical stress fractures, proximal suspensory desmitis, desmitis of the accessory ligament of the DDFT, fractures of the proximal aspect of the splint bones, adhesions between the suspensory ligament and the axial margin of 1 of the splint bones, neuropathy of the deep branch of the lateral plantar nerve, and tendinitis of the SDFT or DDFT. Some of these lameness problems in the proximal metacarpal or metatarsal region have been difficult to diagnose accurately because affected horses frequently have no or equivocal radiological or ultrasonographic signs of disease.

Ultrasonography of the proximal palmar/plantar metacarpal/metatarsal regions may be difficult. The heterogeneous echogenicity of the proximal part of the suspensory ligament reflects its structure, which comprises striated muscle, connective tissue, adipose tissue, and vessels. It may not always be possible to distinguish between normal and structural abnormalities of the suspensory ligament using ultrasonography.[18] In addition, edge shadowing and refraction from the surrounding soft tissue structures as well as the axial aspect of the splint bones frequently causes interference during ultrasonographic examination of the proximal part of the suspensory ligament. Such problems are not encountered with MRI, which produces good soft tissue contrast and detail without superimposition and is able to visualize inflammatory fluid within bone, tendon, or ligaments when gross anatomic change has not yet occurred. Moreover, sectional images allow assessment of size and signal changes within the complex anatomy of this region, which is difficult to evaluate by palpation.

MRI Protocol

A useful high-field protocol for the metacarpal and metatarsal regions is shown in Table 4.7. This protocol consists of sagittal and transverse PD, T2-weighted, and inversion recovery fast spin echo sequences. Image planes extend from the proximal intertarsal/radiocarpal joint to the middle of the metacarpal/metatarsal region. Transverse slices are aligned parallel to the carpometacarpal/tarsometatarsal joint. The dorsal 3-D, T1-weighted, spoiled gradient fast low angle shot sequence (3D FLASH) is aligned perpendicular to the sagittal slices and parallel to the palmar/plantar aspect of the MC3/MT3. The 3-D FLASH sequence is used to evaluate the joint spaces and subchondral bone of the distal tarsal/carpal joints.

Lesion Incidence

The incidence of MRI diagnoses in horses with lameness localized to the proximal palmar/plantar metacarpal/metatarsal region[9,68] is summarized in Table 4.10. The most common cause of lameness in this anatomical region is proximal suspensory desmitis with or without evidence of bone injury at the level of the attachment of the suspensory ligament. Desmitis of the accessory ligament of the SDFT occurred as frequently as proximal suspensory desmitis in 1 report, especially in forelimbs.[9] The diagnosis of abnormalities of the distal tarsal region in horses with lameness localized to the proximal plantar metatarsal region indicates that local anesthetic techniques lack specificity for accurate localization of lameness in this area.[39]

MRI Abnormalities in the Proximal Metacarpal/ Metatarsal Regions

Proximal Suspensory Desmitis

The normal suspensory ligament is a low signal intensity structure of dense collagen fibers interspersed with more centrally located high signal intensity muscle fibers in both the fore- and hindlimbs and surrounded by a high signal intensity border composed of loose connective tissue, neurovascular structures, and adipose tissue.

There is substantial variation between the shape and structure of the suspensory ligament in fore- and hindlimbs.[1] In forelimbs, the suspensory ligament attaches primarily to the proximal palmar aspect of the third metacarpal cortex and to a lesser extent to the distal row of carpal bones. A high signal intensity sagittal dorsal cleft formed by loose connective and adipose tissue nearly divides the suspensory ligament into 2 branches just distal to its origin. The medial portion is mostly flat, while the lateral portion is thicker and rounder on transverse sections.

In hindlimbs, the suspensory ligament attaches mainly to the proximal plantar aspect of the third metatarsal cortex, with a few fibers attaching to the distal row of tarsal bones and a small separate lateral branch to the calcaneus. Near the origin, the suspensory ligament is more rounded and positioned more laterally on the plantar aspect of the MTIII than in forelimbs. The suspensory ligament also has a slightly bi-lobed structure but there is no significant difference between the thickness of the medial and lateral lobes in hindlimbs.[1] Bundles of muscle fibers and adipose tissue are situated centrally in each lobe of the suspensory ligament, starting immediately distal to the most proximal level of the origin and extending distally to the level of the bifurcation of both suspensory branches. Forelimb muscle fibers are initially aligned parallel to the palmar surface

Table 4.10. The primary MRI diagnoses made in horses with lameness localized to the proximal metacarpal/metatarsal region.

Primary MRI diagnosis % incidence	Schramme and Redding 2009[68] N = 56	Brokken et al. 2007[9] N = 45
Proximal suspensory desmitis without bone injury	37	27
Proximal suspensory desmitis and bone injury proximal MC3/MT3, MC4/MT4	11	24
Desmitis of the accessory ligament of the DDFT	—	33
Distal tarsal OA	13	—
Bone injury proximal MC3/MT3, MC4/MT4	9	2
Splint bone injury with focal suspensory desmitis	5	—
Central tarsal bone cyst	5	—
Focal tarsal bone edema	4	—
Enostosis-like lesions MC3/MT3	4	—
Proximal suspensory desmitis and desmitis of the accessory ligament of the DDFT	—	4
Desmitis of the accessory ligament and tendinitis of the DDFT	—	4
Dorsal injury MC3/MT3	2	—
Tendinitis of the DDFT	1	2
Effusion of the distal tarsal sheath		2
No obvious abnormalities	9	2

OA = osteoarthritis, DDFT = deep digital flexor tendon, MC3/MT3 = third metacarpal/metatarsal bone, MC4/MT4 = fourth metacarpal/metatarsal bone (Brokken et al. 2007, Schramme and Redding 2009).

of the MC3/MT3 and then curve roughly into 2 semilunar bundles, the concave sides facing each other. In the hindlimbs, the muscle bundles are more linear shaped and run roughly parallel in a dorsoplantar direction. The normal suspensory ligament does not contact the palmar/plantar metacarpal/metatarsal cortex at any point other than its origin.

Injuries to the origin and body of the suspensory ligament result in disruption of the normal, hypointense collagenous tissue by areas of signal hyperintensity, mainly in the central portion of the ligament (Figure 4.255). Abnormalities of the proximal part of the suspensory ligament are best seen in transverse PD images. Desmitis is usually associated with enlargement of the cross sectional area of the suspensory ligament but this may be mild. Because of the normal variation in both signal composition and size in the proximal part of the suspensory ligament, systematic comparison with the contralateral limb is very important.[9,39]

Lesions can be graded as mild, moderate, or severe, depending on the abnormal signal intensity and the proportion of total cross sectional area of the ligament that is affected. In 1 report, on average, lesions extended 13.2 to 51.1 mm distal to the tarsometatarsal joint with lesion length varying from 4.3 to 107 mm.[39] In many cases, evidence of bone injury at the attachment of the suspensory ligament to the proximal palmar/plantar

aspect of the MC3/MT3 can also be seen (Figure 4.256). Although thickening may result in a decrease of the space between the suspensory ligament and the MC3/MT3, periligamentous fibrosis and adhesion formation are uncommon.

The ability to visualize the margins of the entire suspensory ligament with MRI has enabled definitive diagnosis of adhesions between it and exostoses of the splint bones.[91] Adhesions are visible as low signal tissue connecting the suspensory ligament to the axial aspect of a splint bone exostosis, where ultrasonography is unable to determine the existence of abnormality. Normal horses have a distinct high signal intensity line of division between the suspensory ligament and the splint bones.

Osseous Injury to the Proximal Palmar/Plantar Cortex of the MC3/MT3

The normal proximal palmar/plantar metacarpal/metatarsal cortex has a uniform thickness and smooth periosteal and endosteal surfaces. Bone injury at the site of attachment of the suspensory ligament occurs most frequently in combination with proximal suspensory desmitis but can also be seen as an isolated injury.[9,39] Abnormalities indicative of a bone injury at the origin of the suspensory ligament include abnormal medullary

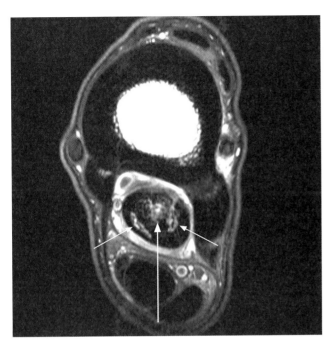

Figure 4.255. Transverse proton density image of the proximal metatarsal region of the right hindlimb of a horse with mild to moderate proximal suspensory desmitis. There is an abnormal area of diffuse signal increase in the central part of the suspensory ligament (long arrow). This must be distinguished from the 2 normal focal areas of high signal intensity associated with 2 muscle bundles in the suspensory ligament (short arrows).

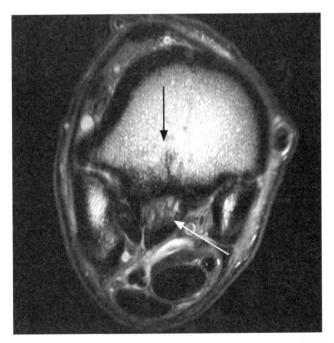

Figure 4.256. Transverse proton density image of the proximal metatarsal region of the left hindlimb of a horse with marked proximal suspensory desmitis and enthesopathy of the proximal plantar metatarsal cortex. There is a large central area of abnormal signal hyperintensity in the suspensory ligament (white arrow). There are irregular areas of low signal in the medullary cavity of the third metatarsal bone reflecting the presence of osteosclerosis (black arrow). The plantar metatarsal cortex is thickened and has an irregular endosteal margin.

signal hypointensity on transverse PD and T2-weighted images indicative of sclerosis (Figure 4.256), medullary STIR signal hyperintensity compatible with the presence of abnormal bone fluid, or a combination of both sclerosis and fluid. Horses with chronic lesions may also have evidence of thickening of the proximal palmar/plantar cortex and an irregular endosteal or periosteal contour (Figure 4.256). The palmar/plantar cortex may further contain focal high intensity signal indicative of trabecular bone loss resulting in an altered contour with a focal concave bone defect. Incomplete hairline stress fractures may also be seen. MRI evidence of bone injury is not limited to the proximal palmar/plantar metacarpal/metatarsal cortex but has also been encountered in the dorsal cortex of the MTIII, as well as the third and fourth tarsal and fourth metatarsal bones.[39]

Desmitis of the Accessory Ligament of the DDFT

The accessory ligament of the DDFT is a homogeneous, low signal structure on all spin echo sequences. This structure may be susceptible to magic angle effect on gradient echo sequences. As the accessory ligament of the DDFT extends proximally to its third carpal bone attachment, its overall signal intensity increases. The normal accessory ligament of the DDFT has clear margins on all sequences.

The transverse PD sequences are most useful in determining alterations in signal and shape of the accessory ligament. Comparison with the contralateral limb is essential to allow detection of subtle changes in signal and size. MRI signs of desmitis are enlargement and focal to diffuse intraligamentous signal hyperintensity. Lesions generally extend from 1 to 4 cm distal to the carpometacarpal joint.[9] Abnormalities of the DDFT may accompany desmitis of the accessory ligament. In horses with chronic desmitis, irregularity of the borders of the ligament and loss of the distinct high signal border between the accessory ligament and the DDFT may occur. Low signal scar tissue bridging the hyperintense space between the ligament and tendon is strongly indicative of adhesion formation.

Other Abnormalities

Other injuries have been reported in horses with lameness localized to the proximal palmar/plantar metacarpal/metatarsal region with a much lower incidence than those listed above (Table 4.10). These lesions usually involve the distal rows of tarsal bones and include focal osteoarthritic change, osseous cyst-like lesions, and bone edema of the third or central tarsal bones.[39] Spraining of the intertarsal ligament between the central and third tarsal bone has also been reported.[61] Occasionally focal fiber disruption without thickening is recognized with MRI in the SDFT and DDFT in the absence of ultrasonographic abnormalities.[39,62] These findings indicate the lack of specificity of diagnostic analgesia in this area.

The use of MRI has not yet been reported for the diagnosis of injuries to the SDFT and DDFT in the metacarpal region. It is becoming clear, however, that abnormal MRI signal may continue to be seen when a tendon has regained normal echogenicity, especially in short echo time sequences.[36,37,67] The clinical significance of this persistence of high signal intensity is still unclear but MRI may be more sensitive than ultrasonography for monitoring tendon repair. The T2 vs. T1 signal differences in healing tendon need further elucidation and may prove to be helpful in planning the rehabilitation of horses with tendon injuries more accurately. The use of a low-field standing magnet would have obvious advantages for repeated follow-up examinations without the need for general anesthesia, if the effect of motion can be adequately eliminated.

In conclusion, MRI is able to reveal more subtle bone and soft tissue changes than ultrasonography, which makes it more sensitive to lesions that have bone edema, mild sclerosis, little fiber disruption, or only mild enlargement. This is particularly useful in an area such as the proximal palmar/plantar metacarpal/metatarsal region where ultrasonographic examination is difficult. The improved diagnostic accuracy of MRI in comparison with ultrasonography should result in selection of a more specifically targeted treatment and a better outcome for horses with proximal palmar/plantar metacarpal/metatarsal pain.

MAGNETIC RESONANCE IMAGING OF THE CARPAL, TARSAL, AND STIFLE REGIONS

Although it is possible to obtain diagnostic MR images of areas proximal to the carpometacarpal and tarsometatarsal joints, few reports are available of *in vivo* results of carpal, tarsal, and stifle MRI in horses.[35,90] This is partly due to the practical problems that may arise when scanning proximal limb areas in horses. Images can potentially be obtained using high-field closed units, low-field open units, or low-field standing systems. The area of interest must be positioned within the isocenter of the magnet, and this creates logistical difficulties in some long, closed-bore, high-field magnets. If the distance from the edge of the magnet to the imaging portion is greater than the distance from the carpus, tarsus, or stifle to the chest or abdomen, then it may be impossible to gain diagnostic images. This problem does not occur with an open magnet, provided that the magnet shape is sufficiently wide to accommodate the area of interest. When MR images are obtained on standing sedated horses, increased movement at more proximal levels of the limb than the foot makes diagnostic quality imaging difficult.

Magnetic Resonance of the Carpal Region

A suitable protocol for MRI of the carpus is shown in Table 4.7. Other protocols with more emphasis on 3-D gradient echo scanning are also used.[52] The normal anatomy of the carpus has been described.[52] Spoiled gradient echo sequences were found to allow accurate measurements of cartilage thickness of the proximal articular surfaces of the proximal carpal bones.[50] In this study, it was more difficult to detect cartilage defects at the palmar aspect of the joint where articular surfaces were in close apposition than on the dorsal aspect where the articular surfaces were separated. There was variable thickness of the subchondral bone in the carpal

bones, most particularly in the medial facet of the third carpal bone. This likely reflects a difference in exercise history between horses, which should be taken into account when interpreting MR images.

Lesions detected with MRI in a cadaver study of horses with carpal lameness included cartilage erosions, subchondral bone fracture, subchondral bone defects, osseous cyst-like lesions, carpal bone chip fractures, intercarpal ligament injuries, hemorrhage, edema and thickening of the joint capsule, and adherence of synovium to the articular surface[52]. Intercarpal ligament damage was seen as loss of the linear structure of the ligaments with either increased signal intensity within the ligament on both T1- and T2- weighted images or low signal intensity on T1-weighted images with high signal intensity on T2-weighted images because of ligament disruption and infiltration of synovial fluid into the defect.

Magnetic Resonance of the Tarsal Region

MRI can be useful for evaluation of distal tarsal pain because there is a lack of correlation between the presence and severity of radiographic changes on the one hand and lameness on the other.[54] Protocols for MRI of the tarsus have been suggested[8] (Table 4.7) and equine tarsal MRI anatomy has been described using both low- and high-field systems.[2,8] In the normal tarsus, articular cartilage of the distal tarsal joints is very thin, which does not allow for distinction of proximal and distal cartilage layers in these joint spaces.[8] Subchondral bone plates of the distal tarsal bones and the MTIII have homogeneous, low signal intensity with a regular

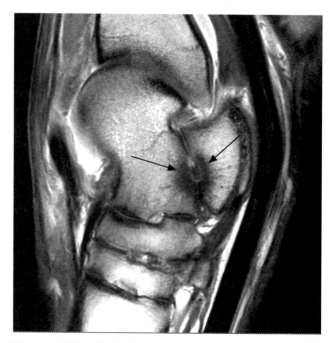

Figure 4.257. Sagittal proton density image of the tarsus of a horse with osteoarthritis of the talocalcaneal joint. There is localized loss of joint space and subchondral bone margins in the center of the joint. This lesion is surrounded by a wide irregular area of signal loss reflecting reactive osteosclerosis in both the talus and the sustentaculum tali of the calcaneus (arrows).

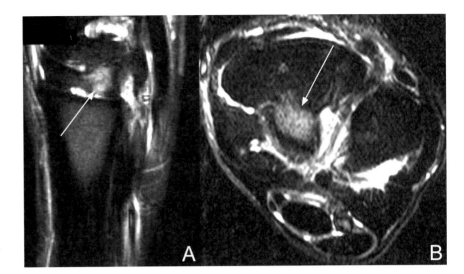

Figure 4.258. Sagittal (A) and transverse (B) STIR images of the right tarsus of a horse with acute onset hindlimb lameness. There is abnormal intra-osseous signal hyperintensity in the plantar aspect of the third tarsal bone (arrows), compatible with bone edema or a bone bruise.

osteochondral junction and a smooth but undulating deep border.[8] In competition horses that undergo high intensity training, subchondral bone thickness is greater medially in the distal intertarsal joint and laterally in the tarsometatarsal joint. This repeatable thickness pattern of subchondral bone is lost in horses with distal tarsal lameness.

There are no reports on the incidence of MRI diagnoses in the tarsus of live horses. In 1 cadaver study, MRI was more sensitive and specific than radiography for detection of all types of pathology of the distal tarsal joints, including intertarsal ligament pathology, cartilage erosion, osseous cyst-like lesions, and subchondral bone irregularity.[54] In live horses with lameness associated with the tarsal region, the presence of abnormal STIR signal hyperintensity compatible with the presence of bone bruising was reported in the central and third tarsal bones, talus, and tibia.[39,90]

In the authors' clinic, MRI of the tarsus has been helpful in the diagnosis of abnormalities that could not be detected radiographically or ultrasonographically. These abnormalities have included subchondral bone injury of the talocalcaneal joint (Figure 4.257), bone bruising of the distal tibia, intertarsal ligament enthesopathy with associated bone edema (Figure 4.258), focal osteoarthritis in the plantar aspect of the distal intertarsal (Figure 4.259) and talocalcaneal joints with localized loss of joint space and subchondral bone sclerosis, desmitis of the collateral ligaments of the tibiotarsal and the proximal intertarsal joints, and tendinitis of the DDFT at the level of the calcaneus.[68]

Magnetic Resonance of the Stifle Region

The MRI anatomy of the stifle has been described in cadaver limbs. MRI with a 1.5-T magnet allowed for detailed evaluation of the cranial and caudal cruciate ligaments, medial and lateral menisci, meniscotibial and meniscofemoral ligaments, long digital extensor tendon, and patellar ligaments.[32] In addition, MR images provided excellent resolution of articular cartilage and subchondral bone.[32]

MRI of the stifle is only rarely possible in live horses. One study reports clinical MRI of the stifle in horses

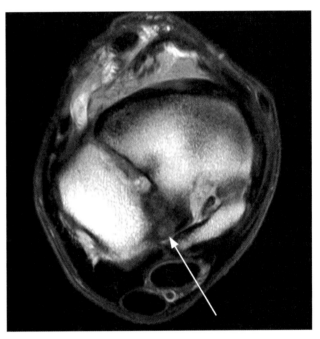

Figure 4.259. Transverse proton density image through the proximal row of tarsal bones of the left tarsus of a horse with focal osteoarthritis of the interosseous articulation between the central and fourth tarsal bones. There is loss of joint space and subchondral bone outline surrounded by a margin of irregular osteosclerosis of the fourth and central tarsal bones (arrow).

with a femur length greater than 44 cm, tibial length greater than 44 cm, and pelvic width less than 62 cm in a 1.5-T ultra-short (95-cm), wide-bore (70-cm) magnet (Siemens Magnetom Espree™, Siemens Medical Solutions Inc., Malvern, PA, USA).[35]

Abnormalities identified on MR images of clinical cases have included tearing of the medial meniscus (Figure 4.260), desmitis of the cranial and caudal cruciate ligaments, desmitis of the patellar ligaments, collateral ligament desmitis, synovitis, synovial effusion, bone bruising of the femur or tibia (Figure 4.260), osteochondral fragmentation, and focal cartilage

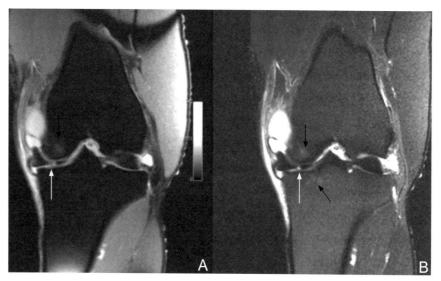

Figure 4.260. Dorsal proton density image with fat saturation (A) and dorsal STIR image (B) of the left stifle of a horse with a tear of the cranial horn of the medial meniscus (white arrows). There is intra-osseous signal hyperintensity in the medial femoral condyle and the axial margin of the medial tibial plateau, suggestive of abnormal bone fluid (black arrows). (Courtesy of Dr. Carter Judy.)

erosions.[35] This technique has enormous potential for diagnosis of complex injuries of the stifle because many of the soft tissue structures of the joint cannot be evaluated comprehensively with any other imaging modality. However, further developments in bore width and length are needed before stifle MRI can become a routine imaging examination for horses.

CONCLUSION

MRI has revolutionized equine diagnostic imaging and clearly highlighted the potential shortfalls of both radiography for bone and ultrasonography for imaging soft tissue lesions. The challenge has now become to select the correct treatment for the specific diagnosis made possible with MRI and to develop improved treatment modalities for those conditions in which MRI has led to a better understanding of the diagnosis, pathogenesis, clinical progression, and outcome.

References

1. Bischofberger AS, Konar M, Ohlertht S, et al. Magnetic resonance imaging, ultrasonography and histology of the suspensory ligament origin: a comparative study of normal anatomy of Warmblood horses. Equine Vet J 2006;38:508–516.
2. Blaik MA, Hanson RR, Kincaid SA, et al. Low-field magnetic resonance imaging of the equine tarsus: normal anatomy. Vet Radiol Ultrasound 2000;41:131–141.
3. Blunden TS, Dyson SJ, Murray RM et al. Histopathology in horses with chronic palmar foot pain and age-matched controls. Part 1: Navicular bone and related structures. Equine Vet J 2006;38:15–22.
4. Blunden TS, Dyson SJ, Murray RM et al. Histopathology in horses with chronic palmar foot pain and age-matched controls. Part 2: The deep digital flexor tendon. Equine Vet J 2006;38:23–27.
5. Blunden A, Murray R, Dyson S. Lesions of the deep digital flexor tendon in the digit: a correlative MRI and post mortem study in control and lame horses. Equine Vet J 2009;41:25–33.
6. Boado A, Kristoffersen M, Dyson S, et al. Use of nuclear scintigraphy and magnetic resonance imaging to diagnose chronic penetrating wounds in the equine foot. Equine Vet Educ 2005;17:62–68.
7. Boswell JC, Schramme MC, Murray RM, et al. Low or high-field MRI in equine lameness diagnosis. In Proceedings European College of Veterinary Surgeons 2005;14:189–194.
8. Branch M, Murray RC, Dyson SJ, et al. Magnetic Resonance Imaging of the Equine Tarsus. Clin Tech Equine Pract 2007;6:96–102.
9. Brokken MT, Schneider RK, Sampson SN, et al. Magnetic resonance imaging features of proximal metacarpal and metatarsal injuries in the horse. Vet Radiol Ultrasound 2007;48:507–517.
10. Busoni V, Snaps F. Effect of deep digital flexor tendon orientation on magnetic resonance imaging signal intensity in isolated equine limbs—the magic angle effect. Vet Radiol Ultrasound 2002;43:428–430.
11. Busoni V, Heimann M, Trenteseaux J, et al. Magnetic resonance imaging findings in the equine deep digital flexor tendon and distal sesamoid bone in advanced navicular disease—an *ex vivo* study. Vet Radiol Ultrasound 2005;46:279–286.
12. Chandnani VP, Ho C, Chu P, et al. Knee hyaline cartilage evaluated with MR imaging: a cadaveric study involving multiple imaging sequences and intra-articular injection of Gadolinium and saline solution. Radiology 1991;178:557–561.
13. Cohen JM, Schneider RK, Zubrod CJ, et al. Desmitis of the distal digital annular ligament in seven horses: MRI diagnosis and surgical treatment. Vet Surg 2008;37:336–44.
14. Cohen ZA, McCarthy DM, Kwak SD, et al. Knee cartilage topography, thickness, and contact areas from MRI: *in-vitro* calibration and *in vivo* measurements. Osteoarth and Cart 1999;7:95–109.
15. Costa-Paz M, Muscolo DL, Ayerza M, et al. Magnetic resonance imaging follow-up study of bone bruises associated with anterior cruciate ligament ruptures. Arthroscopy 2001;17:445–449.
15. Dyson S, Murray R, Schramme M, et al. Magnetic resonance imaging of the equine foot: 15 horses. Equine Vet J 2003;35:18–26.
16. Dyson S, Murray R, Schramme M, et al. Lameness in 46 horses associated with deep digital flexor tendinitis in the digit: diagnosis confirmed with magnetic resonance imaging. Equine Vet J 2003;35:681–690.
17. Dyson S. Proximal metacarpal and metatarsal pain: a diagnostic challenge. Equine Vet Educ 2003;15:134–138.
18. Dyson SJ, Murray RC, Schramme M, et al. Collateral desmitis of the distal interphalangeal joint in 18 horses (2001–2002). Equine Vet J 2004;36:160–166.

19. Dyson S, Murray R. Collateral desmitis of the distal interphalangeal joint in 62 horses (January 2001–December 2003). In Proceedings Am Assoc Equine Pract 2004;50:248–256.

20. Dyson S, Murray R, Schramme M. Lameness associated with foot pain: results of magnetic resonance imaging in 199 horses (January 2001–December 2003) and response to treatment. Equine Vet J 2005;37:113–121.

22. Dyson SJ, Blunden T, Murray RM et al. Current concepts of navicular disease. Equine Vet Educ 2006;18:45–56.

23. Dyson SJ, Murray R. Osseous trauma in the fetlock region of mature sports horses. Proceedings Am Assoc Equine Pract 2006;52:443–456.

24. Dyson SJ, Murray RC. Magnetic resonance imaging evaluation of 264 horses with foot pain: the podotrochlear apparatus, deep digital flexor tendon and collateral ligaments of the distal interphalangeal joint. Equine Vet J 2007;39:340–343.

25. Dyson SJ, Murray RM. Magnetic resonance imaging of the equine fetlock. Clin Tech Equine Pract 2007;6:62–77.

26. Dyson SJ, Blunden T, Murray R. The collateral ligaments of the distal interphalangeal joint: magnetic resonance imaging and post mortem observations in 25 lame and 12 control horses. Equine Vet J 2008;40:538–44.

27. Edelman R, Hessenlink J, Zlatkin M, et al. In Clinical Magnetic Resonance Imaging, 3rd ed. Elsevier Health Sciences, Philadelphia. 2006;358–409.

28. Ferrel EA, Gavin PR, Tucker RL, et al. Magnetic resonance for evaluation of neurologic disease in 12 horses. Vet Radiol Ultrasound 2002;43:510–516.

29. Gonzalez L, Schramme M, Redding WR, et al. MRI features of metacarpo(tarso)phalangeal region lameness in 40 horses. Vet Radiol Ultrasound 2010;51:404–414.

30. Guckel C, Jundt G, Schnabel K, et al. Spin-echo and 3D gradient-echo imaging of the knee joint: a clinical and histopathological comparison. Eur J Radiol 1995;21:25–33.

31. Gutierrez-Nibeyro SD, White NA II, Werpy NM, et al. Magnetic resonance imaging findings of desmopathy of the collateral ligaments of the equine distal interphalangeal joint. Vet Radiol Ultrasound 2009;50:21–31.

32. Holcombe SJ, Bertone AL, Biller DS, Haider V. Magnetic resonance imaging of the equine stifle. Vet Radiol Ultrasound 1995;36:119–125.

33. Holmes SP. MR cartilage imaging. In Proceedings American College of Veterinary Surgeons 2009;19:48–52.

34. Judy CE, Saveraid TC, Rodgers E, et al. Characterization of foot lesions using contrast enhanced equine orthopedic magnetic resonance imaging. In Proceedings Am Assoc Equine Pract 2008;54:459.

35. Judy CE. Magnetic resonance imaging of the equine stifle in a clinical setting. In Proceedings American College of Veterinary Surgeons 2008;18:163–166.

36. Karjaleinen P, Ahovuo J, Pihlajamaki H, et al. Post operative MR imaging and ultrasonography of surgically repaired Achilles tendon ruptures. Acta Radiologica 1996;37:639–646.

37. Kasashima Y, Kuwano A, Katayama Y, et al. Magnetic resonance imaging application to live horse for diagnosis of tendonitis. J Vet Med Sci 2002;64:577–582.

38. Kawahara Y, Uetani M, Nakahara N, et al. Fast spin-echo MR of the articular cartilage in the osteoarthritic knee. Correlation of MR and arthroscopic findings. Acta Radiol 1998;39:120–5.

39. Labens R, Schramme MC, Robertson ID, et al. Clinical, magnetic resonance, and sonographic imaging findings in horses with proximal plantar metatarsal pain. Vet Radiol Ultrasound 2010;51:11–18.

40. Li J, Zheng ZZ, Li X, et al. Three Dimensional Assessment of Knee Cartilage in Cadavers with High Resolution MR-Arthrography and MSCT-Arthrography. Acad Radiol 2009;16:1049–1055.

41. Link TM, Stahl R, Woertler K. Cartilage imaging: motivation, technique, current and future significance. Eur Radiol 2007;17:1135–1146.

42. Maher MC, Werpy NM, Goodrich LR, et al. Distension of the navicular bursa to determine the presence of adhesions using magnetic resonance imaging. In Proceedings Am Assoc Equine Pract 2008;54:460–461.

43. Mair TS, Kinns J, Jones RD et al. Magnetic resonance imaging of the distal limb of the standing horse: Technique and review of 40 Cases of Foot Lameness. In Proceedings Am Assoc Equine Pract 2003;49:29–41.

44. Mair TS, Sherlock CE. Osseous cyst-like lesions in the feet of lame horses: diagnosis by standing low-field magnetic resonance imaging. Equine Vet Educ 2008;20:47–56.

45. Mair TS, Sherlock TE. Collateral desmitis of the distal interphalangeal joint in conjunction with concurrent ossification of the cartilages of the foot in nine horses. Equine Vet Educ 2008;20:485–492.

46. Mitchell RD, Edwards RB, Makkreel LD, et al. Standing MRI lesions identified in jumping and dressage horses with lameness isolated to the foot. Proc Am Assoc Equine Pract 2006;52:422–426.

47. Munk B, Madsen F, Lundorf E, et al. Clinical magnetic resonance imaging and arthroscopic findings in knees: a comparative prospective study of meniscus anterior cruciate ligament and cartilage lesions. Arthroscopy 1998;14:171–5.

48. Murray R, Dyson SJ, Schramme, M. et al. Magnetic resonance imaging of the equine digit with chronic laminitis. Vet Radiol Ultrasound 2003;44:609–617.

49. Murray RC, Roberts BL, Schramme MC, et al. Quantitative evaluation of equine deep digital flexor tendon morphology using magnetic resonance imaging. Vet Radiol Ultrasound 2004;45:103–111.

50. Murray RC, Branch MV, Tranquille C, et al. Validation of magnetic resonance imaging for measurement of equine articular cartilage and subchondral bone thickness. Am J Vet Res 2005;66:1999–2005.

51. Murray RM, Blunden TS, Schramme MC, et al. How does magnetic resonance imaging represent histologic findings in the equine digit? Vet Radiol Ultrasound 2006;47:17–31.

52. Murray RM. Magnetic resonance imaging of the equine carpus. Clin Tech Equine Pract 2007;6:86–95.

53. Murray RM, Dyson SJ. Image interpretation and artifacts. Clin Tech Equine Pract 2007;6:16–25.

54. Murray RM, Dyson S, Branch M, et al. Validation of magnetic resonance imaging use in equine limbs. Clin Tech Equine Pract 2007;6:26–36.

55. Murray RM, Mair TS, Sherlock CE, et al. Comparison of high-field and low-field magnetic resonance images of cadaver limbs of horses. Vet Rec 2009;165:281–288.

56. Nakamae A, Engebretsen L, Bahr R, et al. Natural history of bone bruises after acute knee injury: clinical outcome and histopathological findings. Knee Surg Sports Traumatol Arthrosc 2006;14:1252–1258.

57. Olive J, Mair TS, Charles B. Use of standing low-field magnetic resonance imaging to diagnose middle phalanx bone marrow lesions in horses. Equine Vet Educ 2009;21:116–123.

58. Palmer WE. MR arthrography: Is it worthwhile? Top Magn Res Imaging. 1996;8:24–43.

59. Rangger C, Kathrein A, Freund M, et al. Bone bruise of the knee. Histology and cryosections in 5 cases. Acta Orthop Scand 1998;69:291–294.

60. Rutt BK, Lee DH. The impact of field strength on image quality in MRI. J Magn Reson Imaging 1996;6:57–62.

61. Sampson SN, Schneider RK, Tucker RL. Magnetic resonance imaging of the equine distal limb, In Equine Surgery, 3rd ed. Auer JA, Stick JA, eds. Elsevier, Philadelphia. 2006;946–963.

62. Sampson SN, Tucker RL. Magnetic resonance imaging of the proximal metacarpal and metatarsal regions. Clin Tech Equine Pract 2007;6:78–85.

63. Sampson SN, Schneider RK, Tucker RL, et al. Magnetic resonance imaging features of oblique and straight distal sesamoidean desmitis in 27 horses. Vet Radiol Ultrasound 2007;48:303–311.

64. Sampson SN, Schneider RK, Gavin PR, et al. Magnetic resonance imaging findings in horses with recent onset navicular syndrome but without radiographic abnormalities. Vet Radiol Ultrasound 2009;50:339–346.

65. Schramme MC, Murray RM, Blunden TS, et al. A comparison between magnetic resonance imaging, pathology and radiology in 34 limbs with navicular syndrome and 25 control limbs. In Proceedings Am Assoc Equine Pract 2005;51:348–358.

66. Schramme M, Kerekes Z, Hunter S, et al. Improved identification of the palmar fibrocartilage of the navicular bone with saline magnetic resonance bursography. Vet Radiol Ultrasound 2009;50:606–614.

67. Schramme M, Kerekes Z, Hunter S, et al. Tendon injury and repair evaluated by high-field magnetic resonance imaging in a surgical model of tendinitis of the superficial digital flexor tendon of horses. Vet Radiol Ultrasound 2010;51:280–287.

68. Schramme and Redding (2009) unpublished data.
69. Shalabi A, Kristoffersen-Wiberg M, Aspelin P, et al. MR evaluation of chronic Achilles tendinosis. A longitudinal study of 15 patients preoperatively and two years postoperatively. Acta Radiol 2001;42:269–276.
70. Shalabi A, Kristoffersen-Wiberg M, Papadogiannakis N, et al. Dynamic contrast-enhanced MR imaging and histopathology in chronic Achilles tendinosis. A longitudinal MR study of 15 patients Acta Radiol 2002;43:198–206.
71. Shalabi A. Magnetic resonance imaging in chronic Achilles tendinopathy. Acta Radiol 2004;45:1–45.
72. Sherlock CE, Kinns J, Mair TS. Evaluation of foot pain in the standing horse by magnetic resonance imaging. Vet Rec 2007;161:739–744.
73. Sherlock C, Mair T, Blunden T. Deep erosions of the palmar aspect of the navicular bone diagnosed by standing magnetic resonance imaging. Equine Vet J 2008;40:684–692.
74. Sherlock CE, Mair TS, Braake F. Osseous lesions in the metacarpo(tarso)phalangeal joint diagnosed using low-field magnetic resonance imaging in standing horses. Vet Radiol Ultrasound 2009;50:13–20.
75. Smith MA, Dyson SJ, Murray RC. Is a magic angle effect observed in the collateral ligaments of the distal interphalangeal joint or the oblique sesamoidean ligaments during standing magnetic resonance imaging? Vet Radiol Ultrasound.. 2008;49: 509–515.
76. Smith S, Dyson SJ, Murray RC. Magnetic resonance imaging of distal sesamoidean ligament injury. Vet Radiol Ultrasound 2008;49:516–528.
77. Spriet M, Mai W, McKnight A. Asymmetric signal intensity in normal collateral ligaments of the distal interphalangeal joint in horses with a low-field MRI system due to the magic angle effect. Vet Radiol Ultrasound 2007;48:95–100.
78. Spriet S, McKnight A. Characterization of the magic angle effect in the equine deep digital flexor tendon using a low-field magnetic resonance system. Vet Radiol Ultrasound 2009;50:32–36.
79. Tehranzadeh J, Ashikyan O, Anavim A, et al. Enhanced MR imaging of tenosynovitis of hand and wrist in inflammatory arthritis. Skeletal Radiol 2006;35:814–822.
80. Tucker RL, Sampson SN. Magnetic resonance imaging protocols for the horse. Clin Tech Equine Pract 2007;6:2–15.
81. Werpy NM, Ho CP, Kawcak CE, et al. Review of principles and clinical applications of magnetic resonance imaging in the horse. Proceedings Am Assoc Equine Pract 2006;52:427–440.
82. Werpy NM. Magnetic resonance imaging of the equine patient: A comparison of high- and low-field systems. Clin Tech Equine Pract 2007;6:37–45.
83. Werpy NM, Ho CP, Pease A, et al. Preliminary study on detection of osteochondral defects in the fetlock joint using low and high-field strength resonance imaging. Proc Am Assoc Equine Pract 2008;54:447–451.
84. Werpy NM. Diagnosis of middle phalanx bone marrow lesions in horses using magnetic resonance imaging and identification of phase effect cancellation for proper image interpretation. Equine Vet Educ 2009;21:125–130.
85. Westbrook C, Kraut C. In MRI in Practice, 2nd ed. 1998. Blackwell Scientific Ltd, Oxford.
86. White LM, Sussman MS, Hurtig M, et al. Cartilage T2 assessment: differentiation of normal hyaline cartilage and reparative tissue after arthroscopic cartilage repair in equine subjects. Radiology 2006;241:407–14.
87. Wright I, Kidd L, Thorp B. Gross, histological and histomorphometric features of the navicular bone and related structures in the horse. Equine Vet J 1998;30:220–234.
88. Zanetti M, Bruder E, Romero J, et al. Bone marrow edema pattern in osteoarthritic knees: correlation between MR imaging and histologic findings. Radiology 2000;215:835–840.
89. Zlatkin MB. Techniques for MR imaging of joints in sports medicine. Magnetic Resonance Imaging Clinics of North America 1999;7:1–21.
90. Zubrod CJ, Schneider RK, Tucker RL, et al. Use of magnetic resonance imaging for identifying subchondral bone damage in horses: 11 cases (1999–2003). J Am Vet Med Assoc 2004;224: 411–418.
91. Zubrod CJ, Schneider RK, Tucker RL. Use of magnetic resonance imaging to identify suspensory desmitis and adhesions between exostoses of the second metacarpal bone and the suspensory ligament in four horses. J Am Vet Med Assoc 2004;224: 1815–1820.
92. Zubrod, CJ, Farnsworth KD, Tucker RL, et al. Injury of the collateral ligaments of the distal interphalangeal joint diagnosed by magnetic resonance. Vet Radiol Ultrasound 2005;46:11–16.

COMPUTED TOMOGRAPHY

Anthony P. Pease and W. Rich Redding

INTRODUCTION

Computed tomography (CT) imaging, also known as "CAT" scanning (computerized axial tomography), combines the use of a digital computer with a rotating X-ray generator to create detailed cross sectional images or slices of the different organs and parts of the body. Tomography is from the Greek word "tomos," meaning slice or section, and "graphia," meaning to describe.

Computed tomography is based on the principals of X-ray generation and their interaction with tissue. X-rays are directed through the body and absorbed or attenuated at differing levels, creating a matrix or profile of X-ray beams of different strength. In standard radiographs generated by film-screen systems, the X-ray passes through the body part to an intensifying screen that emits light which interacts with emulsion on film. However, in the case of CT, the film-screen system is replaced by a banana-shaped detector that measures the X-ray profile of the differential X-ray absorption by each tissue. This CT technology allows the detection of thousands of differences of X-ray absorption of tissues, called Hounsfield units or CT numbers, which can be used to differentiate fat from fluid and even soft tissue.

CT is so sensitive that it is capable of discriminating tissues with density differences of as little as 0.5%, whereas at least 10% change in density difference is necessary before radio-opaque differences can be seen radiographically. This ability is termed contrast resolution and it is far superior compared to film-screen combinations. In addition, rather than having a stationary X-ray tube with conventional radiography, the X-ray tube is rotated around the patient to allow for a cross-sectional image to be produced, eliminating superimposition.

IMAGING BENEFITS OF CT

CT is unique in its ability to image a combination of soft tissue, bone, and blood vessels at a high resolution. However, in equine medicine it is probably most frequently used to demonstrate bony abnormalities. For example, conventional X-ray imaging of the head can only show the bone structures of the skull, though all of the structures are superimposed, such as the nasal cavity and sinuses (Figure 4.261).[4–6,10] Therefore, orthogonal radiographs as well as oblique radiographs

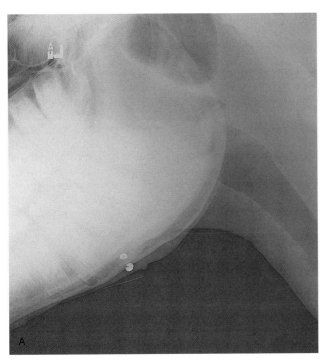
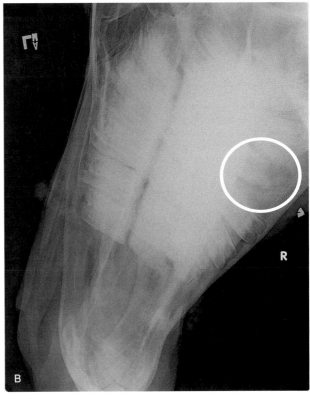

Figure 4.261. Lateral (A) and oblique (B) radiograph of a horse with a mandibular draining tract. Radiopaque markers have been placed at the level of the draining tract in (A). Note that due to superimposition, limited information about the occlusive surface of the bone can be obtained. In (B) the apex of the tooth root has a lucent region (white circle) indicating that a tooth root abscess is present, but the extent cannot be seen.

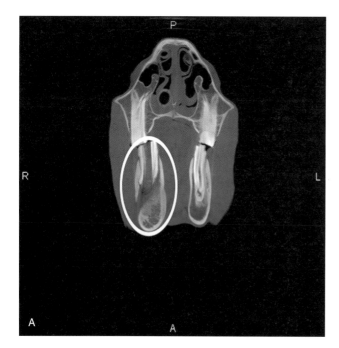

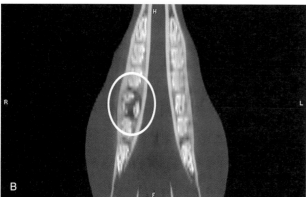

Figure 4.262. A. Transverse CT scan of the same horse as in Figure 4.261. Note the separation of the tooth along the sagittal plane and the communication with the ventral aspect of the mandible (circle). This horse had a sagittal fracture of tooth 408 (fourth right mandibular premolar). A multiplanar reconstruction on the dorsal plane (B) shows the location in relation to the other teeth (circle).

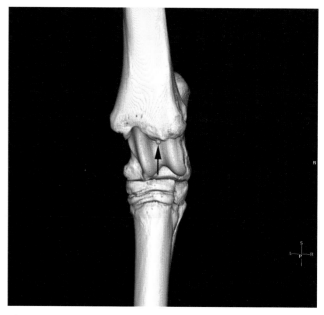

Figure 4.263. 3-D reconstruction of the dorsal aspect of an equine tarsus showing a small osteochondritis dessicans lesion (arrow) that is just distal to the intermediate ridge of the tibia in a horse with a swollen tarsus.

are obtained to help minimize this effect, but it cannot be eliminated. CT also easily shows the bone structure, but this is portrayed in cross section which allows better anatomic definition and delineation of pathological conditions (Figure 4.262). When intravenous contrast medium is used, soft tissue structures can be delineated from fluid.

Magnetic resonance (MR) imaging, which is another cross sectional imaging technique, does an excellent job of showing soft tissue and blood vessels, but does not provide as much bony detail of structures, such as the skull. MRI, when compared to CT, has much better contrast resolution for soft tissues due to the fact that it images hydrogen, does not use ionizing radiation, and its sequences yield additional pathophysiological information. However, the generally poor bone detail (due

to the lack of water in bones) generated by MRI makes CT an extremely valuable diagnostic method in horses.

CT is much less expensive than MRI on a per-case basis, has faster scan times (especially multidetector systems), provides better detection of acute hemorrhage and small calcifications, and provides better spatial resolution because images can be less than 1 mm in thickness without changing the acquisition time. In addition, the images can be reconstructed in any image plane and can be made into 3-D reconstructions (Figure 4.263). Though 3-D reconstructions are possible with MRI, more time is needed to acquire the images as well small image slices. CT also has the ability to image patients with ferrous implants better than MRI.

Cross sectional imaging of a structure eliminates the superimposition of bone and soft tissue, which makes CT especially helpful to examine complex joints such as the foot, fetlock, carpus, and tarsus. The CT examination is made up of multiple parallel cross sectional slices that are acquired in transverse orientation (in the case of an extremity or head, when placed in the gantry of the CT). CT imaging has also been very useful in the evaluation of bone/soft tissue structures of the head of the horse.

Modifications of current computed tomographic systems have allowed evaluations of the horse in a select few institutions. However, CT availability is limited by numerous considerations including purchase price, installation cost, and service contracts, which can be very expensive.

From a practical standpoint, CT requires the patients to move through the gantry as the examination is being performed, unlike MRI, in which the patient is placed in the magnet field and the images are generated. Because of the weight of the horse and the need to move a table through the gantry, use of CT in the horse requires a special table that interfaces with the CT table without hindering the CT table's motor. Some tables have been constructed that are capable of independent, precise, incremental computerized table movements. Some older CT systems do not use an integrated table but instead the gantry interfaces with the standard CT table and therefore the horse table bears the weight while the integrated "human" CT table moves the horse into the gantry. However, depending on the interface with the human CT table, companies can void the warranty on the CT machine due to the modifications that must be made.

In Europe and being developed in the United States, a standing CT has been designed to image a horse's head. In this configuration, the CT gantry is placed on a railing system and moves while the patient remains still or the horse is placed on a stock that floats on an air cushion while the horse's head is strapped to the CT table. This requires heavy sedation and limited numbers are available for use, but efforts are continuing to optimize this technique.

Many human CT systems are available for sale at very affordable prices but these systems should be evaluated in terms of available service and necessary modifications to allow for equine patients to be anesthetized, transported to the CT scanner, and then scanned and recovered.

Though the amount of scatter radiation from CT machines is less than with conventional radiographs, a shielded room with lead-lined doors is still needed. Furthermore, the room must be large enough to allow for anesthesia equipment as well as movement of the equine table into and out of the gantry. These systems should also be evaluated for gantry diameters that physically limit introduction of the proximal limb or caudal cervical area (50 to 60 cm). Smaller orthopedic CT units are available with small gantries (20 to 40 cm in diameter), but these units can only perform studies on the distal limbs and are difficult to impossible to use when imaging the adult equine head.

INTERPRETATION OF CT IMAGES

Interpretation of CT images is relatively straightforward if the clinician has an appreciation of the specific anatomy of the region imaged. CT uses the same technology as conventional X-rays; therefore, the concepts of attenuation (whites and blacks) are similar to those of a radiographic examination. The 5 roentgen opacities (air, fat, soft-tissue/fluid, mineral, and metal) still hold true, but CT allows for a number (called CT number or Hounsfield unit) to be assigned to differentiate fluid and soft tissue. In addition, the IV administration of contrast medium allows for separation of soft-tissue compared to fluid in sinuses, and help to evaluate tendon lesions.

In the examination of the extremities, images of both limbs are usually acquired at the same time, which permits critical comparison of suspected abnormalities. Attempts should be made to place the limbs in such a way as to acquire the slices of both limbs at roughly the same level. Alternatively, each limb can be imaged separately; most imaging viewer programs allow the user to match the images to provide a direct side-by-side comparison.

The original data set can also be digitally manipulated to view the volume of data in any image plane (Figure 4.264). This multiplanar reconstruction (MPR) can be performed with the CT scanner hardware or with most image viewing programs with a slight loss of

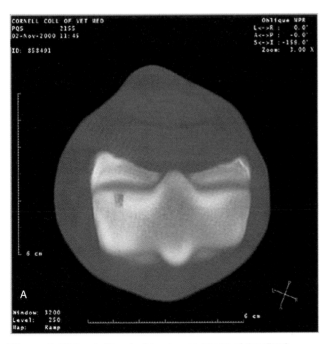 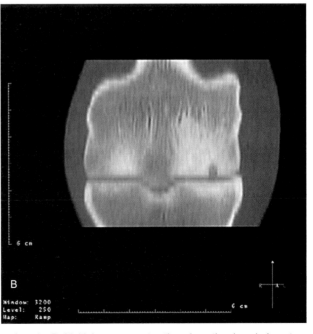

Figure 4.264. A. Standard transverse image of the distal aspect of the third metacarpal bone. Note the region of decreased attenuation surrounded by higher attenuating bone. This is indicative of a subchondral cyst-like lesion with associated sclerosis. B. Multiplanar reconstruction along the dorsal plane to show the cyst communicating with the metacarpophalangeal joint. (Courtesy of Cornell University Hospital for Animals.)

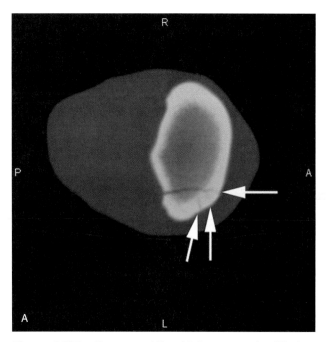

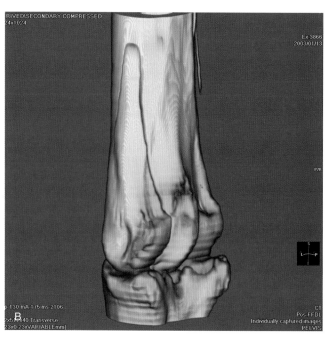

Figure 4.265. Transverse (A) and 3-D reconstruction (B) of a lateral condylar fracture of the distal aspect of the third metacarpal bone. Note that the small fissures identified on the transverse image (white arrows) are not seen in the 3-D reconstruction and the fracture appears incomplete on the 3-D reconstruction. (Courtesy of Cornell University Hospital for Animals.)

resolution, depending on the thickness of the slices used for the reconstruction. This limitation of resolution is being minimized with newer multislice CT scanners and sub-millimeter slice thicknesses.

After image acquisition, the data can be reconstructed and illustrated with a 3-D software program to provide the clinician with a better anatomic orientation of an area and, in the case of an extremity fracture, provide better characterization of fracture orientation (and/or disease extension). The main limitation in 3-D reconstruction of the extremities is that small fracture fragments or fissure lines may be lost because the images are generated by providing smoothing and shading filters to the image, which hide small imperfections (Figure 4.265). These imperfections can be seen on the cross-sectional (transverse) images; therefore, 3-D images are not used as frequently for diagnostic purposes, but rather for evaluation and surgical planning. For PC-based computers, 3-D reconstruction requires more sophisticated software than is present in the CT computer. On Macintosh computers, this is offered as freeware. Regardless of the source, 3-D reconstruction programs are considered very helpful for pre-surgical planning of complex fractures.[9] In middle phalangeal fractures, the use of CT allows for better surgical planning and determination of prognosis due to the lack of superimposition as well as the assessment of joint involvement and direction of fracture lines (Figure 4.266).[9]

The relationships between adjacent structures is easily demonstrated with CT. It is also helpful for the calculation of tumor volumes and for a technique called virtual endoscopy, both of which are more useful in human medicine. Virtual endoscopy allows the radiologist to position the point of view inside any structure

that has been imaged with CT and then travel down the structure as if seeing it with an endoscope (Figure 4.267). In human medicine, this has been used for virtual colonoscopy; however, the images generated only show contour, so a small nodule on the wall of the colon can be a polyp, a mass, or fecal material. There is no way to differentiate it using CT images without the administration of contrast medium.

A recent advancement in technology has combined positron emission tomography (PET) and CT technology to provide functional as well as anatomic information. This technology is mainly being explored in humans to look at myocardial infarctions and in small animals to look at hypoxic regions of tumors for radiation therapy prognosis. The premise of the technology is to inject a radioactive material (much like a bone scan), but this radiopharmaceutical acts like glucose and is taken up by metabolically active cells (such as tumors). Much like bone scintigraphy, the images lack anatomic detail. However, by acquiring a CT at the same time as the PET images, a precise location of the tumor as well as the metabolic characteristics can be obtained. This technology holds vast potential to help with the treatment and monitoring of cancer, but due to the horse's size and the limited occurrence of tumors in the equine population, its use will likely be limited. At this time, the authors know of no facility in the United States or Europe using this technology on horses, nor any publications reporting on its use in horses.

CONTRAST-ENHANCED CT

Contrast medium enhancement is routinely used in equine and human CT examinations. For a standard brain evaluation, approximately 300 mL[10] of contrast

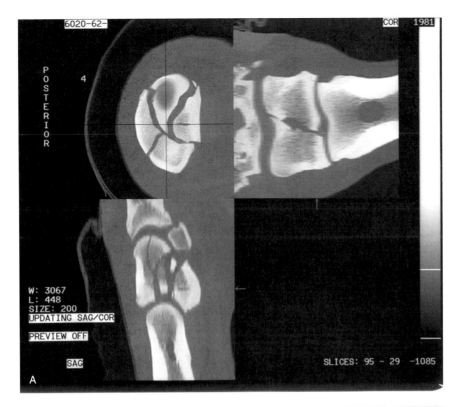

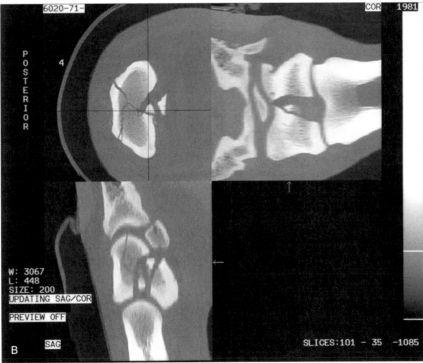

Figure 4.266. CT images of a horse with a comminuted P2 fracture that were obtained just before surgery to help with surgical reconstruction of the fracture. The fracture was repaired with two dorsally applied bone plates. The images are in 3 planes (transverse–upper left image, dorsal–upper right image with proximal to the left of the image, and sagittal–lower left image with proximal at the bottom of the image). (Courtesy of Dr. Gary Baxter.)

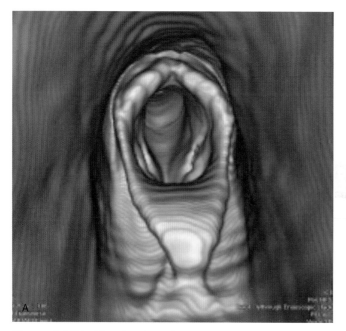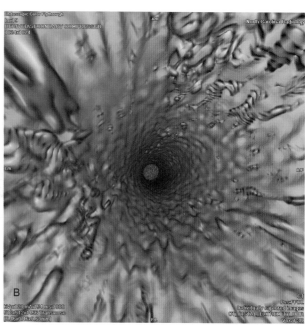

Figure 4.267. Virtual endoscopic images of the larynx (A) and medullary cavity of the third metacarpal bone (B) using CT reconstruction. These images were generated by creating a virtual fly-through of any structure that has a lumen. The clinical relevance of this technique is limited, but provides a unique perspective compared to conventional transverse and the 3-D views.

medium is administered (references give a range of 200 to 500 mL). An ionic, iodinated contrast material generally is used to limit the cost because such a large volume is needed.

Regional perfusion also has been described as a method to increase contrast resolution between the soft tissues of the tendons and the surrounding fluid of the digital sheath when evaluating the normal equine tendons of the distal limbs. This procedure involves using ultrasound to help place a catheter into the metatarsal or metacarpal artery and infusing contrast medium at a rate of 3 mL/second with a power injector.[1,7,8] Lesions were identified in 75% of the limbs evaluated in 151 horses (200 limbs) imaged using this technique.[8] These horses underwent a palmar digital nerve block and distal interphalangeal joint and/or digital tendon sheath anesthesia. DDFT lesions were identified in 77% of the limbs imaged and 49% of those horses had multiple lesions identified on CT.[8] CT has been used more for specific problems of the complex joints (carpus, tarsus [Figure 4.268], fetlock, and occasionally foot) as well as the head and cranial cervical verterbra.[2-6,9-11]

Many equine hospitals now have access to CT and low-field standing or high-field MRI (there are currently approximately 8 high-field magnets in the country that can accommodate horses), so the benefits and disadvantages of each modality must be understood for each to be used appropriately. CT is primarily used for a quick evaluation of complex fractures (Figure 4.269) or other primary bone abnormalities that require further definition before surgery (Figures 4.266 and 4.270). The cost for the CT examination is usually half that of an MR examination. As noted previously, scan times are usually shorter than for MR (about 20 minutes with positioning

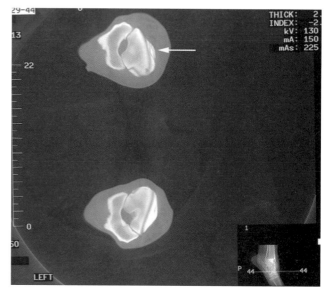

Figure 4.268. CT images of a horse with lameness and effusion of the tarsocrural joint. A fracture of the central tarsal bone was suspected but could not be seen on radiographs, and was confirmed with these CT images. The fracture was comminuted (arrow) and did not extend through the entire aspect of the bone. (Courtesy of Dr. Gary Baxter.)

using CT, compared to MRI imaging procedures that can take up to 90 minutes in a high-field system and 2 to 3 hours in a low-field system).

However, new multislice CT scanners reduce scan times dramatically. An average equine head can be scanned in approximately 2 minutes and the entire distal limb can take less than 5 minutes. This new tech-

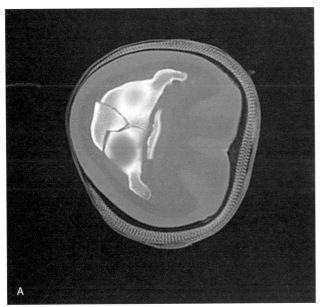
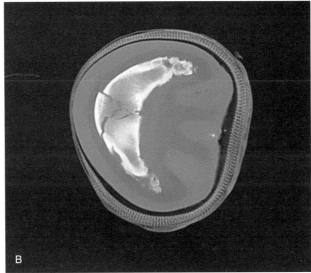
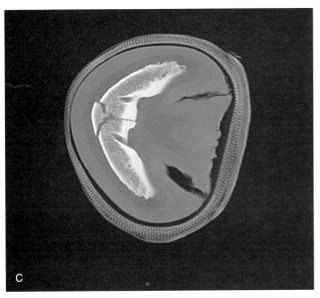

Figure 4.269. Proximal (A), middle (B), and distal (C) CT images of a comminuted fracture of the distal phalanx. The CT was used to rule out the possibility of lag screw repair and further define the extent of comminution. (Courtesy of Dr. Gary Baxter.)

nology is becoming more affordable with the recent invention of the 256-slice CT scanner, making 4-slice and 16-slice CT scanners obsolete in the human market and very affordable in the veterinary market.

The greatest expense (aside from the CT unit itself) is the table that must be built to allow access of the horse into the gantry. For a custom built motorized CT table, the cost can approach $85,000. Other less expensive tables ($20,000 to $40,000) are available but do not include separate motorized systems. These tables are integrated into the CT unit, which can potentially void the service contract if not done to manufacturer specifications. In these instances the CT manufacturer should be contacted.

As noted previously, in most hospitals the largest application of CT is the evaluation of the head, espe-cially sinuses and dental diseases. These cases primarily require assessment of the structural involvement of the bones in the skull and teeth and the extent of sinus involvement before surgery (unilateral vs. bilateral involvement). In horses with an abnormal mentation, the odds of finding a lesion on CT was 30 times higher than that of a horse with normal mentation.[10] If cranial nerve deficits were identified, CT was 11 times more likely to find an abnormality compared to a similar horse without cranial nerve deficits.[10] For a horse with seizure-like activity, the odds of finding an abnormality on CT was only 0.05 times higher than imaging a horse without seizure-like activity.[10] This study was based on 57 cases from 2001 to 2007 and illustrates the benefit of intracranial CT examination compared to MRI.

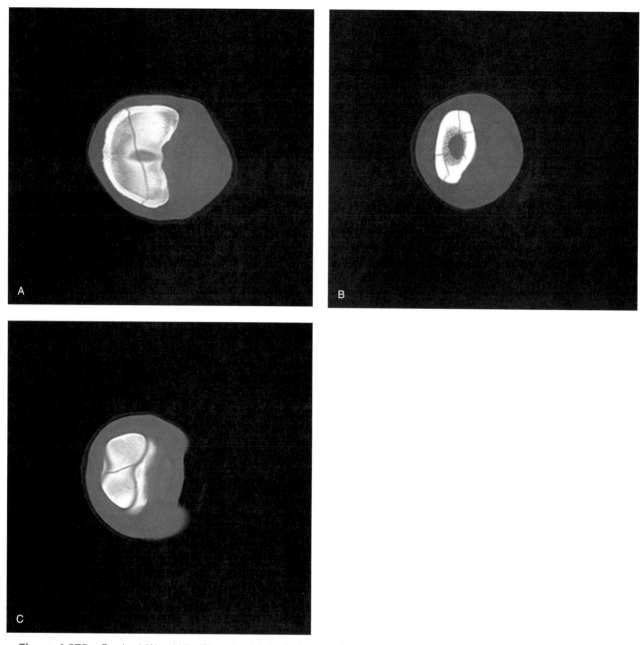

Figure 4.270. Proximal (A), middle (B), and distal (C) CT images of a non-displaced comminuted fracture of the first phalanx that were used to help decide the location and direction for lag screw repair of the fracture. (Courtesy of Dr. Gary Baxter.)

INDICATIONS FOR CT IN EQUINE LAMENESS AND SURGERY

The use of CT in the equine lameness population is underutilized. CT diagnoses, with or without the use of contrast medium, can provide a rapid, highly detailed assessment of the distal limbs. Though CT lacks the ability to identify bone edema or some more subtle tendon lesions, these lesions are generally those that are treated similarly with stall rest and slow return to work. The only benefit of using MRI in these cases is that the lesion is identified and can be monitored.

With injuries that require surgical intervention, CT is proving to be the modality of choice in the equine

patient due to anesthetic time. The average horse can undergo anesthesia for 2 to 3 hours without the risk of muscle damage and with minimal risk at recovery. A standard MR examination of both pelvic limbs requires approximately 1.5 to 2 hours, leaving the surgeon with no option to perform surgery on the same day. In addition, the average MRI requires at least 5 to 10 sequences. Though this provides a large amount of information, it is difficult to interpret in a rapid manner because it is dissimilar to radiographs and the white and dark areas have different diagnoses, depending on the sequence performed.

On the contrary, an average CT examination and contrast administration can be performed in 30 minutes or less. The images are relatively straightforward to interpret and 3-D reconstructions can be made in the time it takes the horse to be prepared for surgery. This leaves the surgeon with 2 hours to perform the surgery and recover the horse.

MRI is far superior for diagnosing subtle lameness or in cases in which radiographs and rest have provided no benefit. However, with the use of contrast medium, the speed of CT as well as the affordability of the equipment compared to MRI makes it a valuable diagnostic tool for equine lameness examination.

References

1. Collins JN, Galuppo LD, Thomas HL, et al. Use of computed tomography angiography to evaluate the vascular anatomy of the distal portion of the forelimb of horses. Am J Vet Res 2004;65(10):1409–1420.
2. Garcia-Lopez JM, Kirker-Head CA. Occult subchondral osseous cyst-like lesions of the equine tarsocrural joint. Vet Surg 2004;33(5):557–564.
3. Hanson JA, Seeherman HJ, Kirker-Head CA, et al. The role of computed tomography in evaluation of subchondral osseous lesions in seven horses with chronic synovitis. Equine Vet J 1996;28(6):480–488.
4. Jose-Cunilleras E, Piercy RJ. Advanced diagnostic imaging options in horses with neurological disease that localizes to the head. Equine Vet Educ 2007;19:179–181.
5. Kinns J, Pease A. Computed tomography in the evaluation of the equine head. Equine Vet Educ 2009;21(6):291–294.
6. Probst A, Henninger W, Willmann M. Communications of normal nasal and paranasal cavities in computed tomography of horses. Vet Radiol and Ultrasound 2005;46(1):44–48.
7. Puchalski SM, Galuppo LG, Hornof WJ, et al. Intraarterial contrast-enhanced computed tomography of the equine distal extremity. Vet Radiol and Ultrasound 2007;48 (1):21–29.
8. Puchalski SM, Schiltz RM, Bell RJK, et al. Intra-arterial contrast enhanced computed tomography in equine foot lameness: 151 horses. Abstract Submission, ACVR Annual Conference, Oct 23, 2009. Memphis, TN.
9. Rose PL, Seeherman H, O'Callaghan M. Computed tomographic evaluation of comminuted middle phalangeal fractures in the horse. V Radiol and Ultrasound 1997;38(6):424–429.
10. Sogaro-Robinson C, Lacombe V, Reed S, et al. Factors predictive of abnormal results for computed tomography of the head in horses affected by neurologic disorders: 57 cases (2001–2007). J Am Vet Med Assoc 2009;235:176–183.
11. Vanderperren K, Ghaye B, Snaps F, et al. Evaluation of computed tomographic anatomy of the equine metacarpophalangeal joint. Am J Vet Res 2008;69:631–638.

ARTHROSCOPY/ENDOSCOPY/BURSOSCOPY

C. Wayne McIlwraith

INTRODUCTION

Arthroscopy in the horse went through a similar evolution as that in humans in that it was initially used as a diagnostic instrument.[10] The procedure of diagnostic arthroscopy initially met with considerable skepticism within human orthopedics, until its value was demonstrated in the total evaluation of the knee.[4,6,20] Diagnostic arthroscopy revolutionized the diagnosis of joint disease in the horse and quickly became the gold standard for definition of changes in the synovial membrane, articular cartilage, subchondral bone, and intra-articular ligaments.[11]

The development of arthroscopic techniques and their usefulness has somewhat overshadowed the use of the arthroscope in diagnostic evaluation of the joint. However, it must be recognized that diagnostic arthroscopy is still commonly done as a sole procedure and a complete diagnostic examination is always part of a planned arthroscopic surgery when other diagnostic techniques have identified a given problem that indicates surgical intervention.

THE USEFULNESS OF DIAGNOSTIC ARTHROSCOPY RELATIVE TO OTHER DIAGNOSTIC METHODS

At the time arthroscopic surgery techniques were developed, neither computer tomography nor MRI were available for the horse. At that time diagnostic abilities consisted of clinical examination, synovial fluid analysis, and radiography. The use of scintigraphy later became routine and while it is sensitive to detect early change in the joint, it is nonspecific. The development of diagnostic arthroscopy enabled visualization of the articular cartilage, subchondral bone (when it was diseased), synovial membrane, and intra-articular ligaments.

The use of magnetic resonance imaging of an osteo-arthritic fetlock joint and comparison to other arthroscopic techniques, including arthroscopy, was described in 1996.[9] An editorial accompanying this article in *The Equine Veterinary Journal* implied that MRI might be the new gold standard, but apparently ignored the fact that the MRI imaging had been done post-mortem with the leg cut off. Since that time, MRI techniques have been developed and the successful use of standing MRI for imaging the distal limb described. Using high-field magnets, MRI has become a technique that enables visualization of the carpus and fetlock, as well as tarsus, but the usefulness of MRI to image the stifle is generally not available for clinical cases.[22,23]

Even when joints can be imaged with a high-field magnet, resolution in the articular cartilage is still a challenge because of the relative thinness of the cartilage in the carpus and fetlock. The arthroscope still gives optimum evaluation of the articular cartilage relative to high-field-strength MRI in these joints. Diagnostic arthroscopy (used in conjunction with diagnostic ultrasound) provides the optimal diagnostic abilities in the femoropatellar and femorotibial joints.

The usefulness of diagnostic arthroscopy in enabling the clinician to make a diagnosis when no other technique can do so is worthy of emphasis. Such conditions include tears in the cruciate ligaments as well as the medial palmar intercarpal ligament, meniscal injuries and radiographically 'silent' osteochondral fragmentation, subchondral bone disease, and various articular cartilage lesions.

PRINCIPLES OF DIAGNOSTIC ARTHROSCOPY

Diagnostic arthroscopy involves visualization as well as palpation of potential lesions, and involves the basic principles of arthroscopic triangulation. This technique brings operating instruments through separate portals to the arthroscopic portal and into the visual field of the arthroscope, with the tips of the instrument and arthroscope forming the apex of the triangle. The principle is illustrated in Figure 4.271. To be able to use this technique effectively, the surgeon must develop the manual psychomotor skills of manipulating two objects in a confined space while using monocular vision, which eliminates the convergence that provides depth perception. The positioning of arthroscopic and instrument portals in the various joints has been described in detail elsewhere.[11] The use of a probe through an instrument portal is critical, both to evaluate defects that cannot be discerned with vision alone and to provide an index of size by comparison of the lesions and the probe (Figure 4.271).

Knowledge of normal arthroscopic anatomy is critical. Before valid interpretations of changes in the joint can be made the surgeon must know the arthroscopic anatomy, which in turn requires re-learning of joint anatomy. For example, in the normal middle carpal joint, polyp-like filamentous villi are typical of the dorsomedial and dorsolateral areas of the joint (Figure 4.272), whereas in the far medial portion of the joint, the synovial membrane is smooth, white, and without villi. The presence and morphology of normal synovial plicae and the normal intra-articular ligaments need to be known (Figure 4.273).

EVALUATION OF SYNOVIAL MEMBRANE AND SYNOVITIS

The morphologic features of the synovial membrane and its villi can be visualized better with arthroscopy than by examination of a gross specimen or during arthrotomy. When arthrotomy is performed villi tend to cling to the synovial membrane and therefore cannot be seen distinctly, whereas with arthroscopy, because of

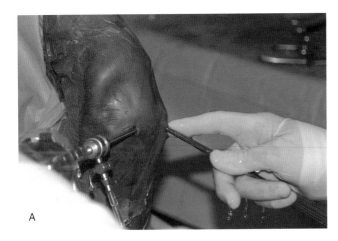

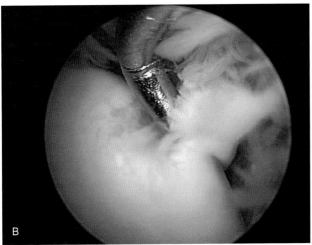

Figure 4.271. Use of a probe to palpate under arthroscopic visualization. A. External view. B. Arthroscopic view.

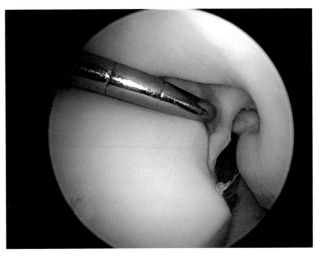

Figure 4.273. The use of the probe to palpate the medial palmar intercarpal ligament to distinguish between the lateral and medial portions.

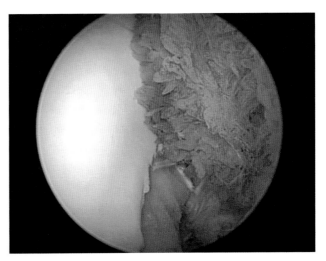

Figure 4.274. Acute synovitis associated with a fresh distal radius chip fracture.

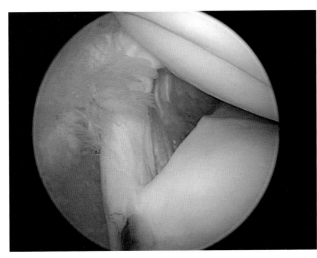

Figure 4.272. Normal synovial membrane in the dorsomedial portion of the middle carpal joint. Notice the villous synovial membrane contrasting with smooth synovial membrane in the more medial aspect of the joint medial to the dorsomedial intercarpal ligament.

the fluid medium, the shape of the villi stand out distinctly and transillumination allows improved visualization of the villous vascularity. The magnification of the arthroscope also facilitates definition but this degree of magnification varies depending on the distance of the object from the end of the arthroscope. hyperemia is typical in acute synovitis (Figure 4.274), whereas proliferation and thickening of synovial villi occur in chronic synovitis (Figure 4.275).

As diagnostic arthroscopy developed, new conditions were recognized. This includes the structures that were normal but had not previously been noted (for example, the dorsomedial intercarpal ligament in the middle carpal joint) and synovial folds were recognized in various locations such as the distal aspect of the medial trochlear ridge in some femoropatellar joints. In humans, "pathologic plicae" have been recognized and associated with a direct blow, repeated activity, or nonspecific synovitis leading to fibrosis and hypertrophy of

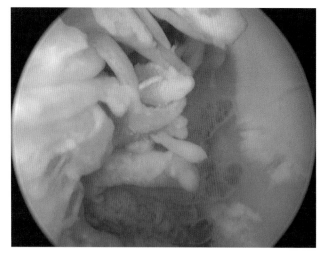

Figure 4.275. More chronic synovitis typified by both proliferation and thickening of synovial villi of the medial middle carpal joint. (Reproduced from McIlwraith et al. 2005, Diagnostic and Surgical Arthroscopy in the Horse, 3rd ed. Figure 3.13.)

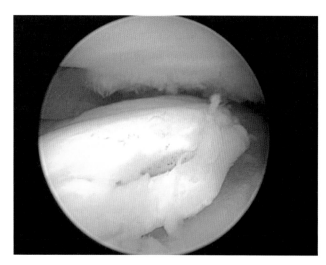

Figure 4.276. Fibrous thickening of the dorsal synovial pad (villonodular pad) above the medial condyle of the metacarpus.

the synovial plica.[11] Hypertrophy or fibrosis of a normal synovial structure is best exemplified in the horse by hypertrophy and fibrosis of the dorsal synovial pad of the fetlock (Figure 4.276).

In some instances resection of synovial membrane (synovectomy) is necessary for optimal observation and thus complete diagnostic examination of the joint. A common example of this is local resection of synovial membrane in the femoropatellar joint where it obscures a complete view of the lateral trochlear ridge in assessment of an OCD lesion.

Evaluation of Intra-articular Ligaments and Menisci

Arthroscopy has enabled veterinarians to diagnose otherwise unrecognized lesions in the medial palmar intercarpal ligament,[13] cranial cruciate ligament,[19] meniscal ligaments,[19] and menisci.[18] While ultrasonog-

raphy can be used to diagnose some tears of the menisci, definitive diagnosis is usually based on diagnostic arthroscopy (Figure 4.277). Arthroscopy is the only way to define partial tearing of the cranial or caudal cruciate ligaments.

EVALUATION OF ARTICULAR CARTILAGE

The other major use of diagnostic arthroscopy is the evaluation of the articular cartilage. Evidence of pathological changes in the cartilage can be recognized radiographically when those lesions extend into the subchondral bone or cover sufficient area to cause loss of joint space. Many instances of cartilage compromise are less severe than this, but still represent a significant clinical problem.

Articular cartilage erosion is very common in the horse, particularly associated with osteochondral chip fragments of the carpus (Figure 4.278) and metacarpophalangeal joint and more recently on diagnostic arthroscopy of the medial femorotibial joint. In most fetlock joints the principle manifestations are wear lines with some focal erosion seen occasionally. Articular cartilage lesions on the medial femoral condyle have been reported as a cause of lameness in 11 horses.[16] Such lesions are increasingly diagnosed as diagnostic arthroscopy of the femorotibial joints becomes routine and an important investigation in many instances where the problem has been localized to the femorotibial joints. Partial-thickness and full-thickness erosions represent more severe changes in the articular cartilage (Figure 4.279). Other instances of cartilage damage are also recognized with the use of diagnostic arthroscopy, including osteochondral erosion in the palmar aspect of the visible articulation in the middle carpal joint, where the indication for diagnostic arthroscopy was localization of the problem with IA analgesia, lack of radiographic changes, and lack of response to repeated intra-articular injections.

Osteochondral fractures or flaps that were not evident on radiographs are found regularly at diagnostic arthroscopy. Disease involving the subchondral bone has been recognized in multiple locations and in all but the proximal third carpal bone.

THE USE OF DIAGNOSTIC TENOSCOPY

Tenoscopic examination of the tendon sheaths is important for the definition of a number of disease processes in the digital flexor tendon sheath, carpal sheath, tarsal sheath, and extensor tendon sheath.[11]

The standard tenoscopic approach to the digital flexor tendon sheath should involve entry outside the manica flexoria, where many of the larger tendon sheath masses develop. The arthroscope can then be withdrawn back into the fetlock canal and inserted beneath the manica flexoria to examine the proximal DDFT. Linear clefts in the DDFT are frequently found at this level, which may correspond to the most constricted region of the fetlock canal when the limb is loaded. Further details are described elsewhere.[11] Conditions diagnosed with endoscopic examination of the digital flexor tendon sheath include tenosynovial masses (Figure 4.280), chronic synovitis and adhesions, con-

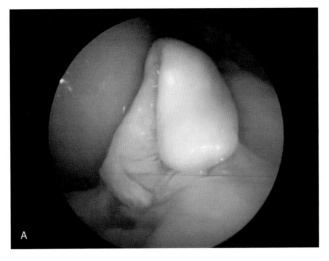

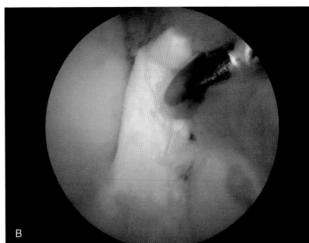

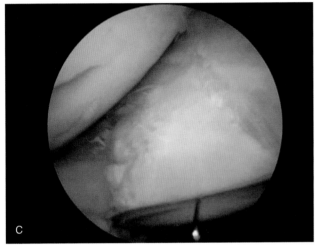

Figure 4.277. A. Longitudinal tear of cranial horn of medial meniscus. The torn portion is folded back on itself. B. A probe has been used to show the base of the torn portion. C. Debridement after removal of the torn portion. (Reproduced from McIlwraith et al. 2005, Diagnostic and Surgical Arthroscopy in the Horse, 3rd ed. Figure 6.77.)

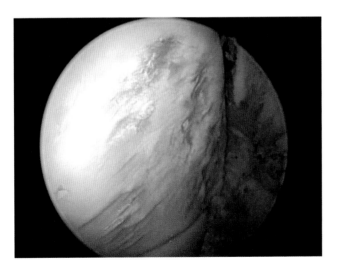

Figure 4.278. Punctate erosions of the articular cartilage on the third carpal bone.

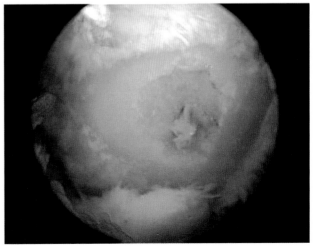

Figure 4.279. Full-thickness erosion on medial femoral condyle. Note central erosion beyond the subchondral bone plate.

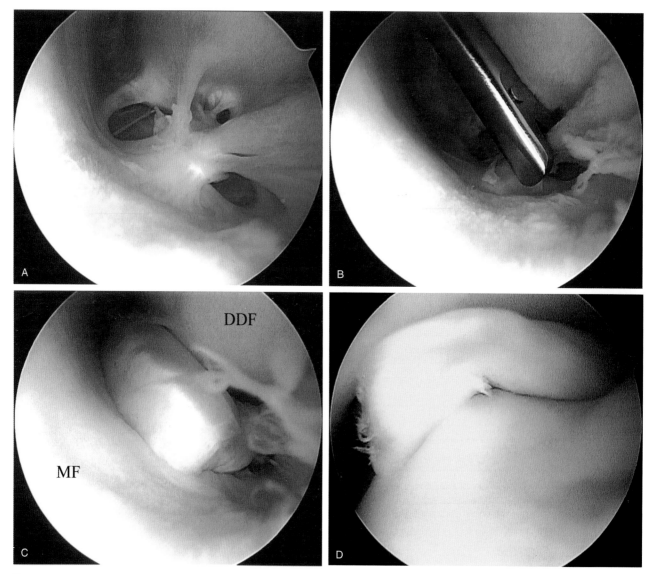

Figure 4.280. A. Adhesions between the flexor tendons and the tendon sheath. B. Arthroscopic biopsy punch ronguers being used to divide and remove adhesions from the sheath. C. Masses protruding between the deep digital flexor tendon (DDF) and the manica flexoria (MF) of the superficial digital flexor tendon (SDFT). D. A semi-detached portion of the DDF protruding between the DDF and MF of the SDFT that was removed. (Reproduced from McIlwraith et al. 2005, Diagnostic and Surgical Arthroscopy in the Horse, 3rd ed. Figure 12.12D.)

striction of the palmar/plantar annular ligament, and linear clefts of the DDFT (less frequently in the SDFT).

Carpal sheath conditions that result in chronic and often insidious lameness have been increasingly recognized and examined by exploratory endoscopy.[11,12,14,17] Radial osteochondroma and radial exostosis, tendinitis, or myotendinitis of the proximal portion of the digital flexors, and idiopathic carpal tunnel syndromes may all result in lameness and/or sheath distention. These conditions frequently have little to differentiate them based on their clinical appearance. Endoscopic examination is useful for assessment and confirmation of the diagnosis of any of these syndromes, which can then be repaired.

Radial osteochondromas as well as protruding bony exostosis from the closed distal physis of the radius can represent diagnostic dilemmas. Asymptomatic protru-

sions can be seen on radiographs; however, failure to identify protrusions radiographically in horses with clinical cases occurs. Some are diagnosed with ultrasonography, but others require arthroscopic confirmation.[11,12,14]

Idiopathic carpal canal syndrome can arise from damage to the carpal retinaculum, carpal sheath, myotendinous junction of the flexor tendon, and fracture of the accessory carpal bone. Tenoscopic division of the carpal retinaculum can be used to open the carpal canal and release pressure on the digital flexor tendon.[17]

Endoscopic examination of the tarsal sheath has been used as indicated for chronic tenosynovitis that is poorly responsive to medical therapy, including masses and adhesions spanning from the tarsal sheath parietal layer to the DDFT as well as chronic synovitis within the tendon sheath, tears of the DDFT, mineralizing masses within the tarsal sheath, and mineralization of the surface and deeper structures of the DDFT.[11] Confirmation of fragmentation of the sustentaculum tali, as well as clarification of the presence of infection, is another indication.[5,8,15,21]

THE USE OF DIAGNOSTIC BURSOSCOPY

Bursoscopy has become an accepted term to described intrathecal endoscopy of synovial bursae. These closed sacs are found interposed between moving parts or at points of unusual pressure and may be congenital or acquired. Congenital bursae develop between bursae and are located in constant positions. The principle congenital bursae of clinical importance (from an endoscopic perspective) are the calcaneal bursa, intertubercular (bicipital) bursa, and podotrochlea (navicular) bursa. Techniques describing their evaluation in horses have been published on the calcaneal bursa,[7] intertubercular bursa,[1] and navicular bursa.[24]

Bursoscopy of the calcaneal bursa has been used to debride osteolysis on the calcaneal tuber,[2,7] diagnose tearing of the medial (most commonly) or lateral retinacular insertions of the SDFT (partial tears of the retaniculi have been identified on endoscopic examination after a tentative diagnosis had been obtained with ultrasonography), and traumatic fragmentation of the calcaneus. Bursoscopy of the bicipital bursa has been used to investigate lameness referable to the site and treat intrathecal fragmentation of the supraglenoid tubercle of the scapula and lateral tuberosity of the humerus together with contaminated and infected bursae. Booth, in 1999,[3] reported a horse with lameness localized to the bicipital bursa that was accompanied by radiologic and ultrasonographic abnormalities. Endoscopy revealed widespread loss of fibrocartilage in the humerus, with adhesions to the bicipital tendon. The extensive nature of the lesions precluded treatment but endoscopy was considered diagnostically useful. Loss of humeral fibrocartilage with fibrillation in the adjacent bicipital tendon and rupture of the lateral wall of the bursa in horses with lameness localized to this site has been seen.[11]

Currently the principle indication for endoscopy of the navicular bursa is evaluation and treatment of contamination and infection resulting from penetrating wounds.[25] Intrathecal lesions have been identified, removed, and debrided.

Endoscopy Examination in the Management of Contamination and Infection of Joints, Tendons, Sheaths and Bursae

Although often diagnosed without endoscopic examination, infections of joints, tendon sheaths, and bursae are more clearly delineated with such examination and treatment procedures are also carried out under endoscopic visualization.[11] The distinct advantage of endoscopy is the ability to see and remove foreign debris that may be present within the synovial cavity.[11]

References

1. Adams MN, Turner TA. Endoscopy of the intertubercular bursa in horses. J Am Vet Med Assoc 1999;214:221–225.
2. Bassage LH II, Garcia-Lopez J, Gurrid EM. Osteolytic lesions of the tuber calcanei in two horses. J Am Vet Med Assoc 2000;217:710–716.
3. Booth TM. Lameness associated with bicipital bursa in an Arab stallion. Vet Rec 1999;145:194–198.
4. Casscells SW. The place of arthroscopy in the diagnosis and treatment of internal derangement of the knee: An analysis of 1,000 cases. Clin Orthop 1980;151:135–142.
5. Cauvin ER, Tapprest J, Munroe JA, et al. Endoscopic examination of the tarsal sheath of the lateral digital flexor tendon in horses. Equine Vet J 1999;31:219–227.
6. Dandy DJ, Jackson RW. The impact of arthroscopy on the management of disorders of the knee. J Bone Joint Surg (Br) 1975;57:346–348.
7. Ingle-Fehr JE, Baxter GM. Endoscopy of the calcaneal bursa in horses. Vet Surg 1998;27:561–567.
8. MacDonald MH, Honnas CM, Meagher DM. Osteomyelitis of the calcaneus in horses: 28 cases. J Am Vet Med Assoc 1989;194:1317–1323.
9. Martinelli MJ, Baker DJ, Clarkson RB, et al. Magnetic resonance imaging of degenerative joint disease in a horse: A comparison of other diagnostic techniques. Equine Vet J 1996;28:410–415.
10. McIlwraith CW, Fessler J. Arthroscopy in the diagnosis of equine joint disease. J Am Vet Med Assoc 1978;172:263–268.
11. McIlwraith CW, Nixon AJ, Wright IM, et al. In Diagnostic and Surgical Arthroscopy of the Horse, 3rd ed. 2005. Mosby Elsevier, Edinborough.
12. McIlwraith CW. Osteochondromas and physeal remnant spikes in the carpal canal. In *Proceedings*. 12th Annual ACVS Symposium 2002;12:168–169.
13. McIlwraith CW. Tearing of the medial palmar intercarpal ligament in the equine mid-carpal joint. Equine Vet J 1992; 24:547–550.
14. Nixon AJ, Schachter BL, Pool RR. Exostosis of the caudal perimeter of the radial physis as a cause of carpal synovial sheath tenosynovitis in horses: 10 cases (1999–2003). J Am Vet Med Assoc 2004;224:264–270.
15. Santschi EM, Adams SB, Fessler JF, et al. Treatment of bacterial tarsal tenosynovitis and osteitis of the sustentaculum tali of the calcaneus in 5 horses. Equine Vet J 1997;29:244–247.
16. Schneider RK, Jenson P, Moore RM. Evaluation of cartilage lesions on the medial femoral condyle as a cause of lameness in horses: 11 cases (1988–1994). J Am Vet Med Assoc 1997;210: 1649–1652.
17. Textor JA, Nixon AJ, Fortier LA. Tenoscopic release of the equine carpal canal. Vet Surg 2003;32:278–284.
18. Walmsley JP, Phillips TJ, Townsend HCG. Meniscal tears in horses: An evaluation of clinical signs and arthroscopic treatment of 80 cases. Equine Vet J 2003;35:402–406.
19. Walmsley JP. Arthroscopic surgery of the femorotibial joint. Clin Tech Equine Pract 2002;1:226–233.
20. Watanabe M, Takeda S, Akeuchis HS. In Atlas of Arthroscopy 3rd ed. 1978. Igakushoin IS, Tokyo.
21. Welch RD, Auer JA, Watkins JP, et al. Surgical treatment of tarsal sheath effusion associated with an exostosis on the calcaneus of the horse. J Am Vet Med Assoc 1990;196:192–194.
22. Werpy NM. MRI for diagnosis of soft tissue and osseous injuries in the horse. Clin Tech in Equine Pract 2005;3:389–398.
23. Werpy NM. Magnetic resonance imaging of the equine patient: Comparison of high-and low-field systems. Clin Tech in Equine Pract 2007;6:37–45.
24. Wright IA, McMahon PJ. Tenosynovitis associated with longitudinal tears of the digital flexor tendon in horses: a report of 20 cases. Equine Vet J 1999;31:12–18.
25. Wright IM, Phillips TJ, Walmsley JP. Endoscopy of the navicular bursa: A new technique for the treatment of contaminated and septic bursae. Equine Vet J 1999;31:5–11.

THERMOGRAPHY

Tracy A. Turner

Thermography is the pictorial representation of the surface temperature of an object.[9,15] It is a noninvasive technique that measures emitted heat. A medical thermogram represents the surface temperatures of skin, making thermography useful for the detection of inflammation. This ability to noninvasively assess inflammatory change makes thermography an ideal imaging tool to aid in the diagnosis of certain lameness conditions in the horse.[1,9,10,12–16,23]

Thermography was first used in veterinary medicine 45 years ago. Originally, its use was limited for the most part to university hospitals or large referral practices. But over the last 20 years, thermography has been used practically in equine medicine. This is a physiological imaging modality that requires a learning curve for interpretation but it offers the operator new insight into his/her patients.

THERMOGRAPHIC INSTRUMENTATION

Thermographic instrumentation in the past has been divided into contacting and non-contacting devices.[17] However, in the 1990s a new technology using focal plane array detectors made all older thermographic devices obsolete with regard to equine veterinary use. Focal plane array detectors are uncooled technology which employs special lenses to focus infrared radiation on a series of detectors. These instruments are self contained and highly portable.

One of the most important factors to consider before purchasing a thermographic camera is the spectral range.[17] For medical use the range of 8 to 14 microns is ideal because this is the peak emissivity of skin. From a practical standpoint, there is also less environmental artifact at this range. The author prefers real-time thermography vs. still thermography because real-time eliminates any problems with motion, makes thermographic assessment more dynamic in that the operator can immediately observe change, and allows for faster imaging. Sensitivity refers to the amount of temperature difference that can be detected; uncooled units can differentiate 0.1°C, which is sensitive enough for medical uses. The final factor is portability and durability. Uncooled cameras using the focal array technology are very portable and durable because they have no moving parts.

PRINCIPLES OF USE

The circulatory pattern and the relative blood flow dictate the thermal pattern, which is the basis for thermographic interpretation.[15] The normal thermal pattern of any area can be predicted on the basis of its vascularity and surface contour. Skin overlying muscle is also subject to temperature increase during muscle activity.

Based on these findings, some generalizations can be made regarding the thermal patterns of a horse: the midline is generally warmer;[9,15] this includes the back, chest, between the rear legs, and along the ventral midline (Figure 4.281). Heat over the legs tends to follow the routes of the major vessels, the cephalic vein in the forelimb, and the saphenous vein in the hindlimb.

On the dorsal view of the distal limb, the metacarpus (metatarsus), fetlock, and pastern appear relatively cool because the image recorded is away from the major blood supply. Thermographically, the warmest area in the distal limb is around the rich arteriovenous plexus of the coronary and laminar corium located proximally on the hoof wall. Normally, there is increased warmth between the third metacarpus and flexor tendons, following the route of the median palmar vein in the forelimb and the metatarsal vein in the hindlimb. Over the foot, the warmest area corresponds to the coronary band. From the palmar/plantar aspect, the tendons are

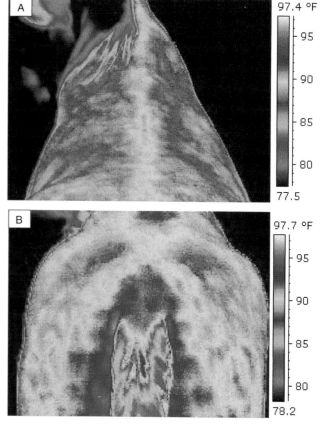

Figure 4.281. Normal back (A) and croup (B) thermograms of a horse. Note the back is warm down the center with isothermic bands around it. The croup forms a "T" of uniform temperature between the tuber coxae and the midline.

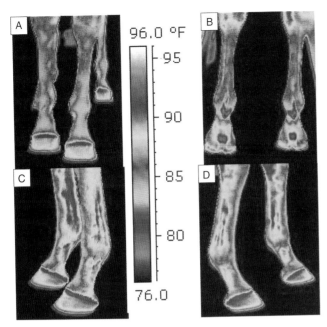

Figure 4.282. Normal distal limb of a horse. The warmest areas follow the vasculature. Abnormalities are heat where it is not expected or changes in the normal thermal pattern. Essentially, if the image is not normal and cannot be explained as an artifact, then it represents abnormal thermography. A. Dorsal view. B. Palmar view. C. Left side. D. Right side.

relatively cool and the warmest area is consistently between the bulbs of the heel along the midline (Figure 4.282).

Injured or diseased tissues invariably have an altered circulation.[15] One of the cardinal signs of inflammation is heat which is due to increased circulation. Thermographically, the "hot spot" associated with the localized inflammation generally is seen in the skin directly overlying the injury.[1,2,4,5,9–16,23–25] However, diseased tissues may in fact have a reduced blood supply either due to swelling, thrombosis of vessels, infarction of tissues, or change in sympathetic tone.[15,16] With such lesions the area of decreased heat is usually surrounded by increased thermal emissions, probably due to shunting of blood.

Certain factors must be controlled to produce reliable thermographic images: motion, extraneous radiant energy, ambient temperature, and artifacts.[17] Motion can be controlled by immobilizing the horse in stocks or using a qualified handler. The use of real-time thermography eliminates the need for complete immobilization. Chemical restraining agents to keep the horse from moving should be avoided because these drugs affect the peripheral circulation and cardiovascular systems, which could cause false thermal patterns to be produced; however, the author has not encountered this.

To reduce the effects of extraneous radiant energy, thermography should be performed under cover shielded from the sun.[15] Preferably, thermography should be done in darkness or low-level lighting. Ideally, ambient temperature should be in the range of 20°C (68°F) but any temperature is acceptable as long as the horse is not sweating. Heat loss from sweating does not occur below 30°C (86°F), because radiation and convection are responsible for heat loss below that temperature. Very cold environmental temperatures may cause vasoconstriction of the lower legs and interfere with imaging. In these cases, low level exercise to stimulate vasodilation is necessary.

The thermographic area ideally should have a steady, uniform airflow so that erroneous cooling does not occur. Practically, the horse should be kept from drafts. Likewise, the horse should be allowed 10 to 20 minutes to acclimate to the environment or room where thermography is performed.

Artifacts are extraneous sources on the skin that can cause irregular images, including debris, scar tissue, hair length, liniments, leg wraps, and equipment.[15] To avoid artifacts, make sure all subjects are groomed and free of leg wraps and equipment for two hours whenever possible. Hair insulates the leg and blocks the emission of infrared radiation. However, as long as the hair is short and of uniform length, the thermal image produced is accurate. The skin should always be evaluated for changes in hair length that may cause false hot spots in the thermogram.

Multiple thermographic images of a suspect area should be made.[24,25] The area in question should be evaluated from at least two directions approximately 90° apart to determine if a hot spot is consistently present. The horse's extremities should be examined from 4 directions (circumferentially).[15] Significant areas of inflammation will appear over the same spot on each replicate thermogram.

There are at least 4 ways in which thermography can be used in equine veterinary practice. The first is as a diagnostic tool. In these cases, thermography is a physiologic imaging method in which a 1°C difference between 2 anatomically symmetrical regions indicates a region of inflammation.[17] A decrease in temperature is just as important as an increase in temperature. The image identifies an area of interest to pursue with an anatomic imaging method such as ultrasonography and/or radiography.

The second method is to enhance the physical examination. In this case, thermography is used to identify changes in heat and therefore locate areas of suspicion.[17] Thermographic cameras are easily 10 times more sensitive than the hand in determining temperature differences. This method simply helps identify asymmetry and then the practitioner must use the information to determine the actual cause and significance of the temperature difference.

The third method of using thermography is in a wellness program. In this method, horses in training are followed on a routine basis, once weekly.[18] In the author's experience, thermographic changes often occur 2 weeks prior to clinical changes. In these cases, thermography can be used to identify subclinical problems and then training alterations can be made so that injury may be avoided altogether.

The fourth method is in the regulation of equine events.[17] Presently, thermography is used by the Federation Equestre Internationale (FEI) and the United States Department of Agriculture (USDA) to enforce regulations. The instrument is used as a screening tool to determine potential misuse. In these cases, the final determination is made by a group of examining veterinarians.

SPECIFIC APPLICATIONS FOR LAMENESS DIAGNOSTICS

The Examination

If thermography is to be used, all bandages and leg wraps should be removed 2 hours before the examination. The horse should be thoroughly brushed to remove any dirt and debris. Thermography is best performed after the clinical examination has been performed (including watching the horse move, palpation, and manipulations) but before nerve or joint diagnostic analgesia. The horse is brought into a covered area away from direct sunlight and any breezes. A 10-minute acclimatization period is allowed and then a systematic examination of the horse is performed using the thermographic camera.[17]

The camera is positioned 90° to the area of interest and the sequential images are taken. The limbs are examined from all 4 directions, the neck from both sides and ventrally, the torso from both sides (dorsally and ventrally), the shoulders from the front and both sides, the hips from both sides and the back, and the head from both sides (dorsally and ventrally). Each of the images is then assessed in relation to the findings of the clinical examination of the horse.

The Foot

Thermography of the hoof has been useful for the diagnosis and evaluation of several conditions of the foot.[9,13,15] Laminitis, palmar foot pain, subsolar or submural abscesses, corns, and any other inflammatory condition of the hoof are specific conditions in which thermography provides valuable information. Obviously, thermography is not needed to definitively diagnose these problems. Thermography does, however, provide additional information that is helpful in localizing the problem, assessing the degree of inflammation associated with it, and deciding the best course of treatment. Thermographic evaluation is particularly helpful with early or occult conditions of the foot, in which the physical and/or radiographic examination findings are inconclusive.

Normally, the coronary band is the warmest area of the leg and therefore, inflammation of this area can be difficult to detect.[9] The hooves should be thermographically compared in several ways. Comparisons should be made between all 4 hooves, front to front and front to rear. A difference of more than 1°C between hooves is significant. In cases in which all 4 feet are involved, comparisons of the hoof temperature with the temperature of the area between the bulbs of the heel should be made.

Laminitis is characterized by inflammation of the laminar structures of the hoof. Laminitis can be divided into 4 phases: developmental, acute, chronic, and post chronic, and each of the phases has characteristic thermal information. The developmental stage has been studied thermographically the least. During the developmental stage there are no clinical signs but the thermal image changes. There are progressive periods of vasoconstriction followed by periods of profound vasodilation; the heat seen gets hotter and broader following each vasoconstrictive period.

During the acute phase a change in the thermal pattern of the hoof wall is useful in recognizing laminitis. Generally, the coronary band is 1° to 2°C warmer than the remainder of the hoof. An inflammatory problem is indicated when the hoof begins to approach the temperature of the coronary band. Thermography can also be very beneficial in the progressive evaluation of the contralateral limb where support limb laminitis is a potential sequela. Thermography makes it possible to detect inflammation in the contralateral foot well before lameness is evident. Preventative therapy can therefore be instituted sooner in the course of disease and hopefully before the laminitis is irreversible.

The chronic phase is characterized by progressive displacement of the third phalanx. The thermal image is the opposite of the acute phase. As the coffin bone displaces, the vasculature is pulled further away from the surface causing the thermal image to appear progressively cooler. That is, the coronary band is more difficult to distinguish from the remainder of the hoof wall.

Finally, the post chronic phase is seen when the laminae have healed but vascular changes (damage) persist secondary to coffin bone displacement. Thermal imaging can be useful to identify the vascular damage that has occurred; this is seen as areas of intense cold which identify the areas of vascular damage.

Thermography is also an excellent method of evaluating the patient with palmar foot pain syndrome.[14] The author has never identified a consistent thermal pattern associated with these cases, but has been able to characterize reduced blood flow to the caudal hoof and to identify thermal stresses associated with hoof imbalance and superficial inflammatory disease. Thermography is one of the few methods that can readily determine the relative blood flow to the palmar foot area. This is accomplished by thermographically evaluating the foot both before and after exercise. The normal horse sustains a 0.5°C increase in temperature of the foot after exercise but about 40% of horses with palmar foot pain syndrome do not sustain this increase in the caudal foot due to the low blood flow. This is in sharp contrast to other focal inflammatory conditions of the hoof, such as bruises or fractures, which are characterized by focal areas of increased temperature that correspond to the site of injury. Exercise in these cases intensifies the hot spot.

Hoof abscesses before they drain are often seen as relatively cold areas. This is due to the pressure caused by the abscess which decreases the circulation to the abscessed area. The hoof capsule is a closed environment, and the swelling that occurs due to the abscess is seen thermographically as an abnormal cold area. Once the abscess opens and the pressure is relieved the cold area changes to a hot area.

Joint Diseases

Joint inflammation produces characteristic thermal patterns. The best view to study most joints is from the

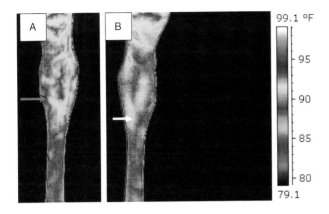

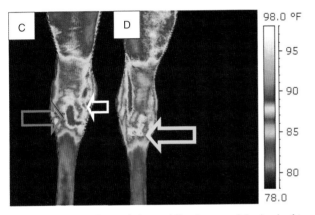

Figure 4.283. Thermal views of the dorsum of the hock of two different horses. A. Right hock of horse 1. B. Left hock of horse 1. C. Right hock of horse 2. D. Left hock of horse 2. (B) is the most normal thermogram; the white arrow indicates the saphenous vein and the warmest area. (A) shows a horizontal line (red arrow) indicating early lower tarsal joint inflammation. (C and D) show variations of distal hock inflammation. (C) shows the horizontal line and area over the central hock, which are hotter (hollow red arrow) than the area of the saphenous (hollow white arrow). (D) shows that the distal hock is a horizontal line (hollow yellow arrow).

dorsal aspect.[13,23] Typically, the normal joint is cool compared to the surrounding structures. An exception to this rule is the hock, which has a vertical hot spot along the medial aspect that corresponds to the saphenous vein (Figure 4.283). As a joint becomes inflamed, the thermal pattern changes to an oval area of increased temperature that is centered over the joint and widest horizontally medial to lateral. The exception to this rule is the joints of the distal limb, where the thermal pattern associated with inflammation of these joints is a circular pattern. The areas of joint capsule attachment tend to be hotter, but the center of the joint is relatively cooler. This may be due to joint swelling or pressure and subsequent loss of microcirculation (Figure 4.284). No specific correlation can be made between heat and joint damage. The temperature of the joint appears to be related to many factors: the chronicity of the problem (the more chronic the problem, the less heat), degree of synovial involvement, actual amount of cartilage damage, and presence or absence of osteochondral fragments. These factors have a complicated interaction and

all affect the inflammatory response of the joint temperature. The degree to which each affects this response has yet to be determined.

Thermal patterns of joints have been shown to change 2 weeks before the onset of clinical signs of lameness.[18,23] In this manner, thermography can be used to assist training and help prevent serious injuries. By locating inflammation before clinical signs are evident, training programs can be changed to reduce stress on the inflamed area, thereby preventing serious injury.

Long Bone Injuries

Thermography is of less value in the diagnosis of most long bone problems. Because thermography evaluates skin temperature, a bone must be in relatively close contact with the skin to affect its temperature.[2] Consequently, bones that are heavily covered with muscle cannot be as accurately assessed by thermography. Thermography is best used to evaluate dorsal metacarpal disease or stress fractures of the radius or tibia.

Dorsal metacarpal disease, the so-called bucked shin complex, is categorized into 3 grades.[7] Grade 1 is characterized by eliciting pain upon palpation of the cannon bone but radiographic evidence of bone pathology cannot be identified. Grade 2 is characterized by pain over the cannon bone and radiographic evidence of subperiosteal callus. Finally, grade 3 is characterized by cannon bone pain and radiographic evidence of a stress or fatigue fracture.

Grades 2 and 3 may be indistinguishable and radiographic confirmation of a stress fracture may not be possible for 2 to 3 weeks. Thermal variations between the latter 2 may help differentiate grade 3 lesions earlier than radiographs. Diseases of grades 1 and 2 are characterized by hot spots located midshaft over the dorsal cannon bone. The hot spot is generally 1° to 2°C warmer than the surrounding tissues. In contrast, the grade 3 disease has hot spots that are not centrally located and are usually seen on the lateral and medial views in addition to the dorsal view. These areas are characteristically 2° to 3°C warmer than the surrounding tissues. Because thermographic changes typically precede radiographic changes by 2 weeks,[13] with accurate thermography, a tentative diagnosis can be made earlier and appropriate treatment measures taken sooner.

Tendon Injuries

Thermal patterns of the normal flexor tendons are bilaterally symmetrical and consist of elliptical isothermic zones.[11,12] The lowest temperature is centered over the palmar aspect of the tendons and the peripheral areas near the carpus and fetlock are approximately 1°C warmer.

Acute tendinitis invariably causes a hot spot over the site of the tendon lesion (Figure 4.285).[12] The hot spot of a tendon lesion usually can be demonstrated up to 2 weeks before physical evidence of swelling and pain around the tendon. Therefore, tendon lesions of potentially clinical significance can be identified and adjustments in the training protocol can be made to prevent further damage to the tendon.

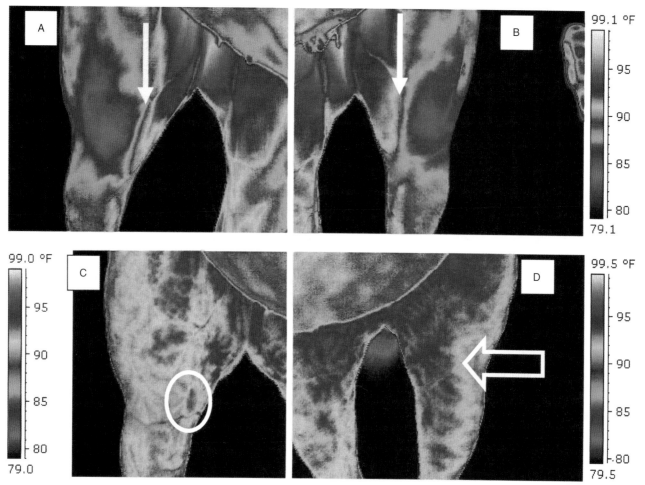

Figure 4.284. Normal right (A) and left (B) cranial stifle thermograms. The thermal pattern on the inside of the stifle is warm and there is a line of demarcation in the area of the medial patellar ligament (arrow) and the front of the stifle is relatively cool. (C and D) represent abnormal thermograms of 2 different horses. Horse (C) shows a focal hot spot (circle) over the distal medial stifle; radiographs revealed a cyst-like lesion in the medial tibial plateau. Horse (D) shows a pattern that has heat from the medial side covering half the cranial aspect (hollow arrow). This horse had very noticeable effusion but no radiographic changes.

As the tendon heals the thermal pattern becomes more uniform but remains abnormally elevated when compared to normal tendon.[12] As the lesion heals and scar tissue is deposited, the skin over the injured area may actually show a decrease in temperature, whereas the remaining neovascularized tendon continues to have increased thermal emissions. During the assessment of healing, the thermal changes do not correlate well to the structural reorganization of the tendon matrix as assessed by ultrasonography.[4] This is because as the tendon undergoes neovascularization, the thermal pattern diffuses so there is no longer a hot spot. However, if one compares healing tendon to a normal tendon, there are overall increased thermal emissions from the damaged tendon. Mechanical stress proximal to the injury can aggravate the existing tendon damage. Again, thermography can detect these areas of proximal stress before they cause a clinical problem, and therefore specific imaging can be used to decide if a therapeutic desmotomy should be performed.

Ligament Injuries

Thermographically, ligament injuries appear very similar to tendon injuries. Hot spots can be expected to be centered over the injured area (Figure 4.285). An exception to this is in some high suspensory injuries of the metacarpi; the dorsal thermal image of the injured leg shows a focal hot spot located proximally on the cannon bone. This is interesting, considering that inflammation and pain would be expected to be on the palmar aspect of the limb. Clinically, thermography is most useful when trying to correlate whether there is heat associated with a sensitive ligament. This is particularly true of the suspensory ligament, where the clinical significance of palpable sensitivity within the body of the ligament can be difficult to determine. Thermography can be used to determine if there is inflammation associated with the sensitivity. In a similar vein, splints or metacarpal callus can cause suspensory desmitis. Thermography can detect whether there is

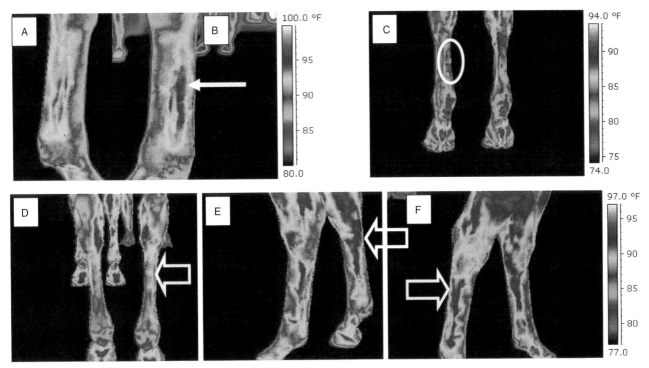

Figure 4.285. Abnormal thermograms. A. Normal medial aspect of the left fore of a horse. B. Abnormal medial aspect of the right fore of the same horse. The hot area (arrow) centered over the suspensory ligament was shown via ultrasonography to be due to suspensory desmitis. C. Superficial digital flexor tendon lesion (circle) was confirmed sonographically. D to F. Three views of the same horse showing a high suspensory ligament lesion confirmed ultrasonographically (hollow arrows).

inflammation associated with the suspensory ligament adjacent to the splint. These indications apply to any ligament.

Muscle Injuries

Thermography may have its greatest clinical application in the assessment of individual muscle injuries, which are difficult to diagnose.[16] While serum muscle enzyme elevation may non-specifically indicate muscle damage, the specific muscle or muscles damaged may be difficult to identify. Thermography offers 2 types of information important in the evaluation of muscle injury: it can locate an area of inflammation associated with a muscle or muscle group and it can illustrate atrophy well before it becomes apparent clinically.

Muscle inflammation is most commonly seen thermographically as a hot spot in the skin directly overlying the affected muscle.[16] On a rare occasion, swelling and edema in the affected muscle are severe enough to inhibit blood flow through the muscle. In this case the injured muscle is seen thermographically as a cold spot. Thermographic evaluation of muscle must be made from the right and left sides. These comparison images should be nearly identical. Consistent variations from side to side indicate muscle damage located at either the hot or cold spot.

The most common cause of muscle inflammation is muscle strain. A classification of first-, second-, or third-degree strain injuries, described in human athletes, has been applied to horses.[16] Muscle strains have not been commonly documented in the forelimb. The author has most commonly identified pectoralis and shoulder extensor myopathies. Thermographic description of muscle strains of the back and hindlimb muscles have been best described.[16] These strains have been termed croup and caudal thigh myopathies. Croup myopathies are actually strains of the longissimus, origin of the gluteus medius (level of the sacroiliac), body of the gluteus medius, and insertion of the gluteals on the greater trochanter and the third trochanter of the femur. Caudal thigh myopathies consist of injuries to the biceps femoris and semitendinosus or semimembranosus muscles. Injuries to the biceps femoris and semimembranosus most commonly are mid body muscle strains, but semitendinosus injuries usually occur at the musculotendinous junction.

Back Problems

Diagnosis of injuries to the vertebral column can be aided through thermography.[13] Many of these injuries are undiagnosed or the diagnosis is delayed because radiography of the equine spine is difficult and/or may require general anesthesia. Thermography offers a distinct advantage because it is best performed on the standing animal, and in suspect cases may be used as a general screening test to determine whether referral for radiography is warranted. Injuries to the vertebral column are characterized by either hot spots, cold spots, or root signatures.

Thermography has been used to identify 6 different back injuries: over-riding dorsal spinous processes (kissing spines), dorsal spinous ligament injuries, muscle pain, withers injuries, sacroiliac problems, and saddle fit problems.[19] The author uses 2 different thermal images to assess the back: a thoracolumbar view and a croup view.[19] The thoracolumbar view shows the withers and the sacrum, and is especially good for looking at the mid back region. The croup view is best for evaluating the sacroiliac region. The thermal pattern is the most important aspect of assessing the thermogram of the back. It must be remembered that thermography establishes the location of a possible problem but does not characterize the lesion. However, there are certain thermal patterns that have been seen consistently with particular back problems.

The normal back thermal pattern is: warmest down the midline, cooling slightly in the lumbar region; warm from tuber coxae to tuber coxae and over the tuber sacrale; and the same warmth down the middle of the croup (Figure 4.281).[19] The warm area has symmetric isothermic bands on either side. Any variation of this pattern is either due to an artifact (thin hair, rubbed area) or pathologic process. If the lesion occurs along the midline of the thoracolumbar area, radiographs of the thoracolumbar spine are indicated. If the lesion occurs off the midline or in the croup region, the area is usually imaged with ultrasonography.

Overriding spinous processes or kissing spine has been associated with 1 of 3 different thermal patterns:[21]

Pattern 1: A hot streak perpendicular to the thoracic spine (Figure 4.286)
Pattern 2: A cold streak perpendicular to the thoracic spine
Pattern 3: a combination hot spot-cold streak pattern over the back; the most common.

The author's practice has evaluated more than 150 cases over a 5-year period and has determined that the sensitivity of thermography to diagnose overriding spinous process is 99%. However, the specificity was only 70%. This resulted in a positive predictive value of 91% compared to the positive predictive value of palpable pain in the thoracolumbar area for kissing spine of 67%.

Dorsal spinous ligament injuries have not presented with that type of pathognomonic thermal pattern.[19] Thermographic changes associated with this injury have been increased heat, decreased heat, or simply an abnormal back thermogram. The lesion has been detected

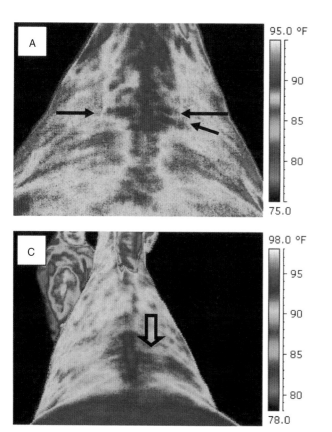

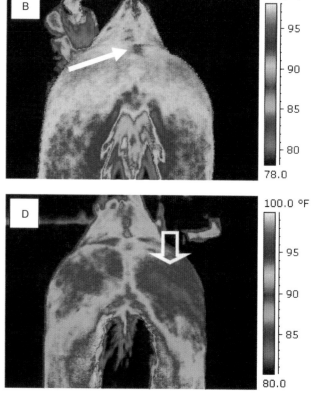

Figure 4.286. A. Thermogram typical of overriding spinous processes in the horse's back. Note the horizontal hot spots (black arrows); overriding spinous process was confirmed radiographically. B. Thermogram depicting a cold area over the tuber sacrale (white arrow). This is seen whenever the horse does not bend its back normally and has been associated with thoracolumbar and sacroiliac pain. This horse had evidence of sacroiliac desmitis on ultrasonography. C. A back with heat over the right epaxial muscles (hollow black arrow), which correlated with palpable pain on the same area. D. Nonspecific thermal pattern over the croup that shows thermal asymmetry with the right side being colder (white hollow arrow). When this pattern is seen the lame leg is the cold leg and is thought to be associated with decreased use.

using ultrasonography after knowing there is an abnormal thermogram.

Muscle injuries of the thoracolumbar region also do not have characteristic thermograms.[19] Typically, however, the thermal patterns show either hot spots or cold spots off the midline (Figure 4.286). It is in these regions that sonography is concentrated to determine whether muscle lesions can be seen. Withers injuries have all shown hot spots in the area of the withers but nothing more characteristic than that. The croup muscles show some specific changes.[16]

Sacroiliac region thermography has shown several different patterns.[19] The most common is a cold area centered over the region of the tuber sacrale (Figure 4.286). This finding of cold is hypothesized to be due to lack of normal movement in the sacroiliac region. This lack of movement can be due to primary pathology or secondary to other causes of the horse not moving normally through the pelvic region. This has been consistent with the author's clinical findings as well. Specifically, the author has found that only about half the horses exhibiting this thermal pattern actually show pain in the sacroiliac area. In addition, sonographic evaluation reveals pathology in only about half the cases and this pathology usually looks chronic in nature. Both thinning and thickening of the cross sectional diameter of the dorsal sacroiliac area has been identified. In cases with a cold area and palpable pain, the sacroiliac region is sonographically examined. On the other hand, if there is no pain or the horse moves normally through the pelvis, other causes of loss of back mobility are sought. Pathology is seen much more commonly if the area over the tuber sacrale is hot or if there is a hot spot centered over one tuber sacrale or the other. The pathology varies from hypoechoic areas within the dorsal sacral ligaments to generalized edema in the region. This thermographic pattern is almost always associated with either pain or marked stiffness in the sacroiliac region.

Saddle fit thermography is very interesting and requires multiple examinations.[20] In evaluating the dynamic interaction between the saddle and the horse's back, thermography shows not only the heat generated in contact areas on the saddle but also the physiologic effects of the saddle on the horse's back. The author's protocol is to perform a baseline thermographic examination of the horse's back and again after the horse has been worked under saddle. The horse should be saddled with a simple cotton pad with the girth tightened as it would be for riding. The horse is then lunged for at least 20 minutes. The horse should be exercised at its normal gaits (walk, trot, canter) and equally in both directions. Both the bottom of the saddle and the horse's back are evaluated. The most important criterion for the saddle is thermal symmetry. In regard to the horse, due to the heat generated by the saddle, its midline is now colder than the other structures under the saddle. In addition, the examiner is looking for focal hot spots, particularly along the spine, or hot or cold spots over the musculature. These abnormalities indicate problems caused by the saddle. The assessment is then repeated after a similar exercise session with the rider mounted. This evaluation allows consideration of the effect of the rider on the horse's back.

References

1. Bowman KF, Purohit RC, Ganjam UK, et al. Thermographic evaluation of corticosteroids efficacy in amphotericin B induced arthritis in ponies. Am J Vet Res 1983;44:51–53.
2. Goodman PH, Healset MW, Pagliano JW, et al. Stress fracture diagnosis by computer-assisted thermography. Phys Sportsmed 1985;13:114–116.
3. Genovese RL, Rantanen NW, Hauser ML, et al. Clinical application of diagnostic ultrasound to the equine limb. In Proceedings Am Assoc Equine Pract 1985;30:701–704.
4. Hall J, Bramlage LR, Kantrowitz BM, et al. Correlation between contact thermography and ultrasonography in the evaluation of experimentally-induced superficial flexor tendonitis. In Proceedings Am Assoc Equine Pract 1987;30:429–431.
5. Lamminen A, Meurman K. Contact thermography in stress fractures. Acta Thermographica 1980;5:89–91.
6. Love TJ. Thermography as an indicator of blood perfusion. Ann NY Acad Sci 1980;335:429–433.
7. Norwood GL, Haynes PF. Dorsal metacarpal disease. In Mansmann RA, McAllister ES, eds. Equine Medicine and Surgery. American Veterinary Publications, Santa Barbara. 1982; 1110–1111.
8. Palmer SE. Use of the portable infrared thermometer as a means of measuring limb surface temperature in the horse. Am J Vet Res 1981;42:105–108.
9. Purohit RC, McCoy MD. Thermography in the diagnosis of inflammatory processes in the horse. Am J Vet Res 1980; 41:1167–1169.
10. Purohit RC, McCoy MD, Bergfeld WA. Thermographic diagnosis of Horner's syndrome in the horse. Am J Vet Res 1980; 41:1180–1181.
11. Stein LE, Pijanowski GJ, Johnson AL, et al. A comparison of steady state and transient thermography techniques using a healing tendon model. Vet Surg 1988;17:90–93.
12. Stromberg B. Morphologic, thermographic and ^{133}Xe clearance studies on normal and diseased superficial digital flexor tendons in race horses. Eq Vet J 1973;5:156–161.
13. Stromberg B. The use of thermography in equine orthopedics. J Vet Radiol 1974;15:94–97.
14. Turner TA, Fessler JF, Lamp M, et al. Thermographic evaluation of podotrochleosis in horses. Am J Vet Res 1983;44:535–538.
15. Turner TA, Purohit RC, Fessler JF. Thermography: A review in equine medicine. Comp Cont Ed 1986;8:855–858.
16. Turner TA. Hindlimb muscle strain as a cause of lameness in horses. In Proceedings Am Assoc Equine Pract 1989;34:281–283.
17. Turner TA. Diagnostic thermography. Vet Clin North Am (Equine Pract) 2001;17:95–114.
18. Turner TA, Pansch J, Wilson JH. Thermographic assessment of racing Thoroughbreds. In Proceedings Am Assoc Equine Pract 2001;47:344–346.
19. Turner TA. Back problems in horses. In Proceedings Am Assoc Equine Pract 2003;49:71–74.
20. Turner TA. How to assess saddle fit in horses. In Proceedings Am Assoc Equine Pract 2004;50:196–201.
21. Turner TA. Thermography In Henson F, ed. Equine Back Pathology: Diagnosis and Treatment. Wiley-Blackwell, Cambridge, 2009;125–132.
22. Ueltschi G. Bone and joint imaging with ^{99m}Tc-labeled phosphates as a new diagnostic aid in veterinary orthopedics. J Am Vet Radiol Soc 1977;18:80–82.
23. Vaden MF, Purohit RC, McCoy MD, et al. Thermography: A technique for subclinical diagnosis of osteoarthritis. Am J Vet Res 1980;41:1175–1178.
24. Weinstein SA, Weinstein G. A review of 500 patients with low back complaints; comparison of five clinically-accepted diagnostic modalities. Proceedings. 2nd Acad Neuro Musc Thermography 1985;40–44.
25. Weinstein SA, Weinstein G. A clinical comparison of cervical thermography with EMG, CT scanning, myelography and surgical procedures in 500 patients. Proceedings 2nd Acad Neuro Musc Thermography 1985;44–48.

Lameness in the Extremities

THE FOOT

GARY M. BAXTER AND TED S. STASHAK; JAMES K. BELKNAP AND ANDREW PARKS (LAMINITIS SECTION)

NAVICULAR DISEASE/SYNDROME

Navicular disease or syndrome remains one of the most controversial and common causes of intermittent forelimb lameness in horses between 4 and 15 years of age.[25,67,74] It is estimated that the syndrome is responsible for one-third of all chronic forelimb lameness in horses.[15,67] Quarter horses, Thoroughbreds, and Warmbloods, particularly geldings, appear to be at greatest risk; whereas the syndrome is rarely diagnosed in ponies or Arabian horses.[25,67] The disease has been shown to have a hereditary predisposition possibly due to limb conformation of the horse or to the specific shape of the navicular bone.[7,22,23] The shape of the proximal border of the navicular bone has been determined to be inherited in Dutch Warmblood horses, and horses with an undulating or concave proximal border are more predisposed to the disease.[22,23,57] Other factors such as faulty conformation, hoof imbalances, improper or irregular shoeing, and exercise on hard surfaces are also believed to predispose and aggravate the condition.[54,67,74] Although the hindlimbs can be affected, it is rare, and navicular disease is primarily considered a problem of the forelimbs.

The definition of navicular disease (or which horses should be labeled as having navicular disease) is controversial and seems to differ among clinicians. The term "disease" implies a known cause and a specific treatment, of which neither are known for navicular disease, and therefore some prefer the term "navicular syndrome."[67] In addition, many horses with bilateral foot pain have concurrent soft tissue and navicular bone abnormalities, suggesting that navicular syndrome may be more appropriate in the majority of horses. "Palmar foot syndrome" has also been recommended to describe these horses because a variety of pathological entities may be identified (Box 5.1).[57] However, the term "navicular disease" is often used when obvious radiographic abnormalities are present within the navicular bone, and the terms "navicular syndrome" or "palmar heel pain" are used to describe horses that block to a low palmar digital (PD) with minimal to no radiographic changes.[1,61] This is somewhat arbitrary but it avoids labeling horses as having navicular disease when the lameness could be due to many other sources in the foot.

Navicular disease/syndrome has been defined as a chronic forelimb lameness associated with pain arising from the navicular bone and closely related structures including the collateral suspensory ligaments (CSLs) of the navicular bone, distal sesamoidean impar ligament (DSIL), navicular bursa, and the deep digital flexor tendon (DDFT).[25,61] Horses with primary DDFT tendinitis within the foot are usually not considered to have navicular disease/syndrome.[25] The disease is characterized by degenerative changes in the structure, composition, and mechanical function of the cartilage, subchondral bone, and surrounding soft tissues of the navicular apparatus.[57] However, documenting many of these abnormalities in horses that do not have radiographic abnormalities requires advanced imaging such as computed tomography or magnetic resonance (MR) imaging. In addition, hoof imbalances, hoof capsule distortion, contracted or sheared heels, etc. may be the sole cause of lameness without abnormalities within the deeper structures of the foot.[18,67]

The bottom line is that not all lameness conditions associated with the palmar aspect of the foot should be labeled as navicular disease or syndrome. Some clinicians feel that navicular disease/syndrome should be reserved for horses with chronic bilateral forelimb lameness that fit a very specific set of diagnostic criteria.[67]

Adams and Stashak's Lameness in Horses, 6e, edited by Gary M. Baxter
© 2011 Blackwell Publishing, Ltd.

Box 5.1.   Abnormalities that may exist in horses classified as having navicular disease, navicular syndrome, palmar foot syndrome, or palmar heel pain.

1. Navicular disease: radiographic, CT, or MRI abnormalities within the navicular bone
2. Desmitis/trauma of the podotrochlear apparatus
   a. Collateral ligaments of the navicular bone
   b. Desmitis of the distal sesamoidean impar ligament
   c. Desmitis of the distal digital annular ligament
3. Tendonitis of the DDFT: usually at 3 locations
   a. The insertion
   b. Palmar to the navicular bone
   c. Proximal to the navicular bone
4. Desmitis of the collateral ligaments of the DIP joint
5. Navicular bursitis
6. Synovitis/capsulitis/OA of the DIP joint
7. Primary hoof imbalances (improper trimming or shoeing)
8. Hoof capsule and/or heel distortions

central to these biomechanical studies. Abnormal forces on the navicular bone could arise from either excessive physiological loads applied to a foot with normal conformation or normal loads applied to a foot with abnormal conformation.[70] Poor hoof conformation and balance, particularly the long toe, low heel hoof conformation accompanied by the broken-back hoof pastern axis, have historically been considered major risk factors for the development of navicular disease. This concept has withstood the test of time, supporting the theory that excessive and repetitive forces applied to the distal third of the navicular bone by the DDFT is a major contributor to the disease. Further supporting this is the finding that the force exerted on the navicular bone is negatively correlated to both the angle between the third phalanx (P3) and the ground and the ratio between heel and toe height.[32] This corresponds to the hoof conformation known as "reverse angle of the distal phalanx" in which the palmar aspect of P3 is lower than the apex (Figure 5.1). This type of conformation greatly increases the contact stress on the navicular bone by the DDFT. In contrast, heel elevation is used to treat horses with navicular disease and is thought to decrease the tension on the DDFT, which reduces the forces applied to the navicular bone.[57,81]

Most horses with true navicular disease have a bilateral forelimb lameness that switches to the opposite limb after a low PD block, pain on hoof testers across the central or cranial aspect of the frog, and some evidence of radiographic abnormalities within the navicular bone. However, hoof tester sensitivity may be variable and based on recent MR imaging studies, the lack of radiographic abnormalities does not rule out navicular bone pathology.[1,25,61]

Etiology

The two proposed causes of navicular disease are vascular compromise and biomechanical abnormalities leading to tissue degeneration.[3,15,42,43,48,54,56,57,67,70,85] With the vascular theory, thrombosis of the navicular arteries within the navicular bone, partial or complete occlusion of the digital arteries at the level of the pastern and fetlock, and a reduction in the distal arterial blood supply due to atherosclerosis was thought to result in ischemia of the navicular bone.[15,43,56] The vascular theory has not withstood scientific scrutiny because of failure either to reproduce the disease by altering blood flow or to identify histological tissue changes compatible with the theory.[56,57,70] In addition, increased bone remodeling/modeling and vascularization have been demonstrated in horses with navicular disease.[43,48,85] The increased vascularization was shown to be a combination of active arterial hyperemia and passive venous congestion. Obstruction of the venous outflow was thought to result in venous congestion, increased bone marrow pressure, and pain.[52,54,68]

There is increasing evidence that abnormal non-physiological biomechanical forces leading to tissue degeneration is the most likely cause of navicular disease.[3,11,42,54,57,70] Forces exerted on, or experienced by, the navicular bone and the podotrochlear apparatus are

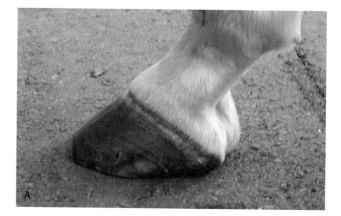

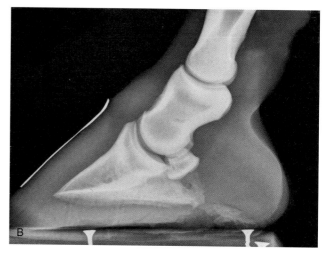

Figure 5.1.   (A) Front foot and (B) lateral radiograph of a horse with a reverse or negative angle of P3 that is thought to predispose to problems in the palmar aspect of the foot.

The location of the navicular bone between P3, the second phalanx (P2), and the DDFT suggests that it functions primarily as a buffer to spread forces among the anatomical structures.[57] It ensures that the DDFT maintains a constant angle of insertion, and the distal aspect of the bone must withstand great forces during the propulsive phase of the stride.[11,12,20] A study in isolated limbs using pressure-sensitive film has documented that the contact load on the navicular bone and associated joints was highest during dorsiflexion (extension) of the limb, which corresponds to the end of the stance phase or the beginning of the propulsion phase.[11] However, in another study, both force and stress on the navicular bone in horses with navicular disease were approximately double those of normal horses during the early stance phase of the stride.[83] This was associated with greater tension on the DDFT, which the authors attributed to contraction of the deep digital flexor muscle in the early stance phase. Contraction of the deep digital flexor muscle was thought to help avoid heel-first landing in an attempt to unload the heels, but this appears to simultaneously increase the forces on the navicular bone.[57,83]

In addition, some horses may be predisposed to navicular disease as a result of an inherent abnormal gait pattern. Horses with navicular disease were found to have abnormal limb-loading force patterns compared to normal horses that were not altered by loss of sensation in the palmar foot region.[82] The authors suggested that analysis of gait patterns could be used for detection and appropriate management of horses susceptible to development of navicular disease.[82]

It has been estimated that the peak forces on the navicular bone approximate $0.67\times$ body weight during the walk and $0.77\times$ body weight at a slow trot.[54,67] However, the forces applied to the navicular region are influenced not only by body weight, but by limb and foot conformation and the type of work performed by the horse. Factors such as excessive body weight, small feet, broken pastern angles, long toes, low heels, hoof imbalances, and work on hard surfaces are likely to increase the forces per unit area of the navicular bone and podotrochlear apparatus (Figures 5.1 to 5.3). Minor conformational abnormalities and other predisposing factors do not cause excessive loading of the navicular bone in most horses, resulting in normal modeling/remodeling of the navicular bone over time without the development of lameness.

In horses with severe or multiple predisposing factors, nonphysiological forces exerted on the navicular bone region begin the pathologic process that can affect the palmar/plantar fibrocartilage, dorsal articular cartilage, underlying bone, navicular bursa, podotrochlear apparatus, and DDFT.[57] Many of the pathologic changes within the navicular bone resemble those seen grossly and microscopically with osteoarthritis (OA) at other locations such as the distal tarsal and proximal interphalangeal joints.[57,67,70] These microscopic changes include focal degeneration, cartilage erosion, subchondral bone sclerosis associated with thickening of the trabeculae, focal areas of lysis, edema, congestion, and fibrosis in the marrow spaces (Figure 5.4).[25,52,54,57,85] Additional abnormalities that have been found on the flexor surface of the navicular bone in lame horses

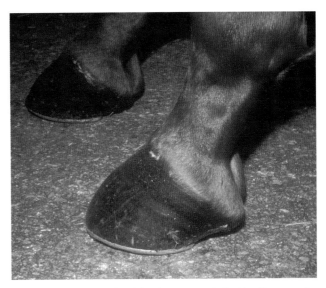

Figure 5.2. Broken back hoof pastern axis that is often seen in horses with navicular disease/syndrome.

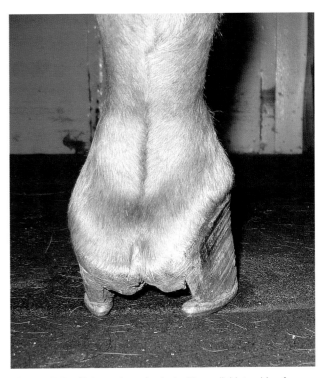

Figure 5.3. Palmar view of a foot with medial-lateral hoof imbalance. The medial hoof wall is longer and more upright than the lateral aspect and the coronary band is displaced proximally on the medial side.

compared to age-matched controls included thinning, crevicing or loss of the fibrocartilage layer, chondrone formation, and subchondral bone necrosis (Figure 5.5).[5] In this study there was no relationship between age and the severity of the histological abnormalities in the navicular bone, but the lesions were more common in lame horses than controls.[5]

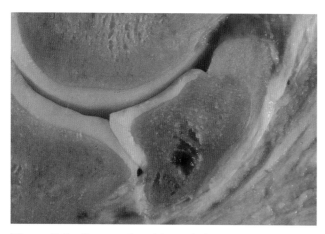

Figure 5.4. Cross section of the navicular bone at necropsy demonstrating cyst-like lesions within the body of the navicular bone.

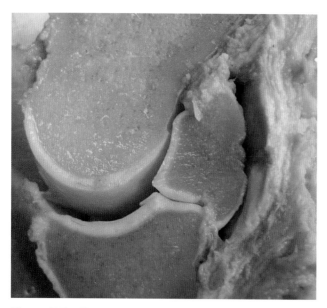

Figure 5.5. Post-mortem view of the navicular bone illustrating degeneration of the flexor cortex. This horse also had surface fibrillation of the DDFT.

Scanning electron microscopy studies of the distal sesamoid bone and DDFT have identified fraying of collagen fibers in the DDFT and fissuring of the fibrocartilage on the flexor surface of the navicular bone.[24,84] Damage to the fibrocartilage together with DDFT fibrillation may predispose to adhesion formation between the tendon and the bone. Other studies have identified superficial or deep sagittal or parasagittal crevices or splits of the DDFT, abrasions or fibrillation on the dorsal surface, focal fibrocartilaginous metaplasia, and focal fibroplasia (Figure 5.5).[6,57] These abnormalities were not related to age, but lesions on the dorsal aspect of the DDFT were significantly more common in lame horses than control horses.[6] In addition, true core lesions appeared to be uncommon, and there was little evidence of acute inflammatory changes within the DDFT.[6] Superficial lesions on the dorsal surface of the

DDFT may occur without detectable lameness but deep sagittal splits are usually related to lameness.[57] Abnormalities within the podotrochlear apparatus (CSL, DSIL) have also been described in horses with navicular disease but their clinical significance is not documented as well.[5,57] Fibrocartilaginous metaplasia, collagen degeneration, and fibroplasia were the most common microscopic findings.[5,6]

The pain and lameness in horses with navicular disease/syndrome presumably comes from within the bone and/or the surrounding supporting soft tissue structures. In most cases, it probably originates from more than 1 site because combination injuries within the foot appear to be most likely. With significant bone degeneration, the origin of pain is probably similar to that of horses with OA. Venous drainage of marrow spaces below lesions of degenerative joint disease is thought to be sluggish, and pain is associated with dilated vessels in the subchondral spongiosa.[54] Human patients experience pain when bone marrow pressure exceeds 40 mm Hg, even in resting positions.[67] Horses with navicular syndrome also have impaired venous drainage[40,52] and have bone marrow pressure exceeding 50 mm Hg, which is significantly higher than that of control horses.[52,68] Therefore, increased intra-osseous pressure associated with venous distention and hypertension may be the cause of bone pain.

Pain from injuries to the supporting ligaments and the DDFT most likely contribute to the lameness in most cases. Significant DDFT lesions (sagittal splits and core lesions) may be very painful, similar to tendinitis at other locations. Enthesiophyte formation on the proximal or distal borders of the navicular bone may represent previous tearing of the CSL attachments, but it is often difficult to determine if these abnormalities actively contribute to the pain.[67] In addition, sensory nerve endings have been identified in the CSL, DSIL, and DDFT at its attachment to the distal phalanx.[8,9] The location where the DSIL and the dorsal aspect of the DDFT insert onto the distal phalanx has been referred to as the "intersection" and is thought to have a rich sensory innervation, particularly of substance P and neuropeptide-producing fibers, and abundant arteriovenous complexes (Figure 5.5).[8,70] This anatomic region may act as an initiation site for many of the more extensive tissue changes that subsequently develop in many horses with navicular disease.[70]

Clinical Signs

Horses with navicular disease/syndrome usually have a history of progressive, chronic, unilateral or bilateral forelimb lameness, which may have an insidious (most common) or acute onset.[67] The history may include a gradual loss of performance, stiffness, shortening of the stride, loss of action, unwillingness to turn, and increased lameness when worked on hard surfaces.[25] Chronic bilateral forelimb lameness is considered the norm and navicular syndrome has been described as heel pain that blocks to a PD nerve block on both forelimbs with or without radiographic abnormalities.[61] However, unilateral lameness can also occur, especially with lesions that involve the flexor surface of the navicular bone and/or the DDFT. Most horses with an acute onset of unilateral

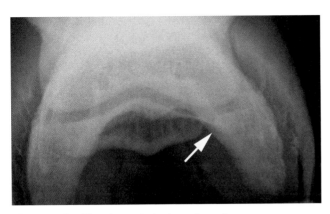

Figure 5.6. Bipartite navicular bone (arrow) as seen on a skyline radiograph in a young horse with lameness isolated to the foot.

lameness that blocks to the foot are not considered to have navicular disease/syndrome and lesions in the DDFT or other problems in the foot should be suspected.

Navicular disease/syndrome is considered to be a degenerative process due to wear and tear similar to OA; therefore, middle-aged to older horses are most commonly affected. Clinical signs usually become apparent in most horses between 7 and 10 years of age, although younger horses can be affected.[25,61,67] Horses with developmental/congenital abnormalities such as bipartite navicular bones can often become lame as early as 2 to 3 years of age (Figure 5.6). Geldings are more commonly affected than mares or stallions and Quarter horses, Warmbloods, and Thoroughbreds seem more predisposed to the disease than other breeds.[25,61] The classic signalment and history for many horses with navicular disease/syndrome is a middle–aged Quarter horse gelding with a history of chronic bilateral fore-limb lameness.

Although navicular disease/syndrome usually affects both front feet, the lameness may initially appear uni-lateral.[67] Greater than 95% incidence of asymmetrical lameness has been reported.[86] Most horses are more lame in 1 forelimb, both at a straight trot and when circled on a hard surface, but often demonstrate lame-ness on the opposite forelimb when circled with that limb on the inside. Bilateral forelimb lameness observed when circled both directions was present in 76% of the horses with less than 6 months' duration of lameness and in 52% in horses with greater than 6 months' dura-tion of lameness in a recent study.[61] The remainder of the horses had a unilateral lameness until a PD nerve block was performed, at which time the lameness switched to the opposite forelimb.[61] However, the true severity of a unilateral lameness at a straight trot may be misinterpreted because of the concurrent lameness in the opposite forelimb. In addition, the horse may tend to point one forelimb or alternate pointing each forelimb.[67,86] Asymmetry in the extensor muscles with atrophy of the muscles associated with the lame limb can often be observed in horses with chronic lameness.[67,86]

Various abnormalities of the hoof can be present in horses with navicular disease/syndrome. It can often be

difficult to determine whether the hoof abnormalities are contributing to the disease or have developed sec-ondary to the lameness and disuse of the foot. For example, both low, collapsed heels typical of Thorough-breds and narrow, upright feet typical of Quarter horses can occur in horses with navicular disease/syndrome. Secondary hoof abnormalities are most likely to develop in horses with a chronic duration of lameness. Common hoof problems seen in horses with navicular disease/syndrome include low, underrun heels, contracted or collapsed heels, medial to lateral imbalances, and long toes (Figures 5.1 to 5.3).[67,74,86] Dorsal to palmar imbal-ances such as the broken back hoof pastern axis is also commonly seen and is considered to be a predisposing factor for development of a multitude of problems in the foot. In one study, a broken back hoof pastern axis occurred in 71% of the horses with navicular disease/syndrome.[86] One forefoot is often smaller, narrower, and more upright (longer heels) than the other, which is presumably from disuse atrophy. In most cases the limb with the more upright hoof conformation is the limb with the greatest lameness.[18,67,86] Angular limb deformities, either valgus or varus, associated with the carpus and fetlock region have also been observed in a small percentage of cases.

At exercise, most horses with navicular disease/syn-drome exhibit a mild to moderate lameness (2 to 3 of 5) that is worse on hard surfaces. Only occasionally is severe lameness encountered. Some clinicians feel that the severity of lameness usually increases with the dura-tion of the lameness.[67] However, in a recent study the mean lameness grade of horses with navicular syndrome was grade 3 for horses with less than 6 months' dura-tion of lameness and grade 2 for horses with more than 6 months' duration of lameness.[61] The severity of lame-ness may be more related to the specific cause(s) of pain rather than the duration of the lameness.

While walking or trotting, many horses tend to land toe first and may occasionally stumble.[43,57,70] At a trot, horses with bilateral lameness tend to have a stiff, shuf-fling gait and often carry their heads and necks rigidly. This stilted gait is usually worsened when circled and has been described as the horse "trotting on egg-shells." This characteristic gait is often misinterpreted by owners as an unwillingness to advance the limbs associated with shoulder pain. When circled in either direction on a hard surface, the lameness is usually exaggerated in the limb that is on the inside of the circle. The lameness and stilted gait often worsens as the size of the circle is reduced. The horse may hold its head and neck to the outside of the circle in an effort to reduce the amount of weight carried on the inside limb.

The characteristic gait of horses with navicular disease/syndrome has historically been considered a compensatory change by the horse to avoid loading the heel region of the foot. However, a recent study dem-onstrated that the force exerted on the navicular bone was actually increased in horses with navicular disease compared to control horses in the early stance phase of the stride.[46,83] This was attributed to a greater force in the DDFT due to contraction of the deep digital flexor muscle in the early stance phase as the horse attempted to unload the heels. This seems contradictory, that in an attempt to avoid landing heel-first, the horse would simultaneously increase the force exerted on the navicular bone.

An additional study found that horses with navicular disease had abnormal limb-loading force patterns that were not altered by loss of sensation in the palmar region.[82] The authors hypothesized that some horses may be predisposed to navicular disease as a result of an inherent abnormal gait pattern. Further investigation into these findings will be necessary to determine their clinical relevance.

Hoof tester examination is considered essential for the clinical diagnosis of navicular disease/syndrome by many clinicians. However, the reliability of this test is somewhat controversial because a negative response to hoof testers over the frog region is not uncommon in horses with navicular syndrome/disease.[25,61,76] In one study, only approximately 50% of the horses with lameness localized to the navicular region responded positively to hoof tester pressure over the central third of the frog.[76] In contrast, a nonfatiguable painful withdrawal to intermittent hoof tester pressure over the central and occasionally the cranial third of the frog is considered a fairly consistent feature of navicular disease/syndrome by others.[67] It is the author's clinical opinion that horses with radiographic abnormalities in the navicular bone are more likely to be painful over the frog region with hoof testers than horses without radiographic changes. In addition, it is important to apply direct compressive pressure to the navicular region rather than simply applying lateral (shearing pressure) across the frog when using the hoof testers.[67] Horses with very thick soles and hard frogs usually do not respond to hoof tester pressure. Hoof tester pain may also be present over the toe secondary to bruising from landing toe-first but is usually of minor clinical significance.

Distention of the distal interphalangeal (DIP) joint may be present in horses with navicular disease but it is not a consistent clinical feature. However, the presence of DIP effusion may be an important finding when developing a treatment plan for an individual horse. In addition, asymmetrical DIP joint effusion is usually clinically relevant and often suggests a secondary problem within the joint. Many horses with navicular disease/syndrome may react positively to a phalangeal flexion test, which often exacerbates the lameness.[67,86] However, a positive phalangeal flexion test is not specific for the navicular region and is usually not that beneficial in localizing the lameness to the foot. A positive phalangeal flexion may suggest a primary or secondary problem within the DIP joint in some horses with foot pain.

Two types of wedge tests have been recommended to aid in the diagnosis of navicular disease/syndrome.[74] The frog wedge test is performed by placing the wedge of wood under the palmar two-thirds of the frog and forcing the horse to stand on that foot for 60 seconds (Figure 3.80 in Chapter 3). The toe extension test is performed by elevating the toe of the hoof with the wedge of wood and forcing the horse to stand on the limb for 60 seconds (Figure 3.81, Chapter 3). Both tests most likely apply compressive forces to the navicular region and a positive response suggests a problem in the area. The wedge test has been reported to suggest a

problem in the navicular bursa and the toe extension test to suggest a problem in the DDFT or the podotrochlear apparatus.[76] However, these interpretations are very subjective and additional diagnostics are always necessary to determine the exact cause of the lameness.

Diagnosis

Local Anesthesia

The diagnosis of navicular disease/syndrome begins with localizing the site of lameness to the foot or more specifically to the palmar aspect of the foot using diagnostic anesthesia. Historically, a PD nerve block was thought to only desensitize the palmar aspect of the foot but it is now known that it is relatively nonspecific and alleviates pain in the navicular bone, podotrochlear apparatus, navicular bursa, distal aspect of the DDFT, distal phalanx, middle phalanx, DIP joint, dorsal aspect of the hoof, and possibly the digital tendon sheath and PIP joint.[57,62] Therefore, a multitude of clinical problems in the foot can be desensitized with a PD block; this has been confirmed in several studies.[27–29,60,61]

Using a small volume of anesthetic (1.0 mL) and performing the PD block as low as possible in the heel region (axial and distal to the proximal limits of the collateral cartilages) is recommended to improve the specificity of the block to the structures within the palmar aspect of the foot.[57,63] However, using this approach does not guarantee that multiple other structures in the foot have not been desensitized. The majority of horses affected with navicular disease/syndrome (80% to 100%) improve substantially following a PD block and the lameness in the opposite forelimb either worsens or becomes apparent if a unilateral lameness was initially found.[61,67] Kinematic gait analysis has found that the mean maximal extension of the fetlock during the stance phase of the stride and the maximum flexion of the carpal joint during swing phase of the stride were significantly increased after PD blocks in horses with navicular disease.[41] In addition, the total stance phase, cranial stance phase, and break-over duration were significantly shorter after the block.[41]

Intrasynovial anesthesia of the DIP joint and the navicular bursa can also be performed to potentially further localize the site of pain. Historically, blocking the DIP joint was thought to help distinguish between problems associated with the joint vs. the navicular region. However, several studies have demonstrated a lack of specificity of intrasynovial anesthesia of the DIP joint due to diffusion of anesthetic and the location of sensory nerves in close approximation to the synovial outpouchings of the DIP joint.[9,10,26,53,64,65] Anesthesia of the DIP joint is known to improve the lameness in a large percentage of horses diagnosed with navicular syndrome.[25,26,67] However, it is the author's opinion that the amount of improvement in lameness following DIP joint anesthesia is less than that following a PD block in most horses with navicular disease/syndrome. Recommended methods to improve the specificity of DIP joint anesthesia are to use no more than 5 to 6 mL of anesthetic and to assess the response to the block within 5 to 10 minutes.[57,63]

Anesthesia of the navicular bursa is probably the most specific nerve block that can be used to help localize the site of pain in horses with navicular disease/syndrome. However, it is not used routinely by the author because of the need for radiographic or fluoroscopic confirmation of the injection. A positive response to intrasynovial anesthesia into the navicular bursa may indicate problems of the navicular bursa, navicular bone, and/or its supporting ligaments, sole, and/or toe, or distal aspect of the DDFT.[63-65] Even though diffusion of local anesthetic into the navicular bursa occurs following DIP joint injection the converse does not occur, and analgesia of the navicular bursa does not usually result in analgesia of the DIP joint.[63,64] Pain from the DIP joint can likely be excluded as a cause of lameness if analgesia of the navicular bursa improves the lameness within 10 minutes.[63,64] In addition, a positive response to intra-articular analgesia of the DIP joint together with a negative response to navicular bursa analgesia incriminates pain within the DIP joint as the cause of lameness.[63]

See Chapter 3 for further information about local anesthesia.

Radiography

Despite its limitations, radiography remains the initial diagnostic tool to assess the navicular bone in most horses with navicular disease/syndrome. However, degenerative changes within the bone can be missed because a 40% change in bone density is required before it can be identified with radiographs.[57] Therefore, the lack of abnormalities in the navicular bone does not eliminate the bone as the site of the pain, and does not necessarily indicate a soft tissue problem in the foot. In a recent study of horses with navicular syndrome that did not have radiographic abnormalities within the navicular bone, the navicular bone was considered to be abnormal in the majority of horses on MRI.[61] However, the navicular bone was considered the primary abnormality in only 33% of horses with a recent onset of lameness and in only 16% of horses with a more chronic duration of lameness.[61]

A complete radiographic evaluation of the navicular bone requires a minimum of lateromedial, 60° dorsoproximal-palmarodistal oblique, and palmaroproximal-palmarodistal oblique (skyline) high-quality views.[30,67] Additional radiographs such as the 60° dorsoproximal-palmarodistal oblique view of the distal phalanx and the weight-bearing dorsopalmar view are often included to completely evaluate all bony structures in the foot. Careful attention to foot preparation (packing the frog), limb position, and centering and directing the x-ray beam according to the hoof capsule conformation is important to avoid artifacts.[30]

Potentially significant radiographic abnormalities include (1) enthesiophytes at the proximomedial and proximolateral aspect of the bone, (2) proximal or distal extension of the flexor border of the bone, (3) distal border fragments, (4) large and variably shaped distal border radiolucent zones, (5) discrete radiolucent areas in the spongiosa with or without detectable communication with the flexor cortex, (6) new bone at the sagittal ridge, (7) increased thickness of the flexor

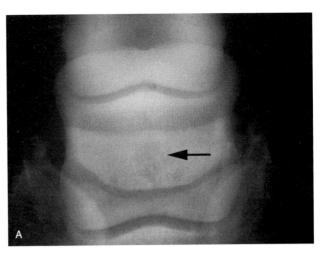

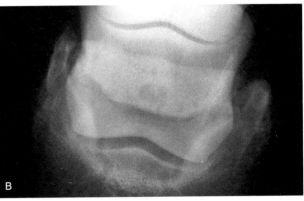

Figure 5.7. A and B. Single large cystic lesions in 2 different horses (arrow in A) within the navicular bone as seen on oblique radiographs.

cortex, (8) sclerosis of the spongiosa, and (9) a bipartite bone.[30] Additional abnormalities that are considered important include flexor cortex defects or erosions, loss of corticomedullary distinction, and mineralization of the supporting ligaments of the navicular bone or the DDFT.[39,76,79]

The radiographic abnormalities that appear to be the most reliable indicators of navicular disease/syndrome are cyst-like lesions within the medullary cavity (Figures 5.7 and 5.8), flexor cortex lesions, and sclerosis of the spongiosa with loss of demarcation of the flexor cortex and medulla (Figures 5.9 and 5.10).[79] Flexor cortex defects were seen in less than 1% of normal horses; they represent lysis of subchondral bone and are linked to fibrocartilage degeneration and damage to the DDFT (Figure 5.11).[39,79] Sclerosis was present in up to 80% of horses with navicular syndrome but in less than 16% of normal horses.[39]

Less reliable radiographic indicators include enthesiophytes at the proximal or distal border of the bone, elongation of the flexor border of the bone, distal border fragments, and enlarged synovial invaginations. All of these abnormalities of the navicular bone can be present in nonlame horses and by themselves may not constitute radiographic evidence of navicular disease.[79] However, distal border fragments appear to be recognized more frequently with digital radiography and are thought to

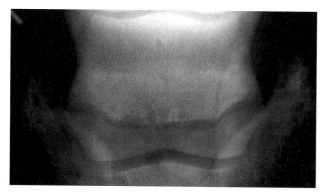

Figure 5.8. Multiple smaller cystic lesions along the distal border of the navicular bone as demonstrated on an oblique radiograph.

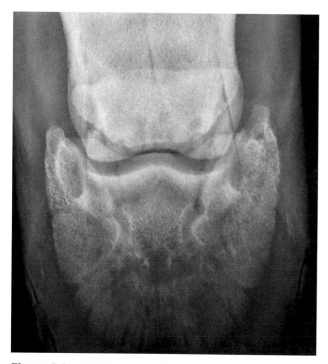

Figure 5.9. Multiple abnormalities within the navicular bone as seen on an oblique radiograph. Abnormalities present include remodeling along the proximal border, multiple cystic lesions along the distal border, and enthesiophytes on the wings of the navicular bone.

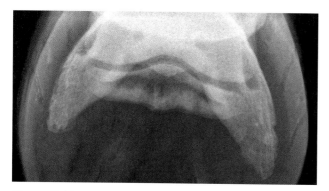

Figure 5.10. Skyline radiograph of the same horse as in Figure 5.9 demonstrating sclerosis of the medullary cavity of the navicular bone and erosions along the flexor surface.

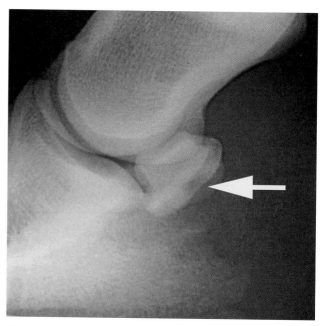

Figure 5.11. Lateral radiograph of the foot in the horse in Figure 5.5. A lytic defect is present in the flexor surface of the navicular bone (arrow).

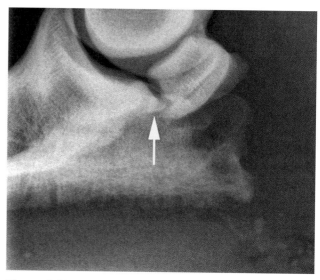

Figure 5.12. An avulsion fracture from the distal border of the navicular bone (arrow) can be seen on this lateral radiograph.

be associated with navicular disease (Figure 5.12).[29,30] These fragments may represent a fracture, enthesiophyte, or dystrophic mineralization within the DSIL. See Chapter 4 for further information on radiography of the navicular bone.

Navicular bursography has been reported as a technique that can provide information regarding pathologic changes associated with the fibrocartilage on the flexor surface of the navicular bone and the DDFT.[77] The authors concluded that navicular bursography identified pathology in the flexor cortex of the navicular bone 60% more often than plain radiography. However, this technique is infrequently used clinically and the development of other imaging techniques to visualize soft tissues of the foot has rendered it relatively absolete.[57]

Ultrasonography

Ultrasound is an economical and readily available diagnostic technique that can be used to help diagnose potential soft tissue injuries within the foot in horses with navicular disease. However, the keratinized hoof wall, frog, and sole all limit contact with the ultrasound probe and prevent good images from being obtained.[13,57] With experience, ultrasound can be used to assess the flexor surface of the navicular bone, distal part of the DDFT, podotrochlear apparatus, CL of the DIP joint, and entheses of the distal phalanx.[13,34,57] A transcutaneous approach either between the heel bulbs and/or through the frog after it has been softened by soaking is usually used. Similar to radiography, the accuracy of ultrasound to document pathology within the foot has been criticized based on results of more advanced imaging such as MRI. Therefore, negative findings with ultrasound do not rule out the presence of abnormalities in the navicular region.

Scintigraphy

Scintigraphy (nuclear imaging) is thought to be able to identify early pathologic changes within the navicular bone. Its sensitivity is related to the ability to identify early alterations in bone metabolism rather than relying on anatomic changes. Scintigraphic is probably most useful in cases where radiographic changes have not developed or they are equivocal.[60,71]

Increased radiopharmaceutical uptake (IRU) has been documented in some horses with navicular disease/syndrome.[27,31,40,60] In one study that evaluated 264 horses with foot pain, IRU was detected in the navicular bone in 36.6% of the limbs and in a very small percentage of limbs with soft tissue injuries within the foot.[31] Scintigraphic assessment of the foot can be helpful to identify the potential source of pain causing lameness but false positive results can occur, especially in horses with low heel conformation.[27,31] Another study concluded that a negative scintigram of the foot does not preclude significant injuries.[31] In addition, scintigraphy does not provide a definitive diagnosis and it may be difficult to localize the area of pathology when a relatively small bone such as the navicular bone is involved.[57] For these reasons, and the economics of performing multiple advanced imaging techniques on the same horse, MRI is usually performed instead of scintigraphy.

Computed Tomography (CT)

Computer tomography is the best modality to detect and assess pathology within the cortex and trabeculae of the navicular bone.[57,69] Many osseous changes seen on CT are not radiographically evident, such as shape changes within the bone, distal border fragments, and intramedullary changes.[57,69] Soft tissue abnormalities within the foot may be detected with CT, but in general, CT is best to assess bone and MRI is best to assess soft tissue lesions.[80] However, intra-arterial contrast-

enhanced CT has been shown to improve the imaging of soft tissue structures within the foot, and may be an alternative to using MRI.[55] The use of CT would facilitate an earlier and more accurate diagnosis of navicular disease in horses; the disadvantages are the cost and the requirement for general anesthesia. In addition, concurrent soft tissue abnormalities appear to be a major component of horses with foot pain[57] and these lesions would be best assessed using MRI vs. CT. See Chapter 4 for more information on CT.

Magnetic Resonance Imaging (MRI)

Magnetic resonance imaging has become increasingly available in recent years and is currently the preferred diagnostic technique to assess most horses with navicular disease/syndrome.[14,28,29,47,61] The different sequences permit accurate evaluation of soft tissues, cartilage, and bone within the digit in near anatomic detail. The MRI technique can be performed in both the standing or recumbent patient but better quality images are thought to be obtained with units that require the horse to be anesthetized.

Numerous pathologic entities have been identified with MRI in horses with navicular disease/syndrome, and many horses appear to have multiple abnormalities present within the same foot.[28,47,61] The most common abnormalities found on MRI involve the navicular bone, CSL, DSIL, DDFT, navicular bursa, CL of the DIP joint, and the DIP joint.[28,47,61] Several studies have documented that the DDFT and the DSIL are commonly abnormal in horses with foot pain (Figures 5.13 and 5.14).[28,47,61] However, the frequency of occurrence of lesions differs among studies in regard to injuries to the CSL and the CL of the DIP joint.

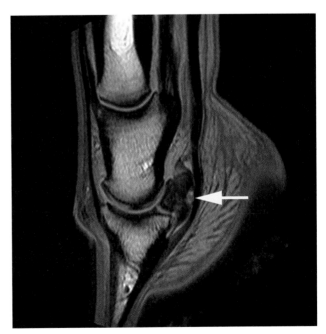

Figure 5.13. A lateral STIR MR image of the horse in Figure 5.11 demonstrating abnormal signal within the navicular bone (arrow).

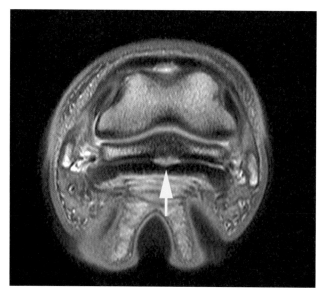

Figure 5.14. Surface damage to the DDFT (arrow) can be seen on this MR image of the same horse as in Figures 5.11 and 5.13.

Certain studies have reported a high frequency of lesions within the CL of the DIP joint and few lesions within the CSL.[28,29] In contrast, another large study indicated a high frequency of lesions within the CSL and few within the CL of the DIP joint.[61] This may represent differences in the population of horses of each group or possibly in the interpretation of the MRI. From a clinical viewpoint, the current difficulty with interpreting the results of MRI is determining what may be the primary abnormality when multiple lesions are found. However, this may be less important if we now assume that multiple abnormalities within the foot most likely contribute to the pain in horses with navicular disease/syndrome. See Chapter 4 for more information on MRI.

Treatment

Multiple factors are involved when deciding on a treatment protocol for horses with navicular disease/syndrome. In most cases the treatment must be tailor made for each individual horse based on the severity of lameness, intended use of the horse, wishes of the owner, results of diagnostics (or lack of diagnostics such as MRI), hoof conformation, previous treatments, and most likely diagnosis.

Realistically, horses with advanced radiographic abnormalities in the navicular bone will be problematic regardless of the treatments employed. Historically, horses with minimal radiographic abnormalities of the navicular bone were thought to respond to therapy better than those with radiographic abnormalities.[67] However, this generalization is debatable because horses with DDFT injuries with or without navicular bone abnormalities tend to do poorly regardless of treatment.[29,57] In addition, developing a treatment protocol for horses without radiographic abnormalities and without performing an MRI can be challenging because

a definitive diagnosis is difficult to make in these horses. The ability to develop a more precise treatment protocol is considered one of the benefits of performing an MRI in horses with foot pain.

A variety of treatment options are available for horses with navicular disease/syndrome with the goal of managing the disease. One of the most important treatments is corrective trimming and shoeing.[57,67,73] Other nonsurgical treatments include rest and controlled exercise and drugs to improve blood flow such as isoxsuprine, nonsteroidal anti-inflammatory drugs (NSAIDs), bisphosphonates such as tiludronate, intrasynovial medications, and medications aimed at preventing OA. Surgical treatments include palmar/plantar digital neurectomy, desmotomy of the CSL, inferior check ligament desmotomy, and endoscopy of the navicular bursa. A brief overview of these treatments is discussed below. See Chapters 8 and 12 for more information.

Rest and Controlled Exercise

In the past, prolonged rest has not been recommended for most horses with navicular disease because the lameness often returns shortly after the horse resumes exercise.[44] However, significant soft tissue injuries within the foot such as DDFT or CSL lesions may warrant a more extended rest and rehabilitation period, similar to that recommended for horses with tendinitis elsewhere in the limb. However, many of the lesions within the DDFT appear to be degenerative and not inflammatory, so it could be debated whether they will respond to rest alone. Nevertheless, a short period of rest is usually recommended for most horses with navicular disease/syndrome to help reduce the soft tissue inflammation and allow the horse to acclimate to corrective trimming and shoeing.[67] This is substantiated by MRI findings that concurrent soft tissue and bone pathology most likely contribute to the pain in many horses with palmar foot pain.[28,47] Although the rest period may vary for individual cases, the author usually recommends no work until at least the first shoeing change in most horses. A period of complete rest for 3 weeks followed by controlled exercise at a walk only for an additional 3 weeks is preferred. A decision is usually made regarding further exercise and continued treatment at the first shoeing change based on the response to treatment.

Corrective Trimming and Shoeing

Corrective trimming and shoeing is the basis for managing most horses with navicular syndrome.[18,57,67,73] Many horses respond favorably to shoeing alone without requiring further medical or surgical therapy. In one study, improvement in clinical signs within 3 months of initiation of treatment was seen, and 86% of the horses remained free of lameness for 1 year.[73,74] In another study, 73% (22 of 30) of horses with signs of navicular syndrome improved 1 grade in lameness after 6 weeks following corrective trimming and shoeing.[50]

The goals of trimming and shoeing are to (1) restore normal foot balance, (2) correct foot problems such as shearing of the quarters and heels, underrun heels, and heel bulb contraction, (3) reduce biomechanical forces on the navicular region, (4) ease break-over, (5) support the heels, and (6) protect the injured areas of the foot.[18,67]

Multiple types of shoes have been used for horses with heel pain and 1 type of shoe cannot be used in every horse. For instance, a horse with the low heel, long toe conformation may benefit from an elevated heel shoe, whereas a horse with a narrow upright foot may actually benefit from heel removal and placement of a flat natural balance or egg-bar shoe. When the heels are long, they tend to grow forward, decreasing heel support and contributing to dorsopalmar hoof imbalance.[18] In general, foot preparation or trimming is more important than the type of shoe used in most horses with navicular disease/syndrome. A well-made shoe placed on an improperly trimmed foot serves little purpose. The heels should be trimmed to the widest aspect of the frog and the toes shortened as much as possible to shift weight-bearing to the back of the foot.[18,49] See Chapter 12 for more information on foot trimming and shoeing.

Much information to aid trimming and shoeing of horses with navicular disease/syndrome can often be obtained from lateral and weight-bearing dorsopalmar radiographs. Medial to lateral and dorsopalmar hoof balance, toe length in relation to the distal phalanx, heel height, sole depth, and solar angle of the distal phalanx are all very important pieces of information that should be used during the shoeing process. A thumbtack placed at the apex of the frog on a lateral radiograph may also be used to approximate the break-over point of the shoe when using the natural balance shoeing approach.[50] The distance from the thumbtack to the designated point of break-over dorsal to the tip of the distal phalanx (one-quarter inch dorsal to the tip of the distal phalanx) can be measured on the radiograph and used as a reference point when placing the shoe (Figure 5.15). Alternatively, the break-over point can be located at the point where a line drawn along the dorsal aspect of the distal phalanx bisects the sole of the hoof.[18]

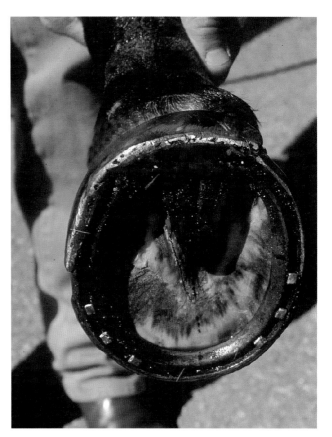

Figure 5.16. Using egg-bar shoes is a common shoeing technique to treat horses with navicular disease/syndrome.

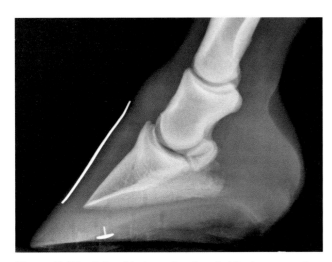

Figure 5.15. A thumbtack can be placed at the true apex of the frog when taking lateral radiographs to identify its location relative to the tip of P3. This can be used to estimate the break-over point on the bottom of the foot.

Several different types of steel or aluminum shoes are thought to be effective in treating horses with heel pain. These include elevated heel shoes such as the Tennessee navicular shoe, regular shoes with heel elevation using a wedge-pad, rolled or rockered toed shoes, egg-bar shoes, natural balance shoes, equine digital support system (EDSS), and full-bar support shoes (Figures 5.16 and 5.17).[18,44,67,73] Rolling, rockering, or squaring the toe of any of these shoes enhances break-over, thus reducing the stress on the DDFT. The goals of any of these shoes should be to ease break-over, support the heels, and reduce the forces acting on the navicular bone by the DDFT.

Heel elevation has repeatedly been shown to decrease tension in the DDFT, reduce pressure applied to the navicular bone, reduce the load to the forelimbs, and reduce the stresses on the hoof capsule (Figure 5.17).[57,58,62,81] The heels are supported for a greater proportion of the stride and the wedge tends to increase the weight transferred through the heels. In addition, heel elevation alone or when combined with phenylbutazone has been shown quantitatively (using a force plate) to improve lameness in clinical cases of horses with navicular syndrome.[62] The disadvantages are that the use of pads in horses with underrun heels may cause further collapse of the poorly supported heels and that heel growth appears to be reduced with wedge-pads.[18] This makes discontinuing the use of the wedge-pads in the future problematic.

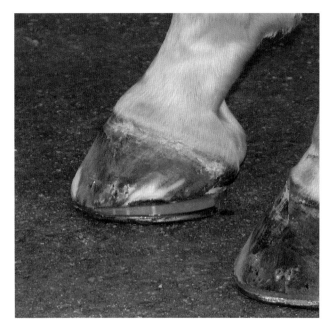

Figure 5.17. Natural balance shoes with a full wedge-pad and dental impression material placed in the palmar aspect of the foot can also be used to treat horses with navicular disease/syndrome.

In contrast, egg-bar shoes and natural balance shoes have not been shown to reduce the forces on the navicular bone as effectively as heel elevation.[57] However, egg-bar shoes increase the length of the toe-heel axis causing the center of pressure to shift caudally.[58] Egg-bar shoes are usually recommended in cases where the hoof capsule is unstable due to shearing or in horses with severely under-run or collapsed heels. The egg-bar shoe increases the surface area of contact and the stability of the hoof. The shoe should be applied so it is clearly visible at the quarters and extends far enough palmarly to cover the heels.[67,73,74] Natural balance shoes, by their design, reduce break-over, and if combined with heel elevation also reduce the forces acting on the navicular bone. See Chapter 12 for more information on corrective trimming and shoeing.

A minimum 2- to 3-week adaptation period is often necessary to achieve pain relief with any type of shoeing.[57,62] In most cases improvement in clinical signs after corrective trimming and shoeing is often seen within 6 weeks; however this depends on the severity of the initial lameness and the specific structures affected. Severe hoof imbalances may require several shoeing intervals to achieve a normal hoof conformation and, in some cases, the underrun heels may persist indefinitely. Additionally, not all horses respond in the same manner to a particular shoeing type, and we as veterinarians should remain flexible in using a different type of shoe if a clinical response is not obtained.

Nonsteroidal Anti-inflammatory Drugs

The use of NSAIDs is a common adjunctive treatment for horses with navicular disease/syndrome. Flunixin meglumine, phenylbutazone, or firocoxib are used most commonly and all should be effective in reducing inflammation and lameness. Horses with navicular disease that were treated with 1.1 mg/kg of flunixin meglumine or 4.4 mg/kg phenylbutazone once daily for 4 days showed significant reduction in lameness scores for 24 hours after the last dose compared to baseline and horses treated with saline.[33] The clinical responses between flunixin meglumine and phenylbutazone were similar and suggest that once-daily dosing of NSAIDs should be effective to control pain in the majority of these horses.

NSAIDs are often used for pain relief if the horse is severely lame or if the horse needs to continue working through the initial treatment period. Phenylbutazone is usually used most frequently because it is less expense than flunixin meglumine. It is usually given at a dose of 4.4 mg/kg PO once daily for 7 to 10 days as the initial treatment. This appears to effectively break the pain cycle and allows for adjustment to corrective trimming and shoeing.[67] NSAIDs may be used intermittently thereafter if they are permitted for the athletic activity of the horse.

Intrasynovial Medication

Injecting medications into the DIP joint or navicular bursa is often used as an adjunctive treatment for horses with navicular disease/syndrome.[18,19,62,78] Injection of medications into the digital flexor tendon sheath (DFTS) may also benefit some horses with more proximal lesions of the DDFT that are documented with MRI. Deciding when to treat horses with navicular disease/syndrome intrasynovially and with what medication(s) is strictly empirical based on many clinical and diagnostic findings. The types of medications used are similar to those used to treat OA/synovitis/capsulitis in joints at other locations, such as corticosteroids alone, corticosteroids combined with hyaluronan (HA), or polysulfated glycosaminoglycans (PSGAGs).

Horses with navicular disease are thought to benefit from intra-articular treatment of the DIP joint by reducing the inflammatory response both within the joint and within the navicular region.[51] A recent study demonstrated that a clinically effective concentration of methylprednisolone acetate (MPA)or triamcinolone (TA) diffused between the DIP joint and navicular bursa after intra-articular or intrabursal injection.[51] Studies have documented the benefit of intrabursal injections in providing substantial but temporary relief of pain in many horses with navicular disease.[19,78] The mean duration of soundness following injection was 4.6 months in one study.[19] The benefit of DIP joint injections is less well documented but anecdotally it is considered effective in many horses.[18] One study did not find a significant reduction in lameness from treating the DIP joint with TA compared to corrective shoeing alone.[62] However, the overall severity of lameness was further reduced following treatment of the DIP joint, although not significantly.

Many clinicians use intrasynovial treatment of the DIP joint as part of the initial treatment regimen, together with corrective trimming and shoeing and phenylbutazone for most horses with navicular disease/syndrome. Others may only use intrasynovial treatment in those cases that do not respond favorably to corrective trimming and shoeing, controlled exercise, and NSAIDs.

In many horses, especially if advanced imaging cannot be performed, there is a step-wise progression of treatment options based on the clinical response. The decision to use intrasynovial treatment is often made at the first or second shoeing interval and is usually based on the clinical improvement in lameness. In most cases, treatment of the DIP joint is performed before treatment of the bursa or DFTS because it is easier to perform and has fewer potential complications. However, horses with radiographic abnormalities confined to the flexor surface of the navicular bone would most likely respond better to treatment of the navicular bursa than the DIP joint, in the author's opinion. Intrasynovial medication strategies may be greatly improved if a complete diagnostic picture of the foot abnormalities can be determined with MRI.

Both TA (5 to 10 mg) and MPA (20 to 60 mg) may be used for intrasynovial treatment, but MPA is usually reserved for use in the navicular bursa rather than the DIP joint. In most cases the corticosteroid is combined with HA, and amikacin is included when injecting the navicular bursa.[18,19] An immediate improvement in lameness is often seen in the majority of cases after intrabursal treatment.[19,78] In one study, 80% of the horses returned to work within 2 weeks of injection and the mean duration of soundness was 4.6 months.[19] In another study of 148 horses with navicular disease that had intrabursal injections, pain was alleviated for at least 2 months in more than 60% of the cases.[78] Intrabursal injections appear to reduce the clinical signs of navicular disease in most horses for several months but repeated injections may predispose to rupture of the DDFT in some horses.[19]

Isoxsuprine

Isoxsuprine hydrochloride has been commonly used to treat horses with navicular syndrome.[59,67,72] It is a β-adrenergic agonist that is thought to have both vasodilatory and rheologic properties, although its mode of action in the treatment of navicular disease is unknown because no measurable cardiovascular effects of isoxsuprine given orally at twice the recommended dosage can be detected in the horse.[37,44] In a clinical trial, horses with navicular syndrome showed significantly greater improvement when treated with isoxsuprine, compared to those treated with a placebo.[72] In that study, isoxsuprine was administered orally at 0.66 mg/kg BID for 3 weeks, followed by 0.66 mg/kg once daily for 2 weeks, followed by every-other-day dosing.[72] Higher doses (1.2 mg/kg) may be used to overcome the poor absorption of the drug, but no studies have documented the clinical efficacy of higher doses of isoxsuprine. Reported success rates range from 40% to 87%, with the best results occurring in horses affected less than 1 year.[72] Improvement in clinical signs may persist for up to 1 year after discontinuing isoxsuprine, especially if other predisposing foot problems have been corrected.

Continuous treatment with isoxsuprine can be used in horses that become painful when taken off of the drug because adverse side effects have not been reported with oral isoxsuprine in the horse. However, the drug has not been proven safe for use in pregnant mares. In general, oral isoxsuprine appears to be most effective clinically in horses with mild radiographic abnormalities of the navicular bone or in the early stages of the disease. The response to treatment in horses with major radiographic abnormalities is generally poor.[44] In addition, the clinical use of isoxsuprine to treat horses with navicular disease appears to have decreased in recent years.

Polysulfated Glycosaminoglycans

Polysulfated glycosaminoglycans have been used in horses with navicular disease/syndrome based on the assumption that the etiology may be similar to that of OA. One double-blinded clinical trial documented a benefit of 500 mg of PSGAG IM at 4-day intervals for 8 treatments compared to saline controls.[16] In addition, PSGAG given weekly or every other week IM was thought to benefit Western performance horses with chronic navicular problems.[18] PSGAG may also be injected intrasynovially into the DIP joint or navicular bursa, similar to corticosteroids, but no studies have documented the benefit in horses with navicular disease with this treatment protocol.

Tiludronate

Bisphosphonates, such as tiludronate, are drugs that reduce bone resorption and have proven very effective in human medicine.[57] Areas of increased bone resorption and formation are often typical of lesions within a diseased navicular bone. In one clinical trial of 73 horses, tiludronate (0.1 mg/kg) given IV once daily for 10 days resulted in a clinical improvement of lameness and horses returned to a normal level of activity 2 to 6 months post treatment.[21] Horses with more recent onset of clinical signs responded better to treatment than those with more chronic disease.

Tiludronate is currently not licensed for use in the United States but is labeled for use in other countries for horses with navicular disease, bone spavin, and fetlock suspensory ligament enthesopathies. The drug is currently recommended at a dose of 1 mg/kg IV over 30 minutes as a single treatment instead of 10 daily treatments. Further studies are necessary to determine its efficacy in treating horses with navicular disease/syndrome. See Chapter 8 for more information on tiludronate.

Surgical Treatments

Palmar Digital Neurectomy

Palmar digital neurectomy remains the most commonly performed surgical technique to manage horses with navicular disease/syndrome. It is usually performed as a last resort after other treatment options have failed. It should be done in conjunction with corrective hoof trimming and shoeing to reduce abnormal forces on the foot, thus slowing the progression of the degenerative changes associated with the navicular syndrome.[67] A PD nerve block should always be performed before the surgery to document how much clinical improvement can be expected following the neurectomy.

Horses with suspected or confirmed abnormalities of the DDFT at the level of the navicular bone are usually not good candidates for a neurectomy because of an increased risk of rupture of the DDFT. However, this has not been documented in any clinical study, to the author's knowledge. The decision of whether to perform a neurectomy is often based on the severity of lameness, age and intended use of the horse, known abnormalities based on imaging results, responses to previous treatments, and the wishes of the owner.

Various methods of PD neurectomy have been described including the guillotine technique (sharp transection of the nerve and a segment of the nerve is removed), laser neurectomy (CO_2 and ND : YAG), the pull-through or stripping technique, epineural (perineural) capping, silicone capping, cyanoacrylate glue capping, radioactive ligature, and intramedullary anchoring of the nerve.[4,17,35,36,38,45,67] All of these proposed techniques have been developed to ensure complete desensitization, prevent painful neuroma formation, and prevent axonal regrowth which may result in reinnervation. In one study of 50 horses with follow-up after a PD neurectomy was performed, recurrence of heel pain was a more common complication (14 of 50) than development of painful neuromas (3 of 50).[38]

Choosing which surgical technique to perform is often a personal preference of the veterinarian as several studies have failed to determine the ideal PD neurectomy technique. Attempts to find a superior technique to the time-honored guillotine approach have failed and currently most surgeons recommend this approach for PD neurectomy. The pull-through or stripping technique is recommended by the author and the clinical results appear to be very good (Figure 5.18).[18,45] The

advantages of the pull-through approach are that no special equipment is needed, it can be easily performed in the standing or recumbent horse, and the end of the transected nerve is not located within the incision. Regardless of the technique used for a PD neurectomy, a clean and atraumatic surgery and diligent postoperative care will minimize complications.[18] Limited activity for 30 to 60 days and careful bandaging of the limbs for at least 3 to 4 weeks is thought to reduce the inflammatory response created by the surgery and reduce scar tissue formation around the nerve stumps.[18]

The prognosis of horses following a PD neurectomy appears to be very good initially but becomes less favorable as time progresses. In a study of 57 horses, 74% of the horses were sound at 1 year, but this decreased to 63% after the second year.[38] In a study of horses that underwent the pull-through neurectomy technique, 88% were free of lameness at 1 year.[45] Survival analysis that was used to assess the time to recurrence of lameness indicated that the mean survival with no lameness after surgery was estimated at 4.14 ± 0.33 years (median, 5 years).[45] The most significant complications after a neurectomy include rupture of the DDFT, regrowth of the nerves resulting in recurrence of the lameness, and severe infection within the foot that goes unnoticed.

Navicular Suspensory Ligament Desmotomy

Navicular suspensory desmotomy has been used in the past as a treatment for horses with navicular disease/syndrome.[2,87] In a review of 118 horses that were treated with navicular suspensory desmotomy, 76% were sound at 6 months and 43% were sound after 36 months.[87] The presence of flexor cortex defects, proximal border enthesophytes, mineralization of the DDFT, and medullary sclerosis were all associated with a diminished response. The ligaments were transected using an open approach in the pastern region below their attachments to the proximal phalanx. This treatment has not gained widespread use over the years and has fallen out of favor as a legitimate treatment for horses with navicular disease.[18]

An arthroscopic approach through the palmar aspect of the DIP joint to transect the CSL is currently being developed. The ligaments are identified along the DIP joint capsule with the arthroscope and transected with a hooked blade. This technique is being used to treat horses with primary lesions within the CSL that have been identified on MRI.[61] Further information will be necessary to determine if this is a viable treatment option for these horses.

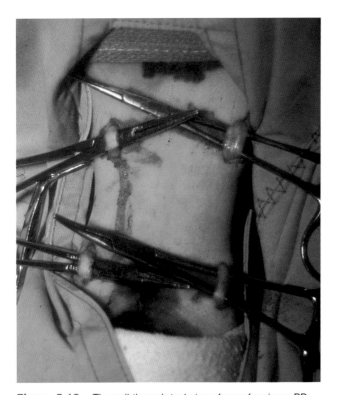

Figure 5.18. The pull-through technique for performing a PD neurectomy. Small skin incisions are made distally and proximally in the pastern region and the PD nerve is transected distally and pulled through the proximal incision.

Inferior Check Ligament Desmotomy

Inferior check ligament desmotomy has been used in selected cases of horses with navicular syndrome in which dorsal palmar hoof imbalance (either broken forward or broken backward axis) appears to be a major contributing factor. In one study, 4 horses with navicular syndrome that were treated with an inferior check ligament desmotomy all returned to full use, and the surgery made it possible to align the hoof pastern axis after surgery.[75] This surgery seems to be most useful in horses with an upright heel conformation and a broken forward hoof pastern axis, as is sometimes seen in Quarter horses with mismatched front feet. In addition, the surgery may help to reduce the compressive forces on the navicular bone generated by contraction of the deep digital flexor muscle that is thought to occur in horses with navicular disease in an attempt to unload the heels.[46,83]

Endoscopy/Bursoscopy

Endoscopy of the navicular bursa has become the preferred surgical treatment of horses with infections or wounds that enter the navicular bursa. Endoscopy of the bursa may also be performed both as a diagnostic and treatment tool in a select group of horses with navicular disease using a modified surgical approach.[66] Horses with known or suspected abnormalities on the flexor surface of the navicular bone (flexor cortex erosions) and those with DDFT lesions (dorsal abrasions) at the level of the navicular bone are the ideal candidates for navicular endoscopy (Figure 5.19). In a recent study, 23 bursae were examined endoscopically in 20 horses and tears of the DDFT were seen in all horses (22 bursae).[66] Cartilage lesions on the flexor surface of the navicular bone were also present in 8 bursae, but were not diagnosed with pre-surgery CT or MRI. Greater than 6-month follow-up information was available for 15 animals, of which 11 were sound and 9 had returned to preoperative levels of performance. Endoscopy of the navicular bursa should be considered as a treatment option for horses with abnormalities that are localized to the navicular bursa region. Advanced imaging with CT or MRI would most likely be necessary prior to endoscopy in most cases to best determine the potential benefit of the surgery.

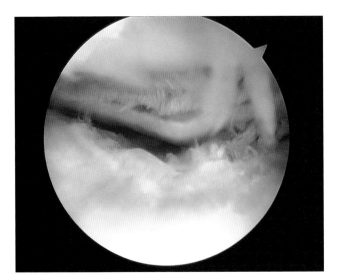

Figure 5.19. Endoscopic view of the flexor cortex lesion and the fibrillation of the DDFT that was present in the horse in Figures 5.13 and 5.14. The navicular bone is at the top of the image and the DDFT is on the bottom.

Prognosis

The prognosis of horses with navicular disease/syndrome is difficult to predict because of the numerous bone and soft tissue abnormalities that can occur concurrently. Radiographs alone are usually not adequate to completely assess the pathology within the foot, and therefore cannot be used alone to determine the prognosis unless the abnormalities are advanced. Based on what has been learned to date from published MRI studies, multiple bone and soft tissue lesions should be suspected, which can greatly alter the prognosis. In addition, most abnormalities are degenerative in nature and worsen with time and continued use of the horse.

There is no cure for the disease and the preceding treatments are probably more appropriately termed management strategies because the disease/syndrome is unlikely to resolve completely. In general, clinical resolution may occur in 40% to 50% of the horses with navicular disease/syndrome but the optimal treatment and prognosis may differ depending on the specific pathologies that may be present.[57] For instance, horses with major radiographic abnormalities most likely will have a worse prognosis than horses with no radiographic changes and minor soft tissue pathology. Horses with navicular bone pathology demonstrated on radiographs or MRI together with concurrent DDFT lesions will also tend to have a poor prognosis. In general, horses with primary soft tissue injuries are thought to have a guarded prognosis for return to full athletic function and horses with lesions in the navicular bone per se have a poor prognosis.[28,29,57] Due to the diversity of underlying problems associated with the disease, the key to controlling navicular disease/syndrome is most likely prevention.[57] Good foot care, proper trimming and shoeing, maintaining correct dorsopalmar hoof balance, and preventing overextension of the palmar aspect of the foot cannot be overemphasized.

References

1. Barber MJ, Sampson SN, Schneider RK, et al. Use of magnetic resonance imaging to diagnose distal sesamoid bone injury in a horse. J Am Vet Med Assoc 2006;229:717–720.
2. Bell BTL, Bridge IS, Sullivan STK. Surgical treatment of navicular syndrome in the horse using navicular suspensory desmotomy. New Zealand Vet J 1996;44:26–30.
3. Bentley VA, Sample SJ, Livesey MA, et al. Morphologic changes associated with functional adaptation of the navicular bone of horses. J Anat 2007;211:662–672.
4. Black JB. Palmar digital neurectomy: an alternative surgical approach. Proceedings Am Assoc Equine Pract 1992;38:429–432.
5. Blunden A, Dyson S, Murray R, et al. Histopathology in horses with chronic palmar foot pain and age-matched controls. Part 1: Navicular bone and related structures. Equine Vet J 2006;38:15–22.
6. Blunden A, Dyson S, Murray R, et al. Histopathology in horses with chronic palmar foot pain and age-matched controls. Part 2: The deep digital flexor tendon. Equine Vet J 2006;38:23–27.
7. Bos H, van der Meij GJ, Dik KJ. Heredity of navicular disease. Vet Q 1986;8:68–72.
8. Bowker RM, Van Wulfen KK. Microanatomy of the intersection of the distal sesamoidean impar ligament and the deep digital flexor tendon: A preliminary report. Pferdeheilkunde, 1996;12:623–627.
9. Bowker RM, Rockershouser SJ, Vex KB, et al. Immunocytochemical and dye distribution studies of nerves potentially desensitized by injection onto the distal interphalangeal joint or the navicular bursa of horses. J Am Vet Med Assoc, 1993;203:1707–1714.

10. Bowker RM, Linder K, Van Wulfen KK. Distribution of local anesthetics injected into the distal interphalangeal joint and podotrochlear bursa: An experimental study. Pferdeheilkunde, 1996;12:609–612.
11. Bowker RM, Atkinson PJ, Atkinson TS, et al. Effect of contact stress in bones of the distal interphalangeal joint on microscopic changes in articular cartilage and ligaments. Am J Vet Res 2001;62:414–424.
12. Bowker RM. Contrasting structural morphologies of "good" and "bad" footed horses. Proceedings Am Assoc Equine Pract 2003;49:186–209.
13. Busoni V, Denoix JM. Ultrasonography of the podotrochlear apparatus in the horse using a transcuneal approach: technique and reference images. Vet Radiol Ultrasound 2001;42:534–540.
14. Busoni V, Heimann M, Trenteseaux J, et al. Magnetic resonance imaging findings in the equine deep digital flexor tendon and distal sesamoid bone in advanced navicular disease—an *ex vivo* study. Vet Radiol Ultrasound 2005;46:279–286.
15. Colles CM. Navicular Disease and its Treatment. In Practice 1982;4:29–36.
16. Crisman MV, Furr MO, Ley WB, et al. Evaluation of polysulfated glycosaminoglycan for the treatment of navicular disease: A double blind study. Proceedings Am Assoc Equine Pract 1993;39:219–220.
17. Dabareiner RM, White NA, Sullins KE. Comparison of current techniques for palmar digital neurectomy in horses. Proceedings Am Assoc Equine Pract 1997;43:231–232.
18. Dabareiner RM, Carter GK. Diagnosis, treatment, and farriery for horses with chronic heel pain. Vet Clin North Am Equine Pract 2003;19:417–441.
19. Dabareiner RM, Carter GK, Honnas CM. Injection of corticosteroids, hyaluronate, and amikacin into the navicular bursa in horses with signs of navicular area pain unresponsive to other treatments: 25 cases (1999–2002). J Am Vet Med Assoc 2003;223:1469–1474.
20. Denoix JM. Functional anatomy of the equine interphalangeal joints. Proceedings Am Assoc Equine Pract 1999;45:174–177.
21. Denoix JM, Thibaud D, Riccio B. Tiludronate as a new therapeutic agent in the treatment of navicular disease: a double-blind placebo-controlled clinical trial. Equine Vet J 2003;35:407–413.
22. Dik KJ, van den Belt AJ, Enzerink E, et al. The radiographic development of the distal and proximal double contours of the equine navicular bone on dorsoproximal-palmarodistal oblique (upright pedal) radiographs, from age 1 to 11 months. Equine Vet J 2001;33:70–74.
23. Dik KJ, van den Broek J. Role of navicular bone shape in the pathogenesis of navicular disease: a radiological study. Equine Vet J 1995;27:390–393.
24. Drommer W, Damsch S, Winkelmeyer S, et al. Scanning electron microscopy of the sesamoid bone and deep flexor tendon of horses with navicular disease. Deutsche- Tierarztliche-Wochenschrift. 1992;99:235.
25. Dyson SJ. Navicular disease and other soft tissue causes of palmar foot pain. In Diagnosis and Management of Lameness in the Horse. Ross MW, Dyson SJ, eds. Saunders, St. Louis, MO 2003;286–298.
26. Dyson SJ. Comparison of responses to analgesia of the navicular bursa and intra-articular analgesia of the distal interphalangeal joint in 102 horses Proceedings Am Assoc Equine Pract 1995;41:234–239.
27. Dyson S, Murray R. Use of concurrent scintigraphic and magnetic resonance imaging evaluation to improve understanding of the pathogenesis of injury of the podotrochlear apparatus. Equine Vet J 2007;39:365–369.
28. Dyson S, Murray R. Magnetic resonance imaging evaluation of 264 horses with foot pain: the podotrochlear apparatus, deep digital flexor tendon and collateral ligaments of the distal interphalangeal joint. Equine Vet J 2007;39:340–343.
29. Dyson SJ, Murray R. Lameness and diagnostic imaging of the sports horse: recent advances related to the digit. In Proceedings Am Assoc Equine Pract 2007;53:262–274.
30. Dyson SJ. Radiological interpretation of the navicular bone. Equine Vet Education 2008;May:268–280.
31. Dyson S, Murray R. Verification of scintigraphic imaging for injury diagnosis in 264 horses with foot pain. Equine Vet J 2007;39:350–355.
32. Eliashar E, McGuigan MP, Wilson AM. Relationship of foot conformation and force applied to the navicular bone of sound horses at the trot. Equine Vet J 2004;36:431–435.
33. Erkert RS, MacAllister CG, Payton ME, et al. Use of force plate analysis to compare the analgesic effects of intravenous administration of phenylbutazone and flunixin meglumine in horses with navicular syndrome. Am J Vet Res 2005;66:284–288.
34. Grewal JS, McClure SR, Booth LC, et al. Assessment of the ultrasonographic characteristics of the podotrochlear apparatus in clinically normal horses and horses with navicular syndrome. J Am Vet Med Assoc 2004;225:1881–1888.
35. Harris JM, Kennedy MA. Modified posterior digital neurectomy for management of chronic heel pain in horses. Proceedings Am Assoc Equine Pract 1994;40:99–100.
36. Haugland LM, Collier MA, Panciera RJ, et al. The effect of CO_2 laser neurectomy on formation and axonal regeneration. Vet Surg 1992;21:351–354.
37. Ingle-Fehr JE, Baxter GM. The effect of oral isoxsuprine and pentoxifylline on digital and laminar blood flow in healthy horses. Vet Surg 1999;28:154–160.
38. Jackman BR, Baxter GM, Doran RE, et al. Palmar digital neurectomy in horses. 57 Cases 1984–1990, Vet Surg 1993;22:285–288.
39. Kaser-Hotz B, Ueltschi G. Radiographic Appearance of the Navicular Bone of Sound Horses. Veterinary Radiology and Ultrasound. 1992, 33:9–17.
40. Keegan KG, Wilson DA, Lattimer JC, et al. Scintigraphic evaluation of 99 mtc-methylene diphosphonate uptake in the navicular area of horses with lameness isolated to the foot by anesthesia of the palmar digital nerves. Am J Vet Res 1996;57:415–421.
41. Keegan KG, Wilson DJ, Frankeny RL, et al. Effects of anesthesia of the palmar digital nerves on kinematic gait analysis in horses with and without navicular disease. Am J Vet Res 1997;58:218–223.
42. Leach DH. Treatment and pathogenesis of navicular disease ("syndrome") in horses. Equine Vet J 1993;25:477–481.
43. MacGregor CM. Studies on the Pathology and Treatment of Equine Navicular Disease. PhD Thesis. University of Edinburgh 1984.
44. Madison JB, Dyson SJ. Treatment and prognosis of horses with navicular disease. In Diagnosis and Management of Lameness in the Horse. Ross MW, Dyson SJ, eds. Saunders, St. Louis, MO 2003;299–303.
45. Maher O, Davis DM, Drake C, et al. Pull-through technique for palmar digital neurectomy: forty-one horses (1998–2004). Vet Surg 2008;37:87–93.
46. McGuigan MP, Wilson AM. The effect of bilateral palmar digital nerve analgesia on the compressive force experienced by the navicular bone in horses with navicular disease. Equine Vet J 2001;33:166–171.
47. Murray RC, Schramme MC, Dyson SJ, et al. Magnetic resonance imaging characteristics of the foot in horses with palmar foot pain and control horses. Vet Radiol Ultrasound 2006;47:1–16.
48. Ostblom L, Lund C, Melsen F. Histological study of navicular bone disease. Equine Vet J 1982;14:199–202.
49. Ovnicek G. New hope for soundness; seen through the window to wild horse hoof patterns. Colombia Falls MT, Equine Digit Support Systems, Inc. 1997.
50. Page BT, Bowker RM, Ovnicek G, et al. How to mark the hoof for radiography to locate the distal phalanx and determine breakover. Proceedings Am Assoc Equine Pract 1999;45:148–150.
51. Pauwels FE, Schumacher J, Castro FA, et al. Evaluation of the diffusion of corticosteroids between the distal interphalangeal joint and navicular bursa in horses. Am J Vet Res 2008;69:611–616.
52. Pleasant RS, Baker GJ, Foreman JH, et al. Intraosseous pressure and pathologic changes in horses with navicular disease. Am J Vet Res 1993;54:7–12.
53. Pleasant RS, et al. Intra-articular anesthesia of the distal interphalangeal joint alleviates lameness associated with the navicular bursa in horses. Vet Surg, 1997;26:137–140.
54. Pool RR, Meagher DM, Stover SM. Pathophysiology of navicular syndrome. Vet Clin North Am Equine Pract 1989;5:109–12.
55. Puchalski SM, Galuppo LD, Hornof WJ, et al. Intraarterial contrast-enhanced computed tomography of the equine distal extremity. Vet Radiol Ultrasound 2007;48:21–29.
56. Rijkenhuizen AB, Nemeth F, Dik KJ, et al. The effect of artificial occlusion of the ramus navicularis and its branching arteries on the navicular bone in horses. An experimental study. Equine Vet J. 1989;21:425–430.
57. Rijkenhuizen AB. Navicular disease: a review of what's new. Equine Vet J 2006;38:82–88.

58. Rogers CW, Back W. The effect of plain, egg-bar and 6 degrees-wedge shoes on the distribution of pressure under the hoof of horses at the walk. N Z Vet J 2007;55:120–124.

59. Rose RJ, Allen JR, Hodgson DR, et al. Studies on isoxsuprine hydrochloride for the treatment of navicular disease. Equine Vet J 1983;15:238–243.

60. Ross MW. Observations in horse with lameness abolished by palmar digital analgesia. Proceedings Am Assoc Equine Pract 1998;44:230–232.

61. Sampson SN, Schneider RK, Gavin PR. Magnetic resonance imaging findings in horses with recent and chronic bilateral forelimb lameness diagnosed as navicular syndrome. Proceedings Am Assoc Equine Pract 2008;54:419–434.

62. Schoonover MJ, Jann HW, Blaik MA. Quantitative comparison of three commonly used treatments for navicular syndrome in horses. Am J Vet Res 2005;66:1247–1251.

63. Schumacher J, Schumacher J, Schramme MC. Diagnostic analgesia of the equine forefoot. Equine Vet Educ 2004; June:199–204.

64. Schumacher J, Gillette R, DeGraves F, et al. The effects of local anesthetic solution in the navicular bursa of horses with lameness caused by distal interphalangeal joint pain. Equine Vet J 2003;35:502–505.

65. Schumacher J, Schramme M, Schumacher J, et al. Abolition of lameness caused by experimentally induced solar pain in horses after analgesia of the distal interphalangeal joint. Proceedings Am Assoc Equine Pract 1999;45:193–194.

66. Smith MR, Wright IM, Smith RK. Endoscopic assessment and treatment of lesions of the deep digital flexor tendon in the navicular bursae of 20 lame horses. Equine Vet J 2007;39:18–24.

67. Stashak, TS. Navicular syndrome (navicular disease). In NA White, JN Moore, 2nd ed. Current techniques in equine surgery and lameness. WB Saunders, Philadelphia, PA. 1998;537–544.

68. Svalastoga E, Smith M. Navicular disease in the horse. The subchondral bone pressure. Nord Vet Med 1983;35:31–37.

69. Tietje S. Computed Tomography of the Navicular Bone Region in the Horse: A Comparison With Radiographic Documentation. PferdeheilKunde 1995;11:51–61.

70. Trotter G. The biomechanics of what really causes navicular disease. Equine Vet J 2001;33:334–336.

71. Trout DR, Hornof WJ, O'Brien TR. Soft tissue- and bone-phase scintigraphy for diagnosis of navicular disease in horses. J Am Vet Med Assoc 1991;198:73–77.

72. Turner AS, Tucker CM. The evaluation of isoxsuprine hydrochloride for the treatment of navicular disease: a double blind study. Equine Vet J 1989;21:338–341.

73. Turner TA. Shoeing principles for the management of navicular disease in horses. J Am Vet Med Assoc 1986;189:298–301.

74. Turner TA. Diagnosis and treatment of the navicular syndrome in horses. Vet Clin North Am Equine Pract 1989;5:131–144.

75. Turner TA, Rosenstein D. Inferior check desmotomy as a treatment for caudal hoof lameness. Proceedings Am Assoc Equine Pract 1992;38:157–163.

76. Turner TA. Predictive value of diagnostic tests for navicular pain. Proceedings Am Assoc Equine Pract 1996;42:201–204.

77. Turner TA. Use of navicular bursography in 97 horses. Proceedings Am Assoc Equine Pract 1998;44:227–229.

78. Verschooten F, Desmet P, Peremans K, et al. Navicular disease in the horse: the effect of controlled intrabursal corticoid injection. J Eq Vet Sci 1990;10:316–320.

79. Widmer WR, Fessler JF. Review: Understanding radiographic changes associated with navicular syndrome—Are we making progress? Proceedings Am Assoc Equine Pract 2002;48:155–159.

80. Widmer WR, Buckwalter KA, Fessler JF, et al. Use of radiography, computed tomography and magnetic resonance imaging for evaluation of navicular syndrome in the horse. Vet Radiol Ultrasound 2000;41:108–116.

81. Willemen MA, Savelberg HH, Barneveld A. The effect of orthopaedic shoeing on the force exerted by the deep digital flexor tendon on the navicular bone in horses. Equine Vet J 1999;31:25–30.

82. Williams GE. Locomotor characteristics of horses with navicular disease. Am J Vet Res 2001;62:206–210.

83. Wilson AM, McGuigan MP, Fouracre L, et al. The force and contact stress on the navicular bone during trot locomotion in sound horses and horses with navicular disease. Equine Vet J 2001;33:159–165.

84. Winkelmeyer S. Histological and scanning electron microscopical findings in deep flexor tendons and the distal sesamoid bone of horses. Correlations with a clinical diagnosis of navicular disease. Tierarztliche Hochschule. 1989;191.

85. Wright IM, Kidd L, Thorp BH. Gross, histological and histomorphometric features of the navicular bone and related structures in the horse. Equine Vet J 1998;30:220–234.

86. Wright IM. A study of 118 cases of navicular disease: clinical feature. Equine Vet J 1993;25:488–492.

87. Wright IM. A study of 118 cases of navicular disease: treatment by navicular suspensory desmotomy. Equine Vet J 1993;25:501–509.

FRACTURES OF THE NAVICULAR (DISTAL SESAMOID) BONE

Fractures of the navicular bone are an uncommon cause of lameness in horses.[5,7,11] They have been reported in many breeds and in horses with varied use.[1,7] Complete fracture can occur after acute trauma or secondary to severe bone demineralization due to navicular disease or osteomyelitis from sepsis.[1,5,10] Avulsion fractures are often associated with navicular disease and occur along the distal border of the navicular bone.[2,13] The forefeet appear to be at a greater risk for fracture.[1,3,7] In one report, 22 of 25 fractures of the navicular bone were in the forelimbs[3] and in another, 15 of 17 were in the forelimbs.[7]

Fractures of the navicular bone have been classified as avulsion fractures/fragments, simple complete fractures (transverse or oblique), comminuted complete fractures, and congenital bipartite navicular bones.[2,13] The latter is not considered a true fracture but can be confused with a chronic fracture based on its radiographic appearance. Avulsion fractures/fragments usually involve the distal border of the navicular bone in the forefeet, and are frequently associated with other radiographic signs of navicular syndrome.[2,13] These fracture fragments vary in shape, are usually small (0.2 to 1.2 cm in size), and occur more commonly in lame horses than clinically normal horses (Figure 5.12).[2,13] Simple complete fractures may be vertical, slightly oblique, or transverse.[2,6,13] The vertical and slightly oblique fractures usually occur medial or lateral but fairly close to the central eminence (sagittal ridge) of the navicular bone. Generally, these fractures are not displaced, but they are usually slightly separated so an obvious fracture line exists on the radiograph (Figure 5.20). Comminuted complete fractures are even more uncommon than simple complete fractures (Figure 5.21).[1,13] In one report 3 of 18 horses with complete navicular bone fractures were comminuted.[1] Rupture of the distal sesamoidean (impar) ligament or DDFT may accompany these fractures.[4,11]

Etiology

Acute trauma (concussion) to the foot is the most likely cause of most simple and comminuted complete navicular bone fractures. However, severe navicular bone osteolysis associated with navicular disease or sepsis may predispose to pathologic fractures. Avulsion fractures are most likely due to pathologic changes occurring within the navicular bone associated with navicular disease, but may also be trauma induced.

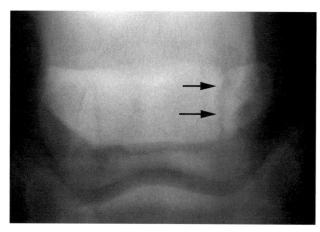

Figure 5.20. A wing fracture of the navicular bone (arrows) as seen on the oblique radiograph of the foot.

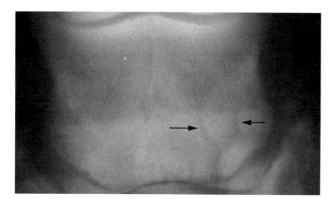

Figure 5.21. A comminuted Y-shaped fracture of the navicular bone (arrows).

Clinical Signs

The severity of lameness and clinical signs in horses with avulsion fractures are similar to those in horses with navicular disease. However, there may be a history of sudden worsening of the lameness in a single limb that responded to rest. Horses with complete navicular bone fractures typically have a history of an acute, severe lameness in 1 limb that improves with time.

One retrospective study found that most horses were severely lame at presentation, and that the less lame horses (2 of 5) were evaluated at a mean time of 90 days after the onset of lameness (range, 30 to 150 days).[7] In another study, the mean duration of lameness before presentation was 4.3 months.[1]

Most horses have a painful response to hoof testers across the frog region and have effusion within the DIP joint. An increased digital pulse may be present in the acute stage, similar to horses with P3 fractures, but is rare in more chronic cases. Horses with significant hindlimb lameness (grade 2 to 3 out of 5) and clinical signs referable to the navicular region should be suspected of having a navicular bone fracture. A PD nerve block should improve the lameness in most cases. However, in one study perineural anesthesia of these nerves did not totally eliminate the lameness and

regional anesthesia at a more proximal level was required.[7] The reason for this is uncertain since the PD block is thought to desensitize most if not all of the foot including the DIP joint. However, the fracture may cause articular pain or pain within the deep digital flexor tendon that is not completely eliminated by a PD nerve block. Intra-articular anesthesia of the DIP joint usually eliminates the lameness associated with navicular bone fractures.[11]

Diagnosis

Radiographic examination of the foot is required to confirm the diagnosis. Careful packing of the frog is necessary to avoid confusing the lines from the lateral sulci of the frog that cross the navicular region with a fracture. If the line extends beyond (above or below) the navicular bone, it is not a fracture. When in doubt, it is best to retake the radiograph at a slightly different angle. Complete simple fractures are typically located in the sagittal plane medial or lateral to the midline (parasagittal).[2,10] Most complete fractures are best identified on the skyline or 60° oblique views of the navicular bone, and should be present on multiple views (Figures 5.20 and 5.21). The fracture line should begin and end at the edges of the navicular bone, and is usually easily visible, especially in chronic fractures. Navicular bone fractures need to be differentiated from congenital bipartite or tripartite separation.[2,7] Bipartite navicular bones are usually symmetric with smooth edges and have a wide radiolucent region (Figure 5.6).[2,9] They are often bilateral so the opposite navicular region can be imaged to confirm the diagnosis.

Avulsion fractures can be difficult to identify on radiographs and close scrutiny is often required. They can often be best seen on the 60° oblique view of the navicular bone but may also be present at the distal aspect of the navicular bone on a lateromedial view (Figure 5.12)or within the medullary cavity of the navicular bone on the skyline view.[2] There is some question as to whether these osseous fragments represent true avulsion fractures of the navicular bone or are ectopic mineralization of the distal sesamoidean impar ligament or a fracture of an enthesiophyte at the origin of the distal sesamoidean impar ligament.[2]

Treatment

There is no known specific treatment for avulsion fractures of the navicular bone. Horses are treated similar to those with navicular syndrome (see Navicular Disease/Syndrome, above) but often benefit from heel elevation (provided the heels are not already too long) to relieve tension on the DSIL and DDFT. Horses with complete navicular bone fractures are usually treated nonsurgically by confinement alone, confinement and corrective shoeing (usually with heel elevation), or external coaptation aimed at reducing hoof expansion.[1,5,7]

In one study, horses were treated with 12° of heel elevation by using 4 3° wedge-pads and a flat shoe.[12] Heel elevation is thought to be an important aspect of treatment but it is unknown if less than 12° of heel elevation (3° to 6°) may also be beneficial. Regardless of the amount of heel elevation used, the horse should be re-shod monthly and gradually returned to normal foot angles over a 4- to 6-month period. A minimum of 4 to 6 months of stall rest has been recommended because these fractures are very slow to heal.[7,12] One study found that a minimum of 6 months of stall rest was necessary before there was resolution of clinical signs.[7]

Surgical repair of simple complete navicular bone fractures using a single cortical bone screw placed in lag fashion has been reported.[8] Intra-operative radiographic monitoring and a specially developed guide apparatus was necessary to implant the screw precisely along the transverse axis of the navicular bone. This technique was reported to be successful in 4 of 5 horses and all fractures healed without excessive callus.[8] This technique is difficult and performed infrequently to the author's knowledge.

Palmar or plantar digital neurectomy can also be performed to relieve pain in cases that have not responded to conservative treatment.[1,7] The navicular bone is very slow to heal and these fractures are invariably associated with damage to the impar ligament, DDFT, and DIP joint.[1,4] Chronic lameness may result from poor fracture healing and adhesions that develop between the DDFT and the navicular bone.[7] Follow-up radiography on 17 horses with complete navicular bone fractures revealed increases in the width of the fracture gap for up to 4 months after injury.[7] A noncalcified fibrous union can still be evident years after the fracture occurred, although some may heal completely (Figure 5.22).[11] Failure of an osseous union may be due to constant motion at the fracture site.[7] A combination of the soft tissue attachments and loading forces presumably serve to continually distract the fracture fragments.[7] Also the navicular bone is located between two synovial spaces, and synovial fluid may also inhibit healing.[9] If a neurectomy is performed, prolonged rest afterward should be considered to permit the fracture to heal and prevent further damage to the surrounding soft tissue structures.[11]

Prognosis

The prognosis is considered guarded to poor for horses with complete navicular bone fractures to return to athletic performance. In general, horses with fractures in the hindlimb are considered to have a better chance to return to performance than those affected in the forelimbs. In one report 3 of 6 horses treated by stall rest alone or stall rest and external coaptation, and 2 of 4 horses treated with stall rest and corrective shoeing returned to their intended use.[7] Also, only 1 of 5 horses that underwent neurectomy returned to its intended use.[7] In another report 3 of 7 horses treated with rest alone returned to performance and 4 remained lame. Of the 6 horses that were treated with a neurectomy 2 of 6 were sound for light riding, 2 of 6 were sound for only 1 year, and 2 of 6 remained lame.[1] In the study that used a 12° elevated heel shoe together with confinement, 4 of 4 horses became serviceably sound for riding and 2 of 4 returned to competition.[12] Although the horses were sound for use, complete radiographic healing did not occur in any case in this study.[12] Important clinical features of these studies include:

1. Heel elevation should be an important aspect of treatment.
2. Four to 6 months of confinement may be necessary.
3. Complete fracture healing is unlikely to occur.
4. Performing a PD neurectomy does not necessarily guarantee a sound horse.

References

1. Baxter GM, Ingle JE, Trotter GW. Complete navicular bone fractures in horses. Proc Am Assoc Equine Pract 1995;41: 243–244.
2. Dyson S. Radiological interpretation of the navicular bone. Equine Vet Educ 2008;May:268–280.
3. Hertsch B, Konigsmann D. Sagittal fracture of the equine navicular bone. Contribution to diagnosis and treatment. Pferdeheilkunde 1993;9:3–13.
4. Hoegaerts M, Pille F, De Clercq T, et al. Comminuted fracture of the navicular bone and distal rupture of the deep digital flexor tendon. Vet Radiol Ultrasound 2005;46:234–237.
5. Honnas CM. Fractures of the distal sesamoid bone. In Equine Surgery, JA Auer, ed. Philadelphia, Saunders 1992; 992–993.
6. Kaser-Hotz B, Ueltschi G, Hess N. Navicular bone fracture in the pelvic limb in two horses. Vet Radiol 1991;32:283–285.
7. Lillich JD, Ruggles AJ, Gabel AA, et al. Fracture of the distal sesamoid bone in horses: 17 cases (1982–1992). J Am Vet Med Assoc 1995;207:924–927.
8. Nemeth F, Dik KJ. Lag screw fixation of sagittal navicular bone fractures in five horses. Equine Vet J 1985;17:137–139.
9. Reeves MJ, Yovich JV, Turner AS. Miscellaneous conditions of the equine foot. Vet Clin North Am Equine Pract 1989;5: 221–242.
10. Rick MC. Navicular bone fractures. In Current Practice of Equine Surgery. Whites NA, Moore JN, eds. Philadelphia, JB Lippincott Co.1990;602–605.
11. Stashak TS. The Foot. In Adams' Lameness in Horses. Stashak TS ed. 5th ed. Lippincott Williams and Wilkins, Philadelphia. 2002;645–733.
12. Turner TA. How to treat navicular bone fractures. Proc Am Assoc Equine Pract 1997;43:370–371.
13. Van De Watering CC, Morgan JP. Chip Fractures as a Radiologic Finding in Navicular Disease of the Horse. J Am Radiol Soc 1975;16:206.

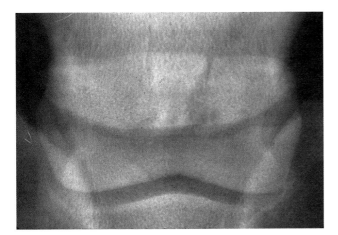

Figure 5.22. This oblique radiograph of the navicular bone was taken 23 months after the fracture occurred.

SOFT TISSUE INJURIES IN THE FOOT

Multiple structures within the foot are desensitized with a PD nerve block.[16] Historically, horses that have improved with a PD nerve block have been diagnosed as having navicular disease, navicular syndrome, or palmar/caudal heel pain. Navicular disease has usually been reserved for those horses with radiographic abnormalities of the navicular bone and navicular syndrome and palmar/caudal heel pain for those horses without radiographic abnormalities of the navicular bone. However, there is lack of agreement as to what constitutes a radiographically "abnormal navicular bone" and radiographically normal navicular bones have been found to be "abnormal" with MRI as indicated by bone edema.[2] To add further confusion, the PD nerve block has been found to desensitize most if not all of the foot including the DIP joint.[16] Designating horses that block to a PD nerve block as having only palmar or caudal heel pain could be interpreted as erroneous.

Soft tissue injuries of the foot have always been suspected in horses with foot pain without radiographic abnormalities, but these abnormalities have been difficult to delineate. Advances in ultrasound, CT, and MR imaging techniques have enabled improved recognition of these potential problems.[6–13,18] These imaging modalities have also helped determine that it is not an "either/or" situation because it appears common for soft tissue and bony abnormalities to co-exist in many lame horses with foot problems. For instance, a recent MRI study revealed a positive association between DDFT lesions and navicular bone pathology involving all aspects of the bone.[10] However, primary tendinitis of the DDFT was found more frequently than concurrent tendinitis and navicular bone pathology (43% vs. 19%) in one MRI study.[8]

Soft tissue structures within the foot that can be desensitized with a PD block include the heel bulbs, digital cushion, collateral cartilages of the distal phalanx, podotrochlear apparatus (DSIL, and CSLs of the navicular bone), DDFT (may only partially improve with a PD block), and CLs of the DIP joint.[5,8,11,16] The navicular bursa and DIP joint are also desensitized with a PD block but are not considered true soft tissue structures for this discussion. In addition, abnormalities of the digital cushion, heel bulbs, and collateral cartilages are often related to poor hoof conformation and foot imbalances, and are addressed in chapter 12. Therefore, this discussion focuses on abnormalities of the podotrochlear apparatus, DDFT, and CLs of the DIP joint.[1–6]

Etiology

The DDFT is the most commonly affected soft tissue structure in the foot and injuries may occur alone, in conjunction with navicular bone pathology, or as one component of a complex of multiple soft tissue injuries in the foot.[8–10,15] The DDFT is bi-lobed within the foot and lesions can occur in either lobe anywhere along its length, from the level of the proximal interphalangeal (PIP) joint distally to its attachment on P3.[15] Abnormalities have been identified at the DDFT insertion to the distal phalanx (least common), the level of the navicular bone or CSLs (most common), more prox-

imally in the pastern, or a combination of sites.[8,10] The most common location is at the level of the navicular bone and CSLs, and can be true core lesions or sagittal splits, erosions, or abrasions (Figure 5.14).[3,4,10,15]

Abnormalities at the level of the proximal phalanx are more typical of true core lesions within the tendon.[10] Abnormalities of the podotrochlear apparatus are often present in association with abnormalities of the navicular bone, especially involving the proximal or distal borders and the medulla.[10] Lesions of the CL of the DIP joint were the second most common soft tissue injury in one MRI study, and they can occur alone or together with other injuries.[9] The medial collateral ligament of the forelimb is the most common site of the injury.[11,14]

Acute-onset or repetitive trauma is considered the most likely cause of most soft tissue injuries within the foot.[5] Concurrent abnormalities of the podotrochlear apparatus and navicular bone suggest that similar biomechanical forces and repetitive trauma to the palmar aspect of the foot likely contribute to both types of injuries.[10] Asymmetrical foot placement or foot imbalances may cause sliding and rotation of the distal phalanx relative to the middle phalanx, contributing to injuries to the CL of the DIP joint.[6]

Horses that jump or have a low heel hoof conformation may be at risk for injuries to the DDFT.[5] Single-event traumatic "tearing" of the DDFT causing a true tendinitis may also occur but is probably less common. Based on MRI studies, this type of lesion is most likely to occur more proximal in the foot at the level of the proximal phalanx.[10] Exceptions to this may be true ruptures of the DDFT, but the location of where these ruptures occur has not been documented. In most cases, however, it would seem likely that previous abnormalities of the DDFT would predispose to complete failure.

Lesions within the CL of the DIP joint have recently been reported to be a primary degenerative process rather than inflammatory.[7] Histology revealed extensive fibrocartilaginous metaplasia and development of multiple, intercommunicating fissures within the degenerate collagen in severe lesions.[7] This was thought to explain the poor response to conservative treatment in many horses with desmitis of the CL of the DIP joint. Similar degenerative abnormalities may also exist within other soft tissue structures of the foot, particularly the DDFT.[3,4,15] Core lesions of the DDFT are often characterized by fiber necrosis and disruption.[15] Ectopic mineralization within the DDFT, which may represent chronic degeneration within the tendon, is occasionally identified radiographically but its clinical significance is often questioned.[5] However, the presence of degenerative processes vs. inflammatory processes histologically may also reflect the stage of the disease because the majority of soft tissue lesions within the digit are most likely chronic in nature.

Clinical Signs

In general, horses that have primary soft tissue injuries in the foot are more likely to have a history on an acute onset of lameness and be unilaterally lame compared to horses with navicular disease. Horses with multiple foot problems and those with concurrent navicular pathology and soft tissue injuries are less likely to conform to this generalization. In addition, horses with flexor cortex erosive lesions of the navicular bone are often unilaterally lame. The majority of horses will improve with a PD nerve block but the lameness will not be completely abolished in many horses with lesions of the DDFT and CL of the DIP joint.[5,8,11] More specific clinical information has been obtained from horses with injuries to the DDFT and CL of the DIP than from horses with injuries to the podotrochlear apparatus. The clinical signs of horses with abnormalities of the podotrochlear apparatus may resemble those with navicular disease because these injuries often occur concurrently with navicular bone pathology.[10] A summary of the clinical findings for horses with injuries to the DDFT and CL of the DIP joint are presented below.

DDFT Injuries

The clinical signs may vary, depending on whether the DDFT lesion is primary or associated with navicular pathology. However, there is often a history of an acute onset of moderate to severe lameness that may improve with rest and worsen with exercise.[5] There may be a history of activity that caused excessive hyperextension of the foot such as working in soft ground and/or jumping. The lameness is usually unilateral and may worsen in a circle or when exercised on soft ground. Occasionally, pain may be elicited with deep palpation of the DDFT between the collateral cartilages of the heels. Hoof tester pain is variable but may be present if a DDFT lesion and navicular pathology are present concurrently. Phalangeal flexion may cause a positive response but is often variable. Increasing tension on the DDFT with the navicular wedge test may accentuate the lameness.[5]

The lameness is not reliably abolished with a PD nerve block in horses with DDFT lesions.[5,8] Horses often improve but in one study only 24% of those with DDF tendinitis responded completely to a PD nerve block.[8] The lameness should respond to basi-sesamoid block and many improve after IA anesthesia of the DIP joint. Anesthesia of the DIP joint was more effective in alleviating the lameness in horses with DDFT lesions than was the PD block in one study.[8] This finding differs from the clinical experience of the author. However, the response to perineural anesthesia may depend on the location of the lesion(s) and whether concurrent problems exist in the foot.

CL Injuries of the DIP Joint

There are often few localizing clinical signs in horses with injuries to the CL of the DIP joint.[6,11,14] Horses often have a history of a chronic forelimb lameness of variable severity that is worse in the circle. Palpable swelling and pain of the medial CL at its proximal attachment to the middle phalanx may be present above the coronary band in severe cases. However, this is uncommon and effusion of the DIP joint is also not a consistent clinical finding. Most horses (87% in one study) improve with a PD nerve block but may not be completely sound until a more proximal block is per-

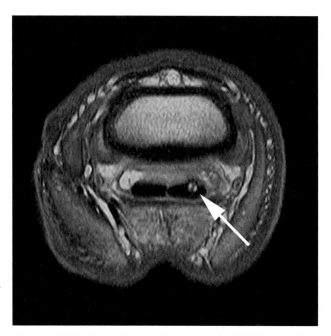

Figure 5.23. A core lesion within lobe of the DDFT above the level of the navicular bone (arrow) can be seen in this PD axial MR image. (Courtesy of Dr. Natasha Werpy.)

formed.[11] Surprisingly, only 40% of horses improved with IA anesthesia of the DIP joint in one study.[11]

Diagnosis

A definitive diagnosis of a soft tissue injury of the foot is best determined with MRI in either the recumbent or standing patient.[6–12,14,15] Tendon damage within the DDFT is often seen as focal signal increase on both the T1- and T2-weighted sequences and swelling of the affected lobe in the acute stages of the disease. There is good correlation between MRI appearance of DDFT lesions and their pathological classification into core lesions, sagittal splits, insertional lesions, and dorsal surface erosions (Figure 5.23).[15] Lesions within the CL of the DIP joint are identified by the alteration in size and signal intensity (Figure 5.24).[11] In addition, some horses may have abnormal mineralization and fluid within the distal phalanx at the insertion of the ligament.[11] See Chapter 4 for more information on MRI.

Typically, horses have minimal to no radiographic abnormalities. Ectopic mineralization may be seen in some horses with DDFT lesions but may not be correlated with tendinitis of the DDFT (Figure 5.25).[5] Bone exostosis, lysis, or sclerosis may occur at the insertion sites of the CL on the distal or middle phalanges but appear to be uncommon (Figure 5.26). In one study of 18 horses with desmitis of the CL of the DIP joint, 16 horses had no radiographic abnormalities.[11] Enthesiophytes involving the podotrochlear apparatus attachments to the navicular bone and other radiographic abnormalities of the navicular bone may suggest damage to this structure but does not provide a definitive diagnosis. Likewise, erosive lesions of the flexor surface of the navicular bone are most likely associated with dorsal abrasions of the DDFT but navicular bursal

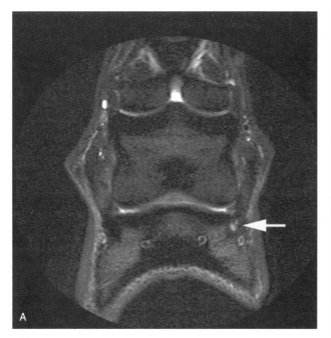
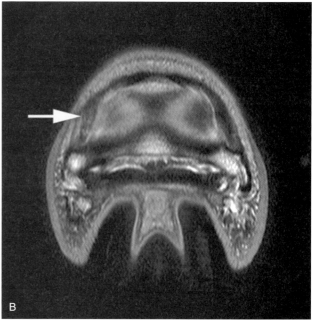

Figure 5.24. Frontal STIR (A) and PD axial (B) MR images of the foot of a 12-year-old Quarter horse with abnormalities within the medial collateral ligament of the DIP joint (arrows).

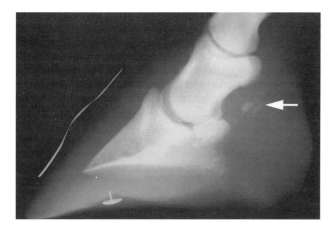

Figure 5.25. Lateral radiograph of a horse with chronic navicular disease that demonstrates calcification within the DDFT proximal to the navicular bone (arrow). A thumbtack was placed at the apex of the frog prior to the radiograph.

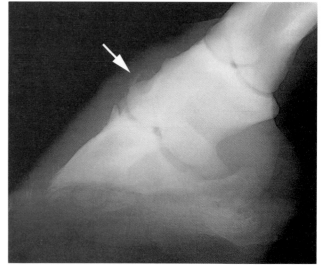

Figure 5.26. Bony proliferation on the dorsolateral aspect of P2 on this oblique radiograph (arrow) is suggestive of an injury to the CL of the DIP joint.

endoscopy or MRI is needed for a definitive diagnosis (Figure 5.27).

Ultrasound can be used to diagnose some injuries to the DDFT, podotrochlear apparatus, and CL of the DIP joint.[1,5,11,13] Ten of 18 horses with desmitis of the CL of the DIP joint were diagnosed with ultrasound in one study[11] and abnormalities within the DDFT, podotrochlear apparatus, and navicular bone have been documented with ultrasound.[13] Ultrasound can be performed either between the heel bulbs and/or through the frog after it has been softened by soaking. However, documenting the lesion may be difficult depending on its location and the skill of the operator. Certain aspects of both the DDFT and the CL of the DIP joint are inac-

cessible with ultrasound, suggesting that negative findings do not rule out the presence of a lesion.[6,8,11]

Nuclear scintigraphy has also been used to help document lesions of the DDFT, CL of the DIP joint, and portions of the podotrochlear apparatus. However, scintigraphy is most helpful to suggest the location of the abnormality within the foot and not make a definitive diagnosis. For instance, 57% of the horses with CL of the DIP joint had focal increased radiopharmaceutical uptake at the insertion site of the CL, suggesting an abnormality in that location.[11] Additional diagnostics such as ultrasound or MRI were needed to actually

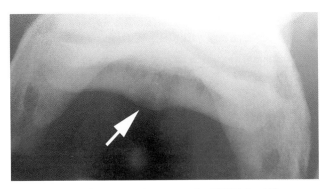

Figure 5.27. Secondary damage to the DDFT should be suspected in horses with erosive lesions on the flexor surface of the navicular bone (arrow).

image the ligament. Computed tomography has also been used to document abnormalities in the DDFT within the hoof capsule but can only be performed under general anesthesia.[1,15,18] See Chapter 4 for further information on diagnostic modalities.

Treatment

The most important aspects of treatment of soft tissue injuries of the foot are rest, rehabilitation, and corrective foot care.[14,15] Foot imbalances that may have contributed to their occurrence such as low heels, long toes, mediolateral imbalance, reverse angle of the distal phalanx, etc. should be corrected if possible. Horses with injuries to the podotrochlear apparatus are usually treated similarly to horses with navicular disease.

Types of shoes that may benefit horses with DDFT injuries include egg-bar shoes and shoes and pads to elevate the heels.[15] Natural balance shoes are also considered beneficial in many cases. Elevation of the heels is usually not recommended for horses with injuries to the CL of the DIP joint. Rest and rehabilitation is usually performed over a minimum of 6 months and may be necessary for even longer. Stall confinement for 6 months with 10 to 15 minutes of daily hand-walking has been recommended for horses with DDFT injuries.[15] Even though rest and rehabilitation is an important aspect of treatment, the prognosis with this therapy alone has not been considered favorable.[5,15] Adjunct treatment approaches for these injuries are discussed below.

DDFT Injuries

Additional treatment options for horses with DDFT lesions often depend on the location of the lesion, but the overall prognosis remains guarded. Lesions at the level of the navicular bone may benefit from endoscopy of the navicular bursa and debridement of any torn tendon fibers.[15,17] Intralesional treatment of the DDFT injury and/or treatment of the navicular bursa can be performed at the time of surgery or subsequent to surgery. Navicular bursoscopy with tendon and fibrocartilage debridement followed by intrabursal or intralesional injection of biological therapeutic compounds combined with rest and rehabilitation is currently con-

sidered the optimal treatment of horses with DDFT lesions.[15] However, lesions in the DDFT proximal or distal to the navicular bursa cannot be treated with this approach.

A technique to inject the insertion of the DDFT at the level of P3 has recently been described.[1] The injections were performed under radiographic guidance in cadaver limbs that simulated the standing horse. An 8.9-cm, 20-g spinal needle was inserted at the depression between the heels bulbs at the level of the coronary band. The needle was directed dorsally and slightly distally at an angle of no greater than 10° to the horizontal toward the solar surface.[1] The needle was advanced until it contacted bone at the interface of the DDFT and P3, which was confirmed radiographically. The authors concluded that this technique could be used to treat insertional injuries of the DDFT in standing horses with intralesional therapies.

Intralesional treatment of DDFT lesions at other locations may be performed with CT guidance but requires the horse to be anesthetized and is not clinically feasible in most cases.[1] Intrabursal injection of medications without navicular bursoscopy can also be performed. Corticosteroids alone or combined with hyaluronan may be used to reduce the inflammation and pain, or biological compounds such as stem cells or platelet rich plasma may be used to hopefully promote tendon healing. Extracorporeal shock wave therapy may also be used in select cases. See Chapter 8 for more detailed information on these treatment modalities.

CL Injuries of the DIP Joint

Additional treatments for desmopathy of the CL of the DIP joint in a recent study included extracorporeal shock wave therapy, application of a half-limb or foot cast, and medication of the DIP.[14] Intralesional therapy with stem cells, platelet rich plasma, and other biological products may also be used, especially if the injury is accessible above the hoof wall. Ultrasound guidance of the injection can be helpful.(See Chapter 8 for more detailed information on these treatment modalities.)

Prognosis

In general the prognosis for horses with soft tissue injuries of the foot is considered to be guarded to poor for return to athletic performance. This is usually worsened if the injury is combined with navicular bone pathology.[9] Injuries to the DDFT are considered to be the most problematic since only 28% of horses returned to performance after 6 months' rest.[9] In the same study, 95% of horses with DDFT injuries and concurrent navicular bone pathology remained lame after 6 months.[9] Horses with DDFT lesions localized to the navicular bursa that were debrided endoscopically appear to have an improved prognosis since 11 of 15 horses with greater than 6 months' follow-up were sound and 9 returned to preoperative levels of performance.[17] However, this is a select group of horses, as many DDFT lesions are not accessible to debridement. Intralesional therapy of these DDFT injuries may be attempted because the response to rest and rehabilitation alone appears to be discouraging.

The reported prognosis for horses with desmopathy of the CL of the DIP joint is variable. Two studies have reported that only 29% of horses treated with rest and rehabilitation returned to athletic function.[6,11] However, a more recent study indicated that 60% of treated horses (12 of 20) returned to their previous level of exercise.[14] Horses with multiple soft tissue injuries would most likely have a lower prognosis than those with single, isolated lesions, but this has not been documented.

References

1. Anderson JDC, Puchalski SM, Larson RF, et al. Injection of the insertion of the deep digital flexor tendon in horses using radiographic guidance. Equine Vet Educ 2008;July:383–388.
2. Barber MJ, Sampson SN, Schneider RK, et al. Use of magnetic resonance imaging to diagnose distal sesamoid bone injury in a horse. J Am Vet Med Assoc 2006;229:717–720.
3. Blunden A, Dyson S, Murray R, et al. Histopathology in horses with chronic palmar foot pain and age-matched controls. Part 2: The deep digital flexor tendon. Equine Vet J 2006;38:23–27.
4. Blunden A, Dyson S, Murray R, et al. Histopathology in horses with chronic palmar foot pain and age-matched controls. Part 1: Navicular bone and related structures. Equine Vet J 2006; 38:15–22.
5. Dyson SJ. Primary lesions of the deep digital flexor tendon within the hoof capsule. In Diagnosis and Management of Lameness in the Horse. Ross MW, Dyson SJ, eds. Saunders, St. Louis, MO 2003;305–309.
6. Dyson SJ. Collateral desmitis of the distal interphalangeal joint in 62 horses (January 2001–December 2003). Proceedings Am Assoc Equine Pract 2004;50:248–256.
7. Dyson S, Blunden T, Murray R. The collateral ligaments of the distal interphalangeal joint: Magnetic resonance imaging and post mortem observations in 25 lame and 12 control horses. Equine Vet J 2008;40:538–544.
8. Dyson S, Murray R, Schramme M, et al. Lameness in 46 horses associated with deep digital flexor tendinitis in the digit: diagnosis confirmed with magnetic resonance imaging. Equine Vet J 2003;35:681–690.
9. Dyson SJ, Murray R, Schramme MC. Lameness associated with foot pain: results of magnetic resonance imaging in 199 horses (January 2001–December 2003) and response to treatment. Equine Vet J 2005;37:113–121.
10. Dyson S, Murray R. Magnetic resonance imaging evaluation of 264 horses with foot pain: the podotrochlear apparatus, deep digital flexor tendon and collateral ligaments of the distal interphalangeal joint. Equine Vet J 2007;39:340–343.
11. Dyson SJ, Murray RC, Schramme M, et al. Collateral desmitis of the distal interphalangeal joint in 18 horses (2001–2002). Equine Vet J 2004;36:160–166.
12. Dyson S, Murray R, Schramme M, et al. Magnetic resonance imaging of the equine foot: 15 horses. Equine Vet J 2003; 35:18–26.
13. Grewal JS, McClure SR, Booth LC, et al. Assessment of the ultrasonographic characteristics of the podotrochlear apparatus in clinically normal horses and horses with navicular syndrome. J Am Vet Med Assoc 2004;225:1881–1888.
14. Gutierrez-Nibeyro SD, White NA, Werpy NM, et al. Magnetic resonance imaging findings of desmopathy of the collateral ligaments of the equine distal interphalangeal joint. Vet Radiol Ultrasound 2009;50:21–31.
15. Schramme MC. Treatment of deep digital flexor tendinitis in the foot. Equine Vet Educ 2008;July:389–391.
16. Schumacher J, Schumacher J, Schramme MC, et al. Diagnostic analgesia of the equine forefoot. Equine Vet Education 2004;June:199–204.
17. Smith MR, Wright IM, Smith RK. Endoscopic assessment and treatment of lesions of the deep digital flexor tendon in the navicular bursa of 20 lame horses. Equine Vet J 2007; 39:18–24.
18. Widmer WR, Buckwalter KA, Fessler JF, et al. Use of radiography, computed tomography and magnetic resonance imaging for evaluation of navicular syndrome in the horse. Vet Radiol Ultrasound 2000;41:108–116.

OSTEOARTHRITIS (OA) OF THE DISTAL INTERPHALANGEAL (DIP) JOINT

Osteoarthritis/synovitis/capsulitis of the DIP joint, or "low ringbone," is a common cause of forelimb lameness in horses. It can be a primary cause of lameness or it may occur concurrently with other lameness conditions of the foot such as navicular disease. Historically, advanced low ringbone has been associated with dorsal exostosis of the extensor process and distal aspect of P2, contributing to an enlargement at the coronary band and pyramidal distortion of the hoof.[8,13] This has been referred to as pyramidal disease or buttress foot (Figure 5.28). Distortion of the hoof secondary to low ringbone occurs uncommonly in the author's experience, and most cases of buttress foot are associated with large extensor process fractures of the distal phalanx.[1] See the section on fractures of the distal phalanx in this chapter for more information.

Etiology

Osteoarthritis/synovitis/capsulitis of the DIP joint may occur as a primary problem or secondary to other injuries within the joint. Primary OA can be due to acute or repetitive trauma to the joint comparable to any articulation in the horse. Horses with a broken pastern axis (forward or backward) and other types of hoof imbalances appear particularly prone to repetitive trauma to the DIP joint and development of OA. Acute or repetitive trauma may cause tearing of the joint capsule or direct damage to the articular cartilage and subchondral bone. Excessive strain of the attachments of the long or common digital extensor tendon to the extensor process may also occur, and contribute to periostitis and enthesiophyte formation along the dorsal aspect of the joint.[13]

Secondary OA can occur from other lameness conditions that involve the DIP joint, either directly or indirectly. These include navicular disease, complete navicular bone fractures, articular fractures of the distal

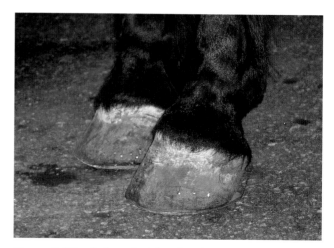

Figure 5.28. Buttress foot describes horses with firm enlargements just proximal to the dorsal hoof wall. This is usually due to fracture of the extensor process but may also be seen in horses with severe OA of the DIP joint.

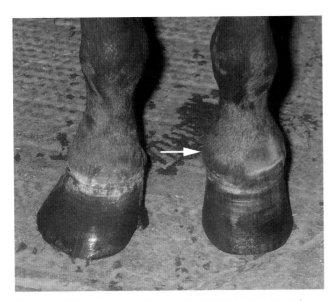

Figure 5.29. Effusion within the DIP joint can be seen and palpated as swelling just above the coronary band (arrow).

phalanx, subchondral cystic lesions (SCL) of the distal phalanx, osteochondral fragmentation within the joint, and desmitis of the CLs of the DIP joint.[2–4,10,13] These abnormalities are thought to directly or indirectly cause pathology to the DIP joint, which leads to the development of OA over time. Prevention of DIP joint OA is often an important aspect of treatment for many of these conditions. See the discussion of each of these conditions in this chapter for more information.

Clinical Signs

Effusion of the DIP joint is usually present in most horses with OA/synovitis/capsulitis of the DIP joint (Figure 5.29). However, effusion can be present in normal horses so this finding is not always indicative of problems within the DIP joint.[2] Normal horses usually have less DIP joint effusion and the effusion is often symmetrical. Most times significant effusion of the DIP joint can be seen as a slight bulging just above the coronary band. The fluid can usually be balloted from medial to lateral along the dorsal midline of the joint. With chronic or advanced disease the joint capsule may become thickened, resulting in a firm swelling just above the dorsal aspect of the coronary band. Digital pressure over the swelling may elicit a painful response.[13] The joint may be painful to flexion and rotation but this is uncommon unless the OA is advanced or secondary to another problem in the joint. Lameness is variable and often depends on the severity of the disease, whether it is primary or secondary, and whether 1 or both limbs are affected.[2] The lameness is often worse on hard ground, when circled, and after distal limb or phalangeal flexion.

Lameness associated with the DIP joint is often improved and sometimes alleviated completely with a PD nerve block.[5,12] However, anesthesia at the base of the sesamoid bones or a pastern ring block may be required for complete resolution of the lameness. Intra-articular (IA) anesthesia of the DIP joint is not specific

for problems within the joint, but using a small volume of anesthetic (6 mL or less) and observing for a change in lameness very soon after the injection (within 10 minutes) can improve the specificity of the block for the joint.[2,12] Most horses with DIP joint pain improve rapidly and substantially after IA anesthesia. If the lameness only partially improves but persists after 10 minutes, the DIP joint is not likely the primary site of the pain.[2] For instance, horses with desmitis of collateral ligaments of the DIP may not improve with DIP joint anesthesia.[4] In addition, a positive response to an IA block combined with a negative response to navicular bursa anesthesia often incriminates the joint as the primary problem area.[5,12] See Chapter 3 for more details about perineural and intrasynovial anesthesia.

Diagnosis

A definitive diagnosis of OA of the DIP joint can often be obtained with radiography of the foot. However, horses with synovitis/capsulitis or early OA of the DIP joint may have no radiographic abnormalities. A complete radiographic study of the foot should be performed to rule out other potential problems because DIP joint OA may be secondary to other conditions, and anesthesia of the DIP joint is not always specific for the joint.

Oblique views of the DIP joint can aid in detecting periarticular new bone formation of the distal aspect of the middle phalanx (Figure 5.30).[2] Close inspection of the extensor process, palmar/plantar aspect of distal P2, and dorsoproximal aspect of the navicular bone for osteophyte and enesthesiophyte formation is important. Joint space congruity and the shape of the proximal surface of the distal phalanx should be assessed carefully.[2] An increase in the size and number of the lucent zones (synovial invaginations) along the distal border

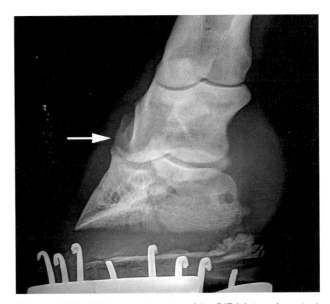

Figure 5.30. Oblique radiographs of the DIP joint are important to document abnormalities. The bony proliferation (arrow) and narrowing of the DIP joint seen on this oblique radiograph was not apparent on other views of the joint.

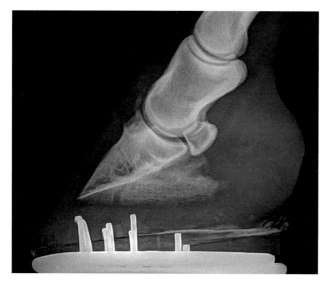

Figure 5.31. The calcification of the extensor tendon seen on this lateral radiograph was not clinically significant in this horse following removal of an extensor process fracture.

of the navicular bone may also be associated with chronic synovitis of the DIP joint.[2] However, the radiographic abnormalities surrounding the DIP joint should not be overinterpreted because there is much variation in the shape of the extensor process among horses and enthesiophytes may not be associated with lameness (Figure 5.31).[2,10] In contrast, the presence of any radiographic abnormalities of the DIP joint was associated with a poor response to treatment in one study.[3]

Additional diagnostics that may be used to confirm the diagnosis of a problem within the DIP joint, particularly if the radiographs are within normal limits, include ultrasound, nuclear scintigraphy, MRI, and diagnostic arthroscopy. Ultrasound can be helpful to document problems within the CLs of the DIP joint proximal to the hoof wall and thickness of the dorsal joint capsule.[2,4] Scintigraphy may be helpful to document subchondral bone trauma and injuries to the CLs of the DIP at their bony attachment, but is usually insensitive to identify OA unless it is advanced.[2,4,11] MRI is the most comprehensive advanced imaging modality that can detect articular cartilage, subchondral bone, and soft tissue abnormalities of the DIP joint if present.[4,6] Arthroscopy may be used to document articular cartilage or subchondral bone damage but much of the joint surface of the DIP joint is not visible.

Treatment

Horses with primary OA/synovitis/capsulitis of the DIP joint are usually treated with a combination of intra-articular medication and corrective shoeing. Predisposing factors such as mediolateral and dorsopalmar hoof imbalances should be corrected to reduce repetitive trauma to the joint. Shortening the toe and moving the break-over further palmarly often helps these horses, and using a rim pad may alleviate concussion to the joint.[13] Direct medication of the DIP joint is

usually more effective than systemic medications to reduce the inflammatory response within the joint. The type(s) of medication chosen may depend on the severity and duration of the lameness and the severity of the radiographic abnormalities. Corticosteroids alone, corticosteroids combined with HA, or PSGAGs are used most frequently. Autogenous serum may also be used if desired.

Typically, the author recommends a combination of hyaluronan and triamcinolone. However, a recent study reported that 3 weekly injections of the DIP joint with PSGAG was more effective in improving lameness associated with the DIP joint than MPA.[7] Horses treated with PSGAG had a 67% successful outcome, compared with 46% of those receiving MPA alone.[7] In addition, a significantly better result was obtained in dressage horses than in jumping horses (eventing and show jumping).[7] This study and the clinical observations of the authors support the rationale for treating horses with DIP joint pain with intra-articular medication. However, horses that block completely with DIP joint anesthesia usually respond better to intra-articular medication than those that only partially improve.[2] Repeat intra-articular injections may be required, depending on the severity of the abnormalities within the joint and the response to treatment.

Treatment of horses with secondary OA of the DIP joint usually focuses on the underlying contributing problem. Treatment of the primary condition is usually beneficial to prevent worsening of the problems within the DIP joint. For instance, extensor process fractures of the distal phalanx should be removed in most cases and other articular distal phalanx fractures should be stabilized with corrective shoeing. Subchondral cystic lesions should be debrided if possible and horses with known trauma to the articular cartilage, subchondral bone, or CLs of the DIP joint should be treated appropriately until healing has occurred. Horses with navicular disease should be shod appropriately to minimize progression of the DIP joint OA. Many of these horses may also benefit from IA medication, depending on the underlying problem. For instance, horses with navicular disease benefit from intra-articular treatment of the DIP joint by reducing the inflammatory response, both within the joint and within the navicular region.[9] A recent study documented that a clinically effective concentration of MPA or TA diffused between the DIP joint and navicular bursa after IA or intrabursal injection.[9] Systemic joint medications such as IM PSGAG, IV hyaluronan, and nutraceuticals may also benefit these horses. See the other sections of this chapter for more detailed information about treating these underlying problems.

Prognosis

Horses with primary synovitis/capsulitis of the DIP joint usually have a very good prognosis to return to performance if the predisposing hoof imbalances can be corrected and maintained. Recurrence is possible but is often related to relapses in the hoof imbalances. However, one study indicated a less optimistic prognosis with only 30% of horses responding to treatment.[3] The prognosis of horses with primary or secondary OA of the DIP joint is usually related to the severity of the radiographic abnormalities.[2,3] Horses with advanced OA often respond less to any form of treatment, or the lameness recurs more quickly. Horses with mild to moderate OA have a good to guarded prognosis to return to performance. Horses with secondary OA of the DIP joint have a variable prognosis depending on the underlying problem. However, the development of radiographic signs of OA within the DIP joint does not preclude athletic performance. For instance, several racehorses with type II fractures of the distal phalanx returned to racing despite radiographic evidence of OA within the DIP joint.[10] It is possible that the radiographic abnormalities within the DIP are overinterpreted as to their influence on lameness.[10]

References

1. Dechant JE, Trotter GW, Stashak TS, et al. Removal of large fragments of the extensor process of the distal phalanx via arthrotomy in horses: 14 cases (1992–1998). J Am Vet Med Assoc 2000;217:1351–1355.
2. Dyson SJ. The distal phalanx and distal interphalangeal joint. In Diagnosis and Management of Lameness in the Horse. Ross MW, Dyson SJ, eds. Saunders, St. Louis, MO 2003;310–316.
3. Dyson SJ. Lameness due to pain associated with the distal interphalangeal joint: 45 cases. Equine Vet J 1991;23:128–135.
4. Dyson SJ, Murray R, Schramme M, et al. Collateral desmitis of the distal interphalangeal joint in 18 horses (2001–2002). Equine Vet J 2004;36:160–166.
5. Dyson S, Marks D. Foot pain and the elusive diagnosis. Vet Clin North Am Equine Pract 2003;19:531–565.
6. Dyson S, Murray R, Schramme M, et al. Magnetic resonance imaging of the equine foot: 15 horses. Equine Vet J 2003; 35:18–26.
7. Kristiansen KK, Kold SE. Multivariable analysis of factors influencing outcome of 2 treatment protocols in 128 cases of horses responding positively to intra-articular analgesia of the distal interphalangeal joint. Equine Vet J 2007;39:150–156.
8. Park A. Chronic foot injury and deformity. In Current Techniques in Equine Surgery. NA White and JN Moore, eds. 2nd ed. WB Saunders, Philadelphia, 1998;534–537.
9. Pauwels FE, Schumacher J, Castro FA, et al. Evaluation of the diffusion of corticosteroids between the distal interphalangeal joint and navicular bursa in horses. Am J Vet Res 2008; 69:611–616.
10. Rabuffo TS, Ross MW. Fractures of the distal phalanx in 72 racehorses: 1990–2001. Proceedings Am Assoc Equine Pract 2002;48:375–377.
11. Ross MW. Observations in horses with lameness abolished by palmar digital analgesia. Proceedings Am Assoc Equine Pract 1998;44:230–232.
12. Schumacher J, Schumacher J, Schramme MC, et al. Diagnostic analgesia of the equine forefoot. Equine Vet Education 2004;June:199–204.
13. Stashak TS. The Foot. In Adams' Lameness in Horses. Stashak TS, ed. 5th ed. Lippincott Williams and Wilkins. Philadelphia. 2002;645–733.

FRACTURES OF THE DISTAL PHALANX (P3, COFFIN BONE)

Fractures of the distal phalanx are an uncommon cause of lameness compared to the numerous other conditions that affect the horse's foot.[28,29] An older report identified 65 cases of P3 fractures in 20,638 cases admitted to a hospital.[28] These fractures can occur in any foot but most commonly affect the lateral aspect of the left forelimb and the medial aspect of the right forelimb in racehorses.[27,29] Type I and II "wing" frac-

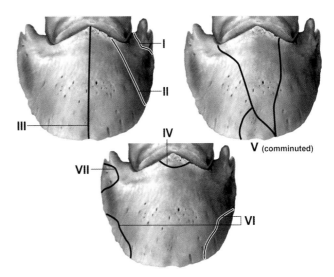

Figure 5.32. Classification of P3 fractures in horses. (Reprinted with permission from Dr. Alicia Bertone, Equine Fracture Repair, Nixon AL, ed.)

tures are most common and the majority of these fractures enter the DIP joint.[27,28] In a recent report of P3 fractures in Thoroughbred and Standardbred racehorses, 71 of 74 fractures were wing fractures (types I and II) and the majority of these were articular.[27] In an older report of 65 cases of P3 fractures, 57 of 65 (89.5%) affected the lateral wing of the left forelimb or the medial wing of the right forelimb, and 53 of 65 (82%) entered the DIP joint.[28] Although all breeds and classes of horses can be affected, there appears to be a higher incidence observed in racing breeds.[27–29]

Although fractures of P3 can assume a variety of configurations, these fractures can be classified into 7 types (Figure 5.32).[5] Type I fractures are nonarticular oblique palmar/plantar process (wing) fractures (Figure 5.33). Type II fractures are articular oblique palmar or plantar process (wing) fractures (Figure 5.34) and are by far the most common type.[27,28] Type III fractures are sagittal articular fractures that roughly divide the distal phalanx into 2 separate halves (Figure 5.35). These fractures are uncommon and represent 3% to 4% of fractures of the distal phalanx[8,27,28] and occur more commonly in the hindlimb than the forelimb.[3] Type IV fractures are articular fractures involving the extensor process. They occur most frequently in the forelimbs and can be bilateral (Figure 5.36).[4,6,8] Type V fractures are comminuted articular or nonarticular fractures and can be a variety of configurations (Figure 5.37). Type VI fractures are nonarticular solar margin fractures of the distal phalanx (Figure 5.38). Type VII fractures are nonarticular fractures of the palmar or plantar process of the distal phalanx in foals (Figure 11.45). These fractures begin and end at the solar margin and are usually triangular or oblong in shape.[8,14,32] Initially they were thought to represent osseous bodies but histologic findings were consistent with a fracture.[14] Frontal fractures of P3 (fracture line runs lateral to medial and splits the bone into dorsal and palmar/plantar halves) occur but are extremely rare.[1,20]

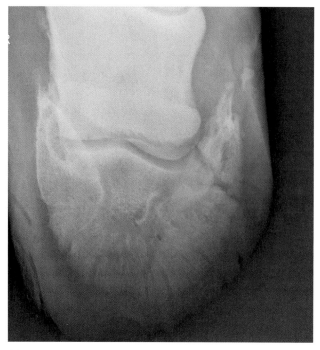

Figure 5.33. Type I fracture of the wing of P3. This fracture is nonarticular but it may be difficult to document this. This particular fracture is larger than most type 1 fractures and may be a type II articular fracture.

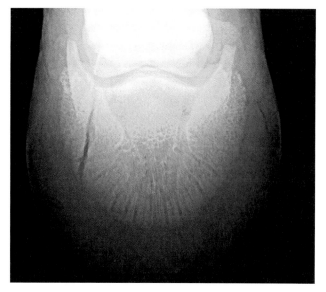

Figure 5.34. Type II articular "wing" fracture. This is the most common type of P3 fracture.

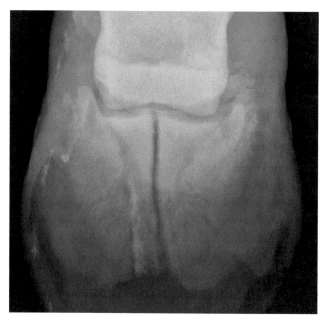

Figure 5.35. Type III sagittal fracture that essentially splits the bone into 2 pieces.

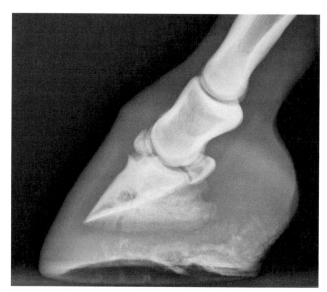

Figure 5.36. Type IV P3 fractures involve the extensor process.

Etiology

Single event trauma appears to be the predominant cause of P3 fractures. However, repetitive trauma leading the stress-related bone injury may be the cause in racehorses.[27] Scintigraphic abnormalities of P3 have been identified in racehorses before radiographic evidence of a fracture was present.[17,27] This suggests that P3 fractures may be similar to other "stress" or "fatigue"

type fractures that occur in racehorses. Acute trauma is often the cause in nonracehorses, especially in those that involve the hindlimb.[3,5] Type III sagittal articular fractures usually result from direct trauma to the hoof from kicking a solid object.[28] Type VI solar margin fractures may be related to the shape and location of the solar margin within the hoof and the tremendous forces the distal phalanx undergoes during weight-bearing and work.[9] These fractures may also occur concurrently with laminitis and pedal osteitis due to resorption of the apex of P3.[29] Type VII fractures in foals are thought to occur from compression either on the solar or dorsal

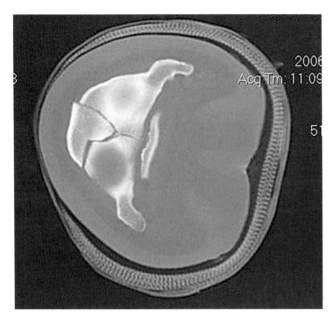

Figure 5.37. CT image of a Type V, comminuted fracture of P3. Fracture lines were present on both the lateral and dorsoplantar radiographs.

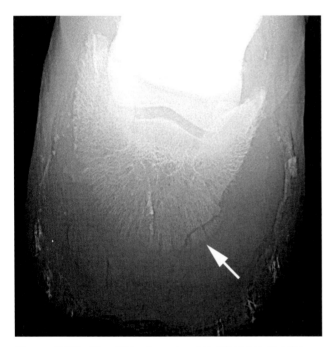

Figure 5.38. Type VI fractures are also referred to as solar margin fractures of P3 (arrow).

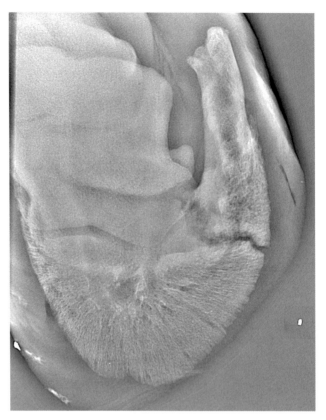

Figure 5.39. Type II articular fracture that was associated with a large sidebone of P3.

cortex of the distal phalanx during weight-bearing or from tension forces generated by the DDFT.[14] Excessive trimming of the heels, sole, and frog in foals does not appear to affect the occurrence of type VII fractures in foals.[16] Occasionally, P3 may be fractured as a result of penetration of a foreign body through the sole. A large sidebone may also serve to predispose to type II fractures due to its lever arm affect on the palmar/plantar process (Figure 5.39.) In either case, the P3 fracture

usually involves one of the lateral processes and is often articular.

Type IV extensor process fractures may occur due to excessive tension on the common digital extensor tendon resulting in an avulsion fracture. Overextension of the DIP joint may cause contact of the extensor process with the middle phalanx, and trauma to the dorsal aspect of the foot has also been proposed as a cause.[9,10,31] The development of a separate center of ossification or an osteochondrosis lesion of the extensor process may also occur.[8,26,28,31] Supporting a theory of a developmental lesion is the fact that lesions are often bilateral, occur in relatively young horses, and can be observed radiographically as an incidental finding in horses that are clinically normal (Figure 5.36).[4,6,8]

Clinical Signs

Generally the clinical signs are similar during the acute phases for all types of P3 fractures. A history of an acute onset of a moderate to severe lameness (grade 4 to 5 out of 5) is common.[5,17,29] In some cases the lameness will worsen within the first 24 hours after injury, presumably due to increased pressure within the hoof capsule secondary to inflammation and swelling. Exceptions to this are solar margin fractures, type VII fractures in foals, and developmental type IV fractures of the extensor process. Horses with these types of P3 fractures are usually only mild to moderately lame and the lameness must be differentiated from the many other potential problems within the foot.[5,10,12,14] In all cases, if the fracture is chronic, the signs of lameness are usually diminished.[29]

With acute fractures, an increased digital pulse may be palpable and heat in the affected foot may be appreciated. With articular fractures DIP joint effusion is often palpable dorsal and proximal to the coronary band. Swelling and edema may also be present above the hoof wall in the pastern region. Hoof tester examination usually reveals pain over the sole region, and focal pressure over the fracture site usually induces a marked painful response. However, a negative hoof tester response does not rule out the presence of a P3 fracture, especially in chronic cases.[10,15,29] Perineural anesthesia of the PD digital nerves or intra-articular anesthesia of the DIP joint may aid in localizing the lameness to the foot region. In general, regional anesthesia is usually unnecessary to diagnose type II and III fractures because the clinical signs are sufficient to localize the pain to the foot region. However, regional anesthesia is often necessary in horses with chronic P3 fractures and those that do not cause severe lameness.

Horses with large chronic extensor process fractures may have enlargement of the dorsal aspect of the coronary band and abnormal growth of the dorsal hoof wall. As the hoof grows, it develops a "V" or triangular shape called a buttress foot.[5,12,29] The abnormal hoof shape eventually will extend from the coronary band to the ground surface. Smaller type IV fractures rarely cause deformity of the dorsal hoof wall, but effusion of the DIP joint is common.

Diagnosis

Radiographic examination (30° dorsopalmar/plantar, 65° dorsoproximal-palmarodistal, lateral, and both obliques) are used to confirm the diagnosis and document the type and location of the fracture (see Chapter 4 for more details on radiographic views). In some cases it may be necessary to take special views of the palmar/plantar processes to identify the fracture. Solar margin fractures are most easily identified on the 60° dorsoproximal-palmarodistal projection using a radiographic technique with approximately one-half the exposure needed to evaluate the navicular bone.[8] Extensor process fractures are usually identified on the lateromedial view.[5,29]

Most P3 fractures are readily apparent on routine radiographic projections. However, nondisplaced or stress-related fractures in racehorses may not be apparent on the initial radiographic examination because of insufficient time for resorption of the bone along the fracture line or because the cast-like effect of the hoof wall may prevent fracture displacement.[8,17,27] In these cases, radiographs should be repeated in 1 to 2 weeks or nuclear scintigraphy can be used to help identify radiographically occult fractures of P3.[17,27,29]

In a scintigraphic study performed on 27 horses with P3 fractures, the palmar scintigraphic views had evidence of focal areas of increased uptake that corresponded to fracture line location on radiography.[17] Lateral views of P3 had a diffuse pattern of uptake. In a more recent study, abnormal uptake was most prominent on lateral views when the fractures were lateral but

dorsal, plantar, or solar views were necessary for diagnosis in horses with medial fractures.[27] Scintigraphic uptake is most intense and focal in acute fractures (less than 10 days) and becomes less intense and diffuse with chronicity. Increased scintigraphic uptake may still be evident 25 months after injury.[17]

Although not usually necessary to diagnose P3 fractures, computer tomography (CT) can be used to document occult fractures in the palmar/plantar processes of P3.[19] In one report, CT found an incomplete oblique fracture of the palmar process that was not evident radiographically 25 days after the injury.[19] The author has also used CT in a horse with a severely comminuted P3 fracture that had fracture lines present in both the lateromedial and dorsoplantar radiographic projections. The CT confirmed the fracture configuration (Figure 5.37).

Treatment

Options for treating horses with P3 fractures include confinement alone, confinement with corrective shoeing or foot casts, lag screw fixation (types II, III, and IV), and surgical removal of the fracture/fragment (type IV only). The decision often depends on the age and intended use of the horse, specific characteristics of the fracture, and financial constraints of the owner. In general, the majority of horses with P3 fractures are treated with confinement and corrective shoeing aimed at immobilizing the fracture and preventing expansion of the hoof wall (Figure 5.40). However, a foot cast may serve the same purpose as the shoe.

Types of shoes that may be used include a bar shoe with clips (Figure 5.41), a continuous rim-type shoe, or the Klimesh contiguous clip shoe (Figure 5.42).[1,11,23,29] All of these approaches appear to effectively prevent

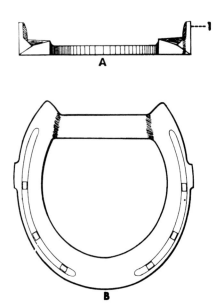

Figure 5.40. Full bar shoe that can be used to treat horses with distal phalanx fractures. A. Rear view of shoe showing quarter clips. B. Ground surface view of the shoe showing full bar and quarter clips welded to the shoe.

expansion of the hoof wall during weight-bearing, thus stabilizing the fracture. Regional anesthesia of the foot often aids application of the shoe and many horses walk more comfortably shortly after the foot is immobilized.[9,29]

One case of a comminuted frontal plane fracture was treated successfully by applying a 3° wedge-pad to the

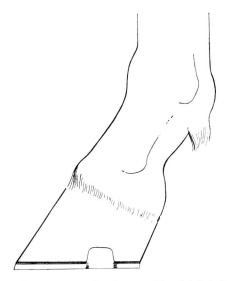

Figure 5.41. Side view of a shoe used for distal phalanx fractures, showing quarter clips in place.

bottom of the foot after which fiberglass hoof tape was applied to restrict hoof expansion and hold the wedge in place. The heel wedge was used to prevent tension in the DDFT from causing distraction of the fracture.[1]

In most cases the foot should remain in one of these shoes for 6 to 8 months, with the shoe reset every 4 to 6 weeks. Once clinical improvement has occurred, a less restrictive type of shoe (bar shoe only or bar shoe with quarter clips) may be used. Horse should not be worked for approximately 8 to 10 months, and in some cases, 1 year of rest may be necessary for clinical improvement.[29] Many P3 fractures are very slow to heal and may never develop radiographic bone union.[7,27,29] Thus, it was previously been thought that horses with P3 fractures may require continued use of bar shoes with quarter clips to ensure working soundness.[29] However, a recent study on nonracehorses found that horses do not need to be shod with bar shoes and clips for the remainder of their athletic career.[24]

Specific treatment of each type of P3 fracture is given below and included in Table 5.1.

Type I

This nonarticular fracture is best treated with confinement and methods to prevent hoof expansion (shoe or foot cast; see above for details). However, it may also respond to confinement and rest alone.

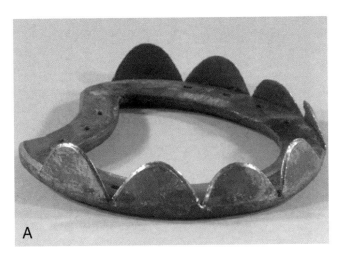

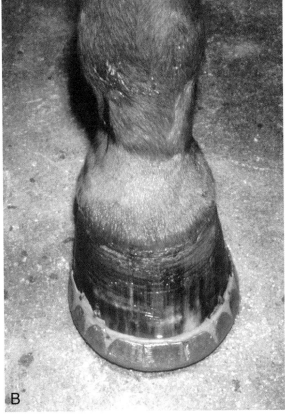

Figure 5.42. A. Contiguous clip shoe. B. Contiguous clip shoe after it has been placed on the foot. It can be held in place with acrylic.

Table 5.1. Types of distal phalanx fractures.

Fracture type	Location	Articular	Recommended treatment	Prognosis
I	Palmar/plantar process	No	Confinement ± shoeing(foot cast instead of shoe)	Very good to excellent
II	Oblique fractures of palmar/ plantar process ("wing" fractures)	Yes	Confinement + shoeing(foot cast instead of shoe) Lag screw repair of large type II fractures	Fair to good
III	Midsagittal fracture	Yes	Confinement + shoeing(foot cast instead of shoe) Best candidate for lag screw repair	Unpredictable; guarded?
IV	Extensor process(variable size)	Yes	Removal in most cases regardless of size: arthroscopy/arthrotomy Lag screw repair; some acute cases	Small: excellent Large: good
V	Comminuted	Yes or no	Confinement + shoeing(foot cast instead of shoe) Removal if secondary to infection	Unpredictable Guarded to good?
VI	Solar margin	No	Confinement + protective shoeing (wide-web shoes or shoes with full or rim pads)	Very good
VII	Palmar/plantar process—begins and ends at solar margin	No	Primarily in foals Confinement alone; no shoeing	Very good to excellent

Type II

Foals less than 6 months of age should be treated with stall confinement.[32] Treatment that restricts the expansion of the hoof is usually unnecessary and may result in severe hoof contraction. Foals should be confined for 6 to 8 weeks and their exercise should be restricted until bony union of the fracture is observed radiographically. Adult horses can be treated with confinement and methods to restrict hoof expansion (see above) or surgically by placing a lag screw. However, most type II fractures are treated nonsurgically because screw placement can be very difficult with this fracture type.[3,27] Surgery is often only considered in horses with large wing fractures because of the risks of the surgery, and it is currently unknown if surgery actually improves the overall prognosis in these horses.[3]

Type III

This is an unusual fracture in foals and adult horses but can be treated similarly to a type II fracture. These fractures tend to cause more severe lameness than type II fractures and foot immobilization is often important to improve weight-bearing on the affected limb to prevent contralateral limb laminitis.

Acute type III fractures in adult horses are usually the best candidates for surgical repair using lag screw fixation (Figure 5.43).[3,5,26] Fractures of greater than a few days duration may fill with granulation/fibrous tissue, making it difficult to reduce the fracture.[26] However, if conservative methods are not considered satisfactory, it is feasible to undertake screw fixation 4 to 6 weeks after the injury, even though the opportunity for interfragmentary compression is minimal.[7]

The correct site for screw placement is midway between the articular surface and solar canal through a hole in the side of the hoof wall.[29] Screw placement for

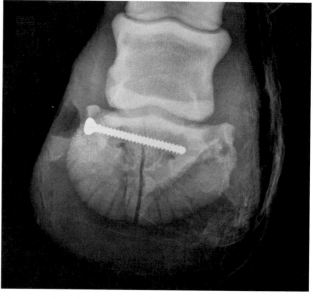

Figure 5.43. Lag screw repair of a type III P3 fracture. The screw must be placed through a hole within the hoof wall.

type III fractures is usually less difficult than for type II fractures because the bone is essentially divided in half and there is less risk of splitting the fracture when the screw is tightened.[5,9,10] The major risks with this procedure are infection developing around the implant, the inability to compress the fracture, incorrect screw placement leading to continued lameness, and overriding of the fracture fragments during compression. The primary advantages are less risk of secondary OA developing in the DIP joint and faster healing of the fracture due to surgical compression.

Complete fracture healing can be expected in 6 to 12 months and the screw may have to be removed if lameness persists or infection around the implant is evident.[3,5,10,26] Recently, a computer-assisted surgery (CAS) technique has been developed to improve accurate screw insertion into sagittal P3 fractures.[2] This technique resulted in greater precision of screw length and placement compared with the conventional technique and may enable placement of 2 screws for improved compression.[2] In addition, using larger diameter screws (6.5 or 5.5 mm) has been shown to increase axial compression of P3 when compared to 4.5-mm screws in an *in vitro* model.[13] Typically, 4.5-mm screws are used because of the small space for screw insertion. However, larger screws may improve interfragmentary compression.

Type IV

Surgical repair with a lag screw or surgical removal of the fracture/fragment is usually the preferred treatment for type IV P3 fractures.[4,6,10,12,18,21,22] Acute extensor process fractures are rare in horses but are the best candidates for lag screw fixation (Figure 5.44). Conservative treatment with prolonged stall rest is often unsuccessful because the extensor process fracture does not heal and horses remain lame.[6,8,26] However, most large type IV fractures are chronic and lag screw repair of these fractures has been reported but is generally not recommended by the author. Surgical removal of the extensor process fractures/fragments with arthroscopy or a dorsal arthrotomy is usually the treatment of choice (Figure 5.45). Arthroscopy using a dorsal approach is the preferred technique for removal of small extensor process fractures.[4,21] Large extensor process fractures (greater than 1 cm) have also been successfully removed with arthroscopy by using a motorized burr to remove the fragment.[6,21] These fractures usually involve a large part of the extensor process and can be challenging to remove (Figure 5.46) The convalescence time after removing large fragments is longer than after removing smaller fragments. In one report of using an arthrotomy to remove large fragments, the mean recovery time before returning to work was 7.5 months.[6]

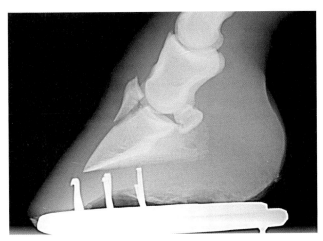

Figure 5.44. A large type IV P3 fracture that may warrant lag screw repair.

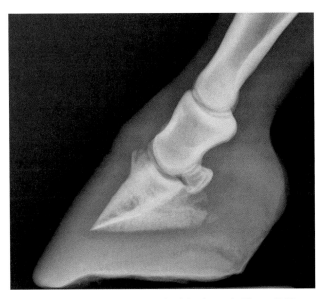

Figure 5.45. Lateral radiograph of the horse in Figure 5.36 following arthroscopic removal of an extensor process fracture.

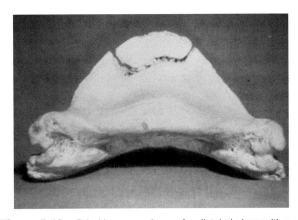

Figure 5.46. Dried bone specimen of a distal phalanx with a fracture of the extensor process. Note the width of the extensor process.

Type V

This fracture may be articular or nonarticular but regardless is best treated with confinement and methods to prevent hoof expansion (shoe or foot cast; see above for details). Confinement alone is usually not recommended for these fractures unless the fracture only involves the apex of P3.

Type VI

Treatment of solar margin fractures depends on whether the condition is primary or secondary to a chronic foot disorder (e.g., laminitis or pedal osteitis). However, primary causes of solar margin fractures are usually treated with corrective shoeing (wide web shoes, shoes and full pads, or shoes with rim pads) and stall or paddock rest for 4 to 12 months.[11,29] Strict immobilization with bar shoes and quarter clips is not necessary. Prolonged rest appears to be required for the best fracture healing but this often depends on the size of the fracture. If the cause is secondary, then treatment is directed at the underlying cause initially, followed by management of the solar margin fracture.[11]

Type VII

Affected foals with this fracture are usually treated satisfactorily with confinement alone for 6 to 8 weeks. Exercise should be restricted until radiographic evidence of bony union is evident, which is usually observed at about 8 weeks after the diagnosis.[16,32] Application of restrictive external coaptation (e.g., bar shoe or acrylic) to the hoof is not recommended because of the severe heel contraction that can occur and the potential for the hoof to slough.[32]

Osteoarthritis of the DIP joint is a common sequelae to articular P3 fractures. All racehorses with articular wing fractures that had follow-up radiographs had evidence of OA on the radiographs.[27] However, this did not preclude horses from racing and the authors warned to not over-interpret radiographic abnormalities within the DIP joint. Nonetheless, secondary abnormalities within the DIP joint subsequent to articular fractures may limit future athletic endeavors.[10,29] Secondary OA of the DIP joint appears to be more likely to develop with type III fractures than type II P3 fractures. If lameness persists, a neurectomy of the PD nerves may permit horses to resume athletic activity. In racehorses with primarily type II fractures, 18% had a PD neurectomy performed which completely resolved the residual lameness and permitted them to race.[27]

Prognosis

In general the prognosis for nonarticular P3 fractures (types I, V, VI, and VII) is usually very good for all ages of horses if sufficient rest is given.[11,16,28,29] For type VI solar margin fractures the prognosis depends on the severity of the primary disease, but 6 of 9 horses returned to soundness in one report.[11] Foals with type VII P3 fractures have an excellent prognosis for return to performance and fracture healing is expected in about 8 weeks.[16,32]

A 50% return to soundness has been reported for horses with type II wing fractures treated conservatively.[8,28,29,32] However, a much better success rate has been recently reported in Standardbred racehorses with 81% returning to training and 63% racing.[25] However, 89% that returned to training without a bar shoe refractured at the same site. Sixty percent of horses returning to training with a bar shoe raced successfully.[25] This is in contrast to nonracehorses, of which 69% returned to their previous level of use and did not wear a bar shoe when they returned to training.[24]

The prognosis for small extensor process fractures treated by arthroscopic removal is excellent. Two reports identified that 88% of the horses treated by this method returned to soundness.[4,22] Removal of chronic large extensor process fragments also results in a good prognosis; 8 of 14 cases returned to their intended use in one report.[6] The author also feels that most horses with large extensor process fractures will do well following removal. The prognosis for large extensor process fractures treated by internal fixation also

appears good in the small number of cases reported.[18,26,29] However, the prognosis is usually reduced if OA of the DIP joint is present.[6,29]

The type of P3 fracture with the most variable prognosis is type III fractures. It remains unknown if affected horses have an improved prognosis with lag screw fixation compared to confinement and corrective shoeing.[3] Variable success of surgical treatment was reported in the most recent report.[3] All fractures healed but only 2 of 4 horses returned to athletic activity and surgery did not reduce the convalescence time required. An older study using internal fixation to treat these fractures reported 11 of 11 horses older than 3 years of age became sound.[26] Regardless of the treatment used, horses with type III fractures have a worse prognosis to return to performance than the other types of P3 fractures, and re-fracture of the bone may occur.[25,26]

References

1. Anderson BH, Turner TA, Kobluk CN. Treatment of a comminuted frontal-plane fracture of the distal phalanx in a horse. J Am Vet Med Assoc 1996;209:1750–1752.
2. Andritzky J, Rossol M, Lischer C, et al. Comparison of computer-assisted surgery with conventional technique for the treatment of axial distal phalanx fractures in horses: an *in vitro* study. Vet Surg 2005;34:120–127.
3. Barr ARS. Internal fixation of fractures of the third phalanx in 4 horses. Equine Vet Educ 1993;5:308–312.
4. Boening KJ et al. Diagnostic and surgical arthroscopy of the equine coffin joint. Proceed Am Assoc Equine Pract 1989; 34:311–317.
5. Bertone AL. Fractures of the distal phalanx. In Equine Fracture Repair. Nixon AJ, ed. WB Saunders Co. Philadelphia, 1996; 146–152.
6. Dechant JE, Trotter GW, Stashak TS, et al. Arthrotomy removal of large extensor process fragments of the distal phalanx in horses: 14 cases (1992–1998). J Am Vet Med Assoc 2000;217: 1351–1355.
7. Gerring EL. Fractures of the third phalanx. Equine Vet Educ 1993;5:324–325.
8. Honnas CM, O'Brien TR, Linford RL. Distal phalanx fractures in horses: A survey of 274 horses with radiographic assessment of healing in 36 horses. Vet Radiol. 1988;29:98–100.
9. Honnas CM, Vacek JR, Schumacher J. Diagnosis and treatment of articular fractures of the equine distal phalanx. Vet Med 1992;87:1208–1214.
10. Honnas CM, Trotter GW. The distal interphalangeal joint. In Current Techniques in Equine Surgery and Lameness. NA White, JN Moore eds., 2nd ed. WB Saunders Co. Philadelphia, 1998;389–397.
11. Honnas CM, O'Brien T, Linford RL. Solar margin fractures of the equine distal phalanx. Proceedings Am Assoc Equine Pract 1987;33:399–410.
12. Honnas CM. Fractures of the extensor process. In JA Auer, ed. Equine Surgery. WB Saunders Co. Philadelphia. 1992;994–995.
13. Johnson KA, Smith FW. Axial compression generated by cortical and cancellous lag screws in the equine distal phalanx. Vet J 2003;166:159–163.
14. Kaneps AJ, O'Brien TR, Redden RF, et al. Characterization of osseous bodies of the distal phalanx of foals. Equine Vet J 1993;25:285–292.
15. Kaneps AJ, O'Brien RF, Stover SM, et al. Characterization of osseous bodies of the distal phalanx of foals. Proceedings Am Assoc Equine Pract 1992;38:283–284.
16. Kaneps AJ, O' Brien RF, Willits NH, et al. Effect of hoof trimming on the occurrence of distal phalangeal palmar process fractures in foals. Proceedings Am Assoc Equine Pract 1995;41:251–252.
17. Keegan KG, Twardock AR, Losonsky JM, et al. Scintigraphic evaluation of fractures of the distal phalanx in horses; 27 cases (1979–1988). J Am Vet Med Assoc 1993;202:1993–1997.
18. MacLellan KNM, MacDonald DG, Crawford WH. Lag screw fixation of extensor process fracture in a foal with a flexural deformity. Can Vet J 1997;38:226–228.

19. Martens P, Ihler CF, Rennesund J. Detection of a radiographically occult fracture of the lateral palmar process of the distal phalanx in a horse using computed tomography. Vet Radiol Ultrasound 1999;40:346–349.
20. McDiarmid AM. An unusual case of distal phalanx fracture in a horse. Vet Rec 1995;137:613–615.
21. McIlwraith CW. Diagnostic and surgical arthroscopy of the phalangeal joints. In Diagnostic and Surgical Arthroscopy in the Horse. McIlwraith CW, Nixon AJ, Wright IM, Boening KJ, eds. Elsevier, Philadelphia, 2005;347–364.
22. Miller SM, Bohanon TC. Arthroscopic surgery for the treatment of extensor process fractures of the distal phalanx in the horse. Vet Comp Orthop Traumat 1994;7:2–6.
23. Moyer W, Sigafoos R. Treatment of distal phalanx fractures in racehorses using a continuous rim-type shoe. Proceedings Am Assoc Equine Pract 1988;34:325–328.
24. Ohlsson J, Jansson N. Conservative treatment of intra-articular distal phalanx fractures in horses not used for racing. Aust Vet J 2005;83:221–223.
25. O'Sullivan CB, Dart AJ, Malikides N, et al. Nonsurgical management of type II fractures of the distal phalanx in 48 standardbred horses. Aust Vet J 1999;77:501–503.
26. Pettersson H. Fractures of the pedal bone in the horse. Equine Vet J 1976;8:104–109.
27. Rabuffo TS, Ross MW. Fractures of the distal phalanx in 72 racehorses: 1990–2001. Proceedings Am Assoc Equine Pract 2002;48:375–377.
28. Scott EA, McDole M, Shires MH. A review of third phalanx fractures in the horse. Sixty-four cases. J Am Vet Med Assoc 1979;174:1337.
29. Stashak TS. The Foot. In Adams' Lameness in Horses. Stashak TS, ed. 5th ed. Lippincott Williams and Wilkins. Philadelphia. 2002;645–733.
30. Yovich JV, Hilbert BJ, McGill, CA. Fractures of the Distal Phalanx in Horses. Aust Vet J 1982;59:180–182.
31. Yovich JV. Fractures of the distal phalanx in the horse. Vet Clin North Am Equine Pract 1989;5:145–160.
32. Yovich JV, Stashak TS, DeBowes RM, et al. Fractures of the distal phalanx of the forelimb in eight foals. J Am Vet Med Assoc 1986;189:550–553.

PEDAL OSTEITIS (PO)

Pedal osteitis (PO) is defined as an inflammatory condition of the foot that results in demineralization of the distal phalanx. Radiographically the condition appears as a focal or diffuse radiolucency of the bone or as new bone formation.[3,8,9,13] The 2 recognized classifications of pedal osteitis are nonseptic and septic.[1,3] The distal phalanx does not have a medullary cavity so inflammation of this bone is referred to as osteitis rather than osteomyelitis.[4]

Etiology

Nonseptic PO is a poorly defined disorder of the distal phalanx that may occur as a primary condition or develop from a secondary cause.[1] Primary PO is usually associated with severe or chronic sole bruising resulting from repeated concussion during exercise on hard surfaces.[9,13] It is believed that the bone and vascular channel changes result from pressure on, and hyperemia of, the solar lamina.[9] Secondary causes of nonseptic PO include persistent corns, laminitis, penetrating wounds, bruised soles, and conformational faults.[1,13] Regardless of the cause, PO is typically associated with persistent, generally chronic inflammation of the foot.[13] Histologically, nonseptic PO appears as a solar variant of laminitis affecting epidermal and corial laminae of the distal wall and sole, primarily in the toe and wing regions.[11]

Septic PO refers to bacterial infection within the distal phalanx. Environmental microbes gain access either by direct introduction of the microbes into the distal phalanx (e.g., deep penetrating wound), extension of infection from the soft tissues of the foot into the distal phalanx, or from hematogenous sources in foals.[6,10,15] Septic PO in foals should be considered as a potential site for hematogenous spread of infection associated with the septic arthritis/joint ill syndrome.[10] A recent study found that 8 of 22 foals with septic PO had multiple other foci of infection, and none of the foals had a history of a penetrating wound or subsolar abscess.[10] Other causes of septic PO in adult horses include chronic severe laminitis, subsolar abscesses (most common), solar margin fractures, deep hoof wall cracks, avulsion hoof injuries, and penetrating wounds of the foot.[2,4,7] A sequestrum may develop in the distal phalanx as the osseous infection progresses.[2,5,6] In a review of 63 horses treated for septic PO, subsolar abscesses were the most common cause (56%) followed by solar margin fractures (25%) and penetrating wounds (13%).[7]

Clinical Signs

Nonseptic PO most commonly affects the forelimbs, and the condition may be unilateral or bilateral. The severity of the lameness is variable and depends on the cause and degree of injury. The lameness may be accentuated after exercise, work on hard surfaces, or directly after trimming and shoeing.[9] Hoof tester examination often reveals focal or diffuse sensitivity of the sole at the toe region. However, the entire sole may be painful. Perineural anesthesia of the PD nerves usually eliminates the lameness.

Septic PO occurs most commonly in the forelimbs in adult horses and in the hindlimbs in foals.[2,10] The forelimbs were affected twice as commonly as the hindlimbs in one study[7] and 11 of 18 cases involved the forelimbs in another study.[2] The severity of lameness in horses with septic PO is usually greater than that seen with nonseptic PO. One study revealed that 53% of the horses were grade 4 of 5 lame and 33% were grade 3 of 5 lame at presentation.[2] The lameness is often chronic; the average duration of lameness prior to presentation in one study was 18.5 days.[7] Increased hoof temperature and prominent digital pulses are common in the affected limb. Hoof tester exam may be beneficial to localize the site of pain as well as to promote abscess drainage in some cases. Perineural anesthesia of the PD nerves may not eliminate the lameness in all horses with septic PO. No or minimal response to PD nerve block was seen in 5 of 5 cases of septic PO, and all 5 cases improved after an abaxial sesamoid nerve block.[2]

Diagnosis

Radiographic assessment of the distal phalanx for the presence of nonseptic PO should include at least three views: 60° dorsopalmar and the medial and lateral oblique projections.[12] The radiographic signs associated with nonseptic PO include demineralization, widening of the nutrient foramina at the solar margin, and irregular bone formation along the solar margins of the distal

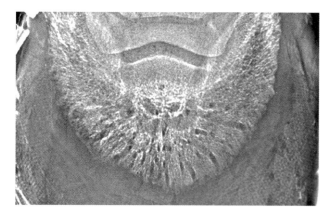

Figure 5.47. Horse with pedal osteitis characterized by demineralization of the distal phalanx.

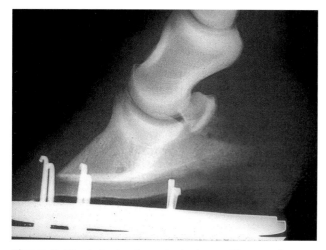

Figure 5.48. Lateral radiograph of a horse with nonseptic pedal osteitis demonstrating osteopenia and remodeling of P3.

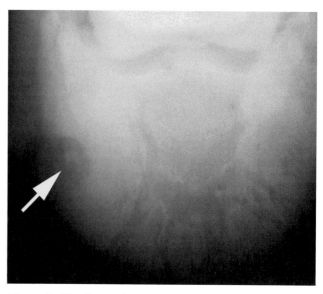

Figure 5.49. Dorsopalmar radiograph of a horse with a chronic draining tract from the solar surface of the foot. Lysis and a sequestrum can be seen along the solar surface of P3 (arrow).

phalanx (Figures 5.47 and 5.48).[13] Osseous proliferation of the solar margin of the distal phalanx is thought to develop secondary to prolonged inflammation. However, there can be wide variation in the radiographic characteristics of the distal phalanx and radiographs alone should not be used to make the diagnosis.[15]

The number and size of the vascular channels vary and the lateral border of the distal phalanx usually appears to be more roughened than the medial on a dorsopalmar projection.[12] The normal notch (crena) at the toe of the distal phalanx should not be interpreted as an abnormality. Radiographic abnormalities of the distal phalanx should not be over-interpreted and the diagnosis of PO should be made only when clinical signs concur with the radiographic findings.[12,15] Scintigraphic abnormalities associated with PO were uncommon in horses whose lameness improved with PD nerve blocks, which suggests that the condition may be overdiagnosed.[14]

Radiographic signs suggestive of septic PO are usually more straightforward than with nonseptic PO and are consistent with areas of bone infection. Generally there is a loss of trabecular detail (osteolysis)

with indistinct margins fading into the surrounding bone.[12] Sequestra may develop but marginal sclerosis is rarely observed in these cases (Figure 5.49).[7] Radiographic examination of 18 horses diagnosed with septic PO revealed discrete osteolysis at the margins of the distal phalanx (13 of 18 cases), gas density adjacent to the bone on 2 different radiographic projections (15 of 15 cases), focal (9 cases) or diffuse (3 cases) decrease in bone density, generalized roughening of the solar margin of the distal phalanx (7 of 18 cases), and widening of the vascular channels (13 of 18 cases).[2] Sequestra were identified in 4 horses.[2] In foals with septic PO, evidence of localized lysis or focal loss of bone density were observed at the toe (14 of 22 cases), extensor process (5 of 22 cases), or the palmar/plantar process (3 of 22 cases) of the distal phalanx.[10]

Treatment

Treatment of nonseptic PO often depends upon the inciting cause, use of the horse, and environmental factors. In general, treatment is aimed at reducing the inflammation within the distal phalanx, minimizing concussion to the foot, and eliminating the inciting cause.[8,9] For example, horses with PO secondary to severe or chronic solar bruising are often treated with corrective shoeing, rest, and oral NSAIDs for variable periods of time. A wide web egg-bar shoe whose solar surface is deeply concaved has been recommended to prevent the injured sole from contacting the ground.[9] Alternatively, shoes with rim pads can be applied to reduce concussion and protect the injured sole. The toe of the shoe can be squared or rolled to enhance break-over.[15]

Thin and soft soles can be medicated topically with equal parts of phenol, formalin, and iodine to "toughen" them.[15] A prolonged rest period is usually only necessary if a solar margin fracture is present or if the lameness is severe. Rest and avoiding exercise on hard

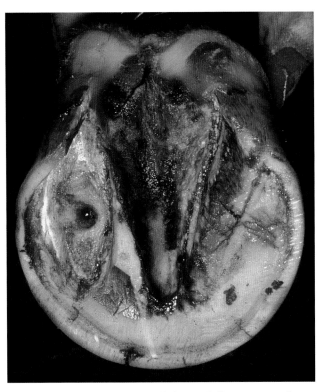

Figure 5.50. The sequestrum in image 5.49 was removed through the solar surface of the foot.

surfaces are usually indicated until the lameness subsides. Exercising on softer track surfaces, such as wood chips, or swimming the horse to maintain fitness may allow the horse to continue training until the lameness resolves.

Treatment of septic PO usually involves systemic and local antimicrobials (regional limb perfusion) and surgical debridement of the infected bone.[1-6,10] Surgical debridement of septic PO of the extensor process was not performed in foals but was recommended at other locations of the bone.[10] Debridement can be performed with the horse standing if the solar surface of the distal phalanx is involved (Figure 5.50). However, general anesthesia is often necessary to permit accurate location of the lesion if a draining tract is not present and for thorough debridement. In most cases the site of infection is approached through the draining tract which is usually located on the sole. The abnormal bone is debrided and a sample submitted for culture and sensitivity. The defect can be packed with gauze soaked in dilute povidone iodine and a protective bandage applied. A shoe with a removable metal plate can be applied to protect the sole once the infection has resolved. Regional IV limb perfusions can be repeated after surgery to help treat the infection (see Chapter 10 for more details). One study found that most of the bacterial isolates associated with septic PO were sensitive to metronidazole and recommended its use in all cases.[2] However, this antimicrobial is not used commonly by the author. Another study found that up to 24% of the distal phalanx could be removed without long-term adverse effects.[4]

Prognosis

The prognosis for nonseptic PO is often very good if the condition is of a relatively short duration and the exercise environment can be controlled. It is less favorable if the disease is chronic and the horse must continue to compete on hard surfaces, or if the condition is secondary to chronic laminitis.

The prognosis for horses with septic PO appears very good to excellent if the infection can be controlled.[1,15] Of 33 cases of septic PO in which follow-up was available, all 33 horses returned to their intended use.[7] In other studies, 7 of 9 horses returned to their intended use,[4] and 13 of 18 had a favorable outcome despite a high incidence of sequestra and fractures.[2] Foals with septic PO also have a good prognosis; 86% of the foals survived, 16 of 22 foals reached racing age, and 11 of these raced.[10]

References

1. Chaffin MK. Pedal osteitis. In Current Techniques in Equine Medicine and Surgery. White NA, Moore JN, eds. 2nd ed. WB Saunders Co. Philadelphia, 1998;530–531.
2. Cauvin ER, Munroe GA. Septic osteitis of the distal phalanx: findings and surgical treatment in 18 cases. Equine Vet J 1998;30:512–519.
3. DeBowes RM, Yovich JV. Penetrating wounds, abscesses, gravel and bruising of the equine foot. Vet Clin North Am Equine Pract 1989;5:179–194.
4. Gaughan EM, Rendano VT, Ducharme NG. Surgical treatment of septic pedal osteitis in horses: nine cases (1980–1987). J Am Vet Med Assoc 1989;195:1131–1134.
5. Honnas CM, Dabareiner RM, McCauley BH. Hoof wall surgery in the horse: approaches to and underlying disorders. Vet Clin North Am Equine Pract 2003;19:479–499.
6. Honnas CM, Peloso JG, Carter GK, et al. Diagnosing and treating septic conditions of the equine foot. Vet Med 1994;89: 1060–1071.
7. Lindford S, Embertson R, Bramlage L. Septic osteitis of the third phalanx: a review of 63 cases. Proceedings Am Assoc Equine Pract, 1994;40:103.
8. Moyer W. Traumatic pedal osteitis (TPO) in racehorses. Proceedings Am Assoc Equine Pract,1989;34:417–419.
9. Moyer W. Non-septic pedal osteitis: A cause of lameness and a diagnosis. Proceedings Am Assoc Equine Pract 1999;45: 178–179.
10. Neil KM, Axon JE, Todhunter PG, et al. Septic osteitis of the distal phalanx in foals: 22 cases (1995–2002). J Am Vet Med Assoc 2007;230:1683–1690.
11. Pool RR. Gross, histologic and ultrastructural pathology of disorders of the distal extremity. Proc of 13th Bain Fallon Memorial Lecture, 1991;25–31.
12. Rendano VT, Grant B. The equine third phalanx: Its radiographic appearance. Am J Vet Rad Soc 1978;19: 125–135.
13. Reeves MJ, Yovich JV, Turner AS. Miscellaneous conditions of the equine foot. Vet Clin North Am Equine Pract 1989;5: 221–242.
14. Ross MW. Observations in horses with lameness abolished by palmar digital analgesia. Proceedings Am Assoc Equine Pract 1998;44:230–232.
15. Stashak TS. The Foot. In Adams' Lameness in Horses. Stashak TS, ed. 5th ed. Lippincott Williams and Wilkins. Philadelphia. 2002;645–733.

SUBCHONDRAL CYSTIC LESIONS OF THE DISTAL PHALANX (P3)

Subchondral cystic lesions (SCLs) of the distal phalanx are uncommon and can affect a wide variety of horse breeds of all ages.[1,5,10] Affected horses are usually intermittently lame, and the forelimbs are more frequently affected than the hindlimbs. Verschooten reported on 15 cases of SCLs involving the distal phalanx, 14 of which were located in the forelimb.[10] In another study 27 of 28 cases involved the forelimbs.[2] Most SCLs communicate with the joint surface,[3,9] although communication with the adjacent joint space can be variable.[5,10]

Etiology

Regardless of their location, the cause of most SCLs in the horse is considered to be either trauma or osteochondrosis.[1,6,7] Damage to the subchondral bone in the stifle has been shown to cause SCLs of the medial femoral condyle and SCLs can occur at sites of previous intra-articular fractures.[1,6] Damage to the cartilage and subchondral bone is thought to permit passage of joint fluid through the opening, resulting in resorption of the subchondral bone.[1,10] Alternatively, a developmental osteochondrosis lesion predisposes to the lesion because SCLs are often found in young horses and are frequently bilateral.[1,7] See Chapter 11 for more information about SCLs and osteochondrosis.

Clinical Signs

A history of an acute onset of lameness may be present but more often the lameness is chronic and intermittent. The lameness may subside with rest and recur with exercise, and the severity can be variable. There are often no palpable abnormalities (including hoof tester examination) but effusion within the DIP joint may be present. The digital pulse rate may be elevated and the phalangeal flexion test is usually positive.[2] A PD nerve block improves the lameness in most cases, but perineural anesthesia at the base of the sesamoid bones may be needed for complete resolution of the lameness. Intrasynovial anesthesia of the DIP joint also eliminates the lameness, especially if the SCL communicates with the joint.[3,10]

Diagnosis

Radiography is necessary for a definitive diagnosis of a SCL of the distal phalanx. The SCLs are variable in size and are usually identified within the body of the distal phalanx (Figure 5.51). The majority of SCLs communicate with the joint.[3,9] In one study, 18 of 27 SCLs were located centrally in the distal phalanx and communication with the DIP joint was observed in all cases.[2] In the more recent study, all 11 horses had SCLs that were intra-articular.[9]

Treatment

Recommended treatments of SCLs of the distal phalanx have included (1) confinement followed by increasing exercise, (2) intra-articular medications, (3) transcortical drilling, (4) extra-articular surgical curettage, and (5) arthroscopic debridement.[3–5,7–10]

Most horses respond only transiently to intra-articular medications, and debridement through hoof wall windows has been complicated by recurrent abscessa-

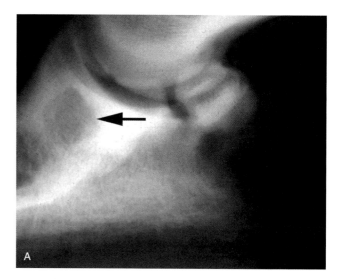

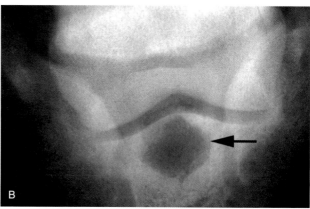

Figure 5.51. Lateral (A) and dorsopalmar (B) radiographs of a horse with SCL of P3 (arrows).

tion and lameness.[4] A dorsal arthroscopic approach for intra-articular debridement recently has been described in 11 horses.[9] This technique is performed with the DIP joint extended and distracted to permit access to the SCL.[9] Because of the morbidity associated with extra-articular debridement techniques, arthroscopic debridement should be considered the treatment of choice.[4,9] However, some SCLs in the distal phalanx may be inaccessible with the arthroscope.[3]

Prognosis

Variable results have been reported with extra-articular debridement of these lesions, and these techniques are often complicated by infection and continued lameness.[3,7] However, there are reports of successful debridement of SCLs through the hoof[5,10] and 1 horse treated with an autogenous bone graft returned to race training after 6 months.[8] Ten of 11 (91%) horses treated with arthroscopic debridement of a distal phalanx SCL returned to athletic soundness.[9] All of these horses were treated between 16 and 33 months of age, so results may vary depending on the age at diagnosis.[9] However, arthroscopic debridement of SCLs of the distal phalanx should provide a superior outcome in any age horse compared to extra-articular approaches.

References

1. Baxter GM. Subchondral cystic lesions in horses. In Joint Disease in the Horse. McIlwraith CW, Trotter GW, eds. WB Saunders, Philadelphia. 1996:384–397.
2. Haack D, Hertsch B, Baez C. Cyst-like defects in the coffin bone of horses. Pferdeheilkunde. 1988; 4:143–148.
3. Honnas CM, Trotter GW. The distal interphalangeal joint. In Current Techniques in Equine Surgery and Lameness. White NA, Moore JN, eds. 2nd ed. WB Saunders Co. Philadelphia, 1998; 389–397.
4. McIlwraith CW. Diagnostic and surgical arthroscopy of the phalangeal joints. In Diagnostic and Surgical Arthroscopy in the Horse. McIlwraith CW, Nixon AJ, Wright IM, Boening KJ, eds. Elsevier. Philadelphia, 2005;347–364.
5. Pettersson H, Sevelius F. Subchondral bone cysts in the horse: clinical study. Equine Vet J 1968;1:75.
6. Ray CS, Baxter GM, McIlwraith CW, et al. Development of subchondral cystic lesions after articular cartilage and subchondral bone damage in young horses. Equine Vet J 1996;28: 225–232.
7. Stashak TS. The Foot. In Adams' Lameness in Horses. Stashak TS, ed. 5th ed. Lippincott Williams and Wilkins, Philadelphia. 2002;645–733.
8. Stanek V, Edinger H. Surgical treatment of a subchondral bone cyst of the third phalanx in a standardbred gelding by use of an autogenous bone graft. Wien Tierärztl Mschr 1990;77:198–202.
9. Story MR, Bramlage LR. Arthroscopic debridement of subchondral bone cysts in the distal phalanx of 11 horses (1994–2000). Equine Vet J 2004;36:356–360.
10. Verschooten F, DeMoor, A. Subchondral cystic and related lesions affecting the equine pedal bone and stifle. Equine Vet J 1982;14:47–54.

OSSIFICATION OF THE COLLATERAL CARTILAGES OF THE DISTAL PHALANX (SIDEBONE)

Ossification of the collateral cartilages of the distal phalanx is relatively common in certain breeds of horses, including most larger breeds such as Warmbloods and draft horses and Finnhorses and Brazilian jumpers.[6,9–12,15] The forefeet appear to be more commonly involved than the hindfeet and the clinical significance of the condition remains questionable.[3,4,13,15] Female horses appear to be more susceptible to development of this condition and the lateral cartilage often shows more ossification than the medial cartilage.[12] The ossification can begin at the base of the cartilage or originate as a separate area in the center of the cartilage.[2,5,6] In Brazilian jumpers, 7% of the horses had no ossification, 86% had ossification beginning at the base, and 7% had a separate center of ossification.[6] In either case the palmar/plantar aspect of the cartilage is likely to be spared from the ossification process.[12]

In a radiographic study of 462 Finnhorses, 80% had evidence of sidebones, and large sidebones or separate centers of ossification were significantly more common in females than males.[11] Ossification of the cartilages in the forefeet was present in 93% of Brazilian jumpers.[6] Ten percent of Warmblood horses and 80% of draft horses had ossification of the cartilages of the distal phalanx and the ossification was more extensive in draft horses than in Warmblood horses.[15] The lateral and medial cartilages were ossified equally in draft horses, but the lateral cartilages were more commonly involved in Warmbloods. In this same study it was concluded that ossification of the cartilage had no clinical significance.[15]

Etiology

The specific cause(s) of sidebones is/are not clear.[11] It has been suggested that the tendency to develop sidebones is partly hereditary in certain horse breeds in Australia, Finland, and Sweden.[11,15] Hoof concussion causing trauma to the cartilage, poor conformation (particularly base narrow), and poor trimming and shoeing have also been proposed as inciting causes.[13] One study documenting the incidence of sidebones in Finnhorses found that very few horses were base narrow and most horses were base wide and toed out.[11] Another study concluded that ossification of the cartilages was neither the cause nor the result of conformational adaptations of the front feet.[9] It has also been suggested that prolonged exercise and or racing may have some preventative influence on ossification of the collateral cartilages.[10] The amount of weight placed on the foot may also be contributory because primarily larger breed horses develop sidebone.

Clinical Signs

Lameness resulting from sidebones is considered rare and the clinical significance of radiographic-apparent ossification is questioned.[4,14] One study found no correlation between the extent of ossification of the collateral cartilages and the onset of lameness.[15] Furthermore, despite the development of large sidebones in many Finnhorses, most horses performed satisfactorily without lameness.[11] However, large sidebones have been seen in horses associated with type II distal phalanx fractures by the author, and were thought to contribute to the fracture and chronic lameness (Figure 5.39 and 5.52).

In a scintigraphic study, a radiographically identified separate center of ossification could be detected with

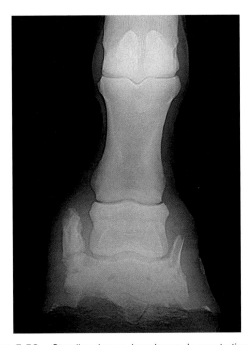

Figure 5.52. Standing dorsopalmar horse demonstrating a large uniaxial sidebone that was thought to contribute to lameness.

scintigraphy in 12 of 17 feet.[7] The authors suggested that scintigraphy may be useful to determine the clinical significance of ossification of the cartilages, prompting further clinical investigation such as uniaxial PD nerve block or advanced imaging.[7] However, another study by the same authors found considerable variation in the radiographic, scintigraphic, and MRI appearance of the palmar processes of the distal phalanx.[8] The study concluded that further investigation was needed to determine the clinical significance of the MRI abnormalities within the palmar processes. Currently, the clinical relevance of ossification of the collateral cartilages has not been documented but should be considered when clinical abnormalities associated with sidebones are found in lame horses.[7,8,14]

Sidebones may be visually apparent as an enlargement of the lateral and medial dimensions of the pastern region if the ossification is extensive. If the ossification involves the proximal extent of the cartilage, palpation may reveal an obvious firmness to the cartilage. Rarely is pain elicited with digital pressure. If present, the enlarged sidebone may contribute to the lameness or may be associated with a secondary fracture of the distal phalanx. A fractured sidebone reportedly causes more acute signs of lameness.[3,14] However, sidebones may accompany other lameness conditions of the palmar heel region (e.g., navicular syndrome) and may be mistaken for the cause. On the other hand, pain in the palmar heel region may originate from the axial projections of the ungual cartilages that extend toward the midline and have an abundant sensory nerve supply.[1]

Diagnosis

Radiographic examination of the foot usually reveals the extent of the ossification of the cartilage or cartilages (Figure 5.52). Occasionally a sidebone may appear fractured; however, the radiolucent defect must be differentiated from the junction between a separate ossification center and that part of the cartilage that is ossifying from the palmar process of the distal phalanx.[12,14] A fracture in the ossified cartilage can occur but is rare.[3,14]

Documenting that sidebone is the cause of lameness in horses can be difficult. Asymmetrical swelling of pastern region, pain on palpation of the collateral cartilage, and improvement of the lameness with a uniaxial PD nerve block is suggestive of a problem in this region. However, the mere presence of an ossified cartilage without any other radiographic abnormalities is not diagnostic. The clinical relevance would probably need to be further documented with scintigraphy and/or MRI.[7,8]

Treatment

If sidebone is suspected as the cause of lameness, conservative treatment with rest, topical 1% diclofenac sodium cream (Surpass®), and oral administration of NSAIDs is recommended initially. Any contributing foot problems such as foot imbalances should be addressed. Surgical removal of suspected fractured sidebones is not recommended. If lameness persists and sidebone is considered the cause of the lameness, a PD neurectomy can be performed but is usually unneces-

sary. Horses with sidebone and a secondary distal phalanx fracture are treated with corrective shoeing and confinement similar to a horse with a distal phalanx fracture alone (see type II P3 fractures).

Prognosis

The prognosis is difficult to predict because this condition is thought to rarely cause lameness.

References

1. Bowker RM, Van Wulfin K, Springer SE, et al. Functional anatomy of the cartilage of the distal phalanx and digital cushion in the equine foot and a hemodynamic flow hypothesis of energy dissipation. Am J Vet Res. 1998;59:961–968.
2. Butler JA, Colles CM, Dyson SJ, et al. Distal phalanx. In Clinical Radiology of the Horse. Blackwell Scientific Publications. Oxford, 1993;25–47.
3. Colles CM. Diseases and injuries of the horse's foot. In J Hickman's Equine Surgery and Medicine, 1st ed. Academic Press Inc. London, 1986;221–223.
4. Johnson JH. The Foot. In Equine Medicine and Surgery. 3rd ed. Mansmann RA, McAllister ES, eds. American Veterinary Publications. Santa Barbara, 1982;1052.
5. McNeel SV. The phalanges. In Textbook of Veterinary Diagnostic Radiology. Thrall DE, ed. 2nd ed. WB Saunders Co. Philadelphia, 1994;190–213.
6. Melo e Silva SR, Vulcano LC. Collateral cartilage ossification of the distal phalanx in the Brazilian Jumper horse. Vet Radiol Ultrasound 2002;43:461–463.
7. Nagy A, Dyson SJ, Murray RM. Scintigraphic examination of the cartilages of the foot. Equine Vet J 2007;39:250–256.
8. Nagy A, Dyson SJ, Murray RM. Radiographic, scintigraphic and magnetic resonance imaging findings in the palmar processes of the distal phalanx. Equine Vet J 2008;40:57–63.
9. Ruohoniemi M, Tulamo RM, Hackzell M. Radiographic evaluation of ossification of the collateral cartilages of the third phalanx in Finnhorses. Equine Vet J 1993;25:453–455.
10. Ruohoniemi M, Ryhanen V, Tulamo RM. Radiographic appearance of the navicular bone and distal interphalangeal joint and their relationship with ossification of the collateral cartilages of the distal phalanx in Finnhorse cadaver forefeet. Vet Rad and Ultrasound. 1998;39:125–132.
11. Ruohoniemi M, Laukkanen H, Okala M, et al. Effects of sex and age on the ossification of the collateral cartilages of the distal phalanx of the Finnhorse and the relationships between ossification and body size and type of horse. Res Vet Sci 1997;62:34–38.
12. Ruohonieme M, Raekallio M, Tulamo RM, et al. Relationship between ossification of the cartilages of the foot and conformation and radiographic measurements of the front feet in Finnhorses. Equine Vet J 1997;29:44–48.
13. Schneider RK, Stickle RL. Orthopedic problems of the foot. In Current Therapy in Equine Medicine, 2nd ed. WB Saunders, Philadelphia. 1987;282–289.
14. Stashak TS. The Foot. In Adams' Lameness in Horses. Stashak TS, ed. 5th ed. Lippincott Williams and Wilkins. Philadelphia, 2002;645–733.
15. Verschooten F, Waerebeek B van, Verbeeck J. The ossification of cartilages of the distal phalanx in the horse: an anatomical, experimental, radiographic and clinical study. J Equine Vet Sci 1996;16:291–305.

QUITTOR (INFECTION AND NECROSIS OF THE COLLATERAL [UNGUAL] CARTILAGE)

Quittor is the term used to describe chronic purulent inflammation of a collateral cartilage of the distal phalanx characterized by cartilage necrosis and multiple fistulous draining tracts proximal to the coronary band. The lateral cartilages of the forelimb are most commonly affected.[1–3,5] In a retrospective study of necrosis of the collateral cartilages, 14 of 16 cases involved the lateral cartilage of the forelimbs and hindlimbs.[1]

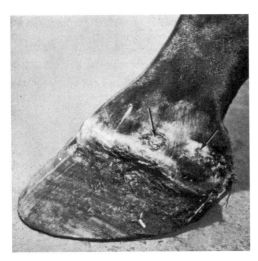

Figure 5.53. Clinical appearance of a horse with quittor. Arrows point to 2 draining tracts located just above the coronary band.

Etiology

Infection and subsequent necrosis of the collateral cartilage is usually caused by a direct injury to the cartilage or to the soft tissues overlying the cartilage. Injuries to the collateral cartilage that predispose to quittor include penetrating wounds and lacerations, external blows that bruise and damage its blood supply (e.g., interference), foot abscesses, chronic ascending infections of the white line in the quarters, and deep hoof cracks that result in localized infection in the collateral cartilage.[1,3,5]

Clinical Signs

Quittor is characterized by the formation of abscesses within the collateral cartilage which break open and drain just proximal to the coronary band (Figure 5.53). A history of recurrent drainage from fistulous tracts overlying the affected cartilage and intermittent severe lameness is common. Swelling, heat, and pain with pressure over the affected cartilage are often present. Pain is usually elicited with hoof testers over the affected quarter. The degree of lameness is usually affected by the patency of the fistulous tract draining the abscesses.[1,3] Lack of drainage increases pressure within the abscess, often resulting in severe lameness. Once the abscess breaks open and drains, the lameness usually subsides. Chronic inflammation of the involved cartilage may cause permanent hoof damage resulting in deformity of the foot and persistent lameness.

Diagnosis

The diagnosis is usually based on a history of recurrent swelling of the affected collateral cartilage, the presence of 1 or more fistulous tracts proximal to the coronary band, and intermittent lameness. Swelling and pain over the affected cartilage supports the diagnosis. Quittor should be differentiated from shallow abscesses and ascending infection of the white line (gravel). The drainage tract associated with gravel is usually located at or just proximal to the coronary band, and the inflammatory process is often localized.[3,5] With quittor there may be multiple fistulous tracts, and the swelling is usually more diffuse and located more proximally over the collateral cartilages.[1–3,5]

Radiographs can be used to rule out bone involvement but lysis of the collateral cartilage associated with infection cannot be seen on radiographs. However, osteomyelitis of an ossified collateral cartilage can occur.[3] The depth and dimension of the draining tract(s) can also be determined with fistulography or by placing a sterile flexible metal probe within the tract.[3,5]

Treatment

The treatment of choice is surgical excision of the fistulous tract(s) and necrotic cartilage.[1–5] Medical management with systemic antibiotics, foot soaks, and injection of the fistulous tracts with antiseptics is usually not effective because of the limited blood supply to the cartilage.[1–3] Medical treatment may temporarily suppress the infection but often just delays the eventual need for surgery. However, improved medical treatment of these infections may be obtained with IV regional perfusion of antimicrobials, and 1 of 3 horses treated conservatively became sound in one study.[1]

At surgery the foot should be held in rigid extension by placing traction with wires placed through holes drilled in the hoof wall. Extending the foot tenses the joint capsule and retracts it from the surgical dissection plane, thus reducing the chance of inadvertent penetration of the DIP joint.[1–3] Access to the cartilage is best achieved through a curved skin incision based proximally, which is dissected from the abaxial surface of the cartilage and reflected proximally.[3] A curved incision beginning just dorsal to the coronary band over the diseased collateral cartilage and reflected distally can also be used.[5] Necrotic cartilage is recognized by its dark blue or reddish blue appearance. Only in advanced cases is the entire cartilage removed.[4] The incision can be closed primarily and the foot and pastern region are protected with either a bandage or a foot cast.

Prognosis

The prognosis for most cases of quittor following complete excision of the necrotic cartilage is good unless the infection is very chronic.[5] Secondary complications such as osteomyelitis of the distal phalanx, septic arthritis of the DIP joint, or infection of the digital cushion or other soft tissues in the foot reduce the prognosis appropriately.[2,5] A retrospective study indicated that 66% of the horses were sound and that horses with drainage of less than 1 months' duration had a better prognosis for return to soundness than horses with drainage of more than 1 months' duration prior to the initiation of treatment.[1]

References

1. Honnas CM, Ragle CA, Meagher DM. Necrosis of the collateral cartilage of the distal phalanx in horses: 16 cases (1970–1988). J Am Vet Med Assoc 1988;193:1303–1307.
2. Honnas CM. The foot. In Equine Surgery, 2nd ed. Auer JA, Stick JA, eds. WB Saunders, Philadelphia, 1999;779–791.

3. Honnas CM, Dabareiner RM, McCauley BH. Hoof wall surgery in the horse: approaches to and underlying disorders. Vet Clin North Am Equine Pract 2003;19:479–499.
4. Johnson JH. The Foot. In Equine Medicine and Surgery, 3rd ed. Mansmann RA, McAllister ES, eds. American Veterinary Publications, Santa Barbara, 1982:1052.
5. Stashak TS. The Foot. In Adams' Lameness in Horses. Stashak TS, ed. 5th ed. Lippincott Williams and Wilkins. Philadelphia, 2002;645–733.

SOLE BRUISES, CORNS, AND ABSCESSES

A bruise results from the rupture of blood vessels in the dermis (corium or sensitive tissue) beneath the sole, frog, or hoof wall. With time the hemorrhage spreads into the deep layers of the epidermis and becomes visible as the hoof grows. Accordingly the discoloration associated with a sole bruise is most often seen several weeks after injury, whereas the same injury occurring in the hoof wall may take months before it becomes apparent.[4] Logically, bruises are most visible when the hemorrhage is superficial and the hoof is nonpigmented. It is likely the pain associated with the injury is due to the inflammatory response as well as the increased subsolar pressure.[5]

A corn is a bruise that involves the tissues of the sole at the angle formed by the wall and the bar (Figure 5.54).[5] This site is often referred to as the seat of the corn. Corns occur most frequently on the inner angle of the front feet and are rarely found in the hindfeet.[5] If the bruised site becomes infected a subsolar abscess may develop.

Sole bruising and corns have been classified into 3 types (dry, moist, or suppurative) depending on their clinical picture.[4,5] Dry bruises appear as red (old hemorrhage) stains on the sole and may not cause any clinical signs. Moist bruises occur when serum accumulates beneath the injured epidermis and may cause mild lameness. Suppurative bruises have become infected and often contribute to severe lameness.

Etiology

Trauma to the sole is the cause of most sole bruising. However, sole bruising at the toe region may be secondary to an underlying condition such as chronic laminitis and flexural deformities.[4] Horses with flat feet, thin soles, and soft soles appear to be predisposed to sole bruising.[1] Also, horses that are barefoot, have their hooves trimmed too short, or have the sole protruding below the hoof wall appear more likely to develop sole bruising. Horses housed in muddy pens in freezing conditions, whether shod or not, often bruise their soles when the lumpy mud freezes hard.[5] Flat-footed horses that have repeated concussion to the sole adjacent to the white line because the sole contacts the inner aspect of the shoe may also develop sole bruises.[3] Any form of shoeing that concentrates weight-bearing on the sole is likely to cause bruising.

Corns usually are caused by pressure from horseshoes or when a stone becomes wedged between the shoe and sole. They are rare among horses that are not shod. When shoes are left on too long, the heel may overgrow the shoe, causing selective pressure on the sole at the angle of the wall and the bar leading to a corn. Additionally, bending the inside branch of the shoe toward the frog to prevent pulling or stepping off the shoe can result in direct pressure to the sole, leading to bruising.[3,5] The application of a shoe that is one-half to one full size too small for the foot also increases the pressure on the sole area at the angle of the heels.[3,5] Heel calks usually enhance this effect.

Clinical Signs

The clinical signs associated with sole bruising or corns are often similar and variable. Most sole bruises occur at the toe or quarter regions and corns occur at the angle of the wall and bar. Occasionally the frog can be bruised as well.[4] The horse may show varying degrees of lameness (usually mild to moderate) depending upon the severity and type of the bruise or corn. The characteristics of the lameness and foot placement vary according to the location of the bruise or corn. If the bruise is acute or infected, the hoof may appear warmer and an increased digital pulse is often present.[4,5] Hoof testers often identify a focal site of pain unless the lesion is underneath the shoe at the white line. Perineural anesthesia may be required in some cases to exclude other sources of pain causing lameness.

Horses with foot abscesses are typically very lame and often nonweight-bearing. Increased heat is often palpable in the foot and distal limb and an increased digital pulse is commonly found. Hoof tester pain is typically severe and in some cases digital pressure at the site of the abscess causes a painful response. Increased swelling at the coronary band (especially at 1 heel bulb) may be present if the abscess has migrated up along the hoof wall.

Diagnosis

A tentative diagnosis can often be made based on the history and clinical signs. If pain is localized to the foot but there are no obvious external abnormalities, the shoe should be removed and the sole explored by removing the exfoliating (flaky) sole with a hoof knife. Acute sole bruises may not be readily apparent because the hemorrhage has not migrated far enough distally.

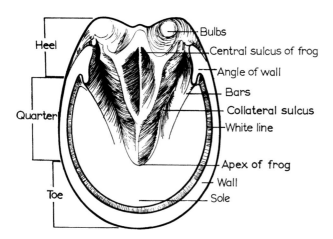

Figure 5.54. Normal forefoot showing anatomic structures.

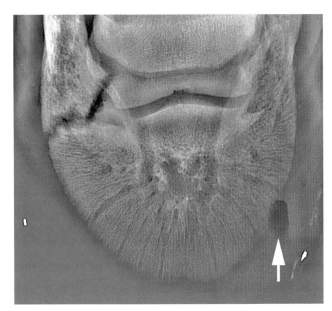

Figure 5.55. This horse with a type 2 P3 fracture became acutely lame 2 months after diagnosis. A dorsopalmar radiograph demonstrated a fluid pocket (arrow) consistent with an abscess.

Drainage is the key to treating suppurative bruises and other subsolar abscesses. A small amount of sole overlying the abscess should be removed to permit ventral drainage. Removing a large amount of sole should be avoided because this is usually not necessary for drainage and prolongs the healing time. The foot can then be soaked in antiseptic solution if desired, and the foot bandaged. Once the abscess has resolved, the sole can be protected with protective boots or shoes until the defect has completely keratinized.

In cases in which shoeing contributes to the bruising, removal of the shoe may be all that is necessary. The horse should be rested and should not be reshod until symptoms disappear. If the horse must be used, the wall and bar in the region of the corn should be removed to prevent pressure by the shoe. A complete support shoe can be applied to allow the frog to absorb the concussion that would normally be distributed to the corn area. Another option is to apply a wide web shoe that has been concaved out at the damaged region to decrease the pressure on the bruised site.[2,3] To prevent shoes from causing corns, the heels of the shoes should extend well back on the buttresses and should fit full on the wall at the quarters and heels.[5]

Prognosis

The prognosis is usually very good for horses suffering from a single traumatic episode and in those with good foot conformation. The prognosis is reduced in horses with poor hoof conformation that are continually worked on hard ground because recurrence is common. Many of these cases develop chronic sole bruising, which eventually may cause osteitis of the distal phalanx (pedal osteitis). Horses with routine foot abscesses also have a very good prognosis provided the infection does not involve deeper structures in the foot. It should always be remembered that subsolar abscesses may be associated with other conditions of the foot such as keratomas, chronic laminitis, and septic pedal osteitis (Figure 5.56).

Chronic bruises are usually visible as a stippled reddened region.[5] In some cases the discoloration may be bluish, especially if a sole abscess is developing. Sole abscesses may have a small defect in the sole where the abscess is trying to break through the sole. Removing a small area of sole around this defect may reveal purulent material, confirming a subsolar abscess. Hoof tester pressure at the site also may cause purulent material to exit the sole defect.

Acute sole bruises may not be evident radiographically unless a serum pocket or abscess has developed. Many subsolar abscesses may be seen radiographically as a gas pocket within the sole (Figure 5.55). However, many are not visible, depending on the radiographic projections, and the lack of radiographic abnormalities does not rule out an abscess. Chronic sole bruising may be associated with demineralization, increased vascular channels, and irregularity of the solar margin of the distal phalanx.[4] Chronic abscessation may be due to an underlying condition such as laminitis and may contribute to osteitis of the distal phalanx and sequestrum formation.

Treatment

Many bruises often resolve without treatment if the source of the trauma is removed. The horse should be rested from heavy work, especially if the soles are abnormally thin. When possible, the environment should be changed so that the horse is not worked on rough ground. If the horse must be used, the sole can be protected with a full pad applied under the shoe. The pad should be placed to avoid pressure to the bruised site. Wide web shoes may also be beneficial to relieve pressure on the sole. Light paring of the sole overlying the bruise often relieves the pressure and makes the horse more comfortable.[4]

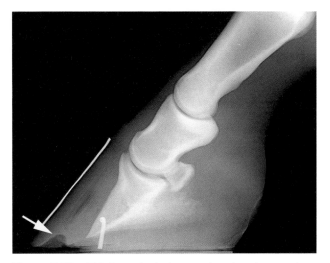

Figure 5.56. This horse had what was thought to be a routine abscess at the toe (arrow) but a lateral radiograph revealed chronic laminitis.

References

1. DeBowes RM, Yovich JV. Penetrating wounds, abscesses, gravel and bruising. Vet Clin North Am Equine Pract 1989;5: 179–194.
2. Moyer W. Therapeutic principles of diseases of the foot. Proceedings Am Assoc Equine Pract 1981;27:453.
3. Moyer W. Corrective shoeing. Vet Clin North Am Large Anim Pract 1980;2:3–24.
4. Parks A. Foot bruises: Diagnosis and treatment. In Current Techniques in Equine Surgery and Lameness. White NA, Moore JN, eds. 2nd ed. WB Saunders. Philadelphia, 1998;528–529.
5. Stashak TS. The Foot. In Adams' Lameness in Horses. Stashak TS, ed. 5th ed. Lippincott Williams and Wilkins. Philadelphia. 2002; 645–733.

GRAVEL (ASCENDING INFECTION OF THE WHITE LINE)

Gravel is the layman's term for what supposedly is the migration of a piece of gravel from the white line proximally to the coronary band, where it is discharged as an abscess.[5] What actually occurs is an opening in the white line at the sole/wall junction that permits infection to invade the laminae, resulting in the development of a submural abscess. The abscess follows the path of least resistance, and eventually breaks and drains at the coronary band.

Etiology

A wound or crack in the white line, a separation in the white line ("seedy toe"), or a subsolar abscess adjacent to the white line may predispose the horse to development of gravel.[7] Horses with white line disease and/or chronic laminitis are usually at greater risk. Trauma and penetrating injuries to the sole/hoof wall junction may also contribute to the disease.

Clinical Signs and Diagnosis

Lameness similar to that observed with subsolar abscesses or a penetrating wound to the foot may be observed in horses with ascending infections of the white line.[1] Moderate to severe lameness usually appears 1 or 2 days before drainage at the coronary band occurs.[1,7] However, the condition may go undiagnosed until drainage at the coronary band is observed. Signs of lameness may also vary depending on the severity and location of the infection. Hoof tester examination is often helpful to determine the approximate location of the ascending infection before it breaks out at the coronary band. Careful examination of the white line and sole in the painful region should be performed. The hoof and sole should be trimmed lightly, and exploration of any black areas (black spots) with a flexible metal probe may reveal the site where the laminae was penetrated.[7] If the probe enters the laminae and exudate is observed this is likely the site of the original defect. Removal of sole and wall at suspicious sites can be performed to help identify the tract but should be kept to a minimum. Diagnostic anesthesia may be helpful in some cases to confirm the location of the lameness to the foot.

A definitive diagnosis often is not made until the abscess breaks out at the coronary band. Purulent drainage at the coronary band confirms the diagnosis, but if the drainage occurs on the lateral or medial aspects of the coronary band it should be distinguished from necrosis of the collateral cartilages of the distal phalanx.[2,3] The tract associated with an ascending infection of the white line is superficial and usually breaks out just proximal to the coronary band. In contrast, draining tracts associated with necrosis of the collateral cartilages erupt from deep within the cartilage, are often multiple, and are usually located 1 to 2 cm proximal to the coronary band. Fistulograms can be helpful to determine whether the tract is deep or superficial.[2,3]

Treatment

If an ascending infection of the white line is suspected but cannot be confirmed (no drainage at the coronary band), soaking or poulticing the foot may draw the infection to the surface. When the abscess comes to a "head" just proximal to the coronary band, drainage can be established by lancing the abscess.[2–4] If a draining tract is present at the time of presentation, flushing the tract with antiseptics to promote drainage and local wound care is usually all that is needed.

If the entry site at the bottom of the foot can be identified, it should be opened and enlarged to permit ventral drainage.[7] Loop hoof knives or hoof curettes are very useful to remove small amounts of sole around a defect. Soaking the foot and irrigating the draining tract usually resolves the infection. Bandaging the foot or using a protective boot to prevent contamination of the tract openings can be beneficial. If the drainage persists for more than 7 to 10 days, further diagnostics should be considered to rule out the possibility of a foreign body, keratoma, or infection of deeper structures.[7]

Chronic cases with a long history of drainage at the coronary band may cause considerable undermining of the hoof wall (Figure 5.57). It may be beneficial in theses cases to create a circular hole in the hoof wall midway between the solar surface and the coronary band. This permits better access to more thoroughly debride the tract of necrotic and infected tissue and provides better drainage.[1] A trephine hole placed at the lowest point of the infected tract in the hoof wall can also be used to provide drainage.[6] Bandaging to protect the foot from contamination should follow until all signs of infection have disappeared. Systemic and local antibiotics may be required if the infection involves the regional soft tissues of the pastern or under the hoof wall.

Prognosis

The prognosis is generally favorable if the condition is diagnosed early and adequate drainage and wound care are provided. The prognosis is guarded if the condition becomes chronic and extensive hoof wall undermining has occurred. However, the majority of these horses also return to complete soundness if treated appropriately. The prognosis is even more guarded if the contamination of the sensitive lamina is secondary to separation of the white line from chronic laminitis.[4,7]

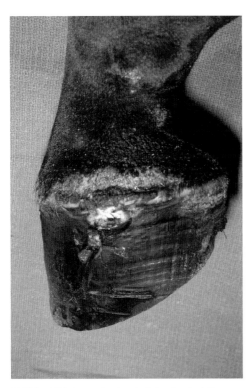

Figure 5.57. This horse had a draining tract at the coronary band but no abnormalities could be found on the solar surface of the foot. Exploration of the tract revealed a small piece of wood.

References

1. DeBowes RM, Yovich JV. Penetrating wounds, abscesses, gravel and bruising. Vet Clin North Am Eq Pract 1989;5:179–194.
2. Honnas CM, Ragle CA, Meagher DM. Necrosis of the collateral cartilage of the distal phalanx in horses: 16 cases (1970–1985). J Am Vet Med Assoc 1988;193:1303–1307.
3. Honnas CM, Dabareiner RM, McCauley BH. Hoof wall surgery in the horse: approaches to and underlying disorders. Vet Clin North Am Equine Pract 2003;19:479–499.
4. Honnas CM, Peloso JG, Carter KG, et al. Managing two infectious diseases of the horse's foot. Vet Med 1994;89:891–896.
5. Johnson J H: The Foot. In Equine Medicine and Surgery, 3rd ed. Mansmann RA, McAllister ES, eds. American Veterinary Publishing. Santa Barbara, 1982;1038.
6. Meagher DM. Ascending infection under the hoof wall (Gravel). In Large Animal Internal Medicine. Smith BP, ed. CV Mosby. Philadelphia, 1990;1178.
7. Stashak TS. The Foot. In Adams' Lameness in Horses. Stashak TS, ed. 5th ed. Lippincott Williams and Wilkins. Philadelphia. 2002; 645–733.

CANKER

Equine canker is described as an infectious process that results in the development of chronic hypertrophy of the horn-producing tissues.[1] It has also been described as a chronic hypertrophic, moist pododermatitis of the epidermal tissues of the foot.[3,6] Canker typically originates in the frog but can invade the adjacent sole, bars, and hoof wall.[1,2] Historically, the disease was primarily observed in the hindfeet of draft breeds and was thought to be due to unhygienic environmental conditions.[5,7] However, more recent reports suggest that the front feet are often involved, any breed or sex of horse can be affected, and horses that are well cared for with routine hoof care can still get canker.[2]

The infection is thought to cause abnormal keratin production or dyskeratosis, which is seen as filamentous fronds of hypertrophic horn.[2,3] The disease is most commonly seen in semitropical areas of the southern states and in the humid environment of the Midwest, and may have a seasonal occurrence.[2] Canker may be misdiagnosed as thrush, particularly in the early course of the disease, and unfortunately the disease seems to flourish in the face of treatment aimed at resolving thrush.[6] The distinguishing feature of thrush being primarily loss of frog tissue can usually be readily differentiated from the proliferative nature of canker.[6]

Etiology

The exact cause of canker is unknown but historically affected horses have a history of being housed on moist pastures year round or in wet, unhygienic conditions.[3,5] Horses standing in urine, feces, or mud-soaked bedding appear to be at risk.[3] However, the most recent study on canker contradicts this risk factor because the majority of horses in that study were well cared for with routine hoof care.[2] Despite this finding, the authors concluded that keeping the foot dry was a crucial aspect of treatment, suggesting that excessive moisture plays some role in the disease.[2] The causative anaerobic Gram-negative organisms are thought to be *Fusobacterium Necrophorum* and one or more *Bacteroides spp*.[2,6,8]

Clinical Signs

Lameness usually is not present in early stages of the disease because the superficial epidermis is primarily involved. Early stages of canker may present as a focal area of granulation tissue in the frog that bleeds easily when abraded (Figure 5.58).[2] However, the disease is

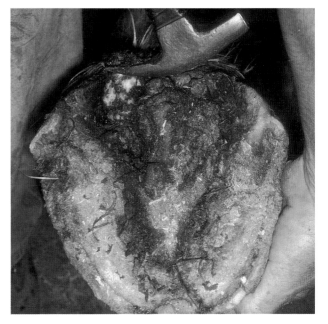

Figure 5.58. Small, pale, demarcated growth along the caudal aspect of the frog that can be consistent with early canker.

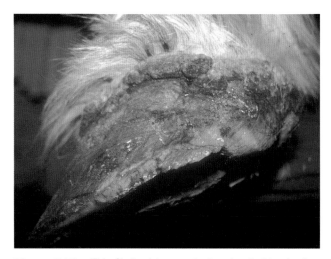

Figure 5.59. This Clydesdale mare had canker that involved the entire frog, heels, and coronary band.

often not be detected until it becomes diffuse and involves the other structures of the hoof (Figure 5.59). Lameness is often present in advanced cases. Examination of the foot usually reveals a fetid odor and the frog, which may appear intact, has a ragged proliferative filamentous appearance. The proliferative frog may have numerous small finger-like papillae of soft, off-white material that have a cauliflower-like appearance.[1,2] The epidermal tissue of the frog is usually friable and may have a white cottage-cheese-like appearance. The affected tissue bleeds easily when abraded and may be extremely painful when touched.[2]

Diagnosis

A presumptive diagnosis can often be made based on the physical findings of a moist exudative pododermatitis with characteristic hypertrophic filamentous fronds involving the frog and surrounding tissue. It can be confirmed with a biopsy but is seldom performed by most clinicians. The histologic findings of proliferative papillary hyperplasia of the epidermis with dyskeratosis, keratolysis, and ballooning degeneration of the outer layers of the epidermis confirm the diagnosis.[2] Although the disease is thought to be infectious, cultures are rarely performed because a mixed population of bacteria are often observed on the epidermis of the frog.

Treatment

Multiple treatment protocols for canker have been described in the literature. No treatment appears to be consistently effective in treating the disease. However, there are several principles for treating canker that should improve resolution of the disease: (1) early recognition of the problem, (2) thorough debridement of the lesion, (3) methodical topical treatment, and (4) keeping the wound clean and dry until the defect begins to cornify.[2] Systemic antimicrobials to treat canker are currently not recommended.

It is important to not confuse canker with thrush so that appropriate treatment is not delayed. There is a

proliferation of tissue with canker and a loss of tissue with thrush. Complete debridement is considered essential by some, whereas only superficial debridement is recommended by others.[2,7] The method of debridement is probably not important; it can be performed with a hoof knife, scalpel blade, electrocautery, or the CO_2 laser. A tourniquet is essential and cryotherapy can be performed after physical debridement if considered necessary.[2] Debridement can be performed in the standing, sedated horse but is often best performed under general anesthesia if the lesion is large. If complete debridement cannot be performed, less aggressive removal is often beneficial and was reported to be superior to complete debridement in one older study of canker.[6]

Topical treatments to treat canker include chloramphenicol; metronidazole powder; 2% metronidazole ointment; a mixture of ketoconazole, rifampin and DMSO; and a mixture of 10% benzoyl peroxide in acetone and metronidazole powder.[2,4,6–8] The latter topical treatment was reported to successfully treat 54 cases of canker with minimal recurrence.[2] These medications are usually applied directly to the debrided area or to gauze sponges that are placed on the wound. Direct contact of the topical medication with the defect is important for success.[2] Keeping the wound clean and dry with bandages or a treatment plate (Figure 5.60) and maintaining the horse in a dry environment are critical to the aftercare.[2] The duration of treatment may be several weeks to months, depending on the stage of the disease. Owner commitment to prolonged treatment is an important part of the aftercare.

Prognosis

The prognosis is favorable for complete resolution of the problem if treatment is instituted early in the course of the disease. However, advanced cases of canker that invade the sole, bars, and hoof wall, and those that involve multiple limbs remain very difficult to treat. Thorough debridement followed by topical medication of either metronidazole powder alone or 10% benzoyl peroxide in acetone plus metronidazole powder is currently the recommended treatment.[2,7,8] Topical treatment with 10% benzoyl peroxide in acetone plus metronidazole powder was very successful in the most recent retrospective study of canker.[2] Keeping the

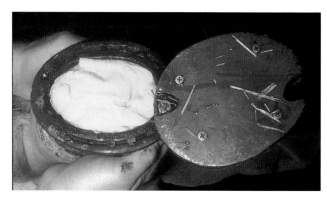

Figure 5.60. Treatment plate that can be very beneficial in treating canker. Keeping the foot clean and dry is a very important aspect of treatment.

wound and foot dry appears to greatly improve the success of any form of treatment.

References

1. Moyer WA, Colohan PT. Canker. In Equine Medicine and Surgery, 5th ed. Mosby. St. Louis, MO, 1999;1544–1546.
2. O'Grady SE, Madison JB. How to treat equine canker. Proceedings Am Assoc Equine Pract 2004;50:202–205.
3. Reeves MJ, Yovich JV, Turner AS. Miscellaneous conditions of the equine foot. Vet Clin North Am 1989;5:221–242.
4. Sherman K, Ginn PE, Brown M. Recurring canker in a shire mare. J Eq Vet Sci 1996;16:322–323.
5. Steckel RR. Puncture wounds, abscesses, thrush, and canker. In Current Therapy in Equine Medicine, 2nd ed. Saunders. Philadelphia, 1987;271.
6. Wilson DG, Calderwood Mays MB, Colahan PT. Treatment of canker in horses. J Am Vet Med Assoc 1989;194:1721–1723.
7. Wilson DG. Topical metronidazole in the treatment of equine canker. Proceedings Am Assoc Equine Pract 1994;40:49–50.
8. Wilson DG. Equine canker. In Current Therapy in Equine Medicine, 4th ed. Robinson NE, ed. Saunders. Philadelphia, 1997;127–128.

THRUSH

Thrush is a degenerative condition of the frog involving the central and lateral sulci, which is characterized by the presence of black necrotic exudate and a foul odor. The hindlimbs are most frequently involved.[3,4] The infection may extend to the dermal laminae and cause lameness if it becomes chronic. In severe cases the infection may undermine the sole and result in swelling of the distal limb (cellulitis) and lameness.[3,4]

Etiology

Contributing factors for thrush are wet, unhygienic stable conditions, especially when horses stand in urine and manure soiled bedding, neglect of daily foot care, and lack of exercise.[3,4] Inadequate or improper trimming and shoeing, which promote long contracted heels and deep sulci, also contributes to the risk of infection. Although no specific organism has been identified as the cause, *Fusobacterium necrophorum* is commonly isolated.

Clinical Signs and Diagnosis

There is usually an increased amount of moisture on the bottom of the foot and a black discharge in the sulci of the frog. This discharge, which varies in quantity, usually has a very offensive odor.[2,4] The affected sulci of the frog are often deeper than normal and may extend into the sensitive tissues of the foot, causing them to be painful. The frog may also be undermined, and large areas can be detached from the underlying tissue.[4] Lameness is present in severe cases that involve the corium and swelling of the distal limb may be seen. The diagnosis is usually based the presence of black, odiferous discharge in the sulci of the frog together with the loss of the frog.[4] The condition should be differentiated from canker.

Treatment

Early cases usually respond to debridement of the diseased tissue and the topical application of an astringent with or without foot bandages.[2,4] Astringents that can be used include copper sulfate, 2% iodine alone or mixed with phenol, methiolate, and 10% formalin.[4] These treatments should be repeated until the infection is controlled. The horse should be kept in a dry, clean stall or in a dry yard. Repeated trimming of the frog may be required before the infection is controlled.

Severe cases of thrush are treated in a similar manner as above except debridement of the diseased undermined tissue is more extensive. Some horses may benefit from daily soaking in supersaturated solutions of magnesium sulphate, after which an astringent is applied and the foot protected in a sterile bandage.[1,4] Prevention is superior to treatment and is most important for horses confined to stalls for prolonged periods. Adequate clean, dry bedding and routine foot care prevent most cases of thrush. Proper hoof trimming and shoeing are also important in prevention because horses with overgrown hooves are more susceptible to the disease.

Prognosis

The prognosis is good if the disease is diagnosed early before the foot has suffered extensive damage. It is guarded if the infection is extensive and involves the corium.[4]

References

1. Johnson JH. The foot. In Mansmann RA, McAllister ES, eds. Equine Medicine and Surgery, 3rd ed. American Veterinary Publications. Santa Barbara, 1982;1033.
2. Parks A. Chronic foot injury and deformity. In White NA, Moore, JN. Current techniques in equine surgery and lameness. WB Saunders Co. Philadelphia, 1998;534–536.
3. Reeves MJ, Yovich JV, Turner AS. Miscellaneous conditions of the equine foot. Vet Clinics of North Am Equine Pract 1989; 5:235–236.
4. Stashak TS. The Foot. In Adams' Lameness in Horses. Stashak TS, ed. 5th ed. Lippincott Williams and Wilkins. Philadelphia. 2002;645–733.

WHITE LINE DISEASE

White line disease has been described as a keratolytic process on the solar surface of the hoof that is characterized by progressive separation of the inner zone of the hoof wall.[2,3] The separation occurs in the nonpigmented horn between the stratum medium and stratum internum. It differs from laminitis in that it does not involve the sensitive tissue beneath the hoof wall. It usually begins at the solar surface of the hoof and most frequently affects the toe region but can originate in the quarter or heel.[3] The disease progresses to varying heights and configurations proximally toward the coronary band but never involves the coronary band. It has numerous other names such as seedy-toe, yeast infection, hoof-wall disease, environmentally induced separations, onychomycosis, and Candida.[1-5]

Etiology

Numerous causes have been proposed for white line disease. These include mechanical stress on the hoof wall associated with long toes and poor hoof conformation, environmental conditions such as excessive moisture or dryness that affect the inner hoof-wall attachment, toxicity associated with selenium, and infection of the white line with bacteria and/or fungi.[1–5] For instance, excessive dryness of the hoof is thought to predispose to hoof cracking, which permits bacteria and fungi to invade the white line area. Pathogens usually isolated include a mixed flora of bacteria and *Pseudoallsheria*, *Scopulariopsis,* and *Aspergillus* fungi. However, it is currently debatable whether bacteria and fungi found with white line disease are the primary cause or simply accumulate within the hoof separation. A variety of bacteria and fungi have been identified and are currently considered secondary opportunists.[3] One reason for this is that many cases of white line disease respond to local debridement alone without antimicrobial or antifungal therapies.[3]

Clinical Signs

Horses with white line disease often have variable to no lameness, and the condition is often only found during routine trimming.[1–3] In the early stages the only noticeable change may be a small powdery area located just dorsal to the hoof wall/sole junction. Other early signs may include sole pain with hoof testers, occasional heat, and increasingly flat soles. With time the hoof separation enlarges and the hoof wall growth may slow and be of poor consistency. Exploration of the inner hoof wall often reveals a separation that is filled with white/gray powdery horn material and debris (Figure 5.61).[3] With time the hoof defect may progress up the dorsal hoof wall. Percussion of the dorsal hoof wall may reveal a hollow sound, suggesting that the hoof wall is undermined. Severe undermining of the hoof wall at the toe region can resemble chronic laminitis but the hoof separation is within the hoof wall and does not involve the sensitive laminae. White line disease can also be a secondary problem following extensive subsolar or submural abscesses that can occur with chronic laminitis.[3]

Diagnosis

The diagnosis is usually made on the basis of clinical findings. Hoof tester pain and lameness are not always present. The sole/wall junction is usually wider than normal and has a chalky texture. Further examination dorsal to the white line will reveal a concavity that contains white/gray powdery horn material and occasionally black serous drainage.[3] Radiographs are always recommended to rule out the possibility of other bony abnormalities such as chronic laminitis or pedal osteitis. A gas line along the dorsal hoof wall may be seen with both white line disease and chronic laminitis. The gas line is located between the layers of the hoof wall and originates at the sole with white line disease; it is located between the inner hoof wall and laminar papillae with laminitis.[3] Radiographs are also beneficial to discern various hoof-capsule distortions that may contribute to the disease. Other diagnostics that can be performed but are typically unrewarding include bacterial or fungal cultures and biopsies of the hoof wall.[3]

Treatment

Therapy for white line disease is directed toward protecting and unloading the damaged section of foot with therapeutic shoeing combined with removing the hoof capsule over the affected area.[1–5] The hoof wall can be removed with hoof knives and nippers and/or a motorized burr.[1–3] The type of therapeutic shoe and its method of attachment are dictated by the extent of damaged hoof wall (Figure 5.62). Topical disinfectants/ astringents are often applied after hoof wall resection. Systemic medical treatment is considered unnecessary in most cases and is of no value without resection of the damaged hoof wall.[3] Correction of predisposing hoof capsule distortions such as long toes and low heels is essential.

In mild to moderate cases, local debridement and regular shoeing to protect the sole are often all that is

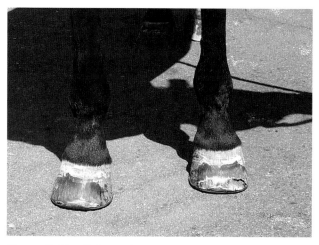

Figure 5.61. Flaky, chalky material beneath the dorsal hoof wall is often characteristic of white line disease.

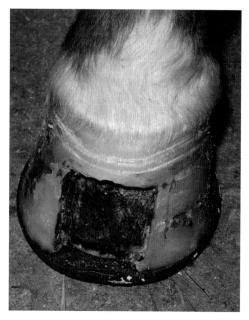

Figure 5.62. Resection of the hoof wall over the diseased portion of the hoof is often performed in horses with white line disease.

required. Moving the break-over back reduces the lever arm placed on the toe and prevents pinching of the laminae at the junction of the normal and resected hoof wall. A full support bar shoe is recommended to protect and unload the damaged section of foot if extensive removal of the hoof wall is required. Acrylic repair should only be considered after all tracts have been removed and the defect is solid to avoid trapping infection beneath the composite.[3] Repeat debridement of the lesions may be required and the shoeing interval should be 4 weeks or less. The feet should be kept as dry as possible and the hoof wall defects should be covered with a light bandage to keep them clean. The duration of treatment depends on the amount of wall removed, but most horses can return to work when the surface of the defect has cornified. Recurrence of white line disease is possible and good foot care helps prevent the disease.[1-3] See Chapter 12 for further information on farriery treatment of white line disease.

Prognosis

Most horses with white line disease have a very good prognosis with local debridement and corrective shoeing. However, many owners are reluctant to have portions of their horse's hooves removed. This has led to a wide variety of medical treatments aimed at treating white line disease. To date, there is no known medical treatment for white line disease and the condition is unlikely to improve unless the affected, undermined hoof wall is removed.[1-3]

References

1. Moyer W. Hoof wall defects: chronic hoof wall separations and hoof wall cracks. Vet Clin North Am Equine Pract 2003;19: 463–477.
2. O'Grady SE. White line disease—an update. Equine Vet Educ 2001;2001:66–72.
3. O'Grady SE. How to manage white line disease. Proceedings Am Assoc Equine Pract 2006;52:520–525.
4. Turner TA. White line disease. Equine Vet Educ 1998;4:73–76.
5. Stashak TS, Hill C, Klimesh R, et al. Cracks. In Adams' Lameness in Horses. Stashak TS, ed. 5th ed. Lippincott Williams and Wilkins. Philadelphia. 2002;1113–1115.

PENETRATING INJURIES OF THE FOOT

Penetrating injuries of the foot are commonly seen in equine practice. The injury is often sustained by the horse stepping on (bottom of the foot) or contacting (coronary band, heel bulbs and pastern region) a sharp object. Although any deep penetrating injury to the foot can potentially be serious, those that penetrate the central third of the frog, the coronary band, and the heel bulbs are at greatest risk to involve deeper vital structures. Structures at risk with injuries to the central third of the frog include the navicular bursa, navicular bone, DDFT, or distal phalanx. Coronary band injuries may involve the DIP joint, distal phalanx, and collateral cartilages of the distal phalanx. Injuries to the heel bulb region are most likely to damage the digital flexor tendon sheath, DDFT, or palmar/plantar aspect of the DIP joint. Injuries elsewhere on the bottom of the foot most likely only damage the digital cushion or the solar surface of the distal phalanx and are usually less prob-

lematic. Early identification of the involvement of a deeper vital structure and aggressive medical and surgical treatment greatly affect the outcome of horses with these injuries.[1-4,9] See Chapter 10 for further information about treating septic synovial structures.

Clinical Signs

The clinical signs caused by penetrating injuries may vary depending on the depth (superficial vs. deep), location (sole vs. coronary band), and duration (acute vs. chronic) of the injury.[9] In general, the more superficial the injury, the less severe the clinical signs. Horses with minor injures to the sole that may remain asymptomatic for several days until a subsolar abscess develops are the exception. These types of injuries penetrate the cornified layer of the sole into the digital cushion but do not cause clinical signs unless an abscess develops. Deep injuries that penetrate completely through the hoof wall and contact a bone, tendon, or synovial cavity typically cause severe and acute lameness. Also, horses with wounds in the frog region that involve vital structures usually become rapidly symptomatic.

Affected horses often point the foot and resist contacting the heel (walk on the toe) when walked.[8,9] Palpation of the hoof in any horse with a penetrating injury may reveal increased heat, and a prominent digital pulse can usually be palpated.[8,9] Careful examination of the sole (visual, hoof tester, and probing) and coronary band is important. It has been stated that any penetrating wound of the foot deeper than 1 cm should be considered serious. The approximate reported depths of a perpendicular penetration before vital structures become involved were 1 cm for the sole, 1.5 cm for the frog, and 1.2 cm for the hoof wall.[9]

If a foreign body such as a nail is present in the bottom of the foot, it is ideal to take a radiograph to determine the exact depth and direction of the nail's path before removing it (Figure 5.63).[1,2,9] However, this

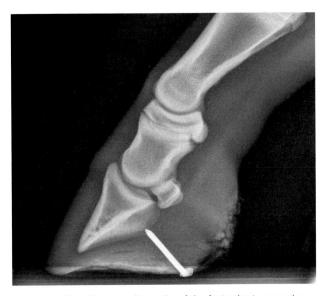

Figure 5.63. Taking radiographs of the foot prior to removing the foreign body can help identify the direction and depth of the puncture.

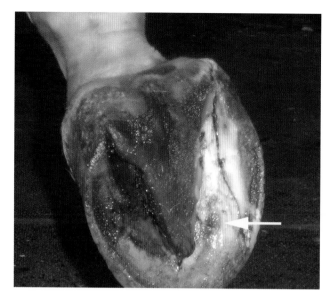

Figure 5.64. Chronic penetrating injuries to the foot may be identified by small areas of granulation tissue on the sole.

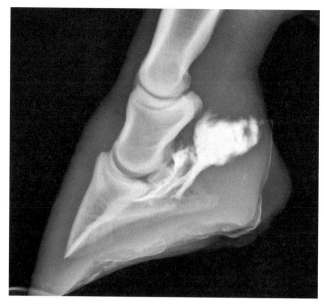

Figure 5.65. Contrast radiography can be helpful to document synovial involvement in horses with chronic penetrating injuries of the frog and sole. The puncture in this horse had completely healed but the horse developed an abscess just above the heel bulb. Contrast injected into the abscess communicated with the navicular bursa.

is not always possible and care should be taken to avoid deeper penetration of the nail during the process. If a wound is not obvious, careful application of hoof testers may help identify focal pain which may indicate the site of penetration. Once a focal site of pain is found in the sole or frog, it is explored with a hoof knife. If the injury is acute (before infection) and involves the sole, a crack or small hole may be the only abnormality found (Figure 5.64).[9] In most cases, puncture wounds of the sole appear black at the entry site.

Wounds that penetrate the frog can be particularly difficult to locate because the softer and more elastic tissues of the frog tend to collapse and fill in the tract. Careful removal of the frog is often required to visualize the entry site. Probing of the tract can help identify both the depth and direction of the injury. A radiograph can be taken with the probe placed into the tract to further verify its location. If infection is present gentle pressure with the thumbs or hoof testers around the entry hole may cause purulent exudate to exit the tract.[9] Perineural anesthesia is usually not needed to localize the site of lameness but is very beneficial to facilitate close examination of the injury site and removal of the frog or sole if needed.

Palpation of the coronary band for heat, pain, and swelling may also be helpful to identify the location of a penetrating wound to this region. A penetrating wound of the coronary band can be overlooked if the hair is long or if local swelling and wound drainage are not present. Once identified, wounds at the coronary band should be carefully probed and explored because they are often caused by a wood splinter (Figure 5.57).[9]

Heat, pain, and swelling of 1 heel bulb are often seen with migration of a subsolar abscess.[9] Effusion of the digital tendon sheath or DIP joint may suggest infectious synovitis.[1,2,5,6] Synovial fluid analysis can usually be used to confirm the diagnosis. An increased white blood cell count (more than 30,000) with neutrophilia, a pH below 6.9, and an increased protein (more than 4.0 g/dl) are highly suggestive of a septic process.[1,2,9]

Diagnosis

Additional diagnostics that can be performed to confirm the location and depth of a penetrating injury include distention of a synovial cavity with saline to detect leakage from the wound, plain radiographs, radiographs with a metallic probe inserted in the wound, contrast radiography (fistulogram), or ultrasound.[1,2] Plain radiographs may reveal the presence of gas which can be seen with a subsolar abscess or penetration of a synovial cavity. Concurrent fractures and osteolysis due to infection may also be visible. Placement of a metallic probe confirms depth and direction of the injury, and contrast radiography often confirms penetration of a synovial cavity (Figure 5.65). Ultrasound may be helpful to document injuries to the DDFT and involvement of the digital flexor tendon sheath.

Treatment

Treatment of superficial penetrating wounds that do not involve vital structures (bone, tendon, or synovial cavities) is generally uncomplicated. Treatment is aimed at providing adequate drainage, removing infected and necrotic tissue, and protecting the site from further contamination.[7,9] The majority of cases can be treated in the standing, sedated horse using the help of perineural anesthesia. Drainage is established by removing a small amount of adjacent sole or frog with a sharp hoof knife (loop hoof knives work well) and/or a hoof groover. Underlying necrotic/infected tissue should be removed with a standard curette, hoof curette, or nail hole curette.[9] An antiseptic dressing is applied and the foot is protected to minimize further contamination. More extensive superficial infections may require periodic

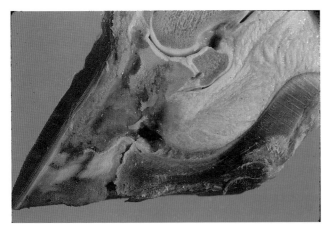

Figure 5.66. Sagittal section of P3 in a horse that sustained a puncture wound to the solar surface of P3. Subsequent infection of P3 contributed to a pathologic fracture of the bone and involvement of the DIP joint.

flushing or soaking of the foot together with bandaging and foot protection.

Penetrating injuries that involve bone, tendon, or synovial cavities require more aggressive treatment depending on the deeper structure that is involved. Typical treatments include both systemic (IV) and local (IV regional perfusion and intrasynovial) antimicrobials, NSAIDs, local debridement of the wound, and lavage, endoscopy or arthroscopy if a synovial cavity is involved. Wound debridement may be performed in the standing patient but it usually best performed with the horse under general anesthesia. Lavage, endoscopy, or arthroscopy of a synovial cavity usually requires general anesthesia. Wounds that penetrate the distal phalanx should be enlarged and the distal phalanx curetted if possible (Figure 5.66). Soaking the foot to lavage deep wounds of the foot is generally not recommended.[7] Involvement of the navicular bursa is best treated with endoscopy or lavage and local debridement of the defect in the frog.[1,2,11,12] A street nail procedure is not recommended as the initial treatment because of the morbidity associated with this procedure. See the section on prevention/treatment of orthopedic infections in Chapter 10 for further information.

Prognosis

Horses with penetrating injuries that do not involve bone, tendon, or a synovial cavity typically do very well. Horses with deep penetrating injuries outside the frog or frog sulci also do well. In a retrospective study of 50 cases with deep puncture wounds of the foot, 95% (21 of 22 cases) of horses with injuries outside the frog or frog sulci regained full athletic soundness.[10] In the same study, only 50% (14 of 28 cases) of horses that sustained deep puncture wounds in the frog region fully recovered from the injury. Horses with septic osteitis of the distal phalanx also have a good prognosis following debridement.[3] Horses with injuries that involve the navicular bursa and DIP joint represent the most difficult challenge to return to performance.[5,6,11,12] Nonetheless, 10 of 16 horses with septic navicular bursitis returned to their pre-injury performance level fol-

lowing endoscopic lavage and debridement.[11] In general, prompt treatment of any penetrating injury to the foot regardless of the structure(s) involved improves the chance of a successful outcome.

References

1. Baxter GM. Treatment of wounds involving synovial structures. Clin Tech Equine Pract 2005;3:204–214.
2. Baxter GM. Management and treatment of wounds involving synovial structures in horses. In Equine Wound Management, 2nd ed. Stashak TS, Theoret CL, eds. Blackwell Publishing, 2008;463–488.
3. Cauvin ER, Munroe GA. Septic osteitis of the distal phalanx: findings and surgical treatment in 18 cases. Equine Vet J 1998;30:512–519.
4. DeBowes RM, Yovich JV. Penetrating wounds, abscesses, gravel, and bruising of the equine foot. Vet Clin North Am Equine Pract 1989;5:179–194.
5. Honnas CM, Welch RD, Ford TS, et al. Septic arthritis of the distal interphalangeal joint in 12 horses. Vet Surgery 1992;21:261.
6. Honnas CM, Trotter GW. The distal interphalangeal joint. In Current techniques in equine surgery and lameness. White NA, Moore JN, eds. 2nd ed. WB Saunders Co. Philadelphia, 1998;389–397.
7. Parks AH. Equine foot wounds: General principles of healing and treatment. Proc Am Assoc Equine Pract 1999;45:180–187.
8. Richardson GL. Surgical management of penetrating wounds to the equine foot. Proc Am Assoc Equine Pract 1999,45:198–189.
9. Stashak TS. The Foot. In Adams' Lameness in Horses. Stashak TS, ed. 5th ed. Lippincott Williams and Wilkins. Philadelphia, 2002;645–733.
10. Steckel RR, Fessler JF, Huston LC. Deep puncture wounds of the equine hoof: A review of 50 cases. Proc Am Assoc Equine Pract 1989,35:167.
11. Wright IM, Phillips TJ, Walmsley JP. Endoscopy of the navicular bursa: A new technique for the treatment of contaminated and septic bursae. Equine Vet J 1999;31:5–11.
12. Wright IM, Smith MR, Humphrey DJ, et al. Endoscopic surgery in the treatment of contaminated and infected synovial cavities. Equine Vet J 2003;35:613–619.

SHEARED HEELS AND/OR QUARTERS

Sheared heels and quarters are descriptive terms for the structural breakdown that occurs between the heel bulbs and hoof capsule with a disproportionate use of one heel and/or quarter.[2,3] Either the lateral or medial heel or quarter may be out of balance and result in the overuse of 1 heel or quarter (Figure 5.67). It is a type of medial-lateral (ML) hoof imbalance. The degree of damage and lameness is usually proportional to the duration and degree of foot imbalance.[1–3] The shearing of the heel and or quarter can result in heel pain (similar to navicular syndrome), hoof cracks in the heel or quarter, and deep thrush in the central sulcus of the frog. Chronic sheared heels may also predispose to navicular syndrome and other painful conditions of the foot.[2,6]

Etiology

Improper trimming and shoeing resulting in one heel and quarter longer than the other is a common cause of this condition.[1,2] Because the heels and quarters are a different length and height, the foot is referred to as being out of ML balance. A disproportionate amount of force is being applied to the longer side of the heels during weight-bearing. This creates abnormal shearing forces between the heel bulbs and quarters during

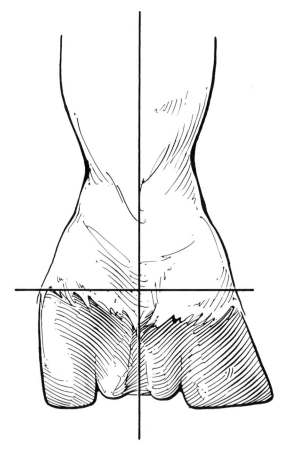

Figure 5.67. Sheared heels. Notice the left heel bulb is higher than the right. The hoof is straighter on the affected side (left side) while the hoof wall associated with the lower heel (right side) is flared.

loading, which results in structural breakdown. Horses with long toes and short heels are thought to be more susceptible to the development of sheared heels.[6]

Corrective trimming that is used to alter conformational defects in young horses may also predispose to sheared heels.[2] For instance, if the lateral heel and quarter is lowered and the medial heel and quarter is raised with a shim placed between the shoe and the hoof wall, a disproportionate force will be applied to the medial quarter of the heel during weight-bearing.[2] This can result in shearing of the heels and quarters. Heel calks ("stickers") may also exaggerate the slightest imbalance in the heels, resulting in a shearing effect.[2]

A diagonal hoof imbalance may also cause an overload of 1 heel. In this condition the hoof lands on 1 front corner (toe) of the foot and weight-bearing then loads the diagonal back corner (heel).[4] Horses with diagonal imbalance usually land on the lateral toe or quarter region and then overload the medial heel or quarter.[4] The excessive weight-bearing of 1 heel or quarter can result in proximal displacement of the region.[4]

Clinical Signs

In most cases of sheared heels, the heel bulb and/or quarter on the affected side is visually higher, the hoof

wall is straighter, and there is an abnormal flare to the hoof wall on the opposite unaffected side (Figure 5.67).[6] The differential height in the heels and/or quarter is best viewed from behind the foot with the horse standing on a hard, flat surface or with the limb hand-held. The accentuated hoof wall flare opposite the affected side is observed by viewing the horse from the front or from above at the shoulder level.[6] The hoof wall on the affected side may be rolled under in very severe chronic cases. This same hoof conformation may be seen with a diagonal imbalance of the hoof.[4]

In horses viewed from the rear as they are walked on a hard surface, the heel of the affected side usually contacts the ground first and a proximal displacement of that heel bulb occurs. Most frequently horses will break over in the short toe region opposite the flare of the unaffected side.[6] The lameness can be variable and depends on the degree of damage from the shearing effect. Horses with a diagonal imbalance usually land on the lateral toe and quarter and then load the medial heel and quarter.[4]

An important finding on palpation and manipulation of the foot is the loss of structural integrity between the heel bulbs.[3] The heel bulbs can be separated more easily and can be displaced in opposite directions (Figure 5.68). Manipulation may also be painful. Pain across the heels and frog is often found with hoof testers similar to navicular syndrome, and a PD nerve block usually eliminates the lameness.

Diagnosis

The diagnosis of sheared heels must be differentiated from navicular syndrome, hoof imbalances, and the

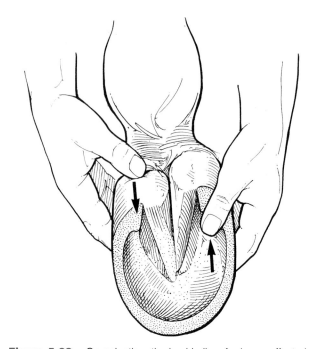

Figure 5.68. On palpation, the heel bulbs of a horse affected with sheared heels may be separated more easily and displaced in opposite directions. The increased movement is caused by a loss of structural integrity between the heel bulbs, and manipulation is often painful.

numerous other conditions of the foot that may cause similar clinical signs.[6] In addition, sheared heels and other hoof imbalances may occur concurrently in many horses with navicular disease. The diagnosis of sheared heels is often made based on the physical examination findings and negative radiographic abnormalities in the foot. However, this does not eliminate another concurrent problem in the foot. Standing horizontal dorsopalmar/plantar radiographs of the feet can be useful to document the severity of the heel distortion and the secondary hoof deformities.

Treatment

Treatment is directed toward bringing the foot, heels, and quarters back into balance and alleviating the pain. The selection of treatment depends on the severity of the sheared heels and the degree of hoof wall distortion.[1–3] Mild cases usually respond to trimming of the longer heel/quarter and allowing free exercise. The foot should be trimmed to correct both medial-lateral and dorsopalmar/plantar imbalances if possible. A full bar shoe is recommended for hoof stability if the horse needs to return to performance immediately.[1,3] See Chapter 12 for more details.

In severe cases the affected heel is displaced sufficiently proximad that a single trimming cannot restore the foot to balance. In these cases, the affected side is trimmed from the heel through the quarter to create a space when the shoe is applied (Figure 5.69). The weight

of the horse and time will permit the heel to drop down into correct alignment. A full bar shoe is recommended because of the instability between the heels. Soaking the foot in hot water and keeping it bandaged for 12 to 24 hours before applying the shoe may permit more rapid correction of the affected heel.[5]

In very severe cases in which considerable structural damage to the heel bulb and/or quarter cracks have developed, a diagonal bar shoe can be added to the full bar shoe. This is applied to the affected side to provide more protection and stability.[2] If the hoof wall on the affected side begins to curl under, the horse can be shod full to the affected side in an attempt to encourage hoof wall growth to that side.[2] Foals with sheared heels are best treated with corrective trimming of the heels/quarters and rounding the toe to encourage proper break-over.

Prognosis

The prognosis is considered good for mildly affected horses. Those presenting with severe sheared heels and secondary hoof wall deformities usually require several shoe resets to bring the heels back into balance. It is thought that some horses with severe structural damage between the heels may benefit from continual use of a full bar shoe.[6]

References

1. Johnson JH. The Foot. In Equine Medicine and Surgery, 3rd ed. Mansmann RA, McAllister ES, eds. American Veterinary Publications, Santa Barbara 1982:1044.
2. Moyer W. Diseases of the Equine Heel. Proceedings Am Assoc Equine Pract 1979;25:21.
3. Moyer W, Anderson JP. Sheared Heels: Diagnosis and Treatment. J Am Vet Med Assoc 1975;166:53.
4. Page B, Anderson GF. Diagonal imbalance of the equine foot: A cause of lameness. Proceedings Am Assoc Equine Pract 1992; 38:413.
5. Snow VE, Birdsall DP. Specific parameters used to evaluate hoof balance and support. Proceedings Am Assoc Equine Pract 1991; 37:299.
6. Stashak TS. The Foot. In Adams' Lameness in Horses. Stashak TS, ed. 5th ed. Lippincott Williams and Wilkins. Philadelphia, 2002; 645–733.

KERATOMA

Keratoma is an uncommon condition of the hoof that is characterized by keratin-containing tissue growing between the hoof wall and the distal phalanx. Although the term implies a neoplastic process, histologic examination reveals abundant keratin, squamous epithelial cells, occasionally granulation tissue, and inflammatory cells.[4,7,12] The growth usually begins near the coronary band, but it may extend to the solar surface anywhere along the white line.[6] A visible deviation of the coronary band and/or hoof wall is often present, and the most commonly affected areas of the foot are the toe and quarter.[12] Occasionally a keratoma may be located at a focal site between the coronary band and sole. Lameness and the radiographic changes are thought to arise from the growth of the keratoma and the subsequent pressure that is applied to the sensitive lamina and distal phalanx.[6,12] Keratomas have been observed in horses ranging from 2 to 20 years of age

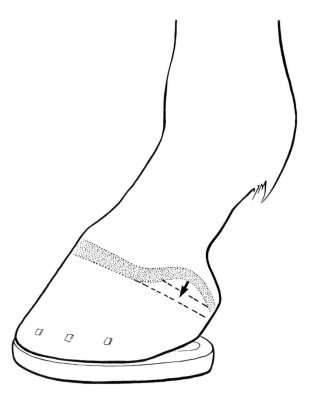

Figure 5.69. Corrective trimming and shoeing of a horse affected with sheared heels. The affected side is trimmed from the heel through the quarter to create a space between the hoof wall and the full bar shoe. The stippled area indicates the level of the coronary band. The arrow is pointing to where the coronary band should be.

and they should be differentiated from other growths that can occur in the hoof such as squamous cell carcinoma, canker, and melanoma.[1,8,9,12,13] In addition, multiple keratomas may be present in the same foot, but this is uncommon.[5]

Etiology

Trauma and chronic irritation in the form of sole abscesses or direct hoof injuries are the cause in the majority of cases.[6,12] However, a keratoma can develop without a history of previous injury and the initiating cause often cannot be determined.[4,6,13]

Clinical Signs

A history of a slow onset of intermittent lameness is common. The lameness is often seen before the distortion at the coronary band and hoof wall becomes obvious. Moderate to severe lameness is commonly observed at presentation.[4,6,12] The coronary band and hoof wall may or may not be abnormally shaped and close examination of the foot may be required to identify any abnormality. In those cases in which the growth has extended from the coronary band to the sole, a bulge in the hoof wall and a deviation in the white line toward the center of the foot may be seen (Figure 5.70). In some cases a fistulous tract may develop in the sole or hoof wall, mimicking a subsolar abscess.[3,4,9,11] Common clinical signs of keratomas in a recent retrospective study were lameness and the presence of a subsolar abscess.[3] Hoof tester examination often elicits a painful response when pressure is applied over the lesion. Although perineural anesthesia of the PD nerves

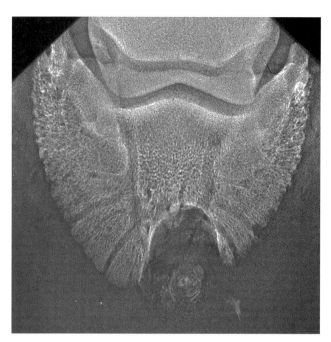

Figure 5.71. Dorsopalmar radiograph of P3 demonstrating a smooth margined lytic defect within the bone that is characteristic of a keratoma.

at or below the level of the collateral cartilages often improves the lameness, a basi-sesamoid or abaxial sesamoid block may be required to completely eliminate the lameness.

Diagnosis

A definitive diagnosis of keratoma is usually made based on the characteristic radiographic features. A discrete semicircular defect in the distal phalanx is often seen (Figure 5.71).[6] However, a discrete radiolucent defect was present in only 3 of 7 horses in one study, indicating that this cannot be used to rule out the presence of a keratoma.[12] The radiographic signs of a keratoma can usually be differentiated from lysis due to infection because of the smooth borders and lack of a sclerotic margin. Ultrasonographic imaging of a keratoma has been reported and a hypoechoic, well-delineated soft tissue mass between the hoof wall and the articulation of the distal and middle phalanges was seen.[14] Only keratomas originating near the coronary band can be imaged ultrasonographically.

Treatment

Treatment involves complete surgical removal of the abnormal growth. Only 42% of horses treated without surgery (12 horses) returned to performance compared to 83% that were treated with surgery (23 horses).[2] Incomplete removal of the keratoma is thought to result in recurrence of the growth.[6,12] Surgery may be performed with the patient under general anesthesia or while the patient is standing using regional anesthesia and sedation.

Two methods of gaining access to the abnormal tissue have been described.[10,11] In one method a hoof

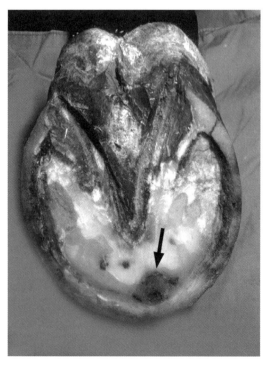

Figure 5.70. Inward deviation of the white line (arrow) caused by a keratoma.

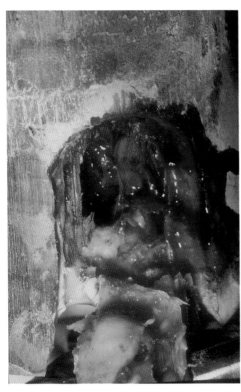

Figure 5.72. Hoof wall removal directly over the keratoma demonstrated in Figure 5.71. The keratoma can be seen beneath the hoof wall.

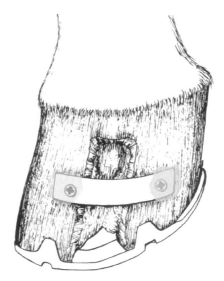

Figure 5.73. Metal strip being used to span a defect in the hoof wall together with a clipped shoe. The metal strip is attached to the hoof wall with screws and acrylic is placed over the screws.

wall flap can be created by making 2 parallel vertical cuts in the hoof wall down to the sensitive lamina on either side the keratoma.[11] A third cut is made distally at the base of the mass and a final cut can be made proximal to the mass (Figure 5.72). The hoof wall cuts can be made with a motorized burr, a cast cutting saw, or an osteotome. Alternatively, the hole in the hoof wall can be made with a large Galt trephine. This technique can be performed in the standing, sedated patient.[11] With this technique, the location of the keratoma must be documented. Multiple trephinations can be performed to adequately expose the lesion. The major advantage to this approach is the relative lack of disruption of the hoof wall.[11] In one study, horses undergoing a partial hoof wall resection for keratoma removal had significantly fewer complications and shorter convalescent times than horses undergoing a complete hoof wall resection.[3] However, the overall prognosis for horses returning to performance was not different.

If hoof stabilization is necessary, a bar shoe with large clips drawn on either side of the defect will prevent independent movement of the two portions of the hoof wall. Drawing clips is usually adequate when the hoof defect is small and located distally. If the hoof wall resection extends proximally toward the coronary band, a metal strip that spans the defect can be attached to the hoof wall to further stabilize the foot (Figure 5.73).[8,9,11] This prevents the hoof wall from becoming unstable which can lead to exuberant granulation tissue and pain.[4,11] However, the goal of surgery should be to remove as little hoof wall as possible to prevent these complications and to shorten the healing time.[3]

Prognosis

The prognosis is generally very good for return to performance if the abnormal tissue is completely removed.[2,3,10] In one study 6 of 7 horses were sound 1 year after surgery with no recurrence of the keratoma.[12] In another, 25 of 26 horses returned to their previous exercise level.[3] Adequate stabilization of the hoof defect and complete removal of the lesion are important for a successful outcome. Performing a partial vs. complete hoof wall resection reduces complications and permits most horses to return to performance more quickly.[3]

References

1. Berry CR, O'Brien TR, Pool RR. Squamous cell carcinoma of the hoof wall in a stallion. J Am Vet Med Assoc 1991; 199:90–92.
2. Bosch G, van Schie MJ, Back W. Retrospective evaluation of surgical versus conservative treatment of keratomas in 41 lame horses (1995–2001). Tijdschr Diergeneeskd 2004;129:700–705.
3. Boys Smith SJ, Clegg PD, Hughes I, et al. Complete and partial hoof wall resection for keratoma removal: post operative complications and final outcome in 26 horses (1994–2004). Equine Vet J 2006;38:127–133.
4. Chaffin MK, Carter GK, Sustaire D. Management of a keratoma in a horse: A case report. J Eq Vet Sci 1989;323–326.
5. Christman C. Multiple keratomas in an equine foot. Can Vet J 2008;49:904–906.
6. Frisbie DD, Trotter GW. Keratomas. In Current Techniques in Equine Surgery and Lameness. White NA, Moore JN, eds. 2nd ed. WB Saunders Company. Philadelphia, 1998;531–533.
7. Hamir AN, Kunz C, Evans LH. Equine keratoma. J Vet Diagn Invest 1992;4:99–100.
8. Honnas CM, Liskey CC, Meagher DM, et al. Malignant melanoma in the foot of a horse. J Am Vet Med Assoc 1990; 197:756–758.
9. Honnas CM, Peloso JG, Carter GK, et al. Surgical management of incomplete avulsion of the coronary band and keratomas in horses. Vet Med 1994;89:984–988.
10. Honnas CM. Keratomas of the equine digit. Eq Vet Edu 1997;9:203–207.
11. Honnas CM, Dabareiner RM, McCauley BH. Hoof wall surgery in the horse: approaches to and underlying disorders. Vet Clin North Am Equine Pract 2003;19:479–499.

12. Lloyd KCK, Peterson PR, Wheat JD, et al. Keratomas in horses: Seven cases (1975–1986). J Am Vet Med Assoc 1988; 193:967–970.
13. Reeves MJ, Yovich JV, Turner AS. Miscellaneous conditions of the equine foot. Vet Clin North Am Eq Pract 1989;5:221–242.
14. Seahorn TL, Sams AE, Honnas CM, et al. Ultrasonographic imaging of a keratoma in a horse. J Am Vet Med Assoc 1992;200:1973–1974.

AVULSION INJURIES OF THE HOOF

Avulsion injuries of the foot region are relatively uncommon in horses but can be very serious and difficult to manage. The injuries can be categorized as complete (when the tissue is totally removed), or partial or incomplete (when the tissue remains intact on at least one border).[5,8] These injuries may involve the hoof wall, coronary band, pastern region, sole, and structures deep to the hoof capsule (e.g., distal phalanx, digital cushion, laminae, synovial cavities). In general, the seriousness of the injury is related to the depth of the avulsion and the amount of tissue that is removed. However, even with significant loss of germinal tissue, the foot has the capacity to heal, although slower than other tissues, with complete reformation of hoof wall structures if treated properly for a long enough period.[2–4,8] The foot region has limited ability for wound contraction; therefore, the wound heals primarily by epithelialization and reformation of the corium.[6,7] These processes require a healthy bed of granulation tissue and a stable, clean environment to prevent permanent hoof defects.

Complete or incomplete avulsion injuries of the coronary region may result in deformities and/or permanent hoof wall defects if not treated properly (Figure 5.74). However, if treated promptly and correctly the majority heal without problems.[1,6,8] In addition, partial loss of the distal phalanx, digital cushion, or collateral cartilages does not appear to reduce the prognosis of affected horses for future soundness.[8] However, secondary infection of deeper hoof tissues usually reduces the chances of a complete recovery. The time required for healing depends on the size and extent of the avulsion injury

and the method of treatment. Generally 3 to 5 months are needed for second intention healing of complete avulsion injuries, compared to 3 to 4 weeks for incomplete avulsions that are surgically repaired.[1,6,8]

Etiology

Incomplete avulsion of the hoof wall of the heel can be caused by vertical tears of the hoof wall, kicking or stepping on sharp objects, continued foot imbalance, and improper shoe removal in which nails are torn out of the heel and quarter regions.[6,8] Other avulsion injuries of the foot and pastern are usually caused by lacerations from sharp objects. The horse either steps on or kicks at a sharp object, or the foot becomes entrapped, resulting in the avulsion. These are commonly seen as heel bulb lacerations that often involve the hoof.

Clinical Signs and Diagnosis

The degree of lameness usually varies with the duration, extent, and location of the avulsion injury. Moderate lameness is usually seen with an acute superficial injury that does not involve deeper structures. More extensive avulsion injuries usually cause severe lameness. Gentle manipulation of the foot and phalanges can provide important information regarding the status of support structures. Involvement of deeper structures such as the DIP joint, navicular bursa, and the digital tendon sheath should be identified. This can often be determined by one or several of the following diagnostic procedures: visual exam of the wound, manipulation of the digit, palpation of the wound with a gloved finger, injection of sterile fluid into a synovial cavity remote from the wound, radiography, contrast radiography, or ultrasonography.[8]

For chronic avulsion injuries, varying degrees of lameness may be present. If the wound heals without problems, lameness usually subsides with time. However, if lameness and purulent exudate persist, further diagnostics such as probing the wound with a sterile probe, radiography, contrast radiography, and ultrasonography should be performed to determine the cause of the continued drainage and lameness.[8] A chronic nonhealing wound with drainage usually suggests continued infection of deeper structures or involvement of a synovial cavity.

Treatment

Incomplete Avulsion (Coronary Band Not Involved)

Incomplete avulsions of the hoof wall at the heel and quarter without involvement of the coronary band are usually best removed.[6,8] Attempts to salvage the hoof wall are often unrewarding and contribute to continued lameness and infection beneath the avulsed hoof wall (Figure 5.75). Removal also prevents the wall from being snagged and continually traumatized, which is often very painful.

The hoof wall can be removed with the horse standing for limited involvement or under general anesthesia for larger lesions. Sharp hoof knives, nippers, and a

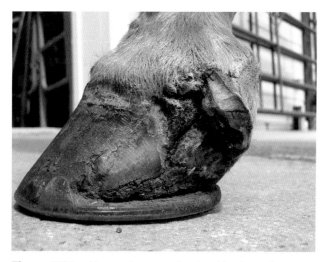

Figure 5.74. Abnormal coronary band and hoof growth associated with a previous injury to the medial aspect of the coronary band.

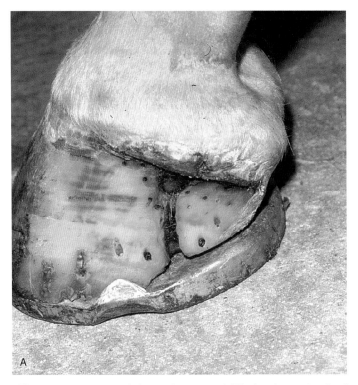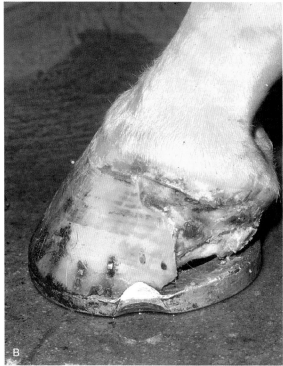

Figure 5.75. Before (A) and after removal (B) of an incomplete hoof avulsion of the medial quarter of the hindfoot. The avulsion was initially repaired by suturing the hoof wall but the horse became lame and therefore it was removed.

hand-held electric drill (Dremel tool) to burr the hoof wall at its attachments may be used for removal.[6,8] The Dremel tool permits more discrete removal of the hoof wall without tearing of healthy hoof wall from the dermal laminae but is time consuming.[8] Hoof knives or nippers may result in tearing of healthy tissues but enable quicker removal of avulsed hoof wall. The dorsal attachment of the unaffected hoof wall should be beveled flush to the wound so there is little tendency for it to be snagged, resulting in further separation. The wound should be bandaged and protected from contamination and trauma until the exposed tissues become keratinized. A full support shoe (egg-bar, heart-bar shoe) can be used to provide hoof wall stability and to reduce weight-bearing on the hoof defect by "floating" the involved heel. A hoof acrylic can be used to fill the defect once it has keratinized but this is often unnecessary.

Incomplete Avulsion (Coronary Band Involved)

Incomplete avulsion injuries of the coronary band alone or the coronary band and hoof wall are best managed by suturing the wound whenever possible. Re-apposition of the coronary band is important to prevent future hoof deformities.[3,5] Often the hoof wall cannot be salvaged and will require removal, but the coronary band should be reconstructed in any way possible (Figure 5.76). Lacerations of the coronary band without loss of hoof wall should be sutured primarily and immobilized in a foot cast (Figure 5.77). Avulsion injuries that affect the coronary band and a small portion of the hoof wall can also be sutured and immo-

bilized. The hoof wall adjacent to the defect can be thinned with a hoof rasp and the separated piece of hoof wall can be thinned with a motorized burr to permit suturing.[6,8] If the blood supply is questionable or excessive contamination exists, delayed closure may be used.[6–8]

When the avulsion injury extends from the solar surface proximally through the coronary band, the majority of the hoof wall can be removed to within 1 cm of the coronary region, and the coronary band and soft tissues sutured if possible. Alternatively, the hoof wall can be included in the closure by thinning the walls adjacent to the defect with a Dremel tool.[6] Regardless of the technique, accurate approximation of the coronary band is important. If left untreated, these incomplete avulsion injuries of the coronary band often remain elevated, eventually producing a horny spur at the distal extremity of the avulsion while the remaining underlying tissue heals by scarring and epithelialization (Figure 5.78).[6–8] Invariably these avulsions protrude above the skin and hoof wall surface, making them susceptible to further trauma and painful to palpation. If the avulsed tissue is just removed, a permanent hoof wall defect will often develop (Figure 5.74).

Complete Avulsion

With complete avulsion injuries of the hoof, there is usually no tissue to appose, and the wound and hoof defect heal by second intention (Figure 5.79). The initial clinical picture is usually that of a hemorrhagic wound with obvious tissue loss.[3] The depth of the defect and potential involvement of other structures should be

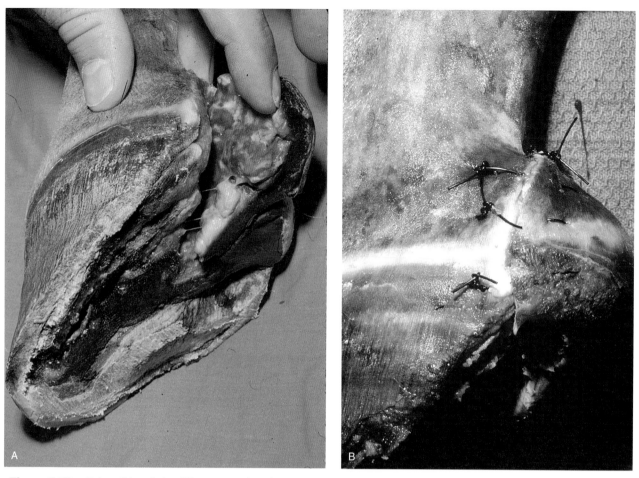

Figure 5.76. Before (A) and after (B) reconstruction of an incomplete hoof avulsion that involved the coronary band, sole, and frog. Realignment of the coronary band should be performed whenever possible.

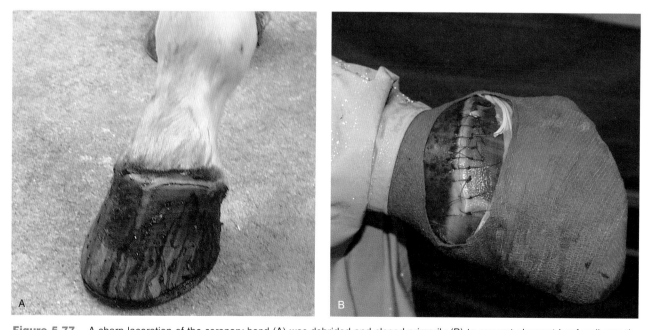

Figure 5.77. A sharp laceration of the coronary band (A) was debrided and closed primarily (B) to prevent aberrant hoof wall growth.

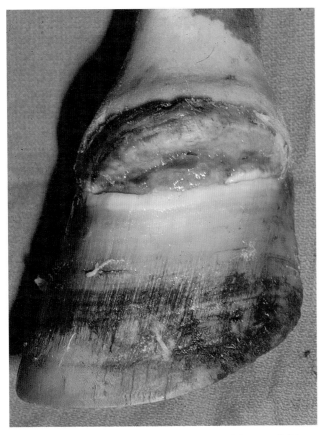

Figure 5.78. Laceration of the coronary band that was left to heal by second intention. The edges of the coronary band have separated and the hoof is growing horizontally rather than downward toward the existing hoof.

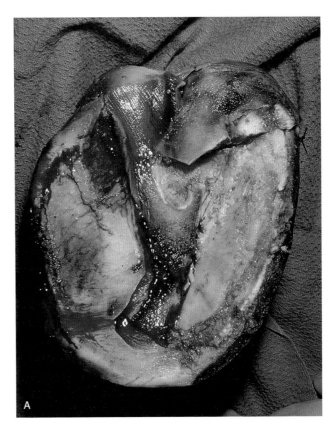

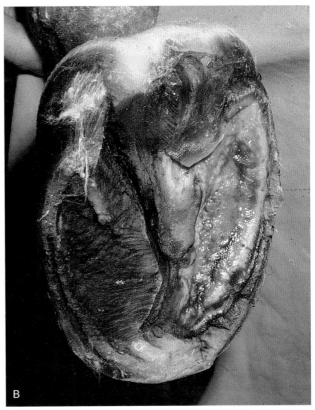

Figure 5.79. Complete avulsion of the sole with exposure of the solar aspect of P3 (A) and the same defect after it has filled with granulation tissue (B).

determined prior to treatment because their involvement affect both the type of treatment recommended and the prognosis. The practical treatment of these wounds in terms of bandaging, the use of systemic and local antimicrobials, and local wound care follow the same guidelines used to treat other limb wounds in horses.[3] Many of these wounds can be bandaged initially to control hemorrhage and permit repeated lavage and debridement of the wound. However, immobilization with a foot cast is often very beneficial in the long-term management of these injuries. Casts are usually left in place for 3 to 4 weeks, and may need to be reapplied depending on the size and location of the avulsion. Wound stability is thought to improve the chances of complete reformation of the hoof wall.[8]

Hoof avulsions heal by similar processes to other open wounds, but healing is often protracted because wound contraction is limited in the foot. Wounds must heal be epithelialization and reformation of the corium which often requires 3 to 5 months, depending on the size of the defect.[6] There are several types of germinal epithelial tissues in the foot (skin, limbic, coronary, parietal, and solar) and all can contribute to epithelialization of the defect.[2–4] The structure and quality of the hoof that forms is related to the type of epidermis that migrates over the surface of the wound.[3] Epithelial cells that migrate aberrantly can lead to hoof deformities.[3,5]

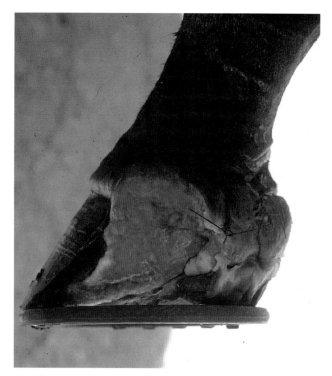

Figure 5.80. Complete avulsion injuries that involve the hoof wall and a large portion of the coronary band can be especially difficult to manage to prevent abnormal hoof growth.

For instance, if epidermis from the parietal integument grows into the space formerly occupied by the coronary band, the wall generated in that location will not resemble wall generated from the coronary integument. If epidermis from the hoof migrates proximally to the coronary band, a horny spur will form in the pastern region.[3,5] One of goals of treating complete hoof avulsion injuries is to prevent aberrant migration of epithelial cells and hoof wall deformities (Figure 5.80).

Prognosis

Generally, incomplete avulsion injuries of the hoof wall alone and/or including the coronary band have a very good functional and cosmetic outcome if they are sutured.[6–8] The prognosis for deeper avulsion injuries is often difficult to predict until complete healing has occurred. Complications such as fracture of the distal phalanx, osteomyelitis, septic arthritis, and OA of a damaged DIP or PIP joint obviously reduce the prognosis for a sound horse. Chronic hoof deformities are one of the most common sequelae of hoof avulsion injuries but do not always cause a clinical problem.[5]

References

1. Markel MD, Richardson GL, Peterson PR, et al. Surgical reconstruction of chronic coronary band avulsion in three horses. J Am Vet Med Assoc 1987;190:687–688.
2. Park AH. Equine foot wounds: general principles of healing and treatment. Proceedings Am Assoc Equine Pract 1999;45: 180–187.
3. Park AH. Hoof avulsions. Equine Vet Educ 2008;August: 411–413.
4. Park AH. Wounds of the equine foot; principles of healing and treatment. Equine Vet Educ 1997;9:317–327.
5. Park AH. Chronic foot injury and deformity. In Current Techniques in Equine Surgery and Lameness. White NA, Moore JN, eds. 2nd ed. WB Saunders. Philadelphia, 1998;534–537.
6. Schumacher J, Stashak TS. Management of wounds of the distal extremities. In Equine Wound Management. Stashak TS, Theoret C, eds. 2nd ed. Wiley-Blackwell. Ames, IA, 2008:375–425.
7. Stashak TS. Management of lacerations and avulsion injuries of the foot and pastern region and hoof wall cracks. Vet Clin North Am Equine Pract 1989;5:195–220.
8. Stashak TS. The Foot. In Adams' Lameness in Horses. Stashak TS, ed. 5th ed. Lippincott Williams and Wilkins. Philadelphia. 2002;645–733.

TOE CRACKS, QUARTER CRACKS, AND HEEL CRACKS (SAND CRACKS)

Hoof wall cracks represent a focal wall failure, and as such, they can occur anywhere on the hoof wall. Most are oriented in the direction of hoof tubule orientation. Hoof wall cracks are generally described by their location (toe, quarter, heel, or bar), length (partial- or full-length), depth (superficial or deep), and the presence or absence of hemorrhage or infection.[1] In most instances, the underlying wall damage is considerably more extensive than that noted from the exterior. These cracks may occur in the front or hind feet and may be superficial (only involve the hoof tissue) or deep (if the crack is full-thickness and involves the sensitive laminae beneath). These cracks may begin at the bearing surface of the wall and extend variable distances up the hoof wall, or they may originate at the coronary band and extend distally (Figure 5.81). Quarter cracks and heel cracks are usually the most severe because they often involve the sensitive laminae (Figure 5.82).[3] Affected horses are usually lame and hemorrhage after exercise may be noticed. Infection within the hoof crack is commonly observed.

Etiology

Excessive growth of the hoof wall from lack of trimming increases the risk of splitting of the wall. Depending

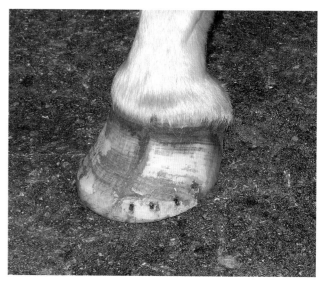

Figure 5.81. A partial-thickness toe crack that developed in a horse with a concavity of the dorsal hoof wall.

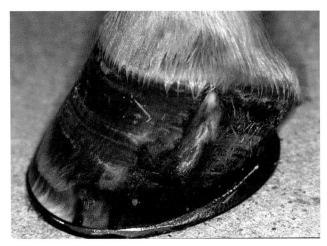

Figure 5.82. A full-thickness quarter crack just after debridement down to the sensitive laminae.

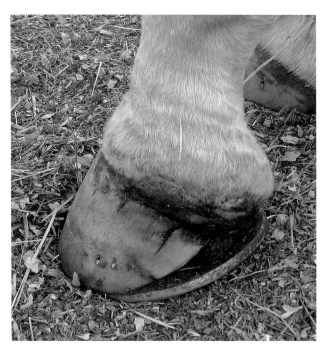

Figure 5.83. These vertical and horizontal hoof cracks involving the medial hoof wall were contributing to significant lameness in this horse.

on its location, the crack may spread proximally along the hoof wall. Previous injuries to the coronary band often cause a weak and deformed hoof wall that grows distally. This hoof wall is more susceptible to normal forces on the foot, predisposing to cracks originating at the coronary band. Weakening of the wall due to excessive drying or excessively thin walls may also contribute to hoof cracks. Moisture is the key to maintaining flexibility of the hoof wall and sole. The normal hoof wall contains about 25% water, the sole about 33%, and the frog 50%. If the foot becomes excessively dry, it becomes brittle and more susceptible to cracking.[2,3] If a full-thickness crack occurs, environmental bacteria may gain entrance into the deeper laminar tissue, causing secondary infection of the crack.

Central toe cracks often show evidence of significant wall separation (chronic laminitis, white line disease, and club foot malformation) that may have contributed to the hoof defect (Figure 5.81).[1] Heel and quarter cracks are frequently associated with underrun heels and long toes.[1,3] Linear cracks parallel to the coronary band invariably represent pre-existing damage to the coronary corium tissues (trauma or infection), interrupting normal wall growth (Figure 5.83). In some instances, the damage to the coronary corium is permanent; thus, the crack/defect remains in place regardless of the technique of repair chosen.

Clinical Signs

The presence of the defect in the hoof wall is usually obvious. Variable lesions may be found above the coronary band in those cases in which the crack is due to a previous injury. However, not all hoof cracks are clinically significant and contribute to lameness. Lameness is often not present with superficial cracks, but is usually obvious with deep cracks because they often pinch the sensitive tissues beneath the hoof wall (Figure 5.83). If secondary infection is present, lameness may be severe and purulent exudate is often seen within the hoof crack. The hoof wall around the crack is usually very sensitive to hoof testers with infected hoof cracks and in those that are contributing to lameness.

Diagnosis

The diagnosis is based on the presence of the crack, which is easily identified, and is classified according to its location and depth. Blood or purulent exudate is only present with full-thickness hoof cracks. Bleeding from the hoof crack after exercise also indicates that the crack is full-thickness and extends to the sensitive laminae. Most clinically significant hoof cracks are painful to hoof testers. Perineural anesthesia can also be helpful in some cases to determine whether the hoof crack is contributing to the lameness.

Treatment

See Chapter 12 for a discussion of the treatment options for hoof cracks

References

1. Moyer W. Hoof wall defects: chronic hoof wall separations and hoof wall cracks. Vet Clin North Am Equine Pract 2003; 19:463–477.
2. Stashak TS. Management of lacerations and avulsion injuries of the foot and pastern region and hoof wall cracks. Vet Clin North Am Equine Pract 1989;5:195–220.
3. Stashak TS. The Foot. In Adams' Lameness in Horses. Stashak TS, ed. 5th ed. Lippincott Williams and Wilkins. Philadelphia, 2002; 645–733.

LAMINITIS

Equine laminitis is a disease in which failure of the soft tissue structure that suspends the distal phalanx within the hoof wall, the interdigitation between the dermal and epidermal laminae of the digit, commonly results in a crippling lameness due to displacement of the distal phalanx within the hoof capsule. Displacement of the distal phalanx can take place as a symmetrical distal displacement or sinking of the phalanx, an asymmetric distal displacement of the phalanx (either medial or lateral), or a rotation of the distal phalanx away from the dorsal hoof wall with or without concurrent flexion of the coffin joint (termed capsular or phalangeal rotation, respectively). Both distal displacement and rotation can occur in the same horse.

Laminitis is not a primary disease, but usually occurs as a sequelae to 4 different clinical entities:

1. Diseases associated with sepsis/endotoxemia
2. Excessive weight placed on a limb due to injury to the opposite limb
3. Cushing's disease in the older horse
4. equine metabolic syndrome (EMS) including pasture-associated laminitis.

Laminitis secondary to consumption of black walnut shavings could be listed as a fifth clinical entity, but is much rarer than the other 4 causes.

The majority of laminitis research up to this point has focused on models of sepsis/endotoxemia, although some headway has been made recently on metabolic syndrome-related laminitis. Very little data are available regarding supporting limb laminitis or laminitis secondary to Cushing's disease. The 2 principal experimental models from which most laminitis reports have emanated are the carbohydrate overload (CHO) models (wood starch model and the oligofructose model) and the black walnut extract (BWE) model. These appear to be models of endotoxemia/sepsis,[15] with a similar systemic inflammation as observed in sepsis being documented in the black walnut extract model,[74] and both systemic inflammation and endotoxemia documented in the carbohydrate overload model.[6] Recent models of pasture-associated laminitis/EMS have involved excessive feed intake over various periods of time.[31]

Laminitis literature usually refers to 3 stages of laminitis: developmental, acute, and chronic. The developmental (also termed "prodromal") stage is the period during which a horse suffering from a disease is at risk of laminitis (i.e., the septic case of enterocolitis or surgical acute abdomen) prior to the onset of clinical signs of laminitis. The acute stage describes the horse exhibiting digital signs of laminitis but no radiographic evidence of displacement of the distal phalanx. The chronic stage refers to the period after displacement of the distal phalanx has occurred. Because displacement of the distal phalanx can occur within days of onset of clinical signs of laminitis, the chronic stage covers a large breadth of clinical presentations ranging from the horse with unstable laminae undergoing active phalangeal displacement early in the disease process to the horse that is several years past the initiating cause of laminitis and now has stable laminae but a chronic lameness due to displacement of the distal phalanx (commonly due to ongoing solar pressure/bruising). The terminology describing the clinical stages of laminitis is varied, but the authors have attempted to conform to that most widely used.[58]

Etiology

Pathogens Involved in Sepsis-related Laminitis

The majority of studies on bacterial toxemia in horses have concentrated on the effect of the Gram-negative bacterial wall component endotoxin. However, it has been well established recently in the human literature that a host of different molecules can result in the same systemic inflammation and tissue/organ injury (through the toll-like receptor signaling) including other bacterial toxins from Gram-negative and Gram-positive bacteria, viral and bacterial DNA components, fungal products, and, most recently, proteins (especially mitochondrial proteins) released by host cells undergoing necrosis, commonly at the original source of sepsis.[15] Thus, it is likely that in diseases such as enterocolitis, other bacterial toxins and even proteins from the injured/necrotic colonic cells may work synergistically with endotoxin to induce systemic inflammation and organ/tissue injury.

There has been long-standing confusion regarding the role of endotoxin/endotoxemia in laminitis, due to the facts that (1) clinical diseases that put a horse at risk of laminitis appear to always have a Gram-negative component, but endotoxemia has been inconsistently reported in studies of laminitis,[6,72] and (2) endotoxin administration results in some abnormalities in digital blood flow but does not result in laminar failure.[37,39] One reason for a lack of detection of endotoxin in the systemic circulation in many studies is the likely clearance of absorbed endotoxins by tissue macrophages in the liver or lung, which then release inflammatory cytokines into the circulation.[5] The likely reason that endotoxin does not result in laminitis is that it is a cocktail of different bacterial toxins, necrotic cell products, and proinflammatory cytokines that the laminae are exposed to in the septic horse, not endotoxin by itself.

In a recent study, the equine epidermal epithelial cell, the cell type at the point of laminar failure, was found to not undergo inflammatory signaling when exposed to toxins more associated with Gram-positive sepsis (lipoteichoic acid and peptidoglycan), whereas the cells did respond to 2 toxins more associated with Gram-negative sepsis, endotoxin, and flagellin.[44] These results, which are different from that reported in human keratinocytes (which respond to both Gram-positive and Gram-negative toxins), may help to explain the need for a Gram-negative component in sepsis-related laminitis.

Recently, *Streptococcus bovis* has been proposed to be the primary source of bacterial toxins in laminitis from research documenting marked proliferation of the bacterium in the intestinal tract of horses in the carbohydrate model of laminitis,[51,61] and induction of separation of the epidermal and dermal components of the laminae upon *in vitro* exposure of hoof explants to S. bovis products.[61] However, although S. bovis may play a role in gastrointestinal disease, it is not likely to be present in other types of laminitis-inducing sepsis such as endometritis or pleuropneumonia. Finally, a fulminant Gram-positive sepsis such as *Streptococcus equi* respiratory infection rarely if ever results in laminitis. Thus, it is likely that endotoxin plays a role in laminitis, but other circulating mediators and/or toxins (i.e., flagellin) are necessary to cause pathophysiological events that result in laminar failure.

Alterations in Laminar Vascular Dynamics

VASOCONSTRICTION

The importance of alterations in the equine digital vasculature in the developmental and acute stages of laminitis has been the subject of intense study in the past 4 decades. Some very early work used contrast radiography of the digit to demonstrate a decrease in perfusion of the digital laminar region at the onset of clinical laminitis.[21] More recently, physiologic studies using an extracorporeal digital perfusion model were used to report marked increases in capillary pressure (most likely due to an increase of up to 20-fold in postcapillary resistance) and concomitant increases in laminar interstitial pressure (indicative of laminar edema) in both the carbohydrate and black walnut extract models of laminitis.[3,27] The investigators concluded that venoconstriction in the digital microvasculature is likely to cause the increased capillary pressure, leading to laminar edema, increased arteriovenous shunting, and possibly capillary collapse due to the inability of edematous laminar tissue to expand against the constraints of the inelastic hoof wall and distal phalanx.

Interestingly, recent work using isolated laminar vessels from the microvasculature have indicated that the laminar venules are much more reactive than the arterioles to vasoactive (vasoconstrictor) agents likely to be present in affected laminae including thromboxane, PGF2α, endothelin-1, and isoprostanes.[53,59] The reported adhesion of leukocytes and platelets to the laminar microvasculature, which occurs preferentially in venules in most studies of sepsis and inflammation in other species, is likely to play a role in this venoconstriction. Platelets release numerous vasoactive substances such as histamine, serotonin, and thromboxane, whereas leukocytes are reportedly potent producers of vasoactive prostanoids.[69] Other studies using laser Doppler flowmetry and hoof wall temperature have presented more conflicting data, most likely due to variability in laminitis models and variability in both Doppler flowmetry and temperature measuring techniques.[2,34,63]

ARTERIOVENOUS (AV) SHUNTING IN THE DIGITAL LAMINAE

A high concentration of arteriovenous anastomoses (AVAs, more than 500 AVA/cm2 in dermal laminae) have been documented in the laminae themselves and at the base of the laminae.[64] One early study provided somewhat compelling evidence of AV shunting in the digit, where isotope-labeled macroaggregated albumin (large enough aggregates to reportedly become trapped in the laminar capillaries) injected into the digital arteries appeared to bypass the laminar capillaries in the acute stage of laminitis, but became lodged in the laminar capillaries when clinical signs of laminitis were not present.[33]

COAGULOPATHY

Although thrombi have been identified in the laminar microcirculation of horses with either naturally occurring or experimentally induced laminitis,[9,82] detection of microthrombi in individual horses in the different models of laminitis has been inconsistent, indicating that there is likely not an ample extent of thrombosis to induce laminar ischemia. However, platelets are likely to play a role in laminar pathology, as indicated by:

1. Reported activation of circulating platelets[6]
2. Platelet localization/adhesion to the digital circulation in the early stages of experimental laminitis[82]
3. A reduction in the incidence of laminitis via administration of an inhibitor of platelet aggregation[81]

Platelets can play an important role in vascular pathology, exacerbating vascular disturbances and inflammatory injury via the release of inflammatory and vasoactive mediators, and by promoting adhesion and activation of leukocytes to the laminar vasculature; platelet-neutrophil aggregates have been reported in the circulation in the early stages of laminitis.[26,80]

Inflammation in Laminitis

A similar inflammatory injury to the laminae in laminitis appears to occur as has been reported to lead to organ injury in human sepsis, in which all types of leukocytes (lymphocytes, monocytes/macrophages/neutrophils) play a role in the inflammatory injury. The laminae normally have a resident population of macrophages and B- and T-lymphocytes.[11] In the early stages of laminitis, there is an activation of the endothelium with concomitant expression of adhesion molecules on the luminal surface, followed by leukocyte adhesion in the laminar venules and emigration into the laminar dermal tissue.[18,47] Although both neutrophils and monocytes emigrate into the laminar tissue in the acute disease process, there is a difference in leukocyte type between the 2 models of laminitis. Whereas the vast majority of cells emigrating into the tissue are neutrophils in the BWE model,[18] monocytes are the principal cell type in the CHO model of laminitis.

The laminar inflammatory response includes an increased laminar expression of central proinflammatory cytokines reported to be involved in human disease, including IL-1β and IL-6; these increases range from a 10-fold increase to greater than a 1,000-fold increase in gene expression.[13,47] There is also a marked increase in expression of chemokines including IL-8, GRO-α, and MCP-1, which play an important role in leukocyte activation and chemotaxis.[29,47] Laminar expression of the inducible cyclooxygenase (COX) gene, COX-2, occurs in both the BWE and CHO models of laminitis,[19,78] indicating that prostaglandins are likely to play a role in laminar dysfunction.

There is a temporal difference in leukocyte emigration and cytokine expression between the BWE model and the two main CHO models, with both leukocyte emigration and cytokine expression occurring in early prodromal stages in the BWE model,[47] but neither occurring until the onset of lameness in the CHO model.[12] Similarly, laminar expression of COX-2 is increased at both the prodromal and lameness stages in the BWE model, but not induced until the onset of lameness in the CHO model.[12]

It has recently been reported that the same degree of inflammatory events (leukocyte emigration, cytokine, chemokine, and COX-2 expression) occurs in the laminae of the hindfeet as occurs in the forelimb laminae, indicating that physical factors (increased weight born on forelimbs) are the likely reason for increased incidence of the disease in the forelimbs.[42]

The inflammatory response in laminitis does not appear to be limited to the laminae; inflammatory changes have also been reported in the lung and liver, target organs injured in human sepsis.[74] Inflammatory changes are much less severe in these organs compared to the laminae in the same horses, indicating that the laminae undergo a unique event (e.g., vascular disturbance) which exacerbates the inflammatory injury in that tissue.

The one cytokine reported to be increased in the visceral organs that is not increased in the laminae is tumor necrosis factor-α (TNF-α), a central cytokine reported to play an important role in sepsis-related organ injury. Increased plasma concentrations of TNF-α have recently been reported in the oligofructose model of laminitis.[6] Thus, because expression of TNF-α most likely occurs in cells exposed to the circulation (fixed macrophages including Kupffer cells in the liver and pulmonary intravascular macrophages [PIMs] in the equine lung),[74] these organs almost certainly provide a source of circulating TNF-α for both activation of circulating leukocytes and activation of host cells within the laminae.

Investigators have presented data indicating that peripheral blood leukocytes are activated during the developmental stage of laminitis.[38] Thus, because clinical laminitis is usually associated with systemic signs of endotoxemia or Gram-negative sepsis, it is possible that, similar to human sepsis, a systemic inflammatory response occurs which results in a simultaneous activation of leukocytes and the vascular endothelium, followed by adhesion to and migration of these cells through the venous endothelial lining into the tissues with the local release of inflammatory mediators.

Failure of the Epidermal/Dermal Laminar Interface at the Level of the Laminar Basal Epithelial Cell and Basement Membrane

Subsequent to histologic studies in which laminar failure was demonstrated to occur at the level of the basement membrane underlying the laminar basal epithelial cells, the toxic/metabolic hypothesis was derived. This suggests that circulating bacterial toxins and other inflammatory proteins induce matrix metalloproteases (MMPs) to cause laminar failure by breaking down the extracellular matrix (ECM) underlying the laminar basal epithelial cells and to which the cells are adhered.[60] Extracellular matrix consists primarily of fibrous structural proteins and proteoglycans, which provide strength and resistance to compression, respectively.[17] The MMP family includes more than 20 proteins that use distinct proteins in the extracellular matrix as their substrates.

MMP expression is induced by many stimuli reported to be present in laminitis including bacterial toxins, inflammatory cytokines, and ischemia. Generally,

MMPs are secreted as inactive proenzymes that require proteolytic cleavage by other MMPs or extracellular proteases (e.g., plasmin, elastase) for activation.[17] Additionally, many inhibitors of MMPs are present in the ECM (i.e., tissue inhibitors of MMPs [TIMPs]), which regulate activity of the MMPs.[17]

MMPs have been proposed to cause degradation of the basement membrane between the dermal and epidermal laminae, thereby disrupting adhesion of the dermal and epidermal laminae resulting in laminar separation and loss of support of the distal phalanx.[60] MMP-2 (a collagenase) and MMP-9 (a gelatinase) are 2 of the most-studied metalloproteases that break down components of the basement membrane. Increased MMP-2 and MMP-9 concentrations have been demonstrated in laminar tissue from horses with either naturally occurring or experimentally induced laminitis.[48] Increased laminar concentrations of MMP-9 and increased mRNA and protein concentration of MMP-2 have been reported in the different models of laminitis.[41,47,54] MMP-9 concentrations have also been correlated with the number of neutrophils infiltrating the laminae (most likely due to MMP-9 being present in neutrophil cytoplasmic granules).[47] However, the recently published facts that (1) MMP-9 is mainly found in the inactive zymogen form,[47-48] and (2) laminar MMP-2 is only minimally active or not active in starch-gruel induced laminitis up to Obel grade 1 lameness (SJ Black, personal communication), suggest that these proteases may not play as central a role as previously proposed in the acute disease process.

A protease gene of the ADAM-TS (a disintegrin and metalloproteinase with thrombospondin motifs) family which degrades proteoglycans, ADAM-TS4, has recently been reported to be expressed in the early stages of laminitis in both experimental models and clinical cases.[17] Elevated laminar gene expression is accompanied by an elevated presence of laminar ADAM-TS4 cleavage neoepitopes on proteoglycan substrates (i.e., sites on the proteoglycan that should be exposed if the proteoglycan were cleaved by ADAMTS-4) during the acute stage of the disease (both OG1 and OG3 lameness, S. Black, personal communication). Thus, ADAMTS-4 and other proteases may play important roles in early laminar injury.

A recently introduced concept which is a more likely process resulting in separation of the LBECs from the basement membrane is the disruption of adhesion of the LBECs to the underlying matrix molecules via loss of function of hemidesmosomes,[30] the integrin complexes responsible for adhesion of epithelial cells to the underlying basement membrane.[52] Because hemidesmosome function depends on cellular processes such as the cell's energy regulation and cytoskeletal dynamics, any injury to the cell that disrupts these processes can result in dysregulation of hemidesmosomes and dysadherence of the epithelial cells from the underlying basement membrane.

Reconsidering the Pathogenesis of Acute Laminitis

Based on evidence presented so far, it appears that the laminar failure is due to a combination of events, including local digital hemodynamic events, inflamma-

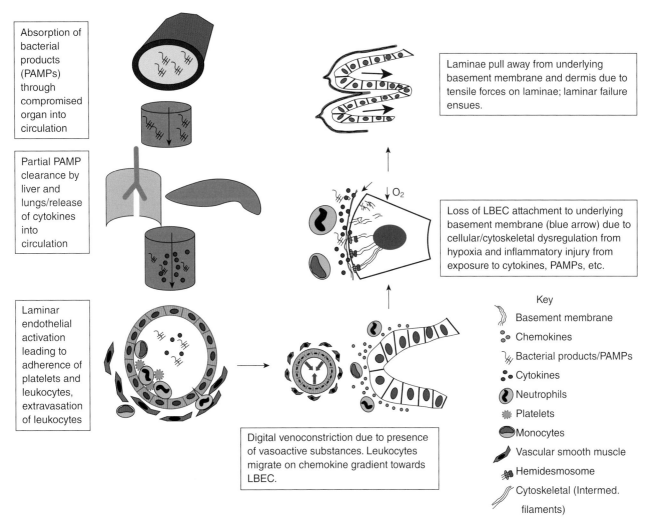

Figure 5.84. This proposed pathogenesis of laminitis incorporates many of the recent findings from laminitis research.

tory events, and prothrombotic events (Figure 5.84). In attempting to coalesce the above data into a unifying pathophysiological mechanism, the recent findings would best support a sequence of events similar to that reported for organ injury in human sepsis. In human bacterial systemic sepsis, bacterial products are absorbed from the local site of infection into the systemic circulation which results in systemic activation of leukocytes, platelets, and the microvascular endothelium, leading to adhesion of platelets and leukocytes to each other and to the endothelium. These responses are then followed by transendothelial migration of the activated leukocytes into the tissues. The leukocytes and platelets then express inflammatory mediators, which induce the further expression of inflammatory mediators and enzymes (e.g., IL-6 and COX-2) by cellular constituents of the laminae.

Production of vasoactive mediators, including prostaglandins and vasoactive amines, by activated leukocytes and platelets may then lead to vascular disturbances including venoconstriction and arteriovenous shunting, possibly limiting the amount of oxygen provided to laminar epithelium by the dermal microvasculature. These changes in blood flow may also amplify the

inflammatory injury by leading to further margination of leukocytes and platelets with attachment to the laminar venous endothelium. Production of oxygen radicals by activated leukocytes may add to the damage, because there appears to be minimal endogenous superoxide dismutase (SOD) in the laminar tissue to neutralize the oxygen radicals.[46] Expression of inflammatory mediators and proteases by the emigrating leukocytes and possibly the resident cells in the laminae may then result in laminar basal epithelial cell injury and dysfunction, leading to dysregulation of the cytoskeleton and adhesion molecules on the basal surface, the hemidesmosomes.

Once there is a critical loss of adhesion of the epidermal laminae to the underlying dermal laminae, the forces upon the hoof wall (discussed below) exceed the support provided by the remaining intact interdigitating dermal and epidermal laminae. This results in tearing of these remaining laminae and displacement of the distal phalanx. The potential space left between the hoof wall and the displaced distal phalanx is likely to fill with blood and necrotic tissue (this area on radiographs may appear radiolucent for a short time after displacement).

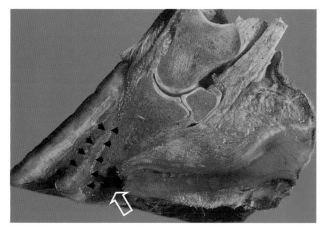

Figure 5.85. A sagittal section of the hoof wall of a horse with capsular rotation of the distal phalanx. Note the lamellar wedge (black arrows) of epithelial tissue that forms from remaining laminar epithelial cells following displacement of the distal phalanx. Also note the penetration of the sole by the dorsodistal tip of the distal phalanx immediately dorsal to the apex of the frog (white arrow).

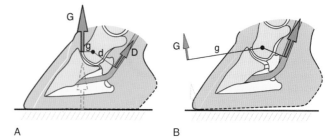

Figure 5.86. A. At rest, the foot is stable with respect to the ground. The ground reaction force is approximately vertical, and positioned approximately in the center of the foot, slightly in front of the center of rotation of the distal interphalangeal joint. The product of the magnitude of the GRF (G, large red arrow) and the length of its moment arm (g) is the extensor moment, which is opposed by the flexor moment, which is the product of the force in the deep digital flexor tendon (D, small red arrow) multiplied by the length of its moment arm (d). B. At break-over, the position of the foot is dynamic, the magnitude of the ground reaction force (G, small red arrow) is decreased as the horse moves off the leg, but the length of the moment arm (g) is increased because the GRF is positioned at the toe. To cause the foot to move from the stable position at rest to the dynamic state, the flexor moment exceeds the extensor moment.

After separation, some germinal epithelial cells remain on the deep surface of the separated epidermal laminae and some remain attached to the surface of the dermal laminae. Similar to wound healing in other tissues, viable germinal epithelial cells proliferate. However, the underlying damaged dermis is unable to exert normal control of epithelial proliferation.[62,79] Therefore, remaining epithelial cells undergo aberrant proliferation in the space created by displacement of the distal phalanx, resulting in a lamellar wedge of disorganized epithelial tissue, the apex of which is proximal and the base distal (Figure 5.85). This wedge most likely impedes the ability of the clinician and farrier to realign the distal phalanx with the dorsal hoof wall.

Pathogenesis: Structural Considerations of the Equine Digit

The stresses on the laminae are related to the stresses born by the 2 anatomical structures to which the laminae attach, the hoof wall and the distal phalanx. Different stresses occur due to both weight-bearing and locomotion. The 3 primary forces affecting the laminae include:

1. The downward force of the horse's weight through the distal phalanx
2. The torque (or moment) around the distal interphalangeal (DIP) joint created by the ground reaction force (the force exerted by the ground on the digit; also termed extensor moment)
3. The tension of the deep digital flexor tendon (DDFT) exerted on the caudal aspect of the distal phalanx (also termed the flexor moment; Figure 5.86).

As it is now accepted that engagement of the solar surface of the digit can provide support to the distal phalanx (i.e., counteracting the downward force on the distal phalanx from the horse's weight), we now realize that the relationship of the foot to the ground surface can greatly affect laminar stress. In the horse shod with standard shoeing that is standing on a firm surface, excessive stress is born by the laminae due to the fact that the only relationship between the foot and the ground surface is through the part of the foot contacting the shoe, the distal hoof wall. The lack of solar support of the distal phalanx is exacerbated by the elevation of the sole off the ground surface due to the thickness of the shoe. In the unshod foot, the character of the ground surface affects the amount of stress born by the laminae. On a hard surface (including those artificial surfaces commonly used in stables), only the distal hoof wall and adjacent sole contact the ground. This results in a similar great degree of stress on the laminae as that of the foot with standard shoes. This is due to the combined effects of concentration of stress through the hoof wall to the laminae and the lack of support of the distal surface of the distal phalanx due to lack of incorporation of the majority of the solar surface. In both of these instances, the distal phalanx can be thought of as being suspended within the foot by the laminar attachments to the hoof wall. When placed on a softer, surface such as sand (or possibly an elastic flooring material), the entire solar surface can be engaged to directly support the distal phalanx in addition to being suspended by the laminar attachments to the hoof wall, distributing the digital support through both anatomic structures and thus decreasing the stress on the laminae.[35] As is discussed later, addition of putty to the solar surface in the shod horse has the same result.

At rest, the center of weight-bearing is approximately at the center of the ground surface of the foot. During the majority of locomotion, the stresses associated with weight-bearing are also centered on the ground surface of the foot. However, during the break-over stage of the stride, ground reaction forces are localized to the toe of the foot, resulting in an increase in the length of the moment arm (and hence the torque or moment; see Figure 5.86) and thus the stress on the laminae.

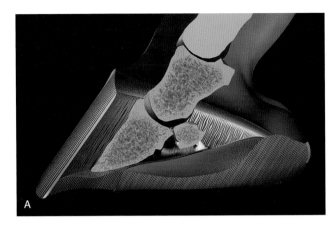

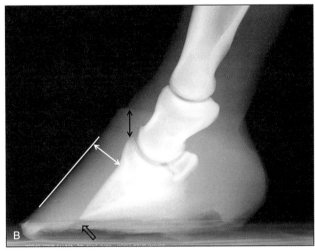

Figure 5.87. In symmetrical distal displacement, the distal phalanx descends within the hoof capsule (A). Therefore, the distal phalanx retains its alignment with the more proximal phalanges and the hoof capsule (B), but the distance between the parietal surface of the distal phalanx and the hoof wall (white arrow) and the distance between the proximal extensor process and the proximal border of hoof wall (black double arrow) increase, and the distance between the distal phalanx and the sole and ground decreases (open arrow).

In a healthy horse, the strength of the laminae greatly exceeds the stresses applied, thereby allowing the distal phalanx to be retained in its normal position. However, in horses with laminitis, the laminar attachments to the distal phalanx are compromised, as discussed above. Partial loss of the laminar attachments causes the remaining intact laminae to endure the entire load of weight-bearing and locomotion, so that the remaining laminae are potentially exposed to a cycle of excessive mechanical stress leading to further dysadhesion or possible tearing and subsequent failure of suspension of the distal phalanx.

The pattern of displacement of the distal phalanx within the hoof capsule varies between horses, and sometimes between an individual horse's feet. The distal phalanx may displace evenly around the circumference of the hoof wall resulting in distal displacement or sinking (Figure 5.87).

Alternatively, the distal phalanx may displace unevenly in relation to the hoof wall. A unilateral distal displacement results in either medial or lateral displacement or sinking of the distal phalanx (Figure 5.88). Although this type of asymmetric displacement is far more uncommon than the dorsal rotational types of distal phalanx displacement, it is important to assess for this because it is a devastating displacement that requires specific foot care.

The most common pattern of asymmetric displacement, rotation of the distal phalanx, occurs when the dorsal distal margin of the distal phalanx moves distally and the dorsal parietal surface of distal phalanx diverges from the dorsal surface of the hoof wall, with the distal aspect of the parietal surface of the phalanx being further displaced from the dorsal hoof wall than the proximal aspect. Rotation is categorized as:

1. Capsular rotation (Figure 5.89): divergence of the parietal surface of the distal phalanx from the dorsal hoof wall (with or without flexion of the DIP joint)

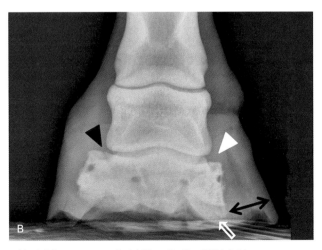

Figure 5.88. In medial or lateral asymmetrical displacement (A), one side of the distal phalanx descends (white open arrow in B). The distance between the wall and the distal phalanx increases (black double arrow), and the distance between the distal phalanx and the sole and ground decreases on the affected side (white open arrow). Additionally, the DIP joint becomes asymmetrical when viewed on a dorsopalmar radiograph; the joint space is increased on the affected side (white arrowhead) and decreased on the unaffected side (black arrowhead).

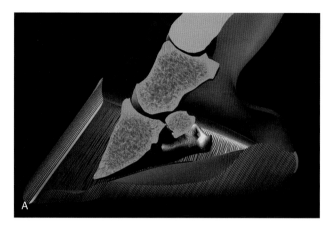
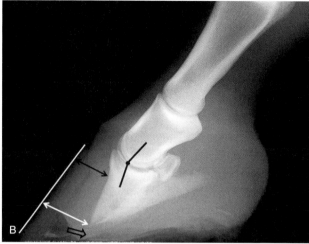

Figure 5.89.   A and B. In horses with early chronic laminitis, the surface of the hoof wall is unchanged, but the distal phalanx rotates about the DIP joint (the joint flexes, black lines in B); consequently, the normal alignment of distal phalanx with the other phalanges is changed (phalangeal rotation). Additionally, the distance between the dorsal distal parietal surface of the distal phalanx and hoof capsule increases (white double arrow) while it remains close to normal proximally (black double arrow); i.e. there is divergence of the surfaces (capsular rotation). Also, the distance between the dorsal margin of the distal phalanx and the sole and ground is decreased (open arrow).

2. Phalangeal rotation (Figure 5.89): Palmar rotation of the distal phalanx (flexion of the DIP joint with or without capsular rotation) in relation to the axis of the phalanges.

In most horses, the pattern of displacement is a combination of distal displacement and rotation of the distal phalanx, although one pattern is usually dominant.

Predisposing Factors

The 3 main presentations of laminitis are those associated with bacterial sepsis, those associated with metabolic/endocrine disorders, and those associated with excessive concussion/weight-bearing. The predisposing diseases associated with bacterial sepsis include retained placenta, surgical acute abdominal cases (usually involving severely compromised segments of the intestine), enterocolitis, pleuropneumonia with a Gram-negative component, and carbohydrate overload (which usually results in a severe transient enterocolitis). Consumption of black walnut shavings may also fit into this group, because a similar systemic inflammation has been reported to occur with the experimental model based on this clinical cause of laminitis. In all of these cases, laminar failure likely results due to systemic and local inflammatory events and related vascular disturbances as detailed earlier in the chapter.

Metabolic/endocrine disorders that predispose to laminitis are primarily associated with equine metabolic syndrome (EMS), also commonly termed "pasture-associated laminitis." Similar to human metabolic syndrome, these animals are commonly obese and insulin resistant (indicated by increased circulating insulin concentrations or abnormal responses to insulin/glucose tolerance tests).[31,76] A low level of systemic inflammation has been reported to be present in horses with EMS (similar to that observed in human metabolic syndrome),[76,77] which may lower their threshold to other insults associated with laminitis. Recent data indicate that other factors of obesity unrelated to insulin resistance may also play a role in EMS. Finally, supporting limb laminitis is a devastating sequela to animals supporting an excessive amount of weight on 1 limb, usually due to an injury to (and commonly orthopedic surgery on) the contralateral limb. Although little is known regarding the pathophysiology of this disease process, there is some evidence that decreased laminar blood flow may play a role in this type of laminar failure.

Clinical Signs

The clinical signs assessed in laminitis mainly refer to the degree of lameness noted and the digital exam. The lameness varies in severity from being barely detectable to an animal that is recumbent the majority of the time due to the digital pain. Due to this variability, more than 60 years ago Obel introduced a grading system to describe the degree of lameness (Table 5.2). Although

Table 5.2.   Obel grades of laminitis.

Grade	Associated lameness and gait abnormalities
1	At rest the horse alternately and incessantly lifts the feet, often at intervals of a few seconds. Lameness is not evident at the walk, but a short stilted gait is noted at the trot
2	The horse moves willingly at a walk, but the gait is stilted. A foot can be lifted off the ground without difficulty.
3	The horse moves very reluctantly, and vigorously resists attempts to have a foot lifted off the ground.
4	The horse refuses to move and will not do so unless forced.

the Obel grading system does not describe all cases of laminitis, it is still used to describe the degree of lameness in both the clinics and when describing time points assessed in laminitis research.

The onset of clinical signs of laminitis commonly occurs 24 to 72 hours following the onset of a septic disease process. The onset of disease in EMS is variable, but commonly occurs in the spring during consumption of lush pasture. In supporting limb laminitis, the onset of disease is also not clear cut, and may occur within days, or occur weeks to months after the onset of excessive weight-bearing in the affected digit. The clinical signs of acute laminitis are characterized by lameness, an increase in the temperature of 1 or more hooves, increased digital pulses, and elicitation of a painful withdrawal response to hoof testers. In EMS and sepsis, the forelimbs are most commonly affected (most likely due to more weight being born by the forelimbs); the hindlimbs may also be involved (usually in severe septic cases). Supporting limb laminitis occurs on the supporting forelimb or hindlimb opposite the nonweight-bearing limb. The characteristic stance of a laminitic horse with both forefeet affected is placement of the forefeet well in front of the normal position and anterior placement of the hind feet in order to shift more weight to the hindlimbs (Figure 5.90).[35]

The characteristic gait of a laminitic horse is stiff limb movement while maintaining the same laminitic posture of both fore- and hindlimbs being placed anteriorly. Horses with distal displacement of the third phalanx more frequently have all 4 feet affected; these horses may have a more normal stance or may appear "camped out" with forelimbs placed more anterior than normal and hindlimbs placed more posterior than normal. The gait may be more normal appearing than with only forelimb involvement (due to all 4 feet being affected), but the animals are usually intensely resistant to movement and more commonly recumbent due to severe pain in all limbs. It is at times difficult to determine whether the forefeet or all 4 feet are affected; short-lived anesthesia (using lidocaine) of the forefeet with abaxial sesamoid nerve blocks helps determine whether any lameness exists in the hindfeet, or if any abnormality noted in hindlimb gait is merely compensation for the painful forelimbs.

Increased hoof temperature and the strength of digital pulses must be interpreted in the context of the lameness and other systemic symptoms, because it is not unusual for an increase in hoof temperature to be transient, and the interpretation of digital pulses is highly subjective. Application of hoof-testers is useful to confirm the presence of pain around the dorsal margins of the sole in cases with mild lameness in which laminitis is suspected. The clinician can also use hoof testers to detect unilateral (more accurately described as uniaxial) pain (medial vs. lateral pain) in unilateral distal displacement. Less commonly, hoof testers can be used to detect heel pain in some chronically affected horses with secondary heel contracture. The veterinarian must keep in mind differential diagnoses such as sole bruising which can present similarly with digital pulses and bilateral pain on hoof testers in the early stages.

Horses with chronic laminitis have different degrees of hoof capsule deformation and lameness. Changes to the hoof capsule vary with the duration of the disease and type of displacement, and may be visible in both the wall and the sole. In the chronic laminitis case with rotation, the wall is unchanged in the immediate period after displacement of the distal phalanx, but commonly assumes a dorsally concave appearance in long-standing cases due to disparate growth between the toes and the heels (slower growth in the toe region). This disparate

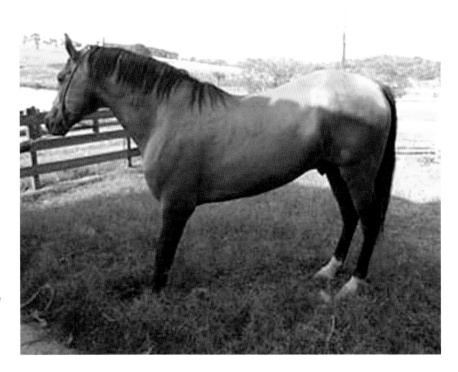

Figure 5.90. Classic stance of a horse with laminitis with the forelimbs placed abnormally far forward and weight shifted toward the hindlimbs. (Courtesy of L. Brandstetter).

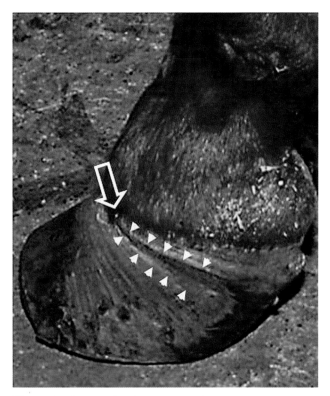

Figure 5.91. This foot from a horse with chronic laminitis demonstrates abnormal hoof growth with wider growth rings at the heel where there is more growth (small arrows), and converging to narrowly placed rings at the toe (large arrow) where minimal hoof growth is occurring. (Courtesy of Dr. Gary Baxter)

growth is also reflected in abnormal growth rings which are more widely spaced in the heel than the toe (Figure 5.91). The sole dorsal to the apex of the frog may be soft and flattened (or convex) due to downward pressure on the sole from the dorsodistal aspect of the displaced distal phalanx secondary to either rotation or distal displacement. The flat, soft character of the sole may lead to bruising around its dorsal margin. The white line may be wider than normal, frequently with elongated keratinized laminae, and show evidence of prior bruising/hemorrhage. In cases of distal displacement of the third phalanx, there may be a palpable (and sometimes visible) groove at the junction of the skin of the pastern and the coronary band. The lameness in the long-standing chronic case is commonly only from excessive sole pressure by the displaced distal phalanx, with no laminar pain present due to healing of the laminae (i.e., the laminae are stable and therefore pain-free even if abnormal morphologically). The most common exception to this is the horse with recurrent laminitis due to either Cushing's syndrome or EMS, in which bouts of laminar injury/instability commonly recur.

Diagnosis

The diagnosis of laminitis may be obvious in acute, severe cases due to the history, characteristic stance, and digital exam. The diagnosis may be much more difficult in chronic mild cases, especially in older horses that may have bilateral distal limb arthropathies contributing to the lameness. In the acute case with severe lameness of the forelimbs, one author (JKB) performs an abaxial sesamoid nerve block with lidocaine (due to the short period of action to limit the possibility of the animal causing further laminar injury by walking excessively on compromised laminae) to:

1. Enable the clinician to rapidly obtain good quality radiographs without undue stress to the horse
2. Enable examination of the solar surface
3. Assess for involvement of the hindlimbs (by limited walking of the horse around the stall in each direction)

In the chronic, mild case, it is best to initially block the digit with a palmar digital (PD) nerve block, which blocks solar pain (a PD nerve block blocks almost all structures within the foot except for the dorsal laminae) due to a displaced distal phalanx,[70,71] but does not appear to block a lameness due to dorsal laminar pain in most horses. Thus, if the PD nerve block abolishes the lameness on the affected digit, it is likely that the pain is entirely due to solar pain and that the laminae are stable. If the PD nerve block does not improve the lameness but an abaxial sesamoid nerve block effectively abolishes it, it is likely that there is still a laminar component to the digital pain (i.e., active laminitis).

In the horse with suspected chronic laminitis in which it is unknown whether the lameness is due to laminitis or other musculoskeletal issues, it is important to perform distal limb flexion prior to nerve blocks; if the horse is severely lame, the response to flexion can be assessed at a walk. A response to flexion usually indicates the presence of an arthropathy unrelated to laminitis, the most common of which is arthropathy of the proximal interphalangeal joint.

To delineate laminar pain from proximal interphalangeal joint pain in the horse that does not respond to a PD nerve block, the clinician can assess laminar pain by performing a modified ring block immediately proximal to the coronary band to block the dorsal branches of the PD nerve. When attempting to rule out the other common cause of bilateral forelimb lameness, navicular syndrome/palmar heel pain, the history, presentation, and radiographs are valuable in addition to the response to nerve blocks. Because both palmar heel pain and solar pain in the chronic laminitis case respond to PD nerve anesthesia, radiographs should be the differentiating factor because displacement of the distal phalanx causes the solar pain in laminitis and should be evident on radiographic imaging. As discussed above, the lameness will usually not block out with PD anesthesia if there is laminar pain present in the chronic laminitis case. In some severely painful cases, the lameness may not block out entirely with local perineural anesthesia.

Radiography

Radiography is not only critical as a diagnostic tool to determine the presence of the disease, but is also critical to monitor progress of the disease and guide treatment. Radiographs should be taken at the first sign of acute laminitis to serve as a baseline for subsequent radiographic comparisons and determine if pre-existing radiographic changes suggestive of previous laminitis are present. The most important views are the lateral and the dorsopalmar/plantar projections (Figures 5.88, 5.92, and 5.93). For both of these projections, it is important that the foot is placed on a block, and that the X-ray beam is centered as close as possible to the solar margin of the distal phalanx (approximately 1.5 cm proximal to the surface of the block).

Early radiographic signs suggestive of distal displacement of the distal phalanx include widening of the distance between the dorsal hoof wall and the parietal surface of the distal phalanx,[23] and increased vertical distance from the proximal aspect of the extensor process to the firm proximal border of the hoof wall located immediately distal to coronary band (sometimes termed the founder surface of the hoof capsule). It is important to ensure that the lateral radiographic view is a true lateral; rotation of the axis of the foot by more than 10° causes the degree of rotation to be underestimated.[40]

A radiopaque object or paste can be applied to the mid-dorsal hoof wall and should end at the level of the coronary band to help identify it (Figure 5.92). The distance between the dorsal surface of the hoof capsule and the parietal surface of the distal phalanx is best measured as a line vertical to the parietal surface of the distal phalanx, and should be measured immediately distal to the base of the extensor process (in Figure 5.92b) to limit the effect of any rotation on the measurement. This calculation is a relatively repeatable measure of the displacement (13 to 20 mm in normal horses, depending on size) in horses in which the distal phalanx has undergone distal displacement. In normal horses (approximately 450 kg), the distance should be less than 18 to 20 mm (reported means of 14.6–16.3 mm).

An accurate measurement that takes into context the magnification and the size of the foot is the ratio between this dorsal measurement and the palmar cortical length of the distal phalanx measured from the dorsodistal tip of the bone to its articulation with the navicular bone (in Figure 5.92c). This ratio, which should be less than 28% in the normal horse, indicates possible distal displacement from 28% to 32%, and indicates likely displacement if greater than 32%. The vertical distance from the extensor process to the firm proximal border of the hoof wall is also well used and is −2–10 mm in normal horses, depending on size (Figure 5.92a).[23] Unilateral distal displacement can only be reliably assessed on a dorsopalmar/dorsoplantar projection (Figure 5.88).

Palmar/plantar rotation of the distal phalanx away from the dorsal hoof wall resulting in an angle greater than 5° confirms the diagnosis of laminitis due to capsular rotation (normal horses can have angles less than 4°). Two types of rotation can be assessed. Capsular rotation, the degree of rotation between the dorsal hoof wall and the parietal surface of the distal phalanx (α in Figure 5.93), is best used in the acute stage because it can be difficult to assess due to deformation of the hoof wall in chronic cases. The angle of solar margin of the distal phalanx to the ground surface (β in Figure 5.93) is a more accurate angle to assess in the chronic case with wall deformation when assessing clinical options. Serial radiographs should be taken to monitor the progression of the disease and determine the success of selected treatments. Digital venography in the standing horse has been developed as a prognostic aid to assess the vasculature of the digit. Venograms, in which there is no filling of contrast of the laminar vessels, the circumflex area, and the terminal arch, are reported to indicate an extremely poor prognosis for recovery.[67]

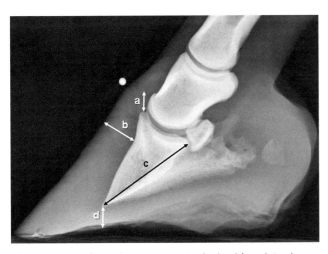

Figure 5.92. Several measurements obtained from lateral radiographs of the digit can be used to assess horses with distal displacement of the distal phalanx. a = distance from the proximal extensor process to the proximal aspect of the hoof wall (immediately distal to coronary band), b = the distance from the dorsal parietal surface of the distal phalanx to the dorsal surface of the hoof capsule, b/c = the ratio of the distance from the dorsal parietal surface of the distal phalanx to the dorsal surface of the hoof capsule (b) to the length of the palmar cortex of the distal phalanx (c), and d = the distance from the dorsodistal tip of the distal phalanx to the ground surface of the sole.

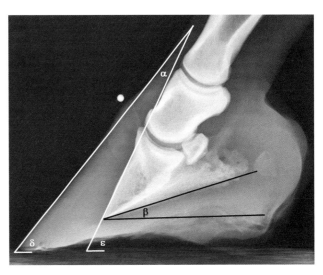

Figure 5.93. For assessment of rotation of the distal phalanx, the clinician can assess the degree of capsular rotation (angle α) at the intersection of the dorsal capsular and dorsal phalangeal lines, or can measure the difference between the dorsal angles δ and ε. The relationship of the solar margin of the distal phalanx to the ground surface of the foot can be assessed by measuring angle β.

Treatment

The goal in the general treatment of the acute laminitis case is to stabilize the digit in the short term regardless of the degree of displacement. In the authors' opinion, if the clinician can attain stabilization of the digital laminae for approximately 3 weeks, distal phalangeal displacement can be addressed with other techniques including corrective shoeing and possibly deep digital flexor tenotomy in nonresponsive cases. In regard to foot support, the veterinarian must be willing to try a variety of techniques (discussed below) in attempt to find the type of digital support that the animal responds to favorably.

Medical Therapy

ANTI-INFLAMMATORY THERAPY

Anti-inflammatory therapy has endured as a central component of laminitis pharmacotherapy over the years. As discussed above, there is compelling evidence to use nonsteroidal anti-inflammatory drugs (NSAIDs) due to marked inflammatory events occurring both prior to and at the onset of lameness in the laminitic horse. Therefore, aggressive, prudent use of NSAIDs is indicated in the horse known to be at risk of laminitis (i.e., colitis, grain overload, etc.) until approximately 48 to 72 hours after the animal is not showing clinical signs of systemic inflammation/toxemia.

In addition to blocking COX enzyme activity, high doses of NSAIDs recently have been found in other species to block other inflammatory pathways including some controlling basic inflammatory gene expression (i.e., NFKB pathway important in proinflammatory cytokine expression), now known to occur in the early stages of laminitis.[15] COX-2 has recently been shown to be an important mediator in the synapses of sensory neurons; therefore, COX-2 inhibition is likely to not only decrease laminar inflammation, but to decrease central pain sensation. Due to the gastrointestinal and renal toxicity caused by NSAIDs, close attention must be paid to the animal's history (i.e., a history of gastric/colon ulcers or renal disease), the animal's hydration status, and laboratory work in the critical case to assess renal function.

The 4 main NSAIDs available to the equine clinician are 3 nonselective COX-1/COX-2 inhibitors (flunixin meglumine, phenylbutazone [PBZ], and ketoprofen) and 1 COX-2 selective NSAID, firocoxib. There is some question whether, during treatment with a COX-2 selective NSAID in the peracute phase of laminitis, the vascular inflammation/injury occurring in the laminae may place the digit at risk of the same vascular accidents (thrombosis leading to myocardial infarction and stroke) that have resulted with the use of COX-2 selective drugs in humans (i.e., the more potent Coxibs such as rofecoxib in humans with compromised vasculature). Thus, until proven otherwise, it may be best to use a nonselective drug in the peracute stage and consider firocoxib in the chronic, long-term case in which the drug's decreased incidence of side effects is more important. Meloxicam is available in countries other than the U.S., and may be of value due to slight COX-2 selectivity (approximately 2- to 3-fold), which appears to make

it a very safe option due to a low incidence of side effects but possibly fewer chances of unwanted vascular events.[16]

In the horse still demonstrating signs of systemic illness with a possible ongoing bacterial toxemia (i.e., colitis), flunixin meglumine is indicated due to its increased efficacy against endotoxemia. In the animal that has a stable hydration status and no indication of renal compromise or intestinal ulceration, the use of high dose (1.1 mg/kg IV TID) flunixin may be indicated for up to 3 to 5 days; the author decreases the dosage after 3 days if the source of bacterial toxemia appears to be resolving. If the lameness does not improve with flunixin, it is indicated to either add other types of analgesics (see CRI, below) or possibly lower the flunixin dosage by half and add 4.4 mg/kg phenylbutazone SID.

In the animal demonstrating renal compromise or clinical signs of gastrointestinal ulceration, ketoprofen is indicated due to its reported efficacy regarding ameliorating endotoxin effects and lameness,[8,57] and a markedly increased margin of safety when compared to flunixin or phenylbutazone.[49] Due to the poor response when the drug is only administered BID and the incredible safety of the drug, the BID dosage of ketoprofen can be administered QID (2.2 mg/kg IV QID). Due to a clinically apparent "peak and trough" analgesic effect between ketoprofen dosages in some animals, it may be indicated to administer 2.2 mg/kg phenylbutazone SID in order to have a more consistent NSAID effect.

Analgesia in the chronic case mainly consists of phenylbutazone (PBZ) therapy, with long-term doses usually in the range of 2 to 3 grams/day to avoid complications. An important reason for PBZ's higher incidence of toxicity when compared to the other NSAIDs (almost every reported case of NSAID-related right dorsal colon ulceration has been due to PBZ) is that the drug has a longer half-life and accumulates in the tissues to a much greater degree than either flunixin or ketoprofen. Therefore, one way to avoid toxicity in animals on long-term PBZ therapy cease administration of the drug for 24 hours once every 5 to 7 days to allow clearance of PBZ from the system. If the animals are too painful to be without an NSAID for 24 hours, either ketoprofen or flunixin may be given without interfering with the clearance of PBZ. Firocoxib has the advantage of once a day treatment, and is much more protective against GI concerns than PBZ; however, it takes several days to obtain effective tissue levels at recommended doses, indicating that another faster acting NSAID should be used in the acute stages.

Pentoxifylline is reported to be anti-inflammatory due to its "anti-TNF" effect;[7] preliminary results from a study using the carbohydrate model indicate a decreased incidence of laminar failure in animals with pentoxifylline therapy initiated at the time of intragastric administration of carbohydrate.[25] It is unknown whether the efficacy is due to inhibition of inflammatory signaling, inhibition of matrix metalloproteases, or any hemorrheologic effect (not likely as requires prolonged therapy to achieve this effect in other species). Digital "cryotherapy" (hypothermia) may possibly address inflammation because it has been shown in one CHO laminitis model (Belknap, Pollitt, and Van Eps, unpublished data) and in some *in vivo* investigations in other species to decrease the expression of genes involved in inflammation.[32,45] Although intravenous lidocaine infusion, similar to that used for treatment of ileus in the equine patient, has been proposed as a treatment to decrease inflammatory signaling in laminitis, a recent study indicated no anti-inflammatory and actually some proinflammatory properties of constant-rate intravenous lidocaine infusion in a laminitis model.[83]

THERAPY REGARDING MATRIX METALLOPROTEASE INHIBITION

Although many practitioners have recently used tetracyclines in laminitis cases based on the drugs' reported MMP inhibitory properties, preliminary data from an equine study indicate that doxycycline is a poor inhibitor of equine MMPs of interest (MMP-2 and MMP-9), and oxytetracycline inhibits MMPs *in vitro* but was ineffective in treating the disease in a model of laminitis.[25] The efficacy of pentoxifylline in ameliorating the severity of laminitis in the CHO model may also be due to its anti-MMP effects. The author of the recent study[48] that questions the role of MMP-2 and -9 due to finding neither protein in the active state in protein extracts of clinical cases of laminitis also states that MMP-2 may be active *in situ* (i.e., MMP2 inhibitors that may inhibit MMP-2 in protein extracts may not have access to the enzyme in the laminar interstitium *in situ*) in the laminae and may still possibly play an important role (Sam Black, University of Massachusetts, personal communication).

DRUGS APPROACHING BLOOD FLOW

The majority of drugs that have been introduced for treatment of possible decreased laminar blood flow have been demonstrated to be ineffective in increasing laminar blood flow in the horse (i.e., isoxsuprine, pentoxifylline, and nitroglycerin paste). The only drug demonstrated to increase digital blood flow is the phenothiazine tranquilizer, acepromazine, which only increases flow for a short period of time (approximately 30 minutes) when administered intramuscularly.[43]

ANTICOAGULANT THERAPY

An area that probably needs revisiting is that of treatments addressing platelet activation and coagulation, with low-molecular-weight heparin (LMWH) likely offering the most advantages. Controversy exists about the use of heparin in horses with laminitis. Whereas heparin was initially used in medicine only as an anticoagulant, it is now realized that this class of drugs also has anti-inflammatory properties (somewhat due to the fact that platelets and factors involved in coagulation can have pro-inflammatory properties). Recently, heparin was reported to have potential anti-inflammatory effects on equine endothelium exposed to the deleterious activity of neutrophil-derived myeloperoxidase (MPO).[65] However, there are confounding data from retrospective clinical studies on the efficacy of heparin as a prophylaxis in horses at risk of laminitis.[14,22] Furthermore, experimental treatment with heparin 24 hours after CHO administration did not ameliorate signs of laminitis or laminar lesions.[50] One problem

with previous heparin studies is that unfractionated heparin was used, which induces autoagglutination of equine red blood cells and become lodged in capillaries (including laminar capillaries); this event may further compromise affected laminar capillaries in laminitis. LMWH may be a valuable alternative because it does not cause equine RBC autoagglutination and has recently been reported to reduce the incidence and severity of laminitis in postoperative colic cases.[24]

ANALGESIC THERAPY

Recently there has been interest in constant-rate infusion (CRI) of analgesic drugs to supplement NSAID therapy in decreasing the level of pain suffered by laminitis patients. A recently presented "Pentafusion" is a combination of ketamine, morphine, lidocaine, detomidine, and acepromazine (Eric Abrahamsen, BEVA Proceedings, 2005).[1] The CRI is a valuable addition to laminitis therapy because it takes some of the humane concerns away from the owner and veterinarian treating an animal in severe pain. Some of these drugs also affect gastrointestinal motility; therefore, the animals must be monitored closely for large intestinal motility/impaction. Additionally, the animals may become unstable or overly sedate if the CRI rate is excessive. Finally, an epidural can be considered for analgesia in hindlimb laminitis.

Hoof Care in the Treatment of Acute and Early Chronic Laminitis

In the acute and early chronic laminitis case, it is likely that laminar instability remains a prominent factor. As discussed previously, one author (JKB) uses a low PD nerve block to assess whether the pain originates from the sole or the dorsal laminae (indicative of ongoing instability). Ideally, in horses with severe acute and early chronic laminitis, the force of the horse's weight on the feet should be reduced. To this end, slings have been used to relieve partial weight-bearing, but availability and inadequate tolerance by the horse frequently result in failure of this effort. Therefore, measures are aimed directly at the foot. The two main objectives of hoof care are to redistribute the force of weight-bearing away from the wall and to decrease the extensor moment about the DIP joint.

Several measures of varying efficacy attempt to redirect weight-bearing away from the wall by recruiting the frog, bars, and all or part of the sole to bear weight. However, as discussed in Chapter 8, it must be remembered that the physiological role of the sole in weight-bearing is undetermined. The amount of the ground surface that can be recruited to bear weight is highly variable between horses. In general, once the distal phalanx has displaced, pressure over the sole under the displaced distal phalanx increases discomfort. Thus, the clinician must weigh the benefits of possibly decreasing laminar stress by applying solar support with the risk of causing excessive solar pressure and worsening the pain (and possibly the pathologic process). Before considering other measures, the clinician must decide whether to leave shoes on the feet if the horse is shod. Shoes on firm surfaces concentrate stress around the perimeter of the foot (e.g., the hoof wall and laminae), and therefore removing them will likely be beneficial by removing this effect. Removing shoes also makes other therapeutic measures more feasible, including recruiting other parts of the ground surface of the foot for weight-bearing and modifying break-over. The potential disadvantage of removing shoes in horses with laminitis is that the removal process itself may cause additional trauma to the laminae.

The simplest way to recruit the sole, frog, and bars for weight-bearing is to place the horse on bedding material that readily conforms to the shape of the foot. In this regard, sand is significantly better than shavings. Peat has also been used. Deep deformable substrates also permit the horse to adjust the angle of its foot to optimize comfort. However, the deep deformable substrates are not selective in how pressure is applied to the ground surface of the foot. Various devices and materials have been placed under the frog, sole, and bars to recruit varying amounts of weight-bearing. These include rolled gauze, Lilly pads, silicone putty, Styrofoam insulation board (usually 2-inch board), closed cell foam (1.5 inches thick, 4 lbs/ft^3 density), and commercial pad systems such as the Soft-Ride boots (Soft-Ride, Inc., Vermillion, OH). The closed cell foam has the advantages of not crushing like Styrofoam does, and it can be cut to bevel the ground surface to move the break-over palmarly. The softer materials may offer the additional advantage of softening impact during locomotion. Rigid materials may transfer weight-bearing more effectively, but are discouraged because they are more likely to cause focal pressure under the margin of the distal phalanx and pain, and should therefore be generally avoided or only used with caution.

The moment or torque about the DIP joint at rest can be decreased by elevating the heels. This decreases the tension in the DDFT, and therefore the tension in the dorsal laminae. This is more likely to benefit horses that have or are about to develop capsular rotation, and is unlikely to help (and may hurt) those that have or are prone to distal displacement. The arm of the extensor moment at break-over can be shortened by moving the point of break-over palmar to the dorsal margin of the toe (Chapter 8). This may be done by rasping the ground surface of the hoof or incorporating it into a supporting device. Commercial plastic cuff and pad combinations conveniently combine a wedged heel and eased break-over (i.e., the Nanric Ultimate, Nanric Co., Lawrenceburg, KY).

Treatment must be titrated to the severity of the disease. Currently it is not routinely possible to assess the degree of injury to the laminae, so the severity of the disease for each type of displacement is usually determined by clinical parameters such as heart rate, the severity of the lameness, response to treatment, and radiographic changes. In the early stages of therapy, the intensity of therapy initiated depends on the severity of clinical signs (i.e., not all horses need all of the measures described). However, in the horse that has undergone treatment and appears to be improving, it is advisable to gradually discontinue treatments, withdrawing 1 treatment measure at a time followed by 2 to 3 days of observation. In more mildly affected horses, treatment may be discontinued over 1 to 2 weeks. However, in severely affected horses, the treatment should be tapered off over 6 to 8 weeks as the treatment switches to that for the chronic laminitic patient.

Treatment of Active and Stable Chronic Laminitis

The objectives for maintaining stability of the distal phalanx and pain control are similar to that of the acute and early laminitic horse. An additional goal is to restore the relationship between the hoof capsule and the distal phalanx. The management varies with the type of displacement, severity of lameness, way in which the horse moves, and stability of the distal phalanx. The treatment of dorsal capsular rotation, symmetrical distal displacement, and asymmetrical displacement are considered separately.

HOOF CARE IN THE TREATMENT OF HORSES WITH ROTATION

The challenge of treating horses with rotation, usually both capsular and phalangeal, is to realign the phalangeal axis while simultaneously realigning the hoof wall with the parietal surface of the distal phalanx (while also controlling pain). Complications are common and must be managed as they occur. The mainstay of treatment is hoof care, but various surgical techniques may be required.

Trimming and shoeing of the foot should be planned based on radiographic observations.[55,66] Dorsopalmar and mediolateral radiographs should both be taken (as described earlier) prior to shoeing. The guiding principles are as follows:

1. Realign the phalangeal axis by trimming
2. Preserve the thickness of the sole
3. Recruit weight-bearing by the ground surface of the foot
4. Move the break-over in a palmar/plantar direction
5. Reduce the tension in the DDFT

The trim should aim to restore the angle that the solar margin of the distal phalanx forms with the ground to between 0° and 5° (in severe cases, it may be preferable to aim for 5° vs. 0°). At the same time, the sole depth should be preserved to at least 15 mm wherever possible. In horses in which the dorsal sole is greater than 15 mm in depth, the trim is along a single plane from the dorsal margin of the sole all the way to the heels (Figure 5.94A). However, in most horses with rotation, the depth of the dorsal sole is significantly less than 15 mm due to the distally displaced dorsodistal aspect of the distal phalanx.

To attempt to realign the distal phalanx with the ground surface with the sole by trimming the ground surface of the foot to one plane would inevitably decrease the thickness of the dorsal sole further. Therefore, only that portion of the foot with greater than 15 mm sole depth is trimmed, which is usually the palmar 50% to 70% of the sole (Figure 5.94B). This results in 2 separate planes for the dorsal and palmar portions of the foot (Figure 5.94B). The dorsal plane of the foot is brought into line with the palmar plane at the time of shoeing, usually by filling the gap with a synthetic polymer. The plane for trimming is identified on the radiograph by drawing a line parallel to and

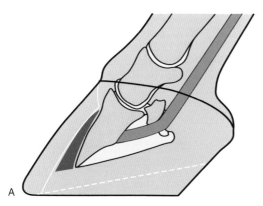 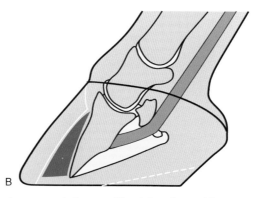

Figure 5.94. A. When the depth of the sole exceeds approximately 15 mm across the sole, the alignment of the distal phalanx with the solar surface of the foot can be achieved by trimming the entire ground surface of the foot on a single plane (dashed line). B. When the dorsal sole is less that 15 mm, which is common in horses with rotation, the goal is to preserve the dorsal sole, yet still realign the distal phalanx for shoeing. The palmar ground surface is trimmed (dashed line) on a different plane to the dorsal half (which is not trimmed).

15 mm distal to the solar margin of the distal phalanx (Figure 5.92).

Some horses, particularly those with mild rotation and sufficient sole depth, may be managed with trimming and maintaining them on a soft ground substrate without shoeing.

Once the foot has been trimmed, the clinician must decide whether or not to shoe the horse, and if so, which type of shoe to use and how to attach it. The shoe may be attached to the foot with nails, directly with glue, with glue and a cuff, or, in some instances, with cast material (i.e., the wooden shoe). Most frequently, shoes are nailed to the foot in the traditional manner. However, when nailing the shoe in place is considered too painful or there is insufficient hoof wall to which to nail, a less traumatic technique using a combination of adhesives, casting tape, and screws may be used. When selecting a shoe, it is important to remember that there are several underlying principles, and numerous ways of achieving them. The underlying principles or goals of shoeing include:

1. Moving the center of pressure
2. Changing the area of distribution of force
3. Decreasing the shock of impact
4. Enhancing ease of movement
5. Protecting parts of the foot

Enhancing ease of movement involves decreasing the moment arm about the DIP joint and smoothing out break-over. This is most beneficial in the dorsopalmar plane, in which the objective is accomplished by rolling the toe, setting the shoe back, squaring the toe, or using an open toe shoe. However, to a lesser extent, break-over in a medial or lateral direction can be eased by the use of rails, rounding the medial and lateral branches of the shoe, or using a Steward clog with beveled sides.

The center of pressure may be moved in relation to the center of the ground surface of the foot and/or the center of rotation of the DIP joint by using extensions (usually the medial or lateral side to address unilateral distal displacement), elevating one side of the foot (usually the palmar aspect/heel in cases of rotation), or recruiting more ground surface to bear weight on one area of the foot than another (usually by filling the palmar ground surface with a resilient putty to support the distal phalanx while protecting the toe from excess pressure). In doing so, weight-bearing can be moved away from the most affected laminae.

Increasing the area of distribution of weight across part or all of ground surface of the foot is theoretically performed to transfer weight-bearing from affected laminae to the sole, bars, and frog to decrease stress in the affected laminae. However, the role of the sole in weight-bearing to spare weight-bearing by the wall has been questioned (See Therapeutic Shoeing in Chapter 8). Regardless of the theoretical considerations, some horses appear to benefit greatly from sole support. Support of the ground surface of the foot is most readily accomplished with the use of synthetic polymers such as polymerized silicone (two-part putties such as the impression material [EDSS, Penrose, CO] or advanced cushion support [NANRIC, Lawrenceburg, KY]) or polyurethane ("pour-in pads") in the space between the branches of the shoe. However, support of the ground surface is also still approached by more traditional means such as pads and heart-bar shoes.

Several shoe types have been used to address these goals including regular keg shoes, egg-bar shoes, reverse shoes, heart-bar shoes, four-point rail shoes, and wooden shoes/clogs. Each deserves consideration to examine how it accomplishes the goals and to discuss its advantages and limitations.

The keg shoe must be modified to be effective in the treatment of active and stable chronic laminitis. Break-over in the dorsopalmar plane can be eased by forging the toe of the shoe to square and roll it, and setting the shoe back. Easing break-over in the medial and lateral directions can be achieved to a limited extent by rounding/beveling the outside rims of the branches of the shoe. Heel elevation can be added as needed by using a shoe with a built-in wedge or using a wedge pad, frequently a wedge rim pad. The wedge rim pad allows incorporation of as much of the ground surface of the foot as needed for weight-bearing using a synthetic polymer in the concavity of the foot between the branches of the shoe (and rim pads).

The egg-bar shoe (Figure 5.95) is probably the most common shoe used because it is readily available and many farriers and veterinarians are familiar with its use in other circumstances. It can be modified in all the same ways as the keg shoe, and it has the added benefit of the bar that extends in a palmar direction. The palmarly extended nature of the bar causes it to act as a mild wedge when the horse stands on a soft surface by acting like a "snowshoe" and inhibiting sinking of the heel. This decreases tension in the DDFT, and hence theoretically decreases the tension placed on the dorsal laminae.

The reverse shoe combines the advantages of the egg-bar shoe with an open toe. The open toe theoretically offers superior easement of break-over in the dorsopalmar plane when compared to a closed toe shoe. However, the open toe also has the potential disadvantages of concentrating stress at the dorsal margin of the branches and not protecting the toe in horses with dorsal solar concerns such as solar prolapse dorsal to the frog. While this shoe currently appears to have fallen out of favor, it may offer a simple solution, particularly when used in horses in which access is needed to the dorsal aspect of the sole.

The heart-bar shoe (Figure 5.96) has been the traditional mainstay in the treatment of horses with laminitis.[20] The heart-bar is a V-shaped piece of bar stock that has been welded between the branches of the shoe to cover the frog. Alternatively, the heart bar may be forged into the shoe, either by hand or during manufacture. As such, it can be modified in the same manner as the keg shoe. The original rationale behind employing this shoe is that it recruits weight-bearing by the frog, and hence decreases weight-bearing by the laminae. An alternative explanation for the effectiveness of this shoe is that it increases the ground surface area of the shoe in the palmar half of the foot and hence either acts as a mild wedge or at least decreases the descent of the heels into a soft substrate.

The overall principles involved in trimming and setting the shoe are similar to those of the keg shoe. However, care must be taken to ensure that there is not undue pressure from the heart-bar on the frog which would result in bruising and increase lameness. Because of this concern, many farriers leave a small space between the frog and heart-bar, and apply a synthetic polymer underneath the heart bar; synthetic polymer can also be placed alongside the heart bar between the branches of the shoe. The heart bar may also be used in conjunction with an open toe or egg-bar shoe.

The four-point rail shoe is based on the pattern of an open-heeled shoe.[66] The toe of the shoe is squared, aggressively rolled, and broadened. Additionally, narrow wedges, called rails, are applied to the axial side of the ground surface of each branch to raise the heels. Thus, this shoe by design incorporates both ease of

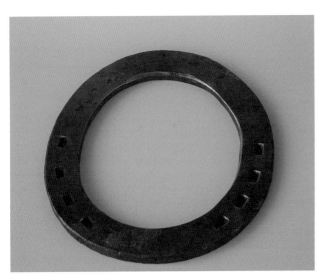

Figure 5.95. Egg-bar shoe.

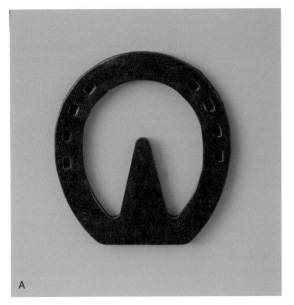
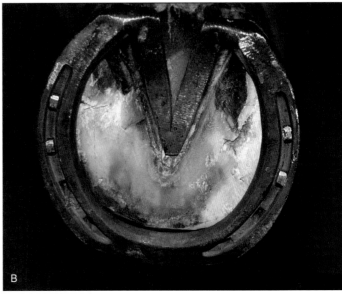

Figure 5.96. Heart bar shoe (A) with correct placement on the foot (B).

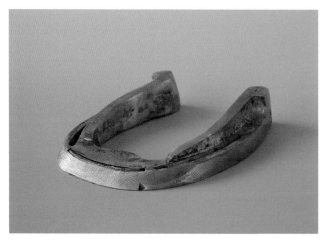

Figure 5.97. A hand-forged aluminum four-point rail shoe. Note the squaring and rolling of the toe (shoe courtesy of Neal Baggett).

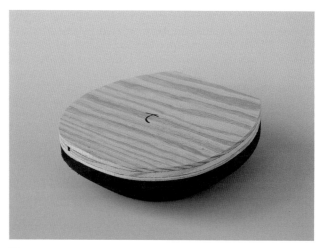

Figure 5.99. A commercially available EVA/wood laminated clog shoe (Equicast, Inc.).

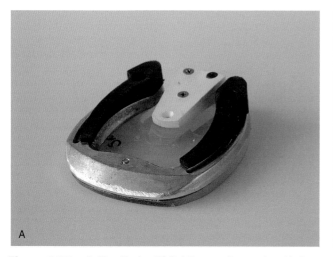

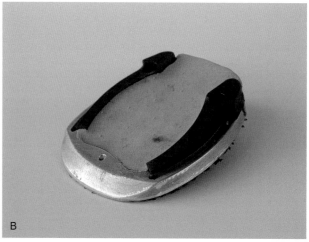

Figure 5.98. A. The Equine Digital Support System is a kit that provides a convenient way to adjust the break-over, support the ground surface of the foot, and elevate the heels.

B. As an alternative to using all the components of the kit, ground support may also be provided with polymerized silicone.

break-over at the toe and elevation of the heel. The use of the rails applied to the axial side of the branch of the shoe also provides improved medial and lateral break-over compared to other designs of shoe used for laminitis.

While the shoe may be hand forged or modified (Figure 5.97), the majority of those used are one of two commercially available designs, the Aluminum Four-Point Rail Shoe and the Equine Digital Support System (EDSS; Figure 5.98). The Aluminum Four-Point Rail Shoe is manufactured to incorporate all the features of the four-point rail shoe in a single unit, with incorporation of the rail into the shoe. The EDSS is marketed in the form of a kit (Figure 5.98). The kit includes a flat shoe with the break-over previously described and a range of rails of different heights that can be attached to the ground surface of the shoe. Additionally, the kit contains pads, frog-shaped inserts, and silicone putty.

The advantage of the Aluminum Four-Point Rail Shoe is simplicity of construction and application;

recruitment of the sole, frog, and bars to bear weight is achieved with a synthetic polymer. The disadvantage of this shoe compared to the EDSS is that the rails are of fixed height (although they can be ground down as needed), and cannot be readily adjusted once the shoe is on the foot. The advantages of the EDSS system are that the rails can be applied after the shoe is on the foot, and the height of the rails can be selected/adjusted. The kit is designed to recruit weight-bearing by applying a pad between the shoe and foot in conjunction with silicone putty placed between the pad and foot; plastic frog inserts can be screwed to the ground surface of the pad. Alternatively, the shoe and rails can be used with a synthetic polymer placed in the concavity of the foot and between the branches of the shoe instead of the pad and frog insert.

The Steward Clog/wooden shoe (Figure 5.99) as originally described is cut from 0.75″ plywood to correspond to the size of the foot, with a squared toe and a 45° degree bevel all around its perimeter so that the ground surface is smaller than the foot surface.[73] The thickness of the shoe may be increased by the addition of an additional three-quarters inch of plywood or rubber similarly beveled and added to the ground surface of the shoe. The shoe is set back from the toe so that the dorsal margin of the shoe is approximately 1.5 inches dorsal to the apex of the frog. Silicone putty is applied between the hoof and the shoe (most attempt to apply caudal to the apex of the frog to avoid excessive toe pressure), and the shoe is attached with screws.

If additional stabilization is needed, an adhesive or a 2-inch roll of casting tape may be applied over the screw heads and distal wall. Furthermore, the shoe is open to almost infinite customization, more common forms of which include adding a wedge or recessing the dorsal solar surface for horses with solar prolapse. This shoe is simple to make and apply. By varying its customization, it can achieve all of the goals previously outlined. In addition, it has been postulated that the thickness of the shoe elevates the forelimbs sufficiently to aid the horse by moving additional weight onto the hindlimbs. Although the shoe is primarily used on forelimbs, Steward has used a shorter variety of the clog on hindlimbs (Mike Steward, personal communication).

The Sigafoos Series II shoe (Figure 5.100) is a kit that is comprised of a cuff bonded to a rim that is attached to an aluminum plate that covers the ground surface of the foot. The aluminum plates may be flat or wedged and have a urethane bonding surface to which additional wedges may be bonded. This shoe can be highly customized to achieve the principal objectives. The attachment of the shoe with a cuff is atraumatic compared with nailing a shoe on, and placement of the acrylic on the outside of the wall causes less harm to the wall than when the acrylic is placed on the ground surface of the wall. Because the cuffed shoes follow the perimeter of the hoof capsule, they may require more extensive modification to set the toe back compared to other methods of shoe application.

The choice of shoe for each case is in large part personal preference based on experience and availability. It is important to emphasize principles over technique.

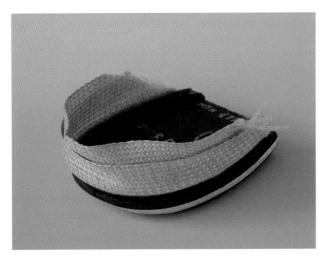

Figure 5.100. Sigafoos Series II Shoe.

There are several complications common to various shoeing techniques. Where weight-bearing has been relieved at the toe and concentrated at the quarters, the wall at the quarters is likely to become thinner and less resilient. Additionally, prolonged heel elevation frequently leads to heel contraction. Finally, prolonged attachment of the shoe with acrylics leads to deterioration in the mechanical properties of the wall, particularly if it is applied to the ground surface of the wall.

The application of the general shoeing principles must be titrated to the specific symptoms of the individual horse. The less damaged the laminae, the less aggressively eased break-over, ground support, and heel elevation are required. Improving the ease of break-over benefits any horse with laminitis. The amount of area across the ground surface of the foot that should be used to distribute weight-bearing is subjective. Pressure should be limited where compression of the underlying dermis may occur between the sole and an unstable or displaced distal phalanx. Otherwise, the comfort of the horse and the perceived instability of the distal phalanx are the best indicators. The requirement for (and degree of) heel elevation is in part similarly determined by the discomfort of the animal, but also by the way the horse lands. Adjusting the heel height so that the horse lands slightly heel first is likely to result in the greatest comfort and stability of the distal phalanx.

The treatment time scale is highly variable and based on the severity of the original disease, recurrence of the disease, and the development of complications. However, some generalizations can be made. A more severely affected horse that is amenable to treatment and improves in an uncomplicated manner is usually shod somewhere between 3 and 6 weeks after the onset of the acute disease with eased break-over, ground surface support, and heel elevation as needed. It is desirable to remove heel elevation as soon as possible after the horse is comfortable landing with a flat foot to limit contraction of the heels, usually between 3 and 6 months. Sole support may be removed, usually in a gradual manner, between 4 and 8 months. The most successful cases may return to near normal shoeing or barefoot trimming between 8 and 12 months. Obviously, less severely affected horses that do not develop complications should recover correspondingly quicker. Horses that suffer recurrent acute episodes or develop complications may take much longer to respond or never respond satisfactorily.

TREATMENT OF CHRONIC LAMINITIS WITH DISTAL DISPLACEMENT

Horses that suffer distal displacement present different challenges from those with dorsal rotation. First, treatment directed at the acute and early chronic disease frequently lasts considerably longer that that for horses with rotation. Easement of break-over and ground surface support are both potentially beneficial and achieved in the same manner as previously described. However, there is no rationale or perceived benefit to elevating the heels; this commonly makes these horses worse. The wooden shoe/clog has gained a great deal of popularity in the treatment of distal displacement in the forelimbs.

TREATMENT OF CHRONIC LAMINITIS WITH UNILATERAL DISTAL DISPLACEMENT (MEDIAL OR LATERAL ROTATION)

The transition between the hoof care used to treat horses with acute and early chronic disease to that of stable chronic laminitis due to unilateral displacement is more blurred than in the previous scenarios because there is much less experience in treating this condition, and complications, particularly separation of the coronary band, are common. However, in line with the overall objective to redirect the load away from the most damaged area of the laminae, the logical approach is to attempt to redirect the load to the opposite side of the foot in conjunction with ground surface support.[56] This can be accomplished by either placing a 4- to 8-mm extension (concentrating ground support on the extended side; Figure 5.101) or placing a thin wedge on the side of the foot opposite the displacement. Of these treatments, the wedge is the most aggressive. Therefore, starting with an extension or modifying ground surface support is suggested. The application of a wedge to the unaffected side of the foot appears counterintuitive if only the radiographic position of the distal phalanx within the hoof capsule is considered because it is natural to try and restore the alignment of the DIP joint. However, consideration of the stresses within the laminae suggests that restoring the symmetry of the DIP joint is likely to be counterproductive. Unilateral distal displacement frequently occurs with some rotation, in which circumstances heel elevation may also be warranted. While this technique has been beneficial in some

horses, more experience is required before firm recommendations are possible.

Casting and Splinting

Casting the distal limb is beneficial in horses with acute and early chronic laminitis, but is particularly valuable in the treatment of chronic cases with unilateral complications such as subsolar abscessation (Figure 5.102). Half-limb casts, half-limb casts with transfixation pins, and open soled half-limb casts have been used (Figure 5.102).[10] However, foot or pastern casts may also provide some stability to the laminae. If fit snugly at the proximal end of the metacarpus, the half-limb casts potentially offer some weight sparing by the digit. However, transfixation pin casts are likely to provide dramatically greater load sparing by the foot. Additionally, by decreasing movement within the distal limb, casts may decrease the pain as the horse moves around a stall. Open soled casts offer the advantage that the ground surface of the foot can be inspected and treated while the foot is in the cast (Figure 5.102B) and that load bearing by the ground surface of the foot may be more selectively applied using synthetic polymers (Figure 5.102 B and C). If casts are only placed on 1 limb, it is important to place some type of support on the contralateral limb (Figure 5.102) to both support the contralateral foot (which is usually also affected with chronic laminitis) and equalize the height of the 2 limbs. Splints offer some of the advantages of immobilization, but offer no relief from load bearing.

Deep Digital Flexor Tenotomy

Tenotomy of the DDFT abolishes or greatly reduces the flexor moment about the DIP joint. The direct result is that the center of pressure should move in a palmar direction to a point directly distal to the center of rotation of the DIP joint. The benefits are that it decreases the tension within the dorsal laminae and compression on the dorsal sole, thus allowing realignment of the distal phalanx with the ground without exacerbating the deleterious forces on the dorsal laminae and sole (Figure 5.103 B and C). This is usually accompanied by decreased pain and increased sole growth dorsally. The disadvantages are that the toe of the foot may become elevated from the ground as the horse rocks back or ambulates, and that mild to moderate subluxation may occur in the DIP joint (Figure 5.103D). Based on these responses, the surgery is primarily indicated in horses with:

1. Early chronic laminitis that continues to rotate despite all other measures taken
2. Intractable pain originating from the dorsal sole and wall despite stabilization and shoeing
3. Secondary flexural deformities

It does not appear to consistently benefit horses with distal displacement, and rarely if ever benefits the horse with unilateral distal displacement of the distal phalanx.

The surgery may be performed in the mid-metacarpal region (Figure 5.103A) or in the mid-pastern region.[4,36] The surgery is easier to perform in the mid-metacarpal region. Additionally, should a second tenotomy be

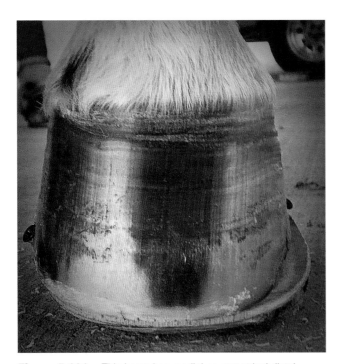

Figure 5.101. This horse has medial asymmetrical distal displacement, evidenced by disparate growth of the medial and lateral walls. A wooden shoe has been positioned to act as a lateral extension to increase weight-bearing by the healthier lateral side of the foot to decrease pain from compression of the sole and tension in the laminae medially. (Courtesy Dr. Stephen O'Grady.)

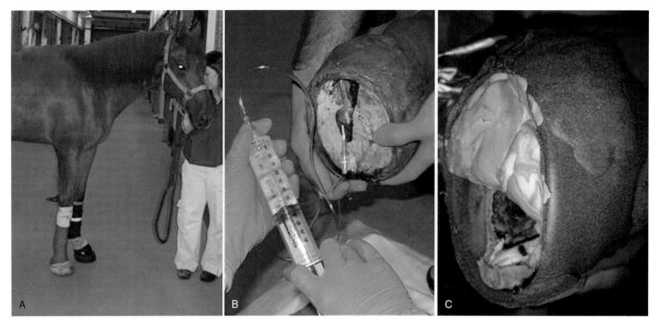

Figure 5.102. This horse with chronic laminitis had a severe abscess on the medial palmar aspect of the right forelimb. An open sole cast was applied to the right forelimb (A and B) with cushion support material applied to the parts of the sole unaffected by the abscess (B). Note the flushing of the abscess with saturated Epsom salts through a 14-g catheter placed through a very small portal made in the solar surface of the affected sole (B). Cushion support material is placed in the palmar aspect of the foot (palmar to the apex of the frog) in the majority of horses (C). A Soft-Ride boot was placed on the contralateral forelimb which was also affected by chronic laminitis (A).

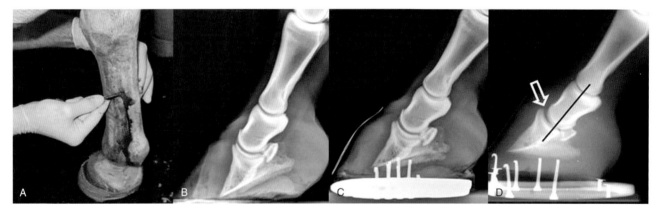

Figure 5.103. Tenotomy of the DDFT is most commonly performed standing at the mid cannon region using a guarded bistoury (A). The tenotomy allows realignment of the rotated distal phalanx (B) with the ground surface (note realignment of the foot in C after 6 weeks). Subluxation of the DIP can occur following the procedure (D), characterized by dorsal displacement of the extensor process of the distal phalanx away from middle phalanx (arrow) and by caudal displacement of the distal articular surface of the middle phalanx so that a line bisecting the middle and proximal phalanges does not bisect the middle of the articular surface of the distal phalanx (black line).

necessary, it is preferable to perform the proximal one first because adhesions may limit the effectiveness of the second surgery in the metacarpal region if the first surgery was performed in the pastern. Tenotomy in the mid pastern appears to provide greater mobility of the foot about the DIP joint, but may also cause more instability of the joint.

The tendon may be cut immediately before or after corrective trimming and shoeing is performed (it is probably best to perform the surgery first to address possible DIP subluxation following DDFT). Because tissue repair at the tenotomy site occurs fairly rapidly and will inhibit any further realignment, it is imperative to obtain the best realignment of the distal phalanx with the ground and phalanges as soon as possible after surgery (i.e., within hours to days). To counter the disadvantages of the surgery, it is advisable to perform radiographs while shoeing immediately following tenotomy of the DDFT to assess both the adequacy of the realignment of the distal phalanx to the ground surface, and, importantly, the degree of subluxation of the DIP joint (indicated by both dorsal displacement of the extensor process of the distal phalanx away from the middle phalanx [arrow, Figure 5.103D], and by palmar displacement of distal articular surface of the middle phalanx in relationship to the articular surface of the distal phalanx [line, Figure 5.103D]). Application of increasing degrees of heel elevation can be assessed radiographically until the subluxation is resolved. If radiographic assessment is not available post tenotomy, the horse should be shod with mild heel extension and elevation.

Drainage and Debridement

Digital sepsis is a well recognized complication associated with laminitis. Drainage may occur at the coronary band or through the dorsal sole. In most horses the infection is confined to the soft tissues of the hoof, but occasionally the infection may involve the distal phalanx. If the hoof capsule of the sole is removed, the solar dermis usually prolapses, and the prolapsed tissue is extremely sensitive to pressure (Figure 5.104). Therefore, when subsolar sepsis is present, it is advisable to create an avenue for drainage through the distal wall rather than the sole whenever possible. If solar drainage is performed, very small portals should be made at the opposite sides of the affected area for drainage and to allow insertion of a catheter or teat cannula (Figure 5.102B) for lavage with saturated Epsom salts (in contrast to the excessive sole removed in Figure 5.104).

Sepsis of the distal phalanx is difficult to both diagnose and treat. It is difficult to diagnose because the radiographic changes in the distal phalanx associated with sepsis closely resemble those associated with prolonged inflammation, and therefore, septic and nonseptic inflammation are very hard to distinguish. In the majority of subsolar sepsis cases, the sepsis does not involve the bone. However, direct contact of bone after inserting a probe in a draining track conclusively identifies exposure of the bone to sepsis and is highly suggestive of septic osteitis (combined with radiographs indicative of severe focal lysis at point of probe contact).

Septic osteitis of the distal phalanx is much more refractory to treatment in horses with laminitis than in horses in which the sepsis occurred for another reason. Additionally, surgery, usually consisting of curettage of the suspect bone, exposes the surface of the distal phalanx in a horse that did not have septic osteitis and increases the likelihood that the horse will develop septic osteitis. Therefore, infection should be treated as superficial unless drainage can be directly linked to the bone or prolonged treatment fails to resolve it and septic osteitis is the best explanation for the continued drainage. In the severely underrun subsolar abscess, one author (JKB) lavages the foot with saturated Epsom salts delivered through a catheter or teat cannula through small portals either in the distal hoof wall (preferred) or sole.

Hoof Wall Resections

Full dorsal hoof wall resections were at one time widely advocated to decrease the pressure of the wall

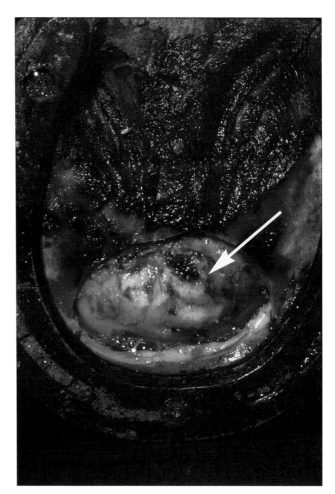

Figure 5.104. Painful granulation tissue (arrow) covered with fibrin exists due to prolapse of the dermis secondary to displacement of the distal phalanx and excessive trimming of the sole. Removal of the sole from the foot in horses with chronic laminitis should be minimized to avoid this painful complication.

on the coronary band, debride necrotic material, and encourage the realignment of the distal phalanx.[20] They accomplish these goals to some degree, including enhancing growth of new wall at the coronary band and increasing the likelihood that the newly formed wall will conform to the parietal surface of the distal phalanx. However, resecting the dorsal wall removes any support that the dorsal wall supplied to the distal phalanx, increases the vertical stresses in the wall at the margins of the resection, and causes further instability by removing circumferential tension that spans the dorsal hoof capsule connecting quarter to quarter. Consequently, the remaining dorsal quarters are more likely to become distracted from the underlying tissues. Therefore, partial hoof wall resections are more commonly performed than total dorsal hoof wall resections to minimize the loss of support to the distal phalanx and stability of the adjacent wall observed in more extensive resections. They are currently most commonly performed to debride necrotic tissues and remove the laminar "wedge" to encourage new hoof wall growth to follow the contour of the distal phalanx.

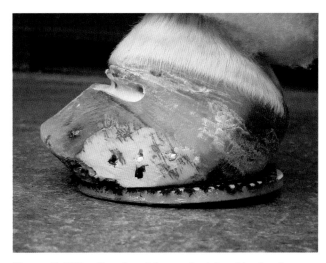

Figure 5.105.   Grooving of the proximal dorsal hoof wall immediately distal to the coronary band to encourage dorsal hoof wall growth and mechanically dissociate new hoof wall growth from the older distal wall.

Coronary Band Grooving and Resection

Coronary band grooving is designed to take pressure off the coronary band to increases the rate of new hoof wall growth (Figure 5.105).[68] It also creates a discontinuity between older, more distal hoof wall and the newer proximal wall so that the distal wall is less likely to distract the new hoof away from the distal phalanx. The groove is created in the dorsal hoof wall at the level of the base of the extensor process, and extends through the full thickness of the stratum medium of the wall from one toe-quarter junction to the other. In the authors' experience, results with this technique are highly variable.

Resection of the cornified layer of the coronary band is probably most frequently performed following separation of the hoof wall from the coronary band. In these circumstances, it is done to decrease the chafing by the separated hoof wall that damages underlying viable germinal tissue and enhance drainage of exudate that has accumulated under the separated tissues. It is advisable to bevel the proximal margin of the remaining tissue so that it is thinnest proximally to avoid a pressure ridge developing that impinges the underlying dermis. The indications and optimal timing for this procedure have not been determined.

More recently, resection of the intact coronary band has been described in a horse with unstable chronic laminitis (referred to as acute founder by the original author) with an intact coronary band that demonstrated reduced hoof wall growth.[28] The hoof capsule overlying the coronary cushion of the dorsal aspect of the hoof was removed, a procedure that required isolating that piece of wall with cuts in the hoof and physically separating the cornified epidermis from the underlying germinal epidermis and dermis. The result was an immediate significant reduction in pain, and as the new coronary hoof capsule formed, and improved alignment of the new horn. The technique offers a potential solution to a difficult problem (realignment of the hoof capsule with the distal phalanx), but more experience is required to validate its effectiveness. If proven successful, the optimal circumstances under which to perform it must be further delineated.

Prognosis

There are numerous reasons why treatment of horses with laminitis is unsuccessful, but the 3 most important reasons are the severity of the original pathology, type of displacement, and severity of the clinical signs.[9,36,56] These factors are likely to determine the continued course of the disease and the development of complications. The prognosis following displacement is always considered guarded to poor.

Regarding the different types of displacement, rotation is considered to have a more favorable prognosis than distal displacement, which in turn is considered to have a more favorable prognosis than unilateral distal displacement. Two criteria have been documented to determine prognosis: the degree of rotation and the distance from the proximal margin of the extensor process of the distal phalanx to the firm proximal margin of the hoof capsule (immediately distal to the coronet, distance also termed the "founder distance").[23,75] Capsular rotation greater than 11.5° predicted poor survival and capsular rotation less than 5.5° predicted return to performance. A coronet-to-extensor-process distance of greater than 15.2 mm is indicative of poor survival. Additionally, the thickness of the sole and the angle that the solar margin of the distal phalanx subtends with the ground may be beneficial in assessing the prognosis for success; thinner soles and greater angles of the solar margin are anecdotally associated with decreased prognosis. Finally, financial constraints of the owner and the failure of the owners to follow recommendations, particularly advice regarding exercise and maintaining appointments, are likely to decrease the success of treatment.

References

1. Abrahamsen EJ. Equine Pain Management. Proc British Equine Vet Assoc 2005;44:241–242.
2. Adair HS, Goble DO, Schmidhammer JL, et al. Laminar microvascular flow, measured by means of laser Doppler flowmetry, during the prodromal stages of black walnut-induced laminitis in horses. American Journal of Veterinary Research 2000;61:862–868.
3. Allen D Jr., Clark ES, Moore JN, et al. Evaluation of equine digital Starling forces and hemodynamics during early laminitis. Am J Vet Res 1990;51:1930–1934.
4. Allen D Jr., White NA 2nd, Foerner JF, et al. Surgical management of chronic laminitis in horses: 13 cases (1983–1985). Journal of the American Veterinary Medical Association 1986;189:1604–1606.
5. Andersen PH, Hesselholt M, Jarlov N. Endotoxin and arachidonic acid metabolites in portal, hepatic and arterial blood of cattle with acute ruminal acidosis. Acta Vet Scand 1994;35:223–234.
6. Bailey SR, Adair HS, Reinemeyer CR, et al. Plasma concentrations of endotoxin and platelet activation in the developmental stage of oligofructose-induced laminitis. Vet Immunol Immunopathol 2009;129:167–173.
7. Barton MH, Moore JN. Pentoxifylline inhibits mediator synthesis in an equine *in vitro* whole blood model of endotoxemia. Circ Shock 1994;44:216–220.
8. Baskett A, Barton MH, Norton N, et al. Effect of pentoxifylline, flunixin meglumine, and their combination on a model of endotoxemia in horses. Am J Vet Res 1997;58:1291–1299.

9. Baxter GM. Equine Laminitis Caused by Distal Displacement of the Distal Phalanx—12 Cases (1976–1985). Journal of the American Veterinary Medical Association 1986;189:326–329.

10. Belknap JK. How to use an open-sole cast in cases of laminitis. Proc Am Assoc Eq Pract 2008;54:219–224.

11. Belknap JK. Inflammatory cells in laminitis: what role do they play? Proceedings of Fifth International Equine Conference on Laminitis 2009:68–69.

12. Belknap JK. Laminitis Research: Ohio State University. Proceedings of the Fifth International Equine Conference on Laminitis 2009:22–23.

13. Belknap JK, Giguere S, Pettigrew A,et al. Lamellar pro-inflammatory cytokine expression patterns in laminitis at the developmental stage and at the onset of lameness: innate vs. adaptive immune response. Equine Vet J 2007;39:42–47.

14. Belknap JK, Moore JN. Evaluation of heparin for prophylaxis of equine laminitis: 71 cases (1980–1986). J Am Vet Med Assoc 1989;195:505–507.

15. Belknap JK, Moore JN, Crouser EC. Sepsis—From human organ failure to laminar failure. Vet Immunol Immunopathol 2009;129:155–157.

16. Beretta C, Garavaglia G, Cavalli M. COX-1 and COX-2 inhibition in horse blood by phenylbutazone, flunixin, carprofen and meloxicam: an in vitro analysis. Pharmacol Res 2005;52:302–306.

17. Black SJ. Extracellular matrix, leukocyte migration and laminitis. Vet Immunol Immunopathol 2009;129:161–163.

18. Black SJ, Lunn DP, Yin C, et al. Leukocyte emigration in the early stages of laminitis. Vet Immunol Immunopathol 2006;109:161–166.

19. Blikslager AT, Yin CL, Cochran AM, et al. Cyclooxygenase expression in the early stages of equine laminitis: A cytologic study. Journal of Veterinary Internal Medicine 2006;20:1191–1196.

20. Chapman B, Platt GW. Laminitis. Am Assoc Equine Pract 1984;13:129.

21. Coffman JR, Johnson JH, Guffy MM, et al. Hoof circulation in equine laminitis. Journal of the American Veterinary Medical Association 1970;156:76–83.

22. Cohen ND, Parson EM, Seahorn TL, et al. Prevalence and factors associated with development of laminitis in horses with duodenitis/proximal jejunitis: 33 cases (1985–1991). Journal of the American Veterinary Medical Association 1994;204:250–254.

23. Cripps PJ, Eustace RA. Factors involved in the prognosis of equine laminitis in the UK. Equine Veterinary Journal 1999;31:433–442.

24. de la Rebiere de Pouyade G, Grulke S, Detilleux J, et al. Evaluation of low-molecular-weight heparin for the prevention of equine laminitis after colic surgery. J Vet Emerg Crit Care (San Antonio) 2009;19:113–119.

25. Eades SC. Laminitis Research: Louisiana State University. Proc Fifth International Equine Conference of Laminitis and Diseases of the Foot 2009:34–35.

26. Eades SC, Stokes AM, Johnson PJ, et al. Serial alterations in digital hemodynamics and endothelin-1 immunoreactivity, platelet-neutrophil aggregation, and concentrations of nitric oxide, insulin, and glucose in blood obtained from horses following carbohydrate overload. Am J Vet Res 2007;68:87–94.

27. Eaton SA, Allen DA, Eades SC, et al. Digital Starling forces and hemodynamics during early laminitis induced by an aqueous extract of black walnut (Juglans nigra) in horses. Veterinary Surgery 1994;23:400–401.

28. Eustace RA, Emery SL. Partial coronary epidermectomy (coronary peel), dorsodistal wall fenestration and deep digital flexor tenotomy to treat severe acute founder in a Connemara pony. Equine Vet Educ 2009;21:91–99.

29. Faleiros RR, Leise BB, Westerman T,et al. In vivo and in vitro evidence of the involvement of CXCL1, a keratinocyte-derived chemokine, in equine laminitis. J Vet Intern Med 2009;23:1086–1096.

30. French KR, Pollitt CC. Equine laminitis: loss of hemidesmosomes in hoof secondary epidermal lamellae correlates to dose in an oligofructose induction model: an ultrastructural study. Equine Vet J 2004;36:230–235.

31. Geor R, Frank N. Metabolic syndrome—From human organ disease to laminar failure in equids. Vet Immunol Immunopathol 2009;129:151–154.

32. Hanusch C, Nowak K, Gill IS, et al. Hypothermic preservation of lung allograft inhibits cytokine-induced chemoattractant-1, endothelial leucocyte adhesion molecule, vascular cell adhesion molecule-1 and intracellular adhesion molecule-1 expression. Clinical and Experimental Immunology 2007;149:364–371.

33. Hood DM, Gremmel SM, Amoss MS, et al. Equine laminitis I: radioisotopic analysis of the hemodynamics of the foot during the acute disease. J Eq Med Surg 1978;2:439–444.

34. Hood DM, Wagner IP, Brumbaugh GW. Evaluation of hoof wall surface temperature as an index of digital vascular perfusion during the prodromal and acute phases of carbohydrate-induced laminitis in horses. Am J Vet Res 2001;62:1167–1172.

35. Hood DM, Wagner IP, Taylor DD, et al. Voluntary limb-load distribution in horses with acute and chronic laminitis. American Journal of Veterinary Research 2001;62:1393–1398.

36. Hunt RJ. A retrospective evaluation of laminitis in horses. Equine Veterinary Journal 1993;25:61–64.

37. Hunt RJ, Allen D, Moore JN. Effect of endotoxin administration on equine digital hemodynamics and starling forces. Am J Vet Res 1990;51:1703–1707.

38. Hurley DJ, Parks RJ, Reber AJ, et al. Dynamic changes in circulating leukocytes during the induction of equine laminitis with black walnut extract. Veterinary Immunology and Immunopathology 2006;110:195–206.

39. Ingle-Fehr JE, Baxter GM. Evaluation of digital and laminar blood flow in horses given a low dose of endotoxin. American Journal of Veterinary Research 1998;59:192–196.

40. Koblik PD, O'Brien TR, Coyne CP. Laminitis. J Am Vet Med Assoc 1988;192:346–349.

41. Kyaw-Tanner M, Pollitt CC. Equine laminitis: increased transcription of matrix metalloproteinase-2 (MMP-2) occurs during the developmental phase. Equine Vet J 2004;36:221–225.

42. Leise BB, Johnson PJ, Faleiros RR, et al. Hind laminar proinflammatory response is present after carbohydrate overload. 2nd AAEP Foundation Equine Laminitis Research Workshop 2009.

43. Leise BS, Fugler LA, Stokes AM, et al. Effects of intramuscular administration of acepromazine on palmar digital blood flow, palmar digital arterial pressure, transverse facial arterial pressure, and packed cell volume in clinically healthy, conscious horses. Veterinary Surgery 2007;36:717–723.

44. Leise BS, Yin C, Pettigrew A, et al. Proinflammatory cytokine responses of equine keratinocytes to bacterial pathogen-associated molecular pattern motifs. Equine Vet J 2010;42:294–303.

45. Lim CM, Kim EK, Koh Y, et al. Hypothermia inhibits cytokine release of alveolar macrophage and activation of nuclear factor kappaB in endotoxemic lung. Intensive Care Med 2004;30:1638–1644.

46. Loftus JP, Belknap JK, Stankiewicz KM, et al. Laminar xanthine oxidase, superoxide dismutase and catalase activities in the prodromal stage of black-walnut-induced equine laminitis. Equine Vet J 2007;39:48–53.

47. Loftus JP, Black SJ, Pettigrew A, et al. Early laminar events involving endothelial activation in horses with black-walnut-induced laminitis. American Journal of Veterinary Research 2007;68:1205–1211.

48. Loftus JP, Johnson PJ, Belknap JK, et al. Leukocyte-derived and endogenous matrix metalloproteinases in the lamellae of horses with naturally acquired and experimentally induced laminitis. Vet Immunol Immunopathol 2009;129:221–230.

49. MacAllister CG, Morgan SJ, Borne AT, et al. Comparison of adverse effects of phenylbutazone, flunixin meglumine, and ketoprofen in horses. Journal of the American Veterinary Medical Association 1993;202:71–77.

50. Martins Filho LP, Fagliari JJ, Moraes JRE, et al. Influence of heparin in occurrence of carbohydrate overload-induced equine laminitis. Arquivo Brasileiro De Medicina Veterinaria E Zootecnia 2008;60:1358–1366.

51. Mungall BA, Kyaw-Tanner M, Pollitt CC. In vitro evidence for a bacterial pathogenesis of equine laminitis. Vet Microbiol 2001;79:209–223.

52. Nievers MG, Schaapveld RQ, Sonnenberg A. Biology and function of hemidesmosomes. Matrix Biology 1999;18:5–17.

53. Noschka E, Moore JN, Peroni JF, et al. Thromboxane and iso-prostanes as inflammatory and vasoactive mediators in black walnut heartwood extract induced equine laminitis. Vet Immunol Immunopathol 2009;129:200–210.

54. Noschka E, Vandenplas ML, Hurley DJ, et al. Temporal aspects of laminar gene expression during the developmental stages of equine laminitis. Vet Immunol Immunopathol 2009;129:242–253.

55. O'Grady SE. How to restore alignment of P3 in horses with chronic laminitis. Proc Am Assoc Eq Pract 2003;49:328–336.
56. O'Grady SE, Parks AH. Farriery options for acute and chronic laminitis. Proc Am Assoc Eq Pract 2008;54:354–363.
57. Owens JG, Kamerling SG, Stanton SR, et al. Effects of ketoprofen and phenylbutazone on chronic hoof pain and lameness in the horse. Equine Veterinary Journal 1995;27:296–300.
58. Parks AH, Mair TS. Laminitis: A call for a unified terminology. Equine Vet Educ 2009;21:102–106.
59. Peroni JF, Moore JN, Noschka E, et al. Predisposition for venoconstriction in the equine laminar dermis: implications in equine laminitis. Journal of Applied Physiology 2006;100:759–763.
60. Pollitt CC. Basement membrane pathology: a feature of acute equine laminitis. Equine Vet J 1996;28:38–46.
61. Pollitt CC. Equine laminitis: a revised pathophysiology. Proc Am Assoc Eq Pract 1999;45:188–192.
62. Pollitt CC, Daradka M. Hoof wall wound repair. Equine Vet J 2004;36:210–215.
63. Pollitt CC, Davies CT. Equine laminitis: its development coincides with increased sublamellar blood flow. Equine Vet J Suppl 1998:125–132.
64. Pollitt CC, Molyneux GS. A scanning electron microscopical study of the dermal microcirculation of the equine foot. Equine Vet J 1990;22:79–87.
65. Rebière G, Franck T, Deby-Dupont G, et al. Effects of unfractionated and fractionated heparins on myeloperoxidase activity and interactions with endothelial cells: possible effects on the pathophysiology of equine laminitis. Veterinary Journal 2008;178:62–69.
66. Redden RF. Shoeing the laminitic horse. Proc Am Assoc Equine Pract 1997;43:356–359.
67. Redden RF. A technique for performing digital venography in the standing horse. Equine Veterinary Education 2001;13:128–134.
68. Ritmeester AM, Blevins WE, Ferguson DW, et al. Digital perfusion, evaluated scintigraphically, and hoof wall growth in horses with chronic laminitis treated with egg bar-heart bar shoeing and coronary grooving. Equine Veterinary Journal Supplement 1998:111–118.
69. Rupp J, Berger M, Reiling N, et al. Cox-2 inhibition abrogates Chlamydia pneumoniae-induced PGE2 and MMP-1 expression. Biochem Biophys Res Commun 2004;320:738–744.
70. Schumacher J, Livesey L, DeGraves FJ, et al. Effect of anaesthesia of the palmar digital nerves on proximal interphalangeal joint pain in the horse. Equine Vet J 2004;36:409–414.
71. Schumacher J, Steiger R, de Graves F, et al. Effects of analgesia of the distal interphalangeal joint or palmar digital nerves on lameness caused by solar pain in horses. Vet Surg 2000;29:54–58.
72. Sprouse RF, Garner HE, Green EM. Plasma endotoxin levels in horses subjected to carbohydrate induced laminitis. Eq Vet J 1987;19:25–28.
73. Steward ML. How to construct and apply atraumatic therapeutic shoes to treat acute or chronic laminitis in the horse. Proc Am Assoc Eq Pract 2003;49:337–346.
74. Stewart AJ, Pettigrew A, Cochran AM, et al. Indices of inflammation in the lung and liver in the early stages of the black walnut extract model of equine laminitis. Vet Immunol Immunopathol 2009;129:254–260.
75. Stick JA, Jann HW, Scott EA, et al. Pedal bone rotation as a prognostic sign in laminitis of horses. Journal of the American Veterinary Medical Association 1982;180:251–253.
76. Treiber K, Carter R, Gay L, et al. Inflammatory and redox status of ponies with a history of pasture-associated laminitis. Vet Immunol Immunopathol 2009;129:216–220.
77. Vick MM, Adams AA, Murphy BA, et al. Relationships among inflammatory cytokines, obesity, and insulin sensitivity in the horse. J Anim Sci 2007;85:1144–1155.
78. Waguespack RW, Cochran A, Belknap JK. Expression of the cyclooxygenase isoforms in the prodromal stage of black walnut-induced laminitis in horses. Am J Vet Res 2004;65:1724–1729.
79. Watt FM, Kubler MD, Hotchin NA, Nicholson LJ, Adams JC. Regulation of keratinocyte terminal differentiation by integrin-extracellular matrix interactions. J Cell Sci 1993;106 (Pt 1):175–182.
80. Weiss DJ, Evanson OA. Detection of activated platelets and platelet-leukocyte aggregates in horses. American Journal of Veterinary Research 1997;58:823–827.
81. Weiss DJ, Evanson OA, McClenahan D, Fagliari JJ, Dunnwiddie CT, Wells RE. Effect of a competitive inhibitor of platelet aggregation on experimentally induced laminitis in ponies. Am J Vet Res 1998;59:814–817.
82. Weiss DJ, Geor RJ, Johnston G, Trent AM. Microvascular thrombosis associated with onset of acute laminitis in ponies. Am J Vet Res 1994;55:606–612.
83. Williams JM, Ravis W, Loftus J, Peroni JF, Hubbell J, Faleiros RR, Black SJ, Belknap JK. Effect of intravenous lidocaine administration on leukocyte emigration in the black walnut extract model of laminitis. J Vet Int Med 2009;23:781.

THE PASTERN

Gary M. Baxter and Ted S. Stashak

The proximal interphalangeal (PIP) joint or pastern joint is a diarthrodial joint, which is formed from the distal aspect of the proximal phalanx (P1) and the proximal aspect of the middle phalanx (P2). The pastern region is bounded dorsally by the common or long digital extensor tendon together with the dorsal branches of the suspensory ligament. Palmar/plantar support structures of the pastern region are formed by the distal sesamoidean ligaments (DSLs; straight, oblique, cruciate, and short), superficial digital flexor tendon (SDFT), deep digital flexor tendon (DDFT), and proximal and distal digital anular ligaments within the digital flexor tendon sheath (DFTS).[21,25] The medial and lateral collateral ligaments provide support in the sagittal plane.

Abnormalities such as dorsal swelling or bony enlargement in the pastern region are often obvious due to minimal soft tissue in the area.[21,25] The severity of lameness from the pastern region ranges from subtle to severe depending on the injury.[21,25] Generally, injuries such as fractures that involve the PIP joint or tendinitis within the DFTS cause obvious lameness, whereas lameness due to early osteoarthritis (OA) of the PIP joint or strains of the DSLs may be mild. Pain and lameness in the pastern region is often exacerbated by distal limb flexion or lunging the horse with the affected limb on the inside of the circle.

Complete analgesia of the pastern region is not always accomplished by perineural analgesia at the level of the basi-sesamoid or abaxial nerve block, and a low 4-point nerve block may be necessary.[21,25] A palmar/plantar digital (PD) nerve block can desensitize the pastern region depending on the location of the block and amount of anesthetic used. However, if the PD block is performed just proximal to the collateral cartilages of the foot, the PIP joint is unlikely to be desensitized.[23] Additionally, horses with suspected stress fractures of P1 should not be blocked to avoid further displacement of the fracture.

Several imaging modalities, such as radiology or ultrasound, are important for the initial characterization of the injury. Ultrasonographic evaluation of the pastern is an integral part of characterizing the extent of any soft tissue injury. Additionally, nuclear scintigraphy, computed tomography (CT), magnetic resonance imaging (MRI), or tenoscopy of the DFTS may all be important to provide additional information necessary for a complete and accurate diagnosis and prognosis.[21,25]

Differential diagnoses for disorders of the pastern region include PIP joint OA, osteochondrosis (OC), fractures, luxation/subluxation of the PIP joint, infection, lacerations, and soft tissue injuries; however, the types of injuries are often breed or use specific.[21,25] For the purposes of this discussion, conditions of the pastern will include bone and joint abnormalities of P1 and P2 and the PIP joint, and soft tissue injuries of the palmar/plantar aspect of the pastern including the distal sesamoidean ligaments (DSL), distal branches of the SDFT, and the DDFT within the distal aspect of the DFTS.

OSTEOARTHRITIS (OA) OF THE PIP JOINT (HIGH RINGBONE)

The term "high ringbone" is often synonymously used with OA of the PIP joint. Historically ringbone has been used to describe any bony enlargement of the phalanges in the pastern region below the fetlock joint.[1,25] If the bony enlargement was associated with the distal aspect of P1 and proximal aspect of P2 with or without PIP joint involvement it was classified as high ringbone. If the bony enlargement was associated with the distal aspect of P2 and the proximal aspect of the distal phalanx with or without distal interphalangeal (DIP) joint involvement it was classified as low ringbone.[1,25] Ringbone has also been classified as articular (involving the joint surface) or periarticular (involving the structures at the perimeter of the joint and the adjacent phalanges).[25] However, most cases present with joint involvement and periarticular pathology, and it is often difficult and unnecessary to differentiate between the two clinically. Therefore, it is suggested that the distinction between articular and periarticular ringbone is probably inappropriate in most cases.[15,25]

Osteoarthritis, or degenerative joint disease or arthrosis, of the PIP joint is an important and common cause of lameness in virtually all breeds and ages of horses.[20,25] Older horses appear to be at greater risk and the forelimbs are more frequently affected than the hindlimbs. Secondary OA from P2 fractures (particularly palmar/plantar eminence fractures) or OC occurs more commonly in the hindlimbs.[10,28] A higher incidence of the disease has also been identified in geldings compared to stallions and mares.[5,10]

Etiology

Chronic overuse or repetitive trauma of the PIP joint and surrounding structures is the most common cause of PIP joint OA. Inherent conformational traits and the type of work the horse performs may also contribute to problems in the PIP joint. For example, horses that are base-narrow and toe-in or toe-out are thought to be predisposed to OA on the lateral side of the joint, whereas horses that are base-wide and toe-in or toe-out are believed to be predisposed to injury on the medial side of the joint.[25] Pasterns that are overly upright may also result in increased concussion to the PIP joint.[1,25] Poor conformation may predispose to pulling/tearing of the soft tissues surrounding the joint or to incongruencies within the joint surfaces.[25] In addition, Western performance horses that are required to start and stop suddenly or twist and turn abruptly appear to be prone to PIP joint damage.

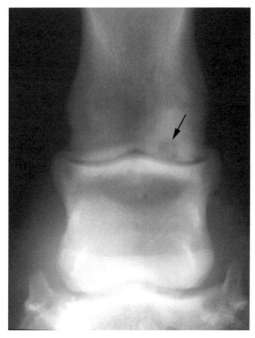

Figure 5.106. Dorsoplantar radiograph of a trauma-induced SCL of the distal aspect of P1 (arrow) that was not apparent radiographically until 3 months after the original injury.

Trauma to the periarticular soft tissues and the PIP joint may be repetitive or occur as a single, high-energy event that does not cause a fracture or joint luxation. Because the PIP joint is considered a low-motion/high-load joint the articular cartilage and subchondral bone are placed under a greater workload, making these structures more susceptible to injury from nonphysiologic loading.[18] Overloading the PIP may cause direct articular cartilage damage and/or subchondral bone bruising (seen primarily in the distal aspect of P1) that may contribute to the development of subchondral cystic lesions (Figure 5.106). The trauma may also cause pulling/tearing of the periosteal attachments of the extensor tendons, ligaments, and joint capsule, resulting in periostitis and new bone formation. In addition, these injuries may cause joint instability or subluxation leading to secondary cartilage damage and OA. The OA may also result from an imbalance between repetitive micro-trauma sustained during athletic performance and the adaptive repair mechanism of the skeletal tissue.[1,18] Whether primary synovitis/capsulitis is a distinct entity involving the PIP joint is uncertain,[15] but it is less commonly recognized than with other joints in the horse. Lame horses that block to intra-articular anesthesia of the PIP joint that do not have radiographic abnormalities may have PIP joint synovitis/capsulitis. However, they may also have subchondral bone bruising or other unrecognized bone damage that would only be recognized with advanced imaging such as CT or MRI (Figure 5.106).

Osteoarthritis of the PIP joint may develop secondarily to a number of abnormalities within the joint. These include OC, unrecognized palmar/plantar eminence fractures of P2, traumatic blows or lacerations, septic arthritis, and selective weight-bearing in young

horses.[6,8,25,28] Osteoarthritis of the PIP joint secondary to OC is usually seen most frequently in the hindlimbs of horses less than 3 years of age and more than one joint can often be affected.[28] Single eminence fractures of P2 also occur most commonly in the hindlimb and can be the cause of chronic hindlimb lameness if unrecognized at the initial injury. Direct blows to the pastern region and lacerations at the margin of the PIP joint or involving the collateral ligaments may contribute to OA of the PIP joint. Infectious arthritis is often associated with an existing laceration or puncture wound that involves the PIP joint but may also develop after a wound has completely healed. Excessive weight-bearing on the contralateral support limb following severe lameness in a rear limb was thought to cause the development of OA in the PIP joint in 6 horses in one report.[6]

Clinical Signs

Focal or diffuse enlargement of the pastern region may be evident visually as well as on palpation (Figure 5.107). Palpable heat and pain with firm digital pressure may be appreciated depending on the duration of the injury. The affected pastern region may feel larger, particularly the dorsolateral and dorsomedial surfaces, than the contralateral joint. In most horses there is pain on flexion and rotation of the pastern region, unless the joint has undergone ankylosis. Obvious enlargement of the pastern and/or varus deformity of the phalanges may be present in horses with advanced disease. Horses with mild disease may have no visual or palpable abnormalities in the pastern region.

Lameness is often variable (2 to 4 out of 5) depending on the severity of the disease. The severity of lameness often correlates with the severity of the OA within the PIP joint. The lameness is usually exacerbated at a

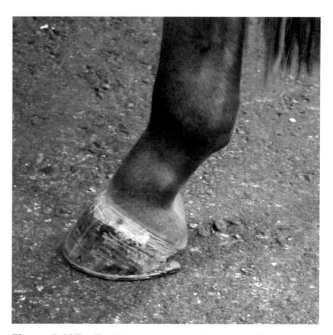

Figure 5.107. Typical enlargement of the pastern that may be visible in horses with OA of the PIP joint. This was a young horse with osteochondrosis of the hindlimb PIP joint.

trot, at exercise on an uneven surface (e.g., slope), or by circling at a trot. Increased lameness is usually seen when the affected limb is on the inside of the circle. In some cases during foot flight, an exaggerated extension of the toe may be seen prior to foot placement.[27]

The lameness should not improve with a PD nerve block if performed very low in the pastern (just above collateral cartilages) with a small volume of anesthetic (1.5 mL).[23] However, some PD nerve blocks may desensitize the PIP joint if performed in the mid-pastern region or if a large volume of anesthetic is used. Most horses improve with a basi-sesamoid or high PD nerve block but may not become completely sound.[25] A pastern ring block is usually effective in completely eliminating the lameness while intrasynovial anesthesia may only block out the intra-articular pain. Response to intra-articular analgesia varies depending on the injury, but improvement of lameness by 50% or more usually implicates the PIP joint as the site of the problem.[21,25] However, most horses with OA of the PIP greatly improve following intra-articular anesthesia. The author prefers the palmar/plantar approach to block and treat the PIP joint because bony proliferation along the dorsal aspect of the pastern often makes the dorsal approaches more difficult.[16]

Diagnosis

A tentative diagnosis of OA of the PIP joint is often made based on physical examination findings combined with the responses to local anesthesia. Radiographic examination of the joint is usually used to confirm the diagnosis. The most common radiographic findings in a study performed on 196 horses (262 joints) with chronic OA of the PIP joint were (1) joint space narrowing or collapse, (2) osteophyte formation, (3) subchondral bone sclerosis, (4) periosteal/periarticular bony proliferation, and (5) deformity/collapse of the joint space (Figures 5.108 to 5.110).[5]

Other radiographic features that may be identified include subchondral bone lysis, subchondral cystic lesions (SCLs; Figure 5.106), and chronic eminence fractures of P2. Periarticular new bone growth associated with lacerations may be limited to the site of trauma unless the joint was invaded and/or infectious arthritis is present. Infectious arthritis of the PIP joint often causes severe periosteal/periarticular bony proliferation, osteophyte formation, and subchondral lysis seen on radiographs. Osteochondrosis of the PIP joint is often characterized by a narrowing of the joint space, marginal osteophytosis, periarticular bone proliferation, and subchondral lucencies within the distal aspect of P1.[25,28] Older horses with trauma-induced OA or young horses with OC should have radiographs of the contralateral PIP joint performed because these disease conditions are often bilateral.

In early acute cases, only soft tissue swelling of the pastern may be present, and radiographic examination may not reveal abnormalities. In addition, radiographic abnormalities may be limited in horses with only mild disease of the PIP joint (Figure 5.108). Repeat radiographic examination should be performed in 3 to 4 weeks because evidence of periostitis (periarticular new bone) and peripheral osteophyte formation may be

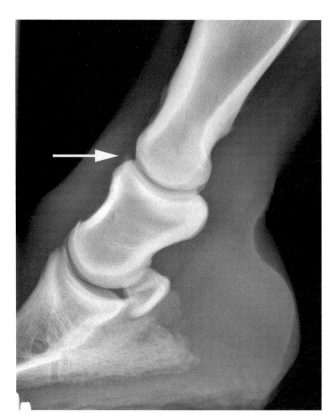

Figure 5.108. Lateral radiograph of the pastern demonstrating a small osteophyte on the dorsal aspect of the joint that may suggest the beginning of OA within the joint (arrow).

present at that time. Subchondral bone lysis associated with bone trauma may not be seen radiographically for 3 to 4 months after injury (Figure 5.106). Alternatively, nuclear scintigraphy can be performed to confirm the region involved in the lameness (Figure 5.111), or an MRI of the pastern region may help reveal subchondral bone and joint abnormalities that are not apparent on radiographs (5.112).[17,30] Bone bruises, contusions or edema, or bone marrow lesions within P1 and P2 are documented causes of lameness in horses and should be suspected in horses that do not have radiographic abnormalities.[17,30] Ultrasonography can also be used to evaluate the PIP joint and other soft tissue support structures in the pastern region.[4]

Treatment

Conservative Management

The decision regarding treatment of horses with OA of the PIP joint depends on the severity of the disease, degree of lameness, age and intended use of the horse, and the owner's expectations and financial constraints. Horses with severe lameness and advanced radiographic abnormalities are usually not good candidates for nonsurgical treatments because their effectiveness is often short-lived. Horses with mild to moderate radiographic abnormalities of the PIP joint may respond well to conservative treatment, depending on the horse's intended use. Horses with a single traumatic injury to the PIP joint may respond well to rest and develop

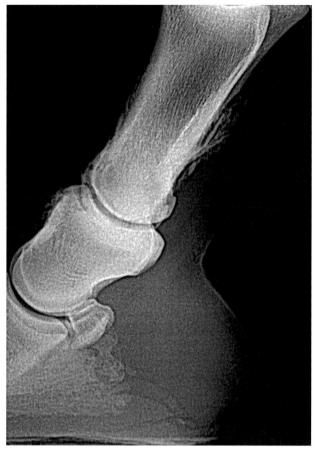

Figure 5.109. Lateral radiograph of the pastern region with a marked periosteal reaction around the PIP joint consistent with advanced OA within the joint.

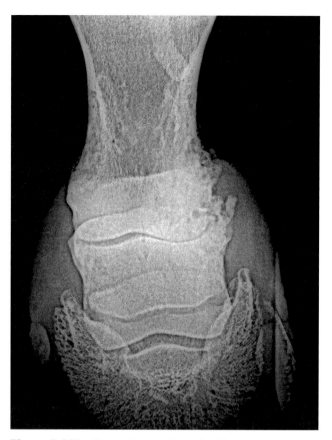

Figure 5.110. Dorsopalmar radiograph of the same horse in Figure 5.109 demonstrating joint space collapse, subchondral lysis, and periosteal reaction around the PIP joint. This horse was lame at the walk and underwent arthrodesis of the joint.

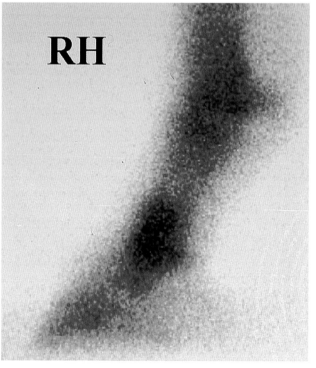

Figure 5.111. Lateral scintigraphic image of the pastern in a horse with lameness isolated to the PIP joint that did not have radiographic abnormalities present.

minimal radiographic abnormalities, depending on the severity of the initial injury. There are numerous treatment options and the decision on how to treat horses with OA of the PIP joint is often made on a case-by-case basis.

Conservative management of PIP OA may involve periods of rest, systemic and/or intra-articular (IA) anti-inflammatory therapy, oral or systemic disease-modifying drugs, trimming and shoeing, and a change in the horse's career. See Chapter 8 for more specific details on these treatment modalities. In acute cases, stall confinement and rest from exercise are important to prevent further trauma, reduce inflammation, and permit healing to occur.[6,27] Rest periods may extend from weeks to months depending on the severity of the injury and the response to treatment. Prolonged rest for 3 to 7 months in foals and weanlings (younger than 7 months of age) with early signs of OA may allow some horses to heal completely and perform at their intended use.[6] In many adult horses the rest and controlled exercise period may be as short as 1 to 2 months before riding can be resumed. Confinement and rest is much less effective in horses with chronic OA of the PIP joint than in horses with acute injuries or mild disease.

Anti-inflammatory treatments are often only palliative but may permit continued use of the horse for variable periods of time. This can be prolonged if it is

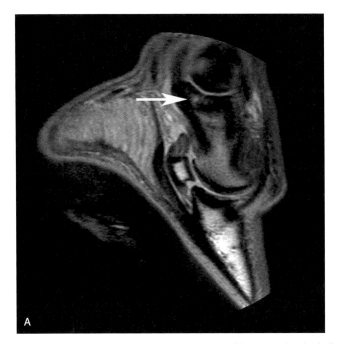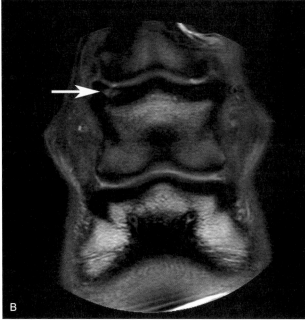

Figure 5.112. Lateral (A) and dorsopalmar (B) proton density (pd) MRI images of a horse with lameness isolated to the pastern region that revealed subchondral bone disease (arrows) of the palmar aspect of P2.

combined with a change in the horse's career to one that is less strenuous. Nonsteroidal anti-inflammatory drugs (NSAIDs) such as phenylbutazone, flunixin meglumine, or firocoxib are still commonly used. Oral phenylbutazone at 2.2 to 4.4 mg/kg every 24 hours for 10 to 14 days is often combined with rest and bandaging for horses with acute PIP joint injuries. For chronic cases, NSAIDs can be given prior to, during the days of performance, and for 1 to 2 days after performance to permit some horses to perform relatively pain free for prolonged periods. Intermittent use of phenylbutazone for a few days at a time is thought to reduce the complications that may be associated with prolonged, continuous use of the drug.

Often oral NSAIDs are combined with IA medication (steroid ± hyaluronan) of the PIP joint in horses with chronic OA to reduce the signs of lameness and improve the effectiveness of both treatments. A combination of a steroid (triamcinolone or methylprednisolone acetate) and hyaluronan (HA) can also be used IA in horses with acute disease to reduce inflammation and slow the progression of the disease. Intramuscularly or IA polysulfated glycosaminoglycans (PSGAGs), IV HA, and oral nutraceutical supplements may be used concurrently but appear to be most beneficial in horses with mild to moderate OA of the PIP joint.

There is some debate as to whether corrective shoeing can benefit horses with PIP joint problems. Changing heel height appears to have much more effect on altering flexion and biomechanical forces of the DIP joint than the PIP joint. In addition, raising the heel decreases the strain on the DDFT but increases strain on the SDFT and the suspensory ligament.[11] Therefore, adjusting heel height may not be beneficial in horses with PIP joint problems. However, the hoof pastern axis should be corrected if abnormal because either a broken-forward

or broken-back hoof-pastern axis can contribute to problems within the PIP joint. In general, the feet should be trimmed and balanced, and shoes applied that minimize break-over forces and provide good lateral and medial support. Horses that are toed-in may benefit from lateral extensions to help reduce compressive forces on the medial aspect of the PIP joint. See Chapters 8 and 12 for more information on corrective shoeing.

Surgical Treatment

Surgical treatment for OA of the PIP joint consists of arthrodesis, which is aimed at eliminating motion within the joint, thereby decreasing pain and lameness. Natural ankylosis of the PIP joint may occur, but it is often a long, painful process with variable results. Surgical arthrodesis is generally considered a better solution with more consistent results. Numerous surgical techniques have been proposed over the years to promote arthrodesis of the PIP joint.[2,3,7–10,12–14,22,24–26] The basic principles include removal of the articular cartilage; internal fixation of P1 and P2 with screws, plates, or a combination of plates and screws; compression across the joint surface; accurate alignment of the phalanges; and variable periods of external immobilization with a half-limb cast.

The surgery is usually performed with an open approach through an incision over the dorsal aspect of the pastern. More recently, less invasive approaches have been reported in which plates and screws are placed through multiple smaller incisions along the dorsal aspect of the pastern.[9,12] These approaches are reportedly less painful and less susceptible to postoperative infection. Cancellous bone grafting is usually unnecessary but forage or osteostixis of the subchondral bone around the joint may promote faster arthrodesis,

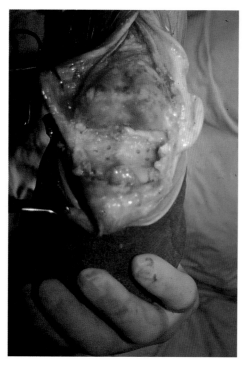

Figure 5.113. Intra-operative view of the PIP joint illustrating osteostixis that is recommended during the arthrodesis procedure in older horses that often have sclerotic bone.

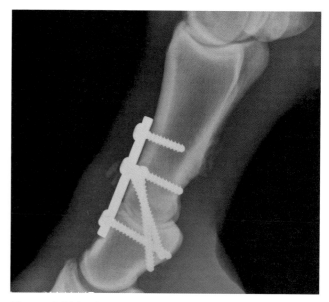

Figure 5.114. Lateral radiograph of the pastern following placement of a 3-hole plate with 2 transarticular 5.5-mm screws for arthrodesis of the PIP joint.

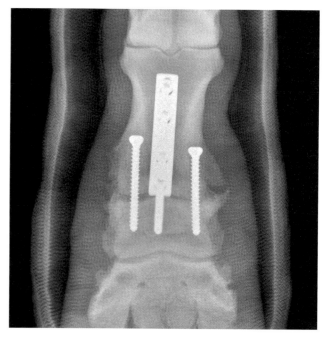

Figure 5.115. Dorsopalmar radiograph following placement of a 4-hole plate with 2 transarticular 5.5-mm screws for arthrodesis of the PIP joint.

especially in older horses that have very dense sclerotic bone (Figure 5.113). Bilateral forelimb or bilateral hindlimb arthrodesis may also be performed successfully.[2,10,20,29]

Many methods to arthrodese the PIP joint have been described and opinions vary as to which technique is preferred. However, the technique of implant placement does not appear to affect the functional outcome of most horses.[22] Current recommended techniques include a single dorsal midline plate with 2 additional transarticular 4.5- or 5.5-mm screws, or 2 dorsally applied plates with or without transarticular screws.[9,10,12,22] Dynamic compression plates (DCP), limited contact dynamic compression plates(LC-DCP), and locking compression plates (LCP) may be used. The author prefers a single dorsally applied 4.5-mm, narrow, 3- or 4-hole plate with 2 5.5-mm transarticular screws (Figures 5.114 and 5.115). This technique is thought to improve the comfort level of horses in the immediate postoperative period, and requires casting for only 2 weeks postoperatively.[10] However, the author typically leaves a half-limb fiberglass cast in place for 3 weeks after surgery in most cases. The plate and two screw method for arthrodesis of the PIP joint can be used for most any reason, including single eminence fractures of P2; however, comminuted P2 fractures are best repaired with 2 dorsally applied plates or specially designed plates such as the spoon plate.[24]

Although the technique for arthrodesis has been adequately described in several reports,[2,3,7–10,12–14,19,22,24–26] a few generalizations about the technique may help minimize complications. In most horses, 5.5-mm screws should be used throughout the repair. This is especially true for heavier horses (over 500 kg). They are substan-

tially stronger than 4.5-mm screws and a more stable fixation often leads to less pain and morbidity when the cast is removed. If using the 2- or 3-lag screw technique, there is no need to make a shelf on the distal aspect of P1. This weakens the bone, predisposing to fracture at this location. Additionally, bone plate(s) should be placed as proximal as possible on P2 to minimize secondary problems with the extensor process of the distal phalanx. This usually means that only 1 screw in the plate can be placed into P2. However, the use of a

4-hole plate with 2 screws placed into P2 has been reported but is not recommended by the author.[9]

The collateral ligaments should be incised just enough to gain adequate exposure of the palmar/plantar joint surfaces for cartilage removal. In cases in which excessive periarticular bone proliferation is present, a chisel or osteotome may be required to adequately open the joint. Alternatively, the PIP joint is not opened and the cartilage is removed by intra-articular drilling or intra-articular laser treatment followed by placement of the implants.[9,12] Arthrodesis using implants without removing the articular cartilage (and without opening the joint) has been used successfully by the author in a small number of horses with advanced OA of the PIP joint.

After surgery the limb is usually immobilized in a lower limb fiberglass cast (just below the carpus or tarsus and incorporating the foot). For horses with routine arthrodesis for OA of the PIP joint, the cast can often be removed after 2 weeks.[10] However, horses that had a PIP joint arthrodesis performed with a minimally invasive procedure were only placed in a bandage and splint after surgery.[12] Arthrodesis procedures associated with phalangeal fractures usually require a longer period of external immobilization. After the cast or bandage and splint are removed stall confinement is recommended for at least another 6 to 8 weeks. Increasing periods of hand-walking exercise can usually begin during this time. Although some horses may be ready to return to performance by 6 months, up to a year of convalescence may be required for others.[2,14,25] One study reported that horses radiographed less than 6 months after surgery had progression of the arthrodesis but it was not yet complete, whereas horses radiographed after 6 months had complete obliteration of the PIP joint space.[10] The implants do not typically need to be removed.

Prognosis

In general, the prognosis for horses following PIP joint arthrodesis is less predictable in the forelimb than in the hindlimb. After arthrodesis of the PIP joint, approximately 89% to 95% of horses with hindlimb and 70% to 85% of horses with forelimb lameness should return to their intended use, and 85% will return to athletic soundness.[10,13,14,22] A successful outcome has also been reported in several horses following bilateral PIP joint arthrodesis.[2,10] Complications that may prevent horses from becoming athletically sound include implant infection, excessive bony proliferation that impinges on the DIP joint, exostosis of the extensor process of the distal phalanx, and soft tissue "irritation" associated with the implants (screws protruding from the palmar/plantar aspect of P1 and P2). In addition, horses treated by PIP joint arthrodesis for chronic infectious arthritis do not have as good of prognosis as those treated for nonseptic conditions.[8,10]

References

1. Adams OR. Lameness in Horses, 3rd ed. Lea and Febiger, Philadelphia, 1974;359.
2. Colahan PT, Wheat JD, Meagher DM. Treatment of middle phalangeal fractures in the horse. J Am Vet Med Assoc 1981;178:1182–1185.
3. Caron JP, Fretz PB, Bailey JV, et al. Proximal interphalangeal arthrodesis in the horse. A retrospective study and a modified screw technique. Vet Surg 1990;19:196–202.
4. Denoix JM. Ultrasound examination of the pastern in horses. In Proceedings Am Assoc Equine Pract 1990;36:363–380.
5. El-Guindy MH, Ali MA, Samy MT. Chronic osteoarthrosis in the equine proximal interphalangeal joint. Equine Pract 1986;8:6–15.
6. Ellis DR, Greenwood ES. Six cases of degenerative joint disease of the proximal interphalangeal joint of young Thoroughbreds. Equine Vet J 1985;17:66–68.
7. Genetzky RM, Schneider EJ, Butler HC, et al. Comparison of two surgical procedures for arthrodesis of the proximal interphalangeal joint in horses. J Am Vet Med Assoc 1981;179:464–468.
8. Groom LJ, Gaughan EM, Lillich JD, et al. Arthrodesis of the proximal interphalangeal joint affected with septic arthritis in 8 horses. Can Vet J 2000;41:117–123.
9. James FM, Richardson DW. Minimally invasive plate fixation of lower limb injury in horses. 32 cases (1999–2003). Equine Vet J 2006;38:246–251.
10. Knox PM, Watkins JP. Proximal interphalangeal joint arthrodesis using a combination plate-screw technique in 53 horses (1994–2003) Equine Vet J 2006;38:538–542.
11. Lawson SE, Chateau H, Pourcelot P, et al. Effect of toe and heel elevation on calculated tendon strains in the horse and the influence of the proximal interphalangeal joint. J Anat 2007;210:583–591.
12. Lescun TB. Minimally invasive pastern arthrodesis in the horse. In Proceedings Am College Vet Surg 2008;36:50–53.
13. MacLellan KN, Crawford WH, MacDonald DG. Proximal interphalangeal joint arthrodesis in 34 horses using two parallel 5.5-mm cortical bone screws. Vet Surg 2001;30:454–459.
14. Martin GS, McIlwraith CW, Turner AS, et al. Long-term results and complications of proximal interphalangeal arthrodesis in horses. J Am Vet Med Assoc 1984;184:1136–1140.
15. McIlwraith CW, Goodman NL. Conditions of the interphalangeal joints. Vet Clin North Am Eq Pract 1989;5:161–178.
16. Miller SM, Stover SM, Taylor KT, et al. Palmaroproximal approach for arthrocentesis of the proximal interphalangeal joint in horses. Equine Vet J 1996;28:376–380.
17. Olive J, Mair TS, Charles B. Use of standing low-field magnetic resonance imaging to diagnose middle phalanx bone marrow lesions in horses. Equine Vet Educ 2009;March:116–123.
18. Pool RR, Meagher DM. Pathologic findings and pathogenesis of racetrack injuries. Vet Clin North Am Equine Pract 1990;6:1–30.
19. Read EK, Chandler D, Wilson DG. Arthrodesis of the equine proximal interphalangeal joint: a mechanical comparison of 2 parallel 5.5-mm cortical screws and 3 parallel 5.5-mm cortical screws. Vet Surg 2005;34:142–147.
20. Rick MC, Herthel D, Boles C. Surgical management of middle phalangeal fractures and high ringbone in the horse: A review of 16 cases. Proceedings Am Assoc Equine Pract 1987;32:315–321.
21. Ruggles AJ. The proximal and middle phalanges and the proximal interphalangeal joint. In Diagnosis and Management of Lameness in the Horse. Ross MW, Dyson SJ, eds. WB Saunders, Philadelphia, 2002;342–348.
22. Schaer TP, Bramlage LR, Embertson RM, et al. Proximal interphalangeal arthrodesis in 22 horses. Equine Vet J 2001;33:360–365.
23. Schumaker J, Livesey F, Degraves, et al. Effect of anaesthesia of the palmar digital nerves on proximal interphalangeal joint pain in the horse. Equine Vet J 2004;36:409–414.
24. Sod GA, Mitchell CF, Hubert JD, et al. In vitro biomechanical comparison of equine proximal interphalangeal joint arthrodesis techniques: prototype equine spoon plate versus axially positioned dynamic compression plate and two abaxial transarticular cortical screws inserted in lag fashion. Vet Surg 2007;36:792–799.
25. Stashak TS. The Pastern. In Adams' Lameness in Horses, 5th ed. Stashak TS, ed. Lippincott Williams and Wilkins, Philadelphia, 2002;733–768.
26. Steenhaut M, Verschooten F, DeMoor A. Arthrodesis of the pastern joint in the horse. Equine Vet J 1985;17:35–40.
27. Swanson TD. Degenerative disease of the proximal interphalangeal joint in performance horses. Proceedings Am Assoc Eq Pract 1989;34:392–397.

28. Trotter GW, McIlwraith CW, Nordin RW, et al. Degenerative joint disease with osteochondrosis of the proximal interphalangeal joint in young horses. J Am Vet Med Assoc 1982;180: 1312–1318.
29. Yovich JV, Stashak TS, Sullins KE. Bilateral pastern arthrodesis in a horse. Equine Vet J 1986;18:79–81.
30. Zubrod CJ, Schneider RK, Tucker RL, et al. Use of magnetic resonance imaging for identifying subchondral bone damage in horses: 11 cases (1999–2003). J Am Vet Med Assoc 2004;224: 411–418.

OSTEOCHONDROSIS (OC) OF THE PIP JOINT

Osteochondrosis of the PIP joint is identified less commonly than other joints in the horse. However, both osteochondral fragmentation and SCLs associated with OC can be seen in the PIP joint.[1,2,4,6,8,9] Osteochondral fragments tend to occur dorsally (usually from the distal aspect of P1; Figure 5.116) or palmarly/plantarly (midline from the eminences of P2; Figure 5.117). Subchondral cystic lesions are usually seen on the distal aspect of P1 do occur rarely in the proximal aspect of P2 (Figures 5.118 and 5.119). Malformation of the condyles of the distal aspect of P1 without fragmentation has also been recognized by the author, and may represent another form of OC that leads to early OA within the PIP joint.

Etiology

The cause of OC within the PIP joint is assumed to be due to similar factors that cause the condition in other locations within the horse. However, traumatic fragmentation and subchondral bone damage leading to SCLs can also occur within the PIP joint, and it may be difficult to differentiate between developmental and traumatic causes. Developmental lesions tend to occur in younger horses, whereas trauma can occur in any age horse. In addition, more severe clinical signs related to the PIP joint may be identified associated with trauma vs. OC.

Clinical Signs

As stated above, developmental lesions tend to occur in young horses and may cause variable signs of lameness. Physical examination findings are similar to other problems within the PIP joint and include no abnormalities, enlargement of the pastern, pain with flexion and manipulation of the pastern region, and positive response to flexion tests. Horses with SCLs of the distal aspect of P1 tend to be more lame than those with osteochondral fragmentation, presumably because the lesion is located on a weight-bearing surface (Figure 5.120).[9] Subchondral cystic lesions are also more common in the hindlimb than in the forelimb.[9] Due to the variable lameness that may be associated with OC in the PIP joint, it is important to identify the true source of lameness using diagnostic anesthesia in many cases.

Diagnosis

The diagnosis of OC is confirmed with radiographs of the pastern region. Osteochondral fragmentation can usually be seen on both lateral and dorsopalmar/plantar

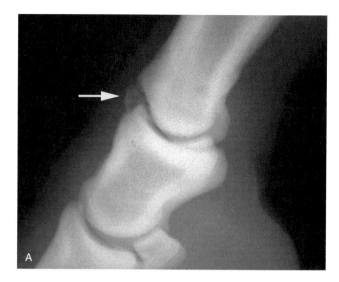

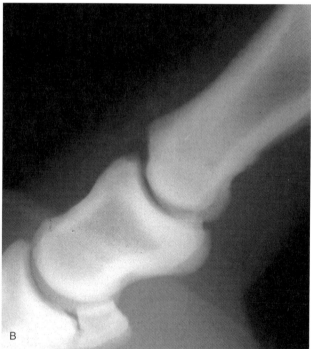

Figure 5.116. Lateral radiographs of a horse before (A) and after arthroscopic surgery (B) to remove a bone fragment (arrow) from the dorsal aspect of the PIP joint.

views (Figure 5.117), whereas SCLs are often only visible on the dorsopalmar/plantar radiographic projection (Figures 5.118 and 5.119). Some lesions, particularly osteochondral fragmentations, may be incidental findings on radiographs. Most SCLs that involve the distal condyle of P1 are clinically significant and often lead to lameness. More often, though, they are accompanied by mild to moderate radiographic changes consistent with OA within the joint.[5,7] Subchondral cystic lesions are usually associated with more secondary OA of the PIP joint.[9] Radiography of the opposite PIP joint should be performed because OC lesions can be bilateral, similar to other locations.

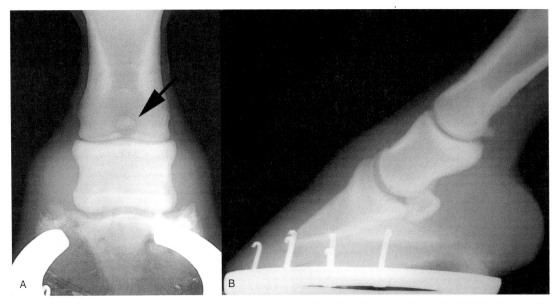

Figure 5.117. Dorsopalmar (A) and lateral (B) radiographs of a horse with palmar fragmentation of the PIP joint (arrow). The fragment was removed with arthroscopy.

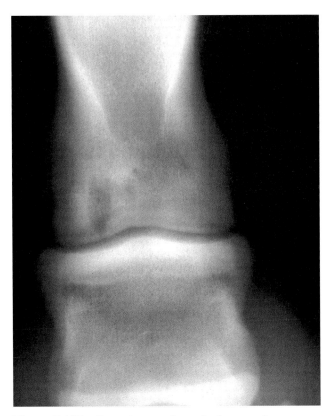

Figure 5.118. Dorsoplantar radiograph of a young horse demonstrating a large SCL of the distal medial condyle of P1. Arthrodesis of the PIP joint was performed in this horse.

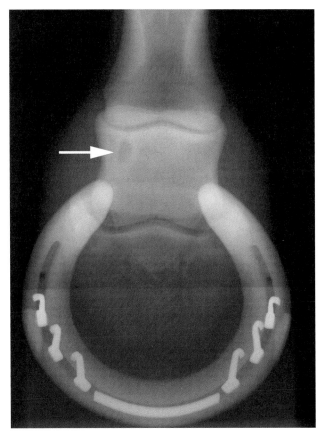

Figure 5.119. Dorsoplantar radiograph of a young horse demonstrating an SCL of the proximal aspect of P2 (arrow). This abnormality was not considered to be the cause of the lameness in this horse.

567

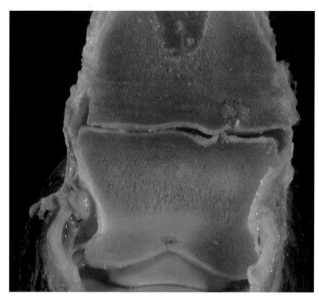

Figure 5.120. Postmortem specimen of a young horse with OC of the rear pastern joint. This horse was affected bilaterally and multiple horses within the same herd had similar lesions.

Treatment

The treatment of choice for osteochondral fragments within the PIP joint that cause clinical problems is arthroscopic removal. Both the dorsal and palmar/plantar pouches of the PIP joint are accessible with the arthroscope but the surgery can be difficult (Figure 5.116).[3,4] An arthrotomy can be performed but is associated with more soft tissue damage and increased likelihood of OA developing within the joint. Subchondral cystic lesions of distal P1 are often clinically significant and can be managed conservatively or surgically, depending on the severity of lameness. Conservative management with NSAIDs and intra-articular medication usually resolves the lameness but recurrence is common. Therefore, most horses with SCLs and PIP joint OA are best treated surgically with arthrodesis of the joint. Please refer to the section on PIP joint OA for information on arthrodesis techniques. Other less utilized surgical treatments include periarticular drilling of the cyst and injection of steroid or cancellous bone into nonarticular lesions, or debridement of the lesion followed by filling the defect with parathyroid hormone peptide (PTH(1–34))-enriched fibrin hydrogel.[2] The latter technique was reported in a single horse but the subchondral lesion healed quickly and may be applicable for treatment of SCLs at other sites in the horse.[2]

Prognosis

The prognosis following removal of OC fragmentation is usually very good and many horses can perform athletically. SCLs of distal P1 typically do well following arthrodesis and these horses can be used as athletes.

References

1. Fjordbakk CT, Strand E, Milde AK, et al. Osteochondral fragments involving the dorsomedial aspect of the proximal interphalangeal joint in young horses: 6 cases (1997–2006). J Am Vet Med Assoc 2007;230:1498–1501.

2. Fuerst A, Derungs S, von Rechenberg B, et al. Use of a parathyroid hormone peptide (PTH(1–34))-enriched fibrin hydrogel for the treatment of a subchondral cystic lesion in the proximal interphalangeal joint of a Warmblood filly. J Vet Med A Physiol Pathol Clin Med 2007;54:107–112.

3. McIlwraith CW. Diagnostic and surgical arthroscopy of the phalangeal joints. In Diagnostic and Surgical Arthroscopy in the Horse. McIlwraith CW, Nixon AJ, Wright IM, Boening KJ, eds. Elsevier, Philadelphia, 2005;347–364.

4. Radcliffe RM, Cheetham J, Bezuidenhout AJ, et al. Arthroscopic removal of palmar/plantar osteochondral fragments from the proximal interphalangeal joint in four horses. Vet Surg 2008; 37:733–740.

5. Ross MW, Dyson SJ. Diagnosis and Management of Lameness in the Horse. WB Saunders, Philadelphia, 2002.

6. Schneider RK, Ragle CA, Carter BG, et al. Arthroscopic removal of osteochondral fragments from the proximal interphalangeal joint of the pelvic limbs in three horses. J Am Vet Med Assoc. 1994;205:79–82.

7. Stashak TS. Adams' Lameness in Horses. JB Lippincott, Philadelphia, 2002.

8. Torre F. Osteochondral chip fractures of the palmar/plantar aspect of the middle phalanx in the horse: 5 cases (1991–1994). Pferdeheilkunde. 1997;13:673–678.

9. Trotter GW, McIlwraith CW, Nordin RW, et al. Degenerative joint disease with osteochondrosis of the proximal interphalangeal joint in young horses. J Am Vet Med Assoc 1982;180: 1312–1318.

LUXATION/SUBLUXATION OF THE PROXIMAL INTERPHALANGEAL (PIP) JOINT

Luxation of the PIP joint is uncommon and can occur in the medial/lateral or palmar/plantar direction. Medial/lateral luxation is usually seen after severe injury to one of the collateral ligaments from external trauma and may be open or closed. Palmar/plantar luxation is usually seen following a severe, traumatic soft tissue injury, such as complete tearing of the straight DSL, branches of the SDFT, or a combination of these injuries (Figure 5.121). Luxation in the medial/lateral and palmar/plantar direction nearly always involves a single limb.

Subluxations of the PIP joint occur most commonly in a dorsal direction and less commonly in a palmar/plantar direction and may involve one or both limbs. The terms dorsal or palmar/plantar refer to the subluxation of the proximal phalanx relative to the position of the middle phalanx. Dorsal subluxations of the PIP joint are most common in young horses and may be secondary to flexural deformities and other developmental orthopedic diseases (Figure 5.122). Although considered to be uncommon, subluxation/luxation of the PIP joint represented 21% of horses that underwent a PIP joint arthrodesis in a recent report.[4]

Etiology

Lateral/medial luxations or subluxations are often caused by severe trauma resulting in joint capsule and ligamentous tearing (e.g., distal limb caught in something and the horse struggles and/or falls) or lacerations that transect the collateral ligament. Palmar/plantar subluxation/luxation generally occurs from acute trauma resulting in overextension of the PIP joint and tearing of the soft tissue support structures (joint capsule, straight DSL, and the insertion of the SDFT). Bilateral palmar/plantar eminence fractures of P2 may cause the same effect due to complete loss of the palmar/plantar supporting soft tissues. Palmar/plantar subluxation can also be seen in foals and weanlings that have

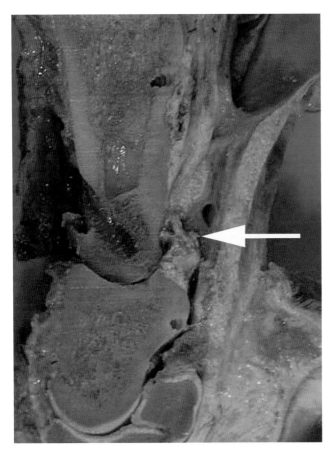

Figure 5.121.   A postmortem specimen from a horse that had complete plantar luxation of the PIP joint. Rupture of the straight DSL can be seen (arrow).

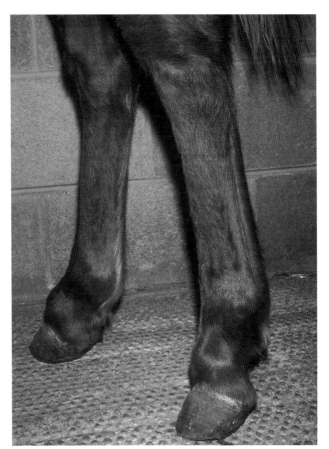

Figure 5.122.   A young horse with bilateral dorsal subluxation of the PIP joints. Dorsal swellings over both rear pastern joints can be seen.

jumped from heights and in foals with flexor tendon laxity that overexert themselves during free exercise.[3] Loss of the ligamentous support of the palmar/plantar aspect of the PIP joint results in subluxation/luxation (Figure 5.123).[2,7]

Dorsal subluxations are thought to be secondary to flexural deformities or limb contracture, and may be seen in foals/weanlings that are rapidly growing with an upright conformation (Figure 5.122). A form of DDFT contracture was responsible for dorsal subluxation of the pastern in the pelvic limbs of 3 horses.[9] Dorsal subluxation may also be seen in horses after traumatic disruption of the suspensory apparatus and arthrodesis of the fetlock joint, or progressive, severe suspensory desmitis.[2,7]

Clinical Signs

The clinical signs associated with complete medial/lateral luxation due to tearing of the collateral ligament are usually obvious. These horses are often nonweight-bearing or lame at the walk, have swelling of the pastern associated with the ligament injury, and a limb deformity may be present. Instability and pain may be identified with rotation or medial/lateral movement of the phalanges. In acute cases, heat, pain, and swelling of the pastern region are usually evident.

Horses with palmar/plantar subluxation/luxation are also often very lame in the acute stage. The lameness may subside over time but most will remain lame at the

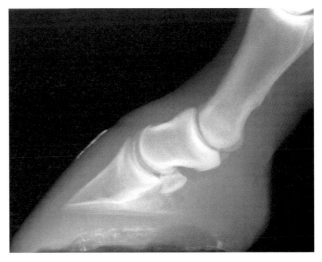

Figure 5.123.   Lateral radiograph of a horse with palmar luxation of the PIP joint. The horse was lame at the walk and had excessive dropping of the fetlock in the affected limb.

walk and the dorsal surface of the pastern will appear concave (dished out) rather than straight or convex as would occur with dorsal subluxation. In chronic cases the heel bulbs may contact the ground and excessive hyperextension of the pastern and sinking of the fetlock is noted when the horse is walked.[6,7]

Dorsal subluxation can occur without any identifiable structural abnormalities of the pastern or metacarpal/metatarsal soft tissue structures. This occurs primarily in the hindlimbs in young horses and lameness is usually absent or mild. A dorsal swelling in the pastern region may be evident when the affected limb is unweighted. This type of subluxation is often dynamic in nature, and usually resolves during full weight-bearing of the PIP joint. An audible clicking sound often accompanies the reduction of the joint. When the pelvic limbs are involved, the condition is often associated with an upright conformation (straighter than normal hocks and stifle angles).[9]

With persistent dorsal subluxation of the PIP joint an obvious swelling over the dorsal aspect of the pastern region is often evident, and the fetlock may appear slightly more extended (dropped) as compared to the contralateral unaffected limb. The dorsal swelling may appear similar to that associated with high ringbone, but on closer observation an abnormal alignment between P1 and P2 is found (Figure 5.122). However, with chronicity, both clinical and radiographic abnormalities consistent with OA of the PIP joint may develop. Lameness is variable and inconsistent in these cases and often depends on the secondary changes that develop within the joint.

Diagnosis

A tentative diagnosis can usually be made from the history and physical examination of the horse. Radiographs should be taken to confirm the diagnosis and identify concurrent abnormalities such as fractures or OA. Stress films may be needed to confirm medial/lateral subluxation because the phalanges can often remain in correct anatomic alignment unless pulled medially or laterally (Figure 5.124). Dorsal and palmar/plantar subluxations/luxations are usually obvious on standing lateral-to-medial views of the pastern (Figure 5.123 and 5.125).

Treatment

The treatment of choice for medial/lateral and palmar/plantar subluxations/luxations of the PIP joint is arthrodesis of the joint.[1,4–8] External coaptation with a cast or Kimzey splint (Kimzey Leg Saver Splint; Kimzey, Inc., Woodland, CA) may be successful in adult horses managed acutely but instability of the PIP joint may preclude successful realignment. Unlike medial/lateral luxations of the fetlock joint, similar luxations of the PIP joint do not respond well to casting alone and often develop secondary OA and persistent lameness. Conservative treatment of palmar/plantar subluxations/luxations is usually unsuccessful and surgery is often the only option to re-align the phalanges (Figure 5.126). Chronic palmar/plantar subluxations/luxations can lead to fibrosis of the PIP joint in an abnormal position, making surgical re-alignment difficult (Figure 5.127). Dorsal subluxations may also be treated with arthrodesis if they fail to respond to other methods of treatment. In most cases the subluxation is best treated surgically before excessive scar tissue has developed to

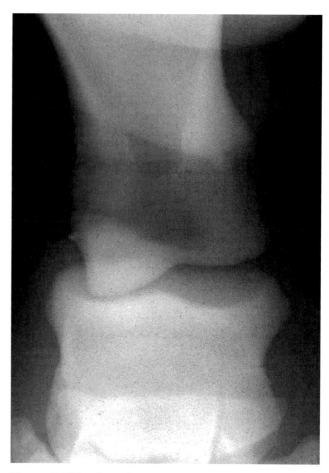

Figure 5.124. Dorsoplantar stress radiograph demonstrating complete rupture of a collateral ligament of the PIP joint. Arthrodesis of the joint is the recommended treatment.

permit more accurate and easier alignment of the joint. Horses with dorsal luxation of the PIP joint with secondary OA are also best treated with arthrodesis. See the section on OA of the PIP joint for more information on arthrodesis.

Horses with intermittent dorsal subluxation with no apparent lameness may be treated conservatively. Horses with bilateral upright hindlimb conformation and dorsal subluxation often respond to anti-inflammatory medication and a controlled exercise program.[6] Horses with intermittent dorsal subluxation of the pelvic limb associated with excessive tension of DDFT have been treated successfully with transection of the medial head of the DDFT.[9] The approach was between the DDFT and the suspensory ligament at the level of the proximal third of the third metatarsal bone, and a 2.5-cm segment of the tendon was removed. Alternatively, it has been suggested that surgical transection of the accessory ligament of the DDFT may be of benefit.[7]

Prognosis

Although there are few reports on long term follow-up, the prognosis appears to be fair to good for horses

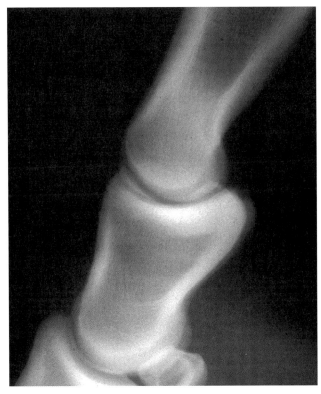

Figure 5.125. Lateral radiograph of the foal in Figure 5.122 demonstrating dorsal subluxation of P1 in relation to P2 within the pastern joint.

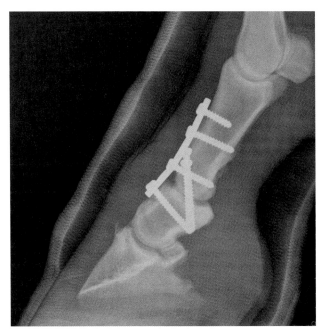

Figure 5.126. Lateral radiograph of a horse with palmar luxation of the PIP joint that was treated with arthrodesis of the joint.

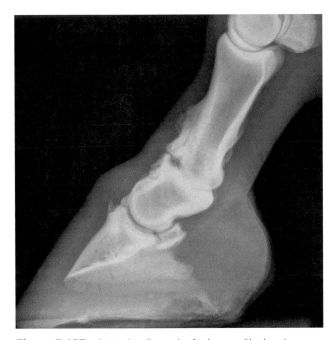

Figure 5.127. Lateral radiograph of a horse with chronic subluxation of the PIP joint and secondary OA. It is much more difficult to properly align the phalanges during surgery for chronic subluxations than for acute luxations.

with luxations/subluxations treated early by arthrodesis in which good reduction and stabilization of the PIP joint was achieved.[1,3–5,8] Convalescence is similar to that of other conditions that require a PIP joint arthrodesis and up to a year may be required before the horse may return to performance. Three cases of bilateral acquired pelvic limb intermittent dorsal subluxation treated by tendonectomy of the medial head of the DDFT responded favorably to the treatment and the subluxation resolved between 1 and 7 days postoperatively.[9] The authors have no experience with this particular surgical technique.

References

1. Adams P, Honnas CM, Ford TS, et al. Arthrodesis of a subluxated proximal interphalangeal joint in a horse. Eq Practice, 1995; 3:26–31.
2. Colahan PT, Wheat JD, Meagher DM. Treatment of middle phalangeal fractures in the horse. J Am Vet Med Assoc 1981,178:1182–1185.
3. Harrison LJ, May SA. Bilateral subluxation of the pastern joint in the forelimbs of a foal. Vet Rec. 1992;131:68–70.
4. Knox PM, Watkins JP. Proximal interphalangeal joint arthrodesis using a combination plate-screw technique in 53 horses (1994–2003) Equine Vet J 2006;38:538–542.
5. Martin GS, McIlwraith CW, Turner AS, et al. Long-term results and complications of proximal interphalangeal arthrodesis in horses. J Am Vet Med Assoc 1984;184:1136–1140.
6. Nixon AJ. Phalanges and the metacarpophalangeal and metatarsophalangeal joints. In Equine Surgery, 3rd ed. Auer JA, Stick JA, eds. Elsevier, Philadelphia, 2006;1217–1238.
7. Stashak TS. The Pastern. In Adams' Lameness in Horses. JB Lippincott, Philadelphia, 2002;741–744.
8. Steenhaut M, Verschooten F, De Moor A. Arthrodesis of the pastern joint in the horse. Equine Vet J 1985;17:35–40.
9. Shiroma JT, Engel HN, Wagner PC, et al. Dorsal subluxation of the pelvic limb of three horses. J Am Vet Med Assoc. 1989;195: 777–780.

FRACTURES OF THE MIDDLE (SECOND) PHALANX (P2)

Fractures of P2 occur most commonly in the hindlimbs of middle-aged Western performance horses used for cutting, roping, barrel racing, pole bending, and reining.[2,3,21] However, these fractures may occur in any horse during lunging, after kicks or falls, or any form of single event trauma. Fractures of P2 can also be seen in foals and usually involve the proximal physis, resulting in subluxation of the PIP joint.[4] Although the fracture is common in Quarter horses, any breed can be affected.[2-4] Based on retrospective studies, the Quarter horse represents approximately 50% of the breeds affected, Western stock is the most common activity contributing to the injury, and the hindlimbs are affected approximately 3 times more frequently than the forelimbs.[2,3]

A variety of fracture types involving P2 have been reported, including osteochondral (chip) fractures, palmar/plantar eminence fractures, axial fractures, and comminuted fractures.[1-3,6-10,12,13,16,17,19,22-24] Osteochondral fractures and axial fractures are rare, whereas eminence and comminuted fractures occur commonly. Thoroughbred and Standardbred racehorses and hunter/jumper horses appear to be at increased risk for osteochondral fractures involving the PIP joint.[11,22] The fracture can either be located dorsally (most common) or on the palmar/plantar aspect lateral or medial to the midline (Figures 5.116 and 5.117).[12,13,16,19,24] Palmar/plantar fractures do not typically involve the attachments of the DSL or the branches of SDFT. Some of these osteochondral fragments may be seen in young horses and may be developmental in origin.[16] Occasionally, multiple fragments may occur on the proximal palmar/plantar aspect of P2 that appear to be avulsion fractures. Despite the size of the fragments, the development of secondary OA appears slow but removal is usually recommended.[13,16,19,22]

Radiographic examination of the opposite PIP joint should be done because palmar/plantar fractures have been reported to occur bilaterally.[12] Osteochondral fractures of P2 involving the DIP joint are uncommon and may be caused by use-related trauma or direct trauma from a penetrating injury.[22,23] Palmar/plantar eminence fractures involving the PIP joint occur frequently. They can either be uniaxial (involving 1 eminence; Figure 5.128) or biaxial (involving both eminences; Figure 5.129). Uniaxial eminence fractures do not result in subluxation of the PIP joint, whereas biaxial fractures can contribute to subluxation or complete luxation of the joint (Figure 5.129).

Simple axial fractures of P2 occur rarely.[13] A misdiagnosis of this fracture can easily be made if the central sulcus of the frog is prominent and it is filled inadequately with packing material prior to the radiographic exam.[21] The fracture should be visible on at least 2 radiographic views to make a definitive diagnosis. This type of fracture may progress to a comminuted fracture under appropriate biomechanical factors.[21]

Comminuted fractures are the most common fracture involving P2. They nearly always involve the PIP joint (uniarticular) but often extend distally into the DIP joint (biarticular).[2,3,7,9,13,21] A variety of fracture configu-

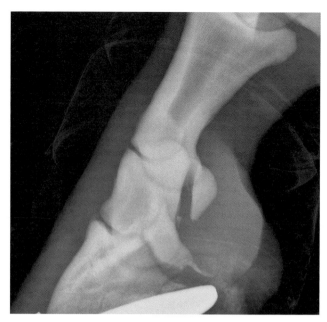

Figure 5.128. Oblique radiograph of the pastern region demonstrating a medial plantar eminence fracture of P2. This horse presented for a hindlimb lameness of 2 weeks' duration.

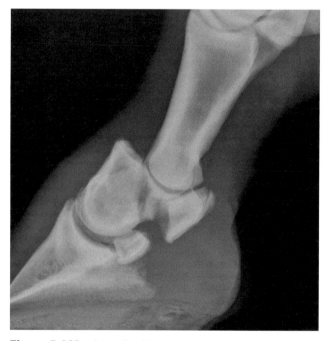

Figure 5.129. Lateral radiograph of the pastern demonstrating biaxial eminence fractures of P2. Internal fixation is recommended for these types of fractures to prevent palmar/plantar luxation of P1.

rations are possible but typically multiple fracture lines oriented in several directions are visible on radiographs (Figure 5.130). In addition, it is not uncommon for these fractures to resemble a "bag of ice" due to the multiple fracture fragments. Although comminuted P2

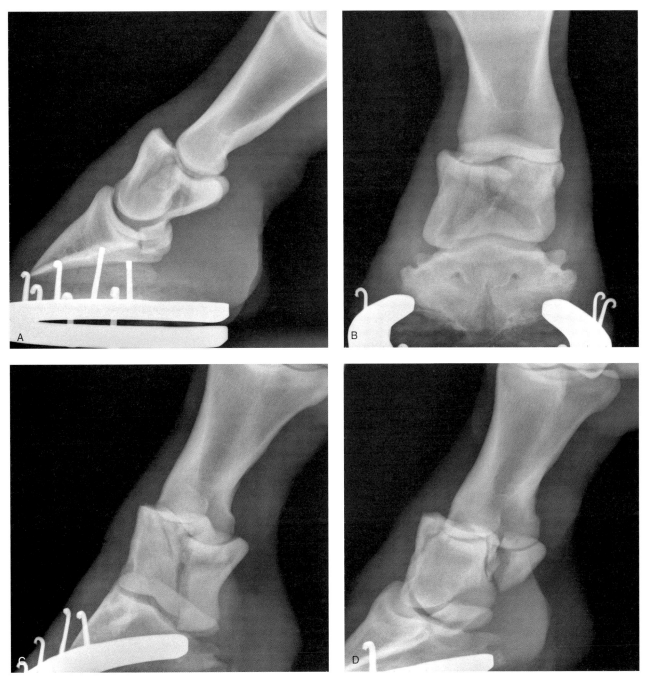

Figure 5.130. Lateral (A), dorsoplantar (B) and two oblique (C and D) radiographic projections of a horse with a comminuted P2 fracture. Multiple fracture lines are commonly seen and most comminuted fractures involve both the PIP and the DIP joint surfaces.

fractures result in marked instability of the pastern region, they are rarely open. Proper immobilization of comminuted P2 fractures prior to transport to a surgical facility is highly recommended.

Etiology

Osteochondral fractures may occur from use, direct trauma to the bone (e.g., a penetrating wound), or avulsion of soft tissue attachments (palmar/plantar aspect), or they may be developmental associated with osteochondrosis. Palmar/plantar eminence fractures may occur from compression and rotation that is associated with sudden stops and short turns. They may also occur during PIP joint overextension which results in excessive tension of the SDFT and straight DSL, causing an avulsion of the eminence(s).[11,13,21]

The cause of simple axial fractures is unknown but may be associated with repetitive trauma. Comminuted fractures are thought to result from external trauma or a combination of compression and torsion (twisting) forces that occur with sudden stops, starts, and short turns.[2,6,13,17,21] Most comminuted P2 fractures are thought to occur as a single-event injury but a history of lameness in the affected limb may precede the fracture in some horses.[21] Horses shod with heel calks are believed to be more prone to comminuted P2 fractures because the calks grip the ground, preventing the normal rotation of the foot and phalanges when the horse rapidly changes directions.[21] These fractures may also occur in horses during light work or unrestrained paddock/pasture exercise due to sudden excessive forces (compression and torsion) placed on the limb ("bad step").[6,21] Horses turned out for exercise after long-term confinement have also been reported to be at risk for comminuted P2 fractures.[6]

Clinical Signs

The clinical signs associated with P2 fractures that do not disrupt the weight-bearing capabilities of P2 (osteochondral fragments, single eminence and simple axial fractures) can be variable. Some horses may have a history of an acute onset of lameness while others may present for a chronic forelimb or hindlimb lameness. In most horses, exercise increases the severity of the lameness. Swelling of the pastern is not a reliable finding but fetlock/phalangeal flexion and rotation of the pastern region often elicit a painful response. Crepitation or instability is generally not appreciated with uniaxial P2 eminence fractures. Circling at a trot usually exacerbates the lameness. Diagnostic anesthesia with either a basi-sesamoid nerve block or intrasynovial anesthesia is often required to localize the lameness to the PIP joint region. However, diagnostic anesthesia is contraindicated with other types of P2 fractures because of the risk of fracture displacement when the horse bears weight on the anesthetized digit.

Horses with comminuted or biaxial P2 eminence fractures often have a history of acute onset of severe lameness. Some owners may report that a loud "pop" was heard just prior to the onset of severe lameness. Horses are usually very lame and painful to manipulation of the pastern, and crepitus may be felt but is not a consistent finding. The pastern may also appear to be unstable during manipulation, and swelling may be present just above the coronary band in horses with comminuted fractures (due to effusion of the DIP joint). With biaxial eminence fractures the swelling is less evident and may not be apparent.

Diagnosis

A definitive diagnosis requires a complete radiographic examination. At least 4 views are recommended: dorsal palmar (DP), lateral medial (LM), dorsal palmar lateral medial oblique (DPLMO), and dorsal palmar medial lateral oblique (DPMLO). Osteochondral fractures are usually easily diagnosed with the routine radiographic views. Additional views may be necessary with comminuted fractures so that the fracture location and configuration can be accurately appreciated. Identification of whether the fracture lines extend into the DIP joint and whether there is an intact "strut" of bone that extends between the PIP and DIP is very important information for comminuted fractures (Figure 5.130). The fracture configuration has considerable

bearing on the treatment method selected as well as the prognosis for future soundness.

Computer tomography (CT) of comminuted P2 fractures has been shown to be helpful in defining the fracture configuration.[18] Imaging with CT produces cross sectional images of the bone which results in spatial separation of superimposed structures that are seen on survey radiographs (Figure 5.131). The use of CT can be especially important if there is doubt whether a comminuted P2 fracture can be repaired and the extent of involvement of the DIP joint. In general, most comminuted P2 fractures appear to have even more fracture fragments on CT than seen on radiographs. However, the location of fracture lines entering the DIP joint and the degree of displacement at the joint surface can be more accurately determined with a CT than conventional radiography. The authors have used CT to assess comminuted P2 fractures more in recent years to aid reconstruction of the DIP joint in an attempt to improve the overall prognosis of these horses.

Treatment

Osteochondral Fractures

Fracture fragments associated with the PIP joint that contribute to lameness are best removed with arthroscopy.[13,16,19,22,23] Both dorsal and palmar/plantar fragments can be removed with arthroscopy, although the maneuverability of the instrumentation is somewhat limited in the dorsal joint pouch due to the extensor tendon attachment immediately distal to the joint.[13,19] The palmar/plantar recess of the PIP joint is larger, which makes surgical manipulation somewhat easier but it is still difficult.[16] Osteochondral fractures involving the DIP joint are also best managed by arthroscopy if possible.

Eminence Fractures

Uniaxial or biaxial eminence fractures of P2 that involve the PIP joint are best treated by arthrodesis of the PIP joint followed by cast application.[8,13,17,21] Lag screw repair of uniaxial eminence fractures has been reported but is not recommended by the author because OA of the PIP joint and continued lameness often develop. A single, narrow, dorsally applied 3- to 4-hole plate with 2 transarticular screws is recommended for horses with uniaxial eminence fractures (Figure 5.132) and 2 3- to 4-hole dorsally applied plates are recommended for biaxial eminence fractures (Figure 5.133).[1,4,8,13] The plates can be positioned so that the most distal screw through the plate(s) can be used to lag or just secure (positional screw only) the palmar/plantar eminence fracture(s) at the time of internal fixation. However, there is debate as to whether securing the eminence fracture(s) is absolutely necessary. For adult horses, 4.5-mm DCP, LC-DCP, or LCP plates may be used, whereas 3.5-mm plates may be suitable for foals. Other plate configurations that have been reported include a single broad DCP, a spoon plate, and a Y plate.[1,5,20] The use of a T plate has been reported but its thin profile usually precludes its use in adult horses.[13] The spoon and Y plates are usually reserved to repair

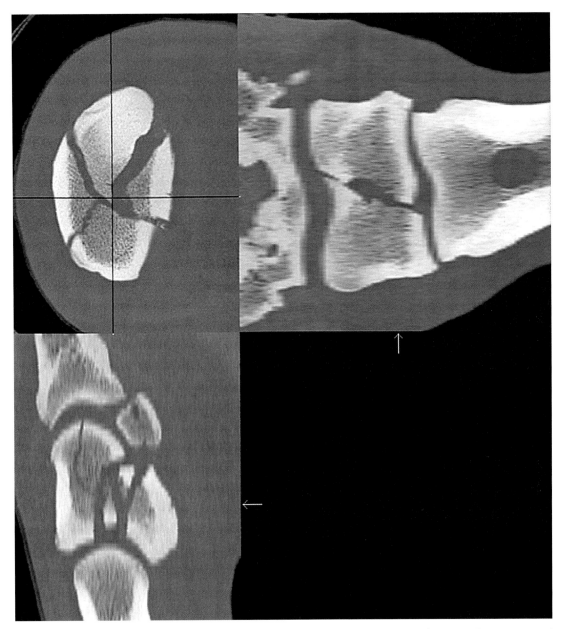

Figure 5.131. CT images of a comminuted P2 fracture that demonstrate the numerous fracture fragments that are present in different orientations. This fracture was repaired with 2 dorsally applied bone plates.

comminuted P2 fractures.[5,20] For more information on PIP joint arthrodesis, see the section on PIP joint OA).

Although casting alone has been reported as an acceptable method of treatment in horses with eminence fractures, it should be reserved for those cases in which pasture or breeding soundness is desired and economic constraints dictate this approach. Single eminence fractures rarely heal back to the parent bone with casting alone and secondary OA of the PIP joint leading to chronic lameness is common. A lower limb (half-limb) fiberglass cast that includes the hoof and extends to the proximal limits of the metacarpus/metatarsus is recommended. The limb should be cast with the phalanges in a relaxed position or with slight flexion to help with fracture reduction.[21]

Horses with biaxial eminence fractures often develop a palmar/plantar subluxation of the PIP joint when casted due to weight-bearing forces pushing P1 distally. If internal fixation of biaxial P2 fractures is not elected, then transfixation pin casts or another type of external fixator is recommended over casting alone to maintain phalangeal alignment (Figure 5.134). The external fixator should be maintained for a minimum of 40 days, and an additional casting period is often needed after removal of the transfixation pin cast depending on the degree of fracture healing.[7] With either casting alone or transfixation pin casts, the initial cost may be less to the owner, but the costs of repeat casting, prolonged confinement, complications, etc. are often not that much less or may be more than what the cost of internal

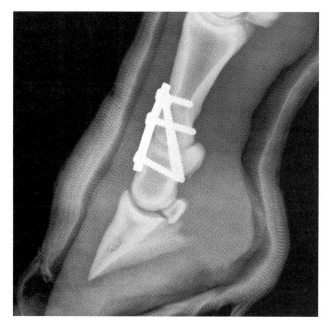

Figure 5.132. Repair method for the horse with a single plantar eminence fracture depicted in Figure 5.128. A single plate and 2 transarticular screws were used.

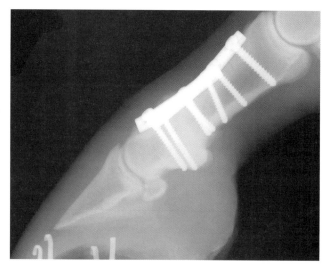

Figure 5.133. Lateral radiograph 1 year after the biaxial eminence fracture of P2 depicted in Figure 5.129 was repaired with 2 plates.

fixation would have been. Therefore, internal fixation of eminence fractures is the preferred method of treatment.

Comminuted P2 Fractures

There are varying degrees of comminution associated with nearly all P2 fractures, which can greatly affect treatment. In general, horses with comminuted P2 fractures should be repaired with some type of internal fixation (bone plating) if at all possible. Horses with an intact strut of bone spanning from the PIP to the DIP joints are ideal candidates for internal fixation. Horses without an intact bony strut yet have large enough bony fragments for screw fixation also often benefit from internal fixation (Figure 5.130). Horses with highly comminuted P2 fractures (so called "bag of ice") that do not have fracture fragments large enough to engage screws are best treated with transfixation pin casts or another type of external fixator.[7,9,14,15] Casting alone can also be used for these highly comminuted fractures but fracture collapse is not uncommon.

The application of dorsal plate(s) combined with PIP joint arthrodesis is recommended for most horses with comminuted P2 fractures for optimal return to performance (Figure 5.135). Plate configurations that can be used depending on the degree of comminution include a single broad DCP, single or double narrow DCP plates, T plates, or a special designed spoon or Y plate.[1,3–5,17,20,24] The newer locking plates may also be used depending on the fracture configuration. Currently, the use of 2 narrow DCP or LCP plates is usually preferred.

Visualization of the fracture configuration at the PIP joint surface is used to determine the best placement of implants (Figure 5.136). Reduction of the palmar/

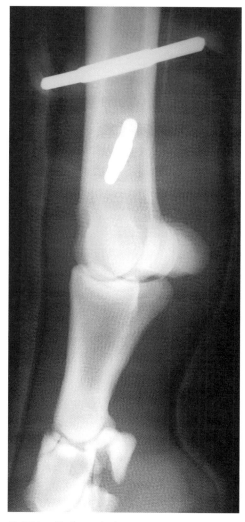

Figure 5.134. Radiograph demonstrating placement of 2 one-quarter-inch centrally threaded transfixation pins within the metatarsus for placement of a transfixation pin cast.

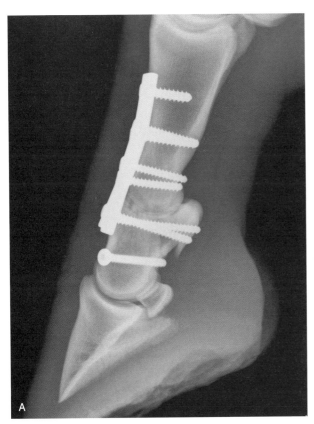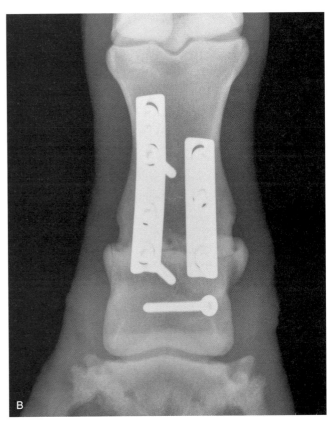

Figure 5.135. Lateral (A) and dorsoplantar (B) radiographs of the repair of the fracture depicted in Figure 5.130. The lag screw within P2 was used to reduce the fracture gag at the DIP joint surface.

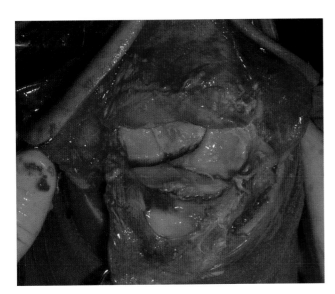

Figure 5.136. Intra-operative view of the proximal articular surface of P2 is used to help decide the location and direction of screw placement during repair of comminuted P2 fractures.

plantar eminences can usually be performed and stabilized by a lag or positional screw placed through the distal plate(s) hole(s). The plates should be placed as far proximally on P2 as possible to avoid impingement of the extensor process of the distal phalanx.[4,21] Individually

placed lag screws independent of the plate(s) can also be used to provide added strength to the repair and to help reduce the fracture gaps at the DIP joint (Figure 5.135). Specially designed spoon plates or Y plates may be comparable biomechanically to double plating with the added benefit of permitting placement of more than 2 screws within the proximal aspect of P2.[5,20] However, they are not used by the author and their availability appears to be limited.

The use of casts, transfixation pin casts, or an external fixator is usually reserved for horses with severely comminuted P2 fractures that cannot be adequately reduced or stabilized by internal fixation, and for which euthanasia is not an option. Economic constraints may also enter into the decision regarding when to use these options, although with the prolonged treatment period, they may not be much less expensive. Pasture soundness for breeding purposes or use as a pet is all that can be expected from horses treated with casts with or without transfixation pins. Traction to the phalanges using wires placed through the hoof wall helps reduce the fracture fragments during cast application. A lower limb cast that incorporates the hoof is mandatory. Some comminuted P2 fractures may be treated successfully using this approach but cast application for a minimum of 8 weeks is usually required.[21]

In the most severely comminuted P2 fractures transfixation pin casts are preferred over casting alone. The transfixation pins are placed into the metaphyseal region of the metacarpus/metatarsus and serve to

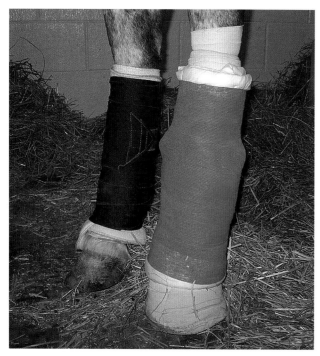

Figure 5.137. Transfixation pin-casts incorporate the foot and extend to the proximal aspect of the metatarsus/metacarpus.

minimize weight-bearing forces through the fracture site. This reduces the chance of fracture collapse within the cast and often makes the horse much more comfortable on the fractured limb compared to casting alone.

Several types of transfixation pins may be used, but centrally threaded pins that engage the metacarpus/metatarsus are preferred over smooth pins. Two pins one-quarter inch in diameter placed 2 cm apart in a divergent fashion are recommended in adult horses (Figure 5.134).[7,9] A distal limb cast incorporating the foot and pins extending to the proximal metacarpus/metatarsus is applied (Figure 5.137). Complications of using transfixation pin casts include lysis/infection around the pins, pin loosening, ring sequestrum of the metacarpus/metatarsus, and fracture of the metacarpus/metatarsus at the site of pin placement.[7,9]

An alternative to transfixation pin casts is a true external fixator designed by Nunamaker. The initial device used a series of large transfixation pins placed through the metacarpus/metatarsus that were incorporated into side connecting bars that attached to a foot plate.[14] More recently, this device has been changed to use tapered-sleeve transcortical pins (7.94 mm in diameter), which reduces the risk of bone fracture at the pin interface.[15] In cases in which casts alone, transfixation pin-casts, or external fixators are used, the damage to the joint surface is usually sufficient to create fusion of the joint with time.

Prognosis

The prognosis of horses with osteochondral fractures treated by arthrotomy or arthroscopy appears to be very good for return to full serviceability.[12,13,16,19,22] In one study 4 of 5 cases with osteochondral fragments (3

involved the PIP joint and 2 involved the DIP joint) treated by arthrotomy returned to their intended use.[22] There are only a few reports of using arthroscopy to remove these fragments but it is the preferred approach with most horses returning to performance.[13,16,19,23]

The prognosis for uniaxial or biaxial palmar/plantar eminence fractures treated by arthrodesis also appears to be very good for return to performance and should be considered similar to that expected for PIP joint arthrodesis used to treat OA of the joint.[8,10] The use of single or double bone plating is considered mandatory for biaxial eminence fractures and will most likely improve the prognosis of these horses returning to function.[4,21]

Horses with comminuted fractures that only involve the PIP joint usually have a good prognosis to return to athletic performance provided they are treated with internal fixation. The prognosis for horses with biarticular comminuted P2 fractures is much reduced because the limiting factor in many cases is related to the health of the DIP joint. Older literature has stated that horses with comminuted biarticular P2 fractures have a 50% survival rate and slightly greater than a 10% chance of returning to athletic performance with casting alone.[2] This remains true today and emphasizes that horses with comminuted P2 fractures treated without internal fixation are very unlikely to be athletically sound.

Internal fixation with bone plates increases both survival and return to athletic function in horses with comminuted P2 fractures.[3] In one report 7 of 8 horses with forelimb involvement were alive 2 years after injury and 4 of 7 horses were being ridden.[3] Of the 2 horses with hindlimb involvement 1 was being ridden and 1 was lost to follow-up.[3] In another report, 2 of 3 mature horses with comminuted fractures that involved the forelimbs returned to athletic performance and 2 of 3 foals with physeal fractures also performed.[4]

The prognosis of these horses is often dictated by the amount of fracture displacement at the DIP joint and the ability to reduce this displacement at the time of surgery. Horses with fractures of the hindlimb are also thought to have an improved prognosis over those affecting the forelimb. In general, horses with biarticular comminuted P2 fractures should be considered to have a 40% to 50% chance of returning to performance after internal fixation, provided complications do not occur.

References

1. Bukowieki CF, Bramlage LR. Treatment of a comminuted middle phalangeal fracture in a horse by use of a broad dynamic compression plate. J Am Vet Med Assoc 1989;194:1731–1733.
2. Colahan PT, Wheat JD, Meagher DM. Treatment of middle phalangeal fractures in the horse. J Am Vet Med Assoc 1981;178:1182–1185.
3. Crabill MR, Watkins JP, Schneider RK, et al. Double plate fixation of comminuted fractures of the second phalanx in horses in 10 cases (1985–1993). J Am Vet Med Assoc 1995;207: 1458–1461.
4. Doran RE, White NA, Allen D. Use of a bone plate for treatment of middle phalangeal fractures in horses: Seven cases (1979–1984). J Am Vet Med Assoc 1987;191:575–578.
5. Galuppo LD, Stover SM, Willits NH. A biomechanical comparison of double-plate and Y plate fixation for comminuted equine second phalanx fractures. Vet Surg 2000;29:152–162.

6. Honnas CM. Surgical treatment of selected musculoskeletal disorders of the forelimb. In Equine Surgery. Auer JA, ed. WB Saunders, Philadelphia, 1992;995–997.
7. Joyce J, Baxter GM, Sarrafian TL, et al. Use of transfixation pin casts to treat adult horses with comminuted phalangeal fractures: 20 cases (1993–2003). J Am Vet Med Assoc 2006;229: 725–730.
8. Knox PM, Watkins JP. Proximal interphalangeal joint arthrodesis using a combination plate-screw technique in 53 horses (1994–2003) Equine Vet J 2006;38:538–542.
9. Lescan TB, McClure SR, Ward MP, et al. Evaluation of transfixation casting for treatment of third metacarpal, third metatarsal, and phalangeal fractures in horses: 37 cases (1994–2004). J Am Vet Med Assoc 2007;230:1340–1349.
10. Martin GS, McIlwraith CW, Turner AS, et al. Long-term results and complications of proximal interphalangeal arthrodesis in horses. J Am Vet Med Assoc 1984;184:1136–1140.
11. McIlwraith CW, Goodman NL. Conditions of the interphalangeal joints. Vet Clin North Am Equine Pract 1989;5: 161–178.
12. Modransky PD, et al. Surgical treatment of a palmar midsagittal fracture of the proximal second phalanx in a horse. Vet Surg 1982;11:129–131.
13. Nixon AJ. Phalanges and the metacarpophalangeal and metatarsophalangeal joints. In Equine Surgery, 3rd ed. Auer JA, Stick JA, eds. Elsevier, Philadelphia, 2006;1217–1238.
14. Nunamaker DM, Richardson DW, Butterweck DM, et al. A new external skeletal fixaton device that allows immediate full-weight-bearing application in the horse. Vet Surg 1986;15:345–355.
15. Nunamaker DM, Nash RA. A tapered-sleeve transcortical pin external skeletal fixation device for use in horses: development, application, and experience. Vet Surg 2008;37:725–732.
16. Radcliffe RM, Cheetham J, Bezuidenhout AJ, et al. Arthroscopic removal of palmar/plantar osteochondral fragments from the proximal interphalangeal joint in four horses. Vet Surg 2008; 37:733–740.
17. Rick MC. Fractures of the middle phalanx. In Current Practice of Equine Surgery. White NA, Moore JN, eds. Lippincott, Philadelphia, 1990;606–609.
18. Rose PL, Seeherman H, O'Callaghan M. Computed tomographic evaluation of comminuted middle phalangeal fractures in the horse. Vet Radiol Ultrasound. 1997;38:424–429.
19. Schneider RK, Ragle CA, Carter BG, et al. Arthroscopic removal of osteochondral fragments from the proximal interphalangeal joint of the pelvic limbs in three horses. J Am Vet Med Assoc 1994;205:79–82.
20. Sod GA, Mitchell CF, Hubert JD, et al. In vitro biomechanical comparison of equine proximal interphalangeal joint arthrodesis techniques: prototype equine spoon plate versus axially positioned dynamic compression plate and two abaxial transarticular cortical screws inserted in lag fashion. Vet Surg 2007; 36:792–799.
21. Stashak TS. The Pastern. In Adams' Lameness in Horses. JB Lippincott, Philadelphia, 2002;744–755.
22. Torre F. Osteochondral chip fractures of the palmar/plantar aspect of the middle phalanx in the horse: 5 cases (199–1994) Pferdeheilkunde 1997;13:673–678.
23. Vail TB, McIlwraith CW. Arthroscopic removal of an osteochondral fragment from the middle phalanx of a horse. Vet Surg 1992;21:260–272.
24. Watkins JP. Fractures of the middle phalanx. In Equine Fracture Repair. Nixon AJ, ed. WB Saunders, Philadelphia, 1996; 129–136.

FRACTURES OF THE PROXIMAL (FIRST) PHALANX (P1)

Fractures of the proximal phalanx (P1) occur frequently and can be broadly categorized into noncomminuted and comminuted fractures.[13] Osteochondral fragmentation of the proximal dorsal or palmar/plantar aspects of P1 are types of noncomminuted fractures and are discussed in the fetlock section. Fracture configurations (excluding osteochondral fragmentation) range from small fissures that enter the metacarpo/metatarso-phalangeal (MCP/MTP) joint to highly comminuted fractures ("bag of ice") that affect both cortices and the proximal and distal joint surfaces. Stress or fatigue-type fractures that may not be identified on routine radiographs may also occur in performance horses. Most P1 fractures are closed, although 8 of 64 comminuted fractures were open at the time of presentation and an additional 4 had extensive bruising with serous fluid oozing through intact skin in a retrospective review.[8]

Noncomminuted P1 fractures have been classified into several types (Figures 5.138 to 5.142):[1,3–6,9,12–14,16,22]

1. Midsagittal or sagittal fractures: exist primarily in the sagittal plane and begin at the proximal articular surface
   a. Short (extend less than 30 mm in length distally)
   b. Long (extend more than 30 mm in length distally; Figure 5.138)
   c. Complete (exit the lateral cortex or span both joint surfaces; Figure 5.139)
2. Dorsal frontal fractures: begin at the MCP/MTP joint in the frontal plane and extend to the dorsal cortex or distally toward the PIP joint; can be incomplete or complete (Figure 5.140)
3. Distal joint fractures: involve the PIP joint (Figure 5.141)
4. Palmar/plantar eminence fractures: involve the MTP/MCP joint (Figure 5.142)
5. Physeal fractures: usually Salter-Harris type 2
6. Oblique or transverse diaphyseal fractures

Comminuted P1 fractures can range from fairly simple 3-piece fractures to the bag of ice type of injury (Figure 5.143).[15,16,19] However, a variety of configurations of comminuted P1 fractures is possible (Figure 5.144). For treatment purposes, they are divided into fractures that have an intact cortex (strut) of P1 from the proximal to distal joint surfaces (moderately comminuted) and fractures that do not have an intact bone strut (severely comminuted).[8,15,19] Less common types of P1 fractures include proximal medial collateral ligament avulsion fractures (Figure 5.145), dorsal nonarticular fractures, and stress or fatigue fractures. Stress or fatigue type fractures may precede sagittal or comminuted P1 fractures and occur almost exclusively in performance horses.[21] Medial collateral ligament avulsion fractures are discussed in the fetlock section.

Sagittal P1 fractures occur most commonly and may be present in the contralateral limb in a small percentage of the cases.[4,14,22] Sagittal and other types of noncomminuted P1 fractures are primarily seen in racing Thoroughbreds and Standardbreds but can also occur in other types of performance horses. They often affect the hindlimbs in Standardbreds and the forelimbs in Thoroughbreds.[4,5,14,22] Dorsal frontal fractures are relatively rare but usually occur in the hindlimb.[1] Comminuted P1 fractures also occur commonly in racing Thoroughbreds and Standardbreds. In a recent report, 72% of horses with comminuted P1 fractures sustained the injury during racing or race training.[8] However, comminuted P1 fractures may occur in other types of performance horses (especially Western performance or polo) and may occur in any horse at pasture

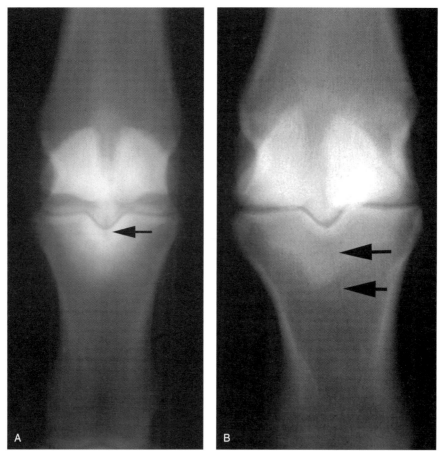

Figure 5.138. Dorsopalmar radiographs of the pastern region revealing short (A) and long (B) incomplete sagittal fractures of P1 (arrows). The fracture in (B) was repaired with 2 lag screws through stab incisions.

or at exercise from a single traumatic event.[8,14,20] In one report 27% of the horses sustained a comminuted fracture while at pasture and a smaller percentage developed the fracture while being used for showing or pleasure riding.[14] In a more recent report, 28% of all comminuted P1 fractures were from nonracing causes.[8]

Etiology

It appears that a combination of longitudinal compression in conjunction with asynchronous lateral-to-medial rotation of P1 or twisting of P1 in relation to the metacarpus/metatarsus may be the cause.[20] During normal weight-bearing, the convex sagittal ridge of the distal end of the third metacarpal or metatarsal bone fits into the concave groove in the proximal surface of P1. If this alignment is not perfect, the convex sagittal ridge may act as a wedge to create the fracture. Also, during limb flexion, there is a lateral-to-medial rotation of P1 around its long axis. If the rotary movement is accelerated, as would occur if the foot slips, a P1 fracture may result.[20] In most cases, a combination of axial weight-bearing and torsional forces usually contributes to P1 fractures.[16]

Nearly all midsagittal fractures begin at the concave groove of the proximal aspect of P1 and tend to be oriented lateral to the midline in the forelimb. This may be due to a smaller lateral articular surface of P1 in the forelimb compared to the hindlimb.[4,20] The consequent position of the center of the sagittal groove lateral to the midline may dictate that fractures propagate down that side of the bone in the forelimb.[4] In contrast, sagittal fractures that extend distal or medial to the midline are approximately twice as common in the hindlimbs than the forelimbs.[4] The relationship between the slope of the proximal and distal articulations of P1 may also account for the different fracture configurations between the fore- and hindlimb.[4]

Stress or fatigue type fractures also occur in P1 and may precede the development of a radiographic apparent sagittal P1 fracture or may predispose to a comminuted fracture. Fatigue fractures are usually only seen in performance horses and often represent an area of bone weakness related to stress remodeling.[21] As microdamage accumulates from repetitive loading of P1, the bone weakens or "fatigues," predisposing to fracture. This same scenario can occur in multiple locations in performance horses (humerus, metacarpus, tibia, pelvis, etc.).[21] Stress fractures tend to occur most commonly in the

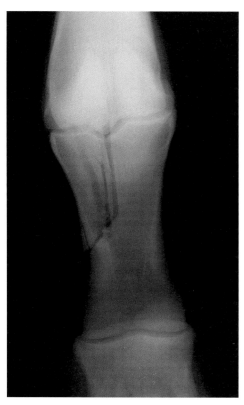

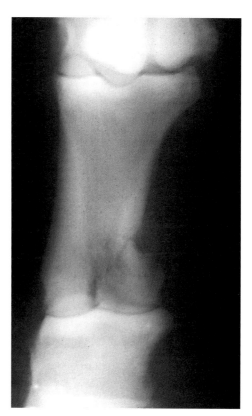

Figure 5.139. Dorsopalmar radiograph of the pastern region demonstrating a complete sagittal fracture of P1 that exists in the lateral cortex. This fracture was repaired with 3 lag screws through an open approach to the fetlock joint. (Courtesy of Dr. Jeremy Hubert.)

Figure 5.141. Dorsopalmar radiograph of the pastern region demonstrating a distal fracture of P1 that communicates with the PIP joint.

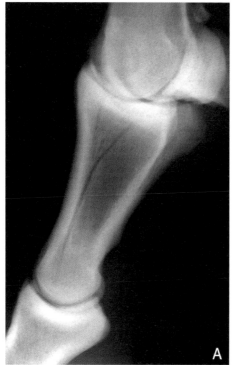

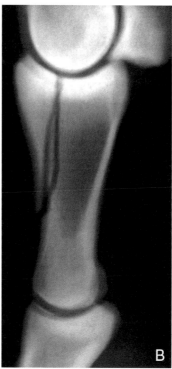

Figure 5.140. A. Oblique view of an incomplete dorsal fracture of P1. B. Lateral view of a complete dorsal fracture of P1 that exits the dorsal cortex. (Courtesy of Dr. Julie Dechant.)

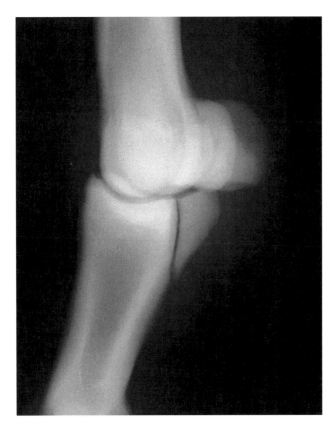

Figure 5.142. Lateral radiograph of the fetlock demonstrating a fracture of the palmar eminence of P1. This fracture was an acute injury and was repaired by lag screw fixation. Smaller, chronic fractures are more common in this location and are often removed if they are problematic.

midsagittal groove at the proximal aspect of the bone, the same area where most P1 fractures originate (Fig 5.138A).

Clinical Signs

The clinical signs associated with P1 fractures are variable and depend on the fracture type and degree of fracture propagation.[16] In most cases there is usually a history of an acute onset of lameness. Horses with incomplete sagittal fractures may demonstrate moderate pain and lameness initially but it may of a short duration. However, fetlock effusion is usually present and a painful response is often elicited with flexion and rotation of the phalanges.[22] Horses with complete sagittal fractures are usually quite lame (grade 3 to 4 of 5) and fetlock effusion and swelling of the pastern region is usually apparent. Horses with comminuted fractures are usually nonweight-bearing and may show signs of physical distress such as sweating.[4,8,19] The pastern region is often obviously swollen, and crepitus and instability is palpable.

Adequate external immobilization of the fracture in these horses is mandatory if they are being transported for surgical repair.[2] Perineural anesthesia is usually unnecessary to make the diagnosis but some horses with short sagittal P1 fractures may present for a routine lameness evaluation. Perineural anesthesia is contraindicated if any type of P1 fracture is suspected because it will increase the risk of fracture propagation.[8,16] Guidelines for transporting horses with comminuted P1 fractures can be found in Chapter 7.

Diagnosis

Radiographs are required to characterize the type of P1 fracture and dictate the appropriate treatment. The radiographic examination should include at least 4 views: dorsal palmar/plantar (DP), lateral medial (LM), dorsal palmar/plantar lateral medial oblique (DPLMO), and dorsal palmar/plantar medial lateral oblique (DPMLO). Additional views at varying angles may be necessary to accurately document the fracture configuration with comminuted fractures as well as the presence or absence of joint involvement.

Midsagittal fractures are often readily apparent on the DP view but some short, incomplete fractures may be difficult to see radiographically. In addition, multiple fracture lines on a single radiographic view do not always indicate more than 1 fracture because of the spiral nature of these fractures. This occurs because the fracture lines are not completely superimposed on the radiographic view.[4,20]

Some P1 fractures may also be misdiagnosed as the nutrient foramen, especially in Standardbreds.[11] In horses with comminuted P1 fractures, the presence or absence of an intact bony strut that spans from the MCP/MTP to the PIP joints is one of the most important radiographic features. In addition, the degree of fracture displacement, presence of comminution at the joint surfaces, and whether the fracture involves the PIP joint are all important radiographic features that may affect treatment. Similar to comminuted P2 fractures, CT can be very beneficial to more accurately assess the degree of comminution of P1 fractures and to aid in preoperative planning for surgery (Figure 5.146).

Treatment

Noncomminuted P1 Fractures

The decision on how to treat horses with noncomminuted fractures usually depends on the fracture type, fracture location and length, degree of displacement, and intended use of the horse. Treatment options include confinement with bandaging, confinement with a distal limb cast, internal fixation with lag screws and/or bone plates, external skeletal fixation alone, or internal fixation combined with external skeletal fixation. In general, most noncomminuted P1 fractures involve an articular surface (MCP/MTP and/or PIP joint) and are best treated with internal fixation using lag screws placed through stab incisions. Horses with displaced fractures that are not treated with internal fixation have a reduced chance of returning to performance.

Short, incomplete sagittal fractures can be treated conservatively with pressure bandaging and stall rest[4] but most are treated with lag screw fixation.[5,8,9] Fracture propagation is a risk of treating short incomplete

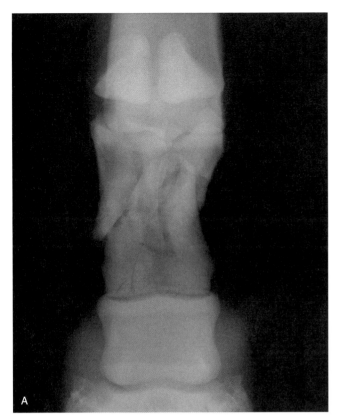 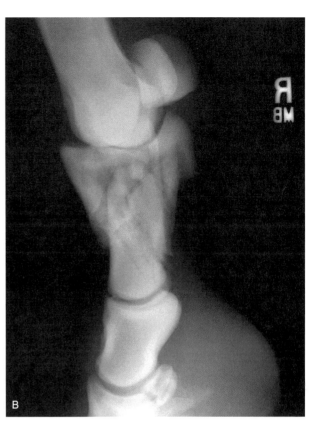

Figure 5.143. Lateral (A) and dorsopalmar (B) radiographs of a horse with a severely comminuted fracture of P1. Internal fixation is not possible with these types of fractures and transfixation pin-casts or external fixators are usually used to attempt salvage of these horses.

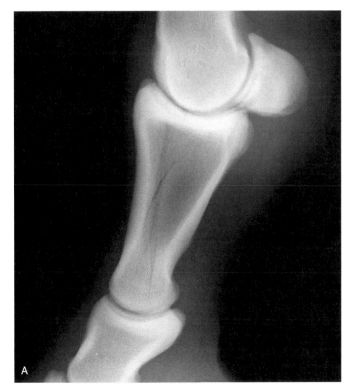 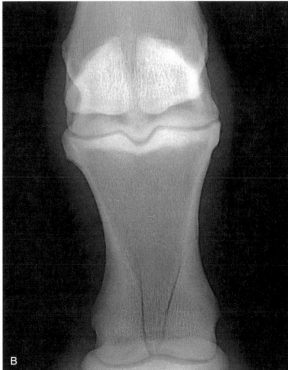

Figure 5.144. Lateral (A) and dorsoplantar radiographs (B) of a nondisplaced, moderately comminuted P1 fracture that was repaired with multiple lag screws placed through stab incisions.

sagittal fractures conservatively, and this occurred in 3 of 85 racehorses in one study.[4] These fractures heal with a periosteal callus over the dorsal aspect of the fracture site which does not appear to limit function.[4,41] If the fracture has not healed after 3 months, lag screw fixation is recommended.[16] However, a recent study found

an improved prognosis in nonracehorses with short, incomplete sagittal fractures that were treated with lag screws.[9] Horses treated conservatively remained lame, only 1 of 4 horses had radiographic evidence of fracture healing, and 2 of 4 horses had catastrophic propagation of the fracture.[9] In addition, another study indicated that all incomplete sagittal fractures greater than 15 mm should be treated surgically.[22]

Horses with long (greater than 30 mm) sagittal incomplete fractures that are to be used for racing should be treated with lag screw fixation placed through stab incisions followed by external coaptation (Figure 5.147).[6,16] Two to three screws placed 20 mm apart are generally used depending on the length of the fracture. The most proximal screw should be placed within 5 mm of the most distal point of the sagittal groove in P1.[16] Radiographic or fluoroscopic monitoring is recommended to ensure that the MCP/MTP joint is not entered and to document fracture compression. If a cast is used postoperatively, it is generally removed after 10 to 14 days. Others prefer bandage support only for recovery from anesthesia.[16]

Complete sagittal fractures that extend distally from the MCP/MTP joint to involve the PIP joint or that exit the lateral cortex are best treated by internal fixation and coaptation.[1,4,14,16,19] These fractures are often displaced and can generally be better reduced with open approaches to P1 followed by lag screw stabilization.[16] Plate fixation may also be used, depending on the fracture configuration.[4,14] However, lag screw fixation through stab incisions similar to incomplete sagittal fractures may be sufficient, depending on the degree of displacement. A distal limb cast is usually recommended after surgery for 2 to 4 weeks, depending on the security of the fixation.

Bandaging and/or external coaptation has been used alone in cases in which breeding soundness is the objective or if there are economic constraints.[1,4] In general,

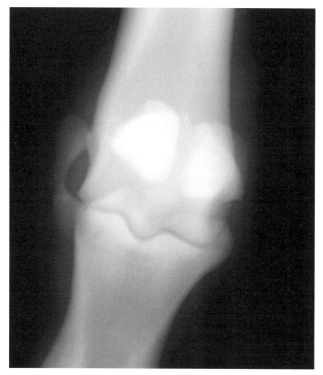

Figure 5.145. Oblique radiograph of the fetlock demonstrating avulsion fractures of the medial collateral ligament from the proximal aspect of P1. An open approach to the fetlock was used to reduce the fractures and repair with lag screws.

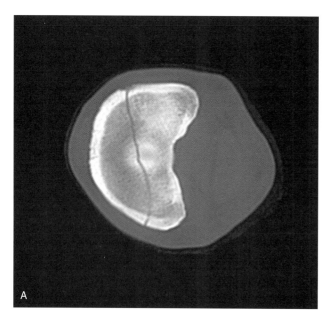
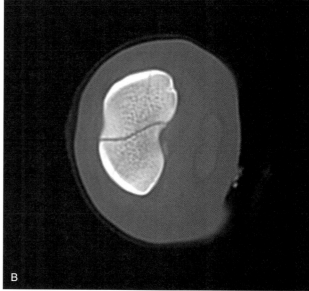

Figure 5.146. These CT images of the proximal (A) and distal (B) aspects of P1 of the fracture in Figure 5.144 helped determine the direction of the fracture lines as they entered the fetlock and PIP joint, respectively.

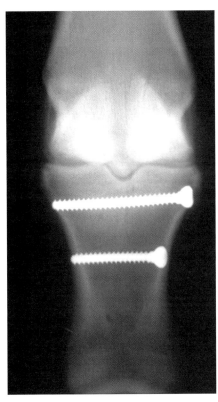

Figure 5.147. Dorsopalmar radiograph of the midsagittal incomplete P1 fracture illustrated in Figure 5.138B that was treated with 2 4.5-mm lag screws placed through stab incisions.

horses that are treated conservatively require about 4 months to become free of pain and lameness.[20] They often develop considerable exostosis at the fracture site and secondary OA of the MCP/MTP joint, which may cause lameness when they resume work.[4,14]

Dorsal frontal incomplete or complete nondisplaced P1 fractures can be treated by rest and bandaging or by internal fixation using lag screws, depending on the fracture size. Needles placed into the MCP/MTP joint during the repair may help determine the proper placement of the screws. Arthroscopic examination of the fetlock joint should be considered to visualize the dorsal articular margin and debride damaged cartilage if needed.[16] A cast or bandage may be used postoperatively.[16] Complete dorsal fractures that extend into the PIP joint are best treated by lag screw fixation using an open approach or through stab incisions and external coaptation.[3] Needles placed in the MCP/MTP and PIP joint help guide the placement of 3 to 4 screws. A half-limb cast is recommended after surgery and is generally removed in 3 weeks. Fracture healing and return to training can be expected earlier following surgical treatment than with nonsurgical treatment of these fractures.[20]

Distal articular fractures occur almost exclusively in the hindlimbs and appear to be more common in foals.[13,14] The acute fracture is generally best treated by lag screw fixation and external coaptation. If the fracture is chronic, secondary OA of the PIP joint is likely and arthrodesis of the PIP joint is recommended.

Physeal fractures are usually Salter-Harris type 2 fractures and are most common in weanlings.[3,14] Minimally displaced fractures are generally best treated conservatively with stall confinement and bandage support. In one report (4 cases) all of these fractures healed with a moderate degree of malunion, but P1 remodeled so that a normal hoof–pastern axis was maintained.[14] If the fracture causes limb deformity and cannot be reduced, internal fixation may be required. If the PIP joint becomes subluxated as a result of the injury, arthrodesis of the PIP joint is recommended to realign the phalanges.

Oblique or transverse fractures are uncommon and do not affect the physis or articular margins. Stabilization of the fracture with lag screws placed through stab incisions has been described.[14] Minimally displaced fractures may heal with external coaptation. Displaced fractures usually require open reduction and internal fixation with bone plates.[20]

Comminuted Fractures

The objective for treatment of most horses with comminuted P1 fractures is usually to preserve the horse for breeding purposes or pasture soundness.[6,8,16,19] Even horses with only moderately comminuted P1 fractures that are repaired surgically rarely return to racing. In the most recent report, zero of 33 Thoroughbred racehorses and 4 of 28 Standardbred racehorses returned to racing after surgery.[8] The goals of surgery are usually to restore the articular congruity of the joint/joints involved and to stabilize the fracture to maintain bone length (Figure 5.148). Methods for treatment of comminuted P1 fractures include:[1,6–8,10,15–20]

1. External coaptation alone
2. External skeletal fixation alone(transfixation pin casts or Nunamaker skeletal fixator)
3. Lag screw fixation through stab incisions ± external skeletal transfixation (Figure 5.148)
4. Open reduction with lag screws and external coaptation
5. Open reduction with plates and screws and external coaptation
6. Open reduction combined with transfixation pin casts (Figure 5.149)

Selection of the specific treatment method often depends on the fracture configuration, intended use of the horse, economic constraints, and preference of the surgeon. If internal fixation is considered, the implants should permit re-apposition of the joint surfaces and provide longitudinal stability of P1.[4] Internal fixation is usually recommended in horses with moderately comminuted P1 fractures that permit fracture realignment (Figure 5.148). With severely comminuted fractures, accurate fracture repair is nearly impossible and the vascular supply to the distal limb and the integrity of the skin overlying the fracture site may be compromised.[8,15]

Horses with an intact cortex (strut of intact fractured P1 that extends from the proximal to distal joint surfaces) should be repaired with internal fixation. These horses have a much greater chance of surviving than do horses without an intact strut of bone. In one study,

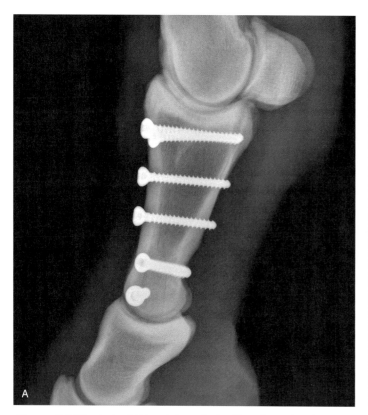
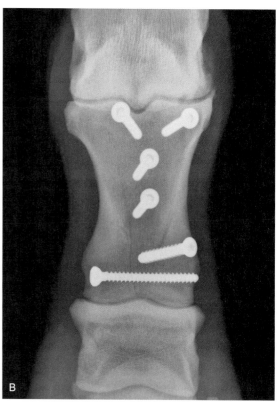

Figure 5.148. Lateral (A) and dorsoplantar (B) radiographs of the fracture in Figure 5.144 that was repaired with multiple lag screws placed through stab incisions.

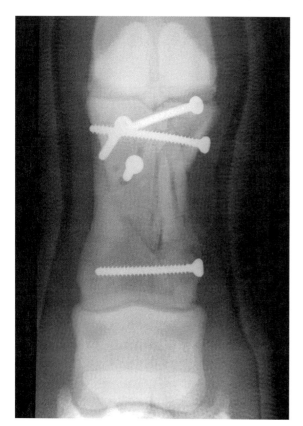

Figure 5.149. Dorsopalmar radiograph of a comminuted P1 fracture that was partially repaired using multiple lag screws. Transfixation pin-casting was used to prevent loading of the fracture during the initial healing period.

92% of horses with moderately comminuted P1 fractures treated with internal fixation had a successful outcome, whereas horses with severely comminuted P1 fractures had a much lower survival rate.[8] The intact strut of bone provides longitudinal stability to the fracture site as well as a solid piece of bone to which fracture fragments can be lagged.

Open approaches for repair of moderately comminuted P1 fractures include straight incisions directly over the fracture site, a lateral or medial curved flap incision that disarticulates the MCP/MTP joint, and H or Y incisions over the dorsal aspect of P1.[6,8,15,16,19] The surgical approach should result in the least soft tissue damage as possible because widely invasive open reduction techniques are associated with a high infection rate.[6,15] Currently, the lateral or medial curved flap incision with MCP/MTP joint luxation or straight incisions directly over the fracture site are recommended for open reduction and internal fixation of moderately comminuted P1 fractures in horses.[8,16,19]

External skeletal fixation is usually the treatment of choice to repair severely comminuted P1 fractures that lack an intact bony strut (Figure 5.143) and for those fractures that are open or have a severely compromised blood supply.[7,8,10,17] External fixation techniques reduce the risk of fracture collapse by using transcortical pins placed in the mid to distal portion of the third metacarpus/metatarsus.[7,8,10] Either transfixation pin casts or the Nunamaker external fixator may be used in these horses.[7,8,10,17,18] Transfixation pin casts are used more frequently because they are easier to apply or more versatile than the Nunamaker external fixator. Centrally threaded positive profile pins are preferred, and 2 pins are usually used. A lower limb fiberglass cast that incorporates the foot and extends to the proximal metacarpus/metatarsus is then applied. Most horses should walk comfortably in the transfixation pin cast after surgery. Pin loosening, bone sequestration, and iatrogenic metacarpal/metatarsal fractures through the pin tracts are complications of using transfixation pin casts.[7,8,10]

Internal fixation with either screws alone or plates and screws may be combined with a transfixation pin cast in horses with comminuted P1 fractures. The transfixation pin cast is used to protect the implants from potential failure in those horses that may not have an intact strut of bone. The lag screws can be placed through stab incisions to improve alignment of the joint surface(s) and in some cases to provide more stability to highly comminuted fractures (Figure 5.149). Transfixation pin casts may also be applied following open reduction and internal fixation of comminuted P1 fractures in which the stability of the fixation is questionable.[7] Transfixation techniques are usually recommended together with internal fixation if 80% of the fragmented cortices cannot be anatomically realigned so that they can support weight.[19]

Casting alone can be used to treat some horses with comminuted P1 fractures but it is less than optimal. Case selection is important and the fracture should be minimally comminuted and relatively stable to prevent axial collapse of the fracture. Additionally, malunion is less likely in those cases in which both joint surfaces are in good alignment prior to the application of the cast.[15]

Complications associated with using a cast alone to treat severely comminuted and unstable P1 fractures include: (1) axial collapse of the fracture, potentially leading to an open fracture, (2) support limb laminitis, (3) excessive callus formation and OA of the MCP/MTP and PIP joints, (4) shortening of the pastern region, and (5) partial ankylosis of the MCP/MTP joint.[4,6,8,16] Because of these numerous complications, external coaptation alone is not recommended for treatment of horses with severely comminuted P1 fractures. In addition, casting or external skeletal fixation is not recommended for horses with moderately comminuted P1 fractures because of the very good success with internal fixation of these fractures.[8]

Prognosis

Noncomminuted Fractures

Horses with noncomminuted fractures generally have a very good prognosis for long-term survival and many return to performance, although often at a reduced level.[1,13,16,22] The prognosis for performance with noncomminuted fractures of P1 often depends on the configuration of the fracture, duration of the fracture until treatment, method of treatment, and breed and intended use of the horse.[1,3–5,16,19,22] In one study in racehorses a significantly lower percentage of horses returned to racing following repair of complete sagittal fractures that extended into the PIP joint(46%) than following repair of short incomplete sagittal fractures (71%), long incomplete sagittal (66%), or complete sagittal fractures that extended to the lateral cortex

(71%).[5] The time from fracture to repair did not affect the outcome. Additionally the median number of races and the median fastest race times before and after surgery were not significantly different.[5] In another study with Standardbred racehorses, 89% of the horses returned to racing, but at significantly decreased performance levels.[22] In another study in young Thoroughbred racehorses, 70% of the horses treated conservatively with short, incomplete sagittal fractures raced and 65% of the horses with long, incomplete sagittal fractures treated conservatively raced.[4] Horses with dorsal frontal fractures treated by lag screw fixation also appear to have favorable prognosis to return to performance.[3,14,19]

Comminuted Fractures

The prognosis for horses with comminuted fractures depends on the severity and configuration of the fracture and the treatment approach selected.[7,8,10,15,19] Horses with open or closed severely comminuted fractures that do not permit reconstruction of the fragments remain difficult to treat and have only a fair prognosis for survival, regardless of the treatment approach used.[8] Moderately comminuted P1 fractures (those with an intact bony strut) can usually be repaired with internal fixation, and a 92% successful outcome has been reported.[8] Reconstruction of the fracture was performed in most of the horses in this study using a long, curved incision, transection of the collateral ligament of the MCP/MTP joint, and open exposure of the proximal articular surface of P1. Reasons for euthanasia of horses with comminuted P1 fractures include economic constraints, fracture collapse, iatrogenic metacarpal/metatarsal fractures, contralateral limb laminitis, and infection of the fracture site.[7,8,10]

References

1. Barr ARS, Deny HR, Waterman AE, et al. Proximal phalangeal fractures in the horse. Vet Comp Orthop Trauma 1988; 2:86–90.
2. Bramlage LR. First aid treatment and transportation of fracture patients. In Equine Fracture Repair. Nixon AJ, ed. WB Saunders. Philadelphia 1996;36–42.
3. Dechant JE, MacDonald DG, Crawford WH. Repair of complete dorsal fracture of the proximal phalanx in two horses. Vet Surg 1998;27:445–449.
4. Ellis DR, Simpson DJ, Greenwood RE, et al. Observations and management of fractures of the proximal phalanx in young Thoroughbreds. Equine Vet J 1987;19:43–49.
5. Holcombe SJ, Schneider RK, Bramlage LR, et al. Lag screw fixation of noncomminuted sagittal fractures of the proximal phalanx in racehorses: 59 cases (1973–1991). J Vet Med Assoc 1995;206:1195–1199.
6. Honnas CM. Fractures of the proximal phalanx. In Equine Surgery. JA Auer, ed. WB Saunders, Philadelphia, 1992; 998–1002.
7. Joyce J, Baxter GM, Sarrafian TL, et al. Use of transfixation pin casts to treat adult horses with comminuted phalangeal fractures: 20 cases (1993–2003). J Am Vet Med Assoc 2006;229: 725–730.
8. Kraus BM, Richardson DW, Nunamaker DM, et al. Management of comminuted fractures of the proximal phalanx in horses: 64 cases (1983–2001). J Am Vet Med Assoc 2004;224:254–263.
9. Kuemmerie JM, Auer JA, Rademacher N, et al. Short incomplete sagittal fractures of the proximal phalanx in ten horses not used for racing. Vet Surg 2008;37:193–200.
10. Lescan TB, McClure SR, Ward MP, et al. Evaluation of transfixation casting for treatment of third metacarpal, third metatarsal, and phalangeal fractures in horses: 37 cases (1994–2004). J Am Vet Med Assoc 2007;230:1340–1349.

11. Losonsky JM, Kneller SK. Variable locations of nutrient foramina of the proximal phalanx in forelimbs of Standardbreds. J Am Vet Med Assoc, 1988;193:671–674.
12. Markel MD, Martin BB, Richardson DW. Dorsal frontal fractures of the first phalanx in the horse. Vet Surg 1985;14:36–40.
13. Markel MD. Fractures of the proximal phalanx. In Current Practice of Equine Surgery. White NA, Moore JN, eds. WB Saunders, Philadelphia, 1990:610–617.
14. Markel MD, Richardson DW. Noncomminuted fractures of the proximal phalanx in 69 horses. J Am Vet Med Assoc 1985; 186:573–589.
15. Markel MD, Richardson DW, Nunamaker DM. Comminuted first phalanx fractures in 30 horses: Surgical vs. nonsurgical treatments. Vet Surg 1985;14:135–140.
16. Nixon AJ. Phalanges and the metacarpophalangeal and metatarsophalangeal joints. In Equine Surgery, 3rd ed. Auer JA, Stick JA, eds. Elsevier, Philadelphia, 2006;1217–1238.
17. Nunamaker DM, Richardson DW, Butterweck DM, et al. A new external skeletal fixation device that allows immediate full weight-bearing: Application in the horse. Vet Surg, 1986, 15: 345–355.
18. Nunamaker DM, Nash RA. A tapered-sleeve transcortical pin external skeletal fixation device for use in horses: development, application, and experience. Vet Surg 2008;37:725–732.
19. Richardson DW. Fractures of the proximal phalanx. In Equine Fracture Repair, Nixon AJ, ed. WB Saunders. Philadelphia 1996;117–128.
20. Stashak TS. The Pastern. In Adams' Lameness in Horses. JB Lippincott, Philadelphia, 2002;733–768.
21. Stover SM. Stress fractures. In Current Techniques in Equine Surgery. White NA, Moore JN, eds. WB Saunders, Philadelphia, 1996:451–459.
22. Tetens J, Ross MW, Lloyd JW. Comparison of racing performance before and after treatment of incomplete, midsagittal fractures of the proximal phalanx in Standardbreds: 49 cases (1986–1992) J Vet Med Assoc 1997;210:82–86.

DESMITIS OF THE DISTAL SESAMOIDEAN LIGAMENTS (DSLs)

There are three DSLs: the straight (superficial), paired oblique (middle), and paired cruciate (deep) (Figure 1.11 in Chapter 1). All of the ligaments originate from the base of the proximal sesamoid bones and intersesamoidean ligament. The straight ligament attaches distally to the proximopalmar/plantar aspect of P2 and the paired oblique ligaments attach to a triangular region on the middle and distal third of P1. The paired cruciate ligaments attach distally to the contralateral eminence of the proximal extremity of P1. There are also paired short ligaments that attach at the proximal articular margins of the metacarpo/metatarsophalangeal (MCP/MTP) joint but are not considered to be part of the DSL complex. See Chapter 1 for further information regarding the anatomy of the DSLs.

Desmitis of the oblique, straight, and cruciate DSLs occurs in all types of performance horses with injury to the oblique DSL being most common.[2,3,7,10,12] Horses that jump (e.g., event horses, show jumpers, field and show hunters, steeplechasers, and timber race horses) and race appear to be particularly prone to these injuries.[2,3,9,10] However, injuries to these ligaments may not be the sole cause of lameness in many horses.[14]

The medial branch of the oblique DSL is more commonly injured than the lateral branch and these injuries are thought to be more common in the forelimb than the hindlimb.[2] However, in a recent report on the use of MRI to diagnose DSL injuries in 27 horses, 10 lesions were in the forelimb and 17 were in the hindlimb.[12] The oblique DSL was injured in 18 horses, the straight DSL

in 3, and both the straight and oblique DSLs in 6 horses.[12] Hindlimb oblique DSL injuries are thought to occur more commonly in horses not used for racing.[11] Horses with a valgus or varus limb conformation or long, sloping pasterns may be at increased risk for injury. Injuries to the straight or cruciate DSL are thought to occur infrequently but 2 recent reports have suggested that injury to the straight DSL proximal to its insertion on P2 should be considered as a possible cause of lameness.[12,13]

Etiology

The DSLs are a functional continuation of the more proximally located suspensory ligament and are an important part of the suspensory apparatus which provides resistance to extension of the MCP/MTP joint during the stance phase. Hyperextension of the MCP/MCT joint can result in supraphysiologic strains in the suspensory apparatus, which may lead to failure of the DSLs. Although the DSLs in total provide this functional counter resistance to extension, each ligament has a separate function which may account for the specific injuries that occur to these structures.[8,15]

The straight DSL is the only unpaired ligament and is thought to contribute to sagittal stabilization of the MCP/MTP and PIP joints. The straight DSL would most likely be injured during hyperextension, but surprisingly, injury to this ligament is less common than to the oblique DSL.[3,8,12] The paired oblique DSLs are thought to play a prominent role in the limitation of rotation and abaxial movements of the MCP/MTP joint.[8,15] Injuries to the oblique DSLs usually occur unilaterally, probably as a result of asymmetric loading caused by abnormal conformation, lateral/medial foot imbalances, a misstep, or poor footing. Injuries to the oblique DSL are more common than those to the straight or cruciate DSLs, although concurrent injuries to the straight and oblique DSLs have been reported.[3,12]

Clinical Signs

Horses with acute desmitis often present with a sudden onset of lameness. Mild swelling of the palmar/plantar surface of the pastern region may be present as a result of digital sheath effusion.[15] The effusion is most commonly seen in acute cases (less than 3 weeks' duration) but soft tissue swelling is usually not apparent in most cases. Heat and pain with digital pressure may also be palpable in acute injuries.[8]

Horses with chronic injuries often present for a routine lameness evaluation. Obvious heat, pain, and swelling are rarely present and the location of the lameness often must be localized with perineural anesthesia. The lameness is usually mild to moderate in severity, positive to fetlock or phalangeal flexion, and worsened when the affected limb is in the inside of the circle. Careful digital palpation dorsal to the flexor tendons midway between the heel bulbs and the proximal sesamoid bones may reveal firm swellings and/or pain in more chronic cases. Palpation of the DSLs is best performed with the foot held off the ground and the MCP/MTP joint flexed so the flexor tendons are relaxed.[15]

Swelling of a DSL must be differentiated from swelling of the medial or lateral branch of the SDFT which is also located in the mid-pastern region. Passive fetlock and phalangeal flexion are commonly painful and direct digital pressure over the swollen region of the DSL for 30 seconds may increase the signs of lameness.[8,15]

Although the clinical findings may indicate a problem in the palmar/plantar pastern region, perineural anesthesia should be performed to rule out concurrent involvement of the foot.[15] Perineural anesthesia of the palmar digital nerve at the base of the sesamoid bone (basi-sesamoid block) should improve the lameness in most cases. However, an abaxial sesamoid or low 4-point block may be necessary if the ligament injury is located proximally in the pastern.[1] In addition, other concurrent problems should be closely evaluated because a recent report suggested that lesions of the DSLs found on MRI were the sole cause of lameness in only 2 of 58 horses.[14] See Chapter 3 for more information on perineural anesthesia.

Diagnosis

Diagnostics that may help document an abnormality to 1 of the DSLs include radiography, ultrasound, and MRI. Radiographic abnormalities that may suggest a previous or concurrent injury of a DSL include: enthesiophyte formation, avulsion fractures/fragments, and dystrophic mineralization within 1 of the DSLs. Enthesiophyte formation at the attachment of the oblique DSL at the palmar/plantar aspect of P1 is a relatively common finding, and may be an incidental finding (Figure 5.151).[3,6] However, these proliferative changes were observed on the medial and lateral aspect of P1 in 31 of 39 horses diagnosed with desmitis of the DSLs.[6] Another study found little correlation between enthesiophyte formation on the back of P1 and ultrasonographic abnormalities in the oblique DSL.[3] Enthesiophyte formation at the proximal aspect of P1 and at the base of the proximal sesamoid bone is also believed to be evidence of injury to the cruciate or short DSL.[15]

Fractures/fragments of the base of the proximal sesamoid bone can involve the DSLs.[1-3] Fragments from either the dorsal aspect of the base of the proximal sesamoid bone or proximal palmar/plantar articular margin of P1 typically involve the short DSL (Figure 5.150).[8] Bone fragments have also been observed on the nonarticular proximal extremity of P1 and at the base of the sesamoid bones.[1,15] These fracture fragments may involve the oblique, cruciate, or short DSLs.[1,8] Dystrophic mineralization associated with the DSLs may also be present radiographically, usually at the base of the sesamoid bones.[6] It is important to differentiate dystrophic mineralization from avulsion fractures at the base of the sesamoid bones because fracture fragments can and should be removed, whereas there is usually no treatment for mineralization.[1]

Sonographic evidence of acute desmitis of the DSLs is manifested by a diffuse increase in ligament size, fiber disruption, discrete core lesions, and peri-ligamentous fluid surrounding the affected ligament.[3,4,7-9] The anechoic space between the ligament and the SDFT is

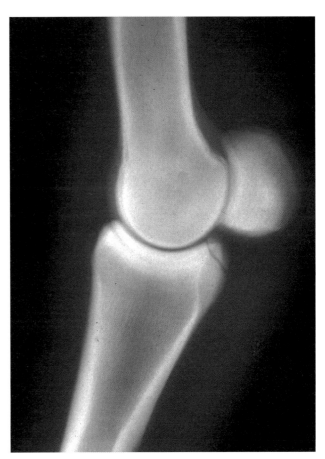

Figure 5.150. Lateral radiograph of the fetlock demonstrating a small palmar eminence fracture that may be associated with the paired short sesamoidean ligaments.

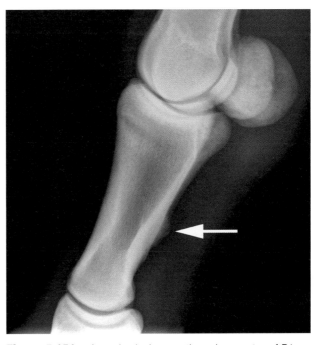

Figure 5.151. An enthesiophyte on the palmar cortex of P1 can be seen on this lateral radiograph of the pastern (arrow). The clinical significance of these lesions is questionable but may suggest a previous injury at the insertion site of one of the DSLs.

often reduced in size with desmitis of the oblique DSL.[3] Chronic sonographic changes may include varying degrees of the acute abnormalities within the ligament, hyperechoic areas consistent with dense scar tissue formation, and dystrophic mineralization.[4,8] Periosteal proliferation in areas of ligament attachments may appear as irregular contours on the bone surface.[8] Basilar sesamoid avulsion fragments, desmitis of the ipsilateral branch of the suspensory ligament in the same limb, and fragments off the proximopalmar/plantar aspect of P1 may occur concurrently in more chronic cases.[2,3] Ultrasonographic identification of cruciate DSL injuries is difficult due to the location of these ligaments, and therefore may be under diagnosed.

Ultrasonography of the palmar/plantar pastern region is difficult to perform and often requires experience to become proficient. There are numerous soft tissue structures that must be ruled out as potential problems. Therefore, only obvious abnormalities within the DSLs may be recognized. In a recent study to describe the normal appearance of the DSLs using MRI, 80% of the lesions found with MRI were not detected with ultrasonography.[14] Although ultrasound can be useful to diagnose problems in the DSLs, lack of ultrasound abnormalities does not rule out a problem within the DSLs. Currently, MRI is the best diagnostic tool to make a definitive diagnosis (Figure 5.152).[12,13] See Chapter 4 for additional information on MRI.

Treatment

In general, injuries to the DSLs are treated very similarly to other soft tissue problems such as tendinitis. In acute cases, confinement, cold therapy, pressure/support wraps, and administration of NSAIDs are recommended. Cold therapy in the form of an ice water slurry applied for 30 minutes twice a day for the first 48 hours

after the acute injury appears to be most beneficial.[15] Pressure/support bandages can be applied in between the cold treatments and maintained for 2 to 3 weeks or as needed. Warm therapy can begin after 48 hours, and NSAIDs can be administered for up to 2 to 3 weeks post injury. Feet and hoof-pastern axis imbalances should be corrected if possible.

Once a definitive diagnosis has been made, a 6-month rest and rehabilitation program is currently recommended.[12,13] This usually involves a short period of stall confinement depending on the severity of the injury (3 to 6 weeks), followed by increasing periods of hand-walking and controlled exercise. Hand-walking exercise usually begins with 5 minutes once or twice a day, 3 to 5 days a week, and then increases 4 to 5 minutes/week. Clinical evaluation should be performed at 4 to 6 weeks, and if the horse has improved, controlled exercise can be increased.

If abnormalities were apparent on ultrasound, re-evaluation is recommended 2 to 3 months post injury. Further controlled or free exercise recommendations are made depending on the ultrasound findings. In one study of 27 horses with DSL injuries, 76% of the horses successfully resumed performance following a 6-month controlled exercise program.[12]

Adjunctive treatments that may be used in addition to the rehabilitation protocol include extracorporeal shockwave,[5] ligament splitting, injection of the DFTS with corticosteroids and hyaluronan,[12] and intralesional treatment of the damaged ligament with stem cells or platelet-rich plasma (PRP). Nonarticular base sesamoid fragments that may be associated with DSL avulsion injuries should be removed using a "keyhole" surgical approach through the DFTS.[1] With this approach, fragments are localized with needles and removed using arthroscopic rongeurs. Nine of 10 surgically treated horses returned to their intended use.[1]

Prognosis

The prognosis for horses with DSL injuries to return to performance has historically been considered to be guarded because of the high probability of re-injury.[3,6,8] However, more recent studies have indicated a much better prognosis. Seventy-six percent, 66%, and 90% of horses with DSL injuries or avulsion fractures of the proximal sesamoid bones returned to performance following treatment.[1,12,13] However, recurrence of DSL desmitis is always a possibility, similar to other soft tissue injuries. In addition, concurrent musculoskeletal problems such PIP joint OA, navicular syndrome, and suspensory desmitis often reduce the prognosis for full recovery.[15]

References

1. Brokken MT, Schneider RK, Tucker RL. Surgical approach for removal of nonarticular base sesamoid fragments of the proximal sesamoid bones in horses. Vet Surg 2008;37:619–624.
2. Denoix JM, Crevier N, Azevedo C. Ultrasound examination of the pastern. Proceedings Am Assoc Eq Pract 1991;37:363–380.
3. Dyson S, Denoix J. Tendon, tendon sheath, and ligament injuries in the pastern. Vet Clin North Am Equine Pract 1995;11:217–233.

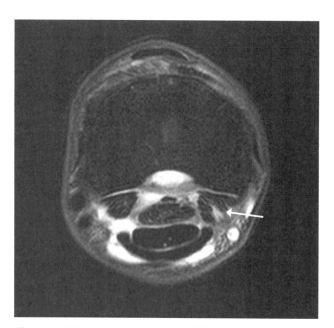

Figure 5.152. Axial proton density MRI image showing high signal intensity (arrow) in the lateral branch of the oblique DSL in the pastern region.

4. Dyson S. Ultrasonographic examination of the pastern region. Equine Vet Educ 1992;4:254.
5. McClure SR, VanSickle D, Evans R, et al. The effects of extracorporeal shock-wave therapy on the ultrasonographic and histologic appearance of collagenase-induced equine forelimb suspensory ligament desmitis. Ultrasound Med Biol 2004;30:461–467.
6. Moyer W. Distal sesamoidean desmitis: Proceedings Am Assoc Equine Pract, 1982;28:245–251.
7. Redding R. Sonographic exam of the digital flexor tendon sheath, distal flexor tendons, and soft tissues of the palmar pastern region. Proceedings Am Assoc Equine Pract 1993;39:11–15.
8. Redding R. Distal sesamoidean ligament injuries and desmitis of the inferior check ligament. Proceedings Dubai International Symp 1996;1:227–240.
9. Reef VB. Ultrasonic evaluation of tendons and ligaments. In Current Practice of Equine Surgery. White NA, Moore JN, eds. JB Lippincott Co., Philadelphia. 1990;425–435.
10. Reef VB. Musculoskeletal Ultrasonography. In Equine Diagnostic Ultrasound. Reef VB, ed. WB Saunders. Philadelphia. 1998;39–186.
11. Ross MW, Dyson SJ. Diagnosis and Management of Lameness in the Horse. WB Saunders, Philadelphia, 2002.
12. Sampson SN, Schneider RK, Tucker RL, et al. Magnetic resonance imaging features of oblique and straight distal sesamoidean desmitis in 27 horses. Vet Radiol Ultrasound 2007;48:303–311.
13. Schneider RK, Tucker RL, Habegger SR, et al. Desmitis of the straight sesamoidean ligament in horses:9 cases (1995–1997). J Am Vet Med Assoc 2003;222:973–977.
14. Smith S, Dyson SJ, Murray RC. Magnetic resonance imaging of distal sesamoidean ligament injury. Vet Radiol Ultrasound 2008;49:516–528.
15. Stashak TS. The Pastern. In Adams' Lameness in Horses. JB Lippincott, Philadelphia, 2002;764–768.

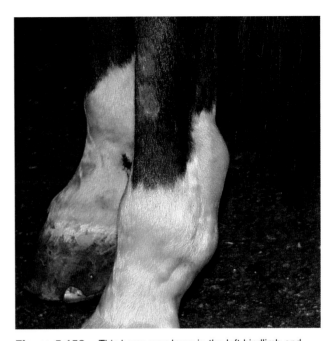

Figure 5.153. This horse was lame in the left hindlimb and had severe effusion of the digital flexor tendon sheath. Lesions of the DDFT within the tendon sheath appear to be more common in the hindlimbs than the forelimbs.

SDFT AND DDFT ABNORMALITIES

In general, injuries to the SDFT in the pastern region occur most frequently in the forelimbs and injuries to the DDFT within the DFTS occur most frequently in the hindlimbs. Injuries to the DDFT that are associated with navicular syndrome are covered under the foot section. Injuries involving the SDFT most commonly involve the branches of the SDFT located outside the DFTS.[1–3,5–7] The SDFT branches at the level of the MCP/MTP joint, giving rise to medial and lateral branches that insert on the palmar/plantar eminences of P2.[9] Abnormal conformation such as a long pastern or an underrun heel may predispose the horse to injury of the SDFT branch. Injuries to the DDFT within the pastern are nearly always within the DFTS, often cause effusion of the sheath, and may contribute to chronic tenosynovitis of the DFTS (Figure 5.153). In one study of horses with DFTS tenosynovitis, injuries to the DDFT were found in 44 of the 76 horses.[8]

Etiology

Injuries to the SDFT in the forelimbs are usually associated with hyperextension of the MCP joint, resulting in nonphysiologic stretching and overload of the SDFT.[5] These injuries occur commonly in racehorses but why some horses get SDFT injuries in the pastern compared to the metacarpal region is unknown. The cause of DDFT injuries within the tendon sheath is unknown but hyperextension of the MCP/MTP joint and overstretching of the tendon are also likely. As with any tendon injury, both SDFT and DDFT damage can occur as a single traumatic event such as a misstep.

Clinical Signs

SDFT Branch Injuries

Lameness usually occurs at the onset of injury with focal heat, swelling, and sensitivity noted on palpation. However, careful palpation and comparison of the medial to lateral branches is important to detect differences in size, heat, and pain because these injuries can be easily missed. Generally, swelling develops within 3 to 4 days and is usually uniaxial on the limb. The medial SDFT branch appears to be more frequently injured than the lateral branch and avulsion fractures of P1 at the insertion of the SDFT branch occur infrequently.[6,7] Some SDFT injuries and damage to the manica flexoria may occur within the DFTS and result in tendon sheath effusion.[4,8]

DDFT

Deep digital flexor tendinitis occurs in a variety of sport horses and typically presents as an acute-onset, unilateral, moderate to severe forelimb or hindlimb lameness that is persistent.[5–7] Heat, pain, and swelling of the DDFT itself are usually not palpable because the damage is often located within the DFTS. Lameness is often worse on a soft surface and generally improves with perineural anesthesia of the palmar/plantar nerves at the level of the proximal sesamoid bones. Distension of the DFTS often occurs in conjunction with the injury and many horses present with chronic tenosynovitis of the DFTS of undetermined cause (Figure 5.153).[8,12] If the DFTS is distended, intrasynovial anesthesia of the sheath is the preferred method to confirm the location of the lameness.

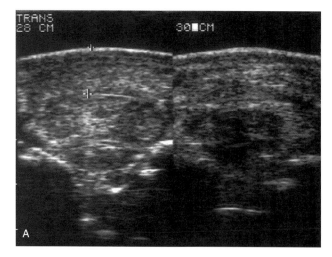

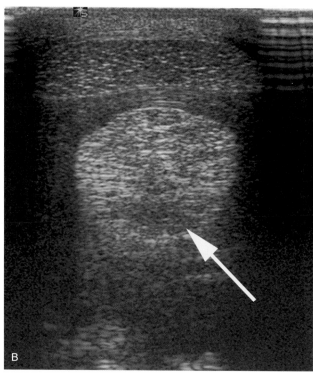

Figure 5.154.   Ultrasound images demonstrating abnormalities of the DDFT within the tendon sheath at the level of the sesamoid bones (A) and above the sesamoid bones (arrow) (B) in 2 different horses.

Diagnosis

Ultrasonography is currently the most commonly used method to diagnose branch lesions of the SDFT and abnormalities within the DDFT. Core lesions, followed by diffuse injury to the affected SDFT branch, are the most common lesions identified with ultrasound.[6,7] However, ultrasonographic examination in the pastern region in the absence of swelling may result in false-negative results in horses with SDFT injuries. The DDFT is bilobed, with each lobe similar in size and shape at the level of the pastern. A lesion may involve one or both lobes and is typically characterized by enlargement and alteration of the tendon with or without a hypoechoic region (Figure 5.154).[7,19] Additionally, different types of lesions within the DDFT have been recognized, depending on the location of the injury in the pastern.[10] Dystrophic mineralization may be seen with chronic injuries.[6,10]

Lesions within the SDFT and DDFT that are visible tenoscopically can be missed with ultrasound.[4] The sensitivity of ultrasound appears to be worse for lesions of the DDFT than the SDFT.[4] However, ultrasonographic evaluation of the DDFT in the pastern region was thought to yield excellent results in another study.[10] Longitudinal tears of the DDFT can be especially difficult to document with ultrasound and these horses often have nonspecific signs of chronic tenosynovitis of the DFTS.[11,12] Because of these limitations, an MRI examination is thought to be superior to an ultrasound examination to characterize the location, type, and severity of damage to both the SDFT and DDFT within the pastern.

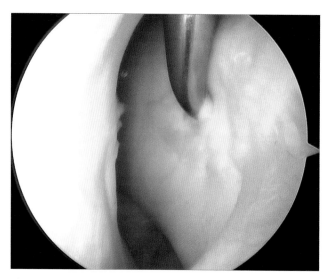

Figure 5.155.   Tenoscopic view of the DFTS showing a longitudinal tear (probe inserted into defect) of the DDFT that was not visualized with ultrasound.

Tenoscopy of the DFTS has become a useful diagnostic tool to document lesions of both SDFT and DDFT that may not be visible with ultrasound (Figure 5.155). In general, branch lesions of the SDFT are usually outside the DFTS, whereas most DDFT lesions are within the DFTS. In one study of horses with tenosynovitis, 19 of 20 horses had lesions involving the DDFT.[12] Therefore, if the lameness is confirmed to the

DFTS and effusion is present, tenoscopy is strongly recommended, especially if the ultrasound findings are equivocal.[4,11] Surgical exploration of the DFTS via tenoscopy is often helpful to identify the extent of the injury, recognize tendon damage often missed with ultrasound, and debride the damaged tendon and any adhesions that may be present.[4,8,11,12]

Treatment

Treatment depends on the location, type, and severity of the lesion. Branch lesions of the SDFT are usually treated with a controlled rehabilitation program similar to any bowed tendon injury; however, 6 to 12 months is typically needed. If the SDFT lesion is within the DFTS or if DFTS effusion is present, surgical exploration via tenoscopy is often helpful to further diagnose the specific problem and debride the damaged tendon.[11,12] Lesions of the DDFT at the level of the pastern are often within the DFTS and tenoscopy is often beneficial because these lesions are often difficult to diagnose and treat.[8,11,12] An anular ligament desmotomy may be performed at the time of surgery if considered appropriate.[11] Additional treatment options include medication of the DFTS with corticosteroids, hyaluronan (HA), or interlukin-1 receptor antagonist protein (IRAP), and intralesional injection of platelet rich plasma (PRP) or stem cells directly into the damaged tendon. See Chapter 8 for more details on these treatments.

Prognosis

In general, soft tissue injures of the SDFT and DDFT in the pastern region can be difficult to diagnose, but affected horses have a reasonable chance of returning to their intended use. However, these injuries are prone to recurrence. Horses with SDFT branch injuries in the pastern region are thought to have a poorer prognosis to return to racing than SDFT injuries in the metacarpal region, with more frequent recurrence of injury.[6,7] Lesions of the DDFT within the DFTS can contribute

to adhesion formation and chronic tenosynovitis, which may result in continued lameness. In one study, 10 of 17 horses with longitudinal tears of the DDFT returned to their previous level of work.[11] In another study of 76 horses with chronic DFTS tenosynovitis, sheath distention was eliminated in 33% and improved in 69% of the horses.[8] In the same study, 68% of the horses were sound and 54% returned to their preoperative level of performance.[8]

References

1. Denoix JM, Crevier N, Azevedo C. Ultrasound examination of the pastern. Proceedings Am Assoc Equine Pract 1991;37:363–380.
2. Dyson S, Denoix J. Tendon, tendon sheath, and ligament injuries in the pastern. Vet Clin North Am Equine Pract 1995;11:217–233.
3. Dyson S. Ultrasonographic examination of the pastern region. Equine Vet Educ 1992;4:254–258.
4. Edinger J, Mobius G, Ferguson J. Comparison of tenoscopic and ultrasonographic methods of examination of the digital flexor tendon sheath in horses. Vet Comp Orthop Traumat 2005;18:209–214.
5. Redding R. Sonographic exam of the digital flexor tendon sheath, distal flexor tendons, and soft tissues of the palmar pastern region. Proc Am Assoc Equine Pract 1993;39:11–15.
6. Reef VB. Equine Diagnostic Ultrasound. WB Saunders, Philadelphia, 1998.
7. Reef VB. Current Practice in Equine Surgery. JB Lippincott, Philadelphia, 1990.
8. Smith MR, Wright IM. Noninfected tenosynovitis of the digital flexor tendon sheath: a retrospective analysis of 76 cases. Equine Vet J 2006;38:134–141.
9. Weaver JC, Stover SM, O'Brien TR. Radiographic anatomy of soft tissue attachments in the equine metacarpophalangeal and proximal phalangeal region. Equine Vet J 1992;24:310–315.
10. Whitcomb MB. Ultrasonographic appearance and distribution of deep digital flexor injuries in the pastern region. Proceedings Am Assoc Equine Pract 2008;54:452–454.
11. Wilderjans H, Boussauw B, Madder K, et al. Tenosynovitis of the digital flexor sheath and anular ligament constriction syndrome caused by longitudinal tears in the deep digital flexor tendon: a clinical and surgical report of 17 cases in Warmblood horses. Equine Vet J 2003;35:270–275.
12. Wright IM, McMahon PJ. Tenosynovitis associated with longitudinal tears of the digital flexor tendons in horses: a report of 20 cases. Equine Vet J 1999;31:12–18.

THE FETLOCK

Alicia L. Bertone

OSTEOCHONDRAL (CHIP) FRACTURES OF THE PROXIMAL (FIRST) PHALANX IN THE METACARPOPHALANGEAL OR METATARSOPHALANGEAL (FETLOCK) JOINT

Osteochondral fractures of the proximal end of the first phalanx (P1) are relatively common in the forelimb of the horse, particularly the racehorse. Most fractures of this type involve the dorsal surface of the proximal eminences, just medial or lateral to the digital extensor tendon. The left forelimb and medial eminence are affected more often than the right forelimb and lateral eminence. Other regions are not so commonly involved. Concussion and overextension of the joint are factors in the production of these fractures. Chip fractures from the distal end of the third metacarpal or metatarsal bone also occur but are less common.

Other less frequently occurring fractures of P1 include fractures of the lateral and medial eminences of the proximopalmar (or proximoplantar) surfaces and avulsion fractures of the midproximal palmar articular margins just below the sesamoid bone. These fractures can be successfully removed with a good prognosis (about 70%) for return to performance.[1,5] Fractures of the proximopalmar (or proximoplantar) surfaces also may be associated with complete or partial tearing of the collateral ligament of the fetlock joint and traumatic subluxation that induces the intra-articular (IA) fracture. These are often referred to as collateral ligament avulsion fractures. Careful evaluation of the joint is indicated to identify this more complex injury.[4]

Etiology

Trauma causes these chip fractures in the horse. From the appearance of the fractures, it seems that excessive overextension of the joint is probably involved (Figure 5.156). Overextension places stress on the dorsal aspect of the proximal end of P1 as it is pressed against the third metacarpal bone. Limb fatigue is a factor in overextension of the fetlock joint, noted at the end of races when the back of the fetlock my contact the ground (running down). Why the fracture most frequently occurs medial to the midline is not fully understood. However, it may be because the medial tuberosity on the proximal dorsal border of the P1 is more prominent and extends slightly more proximad than its lateral counterpart.

Clinical Signs

Signs of chip fractures in the fetlock joint are similar to those of "osselets." Synovitis of the fetlock joint indicated by distention of the joint capsule (between the suspensory ligament and the palmar or plantar surface of the cannon bone) is commonly found. Horses often

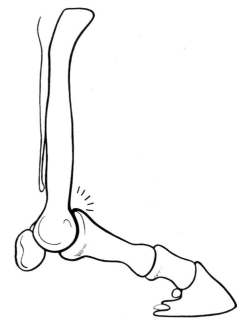

Figure 5.156. Mechanism of chip fractures of the proximal phalanx. (Courtesy of W. Berkeley.)

present with a history of lameness, which increases after exercise, and a workout or a race may cause the horse to be markedly lame. After prolonged rest, the horse may seem to be sound, only to go lame again when returned to training. Occasionally, there may be history of acute lameness followed by dramatic relief when a chip that was caught in the joint is dislodged.

Some horses, particularly in chronic chip fractures, have only a small amount of swelling or lameness to indicate that there is a chip fracture. There may be fibrous enlargement on the dorsal surface of the fetlock joint that is easily palpated. However, dorsal swelling is also often seen in osselets. It is difficult to produce pain in the affected region by digital pressure, but some heat may be detected over the dorsal surface of the joint. Flexion of the affected fetlock often elicits pain and a fetlock flexion test usually exacerbates the lameness. If the examiner is unsure of this response, it should be compared to the opposite fetlock. Lameness is most obvious at the trot during the stance phase.

In most cases it is not necessary to use local anesthesia to identify chip fractures within the fetlock. If the examiner is suspicious that the fetlock is involved, radiographs should be taken. However, if confusion exists regarding the contribution of the fetlock to the lameness, either intrasynovial anesthesia of the fetlock (preferred) or a low 4-point nerve block (proximal to the fetlock) can be performed. See Chapter 3 for more information.

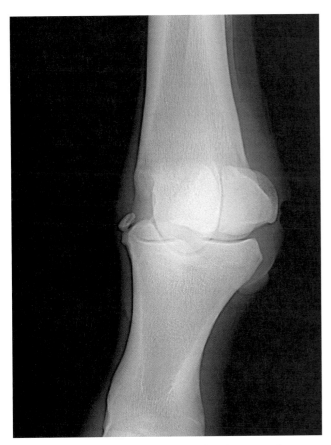

Figure 5.157. An oblique radiograph that documents the medial or lateral location of a proximal P1 osteochondral fracture. (Courtesy of Dr. Gary Baxter.)

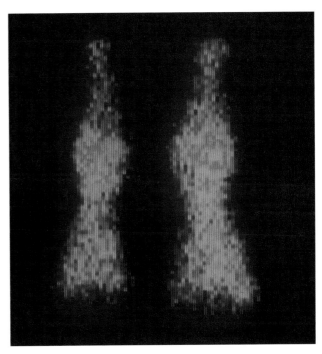

Figure 5.158. Nuclear scintigram demonstrating increased uptake of radiopharmaceutical in the fetlock region in a horse with proximal P1 fractures (right side) compared to the opposite fetlock (left). Scintigraphy is sensitive for bone trauma but nonspecific for the site and structure of the disease. A condylar injury in the distal metacarpus may have a similar appearance.

Diagnosis

A definitive diagnosis is best made with radiographic examination. The lateral radiograph is most revealing diagnostically. Oblique radiographs should be taken to determine whether the chip is on the medial or lateral side of the midline. (Figure 5.157) This is important because the surgical positioning of the arthroscope is opposite the chip fracture. It is important to radiograph the contralateral fetlock, because bilateral fractures are not uncommon, and clinical signs may not appear until the horse is back in training.[1–3,5,8] Ultrasonography also may be used to diagnose chip fractures of the dorsal aspect of P1 and concurrent proliferative synovitis of the fetlock synovial pad if present. Acute proximal eminence fractures are increased in activity on a nuclear bone scan, but nuclear scintigraphy is not usually necessary for diagnosis. (Figure 5.158)

Treatment

Proximal Dorsal Osteochondral (Chip) Fractures

Arthroscopic removal of chip fractures is the treatment of choice for the greatest chance of a quick return to full performance[2,5,6,8] (Figure 5.159). Arthroscopic evaluation permits removal of multiple fragments, visu-alization of the entire joint, and surgical treatment of lesions that may not have been identified on radiographs. Lesions commonly seen in association with P1 chip fracture include proliferative synovitis of the dorsal metacarpal synovial pad (32% of which had chip fractures) and cartilage erosion of the metacarpal condyle.[3,5] It is recognized that some small, nondisplaced fractures can be treated successfully with adequate rest for 120 days. If training continues, these fragments often displace and cause adjacent articular cartilage erosion (Figure 5.159). Arthrotomy for fragment removal from the dorsal fetlock has been abandoned in favor of arthroscopy because of the improved access to the joint with arthroscopy and the complications of arthrotomy wound healing at the dorsal fetlock joint.

The exact location of the chip must be established if surgical removal of the bone fragment is elected (most chips are located medial to the midline). Any other joints indicating soreness or effusion on physical examination should be radiographed to determine whether silent chip fractures could be present in other joints. Carpal or contralateral fetlock chip fractures are common and would most likely be removed at the same surgical procedure. Dorsal recumbency is preferred by many surgeons because it permits multiple joint access without repositioning the horse and it decreases hemorrhage into the joint during surgery. Two to four months' rest is recommended before training is resumed, depending on the degree of joint damage and cartilage debridement.

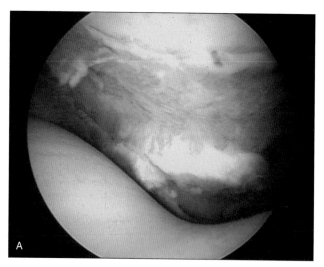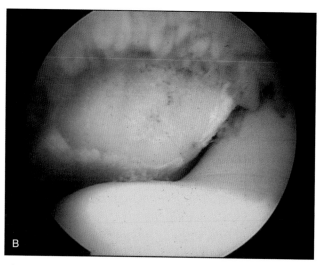

Figure 5.159.   A. Arthroscopic appearance of a fresh nondisplaced medial eminence P1 fracture in a racing Thoroughbred. B. Arthroscopic appearance after removal of the fragment in (A) and debridement of the damaged cartilage. There is little scoring of the articular cartilage on the distal metacarpus which is usually a good prognostic sign.

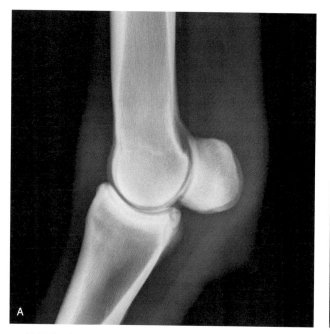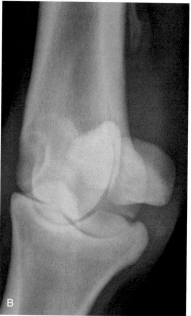

Figure 5.160.   Lateral (A) and oblique (B) radiographs demonstrating a typical palmar/plantar osteochondral fragment of the first phalanx.

Fractures of the Proximal Palmar/Plantar Eminence of P1

Fractures of the medial and lateral palmar/plantar eminences of P1 are not common and should not be confused with osteochondral fragmentation of this site in young growing horses, which is debated to be part of the osteochondrosis syndrome (Figure 5.160).[4] Osteochondral fragmentation of the caudal eminences of the P1 occurs in approximately 5% of Standardbreds and Thoroughbreds without any clinical signs. Fragments are not usually a source of lameness until aggres-sive training. If clinical signs occur, they are mild and consist of a high performance lameness, joint effusion, and mild soreness to flexion. Fractures of the caudal eminences of P1, however, are usually associated with fetlock joint swelling, lameness, and soreness to direct pressure over the eminence.

Joint flexion usually markedly worsens the lameness. Stability of the joint should be assessed in these horses to determine whether collateral ligament damage has also occurred. Horses may respond to stall rest of at least 90 days, but re-injury may occur. Bony healing does not occur in conservatively treated cases because the fracture is distracted by the distal sesamoidean ligament insertions. Nuclear scintigraphy can be used to distinguish fractures from incidental caudal eminence fragments.

Fractures that continue to be a source of pain or are large enough to anchor to the parent bone with a bone screw can be treated surgically. If the fracture has an articular component and is to be removed, arthroscopic removal is possible, but dissection outside the joint capsule is required. Alternatively, or for fractures without an articular component, an incision can be made directly over the fragment and it can be removed with sharp dissection. If compression screw fixation is required, intraoperative monitoring with fluoroscopy or radiographs is needed for proper screw placement. After internal fixation, a cast should be applied for recovery from anesthesia and removed within 48 hours, after which support pressure wraps are applied. Six months' rest is recommended in these cases to allow bone healing and repair of the distal suspensory injury. Bandaging alone can be used for the postoperative case in which chip fractures have been removed.

If collateral ligament injury or instability is noted in the joint, cast support should continue for 1 to 2 months, depending on the severity, to support healing of the ligament and minimize the development of osteoarthritis (OA). Suturing the ligament and removing the caudal eminence proximal phalanx fracture is not necessary for breeding soundness or light athletic soundness. The degree of P1 fracture displacement and avulsion fracture of the collateral ligament determine whether internal fixation repair of the fracture is indicated to maximize joint health during healing and is performed prior to placing the cast.

Prognosis

The prognosis is usually good to excellent for treatment of proximal dorsal chip fractures, but it is somewhat dependent on the size and number of chip fractures, their duration, whether or not steroids have been injected, amount of concomitant articular cartilage damage, and degree of OA (Figure 5.161). Several reports indicate that the prognosis for return to athletic performance, including racing performance, is good to excellent (approximately 80%) with arthroscopic surgery to remove the fragment. The presence of other fetlock lesions noted at arthroscopic surgery decreased the prognosis in racing Thoroughbreds, but success was still good (greater than 70% return to racing).[2,5,6,8]

Small acute, nondisplaced fetlock chip fractures usually have a good prognosis with conservative treatment. Arthroscopic surgical removal may still be elected in these cases because the convalescence is shorter after surgical removal (often under 30 days) than for the bone to heal (90 to 120 days) and the risk of fracture displacement or refracture is eliminated. Factors that lower the prognosis include extreme large size of the fragment, chronicity, degree of synovitis/capsulitis, and amount of OA present. Standardbred racehorses often have chronic joint changes associated with dorsal P1 fractures.

The prognosis for proximal palmar/plantar fractures that require compression screw fixation depends on the

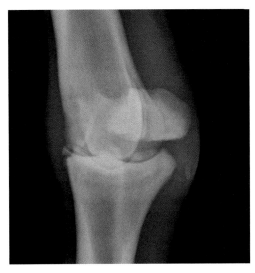

Figure 5.161. This oblique radiograph of the fetlock demonstrated multiple large fragments involving most of the medial eminence of P1 that will most likely decrease the overall prognosis. (Courtesy of Dr. Gary Baxter.)

degree of initial trauma at the time of fracture. Often this is not fully appreciated until the radiographs are taken 3 to 4 months after surgery. The prognosis after removal of smaller proximal palmar fractures is considered to be very good.

References

1. Adams OR. Chip fractures of the first phalanx in the metacarpophalangeal (fetlock) joint. J Am Vet Med Assoc 1966;148:360.
2. Colon JL, Bramlage LR, Hance SR, et al. Qualitative and quantitative documentation of the racing performance of 461 Thoroughbred racehorses after arthroscopic removal of dorsoproximal first phalanx osteochondral fractures (1986–1995). Equine Vet J 2000;32:475.
3. Dabareiner RM, White NA, Sullins KE. Metacarpophalangeal joint synovial pad fibrotic proliferation in 63 horses. Vet Surg 1996;25:199–206.
4. Hubert J, Williams J, Moore RM. What is your diagnosis? Avulsion fracture of the medial plantar eminence of the first phalanx; subluxation of the metatarsophalangeal joint resulting from avulsion of the insertion of the medial collateral ligament. J Am Vet Med Assoc 1998;213:203.
5. Kawcak CE, McIlwraith CW. Proximodorsal first phalanx osteochondral chip fragmentation in 336 horses. Equine Vet J 1994;26:392.
6. McIlwraith CW. Fetlock fractures and luxations. In Equine Fracture Repair. Nixon AJ, ed. WB Saunders, Philadelphia. 1996;153–162.
7. Pettersson H, Ryden G. Avulsion fractures of the caudoproximal extremity of the first phalanx. Equine Vet J 1982;14:333.
8. Yovich JV, McIlwraith CW. Arthroscopic surgery for osteochondral fractures of the proximal phalanx of the metacarpophalangeal and metatarsophalangeal (fetlock) joints in horses. J Am Vet Med Assoc 1986;188:273.

FRACTURES OF THE PROXIMAL SESAMOID BONES

Fractures of the proximal sesamoid bones are common injuries in racing Thoroughbreds, Standardbreds, and Quarter horses[3,7,9,17,19,22–27] and are the most common fatal fracture in racing Thoroughbreds and Quarter horses.[15,20] These fractures take various forms including apical, abaxial (articular and nonarticular), midbody, basilar (articular and nonarticular), sagittal, and comminuted (Figure 5.162). Combinations of fracture types such as apical/abaxial fractures may also occur (Figure 5.163). The forelimbs are most frequently affected in the Thoroughbred (right forelimb) and Quarter horse, whereas the hindlimbs are more fre-

quently affected in the Standardbred (left hindlimb). Most of these fractures distract as a result of the pull of the suspensory ligament proximally and the distal sesamoidean ligaments distally.

Fractures of the apical portion of the sesamoid bone are by far the most common, comprising more than 88% of sesamoid fractures. In Thoroughbred race horses 2 years or older, 64% involve hindlimbs and 36% forelimbs.[22] Sesamoid fractures are most common (53.4%) in 2-year-olds, and then 3-year-olds (23%). Apical fractures are frequently articular, singular, and rarely comminuted, and usually involve less than one-third of the bone (Figure 5.164A). Apical fractures occur most frequently on the lateral sesamoid bones of the left hindlimb (42.8% of fractures) than the right hindlimb (36.6%) in Standardbreds, whereas a more equal distribution is observed in the Thoroughbred.

Basilar fractures are less common than the apical fracture (6% of sesamoid fractures in Standardbreds). They represent an avulsion fracture associated with the distal sesamoidean ligaments and may be comminuted. These fractures are more common in the Thoroughbred than in the Standardbred and can be small articular, transverse articular, or nonarticular (Figure 5.165).

The abaxial fracture is an uncommon sesamoid fracture (3%) in Standardbreds, but it may be more common in Thoroughbreds and Quarter horses.[25,27] It can either be articular or nonarticular. These fractures can be difficult to diagnose and may require an additional tangential projection on the radiographic examination to identify their exact location, or they can be identified on the craniocaudal view.[4,18]

The midbody transverse fracture is seen most frequently in Thoroughbreds, older Standardbreds (mean age 6.5 years) and young foals under 2 months of age. Fractures roughly separate the bone into equal portions and invariably enter the fetlock joint (Figure 5.166). Because of the distractive forces of the suspensory

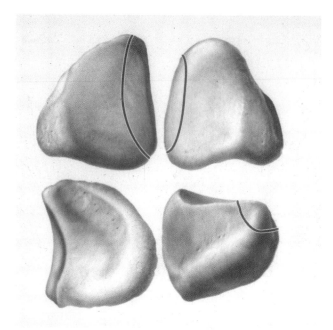

Figure 5.162. Articular abaxial sesamoid fractures. (Reprinted with permission from Bertone AL. Fractures of the Proximal Sesamoid Bones. In Equine Fracture Repair. Nixon A, ed. WB Saunders Company, Philadelphia, 1996;16:163–171.)

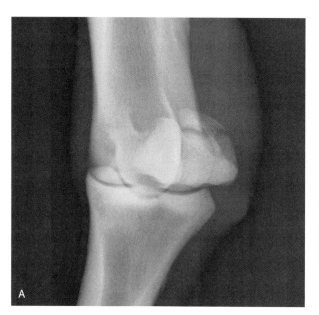
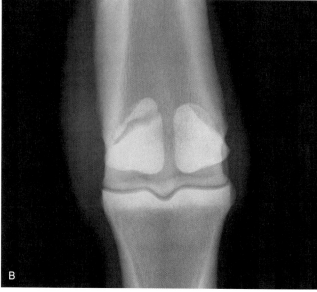

Figure 5.163. Oblique (A) and lateral (B) radiographs of a large apical plus abaxial sesamoid fracture in a Quarter horse mare. (Courtesy of Dr. Gary Baxter.)

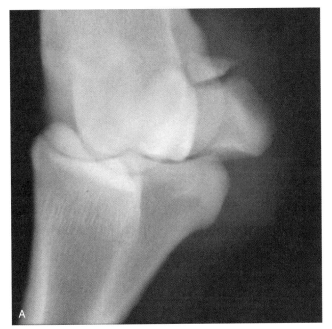

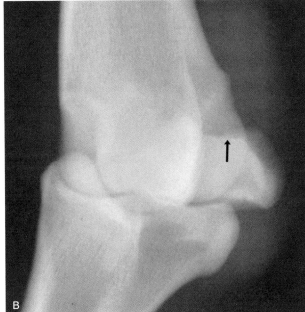

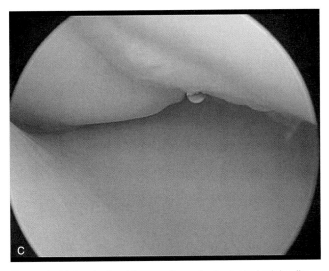

Figure 5.164. A. An oblique radiograph of a typical minimally displaced fresh apical sesamoid fracture in a racing Standardbred that can be removed arthroscopically or with a small arthrotomy. B. After fragment removal, the suspensory ligament will reattach with fibrous tissue to the flat bed of the sesamoid bone (arrow). C. Arthroscopic appearance of a nondisplaced apical sesamoid fracture.

ligament proximally and the distal sesamoidean ligament distally, most of these tend to separate (Figure 5.167). Infrequently, they remain in apposition, but may separate at a later time. If both sesamoid bones are fractured, they usually become distracted and the suspensory support apparatus is lost.

Etiology

The cause of proximal sesamoid bone fractures is excessive tensile forces and direct blunt trauma to the bone. Fetlock extension is greatest at the end of a race due to fatigue of the digital flexor muscles that support the fetlock. This hyperextension maximally loads the sesamoid bones. The bone fails when the sesamoid bone can no longer withstand the distraction forces applied to it by the suspensory ligament and distal sesamoidean ligaments. This muscle fatigue factor is most clearly illustrated when young foals that are placed on pasture fracture their sesamoid bones while running to keep up with the dam.[10,14]

Other factors such as poor conditioning, improper trimming and shoeing, and poor conformation create additional stresses on this bone, as do training and racing schedules.[2,20] Unequal tension applied to the sesamoid bone as the foot strikes the ground in an unbalanced position may also cause these fractures.

During training these bones rapidly remodel, which initially decreases bone porosity and increases bone trabecular width and mineralizing surface, thereby

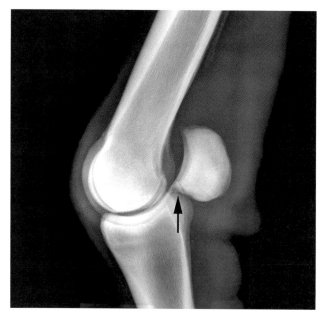

Figure 5.165. Flexed lateral radiograph demonstrating a small articular basilar fracture (arrow) in a Thoroughbred racehorse. This fracture extended across the entire base of the medial sesamoid bone. (Courtesy of Dr. Gary Baxter.)

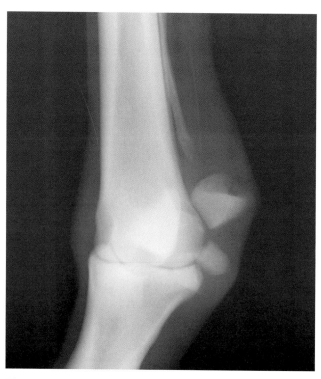

Figure 5.167. Uniaxial comminuted sesamoid fracture that has been distracted by the pull of the suspensory apparatus. (Courtesy of Dr. Gary Baxter.)

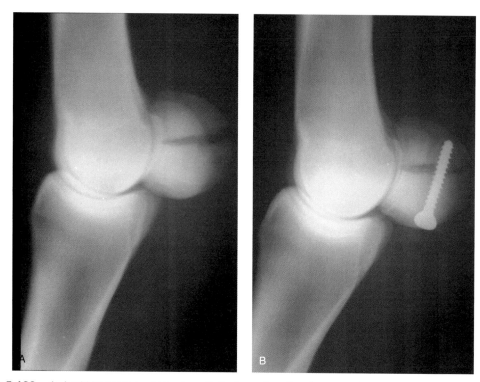

Figure 5.166. A. A mid-body sesamoid fracture. B. Postoperative view demonstrating a single cortical screw that was used to stabilize the fracture.

enhancing the bone's ability to withstand stress.[32] The suspensory ligament also increases in strength with training until its exceeds the strength of the bone, making bone failure the method of suspensory breakdown in racing or heavily training racehorses.[8] The vascular pattern of sesamoid bones may be implicated in site selection of fractures as the orientation and distribution of vessels parallels the radiographic lucencies seen in horses with sesamoiditis and correspond to the configuration of apical fracture patterns.[28]

Direct trauma to the sesamoid bone can cause comminuted fractures and midbody fractures. Direct trauma can occur if the fetlock hits the ground in an athletic event or at the time of a uniaxial sesamoid fracture. It is also possible that a hindlimb could clip the sesamoid, causing fracture and often a wound. The medial sesamoid bone is reported to be the most frequently involved when interference is the cause.[1]

The sesamoid bones also undergo marked bone resorption when the fetlock is immobilized, and pathologic fracture after cast removal has been reported in adult horses.[16]

Clinical Signs

The medial or lateral sesamoid bones, or both, may be fractured. Lameness is very pronounced in acute stages: The horse is reluctant to bear weight on the limb and will not permit the fetlock to descend to a normal position during weight-bearing. Swelling, heat, and pain are marked in the fetlock region. Tenosynovitis or suspensory desmitis, which also may be present, may confuse the diagnosis if radiographs are not taken. The horse evidences pain when pressure is applied to the affected bone or bones. Descent of the fetlock during weight-bearing causes pain. Observation of the gait reveals that the fetlock is held rigid so that it cannot descend as much as the opposite normal fetlock. The fracture in the bone may occur in any area of the sesamoids, but proximal fractures are more common than distal fractures; proximal fractures also are more amenable to treatment. Desmitis of the suspensory ligament and distal sesamoidean ligaments may occur concurrently with fractured sesamoids. Lameness at the walk and trot may not be obvious after 1 to 2 weeks' rest, but joint effusion persists.

A history of galloping to exhaustion in an attempt to keep up with the dam is common for young foals under 2 months of age that have sustained fractures of their sesamoid bones. These fractures often occur in foals that have been confined to a box stall for several days and then turned out for free exercise with the dam.

Diagnosis

Diagnosis is based on radiologic examination of the affected fetlock and the physical changes described. If a fetlock joint is severely swollen and the horse shows pain when pressure is applied over the sesamoid bone(s), radiographs should be taken to rule out the possibility of fracture. Cases of tenosynovitis also should be radiographed to eliminate the possibility of fractured sesamoid bones accompanying this condition. Sesamoiditis may cause similar signs, but radiographs show no frac-

ture, and joint effusion is not a prominent feature of sesamoiditis.

Because the radiodensity and contrast may be poor in radiographs taken in very young foals (due to limited ossification), good-quality radiographs and close scrutiny are required for the diagnosis. In some cases the fracture cannot be diagnosed immediately and may require a few weeks before it becomes apparent. This is also true for hairline nondisplaced fractures that occur in adults. These fractures may be difficult to differentiate from increased vascular channels associated with chronic sesamoiditis.[11,12] Nuclear scintigraphy can be helpful in making the diagnosis in these situations.

Standard radiographic views should include the dorsal palmar (DP), lateral medial (LM), and oblique projections. Occasionally the flexed LM may demonstrate lesions that are not detectable on the other standard projections and estimation of reduction potential of midbody fractures can be made. The addition of the skyline projection of the abaxial surface of the sesamoid bone is helpful in some cases to identify the exact location of fractures on the abaxial surface (Figure 5.168).[18] The radiographs should be closely examined for any signs of OA associated with the fetlock and incomplete fractures that may be confused with increased interosseous vascular channels.

The fracture can be differentiated from the vascular canals by the following criteria: (1) The fracture usually extends to the margin of the abaxial surface of the proximal sesamoid bone, whereas the increased vascular canal does not, and (2) the fracture line frequently

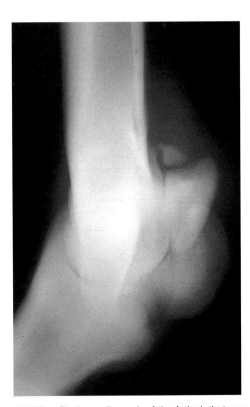

Figure 5.168. Skyline radiograph of the fetlock that was performed to document articular involvement of an abaxial sesamoid fracture. (Courtesy of Dr. Gary Baxter.)

runs in a different direction or plane than the vascular canal. If an incomplete sesamoid bone fracture is suspected, a repeat radiograph should be taken after a period of 2 to 4 weeks of stall rest, or nuclear scintigraphy can be performed. This permits better evaluation of the fracture line because it allows sufficient time for lysis of the bone to occur. A better appreciation for the fibroosseous disruption can be made at this time as well. It should be re-emphasized that if these horses are allowed to exercise, they run a great risk of distracting the fracture and worsening the prognosis. Ultrasonography should be performed on all apical and basilar fractures to identify whether an injury to the supportive ligaments has occurred.

Treatment

The selection of treatment of sesamoid bone fractures is based on the location of the fracture and the intended use of the animal. Treatments include stall rest, cast application, surgical excision, lag screw fixation, circumferential wiring, and bone grafting.

In general, most horses that are not intended for performance and will be relegated to breeding do not require surgery, and simple support, bandaging, or splinting, or casting with stall rest is sufficient.[1] For more severe injuries such as biaxial sesamoid fractures with partial collapse of the suspensory apparatus (identified as a dropped fetlock upon weight-bearing), use of a splint that places the horse on the toe and relieves suspensory tension (e.g., Kimzey Leg Saver) should be used to support fetlock joint ankylosis in a more normal position. The splint can be worn for 2 to 3 months, depending on the severity of the injury.

Stall rest (with or without soft cast or external coaptation) for 3 to 4 months has been successful to obtain fibrous or partial bony union, but management is prolonged, and if casting is used, weakening of the bone is anticipated.[16] This prolonged period of time is needed because the sesamoid bones heal very slowly. The delayed healing may result from limited periosteal covering and the extensive ligamentous attachments that cause distraction and movement. Most fractures that are treated conservatively heal by a weak fibrous union, and the fracture line can be observed on radiographic examination for prolonged periods of time. A portion of these fractures that have apparently healed will separate at a later date and result in pain again. Generally, the conservative approach should be used for those horses that are not going to be used for performance in the future and in young foals without distraction of fracture fragments.

Surgical treatment of sesamoid bone fractures (if indicated) in the horse intended for performance appears to be beneficial and is preferred for the most rapid return to performance with the least risk of future OA or sesamoid re-injury. Surgical removal or stabilization to promote earlier bony union reduces the risk of secondary OA within the fetlock joint.

Apical, articular abaxial, and basilar fractures involving less than one-third of the sesamoid bone are best treated by surgical removal of the fragment (Figures 5.163 to 5.165, 5.168).[4,5,19,22–26] Nonarticular

abaxial fractures may require removal, but horses often perform successfully without surgery. Midbody transverse fractures affecting the middle third and basilar transverse fractures of the proximal sesamoid bones have been treated successfully with lag screw fixation (Figure 5.166) or circumferential wiring to provide postoperative bone compression and immobilization.[4,13,17,31]

Autogenous cancellous bone grafting and cast immobilization has been used with some degree of success but most surgeons prefer to combine autogenous cancellous bone grafting with internal fixation of the fracture for best results. Internal fixation offers the advantage of earlier removal of the cast and earlier weight-bearing.

Fractures through the bodies of both sesamoid bones are a common cause of breakdown in the racing horse.[15] Because the suspensory apparatus is lost and distal limb vascular supply may be disrupted, these horses may be humanely euthanized. However, animals with breeding potential or sentimental value can be salvaged by arthrodesis of the fetlock. See Traumatic Rupture of the Suspensory Apparatus in this chapter.

Surgery is easily performed with the horse in lateral or dorsal recumbency under general anesthesia. Surgical removal of apical sesamoid fractures can be performed by arthroscopy or arthrotomy through the palmar/plantar recess of the fetlock joint. Arthroscopy offers the advantage of very rapid return to performance for small articular fractures without suspensory involvement (3 weeks) and the ability to remove more than 1 fracture from a joint with minimal incisional morbidity. Dorsal P1 fractures or biaxial sesamoid fractures may occur simultaneously. Dorsal recumbency offers the advantage of not having to move the horse to gain access to multiple sites or limbs for surgery, less bleeding, and passive flexion of the joint to enhance visualization and decrease tension of the suspensory ligament. Apical and articular abaxial fractures on both sesamoids can be removed from one arthroscopic portal.

Hemorrhage can limit visualization in fresh fractures that require dissection of the suspensory ligament (apical, articular abaxial fractures and basilar fractures). Use of electrocautery probes for transection of the ligament may enhance precision of separation and less hemorrhage.[5] For classical apical fractures that involve the suspensory ligament, but are smaller than one-third of the length of the bone, arthrotomy or arthroscopy are valid surgical approaches. The arthrotomy can be made small and this joint location heals well.

Casting or splinting is recommended for midbody fractures and comminuted fractures, or if clinical evidence of suspensory disruption accompanies the sesamoid fracture. The horse should be walked daily after 10 days to 2 weeks. Supporting wraps should be kept on for a minimum of 30 days; they are especially important during the 2 weeks following surgery to prevent swelling. Reattachment of the suspensory ligament is slow and 4 to 6 months may be required before returning to training for large fractures.

For basilar fractures, the arthroscope is similarly placed in the fetlock recess, but the instrument portal must be made into the distal fetlock recess such that instruments can be placed parallel to the base of the sesamoid. These fractures are more difficult to remove because of the extent of ligamentous structure attached to the bone. If the fragment cannot be completely removed by arthroscopy the distal instrument portal can be enlarged to allow direct removal by arthrotomy. Blunt dissection between the distal sesamoidean ligaments can retrieve most fragments. Abaxial fragments that lie entirely on the basilar aspect (nonarticular) of the sesamoid bone cannot be reached by any arthroscopic approach and must be removed by incision directly over the fragment. Most of these fractures do not need to be removed and heal by fibrous union. Removal of nonarticular basilar fractures can be performed between the distal sesamoidean ligaments for smaller fragments or through the tendon sheath.[7] Removal of the fragment allows direct healing of the torn ends of the suspensory ligament to the bone, rather than a fibrous union between bones.

Removal of nonarticular basilar sesamoid fractures is performed on the palmar or plantar aspect of the fetlock on the side of the SDFT just distal to the fetlock anular ligament. There is a depression palpable at the base of the sesamoid. The distal sesamoidean ligaments are bluntly dissected and the fragment located with a needle and radiographic imaging if necessary. Once the fragment is located it can be shelled out with a sharp curette or elevator to avoid cutting distal sesamoidean ligament fibers. Alternatively, an approach through the straight DSL and the digital tendon sheath can successfully retrieve fragments.[7] In most instances, nonarticular basilar sesamoid fractures do not require removal and heal with a fibrous union. Chronic pain from recurring tearing of the fibrous tissue can occur and removal seems to improve the outcome.

When a sesamoid fracture involves a third or more of the sesamoid bone, it should be repaired with a lag bone screw directed from distal to proximal (Figure 5.166). The fracture reduction should be assessed with the arthroscope in the palmar or plantar recess of the joint. Fluoroscopic or radiographic examination is necessary to confirm the drilling angulation. Care should be taken not to drill through the proximal portion into the suspensory ligaments, because this may result in dystrophic calcification of this ligament. If the fracture is chronic, the distal fragment may be demineralized and easily fractured. Usually a single 4.5-mm cortical bone screw is selected, although a single or 2 3.5-mm cortical screws have been successful. Placement of the screw from proximal to distal has been described for fractures with a large abaxial component.

Casting is recommended because the forces to bend or cyclically fail the screw at the fracture site are high, particularly if anatomic reduction was not complete. Bone graft can be inserted into the fracture site just prior to tightening the screw. Bony union is expected within 6 months and return to training at about 9 months. The screw does not need to be removed, even if it breaks, as long as it is not infected. Ideally, the fragment should be in 1 piece and should involve at least 30% of the bone for use of screw fixation repair. Approximately 44% of horses repaired with a 4.5-mm

lag screw returned to race.[9] Fractures approaching half of the bone volume are the most favorable. If the fragment does not reduce at surgery or is split, the prognosis is less favorable and additional fragments may make the operation impractical. Circumferential wiring may still contain these fragments and enhance the chance of bony union, and could be elected as an alternative.

Circumferential and transfixation wiring is an alternate approach to internal stabilization of sesamoid fractures that involve more than one-third of the bone. However, in one study none of the horses repaired with this technique returned to racing.[9] Use of polyethylene cable instead of wire could offer better mechanical strength of the repair, but has not been reported clinically.[21]

A palmar or plantar pouch arthrotomy is made to expose the articular surface and apex of the sesamoid bone, and another incision is made into the digital tendon sheath through the anular ligament. Endoscopic visualization in the digital tendon sheath for placing the cable or wire can be performed in preference to opening the tendon sheath. To minimize wire breakage before adequate fracture healing, use of 2 wires or other braided materials not as susceptible to cyclic failure are being investigated. Wire migration after breakage occurs and usually necessitates removal. Casting for a minimum of 30 days is recommended to reduce the risk of wire breakage. The initial breaking strength of the circumferential wiring technique as compared to the screw technique are similar[30] or greater for the circumferential wiring;[29] however, *in vivo* studies or cyclic failure studies have not been performed. The author prefers the screw technique because it has reportedly been more successful than wiring and does not enter the tendon sheath, place foreign material into the tendon sheath, or require implant removal even if implant failure occurs. Additionally if screw placement does not work (i.e., cannot achieve compression or is malpositioned), a wire can subsequently be placed.

When fractures of both bodies of the sesamoid have occurred and the suspensory apparatus is lost, early treatment is required for a successful outcome. Even with early treatment the initial soft tissue trauma may be severe enough that the blood supply to the foot is lost.[6] Management of such injuries is directed toward the support and immobilization of the fetlock joint for a sufficient time period to stabilize soft tissue destruction and then consideration of surgical arthrodesis or conservative ankylosis by soft tissue fibrosis. See the section on traumatic suspensory rupture for more information. A major complication to this "breakdown" injury is support limb laminitis in the contralateral weight-bearing limb.

Fractures of the sesamoid that occur in conjunction with fracture of the metacarpal or metatarsal condyle are serious injuries that should be identified on the radiograph because the prognosis for returning to racing, even with repair of the condylar fracture, is not good.[3] These fractures are usually sagittal and axial and occur with extreme pulling on the intersesamoidean ligament when the condylar fracture displaces. The fractures indicate significant soft tissue injury to the fetlock joint and that OA is likely to ensue.

Prognosis

The reported prognosis for apical sesamoid fractures is good to excellent (88% of Standardbreds[31] and 77% of Thoroughbreds[22] return to racing), for abaxial fractures is good (71% of Thoroughbreds or Quarter horse racehorses returned to racing),[25] for basilar fractures is fair (50% to 60% of Thoroughbreds return to racing),[24] and for midbody fractures repaired by either lag screw fixation or circumferential wiring is fair (44% to 60% return to performance).[13,17] Conservative management reports are not available for comparison, but generally it is presumed that the prognosis is guarded for either basilar or midbody fractures that are not treated. Most of these joints develop significant OA and restricted range of joint motion. If both sesamoids are fractured, the prognosis is less favorable due to the loss of suspensory support.

The prognosis for treatment of fractures of the sesamoid bones that result in loss of the suspensory apparatus is poor and only should be considered for salvage of valuable breeding stock and horses of great sentimental value.

References

1. Adams OR. Lameness in Horses. 3rd ed. Lea and Febiger, Philadelphia, 1974.
2. Anthenill LA, Stover SM, Gardner IA, et al. Risk factors for proximal sesamoid bone fractures associated with exercise history and horseshoe characteristics in Thoroughbred racehorses. Am J Vet Res 2007;68:760–761.
3. Bassage LH, Richardson DW. Longitudinal fractures of the condyles of the third metacarpal and metatarsal bones in racehorses: 224 cases (1986–1995). J Am Vet Med Assoc 1998;212:1757.
4. Bertone AL. Fractures of the proximal sesamoid bones. In Equine Fracture Repair. Nixon AJ, ed. W.B. Saunders, Philadelphia. 1996;163–171.
5. Boure L, Marcoux M, Laverty S, et al. Use of electrocautery probes in arthroscopic removal of apical sesamoid fracture fragments in 18 Standardbred horses. Vet Surg 1999;28:226.
6. Bramlage LR. First aid and transportation of fracture patients. In AJ Nixon's Equine Fracture Repair. WB Saunders Co., Philadelphia, 1996;36–43.
7. Brokken, MT, Schneider RK, Tucker RL. Surgical approach for removal of nonarticular base sesamoid fragments of the proximal sesamoid bones in horses. Vet Surg. 2008;37:619–624.
8. Bukowiecki CF, Bramlage LR, Gabel AA. *In vitro* strength of the suspensory apparatus in training and resting horses. Vet Surg 1987;16:126.
9. Busschers E, Richardson DW, Hogan PM, et al. Surgical repair of mid-body proximal sesamoid bone fractures in 25 horses. Vet Surg 2008;37:771–780.
10. Ellis DR. Fractures of the proximal sesamoid bones in Thoroughbred foals. Equine Vet J 1979;11:48.
11. Grondahl AM, Gaustad G, Engeland A. Progression and association with lameness and racing performance of radiographic changes in the proximal sesamoid bones of young Standardbred trotters. Equine Vet J 1994;26:152.
12. Hardy J, Marcoux M, Breton L. Clinical relevance of radiographic findings in proximal sesamoid bones of two-year-old standardbreds in their first year of race training. J Am Vet Med Assoc 1991;198:2089–94.
13. Henninger RW, Bramlage LR, Schneider RK, et al. Lag screw and cancellous bone graft fixation of transverse proximal sesamoid bone fractures in horses: 25 cases (1983–1989). J Am Vet Med Assoc 1991;199:606.
14. Honnas CM, Snyder JR, Meagher DM, et al. Traumatic disruption of the suspensory apparatus in foals. Cornell Vet 1990;80:123.
15. Johnson BJ, Stover SM, Daft BM, et al. Causes of death in racehorses over a 2-year period. Equine Vet J 1994;26:327.
16. Malone ED, Anderson BH, Turner TA. Proximal sesamoid bone fracture following cast removal in two horses. Equine Vet J 1997;9:185.
17. Martin BB, Nunamaker DM, Evans LH, et al. Circumferential wiring of mid-body and large basilar fractures of the proximal sesamoid bone in 15 horses. Vet Surg 1991;20:9.
18. Palmer SE. Radiography of the abaxial surface of the proximal sesamoid bones of the horse. J Am Vet Med Assoc 1982;181:264.
19. Parente EJ, Richardson DW, Spencer P. Basal sesamoidean fractures in horses: 57 cases (1989–1991). J Am Vet Med Assoc 1993;202:1293.
20. Parkin TD, Clegg PD, French NP, et al. Risk of fatal distal limb fractures among Thoroughbreds involved in the five types of racing in the United Kingdom. Vet Rec. 2004;154:493–497.
21. Rothaug PG, Boston RC, Richardson DW, et al. A comparison of ultra-high-molecular weight polyethylene cable and stainless steel wire using two fixation techniques for repair of equine midbody sesamoid fractures: an *in vitro* biomechanical study. Vet Surg. 2002;31:445–454.
22. Schnabel LV, Bramlage LR, Mohammed HO, et al. Racing performance after arthroscopic removal of apical sesamoid fracture fragments in Thoroughbred horses age > or = 2 years: 84 cases (1989–2002). Equine Vet J 2006;38:446–451.
23. Schnabel LV, Bramlage LR, Mohammed HO, et al. Racing performance after arthroscopic removal of apical sesamoid fracture fragments in Thoroughbred horses age <2 years: 151 cases (1989–2002). Equine Vet J 2007;39:64–68.
24. Southwood LL, McIlwraith CW. Arthroscopic removal of fracture fragments involving a portion of the base of the proximal sesamoid bone in horses: 26 cases (1984–1997). J Am Vet Med 2000;217:236.
25. Southwood LL, Trotter GW, McIlwraith CW. Arthroscopic removal of abaxial fracture fragments of the proximal sesamoid bones in horses: 47 cases (1989–1997). J Am Vet Med Assoc 1998;213:1016.
26. Spurlock GH, Gabel AA. Apical fractures of the proximal sesamoid bones in 109 Standardbred horses. J Am Vet Med Assoc 1983;183:76.
27. Torre K, Motta M. Incidence and distribution of 369 proximal sesamoid bone fractures in 354 Standardbred horses (1984–1995). Equine Pract 1999;21:6.
28. Trumble TN, Arnoczky SP, Stick JA, et al. Clinical relevance of the microvasculature of the equine proximal sesamoid bone. Am J Vet Res 1995;56:720.
29. Wilson DA, Keegan KG, Carson WL. An *in vitro* biomechanical comparison of two fixation methods for transverse osteotomies of the medial proximal forelimb sesamoid bones in horses. Vet Surg 1999;28:355.
30. Woodie JB, Ruggles AJ, Litsky AS. *In vitro* biomechanical properties of 2 compression fixation methods for midbody proximal sesamoid bone fractures in horses. Vet Surg 2000;29:358.
31. Woodie JB, Ruggles AJ, Bertone AL, et al. Apical fracture of the proximal sesamoid bone in standardbred horses: 43 cases (1990–1996). J Am Vet Med Assoc 1999;214:1653.
32. Young DR, Nunamaker DM, Markel MD. Quantitative evaluation of the remodeling response of the proximal sesamoid bones to training-related stimuli in Thoroughbreds. Am J Vet Res 1991;52:1350.

SESAMOIDITIS

Sesamoiditis is observed frequently in racing horses and hunters and jumpers between 2 and 5 years of age.[6–8] The condition is characterized by pain associated with the proximal sesamoid bones and insertions of the suspensory ligament that result in lameness. The pain is thought to result from inflammation at the interface of the suspensory ligament and distal sesamoidean ligaments with the proximal sesamoid bone. Primary disease of the suspensory ligament or distal sesamoidean ligament can also accompany this condition. Pain, heat, and inflammation can be clinically detected at the insertion of the suspensory ligament during the active stages of the disease process, but marked lameness and limita-

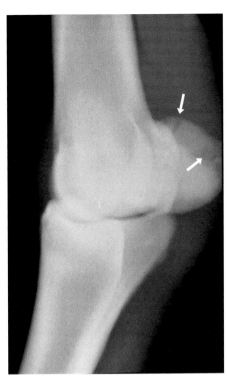

Figure 5.169. Typical findings in sesamoiditis. Note the osteolysis along the vascular channel and bone proliferation at the abaxial edge of the lesion (arrows).

tions on performance can also occur without any clinically detectable signs.[1,4]

Radiographs can reveal a range of changes from accelerated early remodeling response in the bones (increased size and number of vascular canals), to marked proliferation of bone along the abaxial margin of the sesamoid and increased bone density of the sesamoid. The suspensory ligament and the distal sesamoidean ligaments may also be affected and show calcified areas. Demineralization of the sesamoid bone(s) may result from inflammation or direct blunt trauma (Figure 5.169).[8] Impaired blood supply has been proposed as an etiology, but experimental work suggests it is an improbable cause.[2,3] The increased bone production is thought to result from inflammation from tearing of the attachments of either the suspensory ligament or the distal sesamoidean ligament. It is also possible to see radiographic changes indicating chronic sesamoiditis in sound performing horses, suggesting that some horses heal the injury and regain suspensory strength.[4]

Etiology

Any unusual strain to the fetlock region may produce sesamoiditis. Most common in racehorses, hunters, and jumpers, it can affect any type of horse. It is caused by injury to the attachment of the suspensory ligament to the sesamoid bones. This injury to the suspensory ligament attachment may alter blood supply to the sesamoid bone(s). Injury to the distal sesamoidean ligaments may also occur at their attachment to the basilar portion of the sesamoid bones.

The sesamoid bones have a substantial intraosseous blood supply that enters the midportion of the bone through multiple abaxial channels that correspond to the channels that enlarge in sesamoiditis, indicating bone resorption. This may represent the initiation of the remodeling response to bone stress of training or it may reflect an increase in blood flow due to inflammation and injury to the suspensory ligament, or both.[11] The sesamoid bones undergo intense remodeling in response to training[12] and the progression of radiographic changes correlate to bone response to remodeling and injury.

Interestingly, several studies have categorized the radiographic changes in sesamoid bones of young (2- and 3-year-old) racehorses and discovered that many horses have increased size and number of vascular channels without lameness.[4,5] Yearling Thoroughbreds with more than 2 irregular vascular canals had a decrease in number of race starts and earnings at 2 and 3 years of age.[9] This supports the idea that remodeling is a normal response to training and that only if the stresses exceed the bones' capability to strengthen would microfracture and bone damage occur. Although radiographic vascular changes of bone remodeling were not associated with sesamoid fracture, the vascular structures course along known lines of fracture in adult racehorses. The sesamoid bones have an extensive sensory nerve supply that may explain bone pain associated with trabecular bone injury.[3]

Clinical Signs

Symptoms of this condition are similar to those caused by fracture of the sesamoid bone. In the early stage, minimal swelling is observed, but increased heat may be felt over the abaxial surface of the sesamoid bone. As the disease progresses, a visible enlargement of the soft tissues overlying the palmar surface of the fetlock can be seen as fibrosis of the injured suspensory ligament becomes apparent. On palpation, pain withdrawal can usually be elicited by placing pressure over the abaxial surfaces of the sesamoid bone. In more advanced cases, pain may be elicited by applying pressure over the branches of the suspensory ligament and possibly the distal sesamoidean ligament as well. Flexion of the fetlock is also painful.

At exercise the lameness varies considerably and depends on the acuteness of the injury and its degree. In general, the lameness is most evident during the first part of exercise and is more exaggerated when the horse is exercised on hard surfaces. On close observation, a reduction in extension of the fetlock is noticed, and a fetlock flexion test usually exacerbates the lameness.[10] Perineural and/or intrasynovial anesthesia is used infrequently to diagnose this condition. Horses respond to a distal metacarpal nerve block, but not to an intra-articular fetlock block, locating the lameness to the periarticular structures.

Diagnosis

The radiologic changes of true sesamoiditis have been described as bony changes on the abaxial surface or basilar region with increased radiodense buildups, increased number and irregularity of the vascular channels, and increased coarseness and mottling of the bone trabeculation (Figure 5.169). In acute cases radiographs may have to be taken approximately 3 weeks after onset of the condition to determine whether bony changes will occur on the sesamoid bones. The condition may also occur with tenosynovitis, fracture of the sesamoid bones, and injury to the suspensory ligament from which it must be differentiated. Careful radiographic interpretations of the mottled trabecular pattern seen in the proximal sesamoid bone are necessary to differentiate a fracture. Incomplete fracture can be differentiated from these coarse, vascular canals because the fracture usually extends to the abaxial surface and the vascular canals do not. Furthermore, the fracture line frequently runs at different angles than the vascular channels.

Nuclear scintigraphy indicates increased radioactivity in the region of the sesamoid bones, but usually not of fracture activity. Ultrasound of the suspensory and distal sesamoidean ligaments may not be useful because many horses have no abnormalities in the ligaments in the acute phases.

Treatment

If heat, pain, and swelling are detected at the bone or suspensory insertion, then efforts should be made to reduce the inflammation. Alternating cold and hot packs, as well as antiphlogistic packs, should be used. Rest from performance until soundness at the trot is achieved followed by slow convalescent exercise allows the bone to continue to remodel and strengthen. Importantly, the exercise must be kept below the level that would reinjure the bone. Similar to other suspensory ligament injuries, convalescence is long (6 to 8 months) and injury often recurs when horses return to full work. In chronic stages, firing, and blistering have been used but with only limited success. X-ray and gamma-ray radiation, laser heat application, shock wave therapy, and a balanced mineral diet are considered by some to be valuable therapy in this condition, as well as in the treatment of calcification in the suspensory ligament.

Prognosis

The prognosis for return to full athletic performance is guarded to unfavorable, depending upon the amount of periosteal reaction and new bone growth that occurs on the sesamoid bones and the extent of injury to the suspensory ligament and the distal sesamoidean ligaments.

References

1. Clayton HM. Cinematographic analysis of the gait of lame horses II: chronic sesamoiditis. Equine Vet Sci 1986;6:310.
2. Corenelissen BP, Rijkenbuizen AB, Buam P, et al. A study on the pathogenesis of equine sesamoiditis: the effects of experimental occlusion of the sesamoidean artery. J Vet Med A Physiol Pathol Clin Med. 2002;49:244–250.
3. Cornelissen BP. The proximal sesamoid bone of the horse: vascular and neurologic characteristics. Tijdschr Diergeneeskd 1998; 15:123.
4. Grondahl AM, Gaustad G, Engeland A. Progression and association with lameness and racing performance of radiographic changes in the proximal sesamoid bones of young Standardbred trotters. Equine Vet J 1994;26:152.
5. Hardy J, Marcoux M, Breton L. Clinical relevance of radiographic findings in proximal sesamoid bones of two-year-old standardbreds in their first year of race training. J Am Vet Med Assoc 1991;198:2089.
6. Nemeth F. Sesamoiditis in the Horse. Tijdschr. Diergeneesk 1973;98:994.
7. Nemeth F. The pathology of sesamoiditis. Tijdschr. Diergeneesk 1973;98:1003.
8. O'Brien TR, et al. Sesamoiditis in the thoroughbred: a radiographic study. J Am Vet Rad Soc 1971;12:75.
9. Spike-Pierce DL, Bramlage LR. Correlation of racing performance with radiographic changes in the proximal sesamoid bones of 487 Thoroughbred yearlings. Equine Vet J. 2003;35: 350–353.
10. Stashak TS. Sesamoiditis. In Adam's Lameness in Horses, 4th ed. Lea and Febiger, Philadelphia, 1987;582.
11. Trumble TN, Arnoczky SP, Stick JA, et al. Clinical relevance of the microvasculature of the equine proximal sesamoid bone. Am J Vet Res 1995;56:720.
12. Young DR, Nunamaker DM, Markel MD. Quantitative evaluation of the remodeling response of the proximal sesamoid bones to training-related stimuli in Thoroughbreds. Am J Vet Res 1991;52:1350.

OSTEOMYELITIS OF THE AXIAL BORDER OF THE PROXIMAL SESAMOID BONES

Etiology

Osteomyelitis of the axial border of the proximal sesamoid bones is an uncommon cause of lameness in horses. Presumably an injury to the attachment of the intersesamoidean ligament and possibly seeding with bacteria from intra-articular injections may be associated with the condition (Figure 5.170). In one report on

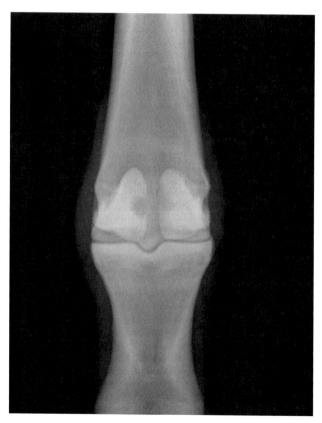

Figure 5.170. Dorsopalmar radiograph of the fetlock illustrating lysis of the axial borders of the sesamoids consistent with osteomyelitis. (Courtesy of Dr. Ellis Farstvedt.)

7 cases, 3 affected horses had a septic tenosynovitis of the digital sheath and 2 of 7 had a fetlock septic arthritis.[2,3] In one report, Aspergillus fungal joint infection accompanied lysis of the axial border of the sesamoid bones.[1] In some cases, even though the clinical signs and radiographic lesions are suggestive of sepsis, histology of lesions revealed infarction and necrosis, not purulent inflammation.

Clinical Signs and Diagnosis

In this condition, horses are quite lame at the walk. In one report lameness ranged from 2 to 5 out of 5 (mean 4 out of 5).[3] Radiographs usually reveal bone lysis at the attachment of the intersesamoidean ligament primarily at the midbody and apical regions (Figure 5.170). A single or both sesamoids may be affected. Some lesions appear cystic, whereas others appear to erode the axial border more diffusely. In one report evidence of acute, subacute, and chronic reparative osteomyelitis was seen in the proximal sesamoid bones in 10 fetlocks of affected horses.

Treatment and Prognosis

Computed tomography of the fetlock can assist with determining the surface location of the lytic areas and assist with the decision for surgery (Figure 5.171). Small lesions that are internal or only open toward the intersesamoidean ligament may be best treated conservatively. Lytic lesions that surface into the joint or tendon sheath have surgical access to the area from the palmar/plantar fetlock joint and/or digital sheath using arthroscopy. Abnormal bone and ligament are debrided if present and samples are submitted for culture and sen-

sitivity. Regional limb perfusion with an antimicrobial offers the advantage of perfusion of multiple affected sites including the fetlock joint, tendon sheath, and sesamoid bones.[1] The prolonged administration (6 to 12 weeks) of broad-spectrum antimicrobials is also recommended.[2]

Although the prognosis for return to performance is considered poor,[3] treatment can result in pasture soundness and, less commonly, return to intended use. If the intersesamoidean ligament is damaged extensively the prognosis for return to performance remains poor.

References

1. Sherman KM, Myhre GD, Heymann EI. Fungal osteomyelitis of the axial border of the proximal sesamoid bones in a horse. J Am Vet Med Assoc. 2006;229:1607–1611.
2. Stashak TS. Personal communication, 2001.
3. Wisner ER, O'Brien TR, Pool RR, et al. Osteomyelitis of the axial border of the proximal sesamoid bones in seven horses. Equine Vet J 1991;23:383.

TRAUMATIC ARTHRITIS/OSTEOARTHRITIS OF THE METACARPOPHALANGEAL (FETLOCK) JOINT (OSSELETS)

Traumatic arthritis includes a diverse collection of pathologic and clinical states that develop after single or repetitive episodes of trauma, and may include synovitis (inflammation of the synovial membrane), capsulitis (inflammation of the fibrous joint capsule), sprain (injury of collateral ligaments associated with the joint), or intra-articular fractures.[1–3,5] Any type of traumatic joint injury can progress to osteoarthritis within the fetlock (Figure 5.172).

Etiology

Soft tissue injury to the joint commonly occurs in horses in full work and represents an overuse of the joint or a single event injury. Joint injury can also occur as a sporadic event due to trauma. In young horses just put into training, fetlock joint soreness and joint effusion can develop and be worked through with a modified exercise plan and medication. Limb conformation may also predispose horses to joint soreness and eventually OA of the fetlock.

Clinical Signs

In mild cases, joint inflammation occurs without lameness and is noted as joint soreness on flexion and joint effusion in a young, recently worked or maximally performing horse. Swelling of the palmar/plantar joint pouches is usually noted first, followed by dorsal pouch effusion in chronic distention. Cases that involve a capsulitis of the fetlock, particularly the dorsal fetlock, often carry heat and a more marked response to flexion. If exercise is sustained, lameness may ensue and is frequently bilateral. In moderate cases and subacute cases, joint soreness and effusion persist and lameness worsens with exercise (Green osselets). In severe cases of injury or advanced joint degeneration, lameness can be severe and obvious joint enlargement and stiffening can ensue.

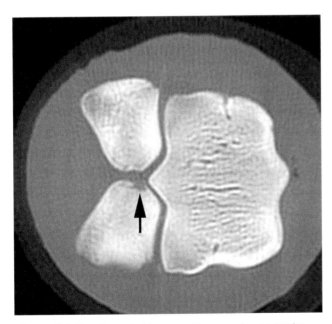

Figure 5.171. Computed tomographic coronal cross section through the metacarpus and proximal sesamoid bones. A focal area of bone lysis is visible on the axial edge of the medial sesamoid bone (arrow) that could not be identified radiographically.

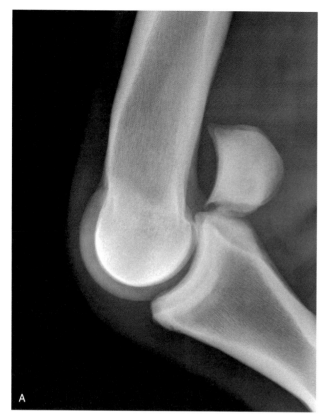

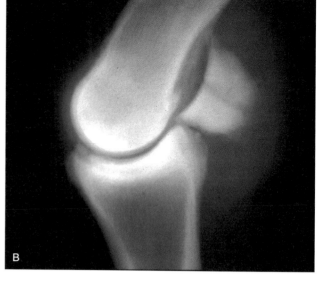

Figure 5.172. Lateral radiographs indicative of mild (A) and severe (B) osteoarthritis of the fetlock joint. The horse in (B) had a chronic midbody sesamoid fracture that was not treated. Secondary OA developed within the fetlock characterized by lipping of the sesamoid bones and osteophytes on the palmar aspect of the metacarpus. (Courtesy of Dr. Gary Baxter.)

Osteoarthritis of the fetlock joint that involves the articular cartilage is more severe because articular cartilage cannot heal and therapies to replace cartilage are only in development.[1-3] Injury or degeneration of articular cartilage should be suspected in horses with subacute or chronic joint synovitis, capsulitis, or sprain; with more severe lameness; and with radiographic evidence of subchondral bone remodeling or injury, such as an intra-articular fracture. In horses with severe or chronic joint injury, lameness may progress and be severe (Figure 5.172B). In horses with a history of an angulation abnormality, a fetlock joint subluxation or luxation should be suspected.

Diagnosis

Clinical examination provides a high degree of suspicion that OA of the fetlock is the cause of lameness. In racehorses, a condylar fracture or P1 fracture may occur along with effusion of the fetlock and pain on flexion. In racehorses, radiographs may be taken before local anesthetic or joint blocks are performed, especially if pain on direct pressure over these bones is present, to avoid worsening the fracture. Both radiographs and nerve blocks or a fetlock joint block can help localize and define the fetlock OA. Radiographs can diagnose an underlying cause in many cases, including intra-articular osteochondral fragments (either as part of

osteochondrosis or as an intra-articular fracture), bone cysts, subchondral bone erosion, osteophytosis, or joint space narrowing. Typically, digital nerve blocks do not block fetlock arthritis, but a distal metacarpal/tarsal nerve block significantly improves the lameness.[1-3] Direct intra-articular anesthesia to the fetlock offers additional benefits of achieving complete resolution of lameness, access to a joint fluid sample for analysis, a direct portal for simultaneous treatment (lavage, intra-articular antibiotics, or steroid), and an assessment of the indication for arthroscopic surgery. If the joint fluid appears hemorrhagic or cloudy, an immediate synovial fluid analysis and culture should be performed to rule out a septic process.

Horses that respond to a direct block to the joint and do not respond to rest or medical therapy are candidates for arthroscopic exploratory. Computed tomography, MRI, and contrast arthrography can offer improved imaging of the cartilage surface over plain radiography. For horses with chronic problems nonresponsive to medication, these further diagnostic techniques may identify an inciting cause or injury.

In horses with chronic fetlock OA, a condition known as proliferative synovitis can occur, particularly in Thoroughbred racehorses.[4] This condition is characterized by enlargement of the synovial pad that is located in the most proximal dorsal joint pouch of the fetlock. Chip fractures of the proximal aspect of P1 are often present concurrently in these horses.[4-6] Bone loss

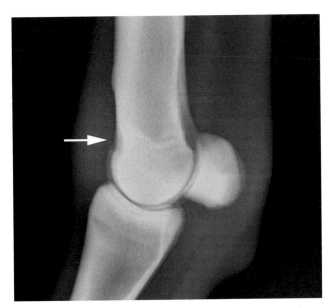

Figure 5.173. Lateral radiograph of the fetlock demonstrating a concave defect in the metacarpus (arrow) at the proximal aspect of the joint consistent with proliferative or villonodular synovitis. (Courtesy of Dr. Gary Baxter.)

or a "cut-back zone" in the distal metacarpus/metatarsus within the fetlock joint on radiographs is suggestive of this condition (Figure 5.173).[4,6] The diagnosis of proliferative synovitis can be confirmed with ultrasound of the dorsal joint capsule, contrast arthrography, or visual assessment of the synovial pad at the time of fetlock arthroscopy.

Treatment

Management of fetlock joint OA should address any primary problem and potentially include the following: rest, physical therapy, bandages, shoeing changes, and systemic and intra-articular joint medications. Arthroscopic surgery is recommended in horses that have concurrent predisposing conditions such as osteochondrosis, fragmentation, or proliferative synovitis. The fetlock joint is a commonly injected joint due to its high rotary motion and distal position within the limb. Intra-articular joint medications are covered in Chapter 8. Horses that are lame from fetlock joint soreness should be rested until lameness resolves, frequently 30 days. Return to work should be gradual and can be supplemented with systemic joint medications and shoeing alterations to promote break-over of the foot and an easy landing (pads, remove caulks and toe grabs, etc). Use of athletic bandages to provide support to the fetlock joint during work can be very helpful and pressure bandages after workouts prevent swelling. Many jumping and race horses are routinely treated with icing and wrapping of the fetlocks after workouts.

Joint medications are popular for horses with osselets or OA of the fetlock. These include systemic nonsteroidal medications to reduce pain and inflammation, systemic polysulfated glycosaminoglycans to manage cartilage health, systemic hyaluronan to reduce synovitis and promote cartilage health, and intra-articular use of these and similar products and/or steroids for maximal relief of pain and inflammation.[1-3] More recently biologic therapies, such as autologous conditioned serum and stem cells, have been promoted for intra-articular treatment of OA. These medications are frequently used after surgery or in OA without a surgical indication. Many show horses, particularly jumping and race horses, have chronic soreness and early degenerative changes in the fetlock joints. Many of these horses are maintained on intra-muscular injection of PSGAGs and intra-venous hyaluronan throughout the show or race season. Physical therapy, such as hydrotherapy boots, is routine for these horses.

The importance of regular and regulated exercise is critical to managing horses with fetlock OA. Confining horses with primary chronic OA often worsens their stiffness and discomfort. Regular exercise and turnout provides the greatest longevity with this condition.

Prognosis

The prognosis for green osselets is good to excellent. Early recognition and management is key to keeping the joint in good health and continuing training. Once degenerative changes in the joint are visible on radiograph, the prognosis is still good with management if the horse is sound enough to perform with treatment. Many horses are maintained in full work with managed fetlock OA. Once horses are no longer sound with the medical management listed, an extended period of rest may permit them to return to training, usually at a reduced expectation. Many top equine athletes can continue to perform at some level of activity with fetlock OA.

References

1. Bertone AL. Distal Limb: Fetlock and Pastern. In Equine Sports Medicine and Surgery. Hinchcliff KW, Kaneps AJ, Goer RJ, eds. Elsevier Science Ltd, Oxford, 2004;289–319.
2. Bertone AL. Joint Physiology: Responses to exercise and training. In Equine Sports Medicine and Surgery. Hinchcliff KW, Kaneps AJ, Goer RJ, eds. Elsevier Science Ltd, Oxford, 2004;152–161.
3. Bertone AL. Noninfectious Arthritis. In Diagnosis and Management of Lameness in Horses. Dyson SJ, Ross MW, eds. WB Saunders, Philadelphia. 2003;606–610.
4. Dabareiner RM, White NA, Sullins KE. Metacarpophalangeal joint synovial pad proliferation in 63 horses. Vet Surg 1996;25:199–206.
5. McIlwraith CW. Diseases of joints, tendons, ligaments and related structures. In Adams' Lameness in Horses, 5th ed. Stashak TS, ed. Lippincott Williams and Wilkins, Philadelphia. 2002;459–644.
6. Murphy DJ, Nixon AJ. Arthroscopic laser extirpation of metacarpophalangeal synovial pad proliferation in eleven horses. Equine Vet J 2000;33:296–301.

FETLOCK SUBCHONDRAL CYSTIC LESIONS (SCLs)

Fetlock subchondral bone cysts (SCLs) occur most commonly on the weight-bearing surface of the metacarpal condyle (Figure 5.174) and less commonly on the weight-bearing surface of proximal P1. Cysts of the distal metacarpus that open into the fetlock joint occur in young horses and are considered part of the developmental osteochondrosis syndrome.[1]

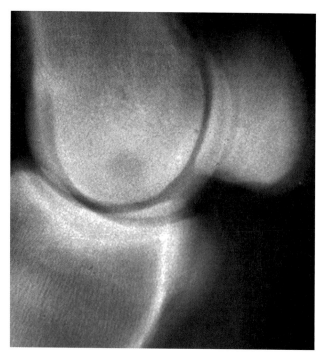

Figure 5.174. Lateral fetlock radiograph with a subchondral bone cyst in the middle of the condyle.

Etiology

Some SCLs are considered part of the developmental orthopedic diseases that occur during growth and the conversion of cartilage to bone. See Chapter 11 for further information on developmental SCLs. Proximal P1 cysts may be traumatically induced. Injury to the articular cartilage and underlying subchondral bone from high impact may allow synovial fluid to enter the fissure and increase intraosseous pressure. The author has seen several of these develop in mature working horses in which the SCL was not initially apparent on radiographs, but developed 30 to 60 days after injury. Typically the lameness and joint inflammation improve as the cyst matures.

Clinical Signs

The average age of horses with clinical signs is 18 months, although the SCL may develop prior to the onset of clinical signs.[2] Proximal P1 SCLs can develop in horses of any age from trauma. Moderate lameness is a feature of the disease that includes soreness to fetlock flexion in most cases and fetlock joint effusion in approximately 50% of the cases. In the author's experience, clinical signs for P1 cysts are an acute onset of lameness, joint heat, and effusion with marked soreness to fetlock flexion in a working horse.

Diagnosis

The diagnosis is made by radiographic evaluation of the joint (Figure 5.174). In the early development of the SCL, it may not be apparent on radiographs and follow-up radiographic examination is recommended if clinical signs that refer to the joint persist. Nuclear scintigraphy identifies a focal area of increased uptake in the bone as the SCL is developing and for several months after it has formed. Chronic SCLs may not have significant bone turnover above the surrounding condyle and may appear quiet on nuclear scan.

Treatment

Surgical debridement of metacarpal SCLs by an arthroscopic approach is the preferable treatment if the diagnosis is made before significant signs of OA have developed.[2] The SCL is approached through the dorsal pouch of the fetlock but some lesions cannot be reached with arthroscopy because the joint cannot be maximally flexed with the arthroscope in place. In these cases, the arthroscope can be removed, the limb forcibly flexed, and a small arthrotomy made directly over the cystic opening into the joint. For SCLs that do not respond to conservative treatment or debridement, osteostixis by extra-articular approach or mosaic autologous osteochondral grafting can be performed.[1]

Proximal P1 cysts cannot be reached by an articular approach because the weight-bearing surface is fully articulating and cannot be exposed by altering the joint position. These cysts can be surgically debrided from an extra-articular approach. A small 2.7-mm drill bit is directed to enter the cyst from the dorsal surface of P1. Radiographic or fluoroscopic control is required to ensure entrance into the cyst and avoidance of the joint. The cyst can be decompressed and debrided from this approach. Relieving the intraosseous pressure has immediate effects of improving lameness in early cases and can produce dramatic clinical improvement. Some articular cartilage damage is expected to remain and an adequate rest period is recommended for cartilage healing. Use of postoperative systemic and follow-up intra-articular medication to support joint healing is indicated.

Prognosis

The prognosis for return to performance appears to be good. In one report, surgical treatment of third metacarpal SCLs resulted in 80% of horses (12 of 15) returning to their intended use.[1] However, horses intended for elite performance, such as racing or national level competition for cutting, western riding, or 3-day eventing, are unlikely to stay sound in the author's opinion. Follow-up radiographs assist with the prognosis because osteophyte formation and signs of OA develop 1 to 2 years after the clinical signs develop.

The prognosis for proximal P1 SCLs is, in the author's opinion, slightly lower than that for metacarpal cysts, particularly if they are traumatically induced. Horses usually dramatically improve in lameness after surgery and usually become sound to the trot, but lameness can recur when returned to heavy training.

References

1. Bodo G, Hangody L, Modis L, et al. Autologous osteochondral grafting (mosaic arthroplasty) for treatment of subchondral cystic lesions in the equine stifle and fetlock joints. Vet Surg. 2004; 33:588–596.

2. Hogan PM, McIlwraith CW, Honnas CM, et al. Surgical treatment of subchondral cystic lesions of the third metacarpal bone: results in 15 horses (1986–1994). Equine Vet J 1997;29:477–82.

TRAUMATIC RUPTURE OF THE SUSPENSORY APPARATUS

Traumatic rupture of the suspensory apparatus with or without fractures of both proximal sesamoid bones is a common cause of acute breakdown in the racing Thoroughbred and often results in humane destruction of the animal.[1,5] Proximal luxations of the sesamoid bone without fracture can also occur with traumatic rupture of the distal sesamoidean ligament (Figure 5.175). Transverse or comminuted fractures of the proximal sesamoid bones can result in distraction of these bones. The apical portions are drawn proximally by the pull of the sesamoidean ligament while the basilar fragments remain attached to the distal sesamoidean ligaments. Occasionally, open luxation of the fetlock joint can occur. Besides the severe trauma sustained by the supporting soft tissues and bone, the adjacent digital arteries are frequently damaged sufficiently to result in ischemic necrosis of the hoof. Treatment of traumatic rupture of suspensory apparatus should only be considered as a salvage procedure for valuable breeding horses or animals with great sentimental value.[1]

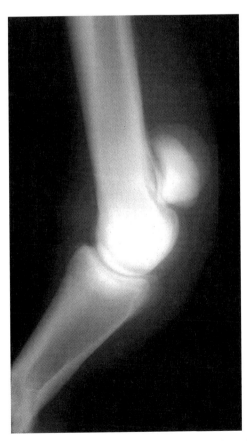

Figure 5.175. Lateral radiograph of a horse with disruption of the distal suspensory apparatus that has permitted the sesamoid bones to luxate proximally. (Courtesy of Dr. Gary Baxter.)

Etiology

The extreme overextension of the fetlock is the likely cause for disruption of the suspensory apparatus. Pre-existing pathology of the bones or suspensory ligament need not be present for this catastrophic failure to occur, but the presence of an abnormal finding in the suspensory ligament on pre-race inspection by a regulatory veterinarian increased the risk of suspensory ligament injury 3.4-fold in future races as compared to a control population.[3] Factors that increase the strain on the flexor surface of the limb would be expected to increase the risk of suspensory apparatus failure. Indeed, Thoroughbred horses racing with low toe grabs were 6.5 times more likely and with full toe grabs 15.6 times more likely to incur a fatal suspensory apparatus injury than horses without toe grabs.[6]

Clinical Signs

On gross observation the affected fetlock is very swollen, and the horse usually bears its entire weight on the unaffected limb. The lameness is obvious, and if the animal transfers its weight to the affected limb, the fetlock will sink to the ground. Palpation often reveals the proximal displacement of either the intact sesamoid bone or the apical fractured fragments. Immediate stabilization of the limb is critical to prevent rupture of the neurovascular bundles. The blood supply to the distal limb can be estimated by palpation of a pulse, presence of distal bleeding and/or use of Doppler devices,[4] or the IV injection of 5 g of sodium fluorescein.[10] A Wood's ultraviolet lamp is required to document fluorescence of viable tissue if the injection of sodium fluorescein is used. The vascular supply is best evaluated after the horse has been treated for shock and the limb stabilized. Intense vasoconstriction initially can be interpreted as lack of blood supply.

Diagnosis

Radiographic examination usually reveals either the proximal displacement of the intact sesamoid bone or proximal displacement of the apical portions of the fractured sesamoid bones (Figures 5.175 and 9.2). Associated swelling of the soft tissues is also quite evident and pre-existing degenerative lesions within the sesamoid bones and fetlock joint may also be present.[11]

Treatment

Treatment should be considered for horses that are to be used for breeding or when there is sentimental value, because a normal gait will not be achieved. Management of the horse on the racetrack is critical for success in treatment. Emergency crews must immediately restrain the horse and apply secure splints, such as a cast or the Leg Saver. Horses should then be moved to a surgical facility for radiographs. Immediate immobilization of the affected limb is required to decrease the chances of further injury to the soft tissue as well as the vascular supply. Maintenance of the splint for a 4- to 5-day period prior to the selection of the final treatment allows the horse to acclimate to the immobilization and

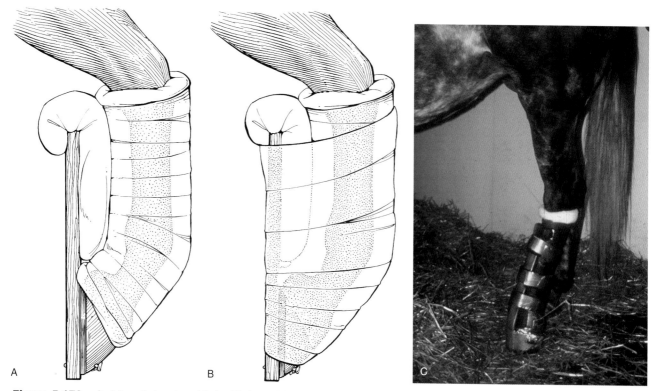

Figure 5.176. A. A heavily bandaged limb with the padded splint brought up to approximate the palmar aspect. B. Complete bandage splint. C. A Kimzey splint, designed for breakdown injuries, including severe sesamoid fractures.

recover from the trauma, and allows definition of the extent of skin necrosis and loss of vascular supply accompanying the injury. The arthrodesis procedure does not need to be done immediately, and the soft tissue injury and permanent deficit and risk of infection must be evaluated to properly predict the outcome with surgery.

Various successful treatments include casting, splinting, and fetlock arthrodesis (Figures 5.176 and 5.177).[1,2,4,11] Casting and splinting are aimed at supporting and immobilizing the fetlock until soft tissues have healed sufficiently to support body weight (ankylosis). The use of a fetlock sling shoe can work in partial breakdown injuries. The Leg Saver splint is not as rigid as a cast, but allows cleaning and treatment of soft tissue injuries and is designed to assist with fetlock joint support in suspensory apparatus injuries (Figure 5.176C). Ankylosis can also be supported with an external fixator placed on the foot and metacarpus to fix the position of the joint during healing. Without other surgical stimulation, fusion will not be complete at removal of the external fixator and continued coaptation is usually necessary. Arthrodesis with implants and bone graft can be used to achieve a pain-free stable fusion of the fetlock joint if the soft tissues are intact and risk of infection is minimal (Figure 5.177). Support limb laminitis of the unaffected foot is also a common sequelae to this injury; therefore, the contralateral foot should be supported to distribute loading along the sole. See the section on laminitis in Chapter 5 for more information.

Although casting the limb in flexion can support and immobilize the fetlock until healing has occurred, it is usually associated with severe pressure sores on the

back of the sesamoids that may result in septic osteomyelitis requiring euthanasia.[11] Casting is also expensive and labor intensive due to the multiple cast changes required and the prolonged duration for fusion. After 8 weeks in a cast, the limb is supported in a bulky bandage and a special shoe is applied to elevate the heel. The height of the heel is gradually lowered in increments over the next 4 weeks until finally only a wedge is required. Other methods of supporting the limb with weight-bearing on the toe (splints) and with sling support shoes can be successful, but continual monitoring and aftercare is required for an extended duration. Of 25 cases managed conservatively, 15 survived. Complications were similar to those from surgical techniques and included pressure sores, osteomyelitis, avascular necrosis, and support limb laminitis.[9]

Surgical arthrodesis of the fetlock should be considered in acute cases with intact skin that have not developed wounds during the initial management of the soft tissues, or in chronic cases that fail to fuse or develop chronic joint pain (Figure 5.177). The goals of surgical arthrodesis are to rigidly stabilize the joint in a neutral position, support osteoinduction, and provide comfort during the healing process. The most popular method to achieve this is use of a single 14-hole broad plate secured with 5.5- and 4.5-mm cortical screws spanning the dorsal surface of the metacarpus, fetlock joint, and proximal phalanx. If the suspensory apparatus is disrupted, the palmar tension band must be re-established or the plate will bend when loaded. The palmar tension band can be re-established by securing dorsal 4.5-mm cortical screws into the sesamoid bones from adjacent to the plate for avulsions proximal to the sesamoid

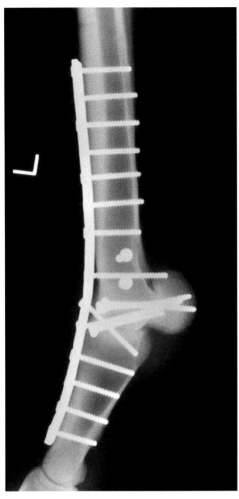

Figure 5.177. Surgical arthrodesis of a fetlock joint with plates and screws to treat a breakdown injury. (courtesy of Dr. Larry Bramlage.)

bones or of the apex of the sesamoid bones. For injuries without intact sesamoid bones or of disruption of the distal sesamoidean ligaments, a tension band wire must be placed around the palmar surface of the joint.[1] Use of locking compression plates for fetlock arthrodesis in Thoroughbreds is likely to produce a more stable repair initially, but is 3 times more expensive than a limited dynamic compression plate with cortical screws.[2]

A cast that includes the foot and extends to just below the carpus or tarsus is applied after surgery. It is removed in 14 days and only reapplied if required. Minimal coaptation is usually needed after cast removal, making the aftercare simple. With this technique the functional length of the limb is slightly increased, but it only takes a short period for the animal to adapt to this. In most cases reported, this technique has provided a pain-free functional limb that can withstand weight-bearing. Horses can be turned out after 4 months of healing. Six to twelve months are required for arthrodesis to be complete.

Use of external fixation to immobilize the fetlock and subsequently allow ankylosis, or combined with bone graft to stimulate ankylosis, is an alternative option to internal fixation for rupture of the suspensory appara-tus. A transfixation device places 3 parallel 9.6-mm threaded transfixation pins in the metacarpus and attaches an aluminum foot plate with a tubular frame distally. The vertical bars are linked to the transfixation pins using a filled polyurethane material that is poured into the tubular frame in liquid form. The dorsal fetlock joint is opened surgically to remove the articular carti-lage and place the bone graft. The construct provides rigid fixation of the fetlock joint for fusion and permits access to wounds and infected tissues. The fixator can be maintained for 6 to 8 weeks; however, fracture through the pin tracts can occur. In 9 horses, 4 were successfully managed with this technique and 2 survived with fair results.[8] This technique offers an advantage over internal fixation for treatment of suspensory appa-ratus ruptures with open wounds or infected ischemic soft tissues. Horses are comfortable in the frame, reduc-ing the risk of supporting limb laminitis.

Techniques and materials to replace the suspensory apparatus have been investigated by placing a thick braided nonabsorbable material secured to the metacar-pus with a screw, tunneled along the back of the fetlock joint, and secured to P1 with a screw.[7] The strength of the repair was significantly lower than control limbs with failure as fracture through the screw holes. The braided material induced significant granulomatous reaction in the tissues caudal to the joint. Other materi-als have not yet been evaluated.

Prognosis

The prognosis appears to be good for pasture and breeding soundness with preselection of cases. With arthrodesis, 32 of 54 horses with arthrodesis of the fetlock survived and were eventually allowed unre-stricted activity.[1] The prognosis is better for horses in which fetlock arthrodesis was elected as the primary treatment rather than as a last resort and was better for horses in which fusion was elected for OA rather than rupture of the suspensory apparatus. Four of 6 Thoroughbreds with breakdown injuries treated with fetlock arthrodesis with the locking compression plate survived.[2] The success rate increases if no signs of sup-porting laminitis are apparent at the time of surgery.

References

1. Bramlage L. Fetlock Arthrodesis. In Equine Fracture Repair, Nixon AJ, ed. WB Saunders Co, Philadelphia 1996;17:172.
2. Carpenter RS, Galuppo LD, Simpson EL, et al. Clinical evalua-tion of the locking compression plate for fetlock arthrodesis in six Thoroughbred racehorses. Vet Surg. 2008;37:263–268.
3. Cohen ND, Peloso JG, Mundy GD, et al. Racing-related factors and results of prerace physical inspection and their association with musculoskeletal injuries incurred in Thoroughbreds during races. J Am Vet Med Assoc 1997;211:454.
4. Haynes PF. Disease of the fetlock and metacarpus. Symposium on Equine Lameness. Vet Clin North Am (Large Anim Pract) 1980;2:43.
5. Johnson BJ, Stover SM, Daft BM, et al. Causes of death in racehorses over a 2-year period. Equine Vet J 1994;26:327–30.
6. Kane AJ, Stover SM, Gardner IA, et al. Horseshoe characteristics as possible risk factors for fatal musculoskeletal injury of Thoroughbred racehorses. Am J Vet R 1996;57:1147.
7. Major MD, Grant BED, White KK, et al. Suspensory apparatus prosthesis in the horse: Part I: in vitro mechanical properties. Vet Surg 1992;21:126.

8. Richardson DW, Nunamaker DM, Sigafoos RD. Use of an external skeletal fixation device and bone graft for arthrodesis of the metacarpophalangeal joint in horses. J Am Vet Med Assoc 1987;191:316.
9. Snyder JR, Wheat JD, Bleifer D. Conservative management of metacarpophalangeal joint instability. Proc Am Assoc Equine Pract 1986;357.
10. Stashak TS. Traumatic rupture of the suspensory apparatus. In Adam's Lameness in Horses, 4th ed. Lea and Febiger, Philadelphia, 1987;pp 584–587.
11. Wheat HD, Pascoe JR. A technique for management of traumatic rupture of the equine suspensory apparatus. J Am Vet Med Assoc 1980;176:205.

LUXATION OF THE METACARPO/METATARSOPHALANGEAL JOINT (FETLOCK LUXATION)

Lateral and medial luxation of the fetlock joint occurs uncommonly, but is a recognized syndrome that can affect all ages and breeds of horses. Usually, either the lateral or medial collateral ligament is ruptured, creating an obvious varus or valgus deformity of the fetlock region.[4,6] Occasionally, avulsion fractures associated with the insertion of these ligaments or joint capsule may occur and be noted on the radiograph proximal to the joint space. Articular fractures of the palmar/plantar eminence may also accompany the luxation.[2] Both forelimbs and hindlimbs can be affected with luxation and the joint was open in half of 10 reported cases.[4,6] The diagnosis is usually quite obvious because an angular deviation of the fetlock joint is present. Occasionally the luxation will reduce spontaneously and only a lateral or medial swelling will be noticed. Immediately after the injury, if the luxation is reduced, some horses will be minimally lame and appear sound at the walk. Reluxation can occur at any moment if the joint is not stabilized until the swelling and pain begin to protect the joint. Physical manipulation of the fetlock in these cases clarifies the suspicion of luxation. Typically, the joint reluxates when it is flexed and abducted away from the side of injury.

Etiology

This injury frequently occurs when the horse steps in a hole or gets a foot caught between 2 immovable objects. The luxation results while the horse attempts to gain freedom. Owners frequently relate the history of finding the horse caught in this situation. Occasionally horses spontaneously luxate their fetlock during high-speed activities (e.g., racing, rodeo eventing) or after running into an object.[4]

Clinical Signs

The clinical signs are usually obvious and are helpful in differentiating this injury from fracture.[1] A varus (outward deviation of the cannon bone and inward deviation of the digit) or valgus (inward deviation of the cannon bone, outward deviation of the digit) angular deformity is usually present (Figure 5.178). Occasionally, the luxation will reduce spontaneously and the remaining evidence of its occurrence will be lameness, joint instability, and swelling over the torn collateral ligament.

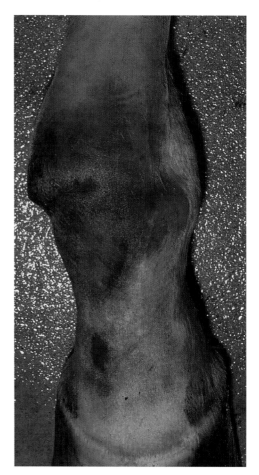

Figure 5.178. Horse with an acute, closed luxation of the fetlock joint with considerable bruising and subcutaneous hemorrhage that often accompanies these injuries. (Courtesy of Dr. Gary Baxter.)

On palpation the fetlock can be reduced and reluxated without the degree of pain or evidence of crepitation associated with fracture. Most frequently the swelling that is present is less than that observed with fracture, and the swelling is located selectively over the lateral or medial surface (Figure 5.178). Although the digital vascular supply is rarely compromised, it should be carefully evaluated, particularly in open luxations.

Diagnosis

Generally, the diagnosis can be made by physical examination alone. However, radiographs should be taken to identify an avulsion fracture, intra-articular fractures, or damage to the articular surface that has entered into the subchondral bone (Figure 5.179). Radiographs are particularly important in young foals to rule out the possibility of growth plate fractures as a primary cause or a secondary contributing cause to the angular deformity.

Treatment

Treatment of simple luxation of the fetlock can be rewarding. In most cases the injury is limited to the

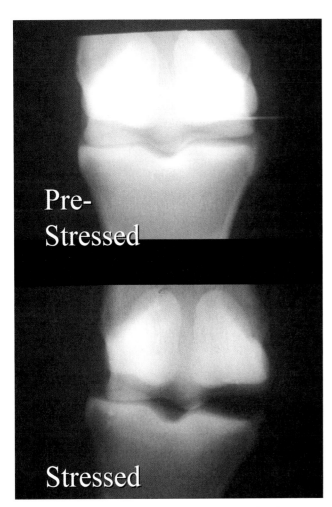

Figure 5.179. Pre-stress and stressed radiographs of a collateral ligament injury demonstrating an increased gap at the medial edge of the joint.

supporting soft tissues, and after the luxation is reduced under anesthesia, good axial alignment can be maintained by casting or splinting the limb until healing occurs. Prior to applying the cast, needle drainage of the hematoma (if present) that overlies the ruptured collateral ligament provides a better fit for the cast. This area should be clipped and shaved and aseptically prepared prior to percutaneous puncture and aspiration. Although centesis of the hematoma and cast application can be performed in the standing horse, general anesthesia and lateral recumbency are preferred. Reduction of the luxation is usually not difficult. A cast is applied that incorporates the foot and extends to just below the carpus or tarsus in the adult. Alternatively, a cast that does not encase the foot can be used. Casts or splints are maintained for 6 weeks with stall rest. After cast or splint removal, bandage support and limited exercise are recommended. Only slight swelling (thickening) will be noticed over the area of collateral ligament rupture and a cosmetic blemish will remain.

Success can be achieved without suture of the collateral ligament, although there are several reports in the literature on open repair. To repair the ligament, the end is located after surgical incision, debrided, and sutured.[6] Alternatively, a polypropylene mesh has been substituted for the ruptured ligament.[5] Arthroscopic removal of the articular fractures should be elected if full athletic performance is a goal. This is not necessary for light riding soundness if the fragments are small and from the palmar/plantar eminence. Occasionally large avulsion fractures associated with the collateral ligament may warrant internal fixation to reconstruct the joint surface and improve the prognosis.

Acute open luxations can also be managed successfully.[4] However, prior to immobilization, thorough debridement of all devitalized soft tissues, bone, and cartilage should be performed. The joint should be thoroughly lavaged and antimicrobials placed within the synovial cavity. IV regional perfusion also is warranted. If the joint is minimally contaminated and was treated immediately, a primary suture apposition of the soft tissues is recommended. A distal limb cast is then applied and removed in 4 to 7 days to permit re-examination of the wound. The decision can then be made regarding the advisability of delayed primary closure or recasting over a sterile bandage and relying on secondary intention healing for wound closure. Casts are required in most cases for at least 6 weeks. The horse should be confined to the stall and treated with the appropriate broad-spectrum antibiotics and analgesics.

Chronic severe injuries such as traumatic rupture of the suspensory apparatus or luxation combined with extensive fracture can best be managed with surgical arthrodesis. An external fixator may be necessary in open fractures/luxations. Immediate bone grafting and removal of cartilage and damaged bone may need to be elected. See Traumatic Rupture of the Suspensory Apparatus section in this chapter.

Prognosis

The prognosis for simple luxation of the fetlock is good for breeding soundness but guarded for athletic performance. In one report, 7 of 10 horses, some with open luxations, could be used for breeding and 1 horse was riding sound.[6] However, the final decision should be made regarding the outcome after follow-up radiographs are taken at 2 months. Immediate stabilization of the joint usually permits healing without the development of OA. Lack of stabilization or unrecognized luxation often results in OA in horses allowed exercise.[3]

Acute open luxations exposing the fetlock joint also respond well to early therapy as described. However, one must always be reserved in giving a good prognosis until joint infection and OA from direct trauma have been ruled out as complications. The long-term outlook for return to serviceability is totally dependent on the degree of initial trauma sustained by the bone. Follow-up radiographs in 3 to 4 months can be helpful in giving a realistic prognosis.

References

1. Fessler JF, Amstutz HE. Fracture repair. In Large Animal Surgery. Oehme FW, Prier JE, eds. Williams and Wilkins Co., Baltimore, 1974.

2. Moore RM, Weisbrode SE, Biller DS, et al. Metacarpal fracture associated with lymphosarcoma-induced osteolysis in a horse. J Am Vet Med Assoc 1995;207:208–210.
3. Simmon EJ, Bertone AL, Weisbrode SE. Instability–induced osteoarthritis in the metacarpophalangeal joint of horses. Am J Vet Res 1999;60:7.
4. Stashak TS. Lateral and medial luxation of the metacarpophalangeal and metatarsophalangeal joints. In Adams' Lameness in Horses. Stashak TS, ed. Lea and Febiger, Philadelphia, 1987; pp 587–589.
5. Van Der Harst MR, Rijkenhuizen AB. The use of polypropylene mesh for treatment of ruptured collateral ligaments of the equine metatarsophalangeal joint: a report of 2 cases. Vet Q 2000; 22(1):57.
6. Yovich JV, Turner AS, Stashak TS, et al. Luxation of the metacarpophalangeal and metatarsophalangeal joints in horses. Equine Vet J 1987;19:295.

CONSTRICTION OF OR BY THE FETLOCK PALMAR/PLANTAR ANULAR LIGAMENT

Constriction of or by the fetlock anular ligament is a relatively common cause of lameness in performance horses. Although all breeds and uses of horses can be affected, sport horses, racehorses, Paso Fino horses, and Warmblood type horses appear to be at a greater risk. In one report desmitis of the fetlock anular ligament was diagnosed mainly in sport horses and less frequently in racehorses.[14] In an unpublished report on 49 horses, Paso Fino horses and Warmblood types were overrepresented (19 times and 5 times, respectively) compared to the normal hospital population.[13] The mean age of horses at presentation was 8.6 years (range 1 to 20 years). There was a significantly smaller portion of horses in the 2- to 4-year age group, and a significantly larger proportion of horses over 10 years of age.

Anular ligaments are tough, fibrous, thickened, relatively inelastic parts of the fascial tendon sheath strategically located to support the tendons as they course around a joint, providing a canal for them to glide through. They are lined with synovia and act to prevent displacement of the tendon, which would reduce its mechanical efficiency. Tendons lying within a tendon sheath and supported by an anular ligament can become enlarged from injury or infection. The anular ligament can also be injured, resulting in thickening (desmitis) and a reduction of the diameter of the canal.[9] As a result of either situation, compression of the tendon and pressure within the canal subsequently restricts the free gliding function of the tendon, inducing pain and possibly ischemia to the tissues within the canal (tunnel syndrome).

The condition can affect any limb. In one report injuries in Quarter horses, Thoroughbreds, and Arabians were distributed evenly between all 4 limbs, whereas Paso Fino and Warmblood type horses were affected in only the hindlimb.[10] In general, hindlimbs are more commonly affected.[10]

Etiology

Constriction of or by the fetlock anular ligament usually occurs as a result of trauma and/or infection. The injury may involve the anular ligament, primarily resulting in inflammation and thickening (desmitis) of the structure and thus producing constriction without abnormalities in other structures within the fetlock canal. Alternatively, the condition may be associated with distal SDFT tendinitis (low bow) or longitudinal tears in the DDFT.[16] Because anular ligaments are minimally elastic, swelling of the digital flexors caused by fibrosis and associated tenosynovitis can cause the signs of constriction of the anular ligament. Inflammation and subsequent scar tissue enlargement often associated with a low flexor tendinitis ("low bowed tendon") may extend to involve the palmar or plantar anular ligament, also resulting in desmitis. Adhesions may form between the SDFT and the anular ligament, further restricting motion. Tendinitis of the DDFT within the fetlock canal also enlarges the tendon within the canal and induces a tenosynovitis and produces the signs of anular ligament constriction (Figure 5.209). Wounds such as wire cuts or nail punctures can occur in the region of the palmar/plantar aspect of the fetlock, producing thickening, tenosynovitis, and constriction. One report on 49 horses revealed that desmitis of the anular ligament was the cause in 55% of the cases, tendinitis was the cause in 31%, and sepsis was the cause in 14% of the cases.[10] Synovial masses within the digital tendon sheath may also produce a constriction of the anular ligament and signs of tenosynovitis.[4]

Clinical Signs

Horses often present with a history of lameness that increases with exercise, resolves with rest, and returns when put back into performance. The most notable feature of anular ligament constriction is swelling of the palmar/plantar soft tissues of the distal limb around the fetlock and a characteristic observable proximal border of the anular ligament ("notching"). This notching is caused by anular ligament constriction (Figure 5.180). In nearly all cases there is distention of the digital tendon sheath proximal to the anular ligament. Palpation of the region usually reveals thickening at the junction of the SDFT and anular ligament.

The lameness is characterized by its persistence, pain on fetlock flexion, and worsening with exercise because of inflammation and increased constriction. Lameness is characterized by a decreased extension (dorsiflexion) of the fetlock during weight-bearing and a shortened caudal phase to the stride. In the most severe cases the horse is reluctant to place the heel on the ground and will accentuate the cranial phase of the stride to compensate. Continued pressure may produce changes in the digital flexor tendons.[9]

Regional perineural anesthesia, first of the foot and subsequently of the distal metacarpus or metatarsus, eliminates the lameness and locates the source to the region of constriction. Direct anesthesia of the tendon sheath is usually not necessary, but may be performed if a fluid sample is being obtained for cytology or if the sheath is injected as a conservative treatment. Most horses improve partially with anesthesia to the sheath, but other structures involved, such as the tendons and anular ligament, may still induce lameness. However, in horses that respond dramatically to tendon sheath anesthesia, endoscopy of the tendon sheath rather than simple anular ligament transection is indicated.

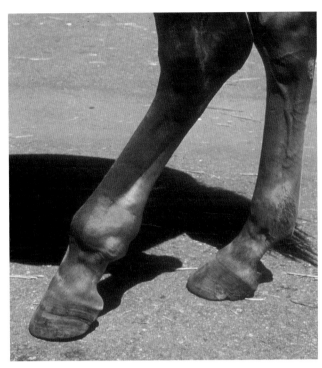

Figure 5.180. This horse had swelling of the digital flexor tendon sheath and evidence of constriction of the fetlock anular ligament of the left hindlimb.

Diagnosis

The physical findings and the results of diagnostic anesthesia provide a presumptive diagnosis. Ultrasonography is indicated to identify the structures involved and assist with the selection of treatment. Normally the anular ligament is thin (less than 2 mm) and cannot be distinguished without contrast agents, such as air tenograms. The distance from the skin surface to the palmar/plantar surface of the SDFT is 3 to 4 mm for the forelimb and 3 to 5 mm for the hindlimb.[8] One study found that measurement from the external skin surface to the internal anular ligament surface was the most reproducible index of anular ligament thickening.[10] One report on 49 horses with constriction of the anular ligament found that the mean anular ligament thickness measured ultrasonographically was 9.1 mm ± 2.3 mm.[13]

Lesions identified at ultrasound vary and can include core tendon lesions or longitudinal tearing of the DDFT and SDFT, fibrosis, tenosynovitis and synovial proliferation, adhesions, and thickening of the anular ligament. In 16 Warmblood horses with fetlock anular ligament constriction, 9 had thickening of the anular ligament and tenosynovitis, 3 were dominated by distention of the sheath, 3 had SDFT injury, and 1 had marked synovial sheath proliferation.[3] In racehorses, SDFT tendinitis may be more commonly associated with fetlock anular ligament constriction.[5] In another report on 49 cases, 27 horses had thickening of the anular ligament and 15 had tendon injuries.[10]

Radiographic evaluation of the fetlock region should always be performed to evaluate bone involvement, particularly of the sesamoids. In lesions associated with wounds or of traumatic origin, an osteomyelitis or sequestrum of the sesamoid bones necessitates additional treatment and reduces the prognosis for soundness or elimination of infection. In 38 cases of anular ligament constriction, 6 horses had proximal sesamoid bone abnormality and 12 horses had bone enthesiophytes at the attachment of the anular ligament (insertion desmopathy).[11] Radiography with the use of air tenograms allows the evaluation of the thickness of the anular ligament and the presence of adhesions, but this technique has generally been replaced by ultrasonographic evaluation.[12]

Treatment

Surgical resection of the palmar or plantar anular ligament is the most effective treatment.[1] Adjunctive surgical procedures to simultaneously treat tendinitis, tendon core lesions, adhesions, and synovial proliferation are indicated if the underlying conditions exist. These procedures include accessory ligament desmotomy of the SDFT, tendon splitting, adhesiolysis, and synovial resection, respectively.[4,6,9,10,16] Three approaches to perform the transection of the anular ligament are described and the decision to select one over the other depends on the presence of concomitant pathology, cost, and surgical facilities available. The three techniques are open transection, tenoscopic release, and percutaneous transection. The originally described open transection technique is rarely elected today unless septic tenosynovitis is present and open drainage and lavage as well as release of the anular ligament are the goals of therapy. Even in those instances, the sheath incision may be made proximal to the anular ligament and the actual transection still performed subcutaneously.[2,7] Tenoscopy of the digital flexor tendon sheath is currently the preferred method to address synovial masses and tendon lesions and perform the anular ligament resection (Figure 5.181).

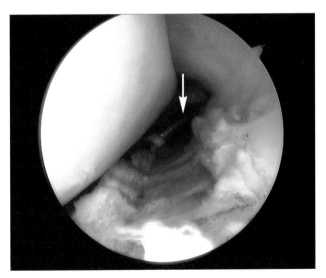

Figure 5.181. Tenoscopic view within the DFTS following transection of the anular ligament with a curved radiofrequency probe (arrow). (Courtesy of Dr. Gary Baxter.)

If tenoscopy is not an option then the percutaneous approach to transaction of the anular ligament can be performed. A small incision (1- to 2-cm long) is made at the proximal limits of the anular ligament down through the ligament to expose the tendon. A straight pair of Mayo scissors is then used to make a subcutaneous tunnel over the ligament and then to cut the ligament, leaving the overlying subcutaneous tissue and skin intact. A curved blunt-tipped bistoury can also be used in place of the Mayo scissors. This technique offers the advantage of low cost and standing if necessary, but visibility of tendon or tendon sheath structures is not attained.

Endoscopic evaluation of the digital tendon sheath and transection of the fetlock anular ligament is the preferred treatment approach (Figure 5.181). Tenoscopy offers the advantage of visualization of the sheath and synovium, and the tendons partially. Resection of adhesions, proliferative synovium, and tendon splitting can be performed as desired.[4,8] The disadvantages of the technique are cost and equipment requirements. Tenoscopy is specifically recommended in horses with adhesions and synovial proliferation noted on ultrasound and in those that respond dramatically to anesthesia of the digital sheath.[8]

Prognosis

If the primary etiology is desmitis of the palmar/plantar anular ligament and is not accompanied by extensive changes in the tendon (bowed tendon), the prognosis following surgical resection is good (84% returned to performance).[5,15] Other studies found that 50% to 87% of the horses with desmitis of the palmar/plantar ligament became sound following anular ligament resection.[9,10] If superficial digital flexor tendinitis is present, the tendinitis rather than the constriction appears to limit the performance. The Standardbreds in which anular ligament desmotomy was performed in addition to other surgical procedures for tendinitis improved and were able to race.[6] Of 13 horses with tendinitis and anular ligament desmitis treated by anular ligament resection, 38% became sound.[13] Of horses with longitudinal tears of the DDFT 58% became sound.[16] Of 25 horses with synovial masses and adhesions, 72% became sound.[4] Some horses with primary desmitis can become sound with rest alone.[9]

References

1. Adams OR. Constriction of the palmar (volar) or plantar anular ligament in horses. VM/SAC 1974;69:327.
2. Bertone A. Infectious Tenosynovitis. Vet Clinics of N America (Equine Practice) 1995;11:2,163–176.
3. Dik KJ, Van Den Belt JM, Keg PR. Ultrasonographic evaluation of fetlock anular ligament constriction in the horse. Equine Vet J 1991;23:4,285–288.
4. Fortier LA, Nixon AJ, Ducharme NG, et al. Tenoscopic examination and proximal anular ligament desmotomy for treatment of equine "complex" digital sheath tenosynovitis. Vet Surg 1999;28:429–435.
5. Gerring EL, Webbon PM. Fetlock anular ligament desmotomy: A report of 24 cases. Equine Vet J 1984;16:113–116.
6. Hawkins JF, Ross MW. Transection of the accessory ligament of the superficial digital flexor muscle for the treatment of superficial

digital flexor tendinitis in Standardbreds: 40 cases (1988–1992). J Am Vet Med Assoc 1995;206:674–678.
7. Honnas CM, Schumacher J, et al. Septic tenosynovitis in horses: 25 cases (1983–1989) J Am Vet Med Assoc 1991;199:1616.
8. Lowery J. Personal communication. 2001.
9. McGhee JD, White NA, Goodrich LR. Primary desmitis of the palmar and plantar anular ligaments in horses: 25 cases (1990–2003). J Am Vet Med Assoc 2005;226:83–86.
10. Owen KR, Dyson SJ, Parkin TD, et al. Retrospective study of palmar/plantar anular ligament injury in 71 horses: 2001–2006. Equine Vet J 2008;40:237–44.
11. Stanek C, Edinger H. Radiographic diagnosis of stricture of, or constriction by the anular ligament of the equine fetlock. Pferdeheilkunde 1990;6:125–128.
12. Stashak TS. Constriction of or by the palmar (volar) or plantar anular ligament. In Adams' Lameness in Horses, 4th ed. Stashak TS, ed. Lea and Febiger, Philadelphia, 1987;pp 593–595.
13. Vail T, Stashak TS, Park RD, et al. Results and prognosis of desmotomy of the equine fetlock anular ligament (49 horses) Unpublished data, 1993.
14. Vandenberg MJ, Rijkenhuizen ABM, Nemeth F. The fetlock tunnel syndrome: a macroscopic and microscopic study. Vet Quarterly 1995;17:138–142.
15. Verschooten F, Picavet TM. Desmitis of the fetlock anular ligament in the horse. Equine Vet J 1986;18:138–142.
16. Wilderjans H, Boussauw B, Mader K, et al. Tenosynovitis of the digital flexor tendon sheath and anular ligament constriction syndrome caused by longitudinal tears in the deep digital flexor tendon: a clinical and surgical report of 17 cases in Warmblood horses. Equine Vet J 2003;35:270–275.

DIGITAL FLEXOR TENDON SHEATH (DFTS) TENOSYNOVITIS

Digital flexor tendon sheath (DFTS) tenosynovitis is often characterized by effusion within the sheath and possibly heat and tenderness of the DFTS around the fetlock joint. The sheath serves to contain fluid around the superficial and deep digital flexor tendons as they glide over the palmar/plantar fetlock joint to provide frictionless movement of this high rotary motion joint. Effusion can be a blemish (windpuffs) or be associated with lameness and disease conditions of the superficial or deep digital flexor tendons, anular ligament, or sheath itself.[3]

Etiology

DFTS tenosynovitis can occur spontaneously, have no identifiable pathology associated with the surrounding structures, and be present without lameness. Presumably this is an early "wear and tear" phenomenon that represents some early biochemical or vascular alterations within the lining of the sheath. In most instances of lameness or marked swelling of the sheath, trauma to the flexor tendons, proximal sesamoid bones, intersesamoidean ligament, digital flexor sheath itself, or anular palmar/plantar ligament is suspected.[2] Septic tenosynovitis must always be considered, particularly if puncture wounds or a history of injection are present. The proximal portion of the sheath is not protected by the anular ligament of the fetlock and therefore direct blunt trauma may cause sheath contusion and subsequent hemorrhage or herniation. In more complicated cases, SDFT or DDFT or suspensory ligament injury may cause swelling or fibrosis of these structures, leading to relative stenosis of the fetlock canal and subsequent contusion of the DFTS. Overstretching or compression of the digital sheath may also cause friction between opposing parietal and visceral layers of the synovial sheath between the normal flexor tendon and digital sheath attachments or in the intimate attachments between the SDFT, digital sheath, and palmar/plantar or proximal digital anular ligaments. Tenosynovitis associated with longitudinal tears of the DDFT in horses has been described. Tendinous defects within the sheath can involve the DDFT, SDFT, and manica flexoria of the SDFT.

Clinical Signs

Effusion of the DFTS is visible and palpable. Fluctuant swelling palmar/plantar to the suspensory ligament and proximal to the sesamoids is present (Figure 5.182). Effusion of the fetlock joint is dorsal to the suspensory ligament and should not be confused with the effusion within DFTS. Confirmation of the effusion can be made by palpation of a small (2-cm) fluctuant swelling on the palmar/plantar mid pastern region, representing the distal most aspect of the DFTS that becomes very superficial at the bifurcations of the distal sesamoidean ligaments. Acute septic tenosynovitis is usually characterized by a sudden onset of mild to severe lameness associated with warm, painful effusion of the DFTS. The distention is most prominent in the proximal portion of the digital sheath but it is also palpable over the palmarodistal aspect of the pastern where the distal portion of the sheath protrudes between the proximal and distal digital anular ligament. Lameness is usually worsened with lower limb flexion.[5]

Diagnosis

Clinical examination is often sufficient to determine the presence of DFTS tenosynovitis, but the severity or association with lameness requires further work-up. Radiographs are usually indicated to determine associated trauma to bony structures, such as sesamoid fracture, dystrophic mineralization of the soft tissue structures around the fetlock, or lysis of the intersesamoidean area. Ultrasound examination of the soft tissue structures on the flexor surface, most notably the DDFT, is paramount to identify DDFT injury, fibrosis of other flexor tendons, anular desmitis, synovial proliferation, synovial adhesions, synovial masses, or flocculent fluid. Centesis of the DFTS can accurately be performed, if needed, with ultrasound guidance, and fluid analyzed for the presence of septic or nonseptic synovitis. Use of computed tomography and/or MRI of the fetlock can reveal subtle lesions of the sesamoid bones and soft tissues not identified by ultrasound. Longitudinal tears of the DDFT are difficult to diagnose by ultrasound examination alone.[1,3,4]

Treatment

Physical and medical management of DFTS tenosynovitis is similar to management of joint synovitis/ osteoarthritis. Treatment includes rest, cold hydrotherapy, bandaging, and topical and systemic NSAIDs medication. Systemic hyaluronan may be used to address the synovitis and provide lubrication. In cases that do not respond within 2 to 3 weeks, and if radiographs and ultrasound examination do not reveal abnormalities, aspiration of fluid and injection of medications may be performed, including the options of hyaluronan, corticosteroids, or autologous conditioned serum. Diagnostic tenoscopic examination can successfully treat synovial masses, adhesions, and tears of the DDFT, and provide lavage and a mechanism to perform anular desmotomy if indicated.

Open surgical drainage of the sheath should be reserved for nonresponding septic tenosynovitis or extensive fibrosis that can not be fully resected by tenoscopy. The digital sheath is a high-motion area and can be difficult to close, and incisional dehiscence is a recognized complication. In addition, synovial fistulae tend to occur more commonly in association with the DFTS than other synovial cavities.

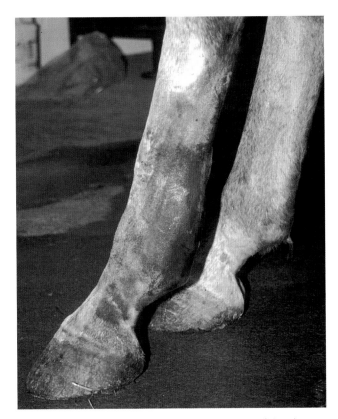

Figure 5.182. This horse had diffuse thickening of the plantar aspect of the fetlock region and effusion of the DFTS that is typical of horses with chronic tenosynovitis. (Courtesy of Dr. Gary Baxter.)

Prognosis

The prognosis for soundness in horses with DFTS tenosynovitis is good, with 68% returning to soundness and 54% returning to levels of previous work.[5] However, the prognosis for cosmetic improvement is guarded. Persistent uninflamed effusion of the DFTS is common. In addition, horses with concurrent lesions of the DDFT often have a guarded prognosis for athletic performance. See the pastern section of this chapter 5 for further information on DFTS tenosynovitis.

References

1. Cohen JM, Schneider RK, Zubrod CJ, et al. Desmitis of the distal digital anular ligament in seven horses: MRI diagnosis and surgical treatment. Vet Surg 2008;37:336–44.
2. Dik KJ, Dyson SJ, Vail TB. Aseptic tenosynovitis of the digital flexor tendon sheath, fetlock and pastern anular ligament constriction. Vet Clin North Am Equine Pract 1995;11:151–162.
3. Edinger J, Mobius G, Ferguson J. Comparison of tenoscopic and ultrasonographic methods of examination of the digital flexor tendon sheath in horses. Vet Comp Orthop Traumatol 2005;18:209–14.
4. Fraser BS, Bladon BM. Tenoscopic surgery for treatment of lacerations of the digital flexor tendon sheath. Equine Vet J 2004; 36:528–31.
5. Smith MR, Wright IM. Noninfected tenosynovitis of the digital flexor tendon sheath: a retrospective analysis of 76 cases. Equine Vet J 2006;38:134–41.

THE METACARPUS AND METATARSUS

Alicia L. Bertone

PERIOSTITIS AND FRACTURE OF THE DORSAL METACARPUS (BUCKED SHINS, SHIN SPLINTS, AND STRESS FRACTURE)

Periostitis and stress fracture of the dorsal surface of the third metacarpal bone constitute a spectrum of diseases that are commonly observed in young (2 to 3 years of age) fast gaited horses. Although the greatest incidence is observed in young racing Thoroughbreds, it also affects young Quarter horses and occasionally racing Standardbreds (Figure 5.183). The hindlimbs are infrequently involved.[16]

Etiology

Different subdivisions of this disease are described later; however, it appears that all clinical syndromes have a common pathogenesis.

In young horses put in training, the metacarpal bone is exposed to new stresses. In younger horses (2-year-olds), the metacarpal bone is less stiff, and therefore, greater strains (bone movement) are measured on the

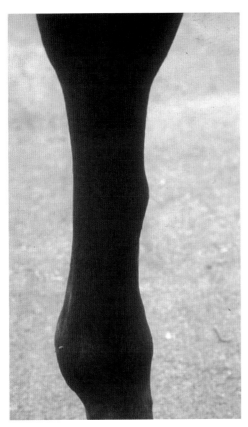

Figure 5.183. A racing Quarter horse with the classical metacarpal profile of a dorsal cortical stress fracture.

dorsal cortex during high-speed exercise than in older horses. These high strains may lead to low cycle fatigue of the bone and subsequent bone pain (bucked shins, sore shins).[19] Dorsal metacarpal strain is even greater in the lead limb (the left limb in racing in the United States), correlating with the most common location of fracture.[6]

During normal maturation of the third metacarpus, horses aged 1 to 2 years normally resorb primary osteons and have a greater amount of resorption cavities and incompletely filled secondary osteons than older horses. This bone structure is more susceptible to fatigue microdamage resulting from training because of higher bone porosity, fewer completed secondary osteons, and a lower proportion of circumferentially oriented collagen fibers.[28] In racing Quarter Horses put in training, the bone density of the medial and lateral dorsal metacarpus significantly decreased during the first 62 days of training, then significantly increased from day 104 to day 244 of training.[7,15] Horses experienced fewer bone-related injuries when they had greater cortical mass in the lateral aspect of the third metacarpus at the commencement of training.[15] The changing shape of the metacarpal bone during maturation[17] and training[5,24] is consistent with lower strains during high-speed exercise in older horses.

The thickening of the dorsal cortex, including diffuse dorsal periosteal new bone seen particularly in horses in training, is likely a natural response to these demands on the bone to withstand stress without developing microfractures or dorsal cortical fractures (Figure 5.184). This has been further confirmed by experimental exercise conditions that induced marked modeling (not remodeling) of the dorsal cortex, particularly subperiosteal bone formation at the mid-shaft of the third metacarpal bone. Additionally, horses completing the full training program had greater mineral bone content despite a lighter body weight.[13] Foals significantly increase metacarpal bone mineral density with age, and lack of exercise retards the normal bone development.[3]

In summary, in horses in race training, high strains can induce low cyclic fatigue of bone, resulting in microdamage or ultimate bone failure. The body responds with bone modeling, but microfracture damage may develop and cause pain. The majority (more than 80%) of 2-year-old racing Thoroughbreds[1] and many racing Quarter Horses[7] demonstrate dorsal cortical pain and it is estimated that approximately 12% go on to develop acute failure or dorsal cortical fracture, usually within 6 months to 1 year of showing dorsal cortical pain.[17] Thoroughbred horses trained on dirt surfaces as compared to wood fiber[14] and 2-year-old horses with faster works (15 m/s)[1] had significantly greater incidence of dorsal metacarpal disease, further supporting this pathogenesis. The incidence of fatigue failure of the

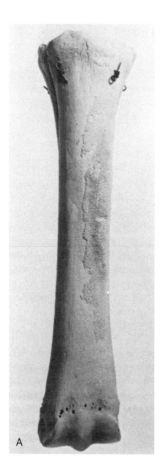
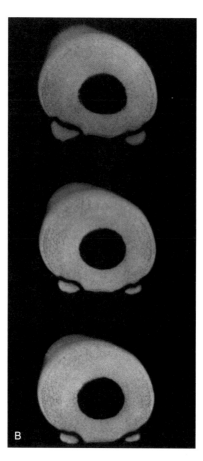

Figure 5.184. A. A macerated specimen of the right third metacarpal bone illustrating a subperiosteal callus on the dorsal medial surface. B. Cross section through the third metacarpal bone of a horse with dorsal metacarpal disease. Note that the dorsal cortex is thicker than the palmar cortex. (Courtesy of Dr. PF Haynes.)

metacarpal dorsal cortex is greater in Thoroughbreds than Standardbreds. This was not attributed to inherent differences in the mechanical properties of the bone, but rather gait differences and resultant bone stresses during training and racing.[18]

Clinical Signs

Early dorsal metacarpal disease is usually observed in young Thoroughbred racehorses (8 to 36 months of age), and occasionally in older horses that have not been strenuously trained or raced as 2-year olds. The disease has an acute onset and is most obvious after intense exercise. There is usually minimal alteration of the horse's gait, particularly after short periods of rest. A visible convex swelling overlying the surface of the affected portion of the cannon bone is common (Figure 5.183). On palpation, the dorsal cortex of the third metacarpal bone is acutely painful to pressure. Frequently the horse will withdraw the limb in response to pain. Radiographs taken at this time are usually negative; however, fractures are occasionally observed as well as a minimal amount of superficial cortical osteolysis.[16]

Subacute to chronic dorsal metacarpal disease invariably develops as a result of acute disease that is unresponsive to therapy or has gone unrecognized. It is most frequently seen in horses 26 to 42 months of age.[16] Only mild degrees of gait deficit may be noticed at exercise. On palpation, varying degrees of pain may be elicited, but a more obvious enlargement is palpable on the dorsomedial cortex (Figure 5.183). The pain response is typically more profound after strenuous exercise and the left limb is usually more severely affected. Periosteal new bone formation is usually observed on radiographic examination (Figures 5.183 and 5.184).[16]

Dorsal metacarpal bone failure results in a fracture of the dorsal or dorsolateral cortex of the third metacarpal bone. It is usually observed in older horses 3 to 5 years of age. As with dorsal metacarpal disease, the lameness may not be prominent while the horse is rested. However, it is usually prominent after strenuous exercise. On palpation, a rather discrete painful area can be palpated on the dorsolateral surface of the left third metacarpal (cannon) bone at the junction of its middle and distal third. Only rarely is the right third metacarpal bone involved. Radiographs usually point to a cortical fracture on the dorsolateral surface (Figure 5.185).[16]

Diagnosis

A tentative diagnosis of metacarpal periostitis or stress fracture can be made from the clinical findings and the age relationship. Little information is derived from local direct infiltration anesthesia of the painful area because it provides only partial relief in the lameness. Median and ulnar nerve perineural anesthesia or proximal metacarpal regional anesthesia with a ring block is required for total relief of pain, but this is rarely indicated.

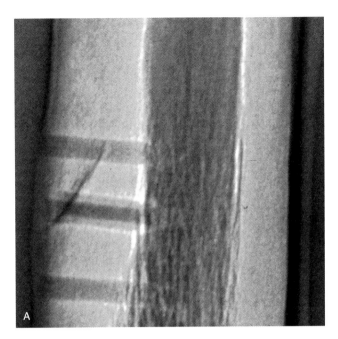

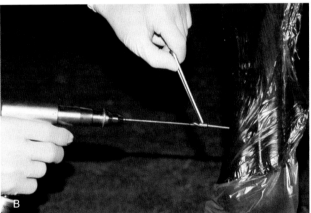

Figure 5.185. Radiograph of a dorsal cortical fracture treated with osteostixis procedure (A) that was performed standing (B).

Radiographs can assist with the diagnosis of dorsal cortical fracture. A series of 4 radiographic views should be taken: dorsopalmar (DP), lateral to medial (LM), dorsal palmar lateral to medial oblique (DPLMO), and dorsal palmar medial to lateral oblique (DPMLO). The DPLMO and the LM best identify the dorsal medial bone proliferation and the DPMLO and LM best identify the dorsal lateral cortical fractures. Horses continuing to train and race with sore shins can be screened for the development of fractures with radiographs.

It is rare to see radiographic abnormalities in acute dorsal metacarpal disease. In subacute dorsal metacarpal disease, periosteal new bone formation (of reduced density compared to underlying cortex) and surface cortical bone resorption may be observed. In chronic disease, a thickening of the dorsomedial cortex with associated periosteal new bone formation is seen. Occasionally an endosteal response may be observed in the advanced cases. Dorsal cortical fractures have a characteristic radiographic appearance and usually enter the cortex distally and progress proximad at a 35° to 45° angle.

Most frequently the fracture appears in radiographs as a straight or slightly concave fracture line (tongue fracture) (Figure 5.185). Occasionally it proceeds proximad to exit through the dorsal cortex (saucer fracture). Rarely, the fracture continues to enter the medullary canal. Multiple fractures may emanate from the distal site of the cortical entry (often termed "fissure fractures"). Periosteal callus is often present at the site of fracture and is a function of the chronicity of the disease. Endosteal proliferation is observed occasionally in fractures that are completely through the cortex. Repeated radiographs at 7- to 10-day intervals may be necessary to identify a fracture that is suspected but not observed on initial radiographic examination.[16]

Nuclear scintigraphy can provide information about the stage of disease in horses showing dorsal cortical pain or in those with undiagnosed forelimb pain. The sensitivity of this technique to identify bone metabolism and turnover is high, and it allows detection of abnormalities in horses in the acute-subacute stages that are still in training. Racehorses may have bone scintigrams performed to determine whether training should continue or to identify focal uptake indicative of impending fracture. In a review of 121 bone scintigrams of racing Thoroughbreds with clinical history of dorsal metacarpal disease, horses without fractures (bucked shins) had a mild to moderate diffuse uptake of radioisotope, unlike the focal intense uptake typical of dorsal cortical fracture. Chronic fractures are less focal and intense because of surrounding bone remodeling; however, they still appear relatively focal compared to early disease.[11]

Use of quantitative computer tomography to measure bone mineral density and 3-dimensional morphologic changes in the metacarpus may provide improvements in identifying risk factors or imminence of fracture.

Treatment

There is no specific medical treatment for dorsal metacarpal disease, necessitating that horses be laid up or put on a convalescent exercise program to provide time for the early acute changes to subside. Many horses with acute bucked shins can continue to train after 5 to 10 days of rest and anti-inflammatory analgesics. Hand walking, ponying, cold water hosing, and bandaging should continue until the dorsal cortex can be palpated without eliciting pain. Speed and distance are introduced slowly, with constant monitoring of dorsal cortical pain. Initially, daily galloping distance is reduced to 50%. If speed is increased, distance should be decreased.[17] The goal is to gradually increase the stress to the dorsal surface of the metacarpal bone at such a rate such that this surface can model according to compressive demands without producing structural damage.

Subacute and chronic dorsal metacarpal disease can be the most difficult to treat. After an exacerbation, many of these horses may not be suitable for the modified training regimen described above and pain immediately returns with any sustained galloping. These horses may have marked periosteal new bone formation. More prolonged rest is usually necessary for bone remodeling of this new periosteal bone and remodeling of fatigued bone. The time required is usually 110 days.

Dorsal cortical fractures in young horses may resolve with the conservative approach outlined above for subacute or chronic bucked shins. Convalescent periods may extend from 4 to 6 months because fracture healing is slow at this site.[16] Older horses often do not respond as well to conservative treatment and surgery is recommended. In either case, serial radiographic studies should be performed at least every 30 to 45 days to assess the bone healing.[16]

Several surgical procedures have been recommended for treatment of dorsal cortical metacarpal fractures, including placement of a unicortical or transcortical screw in lag fashion, placement of a neutral unicortical positional screw, and dorsal cortical drilling (Figure 5.185B and 5.186). Transcortical screws are no longer recommended due to the expected differences in strain between the palmar and dorsal cortices, risk of fracture, and risk of damage to the suspensory ligament. Placement of a dorsal unicortical screw in lag fashion can be technically difficult due to the short depth of the cortex (about 22 mm) and need for radiographic control, but provides the best fracture stability. Placement of a neutral dorsal unicortical screw to help stabilize the fracture, combined with dorsal cortical drilling, is often elected to provide added stability over dorsal cortical drilling alone. For screw fixation, cortical bone screws (4.5 mm or 3.5 mm) are used. Consensus has not occurred on the recommendation for screw removal.

Many horses have and will race successfully with the dorsal cortical screw in place. However, reoccurrence of dorsal cortical pain may occur (regardless of the presence of a screw) and the screw will be presumed to be the cause. If any fracture occurs in this horse in the future, such as condylar fracture or complete metacarpal failure, the screw may be considered a cause. Many surgeons currently recommend removal of the screw after a sufficient time of healing (2 months). Selection of 4.5-mm cortical screws allows for easy removal while standing.[2,4,9,26] Fracture fixation is accomplished under general anesthesia with the aid of precise radiographic or fluoroscopic monitoring.

Postoperative management includes bandaging for 2 to 4 weeks, hand walking after 2 weeks, stall rest for 6 weeks, screw removal at 8 weeks, hand walking for 2 weeks, then limited turnout up to 3 months. Light training can begin as early as 3 months. Greater than 95% of horses can return to racing in approximately 8 months.[4]

Osteostixis can be performed under general anesthesia or in the standing horse (Figure 5.185B). Drill holes (5 to 7) are made in a diamond pattern through the dorsal cortex into the marrow cavity. This procedure can be combined with unicortical screw application. Success for return to racing is similar (greater than 80%) to that recently reported for screw fixation, and a quicker return to racing (4 to 6 months) has been reported.[9] Clustered drill holes act as a stress concentrator and significantly decreases the stress required for metacarpal failure in cadaver limbs, but catastrophic failure through the drill holes is not a reported complication of the procedure *in vivo*.[25]

Other adjunctive treatments have been recommended with or without surgical treatment, including electrical stimulation at the fracture, shock wave therapy, injection of osteogenic substances (sodium oleate), intralesional injection of steroids, thermocautery (pin firing), chemical vesication (blistering), needle drainage of the hematoma, and cryotherapy (point freezing). These treatments have met with varying degrees of success, and no controlled studies have been performed. In all cases, no matter what the treatment, an adequate period of rest combined with a controlled exercise program is required.

In one study of Thoroughbred racehorses, distinct training strategies were used at various stables and the allocation of exercise to breezing (15 m/s), galloping (11 m/s), and jogging (5 m/s) was associated with lack of bucked shins for 1 year (survival of bucked shin syndrome). Survival was significantly reduced by allocation of exercise to breezing, and increased by allocation to galloping. It was recommended that to reduce the incidence of bucked shins trainers should allocate more training effort to regular short-distance breezing and less to long-distance galloping.[1]

Prognosis

The prognosis is good to excellent for return to racing with surgical treatment of dorsal cortical fractures; reports range from 80% to 98%. However, this underestimates the loss of racing days of horses with sore shins that remain in training and recurrence of pain or fracture once subacute or chronic disease occurs. The impact of this syndrome, particularly in 2-year-olds, is evidenced by the observation that if 2-year-old racing Thoroughbreds were not permitted to race for 6 weeks

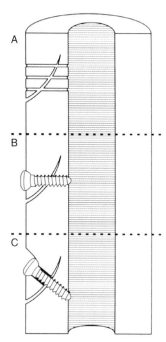

Figure 5.186. A. Dorsal cortical drilling (osteostixis) of a dorsal metacarpal stress fracture. B. Positional unicortical screw placement. C. Unicortical screw placement in lag fashion.

if sore shins are palpated prerace, significant improvements in predictable finishes occurred.[8] Adjustment of training regimens may assist with prevention, and training on grass, wood fiber, or softer surfaces without toe grabs is recommended.

Other Stress Fractures of the Metacarpal

Although dorsal cortical stress fractures are by far the most common location of stress fracture in horses, particularly racehorses, other sites and variations within the metacarpus can occur. Dorsal cortical fractures may extend more proximal than the site of exit from the cortex, and fissure lines can sometimes be identified, most typically in the proximal metacarpus on other views. If a fracture line is noted on the cranio-caudal view, a spiraling fracture or nondisplaced complete metacarpal fracture should be suspected. Fractures may be limited to the dorsal cortex and respond to lag screw fixation. Detailed radiographic investigation should be performed to define the fracture and determine whether confinement to an overhead wire, casting, or surgery and compression of the fracture with screws is recommended.[20,27,29] Similar fractures can occur in the metatarsus of the hindlimb.[20]

Incomplete fractures of the distal palmar condyle have been reported in 5 racehorses; nuclear scintigraphy or the 125° degree dorsoproximal-dorsodistal view were required for identification. Horses returned to their previous level of racing with rest.[10]

Primarily in racing Standardbreds, stress fractures or focal intense radioactive areas of uptake on nuclear scintigraphy can occur in the proximal palmar aspect of the third metacarpus, and is a recognized syndrome. Physical findings are very subtle, but lameness can be blocked to the proximal metacarpus and scintigraphy is diagnostic. Most horses have abnormal radiographs, although high detail film and several projections may be needed to see the fracture. Rest resulted in a 64% return to the previous level of performance.[12,21] Internal screw fixation [23] and surgical drilling[30] also resulted in success. Dorsomedial articular fractures of the third metacarpal bone also can occur in racing Standardbreds. Lameness is abolished with intracarpal anesthesia. Periosteal new bone production can be seen on radiographs near the distal aspect of the fracture. All 7 horses in one study healed and returned to soundness (1 with internal fixation).[22]

References

1. Boston RC, Nunamaker DM. Gait and speed as exercise components of risk factors associated with onset of fatigue injury of the third metacarpal bone in 2-year-old Thoroughbred racehorses. Am J Vet Res 2000;61:602.
2. Cervantes C, Madison JB, Ackerman N, et al. Surgical treatment of dorsal cortical fractures of the third metacarpal bone in thoroughbred racehorses: 53 cases (1985–1989). J Am Vet Med Assoc 1992;200:1997–2000.
3. Cornelissen BP, Vanweeren PR, Ederveen AG, et al. Influence of exercise on bone mineral density of immature cortical and trabecular bone of the equine metacarpus and proximal sesamoid bone. Equine Vet J (Suppl) 1999;31:79.
4. Dallap BL, Bramlage LR, Embertson RM. Results of screw fixation combined with cortical drilling for treatment of dorsal cortical stress fractures of the third metacarpal bone in 56 Thoroughbred racehorses. Equine Vet J 1999;31:252.
5. Davies HM, Gale SM, Baker ID. Radiographic measures of bone shape in young thoroughbreds during training for racing. Equine Vet J (Suppl) 1999;30:262.
6. Davies HM, McCarthy RN, Jeffcott LB. Surface straining on the dorsal metacarpus of thoroughbreds at different speeds and gaits. Acta Anat (Basel) 1993;146:148.
7. Goodman NL, Baker BK. Lameness diagnosis and treatment in the Quarter horse racehorse. Vet Clin North Am: Equine Pract 1990;6:85.
8. Griffiths JB, Steel CM, Symons PJ, et al. Improving the predictability of performance by prerace detection of dorsal metacarpal disease in thoroughbred racehorses. Aust Vet J 2000;78:488.
9. Hanie EA, Sullins KE, White NA. Follow-up of 28 horses with third metacarpal unicortical stress fractures following treatment with osteostixis. Equine Vet J (Suppl) 1992;22:5.
10. Kawcak CE, Bramlage LR, Embertson RM. Diagnosis and management of incomplete fracture of the distal palmar aspect of the third metacarpal bone in five horses. J Am Vet Med Assoc 1995;206:3,335–337.
11. Koblik PD, Hornof WJ, Seeherman HJ. Scintigraphic appearance of stress-induced trauma of the dorsal cortex of the third metacarpal bone in racing Thoroughbred horses: 121 cases (1978–1986). J Am Vet Med Assoc 1988;192:390.
12. Lloyd KE, Koblik P, Ragle C, et al. Incomplete palmar fracture of the proximal extremity of the third metacarpal bone in horses: ten cases (1981–1986). J Am Vet Med Assoc 1988;192:798.
13. McCarthy RN, Jeffcott LB. Effects of treadmill exercise on cortical bone in the third metacarpus of young horses. Res Vet Sci 1992;52(1):28.
14. Moyer W, Spencer PA, Kallish M. Relative incidence of dorsal metacarpal disease in young Thoroughbred racehorses training on two different surfaces. Equine Vet J 1991;23:166.
15. Neilsen BD, Potter GD, Morris EL, et al. Changes in the third metacarpal bone and frequency of bone injuries in young quarter horses during race training—observations and theoretical considerations. J Equine Vet Sci 1997;17:541.
16. Norwood GL, Haynes PF. Dorsal metacarpal disease. In Equine Medicine and Surgery, 3rd ed. Mansmann RA, McAllister ES, eds. American Veterinary Publications, Santa Barbara, 1982; 1110.
17. Nunamaker DM. Metacarpal stress fractures. In: Equine Fracture Repair, Nixon AJ, ed. WB Saunders, Philadelphia. 1996; 195–199.
18. Nunamaker DM, Butterweck DM, Black J. In vitro comparison of Thoroughbred and Standardbred racehorses with regard to local fatigue failure of the third metacarpal bone. Am J Vet Res 1991;52:97.
19. Nunamaker DM, Butterweck DM, Provost MT. Fatigue fractures in thoroughbred racehorses: relationships with age, peak bone strain, and training. J Orthop Res 1990;8(4):604.
20. Pilsworth RC. Incomplete fracture of the dorsal aspect of the proximal cortex of the third metatarsal bone as a cause of hindlimb lameness in the racing thoroughbred: a review of three cases. Equine Vet J 1992;24:147.
21. Pleasant RS, Baker GJ, Muhlbauer MC, et al. Stress reactions and stress fractures of the proximal palmar aspect of the third metacarpal bone in horses: 58 cases (1980–1990). J Am Vet Med Assoc 1992;201:12,1918–1923.
22. Ross MW, Martin BB. Dorsomedial articular fracture of the proximal aspect of the third metacarpal bone in standardbred racehorses: seven cases (1978–1990) J Am Vet Med Assoc 1992;201:2,332–335.
23. Ross MW, Ford TS, Orsini PG. Incomplete longitudinal fracture of the proximal palmar cortex of the third metacarpal bone in horses. Vet Surg 1988;17:2,82–86.
24. Sherman KM, Miller GJ, Wronski TJ, et al. The effect of training on equine metacarpal bone breaking strength. Equine Vet J 1995;27:135.
25. Specht TE, Miller GJ, Colahan PT. Effects of clustered drill holes on the breaking strength of the equine third metacarpal bone. Am J Vet Res 1990;51:1242.
26. Specht TE, Colahan PT. Osteostixis for incomplete cortical fracture of the third metacarpal bone. Results in 11 horses. Vet Surg 1990;19(1):34.
27. Spurlock GH. Propagation of a dorsal cortical fracture of the third metacarpal bone in two horses. J Am Vet Med Assoc 1988;192:1587.
28. Stover SM, Pool RR, Martin RB, et al. Histological features of the dorsal cortex of the third metacarpal bone mid-diaphysis

during postnatal growth in thoroughbred horses. J Anat 1992; 181:45.

29. Watt BC, Foerner JJ, Haines GR. Incomplete oblique sagittal fractures of the dorsal cortex of the third metacarpal bone in six horses. Vet Surg 1998;27:337.

30. Wright IM, Platt D, Houlton JE, et al. Management of intracortical fractures of the palmaroproximal third metacarpal bone in a horse by surgical forage. Equine Vet J 1990;22:2,142–144.

FRACTURES OF THE CONDYLES OF THE THIRD METACARPAL/METATARSAL BONES (CONDYLAR FRACTURES, LONGITUDINAL ARTICULAR FRACTURES)

Fractures of the condyles of the third metacarpal and metatarsal bones occur most frequently in racing Thoroughbreds, less frequently in Standardbreds, and occasionally in Quarter horses and Polo ponies; they comprise a subset of catastrophic breakdowns on race-tracks.[2,11,12] Males are overrepresented (59% in one study and 75% in another) and the distribution of fractures is approximately one-third incomplete-nondisplaced, one-third complete-nondisplaced, and one-third complete-displaced (Figure 5.187).[25] In a study of 145 condylar fractures in mostly Thoroughbreds, forelimbs (81%) and lateral condyles (85%) were more frequently involved. The right and left forelimbs were approximately equally involved. Most fractures (59%) were initiated in the middle of the condyle and extended a mean of 75 mm proximally to exit the cortex. Axial fractures and medial condylar fractures tend to be longer. Articular comminution can occur, usually at the palmar/plantar articular margin, and was identified in 15% of fractures. The more axial fractures were more likely to have articular comminution (23%). Eight of 145 fractures evaluated spiraled proximally. Concurrent lesions included proximal phalanx eminence fractures, sesamoid fractures, and sesamoiditis.[24]

In another study of 233 condylar fractures, Thoroughbreds were overrepresented and Standardbreds underrepresented based on the hospital population. Standardbreds had more metatarsal condylar fractures. Medial metatarsal condylar fractures had a 25% chance of suffering a mid-diaphyseal fracture ("Y" fracture). In this study, the distribution of Thoroughbred condylar fractures was 66% forelimb, with approximately 50% complete. Seventy-nine percent of Thoroughbreds with incomplete lateral condylar fractures (77% treated surgically) returned to racing, whereas a significantly lower percentage (33%) of complete lateral condylar fractures returned to racing (all treated surgically). Eighty percent of Standardbreds (6 of 7 treated surgically) raced after treatment. In summary, return to racing in Thoroughbreds was significantly reduced with complete fractures, forelimb fractures, evidence of sesamoid fracture, or female sex (presumed retired for breeding).[2] Complete condylar fractures tend to be longer (mean 85 mm) than incomplete fractures (mean 57 mm).[16] Axial sesamoid fractures are associated with displaced lateral condylar fractures that disrupt the collateral ligament and avulse the intersesamoidean ligament complex.[1,6]

Another report of 124 condylar fractures in Thoroughbreds corroborates the above findings of the more recent reports. It was noted that 90% of condylar fractures occurred in 2- and 3-year-olds and that most were acquired during training between April and October. In this report, 17% of displaced lateral condylar fractures returned to racing.[4] The variation in successful return to racing of displaced condylar fractures may be related to the duration of fracture prior to surgery. Destruction of the articular surface occurs quickly following a displaced fracture; therefore, immediate immobilization and repair are critical to a successful outcome.[14]

Condylar fractures of the hindlimb are more common in Standardbreds and are more likely to be medial and to not exit the cortex. These fractures can propagate proximally or progress to a complete "Y" fracture, even with stall confinement.[14,15]

Etiology

The etiology includes trauma from high compressive loads, asynchronous longitudinal rotation of the cannon bone, and exercise on uneven surfaces. The risk of fatal condylar fracture in Thoroughbred racehorses is 7 times and 17 times more likely if horses are shod with low or regular toe grabs, respectively.[7] The toe grab changes the hoof angle and presumably places more stress on the suspensory apparatus and plants the foot more securely. This likely alters the compressive and rotatory forces on the distal metacarpus.

Recent structural studies of the distal condyle of unexercised and exercised horses have demonstrated

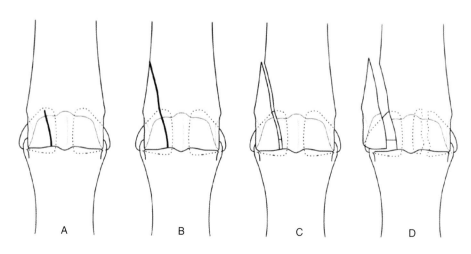

Figure 5.187. Condylar fractures. A. Incomplete. B. Complete nondisplaced. C. Complete separated. D. Complete displaced.

that the normal mineralized articular cartilage tends to cleave in the sagittal plane and that the main subchondral bone trabeculae are columnated and run in the sagittal direction with fewer mediolateral connections. Blood vessel canals lie inside the sagittally oriented structure. The sagittal column orientation provides maximum strength and protection in the sagittal plane in which the joint rotates, but offers minimal resistance to fracture propagation in this plane. The anatomical course of condylar fractures of the third metacarpal bone can be explained by the anisotropic structural arrangement of the mineralized tissues.[3] In horses in race training, densification (sclerosis) of the subchondral bone of the palmar/plantar surface of the condyles was identified by computer tomography techniques,[19] and this correlated with linear defects in the mineralized cartilage and subchondral bone in the same region with intense surrounding bone remodeling.[18] Microcracks in the subchondral bone of the metacarpus may coalesce and represent a pre-existing pathology in horses with catastrophic fracture.[9,11]

In a histopathologic study on North American racehorses, similar palmar condylar cartilage fibrillation with underlying bone sclerosis and areas of bone necrosis were noted. Evidence of active bone remodeling was present around the sclerotic zones with osteocyte necrosis apparent as prominence of subchondral vessels and osteoclastic activity. Fragmentation lines indicating matrix fragility and microfractures were apparent. This area of the condyle was grossly flattened.[10] Similar microdamage including microfractures in regions of osteoporosis and thinning of the zone of calcified cartilage was seen histologically in the bone of lateral condylar fractures obtained from fatal injuries.[22] In an experimental study with controlled training exercise, bone density, particularly in this palmar condyle region, was significantly greater in horses with high intensity exercise.[17] In summary, the palmar condyle is the site of maximum loading in racing and the bone responds by increasing density (sclerosis). Bone fatigue failure occurs and due to the normal columnar arrangement of the bone trabeculae, propagates acute failure in the configuration seen in condylar fractures (Figure 5.188).

Clinical Signs

The clinical signs may vary from a mild lameness that is exacerbated by exercise with little heat or swelling present with nondisplaced, incomplete fractures, to severe lameness with heat, pain, and swelling in the acute displaced fracture. The incomplete nondisplaced fractures are often so subtle they are missed on physical examination, but may be detected by screen radiographs or nuclear scintigraphy. However, fetlock joint effusion is always present because all actual fractures originate at the articular surface. This is best seen in the palmar or plantar recess of the fetlock joint capsule. The external swelling of the lateral side of the large metacarpal or metatarsal bone depends on the degree of separation of the proximal end of the fragment, and is readily palpated in displaced fractures. More swelling is observed with greater separation of the fracture fragment. The degree of pain associated with the palpation

and the amount of heat that is felt depends on the acuteness of the fracture. More heat is palpated with the acute displaced fracture. Fracture movement and crepitation also may be detected.

Increased lameness can be observed in a horse after it has been exercised and when the horse is circled to the affected side. Flexion and rotation of the fetlock usually result in sufficient pain to cause withdrawal of the limb. In the acute displaced fracture, crepitation may be felt with rotation of the fetlock. Increased lameness can be observed when flexion tests are used in cases in which there is a fissure fracture. Preferably, if a fracture is suspected based on history, clinical signs, and joint effusion, radiographs should be immediately taken without further lameness examination or joint manipulations to decrease the risk of propagating the fracture or worsening the articular cartilage injury.

Diagnosis

It is advisable to take radiographs if a condylar fracture is suspected. Perineural and intrasynovial anesthesia should be considered only if a fracture is not present. However, a small percentage of these fissure fractures are difficult to identify radiographically, so it is important to closely scrutinize the radiographs.

Diagnosis is made with a standard series radiographic examination (dorsal palmar [DP], lateral to medial [LM], dorsal palmar lateral to medial oblique [DPLMO], and a dorsal palmar medial to lateral oblique [DPMLO]) plus a 125° caudocranial view to produce a view tangential to the palmar surface of the condyle. Alternatively, this view can be taken palmar to dorsal with the fetlock in flexion, although bone distortion occurs. Long cassettes are recommended so that the fetlock joint as well as the proximal cannon bone can be included in the study (Figure 5.189). Close evaluations of the study should follow to rule out the possibility of other injuries. Lesions that have been associated with condylar fractures include osteochondral fractures of the proximal phalanx (P1), fractures of the proximal sesamoid bone, osteoarthritis (OA) of the fetlock, palmar and plantar erosive lesions of the distal third metacarpal or metatarsal bone, suspensory ligament desmitis,[8] and longitudinal fractures of the metatarsus. These associated lesions may be significant regarding the recommendation of treatment and the prognosis. Nuclear scintigraphy can also be used to locate bone damage prior to fracture or to identify a fracture.

Treatment

The recommended treatment of most condylar fractures is internal fixation with transcortical screws placed in lag fashion for return to full athletic performance and health of the fetlock joint (Figures 5.189 and 5.190).[21] Incomplete, nondisplaced fractures can be treated conservatively with successful return to racing, and surgery is not always required. The advantages of screw fixation include: the original fracture will not become further displaced, shorter convalescence, a reduced incidence of refracture at the same site, and primary bone healing will decrease the risk of OA within the fetlock.

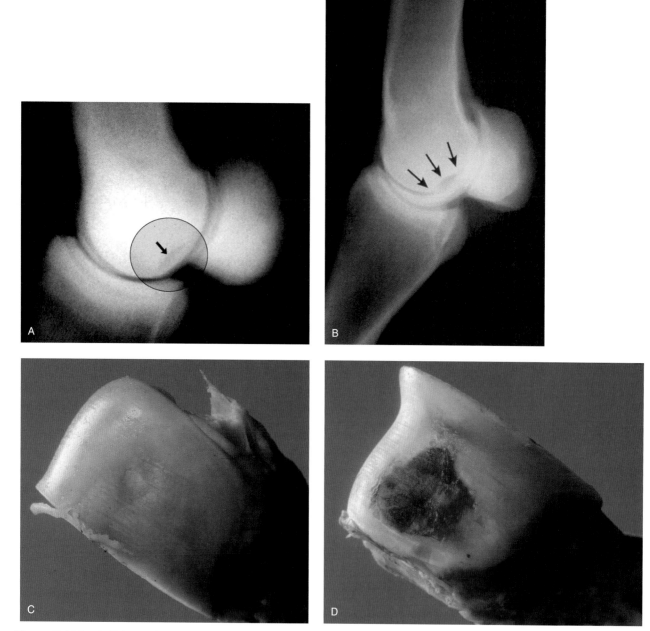

Figure 5.188. A. Palmar subchondral nondisplaced cortical stress fracture seen in racehorses (arrow in circle). B. Palmar subchondral cortical bone lysis seen in racehorses (arrows). C. A Standardbred racehorse's condyle demonstrating the classical appearance of the lesions corresponding to collapse and necrosis of the subchondral bone with secondary distortion of the articular cartilage. D. Severe osteolysis, necrosis, and collapse of the subchondral bone with a complete ulcer through the articular cartilage seen in a racing Standardbred that was lame at the walk.

Articular alignment and minimal cartilage gap is best maintained when compression is used. Arthroscopic evaluation of the articular alignment can be used if necessary in displaced fractures, particularly if other bone fragments must be removed, such as P1 eminence fractures or comminution of the palmar fracture line. Articular damage also can be assessed, which may affect prognosis in displaced fractures, particularly those of more chronic duration (days to weeks). Horses with condylar fractures that spiral proximally, typically in hindlimbs and medial, but also lateral, can be repaired with the horse sedated and standing.[20] This reduces the cost of the procedure and may reduce the risk of catastrophic breakdown on recovery from anesthesia (Figure 5.189). There are also successful reports of repairing spiral fractures by spiraling the plate to follow the fracture line or using screws alone under general anesthesia.[21,23]

Horses with incomplete fractures that are treated with cast or support bandages should be confined to

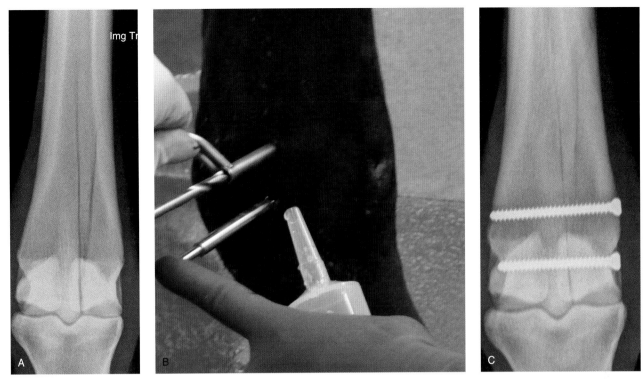

Figure 5.189. Radiograph of a spiraling medial condylar fracture in a racing Standardbred (A) repaired standing (B) with 2 parallel 5.5-mm cortical bone screws. At 4 weeks post operatively, the compression at the screws is apparent and bone healing is progressing (C).

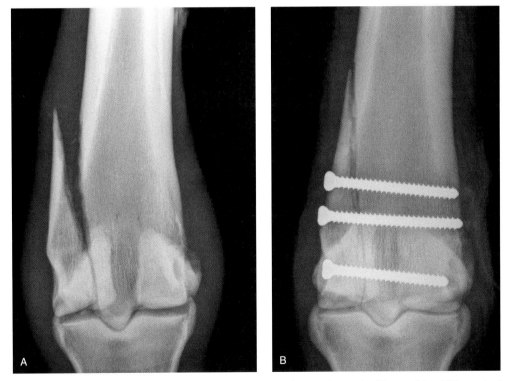

Figure 5.190. Cranio-caudal radiograph of a displaced lateral condylar fracture in a racing Thoroughbred (A) repaired with 3 5.5-mm cortical bone screws (B).

box stalls and observed closely for 2 to 3 weeks for any signs of increased pain and possible displacement. Bandages should be reset at least every other day for limb inspection and maximal support. For conservative management of nondisplaced fractures, stall rest for 2 months followed by 30 days of hand walking and then 30 days of light turnout are recommended. Fractures in young horses can heal by 90 days, but the most articular edge of the fracture often requires additional time. Horses put in training at 90 days are at risk of articular osteolysis upon return to training.

Internal fixation should be used in all complete condylar fractures (nondisplaced and displaced) in horses intended for athletic performance (Figures 5.189 and 5.190). Immediate diagnosis and immobilization of the limb is critical preoperatively to enhance success. Surgery should be performed quickly, but need not be performed on an emergency basis. The horse can be safely transported and permitted to recover from the incident if the limb is immobilized in a cast or complete commercial splint.

For surgery, the horse is positioned in lateral recumbency under general anesthesia with the affected limb up for a lateral condylar fracture. If a nondisplaced condylar fracture is present, the screws can be placed through strategically placed stab incisions in the skin. The location and spacing of the screws can be pre-planned by measurements made on the radiographs; however, the first screw is always located in the condylar fossa and subsequent screws placed 1.5 to 2 cm proximal to the first one. Placement of the most proximal screw can be omitted if comminution of the most proximal tip of the cortical fracture is evident on radiographs. Ideal screw placement is parallel to the joint with the first screw in the condylar fossa, engagement of both cortices without depositing bone material in the opposing collateral ligament, and compression of the fracture so the fracture line is eliminated or barely identifiable on the immediate postoperative radiograph. Increased duration and displacement of the fracture reduce the success in obtaining the latter result. In displaced condylar fractures, 5.5-mm cortical bone screws should be used, whereas in nondisplaced fractures 4.5-mm cortical bone screws or headless titanium compression screws can be successful (Figure 5.190).[5,13] Intraoperative fluoroscopy (preferably) or radiography should be used as needed to obtain the best results. Computed tomography should be performed prior to starting the surgery to understand the fracture propagation if there is any question about the presence of a spiraling component to the fracture. This may affect screw placement and casting the limb for recovery.

Complete or displaced fractures should be compressed with ASIF bone clamps prior to drilling to stabilize the fracture and initiate compression. Reduction of displaced condylar fractures can be a challenge, particularly in the cranial to caudal direction that may not be apparent on craniocaudal radiographs taken at surgery. Arthroscopic inspection of the dorsal articular surface often reveals a 1- to 2-mm step in the cranial direction of the fractured component.

In displaced fractures, an open incision the full length of the fracture, use of multiple bone clamps, and initial focus on the reduction of the most proximal portion of the fracture may help maximize reduction. The longer the duration of displaced fracture prior to surgery, the less likely perfect reduction will be achieved. Screws (5.5-mm cortical bone screws) are tightened distal to proximal and retightened to maximize compression. The head of the most distal screw is not countersunk because it is placed in the condylar fossa and countersinking of the most proximal screw may split the thin proximal portion of the fragment. The number of screws used depends on the length of the fracture fragment. However, in most cases of condylar fracture, only 2 to 3 screws are required. If spiraling of the fracture was identified on radiographs, screws are placed in lag fashion across the fracture for as far as it is identified and a cast is applied for recovery. This is particularly important for medial condylar fractures in the hindlimb.

Currently, displaced condylar fractures should be repaired with 5.5-mm cortical bone screws and nondisplaced fractures can be successfully repaired with 5.5-mm or 4.5-mm cortical bone screws or headless compression screws. Complications of screw pullout or bending have not posed problems with 4.5-mm screw repairs in nondisplaced fractures, but in the author's experience they can fail in severely displaced fractures. Rarely, refracture after return to racing can occur, even with screws in place, and 5.5-mm screws may offer an advantage in this situation. Screw design affects screw stiffness and strength in the equine distal condyle.

Casting usually is not performed for nondisplaced incomplete fractures or in complete fractures if a secure repair was obtained. A complete boot or cast should be used if the repair was less than ideal, in displaced fractures, or in spiraling fractures. A full-limb cast has been recommended for long spiraled fracture repairs, but not all surgeons use this because there is a risk of complications in recovery.[15] More recently, the author has repaired these fractures in the standing horse using a regional intravenous block to the distal limb. Horses are usually comfortable on the limb immediately after repair and walk in the stall without gait deficit when on low doses of phenylbutazone. Continued lameness postoperatively is a red flag for problems and radiographs should be obtained.

Postoperative exercise should be limited for at least 90 days. Stall rest confinement is recommended for this period, and after 6 weeks hand walking exercise can begin. Follow-up radiographs should be taken at this time, and if the healing is progressing normally, the horse can be turned out into a small paddock for an additional 90 days. If the radiographic follow-up shows good healing, the horse can be placed on pasture or in a large paddock. The training schedule depends on the type of fracture, but could begin as early as 4 months or as late as 6 months. In one study horses were more likely to race if the fracture line could no longer be identified at the 2- to 4-month radiographs.[24]

Screws are generally not removed after healing has occurred unless residual lameness results that can be directly attributed to their presence. In a review of 233 cases of condylar fractures, most repaired by interfragmentary compression, screws were only removed in 20 of the cases and there appeared to be no consistent difference in the performance between this group and the group with screws in place.[2] This study noted that horses with screws placed closer to the joint had a lower return to racing. Subchondral sclerosis was proposed as a cause for this pain. In general, removal of screws is not routinely performed for condylar fractures except if screws are placed in the diaphysis such as in medial condylar fractures of the metatarsus or spiraling fractures. Screw removal is easily performed under general anesthesia; the location of the screws can be confirmed with marker needles and radiographs. In most cases the screws can be removed through small stab incisions alone.

Prognosis

The general prognosis for athletic performance and returning to racing is excellent for nondisplaced incomplete fractures, whether treated conservatively (82% and 87% in 2 reports)[2,24] or following internal fixation (74% and 79% in 2 reports) for forelimb fractures,[2,24] and 93% for metatarsal fractures in one report.[2] Prognosis for athletic performance and return to racing is fair for complete displaced and nondisplaced fractures following internal fixation (58% in one report).[24] In 2 other reports, 33% of complete fractures (displaced and nondisplaced)[2] and 19% of displaced fractures[4] returned to racing. Rapid immobilization and repair of displaced fractures probably can dramatically affect outcome. In cases of complete displaced fractures or when there has been a delay in diagnosis and treatment and/or improper immobilization has been selected, a guarded to poor prognosis can be expected.[16] Only 12 of 38 cases in one report were able to return to racing.[16] This prognosis is altered because of increased damage to the articular surface that is likely to result in OA of the fetlock and irritation to the periosteum resulting in increased callus formation. The prognosis for return to racing is considered poor for comminuted fractures or subchondral erosive lesions in the palmar or plantar surface of the distal end of the cannon bone.[16]

References

1. Barclay WP, Foerner JJ, Phillips TN. Axial sesamoid injuries associated with lateral condylar fractures in horses. J Am Vet Med Assoc 1985;186:278.
2. Bassage LH, Richardson DW. Longitudinal fractures of the condyles of the third metacarpal and metatarsal bones in racehorses: 224 cases (1986–1995). J Am Vet Med Assoc 1998;212:1757.
3. Boyde A, Haroon Y, Jones SJ, et al. Three dimensional structure of the distal condyles of the third metacarpal bone of the horse. Equine Vet J 1999;31:122.
4. Ellis DR. Some observations on condylar fractures of the third metacarpus and third metatarsus in young Thoroughbreds. Equine Vet J 1994;26:178.
5. Galuppo LD, Simpson EL, Greenman SL, et al. A clinical evaluation of a headless, titanium, variable-pitched, tapered, compression screw for repair of nondisplaced lateral condylar fractures in Thoroughbred racehorses. Vet Surg 2006;35(5):423–430.
6. Greet TR. Condylar fracture of the cannon bone with axial sesamoid fracture in three horses. Vet Record 1987;120(10):223.
7. Kane AJ, Stover SM, Gardner IA, et al. Horseshoe characteristics as possible risk factors for fatal musculoskeletal injury of Thoroughbred racehorses. Am J Vet Res 1996;57:1147.
8. Le Jeune SS, Macdonald MH, Stover SM, et al. Biomechanical investigation of the association between suspensory ligament injury and lateral condylar fracture in Thoroughbred racehorses. Vet Surg 2003;32(6):585–97.
9. Muir P, McCarthy J, Radtke CL, et al. Role of endochondral ossification of articular cartilage and functional adaptation of the subchondral plate in the development of fatigue microcracking of joints. Bone 2006;38(3):342–349.
10. Nordin RW, Kawcak CE, Capwell BA, et al. Subchondral bone failure in an equine model of overload arthrosis. Bone 1998;22:133.
11. Parkin, TD, Clegg PD, French NP, et al. Catastrophic fracture of the lateral condyle of the third metacarpus/metatarsus in UK racehorses—fracture descriptions and pre-existing pathology. Vet J 2006;171(1):157–165.
12. Parkin TD, Clegg PD, French NP, et al. Risk of fatal distal limb fractures among Thoroughbreds involved in the five types of racing in the United Kingdom. Vet Rec 2004;154(16):493–497.
13. Rahm C, Ito K, Auer J. Screw fixation in lag fashion of equine cadaveric metacarpal and metatarsal condylar bone specimens: a biomechanical comparison of shaft and cortex screws. Vet Surg 2000;29(6):564.
14. Richardson DW. Third metacarpal/metatarsal condylar fractures. In Current Practice of Equine Surgery. White NA, Moore JN, eds. JB Lippincott, Philadelphia. 1990:617–622.
15. Richardson DW. Medial condylar fractures of the third metatarsal bone in horses. J Am Vet Med Assoc 1984;185:761.
16. Rick MC, Obrien TR, Pool RR, et al. Condylar fractures of the third metacarpal bone and third metatarsal bone in 75 horses: Radiographic features, treatments, and outcome. J Am Vet Med Assoc 1983;183:287.
17. Riggs CM, Boyde A. Effect of exercise on bone density in distal regions of the equine third metacarpal bone in 2-year-old Thoroughbreds. Equine Vet J (Suppl) 1999;30:555.
18. Riggs CM, Whitehouse GH, Boyde A. Structural variation of the distal condyles of the third metacarpal and third metatarsal bones in the horse. Equine Vet J 1999;31:130.
19. Riggs CM, Whitehouse GH, Boyde A. Pathology of the distal condyles of the third metacarpal and third metatarsal bones of the horse. Equine Vet J 1999;31:140.
20. Russell TM, MacLean AA. Standing surgical repair of propagating metacarpal and metatarsal condylar fractures in racehorses. Equine Vet J 2006;38(5):423–427.
21. Smith LC, Greet TR, Bathe AP. A lateral approach for screw repair in lag fashion of spiral third metacarpal and metatarsal medial condylar fractures in horses. Vet Surg 2009;38(6):681–688.
22. Stover SM, Deryck HR, Johnson BJ, et al. Lateral condylar fracture histomorphology in racehorses. Proceedings Am Assoc Equine Pract 1994;173.
23. Wright IM, Smith MR. A lateral approach to the repair of propagating fractures of the medial condyle of the third metacarpal and metatarsal bone in 18 racehorses. Vet Surg 2009;38(6):689–695.
24. Zekas LJ, Bramlage LR, Embertson RM, et al. Results of treatment of 145 fractures of the third metacarpal/metatarsal condyles in 135 horses (1986–1994). Equine Vet J 1999;31:309.
25. Zekas LJ, Bramlage LR, Embertson RM, et al. Characterization of the type and location of fractures of the third metacarpal/metatarsal condyles in 135 horses in central Kentucky (1986–1994) Equine Vet J 1999;31(4):304.

FRACTURES OF THE THIRD METACARPAL/ METATARSAL (CANNON) BONE

Fractures of the third metacarpal/metatarsal (cannon) bone occur commonly in all ages, but more commonly in young horses, and all breeds of horses. The metacarpus is particularly susceptible to fracture because of the distal location and because little soft tissue covers the bone to help absorb impact energy in blunt trauma.[23]

Although fractures of the cannon bone can assume a variety of configurations, ranging from a simple fissure to severe comminution, younger horses seem to sustain simpler fractures than adults, possibly because of more elastic and less brittle and shatter-prone bone. The fracture can occur anywhere along the bone length and can enter either the proximal or distal joint. Frequently, distal fractures that involve the growth plate, or rarely persistent proximal physes, in young animals are Salter type II fractures (Figure 11.5, Chapter 11).[16] Because of the minimal soft tissue covering, the fractures are commonly open or become open soon after the injury occurs and more than half of referred metacarpal/metatarsal fractures are open.[18] Concurrent fractures of the small metacarpal bones are common. Stress fractures of the metacarpus and metatarsus in racehorses that can progress to acute and complete failure of the bone are discussed earlier in this chapter. Once catastrophic failure occurs, fractures are treated as discussed below.

Etiology

External trauma in any form can cause fracture of the cannon bone. Injuries that are frequently reported by clients include kicks; halter-breaking injuries; injuries associated with ground holes, fences, or cattle guards; slipping accidents; slipping on ice; and accidents associated with moving vehicles. When foals are affected the dam has often stepped on the limb, causing fracture. Propagation of stress fractures, particularly more uncommon stress fractures, or propagation of forces through screw or pin holes in various other repairs can result in similar complete cannon bone failure. Preexisting bone abnormalities are not typically present because the injury represents a singular overloading event on the metacarpus/metatarsus.

Clinical Signs and Diagnosis

Complete yet nondisplaced fractures of the cannon bone secondary to direct trauma can occur and may be difficult to initially diagnose (Figure 5.191). The lameness may be nonspecific and variable. On gross observation the cannon bone may be enlarged slightly, and on palpation heat, swelling of the soft tissues overlying the fracture, and pain on deep digital palpation are present. Swelling and pain are more diffuse than with stress fractures and a wound at the site of impact is often present. Diagnosis may be delayed if soft tissue injury is evident because the lameness may be attributed to this cause. As lameness persists or worsens, radiographs are often taken and may reveal fracture lines. If the horse is turned out, invariably complete bone failure occurs. If stall confinement is maintained, the diagnosis is often made at the second radiograph when periosteal reaction is noted at sites of cortical exit and bone resorption of the fracture line widens the fractures.

In complete bone failure, the diagnosis of fracture of the cannon bone is obvious (Figure 5.192). An angular limb deformity is usually present, along with nonweight-bearing lameness. In all cases, these fractures should be immediately supported and eventually radiographed to identify the type (simple vs. comminuted) and location in relation to joint surfaces. The limb should not be manipulated excessively during the physical exam because this may lead to penetration of bone fragments through the skin.

If treatment is to be considered or further diagnosis is to be obtained, a cast or PVC full-limb splint should be immediately secured to the limb without moving the horse.[1,3] Loss of lower limb control may cause the horse to panic, and further soft tissue injury and an open fracture may result. Splinting is critical because a poorly applied splint may actually do more harm than good. Cast material can be applied over a light padded bandage for transport to a facility where radiographs and a better cast can be applied. In the forelimb and hindlimb, cast material is the easiest way to immobilize above the carpus and tarsus. If cast material not available, PVC pipe cut in half to create a sleeve can be placed over a tight padded bandage and secured aggressively with nonelastic tape. In the forelimb it should extend to the elbow; in the hindlimb it can extend to the top of the hock and a heavily padded and taped bandage extended proximally to the stifle.[1] Radiographs can often be obtained through the cast material or PVC splint, particularly if euthanasia is likely and final confirmation of the severity is all that is needed for the decision. If, however, surgical repair is anticipated, a full series of high detail radiographs are needed and can be obtained under general anesthesia either as a separate procedure or preferably, just prior to surgery.

Treatment

The selection of treatment of cannon bone fractures depends on the type of fracture (open vs. closed, simple vs. comminuted), location of the fracture (articular vs. nonarticular, proximal vs. distal), animal's age and intended use, presence of wounds, vascular compromise, and economics.

The preferred treatment for most cannon bone fractures is internal fixation with 1 or 2 DCP plates (Figures 5.192 and 5.193) or minimally invasive plate fixation extending the length of the bone[12], combined with individual screws where appropriate. This technique is rec-

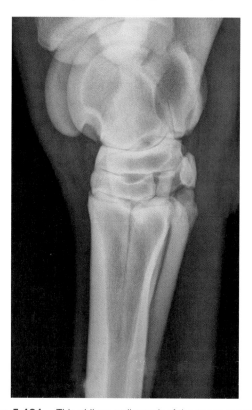

Figure 5.191. This oblique radiograph of the tarsus revealed an incomplete proximal metatarsal fracture. This fracture occurred from an accident at a jump and was initially thought to be a proximal suspensory injury. (Courtesy of Dr. Ty Wallis.)

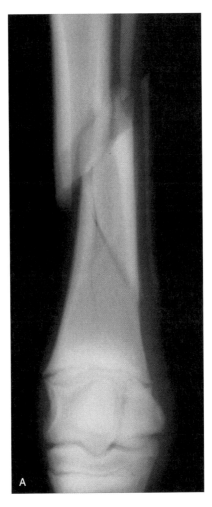
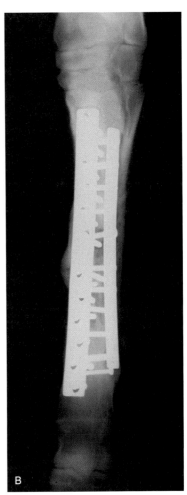

Figure 5.192. A. Open comminuted mid-diaphyseal fracture of the metatarsus in a 7-month-old weanling. B. Postoperative view demonstrating fracture repair with 2 broad dynamic compression plates on the dorsolateral and dorsomedial sides of the metatarsus. Additional screws were placed in lag fashion from outside the plates to secure the butterfly fragments.

ommended even in open fractures, particularly if the wound is minor and represents a puncture of the bone end through the skin and the area was clipped, cleaned, and placed under an antiseptic wrap early in the process. Fracture configuration, such as very proximal or distal comminution or severe comminution with extensive fissuring, as well as more extensive wounds or vascular compromise, may not make this repair the method of choice without a variation of including arthrodesis or combining with external coaptation.[4] These severe fractures may heal with transfixation pins and external fixators or casts. These methods are more successful in foals with rapid healing and low body weight. In adult horses, these severe fractures have a guarded prognosis, but use of external coaptation, plating in the face of open wounds and vascular compromise, or sequential procedures have been successful in rare instances.[2,12,14]

The basic principles of cannon bone fracture repair include:

1. Reconstruct the fracture into 2 fragments (usually with lag screws) before application of plates
2. Anatomically reduce the fracture, particularly articular components
3. Place plates on the tension band side of the cannon bone (dorsal or dorsolateral) and over fragments at 90° to one another
4. Stagger the plates
5. Fill all screw holes if at all possible
6. Use 5.5-mm screws in the metaphyses and adjacent to the fracture ends for maximal pullout and bending strength, respectively
7. Lute the plates with antimicrobial-impregnated polymethylmethacrylate[21]
8. Place autogenous bone graft in most cases
9. Do not end the plates at the top of the cast
10. Apply a cast for recovery and possibly longer

The surgical approach to the metacarpus and metatarsus for bone plate application is through a flaplike incision or the plates can be placed by minimally invasive percutaneous procedure. The flap should be large enough to allow coverage of the plates and to ensure that the suture line is not directly over the plates. Two plates are used, except in small neonates (Figure 5.193). Two narrow plates or 1 narrow and 1 broad DC plate can be used in foals or ponies, depending on size. Two broad DC plates are needed for most horses, including large weanlings and yearlings. The limiting factor is the size of the metacarpus and whether two broad plates can fit on the bone.

In the classic metacarpal fracture with 1 large butterfly fragment, the fragment can be secured to the proximal bone with 2 3.5-mm cortical bone screws. The heads of these screws are small and can be easily countersunk to allow placement under the plate if necessary.

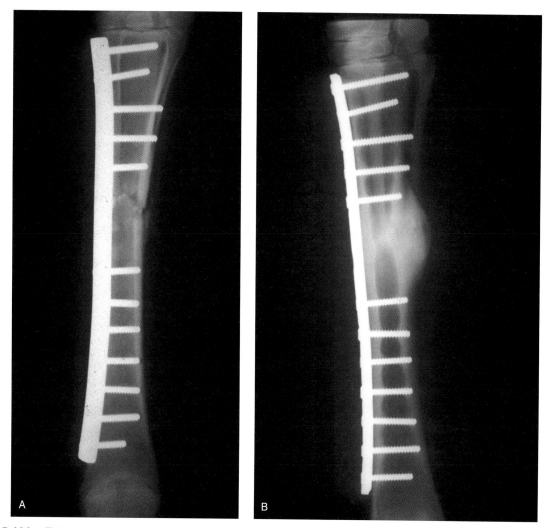

Figure 5.193. This transverse metatarsal fracture in a foal was repaired with a single broad DCP (A) and healed well with a relatively large callus (B). (Courtesy of Dr. Gary Baxter.)

The goal is to achieve the best possible anatomic reduction to minimize the gap for fracture callus to bridge and to produce the most interdigitation for inherent stability.

Autogenous bone graft can be placed into any gaps and around the fracture site after plate luting.[21] Graft can be obtained from the sternum in horses in dorsal recumbency and the tuber coxae in horses in lateral recumbency, and is expected to increase bone density in screw holes during healing.[10] A distal limb cast is usually applied. If the fracture is stable and the animal is young or small, the cast can be removed 10 to 14 days after incisional healing is anticipated. Antimicrobials are discontinued after hemorrhage is anticipated to have ceased (about 24 to 72 hours) and horses should be willing to use the cast within 72 hours postoperatively if not immediately.

Healing of the bone requires 60 to 90 days in foals and 4 to 12 months in adults, depending on severity of the fracture and complications. Stall rest should be anticipated for 4 months in foals and 6 months in adults, although hand walking can begin as soon as

fracture callus bridges the fracture and other complications of implant failure have not occurred or have arrested. An unsuccessful outcome in foals may be due to infection and nonunion, or secondary complications such as cast sores and osteonecrosis or severe tendon laxity. An unsuccessful outcome in adults is usually due to laminitis of the supporting limb, infection or sequestration of large fracture fragments and loss of repair stability, and other secondary complications that prohibitively increase cost.

Use of the interlocking nail system for internal fixation of cannon bone fractures usually is not elected because fractures are commonly comminuted and the interlocking nail system is not as strong as double plating in torsion.[15] The use of external fixators in adult horses usually is not selected because external fixation ring constructs with one-quarter-inch Steinman pins are not stiff enough for repair of an unstable third metacarpal bone fracture in an adult.[7] Fracture through the pin holes can occur in a subset of horses.[14] Other unusual internal fixation methods have been reported to be successful and include use of an Ilizarov ring fixator in a

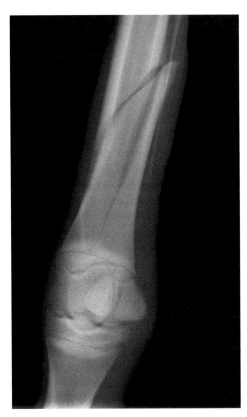

Figure 5.194. Radiograph of a long oblique metatarsal fracture in a foal that entered the distal physis. (Courtesy of Dr. Gary Baxter.)

metacarpal fracture in a foal[13] and use of a cortical allograft under 2 plates to replace a large portion of sequestered bone in a metatarsal fracture of a foal.[6]

In young foals sustaining fractures that have extended into the growth plate, it may be necessary to bridge the growth plate with an implant to achieve stability of the fracture (Figure 5.194). In very young foals, from birth to 6 weeks, this may alter limb growth sufficiently to cause shortening or an angular limb deformity may develop. The majority of the growth from the physis (growth plate) occurs prior to 2.5 or 3 months of age; therefore, there is little chance of altering or arresting growth after this age. Alignment of the limb is critical during repair, and closure of the distal growth plate to prevent asymmetric growth can be a goal in the repair. The slightly shorter cannon bone is often compensated for with fetlock angle and hoof growth.

The decision to remove bone plates depends on the animal's age and intended use, and whether draining fistulae are present. In general, horses that are to be used in athletic competition should have their plates removed in stages, 3 months apart. After plate removal, the limb is supported in a cast for a short time and exercise is slowly initiated. If draining fistulae are present, fracture healing should be complete before plate removal. Removing all plates and screws usually resolves the infection.

External coaptation alone has been used successfully to treat many cases of nondisplaced cannon bone fractures,[3,9] but is not optimal for complete fractures. In complete fractures, the healed result is likely to be a malunion, if the horse survives the prolonged healing time and discomfort. Standard casts do not adequately decrease axial loading or movement of the fracture ends, even if applied up to the elbow or stifle. Axial alignment is better than a bandage, but nonunion or failure due to secondary complications of a prolonged healing time and lameness are likely.

Cast application often becomes as expensive as internal fixation due the multiple applications and prolonged healing time. Simple distal fractures in foals may be successfully treated with casts, but internal fixation is still preferred for early weight-bearing and reduction in secondary complications, such as poor reduction, tendon laxity, cast sores, or nonunion. A full-limb cast will reduce metacarpal bone strain but a full-limb walking cast more consistently reduced metacarpal bone strains to 11% of baseline and neutralized bending and torsional forces in one study.[5] A half-limb cast or half-limb transfixation pin cast does not significantly reduce metacarpal bone strain as it does on the phalanges, and therefore probably does not provide adequate immobilization or load sharing for metacarpal fractures.[22]

Casts in conjunction with transfixation pinning have been successful in a limited number of cases in foals and adults that have sustained proximal comminuted fractures of the cannon bone. Pinning provides significantly greater resistance than standard casts against the axial collapse of metacarpal fractures.[11] These fractures are so proximal that they are not amenable to routine techniques of internal fixation (e.g., bone plating).

In most cases 2 large-diameter pins (6-mm) are placed transversely from lateral to medial through the distal end of the radius, and the other 2 pins are placed in a similar fashion below the fracture site in the third metacarpal bone. A full-limb cast is applied over the pins. Divergent transfixation pins are a stronger configuration under torsional strain.[19] Holes drilled in the metacarpus significantly reduce the metacarpal strength over intact bone,[24] and centrally threaded, positive-profile transfixation pin designs provide greater strength over negative profile pins and should not be self tapped for maximal pull-out strength and the least bone damage on insertion.[20] A cast is then applied over and around the pins. Very strong, lightweight external support can be applied with the new fiberglass casting materials. The pins are used to further stabilize the very unstable comminuted fracture. Foals can be maintained in stall confinement, whereas adults may require slinging. Other forms of coaptation, such as leg braces in many forms, and splints, have been used to successfully treat cannon bone fractures in a limited number of cases but are not the recommended treatment of first choice.[9]

Open fractures associated with moderate to severe contamination and increased soft tissue inflammation may be treated by temporary casting or pin casting for periods of 7 to 10 days, after which internal fixation can be applied. This delayed approach is only recommended if reasonable stabilization of the fracture can be achieved. The cast is removed after 3 to 4 days, the wound is examined, deep samples for culture and sensitivity are taken, further debridement and lavage may be performed if indicated, and a sterile bandage and cast are reapplied. Depending on the state of the wound, the cast is removed in 7 to 10 days and a final decision is made regarding the application of internal fixation. If the wound is obviously infected, euthanasia may be advised.

This delay provides sufficient time to identify whether infection will be a problem before committing the client to the expense of internal fixation. The delay also allows the process of autodebridement to occur and minimizes the chances of infection locally. Foals may have success with this method; adults rarely survive. If the fracture line extends into the nutrient foramen of the cannon bone, attempt at repair may be futile because ischemic necrosis and sequestrum may result.[23] Serial use of nuclear scintigraphy can detect loss of cortical bone vascularity, but in one study did not predict successful healing in the 2 cases reported, as 1 case revascularized.[17]

Prognosis

The prognosis for successful treatment of third metacarpal and metatarsal bone fractures depends on multiple factors, so an individual assessment of each case is warranted. In a study of 25 complete fractures of the metacarpal or metatarsal bones of horses that were treated, age, sex, weight, and limb did not affect the outcome, but case selection had already occurred. Seventeen of the 25 cases had an open fracture, and nonunion in an infected fracture was the most common cause of postoperative failure in 7 cases. Eleven horses had no complications related to the surgical repair.

In general, transverse, slightly oblique, and minorly comminuted (1 butterfly fragment) fractures in the mid-cannon bone region in foals under 7 months of age have a good to excellent prognosis with internal fixation. Older horses with similar fractures have a more guarded prognosis due to their size and the risk of supporting limb laminitis, but in general have a fair to good prognosis. Older horses with open, comminuted, or articular fractures have a guarded to poor prognosis for recovery. Unfortunately, older horses have a greater risk of comminuted open fractures that involve the nutrient foramen.[18]

References

1. Bertone AL. Management of Orthopedic Emergencies. In Vet Clin N Am (Equine Pract) 1994;10:603.
2. Bischofberger AS, Furst A, Auer J, et al. Surgical management of complete diaphyseal third metacarpal and metatarsal bone fracture: clinical outcome in 10 mature horses and 11 foals. Equine Vet J 2009;41:465–473.
3. Bowman KF, Fackleman GE. Management of comminuted fractures in the horse. Comp Cont Ed 1980;11:298.
4. Bramlage LR. Fetlock arthrodesis. In Equine Fracture Repair. Nixon AJ, ed. WB Saunders, Philadelphia. 1996;172–178.
5. Brommer H, Back W, Schamhardt HC, et al. In vitro determination of equine third metacarpal bone unloading, using a full limb cast and a walking cast. Am J Vet Res 1996;57:1386.
6. Cassotis NJ, Stick JA, Arnoczky SP. Use of full cortical allograft to repair a metatarsal fracture in a foal. J Am Vet Med Assoc 1997;211:1155.
7. Cervantes C, Madison JB, Miller GJ, et al. An in vitro biomechanical study of a multiplanar circular external fixator applied to equine third metacarpal bones. Vet Surg 1996;25:1–5.
8. Colgan SA, Hecker AT, Kirker-Head CA, et al. A comparison of the Synthes 4.5-mm cannulated screw and the Synthes 4.5-mm standard cortex screw systems in equine bone. Vet Surg 1998; 27:540.
9. Fessler JF, Amstutz HE. Fracture repair in large animals. In Large Animal Surgery. Oehme FW, Prier JE, eds. Williams and Wilkins Co., Baltimore, 1974;301.
10. Hanie EA, Sullins KE, Powers BE. Comparison of two grafting methods in 4.0-mm drill defects in the third metacarpal bone of horses. Equine Vet J 1992;24:387.
11. Hopper SA, Schneider RK, Johnson CH, et al. In vitro comparison of transfixation and standard full-limb cases for prevention of displacement of a mid-diaphyseal third metacarpal osteotomy site in horses. Am J Vet Res 2000;61:1633.
12. James FM, Richardson DW. Minimally invasive plate fixation of lower limb injury in horses: 32 cases (1999–2003). Equine Vet J. 2006;38:246–251.
13. Jukema GN, Settner M, Dunkelmann G, et al. High stability of the Ilizarov ring fixator in a metacarpal fracture of an Arabian foal. Arch Orthop Trauma Surg 1997;116(5):287.
14. Lescun, TB, McClure SR, Ward MP, et al. Evaluation of transfixation casting for treatment of third metacarpal, third metatarsal, and phalangeal fractures in horses: 37 cases (1994–2004). J Am Vet Med Assoc. 2007;230:1340–1349.
15. Lopez MJ, Wilson DG, Vanderby R, et al. An in vitro biomechanical comparison of an interlocking nail system and dynamic compression plate fixation of ostectomized equine third metacarpal bones. Vet Surg 1999;28:333.
16. Lumsden JM, Caron JP, Stickle RL. Repair of a proximal metatarsal Salter type-II fracture in a foal. J Am Vet Med Assoc 1993; 202(5):765.
17. Markel MD, Snyder JR, Hornof WJ, et al. Nuclear scintigraphic evaluation of third metacarpal and metatarsal bone fractures in three horses. J Am Vet Med Assoc 1987;191:75.
18. McClure SR, Watkins JP, Glickman NW, et al. Complete fractures of the third metacarpal or metatarsal bone in horses: 25 cases (1980–1996). J Am Vet Med Assoc 1998;213:847.
19. McClure SR, Watkins JP, Ashman RB. A in vitro comparison of the effect of parallel and divergent transfixation pins on the breaking strength of the equine third metacarpal bone. Vet Surg 1993;389.
20. Morisset S, McClure SR, Hillberry BM, et al. In vitro comparison of the use of two large-animal, centrally threaded, positive-profile transfixation pin designs in the equine third metacarpal bone. Am J Vet Res 2000;61:1298.
21. Nunamaker DM, Richardson DW, Butterweck DM. Mechanical and biological effects of plate luting. J Orthop Trauma 1991; 5(2):138.
22. Schneider RK, Ratzlaff MC, White KK, et al. Effect of three types of half-limb cases on in vitro bone strain recorded from the third metacarpal bone and proximal phalanx in equine cadaver limbs. Am J Vet Res 1998;59:1188.
23. Schneider RK, Jackman BR. Fractures of the third metacarpus and metatarsus. In Equine Fracture Repair. Nixon AJ, ed. WB Saunders, Philadelphia. 1996;179–194.
24. Seltzer KL, Stover SM, Taylor KT, et al. The effect of hole diameter on the torsional mechanical properties of the equine third metacarpal bone. Vet Surg 1996;25:371.

DIAPHYSEAL ANGULAR LIMB DEFORMITIES OF THE THIRD METACARPAL/METATARSAL BONES (CANNON BONE)

Angular limb deformities (ALD) associated with the diaphysis of the third metacarpal/metatarsal bones are a congenital anomaly that rarely affect foals.[2] In most cases the angular deformity is noticed shortly after birth. Although the deviation is centered on the mid to proximal portion of the metacarpus or metatarsus rather than the distal extremity, the fetlock joint may be involved secondarily. Both varus (outward bowing of the cannon) and valgus (inward deviation of the cannon) have been seen[2] in addition to dorsal to plantar deviations (Figure 5.195).

Etiology

The etiology is unknown. However, it has been conjectured that a maldevelopment of the cartilaginous

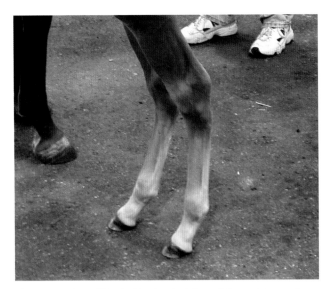

Figure 5.195. This foal had a deviation of the metatarsus in a dorsal-plantar orientation, illustrated by bowing of the metatarsus, and was corrected with an osteotomy. (Courtesy of Dr. Gary Baxter.)

bone precursor may occur from abnormal positioning of the fetus in the uterus.[2] Because the deviations are closely related to the nutrient foramen, it also has been suggested that a vascular aberration may be present during the early period of bone development.[2]

Clinical Signs and Diagnosis

At first glance, the angular deformity may appear similar to the angular deformity associated with the fetlock joint. However, on closer observation it is obvious that the pivotal point (axis of deviation) is located more proximal in the diaphysis of the bone.[1] Observing the limb from above the shoulder and/or hip and looking downward is most informative. The diagnosis is more difficult if the fetlock joint is secondarily involved. Most foals appear quite vigorous and show no signs of lameness. On palpation, mild pain may be elicited from rotation and flexion of the fetlock.[1] On direct palpation of the cannon bone, no heat, swelling, nor pain with pressure is elicited.

A definitive diagnosis is made from the radiographic examination. In most cases a dorsal palmar (DP) and a lateral medial (LM) suffice. An increased thickening of the cortex on the concave side is usually noted.[1,2] This is felt to be attributed to Wolf's law of bone remodeling. The pivotal angle can be identified by placing an overlay of acetate or an undeveloped X-ray film over the DP view. Lines are drawn axially to bisect the cannon bone and fetlock joint. The pivot point (axis of deviation) is where these lines intersect. The degrees of deviation can be recorded with a protractor. This information is particularly important if surgery is contemplated.

Treatment

If the condition is identified by 1 month of age, periosteal transection and stripping of the distal metacarpal/

metatarsal growth plate and the entire concave surface of the cannon bone will help correct the angulation and stimulate modeling of the cannon bone to fill in the concavity. If the metacarpal/metatarsal growth plate is closed, a wedge ostectomy and double plating can be performed to straighten the limb with a good prognosis.[2]

The ostectomy is performed on the convex surface. The exact site and degree of ostectomy is predicted from drawings made on acetate overlays over the DP view. Ideally the ostectomy should be made directly over the center of the pivot point. However, the nutrient foramen vascular supply should be avoided. The widest point of the ostectomy should be at the convex surface, and ideally no bone or very little bone should be removed from the concave side. An oscillating saw is used to make the wedge, after which 2 bone plates are applied according to the Association for the Study of Internal Fixation (ASIF) principles. A cast or a Robert-Jones bandage is applied and removed 2 to 4 weeks after surgery. The bone plates can be removed later in a staggered fashion after complete radiographic healing is evident, if desired.

Prognosis

The prognosis is good because the procedure is elective, the foals are young, and no initial bone and soft tissue trauma have occurred.

References

1. Stashak TS. Angular limb deformities associated with the diaphysis of the third metacarpal and metatarsal bones. In Adams' Lameness in Horses, 4th ed. Stashak TS, ed. Lea and Febiger, Philadelphia. 1987;pp 610–612.
2. White KK. Diaphyseal angular deformities in three foals. J Am Vet Med Assoc 1983;182:272.

METACARPAL/METATARSAL EXOSTOSIS (SPLINTS)

"Splints," a condition of young horses, most commonly affects the proximal medial aspect of the limb between the second and third metacarpal bones (Figure 5.196). The condition is associated with training and subsequent injury between the small metacarpals/metatarsal (MC/MT) bones and cannon bone, resulting in inflammation or tearing of the interosseus ligament. Conformation abnormalities such as offset carpi, improper hoof care, and mineral imbalances may exacerbate the condition.[1,4]

The second and fourth MC/MT bones are commonly called splint bones. Each is attached intimately to the respective third MC/MT bone by an interosseous ligament, thus splinting the large bone. The splint bones articulate with the carpometacarpal joint or tarsometatarsal joint and are exposed to loads on weight-bearing. The interosseus ligament consists of dense fibrous tissue that can tear with the strains applied during independent motion of the splint bones and the cannon bone. Initially, inflammatory desmitis and periostitis develop. Subsequently, new bone is produced to fuse the splints to the cannon bone and stabilize the source of irritation.

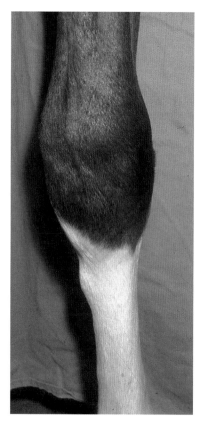

Figure 5.196. Visible enlargement of the medial splint area just distal to the carpus typical of horses with "splints." (Courtesy of Dr. Gary Baxter.)

The terminology used to identify the condition is variable. A true splint refers to a sprain or tear of the interosseous ligament. The resultant enlargement is most frequently observed 6 to 7 cm below the carpus on the medial side at the junction of the second and third metacarpal bones (Figure 5.196). Blind splint refers to an inflammatory process of the interosseous ligament that is difficult to detect on physical examination because the swelling occurs on the axial (inner) side of the splint, between the small metacarpal bone and the suspensory ligament. Osteolysis between the second and third metacarpal bones may be observed on radiographic examination. Periostitis of the splint bones results from superficial trauma to the periosteum, which, in turn, causes a proliferative periostitis. Although a residual blemish remains, the horse is usually not lame. A knee splint is the enlargement of the proximal portion of the splint bone that may lead to OA within the carpometacarpal joint.

Etiology

The enlargement of the splint bones associated with this disease results from proliferation of fibrous tissue and osteoperostitis. The causes are tearing of the interosseous ligament that binds a small metacarpal bone to the large metacarpal/metatarsal bone, external trauma, or healing of a transverse or longitudinal fracture. If the inflammation associated with the periosteum is suffi-

cient, over time it will result in ossification (proliferative exostosis) of the splint bone. The size of the splint is usually depends on the degree of inflammation and the surface area involved. In any case, the splint usually assumes an elongated form, lying parallel to the small metacarpal bone.

The second metacarpal is more frequently involved because of the difference in its articulation with the carpus. The second metacarpus is entirely articular and its articulation is flatter than that of the fourth metacarpal bone. When mechanical load tests were performed on ligamentous preparations of the carpus and metacarpus, it was noted that the carpal bones pushed the small metacarpal bones distad.[5] It is proposed that excessive loading can lead to tearing of the interosseous ligament in the region that is most frequently affected. Metacarpal fusion progresses normally with aging, and 78% of all horses 2 years old and older had 2 or more sites of fusion. The rate of metacarpal fusion/horse/year appeared to be at least 10 times higher than the rate of painful exostoses causing fusion, indicating that this process occurs subclinically in most horses.[3]

Conformation abnormalities that increase the stress on the small metacarpal bones also increase the incidence of this disease.[4] Offset carpi (bench knees) is an example of a conformational abnormality that predisposes to splints on the medial small metacarpal bones. Furthermore, horses that have a base-narrow, toe-out conformation may cause external trauma to the splint bone by hitting it with the opposite limb (interference). See Chapter 2 for examples of these conformation abnormalities. Improper shoeing and trimming also can alter the foot flight enough that the horse may interfere. All can cause either a tearing of the interosseous ligament or a proliferative periostitis of the second and/or third metacarpal bone. The fourth metacarpal bone may be affected by external blows (hitting objects or being kicked). A higher incidence of this type of injury has been observed in the fourth metatarsal bone.

Imbalanced nutrition or overnutrition in young horses has also been implicated in the development of splints.[4] Imbalances and deficiencies in calcium and phosphorus have been associated with an increased incidence of splints. However, no well-documented studies have proven this to be true. In many cases horses that are suspected of having a calcium and phosphorus imbalance also grow rapidly. It may be that their increased weight causes sufficient compressive forces so that splints develop as a result of this, rather than the imbalance. In general, young horses that are poorly conformed, overweight, and overexercised have a greater chance of tearing the interosseous ligament before metacarpal fusion is complete.

Clinical Signs

The condition is most common in 2-year-old horses undergoing heavy training, but cases occasionally occur among 3- or 4-year-olds. Splints most often are found on the medial aspect of the limb, and lameness is usually most obvious in the trot. Heat, pain, and swelling over the affected region may occur anywhere along the length of the splint bone. Splints most commonly occur about 3 inches below the carpal joint (Figure 5.196). One large swelling or a number of smaller enlargements may occur along the length of the splint bone at its junction with the third MC/MT bone.

New bone growth that occurs near the carpal joint may cause carpal OA (knee splints). Extensive new bone formation on a splint bone may also encroach on the suspensory ligament and cause chronic lameness unless it is removed. Growths of this kind can be determined by palpation and radiographic and ultrasound examination. Splint lameness becomes more marked with exercise on hard ground. In mild cases no lameness may be evident at the walk, but lameness is exhibited during the trot. After the original inflammation subsides, the enlargements usually become smaller but firmer as a result of the ossification. The reduction in swelling is usually the result of resolution of fibrous tissue, rather than a decrease in size of the actual bone formation. In the early stages, the greatest bulk of the swelling is from inflammation, and this normally resolves to a much smaller size. Some cases of splints may not cause lameness.

Diagnosis

The obvious signs lead to a diagnosis when the affected limb is examined carefully. Heat, pain, and swelling over the regions mentioned, plus lameness, are enough to make the diagnosis. However, the diagnosis should be confirmed with a radiograph (Figure 5.197). Fracture of the splint bone can be confused with splints. Ultrasonographic examination can demonstrate concomitant injury to the suspensory and possible ligament impingement. In some cases nuclear scintigraphy may be needed to confirm a blind splint. New bone growth resulting from trauma may occur on the third metacarpal or third metatarsal bones, close to the splint bone, and may be mistaken for splints. Palpation and radiographs, however, show that these swellings are dorsal to the junction with the splint bones. This type of new bone growth is most often caused by interference.

Treatment

Treatment for splints includes anti-inflammatory agents and rest for the acute phase, and occasionally surgery in the more chronic stages. Counterirritation is still practiced for the chronic phases, but is of unknown significance. Other treatments include shock wave therapy, icing, topical diclofenac liposomal cream (Surpass), acupuncture, and massage.

Inflammation and swelling are the hallmark of this disease in the acute phase. The administration of non-steroidal anti-inflammatory drugs (NSAIDs) coupled with the application of hypothermia and pressure support wraps appears to be most beneficial to decrease the heat, pain, and swelling. Hypothermia can be attained with ice or ice/water packs or whirlpool boots. They should be applied for 30 minutes 2 to 3 times a day for at least 2 to 3 days. Some recommend hand massage for 10 minutes after each treatment, after which a support bandage is applied. The topical application of dimethyl sulfoxide (DMSO)/Furacin or

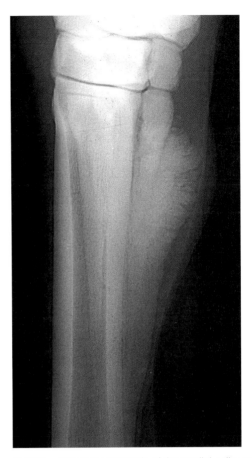

Figure 5.197. This large exostosis of the medial splint was contributing to lameness and was removed surgically. Just the exostosis was removed and the underlying splint bone was left intact. (Courtesy of Dr. Gary Baxter.)

DMSO/steroid sweats or Surpass is also logical. Affected horses should be confined to a stall for at least 30 to 45 days, and hand-walking exercise for 15 to 20 minutes twice a day should be begun after the acute inflammation subsides.[4]

Intralesional corticosteroid can reduce inflammation and may help prevent excessive bone growth. Corticoid therapy should be accompanied by counterpressure bandage. In this case the horse is generally rested longer than 30 days and should not resume training as rapidly as when counter-irritation is used. However, the swelling may be considerably less. It is also true that splints will heal without therapy, provided adequate rest is given.[4] If the splint results from interference, splint or shin boots (guards) may help prevent further trauma. If the horse interferes because of improper trimming and shoeing, this should be corrected.

If the proliferative bone is excessive, surgery may be indicated in a very small percentage of the cases (Figure 5.197). Surgery to remove exostoses for medical or cosmetic reasons has resulted in fair to good success. In one study, 15 exostoses removed for cosmetics or lameness resulted in minimal recurrence of the bone proliferation.[2] In a larger study of 95 Standardbreds, the splint bones were amputated to remove excessive bone callus. In horses with proximal splint bone removal in which the proximal portion was stabilized with screws or bone plates, horses were still limited in performance at 12 weeks. Horses in which a subperiosteal removal of the exostosis was performed were sound 12 weeks postoperatively.[6]

It is recommended to retain the splint bone lever arm by reflecting the periosteum to prevent formation of excessive new bone and associated irritation of the suspensory ligament. In some cases it is necessary to surgically remove a bony exostosis that interferes with the action of the suspensory ligament or the carpal joint or one that is so large that it is hit repeatedly by the opposite foot. These require care in dissection of the proximal structures, including ligaments of the palmar carpal support. If the bone growth has been caused by trauma from interference, the surgery will not be successful unless corrective shoeing or use of splint boots will stop the interference.

Prognosis

Prognosis is good to excellent for soundness except for those in which the exostosis is large and encroaches on the suspensory ligament or the carpal joint. Chronic recurring lameness can occur in horses that are not rested long enough, which can be 5 to 6 months. Surgery to remove the excess bone callus can successfully alleviate lameness and recurrence does not occur in most cases. Surgery may speed up the return to athletic soundness and improve the cosmetic blemish.

References

1. Adams OR. Lameness in Horses, 3rd ed. Williams and Wilkins Co., Baltimore, 1974;207.
2. Barber SM, Caron J, Pharr J. Metatarsal/metacarpal exostosis removal—a prospective study. Vet Surg 1987;16:82.
3. Les CM, Stover SM, Willits NH. Necropsy survey of metacarpal fusion in the horse. Am J Vet Res 1995;56:1421.
4. Ray C, Baxter GM. Splint bone injuries in horses. Comp Contin Educ Vet Prac 1995;17:723.
5. Rooney JR. Biomechanics of Lameness in Horses. Williams and Wilkins Co., Baltimore, 1969;143.
6. Welling EK. Evaluation of the efficacy of surgical intervention on middle and proximal splint bone injuries in 95 Standardbred horses. Vet Surg 1993;253.

FRACTURES OF THE SMALL METACARPAL AND METATARSAL (SPLINT) BONES

Fractures of the small metacarpal and metatarsal bones (splint bones) can occur anywhere along their length but they are most commonly located at the distal third.[1,3,5–7,11] In most cases fractures located at the distal third are simple fractures (Figure 5.198), in contrast to fractures of the middle and proximal portion, which are often complicated by comminution, osteomyelitis, and bone sequestration (Figure 5.199).[2,6,8,10]

Fractures of the distal part of a small metacarpal or metatarsal bone usually occur in older horses (5 to 7 years of age) and only rarely occur in horses under 2 years of age.[3] This is thought to occur as a result of decreased pliability in the interosseous ligament and more strenuous training programs in older horses.[3] In contrast, younger horses tend to sustain damage to the

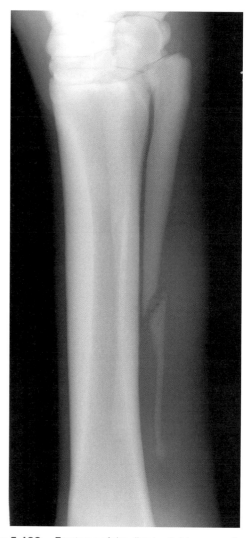

Figure 5.198. Fractures of the distal splint bones such as this rarely heal and are usually removed. (Courtesy of Dr. Gary Baxter.)

interosseous ligament supporting the small metacarpal bones, resulting in the condition referred to as splints. The forelimbs are more frequently involved than the hindlimbs; the left forelimb with the lateral splint is affected more commonly than the hindlimb.[3,11] The relationship between suspensory ligament desmitis, sesamoiditis, and fetlock OA or arthrosis is more than casual. It appears that the enlarged fibrotic suspensory ligament decreases the absorptive capacity of the fetlock and creates a space-occupying mass that may cause the fracture and further displacement of that fractured small metacarpal bone. It is assumed that the decreased ability to extend the fetlock contributes to the arthrosis.

Fractures of the proximal half of the small metacarpal or metatarsal bone are often comminuted, and osteomyelitis with or without sequestrum is a complicating feature. The lateral surface of these bones is most frequently involved and it is thought to result from direct trauma (Figure 5.199).[2,8,10]

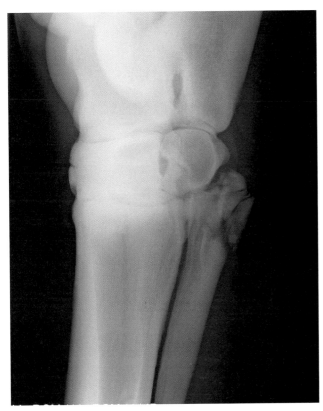

Figure 5.199. Proximal fractures of the fourth metatarsal bone are often comminuted and open and are due to traumatic injuries. (Courtesy of Dr. Gary Baxter.)

Etiology

Fractures of the distal part of the small metacarpal or metatarsal bone result from external and internal trauma. External trauma can result from a kick from another horse, interference, direct blows from hitting another object, or puncture wounds. Internal trauma occurs from increased axial compression forces on these bones during races or from pressure from the suspensory ligament, or increased tension from the fascial attachments. It is conjectured that the increased incidence of left fourth metacarpal bone and right second metacarpal bone fractures observed in Thoroughbreds may be the result of increased weight-bearing on the bones when they are racing in a counterclockwise direction. In contrast, the suspensory ligament and supporting fascia may put these bones under tension sufficient to cause fracture in the hindlimbs.[1,3,5–7,11] Because there is an increase in incidence of left second metatarsal bone and right fourth metatarsal bone, which is the tension side of the hindlimb in horses that run counterclockwise, it is logical to assume that tension created by the bow-string effect of the suspensory ligament or increased tension developed by the internal fascia may lead to fracture.

It is difficult to decide whether the incidence of suspensory ligament desmitis is a result of distal splint bone fractures that may cause irritation to this structure, or, conversely, that the swollen suspensory ligament becomes space occupying enough to cause these frac-

tures. Whatever the case, a higher incidence of suspensory ligament desmitis is noted in the forelimb in association with distal splint bone fractures.[1,3,5–7,11]

More complicated fractures of the proximal part of the small metacarpal or metatarsal bones result from direct trauma, either from interference or direct blows to the surface. These fractures are often open initially, which frequently results in osteomyelitis. In some cases there is not a break in the skin initially, but the comminuted fractures become sequestered and result in recurrent draining tracts. Fractures of the second metacarpal bone of racehorses also have been associated with excessive torsional forces that may occur in the starting gate.

Clinical Signs

On visual observation, swelling is usually a prominent feature of proximal splint fractures, but it may or may not be present with distal splint fractures. In general, the degree of swelling associated with the distal splint fracture depends on the acuteness of the fracture. The more acute the fracture, the more swelling. Associated swelling in the suspensory ligament as well as the fetlock joint may also be observed.

In the acute case, in both instances, horses frequently point their foot. Trotting exercises may or may not cause lameness, but this is totally dependent on the acuteness and type of fracture that has resulted. Circling or fast work may be required to cause sufficient lameness to be observed.

On palpation, heat, pain, and swelling are obvious features of acute fractures, and in some cases draining tracts are also present. The pain and heat decrease with time. However, because callus formation is a frequent sequelae to the nonsurgically treated fracture, the fracture site will become enlarged over time (Figure 5.200). In cases in which only mild pain is evidenced with palpation, yet the horse is quite lame, the limiting features of this horse resuming performance may be associated with suspensory ligament desmitis or fetlock arthrosis.[1,3,5–7,11] To gain a full appreciation of the involvement of the small metacarpal or metatarsal bone, the limb is flexed so the full extent of this bone can be palpated. A thorough physical examination of the suspensory ligament should follow.

Diagnosis

A persistent swelling over the affected splint bone, exhibiting heat and pain when pressure is applied, should lead one to suspect a fractured splint bone. Some fractured splint bones closely resemble the disease called splints. Some such fractures heal, but the bony swelling is confused with "splints". Radiographs are necessary for a positive diagnosis of a fractured splint bone and to differentiate between a fracture of the splint bone and splints or soft tissue injury. Direct infiltration anesthesia of the fractured small metacarpal or metatarsal bone may be used in cases in which a concomitant suspensory ligament desmitis or fetlock arthrosis is present. This helps to define the contribution of the fractured splint to the lameness. This is particularly

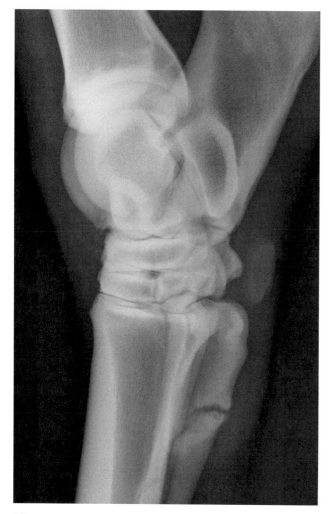

Figure 5.200. This lateral radiograph was taken 3 months after occurrence of a fourth metatarsal fracture. A large callus had developed and there is minimal bridging of the fracture line. (Courtesy of Dr. Gary Baxter.)

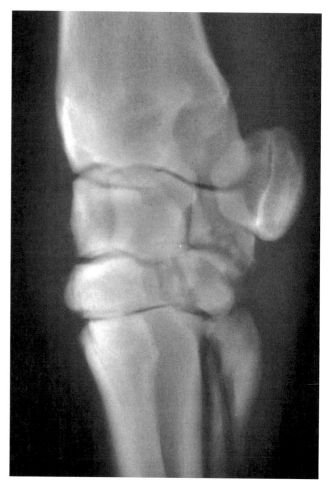

Figure 5.201. Dorsopalmar medial-to-lateral oblique radiograph of the carpus showing an oblique articular fracture of the fourth metacarpal bone.

important in cases in which minimal pain is elicited on deep palpation of the bone but the horse is quite lame.

Radiographs should be taken in all cases to identify the fracture, its limits, and whether sequestration and osteomyelitis exist in association with a complicated fracture. The proximal fractures may extend toward or into the carpometacarpal or tarsometatarsal joint (Figure 5.201).

Treatment

Small Distal Fractures

Small distal fractures of the splint bones are traditionally treated by removing the distal fragment, but this approach is not universally recommended.[7,11] Up to two-thirds of the length of the splint can be removed without untoward sequelae; however, distal splint fractures can heal spontaneously and are not usually the continued cause of lameness. Nonunion distal splint fractures are frequently not the cause of lameness and evaluation of the concomitant suspensory desmitis is warranted. In conclusion, surgical removal of these

distal splint fractures is often not necessary, but may be performed, particularly for persistent fractures. At least 70% of horses with distal splint fractures have suspensory desmitis, which is generally agreed to be the cause of continued lameness.[11]

Closed Nonarticular and Nondistracted Proximal Comminuted Fractures

Closed nonarticular and nondistracted proximal comminuted fractures of the splint bones may heal successfully with 2 to 4 months of rest. In hindlimb lateral metatarsal fractures, the horses will be minimally lame and training can continue after the acute inflammation is resolved (approximately 30 days). Surgery may become necessary if:

1. Draining tracts develop
2. Lameness and pain associated with the fracture are moderate to marked
3. Exuberant bony callus impinges on the suspensory ligament
4. Infection is present
5. A nonunion or sequestra is developing on follow-up radiographs

6. A faster recovery and return to performance is desired

If surgery is required, it should be performed aseptically with the horse placed in lateral or dorsal recumbency.

Two surgical approaches have been successful: removal of the fractured fragments only or removal of the fracture and distal splint bone. If the fracture is in the proximal third, any contiguous piece of bone present should remain to stabilize the proximal component. In closed fractures in which more than two-thirds of the splint bone is to be removed, a small bone plate is recommended to stabilize the remaining proximal fragment.[4,10] If the proximal fragment is not anchored, excessive movement of this fragment may occur and result in interosseous desmitis, degenerative OA of the carpometacarpal or tarsometatarsal joints, or avulsion of the proximal fragment. Screw fixation is less frequently successful. The small metacarpal bones appear to be more predisposed to avulsion after proximal fractures than the metatarsal bones because of the major attachments of the collateral ligaments.

Open Distal and Middle Fractures

Open distal and middle fractures of the splint bone often lead to draining tracts or sequestra, so it is recommended to treat these surgically with open removal of the fracture with or without the distal splint. The distal splint bone is left if it seems to provide some stability to the proximal fragment.

Open Proximal Fractures

Open proximal fractures of the splint bones have a more guarded prognosis, but most require surgery due to draining tracts, sequestra, infectious arthritis, and unstable proximal fragments. The fracture can be stabilized with bone plates[10] or extirpated completely if it involves the fourth metatarsal bone[2] with 60% success (Figure 5.202). It is possible to treat open comminuted fractures with antimicrobials and lavage of the wound after removal of any loose fragments. This technique can be successful if the proximal fragment is not avulsed (displaced) and if septic arthritis has not occurred. Retained sequestra are a frequent consequence and may result in recurrence of swelling and drainage months later. Open surgical treatment is optimal to address all damaged tissue and remove all fragments.

If more than two-thirds of the splint bone is removed and it appears unstable and active infection is not present, a small bone plate can be secured to the proximal portion of the splint and the cannon bone using 3.5-mm screws. If the fourth metatarsal bone is involved, bone plates may be abandoned for complete removal of the splint bone. If placement of a plate is felt to result in implant infection, the proximal portion can just be left and if luxation occurs, can be addressed at that time. This may give adequate time for the wound to clean up and decrease the chance of infecting the repair.

For an optimal cosmetic end result, bandages are maintained for a minimum of 6 weeks postoperatively. The horse should be maintained in a stall for at least a

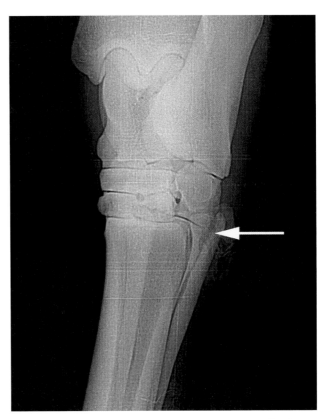

Figure 5.202. Open, articular, comminuted proximal fourth metatarsal fracture (arrow) that was initially debrided and treated conservatively. Infection persisted and the entire fourth metatarsus was removed. (Courtesy of Dr. Gary Baxter.)

total of 6 weeks. Hand walking exercise can begin at about the second week after surgery and free exercise can begin after 6 weeks. Training is usually initiated after 2 to 3 months of rest and is totally dependent on the degree of soft tissue damage associated with the fracture site.

Prognosis

For distal splint bone fractures, the prognosis for return to performance depends on the severity of suspensory desmitis, not on the radiographic healing of the fracture.[3] In a retrospective study of 34 cases of distal splint fractures without suspensory ligament desmitis, 75.3% of the horses returned to previous levels of performance, and only 50% of the horses with suspensory ligament desmitis accompanied by the fractured splint resumed to previous levels of performance.[9] In another series with an increased percentage of suspensory ligament desmitis, only 25% of the horses returned to previous levels of performance.[3]

The prognosis for comminuted closed splint bone fractures is good to excellent with or without surgery, particularly if the horse is used for performances other than racing.[4] The prognosis for open comminuted splint bone fractures is good to excellent with surgery if approximately one-third of the proximal splint remains. The prognosis for open comminuted fractures of the proximal splint is more guarded and about 60% return to performance without lameness. Surgery is necessary in these cases or sequestration, osteomyelitis, and infectious arthritis may persist.

References

1. Allen D, White NA. Management of fractures and exostosis of the metacarpals and metatarsals II and IV in 25 horses. Equine Vet J 1987;19:326.
2. Baxter GM, Doran RE, Allen D. Complete excision of a fractured fourth metatarsal bone in eight horses. Vet Surg 1992;21:273.
3. Bowman KF, Evans LH, Herring ME. Evaluation of surgical removal of fractured distal splint bones in the horse. J Vet Surg 1982;11:116.
4. Bowman KF, Fackleman GE. Surgical treatment of complicated fractures of splint bones in the horse. J Vet Surg 1982;11:121.
5. Doran R. Fractures of the small metacarpal and metatarsal (splint) bones. In Equine Fracture Repair. Nixon AJ, ed. WB Saunders, Philadelphia. 1996;200–207.
6. Doran R. Management of simple and complicated splint bone fractures in horses. Equine Pract 1994;16:29.
7. Duprezz P. Fractures of the small metacarpal and metatarsal bones (Splint bones). Equine Vet Ed 1994;6:279.
8. Harrison LJ, May SA, Edwards GB. Surgical treatment of open splint bone fractures in 26 horses. Veterinary Record 1991;128:606.
9. Jones RD, Fessler TF. Observations on small metacarpal and metatarsal fractures with or without associated suspensory desmitis in standardbred horses. Can Vet J 1977;18:29.
10. Peterson PR, Pascoe JR, Wheat JD. Surgical management of proximal splint bone fractures in the horse. Vet Surg 1987;16:367.
11. Verschooten F, Gasthuys F, De Moor A. Distal splint bone fractures in the horse: An experimental and clinical study. Equine Vet J 1984;16:532.

SUSPENSORY LIGAMENT DESMITIS

The suspensory ligament is predominantly a strong, tendinous band containing variable amounts of muscular tissue.[10] It originates from the palmar carpal ligament and the proximal palmar surface of the third metacarpal bone in the forelimb and descends between the second and fourth metacarpal bones. In the distal metacarpus it divides into 2 branches that insert on the proximal sesamoid bones. The extensor branches pass obliquely dorsad to join the common digital extensor tendon in the proximal phalangeal region. The suspensory apparatus is continued distally as the straight, oblique, cruciate, and short distal sesamoidean ligaments. The suspensory ligament phylogenetically represents the median interosseous muscle and is also known as the interosseous muscle or proximal (superior) sesamoidean ligament.[6–8]

The percentage of muscle in each region has been identified; Standardbreds had 40% more muscle in their suspensory ligament than did Thoroughbreds, and it has been suggested that this may be associated with biomechanical differences in gait between the 2 breeds or genetic factors. *In vitro* strength testing of the suspensory apparatus in training and resting horses suggests that there is an increase of strength with training. The absolute load to failure in a single load-to-failure compression test was higher in horses that had been in racehorse training, and failure in the trained group was usually by fracture of a proximal sesamoid bone. In the untrained group, the suspensory ligament failed.[2]

Injuries to the suspensory ligament can be divided into 3 areas:

1. Lesions restricted to the proximal one-third (proximal suspensory desmitis)
2. Lesions in the middle one-third, sometimes extending into the proximal third (body lesions)
3. Lesions in the medial and/or lateral branch (branch lesions)

Proximal suspensory desmitis (PSD), or inflammation of the origin of the suspensory ligament, is the most common cause of soft tissue injury to the limbs, comprising approximately 30% of tendon/ligament injuries[24] and approximately 60% of soft tissue injuries that localize to the proximal metacarpus/metatarsus (MC/MT).[2] Proximal suspensory desmitis occurs most commonly in sport horses, such as event horses, jumpers, and racehorses. The hindlimbs are more frequently affected that forelimbs and have a lower success rate of returning to performance after rest and convalescence; 69% for hindlimbs vs. 80% for forelimbs.[2] Overall, lameness associated with the origin of the suspensory ligament occurs in about 5% of horses (36 of 1,094 horses and 31 of 638 horses) with a forelimb lameness.[6,7,8]

Injury can be exclusively within the ligament, involve tearing of the Sharpey fibers at the origin of the suspensory ligament, or be associated with avulsion fracture(s) of the origin of the suspensory ligament that involve the proximal MC/MT. High PSD and acute tearing of Sharpey fibers may present with similar signs as those described for blind splints and desmitis of the carpal (distal) check ligament.[20] In chronic cases of tearing of the origin of the suspensory ligament, radiographic evidence of bone resorption and surrounding sclerosis is present. With avulsion fracture of the origin of the suspensory ligament, either the lateral or medial branch may be involved in 1 or both limbs and will likely be noted on radiographs or seen as a displaced piece of bone on ultrasound (Figure 5.203). This lameness most frequently occurs in Standardbreds, hunters and jumpers, and polo ponies, but other breeds are affected as well.[21]

Injury to the body of the suspensory ligament is less common and occurs most frequently in racehorses, specifically Standardbred racehorses. The body of the ligament also is usually involved in cases of degenerative suspensory ligament desmitis (DSLD).[13] In general, lesions of the body of the suspensory have a more guarded prognosis for return to full athletic work than proximal injury or injury of the branches of the suspensory.[25]

Injury to the suspensory ligament branches occurs most commonly in Standardbred racehorses or jumping horses. Frequently, disease of the fetlock joint, such as OA or dorsal proximal phalanx fracture, occurs concomitantly. "Bowing" or "springing" of the distal ends of the splint bones and fracture of the distal splint bones is associated with desmitis of the branches of the suspensory. This finding is considered a result of the enlargement of the branches physically forcing the ends of the splint bones abaxially. This predisposes the splint bones to fail or fracture at their thinnest point. These fractures do not heal spontaneously because the splint bones are under tension. Lameness is often due to the suspensory problem and not the fracture.

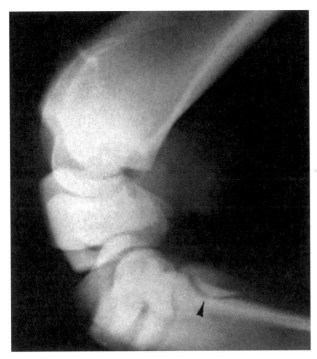

Figure 5.203. Lateral radiograph of the carpus and proximal metacarpus demonstrating a saucer-shaped avulsion fracture (arrow) of the metacarpus at the origin of the suspensory ligament. (Courtesy of Dr. Ted Stashak.)

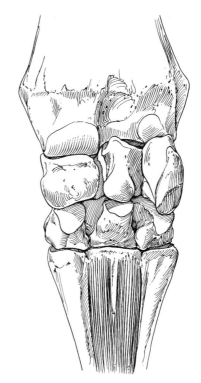

Figure 5.204. The attachments of the suspensory ligament at the proximal palmar surface of the third metacarpal bone. (Courtesy of Dr. Ted Stashak.)

Etiology

The suspensory ligament (SL) is primarily made up of dense white fibrous connective tissue. Proximally, the body of the suspensory ligament separates and attaches into 2 palmar depressions just distal to the carpometacarpal or tarsometatarsal joints (Figure 5.204). Overloading of the SL may cause sprain trauma to any portion of the ligament, but origin injuries are seen more commonly in sport horses. Hyperextension of the carpus/tarsus in conjunction with severe overextension of the fetlock joint has been proposed to cause proximal lesions. In general, the more severe the sprain trauma, the more severe the ligamentous lesion. Working horses in deep, soft arenas or in eventing where there is excessive rotational movement of the limbs may increase the risk of injuries. Lesions in the body or branches of the suspensory also occur in sport horses worked in soft ground. Therefore, soft tissue injuries, including suspensory injuries, occur more frequently in Europe where horses race and train on turf. Lesions within the branches are also associated with fetlock lameness and suggest that high rotary motion of the fetlock may predispose to suspensory branch injury as may occur in racehorses and animals with dropped fetlock conformation.

Clinical Signs

Most horses with PSD present with a history of intermittent lameness of several days' or week's duration that is exacerbated by resumed exercise. The onset may be acute or insidious. Generally, heat and swelling are palpable on the proximal aspect of the limb only in

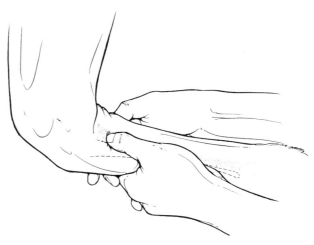

Figure 5.205. Location for digital palpation of the origin of the suspensory ligament in the forelimb. The origin is easier to palpate in the forelimb than in the hindlimb.

acute cases. In chronic, intermittent cases, physical findings are less obvious or may not be present to assist with a diagnosis. However, slight proximal swelling may be felt on the medial side between the suspensory ligament and deep digital flexor tendon in some cases.[4–10,15] Additionally, firm digital pressure overlying the proximal suspensory ligament in these cases usually elicits a nonfatiguable painful response (Figure 5.205). The lameness is generally mild to moderate (1 to 2+ out of 5) at a trot and may be more obvious when the horse is circled at a trot with the affected limb on the outside of the circle. Lower limb flexion exacerbates the lameness in 50% of horses with forelimb suspensory problems, and hock flexion exacerbates the lameness in 85% of horses with hindlimb suspensory pain.[7]

Horses with tearing of the Sharpey fibers at the origin of the suspensory ligament or avulsion fractures most frequently present with a history of acute onset of moderate to severe lameness. Horses sustaining a fracture of the origin of the suspensory ligament often have attained racing speeds in their workouts. Digital pressure at the origin of the suspensory may induce a painful response and exacerbate the lameness (Figure 5.205).

Horses with injury to the body or branches of the suspensory ligament usually have visible and palpable swelling and signs of acute inflammation at the site of injury. In more insidious onset cases, the enlarged ligament has less inflammation and is more firm. Pain on digital pressure and a positive response to fetlock flexion are common in affected horses.

Diagnosis

Proximal suspensory injury is being recognized more frequently with better use of local anesthesia techniques and the advent of diagnostic ultrasonography, nuclear scintigraphy, computed tomography, and magnetic resonance imaging (Figure 5.206).[2,4,9,11,18,25] Nuclear scintigraphy only identified hindlimb origin of suspensory abnormality when a specific region of interest was further analyzed. Subjectively, the nuclear scans appeared normal.[4] Pain withdrawal after selective digital palpation over the origin of the suspensory ligament should direct the examiner to this injury, but may not be present in some cases.

A presumptive diagnosis of proximal suspensory ligament problems can be made with physical finding and with the elimination of the lameness following direct infiltration of the origin of the suspensory ligament or perineural anesthesia. Perineural analgesia of the palmar/plantar nerves and palmar/plantar metacarpal/metatarsal nerves (high 4 point) may not eliminate the lameness because the blocks are often performed too distally. Perineural anesthesia of the lateral palmar nerve usually improves forelimb lameness (preferred technique) and can be performed just below the accessory carpal bone from the lateral aspect of the limb or on the medial aspect of the accessory carpal bone. The ulnar nerve can also be blocked to eliminate the lameness in the forelimb, and intrasynovial anesthesia of the middle carpal joint may eliminate lameness associated with the proximal suspensory ligament due to the distal outpouching of the carpometacarpal joint.[12] The deep branch of the lateral plantar nerve is desensitized to block the proximal suspensory region in the hindlimb. This block can be performed just distal to the head of the lateral splint bone and the needle directed axial to the splint. Direct infiltration of the ligament can be performed in either the forelimb or hindlimb but may interfere with subsequent ultrasound evaluation. See Chapter 3 for more information on nerve blocks.

In the forelimbs, desmitis of the distal accessory ligament of the deep digital flexor tendon also must be

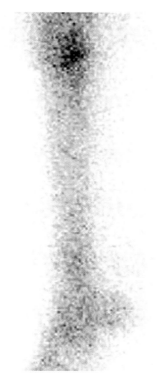
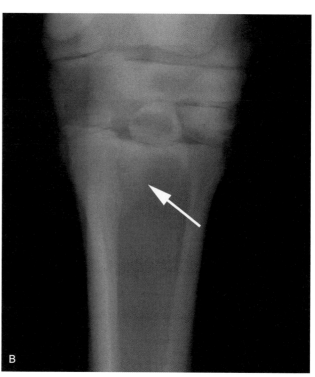

Figure 5.206. Nuclear scintigraphy can identify bone injury at the origin of the suspensory ligament (A). Radiographic lesions such as sclerosis (arrow) can be subtle (B) and usually only identified on the cranio-caudal view due to the overlap with the splint bones on the lateral view.

considered.[2] In one study, lameness due to lesions created in the flexor tendons or proximal suspensory ligament with collagenase injection was not reliably abolished until the ulnar block was added.[17] Similar results were obtained with hindlimb blocks.[14,16] Care must be taken when performing the ulnar nerve block or the lateral palmar nerve block just below the accessory carpal bone because the carpal sheath is entered 68% of the time.[12] Care also must be taken when direct infiltration of the origin of the suspensory ligament of the forelimb is done because the distal reflection of the carpometacarpal joint capsules that lie axial to the small metacarpal bone and extend distad for approximately 4 cm may be injected.

Radiographic examination may be negative for acute high suspensory ligament desmitis and tearing of Sharpey fibers. However, bone sclerosis of the trabecular pattern of the proximal plantar cannon bone, alteration of the plantar subcortical trabecular pattern, and enthesiophyte formation were noted in 23 of 47 horses diagnosed with hindlimb proximal suspensory desmitis (Figure 5.206).[7] Computed tomography can be used to better define this proliferation.[18] Early bone resorption can occur at the origin of the heads of the suspensory ligament. A fracture associated with the origin of the suspensory ligament can also be observed on radiographic examination.

Ultrasonographic examination, magnetic resonance imaging, and to some degree, computed tomography, particularly contrast CT, are the current methods for determining the damage within the origin of the suspensory ligament.[2,6,18,24,25] Computed tomography can identify enthesiophytes that surround the ligament that are not well delineated on radiographs. Nuclear scintigraphy can diagnose cases with bone involvement or remodeling, but in horses with confirmed origin of suspensory lesions has been shown to be less sensitive than expected and cannot reliably diagnose the condition.[4] Ultrasound examinations are the simplest and least expensive method and should be performed every 60 days until the ligament has healed. Morphologic abnormalities of the suspensory that are often identified include: enlargement of the ligament (linear width and circumference), poor definition of margins, hypoechoic areas central or peripheral, diffuse reduction in echogenicity, hyperechogenic foci, and irregularity of the plantar cortex of the third metatarsal bone (enthesiophyte formation).[6,8] Normally, the suspensory ligament is the most echodense structure in the palmar or plantar MC/MT.[8,24] Comparison to the contralateral limb should be performed, but the disease condition can be bilateral in 18% of horses,[8] so standardized normals should also be used.

Ultrasound and radiographic examination of the region should be followed to document and specify the type of injury. However, the lack of ultrasonographic abnormalities in the proximal suspensory ligament does not necessarily rule out a problem. Magnetic resonance imaging of horses diagnosed with proximal suspensory desmitis demonstrated abnormal high signal and enlargement or alteration in shape of the origin.[2]

Desmitis of the body and branches of the suspensory can be diagnosed with a combination of radiography and ultrasonography. Radiographs should be included to identify the concomitant bone abnormalities such as distal splint bone fractures and proximal phalangeal fractures. Ultrasonography commonly identifies enlargement and hypoechoic areas within the body or branches of the ligament.

Treatment

Treatment for horses with a structural abnormality on ultrasound and/or radiography consists of a convalescence program of confinement and slow return to exercise. Immediate medical management, including anti-inflammatories, hydrotherapy, and bandaging, is recommended to reduce any swelling that may occur and to support the fetlock. If a lesion is present on ultrasound, initially, stall rest for 2 months followed by repeat ultrasound is recommended. Hand walking for 15 minutes twice daily for the first 4 weeks and for 20 minutes twice daily for the last 4 weeks can be performed if the horse is sound at the walk, the origin lesion is not greater than 50% of the cross sectional area, and straight hindlimb conformation is not present in a hindlimb injury.[9] Trotting can begin after 8 weeks if the lesion is reasonably improved on ultrasound and the horse is sound at the trot in hand. A slow and controlled (saddle) or rein lunging exercise program can continue until 16 weeks, when another ultrasound is performed. If soundness persists and the lesion appears healed on the 16-week ultrasound exams, the horse's exercise can increase. Total healing time is 8 months and return to full competitive performance may not be possible for 1 year.

Recurrence of injury is greater in horses that have been inadequately rested and for abnormalities within the hindlimbs. Balancing the foot, shoeing with egg-bar shoes, and using sport fetlock support bandages can improve the flexor surface support. A more prolonged convalescent period is required if pain returns after exercise has begun. Use of oral glycosaminoglycans, systemic polysulfated glycosaminoglycans, and systemic hyaluronic acid may have benefit, although unproven. Use of internal blisters, intralesional steroids, and mineralizing agents are contraindicated.

Injection of bone marrow or autologous platelet concentrates,[1,23] ultrasound-guided desmotomy and fasciotomy,[14] and shock wave therapy[15,19] have been described for PSD injury that has significant lesions on ultrasound or does not respond as expected to confinement and medical management. Improvement in most horses occurs over 6 months of treatment. Compressive damage to the lateral plantar nerve in hindlimb proximal suspensory desmitis can confound persistent lameness, and neurectomy of the deep branch of the lateral plantar nerve may improve the lameness in these horses.[22]

In one study of suspensory desmitis of the body, autologous platelet concentrate injection in Standardbred racehorses resulted in all 9 cases returning to racing with good performance, equal to peers in money earned.[23]

In suspensory desmitis of the branches, treatment of concomitant disease of the fetlock, support bandaging, and a modified training program permits many horses to continue performing. Intralesional medical therapies described previously are also frequently performed. Surgical removal of the distal splint fractures is controversial and may not address the primary cause of lameness. In addition, core lesions of the branches of the suspensory ligaments may benefit from ligament splitting similar to that which is advocated for tendon lesions.

Horses with a dropped fetlock conformation have lost suspensory support to the limb and are at high risk of re-injury or complete suspensory ligament breakdown. Use of support bandages and heel extension shoes, such as an egg-bar, are recommended. Many of these horses are retired. In addition, horses with DSLD often have a bilaterally dropped fetlock conformation as part of the presenting clinical picture, suggesting severe damage to the suspensory ligaments.

Prognosis

The prognosis for PSD is good (greater than 80%) for return to full work in sport horses with forelimb PSD following 3 to 6 months of rest and controlled exercise.[2,10,21] For hindlimb lameness, 14% to 69% of horses returned to full athletic function without detectable lameness.[2,5] The wide variety of outcome with hindlimb PSD may be related to the greater range and tendency for more severe lesions, concomitant neuropathy and compartment syndrome, and conformational issues that predispose the suspensory ligament to greater stresses, such as dropped fetlocks and straight hocks. Recently, it was reported that neurectomy of the lateral plantar nerve resulted in an 80% return to performance for hindlimb PSD.[22] Osteostixis of the proximal metatarsus at the origin of the PSD in hindlimbs has also been reported.[14] The presence of upright hindlimb (straight hock) conformation is overrepresented in

horses with hindlimb suspensory injury and may predispose the ligament to injury and recurrence; hence, the poor success rate for permanent resolution of lameness. Another proposed reason for the poor prognosis associated with hindlimb PSD is the development of a "compartmental syndrome" resulting from the limited space available between the prominent splint bones into which the inflamed suspensory ligament can expand.[7]

Recurrence of PSD also relates to use. In one study dressage and show jumping horses had the highest recurrence rate of PSD, 37% and 46%, respectively, compared to racehorses (27%), show hunters (19%), and field hunters (18%).[3] In addition, the larger the suspensory ligament lesion, the greater the chance of recurrence. Generally, the recurrence of PSD after 1 year following successful treatment is low, but when it does occur the prognosis is guarded for return to performance. The prognosis is also reduced when PSD is associated with other lesions such as tendinitis of the superficial and deep digital flexor tendons or desmitis of the radial check ligament.[7]

The prognosis for avulsion fracture associated with the origin of the suspensory ligament appears good for uneventful recovery to full work after 3 to 6 months of rest and controlled exercise. A good blood supply is thought to be the reason for these fractures healing so readily. Horses with evidence of exostoses developing around the splint bones, but in association with PSD, may benefit from bone debridement after computed tomography.[18]

Degenerative Suspensory Ligament Desmitis (DSLD)

Degenerative suspensory ligament desmitis is a debilitating disorder thought to be limited to the suspensory

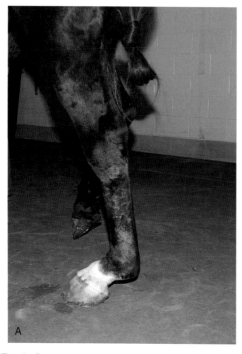
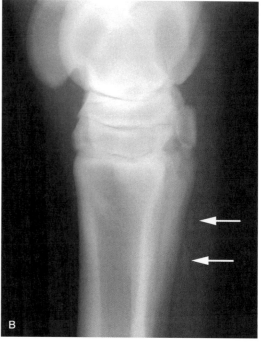

Figure 5.207. A. Severe dropping of the fetlock together with a straight hock conformation is typical of horses with DSLD. B. Dystrophic mineralization of the suspensory ligament (arrows) can sometimes be identified radiographically. (Courtesy of Dr. Gary Baxter.)

ligaments of Peruvian Pasos, Peruvian Paso crosses, Arabians, American Saddlebreds, Quarter horses, Thoroughbreds, and some European breeds. It primarily affects the body and proximal aspects of the ligament and is often bilateral. Both forelimbs or both hindlimbs can be involved and frequently the disorder leads to persistent incurable lameness requiring euthanasia. Many horses have excessive fetlock extension (dropping) on presentation and horses with hindlimb involvement often have the combination of straight hocks and fetlock hyperextension (Figure 5.207). Affected horses often have palpable enlargement and pain of the suspensory ligament. The diagnosis is usually made based on patient signalment and history, clinical examination, and ultrasonographic abnormalities within the affected suspensory ligaments. Treatment is empirical and supportive but often not effective in altering progression of the disease. Horses often remain lame or worsen, and the prognosis is poor for recovery.

The etiology of DSLD is unknown, but the disease tends to run in families, suggesting hereditary influences. However, a recent study suggests that the disease may be due to excessive accumulation of proteoglycans within the suspensory ligaments and other tissues in affected horses.[13] Histopathologic examination of horses affected with DSLD revealed increased accumulation of proteoglycans within the suspensory ligaments, superficial and deep digital flexor tendons, patellar and nuchal ligaments, cardiovascular system, and sclerae, compared to control horses. This study indicated that the abnormalities associated with DSLD are not limited to the suspensory ligaments, but affect many other tissues and organs with significant connective tissue. The authors suggested that DSLD is actually a systemic disorder of proteoglycan accumulation and propose the term equine systemic proteoglycan accumulation (ESPA) as a more appropriate name for the condition.[13]

References

1. Aquelles D, Carmona JU, Climent F, et al. Autologous platelet concentrates as a treatment for musculoskeletal lesions in five horses. Vet Rec 2008;162:208–211.
2. Brokken MT, Schneider RK, Sampson SN, et al. Magnetic resonance imaging features of proximal metacarpal and metatarsal injuries in the horse. Vet Radiol Ultrasound 2007;48:507–517.
3. Cowles RR, Johnson LD, Holloway PM. Proximal suspensory desmitis: A retrospective study. Proceed Am Assoc Eq Pract 1994;4:183–185.
4. Dyson SJ, Weekes JS, Murray RC. Scintigraphic evaluation of the proximal metacarpal and metatarsal regions of horses with proximal suspensory desmitis. Vet Radiol Ultrasound 2007;48:78–85.
5. Dyson S. Proximal suspensory desmitis in the hindlimb: 42 cases. Br Vet J 1994;150:279.
6. Dyson S. Proximal suspensory desmitis: clinical, ultrasonographic and radiographic features. Equine Vet J 1991;23:25.
7. Dyson SJ. Proximal suspensory desmitis in the hindlimb. Equine Vet J 1995;7:275.
8. Dyson SJ. Some observations on lameness associated with pain in the proximal metacarpal region. Equine Vet J (suppl) Orthopedics 1992;6:43.
9. Dyson SJ. Some observations on lameness associated with pain in the proximal metacarpal region. Equine Vet J (Suppl) 1988;6:43.
10. Dyson SJ, Arthur RM, Palmer SC, et al. Suspensory ligament desmitis. Vet Clin N Am 1995;11:177.
11. Edwards RB, Ducharme NG, Fubini SL, et al. Scintigraphy for diagnosis of avulsions of the origin of the suspensory ligament in horses: 51 cases (1980–1993) J Am Vet Med Assoc 1995;207:608.
12. Ford TS, Ross MW, Orsini PG. A comparison of methods for proximal palmar metacarpal analgesia in horses. Vet Surg 1989;18:146.
13. Halper J, Kim B, Khan A, et al. Degenerative suspensory ligament desmitis as a systemic disorder characterized by proteoglycan accumulation. BMC Vet Res 2006;12:2–12.
14. Hewes CA, White NA. Outcome of desmoplasty and fasciotomy for desmitis involving the origin of the suspensory ligament in horses: 27 cases (1995–2004). J Am Vet Med Assoc 2006; 229:407–412.
15. Imboden I, Waldern NM, Wiestner T, et al. Short-term analgesic effect of extracorporeal shock wave therapy in horses with proximal palmar metacarpal/plantar metatarsal pain. Vet J 2008;179:50–59.
16. Keg PR, Barneveld A, Schamhardt HC, et al. Clinical and force plate evaluation of the effect of a high plantar nerve block in lameness caused by induced mid-metatarsal tendinitis. Vet Q (16) Suppl 1994;2:S70.
17. Keg PR, Van Den Belt AJ, Merkens HW, et al. The effect of regional nerve blocks on the lameness caused by collagenase induced tendinitis in the midmetacarpal region of the horse: a study using gait analysis, and ultrasonography to determine tendon healing. Zentralbl Veterinarmed A 1992;39:349.
18. Launois MT, Vandeweerd JM, Perrrin RA, et al. Use of computed tomography to diagnose new bone formation associated with desmitis of the proximal aspect of the suspensory ligament in third metacarpal or third metatarsal bones of three horses. J Am Vet Med Assoc 2009;234:514–518.
19. Lischer CJ, Ringer SK, Schnewlin M, et al. Treatment of chronic proximal suspensory desmitis in horses using focused electro hydraulic shockwave therapy. Schweiz Arch Tierheikd 2006; 148:561–568.
20. Marks D, MacKay-Smith MP, Leslie JA, Soule SG. Lameness resulting from high suspensory disease (HSD) in the horse. Proc Am Assoc Equine Pract 1981;27:493–498.
21. Personett LA, McAllister ES, Mansmann RA. Proximal Suspensory Desmitis. Mod Vet Pract 1983;541–545.
22. Toth F, Schumacher J, Schramme M, et al. Compressive damage to the deep branch of the lateral plantar nerve associated with lameness caused by proximal suspensory desmitis. Vet Surg 2008;37:328–335.
23. Waslelau M, Wutter WW, Genovese RL, Bertone AL. Intralesional injection of platelet-rich plasma followed by controlled exercise for treatment of midbody suspensory ligament desmitis in Standardbred racehorses. J Am Vet Med Assoc 2008; 232:1515–1520.
24. Wood AK, Sehgal Cm, Polansky M. Sonographic brightness of the flexor tendons and ligaments in the metacarpal region of horses. Am J Vet Res 1993;54:1969–1974.
25. Zubrod CJ, Schneider RK, Tucker RL. Use of magnetic resonance imaging to identify suspensory desmitis and adhesions between exostoses of the second metacarpal bone and the suspensory ligament in four horses. J Am Vet Med Assoc 2004;224: 1815–1820.

SUPERFICIAL DIGITAL FLEXOR (SDF) TENDINITIS (BOWED TENDON)

Tendinitis of the superficial digital flexor tendon (SDFT) comprised 29% of soft tissue injuries in Warmbloods and Standardbred racehorses, just behind 32% for suspensory ligament injuries, in one study.[26] Unlike suspensory ligament injury, SDFT injury is almost exclusively a forelimb problem. Lesions can range from peritendinous inflammation and pain without structural damage to complete tendon rupture. Tendinitis usually results in a high degree of morbidity with prolonged periods out of work.

Classical SDF tendinitis is localized to the mid metacarpal region in the forelimb and appears as a convex "bow" to the visual profile of the metacarpus on the side view, hence the term "bowed tendon" (Figure 5.208). Anatomically, the SDFT is the most superficial of the flexor tendons/suspensory ligament and therefore

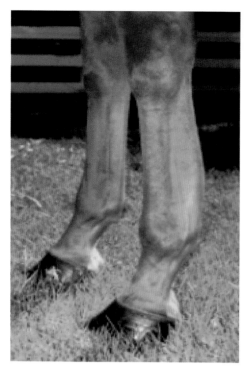

Figure 5.208. Classic appearance of SDF tendinitis of the left forelimb. Note the convex palmar surface to the middle region of the metacarpus.

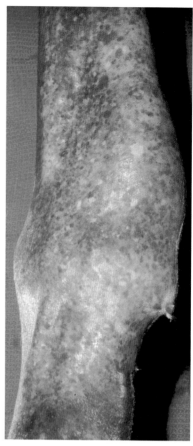

Figure 5.209. A "low bow" of the SDFT as illustrated in this image can be associated with concurrent digital tendon sheath tenosynovitis. (Courtesy of Dr. Gary Baxter.)

enlargement is readily visible and palpable.[17] In normal horses, the SDFT develops in size and tensile strength with training. The SDFT musculotendinous unit originates on the caudal humerus and extends to a bivalved attachment on the caudal eminences of the second phalanx. Therefore, complete disruption of the SDFT can be associated with dorsal subluxation of the distal first phalanx as well as dropping of the fetlock. In the author's experience, rupture of the SDFT is uncommon, but occurs most frequently in eventing horses and geriatric horses that run in pasture.

Less common locations for injuries to the SDFT are the distal MC/MT, the branches of the SDFT in the pastern region, and the caudal aspect of the carpus. Lesions in the distal cannon bone are often referred to as "low bows" and can be associated with digital sheath tenosynovitis or constriction of the anular ligament (Figure 5.209). Tendinitis of the branches of the SDFT can be difficult to diagnose because this is not a common location of injury and the classical swelling seen at other locations may not be present. See the pastern section earlier in this chapter for more details.

Damage to the SDFT in its proximal aspect is a recently reported syndrome that affects older nonrace-horses.[4] In this study, the mean age of affected horses was 18 years (range of 11 to 23 years) and Quarter horses (9 of 12 horses) were the predominant breed. Most horses had positive reactions to carpal flexion and the majority required an ulnar nerve block to alleviate the lameness (9 of 12 horses). The study concluded that tendinitis of the proximal portion of the SDFT was a cause of lameness in aged performance horses and that the prognosis for return to previous use was poor.[4]

Etiology

As the forelimb contacts the ground at the gallop, the fetlock is hyperextended and the flexor tendons placed under very high tensile loads.[12] Tendons are elastic and can store kinetic energy upon loading that assist with propulsion and support of the large body loads in a "bungee cord" effect. In the Thoroughbred racehorse, the tendon strain (elongation) can be as great as 16%, putting this structure close to its physiologic limit during maximal exercise.[26] The theory proposed for the mid-metacarpal location of lesions is that it is the central position of the "tied down" section of the tendon. Repetitive trauma to the SDFT can also result in microdamage to the collagen structure that contributes to final failure of fibrils. The proximal accessory ligament of the SDFT binds the SDFT to the caudal radius and the palmar fetlock joint tethers the ligament during maximal fetlock hyperextension. The accessory ligament of the SDFT is relatively inelastic and serves to provide support to the muscle origin during maximal loading and help prevent avulsion of the proximal muscle unit.

Clinical Signs and Diagnosis

Diagnostic advances, particularly with ultrasonography and magnetic resonance imaging (MRI), have

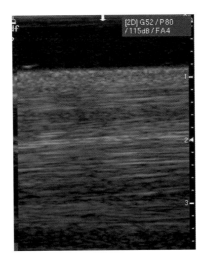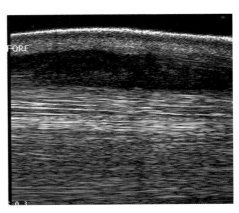

Figure 5.210. Ultrasound longitudinal sections through the midportion of a normal SDFT (left) and SDFT with acute tendinitis. Note the hypoechoic area (black) in the middle of the SDFT that usually corresponds to edema or hemorrhage in acute cases.

greatly enhanced our ability to diagnose and define the degree and extent of damage in SDFT injuries. However, a careful clinical examination can identify early focal swelling and tenderness well before a detectable lameness occurs. Intervention at this early phase can prevent structural damage to the tendon. Excellent husbandry and observant animal caretakers are keys to this early recognition.

In more significant SDFT injuries, a more diffuse enlargement, tendon thickening, and local heat with lameness after exercise occur. Severe tendon injuries are recognized clinically as horses that do not want to put the hoof flat on the ground, thereby putting tension on the flexor surface of the limb. The acute phase of SDF tendinitis can last 2 to 7 days, the subacute phase 1 to 3 weeks. Aggressive treatment of the inflammation and swelling is paramount to limiting the fibrosis and tendon disfiguration that can be permanent.

Chronic SDF tendinitis is manifested by fibrosis and firm swelling on the palmar or plantar (flexor) surface of the limb (Figure 5.208). Chronic SDF tendinitis may not have heat or edema associated with the condition, yet lameness may be present. The use of diagnostic ultrasonography enables initial and reasonably accurate determination of the extent and location of the lesions.

Skill as an ultrasonographer is important to correctly identify lesions. The increased availability of MRI has revealed some of the limitations of ultrasonography to correctly categorize lesions. A complete ultrasound examination extends from proximal to metacarpus/metatarsus, to the heel bulbs, and determines the cross-sectional area of the SDFT and the lesions at multiple locations from proximal to distal. Comparison to the contralateral side may provide a comparison and possibly identify a subclinical condition. Longitudinal scans permit the validation of structural lesions and the assessment of fiber alignment. Loss of the normal intense echogenicity (hypoechoic areas) can be caused by fibrillar disruption and/or inflammatory processes (hemorrhage, edema, and cellular infiltration in the early stages).[20,21] Ultrasound images correlate to histologic lesions. If an SDFT injury is acute/subacute and has clinical signs of inflammation, a repeat ultrasound within 2 weeks is indicated after the inflammation has subsided. Hypoechoic areas within the SDFT can be edema fluid or hemorrhage early on after the injury and may not necessarily be fiber disruption or structural damage (Figure 5.210). If the acute signs of injury have resolved, and hypoechoic areas within the SDFT persist, they likely represent fiber disruption (Figure 5.211). MRI has demonstrated an advantage over ultrasound for distinguishing fibrosis from normal tendon in chronic tendinitis.[15]

Treatment

Immediate medical and physical treatment of SDF tendinitis is recommended to reduce or eliminate the acute swelling and inflammation as rapidly as possible to prevent fiber damage or early fibrous tissue formation. Routine physical therapy such as icing, cold water hydrotherapy, massage, pressure wraps, and topical hyperosmotic sweats or diclofenac liposomal cream, along with systemic NSAIDs, is instituted along with rest until the ultrasound can be performed. In acute, severe injury such as rupture, a soft cast or resin cast may be indicated until radiographs or ultrasound can occur. The application of topical steroids ± dimethylsulfoxide is controversial, but can be very effective at eliminating signs of inflammation. Systemic steroids are generally not recommended because they may impair the early healing response. Local injections in or around the tendon are usually considered after the results of the ultrasound examination at 1 to 2 weeks, when most of the fluid accumulations (edema, blood) have resolved and the extent of fiber damage can be accurately determined.

If ultrasound examination is normal and the acute inflammation surrounding the tendon resolves within 1 to 2 weeks, then hand walking followed by a return to exercise in 30 days or so may be effective. A cautionary re-ultrasound prior to work is indicated to be certain the original ultrasound is still normal, or further damage did not occur upon retraining. If areas of hypoechoic density are noted within the tendon at ultrasound, then additional medication and rest are indicated. Lesions should be quantified and horses rested at least until follow-up ultrasounds at 60-day intervals.[18]

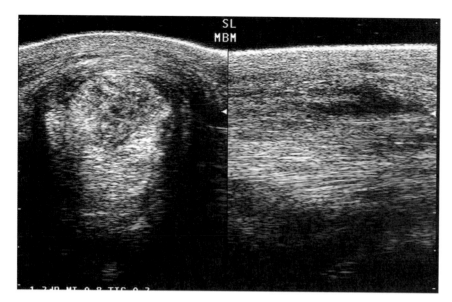

Figure 5.211. Ultrasound cross section (left) and longitudinal section (right) through an affected area of chronic SDF tendinitis. Note the hypoechoic areas (black) that usually correspond to fiber damage in chronic cases.

Many medical treatments for SDF tendinitis are used in practice. Systemic hyaluronan and polysulfated glycosaminoglycans may be used to reduce adhesions and promote extracellular matrix quality, even though they have lower levels of evidence for success; they also carry a low risk of complications.[7–9,18] Intra- or peri-lesional injection of these same drugs is used less often, and controlled experimental studies have been unable to confirm a benefit. Intra-lesional injection carries the risk of introducing infection, trauma, or further inflammation, and therefore is often not elected.

Several medical therapies have been developed specifically for tendon or ligament injuries. Injectable autologous biologic therapies such as blood, bone marrow, acellular collagen, platelet-rich plasma (PRP), and concentrated plasma were initially used for suspensory ligament injuries, but as the treatments have appeared safe in horses, many have extended their use in tendinitis. Currently, subacute or chronic tendinitis with a persistent centralized hypoechoic area may be injected with PRP or acellular collagen (Figures 5.212 and 5.213).[2] Intra-lesional injection of stem cells is most frequently used in tendinitis, and in both clinical uses of bone-marrow derived stem cells,[16,24] adipose-derived stem cells in PRP[5] and experimental use of adipose-derived stem cells[19] have shown improved tendon organization and decreased re-injury rates in racehorses. Use of ultrasound guidance for injection facilitates the injection into the lesion (Figure 5.214). Although these exogenous materials may aid tendon healing, proper rehabilitation and a convalescent exercise program remain paramount to success with any treatment.

Electromagnetic and electroshock stimulations have been proposed as treatments for tendon injury. Studies may suggest that these techniques should be used with caution because they can cause physical damage to the tissue. In a controlled study on healing of surgically created defects in equine superficial digital flexor tendons in the horse, exposure to pulsed electromagnetic field therapy for 2 hours daily significantly delayed the maturation of the tissue formed within the defect.[25]

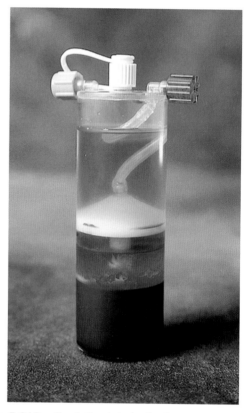

Figure 5.212. Gravitational device for the isolation of platelet-rich plasma and platelet-poor plasma.

Similarly, low-level laser therapy (also called soft or cold laser therapy) has not substantiated clinical claims of benefit.

Surgical Management of SDF Tendinitis

Two surgical procedures are described for treatment of SDF tendinitis: a tendon splitting procedure and

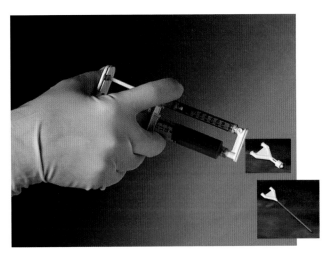

Figure 5.213. A dual port injection syringe that permits the simultaneous injection of platelet-rich plasma (PRP: red) and thrombin (clear) into SDFT core lesions. The thrombin serves to clot the PRP.

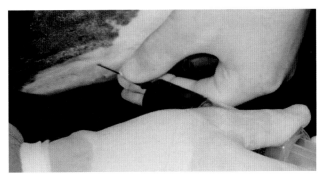

Figure 5.214. Injection of PRP into an SDFT after ultrasound identification of the site of the lesion. Small aliquots (less than 0.5 ml) of PRP can be injected 0.5 cm apart throughout the length of the lesion.

proximal accessory ligament transection on the affected forelimb (frequently both, including the unaffected limb). The surgical technique of longitudinal tendon splitting was advocated to decompress the lesion (relieve the hematoma), provide a vascularization channel to central lesions, and consequently promote healing, particularly of core lesions in injured SDF tendons. This technique is recommended for tendons with a static core lesion that is not healing. In experimental and clinical studies, tendon splitting decreased the core lesion size within 8 weeks.[1,14] Importantly, tendon fibers are separated in the longitudinal plane and not transected, with this procedure, or more fiber damage could occur.

Transection of the accessory ligament (superior check) of the SDFT has been reported to drop the fetlock angle (increase hyperextension) in normal horses[22] and has been used as a successful surgical therapy for flexural deformity of the fetlock for many decades. Transection of this ligament releases the SDFT and a gap forms at the transection site, altering the biomechanical forces on the SDFT.[22] It was theorized that transection of this ligament may alter the strain on the SDFT or the site of strain such that the technique

may be beneficial in horses with SDF tendinitis. In a retrospective study in 62 Thoroughbreds, 92% of the horses were able to train and race after proximal check ligament surgery and 66% started at least 5 races.[3] Another study in Standardbred racehorses reported that 92% of horses raced at least once after surgery and 87% raced at least 5 races, with most having had a bilateral procedure.[13] The evidence for efficacy of proximal check ligament surgery in treating or preventing re-injury in horses with SDF tendinitis may be limited, but lower re-injury rates have been reported. However, one study showed no difference from horses treated conservatively.[10]

Prognosis

Incidence of re-injury is an outcome measure of successful management of SDF tendinitis. Published reports of re-injury in horses treated conservatively with rest alone are 48%[21] and 56%.[23,24] Medical therapies such as hyaluronan, PSGAGs, or BAPTN did not show a difference in re-injury rate.[7] Stem cell therapy reports a significantly reduced re-injury rate of 18%.[24] Surgical transection of the accessory ligament of the SDFT reports a reduced re-injury rate of 25%.[13]

Rehabilitation

The value of a carefully controlled rehabilitation program combined with regular ultrasound examination has been documented as providing the best chance for an equine athlete to return to full performance following SDFT (or suspensory ligament or biceps tendon) injury.[20,] Most structural lesions need a minimum of 6 months of restricted athletic activity to allow for the majority of healing to occur, and clinical signs of lameness should be absent after a short period of rest and before any forced exercise. Tendon rehabilitation protocols are tailored according to whether the structural damage is graded as mild, moderate, or severe. In mild structural injury, the SDF has a tendon cross-sectional area (CSA) that is less than 20% greater than normal SDFT, a core lesion of 15% or less of the total tendon CSA, or a longitudinal lesion of 20% or less of the total length of the tendon. A moderate structural injury has a 20% to 35% greater CSA, a core lesion of 15% to 30% of the total tendon CSA, or a longitudinal lesion of 20% to 35% of the length of the tendon. A severe structural injury has a 35% greater CSA that normal, a core lesion greater than 30% of the total tendon CSA, and a longitudinal lesion greater than 35% of the length of the tendon.

All cases with structural injury to the tendon or suspicion of a structural injury should have an initial period of stall confinement and hand walking after acute inflammation subsides, usually a minimum of 30 days. Hand walking is generally 15 minutes twice daily from zero to 30 days. Many mild tendinitis cases can begin riding at the walk at 30 days, but most moderate and severe injuries require at least 60 days of hand walking.

A second ultrasonographic examination is made at 30 and 90 days and the tendon lesion compared to original scans. In horses with poorly healing lesions or continued lameness, other treatment modalities such as injections or surgery are considered. Horses without lameness and good grades of lesion can increase the rehabilitation exercise to include riding at a walk 30 minutes daily from 90 to 120 days, increasing over the next several months. After several months of walking, and in horses without lameness and improvement in ultrasound grade, horses can begin trotting under control. One method is to have horses trot under saddle only on the straight portions of the ring to avoid asymmetric loading on the limbs. The number of laps and times per day can be increased, gauged by the progress of the horse and tendon healing on ultrasound. Cantering can be added for 5 minutes every 2 weeks for 120 days for good and fair cases, whereas poor cases have a re-evaluation and discussion of further treatment options. No active race or jump training should begin for at least 6 months from the injury.

Arguably, a controlled exercise program may be preferable to turnout after 60 days. This statement is supported by the results of a retrospective study of 50 Thoroughbred racehorses with SDF tendinitis.[11] The severity of the lesion and type of rehabilitation were significant. Of 16 horses kept in pasture, 2 of 8 raced. Of 28 horses kept in a controlled exercise regimen, 20 of 28 raced. Successful cases usually require 8 to 9 months of rest and rehabilitation to return to their previous full workload. Shortening this period or advancing too quickly often results in worsening of the tendon lesions. The premise for use of controlled exercise is to initially reduce inflammation, maintain gliding function, and improve healing.

Prevention

Based on changes seen in tendon matrix associated with development, aging, function, and exercise, it has been hypothesized that immature tendon may have a greater adaptive ability and may respond to an appropriate exercise regimen to produce a more functionally adapted tendon.[10] Recent studies suggest that foals allowed free pasture exercise develop a larger, stronger, more elastic tendon compared to those that were confined or subjected to a training program. Effects on the noncollagenous matrix appear to be responsible for these differences. In contrast, training or excess exercise may have permanent detrimental effects on the biomechanical and functional properties of the SDFT in the foal. The implication is that the determination of optimum exercise intensity and timing and the role of the noncollagenous matrix in tendon physiology in the young horse may hold the key to developing tendons that are more capable of resisting injury. Optimal conditioning of a young horse may result in improved performance and reduced tendon injury later in life.[6,23]

References

1. Allen AK. Experience with ultrasound-guided tendon puncture or splitting. In Proceed Am Assoc Equine Pract 1992;38: 273–277.
2. Arquelles D, Carmona JU, Climent F, et al. Autologous platelet concentrates as a treatment for musculoskeletal lesions in five horses. Vet Rec 2008;162:208–211.
3. Bramlage LR, Rantanen NW, Genovese RL, et al. Long term effects of surgical treatment of superficial digital flexor tendinitis by superior check desmotomy. In Proceed Am Assoc Equine Pract 1988;34:655–656.
4. Chesen AB, Dabareiner RM, Chaffin MK, et al. Tendinitis of the proximal aspect of the superficial digital flexor tendon in horses: 12 cases (2000–2006) J Am Vet Med Assoc 2009;234: 1432–1436.
5. Del Bue M, Ricco S, Ramoni R et al. Equine adipose-tissue derived mesenchymal stem cells and platelet concentrates: their association in vitro and in vivo. Vet Res Commun 2008;Suppl 1:S51.
6. Dowling BA, Dart AJ. Mechanical and functional properties of the equine superficial digital flexor tendon. Vet J 2005; 170:184–192.
7. Dyson SJ. Medical management of superficial digital flexor tendinitis: a comparative study in 219 horses (1992–2000). Equine Vet J 2004;36:415–19.
8. Foland JW, Trotter GW, Powers BE, et al. Effect of sodium hyaluronate in collagenase-induced superficial digital flexor tendinitis in horses. Am J Vet Res 1992;53:2371–2376.
9. Gaughan EM, Gift LJ, DeBowes RM. The influence of sequential intratendinous sodium hyaluronate on tendon healing in horses. VCOT 1995;8:40–45.
10. Gibson KT, Burbidge HM, Pfeiffer DU. Superficial digital flexor tendinitis in thoroughbred race horses: outcome following non-surgical treatment and superior check desmotomy. Aust Vet J 1997;75:631–5.
11. Gillis CL, Meagher DM, Peal RR, et al. Ultrasonographically detected changes in the equine superficial digital flexor tendon during the first month of race training. Am J Vet Res 1993;54:1797–1802.
12. Goodship AE. The pathophysiology of flexor tendon injury in the horse. Equine Vet Educ 1993;5:23–2986.
13. Hawkins JF, Ross MW. Transection of the accessory ligament of the superficial digital flexor muscle for the treatment of superficial digital flexor tendinitis in the Standardbred: 40 cases (1988–1992). J Am Vet Med Assoc 1995;206:674–678.
14. Henninger RW, Bramlage LR, Bailey M, et al. Effects of tendon splitting on experimentally-induced acute equine tendinitis. VCOT 1992;5:1–9.
15. Kasashima Y, Kuwano A, Katayama Y, et al. Magnetic resonance imaging application to live horse for diagnosis of tendinitis. J Vet Med Sci 2002;64:577–82.
16. Lacitiqnola L, Crovace A, Rossi G, et al. Cell therapy for tendinitis, experimental and clinical report. Vet Res Commun 2008;Suppl 1:S33–8.
17. Madison JB. Acute and chronic tendinitis in horses. Compend Contin Educ 1995;853–856.
18. Marr CM, Love S, Boyd JS, et al. Factors affecting the clinical outcome of injuries to the superficial digital flexor tendon in National Hunt and Point-2-Point racehorses. Vet Rec 1993; 132:476–479.
19. Nixon AJ, Dahlgren LA, Haupt JL, et al. Effect of adipose-derived nucleated cell fractions on tendon repair in horses with collagenase-induced tendinitis. Am J Vet Res 2008; 69:928–37.
20. Rantanen NW, McKinnon AO. Equine Diagnostic Ultrasonography. Williams and Wilkins, Baltimore, 1998.
21. Rooney JR, Genovese RL. A survey and analysis of bowed tendon in Thoroughbred racehorses. Equine Vet Sci 1981; 1:49–53.
22. Shoemaker RS, Bertone AL, Mohammad LN, et al. Desmotomy of the accessory ligament of the superficial digital flexor muscle in equine cadaver limbs. Vet Surg 1991;4:245–252.
23. Smith RK, Birch LH, Patterson-Kane J, et al. Should equine athletes commence training during skeletal development? Changes in tendon matrix associated with development, aging, function and exercise. Equine Vet J 1999;S30:201–209.
24. Smith RK. Mesenchymal stem cell therapy for equine tendinopathy. Disabil Rehabil 2008;30:1752–8.
25. Stevens PR, Nunamaker DM, Butterweck DM. Application of a Hall-effect transducer for measurement of tendon strains in horses. Am J Vet Res 1989;50:1089–1095.
26. Watkins JP, Auer JA, Morgan SJ, Gay S. Healing of surgically created defects in the equine superficial digital flexor tendon: effects of pulsing electromagnetic field therapy on collagen-type transformation and tissue morphologic reorganization. Am J Vet Res 1985;46:2097–2103.

DEEP DIGITAL FLEXOR TENDINITIS

Strain injuries of the deep digital flexor tendon (DDFT) in the metacarpal or metatarsal region are uncommon compared to injuries of the superficial digital flexor tendon (SDFT), accessory ligament of the deep digital flexor tendon (ALDDFT), or suspensory ligament (SL) on the basis of both postmortem surveys[8] and ultrasonographic examinations.[3,6] However, many DDFT lesions are within the hoof and cannot be seen with ultrasound.

Etiology

Classic deep digital flexor (DDF) tendinitis in the distal metacarpal/tarsal area is usually traumatic in origin, but direct blunt trauma may be a more common cause than with SDF tendinitis. Excessive strain (stretch) of the tendon, usually as it passes over the fetlock, can induce inflammation or structural damage. The anatomic confluence with the digital sheath and anular ligament relatively immobilize the DDFT at this site, possibly predisposing this area to injury. Horses that hit themselves around the fetlock region with other limbs during exercise can induce a DDF tendinitis. DDF tendinitis can be confused with SDF tendinitis and distal accessory desmitis based on visual appearance (Figure 5.215).[7]

Many, if not most, DDFT abnormalities are degenerative in nature and are located in the distal phalangeal region of the forelimb. Distal injuries of the DDFT caudal to the flexor cortex of the navicular bone are a well recognized postmortem and MRI finding and are considered part of the heel pain syndrome.[4] Fraying of the dorsal DDFT is theorized to cause friction on the proximal sesamoid bone and intersesamoidean ligament.[4,5]

Clinical Signs

DDF tendinitis is suspected with careful physical and lameness examination. It can be confused with distal SDF tendinitis (low bow) or desmitis of the distal accessory ligament of the DDFT (distal check desmitis) on visual examination and palpation, especially if edema or hemorrhage blend the structures (Figure 5.215). Limbs should be palpated both with load on and off the limb. In unloaded limbs, the SDFT can be moved off of the DDFT permitting better palpation. If injury of the DDFT has occurred within the digital sheath, sheath distention can also make palpation of the structures more difficult. In both SDF low bow and DDF tendinitis, a convex appearance to the caudal limb just above the proximal aspect of the anular ligament occurs, suggesting a relative anular ligament constriction.

Horses with acute injury to the DDFT are usually lame, and lameness recurs after rest of less than 30 days. Any soft tissue injury to the limbs that does not resolve within 30 days or is associated with lameness should have an ultrasound examination and/or MRI to determine the structures involved and the extent of structural damage. If ultrasound does not reveal any lesions at the 60-day follow-up and lameness persists, MRI should be performed. Contrast CT has been used to assess angiogenesis of DDF tendinitis and can be used as an alternative to MRI.[5]

In one study, classic traumatic induced DDF tendinitis was seen in 24 cases with ultrasonographic lesions in the DDFT in the metacarpo-metatarsal region.[1] Clinical signs included a sudden onset of mild to moderate lameness associated with filling of the digital flexor tendon sheath. Intrasynovial analgesia of the DFTS consistently improved the degree of lameness in all cases. Regional 4-point blocks also produced a significant improvement but there was a less consistent response to abaxial sesamoid nerve blocks. On ultrasound examination, 20 of 24 cases had small, distinct, often circular focal hypoechoic areas within the DDFT in the distal metacarpus/metatarsus, usually within the digital sheath and proximal to the proximal sesamoid bones. These hypoechoic areas tended to be localized and extended only a short distance proximodistally (usually less than 1 cm). The lesions were considered focal rather than true "core" lesions as seen in the SDFT and could be easily missed if not carefully examined through the digital sheath. All cases had an increase in the amount of fluid in the DFTS.

Longitudinal tears of the DDFT in racehorses have been reported and can be initially thought to be DDF tendinitis. Ultrasound examination has failed to identify the tears in a significant number of horses. Most longitudinal tears occur within the sheath, and effusion should direct the clinician to further investigation of the digital tendon sheath. See the section on digital flexor tendon sheath tenosynovitis.

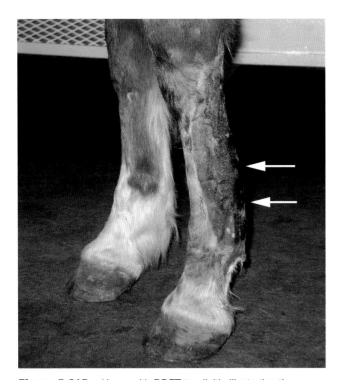

Figure 5.215. Horse with DDFT tendinitis illustrating the location of many of these lesions in the distal aspect of the metacarpus (arrows). However, the swelling can appear similar to SDF tendinitis. (Courtesy of Dr. Gary Baxter.)

Treatment

Treatment of DDF tendinitis is similar to that of SDF tendinitis in terms of physical therapy, systemic medical management, and convalescence. DDF tendinitis may be treated surgically with distal accessory desmotomy for the same reasons that SDF tendinitis may be treated with proximal accessory desmotomy, to relieve tension on the DDFT.[2] Literature supporting this treatment is limited, partly due to the rarity of the condition. Injuries to the DDFT within the sheath are frequently treated as a DDF tenosynovitis, in addition to treatment of the tendon injury. See the digital tenosynovitis in the the pastern section.

Prognosis

The prognosis for DDF tendinitis is guarded, depending on severity. In one study of 24 cases,[7] only 7 returned to athletic use.

References

1. Barr ARS, Dyson SJ, Barr FJ, O'Brien JK. Tendinitis of the deep digital flexor tendon in the distal metacarpal/metatarsal region associated with tendinitis of the digital sheath in the horse. Equine Vet J 1995;27:348–355.
2. Becker CK, Sabelberg HHCM, Buchner HHF, Barneveld A. Long-term consequences of experimental desmotomy of the accessory ligament of the deep digital flexor tendon in adult horses. Am J Vet Res 1998;59:347–351.
3. Genovese RL, Rantanen NW, Hauser ML, et al. Diagnostic ultrasonography of equine limbs. Vet Clin North Am Equine Pract 1986;2:145–226.
4. Mair TS, Kinns J. Deep digital flexor tendinitis in the equine foot diagnosed by low-field magnetic resonance imaging in the standing patient: 18 cases. Vet Radiol Ultrasound 2005;46:458–66.
5. Puchalski SM, Galuppo LD, Drew CP et al. Use of contrast-enhanced computed tomography to assess angiogenesis in deep digital flexor tendonopathy in a horse. Vet Radiol Ultrasound 2009;50:292–7.
6. Reif VB, Martin BB, Elser A. Types of tendon and ligament injuries detected with diagnostic ultrasound: description and follow-up. In Proceedings Am Assoc Equine Pract 1988;245–247.
7. Webbon PM. The racing performance of horses with tendon lesions treated by percutaneous tendon splitting. Equine Vet J 1979;1:264–265.
8. Webbon PM. A histological study of macroscopically normal equine digital flexor tendons. Equine Vet J 1978;10:253–259.

DESMITIS OF THE ACCESSORY LIGAMENT OF THE DEEP DIGITAL FLEXOR TENDON (DISTAL CHECK LIGAMENT)

The accessory ligament of the deep digital flexor tendon (ALDDFT) (distal or inferior check ligament) is a direct continuation of the palmar carpal ligament and fuses to the DDFT in the proximal metacarpus.

Etiology

The ALDDFT provides stability to the hyperextended carpus in the midstance phase of the stride because it shares tensile load with the DDFT.[3] Desmitis of the ALDDFT has been reported as a fairly common forelimb injury, third behind suspensory desmitis and SDF tendinitis. This condition is reported in pleasure horses, ponies, and show jumpers; is less frequent in racehorses and event horses;[2] and may not be recognized as a serious problem initially.[4]

Clinical Signs

Lameness occurs suddenly after work and is associated with visual and palpable swelling in the proximal metacarpus of often older horses (older than 10 years) within 24 hours.[4] Ultrasound examination reveals enlargement of the diameter of the accessory ligament and hypoechoic areas indicating edema, hemorrhage, or fiber damage. Swelling in this region tends to persist and progress to a firm fibrosis. Lameness is consistent and improves with rest, but recurs with resumed exercise, similar to other soft tissue injuries to the flexor surface of the forelimb.

Treatment

Treatment of ALDDFT differs from that of SDF or DDF tendinitis in that the accessory ligament structure is not considered paramount to supporting the load in the working horse. Therefore, treatments may be more geared toward eliminating pain and lameness. Treatment has empirically included oral nonsteroidal medication, intralesional hyaluronan injection to reduce adhesions, and intralesional injection of steroid to reduce pain and inflammation as well as to reduce fibrosis.

Desmotomy of the ALDDFT may relieve excessive tension on a fibrotic ALDDFT in chronic cases (greater than 3 months); in one study, only 14% to 18% made a full recovery.[5] It has been suggested that desmotomy may prevent re-injury.[1] Horses that have received a desmotomy of the ALDDFT as a treatment for chronic rotation of the third phalanx can have pain at the desmotomy site when returned to full work. Similar medical treatment as described above can be effective in eliminating pain. Topical nonsteroidal and steroidal mediations can be effective.

As with all other soft tissue injuries to the flexor surface of the metacarpus/metatarsus, a controlled convalescent exercise program should be followed based on lameness and ultrasound examination at 60-day intervals.

Prognosis

The reported prognosis for resolution of pain and return to work is guarded. In one study of 27 horses, 12 (44%) resumed work within 5 months and 10 (37%) eventually resumed full work. It is strongly recommended that controlled exercise be used, rather than pasture turnout, and that lameness is resolved long before healing is complete. The horse's return to work should be based on the results of serial ultrasonographic appearance.

References

1. Becker CK, Sabelberg HHCM, Buchner HHF, Barneveld A. Long-term consequences of experimental desmotomy of the accessory ligament of the deep digital flexor tendon in adult horses. Am J Vet Res 1998;59:347–351.
2. Dyson SJ. Desmitis of the accessory ligament of the deep digital flexor tendon: 27 cases (1986–1990). Equine Vet J 1991; 23:438–444.
3. Leach D, Harland R, Burko B. The anatomy of the carpal tendon sheath of the horse. J Anatomy 1981;133:301–307.

4. McDiarmid AM. Eighteen cases of desmitis of the accessory ligament of the deep digital flexor tendon. Equine Vet Educ 1994;6:49–56.
5. Van den Belt AJM, Becker CK, Dik KJ. Desmitis of the accessory ligament of the deep digital flexor tendon in the horse: clinical and ultrasonographic features. A report of 24 cases. Zentralbl. Veterinarmed (A) 1993;40:492–500.

TENDON LACERATIONS

Etiology

Tendon lacerations in the MC/MT regions occur more commonly to the extensor tendons than flexor tendons due to the dorsal location and vulnerability to trauma. They also occur more commonly in the hindlimbs than forelimbs. Horses are prone to deep lacerations that may involve tendons, due to their flight response, kicking defense, and high speeds. Horses may jump sharp objects or fences, or often pull excessively if their lower limb is trapped, inciting significant tendon injury.

Clinical Signs

Complete severance of tendons may result in a characteristic gait deficit. If the extensor tendons are severed, the lower foot may move more freely and the horse may intermittently knuckle at the fetlock due to failure to extend the digit during limb placement (Figure 5.216). Horses are often not lame on weight-bearing with extensor tendon injuries.[3] Complete severance of both the DDFT and SDFT results in hyperextension of the fetlock and the toe coming off the ground during limb placement (Figure 5.217). Laceration of just the SDFT causes the fetlock to drop with normal foot placement (Figure 5.217). If the suspensory ligament is still intact, the fetlock provides some support. If the suspensory ligament is also severed, the fetlock drops almost to the ground. Weight-bearing lameness accompanies flexor tendon lacerations.[1] Immobilization of limbs with lacerated DDFT and SDFT to support the fetlock and prevent further injury should be performed similar as with fractures.

Diagnosis

Digital palpation of the wound can reveal the extent of the laceration to the tendons in most cases (Figure 5.218). Wounds should be prepared aseptically prior to digital exploration and sterile gloves should be worn. Care should be taken to not push foreign material deeper into the wound and to not separate soft tissues, because vital structures such as an artery, tendon sheath, or joint could be damaged or entered. Extensor tendon injuries are often avulsion type trauma with loss of skin over the dorsal aspect of the cannon bone (Figure 5.216). Secondary bone trauma and sequestration of the cannon bone often accompany these severe injuries. Ultrasound examination also defines partial tears and possibly locates foreign material. Systemic assessment is critical because these horses may have lost significant blood or have other injuries and be in a state of shock.

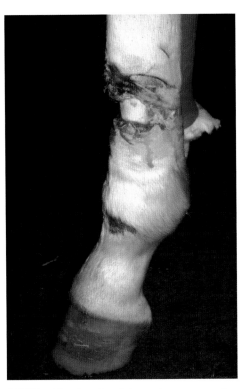

Figure 5.216. The dorsal metatarsus is a common location for extensor tendon lacerations and many injuries also involve the metatarsus. (Courtesy of Dr. Gary Baxter.)

Treatment

Routine first aid management of all wounds is recommended initially. For complete extensor tendon lacerations, and if indicated by duration of injury and other criteria, the optimal approach is to close the wound, reappose the tendon ends, and provide support to the fetlock to prevent knuckling for at least the first 6 weeks of healing. This results in the most rapid healing and return to function, and best cosmetic outcome. However, many extensor tendon lacerations cannot be closed due to the severity of the trauma and are treated with second intention healing. Weight-bearing can be permitted for extensor tendon lacerations, so splints, soft casts, or resin-reinforced bandages can suffice for the fetlock support. The primary goal of immobilization is to prevent dorsal knuckling of the fetlock. Suture reapposition of the extensor tendon ends is not required for successful outcome. Conservative management of the wound and extensor tendon laceration can result in complete return to athletic use. Removal of sequestra from the dorsal cannon bone may need to be performed to permit healing in severe injuries.

In general, flexor tendon lacerations are a more serious injury than lacerations of the extensor tendons and are therefore more difficult to treat. For flexor tendon lacerations, the optimal approach is wound debridement and closure, tendon apposition with suture, and cast application for approximately 4 to 6 weeks (Figure 5.218). Double locking loop or the

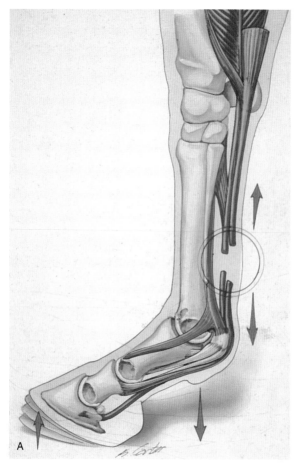
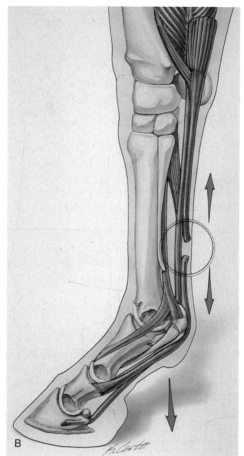

Figure 5.217. Illustration of the biomechanical effects of lacerations of both the SDFT and DDFT (A) and just the SDFT (B) in horses with flexor tendon lacerations. Arrows indicate distractive forces on the tendon ends, dropping of the fetlock, and elevation of the toe. (Courtesy of Dr. Gary Baxter.)

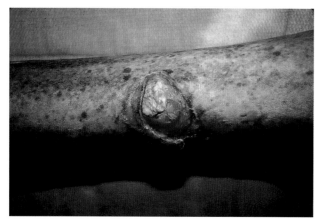

Figure 5.218. Typical location and appearance of a laceration of the flexor tendons in the mid-metatarsal region. The SDFT can be seen outside the wound and digital palpation revealed a lacerated DDFT as well. (Courtesy of Dr. Gary Baxter.)

three-loop pulley suture patterns are recommended for repair of the flexor tendons. Occasionally the tendon ends cannot be re-apposed for a variety of reasons. Wound debridement and closure can still be performed because the tendons will heal with gap healing, provided they are adequately immobilized with a half-limb cast. For wounds that cannot be closed, use of boots and immobilizing splints (Kimzey splint) can achieve acceptable results, but management of these wounds is much more difficult than if casts are used.[1] If the digital sheath is concurrently involved with the laceration, tenoscopic exploratory of the digital sheath or lavage of the sheath should be performed to improve the prognosis.[2] Closure of the tendon laceration together with the digital sheath are indicated in most cases unless gross contamination is present.

Prognosis

Extensor tendon lacerations have a good to excellent prognosis (better than 70%)[3] for return to full function with minimal intervention. Complications include prolonged healing and recurrent treatment of wounds and excessive granulation tissue and scar. Horses that are left untreated or turned out without fetlock support can develop permanent flexural deformity of the fetlock.

Flexor tendon lacerations have a good prognosis for pasture or breeding soundness and a guarded to fair prognosis for athletic soundness. Complications include restrictive fibrosis, infection, and chronic delayed healing due to tendon sheath involvement. Management of flexor tendon lacerations is an expensive proposition due to the long-term care and continual shoe support out to 6 months after surgery. Details on the surgical technique can be found in other texts.[1]

References

1. Dyson S, Bertone AL. Tendon Lacerations and Repair. In Diagnosis and Management of Lameness in Horses. Dyson SJ, Ross MW, eds. WB Saunders, Philadelphia. Part VIII:2003;712–716.
2. Fraser BS, Bladon BM. Tenoscopic surgery for treatment of lacerations of the digital flexor tendon sheath. Equine Vet J 2004; 36:528–31.
3. Mespoulhes-Riviere C, Martens A, Bogaert L, et al. Factors affecting outcome of extensor tendon lacerations in the distal limb of horses. A retrospective study of 156 cases (1994–2003). Vet Comp Orthop Traumatol 2008;21:358–64.

THE CARPUS

Chris Kawcak

The carpus is composed of 3 joints: the antebrachio-carpal (radiocarpal) joint lies between the distal radius and the proximal row of carpal bones, the middle carpal (intercarpal) joint lies between the proximal and distal row of carpal bones, and the carpometacarpal joint lies between the distal row of carpal bones and the proximal third metacarpus (Figure 5.219). The proximal row of carpal bones is comprised of the radiocarpal bone, intermediate carpal bone, ulnar carpal bone, and accessory carpal bone. The distal row of carpal bones is comprised of the second, third, and fourth carpal bones, and occasionally the first carpal bone. These bones have been shown to move independently through strong intercarpal ligaments that help to dissipate the axial stress through the carpus.

Although the antebrachiocarpal joint is usually isolated from the other carpal joints, one report has documented a communication to the middle carpal and carpometacarpal joints.[32] The middle carpal and carpometacarpal joints communicate routinely and on occasion the antebrachial carpal joint and the carpal sheath can communicate.[87] Of clinical significance is the fact that the carpometacarpal joint has distal palmar outpouchings that extend distally to the axial side of the second and fourth metacarpal bones. This area interdigitates with the proximal suspensory ligament; therefore, infusion of anesthetic into this area may inadvertently lead to anesthesia of the carpometacarpal and middle carpal joints. Conversely, injection of the middle carpal joint may lead to inadvertent desensitization of the proximal suspensory ligament area.[33]

Disease within the carpus often results from stress-induced fatigue damage that leads to osteochondral damage at consistent sites, especially in racehorses. Carpal disease can also result from acute damage that can lead to osteochondral damage at inconsistent sites or damage to the soft tissues, which typically occurs in nonracehorses and as acute traumatic incidences in all horses. Because of the consistency of stress-induced damage within racehorses, clinicians are more likely to give a reliable prognosis based on large retrospective studies of these problems. However, acute lesions in unusual sites are often difficult to treat, and it is difficult to give an accurate prognosis. In addition, osteoarthritis is common in the carpus in all breeds and can either result from progression of obvious damage early in life or can be insidious in onset later in life.

Osteoarthritic carpi typically manifest into progressive joint space narrowing, osteophyte and enthesiophyte formation, and restricted range of motion. Often there is varus deformity due to medial collapse of the joints. Regardless of the site of pain within the carpus, horses with carpal pain typically show limb abduction while moving at both the trot and the walk, and consequently have a very short gait. Although synovial effusion of the carpal joints is usually indicative of primary carpal pain, a lack of effusion can occur in cases of primary subchondral bone pain. Conversely, veterinarians must also be careful of swelling in structures other than the carpal joints such as the extensor tendon sheaths and acquired bursitis lesions such as hygromas. Effusion in either structure can be mistaken for synovial effusion of the dorsal aspect of the carpal joints.

DEVELOPMENTAL ABNORMALITIES OF THE CARPUS

Developmental abnormalities of the carpus are one of the most common problems at birth in young horses. The types of developmental problems can be classified into 3 categories:

1. Angular limb deformities or deviation in the frontal plane are defined by the joint and/or bone at the center of the deviation and further defined by the placement of the distal limb in reference to that

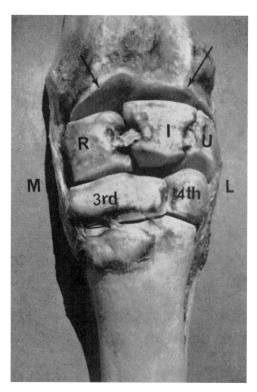

Figure 5.219. Normal left bony carpus. The joints (from proximal to distal) are the antebrachiocarpal (radiocarpal), middle carpal (intercarpal), and carpometacarpal. Arrows, areas where chip fractures may occur on the radius; M, medial; L, lateral; R, radial carpal bone; I, intermediate carpal bone; U, ulnar carpal bone; 3rd, third carpal bone; 4th, fourth carpal bone.

center.[9] For instance, in the carpus the distal limb is medial to the carpus in foals that have carpal varus and the distal limb is lateral to the carpus in those that have carpal valgus. It should be noted that most foals are born slightly carpal valgus because there is greater musculature on the lateral aspect of the distal radius compared to the medial, thus providing increased tension across the carpus on the lateral side of the limb. However, with birth and growth, this usually self resolves to a normally straight limb.

2. Flexural deformities are defined as deviations in the sagittal plane of the knee so that the joint of reference is cranial or caudal to a line drawn down the center of the limb from the lateral side.[9]

3. Rotational deformities occur when the limb distal to the point of origin rotates outward or inward from the normal axis.[9]

Angular and flexural deformities are usually pathologic in origin and often require prompt therapy. However, rotational deformities are often conformational and the origin often occurs proximal to the carpus. In those foals in which angular and flexural deformities are deemed to be of clinical significance, prompt therapy is needed to prevent lameness and loss of future athletic performance.

Angular Limb Deformity

Angular limb deformities (ALD) in general are discussed in Chapter 11, but more detail is provided here on ALD of the carpus. Angular limb deformities of the carpus are one of the most commonly treated problems in equine medicine. However, mistakes are often made using both over-conservative and over-aggressive approaches to treatment. An understanding of the normal developmental patterns of the limbs is essential to avoid these mistakes.

Etiology

Angular limb deformities can result from asymmetric growth in the distal radial metaphysis, asymmetric growth of the distal radial epiphysis, incomplete ossification of the cuboidal bones or the proximal aspect of the second and fourth metacarpal bones, and/or joint laxity. Angular limb deformities are typically congenital or acquired in nature.

Congenital abnormalities such as incomplete ossification of the cuboidal bones and collateral ligament laxity are not uncommon. It is hypothesized that uterine malpositioning or stagnant movement within the uterus can lead to decreased growth. Some feel that this is more common in overweight brood mares;[69] however, this has been subjectively noticed within small mares as well. Over nutrition of the mares in the latter part of the pregnancy has also been of concern and it is important that a nutritionist be consulted during this time frame in pregnancy.

Toxic chemicals and other possible endocrine influences have also been linked to congenital angular limb deformities.[2,34,74] As an example, in a study in which foals were fed low copper levels in their diets, their incidence of angular limb deformities was significantly higher than those fed normal copper levels.[43] In addition, hypothyroidism in foals, possibly due to low iodine, has also been linked to angular limb deformities.[73]

Some foals are born somewhat dysmature and may have joint laxity in general in the carpus. Constant monitoring and reassessment is needed in these cases because sometimes the stress of turnout or small pen exercise is enough to strengthen those tissues and self correct the problem. However, in these individuals, care must be taken to avoid excessive exercise, which could lead to progressive angular limb deformity. In these latter cases, progressive laxity can lead to pathologic stress levels within the carpal bones, possibly leading to carpal bone malformation.

Acquired angular limb deformities often result from developmental orthopedic disease in which a change in endochondral ossification of the long bones and cuboidal bones can occur. This often occurs within the first 3 to 6 months of life and is commonly found in foals that are heavy in size, on high energy nutrition, have a mineral imbalance, (such as low copper and calcium and high phosphorous), genetically susceptible due to a heritable trait, suffer from asymmetric limb loading induced by poor foot care, or suffer from excessive exercise or lack of exercise. The problem has been reported to be over represented in males compared to females.[9]

Foals that have acquired ALD are usually born normal but the limb starts to deviate with time. This can be caused by unrecognized congenital ALD that worsens, trauma to the physis or the epiphysis, lameness on a contralateral limb, over nutrition as a foal which induces large body mass, inappropriate exercise, lack of exercise, excess exercise, or poor conformation with growth.[9] As an example, foals that have narrow chests at birth and yet straight limbs have a propensity to develop a wide chest that may lead to carpal varus in the future. In these cases it is good to examine the mare and possibly the stallion to try to determine the type of conformation that may influence the joints in the future. If trauma to the physis or epiphysis is severe enough, the growth may actually stop on that side due to damage to the physeal cartilage, sometimes leading to bone bridging across the physis.[34]

Regardless of the cause of the deformity, understanding the role of the common stresses through the joint is key to developing a diagnostic and treatment plan. The rate and magnitude of physeal and epiphyseal growth are dictated by the stresses experienced within those areas. For instance, in mild cases of angular limb deformity, the increased stress on the concave side of the joint can stimulate growth and therefore help in self correction. However, if a critical threshold is reached in which that part of the physis is either overstimulated or understimulated, the deformity can either become worse or static in nature, respectively. Super physiologic stresses often lead to complete stoppage of growth and sometimes bridging of bone across the physis.

Clinical Signs and Diagnosis

The most important information that a veterinarian can give an owner about foals is that they require constant monitoring during growth. Foals can be considered to be easily deformable due to a number of factors during growth, as mentioned above, and they require at least weekly monitoring to stay ahead of rapid changes. For instance, a lameness of any cause in any limb may cause secondary angular limb deformities in other limbs. Therefore, during history taking it is important to know how often the foal has been monitored and the changes noted by the owner since birth. The history should reveal whether these foals were normal at birth, if they were premature, the diet of the mare and foal, and when the ALD was first noticed.

The foal should be examined both statically and dynamically. It should be allowed to freely walk around in order to not induce an abnormal stance through handling (Figure 5.220). This should be done for several minutes because clinical impressions can easily change

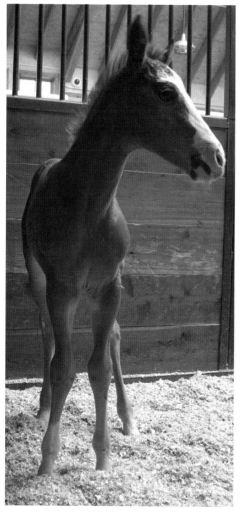

Figure 5.220. A foal demonstrating normal degree of carpal valgus expected after birth in the left forelimb and a moderate carpal valgus of the right forelimb. Notice that the foal is standing fairly square on its own, providing a good examination. However, the examination findings should be an assessment based on several minutes of examination.

based on how the foal is standing. It is also common to examine the limb with the veterinarian standing at the foal's shoulder, looking straight down through the radius, carpus, and third metacarpus to assess angular limb deformity. In addition, because rotational deformities are common with carpal ALD, care must be taken not to overinterpret the severity. For instance, it is common to see outward rotation of the limb in addition to a carpal valgus deformity. If the foal is examined from directly in front of the foal then this rotational deformity can make the ALD look worse than it really is. It is important to remember to stand directly in front of the face of the particular carpus. In the case of the previous example, the examiner must stand dorsolateral to the midline plane of the foal to accurately assess each carpus.

In some instances the author recommends that periodic photographs be e-mailed for review and in these cases it is important to remind the owner that the photographs must be taken directly in front of the face of the carpus. It is common to recommend taking several photographs starting at the very front of the foal and rotating laterally right and left in front of the knee.

During physical examination, the foal can be manually "squared up" if needed; however, that must be taken into consideration along with assessment of the foal moving around freely and standing freely. The foal should also be walked to characterize foot flight. For instance, it is not uncommon in foals with carpal varus to break over the dorsolateral aspect of the foot, in which case they may actually swing the limb out. The same is true with carpal valgus, in which the foal may swing the leg medially due to dorsomedial break-over. The conformation of the hoof can often help in determining break-over, because the site of break-over—either dorsolateral or dorsomedial—will be worn compared to the other side.

During physical examination it is important to identify the site of deformity and estimate its severity, characterizing it as mild, moderate, or severe. Some people advocate the use of a goniometer; however, classifying these into mild, moderate, and severe is sometimes just as effective. It is important to jog these foals or let them run free in a small pen to determine whether a subtle lameness is present, especially in an opposing limb, and to palpate the limbs for effusion, physeal pain, and swelling (Figure 5.221). It is also important to manipulate the limb to characterize any joint laxity. Physeal swelling in particular should be palpated for pain because septic physitis can be insidious in onset and severity.

The above physical examination techniques can only be performed if the foal is sound and standing. When which the foal is recumbent, it can be observed while trying to stand. If this cannot be accomplished and if the owner has not seen the foal stand and nurse, then serum IgG concentrations in the foal should be assessed. If the foal is lying down, joint laxity must be assessed and if there is severe ALD it is important to assess whether this is reducible and if swelling is present anywhere on the limb. The limb should be put through a full range of motion to assess whether pain is involved and to assess the full range of extension and flexion.

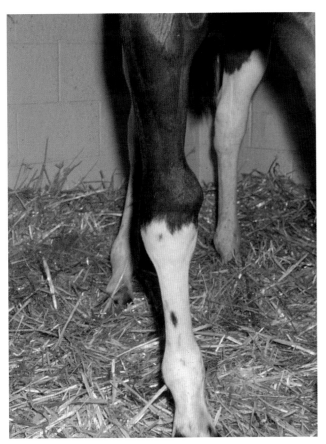

Figure 5.221. A weanling's limb showing mild carpal varus deformity and physeal swelling on the medial aspect of the distal radius.

DIAGNOSTIC IMAGING

Radiographs of the carpus should be performed on long films to include the distal radius and proximal cannon bone for points of reference for measuring ALD. It is important to remember that the growth status of the physes often cannot be accurately assessed radiographically. For instance, characterizing a physis as open or closed is difficult radiographically, since growth stops well before radiographic evidence is seen. In particular, assessment of distal radial physeal closure cannot be accurately estimated with radiographs, because it is not uncommon for the physis to remain visible even after growth has stopped.

Both dorsopalmar and lateromedial views are necessary. On the dorsopalmar views, lines are drawn dissecting both the distal radius and the proximal third metacarpal bone; the area where the lines intersect helps to describe the location within the joint in which the deviation is occurring (Figures 5.222 and 5.223).[15] For instance, if the intersection occurs within the joints, then cuboidal bone malformation often is to blame for the ALD. A goniometer can be used to measure the severity of angulation. In addition, lines can be drawn through the joint surfaces and distal radial physis, and the line or lines that deviate from perpendicular to the third metacarpal bone can be identified as the site of deviation.

Care must be taken not to overinterpret these results. It is not uncommon to have to sedate foals to acquire radiographs, and the sedated stance may not truly represent the severity of deformity. In most cases sedation can make any degree of joint laxity worsen the radiographic findings.

In addition to measuring angles, the degree of ossification, malformation, and damage to the joint must be characterized. It is recommended that a full series of carpal radiographs be taken if initial films show any signs of damage, because subtle damage can affect the prognosis. It is not uncommon in the physes to see metaphyseal flare, asymmetrical widening of the physes, sclerosis of the physes (which usually occurs on the concave surface), physeal widening (which usually occurs on the convex side of the deformity), epiphyseal wedging, carpal bone wedging (which primarily occurs in the third carpal bone), distal displacement of the ulnar carpal bone or the fourth metacarpal bone, and increased angulation of the head of the fourth metacarpal bone.[10,12,83] Although it is important to characterize these findings, their significance on prognosis is questionable. In addition, any osteochondral fragments, signs of physeal trauma, septic physitis, osteomyelitis, or arthritis must be taken into consideration because their presence significantly affects the prognosis. In general, most people characterize the degree of angulation as mild (5° to 10°), moderate (15° to 25°), or severe (more than 25°).

Treatment

Treatment of angular limb deformities of the carpus depends on the severity and type of deformity that is present. Conservative therapy is often used for most congenital causes of ALD. Sometimes, in mild cases of deformity, this is as simple as stall rest in addition to proper trimming for normal break-over of the hoof. In foals with carpal valgus, the dorsomedial aspect of the foot is typically worn because the foal will break over in that location. Therefore, the dorsolateral aspect should be trimmed to achieve a normal appearing foot. Some advocate medial extension, although there is concern that this could lead to angular limb deformities in the fetlock joint, and some advocate the use of excessive dorsolateral trimming. The author prefers to use extensions instead of excessive trimming, especially in foals that are toed out in addition to being carpal valgus. In the author's experience, prolonged use of medial or lateral extensions can lead to abnormal changes in the growth of the fetlock joint, at least until the time of distal third metacarpal physeal closure (3 to 4 months).

Nutritional status of the foals should also be assessed and corrected if abnormalities are detected.

If the degree of palpable joint laxity is significant, the angulation is severe, and/or there is decreased ossification of the cuboidal bones, then a tube cast or splints may be necessary to axially align the joints (Figure 5.224). A tube cast or splint is usually applied from the proximal radius distally to the level of the fetlock joint. It is important to leave the foot out so stimulation of muscle contraction of the forelimb can be continued to minimize limb weakening.

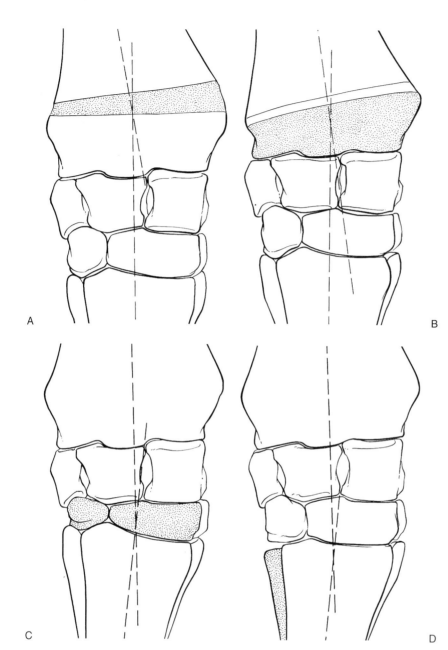

Figure 5.222. Front view of the distal radius carpus. Stippling indicates problem areas. A. The pivot point is centered over the physis, which is caused by asynchronous growth of the distal radial metaphysis. B. The pivot point is centered over the distal epiphysis of the radius, which is caused by wedging of the epiphysis. C. The pivot point is centered over the carpal joints, which is caused by wedging of the third carpal bone and hypoplasia of the fourth carpal bone. D. The pivot point is centered over the distal carpal joints, which is caused by incomplete development of the lateral small metacarpal bone. (Courtesy of Dr. Ted Stashak.)

The techniques for applying tube casts and splints include a bandage alone, bandage plus PVC pipe placed on the caudal aspect of the limb, and bandage plus a cast which is either placed on the caudal aspect of the limb or a true tube cast that surrounds the limb. Regardless of the type of application, these should be changed every 7 to 10 days and usually are needed for approximately 14 days. The author tries to minimize external coaptation, which weakens the limb and can cause significant sores.

Keep in mind that significant problems can result in a foal in a tube cast or in a splint, particularly slippage of the cast or the foal outgrowing the cast. Cast sores are a major problem in foals; if there is any concern about the foal's use of the limb or if heat is detected in the cast, it is best to change it at that time.[89] It is recommended that tube casts and splints be applied under

general anesthesia after physically straightening the limb. The author has successfully used a customized sling and buggy system, especially in foals that have incomplete ossification of their carpal and tarsal bones.

In some cases of mild ALD, brief turn-out may be helpful when the foal is thought to be strong enough. However, close observation is needed, especially in the first few days. It is important to observe the foal before it goes out and assess the degree of angular limb deformity. The typical recommendation is to turn the foal out for a couple of hours initially, and reassess the degree of deformity when the foal comes back in. It is not uncommon to see the ALD worsen and/or the foal develop a mild flexural deformity and/or shaking in the carpal joints when it comes in. If this occurs, the foal's amount of turn-out should be decreased until these

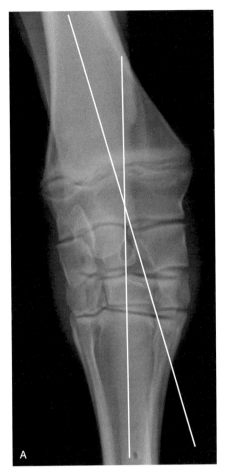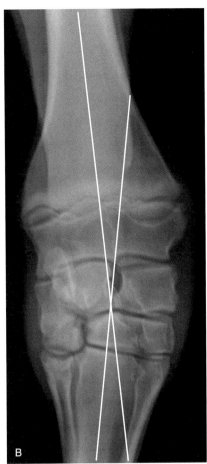

Figure 5.223. Radiographs demonstrating how lines can be used to determine the site of angulation in carpal ALD cases. A. Distal radial epiphysis. B. Intra-articular.

signs cease. Foals usually respond quite rapidly, reaching significant or even full turn-out within 7 to 14 days. Increased turn-out may help strengthen and broaden the chest in narrow-chested foals in which carpal angular limb deformity and external limb rotation are concerns, resulting in a more normal limb conformation. A varus deformity can develop if these cases are operated on too soon, with the chest widening later.

Surgical options are used when the foal either fails to respond to conservative therapy or the angulation is severe enough that it is unlikely to correct on its own. Periosteal transection has been used for decades to help correct angular limb deformities.[3,41] The rationale is that endochondral ossification is stimulated on the side in which the periosteum is transected and elevated (Figure 5.225).[3,20] In the carpus this is typically done on the concave side of the distal radial metaphysis 3 cm proximal the physis.

There are several techniques for doing this. The author prefers to make an incision down to and through the periosteum, approximately 2 to 3 cm proximal to the physis. The soft tissues are elevated and a curved blade is used to transect the periosteum in a cruciate pattern. Care must be taken not to enter the carpal canal or the tendon sheaths in that area.[39] The edges of the flap are elevated. It is important to resect the distal ulnar remnant at this time. Specifically, 1 to 2 cm length of the ulnar is removed with rongeurs. Subcutaneous

tissues are then closed and absorbable sutures are typically placed in the intradermal layer for closure. Limbs are bandaged for approximately 7 days, and depending on the degree of severity, foals can be turned out after bandage removal. Turn-out sometimes helps to further stimulate the effect of the periosteal transection.

The efficacy of periosteal stripping has come under debate in recent years.[85,91] Although some clinicians feel that it still has merit, two studies demonstrated its lack of efficacy.[85,91] The studies are that the limb will correct on its own with proper foot trimming. Slone found that there was no difference between horses that underwent the procedure and those that had stall rest and appropriate hoof manipulation.[91]

Transphyseal bridging, which retards growth on the convex side of the limb, is more predictably effective than periosteal transection for correcting angular limb deformity.[36] The procedures include:

1. Placing 2 screws and a figure-8 wire on the convex side, in which a screw is placed proximal and distal to the physis and wire interlaced between the screws to stop the growth on that side
2. Placing a staple or plate across the physis[9]
3. Placing a transphyseal screw at an angle across the physis on the convex side (recently advocated procedure)

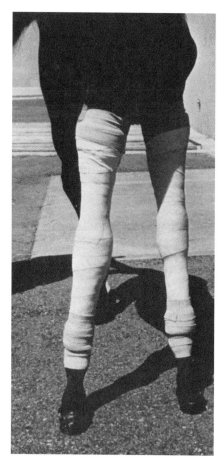

Figure 5.224. Front view of sleeve casts applied to both forelimbs. (Courtesy of Dr. Ted Stashak.)

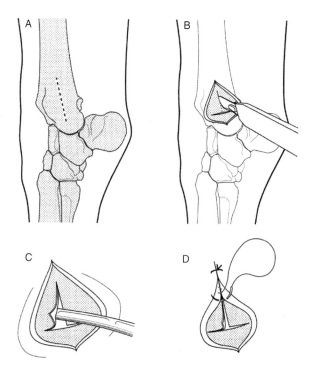

Figure 5.225. A. Incision for hemicircumferential transection of the periosteum. B. Transverse incision in the periosteum 2.5 cm proximal to create an inverted "T." C. The periosteum is elevated. D. Suture apposition of the subcutaneous tissue. Note that the incised periosteum is left open.

Significant growth does not slow in the distal radial physis until approximately 16 months of age; therefore, transphyseal bridges can be used out to 16 to 20 months of age in the carpus.[35] These bridges are most effective between zero and 8 months of age, when the most rapid growth occurs. Bridges also can be used in severe cases younger than 6 months of age or in older cases that are nonresponsive. The author prefers to use the screw and wire technique in foals less than 6 months of age[107] and a transphyseal screw in those older than 6 months because there is concern that bone bridging can occur across the physis and overcorrect the deformity after removal of the transphyseal screw. However, Witte and Hunt[107] have not seen this as a problem.

The concern with the transphyseal screw technique is that although it is simple and quick, the effects of the screw on normal physeal physiology are not completely understood. The screw and wire technique can be used through 2 stab incisions and then the tissues in between undermined to place the wire to minimize scarring and potential soft tissue complications. It is not necessary to countersink the screws because that makes removal more difficult. In addition, some surgeons feel that the screws can be offset in the cranial-to-caudal direction to address rotational abnormalities that may originate at the carpus (Figure 5.226).

Screw removal can generally be done standing or under a quick general anesthesia in more difficult foals. An 18-gauge needle can be used to find the distal most screw in the epiphysis—this screw is subjectively more difficult to find and remove. Once identified, a stab incision can be made. It is important to remove all soft tissues from the screw head before removing the screw. The proximal screw is more easily palpable, but if not, the 18-gauge needle can be used to identify it and the same technique used. The wire or wires can then be grasped and pulled out through the proximal incision. The skin is sutured and a bandage placed for approximately 7 days.

In some cases a dorsomedial toe extension is preferred to help further stimulate growth correction, although it is reserved for foals older than 3 to 4 months of age to avoid problems with fetlock ALD.

Complications can include infection, screw breakage, wire breakage, and overcorrection.

In addition to fixation, in severe cases in which bone bridging is thought to occur, the physis can be resected and fat graft interposed to keep the physis open.[38]

Prognosis

The prognosis is good to excellent in more than 80% of the cases.[3,10,12,36] However, Mitten, et al. found that in 199 racehorses, although there was no significant difference in the ability to start, foals that had periosteal transection experienced a slight decrease in the percentage of starts, a slight decrease in the number of 2-year-

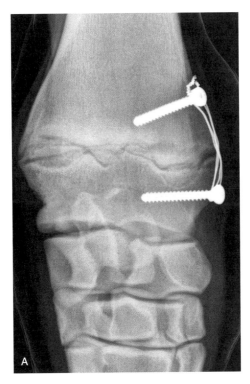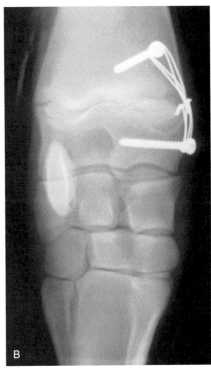

Figure 5.226. Postoperative radiographs from a normally placed transphyseal bridge using the screw-and-wire technique (A), and one in which the screws are offset in the cranial-to-caudal direction to try to manipulate a rotational deformity in the limb (B).

old starts, and a slight decrease in the starts percentile ranking number compared to a nontreated group. Although the limbs were deemed to be straight, the investigator concluded that other factors in the carpus could have led to these reduced outcome parameters in cases treated with periosteal transection.[76] There is concern that significant ALD of the carpus could lead to subtle but permanent deformity within the carpal bones. This could theoretically lead to abnormal forces within the carpus, which is another reason to address these promptly.

Flexural Deformity

Flexural deformity, commonly known as bucked knees, is thought by some to occur in 3% to 4% of foals.[9] While mild cases are typically uneventful (Figure 5.227), severe cases can result in dystocia during birth. The deformities, characterized by a disparity in length between the muscle-tendon unit and bone, can be congenital or acquired. Acquired deformities occur between 1 and 6 months of age.

Etiology

The pathogenesis of flexural deformity is unknown. Autosomal trisomy in 2 foals has been associated with this problem.[17] It has been hypothesized that the more common congenital occurrences are due to uterine malpositioning; poor mare nutrition; exposure of the mare to influenza, Sudan grass, locoweed, or other agents; and trauma to the limb, in which increased flexor tone and decreased extensor tone are noted.[71,72]

Acquired flexural deformity can be induced by rapid growth, overnutrition, or pain in the limb. Rapid growth

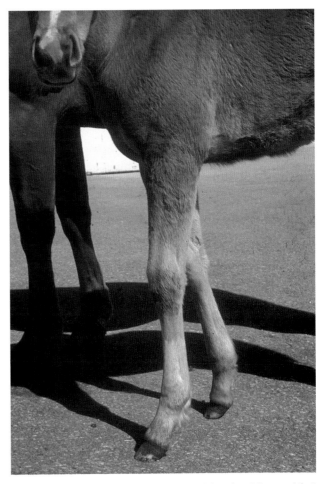

Figure 5.227. A foal with mild flexural deformity of the carpi that did not require treatment because it self-corrected over a few days.

is thought to induce physeal pain and consequently some of these foals stand with their carpi flexed to relieve the pain. In addition, damage to the suspensory ligament, superficial digital flexor tendon, or deep digital flexor tendon, or injury to the heel or carpal pain can cause the foal to rest the limb in a flexed fashion, leading to contracture of those tissues.

It is not uncommon to see mild flexural deformity in foals that have been turned out soon after birth. In these cases it is thought that the normal exercise, especially in those foals that may be slightly dysmature, can lead to microdamage within the physes and consequently pain. This tends to improve on its own within a couple of hours of rest. In addition, rupture of the common digital extensor tendon can lead to flexural deformity; however, it is unknown whether the rupture causes the deformity or vice versa.

Clinical Signs

The degree of flexural deformity is variable and usually involves both front limbs. In mild cases it may only occur after turn-out or when the foal is newborn. In these cases improvement usually occurs within days, with or without rest. In foals with significant flexural deformity, the gait is often significantly affected and it becomes very difficult for the foal to move around. In addition, the fetlock joint may become involved in the deformity and make it difficult for the foal to rise. It is not uncommon to see skin trauma to the fetlock in these foals.

Diagnostic Imaging

Radiographs should be taken in cases that are deemed to be clinically significant. Lateromedial and dorsopalmar views are needed to assess for incomplete ossification of the bones, cuboidal bone malformation, or damage in the carpus. A complete series of radiographs should be taken if abnormalities are detected on initial views.

Treatment

Treatment depends on the severity of the flexural deformity. In cases of acquired deformity in which rapid growth and pain is thought to play a role, the foal can be weaned to decrease the energy intake from the mare's milk or a muzzle can be applied to the foal to reduce nursing. In addition, the foal's nutrition must be reassessed, turn-out can be reduced, and low levels of nonsteroidal anti-inflammatory drugs can be used to reduce the inflammation that is thought to occur in the physis. In mild cases or those that only occur with exercise, turn-out can be reduced. In some mild cases, physical therapy in the form of 15 minutes of manual extension every 4 to 6 hours can also be used.[42]

Oxytetracycline can be administered in most cases with good results.[50,60,64] The typical protocol is 3 gm oxytetracycline mixed in a 1-liter bag of balanced electrolyte solution once daily for 3 days. This should be given over 30 minutes to minimize any possible problems. The effects of oxytetracycline typically occur 3 days beyond the last administration.

If the deformity is severe at birth and the foal cannot stand, casts should be applied immediately and changed every 24 hours. Foals have been shown to respond well to this.[42] Several commercially available braces can also be used. Regardless of the type of external coaptation used, close observation and monitoring are essential.

If the case is severe enough, a splint can be applied. A bandage with a caudal splint is usually sufficient because the flexural deformity is in the cranial-to-caudal.[54] Again, the splint should only extend to the fetlock joint to maintain muscle strength.

Because of the potential of sores from casts and splints, it is not uncommon to use these for several hours a day and rotate their application. The author typically anesthetizes the foal, applies a thin bandage from the fetlock joint to the proximal radius, and molds a 4-inch cast material lengthwise from proximal to distal across the caudal aspect of the limb. Vet wrap can then be applied to stabilize the leg. Once this is set, it can be reused several times in daily bandage changes.

If contralateral limb lameness is present, it must be addressed to prevent and/or treat flexural deformity in the secondary limb.

Medical management of flexural deformities carries a good prognosis if the foal shows improvement within a few weeks. Carpi may buckle or shake slightly for several months; however, that appears to resolve on its own. This appears to vary with turn-out and rest, which can be managed effectively.

Surgical options, while available, are of questionable efficacy. In mild cases, desmotomy of the superior check ligament and/or inferior check ligament can be done to help relax the stress in the caudal aspect of the limb. In congenital forms of flexural deformity, radiographs may indicate cuboidal bone malformation. In these cases, musculotendinous unit contracture of the superficial digital flexor tendon, deep digital flexor tendon, ulnaris lateralis, flexor carpi ulnaris, and possibly the suspensory ligament can occur. Therefore, the ulnaris lateralis and flexor carpi ulnaris insertions on the accessory carpal bone may need to be severed to improve the condition.[9] In addition, it may be necessary to cut the superficial digital flexor tendon, deep digital flexor tendon, or suspensory ligament to resolve the problem. However, all 3 should not be cut because fetlock joint breakdown could occur. The author has performed this in some cases with no improvement. The concern in those cases is that the caudal fascia and joint capsule are fibrosed, which has been seen postmortem.

Prognosis

The prognosis is good for cases of mild flexural deformity that respond well to therapy. However, for those that fail to respond or are severe in nature, the prognosis is often poor.

MISCELLANEOUS CARPAL SWELLINGS

Extensor Carpi Radialis Tendon Damage

Etiology

Rupture or tearing of the extensor carpi radialis tendon occurs rarely in both adults and foals. Although

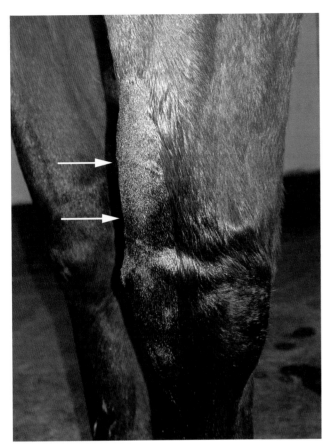

Figure 5.228. An adult horse with synovial effusion of the extensor carpi radialis tendon sheath proximal to the carpal joints (arrows). (Courtesy of Dr. Ty Wallis.)

the etiology is unknown, it has been reported in adults to occur mostly in jumpers and in horses that have exostoses on their distal radius.[18,68,95,100] This is typically traumatic in origin in foals and adults.

Clinical Signs and Diagnosis

On physical examination there is swelling of the sheath over the carpus (Figure 5.228). For those with complete rupture, overflexion of the carpus occurs as the foal or horse walks. There may or may not be extensor carpi radialis muscle atrophy, and a palpable defect is often detected within the swelling of the extensor carpi radialis tendon sheath.

Treatment

Rest is often necessary. Surgical repair of complete rupture in the acute stages in adults has been advocated, with casting for 2 to 4 weeks after surgery. Tenoscopy and debridement of the ruptured ends has also been advocated, along with casting for 2 to 4 weeks.

Prognosis

Overall, the prognosis for complete rupture of the extensor carpi radialis tendon in an adult is poor for

athletic use, but guarded to good for those that have partial tears. Ruptures in foals are thought to carry a good prognosis.

Common Digital Extensor Tendon Rupture

Etiology

Usually both common digital extensor tendons are ruptured, although this can occur in a single limb. The rupture typically occurs shortly after birth. This problem has been reported to occur with other signs such as decreased endochondral ossification at other sites, decreased pectoral muscle mass, and prognathic conformation to the jaw.[75] It is overrepresented in Arabian horses, Quarter horses, and Arab-Quarter horse crosses.[75] Some have speculated that this is heritable, especially if other congenital defects are present. It is often uncertain as to which came first, rupture of the common digital extensor tendon, or the flexural deformity. Historically, these foals often demonstrate some shaking at the carpi and possible buckling. It is interesting to note that one study showed that there were histologic signs of chronic changes in the tendons in a newborn foal that had ruptured; the investigators hypothesized that the chronic changes could have occurred in utero before birth.[9,109]

Clinical Signs and Diagnosis

Clinical signs include swelling on the dorsolateral aspect of the carpus, mainly in the form of effusion in the common digital extensor tendon sheath, occasional fetlock knuckling, possible palpable separation of the tendon, and variable lameness (Figure 5.229). In Meyer's report of 10 cases, 4 foals had severe flexural deformity, 3 had mild flexural deformity, and 3 had no flexural deformity. Thus, the degree of flexural deformity can be variable. These foals must be palpated because they can be easily confused with simple flexural deformities. Radiographs and ultrasound of the carpi can be performed to check for other problems and document the amount of separation.

Treatment and Prognosis

Treatment commonly includes stall rest with or without bandaging. Bandaging is recommended to help protect scraping of the dorsal aspect of the fetlock joint that may occur due to hyperflexion of the carpus. Suturing has been advocated by some,[49] although it is not necessary because the tendon ends are unlikely to heal primarily and rather adhere to the sheath. Splints or casting can be used if a persistent flexural deformity results. Fetlock joint contracture can sometimes occur, and in these cases an inferior check ligament and/or superior check ligament desmotomy can be performed.

In uncomplicated forms of rupture of the common digital extensor tendon, the prognosis is often good, although it is guarded if significant contracture is present.

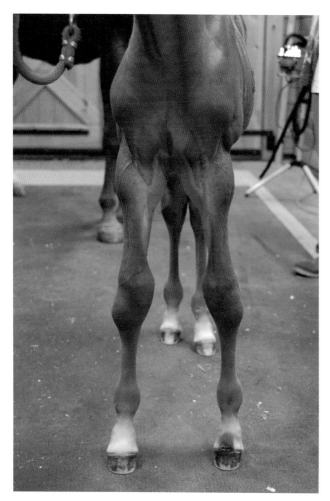

Figure 5.229. A foal showing bilateral effusion of the common digital extensor tendon sheaths due to rupture of the tendons.

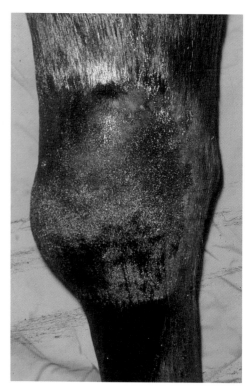

Figure 5.230. Hygroma of the carpus. Notice the diffuse swelling isolated over the dorsum of the carpus. (Courtesy of Dr. Gary Baxter.)

DORSAL CARPAL SWELLING

Hygroma

Etiology

A hygroma is an acquired bursa on the dorsum of the carpus caused by trauma from falling, getting up and down, hitting a fence, or chronically pawing and hitting the dorsum of the carpus, such as on a feeder or water trough.[84,95,99]

Clinical Signs and Diagnosis

Nonpainful, fluctuant, uniform soft tissue swelling occurs on the dorsal aspect of the carpus (Figure 5.230). Pressure does not induce swelling in any associated joints or tendon sheaths. Range of motion of the carpus may be reduced, but lameness is unusual. However, lameness can be severe if the hygroma is infected. Injection of radiopaque contrast agent into the hygroma confirms its extra-articular position. If a hygroma is suspected of being infected, then a fluid sample should be submitted for cytology and culture, similar to the procedures performed for septic arthritis.

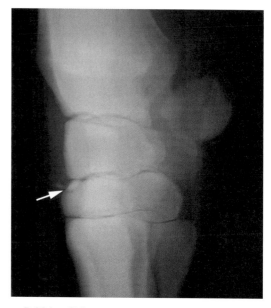

Figure 5.231. Oblique radiograph of the carpus demonstrating osteochondral fragmentation of the proximal third carpal bone (white arrow). Although this site of damage is seen more commonly in Standardbreds, this was a racing Quarter horse. (Courtesy of Dr. Gary Baxter.)

Treatment

Some hygromas may resolve on their own, but in most cases drainage and injection of anti-inflammatory agents can be used; repeated injection is necessary in many horses (Figure 5.231).[95,99] Spontaneous resolution has been seen after injection of an iodine-containing contrast agent. Injection of atropine (7 mg total dose) may also help to resolve the swelling. Owners should be warned that bandaging is an essential component of treatment and that long-term chronic thickening may occur. Other treatments include incisional drainage, injection of irritants such as Lugol's solution, and blistering.[95,99]

Contrast radiography should be performed to ensure that the hygroma is an isolated structure. Although preoperative contrast radiographs may show no communication between a hygroma and a joint or tendon sheath, it is possible that one exists in the form of a one-way valve from the joint into the mass.[45,84] Drainage of the mass with a Penrose drain and bandaging has been used successfully for treatment of recurrent hygromas.[1] However, the author has found the effectiveness of this to be limited.

Surgical excision can be performed in horses with chronic hygroma, and is best accomplished if the fluid sac is left intact and dissected from the other tissues.[93] Soft tissue and skin closure are routine, and a splint or sleeve cast can be used to prevent flexion for better healing. Prognosis for resolution of hygroma is often good, although some degree of thickening usually persists and the owner should be warned of a likely cosmetic blemish.

Synovial Hernia

A synovial hernia is a defect in a joint capsule or tendon sheath through which the synovial membrane can protrude. The condition is uncommon and rarely causes lameness, but it is a cosmetic blemish. A soft tissue mass can be palpated over a joint, and often can be moved between the hernia and the underlying joint or tendon sheath. Synovial hernias can occur between the mass and either the palpable carpal joint or extensor tendon sheaths. Unlike synovial effusion, synovial hernias seem to have a larger outpouching of fluid, and may disappear with joint flexion. Contrast agent injected into the hernial sac is detected in the underlying joint or tendon sheath, although a one-way valve may be present, limiting movement of contrast material. If the synovial hernia is of cosmetic concern, surgical excision can be performed, with a good prognosis for soundness provided no other joint diseases are present.[51]

Ganglion

A ganglion is a fluid-filled structure that connects to a joint or tendon sheath through a one-way tract from the joint into the mass. Unlike a synovial hernia, the mass lacks a synovial lining and often is filled with mucin. Ganglions, although common in humans, are rare in horses, and they have been reported around the stifle and the carpus.[84,67] Demonstrating a connection between a ganglion and an adjacent joint by injection of radiographic contrast agent into the mass may or may not be possible.[1]

Synovial Fistula

Synovial fistulae are communications between two synovial structures, usually a joint and tendon sheath. They have occurred between the antebrachiocarpal joint and the common digital extensor tendon, the middle carpal joint and the extensor carpi radialis tendon sheath or the common digital extensor tendon sheath, and the extensor carpi radialis tendon sheath and a carpal hygroma.[45,47,59,72] Additional joint damage is often present in association with the fistula, causing lameness referable to the area.[59] Swelling in the joint and nearby tendon sheath occurs, and fluid often moves between the structures. Radiography may reveal additional joint or tendon sheath damage, and contrast agent injected into one of the structures is visible in the other.

Occasionally a fistula can be seen during arthroscopic surgery, but closure of the fistula requires an arthrotomy. Arthroscopic surgery for treatment of a primary problem, without repair of the fistula, has resulted in resolution of lameness without resolution of the swelling. Fistulae are typically not repaired unless a cosmetic effect is important, if the swelling itself is impeding performance, or if medical therapy fails to alleviate lameness.

INTRA-ARTICULAR FRACTURES

Although most horses with intra-articular fracture of the carpus display acute onset of clinical signs, the damage is chronic in nature, at least in racehorses, and occurs at consistent sites in the dorsal aspect of the joints. The damage is the end result of a chronic process in which stress-related subchondral bone damage occurs.[53] Acute fracture and fragmentation of the carpus can occur, but this is typically in unusual locations, especially in the palmar aspect of the joints. Therefore, in equine athletes, and particularly racehorses, the damage occurs in predictable sites that lend themselves to more accurate prognosis with treatment.

Three types of fractures can occur within the carpal joints of the horse: osteochondral fragmentation, slab fracture, and comminuted fracture.

Osteochondral fragmentation occurs on a single articular surface and is commonly found on the radial carpal, third carpal, intermediate carpal bones, and distal radius. The fragments can be attached with fibrous tissue, loose, or free within the joint, and are categorized as: (1) recent and complete fragment, (2) fragment with capsule attachment, (3) chronic fragment with bone attachment, usually by fibrous tissue, or (4) fragment with extensive attachment to the bone.[9]

Regardless of the type of fragmentation, osteochondral fragmentation typically occurs at consistent locations; again, this reflects the chronic nature of the disease. Thoroughbreds and Quarter horses commonly show fragments within the radiocarpal and middle carpal joints. In Thoroughbreds, fragmentation commonly occurs off the distal aspect of the radiocarpal bone, distal lateral radius, and proximal aspect of the intermediate carpal bone. In Japan, the most common sites for fragments to occur in Thoroughbred racehorses are the distal lateral radius, proximal aspect of the third carpal bone, and distal aspect of the radiocarpal bone.[77] In racing Quarter horses, fragmentation occurs off the distal aspect of the radiocarpal bone, proximal aspect of the intermediate carpal bone, and distal lateral radius.[72] In Standardbreds, the fragmentation typically occurs in the middle carpal joint, especially on the third carpal bone (Figure 5.231).[61,82,88] It is important not to rely on these generalizations because fragmentation can occur anywhere within the carpi and the distribution may differ with different population bases.

Slab fractures of the carpus usually occur completely through the bone, and although they are most common in the third carpal bone, they can occur in the intermediate and radial carpal bones as well. In Thoroughbreds and Standardbreds, slab fractures commonly occur on the third carpal bone and primarily affect the radial facet. These fractures can also occur on the intermediate facet, both facets, or in a sagittal orientation.[67,88,96]

Comminuted fractures of the carpus occasionally occur, and although they primarily involve the third carpal bone, they can also involve the radial carpal, intermediate carpal, and fourth carpal bones. Horses that suffer these fractures are usually axially unstable. They require emergency stabilization and usually surgery to be sound for breeding.

In addition to fragmentation and fracture of the carpus, it is not unusual to find subchondral bone lysis that leads to pain, typically in racehorses. This primarily occurs in older Standardbred racehorses due to chronic stress-induced disease within the subchondral bone.[87] This syndrome is discussed in the osteoarthritis section of this chapter.

Etiology

The biomechanical forces that occur in the carpus and lead to fracture are difficult to characterize due to the large number of bones and soft tissues involved. The carpal bones are not in direct contact with their opposing surfaces during the flight phase of the gait. However, with weight-bearing and full extension, it is hypothesized that the carpal bones assume a congruent articulation with their opposing bones.[2,4] It is also hypothesized that this level of congruity can change with fatigue, increased speed, poor racing surface, poor trimming, possibly uncoordinated movement, and variability in racing surfaces, perhaps leading to fracture.

Subtle geometric abnormalities that may be within these joints also could predispose these horses to fracture. Considering the incidence of angular limb disease in the carpus, it is likely that these subtle geometric abnormalities occur, causing problems at speed. This is a known occurrence in the distal third metacarpus in the fetlock joint. Pathologic studies that have been performed in an effort to determine the cause of these fractures have led to the observation that many are chronic in nature in racehorses.

It is known that increased axial loading leads to increased dorsal compression between opposing carpal bones. Therefore, chronic high loads and the instantaneous maximum loads likely lead to disease.[80] Although these horses typically present with acute lameness and swelling, histopathologic observations have demonstrated a chronic disease process that not only leads to

bone microdamage but attempts at bone remodeling and healing as described in Chapter 7.[29,30,79,81,108] It has been shown repeatedly that intense bone modeling and remodeling occur at the sites at which osteochondral fracture occurs.[53] It is likely, then, that some of these fractures may in fact occur during the peak bone remodeling phase, which includes intense osteoclastic bone resorption. Not unlike dorsal metacarpal disease, some of these horses may be predisposed to fracture during these intense remodeling periods. Therefore, it is likely that chronic repetitive stress can lead to a chronic pathologic process that ultimately leads to bone failure and demonstration of clinical signs.

Soft tissue fatigue that can occur within the joints includes a decrease in soft tissue support of the joint capsule and the surrounding tendons and ligaments. This is compounded by the hypothesis that the hoof often impacts the ground before maximum extension occurs, thereby causing the joint to snap shut, and leading to the assumption that these intensive, pinpoint stresses can occur at these sites[2,4] and may lead to damage. In addition, it has been observed that fatigue of the flexor tendons and muscles in the caudal aspect of the leg can lead to hyperextension, as has been observed in many horses at the end of the race. Because of the prevalence of damage that occurs dorsally, several investigators have hypothesized that a back-at-the-knee conformation can lead to increased incidence of disease.[2,87] However, Barr, et al. showed that there was no correlation to the incidence of carpal damage when this conformation was evaluated.[5] Others have observed that most horses in Europe are "over at the knee" and therefore likely have a decreased incidence of this problem, although this has not be substantiated.[2]

Clinical Signs

Horses with fracture in the carpus can appear with various degrees of lameness, synovial effusion, soft tissue swelling, and carpal flexion during standing. If osteochondral damage is complete and enters the joint, synovitis typically results, which leads to clinical signs of joint effusion and pain. However, on rare occasions when subchondral bone damage alone occurs, synovitis leading to joint effusion may not be appreciated and the horse may or may not be positive to carpal flexion. Horses with small osteochondral carpal fragments are often only subtly lame with mild amounts of effusion and soft tissue swelling.

The common characteristic of their movement is abduction of the forelimbs, which some have hypothesized is an attempt to minimize carpal flexion. Consequently, this decreases hoof height during flight. Horses with osteochondral damage are often flexion positive, and with some fractures, horses have intense pain even with passive flexion. Horses with fracture or fragmentation of the palmar aspect of the joints are often significantly responsive to flexion, which reflects the extensive soft tissue damage that can occur in this area. In more chronic stages of osteochondral fracture there may be physical limitations to the amount of flexion in the carpus, with or without pain.

Horses with comminuted fractures of the carpus are often axially unstable and effusion may be associated

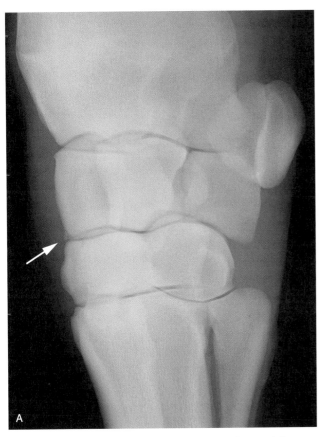

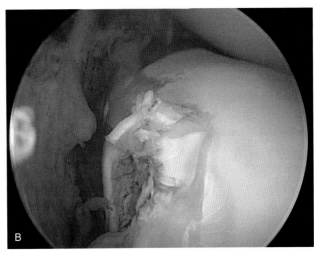

Figure 5.232. A radiographic image (A) showing a subtle fragment on the distal aspect of the radial carpal bone (arrow). The corresponding surgical image (B) is shown as well. This demonstrates how radiographs typically underestimate the severity of articular cartilage damage within the joint.

with subcutaneous swelling. If the horse can tolerate it, it is a good practice to palpate the dorsal aspect of the carpal bones while flexed, because horses with osteochondral damage often demonstrate pain on palpation of certain bones. Often, fibrous thickening of the joint capsule can be appreciated if a significant amount of joint capsule is involved in the fragmentation. However, in these cases, the presence of a hygroma or extensor sheath swelling must be ruled out.

If there are obvious signs of osteochondral fracture it is often a good idea to perform a radiographic examination prior to performing intrasynovial analgesia because with loss of pain, the horse no longer protects the limb, possibly leading to worsened damage. If a subtle lameness is present or radiographs are inconclusive, then intra-articular analgesia is often needed to confirm the site of pain. For intra-articular analgesia of the carpal joints, 5 to 7 mL of anesthetic are injected into the joint and the horse checked after 10 minutes and again at 30 minutes. Horses that have incomplete slab fractures that have not broken into the joint may not respond significantly to intra-articular anesthesia. The same may be true of horses that suffer from subchondral bone disease of the middle carpal joint. However, in these horses, there may be subtle preexisting lameness that prompts further diagnostic imaging.

Diagnostic Imaging

A minimum of 6 radiographic images are needed to fully characterize the carpal joints, especially those with small fragmentation (Figure 5.232). Most of the fragments are on the very dorsal aspect of the bones; therefore, some practitioners recommend that oblique views be taken more parallel with the lateromedial view to fully characterize the damage and detect subtle lesions. Images should be evaluated for osteochondral damage that can be surgically addressed, as well as osteoarthritic changes such as osteophyte, enthesiophyte, and joint space narrowing that can affect the prognosis for any surgical outcome.

Both limbs should be radiographed, because more than 50% of all horses with osteochondral fragments have them in both carpi.[72] In addition, the third carpal skyline view is important for detecting sclerosis, lysis, and fracture, and has been shown to give a good impression of third carpal bone density.[98] Some surgeons believe there is a correlation between the amount of pain and the duration and displacement of the fragment, but no objective studies have characterized this.

Mineralization in the palmar aspect of the carpal joints is often appreciated. Some clinicians have attributed this to chronic corticosteroid injection; however, there is evidence that sometimes this is due to chronic

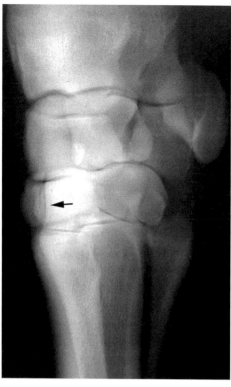

Figure 5.233. A radiograph demonstrating a slab fracture of the third carpal bone (arrow).

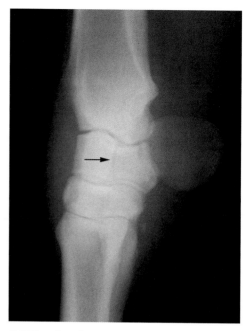

Figure 5.234. A radiograph demonstrating a slab fracture of the radial carpal bone (arrow).

damage within the dorsal aspect of the joints that leads to maceration of the fragments and migration to the palmar aspect of the joint. Sometimes significant osteoarthritis and articular cartilage loss are present in these horses. In addition, in cases of comminuted osteochondral fracture of the carpus, the third carpal bone is usually involved, along with the radiocarpal and/or intermediate carpal bone. These can be difficult to characterize and subtle changes in the angles of the radiographic images may be needed.

Slab fractures of the carpus are usually most easily seen on the standing lateromedial projection because these fractures often reduce in a flexed lateral position (Figures 5.233 and 5.234). Sagittal slab fractures typically occur on the medial aspect of the radial fossa of the third carpal bone, and either a third carpal bone skyline projection or a dorsomedial-palmar lateral oblique projection is needed to see this. In addition, subchondral bone lysis within a third carpal bone may not initially be present on radiographs, which justifies the use of subsequent radiographs to diagnose this problem once the bone in that area has resorbed.

Nuclear scintigraphy is beneficial, especially in racehorses, due to intense remodeling of the carpal bones. Furthermore, scintigraphy can best characterize the intense sclerosis and lysis that can result and may cause pain. A study of Standardbreds showed that increased uptake was common in the middle carpal joint, and most of this reaction was thought to be clinically significant.[28] In addition, intense uptake has been observed in 2-year-old Quarter horses that were worked on a treadmill for 6 months.[53] Therefore, it is important not to overinterpret the findings because uptake can occur in horses that are undergoing active exercise.

Magnetic resonance imaging and computed tomography have also been used to characterize subtle lesions in the carpus. Computed tomography has higher resolution and can be used to detect both subtle lesions and bone mineral density abnormalities. Magnetic resonance imaging is useful for detecting soft tissue damage and bone edema. Edema in the subchondral bone has been seen in joints with damage, but its cause and consequences are unknown. Ultimately, arthroscopic surgery is usually the best diagnostic tool to characterize and treat the problem in the carpus. The exception to this may be cases in which subchondral bone pain is a primary problem without the overlying articular cartilage damage.

Treatment

While some clinicians recommend rest for treatment of osteochondral fragmentation of the carpus, most surgeons believe that arthroscopic removal of the fragments and the resultant reduction of synovitis induced by the instability provide a more predictable outcome. Most surgeons feel that in horses that are conservatively treated, if these fragments are allowed to heal in an incongruent fashion the fragment of bone can break away later with training, again leading to clinical signs. Arthroscopic surgery is the best method to fully characterize the disease process, treat the primary problem, and give an accurate prognosis for return to athletic use.

Degeneration of articular cartilage and bone have been graded for severity and correlated with outcome:[72]

Grade 1: Minimal fibrillation or fragmentation at the edge of the defect left by the fragment, extending no more than 5 mm from the fracture line.

Grade 2: Articular cartilage degeneration extending more than 5 mm back from the defect and including up to 30% of the articular surface of that bone.

Grade 3: Loss of 50% or more of the articular cartilage from the affected carpal bone.

Grade 4: Significant loss of subchondral bone (usually distal radial carpal bone lesions).

After osteochondral fragments have been removed, augmentative therapy such as microfracture or various intra-articular medications can be used if the lesions are severe. There has been concern about operating horses after they have been recently injected with corticosteroids because the horses may be predisposed to postoperative synovial sepsis; however, this has not been shown to be of major concern.

Arthroscopic surgery of the carpus is typically performed in lateral or dorsal recumbency and the goal is to use triangulation to identify and remove the fragmentation or repair the fracture. This allows for the damage to be better visualized and the joint capsule can heal better. Once the damage is identified, the area is debrided and/or repaired. Augmentative procedures such as microfracture may be used, and the amount of damage graded. This provides details about the prognosis and helps in developing a management plan for the horse. For more details on arthroscopic surgery of the carpus, see McIlwraith, et al.[61,70]

While the majority of arthroscopic surgery is performed in the dorsal aspect of the joint, occasionally fragmentation of the palmar aspect of the joint can be removed with relatively good success.[21] This surgery is difficult and should be performed by an experienced surgeon. The same triangulation techniques are used. In some cases, mineralization may be within the joint capsule, making removal impossible. These cases may have extensive osteoarthritis, and the dorsal aspect also should be evaluated to address any concerns.

Slab fractures usually require internal fixation, such as lag screw fixation, to provide the best chance of achieving athletic soundness. However, thin slab fractures (less than 5 mm) can be removed because often they will not support lag screw repair.

Although surgery may not initially be considered for horses intended for retirement or breeding, it is possible that some cases may degenerate and later become unstable or see advanced progression of osteoarthritis if the fracture is not stabilized. The degree of joint surface damage, which is common with slab fractures, often dictates the prognosis of return to athletic use (Figure 5.235). Stephens, et al. showed that complete displaced fractures can be repaired through internal fixation, and incomplete and/or nondisplaced fractures can be treated with rest and conservative therapy.[96]

Sagittal slab fractures also are seen. In a retrospective study, 7 of 12 horses treated conservatively for sagittal fractures raced; however, most experienced surgeons believe that internal fixation is needed for the best prognosis.[31,87] Details of arthroscopic repair of slab fractures can be found in McIlwraith, et al.[67]

Methods to repair slab fractures vary according to surgeons. Some prefer single 4.5-mm or 3.5-mm cortical screws placed through the radial facet via arthroscopic guidance (Figure 5.236). After debridement of the fracture, needles are used to identify the appropriate area

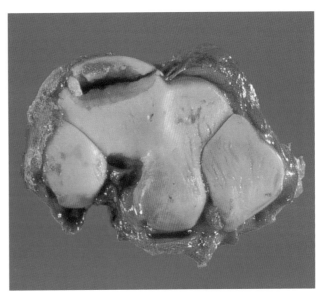

Figure 5.235. Gross image of a slab fracture of the radial facet of the third carpal bone. Notice the degeneration of articular cartilage and subchondral bone that can occur. Even with good reduction, this joint surface defect can worsen the prognosis for return to athletic function.

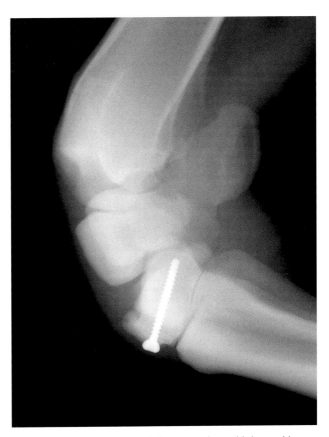

Figure 5.236. A radiograph demonstrating a third carpal bone slab fracture repaired with a lag screw.

for screw placement. The screw is placed using the lag screw technique. Fractures through the radial and intermediate facets require 2 screws. A headless, variable pitch screw has been used, and experimental evidence shows this to be equivalent to cortical screws for holding strength. This type of screw eliminates pain caused by a cortical screw head.[16]

Comminuted fractures require internal fixation or arthrodesis to restore axial stability to the limb and give the horse a chance to become pasture sound.[11,56] The immediate stability gained from internal fixation improves the time to pain-free limb use and prevents overuse and consequent laminitis in the opposing limb. Conservative therapy with casting and/or splints results in more prolonged lameness, which can lead to cast sores within the limb and often laminitis within the opposing limb. Conservatively treated horses sometimes heal with a deviation and significant chronic pain in the limb. It is unusual for a horse to achieve athletic soundness after such an injury because the joint surface damage is often severe. Lag screw fixation can be used to stabilize individual fractures; however, in severely comminuted injuries internal fixation with plates may be necessary and partial or full arthrodesis needed.

Postoperative Care

For osteochondral fragmentation, sutures are removed at 10 days and horses maintained in a bandage for 10 days. One common sequelae to carpal bandages is the creation of sores over the accessory carpal bone and the medial distal condyle of the radius. There are several ways to prevent these, including padding on either side of the structures, creating a window in the bandage for these areas to be exposed, or using super glue or adherent drapes over the incision sites without a bandage. Most clinicians prefer bandages because the compression helps decrease postoperative swelling; however, it has been observed that super glue has worked well.

The time needed for rehabilitation depends on the amount of damage, and the intensity of postoperative rehabilitation depends on the amount of articular cartilage damage and where the damage occurred. Rehabilitation is faster for the antebrachial carpal joint than the middle carpal joint because damage in the former is less common on the weight-bearing joint surface and consequently suffers minimal stress-induced damage. In general, most surgeons recommend 2 weeks of stall rest followed by 2 to 4 weeks of stall rest and hand walking, and then 2 to 4 additional weeks of turnout or swimming for problems within the antebrachial joint.[87] For mild to moderate damage within the middle carpal joint, the recommendation is 2 to 4 weeks of stall rest, 4 weeks of stall rest and hand walking, and 8 weeks of turn-out or swimming; for severe middle carpal joint lesions or global articular cartilage damage, 4 to 6 months of rest are often recommended.[87] Typically horses with slab fractures require 4 weeks of stall rest, 8 weeks of stall rest and hand walking, and 2 to 3 months of paddock turn-out. Horses should be radiographed prior to training, and rarely will the screw need to be removed.[87]

In addition to rehabilitation, some form of intra-articular therapy is recommended to reduce inflammation and speed healing, especially of articular cartilage. If intra-articular medication is needed, the horses can be injected at the time of suture removal or after. The author prefers interleukin-1 receptor antagonist protein (IRAP) or polysulfated glycosaminoglycan/hyaluronic acid combination (with amikacin) once weekly for 3 weeks, starting 2 weeks after surgery. Treatment with IRAP is not uncommon, especially for severe joint damage, because the growth factor content within this product can be significant and theoretically help with articular cartilage healing. Intra-articular hyaluronic acid and polysulfated glycosaminoglycan are thought to promote healing and decrease inflammation.[52] Some surgeons find intra-articular stem cell therapy to be beneficial, although a study showed minimal benefit in experimental osteochondral fragmentation. Theoretically, the stem cells could promote release of growth factors into the joint, affecting on articular cartilage healing of a defect.[52]

Some surgeons use systemic nonsteroidal anti-inflammatory medications for horses with carpal fractures, either phenylbutazone or Equioxx therapy. Local application of Surpass has also been shown to be beneficial both clinically and in experimental studies.[52] Although systemic polysulfated glycosaminoglycan and intravenous hyaluronic acid therapies generally have shown modest effects, they may help maintain horses with carpal damage. The author recommends the use of passive range of motion and swimming if significant joint capsule damage is noted at the time of surgery.

Potential postoperative problems include sepsis and subcutaneous infection. Problems such as persistent effusion and osteophyte formation are usually a result of the primary disease process, although excessive debridement of the joint capsule can lead to enthesiophyte formation.

Prognosis

The prognosis for osteochondral fragmentation is variable depending on the breed. For Thoroughbreds and Quarter horses the chance of racing at the same or increased level is approximately 68%.[72,77] McIlwraith, et al. found that horses with grade 1 or 2 damage were more likely to return to racing than those with grade 3 or grade 4 damage (74% vs. 54%, respectively). However, Lucus, et al. found that in Standardbreds, 74% raced at least 1 start, although most had decreased earnings and numbers of starts.[61] For slab fractures, 65% to 77% of horses raced. Martin, et al. found that 68% of horses raced post surgically, although they had significantly decreased value.[67] Stephens, et al. found that 65% of Thoroughbreds raced but decreased their earnings per start and that 77% of Standardbreds raced, 100% if they had raced before.[96] The prognosis is good for riding or breeding.[57]

ACCESSORY CARPAL BONE FRACTURE

Fracture of the accessory carpal bone can occur in any breed and primarily occurs in the frontal plane through the lateral groove of the bone (Figure 5.237). It is hypothesized that most of these fractures heal by fibrocartilaginous nonunion due to the constant pull from the flexor muscles.[6,26]

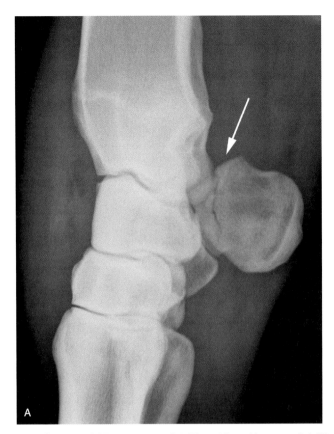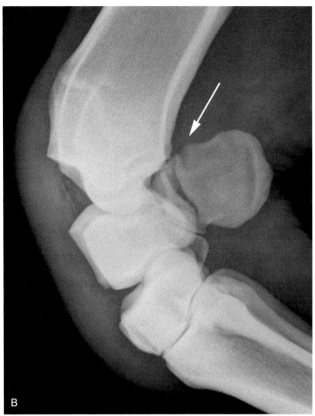

Figure 5.237. Lateromedial (A) and flexed lateromedial (B) radiographs of a fracture of the accessory carpal bone (arrows).

Etiology

These fractures are thought to result from external trauma; however, it is very rare to see primary skin damage over these sites. Some clinicians have hypothesized that the cause may be extreme internal forces such as asynchronous contraction of the flexor carpi ulnaris and ulnaris lateralis muscles,[4] horses landing partially flexed, leading to a bowstring effect of the flexor carpi ulnaris lateralis and flexor tendons,[63] or extreme stress induced by the bone being caught between the third metacarpal bone and the radius, because concurrent lesions have been seen in the caudal radius.[86]

Clinical Signs and Diagnosis

Horses with fractured accessory carpal bone typically have acute lameness with or without dorsal carpal or carpal canal swelling. There is often palpable pain over the accessory carpal bone, crepitus is sometimes felt, and sometimes with flexion, lateral to medial instability can be palpated. Care must be taken in examining these horses because they are very painful with flexion and may stand with their carpus flexed. One frequent clinical sign is a decrease in digital pulses with flexion.[9] Radiographs are often sufficient; however, ultrasound examination of the carpal canal can help to characterize the extent of damage. Ultrasound examination should be repeated during the healing process because fibrous union is common, and expansion of this fibrous response

could impinge the carpal canal, leading to pain. It is thought that severely comminuted fractures could increase the chance of carpal canal involvement, but large retrospective studies are lacking.

Treatment and Prognosis

Three to 6 months of rest or lag screw fixation are recommended.[26] Ulnar neurectomy and arthroscopic surgery and debridement have also been recommended, but subtotal resection is no longer advocated. Small fragments involving the proximal dorsal aspect of the accessory carpal bone may involve the palmar aspect of the antebrachiocarpal joint and can be removed arthroscopically. However, because involvement of the carpal canal is often delayed until well into the healing phase, tenoscopic examination and retinacular release, if needed, also may be delayed. Periodic radiographs should follow treatment; distraction and further lysis of the fracture due to the fibrocartilaginous nonunion may be seen over time. Prognosis for healing is good. Although return to soundness is generally good, it can be reduced if significant carpal canal involvement is evident.

CARPAL LUXATIONS

Luxation of the carpal joints is rare but can occur in any of the 3 joints. The medial collateral ligament is reportedly most commonly ruptured; however, the lateral collateral ligament can be affected with or without carpal bone comminution. Avulsion fractures can also occur as a result of external trauma such as foaling, jumping, falling, slipping, or from kicks.

Clinical Signs and Diagnosis

Clinically, the horses are acutely lame with swelling around the joint and there may or may not be an angular limb deformity present, depending on the severity of damage. These luxations are rarely open; in the author's experience this occurs mostly in racehorses with catastrophic injuries to the carpus. Horses with carpal luxations may be axially unstable and crepitus may be palpable during manual deviation of the joint (Figures 5.238 and 5.239). Damage to the collateral ligament can also occur on its own.[25]

Radiographs and ultrasound are often diagnostic, although in some partial tears the horse must be sedated and manual deviation of the carpus imposed to see the subluxation on radiographs (stress radiographs). In addition, dorsopalmar luxations can occur and radiographs should be assessed closely. Ultrasound is the best diagnostic method for characterizing full- and partial-thickness tears in the collateral ligaments, although with time, enthesiophyte formation is usually appreciated radiographically.

Treatment and Prognosis

Treatment for complete luxations often involves placing the horse under general anesthesia to achieve

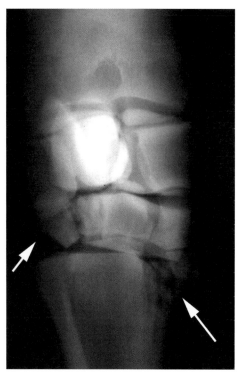

Figure 5.238. Radiograph of a carpus showing luxation of the carpometacarpal joint and multiple sites of osteochondral damage (arrows). This leg was axially unstable and required emergency support for transport.

reduction. Arthroscopic surgery may be helpful to debride damaged tissues if joint damage occurs. The luxation can be reduced if the carpal bones are not involved; otherwise, fractures may need to be debrided to facilitate reduction. Dorsopalmar luxations can be difficult to reduce, and sometimes manual fatiguing of the limb or surgery are needed to reduce the luxations. Once reduced, the limb can be put through rotational manipulation.

If the limb is deemed to be rotationally stable, then a tube cast can be applied from the proximal aspect of the radius to the distal third metacarpus.[9] If the limb is deemed to be rotationally unstable, a full-limb cast should be used. Foals are usually casted for approximately 4 weeks and adults for 6 weeks to allow fibrosis to occur in the collateral ligament area and joint capsule. The horse may be transferred to a bandage and/or splint for several weeks, but stall confinement for several months is necessary.

Partial or pancarpal arthrodesis may be needed to stabilize the limb for breeding and pasture soundness if multiple fractures are present (Figures 5.240). However, even if the limb can be reduced adequately, chronic osteoarthritis and pain may necessitate arthrodesis to control pain and prevent contralateral limb laminitis. Soft tissue lesions can be augmented with stem cells, platelet rich plasma, or extracorporeal shockwave therapy to help stimulate healing. The prognosis is good for healing but guarded for athletic use.

SOFT TISSUE DAMAGE TO THE CARPUS

Collateral ligament injury is sometimes seen in the carpus. Although these may be difficult to diagnose acutely, improvement in ultrasound examination of these structures and the use of MRI have helped with early diagnosis. Some have described collateral ligament abnormalities in the carpus closely associated with osteoarthritis;[25] so the problem is sometimes diagnosed well after osteoarthritis has already been established.

Injury to the intercarpal ligaments is common, especially in cases with osteochondral damage. The dorsomedial intercarpal ligament attaches to the distal radiocarpal bone in the area where osteochondral fragmentation typically occurs. Whitton, et al. have shown that the dorsomedial intercarpal ligament resists dorsomedial displacement of the radiocarpal bone; therefore, it is likely that the stress at this site makes this area prone to damage.[104,105] Selway proposed that hypertrophy of this ligament could lead to disease, but Whitton, et al. have shown no correlation between dorsomedial intercarpal ligament hypertrophy and osteochondral damage.[102,103,106]

The palmar intercarpal ligaments have been shown to provide considerable stability to the carpus. The medial and lateral palmar intercarpal ligaments allow abaxial translation of the carpal bones to dissipate axial forces through the carpus.[14] Whitton, et al. found no correlation of tearing of the palmar intercarpal ligaments with the severity of disease other than the fact that severe tearing of these ligaments can lead to instability of the joint and hemarthrosis. Beinlich and Nixon reviewed the diagnosis and treatment of horses with avulsion fracture of the lateral palmar intercarpal liga-

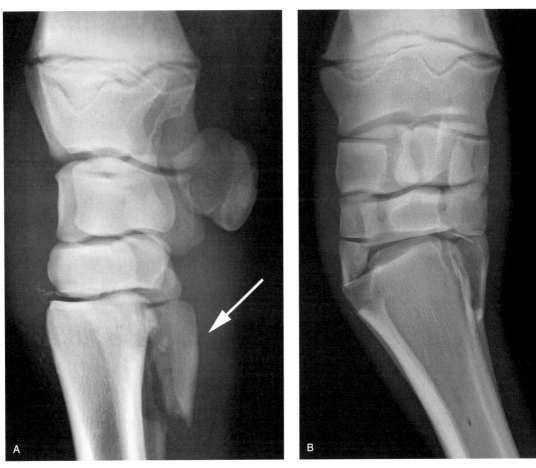

Figure 5.239. Radiographic images showing biaxial splint bone fractures (A, arrow) that led to instability and luxation of the carpus (B). (Courtesy of Dr. Gary Baxter.)

ment from the ulnar carpal bone[7,8] and found that the fragments were best demonstrated on the dorsopalmar and especially the dorsolateral palmar medial projections, which corresponded with arthroscopic findings in this group of horses. In addition, they found that arthroscopic removal of these fragments was more beneficial than rest alone, with 91% of those horses returning to their intended use.[7,8]

OSTEOARTHRITIS

Etiology

Osteoarthritis (OA) is common in the carpus and can result from 1 of 2 syndromes. In young horses that are athletes, such as racehorses, stress-related bone damage—especially that which causes physical damage to the joint—can result in secondary osteoarthritis; see Chapter 7 for details on stress related bone damage. It is likely that the pathologic process that leads to this disease progresses to the point of articular cartilage damage and osteoarthritis. The other form of osteoarthritis occurs in horses that demonstrate insidious, progressive onset of disease regardless of their previous history. In either case, if the severity of damage can be stabilized, these horses are often clinically manageable

for nonracehorse type of work. However, when the damage is progressive, it is possible that even pasture soundness is questionable.

Clinical Signs and Diagnosis

Whether the OA is due to previous injury or insidious in onset, the clinical response is similar. Horses with a previous history of disease can be monitored closely for radiographic evidence of advancing OA and treated. In insidious cases, often no problems are noticed until the limb begins to swell and lameness becomes obvious. In the latter cases, the farrier will often note that the horse begins to resent flexion and manipulation of the limb. Radiographs taken at this point often show some signs, and treatment can be helpful if started at that time.

Radiographic signs of osteoarthritis may include mild osteophytes, enthesiophytes, and osteochondral fragmentation early in the disease process (Figure 5.241). Subchondral bone sclerosis may be identified and mild joint space narrowing may be present. Severe changes can result from the progression of osteoarthritis, leading to combinations of subchondral bone sclerosis and lysis.

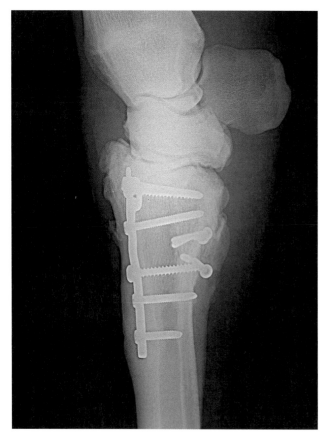

Figure 5.240. Lateral radiograph 1.5 years after the horse in Figure 5.239 underwent arthrodesis of the carpometacarpal joint using a locking plate. (Courtesy of Dr. Gary Baxter.)

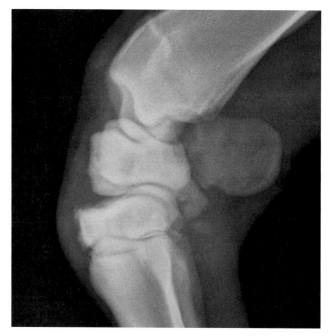

Figure 5.241. Flexed lateral radiograph demonstrating the characteristic osteophyte production along the dorsal aspect of the carpus that is often seen with carpal OA.

Treatment and Prognosis

Some early forms of osteoarthritis can be treated with rest and systemic nonsteroidal anti-inflammatory treatment. Stall confinement is rarely helpful in management of horses with carpal osteoarthritis; in other species, including humans, strengthening of periarticular soft tissues is beneficial.[13] Paddock turn-out seems to help these horses, although it is important to monitor their activity and limit their exposure to other horses that may stimulate excessive exercise.

Surgery can be performed to remove osteochondral fragments or for augmentative therapies such as microfracture and resurfacing; however, the disease process will likely continue to progress postoperatively and in most cases the goal of surgery is to help relieve pain and the severity of the disease.

Intra-articular medication is meant to treat the synovitis component that often leads to pain, but its efficacy for treating subchondral bone damage is questionable. Intra-articular corticosteroid and hyaluronic acid combinations may work for a short period of time but often stop working. Intra-articular hyaluronic acid and polysulfated glycosaminoglycan combinations or IRAP may be considered. Although it is thought that only triamcinolone acetonide or betamethasone should be used in high-motion joints such as the carpus, methylprednisolone acetate may be the only thing that is effective in some cases of severe osteoarthritis. Although this has been shown experimentally to result in progressive articular cartilage damage, in these cases management of pain is often considered the priority.

Medial collapse of the carpal joints is not uncommon in severe cases of osteoarthritis, and often dorsolateral break-over of the hoof in that limb is noticeable. This progressively worsens between trimmings; it is a subjective opinion that this can lead to worsening of pain. A mild lateral extension or a full shoe itself may help to alleviate some of this pain by slowing the dorsolateral break-over that occurs. In severe cases of osteoarthritis, partial or pancarpal arthrodesis is often advocated to reduce the amount of chronic pain in the limb and prevent laminitis in the opposing limb.

CARPOMETACARPAL OSTEOARTHRITIS

Osteoarthritis of the carpometacarpal joint is a separate syndrome that predominantly involves older Arabian horses.[65] The osteoarthritic changes manifest mostly at the articulation between the second carpal and second metacarpal bones, and radiographically show osteoproliferative changes and joint space narrowing medially (Figure 5.242). Lameness is insidious in onset, but can progress rapidly. The etiology of this problem is unknown, but it has been suggested that an anatomic abnormality may exist between the second and third carpal bones.[65] Medical management of these cases can be frustrating over time because they typically become less responsive to treatment. Similar to OA at other sites, medical management is worth attempting until there is concern that the lameness could contribute to opposing limb laminitis. At this point, a partial carpal arthrodesis could be performed.

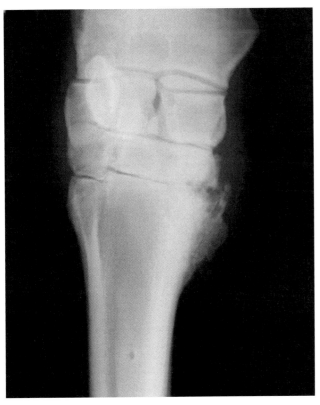

Figure 5.242. A radiograph demonstrating collapse of the medial aspect of the joint space and osteoproliferation typical of OA of the carpometacarpal joint. (Courtesy of Dr. Gary Baxter.)

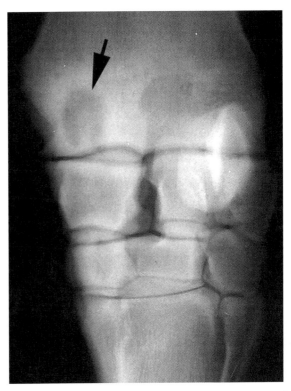

Figure 5.243. A radiograph of a subchondral cystic lesion of the distal radius (arrow). (Courtesy of Dr. Gary Baxter.)

OSTEOCHONDROSIS OF THE CARPUS

Osteochondritis dissecans has been reported in the carpal bones, although it is uncommon compared to other joints in the horse. Subchondral cystic lesions in some carpal bones are incidental and are often of questionable clinical significance. This is especially true with cysts within the second carpal bone in association with the presence of the first carpal bone and in the proximal aspect of the second metacarpal bone. However, subchondral cystic lesions in the radiocarpal bone and the distal aspect of the radius (Figure 5.243) are often clinically significant, and arthroscopic surgery and debridement are warranted if they are felt to communicate with the carpal joints.

OSTEOCHONDROMA OF THE DISTAL RADIUS

Osteochondroma (OC) formation at the distal end of the radius is an uncommon condition causing lameness in the horse.[46,55,62,94] The growth most commonly occurs in adult horses adjacent to the physis at the caudal distal aspect of the radius.[40,92,93] Although very uncommon, the cranial aspect of the radius also can be involved. Radiographically and histologically, these new bone growths appear much like those reported for hereditary multiple exostosis. However, unlike hereditary multiple exostosis, they appear as singular lesions or affect only a few other long bones, rather than numerous growing bones. See Chapter 7. Solitary OCs

have been reported in 2 foals; the distal palmar aspect of the middle phalanx was affected in one, and in the other the calcaneus was involved.[19,27]

Etiology

Although a single dominant autosomal gene is responsible for the development of multiple exostosis in humans and horses,[90] the genetic implications for isolated OC remains unclear. In humans, solitary OCs are not considered to be inherited.[44] It is postulated that metaplastic cartilage foci develop in the metaphysis and distal diaphysis from abnormal growth of the periosteum. As the cartilage grows it undergoes endochondral ossification similar to that occurring at the physis. The developing exostosis, which is continuous with the cortex of the bone and surrounded by a cartilage cap, is called an osteochondroma.

Nixon, et al. have reported on a series of cases in which exostoses of the palmar aspect of the closed physis were removed arthroscopically. In these cases, although they appeared similar to OC, they were histologically different.[78]

Clinical Signs

Affected horses often present with a history of intermittent lameness that increases with exercise. An obvious swelling of the carpal canal sheath cranial to the ulnaris lateralis is often present (Figure 5.244). In some cases the swelling can be extensive. At exercise a moderate lameness graded 1 to 2 out of 5 is commonly

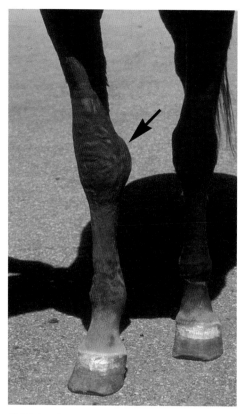

Figure 5.244. Carpal canal swelling (arrow) appreciated on the medial aspect of the limb. (Courtesy of Dr. Gary Baxter.)

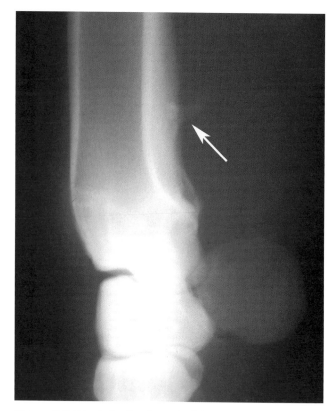

Figure 5.245. Lateral radiograph of the carpus demonstrating an osteochondroma on the caudal aspect of the distal radius (arrow).

observed.[92] Palpation of the caudodistal aspect of the radius with the limb held flexed at the carpus allows the examiner to feel the bony protuberance in some cases. Deep palpation of the site is often painful, resulting in limb withdrawal from the pressure. The range of carpal flexion is usually less than normal and considerable pain is elicited with rapid carpal flexion. A carpal flexion test usually exacerbates the lameness.

Diagnosis

Radiography is necessary to diagnose the condition and its location. In most cases the OC is located on the caudomedial aspect of the distal radius adjacent to the physis; however, smaller OCs have been observed on the caudolateral aspect of the distal radius as well. Radiographically, these lesions appear as conically shaped bony protuberances with an outer cortex and inner medullary cavity (Figure 5.245). The size of the OC and degree of ossification is variable. Ultrasonography can also be used to determine the presence of deep digital flexor tendinitis.[101] Intrathecal anesthesia is occasionally needed to confirm the clinical significance of the lesions.

Treatment

Although the instillation of corticosteroids into the tendon sheath temporarily resolves the tenosynovitis, the clinical signs usually reoccur.[101] Presently surgical excision of the OC is the treatment of choice and it is curative in most cases. Although excision of the OC via an open lateral or medial approach has been described,[40,55,62] the removal using an arthroscopic technique is currently recommended.[92,93] Both lateral and medial endoscopic approaches have been described; the author prefers the lateral approach. With this approach, the surgeon is less likely to injure the medially positioned median artery, vein, and nerve, and it is technically easier to manipulate the scope and instruments without interference from the opposite limb. A brief description of the lateral arthroscopic approach follows.

Some surgeons prefer to perform the surgery in lateral recumbency, although dorsal recumbency allows easier access to both forelimbs if needed and maintains better hemostasis for visualization. The carpal sheath is distended with 20 mL of sterile isotonic polyionic fluid. The arthroscope is inserted into the proximal aspect of the carpal canal through a stab incision located 3.5 cm proximal to the distal radial physis between the tendons of the lateral digital extensor and ulnaris lateralis muscles. Once the arthroscope is in the carpal canal, the sheath is distended with fluid and the OC is readily identified. The exostosis is removed from its attachment to bone at the base with an osteotome placed through a small portal distal to the arthroscopic portal. After the OC is removed the bone bed is curetted, the sheath is lavaged, and the portals are closed routinely. At the same time, any lesions in the deep digital flexor tendon can be addressed.

Support pressure bandages are applied and maintained for 2 weeks. Stall rest is recommended for 2 weeks, with hand walking exercise for an additional 2 to 4 weeks. In most cases the carpal canal distension resolves without further treatment; however, in some horses, intrasynovial treatment with anti-inflammatory agents is required. The significance of damage to the deep digital flexor tendon must be considered for postoperative rehabilitation; significant damage requires prolonged rest and follow-up ultrasonographic assessment.

Prognosis

The prognosis for surgical excision of solitary OCs is good for return to performance. In one report, follow-up on 2 horses after 1 and 2 years found that the horses were free of lameness and no distension of the sheath was apparent.[92] In another report, follow-up 4 months after surgery found the horse to be free of lameness and no swelling in the carpal canal.[93] No lameness has been observed in 2 other cases at 4- and 12-year follow-up, and the bone excision sites remained nonreactive radiographically. Nixon, et al. found that all 10 horses in their series of exostoses returned to intended use, with only 1 horse requiring additional medical therapy.[78]

DESMITIS OF THE ACCESSORY LIGAMENT (RADIAL OR SUPERIOR CHECK LIGAMENT) OF THE SUPERFICIAL DIGITAL FLEXOR TENDON

Etiology

The accessory ligament of the superficial digital flexor tendon (AL-SDFT) is a strong, fibrous band that originates from the distal caudomedial surface of the radius and joins the superficial digital flexor tendon at that level.[37] Until recently sprain to this structure has been poorly defined and many conditions associated with the caudal aspect of the radius and carpus were attributed to this condition including (1) lowering of the angulation of the accessory carpal bone, (2) enthesiophyte formation at the distal caudomedial aspect of the radius, (3) cranial displacement of the proximal end of the radius, and (4) alterations in the antebrachiocarpal (radiocarpal) joint capsule on its dorsal surface.[37,66]

Sprain of the AL-SDFT has been more clearly defined with the improvements in ultrasound resolution and the advent of MRI.[22,24] The condition occurs most commonly in young adult horses with a high level of physical activity. In a report on 23 horses with abnormal ultrasonographic findings in the AL-SDFT, 11 of 23 were racehorses, 9 of 11 were sport horses, and the remaining were pleasure or instruction horses.[22] Presumably, extreme hyperextension of the fetlock in conjunction with hyperextension of the carpus can cause a sprain of the AL-SDFT.[58,66]

Clinical Signs

Affected horses have a history of starting races and workouts quite well but are reluctant to really sprint out. Rarely do they attain their previous performance levels.[37,66] A visible swelling of the carpal sheath is observed in some cases (Figure 5.244). At a walk, a gait impediment characterized by a lateral floating placement of the foot just before it contacts the ground may be observed. The toe and heel are placed on the ground at the same time, much like a horse walking down an incline. In a review of 30 cases, this gait alteration was most commonly observed with radiographic lesions on the caudomedial distal aspect of the radius associated with the origin of the AL.[37] In acute cases the carpal sheath is frequently distended and variably painful to digital palpation.[37] Simultaneous trauma to the superficial digital flexor tendon may also occur, resulting in a painful swelling.[48]

Diagnosis

In acute cases, radiographs of the caudal aspect of the distal end of the radius are usually negative. However, in chronic cases, radiographs of the distal radius may reveal enthesiophytes associated with the attachment of the AL-SDFT. Interestingly, in a study in which radiographs were taken on horses with abnormal ultrasonographic findings in AL-SDFT, only 4 of 18 had an abnormal profile at the caudal distal aspect of the radius and 14 of 18 were considered normal.[24] This underscores the value of ultrasound examination in the diagnosis of desmitis of the AL-SDFT.

Ultrasound findings associated with injury of the AL-SDFT include thickening, hypoechoic defects, and alteration in fiber pattern alignment.[24] Injury to the AL-SDFT can also be accompanied by abnormal findings involving one or more of the structures in the carpal canal such as synovial effusion within the carpal sheath, tendinitis of the SDFT, distension and thickening of the retinaculum flexorum, tenosynovitis of the sheath of the tendon of the flexor carpi radialis muscle, and/or injury to the proximal attachment of the suspensory ligament (third interosseous muscle). Characterization of this additional damage is important for determining therapy and prognosis.

Treatment

In the acute cases exhibiting carpal sheath distention, needle drainage and the injection of a corticosteroid and hyaluronic acid is recommended.[22,24] Rest in a stall for 4 to 6 weeks is recommended with hand walking exercise beginning at the third week. Systemic nonsteroidal anti-inflammatory drugs may be indicated for associated problems and are administered as needed. Pressure support wraps are applied and maintained for 2 to 3 weeks. Following stall rest the horse should be confined to a small run for another 6 weeks. Recheck ultrasound examination should be done at this time to assess healing. Generally, affected horses can return to performance in 4 to 6 months.[22] Arthroscopic examination of the carpal canal can be performed to aid in characterization of the damage and treatment if necessary, and tenoscopic release of the carpal flexor retinaculum can be performed if needed.

Prognosis

The prognosis appears to depend on the severity of the injury, the intended use of the horse, and whether the SDFT is involved. In one study, 8 of 13 sport horses were able to return to their previous level of activity, whereas only 7 of 16 racehorses returned to racing at their previous level.[23] In another report, of 8 horses suffering from injury to the AL-SDFT alone, without tendinitis of the superficial flexor tendon, 6 returned to their previous level of performance within 4 to 6 months.[22] Tenoscopic release of the carpal flexor retinaculum has been useful for resolving lameness in 2 horses.[97]

References

1. Andren L, Eiken O. Arthrographic studies of risk ganglions. J Bone Joint Surg Am 1971;53:299.
2. Auer J. Diseases of the carpus. Vet Clin North Am Large Anim Pract 1980;2:81–99.
3. Auer JA, Martens RJ. Periosteal transection and periosteal stripping for correction of angular limb deformities in foals. Am J Vet Res 1982;43:1530–1534.
4. Auer JA, Watkins JP, White NA, et al. Slab fractures of the fourth and intermediate carpal bones in five horses. J Am Vet Med Assoc 1986;188:595–601.
5. Barr AR. Carpal conformation in relation to carpal chip fracture. Vet Rec 1994;134:646–650.
6. Barr AR, Sinnott MJ, Denny HR. Fractures of the accessory carpal bone in the horse. Vet Rec 1990;126:432–434.
7. Beinlich CP, Nixon AJ. Prevalence and response to surgical treatment of lateral palmar intercarpal ligament avulsion in horses: 37 cases (1990–2001). J Am Vet Med Assoc 2005;226:760–766.
8. Beinlich CP, Nixon AJ. Radiographic and pathologic characterization of lateral palmar intercarpal ligament avulsion fractures in the horse. Vet Radiol Ultrasound 2004;45:532–537.
9. Bertone AL. The carpus. In Adams' Lameness in Horses, 5th ed. Stashak TS, ed. Lippincott Williams and Wilkins, Philadelphia, 2002;830–863.
10. Bertone AL, Park RD, Turner AS. Periosteal transection and stripping for treatment of angular limb deformities in foals: radiographic observations. J Am Vet Med Assoc 1985;187:153–156.
11. Bertone AL, Schneiter HL, Turner AS, et al. Pancarpal arthrodesis for treatment of carpal collapse in the adult horse. A report of two cases. Vet Surg 1989;18:353–359.
12. Bertone AL, Turner AS, Park RD. Periosteal transection and stripping for treatment of angular limb deformities in foals: clinical observations. J Am Vet Med Assoc 1985;187:145–152.
13. Bliddal H, Christensen R. The treatment and prevention of knee osteoarthritis: a tool for clinical decision-making. Expert Opin Pharmacother 2009;10:1793–1804.
14. Bramlage LR, Schneider RK, Gabel AA. A clinical perspective on lameness originating in the carpus. Equine Vet J Suppl 1988;12–18.
15. Brauer TS, Booth TS, Riedesel E. Physeal growth retardation leads to correction of intracarpal angular deviations as well as physeal valgus deformity. Equine Vet J 1999;31:193–196.
16. Bueno AC, Galuppo LD, Taylor KT, et al. A biomechanical comparison of headless tapered variable pitch and AO cortical bone screws for fixation of a simulated slab fracture in equine third carpal bones. Vet Surg 2003;32:167–177.
17. Buoen LC, Zhang TQ, Weber AF, et al. Arthrogryposis in the foal and its possible relation to autosomal trisomy. Equine Vet J 1997;29:60–62.
18. Catlin JE. Rupture of the extensor carpi radialis tendon. VM/SAC 1964;59:1778.
19. Chan CC-H, Munroe GA, Callanan JJ. Congenital solitary osteochondroma affecting the tarsus in a filly foal. Equine Vet Educ 1996;8:153.
20. Crilly RG. Longitudinal overgrowth of chicken radius. J Anat 1972;112:11–18.
21. Dabareiner RM, White NA, Sullins KE. Radiographic and arthroscopic findings associated with subchondral lucency of the distal radial carpal bone in 71 horses. Equine Vet J 1996;28:93–97.
22. Denoix JM, Guiizien I, Perrot P, et al. Ultrasonographic diagnosis of spontaneous injuries of the accessory ligament of the superficial digital flexor tendon (proximal check ligament) in 23 horses. Proceedings Am Assoc Equine Pract 1995;142–143.
23. Denoix JM, Guizien I, Perrot P. Injuries of the accessory ligament of the superficial digital flexor tendon (proximal check ligament) in sport and race horses. Pferdeheilkunde 1996;12:613–616.
24. Denoix JM, Yousfi S. Spontaneous injury of the accessory ligament of the superficial digital flexor tendon (Proximal check ligament): A new ultrasonographic diagnosis. J Equine Vet Sci 1996;16:191–194.
25. Desmaizieres LM, Cauvin ER. Carpal collateral ligament desmopathy in three horses. Vet Rec 2005;157:197–201.
26. Easley KJ, Schneider JE. Evaluation of a surgical technique for repair of equine accessory carpal bone fractures. J Am Vet Med Assoc 1981;178:219–223.
27. Easter JL, Watkins JP, Berridge B, et al. A digital osteochondroma as the cause of lameness in a foal. Vet Comp Orthop Traumatol 1998;11:44.
28. Ehrlich PJ, Dohoo IR, O'Callaghan MW. Results of bone scintigraphy in racing standardbred horses: 64 cases (1992–1994). J Am Vet Med Assoc 1999;215:982–991.
29. Firth EC, Delahunt J, Wichtel JW, et al. Galloping exercise induces regional changes in bone density within the third and radial carpal bones of Thoroughbred horses. Equine Vet J 1999;31:111–115.
30. Firth EC, Goodship AE, Delahunt J, et al. Osteoinductive response in the dorsal aspect of the carpus of young thoroughbreds in training occurs within months. Equine Vet J Suppl 1999;30:552–554.
31. Fischer AT Jr, Stover SM. Sagittal fractures of the third carpal bone in horses: 12 cases (1977–1985). J Am Vet Med Assoc 1987;191:106–108.
32. Ford TS, Ross MW, Orsini PG. Communications and boundaries of the middle carpal and carpometacarpal joints in horses. Am J Vet Res 1988;49:2161–2164.
33. Ford TS, Ross MW, Orsini PG. A comparison of methods for proximal palmar metacarpal analgesia in horses. Vet Surg 1989;18:146–150.
34. Fretz PB. Angular limb deformities in foals. Vet Clin North Am Large Anim Pract 1980;2:125.
35. Fretz PB, Cymbaluk NF, Pharr JW. Quantitative analysis of long-bone growth in the horse. Am J Vet Res 1984;45:1602–1609.
36. Fretz PB, Donecker JM. Surgical correction of angular limb deformities in foals: a retrospective study. J Am Vet Med Assoc 1983;183:529–532.
37. Garner HE, St. Clair LE, Hardenbrook HJ. Clinical and radiographic studies of the distal portion of the radius in race horses. J Am Vet Med Assoc 1966;149:1536.
38. Gaughan EM, Bene DJ, Hoskinson JJ. Partial physiolysis with temporary transphyseal bridging for correction of physeal dysplasia and angular limb deformity in two yearling horses. Vet Comp Orthop and Traumatol 1996;9:101.
39. Hawkins JF, Lescun TB. Sepsis of the common digital extensor tendon sheath secondary to hemicircumferential periosteal transection in a foal. J Am Vet Med Assoc 1997;211:331–332.
40. Held HP, Patton CS, Shires M. Solitary osteochondroma of the radius in three horses. J Am Vet Med Assoc 1988;193:563.
41. Hongaten GR, Rooker GD. The role of the periosteum in growth of long bones. J Bone Joint Surg 1979;61B:218.
42. Hunt RJ. Flexural limb deformity in foals. In Diagnosis and Management of Lameness in Horses. Ross MW, Dyson SJ, eds. WB Saunders, Philadelphia, 2003;562–565.
43. Hurtig MB, Green SL, Dobson H, et al. Defective bone and cartilage in foals fed a low copper diet. Proceedings Am Assoc Equine Pract 1991;637–644.
44. Jaffe HL. Tumors and Tumorous Conditions of Bones and Joints. Lea and Febiger, Philadelphia, 1958;143–160.
45. Jann H. Treatment of acquired bursitis (hygroma) by en-bloc resection. Vet Clin North Am Equine Pract 1990;12:8.
46. Jansson N. Osteochondroma at the distal radial metaphysis in a horse. Pferdeheilkunde 1998;14:151–154.
47. Johnson JE, Ryan GD. Intersynovial fistula in the carpus of a horse. Cornell Vet 1975;65:84–89.

48. Johnson JH. Conditions of the forelimbs. In Equine Medicine and Surgery, 2nd ed. Catcott EJ, Smithcors JF, eds. American Veterinary Publications, Inc. 1972;559.

49. Johnson JH, Lowe JE. Rupture of the common digital extensor tendon. In Textbook of Large Animal Surgery. Oehme FW, Prier JE, eds. Williams and Wilkins Co., Baltimore, 1974.

50. Kasper CA, Clayton HM, Wright AK, et al. Effects of high doses of oxytetracycline on metacarpophalangeal joint kinematics in neonatal foals. J Am Vet Med Assoc 1995;207:71–73.

51. Kawcak C, Trotter G. Other conditions affecting equine joints. In Joint Disease in the Horse. McIlwraith CW, Trotter G, eds. WB Saunders, Philadelphia, 1996.

52. Kawcak CE, Frisbie DD, Werpy NM, et al. Effects of exercise vs experimental osteoarthritis on imaging outcomes. Osteoarthritis Cartilage 2008;16:1519–1525.

53. Kawcak CE, McIlwraith CW, Norrdin RW, et al. Clinical effects of exercise on subchondral bone of carpal and metacarpophalangeal joints in horses. Am J Vet Res 2000;61:1252–1258.

54. Kelly NJ, Watrous BJ, Wagner PC. Comparison of splinting and casting on the degree of laxity induced in thoracic limbs in young horses. Vet Clin North Am Equine Pract 1987;9:10.

55. Lee HA, Grant BD, Gallina AM. Solitary osteochondroma in a horse: a case report. J Equine Med Surg 1979;3:113.

56. Levine DG, Richardson DW. Clinical use of the locking compression plate (LCP) in horses: a retrospective study of 31 cases (2004–2006). Equine Vet J 2007;39:401–406.

57. Lindsay WA, Horney FD. Equine carpal surgery: A review of 89 cases and evaluation of return to function. J Am Vet Med Assoc 1981;179:682–685.

58. Lingard D. Strain of the superior check ligament of the horse. J Am Vet Med Assoc 1996;148:364.

59. Llewellyan HR. A case of carpal intersynovial fistula in a horse. Equine Vet J 1979;11:90.

60. Lokai MD, Meyer RJ. Preliminary observation on oxytetracycline treatment of congenital flexural deformities in foals. Modern Vet Pract 1985;66:237.

61. Lucas JM, Ross MW, Richardson DW. Post operative performance of racing Standardbreds treated arthroscopically for carpal chip fractures: 176 cases (1986–1993). Equine Vet J 1999;31:48–52.

62. Lundvall RL. Periosteal new bone formation of the radius as a cause of lameness in two horses. J Am Vet Med Assoc 1976;168:612–613.

63. Mackay-Smith MP, Cushing LS, Leslie JA. "Carpal canal" syndrome in horses. J Am Vet Med Assoc 1972;160:993–997.

64. Madison JB, Garber JL, Rice B, et al. Effect of oxytetracycline on metacarpophalangeal and distal interphalangeal joint angles in newborn foals. J Am Vet Med Assoc 1994;204:246–249.

65. Malone ED, Les CM, Turner TA. Severe carpometacarpal osteoarthritis in older Arabian horses. Vet Surg 2003;32:191–195.

66. Manning JP, St. Clair LE. Carpal hyperextension and arthrosis in the horse. Proceedings Am Assoc Equine Pract 1972;173.

67. Martin GS, Haynes PF, McClure JR. Effect of third carpal slab fracture and repair on racing performance in Thoroughbred horses: 31 cases (1977–1984). J Am Vet Med Assoc 1988;193:107–110.

68. Mason TA. Chronic tenosynovitis of the extensor tendons and tendon sheaths of the carpal region in the horse. Equine Vet J 1977;9:186–188.

69. Mason TA. A high incidence of congenital angular limb deformities in a group of foals. Vet Rec 1981;109:93.

70. McIlwraith CW. Diagnostic and surgical arthroscopy of the carpal joint. Diagnostic and Surgical Arthroscopy in the Horse, 3rd ed. In McIlwraith CW, Nixon AJ, Wright IM, et al., eds. Mosby Elsevier, Edinburgh, 2005.

71. McIlwraith CW, James LF. Limb deformities in foals associated with ingestion of locoweed by mares. J Am Vet Med Assoc 1982;181:255–258.

72. McIlwraith CW, Yovich JV, Martin GS. Arthroscopic surgery for the treatment of osteochondral chip fractures in the equine carpus. J Am Vet Med Assoc 1987;191:531–540.

73. McLaughlin BG, Doige CE. A study of ossification of carpal and tarsal bones in normal and hypothyroid foals. Can Vet J 1982;23:164–168.

74. McLaughlin BG, Doige CE, Fretz PB, et al. Carpal bone lesions associated with angular limb deformities in foals. J Am Vet Med Assoc 1981;178:224–230.

75. Meyers VS, Gordon GW. Ruptured common digital extensor tendon associated with contracted flexor tendon in foals. Proceedings Am Assoc Equine Pract 1975;67.

76. Mitten LA, Bramlage LR, Embertson RM. Racing performance after hemicircumferential periosteal transection for angular limb deformities in thoroughbreds: 199 cases (1987–1989). J Am Vet Med Assoc 1995;207:746–750.

77. Mizuno Y. Fractures of the carpus in racing Thoroughbreds of the Japan Racing Association: Prevalence, location and current modes of surgical therapy. J Equine Vet Sci 1996;16:25.

78. Nixon AJ, Schachter BL, Pool RR. Exostoses of the caudal perimeter of the radial physis as a cause of carpal synovial sheath tenosynovitis and lameness in horses: 10 cases (1999–2003). J Am Vet Med Assoc 2004;224:264–270.

79. Norrdin RW, Kawcak CE, Capwell BA, et al. Calcified cartilage morphometry and its relation to subchondral bone remodeling in equine arthrosis. Bone 1999;24:109–114.

80. Palmer JL, Bertone AL, Litsky AS. Contact area and pressure distribution changes of the equine third carpal bone during loading. Equine Vet J 1994;26:197–202.

81. Palmer JL, Bertone AL, Mansour J, et al. Biomechanical properties of third carpal articular cartilage in exercised and nonexercised horses. J Orthop Res 1995;13:854–860.

82. Palmer SE. Prevalence of carpal fractures in thoroughbred and standardbred racehorses. J Am Vet Med Assoc 1986;188:1171–1173.

83. Pharr JW, Fretz PB. Radiographic findings in foals with angular limb deformities. J Am Vet Med Assoc 1981;179:812–817.

84. Poole R. Tumors and tumor like lesions of joints and adjacent soft tissues. In Tumors in Domestic Animals. 3rd ed. Moulton JE, ed. University of California Press, Berkley, 1990.

85. Read EK, Read MR, Townsend HG, et al. Effect of hemi-circumferential periosteal transection and elevation in foals with experimentally induced angular limb deformities. J Am Vet Med Assoc 2002;221:536–540.

86. Roberts EJ. Carpal lameness. British Equine Veterinary Association Annual Conference 1964;181.

87. Ross MW. The Carpus. In Diagnosis and Management of Lameness Horses. Ross MW, Dyson SJ, eds. Saunders, Philadelphia, 2003;376–393.

88. Schneider RK, Bramlage LR, Gabel AA, et al. Incidence, location and classification of 371 third carpal bone fractures in 313 horses. Equine Vet J Suppl 1988;33–42.

89. Sedrish SA, Moore RM. Diagnosis and management of incomplete ossification of the cuboidal bones in foals. Vet Clin North Am Equine Pract 1997;19:16.

90. Shupe JL, Leone NC, Olson AE, et al. Hereditary multiple exostoses: clinicopathologic features of a comparative study in horses and man. Am J Vet Res 1979;40:751–757.

91. Slone DE, Roberts CT, Hughes FE. Restricted exercise and transphyseal bridging for correction of angular limb deformities. Proceedings Am Assoc Equine Pract 2000;126–127.

92. Southwood LL, Stashak TS, Fehr JE, et al. Lateral approach for endoscopic removal of solitary osteochondromas from the distal radial metaphysis in three horses. J Am Vet Med Assoc 1997;210:1166–1168.

93. Squire KR, Adams SB, Widmer WR, et al. Arthroscopic removal of a palmar radial osteochondroma causing carpal canal syndrome in a horse. J Am Vet Med Assoc 1992;201:1216–1218.

94. Stahre L, Tufvesson G. Volar, supracarpal exostoses as causes of lameness in the horse. Nord Vet Med 1967;19:356.

95. Stashak TS. Lameness. In Adams' Lameness in Horses. Stashak TS, ed. Lea and Febiger, Philadelphia, 1987.

96. Stephens PR, Richardson DW, Spencer PA. Slab fractures of the third carpal bone in standardbreds and thoroughbreds: 155 cases (1977–1984). J Am Vet Med Assoc 1988;193:353–358.

97. Textor JA, Nixon AJ, Fortier LA. Tenoscopic release of the equine carpal canal. Vet Surg 2003;32:278–284.

98. Uhlhorn H, Ekman S, Haglund A, et al. The accuracy of the dorsoproximal-dorsodistal projection in assessing third carpal bone sclerosis in standardbred trotters. Vet Radiol Ultrasound 1998;39:412–417.

99. van Veenendaal JC, Speirs VC, Harrison I. Treatment of hygromata in horses. Aust Vet J 1981;57:513–514.

100. Wallace CE. Chronic tendosynovitis of the extensor carpi radialis tendon in the horse. Aust Vet J 1972;48:585–587.

101. Watkins JP. Osteochondroma. In Equine Surgery, 2nd ed. Auer JA, Stick JA, eds. WB Saunders Co., Philadelphia, 1999; 840–841.

102. Whitton RC, Kannegieter NJ, Rose RJ. The intercarpal liga-ments of the equine midcarpal joint, Part 3: Clinical observa-tions in 32 racing horses with midcarpal joint disease. Vet Surg 1997;26:374–381.

103. Whitton RC, Kannegieter NJ, Rose RJ. Postoperative perfor-mance of racing horses with tearing of the medial palmar inter-carpal ligament. Aust Vet J 1999;77:713–717.

104. Whitton RC, McCarthy PH, Rose RJ. The intercarpal ligaments of the equine midcarpal joint, Part 1: The anatomy of the palmar and dorsomedial intercarpal ligaments of the midcarpal joint. Vet Surg 1997;26:359–366.

105. Whitton RC, Rose RJ. The intercarpal ligaments of the equine midcarpal joint, Part 2: The role of the palmar intercarpal liga-ments in the restraint of dorsal displacement of the proximal row of carpal bones. Vet Surg 1997;26:367–373.

106. Whitton RC, Rose RJ. Postmortem lesions in the intercarpal ligaments of the equine midcarpal joint. Aust Vet J 1997;75:746–750.

107. Witte S, Rodgerson DH. What is your diagnosis? Swelling of the soft tissue around the carpal joint. Osteomyelitis of the accessory carpal bone. J Am Vet Med Assoc 2005;227:551–552.

108. Young DR, Nunamaker DM, Markel MD. Quantitative evalu-ation of the remodeling response of the proximal sesamoid bones to training-related stimuli in Thoroughbreds. Am J Vet Res 1991;52:1350–1356.

109. Yovich JV, Stashak TS, McIlwraith CW. Rupture of the common digital extensor tendon in foals. Compend Cont Educ 1984;6:S373.

THE ANTEBRACHIUM, ELBOW, AND HUMERUS

Jeremy Hubert and Ted S. Stashak

FRACTURES OF THE RADIUS

In 2 older retrospectives studies, fractures of the radius represented from 8% to 14% of all fractures in horses.[10,19] Of the fracture configurations that were reported in a large retrospective study, comminuted fractures were most common (21 of 47), followed by oblique fractures (12 of 47), transverse fractures (7 of 47), and physeal fractures (7 of 47).[17] Open fractures usually involve the medial surface of the antebrachium, where there is minimal soft tissue covering (Figures 5.246 to 5.248).[17] Incomplete or fissure fractures are relatively common fractures of the radius; a retrospective study of incomplete or fissure fractures showed that the majority of these fractures occurred along the longitudinal plane.[7] Other uncommon radial fractures include stress fractures and smaller articular fractures involving either the proximal or distal articulation (Figure 5.249).[14]

Etiology

Radial fractures usually result from a high-impact blunt trauma such as a kick from another horse. A controlled postmortem study to evaluate fracture configurations of the radius after a simulated kick on the medial aspect of the radius resulted in the majority of the bones sustaining a fissure fracture (incomplete fracture) that ran longitudinally along the diaphysis. The next most common configuration was an oblique fracture, sometimes with a fissure component, followed by a butterfly fragment fracture.[11] The medial aspect of the bone was chosen in the postmortem study to emulate the more common finding of a kick to the medial side; a smaller retrospective study of radial fractures revealed the majority occurred from a kick to the medial aspect of the bone.[7] Age may play a role in fracture configuration; comminuted or butterfly fragment fractures are usually noted in older horses (older than 2 years), whereas simple oblique fractures occurred in younger horses. Transverse fractures were exclusive to foals less than 6 months of age.[17]

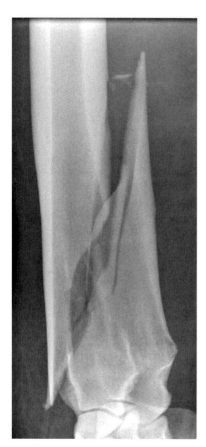

Figure 5.246. A complete oblique fracture of the radius extending from the mid-diaphysis to the metaphysis. (Courtesy of Dr. Andrew Lewis.)

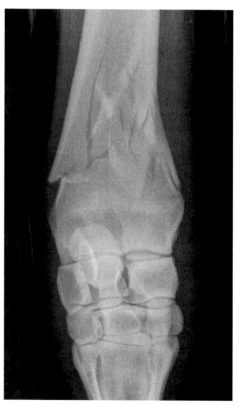

Figure 5.247. A cranial-caudal view of a distal diaphyseal comminuted fracture of the radius. (Courtesy of Dr. Martin Waselau.)

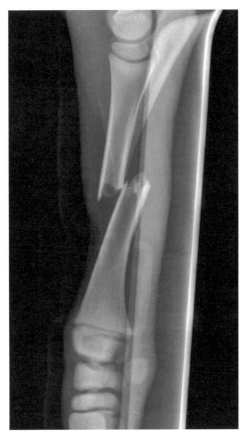

Figure 5.248. A transverse complete midshaft fracture of the radius of a foal. (Courtesy of Dr. Martin Waselau.)

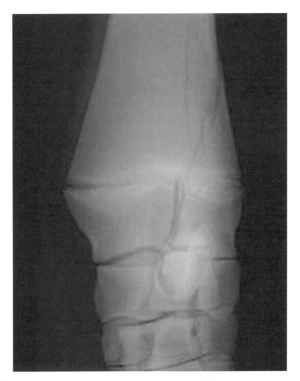

Figure 5.249. A distal articular fracture of the radius entering the radiocarpal joint. (Courtesy of Dr. Markus Wilke.)

Clinical Signs

Complete displaced fractures of the radius are easily identified on physical examination alone. Horses present with a nonweight-bearing lameness, varying degrees of swelling in the antebrachium, and instability associated with the fracture site. Crepitation may be felt and pain elicited when the distal limb is manipulated. Wounds or penetration of the skin from the fracture on the distal medial side of the antebrachium are common.

Complete or incomplete nondisplaced fracture of the radius can be more difficult to identify. Horses that present with this injury are usually very lame but are willing to bear some weight on the limb. Instability and crepitation are not present; however, there is usually some swelling of the antebrachium and pressure applied to the region is often painful.[1,3] Wounds at the site of traumatic impact are often present on the medial distal aspect of the antebrachium.

Stress fractures are difficult to identify on physical signs alone. Horses generally present with a history of an acute onset of lameness that subsides with rest and reoccurs with exercise. Horses are often mildly lame at examination and shoulder flexion may worsen the lameness. These fractures can also occur bilaterally.[14]

Diagnosis

The presence of a displaced radial fracture is confirmed on radiographic examination. Several views are often needed to evaluate the configuration and extent of the fracture. Computerized tomography (CT) may be useful to assist in determining the ideal internal repair method if a complex comminuted fracture is to be assessed completely.

Acute nondisplaced fractures may be difficult to diagnose initially on radiographic exam. If a nondisplaced fracture is suspected, the horse should be cross-tied in a stall to prevent it from lying down and repeat radiographs should be taken in 2 to 4 days.[1] This time period usually allows recognition of the fractures lines. Alternatively, nuclear scintigraphy can be used to assist in the diagnosis.

Stress fractures are usually best diagnosed by nuclear scintigraphy (Figure 5.250); a focal increased uptake of the radionuclide in the midshaft of the radius is usually found.[14] Confirmation with radiography can be performed at a later date (Figure 5.251). Evidence of focal endosteal or periosteal reaction indicates a healing stress fracture that will correlate with the focal area of increased uptake. Alternatively, quantitative scintigraphy can be performed.[20] This enables the clinician to assess the degree of injury if there are no initial radiographic findings as well as later during the convalescent period when the quantitative findings can be used to accurately determine a date to return to training or work.

Treatment

First Aid

The first aid management of horses sustaining a complete displaced fracture of the radius has an important bearing on the outcome. Minimizing further soft tissue injury is paramount. Open wounds associated with

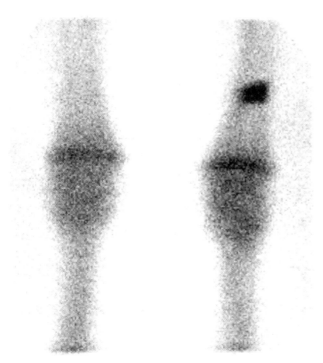

Figure 5.250. A nuclear scintigraphic examination of increased uptake of radioactive isotope in the distal radius, indicating a stress fracture of the metaphysis. (Courtesy of Dr. Dan Burba.)

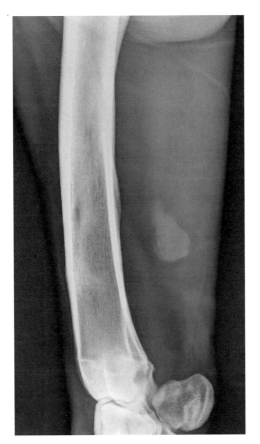

Figure 5.251. Healing stress fracture of the radius evidenced by the extensive remodeling. (Courtesy of Dr. Lorrie Gaschen.)

radial fractures should be treated immediately. Wounds from a kick or from the fracture penetrating the skin are most common on the medial surface of the antebrachium, and they most often communicate directly with the fracture. Initial wound management includes hair removal, thorough cleansing and debridement of the wound, application of a topical antiseptic or antimicrobial, wound protection, and the systemic administration of broad-spectrum antimicrobials.

Immediate immobilization of a displaced radial fracture is very important (Figure 5.252). With closed displaced fractures, application of appropriate external coaptation can prevent the fracture from becoming open. A heavy layered cotton bandage is firmly applied from the hoof to as far proximal on the antebrachium as possible. Two splints, one placed lateral and one placed caudal to the limb, with the lateral splint extending from the ground to the withers and the caudal splint extending from the ground to the olecranon process, is recommended.[5] Nonelastic adhesive tape or 1 to 2 rolls of fiberglass cast material are used to affix the splints to the bandage. The portion of the lateral splint that extends proximal to the bandage should contact the brachium when the limb is in a weight-bearing position.[21] This proximal application of the lateral splint provides counter-pressure to prevent the limb from abducting with weight-bearing. This approach generally stabilizes the limb enough to allow the patient to be transported for treatment without running the risk of further injury to the fracture site.

Displaced Fractures

Internal fixation of complete displaced fractures of the radius is the preferred method of treatment. The use of transfixation casts is generally considered for open contaminated fractures in which the chances of successful plate fixation are poor because of the risk of infection or when there are economic constraints. The application of a full-limb cast alone for displaced fractures of the radius is not acceptable in most cases because the humeroradial joint cannot be adequately immobilized. If a cast is applied, it frequently results in increased rotational forces on and movement at the fracture site. In addition, the more proximal the fracture, the greater the chances that the cast will cause a pendulum effect to the distal limb. This causes more tissue damage and results in a failure of the fracture to heal.[9] However, cast application alone has been used to successfully treat some distal radial fractures when there are economic constraints.

A combination of a full-limb cast and Thomas splint has also been recommended for some uncomplicated midshaft radius fractures in young horses.[9,15] Bandage splints have been used to treat a few horses with complete fractures of the distal radius. In one report, 2 horses with complete fractures (1 nondisplaced, 1 displaced) involving the distal half of the radius were treated successfully with a modified Robert-Jones bandage with the addition of light strong splints.[16] Healing occurred in 14 to 16 weeks and both horses were able to return to usefulness.

A transfixation pin cast using positive profile, centrally threaded, one-fourth-inch stainless steel pins

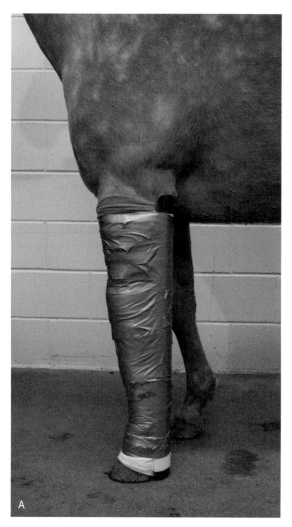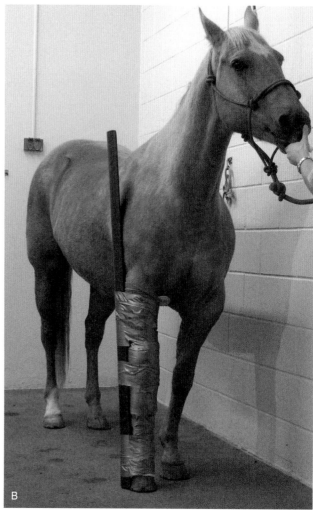

Figure 5.252. Proper bandaging and splinting a horse with a radial fracture. A bandage and caudal splint are applied (A) and then a lateral splint extending proximal to the shoulder is used to help prevent limb abduction (B).

placed transcortically is best suited for fractures in the distal third of the radius (Figure 5.253). Two transfixation pins are placed proximal to the fracture to support some of the horses' weight and stabilize the fracture against torsional forces. The pins are preferentially placed in the sagittal plane at 30° to each other. After the pins are placed, a cast incorporating the pins is applied. Biomechanical studies have been undertaken to compare traditional transfixation pin casts as described above with novel tapered sleeve pins in a transfixation cast; the novel tapered sleeve pins were shown to provide a significantly greater mean load to failure in an *ex-vivo* study.[8]

A single-plate application on the cranial or craniolateral surface is only recommended in foals less than 250 kg that have a transverse mid-diaphyseal fracture with an intact caudal cortex (Figure 5.254).[21] However, internal fixation in adult horses for displaced fractures still carries an unfavorable prognosis. In larger foals and adults, 2 plates are used; one is placed as a tension band on the cranial surface and the other is placed as a neutralization plate on the lateral or medial surface 90° to the other plate.[2] The use of a 5-mm locking compression plate (LCP) or a dynamic condylar plate (DCP) as one of the plates is recommended.[13,21] If a DCP is used, the condylar screw should be placed in the smaller fragment.[21] The plates should be staggered and span as much of the bone as possible. The lateral plate placement is technically demanding; the bone is approached between the extensor carpi radialis and the common digital extensor tendon (Figure 5.255). Lateral placement has an advantage in that it avoids positioning the implant subcutaneously and avoids the often open contaminated medial aspect. In foals, it is preferential not to bridge the physes and to not engage the ulna because it could result in elbow dysplasia and arthritis due to the differential growth rate of the ulna and radius.[18]

Other reported techniques for internal fixation include the use of a cobra head plate for distal fractures[12] as well as the combined use of plates and cerclage wires or cables for minimally displaced fractures.[4] For comminuted fractures, the larger fragments are generally attached to the proximal and distal extent of the radius with lag screws, creating 2 large fragments which

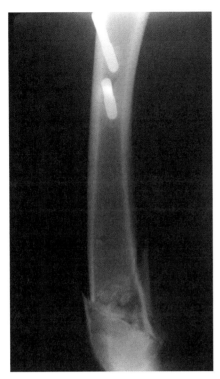

Figure 5.253. Transfixation pins applied to the proximal radius prior to applying a full-limb cast to treat a comminuted distal radial fracture.

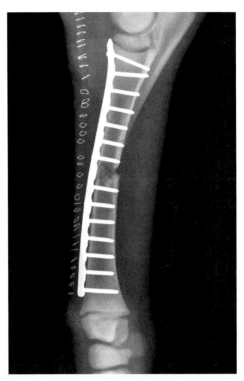

Figure 5.254. Single DCP plate application on the cranial surface of the radius to repair a transverse mid-diaphyseal fracture in a foal weighing less than 250kg.

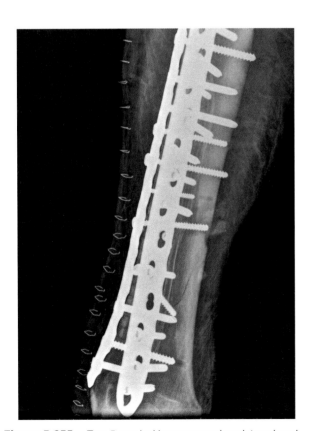

Figure 5.255. Two 5-mm locking compression plates placed on the dorsal and lateral aspects of an obliquely fractured radius. (Courtesy of Dr. Dan Burba.)

are then reduced.[6] 5.5-mm cortical screws are recommended for all holes where possible and compression is applied where possible.[21] Plate luting with antimicrobial–impregnated PMMA and bone graft application is advisable.[21]

Once the fracture is healed, plates are removed in all horses that are to be used as athletes. Removal of the plates should be staged by 60 days to minimize weakening of the bone due to the stress-concentrating affect of empty screw holes.[6] Following this the horse is rested in a box stall until healing is evident.[6]

Nondisplaced Fractures

Fractures that are nondisplaced or incomplete with minimal displacement are often candidates for conservative treatment. This involves stall confinement for up to 3 to 4 months.[3,7] It may be necessary to attach the horse to a wire to ensure it will not be able to lie down to initially prevent catastrophic breakdown of the fracture. Horses should be closely watched for tolerance of being tied. NSAIDs are initially administered; these can be weaned off over time. Short hand walks can be initiated after 90 days. A total of at least 6 months before a return to intended use should be considered.

Physeal Fractures

Salter-Harris type 1 and 2 fractures of the proximal physis are encountered (Figure 5.256). They may be accompanied by a fracture of the ulna, and a degree of radial nerve trauma may be encountered. Repair

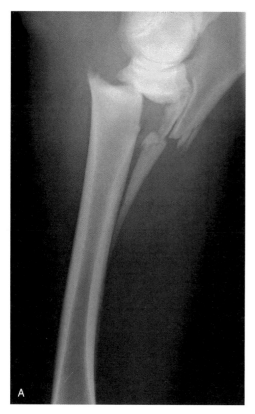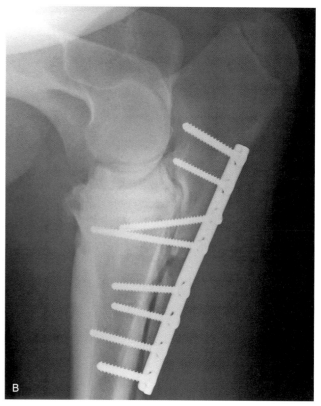

Figure 5.256. A. A Salter-Harris type 2 fracture of the proximal radius combined with fracture of the ulna. The fracture was repaired with a single DCP along the caudal aspect of the ulna with the screws incorporating the radius (B). (Courtesy of Dr. Gary Baxter.)

generally involves a single-plate fixation of the ulna with the screws at the level of the proximal physis and lower, engaging both cortices of the radius. A second plate can be placed laterally with the proximal screw in the physis.[21] In smaller foals, the repair can be performed by transphyseal screws, and a wire fixation instead of a lateral plate can be placed alone. There is minimal growth from the proximal physis due to the damage, and luxation of the elbow joint is unlikely. Type 3 fractures that are nondisplaced are rested, whereas displaced type 3 fractures are repaired with screws placed in lag fashion in combination with a tension band application.[17,21]

The distal radial physis in foals may involve Salter-Harris type 1 fractures with medial displacement of the physis. A transphyseal bridge or T-plate application or Steinmann pins placed across the physis in a cruciate pattern should suffice. Distal type 2 fractures may occur in older horses with considerable displacement. A cast application alone can be considered as can a 2-plate application with the distal screws engaging the epiphysis.

Prognosis

The prognosis for displaced radial fractures depends on the age and weight of the horse, its temperament, and the fracture type. In one report on 47 cases of radial fractures, successful treatment (82%) only occurred in horses younger than 2 years of age.[17] Although there are a few reports of successful treatment of displaced radial fractures with internal fixation in mature horses, most adult horses have an unfavorable prognosis for survival regardless of the treatment selected.[17,21] In one retrospective study of horses weighing more than 300 kg presenting with radial fracture, 9 of 15 were treated with internal fixation and only 2 horses were discharged from the hospital to resume their former activities.[2] In another report, internal fixation was attempted in 6 adult horses and none survived.[17] Reasons for nonsurvival included primary implant failure, infection causing implant failure, and support limb laminitis. Comminuted fractures were associated with the highest incidence of fatal complications.

Displaced closed simple fractures of the radius in foals have a favorable prognosis. Physeal and transverse mid-diaphyseal fractures have an excellent prognosis. In one report 2 of 2 foals with Salter-Harris type I and II proximal physeal fractures and 6 of 7 foals with mid-diaphyseal transverse fractures were treated successfully. Treatment of proximal oblique fractures in 3 of 4 foals also had an excellent outcome.[17]

Nondisplaced complete and incomplete fractures appear to have a good prognosis with conservative treatment.[3,7,16] Stress fractures of the radius are expected to have a good prognosis if adequately rested, similar to reported results of tibial and humeral stress fractures.[15]

References

1. Auer J. Equine fracture repair. In Fractures of the Radius. Nixon A, ed. WB Saunders, Philadelphia, 1996;222–230.

2. Auer JA, Watkins JP. Treatment of radial fractures in adult horses: an analysis of 15 clinical cases. Equine Vet J 1987;19:103–110.
3. Barr AR, Denny HR. Three cases of non-displaced radial fracture in horses. Vet Rec 1989;125:35–37.
4. Bolt DM, Burba DJ. Use of a dynamic compression plate and a cable cerclage system for repair of a fracture of the radius in a horse. J Am Vet Med Assoc 2003;223:89–92.
5. Bramlage L. Current concepts of emergency first aid treatment and transportation of equine fracture patients. Comp Cont Edu 1983;5S:564.
6. Carter BG, Schneider RK, Hardy J, et al. Assessment and treatment of equine humeral fractures: retrospective study of 54 cases (1972–1990). Equine Vet J 1993;25:203–207.
7. Derungs S, Furst A, Haas C, et al. Fissure fractures of the radius and tibia in 23 horses: a retrospective study. Equine Veterinary Education 2001;13:313–318.
8. Elce YA, Southwood LL, Nutt JN, et al. *Ex vivo* comparison of a novel tapered-sleeve and traditional full-limb transfixation pin cast for distal radial fracture stabilization in the horse. Vet Comp Orthop Traumatol 2006;19:93–97.
9. Fessler J, Amstutz H. Ulna. In Large Animal Surgery. Oehme F, Prier J, eds. Williams and Wilkins, Baltimore, 1974;312–316.
10. Frohner E. General Surgery, 3rd edition. Taylor and Carpenter, Ithaca, 1906.
11. Fuerst AE, Oswald S, Jaggin S, et al. Fracture configurations of the equine radius and tibia after a simulated kick. Vet Comp Orthop Traumatol 2008;21:49–58.
12. Kirker-Head CA, Fackelman GE. Use of the cobra head bone plate for distal long bone fractures in large animals. A report of four cases. Vet Surg 1989;18:227–234.
13. Levine DG, Richardson DW. Clinical use of the locking compression plate (LCP) in horses: a retrospective study of 31 cases (2004–2006). Equine Vet J 2007;39:401–406.
14. Mackey V, Trout D, Meagher D, et al. Stress fractures of the humerus, radius, and tibia in horses. Clinical features and radiographic and/or scintigraphic appearance. Veterinary Radiology 1987;28:26–31.
15. O'Sullivan CB, Lumsden JM. Stress fractures of the tibia and humerus in Thoroughbred racehorses: 99 cases (1992–2000). J Am Vet Med Assoc 2003;222:491–498.
16. Pallaoro D. Successful treatment of complete radial fractures in aged horses using external coaptation: Two cases. Equine Practice 1998;20:16–18.
17. Sanders-Shamis M, Bramlage LR, Gable AA. Radius fractures in the horse: a retrospective study of 47 cases. Equine Vet J 1986;18:432–437.
18. Stover R, Rick M. Ulnar luxation following repair of a fractured radius in a foal. Veterinary Surgery 1985;14:27–31.
19. Trum B. Fractures. The Veterinary Bulletin Supplement to the Army Medical Bulletin 1939;33.
20. Valdes-Martinez A, Seiler G, Mai W, et al. Quantitative analysis of scintigraphic findings in tibial stress fractures in Thoroughbred racehorses. Am J Vet Res 2008;69:886–890.
21. Watkins JP. The radius and ulna. In Equine Surgery, 3rd ed., Auer J, Stick J, eds. WB Saunders Co, Philadelphia, 2006;1267–1279.

THE ELBOW

Fractures of the Ulna

The ulna is a very commonly fractured equine long bone; in one report it accounts for 5.2% of all fractures in a 30-year period.[9] It is a relatively common fracture in younger horses. In a retrospective study of 49 ulnar fractures, 79% occurred in horses less than 2 years of age.[18]

Ulnar fractures are classified as types I through VI (Figure 5.257). Types I and II are Salter-Harris types, fracturing through the apophysis of the olecranon tuberosity in horses that are usually less than a year old. Type I is more common in neonates, whereas type II is more common in older foals. The incidence of these fractures is reduced as this physis closes, starting around

15 months of age. Types III through VI involve the diaphysis of the olecranon (Figure 5.258). In adults the fractures often involve the articular surface and are displaced due to contracture of the triceps apparatus.[5–7,18] Displacement is relative to the level of fracture on the ulna; fractures distal to the level of the elbow joint have less distraction due to the ligaments between the radius and ulna.

Etiology

Direct impact or trauma is the most common cause; however, in foals, type I and II fractures can occur from excessive tensile load of the triceps apparatus. Kick injuries appear to be a common cause of ulna fractures in adults and may be associated with wounds on the lateral aspect of the elbow.

Clinical Signs

Fractures of the ulna usually result in an acute non-weight-bearing lameness with a classic dropped elbow appearance (with the carpus flexed and the horse not bearing any weight on the limb; Figure 5.259). Nondisplaced fractures may initially show the dropped elbow appearance but will show progressive weight-bearing of the limb. Varying degrees of soft tissue swelling, crepitation, and skin wounds are apparent. Limb manipulation is resisted and efforts to get the horse to load the leg, even with a splint in place, are unsuccessful until the triceps apparatus has been repaired.

Diagnosis

Diagnosis is based upon the appearance of the horse, limb palpation, and radiographs. Differential diagnoses may include radial or humeral fractures, radial nerve paresis, or joint sepsis until a radiographic study has been performed. This should include lateral and cranio-caudal views to provide the configuration of the fracture. In cases of a type I fracture in foals, it may be necessary to take a flexed view to provide distraction of the fragment to identify the fracture correctly.[16]

Treatment

Fracture cases that include nondisplaced, nonarticular ulna fractures are candidates for conservative treatment. Horses with articular fractures with minimal displacement also may be treated conservatively; however, better results are obtained with internal fixation to maintain joint congruity. Conservative treatment includes bandaging the limb with a caudal splint incorporated to the level of the proximal antebrachium (Figure 5.260). Complete stall rest for at least 6 weeks, along with the possibility of a tethering to a wire in the initial stages, is necessary. The bandage and splint are maintained for several weeks until a substantial improvement in the lameness is noted. NSAIDs are administered in the early stages. Repeated radiographic studies can be performed to ensure fracture healing and that progressive displacement is not occurring.[18]

Anecdotal experience of nonunions occurring in cases treated conservatively have been reported, most

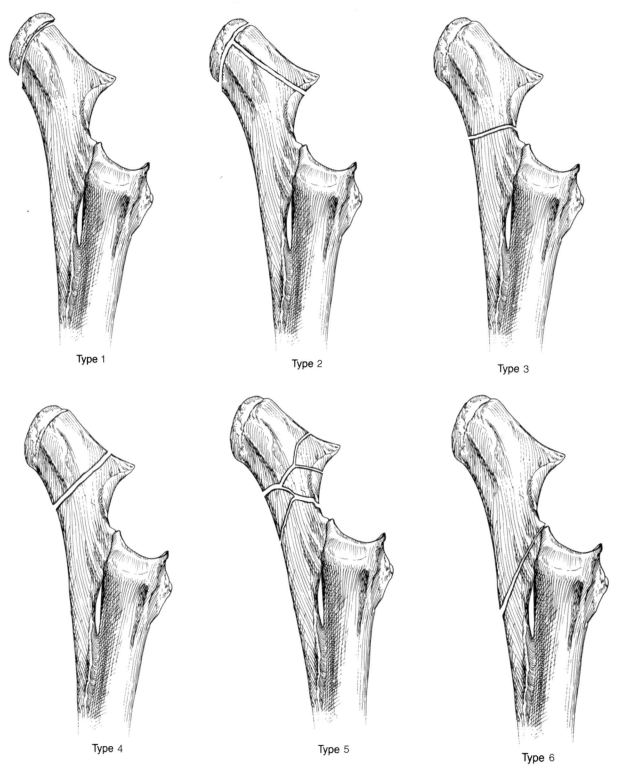

Type 1 Type 2 Type 3

Type 4 Type 5 Type 6

Figure 5.257. Classification of equine ulnar fractures.

likely due to the lack of fracture stability. Nondisplaced fractures with concurrent wounds to the olecranon that are candidates for conservative treatment should be carefully examined to ensure that the wound does not communicate with the fracture and the joint itself. Contrast studies can be performed after adequate debridement to ensure there is no communication.

Internal fixation of ulna fractures are performed in 2 basic manners. In young horses (younger than 6 months), the repair may be performed using a combination of screws, pins, and tension band wires, or plating (Figure 5.261). However, in older horses, a caudal application of a plate using the tension band principle is necessary (Figure 5.262).[2–4,12] A controlled study of

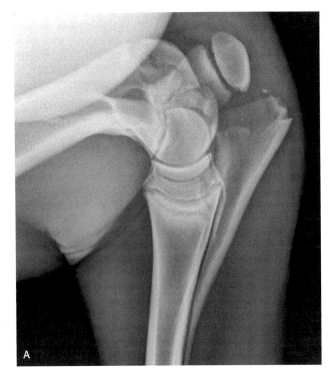
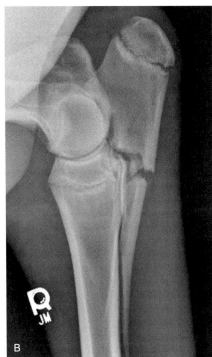

Figure 5.258. A. Type III ulnar fracture. (Courtesy of Dr. Lori Gaschen.) B. Type VI ulnar fracture. (Courtesy of Dr. Martin Waselau.)

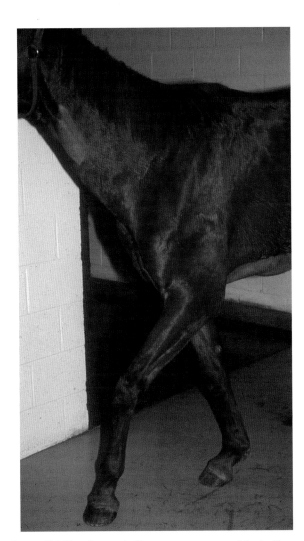

Figure 5.259. Dropped elbow appearance consistent with an elbow fracture. (Courtesy of Dr. Gary Baxter.)

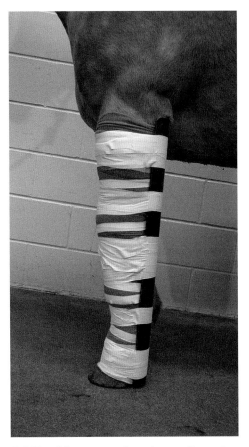

Figure 5.260. When transporting a horse with an ulnar fracture a caudal splint applied from the proximal olecranon to the heel bulbs is the preferred method of stabilizing the limb.

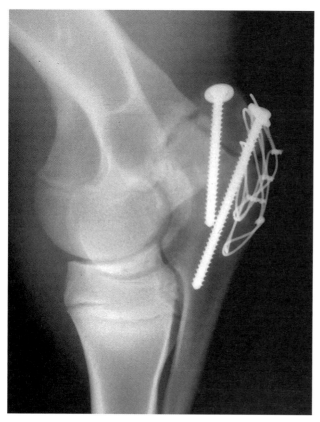

Figure 5.261. Two 4.5-mm cortical screws with washers and figure-8 wires used to create a tension band for a type I ulnar fracture. (Courtesy of Dr. Gary Baxter.)

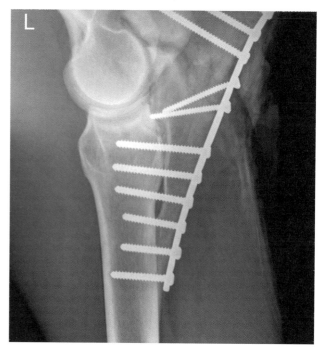

Figure 5.262. Type III ulnar fracture repaired with a narrow DCP applied to the caudal aspect of the ulna. The fracture is in an older horse; therefore, the distal screws penetrate the radius. (Courtesy of Dr. Katie Amend.)

different repair types in adult cadaver limbs showed that DCP plate application was more biomechanically sound than pins and wires.[8] Plates are applied to the caudal aspect of the olecranon and ulna to counteract the tension of the triceps brachii muscle. The plate may be contoured over the top of the olecranon if the fracture is proximally located.[4]

The approach to the ulna is described elsewhere.[13] Depending upon the size of the horse, a narrow or wide DCP can be applied; a broad DCP is applied in horses greater than 500kg.[15] More recently the locking compression plate (LCP) has been used in repairs of the olecranon and may be indicated if possible.[11] There are variable sizes of this plate, and again, the most suitable can be applied. In most adult horses the 4.5-mm narrow LCP is likely to be adequate. It can be useful to flatten the caudal surfaces of the olecranon with an osteotome as well as the proximal eminence if the fracture is located more proximally. Compression can be applied through the plates for oblique fractures and compression can also be applied across the fracture line by applying a tension device to the plate or with the initial 2 screws applied in compression (Figure 5.262). With a highly comminuted fracture the plate should be applied in a neutral fashion. Screws should only penetrate the caudal aspect of the radius in older horses (2 years and older); in younger horses the proximal radius physis is still active and this can result in subluxation of the radiohumeral joint. If it is necessary to place screws into

the caudal radius in younger horses, these screws must be removed as soon as possible. With severely comminuted fractures it may be necessary to place a second, shorter plate along the lateral aspect of the ulna to aid in stabilization.[11]

Articulation of the anconeal process is important for a good result. There are reports of removal of the anconeal process to improve the articulation between the olecranon fossa and the humeral condyles.[15] The prognosis has been good when the anconeal process has fragmented and been removed.[1,10]

Distracted type I and II fractures require contouring the plate over the top of the olecranon. In younger foals a hook plate can be applied, or in even younger foals a tension band device with a pin or screw can be placed through the proximal epiphysis of the olecranon and a tension band of wire applied and twisted about a screw placed caudally and distally in the ulna.[14]

Closure is routine, with application of a stent bandage to protect the incision, and assisted recovery is advised. Perioperative antibiotics are indicated for the duration, depending upon the initial presentation of the fracture and the degree of contamination. Generally, once the triceps apparatus is intact these horses will bear weight immediately and weight-bearing will improve rapidly over the next 10 days. Stall rest for up to 3 months is necessary, and return to exercise usually requires 6 months. The implants are left in place unless infection of the implant develops.

Prognosis

The prognosis for conservative management of nondisplaced fractures and nonarticular fracture types I and

IV of the ulna is considered good.[18] Nondisplaced artic-ular fractures, especially the type VI fracture, also respond well to conservative treatment. One retrospec-tive study reported 70% of affected horses becoming sound.[18]

The prognosis for internal fixation of displaced types III, IV, V, and VI is also considered to be good.[5–7] Internal fixation of type I and II fractures in younger foals has a good prognosis when a hook plate is used, with 7 of 10 foals becoming athletes.[14] Type II fractures in young horses also do very well when repaired with DCP plates, with 16 out of 24 horses returning to ath-leticism.[17] In another study of pins and tension band wiring, 13 of 22 horses were reported to be athletically sound and 18 fractures were considered to be repaired successfully.[12]

References

1. Anderson DE. Comminuted, articular fractures of the olecranon process in horses: 17 cases. Vet Comp Orthop Trauma 1995; 8:141–145.
2. Brown M, Norrie R. Surgical repair of the olecranon in young horses. Journal of Equine Medicine and Surgery 1978;2:545.
3. Colahan P, Meagher D. Repair of comminuted fracture of the proximal ulna and olecranon in young horses using tension band plating. Veterinary Surgery 1979;8:105.
4. Denny HR. The surgical treatment of fractures of the olecranon in the horse. Equine Vet J 1976;8:20–25.
5. Denny HR, Barr AR, Waterman A. Surgical treatment of frac-tures of the olecranon in the horse: a comparative review of 25 cases. Equine Vet J 1987;19:319–325.
6. Donecker JM, Bramlage LR, Gabel AA. Retrospective analysis of 29 fractures of the olecranon process of the equine ulna. J Am Vet Med Assoc 1984;185:183–189.
7. Easley K, Schneider J, Guffy M, et al. Equine ulnar fractures: a review of twenty-five clinical cases. Journal of Equine Veterinary Science 1983;3:5–12.
8. Hanson PD, Hartwig H, Markel MD. Comparison of three methods of ulnar fixation in horses. Vet Surg 1997; 26:165–171.
9. Hertsch B, Abdin-Bey M. Ulna fractures in horses: retrospective analysis of 66 horses. Pferdeheilkunde 1993;9:327–339.
10. Jansson N. Surgical treatment of an ulnar fracture complicated by anconeal process fragmentation. Compendium of Continuing Education for the Veterinary Practitioner 2008;3:144–147.
11. Levine DG, Richardson DW. Clinical use of the locking compres-sion plate (LCP) in horses: a retrospective study of 31 cases (2004–2006). Equine Vet J 2007;39:401–406.
12. Martin F, Richardson DW, Nunamaker DM, et al. Use of tension band wires in horses with fractures of the ulna: 22 cases (1980–1992). J Am Vet Med Assoc 1995;207:1085–1089.
13. Milne D, Turner A. An Atlas of Surgical Approaches to the Bones of Horses. WB Saunders and Co., Philadelphia, 1979.
14. Murray RC, DeBowes RM, Gaughan EM, et al. Application of a hook plate for management of equine ulnar fractures. Vet Surg 1996;25:207–212.
15. Nixon A. Fractures of the ulna. In Equine Fracture Repair. Nixon A, ed. WB Saunders, Philadelphia, 1996;222–230.
16. Richardson DW. Ulnar fractures. In Current Practice in Equine Surgery. White H, Moore J, eds. JB Lippincott, Philadelphia, 1990;641–646.
17. Swor TM, Watkins JP, Bahr A, et al. Results of plate fixation of type 1b olecranon fractures in 24 horses. Equine Vet J 2003;35:670–675.
18. Wilson D, Riedesel E. Nonsurgical management of ulnar frac-tures in the horse. Veterinary Surgery 1985;14:283–286.

Luxation and Subluxation of the Elbow Joint

Subluxation or luxation of the radiohumeral joint with or without a concomitant fracture have been reported, although it is an uncommon injury.[2,4,6,7,9]

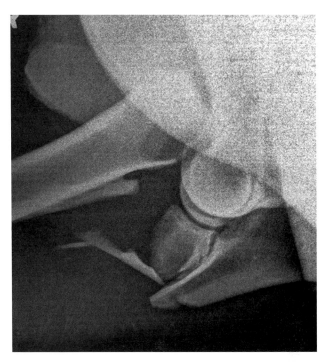

Figure 5.263. Luxation of the elbow joint in conjunction with fracture of both the radius and ulna.

Subluxation commonly occurs with rupture or partial tear of the medial collateral ligament.[8] Complete luxa-tions often occur in conjunction with a fracture[5,9] (Figure 5.263), but luxation without fracture has also been reported (Figure 5.264).[2,4]

Etiology

Severe, forceful limb abduction such as getting a leg caught in a fence is often associated with subluxations of the elbow, whereas severe falls have been reported to cause complete luxations.[2,8]

Clinical Signs

Swelling in the axilla of the affected side with a nonweight-bearing lameness are the commonly reported signs for a subluxation. Palpation of the medial aspect of the joint as well as manipulation elicit a painful response, and limb instability may be noticeable. Signs associated with partial rupture of the medial collateral ligament may be less obvious because there is less inher-ent instability. Swelling may still be noticeable on the medial aspect of the joint. Joint effusion is usually noticeable laterally along with a grade 2 to 3 of 5 lame-ness. Flexion or abduction exacerbate the lameness.[2,8]

A complete luxation usually causes severe swelling and discomfort, with horses unable to bear weight nor extend their limb. This will not resolve until correct alignment and stabilization is established.[8]

Diagnosis

A definitive diagnosis is made with a radiographic examination. Subluxation may require stressed views,

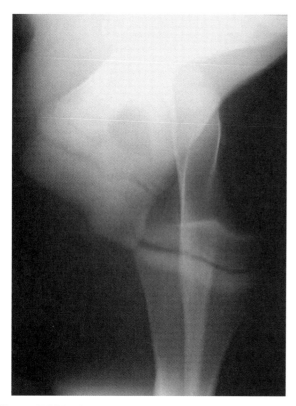

Figure 5.264. Luxation of the elbow joint with the humerus displaced medially. No fracture was present. (Reprinted with permission from Rubio-Martinez LM, Vazquez FJ, Romero A. Elbow luxation in a 1-month old foal. Australian Vet J 2008:86:56–59.)

and chronic cases may reveal evidence of osteoarthritis and an enthesiopathy of the medial collateral ligament. Stressed views are performed by manipulating the limb to exacerbate the subluxation, in this case by stabilizing the humerus and applying pressure to the radius in a medial or lateral direction.

Treatment

Closed reduction and conservative management has been achieved in select cases,[2,4] but more commonly, internal fixation is required because conservative management fails. Conservative management usually results in continued instability and resultant osteoarthritis.[4] Attempts to repair the collateral ligaments in complete luxations have been attempted.[6] Prosthetic collateral ligaments have been made by placing screws in the medial and lateral epicondyles of the distal humerus and the proximal tuberosities of the radius near the attachment of the collateral ligaments and wrapping surgical wire around them in a figure-8 pattern to emulate the ligament.[6]

Luxations in conjunction with an ulna fracture have been reported with no attempt to repair the collateral ligaments. The fracture was repaired with a broad DCP plate placed on the caudal surface of the ulna. Stability was attributed to the interdigitation of the 3 bones of the elbow joint.[9] With any repair attempt, significant distraction is necessary to aid the replacement of the

luxation; in one case a small (1 cm) piece of the anconeal process was removed to assist in reduction.[6] Removal of the anconeal process should not affect prognosis.[1,3]

Prognosis

The prognosis for subluxation of the elbow appears to be guarded to unfavorable to return to performance, depending on the degree of injury to the medial collateral ligament.[8] Generally, a partial tear injury is expected to have a better prognosis and some of these horses may be able to return to light work.

The prognosis for complete luxation is generally considered guarded;[6–8] however, there are at least 2 reports of repairs and the horses were considered sound 6 and 14 months after surgery; the former horse had a concomitant ulna fracture.[2,9]

References

1. Anderson DE. Comminuted, articular fractures of the olecranon process in horses: 17 cases. Vet Comp Orthop Trauma 1995;8: 141–145.
2. Crawley G, Grant B. Repair of elbow joint luxation without concomitant fracture in a horse. Equine Practice 1986;8:19–26.
3. Jansson N. Surgical treatment of an ulnar fracture complicated by anconeal process fragmentation. Compendium of Continuing Education for the Veterinary Practitioner 2008;3:144–147.
4. Jones D. Closed reduction of a radiohumeral luxation in a mule. Equine practice 1995;17:33–36.
5. Levine S, Meagher D. Repair of an ulnar fracture with radial luxation. Veterinary Surgery 1980;9:58–60.
6. Rubio-Martinez LM, Vazquez FJ, Romero A, et al. Elbow joint luxation in a 1-month-old foal. Aust Vet J 2008;86:56–59.
7. Senior M, Smith M, Clegg P. Subluxation of the left elbow joint in a pony at induction of general anaesthesia. Vet Rec 2002;151: 183–184.
8. Stashak T. The Elbow. In Adams' Lameness in Horses. Stashak T, ed. Lippincott Williams and Wilkins, Philadelphia, 2002; 888–890.
9. Trostle SS, Peavey CL, King DS, et al. Treatment of methicillin-resistant Staphylococcus epidermidis infection following repair of an ulnar fracture and humeroradial joint luxation in a horse. J Am Vet Med Assoc 2001;218:554–559, 527.

Subchondral Defects and Subchondral Cystic Lesions (SCL) of the Elbow

Subchondral defects and subchondral cystic lesions (SCL) of the elbow joint are uncommon, although they have been observed in a wide variety of horse breeds of all ages.[1,3,4,8] Subchondral cystic lesions typically communicate with the joint and they most commonly occur on the medial side, involving either the proximal medial radius or distal medial condyle of the humerus (Figure 5.265).[3] Although uncommon, SCLs can occur bilaterally.

Etiology

Proposed causes for subchondral defects and SCLs include osteochondrosis at a weight-bearing location in the joint and trauma. Trauma is perceived to occur by a concussive event, causing damage to the cartilage and subchondral bone plate, and the resultant pressure and presence of synovial fluid developing a cystic lesion.

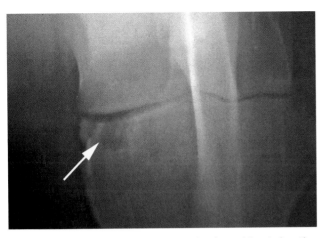

Figure 5.265. Subchondral cystic lesion (arrow) located on the medial aspect of the proximal radius. (Courtesy of Dr. Gary Baxter.)

Clinical Signs

Horses often present with a history of an acute onset of lameness that may wax and wane with use.[1,3] On physical examination there are usually no localizing signs other than lameness. Palpation of the caudal aspect of the elbow joint capsule may reveal fluid distension and some thickening. Flexion and extension of the elbow region often elicits a painful response and a flexion test usually exacerbates the lameness.[3] Horses usually present with lameness graded 2 to 4 out of 5 and the size of the SCL or its location does not appear to influence the degree of lameness. Intrasynovial anesthesia eliminates the lameness in most cases.[1,3,4]

Diagnosis

Radiographs are required to make the diagnosis. In one study, 4 of 7 of the SCLs were located in the proximal medial radius and 3 of 7 were located in the distal medial condyle of the humerus.[3] In another study, the SCLs were located primarily in the proximal medial radius (5 of 6), and the remaining 1 of 6 was located in the distal medial condyle of the humerus.[1] Defects in the subchondral bone were not identified. In general, most SCL appear to occur on the proximal medial aspect of the radius.

Treatment

Subchondral defects are generally treated conservatively, whereas SCLs can be treated either conservatively or surgically.[1,3,8] Both have been treated successfully with prolonged rest and the administration of an anti-inflamatories.[3,8] Initially, rest with concurrent intrasynovial treatment of triamcinolone and hyaluronic acid may be indicated. If the lesions do not appear to be resolving or the lameness does not improve, surgical intervention may be advised. Contrary to the recommendation for conservative treatment, in another study done on 6 horses with SCLs in which conservative (3 of 6) and surgical (3 of 6) treatments were compared[1] surgical extra-articular enucleation of the cyst provided better long-term success (determined by return to athletic function) with less evidence of osteoarthritis.

While extra-articular access of the cyst is the recommended surgical approach, a complete treatment via arthroscopic approach to this joint is limited due to the cyst location. Lesions located in the proximal radius are generally not amenable to an arthroscopic approach; however, lesions located in the medial or lateral humeral condyles may be accessed more easily arthroscopically. Often the lesions are visualized with arthroscope yet adequate debridement is difficult.[6] For a medially located lesion, the surgery is performed with the horse positioned in lateral recumbency with the affected limb down. Care is taken to identify but not disturb the neurovascular plexus, a known complication of this approach, and the humeroradial joint identified with needle placement. The relative location of the cyst is then identified radiographically; extra-articular osteostixis and/or arthroscopically guided intra-lesional or extra-articular steroid injection is performed.

Prognosis

The prognosis appears to be good for conservative treatment of SCLs as long as there is no radiographic evidence of osteoarthritis. Supporting the conservative approach for the treatment of SCLs is one report in which 6 of 7 horses treated with rest and the administration of anti-inflammatory agents returned to their intended use.[3] Five of the 6 horses returned to intense athletic performance, 4 flat racing, and 1 barrel racing. The recommendations from this report were that nonsurgical treatment should be considered in horses without radiographic signs of osteoarthritis and that surgery could be considered as an option if the horse remains lame at the 90-day follow-up examination.

The outcome of surgery on 3 horses with SCLs resulted in 2 of the 3 returning to their intended use. The other horse sustained a comminuted fracture of the radius during recovery from anesthesia.[1] More recently, there is evidence that if accessible, injection of the cyst itself with triamcinolone has shown favorable results in other joints.[5,7] Although there is one report of a successful elbow cyst injection[2]; this is far less invasive in comparison to open extra-articular enucleation of the cyst. Injection of the cyst with steroids either via arthroscopic guidance or in an extra-articular manner is recommended.

References

1. Bertone AL, McIlwraith CW, Powers BE, et al. Subchondral osseous cystic lesions of the elbow of horses: conservative versus surgical treatment. J Am Vet Med Assoc 1986;189:540–546.
2. Foerner J, Rick M, Juzwiak J, et al. Injection of equine subchondral bone cysts with triamcinolone: 73 horses (1999–2005). AAEP Congress 2006, San Antonio, Texas, 2006;412–413.
3. Hopen LA, Colahan PT, Turner TA, et al. Nonsurgical treatment of cubital subchondral cyst-like lesions in horses: seven cases (1983–1987). J Am Vet Med Assoc 1992;200:527–530.
4. Jann H, Koblik P, Fackelman G. What is your diagnosis? J Am Vet Med Assoc 1986;188:1069–1070.
5. Jenner F, Ross MW, Martin BB, et al. Scapulohumeral osteochondrosis. A retrospective study of 32 horses. Vet Comp Orthop Traumatol 2008;21:406–412.

6. McIlwraith C. Diagnostic and surgical arthroscopy of the cubital (elbow) joint. In Diagnostic and Surgical Arthroscopy in the Horse, 3rd ed. McIlwraith CW, Nixon AJ, Wright IM, et al., eds. Philadelphia: Elsevier, 2006;327–336.
7. Wallis TW, Goodrich LR, McIlwraith CW, et al. Arthroscopic injection of corticosteroids into the fibrous tissue of subchondral cystic lesions of the medial femoral condyle in horses: a retrospective study of 52 cases (2001–2006). Equine Vet J 2008; 40:461–467.
8. Yovich JV, Stashak TS. Subchondral osseous cyst formation after an intra-articular fracture in a filly. Equine Vet J 1989; 21:72–74.

Bursitis of the Elbow (Olecranon Bursitis)

Shoe boil or capped elbows are 2 common names for bursitis of the elbow.[3] Historically regarded as a problem in draft breeds, a recent report details 10 cases in Quarter horses.[1] It may occur on one or both elbows and is a characteristic movable swelling over the point of the olecranon tuberosity, usually developing from trauma. The trauma results in a transudative fluid accumulating in the subcutaneous tissue, which becomes encapsulated by fibrous tissue. Ultimately a synovial like membrane develops, producing fluid that is similar to joint fluid although it differs in viscosity and mucin clot.[2]

Chronic bursitis is characterized by the accumulation of bursal fluid and thickening of the bursal wall by fibrous tissue; fibrous bands and septa may develop in the bursal cavity and the subcutaneous tissues around the bursa continue to thicken.[1] Bursal enlargement usually develops as a painless swelling that does not typically interfere with function unless it becomes greatly enlarged. In most cases, the acquired bursa is only a cosmetic blemish unless it becomes infected. An infected bursa is painful, causes lameness, and may break open to drain. The small true bursa that underlies the insertion of the triceps brachii muscle is rarely involved.

Etiology

Acquired bursitis is commonly caused by trauma from the shoe of the affected limb hitting the point of the elbow during motion or more commonly when the horse is lying down. American Saddlebreds and Standardbreds may hit their elbows during exercise. The bursae may become infected by a puncture or iatrogenically.[1]

Clinical Signs

The condition is characterized by a prominent, often freely movable swelling over the point of the elbow, which may contain fluid or may be comprised primarily of fibrous tissue in the chronic stages. Lameness is usually not present unless the bursa is greatly enlarged or infected. Infected bursae feel warm, and firm pressure causes pain (Figure 5.266).

Diagnosis

The diagnosis can usually be made on physical findings alone. However, if the bursa appears infected, radiographs can be taken to rule out trauma or infection

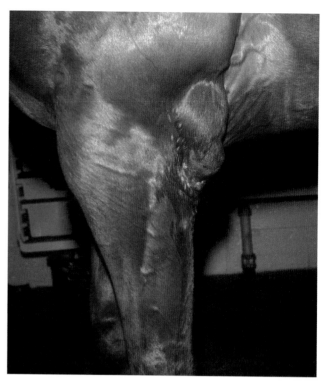

Figure 5.266.   A chronic, infected, acquired capped elbow of the right forelimb. (Courtesy of Dr. Gary Baxter.)

involving the olecranon process. If a draining tract is present, contrast material may be injected into the tract to identify its depth and course. Ultrasound can also be used to determine whether deeper structures are involved.

Treatment

In the acute stage, the condition may resolve by preventing further trauma to the region with a shoe boil roll or boot. The fluid can adjunctively be removed aseptically and corticosteroids injected after the fluid is removed.[1] The lesion can be injected more than once. If the initiating cause is removed and the lesion is treated before extensive fibrosis occurs, it may resolve. However, in one report 7 out of 10 horses were treated with intrabursal steroids and none resolved.[1]

There are reports of other substances being injected into affected bursae with varying success. Orgotein has been used, resulting in reduction but not resolution, as have short–lived radionucleides such as dysprosium-165.[1] Anecdotally, intralesional injection of 7% iodine or iodine-based radiographic contrast material, or packing the incised bursa with iodine-soaked gauze has also been recommended with variable success.

Surgical intervention either by placing drains or en bloc resection appears to have the greatest success.[1,4] Open drainage and application of penrose drains and pressure bandages over periods of up to 8 weeks was successful in 3 horses.[4] En bloc resection is the treatment of choice for large and mature acquired olecranon bursae. Preferentially, the procedure is performed standing. Local anesthesia is administered and a curved skin incision is made over the lateral aspect. A plane of dissection is made to remove the mass in its entirety. Excess skin is removed as needed and the deep and subcutaneous layers are closed with absorbable sutures. The skin is then closed in a tension reducing manner such as widely placed vertical mattress sutures. A stent bandage is placed to protect the suture line and provide some compression. The horse can be maintained in cross-ties or an overhead wire until satisfactory healing is attained, usually 2 to 3 weeks.[1]

Prognosis

Conservative treatment of an acquired bursa to achieve acceptable cosmetic outcome is guarded. En bloc resection is regarded as a superior way to manage the lesion with good cosmesis.[1]

References

1. Honnas CM, Schumacher J, McClure SR, et al. Treatment of olecranon bursitis in horses: 10 cases (1986–1993). J Am Vet Med Assoc 1995;206:1022–1026.
2. McIlwraith C. Diseases of joints, tendons, ligaments and related structures. In Adams' Lameness in Horses. Stashak T, ed. Lippincott Williams and Wilkins, Philadelphia, 2002;640–644.
3. Stashak T. The Elbow. In Adams' Lameness in Horses. Stashak T, ed. Lippincott Williams and Wilkins, Philadelphia, 2002; 888–890.
4. Van Veenendaal J, Speirs V, Harrison I. Treatment of hygromata in horses. Australian Veterinary Journal 1981;57:513–514.

FRACTURES OF THE HUMERUS

Fractures of the humerus are relatively uncommon in horses, possibly because of the short, thick configuration of this bone and the prominent surrounding heavy musculature. The fracture can occur in horses of any age, breed, or sex, but most often affects foals less than 1 year of age, racing or race training Thoroughbreds, and horses that are used for jumping or steeplechase events.[10,20,22,39] In a study done on 54 horses with humeral fractures, the mean age for fracture occurrence was 3 years, and 28 of 54 (52%) were less than 6 months of age.[10]

Humeral fractures are classified as incomplete or complete, open or closed, simple or comminuted, and nondisplaced or displaced. Most are complete, closed, and displaced. Comminution occurs occasionally. Humeral fractures can also be classified by location: (1) proximal humeral head (epiphysis and metaphysis in foals), (2) greater tubercle, (3) deltoid tuberosity, (4) mid-diaphyseal, (5) distal metaphyseal and epiphyseal, and (6) distal condylar and epicondylar (Figures 5.267 and 5.268).[10,14,22,26,30,38] Most fractures are reported to involve the middle third of the diaphysis, either oblique or transverse or spiral configuration and almost never open.[8,21] A study on 54 horses with humeral fractures reported that 9 of 54 (17%) involved the physis (1 proximal and 8 distal), 8 of 54 (15%) occurred in the proximal metaphysis (4 oblique and 4 transverse), 11 of 54 (20.4%) were distal metaphyseal fractures, 26 of 54 (48%) were diaphyseal (2 short oblique, 4 transverse, 20 long oblique or spiral), and 1 of 54 was open.[10] In another study done on 22 horses with humeral fractures, 14 of 22 fractures were spiral in configura-

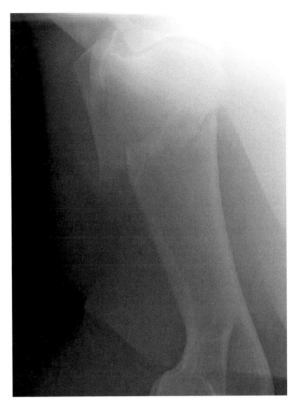

Figure 5.267. Proximal metaphyseal transverse humeral fracture. (Courtesy of Dr. Martin Waselau.)

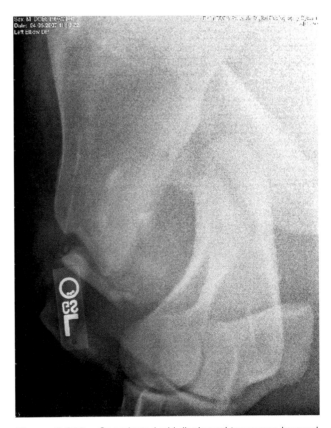

Figure 5.268. Comminuted mid-diaphyseal transverse humeral fracture. (Courtesy of Dr. Martin Waselau.)

tion.[39] Uncommonly foals will sustain multiple fractures involving the elbow region.[5,24] Fractures of the greater tubercle can involve either the caudal or cranial aspect[30,38] and occasionally are comminuted.[22]

Because of the large muscular attachments to the humerus, there is often considerable overriding with displaced fractures (the distal fragment being displaced caudad and the proximal fragment being displaced craniad). However, it is uncommon for proximal complete humeral fractures to become displaced because of the stability provided by the surrounding muscles (supraspinatus, infraspinatus, subscapular, and deltoid), biceps tendinous insertions, and periarticular capsular attachments of the shoulder.[26] Incomplete stress fractures occur in 2 typical locations,; the proximal caudal lateral cortex and the distal cranial medial cortex.[21]

The radial nerve courses in the musculospiral groove of the humerus and may be traumatized to varying degrees as a result of complete displaced diaphyseal or metaphyseal humeral fractures.[8,20] The damage may range from a minor neuropraxia to a complete severance of the nerve.[15] Because of the profound effect on prognosis, it is important to evaluate the degree of nerve dysfunction early in the convalescent period.

Etiology

Humeral fractures frequently occur in foals, in weanlings secondary to falls or other impact injuries, and in racing breeds as either catastrophic failure during race falls or failure as a result of accumulated stress and microfracture.[8,9,17,21,22,29,36,39] In a study of 54 horses with humeral fractures, falls on hard surfaces or related to racing were responsible for fractures in 11 horses, kicks in 2 horses, post-anesthetic recovery in 2 horses, collisions with fences or another horse in 3 horses, and car collision in 1 horse.[10] Trauma is the cause of most fractures of the deltoid tuberosity or greater tubercle.[22]

In an *in vitro* model, the configuration of the fracture was predictable and depended on the direction from which the insult originated. When the force was applied in a craniocaudal direction, the humerus fractured transversally; when the force was applied in lateral to medial direction, the humerus fractured obliquely.[21]

Horses sustaining stress fractures are at an increased risk to develop a complete fracture if they are not managed properly. A study of 34 Thoroughbred racehorses with humeral stress fractures found an increased risk of complete fracture in horses that returned to racing after a short 2-month lay-up period.[9] In one study that did not have any horses develop complete fractures during rehabilitation, the mean time to return to racing for horses with humeral fractures was 7.5 months.[27] Radiographic and scintigraphic re-examination allows for more accurate assessment of recovery.[32]

Clinical Signs

Horses with nondisplaced or minimally displaced proximal fractures (Salter-Harris type I epiphyseal, greater tubercle, or deltoid tuberosity) and nondisplaced mid-shaft fractures often present with a history of a marked lameness that improves over a 24- to 48-hour period. Moderate swelling may be present at the site of injury for a proximal fracture or over the lateral muscles for a mid-shaft fracture. Pain is often present with pressure applied over the fracture and on limb manipulation. If several days have passed, the swelling may be most prominent in a site distal to the fracture. At exercise a moderate (2 to 3 out of 5) lameness is most often seen. Radiology often provides a definitive diagnosis.

Incomplete fractures and stress fractures resulting in lameness can be most difficult to diagnose.[19,21,27,29,36] In some cases lameness and mild swelling may be adequate to lead to a tentative diagnosis of a fracture, but the definitive diagnosis often requires nuclear imaging.[27]

Horses with complete displaced fractures often present with a history of an acute onset of a severe nonweight-bearing lameness. Marked to moderate swelling of the muscles overlying the region is often seen and the elbow is usually dropped. The dropped elbow may be due to the overriding of the fracture segments resulting in functional limb shortening or from the varying degrees of damage to the radial nerve.[1,10] Limb manipulation usually causes increased pain and an increased range of motion when the limb is adducted and abducted. Crepitation is often difficult to appreciate, particularly in heavy muscled horses, because of the degree of fragment displacement and the muffling effect of the swollen musculature. Limited manipulation should be done because it may result in further trauma to the radial nerve. Radiographs will identify the fracture, but evaluation of radial nerve damage is more difficult. Electromyography (EMG) of the antebrachial extensor muscles can be used after 2 weeks to evaluate radial nerve damage. In one study 4 of 40 horses treated for fractures of the humerus were destroyed because of loss of radial nerve function.[10]

Fractures of the distal epiphysis, condyles, and epicondylar region are very uncommon.[24,34] When they do occur they often present with a history of marked lameness of a short duration. Swelling associated with the elbow region may be apparent, including joint effusion if the fracture is articular. Direct pressure on the affected site and limb manipulation often results in a painful response. Radiography is required to document the fracture.

Diagnosis

Radiography is used in most cases to confirm the fracture and define the configuration. A slightly oblique medial lateral projection with the limb held in extension usually provides the information needed for epiphyseal and shaft fractures. In most cases the study can be done in the standing sedated horse. Foals can be restrained in lateral recumbency with the affected limb down to obtain a diagnostic lateral projection. Cranial caudal views of the distal humerus and oblique views of the proximal humerus can be obtained in most standing sedated horses and foals. Cranial caudal views of the entire proximal humerus are more difficult to obtain and general anesthesia may be required.

Multiple radiographic views may be needed to identify fractures of the greater tubercle and deltoid tuberosity.[7] Obtaining a cranioproximal-craniodistal oblique projection of the proximal portion of the humerus in a standing horse often highlights the long oblique fractures of the greater tubercle that are not evident on a mediolateral view.[22]

Horses with stress fractures often have a grade 3 of 5 lameness in the affected limb that improves quickly after the initial injury. Manipulation of the elbow and shoulder often exacerbate the lameness, yet diagnostic anesthesia is not useful.[27] A definitive diagnosis of stress injuries requires nuclear scintigraphic as well as radiographic examination (Figure 5.269). The caudodistal cortex or the caudoproximal cortex are most commonly affected, but fractures of the cranioproximal and craniodistal cortexes also may occur.[4,19,27,29] Radiography may identify callus formation along the affected cortex, particularly in chronic cases.

Treatment

Currently three options are considered when managing a horse with a humeral fracture: nonsurgical (conservative) management with prolonged stall rest, surgical reduction followed by stabilization, and euthanasia.[8,10,20,26,29,31] Of the two treatment approaches, nonsurgical management appears to provide the best outcome compared to surgical approaches for most nonarticular incomplete or complete humeral fractures, no matter what the age of the horse (Figure 5.270).[10,39]

In one report, 7 of 10 horses treated nonsurgically were able to be ridden 5 to 12 months after the diagnosis was made and only 1 of 3 surgically treated (2 Rush pins, 1 lag screws) cases was considered sound for riding.[39] Interestingly, 2 of the nonsurgical cases

were lost to follow-up and therefore were included in the group of unsuccessful cases. The ages of the horses that were treated nonsurgically ranged from 2 to 60 months (mean 21 months). In another study, conservative treatment resulted in 9 of 17 cases being considered

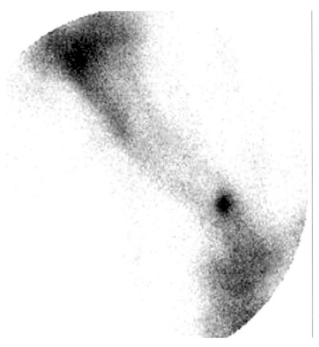

Figure 5.269. Nuclear scintigraphic examination of the humerus with increased isotope uptake indicative of a distal metaphyseal stress fracture. (Courtesy of Dr. Dan Burba.)

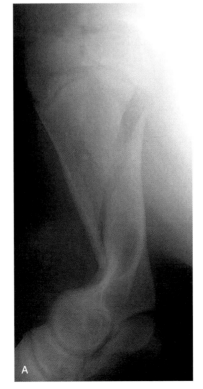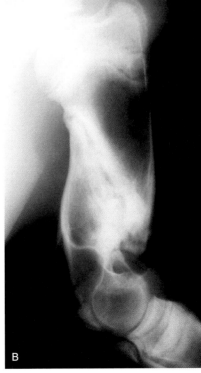

Figure 5.270. A. An oblique lateral view of a spiral nonarticular fracture of the midhumerus. B. Lateral view of a healing spiral nonarticular fracture of the midhumerus treated conservatively for 5 months. (Courtesy of Dr. Gary Baxter.)

successful; 4 became athletically sound and 5 were pasture sound.[10] The horses that were treated nonsurgically ranged in age from 1 week to 15 years (mean 3 years). Euthanasia still remains a commonly selected option. In a retrospective study done on 54 horses with humeral fractures, more horses were euthanized (44.4%) than treated with surgical (24%) or conservative (32%) management.[10] In the other retrospective, 9 of 22 humeral fracture cases were euthanized.[39]

Nonsurgical Management

Nonsurgical management has been used successfully to treat stress fractures; incomplete or complete nondisplaced or minimally displaced nonarticular fractures; minimally displaced Salter-Harris type I and II fractures of the proximal and distal physis; complete displaced proximal and distal transverse and oblique fractures; and complete displaced diaphyseal transverse, short, and spiral oblique fractures.[6,10,21,26,39] In 2 reports a better outcome was obtained in foals compared with adults.[10,39] Long transverse and oblique fractures can be reasonably stable when the caudodistal aspect of the proximal fragment rests within the epicondylar groove. Shorter oblique fractures have less stability and usually require internal fixation. Contraction of the heavy musculature surrounding the humerus also helps stabilize the fracture while it heals.

Nonsurgical management consists of 3 to 6 months' stall rest, with periodic radiographic or nuclear imaging re-evaluation of the fracture for healing.[26,29] Initially, incomplete or complete nondisplaced fractures can be maintained on an overhead wire to minimize the chance of developing a complete fracture.[21,26,29]

Complications are not common but may include contra-limb laminitis and angular limb deformity, radial nerve damage, and nonunion.[10,39] No adverse affects attributable to shortening of the humerus, such as a shortened stride or a straightened elbow joint, were reported in successfully treated horses in this study.

Surgical Management

Various internal fixation techniques have been described for treatment of humeral fractures. Fixation devices have included stacked intramedullary pins,[8,10,13] Rush pins,[16] ASIF (Kuntscher) nails,[19] 1 or more dynamic compression plates,[1,18,20,21,26,28,31,33] interlocking intramedullary nails,[1,18,20,21,26,28,31,33-37] cortical screws and washers for greater tubercle fractures,[22] and a combination of intramedullary pins and cerclage bands or wires.[20] Unfortunately, the current techniques of dynamic compression plating, intramedullary fixations, and cerclage bands or wires do not have sufficient strength to provide adequate stability in adult horses.[8,20,21]

Intramedullary pinning, bone plating, and ASIF or interlocking intramedullary nailing or Rush pins have been used to successfully treat foals and ponies with humeral fractures.[1,10,15,23,26,35] Bone plates have been applied to repair nonarticular humeral fractures in foals and yearlings.[10,23,33] Both lateral and cranial surgical approaches for plate application have been described.[1,10,15,23,26,28] The cranial approach allows access to most regions of the humeral shaft and is preferred over the lateral approach.[26,28] The flat, smooth cranial surface of the bone is ideal for placement of a broad DCP plate. An added benefit to the cranial approach is that a second plate placed laterally can be used in more mature horses to provide greater stability to the repair. At present most reports describe the use of DCP or LC-DCP plates; there are few if any reports of the use of locking compression plates (LCP) for humeral repairs.

Stacked intramedullary pinning with or without cerclage wires or bands appears to be a viable method of repairing humeral fractures compared with dynamic compression plates in young foals.[10] Intramedullary pinning has an advantage over plating in that there is less soft tissue disruption in the surgical approach.[28]

The interlocking intramedullary pin has been used successfully in foals weighing up to 220 kg.[35] In larger foals a cranial plate is also applied to augment the reduction.[35] Although the interlocking nail system provides good axial stability to the fracture repair, the fact that the endosteal blood supply is destroyed when the marrow cavity is reamed out to apply the system may result in delayed fracture healing, although there does not appear to be any effect on foal growth or development.[36]

Unstable and extensive greater tubercle fractures of the proximal humerus may require removal or internal fixation with lag screws.[2,3,22,38] Fragment removal is usually relegated for smaller, displaced, unstable fragments that result in continued chronic lameness.[2,7,22] Larger fragments are treated with internal fixation using 5.5-mm or 6.5-mm lag screws that engage the distomedial cortex of the humeral diaphysis.[26] Screws placed in this fashion usually are enough to counteract the pull (tension forces) of the infraspinatus tendon.

Extensive fractures of the deltoid tuberosity, although uncommon, also can involve the greater tubercle of the proximal humerus. Surgical intervention is required to re-establish cortical continuity of the bicipital groove and re-establish the tensional support of the tendinous insertions of the deltoid, brachiocephalicus, supraspinatus, and occasionally the infraspinatus muscles.[7,26] Generally all that is needed are 2 to 3 4.5-mm or 5.5-mm cortical or 6.5-mm cancellous screws placed in lag fashion that engage the transcortex.[13] In heavy horses a narrow DCP plate may be used to provide a tension band effect.[26]

Fractures of the condyles or epicondyles of the distal humerus occur infrequently in horses but small, articular fragments involving the condyles should be removed arthroscopically.[24,25] More extensive fractures of the condyles or epicondylar region may require internal fixation with lag screws.

Prognosis

The prognosis for stress fractures, nondisplaced complete or incomplete fractures, or minimally displaced complete nonarticular fractures managed conservatively appears very good.[10,20,29,39]

The prognosis for complete displaced nonarticular fractures is guarded but appears better for horses managed conservatively. In one study in which conservative management was used in 17 horses, 9 (53.9%)

were considered successful, 4 horses became athletically sound, and 5 horses became pasture sound; younger horses may do better.[10] In this same study, 13 horses were treated surgically with a variety of internal fixation methods including DCP plate; 3 of 13 horses survived and became athletically sound. The successful outcomes were all surgically treated with stacked pinning and all were young foals. In another study, conservative management was used in 10 horses, 7 of which were able to be ridden 5 to 12 months after the diagnosis was made.[39] The horses' ages in the successful group ranged from 2 to 60 months. Of the 3 horses treated surgically, 1 became pasture sound 10 months after surgery. The conclusion was that the best candidates for nonsurgical treatment are nonarticular humeral fractures with minimal displacement that involve the midshaft and are spiral and oblique with minimal overriding of the ends of the bone.

For fractures involving the greater tubercle and deltoid tuberosity, the prognosis appears good for conservative management of nondisplaced and surgically treated displaced greater tubercle and deltoid tuberosity fractures.[7,11,12,22] In one report, 9 out of 10 horses with greater tubercle fractures treated surgically returned to athletic use. Of these, 7 had the fragment removed and 2 had internal fixation.[22] There are few reports of epicondylar fractures but in one case of a fracture of the epicondyle and supracondylar crest, the horse returned to athletic use after the fracture fragments were removed.[24]

References

1. Adams O. Lameness in Horses, 3rd ed. Lea and Febiger, Philadelphia, 1974.
2. Adams R, Turner T. Internal fixation of a greater tubercle fracture in an adolescent horse: A case report. Journal of Equine Veterinary Science 1987;7:174–176.
3. Allen D, White N. Chip fracture of the greater tubercle of a horse. Compendium of Continuing Education 1984;6:39–41.
4. Arthur R, Constantinide D. Results of 428 nuclear scintigraphic examinations of the musculoskeletal system at a Thoroughbred race track. Proceedings Am Assoc Equine Pract 1995;41:280–281.
5. Auer JA, Struchen CH, Weidmann CH. Surgical management of a foal with a humerus-radius-ulna fracture. Equine Vet J 1996;28:416–420.
6. Baxter G. What is your diagnosis? J Am Vet Med Assoc 1989;195:523–524.
7. Bleyaert H. Shoulder injuries. In White N, Moore J, eds. Current Techniques of Equine Surgery and Lameness. WB Saunders and Co., Philadelphia, 1998;422–423.
8. Bramlage LR. Long bone fractures. Vet Clin North Am Large Anim Pract 1983;5:225–310.
9. Carrier TK, Estberg L, Stover SM, et al. Association between long periods without high-speed workouts and risk of complete humeral or pelvic fracture in thoroughbred racehorses: 54 cases (1991–1994). J Am Vet Med Assoc 1998;212:1582–1587.
10. Carter BG, Schneider RK, Hardy J, et al. Assessment and treatment of equine humeral fractures: retrospective study of 54 cases (1972–1990). Equine Vet J 1993;25:203–207.
11. Dyson SJ. Diagnostic techniques in the investigation of shoulder lameness. Pferdeheilkunde 1986;2:221–226.
12. Dyson SJ. Sixteen fractures of the shoulder region in the horse. Equine Vet J 1985;17:104–110.
13. Dyson SJ, Greet TR. Repair of a fracture of the deltoid tuberosity of the humerus in a pony. Equine Vet J 1986;18:230–232.
14. Embertson R, Bramlage L, Herring D, et al. Physeal fractures in the horse: Classification and incidence. Veterinary Surgery 1986;15:223–227.
15. Fessler J, Amstutz H. Fracture repair. In Large Animal Surgery. Oehme F, Prier J, eds. Williams and Wilkins, Baltimore, 1974;309.
16. Foerner J. The use of rush pins in long bone fractures. Proceedings Am Assoc Equine Pract 1977;223–227.
17. Honnas C. Humerus fractures. In Equine Surgery. Auer J, ed. WB Saunders and Co., Philadelphia, 1992;1044–1045.
18. Kelman D. Surgical repair of a spiral fracture of a humerus in a foal. Australian Veterinary Journal 1980;10:257–259.
19. Mackey V, Trout D, Meagher D, et al. Stress fractures of the humerus, radius, and tibia in horses. Clinical features and radiographic and/or scintigraphic appearance. Veterinary Radiology 1987;28:26–31.
20. Markel M. Fracture of the humerus. In Current Practice of Equine Surgery. White N, Moore J, eds. JB Lippincott, Philadelphia, 1990;652–657.
21. Markel MD, Nunamaker DM, Wheat JD, et al. In vitro comparison of three fixation methods for humeral fracture repair in adult horses. Am J Vet Res 1988;49:586–593.
22. Mez JC, Dabareiner RM, Cole RC, et al. Fractures of the greater tubercle of the humerus in horses: 15 cases (1986–2004). J Am Vet Med Assoc 2007;230:1350–1355.
23. Milne D, Turner A. An Atlas of Surgical Approaches to the Bones of Horses. WB Saunders and Co., Philadelphia, 1979.
24. Mitchell C, Riley CB. Evaluation and treatment of an adult quarter horse with an unusual fracture of the humerus and septic arthritis. Can Vet J 2002;43:120–122.
25. Nixon AJ. Arthroscopic approaches and intra-articular anatomy of the equine elbow. Vet Surg 1990;19:93–101.
26. Nixon AJ. Fractures of the humerus. In Equine Fracture Repair. Nixon A, ed. WB Saunders and Co., Philadelphia, 1996;242–253.
27. O'Sullivan CB, Lumsden JM. Stress fractures of the tibia and humerus in Thoroughbred racehorses: 99 cases (1992–2000). J Am Vet Med Assoc 2003;222:491–498.
28. Rakestraw PC, Nixon AJ, Kaderly RE, et al. Cranial approach to the humerus for repair of fractures in horses and cattle. Vet Surg 1991;20:1–8.
29. Stover SM, Johnson BJ, Daft BM, et al. An association between complete and incomplete stress fractures of the humerus in racehorses. Equine Vet J 1992;24:260–263.
30. Tudor R, Crosier M, Bowman KF. Radiographic diagnosis: fracture of the caudal aspect of the greater tubercle of the humerus in a horse. Vet Radiol Ultrasound 2001;42:244–245.
31. Turner A. Fractures of the humerus. In The Practice of Large Animal Surgery. Jennings P, ed. WB Saunders and Co., Philadelphia, 1984;708–800.
32. Valdes-Martinez A, Seiler G, Mai W, et al. Quantitative analysis of scintigraphic findings in tibial stress fractures in Thoroughbred racehorses. Am J Vet Res 2008;69:886–890.
33. Valdes H, Morris D, Auer J. Compression Plating of long bone fractures in foals. Journal of Veterinary Orthopedics 1979;1.
34. Watkins J. Fractures of the Humerus. In Equine Medicine and Surgery, 4th ed. Colahan P, Mayhew I, Merritt A, et al., eds. American Veterinary Publications, Goleta, CA, 1991;1450–1451.
35. Watkins J. Intramedullary, interlocking nail fixation of humeral fractures: results in 10 foals. Proceedings Am Assoc Equine Pract 1996;42:172–173.
36. Watkins JP, Ashman R. Intramedullary interlocking nail fixation in foals: Effects on normal growth and development of the humerus. Veterinary Surgery 1990;19:80.
37. Watkins JP, Ashman R. Intramedullary interlocking nail fixation in transverse humeral fractures: An in-vitro comparison with stacked pin fixation. Proceedings Vet Orthoped Soc 1991;18:54.
38. Yovich J. Fracture of the greater tubercle of the humerus in a filly. J Am Vet Med Assoc 1985;187:74–75.
39. Zamos DT, Parks AH. Comparison of surgical and nonsurgical treatment of humeral fractures in horses: 22 cases (1980–1989). J Am Vet Med Assoc 1992;201:114–116.

PARALYSIS OF THE RADIAL NERVE

Paralysis of the radial nerve as a primary cause of lameness is an uncommon condition that results in the inability to extend the elbow, carpus and digit. Similar dysfunction may also be observed with other conditions involving the upper forelimb; therefore, differentiation can be difficult, particularly shortly after injury occurs.

The radial nerve, often the largest branch of the brachial plexus, derives its origin chiefly from the eighth cervical and first thoracic nerve roots of the plexus. In 10% of horses the seventh cervical nerve root contributes to the radial nerve.[6] The radial nerve innervates the extensor muscles of the elbow, carpus, and digit, and supplies the lateral flexor of the carpus (ulnaris lateralis). It also gives off a superficial sensory branch to the lateral cutaneous brachial nerve. Paralysis of the radial nerve inactivates these muscles and may result in some loss of sensation to the craniolateral aspect of the forearm.

Etiology

In most cases, paralysis of the radial nerve is due to trauma of the shoulder region caused by hyperextension of the forelimb or extreme abduction of the shoulder.[1,12] Fractures of the humerus, the seventh cervical, and first thoracic vertebrae can result in radial nerve paralysis.[1,9] Tumors, abscesses, and enlarged axillary lymph nodes that occur in the cranial thoracic region along the course of the nerve and tumors of the brachial plexus and radial nerve themselves may also result in radial nerve paralysis.[11] There have been isolated reports of radial nerve paralysis included in a generalized distal axonalopathy.[5]

Prolonged lateral recumbency while under general anesthesia on an operating table or while on the ground may also produce a radial-paralysis-like syndrome in the forelimb next to a hard surface.[8,10] Episodes of ischemia are likely to cause neuropractic conduction changes and permanent nerve changes if prolonged.[10]

Clinical Signs

The signs vary depending upon the extent or degree and location of paralysis. When the portion of the radial nerve supplying the extensors of the digit is affected, the signs are characteristic. In the acute phase the horse is unable to bear weight because of the inability to extend the elbow, carpal, and phalangeal joints. If the limb is placed under the horse and fixed in place, it can bear weight passively.[12] While the horse is standing the shoulder is extended and the elbow is dropped (dropped elbow appearance) and extended while the carpus and digits are flexed. The muscles of the elbow and the extensors of the carpus and digit appear relaxed, and the limb appears longer than normal. The "dropped elbow" appearance is not specific for radial nerve paralysis; this appearance can be seen with many other conditions associated with the elbow, humerus, and shoulder regions (Figure 5.271). Occasionally, radial nerve paralysis is accompanied by paralysis of the entire brachial plexus. In this case, the limb shows paralysis of the flexor and extensor muscles and is unable to bear weight.

With complete radial nerve paresis the horse is generally reluctant to move, and at a walk the limb is dragged forward passively by the action of the proximal pectoral, biceps brachii, and coracobrachialis muscles, with

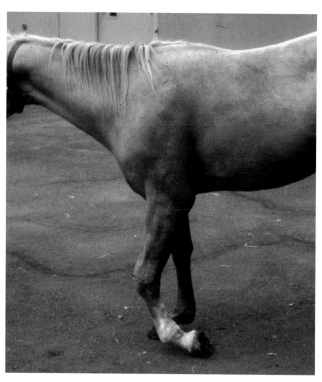

Figure 5.271. Radial nerve paralysis, evidenced by the classic dropped elbow stance. (Courtesy of Dr. Gary Baxter.)

the dorsal surface of the hoof in contact with the ground. Due to the physical stress associated with radial nerve paralysis, some horses may sweat profusely and have an elevated pulse and respiration.[12] Milder cases of radial nerve paralysis present with varying degrees of nonweight-bearing lameness and a dropped elbow with mild flexion of the carpal, fetlock, and phalangeal joints. At a walk the lameness is often characterized by a lowered foot flight arch and a shortened cranial phase of the stride.[4]

Diagnosis

Many cases of radial paralysis are due to external trauma; therefore, the scapula, humerus, radius, and olecranon process should be examined radiographically.[11] Radial nerve paralysis must be further differentiated from rupture of the medial collateral ligament of the elbow; elbow arthritis; and myopathy of the biceps brachii, triceps brachii, anconeus, and extensor carpi radialis muscles.[12]

It previously was believed that cutaneous sensation to the craniolateral aspect of the antebrachium is lost with complete loss of nerve conduction of the radial nerve or brachial plexus, and that if the sensation is present it indicates the lesion selectively affects the motor fibers.[12] However, studies done in horses indicate there are no areas of skin innervated only by either the radial or the axillary nerves—the ulnar, median and musculocutaneous nerves can be related to such areas.[3]

Electrophysiological studies can be helpful in characterizing the extent of nerve damage. Electromyography can be used to determine selective denervation of the extensor muscles. However, because it takes approximately 7 days for the axon distal to the site of the damage to degenerate, electromyography done before this time has limited usefulness.[2] Alternatively, faradic stimulation done 7 days after clinical signs develop can be used to differentiate between neuropraxia and axonotmesis or neurotmesis.[12] Radiography, ultrasonography, and laboratory analysis of muscle enzymes may be needed in some cases to make an accurate diagnosis of radial nerve paralysis.

Treatment

Treatment consists of anti-inflammatory therapy, stall rest, application of a bandage splint, and controlled exercise. NSAIDs are administered in acute cases to reduce inflammation and pain. A low dose of a corticosteroid can be also be administered during the acute phase. Topical application of cold therapy, DMSO, or Surpass may be indicated in some cases if external swelling is obvious. The stall should be bedded deep enough to allow the horse to comfortably assume lateral recumbency. A PVC bandage splint applied to the caudal aspect of the limb from the proximal antebrachium to the fetlock will maintain the limb in extension, permitting the horse to bear weight comfortably. The splint is maintained until the horse can place the limb in extension without support. Controlled exercise can be started when clinical signs (neurologic function) begin to improve. The amount of exercise is dictated by the horses' capabilities. Electromyographic studies can be done at 4- to 6-week intervals to access return of nerve function.

Prognosis

Electromyography has been found to have a good prognostic value in assessing the extent of the injury in a small number of cases.[4] In most cases a guarded to poor prognosis is given,[4,7] but compression and entrapment injuries often lead to partial or complete recovery.[13] Recovery may take a few weeks in pure neuropraxia to several months or years in axonotmesis.[7,11] Reinnervation is, however, unlikely with more severe nerve damage.[4]

References

1. Adams O. Lameness in Horses, 3rd ed. Lea and Febiger, Philadelphia, 1974.
2. Andrews F, Reed S. Diagnosis of muscle disease in the horse. Proceedings Am Assoc Equine Pract 1986;95–100.
3. Blythe LL, Kitchell RL. Electrophysiologic studies of the thoracic limb of the horse. Am J Vet Res 1982;43:1511–1524.
4. Cauvin E, Munroe G, Mitsopoulos A. Peripheral neuropathy involving the brachial plexus nerves in two horses. Equine Veterinary Education 1993;5:90–94.
5. Furuoka H, Okamoto R, Kitayama S, et al. Idiopathic peripheral neuropathy in the horse with knuckling: muscle and nerve lesions in additional cases. Acta Neuropathol 1998;96:431–437.
6. Goshal N. Sisson and Grossman's The Anatomy of the Domestic Animals, 5th ed. WB Saunders and Co., Philadelphia, 1975; 665–688.
7. Lahunta D. Veterinary Neuroanatomy and Clinical Neurology, 2nd ed. WB Saunders and Co, Philadelphia, 1987.
8. Lindsey W, McDonell W, Bignell W. Equine postanesthetic forelimb lameness: intracompartmental muscle pressure changes and biochemical patterns. Am J Vet Res 1980;41:1919.
9. Lopez MJ, Nordberg C, Trostle S. Fracture of the 7th cervical and 1st thoracic vertebrae presenting as radial nerve paralysis in a horse. Can Vet J 1997;38:112.
10. Mackay R. Peripheral Nerve Injury. In Equine Surgery, 3rd ed. Auer J, Stick J, eds. Saunders Elsevier, St. Louis, 2006; 684–691.
11. Mayhew I. Paresis or Paralysis of One Limb. In Large Animal Neurology. A Handbook for Veterinary Clinicians. Mayhew I, ed. Lea and Febiger, Philadelphia, 1989;335–347.
12. Rijkenhuizen A, Keg P, Dik K. True or false radial nerve paralysis in the horse. Veterinary Annual 1994;34:126–133.
13. Stewart J, Aguayo A. Compression and entrapment neuropathies. In Peripheral Neuropathy. Dyck P, Thomas P, Lambert E, et al., eds. WB Saunders and Co., Philadelphia, 1984;1435–1457.

THE SHOULDER AND SCAPULA

Jeremy Hubert and Ted S. Stashak

INFLAMMATION OF THE INTERTUBERCULAR BURSA (BICIPITAL BURSITIS)

Inflammation of the intertubercular (bicipital) bursa as a primary cause of lameness is uncommon, even though the condition can occur in horses of any age, breed, or sex.[2,8,15] It can present as septic or nonseptic.[2,9,15,36] Several case studies have identified a very low incidence of the problem.[5,10,14,20] In 2 reports the condition was responsible for lameness in 1 of 54 and 1 of 41 horses suspected of having shoulder lameness.[9,20]

The bicipital bursa is located between the bilobed tendon of the origin of biceps brachii muscle and the M-shaped tubercles at the cranioproximal aspect of the humerus. The synovial membrane of the bursa extends around the axial and abaxial limits of the tendon and onto the margins of its cranial surface. Although uncommon, communication can exist between the shoulder joint and the bicipital bursa.

Etiology

Trauma to the cranial surface of the shoulder region is believed to be the most common cause of a primary bursitis.[2,9,15,36] Other suggested causes include stretching or tearing of the bursa or biceps tendon during the cranial phase of the stride with the limb in full extension or by a fall or slip that results in flexion of the shoulder with extension of the elbow.[29,35] Inflammation of this bursa can also be caused by dislocation of the biceps brachii tendon that may be associated with congenital abnormality of hypoplasia of the minor tubercle.[6,17,21]

Infection, either from an open or penetrating wound or from hematogenous spread to the bursa has also been reported.[9,28,36] At least 2 reports have implicated *Brucella abortus* as a cause.[5,20] Inflammation of the bicipital bursa has also been reported to occur following influenza or other viral respiratory disease outbreaks, and in one case following a long trailer ride.[1,36] Cases of septic bursitis concurrent with septic tendinitis and arthritis of the scapulohumeral joint or bursitis with associated tendinitis and humeral osteitis have been reported.[11,12]

Clinical Signs

A history of trauma to the shoulder region is the most common factor; the signs of lameness usually have an acute onset which is most obvious during the stance and swing phases of the stride. On physical examination swelling over the cranial aspect of the shoulder region may be evident with or without a wound being present. Generalized shoulder and pectoral muscle atrophy may be seen in more chronic cases.[9,15,36] Pressure applied over the biceps tendon and bursal region and manipulation of the shoulder region in flexion and extension

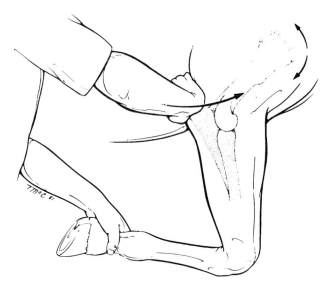

Figure 5.272. As the shoulder is flexed, tension is created in the tendon of the biceps brachii muscle. If the horse has bicipital bursitis or ossification of the tendon, a painful response is elicited.

usually result in a prominent painful response (Figure 5.272). The responses to pressure and limb manipulation should be compared to those found on the contralateral unaffected limb.[15]

The lameness is often marked. At exercise, a lameness of 3 to 4 out of 5 is generally seen (greater if septic), with the swing and stance phases being altered. The lameness is often characterized by a shortened cranial phase of the stride, a decrease in the height of the foot flight arc, reduced carpal flexion, and a fixed shoulder appearance during movement. The horse is often reluctant to bear full weight on the affected limb while standing.[15]

Diagnosis

Radiographs of the shoulder and ultrasound examination are performed if the physical examination localizes the pain causing lameness to the bursal region. Manipulation of the elbow into hyperextension may stress the biceps brachii tendon, helping to localize the lesion.[24] However, if the localizing signs are not obvious, bursitis is confirmed by centesis and local anesthesia of the bursa. A proximal approach to the bursa is considered to be the most successful for bursal centesis.[33] Addition of contrast material and radiographic exam may be necessary to assess the success of centesis.[22]

If there is a history of access to cattle, serum samples should be submitted for *Brucella abortus* titers. Serum titers greater than 40 U/ml have been reported in 42 horses with bursal or tendon sheath infections, includ-

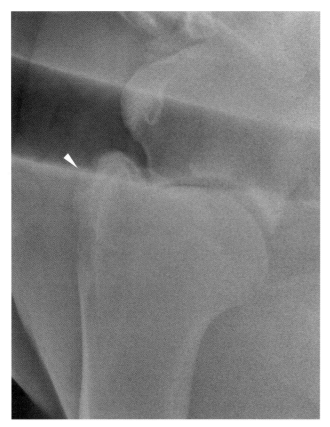

Figure 5.273. Osseous changes on the tubercles of the cranio-proximal humerus (arrowhead). Infiltration of lidocaine into the bursa resolved the lameness in this case.

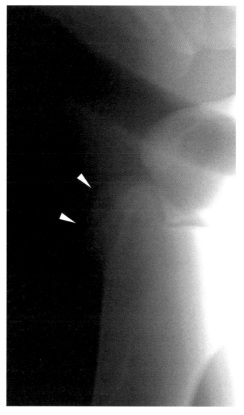

Figure 5.274. An osseous cyst located in the lateral bicipital groove in the cranio-proximal humerus (arrowheads). (Courtesy of Dr. Johan Marais.)

ing 2 horses with infectious bicipital bursitis.[5,20] In another report on 4 horses with septic bicipital bursitis, 1 horse had a titer to *B. abortus* of 13 U/ml, and the other 3 horses did not have titers taken.[36] The recommendation was to obtain serum for determination of titers to *B. abortus* from all horses suspected of having infectious bicipital bursitis not caused by a wound.

Radiographs of the shoulder region are taken to identify any osseous changes in the tubercles or bicipital groove or bursa and to rule out the possibility of fractures of the supraglenoid tuberosity or proximal humerus or ossification of the biceps tendon (Figures 5.273 and 5.274).[2,9,15,26,36] Generally, only mediolateral, craniomedial-caudolateral oblique, and flexed cranio-proximal-craniodistal (skyline) radiograph are taken in adult horses. The flexed cranioproximal-caudoproximal (skyline) projection of the cranial shoulder region has proven useful in identifying lesions associated with the tubercles of the proximal humerus. Radiographic changes associated with bursitis include mottled changes in the tubercle, demineralization of the greater tubercle, osseous densities in the periarticular region, osseous cysts in the cranio-proximal humerus, osteitis in the bicipital groove, ossification of the tendon, and calcification of the bursa.[15,18] Radiographs may appear normal if the disease only involves the bursa. If a wound or draining tract is present, centesis with contrast material assesses communication with the bursa.

Ultrasound examination of the biceps tendon, bursa, and bicipital groove can be very informative, even when radiographs appear normal.[3,16,27] Ultrasound changes associated with bursitis have included edema or hemorrhage in the biceps tendon or bursa, disruption of the tendon architecture with peritendinous thickening, an irregular surface of the bicipital groove, and hyperechoic material in the bicipital bursa.[7,36] Infection must be ruled out if hyperechoic material is seen in the bursa (Figure 5.275).[36] Nuclear medicine may be useful in some cases to detect early infected or actively remodeling bone adjacent to the bursal region when ultrasound and radiography appear normal (Figure 5.276).[15]

Treatment

Conservative Treatment

Noninfectious bursitis without radiographic evidence of a fracture or pathology on the cranioproximal aspect of the humerus may respond favorably to rest, parenteral and/or topical administration of nonsteroidal anti-inflammatory drugs (NSAIDs), and in some cases intrasynovial injection of the bursa with corticoids and HA.[8,9,30]

The duration of the rest generally depends on the nature of the injury, the patient's clinical response to rest, and whether or not the biceps tendon was damaged.

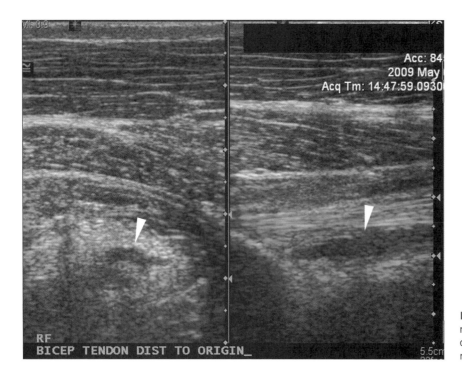

Figure 5.275. Core lesion of the medial branch of the biceps tendon just distal to the origin of the biceps brachii muscle (arrowheads).

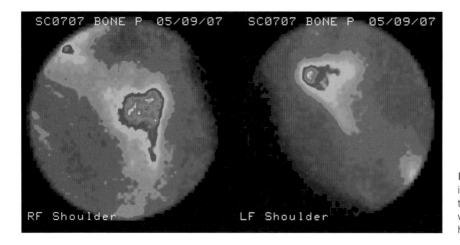

Figure 5.276. Nuclear scintigraphic image of a horse with bicipital bursitis in the right shoulder, whose underlying lesion was an osseous cyst in the proximal humerus. (Courtesy of Dr. Johan Marais.)

NSAIDs are generally administered for 10 to 14 days and hand walking exercise is begun after that. Manipulating the limb passively through a range of motion may also be helpful.[8,9,15,30] When the tendon has been injured, rest periods for up to 3 months followed by paddock rest for another 3 months may be required to allow healing of the tendon.

When the tendon has ossified, extracorporeal shock-wave therapy (ESWT) may be indicated. In humans, calcifying tendinitis is commonly treated with ESWT[13,19,31] and has been used with fair success in horses with calcifying tenopathies of the deep digital flexor tendon.[32] Additional therapy could include stem cell, IRAP, and PRP therapy, depending upon the lesion. ESWT applied to tendon lesions is still controversial; however, anecdotal reports appear to be encouraging.[4] In these horses, controlled exercise is begun as early as possible, generally after 2 to 3 weeks of confinement to improve range of motion and healing. The patient's clinical response and ultrasound findings should be used to determine progress in healing.

Surgical Treatment

Bursitis that results from a displaced fracture, from osseous changes associated with the proximocranial aspect of the humerus, or from sepsis generally requires surgery to resolve the problem. Incisional as well as arthroscopic approaches to the intertubercular bursa have been used and described.[2,9,15,25,34] If a fracture is present the fragment is removed and the bed debrided and smoothed.[15] Controlled exercise as described for the conservative approach is begun at the time of suture removal in most cases.

In the rare event of calcification of the bicipital tendon, surgical removal of the calcific mass may be attempted. In a report on calcifying tendinopathy of the biceps brachii resulting in lameness in a dog, the dog responded favorably to the surgical removal of the calcificied mass followed by longitudinal suture of the transected tendon fibers.[23] Anecdotally, removal of large ossified sections of the biceps tendon removed surgically has resulted in resolution of lameness.

In cases in which infection appears to be the cause, centesis of the bursa should be done to collect fluid for culture and cytology. Next, the bursa should be drained and then debrided and lavaged copiously under arthroscopic guidance followed by instillation of a broad-spectrum antimicrobial into the synovial cavity.[34] Parenteral administrations of broad-spectrum antibiotics and NSAIDs are required. The application of drains and/or an ingress/egress system for lavage postoperatively is done according to the surgeon's preference. In some cases the bursa is left open to drain and heal by second intention. Antimicrobial therapy is generally prolonged, lasting 3 to 4 weeks. Controlled exercise and moving the affected limb through a passive range of motion is advocated to reduce restrictive adhesion formation.[2]

Prognosis

Acute cases of nonseptic bursitis when a fracture is not the cause often respond favorably to conservative treatment.[18] Conservative therapy for more chronic cases of nonseptic or septic bursitis appears less satisfactory.[2,9,15,36] In one report of 3 horses with chronic nonseptic bicipital bursitis that were treated surgically, all became pasture sound.[15]

In chronic septic bursitis cases treated conservatively the prognosis appears poor for return to performance unless surgery is performed. Surgical intervention with debridement, lavage, and appropriate antimicrobial therapy and rest gives a favorable prognosis.[9,11,12,20,28,36]

References

1. Adams O. Lameness in Horses, 3rd ed. Lea and Febiger, Philadelphia, 1974.
2. Blaeyert H. Bicipital bursitis/tenosynovitis and humeral osteitis. In Current Techniques of Equine Surgery And Lameness. White N, Moore J, eds. WB Saunders and Co., Philadelphia, 1998; 424–426.
3. Bohn A, Papageorges M, Grant BD. Ultrasonographic evaluation and surgical treatment of humeral osteitis and bicipital tenosynovitis in a horse. J Am Vet Med Assoc 1992;201:305–306.
4. Bosch G, de Mos M, van Binsbergen R, et al. The effect of focused extracorporeal shock wave therapy on collagen matrix and gene expression in normal tendons and ligaments. Equine Vet J 2009; 41:335–341.
5. Cosgrove J. Symposium on equine practice 2: Clinical aspects of equine brucellosis. Veterinary Record 1961;73:1377.
6. Coudry V, Allen AK, Denoix JM. Congenital abnormalities of the bicipital apparatus in four mature horses. Equine Vet J 2005;37:272–275.
7. Crabill MR, Chaffin MK, Schmitz DG. Ultrasonographic morphology of the bicipital tendon and bursa in clinically normal quarter horses. Am J Vet Res 1995;56:5–10.
8. Dyson S. Intertuberal (bicipital) bursitis. In Equine Medicine and Surgery. Colahan P, Mayhew IG, Merritt A, et al., eds. American Veterinary Publications, Goleta, CA, 1991;1456–1457.
9. Dyson S. Shoulder lameness in horses: An analysis of 58 suspected cases. Equine Vet J 1986;18:29–36.
10. Dyson S. Shoulder lameness in horses: diagnosis and differential diagnosis. Proceedings Am Assoc Equine Pract 1986; 461–480.
11. Forresu D, Lepage OM, Cauvin E. Septic bicipital bursitis, tendinitis and arthritis of the scapulohumeral joint in a mare. Vet Rec 2006;159:352–354.
12. Fugaro MN, Adams SB. Biceps brachii tenotomy or tenectomy for the treatment of bicipital bursitis, tendinitis, and humeral osteitis in 3 horses. J Am Vet Med Assoc 2002;220:1508–1511, 1475.
13. Gerdesmeyer L, Wagenpfeil S, Haake M, et al. Extracorporeal shock wave therapy for the treatment of chronic calcifying tendinitis of the rotator cuff: a randomized controlled trial. J Am Vet Med Assoc 2003;290:2573–2580.
14. Gough M, McDiarmid AM. Septic intertuberal (bicipital) bursitis in a horse. Equine Veterinary Education 1998;10:66–69.
15. Grant BD, Peterson P, Bohn A, et al. Diagnosis and surgical treatment of traumatic bicipital bursitis in the horse. Proceedings Am Assoc Equine Pract 1992;350–354.
16. Hamelin A, Denoix A, Bousseau B, et al. Ultrasonographic examination of the proximal part of the biceps brachii in horses. Practicing Veterinarian Equine 1994;26:41–47.
17. Heinen M, Busoni V, Petite A, et al. Bicipital groove dysplasia and medial dislocation of the biceps brachii tendon in a Welsh pony. Veterinary Radiology and Ultrasound 2002;44:235.
18. Leitch M. The Upper Forearm. In Equine Medicine and Surgery. Mansmann R, McAllister E, eds. American Veterinary Publications, Santa Barbara, CA, 1982;1131–1134.
19. Loew M, Daecke W, Kusnierczak D, et al. Shock-wave therapy is effective for chronic calcifying tendinitis of the shoulder. J Bone Joint Surg Br 1999;81:863–867.
20. Mason TA. Bicipital bursitis in a mare. Vet Rec 1980;107: 330–331.
21. McDiarmid A. Medial displacement of the biceps brachii in a foal: clinical, pathological and comparative aspects. Equine Vet J 1997;29:156–159.
22. Moyer W, Schumacher J, Schumacher J. A Guide to Equine Joint Injection and Regional Anesthesia, 1st ed. Veterinary Learning Systems. Yardley. 2007;44–47.
23. Muir P, Goldsmidt S, Rothwell T, et al. Calcifying tendinopathy of the biceps brachii in a dog. Journal of the American Veterinary Medical Society 1992;201:1747–1749.
24. Nevens AL, Stover SM, Hawkins DA. Evaluation of the passive function of the biceps brachii muscle-tendon unit in limitation of shoulder and elbow joint ranges of motion in horses. Am J Vet Res 2005;66:391–400.
25. Norris Adams M, Turner TA. Endoscopy of the intertubercular bursa in horses. J Am Vet Med Assoc 1999;214:221–225, 205.
26. Pankowski R, Grant BD, Sande R, et al. Fracture of the supraglenoid tubercle: treatment and results in five horses. Veterinary Surgery 1986;15:33–39.
27. Pugh C, Johnson P, Crawley G, et al. Ultrasonography of the equine bicipital tendon region: a case history report and review of anatomy. Veterinary Radiology and Ultrasound 1994;35: 183–188.
28. Riggs C, Rice Y, Patteson M. Infection of the intertuberal (bicipital) bursa in seven horses. 34th BEVA Congress, 1995;46–48.
29. Rooney J. Biomechanics of Lameness in Horses. Williams and Wilkins, Baltimore, 1969.
30. Rose R, Hodgson D. Bicipital Bursitis. In Manual of Equine Practice. Rose R, Hodgson D, eds. WB Sanders and Co., London, 1993;109.
31. Sabeti-Aschraf M, Dorotka R, Goll A, et al. Extracorporeal shock wave therapy in the treatment of calcific tendinitis of the rotator cuff. Am J Sports Med 2005;33:1365–1368.
32. Scheuch B, Whitcomb M, Galuppo L, et al. Clinical evaluation of high-energy extracorporeal shock waves on equine orthopedic injuries. 20th Annual Meeting of the Association for Equine Sports Medicine (AESM), New Brunswick, New Jersey, 2000.
33. Schumacher J, Livesey L, Brawner W, et al. Comparison of 2 methods of centesis of the bursa of the biceps brachii tendon of horses. Equine Vet J 2007;39:356–359.
34. Tudor RA, Bowman KF, Redding WR, et al. Endoscopic treatment of suspected infectious intertubercular bursitis in a horse. J Am Vet Med Assoc 1998;213:1584–1585, 1570.
35. Tulleners EP, Divers TJ, Evans LH. Bilateral bicipital bursitis in a cow. J Am Vet Med Assoc 1985;186:604.
36. Vatistas NJ, Pascoe JR, Wright IM, et al. Infection of the intertubercular bursa in horses: four cases (1978–1991). J Am Vet Med Assoc 1996;208:1434–1437.

INFLAMMATION OF THE INFRASPINATUS BURSA

The infraspinatus bursa is located between the tendon of the infraspinatus muscle and the caudal eminence of the greater tubercle of the proximal humerus. The bursa is not visible in most horses except when inflamed or septic.[2] This is an uncommonly reported cause of lameness.

Etiology

Severe adduction of the forelimb and/or the possibility of direct trauma to this region is considered to be the cause (Figure 5.277).[1,2]

Clinical Signs

The involved forelimb maybe held in an abducted position, presumably in an attempt to reduce the pressure on the infraspinatus bursa. During exercise, a moderate lameness is present with an obvious decreased cranial stride.[1,2] Adduction of the limb reportedly elicits a painful response and results in increased signs of lameness at exercise (Figure 5.278).[1] If the bursa is septic the lameness exhibited is severe.[2]

Diagnosis

Ultrasonographic evaluation and comparison with the opposite limb may be required, along with ultra-

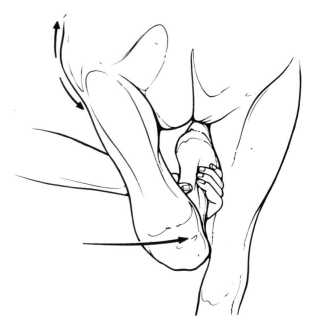

Figure 5.278. Adduction of the limb may result in a painful response in horses with infraspinatus bursitis.

sound-guided centesis and local analgesia, for a definitive diagnosis.[2]

Treatment

In the acute stage, synoviocentesis and the administration of corticosteroids into the bursa is recommended. With sufficient stall rest (6 weeks or more) and the parenteral administration of NSAIDs, a good end result can be expected. Varying degrees of lameness may remain with chronic cases.[1] Septic involvement of the bursa requires endoscopic debridement and flushing. The initial distension of the bursa may require distension with fluid by ultrasonographic guidance to place the needle. The bursa is small and movement of instruments is restricted by the overlying muscle and infraspinatus tendon.[2]

Prognosis

In one report 3 horses returned to soundness after surgical treatment of septic infraspinatus bursae. There are few other reports, however.[2]

References

1. Rooney J. Biomechanics of Lameness in Horses. Williams and Wilkins, Baltimore, 1969.
2. Whitcomb MB, le Jeune SS, MacDonald MM, et al. Disorders of the infraspinatus tendon and bursa in three horses. J Am Vet Med Assoc 2006;229:549–556.

OSTEOCHONDROSIS (OC) OF THE SCAPULOHUMERAL JOINT (SHJ) OR SHOULDER

Osteochondrosis of the scapulohumeral joint or shoulder is most frequently diagnosed in weanlings and

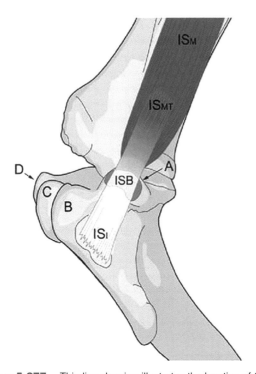

Figure 5.277. This line drawing illustrates the location of the infraspinatus bursa underlying the infraspinatus tendon. A, caudal eminence of greater tubercle (GT); B, cranial eminence of the GT; C, intermediate tubercle; D, lesser tubercle; IS_M, infraspinatus muscle; IS_MT, musculotendinous junction of the infraspinatous muscle; IS_I, infraspinatus tendon insertion; ISB, infraspinatus bursa. (Reprinted with permission from Whitcomb MB, et al. J Am Vet Med Assoc 2006;229:549–556)

yearlings 6 to 12 months of age, but it has been reported in foals younger than 5 months and in horses up to 8 years old.[3,5,8–10,12,14–16] Although it has been suggested that the incidence of OC is related to the rate of skeletal growth and body size, many affected horses appear normal sized for the breed and age and some may be smaller and lighter in weight than expected.[15] Males appear to be more commonly affected than females, and no specific breed predilection has been identified. The incidence of the disease varies; one study reported diagnosing OC of the shoulder in 54 joints of 38 young horses radiographed for shoulder problems,[16] and in another study OC and subchondral bone cysts were observed in 6 of 29 diagnosed shoulder problems.[5] The condition is considered the most debilitating form of osteochondritis dissecans (OCD), and when it is diagnosed in older yearlings, chronic manifestation of secondary degenerative joint changes are usually present.[16]

The primary cartilage lesion is located in the glenoid, humeral head, or both (most common), and the disease often affects a major part of the joint surface.[16] Regardless of the site of the lesion, secondary degenerative changes in the joint are prominent features of this disease. An exception is the solitary subchondral cystic lesions that are occasionally seen in the glenoid cavity.[5,9]

Etiology

Over nutrition, imbalanced nutrition, or a genetic predisposition to rapid growth at some stage of the development still appear to be reasonable hypotheses for most young affected horses. The secondary degenerative changes within the joint are exacerbated by the resultant instability.[16]

Occasionally, subchondral bone cysts are seen in the glenoid without cartilage changes in the humeral head, alterations of the contour of the articulations of the shoulder, or signs of secondary osteoarthritis.[5,9] Thus, it has been suggested that subchondral bone cysts may not be a manifestation of OC in the SHJ.[5] A traumatic etiology is often suspected in such cases of subchondral bone cysts.[9]

Clinical Signs

Most cases present with a history of mild to moderate intermittent forelimb lameness with insidious onset. Atrophy of the muscles associated with the shoulder region is a common finding in chronic cases. A smaller foot with a higher heel and excessive toe wear is also commonly observed in the foot of the affected limb. Direct firm pressure with the thumb just cranial to the tendon of the infraspinatus muscle over the cranial lateral aspect of the shoulder joint may elicit a painful response, particularly in younger horses (Figure 5.279).

Exercise usually results in a moderate to severe lameness that is characterized by a shortened cranial (extension) phase of the stride and a delay in limb protraction. Stumbling may occur in some cases due to inadequate foot clearance. A prominent shoulder lift, reduced carpal flexion, and limb circumduction is often seen in the most severely affected horses. Manipulation of the affected limb in extension and flexion and abduction may cause pain, and often increases the signs of lame-

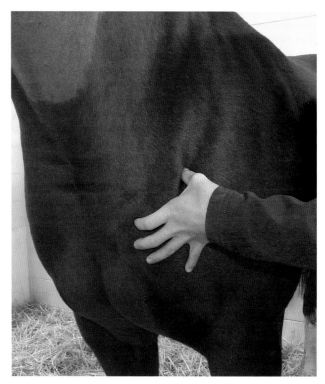

Figure 5.279. Thumb pressure applied just cranial to the infraspinatous tendon may elicit a painful response in horses with shoulder osteochondrosis.

ness. Intrasynovial anesthesia is used to localize the lameness to the shoulder region; 10 to 15 ml of a local anesthetic should improve or eliminate the lameness in most cases[5], and it might be necessary to wait as long as 60 minutes after instillation to note improvement.[7]

Diagnosis

Radiographs are necessary to definitively diagnose the lesion. The most common radiographic findings include:

1. Flattening and indentation of the caudal aspect of the humeral head
2. Alterations in the contour of the glenoid cavity with a subchondral cystic radiolucency
3. Osteophytes at the caudal and cranial aspect of the glenoid cavity (Figure 5.280)
4. Subchondral bone sclerosis
5. Remodeling of the humeral head and glenoid cavity (Figure 5.280).[12]

Less common findings include osteophytes and subchondral bone cysts associated with the humeral head.[16] Intra-articular free bodies are uncommon, but when present they settle in the cranial and caudal cul-de-sacs of the joint.[15] Centrally located glenoid sclerosis and small glenoid cysts can easily be overlooked (Figure 5.281).[4] A contrast arthrogram can confirm the presence or outline the extent of the lesion if the lesion is difficult to identify on plain films.

The normal ultrasonographic anatomy of the SHJ has been described and humeral head osteochondrosis

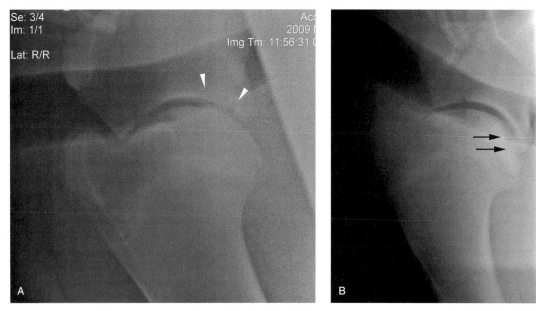

Figure 5.280.   A. An OC lesion of the caudal aspect of the glenoid cavity (arrowheads). This horse was grade 3 out of 5 lame. B. An OC lesion on the caudal humeral head (arrows). This horse was lame at the walk and had significant muscle atrophy.

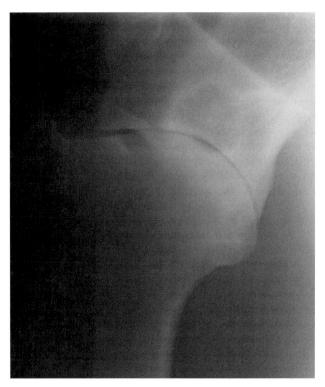

Figure 5.281.   A large articular subchondral cystic lesion located in the glenoid. (Courtesy of Dr. Gary Baxter.)

has been diagnosed using ultrasonography; however, the evaluation of the glenoid is difficult.[18] Nuclear scintigraphy may be used to identify subtle lesions.[4,9]

Arthroscopy may be useful to make a definitive diagnosis in cases in which the lameness is localized to the SHJ with intrasynovial anesthesia but a lesion is not identified on radiography or scintigraphy. The conclusions drawn in one retrospective study of 15 horses with subtle osteochondral lesions in the SHJ suggested that a combination of the physical examination, radiology, scintigraphy, and arthroscopy may be necessary to diagnose subtle osteochondral lesions of the SHJ.[4]

Treatment

Rest and confinement may be considered for horses with have mild to moderate radiographic changes that are not intended for athletic performance.[8,12,16] Of the 17 horses treated with rest, the treatment was considered moderately successful in 7 cases.[16] In another case series of 3 horses with isolated subchondral cysts in the glenoid, sodium hyaluronate was injected into the affected joint with moderate success.[5] In a more recent report of 14 horses treated conservatively, 7 became sound with conservative treatment.[8]

Although both arthrotomy and arthroscopic approaches have been described for the surgical treatment of shoulder OC,[1–3,10,11,15,17] arthrotomies are no longer performed. Surgical cases should be selected carefully because of the generalized pathologic changes that are present in many cases. However, surgery benefits some horses even when secondary changes are present.[2,3] With very severe degenerative changes the prognosis is poor and surgery is not recommended.

While arthroscopic surgery is the preferred approach for treating these lesions,[1,2,11,13] the technique is not easy and it is particularly difficult in adult horses. In most instances the cartilaginous changes extend beyond the limits of the subchondral abnormalities seen on radiographic examination (Figure 5.282). Problems associated with arthroscopic surgery in the shoulder usually involve inadequate access to medially located lesions and debridement of large lesions.

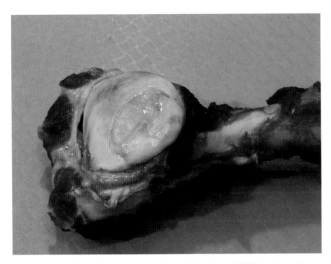

Figure 5.282. Postmortem view of the large OCD lesion of the caudal humeral head depicted radiographically in Figure 5.280B. Arthroscopic access to medially-located lesions or debridement of large lesions such as this can be difficult and often results in a poor prognosis. (Courtesy of Dr. Gary Baxter.)

Prognosis

Generally the prognosis with rest or surgery is considered guarded, but this is somewhat dependent on the horse's intended use and the severity of the OC lesion. Horses with mild to moderate OC have the best prognosis and those with severe lesions usually remain lame. In one report on the outcome of arthroscopic surgery on 11 horses, 7 became athletically sound,[2] and follow-up radiographic examinations on those 7 indicated remodeling and improved contour of the glenoid and humeral head. In another study, a long-term follow-up on 35 horses with OC of the shoulder treated arthroscopically found that 16 of 35 were successful.[6] A more recent study of 32 horses with shoulder OC (16 with bilateral lesions) also reported a poor outcome. In this study, the lesions were graded mild, moderate, or severe using a system that took into account lesion size and lesion severity.[8] However, there was no difference in conservative versus arthroscopic treatment.

References

1. Bertone A, McIlwraith C. Osteochondrosis of the equine shoulder: Treatment with arthroscopic surgery. Proceedings Am Assoc Equine Pract 1987;33:683–688.
2. Bertone AL, McIlwraith CW, Powers BE, et al. Arthroscopic surgery for the treatment of osteochondrosis in the equine shoulder joint. Vet Surg 1987;16:303–311.
3. DeBowes R, Wagner D, Grant B. Surgical approach to the equine scapulohumeral joint through a longitudinal infraspinatous tenotomy. Veterinary Surgery 1982;11:125.
4. Doyle PS, White NA 2nd. Diagnostic findings and prognosis following arthroscopic treatment of subtle osteochondral lesions in the shoulder joint of horses: 15 cases (1996–1999). J Am Vet Med Assoc 2000;217:1878–1882.
5. Dyson S. Diagnostic techniques in the investigation of shoulder lameness. Equine Vet J 1986.
6. Dyson S. Shoulder lameness in horses: An analysis of 58 suspected cases. Equine Vet J 1986;18:29–36.
7. Dyson S. Shoulder lameness in horses: Diagnosis and differential diagnosis. Proceedings Am Assoc Equine Pract 1986; 461–480.
8. Jenner F, Ross MW, Martin BB, et al. Scapulohumeral osteochondrosis. A retrospective study of 32 horses. Vet Comp Orthop Traumatol 2008;21:406–412.
9. Kay A. An acute subchondral cystic lesion of the equine shoulder causing lameness. Equine Veterinary Education 2006;18: 316–319.
10. Mason TA, Maclean AA. Osteochondrosis dissecans of the head of the humerus in two foals. Equine Vet J 1977;9:189–191.
11. McIlwraith C. Diagnostic and surgical arthroscopy of the scapulohumeral (shoulder) joint. In Diagnostic and Surgical Arthroscopy in the Horse, 3rd ed. McIlwraith CW, Nixon AJ, Wright IM, et al., eds. Elsevier, Philadelphia, 2006;307–326.
12. Meagher D, Pool R, O'Brien T. Osteochondrosis of the shoulder joint in the horse. Proceedings Am Assoc Equine Pract 1977; 247.
13. Nixon A. Diagnostic and surgical arthroscopy of the equine shoulder joint. Veterinary Surgery 1987;16:44–52.
14. Nixon A, Stashak T, McIlwraith C. A muscle separating approach to the equine shoulder joint for the treatment of osteochondritis dissecans. Veterinary Surgery 1984;13:247.
15. Nixon AJ. Osteochondrosis of the shoulder and elbow. In Current Practice of Equine Surgery. White N, Moore J, eds. JB Lippincott, Philadelphia, 1990;512–526.
16. Nyack B, Morgan J, Pool R. Osteochondrosis of the shoulder joint of the horse. Cornell Vet 1981;71:149.
17. Schmidt G, Dueland R, Vaughn J. Osteochondrosis dessicans of the equine shoulder joint. Vet Med Small Anim Clin 1975;70: 542.
18. Tnibar M, Auer J, Bakkali S. Ultrasonography of the equine shoulder: Technique and normal appearance. Veterinary Radiology and Ultrasound 1999;40:44–57.

OSTEOARTHRITIS (OA) OF THE SCAPULOHUMERAL JOINT

Arthritis of the scapulohumeral joint (SHJ) is a relatively uncommon condition that can affect a variety of breeds, ages, and uses of horses.[5,7] Reports found a higher incidence of OA in Shetland ponies, miniature horses, and Falabella ponies, with a possible congenital cause.[2,3,9,11]

Although the recognition and treatment of conditions associated with SHJ have improved, the diagnosis of specific problems related to this joint remain a challenge.[5] As a result, some may require extensive diagnostic imaging, including arthroscopy, to make a definitive diagnosis. Unfortunately, the delay in recognition of the cause may increase the likelihood of the development of secondary OA.[10,13]

Etiology

Osteoarthritis of the SHJ can have multiple causes. In younger horses a developmental role due to OC may be the cause, whereas in older horses trauma may be causative.[5] A radiographic study comparing Shetland ponies diagnosed with OA, skeletally mature Shetland ponies without a history of lameness, and skeletally mature horses found that ponies had a flattening (dysplasia) of the glenoid contour, which was thought to make them more susceptible to the development of OA.[2] A recent study showed that 6 of 20 ponies had radiographic evidence of dysplasia with diagnosed shoulder OA.[3] Other case reports of SHJ OA have indicated that the glenoid cavity is relatively dysplastic in Shetland ponies.[9] Other causes of arthritis include intra-articular fracture and injury to the joint capsule resulting in a synovitis and capsulitis.

Clinical Signs

A history of trauma is relatively common. In one report, 8 of 15 horses that had subtle OC lesions in the SHJ had a history of a traumatic insult.[5] Where mild swelling may be apparent over the shoulder region in the acute case, muscle atrophy is variable and may not reflect chronicity or severity of the lameness.[6,8] Disuse atrophy of the extensor carpi radialis muscle may be apparent in the affected limb in some cases, and an upright narrow foot may also be observed in the affected limb.[5] In contrast, in another study only a small proportion (fewer than 5%) of the cases with shoulder problems had a smaller foot on the affected limb, although a severely lame horse may have abnormal toe wear.[6,8] Deep thumb pressure applied just cranial to the tendon of the infraspinatus muscle may elicit a painful response in young and light muscled mature horses. Upper limb manipulation (flexion, extension, adduction, and abduction) may also result in a painful response.[8]

In general, the signs of lameness are typical of shoulder lameness and the degree depends on the severity of the problem. At a trot, the height of the foot flight and the flexion of the carpus is decreased during the swing phase of the stride compared to the contralateral limb. The cranial phase of the stride of the lame limb is often shortened and as the lame limb is advanced a prominent lifting of the head and neck occurs on the affected side.[8] Additionally, the horse appears to "fix" the SHJ on the affected side. The lameness grade in one study ranged from subtle and intermittent to 4 on a scale of 5.[5]

Diagnosis

Diagnostic anesthesia can assist in localizing the problem to the shoulder region.[5,6,8] Radiography, ultrasound, nuclear medicine, and/or arthroscopy may be required to make a definitive diagnosis of the problem.[5,6] Radiography, although important in evaluating abnormalities of the shoulder joint, often underestimates the full extent of the changes involving the glenoid cavity and the humeral head.[6,7] Radiographic changes identified in one report in horses with subtle lesions in the SHJ included glenoid sclerosis, focal glenoid lysis, glenoid cysts, and alteration in the humeral head contour.[5] In another report a flattening of the glenoid without changes in the contour of the humeral head was seen in Shetland ponies.[2] Other radiographic changes associated with OA include osteophyte and enthesiophyte formation (Figure 5.280 B). Contrast arthrography may improve the chances of identifying a SHJ lesion.[8,10]

The normal ultrasonographic anatomy of the shoulder region has been described.[14] Although the detection of humeral head OC has been reported, its major value appears to be in identifying injury to the soft tissue support structures surrounding the SHJ.[6,14] Evaluation of the glenoid cavity with ultrasound also appears limited.[5] Ultrasonography has been used to diagnose the condition in Shetland ponies when radiographs were nondiagnostic and only revealed dysplasia or flattening of the glenoid cavity. Joint distension and capsulitis provides the diagnosis.[9]

Nuclear medicine may be useful to diagnose a subtle shoulder lameness with focal intense uptake of the radioisotope, most commonly in the humeral head.[4,5]

Treatment

Conservative treatment may be indicated in horses that have no radiographic lesions and that respond favorably to intrasynovial anesthesia. Treatment involves rest; controlled exercise; anti-inflammatory drugs; and relevant intra-articular therapy including corticosteroids, hyaluronic acid, and IRAP. Rest periods may be as short as a few weeks to 3 months.

Horses that do not respond to the conservative treatment or have radiographic or scintigraphic changes and have responded favorably to intrasynovial anesthesia are candidates for arthroscopy.[5] Localized cartilage damage is debrided down to healthy subchondral bone, and osteochondral fragments are removed if they are loose.

There are reports of performing scapulohumeral arthrodesis in miniature horses to reduce morbidity in those with severe shoulder dysfunction.[1,12] A narrow DCP plate was placed across the cranial surface of the scapula and the humerus with screws placed in lag fashion across the joint through the plate.[12] This procedure improved the horses' lameness by several grades, improving morbidity.

Prognosis

The prognosis appears favorable for horses without radiographic-apparent lesions that respond favorably to intra-articular anesthesia and are treated conservatively with rest and intra-articular therapy.[7] Those with obvious radiographic evidence of OA generally do not respond well.

The prognosis for horses treated by arthroscopy appears good for subtle cartilage lesion. In the case of SHJ OA due to shoulder dysplasia in ponies, the prognosis does not appear as favorable. In a report of 20 ponies, 6 were euthanized for continuing severe lameness and the other 14 remained lame.[3] In 2 other case reports ponies remained lame despite concurrent conservative treatments.[9,11]

References

1. Arighi M, Miller CR, Pennock PW. Arthrodesis of the scapulohumeral joint in a miniature horse. J Am Vet Med Assoc 1987; 191:713–714.
2. Boswell J, Schramme M, Wilson A. A radiological study to evaluate suspected scapulohumeral joint dysplasia in Shetland ponies. 8th Annual ECVS Meeting, Brugge, Belgium, 1999;51–53.
3. Clegg PD, Dyson SJ, Summerhays GE, et al. Scapulohumeral osteoarthritis in 20 Shetland ponies, miniature horses and falabella ponies. Vet Rec 2001;148:175–179.
4. Devous MD, Twardock AR. Techniques and application of nuclear medicine in the diagnosis of equine lameness. J Am Vet Med Assoc 1984;184:318–325.
5. Doyle PS, White NA 2nd. Diagnostic findings and prognosis following arthroscopic treatment of subtle osteochondral lesions in the shoulder joint of horses: 15 cases (1996–1999). J Am Vet Med Assoc 2000;217:1878–1882.
6. Dyson S. Diagnostic techniques in the investigation of shoulder lameness. Equine Vet J 1986.
7. Dyson S. Shoulder lameness in horses: An analysis of 58 suspected cases. Equine Vet J 1986;18:29–36.

8. Dyson S. Shoulder lameness in horses: diagnosis and differential diagnosis, Proceedings Am Assoc Equine Pract 1986; 461–480.
9. Jones E, McDiarmid A. Diagnosis of scapulohumeral joint osteoarthritis in a Shetland pony by ultrasonography. Vet Rec 2004;154:178–180.
10. Nixon AJ. Osteochondrosis of the shoulder and elbow. In Current Practice of Equine Surgery. White N, Moore J, eds. JB Lippincott, Philadelphia, 1990;512–526.
11. Parth RA, Svalbe LS, Hazard GH, et al. Suspected primary scapulohumeral osteoarthritis in two Miniature ponies. Aust Vet J 2008;86:153–156.
12. Semevolos SA, Watkins JP, Auer JA. Scapulohumeral arthrodesis in miniature horses. Vet Surg 2003;32:416–420.
13. Trotter G, McIlwraith CW. Osteochondrosis dessicans and subchondral bone cysts and their relationship to osteochondrosis in the horse. Journal of Equine Veterinary Science 1981;1:157–162.
14. Williams J, Miyabayashi T, Ruggles A, et al. Scintigraphic and ultrasonographic diagnosis of soft tissue injury in a thoroughbred horse. J Vet Med Sci 1994;56:169–172.

LUXATION OF THE SCAPULOHUMERAL (SHOULDER) JOINT

Luxation or subluxation of the SHJ is uncommon in horses. In a survey of 128 cases of suspected shoulder lameness in horses, only 2 cases had shoulder luxation.[6] Ponies appear to be at a greater risk for this condition.[3,5,7,8,10] The head of the humerus can displace in several directions, including cranial,[9,10] craniolateral, lateral, craniomedial, and medial (Figure 5.283).[3,5,7] When the humerus becomes luxated it displaces proximad due to the contraction of the muscles surrounding

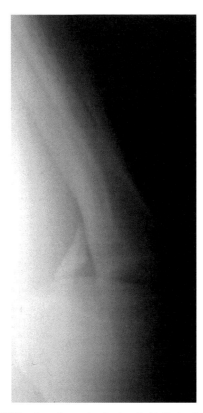

Figure 5.283. A radiograph of a luxated left shoulder. The scapula has luxated laterally. (Courtesy of Dr. Gary Baxter.)

the SHJ, and the direction of the luxation appears to depend on the direction of the inciting injury.

Of the cases presented in which the direction of the luxation was documented, lateral luxation with proximal displacement was most common.[5,8,9] Because the equine SHJ is stabilized by a ball-and-socket articulation, the tendons from surrounding muscles, and the glenohumeral ligaments within the joint capsule, it is not surprising that luxation of the joint results in considerable damage to these structures.[3,5] In one report arthroscopic examination following closed reduction of a luxated SHJ of 2-weeks' duration revealed bony and soft tissue debris, a cartilage defect, and a tear in the joint capsule.[9]

Etiology

Luxation of the SHJ generally occurs following excessive (forceful) trauma to the shoulder region such as may occur from a fall, while a horse is attempting to jump a fence, or as a result of a horse pulling and twisting a flexed limb while the foot is caught fast.[3,8–10] A report documented SHJ luxation in a septicemic foal with multiple joint laxity,[7] another cause was a rough recovery from general anesthesia,[11] and luxation of the SHJ has occurred following removal of a large supraglenoid tubercle fragment.[1,2]

Clinical Signs

A history of trauma with an acute onset of severe lameness is common.[1,2,4,8,10] At presentation, horses typically exhibit a nonweight-bearing lameness. An abnormal stance may also be apparent with the elbow and carpus held semiflexed and the distal limb adducted or abducted, depending on the direction of the luxation. The distal limb is adducted when the humerus is luxated laterally, craniolaterally, or cranially, is slightly abducted if the humerus is luxated medially. A variable amount of swelling is present in the shoulder region, depending on the length of time since injury.

Muscle atrophy may be most prominent in chronic cases. One report found prominent muscle atrophy of the infraspinatus and supraspinatus muscles 2 weeks following luxation of the SHJ.[9] Distortion of the normal anatomic landmarks at the shoulder region may be apparent if swelling is not excessive, which may aid in determining the direction of the luxation. With lateral or cranial luxation the greater tubercle and head of the humerus may be most prominent, and with medial displacement the lateral lip of the glenoid cavity can be felt.[9] Affected horses generally violently oppose upper limb manipulation.[3,8]

Diagnosis

Radiographs should be taken to confirm the diagnosis and rule out fracture. Generally an adequate study can be obtained in the standing horse and the mediolateral view is thought to be the most informative.[6] The addition of the craniocaudal oblique projection will allow a better assessment of the direction of the luxation.[4] Stressed views may assist in diagnosis. Ultrasound examination may also be used to assess the extent of injury to the soft tissues supporting the SHJ.

Treatment

Ideally, the luxation should be corrected as soon as possible. General anesthesia is required in most cases, although there is one report of correction of an SHJ luxation using sedation in a 5-day-old foal with multiple joint laxity.[7] In all cases the anesthetic induction should be assisted to avoid further damage to the soft tissues or joint. In foals, pulling the affected limb into extension while an assistant pushes or pulls the humeral head back into position will generally suffice. The foal may have to be stabilized with counter pressure applied the chest or axilla.

In the mature horse, the patient can be placed in lateral or dorsal recumbency. In lateral recumbency the body can be anchored to a fixed object, and a tension-creating device that is attached to the radius or pastern region to apply traction is used while the operator forces the shoulder back into position. If the horse is placed in dorsal recumbency, a hoist can be used to apply traction and the body weight is sufficient to provide counter weight.[10] An audible click may be heard when the humeral head reduced, after which it should be possible to freely manipulate the joint.[3,8] In acute cases, reduction may be accomplished very quickly. In more chronic cases, gradually increasing traction may be required with limb manipulation before reduction is achieved.[9] Arthroscopic examination of the SHJ following closed reduction may improve the outcome particularly if there is evidence of bony debris within the joint on radiography.[9] As such a radiograph should be taken of the SHJ after the reduction is complete.

Recovery from anesthesia should be assisted in all cases. Following recovery the horse should have strict stall rest for 2 months to allow healing of the joint capsule and surrounding soft tissue structures.[3] Anti-inflammatories and intra-articular therapies are indicated. Reoccurrence of the luxation does not appear to be a problem in the horse.[10]

Prognosis

The prognosis for SHJ luxation is considered good for return to soundness following closed reduction and an adequate rest period, in cases in which there is not a complicating fracture. In one study, all 6 cases reported with SHJ luxation treated by closed reduction returned to soundness.[1–3,5,8–11] The prognosis for larger horses may also be good. One report of shoulder luxation in a Thoroughbred filly has been described.[9] The filly was sound for light work 8 months after closed reduction and arthroscopic examination of the joint. It has been suggested that the prognosis may be improved and more accurately predicted if arthroscopy is used following closed reduction.[3]

References

1. Blaeyert H. Scapulohumeral joint luxations. In Current Techniques of Equine Surgery And Lameness. White N, Moore J, eds. WB Saunders and Co., Philadelphia, 1998;423–424.
2. Bleyaert H, Sullins K, White N. Supraglenoid tubercle fractures in horses. Compendium of Continuing Education for the Veterinary Practitioner 1994;16:531–536.
3. Colbourne C, Yovich J, Bolton J. The diagnosis and successful treatment of shoulder luxation in a pony. Australian Equine Veterinarian 1991 9:100–102.
4. Dyson S. Interpreting radiographs 7: radiology of the equine shoulder and elbow. Equine Vet J 1986;18:352–361.
5. Dyson S. Shoulder lameness in horses: An analysis of 58 suspected cases. Equine Vet J 1986;18:29–36.
6. Dyson S. Shoulder lameness in horses: diagnosis and differential diagnosis. Proceedings Am Assoc Equine Pract 1986; 461–480.
7. Hardy J, Marohn MA. What is your diagnosis? Scapulohumeral luxation. J Am Vet Med Assoc 1989;195:1773–1774.
8. Littlejohn A. Dislocation of the shoulder of a mare. South African Veterinary Medical Association 1954:46.
9. Madison JB, Young D, Richardson D. Repair of shoulder luxation in a horse. J Am Vet Med Assoc 1991;198:455–456.
10. Wilson RG, Reynolds WT. Scapulohumeral luxation with treatment by closed reduction in a horse. Aust Vet J 1984;61: 300–301.
11. Zilberstein LF, Tnibar A, Coudry V, et al. Luxation of the shoulder joint in a horse recovering from general anaesthesia. Vet Rec 2005;157:748–749.

SUPRASCAPULAR NERVE INJURY (SWEENY)

Suprascapular nerve injury resulting in atrophy of the supraspinatus and infraspinatus muscles and shoulder joint instability can affect any age or breed of horse.[3,6] The condition was originally reported as most commonly affecting draft breeds and was believed to be associated with repeated trauma to the shoulder region from poorly fitted harness collars. With the decline in draft breeds the condition is most commonly seen in horses as result of trauma to the shoulder region. The term "sweeny" has been defined as atrophy of the shoulder muscles in horses and is a commonly used synonym for suprascapular nerve paralysis.[3]

Etiology

Trauma to the suprascapular nerve as it passes over the cranial thin border of the scapula is believed to be the cause.[5,6,12] The suprascapular nerve originates from the 6th and 7th cervical spinal segments and passes via the brachial plexus to innervate the supraspinatus and infraspinatus muscles that overlie the scapula.[8] As the nerve reflects around the cranial edge of the scapula, it passes beneath a small but strong tendinous band. In this position the nerve appears to be most susceptible to direct trauma and compression against the underlying bone.[5–7] In horses without clinical evidence of muscle atrophy, there is also histologic evidence of chronic demyelination and remyelination at the point where the suprascapular nerve reflects over the cranial edge of the scapula. These findings suggest there may be chronic nerve compression caused by constriction of the small tendinous band resulting in subclinical neuropathy. It has been suggested that the chronic neuronal injury may make the suprascapular nerve more susceptible to acute trauma and the development of clinical signs or that spontaneous development of the condition, without a traumatic insult, may be possible.[5–7]

Clinical Signs

A history of trauma to the shoulder region is relatively common. The clinical signs vary depending on the extent of the nerve damage and the duration of the condition prior to examination. Shortly after the injury, horses often exhibit severe pain and are reluctant to bear weight on the affected limb.[7] As the pain subsides and the horse begins to bear weight, a pronounced lateral instability (excursion) of the shoulder joint (shoulder slip) during weight-bearing is observed. This sign is usually seen within 24 hours of injury and is most apparent as the horse is walked slowly toward the examiner.[7] The instability is the result of loss of the stabilizing function of the supraspinatus and infraspinatus muscles which serve as the major lateral support for the shoulder.[10,12] It has been suggested that this outward excursion of the scapula during weight-bearing may cause intermittent stretching of the suprascapular nerve leading to continued trauma and perpetuation of the paralysis.[1] The acute lameness may be followed by complete recovery over a 2- 3-month period, or denervation atrophy of the supraspinatus and infraspinatus muscles may become evident. Following injury to the nerve, muscle atrophy usually becomes apparent as early as 10 to 14 days after injury.[5] Once atrophy begins, the scapular spine becomes more prominent due to the loss of the muscles cranial and caudal to it (Figure 5.284).

Diagnosis

A presumptive diagnosis of suprascapular nerve injury can be made from the clinical signs and the history of trauma to the region. Radiographs of the region should be obtained to rule out a fracture or OA of the shoulder joint. Electromyographic evaluation (EMGs) of the supraspinatus and infraspinatus muscles confirm selective suprascapular nerve injury.[9] For the EMG studies to be most meaningful they should be performed a minimum of 7 days after injury. EMG findings of denervation of muscles supplied by other branches of the brachial plexus should prompt further neurologic evaluation to rule out injuries to the brachial plexus, spinal cord disease at the 6th and 7th cervical

segments, and other diseases such as equine protozoal myelitis.[3,5]

Treatment

Both conservative and surgical treatments have been described for management of horses with suprascapular nerve injury.[2,4,7,13,14,16] Initial treatment in all cases is directed toward reducing inflammation in the region of the suprascapular nerve. Stall rest with the administration of NSAIDs and the topical application of cold hydrotherapy or ice packs and topical anti-inflammatories may produce a resolution of the clinical signs.

Conservative Treatment

When conservative treatment is selected stall rest is continued until shoulder joint stability returns, followed by confinement to a pasture for an additional 2 to 4 months. In one study the mean time for resolution of the gait abnormality was 7.4 months and 7 of 8 horses evaluated had a complete resolution of the joint instability.[7] The conclusions from this study were that stall rest appeared to be a viable alternative to surgery for the treatment of suprascapular nerve injury. It can be speculated that surgical decompression may result in a faster return to athletic function.

Injection of a corticosteroid into the shoulder joint may also be beneficial. In one report, 6 horses with suspected suprascapular nerve injury were treated successfully with intra-articular corticosteriods.[13] However, it is uncertain whether these horses had a true neuropraxia of the suprascapular nerve or scapulohumeral joint inflammation that caused disuse muscle atrophy, or both. Anti-inflammatory therapy is recommended. Therapeutic ultrasound has also been suggested as a treatment.[4]

Surgical Treatment

Surgical decompression of the nerve can be considered in patients that continue to exhibit signs of suprascapular nerve dysfunction for 10 to 12 weeks. This time frame is based on the rate of peripheral nerve regeneration (1 mm/day) and the distance from the site of nerve injury on the cranial border of the scapula to the infraspinatus muscle (7 to 8 cm). Using these parameters nerve function should return in 10 to 12 weeks.[14] In horses that show no improvement after 12 weeks or more of rest, entrapment of the suprascapular nerve by scar tissue between the overlying ligament and the cranial border of the scapula is likely. Although the time frame for reversing neurogenic muscle atrophy in large animals is not known, in humans, neurogenic muscle atrophy becomes dramatic after 4 months with loss of up to 80% of muscle fiber volume. It is generally accepted that functional reinnervation is unlikely after 12 months.[11,16] After that, irreversible changes within the muscle occur, and it is replaced by fibrous tissue.

Surgical decompression involves removing a small piece of bone from the cranial border of the scapula underlying the nerve (Figure 5.285).[14] By removing the notch of bone it is thought that the nerve is

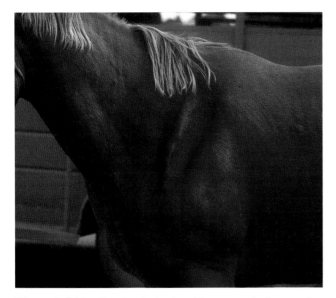

Figure 5.284. Prominent atrophy of the supraspinatus muscle is evident in this horse with suprascapular nerve injury.

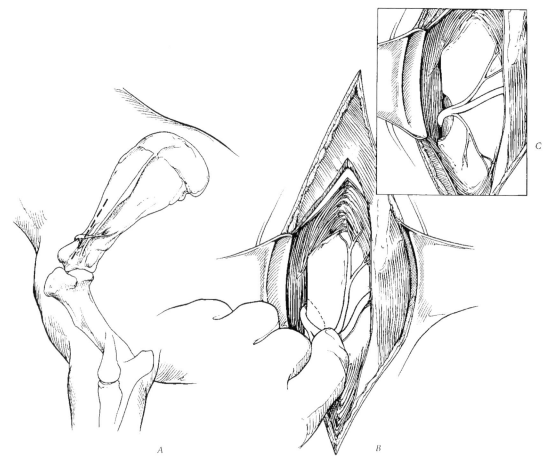

Figure 5.285. A. Location of the skin incision (dotted line), centered over the suprascapular nerve and cranial to scapular spine. B. The suprascapular nerve is identified and a small crescent-shaped piece of bone is removed from the cranial border of the scapula (dotted line). C. The bone has been removed and tendinous band resected.

decompressed, allowing for reinnervation. Complications of the surgery include the possibility of a glenoid fracture arising from the notched bone.

Prognosis

The prognosis for return to soundness in horses with suprascapular nerve injury is favorable for both conservative and surgical treatments. In one report 7 of 8 horses with suprascapular nerve injury treated conservatively were able to return to their intended use.[7] All 8 initially had pronounced shoulder joint instability during weight-bearing, and joint stability returned within 3 to 12 months. The conclusion was that rest alone carries a good prognosis for recovery of a normal gait and return to performance; however, the recovery period may be prolonged.

A high percentage of surgically treated horses are expected to return to performance. In one report 18 of 20 horses with suprascapular nerve injury returned to soundness.[15] An important and severe complication associated with the surgery is the postoperative occurrence of fracture of the supraglenoid tubercle and complete subluxation of the scapulohumeral joint during anesthetic recovery.[14] Horses that develop severe atrophy of the supraspinatus and infraspinatus muscles prior to surgery may not regain normal muscle mass, and some atrophy will remain in the proximal one-third of the scapula.

References

1. Adams O. Lameness in Horses, 3rd ed. Lea and Febiger, Philadelphia, 1974.
2. Adams OR, Schneider RK, Bramlage LR, et al. A surgical approach to treatment of suprascapular nerve injury in the horse. J Am Vet Med Assoc 1985;187:1016–1018.
3. Bleyaert H. Suprascapular nerve injury. In Current Techniques in Equine Surgery. White N, Moore J, eds. WB Saunders, Philadelphia, 1998;426–428.
4. Bleyaert HF, Madison JB. Complete biceps brachii tenotomy to facilitate internal fixation of supraglenoid tubercle fractures in three horses. Vet Surg 1999;28:48–53.
5. Duncan I, Schneider R. Equine suprascapular neuropathy (Sweeny): Clinical and pathologic observations. Proceedings Am Assoc Equine Pract 1985;415–428.
6. Duncan ID, Schneider RK, Hammang JP. Subclinical entrapment neuropathy of the equine suprascapular nerve. Acta Neuropathol 1987;74:53–61.
7. Dutton DM, Honnas CM, Watkins JP. Nonsurgical treatment of suprascapular nerve injury in horses: 8 cases (1988–1998). J Am Vet Med Assoc 1999;214:1657–1659.
8. Dyce K, Sack W, Wensing C. The forelimb of the horse. In Dyce S, Sack W, Wensing C, eds. Textbook of Veterinary Anatomy. WB Saunders, Philadelphia, 1987;542–575.
9. Dyson S. Shoulder lameness in horses: An analysis of 58 suspected cases. Equine Vet J 1986;18:29–36.

10. Hahn C, Mayhew IG, Mackay R. Diseases of the peripheral (spinal) nerves. In Equine Medicine and Surgery, 5th edition. Colahan P, Mayhew IG, Merritt A, et al., eds. Mosby, St. Louis, 1999.
11. Lee SK, Wolfe SW. Peripheral nerve injury and repair. J Am Acad Orthop Surg 2000;8:243–252.
12. Mackay R. Peripheral Nerve Injury. In Equine Surgery, 3rd ed. Auer JA, Stick J, eds. Saunders, Elsevier, St. Louis, 2006; 685–686.
13. Miller R, Dresher L. Treatment of Equine Shoulder Sweeny with intra-articular corticosteroids. Vet Med Small Animal Clinics 1977;72:1077–1079.
14. Schneider JE, Adams OR, Easley KJ, et al. Scapular notch resection for suprascapular nerve decompression in 12 horses. J Am Vet Med Assoc 1985;187:1019–1020.
15. Schneider R, Bramlage LR. Suprascapular nerve injury in horses. Compendium of Continuing Education for Veterinary Practitioners 1990;12:1783–1789.
16. Winberg F. Surgical treatment of suprascapular nerve entrapment—current techniques. 8th Annual ECVS Meeting, Brugge, Belgium, 1999;103–104.

FRACTURES OF THE SCAPULA

Fractures of the scapula are uncommon in horses. This is in part due to the scapula's proximal location, its close proximity to the ribs, and the large protective muscle mass overlying the region.[1] Although scapular fractures occur in all ages and breeds of horses, young (less than 4 years) intact males appear more prone to sustain the fracture.[1]

Fractures of the scapula can involve the spine, supraglenoid tubercle (SGT), body, neck, and glenoid cavity. Of these, fracture of the supraglenoid tubercle is most common. Although simple scapular fractures are most common, comminuted fractures also occur. Bone sequestra may also develop following fractures of the scapular spine, particularly in when a penetrating wound results in a comminuted fracture.[2,8] Stress fractures of the scapula have been recently described in Thoroughbred racehorses.[5] A high incidence of suprascapular nerve injury occurs following fractures of the neck of the scapula. Injury to the subscapularis nerve and brachial plexus is a rare complication associated with fractures of the scapula.

Etiology

Scapular fractures are usually caused by direct trauma or following falls during racing or jumping.[6,8] Scapular fractures resulting from race falls at high speeds tend to be comminuted.[6] Penetrating wounds to the lateral shoulder region can also cause fractures of the spine.[6,8]

Clinical Signs

Horses frequently present with a history of trauma and signs of lameness ranging from mild to nonweight-bearing.[1,2,7] Horses with an acute fracture of the scapular spine usually exhibit focal swelling, they will bear weight, and usually exhibit a mild to moderate lameness at exercise (Figure 5.286). Deep palpation over the fracture site usually elicits a painful response.

Evidence of penetrating wounds may be present. Chronic cases of scapular spine fractures may present with a draining tract or a history of the development of a recurrent draining tract as a result of a penetrating wound and sequestration of bone fragments.[2,8] Horses with fractures of the body or neck of the scapula are

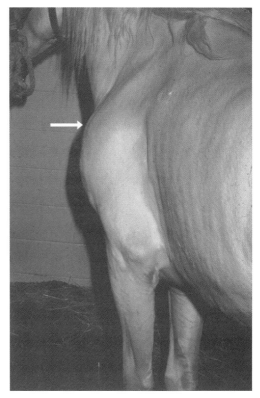

Figure 5.286. Prominent swelling (arrow) over the lateral shoulder region of a horse with a fracture of the body of the scapula.

usually reluctant to bear weight initially, have difficulty advancing the affected limb, and often have swelling over the fracture site. Deep palpation and limb manipulation usually elicits a painful response.[1,4] Fractures of the scapular neck may also result in secondary suprascapular nerve injury and signs of paresis in some cases. Chronic cases of more than 3 weeks' duration usually exhibit varying degrees of atrophy of the muscles in the shoulder region and proximal antebrachium.[7] As time passes swelling may become more apparent in the lateral shoulder region as a result of muscle atrophy, healing soft tissues, and callus formation. A swinging and support limb lameness is observed at a trot. Horses sustaining these fractures should also be assessed for other problems such as fractured ribs and intrathoracic trauma.[4]

Diagnosis

Radiographs of the region are needed for a definitive diagnosis. Medial to lateral, ventrodorsal, and oblique cranial to caudal radiographic projections reveal most fractures of the scapula (Figure 5.287). The study can be done while the horse is standing in most cases. Some fractures through the body of the scapula can be difficult to image because of the superimposition of the ribs and vertebrae over the scapula; in these cases the limb must be protracted to obtain a diagnostic film.[7] If a fracture is suspected but not observed, the horse should be confined to a stall and radiographed again 10 to 14 days after injury.[8] A scintigraphic exam can be

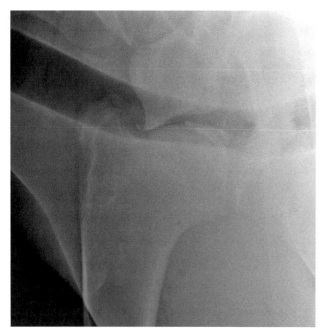

Figure 5.287. Comminuted articular fracture of the glenoid tuberosity and neck of the scapula.

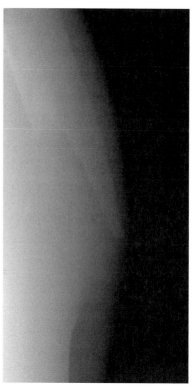

Figure 5.288. Skyline view of a scapula body fracture. The proximal fragment is displaced abaxially. (Courtesy of Dr. Ellis Farstvedt.)

performed prior to this to assist in the diagnosis. Some large, heavily muscled horses in severe pain may require general anesthesia to obtain diagnostic radiographs. Stress fractures of the scapula are diagnosed by nuclear scintigraphic exam and ultrasonography after lower limb analgesia has been performed to rule out a lower limb issue in racehorses that are acutely lame after racing.[5]

Suprascapular nerve injury can be difficult to detect by physical exam alone in the nonweight-bearing limb. Electromyography (EMG) can be helpful in assessing nerve damage at least 7 days after the injury has occurred.[4]

Treatment

Conservative Treatment

Fractures of the scapular spine generally do not require surgical intervention, and most heal by bone union. On the other hand, fractures following a penetrating wound may develop bone sequestra; in these cases surgery is recommended. Some minimally displaced nonarticular fractures of the scapular body and neck or stress fractures may also be treated conservatively with a good result.[3,5,7] Providing stall rest for several months, taping the shoulder to the body wall to prevent abduction of the limb, and slinging cooperative animals has been used successfully in some cases without articular involvement.[5,7,8]

Surgical Treatment

Transverse fractures of the body and proximal neck can be surgically treated with internal fixation in young animals.[4,9,11] Stabilization is achieved with 2 dynamic compression (DCP) bone plates applied cranial and caudal to the scapular spine in the angle formed by the spine and the body (Figures 5.288 and 5.289).[4,9,11] Longitudinal fractures have been repaired using several narrow DCP plates placed across the fracture line staggered along the scapula.[10]

Severely comminuted fractures or fractures of the distal neck and those extending into the glenoid are very difficult to treat surgically with internal fixation. The configuration of the fracture and its close proximity to the shoulder joint do not permit application of orthopedic implants. Euthanasia is recommended in horses with extensive joint involvement and/or severe joint instability.[3]

Prognosis

The prognosis is good for fractures involving the scapular spine with or without surgery for removal of a sequestrum, and most horses can return to performance after an adequate rest period. Young horses with nonarticular simple or minimally comminuted fractures of the body and proximal neck have a good prognosis for soundness after application of internal fixation. At the 1-year follow-up of 2 horses that underwent internal fixation complete healing and return to full function were noted.[4,9] A longitudinal fracture of the scapula in a young horse resulted in soundness at 6 months after internal fixation.[10] In adults, nondisplaced fractures of the body or neck may heal satisfactorily with conservative therapy.[7] Horses with complete fractures in the distal neck, articular fractures, and severely comminuted fractures all have a poor prognosis for return to performance.[3,8]

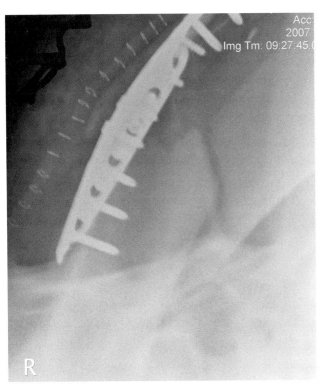

Figure 5.289. Same fracture as in Figure 5.288 after repair with two LCP plates. (Courtesy of Dr. Ellis Farstvedt.)

References

1. Adams S. Fractures of the scapula. In Equine Fracture Repair. Nixon AJ, ed. WB Saunders, Philadelphia, 1996;254–258.
2. Babinski J, Richter W. Fractures of the scapula in sporting horses. Monatshefte Veterinarmed 1990;45:93–94.
3. Bleyaert H. Shoulder injuries. In Current Techniques of Equine Surgery and Lameness. White N, Moore J, eds. WB Saunders and Co., Philadelphia, 1998;422–423.
4. Bukowiecki CF, van Fe RT, Schneiter HL. Internal fixation of comminuted transverse scapular fracture in a foal. J Am Vet Med Assoc 1989;195:781–783.
5. Davidson EJ, Martin BB Jr. Stress fracture of the scapula in two horses. Vet Radiol Ultrasound 2004;45:407–410.
6. Denny HR. Fractures of the scapula. In Treatment of Equine Fractures. Denny HR, ed. Wright, London, 1989;28–33.
7. Dyson S. Shoulder lameness in horses: An analysis of 58 suspected cases. Equine Vet J 1986;18:29–36.
8. Dyson S. Sixteen fractures of the shoulder region in the horse. Equine Vet J 1985;17:104–110.
9. Gobel DO, Brinker WO. Internal fixation of the equine scapula: a case report. Journal of Equine Medicine and Surgery 1977;1:341.
10. Kidd JA, Lamas L, Henson FM. Repair of a longitudinal scapular fracture in a horse. Vet Surg 2007;36:378–381.
11. Shamis LD, Sanders-Shamis M, Bramlage LR. Internal fixation of a transverse scapular neck fracture in a filly. J Am Vet Med Assoc 1989;195:1391–1392.

FRACTURES OF THE SUPRAGLENOID TUBERCLE (TUBEROSITY)

Fractures of the supraglenoid tubercle (SGT) can occur in a variety of breeds of horses and horses with a variety of uses.[2–4,8] They are relatively common, accounting for about 30% to 50% of reported scapula fractures.[5,7] Fractures of the SGT are often simple, intra-articular, and usually affect horses less than 2 years of age.[3,7,8] In contrast, one report on STG fractures in 9 horses found 4 with comminuted fractures and 6 of the 9 were in horses 3 years or older (range 3 to 13 years).[5]

Anatomically, the supraglenoid tubercle serves as the proximal attachment for the biceps brachii muscle and 2 glenohumeral ligaments which support the scapulohumeral joint. The coracoid process, which is the medial projection of the tubercle, serves as an attachment for the coracobrachialis muscle. The SGT and the coracoid process develop from a single center of ossification and fuse with the cranial portion of the glenoid cavity and the main body of the scapula at about 10 to 12 months of age.[6] Because the fracture plane often courses along this growth plate, it has been suggested that this fracture may result from a separation of the physis of the supraglenoid tubercle in young horses.[7]

Etiology

Fracture of the SGT is most frequently associated with trauma to the cranial shoulder region. Because of its superficial location, it appears that the SGT is most susceptible to injury. In 2 reports most horses with supraglenoid tubercle fracture had a history of falling or direct trauma to the shoulder.[5,8] Overflexion of the shoulder leading to increased tension on the biceps brachii and coracobrachialis tendons that attach to the SGT has also been proposed as a mechanism for this fracture.[1] Fracture of the SGT has occurred in several horses with suprascapular nerve paralysis following surgical removal of a piece of bone from the cranial border of the scapula.[2,3]

Clinical Signs

A history of trauma resulting in severe lameness that improves rapidly is common.[2,5,8] This rapid improvement may be the reason that this fracture is not initially diagnosed in some instances, and that recognition of the problem only occurs after the horse remains lame longer than expected or when muscle atrophy becomes prominent.[5,8]

In acute cases swelling is usually apparent over the point of the shoulder and palpation generally elicits a painful response. Crepitation may also be appreciated in some cases. At a walk, the horse typically retains the ability to extend the scapulohumeral joint but the cranial phase of the stride is markedly shortened. A lameness score of 3 to 4 out of 5 is typical in the acute phase. As time passes, swelling over the point of the shoulder diminishes and palpation may reveal a firm, non-painful swelling over the point of the shoulder.[5] Movement of the tubercle can be perceived in some cases. Varying degrees of muscle atrophy are usually apparent in chronic cases.[5] Some horses may also exhibit signs of suprascapular or radial nerve paralysis. Intra-articular anesthesia of the scapulohumeral joint may not improve the lameness.[5]

Diagnosis

Radiography is required to make a definitive diagnosis of the fracture (Figure 5.290). Generally, the fracture is simple or comminuted and intra-articular.[3,5,8] Calcification of the biceps tendon may also be associated with fracture of the SGT.[5] Electromyographic studies are sometimes needed to rule out neurogenic atrophy of the affected muscles.

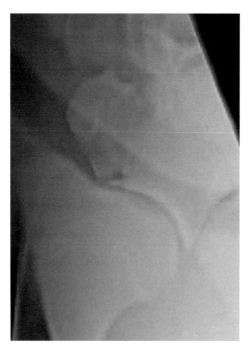

Figure 5.290.   Fracture of the supraglenoid tubercle of the scapula with moderate displacement.

Treatment

Several options can be considered for management of supraglenoid tubercle fractures. The selection of the management approach depends on the nature and duration of the fracture, economics, and the expectation of performance level.

Conservative management consisting of the administration of NSAIDs and prolonged stall rest for 3 to 4 months followed by pasture turn-out for 6 to 9 months may be selected in some cases. Horses with nonarticular or minimally displaced intra-articular fractures respond best to this approach and may be able to return to their intended use, depending upon the degree of OA that may develop.[2,5,8]

Surgical management of horses with SGT fractures consists of either surgical removal of the SGT fragment or internal fixation with or without transection of the biceps brachii tendon. The goal of surgery is to prevent the development of secondary OA caused by joint incongruity.

Removal of the fragment involves dissection of the tendinous attachments of the biceps brachii and coracobrachialis muscles of the SGT. Excising the fractured SGT decreases the pain created by fracture movement and prevents further joint damage that develops from impingement of the fragment on the articular surface of the humeral head.[9] Surgical excision of the SGT appears to be best suited for most chronic cases and for comminuted articular fractures.[8,9] In one report, 4 of 7 horses returned to performance, including 1 racing Thoroughbred that had a successful career at a reduced performance level.[3] Caudal luxation of the scapula can occur with excision of the fractured SGT.[3]

Several methods of internal fixation consisting of various combinations of interfragmentary compression with lag screws and tension band wires have been used.

Cancellous bone screws placed in lag fashion across the fracture gap was reported to be unsuccessful in 2 horses.[7] Internal fixation using Kirschner wires in combination with cerclage wire placed in a figure-8 pattern to stabilize the fracture fragment was used successfully in 1 case.[7] Stab incisions made through the tendon of the biceps brachii muscle to place bone screws in a lag fashion was also used successfully in 1 report.[4] Internal fixation has limited success, particularly in heavily muscled horses; the porous bone in the scapular neck does not hold screws adequately, fracture reduction is difficult, and fixation fails due to the tension exerted by the biceps brachii tendon.[1-3] Partial or complete transection of the biceps tendon has been advocated to eliminate the tension on the fracture fragment and prevent implant and bone failure.[1,3] Trauma and damage to the suprascapular nerve can occur due to the surgical procedures mentioned.

Prognosis

A good prognosis for return to performance can be expected for conservative management of horses that have nonarticular fractures or minimally displaced articular fractures of the SGT.[2] The prognosis for return to athletic soundness is poor for conservative management of horses that sustain simple or comminuted displaced articular fractures, but pasture soundness is possible in some.[3,5]

The prognosis following surgical excision of the fractured SGT is better than that achieved with conservative management for return to performance in horses with displaced simple or comminuted articular fractures and for chronic articular fractures.[2,5,8,9] In one report, 4 of 7 horses treated with surgical excision of the fractured tubercle returned to performance, including one racing Thoroughbred that had a successful career at a reduced performance level.[2]

Presently the prognosis for internal fixation appears best if a combination of internal fixation and complete transection of the biceps brachii tendon is used for simple acute fractures.[1,2,4] In one report, 3 of 3 horses treated by this method were sound for their intended use.[2]

References

1. Adams SB. Surgical repair of a supraglenoid tubercle fracture in a horse. J Am Vet Med Assoc 1987;191:332–334.
2. Bleyaert H, Sullins K, White N. Supraglenoid tubercle fractures in horses. Compendium of Continuing Education for the Veterinary Practitioner 1994;16:531–536.
3. Bleyaert HF, Madison JB. Complete biceps brachii tenotomy to facilitate internal fixation of supraglenoid tubercle fractures in three horses. Vet Surg 1999;28:48–53.
4. Dart AJ, Snyder JR. Repair of a supraglenoid tuberosity fracture in a horse. J Am Vet Med Assoc 1992;201:95–96.
5. Dyson S. Sixteen fractures of the shoulder region in the horse. Equine Vet J 1985;17:104–110.
6. Getty R. Sisson and Grossman's The Anatomy of Domestic Animals, 5th ed. WB Saunders, Philadelphia, 1975.
7. Leitch M. A review of the treatment of tuber scapulae fractures in the horse. Journal of Equine Medicine and Surgery 1977;1:234.
8. Pankowski R, Grant BD, Sande R, et al. Fracture of the supraglenoid tubercle: treatment and results in five horses. Veterinary Surgery 1986;15:33–39.
9. Wagner PC. Resection of the supraglenoid tubercle of the scapula in a colt. Compendium of Continuing Education for Veterinary Practitioners 1985;7:36–41.

The Tarsus and Tibia

Kenneth E. Sullins

THE TARSUS

The tarsus accounts for much of the hindlimb lameness in performance horses, which is often bilateral. Symmetric lameness often obscures the typical clinical signs, and unilateral local anesthesia typically causes the contralateral lameness to become more apparent. Performance horses, especially those that must work while collected, may exhibit secondary soft tissue back pain due to a functional spasm from the altered gait that results from hindlimb pain. It may even be necessary to rest the horse and treat the back pain before a lameness examination is possible. Excessively straight or "curby" conformation or angular deformity could make the tarsus the first rule-out in younger horses as well. Substantial pathology can exist in the distal tarsal joints in spite of an outwardly normal appearance. Conversely, significant lameness emanating from the distal tarsal joints can be present without radiographic abnormalities.

Tarsal lameness is usually exacerbated by hindlimb flexion (spavin test). Ideally, digital flexion and stifle flexion tests (see Chapter 3 and the accompanying DVD) are performed to ascertain that component of the pain, because all the joints of the hindlimb are flexed along with the tarsus. When performing the hindlimb flexion test, some clinicians prefer to hold the foot to prevent pressure on the fetlock, whereas others passively cradle the fetlock to prevent pressure on the metatarsal flexor structures and avoid excessive digital flexion (Figures 3.75 and 3.76 in Chapter 3). Consistency is the most important consideration. Lameness examination is covered more completely in Chapter 3.

Tarsometatarsal (TMT) or distal intertarsal (DIT) joint synovitis does not result in externally visible synovial effusion due to their tight soft tissue investment. Synovial effusion may be inferred by release of watery synovial fluid under pressure when a needle is placed for intra-articular anesthesia. However, the ensuing intra-articular anesthesia may not completely relieve the lameness, casting doubt on the clinical significance of the increased synovial fluid. The TMT and DIT joints should be anesthetized separately because they do not always communicate, and lameness may be emanating from only one of the joints.

The proximal intertarsal (PIT) joint is located within a common joint capsule with the tarsocrural (TC) joint; it is an uncommon singular cause of lameness. Proximal intertarsal joint inflammation should be reflected in TC effusion; persisting PIT synovitis places the more mobile TC joint at risk of OA. However, TC effusion doesn't always accompany PIT disease, so radiographic signs of PIT disease without TC effusion may require closer evaluation.

Most TC joint pathology produces synovial effusion (bog spavin). The "bog" may persist for years in successfully working horses that may or may not have radiographic signs of disease. Some such horses actually have no grossly apparent pathology and may or may not remain sound. Those that have mild but clinically significant disease that they have been working through eventually become lamer as the OA advances.

It is important to differentiate between TC synovial effusion and periarticular edema. Although the two may exist concurrently, they signal different situations. Congruity of the tibial tarsal bone with the distal tibia may allow weight-bearing despite substantial supporting soft tissue damage. Swelling and lameness excessive for their apparent anatomic explanations should be critically evaluated for collateral ligament integrity. Ultrasound and radiographs taken while stressing the medial and lateral collateral ligaments may be necessary.

A routine radiographic examination of the tarsus should include the dorsal plantar (DP), dorsolateral-plantaromedial oblique (DLPLMO), dorsomedial-plantarolateral oblique (DMPLLO), lateral medial (LM), and flexed lateral to medial (FLM) views. Some recommend 2 DP views. In one, the beam is centered on the tibial tarsal bone; in the other, the beam is centered on the central tarsal bone, permitting better evaluation at each level.[7] Depending upon history or clinical signs, flexed tangential or oblique flexed tangential views are required to demonstrate lesions on the caudal extremes of the trochlear ridges or margin of the tarsal canal.

Most of the tarsus is accessible by ultrasound, which is quite useful for imaging a variety of conditions.[9] The author has found ultrasound to be particularly useful for determining the character of increased synovial fluid and evaluating the collateral ligaments and flexor tendons. Lesions identified by MRI may sometimes be monitored by ultrasound as well.

Nuclear scintigraphy can be useful in some cases to confirm distal tarsal joint involvement, particularly in cases in which only partial relief of lameness followed intra-articular analgesia of the distal tarsal joints and there are no apparent radiographic changes.[3] The distribution of inflammation can be demonstrated,[6] which may bear prognostic value as well.

The normal structure of the equine tarsus as demonstrated by computed tomography (CT) has been reported.[8] Detail superior to radiographs facilitated diagnosis of a minimally-displaced comminuted central tarsal bone fracture[4] and clarified radiographically inapparent lesions demonstrated by scintigraphy.[3]

Magnetic resonance imaging (MRI) details the structure and physical status of the tissues; normal appearances of the equine tarsus have been reported.[1,5] A series of cadaveric tarsi from horses with histories of distal tarsal pain revealed variations in subchondral thickness compared to horses without histories of distal tarsal pain.[2] The strength of MRI is detection and

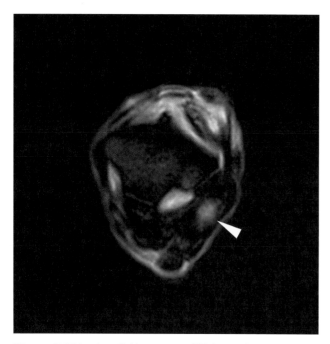

Figure 5.291. Low field transverse MR image that was taken in a standing horse with lameness isolated to the tarsus without radiographic changes. The arrow indicates fluid signal in the calcaneus, signifying active inflammation.

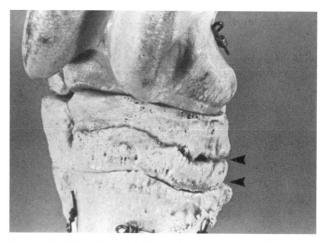

Figure 5.292. Right distal tarsal joints of a horse with bone spavin, dorsal view. The black arrows point to the medial aspects of the distal intertarsal and tarsometatarsal joints. The osteophytes and loss of joint definition occur more severely on the dorsomedial and dorsal aspects of the distal tarsal joints. (Courtesy of Dr. Ted Stashak.)

characterization of radiographically inapparent lesions that have been localized by diagnostic anesthesia (Figure 5.291).

References

1. Blaik MA, Hanson RR, Kincaid SA, et al. Low-field magnetic resonance imaging of the equine tarsus: Normal anatomy. Vet Rad Ultra 2000;41:131–141.
2. Branch MV, Murray RC, Dyson SJ, et al. Alteration of distal tarsal subchondral bone thickness pattern in horses with tarsal pain. Equine Vet J 2007;39:101–105.
3. Garcia-Lopez JM, Kirker-Head CA. Occult subchondral osseous cyst-like lesions of the equine tarsocrural joint. Vet Surg 2004;33:557–564.
4. Kelmer G, Wilson DA, Essman SC. Computed tomography assisted repair of a central tarsal bone slab fracture in a horse. Eq Vet Educ 2008;20:284–287.
5. Latorre R, Arencibia A, Gil F, et al. Correlation of magnetic resonance images with anatomic features of the equine tarsus. Am J Vet Res 2006;67:756–761.
6. Murray RC, Dyson SJ, Weekes JS, et al. Scintigraphic evaluation of the distal tarsal region in horses with distal tarsal pain. Vet Rad Ultra 2005;46:171–178.
7. O'Brien T. Radiographic interpretation of the equine tarsus. Proceedings Am Assoc Equine Pract 1973;19:289.
8. Tomlinson JE, Redding WR, Berry C, et al. Computed tomographic anatomy of the equine tarsus. Vet Rad Ultra 2003;44:174–178.
9. Whitcomb MB. Ultrasonography of the equine tarsus. Proceedings Am Assoc Equine Pract 2006;52:13–30.

DISTAL TARSAL JOINT SYNOVITIS AND OSTEOARTHRITIS (OA) (BONE SPAVIN)

Bone spavin (true spavin or jack spavin) is OA that involves the DIT, TMT, and occasionally the PIT joints (Figure 5.292). Distal tarsal OA more accurately describes the condition and is considered to be the most common cause of tarsal lameness.[1,22,25,30,33,50–52,54,62,64,84] Only 7.2% of a series of 3,566 horses failed to possess distal tarsal radiographic indicators of OA.[86] However, these radiographic signs did not correlate to lameness or athletic ability, a fact that may confound prepurchase examinations. Of 119 horses undergoing scintigraphy for lameness, 44% demonstrated distal tarsal activity.[61] Half of 52 horses diagnosed with distal tarsal OA as the primary problem demonstrated uptake bilaterally. An additional 21% had distal tarsal uptake considered additional to the primary lameness.

Occult spavin (blind spavin or jack spavin) has the same clinical features of OA but lacks radiographic evidence, although scintigraphic evidence of distal tarsal inflammation may be present.[61] Occult or blind spavin and distal tarsal OA should be considered as different stages of the same disease process in which synovitis results from radiographically inapparent cartilage lesions which may be found at necropsy.[1,68] Support for this is provided by observation of increasing radiographic signs correlating with the degree of physical deformity and lameness.[7] Additionally, desmitis of the intratarsal ligaments can produce lameness.[1] However, in spite of persistent lameness, some horses fail to develop the radiographic signs of OA.[1,30] Horses diagnosed with blind/occult spavin may recover completely once treated appropriately.

Distal tarsal disease is observed most frequently in mature horses that are ridden at a gallop and canter, including horses that jump and Western horses used for reining, roping, and cutting.[1,30] Of 112 racing Standardbreds that had scintigraphy for hindlimb lameness, 33% demonstrated distal tarsal inflammation.[26] True distal tarsal OA is uncommon in harness horses but occasionally is observed in the aged trotter.[30] Icelandic horses may have a predisposition for the disease. In a series of 379 horses, 12% were lame in the hindlimb and 25% were lame after hindlimb flexion.[7] Radiographically evident OA was present in 23% of the horses, but only half of those horses were lame. Restated, twice as many horses than were lame had radiographic changes. No diagnostic anesthesia was reported. A survey of 774 Warmbloods less than 5 years of age revealed 50 (6.5%) affected individuals.[36]

Etiology

Repeated compression and rotation of the tarsal bones and excessive tension on the attachment of the major dorsal ligaments are thought to be prominent in the development of this disease.[72,73] Rooney suggested that shear forces due to asynchronous movement of the tarsal bones predisposes the animal to distal tarsal OA.[69] He further suggests a difference in pathophysiology between DIT and TMT disease. Horses working routinely with the hocks in a flexed position (i.e., jumpers and pulling horses) are proposed to develop DIT arthrosis, whereas horses working in a more straight-legged position (i.e., Thoroughbreds or horses short-strided due to lameness) are proposed to be prone to TMT disease. Forelimb lameness may result in the horse carrying more weight on its hindlimbs.[30]

A review of distal tarsal OA in horses that jump made no distinction between DIT and TMT disease.[58] A study in Icelandic horses reports environmental factors such as type and severity of work do not affect the incidence, whereas tarsal angle and age were more important. Incidence was also related to certain sires.[6]

Conditions that disrupt the most fluid motion possible for a horse can cause shear and rotation within the limb. Of 42 racing Thoroughbreds diagnosed with tarsal OA, 85% wore shoes with elevations of the lateral or both heels, and hoof balance and flat shoes were a component of the treatment in 27 that improved noticeably. Many of the horses in the study were affected with more than spavin.[58]

Sickle and cow-hocked conformation predisposes a horse to OA.[28,69] These conformations produce greater stress in the medial aspect of the hock joint. These two often-coexisting conformations, and perhaps others, make predisposition to distal tarsal OA heritable. Horses with narrow, thin hocks are more prone to the disease than those with full, well-developed hocks. However, many affected horses have none of these conformational defects. The author agrees with Moyer and others in that the local stresses from the type and difficulty of the work play an equal or overriding role in the pathogenesis of OA.[57,85] Additionally, specific injury affecting the distal tarsal joints unrelated to type of work or conformation must be considered. Unilaterally affected horses in particular may fall into this category. Once acquired, treatment and outcome of injured horses may not differ from those affected from any other cause. However, such horses that have not sustained articular cartilage damage tend to recover well because their work routine may not continue to aggravate the situation.

Clinical Signs

There is usually a history of gradual onset of lameness. However, bilateral lameness may have been progressing for some time before a problem is noticed. The lameness usually worsens if the horse is worked hard for several days, and may improve with rest. Hunters may begin to jump poorly or refuse to jump at all.[57] Reining horses begin to pivot and stop poorly. In some cases horses refuse to pivot to the affected side and exhibit their objection by laying their ears back or beginning to buck. While horses that must stop quickly often cheat by placing the greatest amount of weight on the least affected limb, this often results in a jerky slide stop because of reluctance to firmly plant their feet. The horse may feel stiff or jerky when circled to the affected side, and it may refuse to go on the opposite lead.[57]

Lameness tends to be worse when the horse is first used; horses with mild spavin tend to warm out of the lameness after working a short time. However, in severe cases, exercise may aggravate the lameness. Racing Thoroughbreds frequently present slightly younger (3-year-olds) than other breeds and with multiple problems that are probably related to the stresses of the speed at which they work. Most of a series of 89 horses eventually diagnosed with distal tarsal OA presented with a primary complaint other than hindlimb lameness.[58] Associated findings included front fetlock and carpal disease, back pain, and front foot pain. It could be argued that the high incidence of forelimb problems occurred secondarily to hindlimb pain. Only 20% of the horses with distal tarsal OA were unaffected with other sources of lameness.

Standardbreds frequently carry their hindquarters to the opposite side of the jog cart from the lame limb, preferring to hold the head to the side of lameness. Lameness diagnosis in a Standardbred racehorse in hand can be challenging and it may be necessary to observe the horse in harness.[29]

Distal tarsal OA often causes an enlargement of variable size on the medial aspect of the hock (Figures 5.293 and 3.49). This enlargement sometimes can be difficult to detect visually, especially if bilateral spavin is present or if a horse normally has large, boxy hocks. When standing, the horse may flex the hock periodically in a spasmodic manner. A mild to moderate hindlimb lameness is usually observed, which worsens following hindlimb flexion (spavin test) (Figures 3.75 and 3.76). The horse is often unwilling to flex the hock in its normal gait, causing a reduction in the height of the foot flight arc and a shortening of the cranial phase of the stride. The foot lands on the toe and, over time, the toe becomes too short and the heel too high. Because of the lower arc of the foot flight, some horses may drag the toe, causing it to wear on its dorsal edge. Possibly due to dorsomedial pathology associated with the distal tarsal joints, some horses swing the foot axially and land on the lateral hoof wall in a "tightrope" fashion, which tends to reduce dorsomedial compression of the limb.

It is advisable to conduct the flexion test on both hindlimbs for comparison or for diagnosis of bilateral OA. The author prefers to flex the least affected hindlimb first, because the more severely affected limb may retain the inflicted lameness, complicating further exam. The disease is often bilateral, and flexing the unaffected limb may be quite positive or it may cause the hindlimb gait to even out because the pain is distributed more evenly behind.

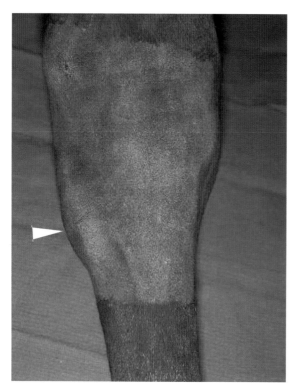

Figure 5.293. Tarsus of a horse with bone spavin; the area is being prepared for surgery. The arrow indicates thickening on the dorsomedial aspect of the tarsus, which is caused by osteophyte and fibrous tissue production. The radiographic changes may or may not be as large as the external growth.

Diagnosis

Horses that have swelling due to periarticular changes from OA are likely to be clinically affected unless the joints have ankylosed; however, reliance on external appearance and response to flexion test alone is ill advised. The hindlimb lameness, positive flexion tests, reduced arc of the foot flight, reduced flexion of the hock, and wearing of the toe are used in diagnosis. Infusion of the distal tarsal joints with local anesthetics is the most helpful procedure for localizing the source of the lameness. It may be expedient to evaluate the hocks first in horses displaying bilateral hindlimb lameness and predisposed to distal tarsal lameness by their breed and line of work. Intra-articular anesthesia of the distal tarsal joints will not obscure the remainder of the lameness examination if it proves to have no effect.

Communication between a substantial percentage of the TMT and DIT joints has been demonstrated.[31,47,70] However, that is unknown in the individual being examined at the time. Because treatment of distal tarsal inflammation may be required for a protracted period of time, it is desirable to know exactly which joints are causing pain. If there is doubt that both distal tarsal joints are involved, separate intra-articular anesthesia facilitates design of a long-term treatment plan. Although diffusion of local anesthetic occurs between the tarsal joints,[35] medication of joints demonstrated to be causing pain by this method should demonstrate what is necessary to alleviate the lameness.

Injection of the TMT and DIT joints is described in Chapter 3 and the accompanying DVD. Each joint typically holds 4 to 6 mL before resistance is encountered and the horse begins to object. Severely degenerative joints are difficult to enter with the needle and diffusion of the anesthetic may be impaired due to obliteration of the joint spaces, which may cause the response to intra-articular anesthesia to be incomplete. Observing the horse again after 30 to 45 minutes may demonstrate a more positive response to the block. Cunean bursal anesthesia may result in partial improvement, but more significant improvement usually follows intrasynovial anesthesia of the distal tarsal joints.[29] In the absence of other findings, the final diagnosis may have to be postponed pending response to therapy.

Blocking of the caudal tibial and deep peroneal nerves is a reasonably accurate diagnostic method. However, other structures in addition to the distal tarsal joints are blocked, and the effect of this block may not be complete. Further, confirmation of complete analgesia is difficult, and desensitization of such a large portion of the limb occasionally alters the horse's movement. The author prefers to jog (or at least stop) horses with tibial and peroneal analgesia on grass for surer footing. If the blocks in and above the tarsal region follow a complete step-wise distal to proximal blocking session, it is advisable to perform the high metatarsal block using a long-acting local anesthetic such as bupivacaine. Pain or dysesthesia from blocks wearing off and pain from those injections renders the lameness exam worthless.

In practice, a substantial number of horses that aren't (and some that are) performing as expected have their distal tarsal joints medicated without specific localization of a problem. On the one hand, there are so many cases of lameness due to distal tarsal synovitis that medication may have an expedient diagnostic value. However, horses with recurrent hindlimb lameness should have definitive diagnoses made before permanent medication plans are made.

To evaluate the distal tarsal joints, the X-ray beam must be centered on the distal tarsal joint spaces. Early radiographic changes may include marginal bone lysis or cyst formation in the adjacent subchondral bone (Figure 5.294). As the lesion progresses, irregular subchondral bone atrophy may cause the joint spaces to appear widened. Some believe that horses with cystic lucency in their radiographs are lamer (Figure 5.295B). As the cartilage degenerates, the joint spaces narrow and marginal osteophytes and subchondral sclerosis develop (Figure 5.295A). After several months, complete ankylosis may occur. In others, even after prolonged periods of time, only minimal degenerative change is observed.[25] If ankylosis occurs, the lameness may be abolished. Some horses with few radiographic signs are problematic in that degeneration never progresses, and they remain lame.

Radiographic evidence of OA usually begins on the dorsomedial surfaces of the TMT and DIT joints, but destructive changes often eventually involve the dorsal surface of these joints. However, in one study Warmbloods less than 5 years old were most frequently affected dorsolaterally on the DIT joint.[36] Subchondral bone thickness may follow a similar progression of

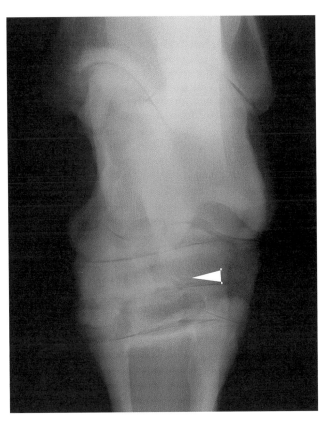

Figure 5.294. Dorsoplantar radiograph of the tarsus of a horse with DIT joint OA (bone spavin). The arrow indicates DIT joint narrowing and in the center of the joint closer to the arrow there is subchondral lysis surrounded by sclerosis.

change.[14] The PIT joint is less commonly affected, but radiographic changes may be reflected more often medially. The most severely lame 25% of a series of 60 cases in Icelandic horses with distal tarsal OA had PIT joint disease.[79]

Few adult performance horses have normal tarsal radiographs, and horses with significant radiographic changes may not be lame (Figure 5.296).[7,16,63] Conversely, significant lameness can emanate from radiographically normal hocks.[16] A series of 4,186 Warmblood and Standardbred horses revealed sufficient radiographic changes in sound horses to cause the authors to rely heavily on the clinical signs.[42] There was no association between duration and degree of lameness, response to IA anesthesia, and radiographic findings in a series of 91 horses confirmed to have pain associated with the distal tarsal joints.[16] However, horses with less severe radiographic changes generally responded better to treatment.

Scintigraphy generally accurately detects distal tarsal inflammation (Figure 5.297)[82] and is quite useful when the diagnosis is complicated by multiple problems or difficulty blocking the joints. Scintigraphic patterns in sound horses reflected activity in the dorsal and lateral aspects of the distal tarsus.[59] Of 99 horses that had scintigraphic examinations for hindlimb lameness, 85 demonstrated distal tarsal uptake.[27] Horses with diffuse radiopharmaceutical uptake tended to respond to treatment better than those with focal uptake;[49] diffuse uptake possibly indicates more generalized inflammation from use as compared to focal articular degeneration demonstrated by focal peaks of uptake.[60] Substantiation of the diagnosis with intra-articular anesthesia and critical evaluation of the response to therapy are the most reliable diagnostic criteria.

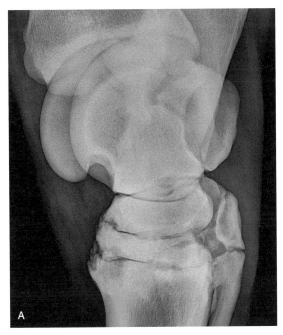

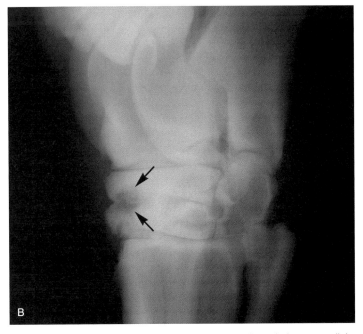

Figure 5.295. A. Dorsomedial to plantarolateral oblique radiograph of a horse with severe OA of the TMT and DIT joints where the horse is most likely lame. These joints do not appear to be progressing toward ankylosis. B. Dorsolateral-plantaromedial oblique radiograph of a horse with subchondral bone lysis (arrows) of the DIT joint that is causing significant lameness.

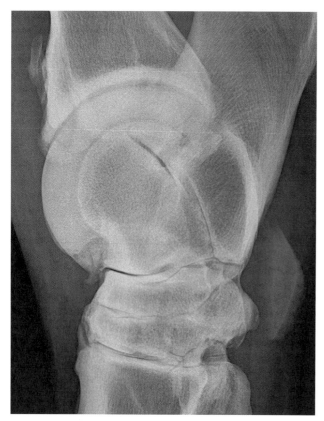

Figure 5.296. Lateromedial radiograph of a tarsus with a large osteophyte on the dorsal aspect of proximal MTIII; the changes involve the TMT and DIT joints. These changes may or may not cause lameness.

Treatment

The goal of the initial treatment often is affected by the radiographic signs but may change depending upon degree and duration of response to that treatment. Horses with minimal to no distal tarsal radiographic changes may respond favorably to a short period of reduced activity, corrective shoeing, and intra-articular medication (see below), and the lameness may subside permanently. If the history indicates that a specific injury may have occurred, more rest for soft tissue healing is warranted. Some horses without radiographic changes have cartilage lesions that cause synovitis to return and the lameness to persist.

Hoof management is aimed toward reducing the rotation/shear forces by easing break-over. The author's preference is to balance the foot and achieve a dorsal hoof angle 1° to 2° steeper than the pastern and square or roll the toe. As much foot as possible should be removed in the process to improve stability. Particularly in show horses, wide-webbed wedged (flat) aluminum shoes help achieve the angle and support the foot that may tend to land unevenly. Some prefer to place a lateral extension on the shoe to minimize the axial swing of the foot.[34,57] Others believe that the presence of anything that alters the landing of the foot increases shear forces; this may be more significant in race horses.[31,58]

Once degenerative changes have begun, the goal of treatment becomes pain management until the distal joints ankylose, if possible. In this case, extended rest

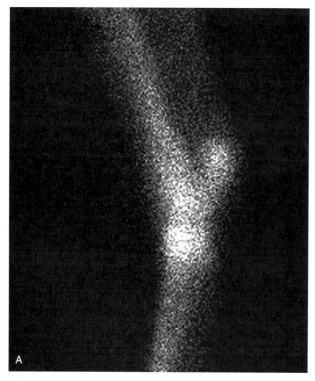
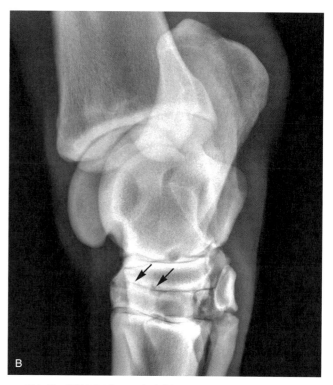

Figure 5.297. Lateral scintigram (A) and radiograph (B) of the tarsus of a horse with distal tarsal OA. There is diffuse uptake within the distal tarsal joints and joint space narrowing and lysis within the DIT joint (arrows) visible on the radiograph. (Courtesy of Dr. Jeremy Hubert.)

beyond a limited period to allow medication to take effect is useless. Further, exercise may facilitate the degeneration to lead to subsequent ankylosis, but most cases will not ankylose spontaneously. For horses with multiple problems possibly caused or aggravated by tarsal pain, more rest may be indicated.[58] If the PIT joint is involved, control of synovitis is critical to preserving TC joint integrity. In spite of numerous types of therapy for treatment of distal tarsal OA, some affected horses remain lame.

Anti-inflammatory therapy is required to resolve or control the pain resulting in lameness. Some horses with distal tarsal pain confirmed by intra-articular anesthesia without radiographic changes can be cured with short-acting intra-articular medication, often consisting of triamcinolone (4 mg/joint) and sodium hyaluronate (HA), and corrective shoeing. Corrective shoeing can be surprisingly effective for many horses once the acute inflammation is relieved.

Some cases appear at the beginning of the chronic problem and can be among the most difficult to treat. Ankylosis occurs faster without the influence of intra-articular corticosteroids; although cartilage degeneration is hastened, healing is impaired. Generally, the best plan is to do the minimum required to keep the horse effectively in work, because more treatment will probably be required eventually. A starting point includes systemic phenylbutazone (2.2 mg/kg, BID), which can be continued for an extended period of time in most horses or given only when the horse is worked. Supporting systemic therapies that may reduce the need for IA medication include intramuscular polysulfated glycosaminoglycans, IV HA, or oral nutraceuticals with a combination of chondroitin sulfate and glucosamine.[18,41,66] Each horse is different and requires discovery of an effective treatment schedule.

Intra-articular corticosteroids are often required to return the horse to work. Many prefer methylprednisolone acetate (80 mg/joint). The duration of effect varies with the individual. Continuing systemic therapy is important because it maximizes the effect and reduces the required frequency of intra-articular therapy. When the horse responds poorly to initial treatment with intra-articular steroids, a second injection 3 to 4 weeks later is often more effective. Using triamcinolone (6 mg/joint) for the first injection and scheduling a second injection with a repositol product makes sense in horses for which long-term pain control is needed; combining the two in a single injection is another approach. The addition of HA may prolong the duration of effect but adds significant cost for multiple IA treatments; systemic treatment often makes more sense.

A period of reduced (but continued) activity after medication usually improves the result; an exception is a fit horse in work with a history of response to a specific therapy. This rest could be interpreted to allow the medication to reduce the inflammation or facilitate conditioning of the supporting soft tissue structures.[31] The rest period has subjectively varied from 5 to 14 days in show horses, or until the lameness improves. Longer periods of up to a month were reported to be effective in racing Thoroughbreds.[58] In that report of 89 horses, the combination of reduced training schedule, corrective shoeing, and local and systemic anti-inflammatory

drugs was more effective than any of the measures alone.

Tiludronate inhibits osteoclast activity and has been used in horses with distal tarsal pain. In a limited double-blind clinical trial of 8 horses with lameness confirmed to originate in the distal tarsal joints given 1 or 2 single IV doses, 1 horse improved.[23] Anecdotally, tiludronate has been used when conventional IA medications begin to lose effect to lengthen the treatment interval with 60% to 70% improvement.[3]

Failing the above conservative measures, a more aggressive approach is required. The goal has been ankylosis/arthrodesis of the distal tarsal joints with the thought that elimination of the motion would eliminate the synovitis and lameness. Synovitis is the logical source of lameness because distal tarsal IA anesthesia usually eliminates the lameness. Aside from cunean tenectomy, the first surgical procedures were aimed at arthrodesis of the joints by removing most or part of the articular cartilage and superficial subchondral bone. Although not technically difficult, arthrodesis and eventual soundness were inconsistent enough to look for other methods. Because horses can become sound without radiographic ankylosis of the joints, and other horses with apparent ankylosis remain lame, the role of physical fusion of the joints is a question.

Cunean Tenectomy

Horses that fail to respond to nonsurgical measures require further intervention. Cunean tenectomy is technically simple and can be performed with the horse standing. Documented results are few, but one series contained positive reports from horse owners.[24] Some perform the procedure only in horses in which the lameness has improved following local anesthesia of the cunean bursa.[31] Even so, anesthetic infiltration of the cunean bursa is likely to anesthetize the adjacent joint capsules and communication between the bursa and the DIT joint may exist. The effectiveness of this procedure appears to depend on the early return to exercise before the scar tissue replacement becomes restrictive. Calling the procedure into question is a report describing similar results between 2 groups of racing Thoroughbreds. One group was treated with cunean tenectomy in addition to other medical therapy and shoeing changes, and the other group had the same measures without surgery.[58] No significant difference in racing performance was observed between a group of Standardbreds of which 27 were operated and 43 were not.[32] Other treatments such as firing and Wamberg's operation have little to recommend them.[30]

Although cunean tenectomy is easily performed with the horse standing, general anesthesia may be necessary for some horses. Local anesthetic is injected over the tendon after which a 3- 4-cm incision is made over the center of the longitudinal axis of the cunean tendon where it crosses the medial aspect of the hock (Figure 5.298). A 3- 4-cm section of the tendon is removed. Pressure bandaging and stall rest improves the cosmetic result. Bohanon described a stepwise return to activity beginning when the skin has healed, consisting of hand walking then riding over poles and progressing to complete return to work after 6 weeks, which is thought to

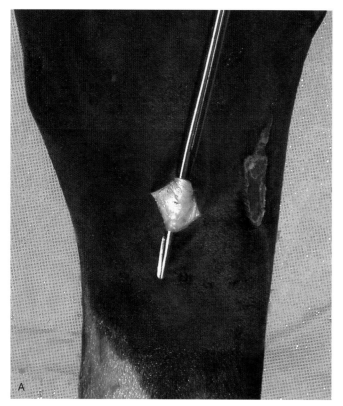 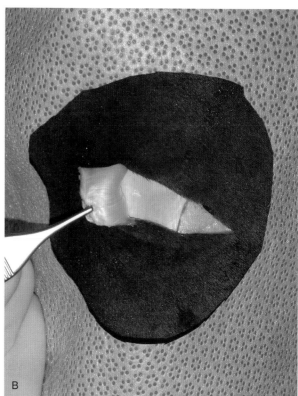

Figure 5.298. Cunean tenectomy can be performed on the medial aspect of the tarsus in the standing horse by isolating the tendon (A) and transecting a small segment (B).

prevent adhesion of the tendon ends to the bursal surface.[12]

A histologic and histochemical study of bursal and tendinous tissues from horses affected with distal tarsal OA revealed that the cunean tendons were markedly unaffected. However, the bursal tissues were inflamed and active as evidenced by granulation response and fibrous tissue production.[10] Apparently the tissue adjacent to the active distal tarsal synovitis is affected, but the tendon is not. These results contrasted findings from a similar study in horses unaffected with distal tarsal OA.[15]

Drilling of the Tarsometatarsal and Distal Intertarsal Joints

A technique of surgical destruction of the joint surfaces was developed by Adams which consisted of destruction of 60% or more of the articular cartilage of the DIT and TMT joints.[1] The degree and duration of postoperative pain rendered the technique impractical. Further evaluation of the technique by Barber again resulted in unacceptable postoperative morbidity and complications.[8] The drilling in these procedures was done in a fan shaped, router fashion that removed substantial amounts of subchondral bone leaving a space that resulted in instability due to loss of joint congruity.

Internal fixation was successful following aggressive articular debridement in a unilaterally affected breeding stallion.[50] The horse recovered from barely weight-bearing to walking well. Although presently not advisable or necessary, this result illustrates the value of stabilization in the face of overly aggressive articular drilling.

More recently, techniques creating single distinct drill paths have proven to cause minimal postoperative morbidity with generally good outcomes.[25,38,55] These techniques include 3 to 4 drill paths with no fanning. It appears that the morbidity is reduced if buttresses between drill paths are left to maintain the structural integrity of the joints. Drill size varies from 2.7 to 4.5 mm with similar results. A 3.2-mm drill bit compromises nicely between sufficient rigidity to drill without breaking while having just enough flexibility to follow the joint space without bypassing islands of cartilage, and 3 drill paths seem to suffice (Figure 5.299).

The success of the procedure depends upon creating solid spot welds of bony bridging to immobilize the joints. Most consider it only a matter of time until both the TMT and DIT joints are involved and treat both regardless of diagnostic indications of the source of pain. Ideally, the drill stays within the joint space. While minor distal penetrations do not affect the outcome, damage to the margins of the joints may cause exostoses, enlargement, and potential gait compromise.[8] Some enlargement at the surgical site may occur, but the procedure should not affect the horse's movement (Figure 5.299C).

The horse is stall rested until the skin sutures are removed and hand walking is allowed for an additional 2 weeks, when light riding is begun; some cases have

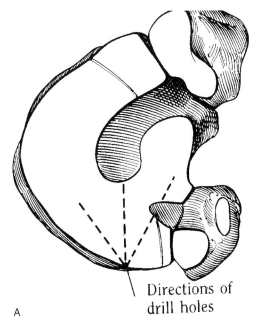

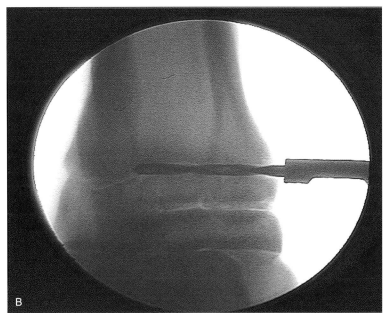

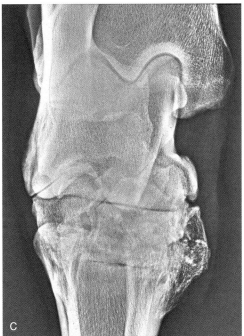

Figure 5.299. DIT joint surface of the central tarsal bone illustrating the 3-drill path technique for distal tarsal arthrodesis. (Courtesy of J.D. Sullins.) The drill is inserted through a single hole, passed in 3 different directions, and can be monitored with radiography or fluoroscopy. (Image is with horse in dorsal recumbency.) (B). A significant amount of joint surface is undisturbed which preserves stability but promotes arthrodesis of the distal 2 tarsal joints (C). (Courtesy of Dr. Gary Baxter.)

shown more rapid improvement. Exercise seems to be important in production of the desired fusion. Some horses require 1 year or longer for recovery and complete ankylosis of the involved joints, but most recover in 4 to 5 months. Systemic analgesia should be administered if required to keep the horse active.

In one report on 20 cases of distal tarsal OA in which arthrodesis of the DIT and TMT joints was performed using the 3-drill-passage technique, 17 of the cases became sound between 3.5 and 10 months after surgery.[25] In another report, 17 of 22 cases had success-

ful outcomes using the procedure.[38,55] In a series of 29 horses with follow-up, 66% returned to performance. Another 14% improved but did not regain their original status. The remaining 20.7% did not improve their status.[19] Subchondral bone lysis (indicating activity) tended to be associated with a better outcome, and joint narrowing was a detractor. Stanger reported success in 26 of 32 horses between 6 and 9 months after surgery; interestingly, only one-third of those had negative hindlimb flexion tests in the same time period. Smaller horses tended to recover faster. Barneveld reported success in 36 of 45 horses using the 3-drill path technique.[9,81]

If the PIT joint is involved, the prognosis is less favorable,[87] but it too should be operated, because this offers the best hope of a complete recovery. Local and systemic anti-inflammatory therapy to protect the TC joint is logical.

Wyn-Jones and May reported a series of 30 horses treated for TMT/DIT or TMT/DIT/PIT disease. A variety of surgical methods, including some with internal fixation, were used. Horses with disease confined to the TMT and DIT joints did better in that drilling alone was more successful in a shorter period of time (78% recovery in 3 to 6 months) when compared to horses that also had PIT disease (55% recovery in 8 months). Lag screws placed obliquely across the affected joint spaces or bone plates were applied in some horses. Recovery was not hastened by using internal fixation in horses with TMT and DIT disease, but the rate of success was slightly improved. The reduced success in horses with PIT disease was not improved by using implants. Postoperative exercise described was similar to that of other reports. Because internal fixation was applied to stabilize the joint spaces for fusion, the question arises whether more rest after surgery instead of the typical return to activity after drilling alone would improve the results. Particularly in horses affected with PIT disease that were treated with internal fixation, it may have been beneficial to restrict exercise to allow the drill paths to heal without stimulating further OA. When bone plates are applied, 5.5-mm screws are recommended, because there is a risk of implant failure with smaller screws in adult horses.[5] In addition to drilling, cancellous bone grafting and compression of the joint spaces using a tension device is suggested. The success rate using this approach is approximately 80% within 6 to 12 months.[5]

Another method of surgical arthrodesis that has been attempted is implanting stainless steel Bagby baskets into large drill holes between the joints.[4,75] Archer, et al. reported that horses became sound after 9 months, but 1 horse that fractured a third tarsal bone remained lame.[4] This technique has not become widely used.

Elevated intramedullary bone pressure has been proposed as a source of lameness in horses with OA; pressure in horses with diseased tarsi approximated 50% more than that from normal horses.[48] A modified drilling procedure coursing obliquely distad to proximad through MT3, DIT, and TMT joints terminating within the central tarsal bone has been described.[80] Diagnostic local anesthesia was not described. Twenty-five of 40 horses regained full working capacity, 13 were considered unsuccessful, and 2 were lost to follow-up. A later series reported 28 of 56 successful cases.[45] Although it is not possible to separate the effect of medullary decompression from immobilization due to bone healing across the drill sites, this technique appears to be approximately as effective as other techniques described.

Chemically Induced Arthrodesis

Intra-articular sodium monoiodioacetate (MIA) or ethanol have been used to induce cartilage necrosis,

presumably leading to ankylosis of the DIT and TMT joints.[13,17,78] Although ankylosis may occur, improvement in the lameness may occur without it. The use of MIA has not been approved by the US Food and Drug Administration (FDA). For legal purchase and clinical use in the US, an Investigational New Animal Drug number must be issued by the FDA for each specified treatment. Sodium monoiodioacetate induces chondrocyte necrosis so that normal use eventually causes the cartilage to break down and allow bone to contact bone.[13]

Soundness in horses 12 months after MIA injection of the distal tarsal joints has been reported in several studies (27 of 29 horses,[11] 2 of 5 horses that had only the TMT joint treated,[71] and 41 of 50 horses[21]). The results seem to be somewhat dose-related, and reported doses include 100 mg/joint,[11] 150 mg/TMT joint once,[71] and mean dosages of 144 mg/PIT and 238 mg/TMT joints,[21] respectively. In the latter series, horses with poorer outcomes received mean doses per joint of 250 mg,[21] whereas a maximum of approximately 80 mg produced a less profound effect in carpi.[39] Another series reported that 5 of 23 examined horses were sound after 12 months, but the dose was not stated.[76]

Postoperative exercise seems to be another important variable. Horses that are returned to activity sooner after treatment seem to become more consistently sound and they more consistently demonstrate radiographic ankylosis of the joints. This is not surprising because MIA is an accelerant of sorts in the natural degradation of chondrocytes in an inflamed joint.[13,21] However, not all horses with complete ankylosis were sound. Notably, in one study, 2 of 6 normal horses treated with MIA remained lame after 6 months.[88]

Horses should be hospitalized for the procedure and should be pretreated with phenylbutazone. In the author's opinion, prophylactic broad-spectrum antimicrobial therapy is advisable. Many perform the procedure on standing horses, but if the horse is at all recalcitrant, general anesthesia should be considered. Inflammation following injection may cause severe lameness for approximately 24 hours, and tibial and peroneal nerve blocks or epidural analgesia may be considered during that period.

Contrast arthrograms must be performed to confirm location of the needle and to rule out communication of the TMT or DIT joint with the PIT/TC joint or the tarsal canal. The contrast study of the TMT joints was omitted in one case series without incident.[21] In that series of 104 horses, DIT-PIT communication was identified in 12 horses, and none of the DIT joints communicated with the TMT joints or the tarsal canal.

If the arthrogram reveals contrast in the PIT/TC joints or tarsal canal or failure to fill the intended joint, the procedure is aborted. Leakage of MIA into the subcutaneous space also produces noticeable inflammation that may lead to a tissue slough. Injection under pressure increases the possibility of leakage. Pain in the immediate post-injection period can be profound but varies among reports. The series reporting the least postoperative pain used 23-gauge needles, aspirated all possible fluid from the joints following the contrast study, and stopped injecting whenever resistance was met.[21]

Complications that have been observed include soft tissue necrosis at the injection site, septic arthritis, unexplained increased lameness, and delayed PIT/TC joint OA. This potential for serious complications must be weighed against the appeal of the simplicity and minimal cost of the procedure. The author believes there are safer ways to approach the problem.

The effect of IA ethanol (70% and 90%) on normal TMT joints has been reported,[78] as has its use in horses clinically affected with distal tarsal OA.[17] Ethanol solubilizes lipids and induces nonspecific protein denaturation, cellular dehydration, and precipitation of protoplasm.[65] As such, it affects chondrocytes in a similar manner as MIA. Ethanol has neurolytic properties that could contribute to its reported early resolution of lameness.[17] In normal horses, no significant postinjection local reaction occurred and no persisting lameness was induced. After 12 months, the TMT joints were largely ankylosed and the horses were not lame. Eleven horses with confirmed distal tarsal OA were treated with 3 mL of 70% ethanol. There were no significant local reactions and all horses demonstrated reduction in lameness. None of the joints appeared completely radiographically ankylosed.[17]

Lavage of fresh cadaveric MCP/MTP joints for 10 minutes with sterile saline heated to 80° C was shown to induce widespread chondrocyte death compared to sham treated joints.[46] Presumably the *in vivo* effect on a joint would be similar to that of MIA or ethanol. Although not reported, capsular neurolysis could also occur. Horses would likely require protective cooling of the periarticular soft tissue.

Treating horses with active distal tarsal OA with any fluid will never be the same as treating normal experimental horses. Affected joints are often difficult to access and uniform distribution of any injected substance is unlikely. This may contribute to the reduced radiographically evident ankylosis in clinical cases compared to research horses.

Laser Treatment of the Distal Tarsal Joints

Laser energy (Nd : YAG or 980-nm gallium-aluminum-arsenide diode laser) applied to the TMT and DIT joints has been reported to relieve distal tarsal pain.[40] All horses in a series of 24 Standardbreds and Western performance horses improved.[40] Stall confinement was enforced for 2 days followed by progressive return to full activity in approximately 2 weeks. The horses were reported to become sound before fusion could have occurred.

The term arthrodesis is not used here because radiographic or physical arthrodesis does not often follow the procedure.[77,88] Experimental laser treatment of normal distal tarsal joints produced minimal localized cartilage necrosis and the defects eventually filled with mostly fibrous tissue.[77]

The results of 2 experimental investigations caused speculation that the clinical effect of laser treatment of the distal tarsal joints is other than stabilizing the joint surfaces.[77,88] The laser fiber penetrates only a short distance into the joint;[77] the rigidity of the quartz does not follow the contour of the joint and the near-infrared

lasers do not penetrate bone. The author agrees with some that the mechanism of action is elimination of sensation in the fibrous joint capsule from "boiling" of intrasynovial fluid. Experimental laser treatment of the pastern produced temperatures of 100°C.[83] This temperature exceeds the 80°C reported to induce chondrocytes necrosis from saline lavage for 10 minutes.[46] However, it takes less than a minute to reach the specified amount of laser energy.

The advantage of laser treatment compared to surgical drilling of the joint spaces is a more rapid return to activity, which is also comparable to that of the chemical treatments described above. Horses treated with the laser returned to normal activity in a few weeks[40] compared to 6 to 17 months after surgical drilling.[2] In a study comparing laser treatment to MIA injection and surgical drilling, the most comfortable horses were those having laser treatment.[88]

Hague reports overall success in clinical cases following laser treatment of the distal tarsal joints, which is in agreement with the author's clinical experience.[40] However, anecdotally, occasional clinical cases have become lame postoperatively for an extended period of time. If the nerve endings are incapacitated as theorized, periarticular soft tissue or subchondral bone pain are the only remaining possibilities. As described below, the needles and skin should be cooled with a slurry of frozen sterile saline to prevent soft tissue necrosis from the heat. Capsular or subcutaneous tissue necrosis likely causes pain. Most laser-treated joints have limited cartilage and subchondral bone necrosis,[77,88] but those that were more lame had more extensive subchondral bone necrosis.[88] The author has observed prolonged postoperative lameness following laser treatment of a tarsus that eventually improved beyond preoperative lameness.

In 2 experimental studies comparing laser treatment to surgical drilling[77] and both laser treatment and drilling to MIA injection,[88] a number of the horses were lame at the respective conclusions. Although not severe, lameness appeared to increase with time over 5 to 12 months. Perhaps this lameness would have abated in time, as has been reported in some clinical cases.[21] Horses with clinically evident distal tarsal disease seem to respond differently to laser treatment than horses with normal hocks.

The procedure for laser treatment of the distal tarsal joints is not difficult but details are important. The author finds dorsal recumbency is more efficient and cooling the surgical sites is more effective. Using radiographic/fluoroscopic control, at least 2 needles are inserted into each tarsal joint so that sterile saline will flush through. Horses with periarticular changes present a challenge in placing needles into the joints, and collapsing joints may have adhesions preventing fluid from flowing through. In contrast with experimental reports, fluid rarely flows across the entire joint in affected joints; location of 2 needles on the medial and lateral side, respectively, is often required to treat the majority of the joint (Figure 5.300). The procedure should not be performed without at least 1 patent lavage portal from the laser entry portal to prevent superheating; there may be more than 1 point of exhaust. A 600-micron quartz fiber is inserted through a 16-gauge

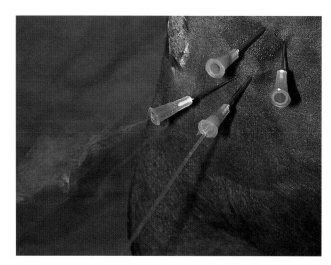

Figure 5.300. Diode laser treatment of the distal tarsal joints (for demonstration). Two needles are placed in the TMT and DIT joints respectively; the blue 16-gauge needles accommodate the laser fiber while 20-gauge needles penetrate into the joint more easily. There is a plume emanating from the exhaust portal in the DIT joint.

needle and is kept in contact with the cartilage with 2-finger pressure as the energy is applied and the fiber burns away; the fiber does not actually travel far into the joint. The power setting varies between 15 and 25 watts and generates total energies of 800 to 1,000 joules.[40] If only the medial or lateral aspect of a joint is being treated, the total energy is divided. The needles and skin must be kept cold with a slurry of frozen sterile saline to avoid skin or deeper necrosis. If the fiber is withdrawn still firing or before it cools, it is less likely to adhere to the joint tissue or to break off the tip in the needle/joint.

Extracorporeal Shock Wave Therapy (ESWT)

Although the technology is not new, ESWT has recently been used as a means to treat equine soft tissue and orthopedic conditions. The principle of the procedure is that an energy wave is produced under water (invisible) by various means and is focused at the anatomic site of concern. Instruments often have radiographic or ultrasonographic means of directing the shock wave specifically at the necessary anatomy. A compressive force is created when the shock wave encounters tissue of different impedances such as soft tissue-bone interfaces. This compression is thought to produce microfractures in the bone, which result in noticeable remodeling during subsequent weeks. No controlled equine studies are available, but profound osseous effects have been demonstrated in rabbit femurs.[20] Importantly, more than one type of ESW-generating machine is available, and no objective evidence of comparative benefits is available.

A series of 74 predominately Western horses (130 joints) were treated for distal tarsal OA using ESWT.[53] The horses had been treated by conservative medical means and had either become nonresponsive or the response had reached an unacceptably short duration. The horses received 2,000 pulses at 22 kV. Ninety days after treatment, 38% had improved 1 lameness grade (scale of 1 to 5) and 42% had improved 2 lameness grades. Eighteen percent became sound, all of which improved 2 lameness grades. Eight of 15 horses that failed to improve became better after a second treatment. No radiographic differences were detectable between pre- and 90-day post-treatment evaluations. Another report relates ESWT treatment of one horse with distal tarsal OA.[74] Improvement was immediate but lasted only 90 days.

An analgesic effect of ESWT has been documented.[67] The fact that ESWT stimulated no further ankylosis in the large series of horses with distal tarsal OA[53] causes one to more strongly consider pain relief as a significant component of the mode of action. Anecdotally, immediate but temporary relief of heel pain and other conditions has been reported in horses; some believe that analgesia may be of longer duration after multiple treatments. Distal tarsal OA is a condition in which pain relief alone is a benefit. Provided no soft tissue compromise occurs, soundness and continued exercise may facilitate eventual ankylosis. Recognizing the density difference between rabbit long bone and equine cuboidal bone, the induced osseous changes may eventually facilitate ankylosis. Aside from distal tarsal disease, there is cause for concern when inducing analgesia in injuries of support structures of horses.

Neurectomy of the Tibial and Deep Peroneal Nerves

The results of an improved method of partial tibial and deep peroneal neurectomy were reported in 24 Warmblood horses.[44] The horses had been affected with OA from 2 months to 7 years. Diagnostic intra-articular or regional anesthesia was not performed. Complete tibial and peroneal neurectomy as previously reported[56] is said to have caused proprioceptive, sensory, and trophic complications and hyperextension of the tarsus.[43]

The revised procedure is performed with the horse in lateral recumbency, rolling the horse when the first side has been completed. Using a tourniquet proximally, 3 15-cm medial skin incisions are used to expose the tibial nerve and its branches into the medial and lateral plantar nerves. All the branches from the exposed nerves are transected. After rolling the horse, another incision is created between the long and lateral digital extensor muscles proximal to the tarsus to expose and resect a 3- 4-cm segment of the deep peroneal nerve.

Postoperative care includes stall rest for 2 months with progressive increases in hand walking after the incisions have healed. Deficits from denervation were not observed. Results were gathered 1 to 3 years after surgery from telephone conversations with owners. Of 21 horses to follow up, 14 were used for dressage, riding, jumping, or eventing for 14 to 36 months. Five horses relapsed 6 to 14 months after surgery, and 2 failed to improve. Radiographic follow-up revealed variable stasis or progression of the OA. The authors' conclusion was that the convalescence was shorter than that following surgical arthrodesis, but that the surgery time was long due to the sizeable incisions that must be closed. A blemish usually developed at the lateral incision site.

Prognosis

The prognosis for bone spavin is always guarded. Horses treated medically and with corrective shoeing respond as individuals. Some horses that have been lame for a shorter period of time respond better. A prognosis usually should be withheld until response to the first line method of therapy is known. Of 29 Warmbloods diagnosed with distal tarsal arthrosis before the age of 5 years, only 5 had become lame and a total of 25 had competed.[37] This illustrates the necessity of making a clinical diagnosis on every horse.

References

1. Adams OR. Surgical arthrodesis for the treatment of bone spavin. J Am Vet Med Assoc 1970;157:1480.
2. Adkins AR, Yovich JV, Steel CM. Surgical arthrodesis of distal tarsal joints in 17 horses clinically affected with osteoarthritis. Aust Vet J 2001;79:26–29.
3. Allen K. Personal communication. 2010.
4. Archer RM, Schneider RK, Lindsay WA, et al. Arthrodesis of the equine distal tarsal joints by perforated stainless steel cylinders. Eq Vet J Supp 1988;125–130.
5. Auer JA. Arthrodesis techniques. In Equine Surgery, 2nd ed. Auer JA, Stick JA, eds. W.B. Saunders, Philadelphia, 1999;696–704.
6. Axelsson M, Bjornsdottir S, Eksell P, et al. Risk factors associated with hindlimb lameness and degenerative joint disease in the distal tarsus of Icelandic horses. Equine Vet J 2001;33:84–90.
7. Axelsson M, Eksell P, Roneus B, et al. Relationship between hind limb lameness and radiographic signs of bone spavin in Icelandic horses in Sweden. Acta Vet Scand 1998;39:349–357.
8. Barber SM. Arthrodesis of the distal intertarsal and tarsometatarsal joints in the horse. Vet Surg 1984;13:227–235.
9. Barneveld A. Arthrodesis of the distal tarsal joint (in horses with spavin). Pferdekrankheiten 1985;29:209–219.
10. Bogner B, Bock P, Stanek C. Correlation of radiological and histological changes of the medial tendon attachment and the related subtendinous bursa of the cranial tibialis muscle in horses affected with spavin. Pferd 1998;14:197–204.
11. Bohanon T. Chemical fusion of the distal tarsal joints with sodium monoiodoacetate in 38 horses clinically affected with bone spavin (abstract). Vet Surg 1995;24:421.
12. Bohanon TC. The tarsus. In Equine Surgery, 2nd ed. Auer JA, Stick JA, eds. W.B. Saunders, Philadelphia: 1999;848–862.
13. Bohanon TC, Schneider RK, Weisbrode SE. Fusion of the distal intertarsal and tarsometatarsal joints in the horse using intra-articular sodium monoiodoacetate. Equine Vet J 1991;23:289–295.
14. Branch MV, Murray RC, Dyson SJ, et al. Alteration of distal tarsal subchondral bone thickness pattern in horses with tarsal pain. Equine Vet J 2007;39:101–105.
15. Burtscher WO, Bock P, Stanek C. The subtendinous bursa of the musculus tibialis cranialis—a histological study. Pferd 1996;12:823–829.
16. Byam-Cook KL, Singer ER. Is there a relationship between clinical presentation, diagnostic and radiographic findings and outcome in horses with osteoarthritis of the small tarsal joints? Equine Vet J 2009;41:118–123.
17. Carmalt JL, Wilson DG. Alcohol facilitated ankylosis of the distal intertarsal and tarsometatarsal joints in the horse. Vet Surg 2009;38:E28.
18. Clayton HM, Almeida PE, Prades M, et al. Double-blind study of the effects of an oral supplement intended to support joint health in horses with tarsal degenerative joint disease. Proceedings Am Assoc Equine Pract 2002;314–317.
19. Dechant JE, Southwood LL, Baxter GM, et al. Treatment of distal tarsal osteoarthritis using a 3-drill technique in 36 horses. Proceedings Am Assoc Eq Pract 1999;45:160–161.
20. Delius M, Draenert K, Al Diek Y, et al. Biological effects of shock waves: In vivo effect of high energy pulses on rabbit bone. Ultrasound Med Biol 1995;21:1219–1225.
21. Dowling BA, Dart AJ, Matthews SM. Chemical arthrodesis of the distal tarsal joints using sodium monoiodoacetate in 104 horses. Aust Vet J 2004;82:38–42.
22. Dykstra RR. Bone spavin. J Am Vet Med Assoc 1913;8:143.
23. Dyson S. Are there any advances in the treatment of distal hock joint pain? Int Symp on Dis of the Icelandic Horse 2004;1111.0604.
24. Eastman T, Bohanon T, Beeman G, et al. Owner survey on cunean tenectomy as a treatment for bone spavin in performance horses. Proceedings Am Assoc Eq Pract 1997;43:121–122.
25. Edwards GB. Surgical arthrodesis for the treatment of bone spavin in 20 horses. Equine Vet J 1982;14:117–121.
26. Ehrlich PJ, Dohoo IR, MW OC. Results of bone scintigraphy in racing standardbred horses: 64 cases (1992–1994). J Am Vet Med Assoc 1999;215:982–991.
27. Ehrlich PJ, Seeherman HJ, O'Callaghan MW, et al. Results of bone scintigraphy in horses used for show jumping, hunting, or eventing: 141 cases (1988–1994). J Am Vet Med Assoc 1998;213:1460–1467.
28. Eksell P, Axelsson M, Brostrom H, et al. Prevalence and risk factors of bone spavin in Icelandic horses in Sweden: A radiographic field study. Acta Vet Scand 1998;39:339–348.
29. Gabel AA. Diagnosis, relative incidence, and probable cause of cunean tendon bursitis-tarsitis of standardbred horses. J Am Vet Med Assoc 1979;175:1079–1085.
30. Gabel AA. Lameness caused by inflammation in the distal hock. Vet Clin N Am 1980;2:101–124.
31. Gabel AA. Prevention, diagnosis and treatment of inflammation of the distal hock horses, joints. Proceed Am Assoc Eq Pract 1983;28:287–298.
32. Gabel AA. Treatment and prognosis for cunean tendon bursitis-tarsitis of standardbred horses. J Am Vet Med Assoc 1979;175:1086–1088.
33. Goldberg SA. Historical facts concerning pathology of spavin. J Am Vet Med Assoc 1918;53:745.
34. Gough M, Munroe GA. Decision making in the management of bone spavin in horses. In Pract 1998;20:252–259.
35. Gough MR, Munroe GA, Mayhew IG. Diffusion of mepivacaine between adjacent synovial structures in the horse. Part 2: Tarsus and stifle. Equine Vet J 2002;34:85–90.
36. Greve J. Juvenile osteoarthrosis in horses, part 1: Prevalence and radiographic changes. Dansk Veterin Nfrtidsskrift, 2008;91:20–25.
37. Greve J. Juvenile osteoarthrosis in the distal tarsal joints of Warmblood horses. Dansk Veterin Nfrtidsskrift, 2008;91:26–28.
38. Gustafson SB. Distal tarsal arthrodesis using 3-drill tracts for treatment of bone spavin in the equine. Colorado State University, Ft. Collins, CO, 1987.
39. Gustafson SB, Trotter GW, Norrdin RW, et al. Evaluation of intra-articularly administered sodium monoiodoacetate-induced chemical injury to articular cartilage of horses. Am J Vet Res 1992;53:1193–1202.
40. Hague BA, Guccione A. Clinical impression of a new technique utilizing a nd : Yag laser to arthrodese the distal tarsal joints. Vet Surg 2000;29:464.
41. Hanson RR, Smalley LR, Huff GK, et al. Oral treatment with a glucosamine-chondroitin sulfate compound for degenerative joint disease in horses: 25 cases. Eq Pract 1997;19:16–22.
42. Hertsch B, Hoppner S, Leonhardt KM, et al. Radiographical examination of German standardbred horses. Pferd 1997;13:97–109.
43. Imschoot J. Unpublished data, 1988.
44. Imschoot J, Verschooten F, Moor Ad, et al. Partial tibial neurectomy and neurectomy of the deep peroneal nerve as a treatment for bone spavin in the horse. Vla Dierg Tijd 1990;59:222–224.
45. Jansson N, Sonnichesen H, Hansen E. Bone spavin in the horse: Fenestration technique. A retrospective study. Pferd 1995;11:97–100.
46. Jenner F, Edwards RB, III, Voss JR, et al. Ex vivo investigation of the use of hydrothermal energy to induce chondrocyte necrosis in articular cartilage of the metacarpophalangeal and metatarsophalangeal joints of horses. Am J Vet Res 2005;66:36–42.
47. Kraus-Hansen AE, Jann HW, Kerr DV, et al. Arthrographic analysis of communication between the tarsometatarsal and distal intertarsal joints of the horse. Vet Surg 1992;21:139–144.

48. Kristoffersen K. Investigations of aseptic hock diseases in the horse. Copenhagen: The Royal Veterinary and Agricultural University, 1981.
49. Labens R, Mellor DJ, Voute LC. Retrospective study of the effect of intra-articular treatment of osteoarthritis of the distal tarsal joints in 51 horses. Vet Rec 2007;161:611–616.
50. Mackay RCJ, Liddell WA. Arthrodesis in the treatment of bone spavin. (Short communication). Equine Vet J 1972;4:34–36.
51. Manning JP. Diagnosis of occult spavin. Illinois Veterinarian 1964;7:26.
52. Martin WJ. Spavin, etiology and treatment. Am Vet Rev 1900;24:464.
53. McCarroll G, McClure S. Extracorporeal shock wave therapy for treatment of osteoarthritis of the tarsometatarsal and distal intertarsal joints. Proceedings Am Assoc Eq Pract 2000;46:200–202.
54. McDonough J. Hock joint lameness. Am Vet Rev 1913;43:629.
55. McIlwraith CW, Robertson JT. Arthrodesis of the distal tarsal joints. McIlwraith and Turner's Equine Surgery: Advanced Techniques, 2nd ed. Williams and Wilkins, Baltimore, 1998;193–197.
56. Merillat L. Veterinary Surgical Operations. A. Eger Publishing, Chicago, 1929.
57. Moyer W. Bone spavin: A clinical review. J Eq Med Surg 1978;2:362.
58. Moyer W, Brokken TD, Raker CW. Bone spavin in throughbread race horses. Proceedings Am Assoc Equine Pract 1983;29:81–92.
59. Murray RC, Dyson SJ, Weekes JS, et al. Nuclear scintigraphic evaluation of the distal tarsal region in normal horses. Vet Rad Ultra 2004;45:345–351.
60. Murray RC, Dyson SJ, Weekes JS, et al. Scintigraphic evaluation of the distal tarsal region in horses with distal tarsal pain. Vet Rad Ultra 2005;46:171–178.
61. Myhre GD, Boucher N, Aiken L. Incidence and correlation of scintigraphic findings to referral lameness at a private hospital. Proceedings Am Assoc Eq Pract 1998;44:218–221.
62. Norrie RD. Diseases of the rear legs. In Equine Medicine and Surgery, 3rd ed. Mansmann RA, McAllister ES, eds. American Veterinary Publications, Santa Barbara, 1982;1141.
63. Novales M, Lucena R, Martin E, et al. Absence of lameness in horses with signs of pathology demonstrated by radiography. Pratique Veterinaire Equine 1997;29:41–45.
64. O'Brien T. Radiographic interpretation of the equine tarsus. Proceedings Am Assoc Eq Pract 1973;19:289.
65. Ritchie JM. The aliphatic alcohols. In The Pharmacological Basis of Therapeutics. Goodman LS, Gilman A, eds. MacMillan Publishers Ltd, New York, 1980;376–390.
66. Rodgers MR. Effects of oral glucosamine and chondroitin sulfates supplementation on frequency of intra-articular therapy of the horse tarsus. International Journal of Applied Research in Veterinary Medicine 2006;4:155–162.
67. Rompe JD, Hope C, Kullmer K, et al. Analgesic effect of extracorporeal shock-wave therapy on chronic tennis elbow. J Bone Joint Surg Br 1996;78:233–237.
68. Rooney JR. Biomechanics of Lameness in Horses. Williams and Wilkins Co., Baltimore, 1969.
69. Rooney JR, Turner LW. The mechanisms of horses pulling loads. J Equine Vet Sci 1985;5:355–359.
70. Sack WO, Orsini PG. Distal intertarsal and tarsometatarsal joints in the horse: Communication and injection sites. J Am Vet Med Assoc 1981;179:355–359.
71. Sammut EB, Kannegieter NJ. Use of sodium monoiodoacetate to fuse the distal hock joints in horses. Aust Vet J 1995;72:25–28.
72. Schebitz H. Spavin: Radiographic diagnosis and treatment. Proceedings Am Assoc Equine Pract 1965;11:207.
73. Schebitz H, Wilkins H. Bone spavin diagnosis and therapy. Munch Tierarztl Wschr 1967;80:385.
74. Scheuch B, Whitcomb M, Galuppo L, et al. Clinical evaluation of high-energy extracorporeal shock waves on equine orthopedic injuries. Equine musculoskeletal high-energy shock wave therapy symposium 2001.
75. Schneider RK, Archer RM. Arthrodesis of the distal two tarsal joints in the horse using perforated stainless steel cylinders and cancellous bone graft. Vet Comp Orth Traum 1991;4:21–27.
76. Schramme M, Platt D, Smith RK. Treatment of osteoarthritis of the tarsometatarsal and distal intertarsal joints of the horse (spavin) with monoiodoacetate: Preliminary results. Vet Surg 1998;27:296.
77. Scruton C, Baxter GM, Cross MW, et al. Comparison of intra-articular drilling and diode laser treatment for arthrodesis of the distal tarsal joints in normal horses. Equine Vet J 2005;37:81–86.
78. Shoemaker RW, Allen AL, Richardson CE, et al. Use of intra-articular administration of ethyl alcohol for arthrodesis of the tarsometatarsal joint in healthy horses. Am J Vet Res 2006;67:850–857.
79. Sigurdsson H. Diagnosis and radiographic examination of spavin in 60 Icelandic horses. Buvisindi 1991;5:33–38.
80. Sonnichsen HV, Svalastoga E. Surgical treatment of bone spavin in the horse. Eq Pract 1985;7:6–9.
81. Stanger P, Lauk HD, Plocki KA, et al. Treatment of spavin by arthrodesis of the distal tarsal joint: Long-term results. Pferd 1994;10:75–79.
82. Stover SM, Hornof WJ, Richardson GL, et al. Bone scintigraphy as an aid in the diagnosis of occult distal tarsal bone trauma in three horses. J Am Vet Med Assoc 1986;188:624–628.
83. Sullins KE. Unpublished data.
84. Vaughan JT. Analysis of lameness in the pelvic limb and selected cases. Proc Am Assoc Eq Pract 1965;11:223.
85. Williams F, Rohe REK. Significance of genetic aspects of bone diseases in horses. Pferd 1996;12:345–346.
86. Winter D, Bruns E, Glodek P, et al. Genetic disposition of bone diseases in sport horses. Zuchtungskunde 1996;68:92–108.
87. Wyn-Jones G, May SA. Surgical arthrodesis for the treatment of osteoarthrosis of the proximal intertarsal, distal intertarsal and tarsometatarsal joints in 30 horses: A comparison of four different techniques. Equine Vet J 1986;18:59–64.
88. Zubrod CJ, Schneider RK, Hague BA, et al. Comparison of three methods for arthrodesis of the distal intertarsal and tarsometatarsal joints in horses. Vet Surg 2005;34:372–382.

BOG SPAVIN (IDIOPATHIC SYNOVITIS/ TARSOCRURAL EFFUSION)

Strictly speaking, bog spavin is a clinical sign and not a diagnosis. It is a descriptive term for synovial effusion of the tarsocrural joint. The effusion is due to an acute or chronic low-grade synovitis which can come from any of several causes.[3] As a primary condition, the term should be limited to situations in which the inciting cause (e.g., OCD or OA) truly cannot be identified. Lameness is variable and depends upon the severity of the synovitis. In spite of potential clinical insignificance, a bog becomes an important cosmetic issue in certain show situations. The dorsomedial enlargement is commonly more visible, but distention of the dorsolateral, plantarolateral, and plantaromedial joint pouches may also be present or produced when the fluid is manually pushed around the joint (Figures 5.301 and 3.46).

Etiology

A significant proportion of affected horses do not have idiopathic synovitis, but have an articular lesion that could be discovered radiographically or arthroscopically. The author's opinion is that the incidence of bog spavin without diagnoses will diminish as imaging improves. Allowed to persist through years of work, this chronic synovitis can lead to cartilage loss and eventual OA and a fibrotic joint capsule. A few individuals experience TC joint filling when they are confined to a stall or are inactive. This effusion disappears with exercise.

The author has treated several cases of idiopathic tarsocrural septic arthritis. The affected horses were all athletes without a history of intra-articular therapy or injury. In one report of 192 horses affected with septic arthritis, 12 had no history to explain the problem.[8]

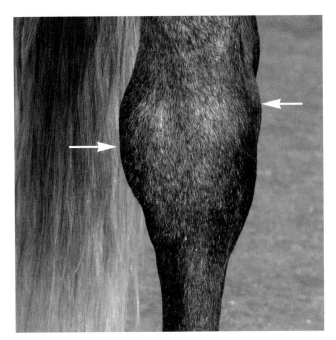

Figure 5.301. Tarsocrural joint effusion (bog spavin). The arrows indicate significant effusion of the dorsomedial and plantarolateral joint pouches.

Seven of those 12 were affected in the tarsocrural joint. The bacteria cultured were more diverse than would be expected following joint invasion. Eighty-three percent of those 12 horses survived to be released from the hospital. For more information on septic arthritis, see Chapter 10.

A horse that is too straight in the hock joint is predisposed to bog spavin, presumably due to continuous trauma to the articular cartilage. If a horse with straight limbs is not affected as a young horse, it may develop the condition after training begins. This could be due to cartilage trauma due to straight conformation, or it could be temporary synovitis/capsulitis typical of young horses beginning training. Depending upon severity and activity of the horse, these subtle cartilage lesions can worsen with time due to the persisting synovitis, leading to OA. Thus, idiopathic synovitis can eventually become OA as could be observed in any other joint. At necropsy, Rooney associated articular wear lines in the distal tibia and erosive lesions on the dorsal edge of the medial and lateral grooves of the distal tibia with TC joint effusion.[7] Although frequently associated with primary pathology such as osteochondrosis, these are examples of OA due to chronic synovitis.

Injury to the hock joint as a result of quick stops, quick turns, or other trauma causes effusion due to injury of the joint capsule. Occasionally, performance horses develop acute TC effusion and lameness approaching that of sepsis. A severe capsulitis is probably the main component. Radiographic signs being absent, horses are treated with rest and local and systemic anti-inflammatory therapy. Response to therapy can be profound and rapid. Structural damage such as collateral ligament sprain or non-displaced fracture should be ruled out before returning the horse to work (Figure 3.47).

Deficiencies of calcium, phosphorus, vitamin A, or vitamin D, alone, or in any combination, apparently can produce bog spavin. Chronic zinc intoxication has also been implicated in TC effusion.[5]

Uncommonly, horses that have had acute progressing to chronic synovitis such as may follow septic arthritis retain the effusion after the original cause has been resolved. The persistence appears to be due to permanent synovial membrane changes or fibrous joint capsule distortion. Regeneration of the synovial membrane takes at least a month and the villi may never regenerate.[2]

Clinical Signs

By definition, the only clinical sign required is TC effusion. There are 3 characteristic fluctuant swellings, the largest of which is located at the dorsomedial aspect of the hock joint (Figures 5.301, 3.46, and 3.47). Two smaller swellings occasionally occur on either side of the surface of the hock joint at the junction of the tibial tarsal and fibular tarsal bones. However, severe effusion can produce distention of all 4 corners of the joint. These plantar swellings are lower (more distal) than the swellings of thoroughpin. When pressure is exerted on any one of these swellings, the other enlargements show an increase in size and an increase of tension of the joint capsule if held. This fluctuant, moveable swelling must be differentiated from periarticular edema, which signals an extra-articular problem.

When present, lameness is due to synovitis. The pain of synovitis is sensed by nerve endings located in the fibrous joint capsule. If the TC synovitis is severe enough to irritate those nerve endings, the horse is lame to some degree. Hindlimb flexion, specifically meant to diagnostically exacerbate that inflammation, may be required to see any lameness. If the seat of the problem is capsulitis, the response could be very positive. More severe inflammatory situations may bring local heat, pain, and swelling. No radiographic changes are evident in uncomplicated bog spavin. There is one report of effusion that apparently became severe enough to rupture the fibrous joint capsule and create a synovial hernia.[4]

Diagnosis

The presence of bog spavin is diagnostic. In most cases the dorsomedial swelling is the largest, but in some horses the 2 plantar swellings are more prominent. In some cases, the location of the primary source of the synovitis may dictate the location of the largest point of effusion. The most important factor in diagnosis is to determine the true etiology if possible.

All diagnostic capabilities should be used to rule out any correctable lesion. Ultrasound is extremely valuable for demonstrating the character of the synovial fluid, synovial membrane, and joint capsule. Computed tomography or magnetic resonance imaging may also be useful. Depending upon degree of lameness, scintigraphy may be considered.

With chronic bogs, synovial fluid changes are commonly unremarkable. Acute injuries may cause hemarthrosis or a rise in WBC and total protein. However, when lameness is severe, septic arthritis must be ruled out, and synovial fluid analysis is important. Synovial fluid analysis of TC effusion due to synovitis from an adjacent or impending septic process usually reflects an elevated total protein without the expected WBC increase. This situation should be monitored closely.

Treatment

Treatment can be part of a diagnostic progression. Presented with a horse with TC effusion, lameness and radiographic examinations are indicated. Still faced with effusion of unknown etiology, intra-articular therapy can be administered.

Young horses should not be treated aggressively. With the needle placed in the TC joint, as much synovial fluid as possible is removed, after which sodium hyaluronate is injected. Particularly when repeated, steroids have been known to cause cartilage exfoliation from the joint surface in young horses. A support bandage is applied to prevent return of the effusion. The joint capsule in foals can become thinned and may have difficulty regaining its normal integrity, even after the synovitis has resolved. Activity is restricted to a stall for a few days then a small paddock. The bandage should be maintained for 2 to 3 weeks to allow the capsule to strengthen. If bandaging becomes difficult to maintain or the skin becomes irritated, elastic stockinet provides substantial support. Nothing further is necessary if the bog is resolved. Diagnostic arthroscopy is indicated if it fails to resolve or returns. Repeat radiographs are also indicated, but often remain negative.

Still assuming no radiographic changes are present, the same plan described above for young horses can be followed for adults, although a steroid could be added to the hyaluronic acid. If the bog returns, further diagnostics, including arthroscopy, are indicated. Continuous steroid injections have an eventual negative effect, and the risk of sepsis increases with each treatment.

Intra-articular atropine has been anecdotally used to treat refractory TC effusion. There is no known pharmaceutical mechanism of action, but 4 to 6 mg is being used with noticeable success. It is wise to purchase atropine in single-use sizes to preserve sterility. Although the mechanism of action is unknown, there is also no information about any negative effect. However, excessive dosage of atropine can contribute to signs of colic. Intra-articular injection is an off-label application of the drug.

Treatment of bog spavin caused by nutritional deficiencies is usually of no avail unless proper corrections are made in the diet. If the deficient mineral(s) and/or vitamin(s) are added to the diet, the overall nutrition regulated, and the horse freed from internal parasites, bog spavins usually disappear in 4 to 6 weeks. Bog spavin resulting from nutritional causes is most common in horses 6 months to 2 years of age.

Tarsocrural effusion due to chronic intoxication with zinc appears to respond to removal of the horse from the source of zinc and feeding a balanced ration supplemented with 60 grams of calcium carbonate/day.[5]

Synovectomy may be useful when irreversible synovial membrane changes have occurred. The author has resolved persistent bog spavin in one horse using synovectomy long after septic arthritis had resolved.

Motorized equipment is required to do a complete job, and the caudal compartment of the tarsocrural joint should be treated as well. Intimal regeneration requires approximately a month, and the villi will not regenerate.[1,6] The functional significance of the loss of the villous surface area is unknown. In the author's experience, horses treated by synovectomy for acute septic arthritis have not demonstrated a negative clinical effect.

One reported case of synovial hernia following chronic TC effusion responded favorably to surgical resection of the hernia.[4] This procedure should not be taken lightly. Support bandaging and prolonged stall rest are necessary to prevent dehiscence and the creation of a much worse problem. The reported case was stall confined for 3.5 months.

Prognosis

The prognosis is guarded if the cause is traumatic or nutritional. It is unfavorable if it is due to conformation, although it must be remembered that in the majority of cases, horses can continue to perform without an obvious lameness.

References

1. Doyle PS, Sullins KE, Saunders GK. Synovial regeneration in the equine carpus after arthroscopic mechanical or CO_2 laser synovectomy. Submitted for publication.
2. Doyle-Jones PS, Sullins KE, Saunders GK. Synovial regeneration in the equine carpus after arthroscopic mechanical or carbon dioxide laser synovectomy. Vet Surg 2002;31:331–343.
3. Gill HE. Diagnosis and treatment of hock lameness. Proc Am Assoc Eq Pract 1973;19:257.
4. Martens A, Steenhaut M, Sercu K, et al. Surgical treatment of a synovial hernia of the tarsocrural joint in a horse. Vet Surg 1997;26:259–260.
5. Messer NT. Tibiotarsal effusion associated with chronic zinc intoxication in three horses. J Am Vet Med Assoc 1981;178:294–297.
6. Palmer JL, Bertone AL, Weisbrode SE. Histological and ultrastructural synovial membrane characteristics following surgical synovectomy. Vet Surg 1994;23:413.
7. Rooney JR. Bog spavin and tibiotarsal joint lesions in the horse. Mod Vet Pract 1973;54:43–44.
8. Schneider RK, Bramlage LR, Moore RM, et al. A retrospective study of 192 horses affected with septic arthritis/tenosynovitis. Equine Vet J 1992;24:436–442.

OSTEOCHONDRITIS DISSECANS (OCD) OF THE TARSOCRURAL JOINT

Horses with tarsocrural OCD usually present for joint effusion (bog spavin). These animals are often presented prior to training and are frequently not lame unless a flexion test is performed. The other common scenario is the discovery of the lesion from routine radiographs taken before a sale. If clinical signs appear after training has begun, lameness is more likely.

Tarsocrural OCD is quite common in Standardbreds, as evidenced by the number of reports in which that breed is common.[2,3,5,8,21,30] Sixty-one joints in 49 Standardbred horses were reported early.[28] A large series that included 154 race horses contained 106 Standardbreds.[14] Additionally, a long-term study revealed 117 joints were affected in 764 yearlings from 3 breeding years.[30]

Tarsocrural fragments were detected in 9.6% of 3,749 Warmblood horses radiographed for sale during a 7-year period.[26] Tarsocrural osteochondrosis is a very common condition found in many breeds.[1,14,19] Subchondral cystic lesions of the proximal trochlear ridges have been reported and accompanied OCD lesions of the distal intermediate ridge of the tibia (DIRT).[15]

Etiology

See Chapter 11 for details regarding potential causes of this condition.

Clinical Signs

Synovial effusion (bog spavin) is by far the most common presenting complaint.[11] Palpation of the TC joint capsule reveals effusion without a painful swelling. Horses with a long-standing bog may have palpable capsular thickening. However, if periarticular or regional edema or swelling beyond the TC joint is present, another problem should be suspected. Lameness may be absent or mild; severe lameness is not consistent with this diagnosis. A reduced flexion angle of the tarsus is observed in horses with excessive synovial effusion. A hindlimb flexion test may increase the lameness slightly. Horses presented after beginning training are more likely to be lame.[14]

Diagnosis

Tarsocrural OCD should be considered whenever a horse presents with spontaneous or traumatically induced joint effusion. Affected horses without clinical signs may develop effusion after some type of incident apparently destabilizes an OCD lesion, causing synovitis, including normal training of young athletes. Synovial fluid analysis is usually unremarkable. One study demonstrated decreased viscosity that normalized with rest.[16]

The most commonly affected sites within the TC joint (in decreasing order of incidence) include the distal (dorsal) intermediate ridge of the tibia (DIRT) (Figure 5.302), lateral trochlear ridge of the tibiotarsal bone (Figure 5.303), medial malleolus of the distal tibia (Figure 5.304), medial trochlear ridge of the tibiotarsal bone, and proportionate combinations of these.[4,12,14,17,30]

The radiographic lesion can consist of subchondral bone lucency, a partially ossified flap, or a larger fragment. All radiographic views of the both hocks should be taken, because at least one of the typically-affected sites is demonstrated by each.[31] Each location has its typical appearance, but OCD also appears in other locations, so a complete evaluation must be made in every case.[18] Approximately half of affected horses have similar contralateral lesions.[2,8,10,32] Though less common, multiple lesions or loose bodies may also be present.[14,25] Typical lesions can be discovered during routine radiography for sale in horses without clinical signs (Figure 5.305).[29] A small percentage of horses with tarsocrural OCD and joint effusion do not have radiographically apparent subchondral bone involvement and require arthroscopy to make the diagnosis.

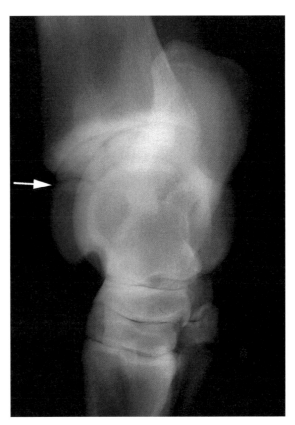

Figure 5.302. Dorsomedial plantarolateral radiograph demonstrating an OCD lesion of the distal intermediate ridge of the tibia (DIRT). This view projects the typical fragment (arrow) well. The lateromedial projection also demonstrates the lesion.

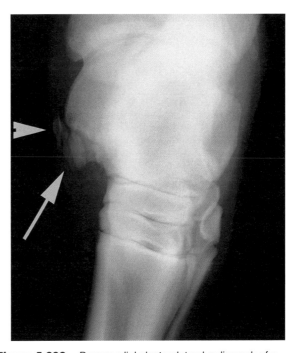

Figure 5.303. Dorsomedial-plantarolateral radiograph of a tarsus with a large distal lateral trochlear ridge OCD lesion (lower arrow). An earlier fragment had dislodged and became embedded in the joint capsule (upper arrow). Extra-articular osseous densities such as the latter fragment are unlikely to affect soundness but are a concern for sale.

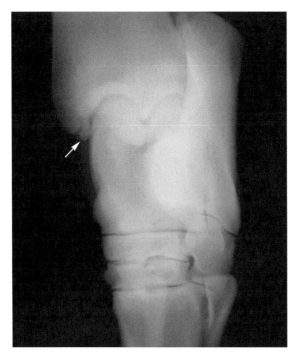

Figure 5.304. Dorsolateral-plantaromedial radiograph of the tarsus demonstrating a medial malleolar OCD lesion (arrow). The fragment is often located on the axial surface of the medial malleolus adjacent to the medial trochlear ridge.

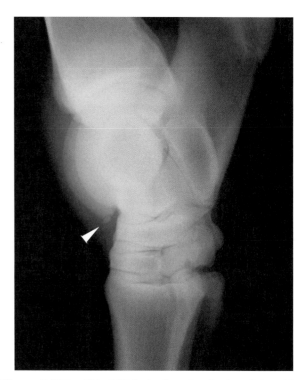

Figure 5.305. This OCD lesion from the distal medial trochlear ridge (arrow) is unlikely to cause clinical signs and may be located outside the joint within the capsule. Without clinical signs, it may not need to be removed.

Foals should be treated conservatively (if clinical signs appear) if early radiographs demonstrate OCD. The majority of typical DIRT and lateral trochlear ridge lesions in Warmblood foals resolved by 5 months of age and those remaining were considered permanent.[7]

The distal tibial lesion is commonly an osteochondral fragment (Figure 11.40 in Chapter 11). Fragment size has been classified, but no correlation to clinical significance or surgical outcome was shown.[14] Lateral trochlear ridge lesions may appear as lucent defects or as partially calcified "bone flaps." Larger lesions may comprise the majority of the distal lateral trochlear ridge (Figure 11.41). Probably because of close joint capsule contact, fragments may become displaced and lodge elsewhere in the TC joint or adjacent to the PIT joint.[25] Medial malleolus lesions are usually straightforward, but should always be checked for radiographically inapparent cartilage defects.[31] Some medial malleolar lesions are axial and must be removed from the abaxial surface of the medial trochlear ridge.[31] Much of the lateral malleolus is extra-articular, and it is an uncommon site for OCD. However, a lateral malleolar subchondral cystic lesion accompanying distal tibial OCD has been reported.[33] Subchondral cystic lesions may also occur in the trochlear ridges.

Radiographic findings that usually do not cause clinical signs include small "buttons" without osseous union to the parent bone or dewdrop lesions on the distal end and a flattening of the ridge of the medial trochlear ridge.[11,23] However, these lesions may be arthroscopically evaluated or addressed in some cases due to the owner's request for the sake of future sale or if the joint is being operated for another reason. Intra-capsular osseous densities may be calcification or early fragments that displaced from OCD lesions and became embedded in the synovial membrane. If they are extra-synovial, they are usually clinically insignificant. True distal medial trochlear ridge fractures may cause lameness,[25] and joints containing questionable findings should be evaluated if lameness is present. Synovial effusion accompanying such lesions may be due to intra-articular lesions that are radiographically inapparent and warrants investigation.

Two reports of tarsal radiographic monitoring, one on 77 Standardbred foals[21] and another on 753 Standardbred yearlings,[8] revealed that clinically significant lesions are generally present at 1 year of age and very rarely appear later. Some of these horses had lesions present at 1 to 3 months of age. However, typical lesions identified early in 11 foals reverted to normal by 7 to 8 months of age.[21] The usual cause for discovering a lesion in a foal is a bog. However, these results indicate that it may be advisable to observe nondisplaced lesions in foals until the late weanling stage, when the situation allows. Control of synovitis (and exercise) is advisable in the interim.

Radiographs are usually adequate for imaging and clinical signs often dictate the need for further diagnostics without the expense of more advanced imaging. Scintigraphy may be limited by lack of increased blood flow to the lesion or normal intense activity of bone in the young animals.[20] Imaging findings should always be considered along with the clinical signs.

Treatment

Horses with radiographic lesions but no clinical signs may have no immediate problem, but clinical signs can always appear during training, disrupting the schedule. In a series of horses with figures adjusted for problems unrelated to OCD, conservative therapy without medication was considered successful in 80% of 71 3- to 5-year-old Warmbloods and 23% of 75 2- 4-year-old Standardbreds.[17] Half of each group presented with tarsocrural effusion. Because lesion location or type has not been correlated to differences in outcome, it seems that training at speed exacerbates lameness. However, it is also disappointing to find advanced OA in experienced horses that have worked with TC joint effusion all their lives when it could have been prevented by early surgery.

Even without severe lameness, the synovitis producing the joint effusion is likely to eventually lead to OA in athletes. Studies have demonstrated better results in athletes with surgical removal and debridement of the lesions when compared to nonsurgical treatment.[9,28,12,14] A retrospective study in 114 Standardbreds revealed similar numbers racing between surgically and conservatively treated horses.[10] Surgically treated horses had fewer total starts but equivalent earnings. Surgery produced better results than nonsurgical treatment in draft horses.[19] In another report, only 2 of 10 horses treated conservatively with intra-articular steroids and systemic supplements remained sound. No mention was made of those 2 horses' presenting or radiographic signs.[6]

With foals, some radiographically evident lesions do not actually disrupt the joint surface and correct themselves with age.[5,24] In a series of 77 Standardbred foals, all ossification and subchondral bone abnormalities observed before 8 months of age resolved spontaneously. Distal tibial and lateral trochlear ridge fragments tended to increase in incidence at approximately the same time and remained unresolved.[5] Some foals may develop synovial effusion without radiographic signs. It is advisable to treat the synovitis to reduce the effusion and wait and see if the situation resolves, because surgery may not be required.

Arthroscopy facilitates exploration and visualization of the tarsocrural joint and provides extensive beneficial lavage in the process. The typical dorsomedial arthroscope placement allows visualization of the entire dorsal aspect of the joint. Instrument access can be varied to reach any of the affected locations or the PIT joint.[12] Exceptionally large fragments cannot be removed through the typical instrument portal, but the incision can be enlarged slightly or the fragment size can be reduced with an osteotome so the incision does not usually require conversion to an arthrotomy.

Subchondral cystic lesions of the proximal trochlear ridges have been successfully injected arthroscopically with steroid[15] or debrided arthroscopically.[13]

Prognosis

The prognosis for athletic activity after arthroscopic debridement of tarsocrural OCD is good.[10] In a series of 183 horses, 76.5% performed successfully after arthroscopic surgery.[14] Tarsocrural effusion resolved after surgery in 89% of racehorses and 74% of nonrace horses. However, effusion was less likely to resolve following surgery on lateral trochlear ridge or medial malleolus lesions. There was no correlation between resolution of effusion and athletic performance.[14] When compared to unaffected siblings, Thoroughbreds and Standardbreds having arthroscopic removal of tarsocrural OCD fragments started at the same rate. However, affected horses were less likely to race as 2-year-olds.[1] Lesion location and unilateral vs. bilateral lesions had no effect on ability to start. Although the trend was present in all groups, only 2-year-old Standardbreds were significantly less likely to start a race when multiple sites within the tarsocrural joint were affected.[1,14,27]

In a series of 143 French trotters undergoing arthroscopy for tarsocrural OCD (predominately DIRT), the success rate was 77% with no difference among horses that raced before or after surgery, with uni- or bilateral lesions or with multiple lesions per joint.[2]

Some surveys of Standardbred racehorses conclude performances of horses with radiographic signs of OCD but not having surgery are equal to or better than performances of normal horses.[3,27] However, no figures on the incidence of clinical signs or therapy during the careers of the horses could be given. Some horses had surgery.[27] Long-term and individual evaluations are required to fully evaluate the effect of racing with tarsocrural OCD lesions.

A survey of radiographic lesions of OCD in 3 yearling crops of Standardbreds (764 horses) revealed that horses with tarsocrural radiographic lesions earned less but comparable amounts to the entire group.[30] The study gives no specifics, but included horses that underwent arthroscopy. The implication is that arthroscopic surgery made no significant difference in racing success. One study revealed that horses affected with OCD were larger and more substantially-built.[22] Aside from surgery not impairing athletic ability, the observation that OCD affects the best individuals may be true.[27]

Intra-operative findings of superficial cartilage fibrillation apparently had no effect upon outcome. However, further cartilage degeneration or erosion decreased success by 30%. Osseous densities that cannot be identified arthroscopically are also unlikely to cause lameness.[25]

References

1. Beard WL, Bramlage LR, Schneider RK, et al. Postoperative racing performance in standardbreds and thoroughbreds with osteochondrosis of the tarsocrural joint: 109 cases (1984–1990). J Am Vet Med Assoc 1994;204:1655–1659.
2. Betsch JM, Albert N, Lienasson D. Retrospective study of 143 cases of osteochondritis of the distal tibia in French trotter horses. (Étude rètrospective de 143 cas d'ostèochondrose du tibia distal chez le trotteur Franáais). 2006;38:41–45.
3. Brehm W, Staecker W. Osteochondrosis (OCD) in the tarsocrural joint of standardbred trotters—correlation between radiographic findings and racing performance. Proc Am Assoc Eq Pract 1999;45:164–166.
4. Canonici F, Serata V, Buldinin A, et al. 134 horses with osteochondritis dissecans of the tarso-crural joint: Clinical considerations and results following arthroscopic surgery. J Eq Vet Sci 1996;16:345–348.
5. Carlsten J, Sandgren B, Dalin G. Development of osteochondrosis in the tarsocrural joint and osteochondral fragments in the fetlock joints of standardbred trotters. I. A radiological survey. Equine Vet J 1993;Suppl. 16:42–47.

6. De Moor A, Verschooten F, Desmet P, et al. Osteochondritis dissecans of the tibio-tarsal joint in the horse. Equine Vet J 1972;4:139–143.
7. Dik KJ, Enzerink E, Weeren PR. Radiographic development of osteochondral abnormalities, in the hock and stifle of dutch warmblood foals, from age 1 to 11 months. Equine Vet J 1999:9–15.
8. Grondahl AM. The incidence of osteochondrosis in the tibiotarsal joint of Norwegian standardbred trotters: A radiographic study. J Equine Vet Sci 1991;11:272–274.
9. Hoppe F, Philipsson J. Racing performance of trotting horses with osteochondrosis of the hock. Svensk Veterinartidning 1984;36:285–288.
10. Laws EG, Richardson DW, Ross MW, et al. Racing performance of standardbreds after conservative and surgical treatment for tarsocrural osteochondrosis. Equine Vet J 1993;25:199–202.
11. McIlwraith CW. Clinical aspects of osteochondrosis dissecans. Osteochondrosis dissecans of the tarsocrural joint. In Joint Disease in the Horse. McIllwraith CW, Trotter GW, eds. WB Saunders, Philadelphia, 1996;369–374.
12. McIlwraith CW, Nixon AJ, Wright IM, et al. Arthroscopic surgery of the tarsocrural joint. In Diagnostic and Surgical Arthroscopy in the Horse, 3rd ed. Elsevier, Philadelphia, 2005; 280–294.
13. McIlwraith CW, Nixon AJ, Wright IM, et al. Arthroscopic surgery of the tarsocrural joint. In Diagnostic and Surgical Arthroscopy in the Horse. 3rd ed. Elsevier, Philadelphia, 2005;294–295.
14. McIlwraith CW, Foerner JJ, Davis DM. Osteochondritis dissecans of the tarsocrural joint: Results of treatment with arthroscopic surgery. Equine Vet J 1991;23:155–162.
15. Montgomery LJ, Juzwiak JS. Subchondral cyst-like lesions in the talus of four horses. Eq Vet Educ 2009;21:629–637.
16. Muttini A, Petrizzi L, Tinti A, et al. Synovial fluid parameters in normal and osteochondritic hocks of horses with open physis. Boll Soc Ital Biol Sper 1994;70:337–344.
17. Peremans K, Verschooten F. Results of conservative treatment of osteochondrosis of the tibiotarsal joint in the horse. J Eq Vet Sci 1997;17:322–326.
18. Ribot X, Lions JA, Leroux D, et al. Osteochondrosis dissecans (ocd) in an unusual site. Pratique Veterinaire Equine 1998;30:235–239.
19. Riley CB, Scott WM, Caron JP, et al. Osteochondritis dessicans [dissecans] and subchondral cystic lesions in draft horses: A retrospective study. Can Vet J 1998;39:627–633.
20. Ross MW. Bone scintigraphy: Lessons learned from 5,000 horses. Proceedings Am Assoc Equine Pract 2005;51:6–20.
21. Sandgren B. Bony fragments in the tarsocrural and metacarpo- or metatarsophalangeal joints in the standardbred horse—a radiographic survey. Equine Vet J 1988;Supplement 6:66–70.
22. Sandgren B, Dalin G, Carlsten J. Osteochondrosis in the tarsocrural joint and osteochondral fragments in the fetlock joints in standardbred trotters. I. Epidemiology. Equine Vet J 1993;Suppl. 16:31–37.
23. Shelley J, Dyson S. Interpreting radiographs 5: Radiology of the equine hock. Equine Vet J 1984;16:488–495.
24. Smallwood JE, Auer JA, Martens RJ, et al. The developing equine tarsus from birth to six months of age. Eq Pract 1984;6:7–48.
25. Stephens PR, Richardson DW, Ross MW, et al. Osteochondral fragments within the dorsal pouch or dorsal joint capsule of the proximal intertarsal joint of the horse. Vet Surg 1989;18:151–157.
26. Stock KF, Hamann H, Distl O. Prevalence of osseous fragments in distal and proximal interphalangeal, metacarpo- and metatarsophalangeal and tarsocrural joints of Hanoverian Warmblood horses. Journal of Veterinary Medicine Series A 2005;52:388–394.
27. Storgaard Jorgensen H, Proschowsky H, Falk Ronne J, et al. The significance of routine radiographic findings with respect to subsequent racing performance and longevity in standardbred trotters. Equine Vet J 1997;29:55–59.
28. Stromberg B, Rejno S. Osteochondrosis in the horse. I. A clinical and radiologic investigation of osteochondritis dissecans of the knee and hock joint. Acta Radiol Suppl (Stockh) 1978;358:139–152.
29. Torre F, Fadiga G. A radiological investigation on metacarpal/tarsal-phalangeal and tibio-tarsal joints in a selected group of standardbred yearlings. Ippologia 1993;4:37–41.
30. Torre F, Motta M. Osteochondrosis of the tarsocrural joint and osteochondral fragments in the fetlock joints: Incidence and influence on racing performance in a selected group of standardbred trotters. Proc Am Assoc Eq Pract 2000;46:287–294.
31. Torre F, Toniato M. Osteochondral fragments from the medial malleolus in horses: A comparison between radiographic and arthroscopic findings. Proc Am Assoc Eq Pract 1999;45:167–171.
32. Tourtoulou G, Caure S, Domaingue MC. Incidence of osteochondrosis in the trotter foals. Pratique Veterinaire Equine 1997;29:237–244.
33. van Duin Y, Hurtig MB. Subchondral bone cysts in the distal aspect of the tibia of three horses. Can Vet J 1996;37:429–431.

ACQUIRED BONE CYSTS OF THE TARSUS

Atypical bone cysts with apparently mixed etiologies have been reported in the distal tibia,[5] distal talus adjoining the PIT joint,[2] and proximal talus.[4] A series of 12 horses with occult subchondral cyst-like lesions of various sites in the tarsocrural joint occurred over a period of several years as well.[1]

Etiology

At least some of the cases appear related to a persistent septic process not as fulminant as most bacterial infections but in which OA is the end result.[1,4,5] Others seem to be related to developmental orthopedic disease (DOD) and respond to routine treatments for OCD or subchondral cystic lesions.[2,4,5] Simultaneous typical lesions of OCD occur with many of the cases. It seems apparent that these are 2 different types of cases, but they have been reported together.

For the more lame and typically older cases, a consistent feature is severe aseptic synovitis usually not seen in horses with acute or long-standing DOD.

Clinical Signs and Diagnosis

In one study affected horses ranged in age from 38 days to 29 years. The horses with apparent or obscure subchondral bone cysts with or without accompanying DIRT OCD lesions presented with synovial effusion and mild or no lameness.[4,5] Horses with more severe clinical signs exhibit mild to severe lameness and synovial effusion. The synovial fluid values, when given, are inflammatory, but less so than in the typical septic joint. Neutrophils are prominent in some but mononuclear cells have been more evident in others, and bacteria have been isolated in a minority of the cases. Fibrin production has been a prominent feature in the synovial fluid of some of the cases. The cystic lesions may be radiographically apparent;[2] scintigraphy or computed tomography has been required to localize some lesions (Figure 5.306).[1]

Treatment

Horses with lesions resembling DOD respond to the same treatments as described for those cases. The DIRT lesions are removed. Arthroscopically, the cysts have been successfully debrided[3] or injected with a steroid.[4] These cases have all progressed to athletic soundness.

The horses with more severe clinical signs have not become sound without arthroscopic exploration and

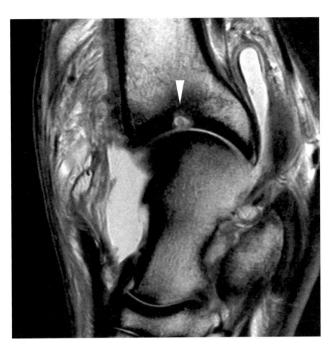

Figure 5.306. Sagittal T2 MR sequence identifying a subchondral cystic lesion (white arrow) in the distal tibia overlying the trochlear ridge. (Courtesy of Dr. Rich Redding.)

debridement. Some were obviously destined to become cripples and euthanatized, but others simply remained lame after conservative therapy. Five of 8 horses treated arthroscopically became sound.[1,2,4]

Prognosis

These cases vary widely in their presentation and outcome; therefore, each case must be regarded individually. The prognosis depends upon the complete clinical picture. More serious cases strongly resemble cases of fungal arthritis that the author has treated, but cystic lesions have not occurred.

References

1. Garcia-Lopez JM, Kirker-Head CA. Occult subchondral osseous cyst-like lesions of the equine tarsocrural joint. Vet Surg 2004;33:557–564.
2. Hawkins JF. Subchondral cystic lesion of the talus in a foal. Eq Pract 1998;20:8–9.
3. McIlwraith CW, Nixon AJ, Wright IM, et al. Arthroscopic surgery of the tarsocrural joint. In Diagnostic and Surgical Arthroscopy in the Horse. 3rd ed. Elsevier, Philadelphia, 2005;294–295.
4. Montgomery LJ, Juzwiak JS. Subchondral cyst-like lesions in the talus of four horses. Eq Vet Educ 2009;21:629–637.
5. van Duin Y, Hurtig MB. Subchondral bone cysts in the distal aspect of the tibia of three horses. Can Vet J 1996;37:429–431.

SLAB AND SAGITTAL FRACTURES OF THE CENTRAL AND THIRD TARSAL BONES

Slab and sagittal fractures of the central and third tarsal bones are most commonly a racing injury, with Standardbreds overrepresented,[21,24] but the condition also has been reported in Thoroughbreds, Quarter horses, Warmbloods, and an Arabian.[8,10,13,16] The left hindlimb of Standardbreds is affected more commonly[13] but there is no predisposition in other breeds.

Etiology

The distal tarsal bones are subjected to axial compression, torsional forces, and tensile forces during exercise. Their main function is, as reported, to absorb concussion and neutralize these twisting forces.[19] When these bones are subjected to the even greater stress of racing speeds, fracture can occur.[21] Rooney described the normal biomechanics of the hock and concluded that asynchronous movement of these tarsal bones due to ligament damage or rapid changes in lead may result in the fracture.[17] A similar fracture that occurs in the right tarsus in racing Greyhounds is thought to result from an overstress mechanism[4] which may also occur in horses. The excessive medial stress that focuses on the right tarsus during counterclockwise racing is thought to result in the fracture. Although a similar mechanism has been considered in the horse,[8] it has not been substantiated in the review of 11 cases in which the right and left tarsus were almost equally affected.[21] No training effect on bone density was demonstrated after 19 weeks of progressive training in a group of Thoroughbreds compared to others that walked for 40 minutes daily.[22] Possibly the treadmill fails to duplicate training stresses, or the incidence of fracture is related more to conformation or incident than training.

Collapse of the dorsal or dorsolateral portion of the third tarsal bone has been described in foals, but the predisposition of this injury is thought to be the lack of bone strength related to a dysmaturity or metabolic or endocrine disorder.[9,11] Younger foals tend to "wedge" the dorsal margins of the central and third tarsal bones, whereas older (or more mature) foals may collapse the more plantar portion of the bone, producing an hourglass shape in the lateromedial or dorsoplantar medial to lateral oblique radiograph.[2,18] Once mature, horses with third tarsal bones with the hourglass-shape tend to fracture at the narrowest point (Figure 5.307).[3] If they separate completely, and the fragment becomes displaced, an angular limb deformity may result.

Clinical Signs

The diagnosis of central and third tarsal bone fractures can be difficult, especially when swelling is minimal and a nondisplaced slab fracture exists.[21] Horses typically present with a history of acute onset of severe lameness that diminishes relatively quickly. However, more lameness can be expected with extremely comminuted fractures. Distal tarsal fractures do not exhibit external swelling, even when they are displaced dorsally. Because there is a communication between the PIT joint and the TC joint, tarsocrural joint effusion is usually seen with slab fractures of the central tarsal bone.[21] On palpation, heat and pain leading to discomfort may be appreciated when pressure is applied to the dorsolateral aspect of the distal row of tarsal bones.[8] A marked reaction to the hock flexion test is usually observed. If bilateral fractures are present, the horse has a wide-based "crabby" way of moving at a jog.

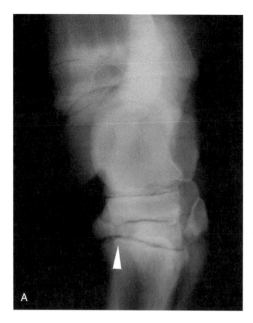
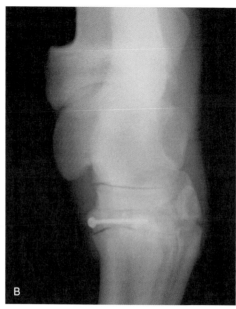

Figure 5.307. A. Radiograph showing slab fracture of the 3rd tarsal bone (arrow) at the point of previous collapse of the bone as a foal. B. Postoperative radiograph of the same horse after placement of a lag screw.

Diagnosis

The lameness does not specifically incriminate the distal tarsus. Intrasynovial anesthesia of the proximal and distal intertarsal joints or (if distended) tarsocrural joint may be helpful.

Although the dorsoplantar and lateral projections are informative, the oblique projections are helpful to identify fragmentation and the specific position of these fractures.[8,10,15,21] The central tarsal bone tends to fracture along the dorsomedial aspect, whereas the third tarsal bone is more often affected dorsally or dorsolaterally.[8,21] Central tarsal fractures may be comminuted in a more plantar location, and the dorsoplantar view should be examined for a sagittal fracture. The dorsomedial-plantarolateral 25° oblique view often demonstrates the fracture line well.[6] Comminution or fractures in the sagittal plane may not appear in routine radiographic projection. In some cases, projection 5° to 10° to either side of the normal angle of projection may reveal the fracture (Figure 5.308). Radiographic evidence of OA usually appears with tarsal bone fractures of long duration.[1,5,11,12]

Radiographic evidence of the fracture may not appear for some time after injury if the fracture is nondisplaced.[20] With localization of the source of the lameness and no definitive radiographic lesion, scintigraphy or computed tomography may be helpful.[7,10,20] Computed tomography can also be helpful to determine if a fracture is a single slab that is repairable or comminuted and not repairable (Figure 4.268 in Chapter 4).

Treatment

Acute fractures should be repaired quickly to facilitate reduction and prevent degenerative changes in the joint. Lag screw fixation has been reported to provide the best chance for the horse to return to performance (Figure 5.308).[8,21,23,24] Reports include 15 of 18, 1 of 1 (2 reports), 4 of 4, and 2 of 2 horses with surgically

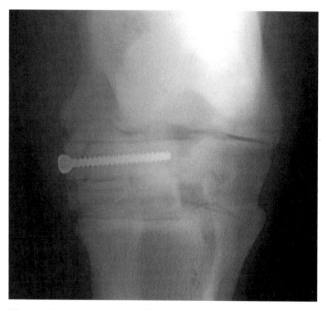

Figure 5.308. A slightly offset dorsoplantar radiograph of the tarsus after lag screw repair of a central tarsal bone fracture. (Courtesy of Dr. Gary Baxter.)

repaired fractures returning to work.[8,10,16,21,24] Surgical repair by lag screw fixation requires radiographic or fluoroscopic imaging. Fluoroscopy facilitates efficient, accurate placement of the drill. Placing the X-ray beam in the same plane of the fracture and centered on the fractured bone is critical for accurate placement of the screw in the parent bone. Third tarsal bones with hourglass compressions are more challenging for central screw placement,[21] and the shape of the bone is permanent.[3]

Successful repairs have been reported using ASIF 4.5- and 3.5-mm cortical screws and 4.5-mm Herbert cannulated compressing screws.[8,10,16,21,24] Each requires a slightly different progression of drilling. Regardless of size or type, cannulated screws work nicely in this type of situation. Where possible, 2 screws may improve stability.[14] In the third tarsal bone, the screws must diverge to miss the notch in the plantar aspect of the bone. If prolonged lameness persists in spite of apparently successful repair, removal of the screw may be necessary.

Some reports indicate satisfactory results without surgery.[13,20] In one series of 25 cases, horses that recovered were restricted to the stall for 6 to 8 months.[13] The fracture line remained radiographically visible in each of 5 horses for which follow-up films were taken, but this was not correlated to a negative result. Ten of 12 Standardbreds with available race records completed at least 5 races after the injury; the median number of starts was 47. Two of 6 Thoroughbreds and 4 of 5 Quarter horses returned to work. Although thickness of the fragment was not correlated to starts, earnings decreased for horses with fragments more than 8 mm thick. The proportion of successful cases with central tarsal bone fractures (2 of 7) was significantly less than those with third tarsal bone fractures (10 of 13).[13] All 3 horses that were treated conservatively in one report were unable to return to training due to persistent lameness.[8]

Prognosis

With surgical repair, a combined 22 of 28 horses returned to performance.[8,10,16,24] Convalescence varied between 3 and 8 months. Presence of OA at presentation diminishes the prognosis for athletic function. Accurate prognosis depends upon detection of all of the fracture lines, particularly with central tarsal bone fractures. The proportion of successful cases with central tarsal bone fractures was less than those with third tarsal bone fractures. This could be due to nonunion of comminuted fragments or tarsocrural OA. Mares treated conservatively are usually sound enough for breeding.

Not all horses are candidates for surgical repair.[8,21] Some comminuted central tarsal bone fractures are impossible to repair, and some comminution is never seen on radiographs before surgery. Winberg reported that zero of 2 horses with plantar central tarsal bone fractures returned to athletic activity.[24]

Successful conservative therapy in a recent series was likely due to the 6- to 8-month period of stall confinement to allow a firm fibrous union; convalescence time ranged from 2 to 44 months.[13] Ten of 12 horses raced successfully.[20] The presence of degenerative changes at the time of diagnosis may not preclude a successful outcome with sufficient stall rest.[13,21]

References

1. Adams OR. Lameness in Horses. 3rd ed. Lea and Febiger, Philadelphia, 1974.
2. Auer JA. Angular limb deformities. In Equine Medicine and Surgery, Vol. II, 5th ed. Colahan PT, Mayhew IG, Merritt AM, et al., eds. Santa Barbara, American Veterinary Publications, 1999;1691.
3. Baird DH, Pilsworth RC. Wedge-shaped conformation of the dorsolateral aspect of the third tarsal bone in the thoroughbred racehorse is associated with development of slab fractures in this site. Equine Veterinary Journal 2001;33:617–620.
4. Dee JF, Dee J, Piermattei DL. Classification, management and repair of central tarsal fractures in the racing greyhound. J Am Anim Hosp Assoc 1976;12:398.
5. Gill HE. Diagnosis and treatment of hock lameness. Proc Am Assoc Eq Pract 1973;19:257.
6. Greet G, Greet TRC. The use of specific radiographic projections to demonstrate three intra-articular fractures. Eq Vet Educ 1996;8:208–211.
7. Kelmer G, Wilson DA, Essman SC. Computed tomography assisted repair of a central tarsal bone slab fracture in a horse. Eq Vet Educ 2008;20:284–287.
8. Lindsay WA, McMartin RB, McClure JR. Management of slab fractures of the third tarsal bone in 5 horses. Eq Vet J 1982;14:55–58.
9. Lokai MD, Ford J. Disorders of endochondral ossification. Eq Pract 1981;3:48.
10. Martin F, Herthel DJ. Central tarsal bone fractures in six horses: Report on the use of a cannulated compression bone screw. Eq Pract 1992;14:23–27.
11. Morgan JP. Necrosis of the third tarsal bone of the horse. J Am Vet Med Assoc 1967;151:1334–1342.
12. Moyer W. Bone spavin: A clinical review. J Eq Med Surg 1978; 2:362.
13. Murphey ED, Schneider RK, Adams SB, et al. Long-term outcome of horses with a slab fracture of the central or third tarsal bone treated conservatively: 25 cases (1976–1993). J Am Vet Med Assoc 2000;216:1949–1954.
14. Nixon A. Fractures of specific tarsal bones. In Equine Fracture Repair. Nixon A, ed. WB Saunders, Philadelphia, 1996; 260–267.
15. O'Brien T. Radiographic interpretation of the equine tarsus. Proc Am Assoc Eq Pract 1973;19:289.
16. Ramey DW. Use of lag screw fixation for repair of a central tarsal bone fracture in a horse. J Am Vet Med Assoc 1988;192: 1451–1452.
17. Rooney JR. Biomechanics of Lameness in Horses. Williams and Wilkins Co., Baltimore, 1969.
18. Ruohoniemi M, Hilden L, Salo L, et al. Monitoring the progression of tarsal ossification with ultrasonography and radiography in three immature foals. Vet Radiol Ultra 1995;36:402–410.
19. Schebitz H. Spavin: Radiographic diagnosis and treatment. Proc Am Assoc Eq Pract 1965;11:207.
20. Stover SM, Hornof WJ, Richardson GL, et al. Bone scintigraphy as an aid in the diagnosis of occult distal tarsal bone trauma in three horses. J Am Vet Med Assoc 1986;188:624–628.
21. Tulamo RM, Bramlage LR, Gabel AA. Fractures of the central and third tarsal bones in horses. J Am Vet Med Assoc 1983;182:1234–1238.
22. Whitton RC, Murray RC, Buckley C, et al. An MRI study of the effect of treadmill training on bone morphology of the central and third tarsal bones of young thoroughbred horses. Eq Vet J Supp 1999;30:258–261.
23. Winberg EG, Pettersson H. Internal fixation of third and central tarsal bone fractures in the horse: A review. Vet Surg 1993;22:252.
24. Winberg FG, Pettersson H. Outcome and racing performance after internal fixation of third and central tarsal bone slab fractures in horses. A review of 20 cases. Acta Vet Scand 1999; 40:173–180.

INTRA-ARTICULAR FRACTURES OF THE TARSOCRURAL JOINT

Intra-articular fractures of the tarsocrural joint are relatively uncommon. In a study of 125 fatal racing accidents, 31 horses had fractures and other injuries of the hindlimb and the tarsal joint was only involved in 2 of these.[11] Baker recorded 1 fracture of the tarsus out of a total of 35 fractures in a survey of 480 cases.[1] Jakovljevic reported 13 cases of traumatic fractures of the tarsal bones, which represented 5.8% of all the horses subjected to radiographs of the hock.[4] One report lists an order of decreasing frequency in 13 cases: tibial malleoli, 5 (4 lateral, 1 medial); fibular tarsal bone, 4 (3 sustentaculum tali, 1 calcaneus); tibial tarsal bone, 3 (2 medial condyle, 1 both condyles); and the fourth metatarsal bone, 1.[4] Fractures of the tibiotarsal bone involve the trochlear ridges or the body of the talus. Older literature often refers to fragments of the distal intermediate ridge of the tibia and distal lateral trochlear ridge as fractures; they are most often OCD.

Clinical Signs

Intra-articular fractures cause tarsocrural effusion, and lameness is usually exacerbated by hindlimb flexion. Although usually not necessary, intra-articular local anesthesia relieves the lameness and response to flexion. If blood is retrieved when the needle enters the joint, the local anesthetic should not be injected, and the hock radiographed at that time. Radiographic examination is required to make a definitive diagnosis.

Trochlear Ridge Fractures

The trochlear ridges are affected by direct trauma, the proximal (caudal) medial ridge is exposed when the limb is flexed, and the distal lateral trochlear ridge is exposed when the limb is extended.[2] Horses are kicked while preparing to kick another horse, resulting in a fracture of the proximal medial trochlear ridge (Figure 5.309).[8–10]

The diagnosis is made based upon the clinical signs and radiographic findings. Proximal medial trochlear ridge fragments appear in routine radiographic projections, but they are often superimposed upon the tibia or tibial tarsal bone. The flexed lateromedial, flexed proximal-distal tangential, or flexed dorsolateral to ventromedial oblique views demonstrate the lesions (Figure 5.309). Distal lateral trochlear ridge fragments should be differentiated from OCD, which is much

more common. The history, shape of the lesion, and degree of lameness are most helpful in making a differentiation.

Proximal medial trochlear ridge lesions can be removed arthroscopically using a plantar approach.[7,13] Distal lateral trochlear ridge lesions are addressed using the routine tarsal arthroscopic approach.[5] Provided OA has not begun or associated soft tissue injury is not limiting, the prognosis is good after fragment removal. Before any horse suffering tarsal trauma is anesthetized, integrity of the collateral ligaments should be confirmed by physical or ultrasound examination.

Sagittal or Comminuted Fractures Of The Talus

Sagittal fractures of the talus may be nondisplaced (at least early) and can be difficult to identify radiographically. The dorsoplantar radiographic projection is the most useful, but slightly oblique variations may better demonstrate the fracture line.[7]

In a series of 11 horses with incomplete sagittal talus fractures, Standardbred racehorses were overrepresented.[3] All horses had a history of chronic hindlimb lameness that became an acute grade 2 to 4 of 5 lameness. Tarsocrural effusion varied from absent to moderate, and hindlimb flexion was markedly positive in 6 of the 7 horses in which flexion was performed. A dorsoplantar or radiographic projection 10° to 20° off dorsoplantar toward dorsolateral-plantaromedial has been described as best.[3] Digital radiographs or scintigraphy may be required to make the diagnosis. Scintigraphy revealed moderate to intense uptake in the proximal aspect of the talus of all 11 horses, 6 of which were radiographically negative. The flexed lateral scintigram was useful because it separates the proximal talus from the distal tibia. All horses were treated conservatively with a month or more of stall rest and a month or more of small paddock turnout. Seven horses returned to racing 115 to 341 days after the injury.

Displaced, noncomminuted sagittal fractures can be repaired using lag screws.[4,6,7] These fractures generally occur toward the medial aspect of the trochlea. Successful lag screw fixation from the lateral[6] and medial[7] approaches have been described. The medial approach provides more bone for the screw to purchase for compression of the fracture line.

Radiographic or fluoroscopic guidance is necessary, and for displaced fractures, arthroscopic observation of reduction is advisable. With accurate reduction and no degenerative changes, the outcome reported has been good.[6,7]

Comminuted fractures are not as challenging to diagnose but are often irreparable. Osteoarthritis and/or instability usually require horses to be euthanatized.

Fractures of the Tibial Malleoli

The tibial malleoli are fractured by direct trauma or avulsion of the collateral ligaments. The majority of horses in 2 reports acquired the injuries in a fall, and the lateral malleolus was affected most commonly. A kick from another horse can also result in this fracture.[4,12] The fractures are demonstrated well in dorsoplantar or oblique radiographs; the entire joint should

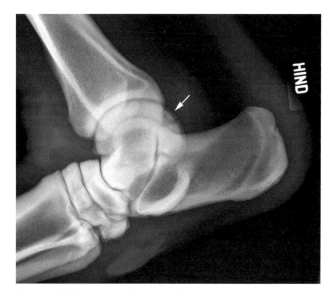

Figure 5.309. Flexed lateromedial radiograph of the tarsus of a horse with a 2-month history of lameness. A large fracture fragment can be seen on the plantar aspect of the medial trochlear ridge of the talus (arrow). (Courtesy of Dr. Gary Baxter.)

be scrutinized for migrating loose bodies. The oblique films should be evaluated to determine the total size of the fragment, which may be misleading. Concurrent collateral ligament injury is a vital consideration and is discussed more extensively later. If collateral ligament damage has occurred, general anesthesia can result in catastrophic luxation. Either a cast can be employed to protect the horse or surgery can be delayed until the soft tissue has healed. Intra-articular sodium hyaluronate is indicated to control synovitis if effusion is present and surgery is delayed.

Treatment

The medial malleolus is affected less often, but the fragment tends to be large enough for lag-screw repair (Figure 5.310). The articular surface must be reconstructed accurately to prevent subsequent OA. Provided stability is attained, perfect reduction of the remainder of the fracture line is less important.[7] Radiographic or fluoroscopic monitoring of screw placement is important to avoid contacting the medial trochlear ridge with hardware. Return to soundness is possible provided that the above complications are avoided.[7] Much of the medial malleolus is well within the tarsocrural joint and accessible arthroscopically for removal of smaller fragments. One medial malleolar fracture treated by stall rest recovered to pleasure horse status.[4]

The lateral malleolus is largely invested in the joint capsule and collateral ligament. The intra-articular portion is limited to the actual joint surface. Many fractures affect the most dorsal portion where the short collateral ligament attaches, but some affect the entire malleolus through to the caudal compartment of the joint. When the fragments are small or comminuted, removal is indicated. The collateral ligament and some small fragments may retract into the periarticular soft tissue, making removal of the fragments inadvisable and

unnecessary. Although unproven, the author's experience indicates that bone fragments may slow the healing of the collateral ligament fibers back to the fracture site, so time and ultrasonographic monitoring are important.

Marginally sized fragments that are repaired by internal fixation may split during the convalescent period and require removal. Three of 4 lateral malleolar fractures treated by stall rest returned to athletic activity.[4]

Prognosis

One author reports 50% return to performance following surgical repair with internal fixation of lateral malleolar fractures.[2] Overall good results are reported after removal of relatively small fragments.[12] Many of these fragments can be removed arthroscopically with minimal dissection into the joint capsule. In summary, the importance of the fragment to the integrity of the joint and the ability to repair it should be considered. The persistence of tarsocrural effusion following anti-inflammatory therapy is an indication for arthroscopic exploration.

References

1. Baker JR, Ellis CE. A survey of post mortem findings in 480 horses 1958 to 1980: (2) Disease processes not directly related to the cause of death. Equine Vet J 1981;13:47–50.
2. Foerner JJ. Surgical treatment of selected musculoskeletal disorders of the rear limb. In Equine Surgery, 1st ed. Auer JA, ed. Saunders, Philadelphia, 1992;1055–1075.
3. Hammer EJ, Ross MW, Parente EJ. Incomplete sagittal fracture of the talus in 11 racehorses. Proc Am Assoc Eq Pract 1999;45:162–163.
4. Jakovljevic S, Gibbs C, Yeats JJ. Traumatic fractures of the equine hock: A report of 13 cases. Eq Vet J 1982;14:62–68.
5. McIlwraith CW, Nixon AJ, Wright IM, et al. Arthroscopic surgery of the tarsocrural joint. In Diagnostic and Surgical Arthroscopy in the horse. 3rd ed. Elsevier, Philadelphia, 2005; 280–294.
6. Meagher DM, Mackey VS. Lag screw fixation of a sagittal fracture of the talus in the horse. J Equine Vet Sci 1991; 10:108–112.
7. Nixon A. Fractures of specific tarsal bones. In Equine Fracture Repair. Nixon A, ed. WB Saunders, Philadelphia, 1996; 260–267.
8. Specht TE, Moran A. What is your diagnosis? J Am Vet Med Assoc 1990;196:1307–1308.
9. Sullins KE, Stashak TS. An unusual fracture of the tibiotarsal bone in a mare. J Am Vet Med Assoc 1983;182:1395–1396.
10. Tulleners EP, Reid CF. An unusual fracture of the tarsus in two horses. J Am Vet Med Assoc 1981;178:291–294.
11. Vaughan LC, Mason BJE. A clinicopathologic study of racing accidents in horses. Adlard and Son, Ltd., Dorking, Surrey, 1975;70.
12. Wright IM. Fractures of the lateral malleolus of the tibia in 16 horses. Equine Vet J 1992;24:424–429.
13. Zamos DT, Honnas CM, Hoffman AG. Arthroscopic and intra-articular anatomy of the plantar pouch of the equine tarsocrural joint. Vet Surg 1994;23:161–166.

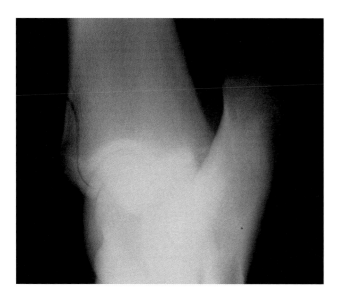

Figure 5.310. Oblique radiograph of a horse that had been kicked on the medial aspect of the tarsus. This articular fracture of the medial malleolus was repaired with lag screws. (Courtesy of Dr. Gary Baxter.)

FRACTURES OF THE FIBULAR TARSAL BONE (CALCANEUS)

Fractures of the fibular tarsal bone (calcaneus) are relatively uncommon.[8] The fractures can either be simple chip fractures involving the plantar surface, or extend completely through the growth plate in foals or through the body in mature horses (Figure 5.311).[7,12,16] Chip fractures involving the plantar surface can be easily missed. In some cases, however, they go on to form sequestra. Physeal fractures and fractures through the body of the bone are often open and are not difficult to diagnose because of the obvious loss of flexor support (Figure 5.312).[7,12]

The sustentaculum also can be injured, resulting in either a fracture or delayed exostosis that produces synovitis of the tarsal sheath (Figure 5.313).[6,10,20] The significance of the lesion is the resultant abrasion injury

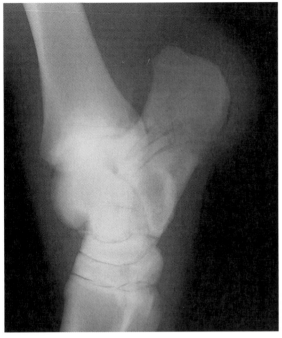

Figure 5.311. A mid-body fracture of the calcaneus is seen on this lateral radiograph. The fracture is not displaced and potentially could be repaired with a tension-band plate applied along the caudal aspect of the calcaneus. (Courtesy of Dr. Dan Burba.)

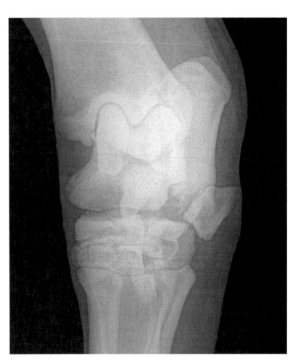

Figure 5.312. Slightly oblique radiograph of an aged Quarter horse mare with a comminuted fracture of the distal aspect of the calcaneus. There is also luxation of the PIT joint secondary to the trauma. (Courtesy of Dr. Gary Baxter.)

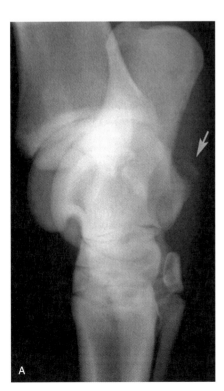

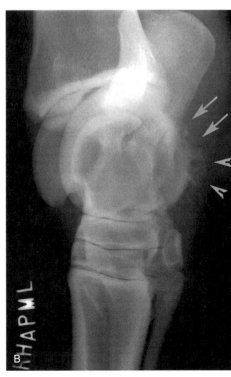

Figure 5.313. A. Dorsomedial-plantarolateral view of a horse that sustained an injury to the sustentaculum tali. At presentation, a draining tract was present and a sequestrum could be seen (arrow). B. Months after surgical debridement and healing of the wound, a large exostosis was noted on the gliding surface of the DDFT (arrows). The horse retained an abnormal gait that could not be changed with local analgesia, likely caused by mechanical interference from adhesions.

to the deep digital flexor tendon; the tendon sheath also may undergo dystrophic calcification.[6] Infection sometimes complicates the situation in this location as well.[9,14,18]

Etiology and Diagnosis

In most cases these fractures occur from external trauma, either from being kicked by another horse or from the affected horse kicking a solid object. The affected areas include the body or proximal epiphysis in foals and the sustentaculum tali. Penetrating wounds have also been implicated in sustentaculum injuries.

Nondisplaced fractures of the body may be difficult to diagnose on physical examination unless an obvious swelling is present or a draining tract associated with sequestration is observed. On the other hand, displaced fractures through the body or epiphysis are easily diagnosed because there is an obvious loss of function of the gastrocnemius muscle, and the horse will assume a dropped hock appearance.[7] The definitive diagnosis is made on radiographic examination. The lateromedial and oblique views are most important to identify the exact location and extent of the fracture (Figures 5.311 and 5.312).

Lesions on the sustentaculum may appear on the lateromedial or dorsomedial-plantarolateral oblique projections. However, the gliding surface is best demonstrated in a flexed tangential (skyline) projection.[15] Contrast arthrography has been described;[3,4] however, sustentaculum lesions may be more efficiently evaluated (and treated) tenoscopically.[1] Ultrasound also may be helpful in predicting and giving a prognosis for the tenoscopic findings.[13] Some sustentacular injuries may result in a sequestrum or septic tenosynovitis and drainage.[9,14,18]

Treatment

Surgical excision of the chip fractures of the fibular tarsal bone may not be necessary unless they enter the tarsocrural joint or become sequestered and are accessible to surgical excision.[11]

Although fractures through the calcaneal tuber can be difficult to reduce and stabilize, they have been treated successfully with bone plates using the tension-band principle, with the additional support of a full-limb cast.[7,16] A tension-band plate is placed on the plantar aspect of the calcaneus beneath the tendon of the superficial flexor tendon to neutralize the distracting forces (Figure 5.311). The surgeons in 2 studies believe it is important to remove the plate to re-establish tarsal mobility.[7,16] Recovery from anesthesia is safer in a cast, which can be removed immediately if desired. In another report on surgical treatment of this fracture, one case involved a combination of internal fixation and external coaptation.[17] The treatment was successful. Conservative approaches using casting alone have not proven to be rewarding.[8] Presumably due to the tension from the tendon of the gastrocnemius, severely comminuted fractures of the tuber calcis fail to heal in spite of immobilization in a cast.

Fractures through the growth plate in young horses are rare in the author's experience. An attempt to treat an open fracture resulted in osteomyelitis. The apophysis in a foal is small and mostly cartilaginous; it is incapable of supporting the distraction by means of a single screw. Shaping the plate to cover the apophysis or using a hooked plate adds support similar to that used for olecranon fractures in foals. A cast lends further stability.

Treatment of lesions of the sustentaculum must leave a smooth surface to prevent damage to the tendon and recurrent synovitis. When a surface lesion of the bone or sepsis cannot be confirmed, intra-synovial anti-inflammatory therapy may be successful. Tenoscopy is a more accurate procedure.[1] Although successful treatment has been reported after a long delay,[19] early treatment minimizes permanent damage. The overall outcome for chronically affected horses is poor.[5,6,20] If the wound is acute and open, it is a surgical emergency. The goal of surgical therapy is debridement of the bony lesion and associated changes within the tendon sheath; septic lesions require lavage and drainage. Successes are reported after conventional open surgery;[2,9,15,18] however, tenoscopy disrupts less tissue and is preferred when possible.[1] See Osteomyelitis of the Sustentaculum Tali, below.

Prognosis

The prognosis for chip fracture of the calcaneus is considered good to guarded, depending on its location (intra-articular vs. extra-articular), the size of the fragment, and whether it has become a sequestrum.

The prognosis for fractures of the growth plate and through the body is considered poor for return to full function. The outcome of fractures of the body of the calcaneus depends upon the ability to stabilize the fragments.[7,16,17] Distraction from pull of the gastrocnemius precludes successful conservative therapy of unstable fractures.

The prognosis must be guarded to poor until proven otherwise for lesions in the tarsal canal. However, favorable results have been reported, making the attempt worthwhile.[9,20] See Osteomyelitis of the Sustentaculum Tali below.

References

1. Cauvin ER, Tapprest J, Munroe GA, et al. Endoscopic examination of the tarsal sheath of the lateral digital flexor tendon in horses. Equine Vet J 1999;31:219–227.
2. Dart AJ, Hodgson DR. Surgical management of osteomyelitis of the sustentaculum tali in a horse. Aust Vet J 1996;73:73–74.
3. Dik KJ, Keg PR. The efficacy of contrast radiography to demonstrate "false thoroughpins" in five horses. Equine Vet J 1990;22:223–225.
4. Dik KJ, Leitch M. Soft tissue injuries of the tarsus. Vet Clin NA Eq Pract 1995;11:235–247.
5. Dik KJ, Merkens HW. Unilateral distension of the tarsal sheath in the horse: A report of 11 cases. Equine Vet J 1987;19:307–313.
6. Edwards GB. Changes in the sustentaculum tali associated with distension of the tarsal sheath (thoroughpin). Equine Vet J 1978;10:97–102.
7. Ferguson JG, Presnell KR. Tension band plating of a fractured equine fibular tarsal bone. Can Vet J 1976;17:314–317.
8. Fessler JF, Amstutz HE. Fracture repair. In Lea and Febiger, Philadelphia, Williams and Wilkins Co., Baltimore, 1974.

9. Hand R, Watkins JP, Honnas CM, et al. Treatment of osteomyelitis of the sustentaculum tali and associated tenosynovitis in horses: 10 cases (1992–1998). Proc Am Assoc Eq Pract 1999; 45:158–159.

10. Hilbert BJ, Jenkinson G. Exostosis on the medial border of the calcaneus. J Am Vet Med Assoc 1984;184:1403–1404.

11. Jakovljevic S, Gibbs C, Yeats JJ. Traumatic fractures of the equine hock: A report of 13 cases. Eq Vet J 1982;14:62–68.

12. O'Brien T. Radiographic interpretation of the equine tarsus. Proc Am Assoc Eq Pract 1973;19:289.

13. Reef VB. Equine Diagnostic Ultrasound. WB Saunders Co., Philadelphia, 1998.

14. Santschi EM, Adams SB, Fessler JF, et al. Treatment of lesions of the sustentaculum of the calcaneus accompanied by tarsal sheath synovitis. Proceedings Am Assoc Equine Pract 1993;39: 249–250.

15. Santschi EM, Adams SB, Fessler JF, et al. Treatment of bacterial tarsal tenosynovitis and osteitis of the sustentaculum tali of the calcaneus in five horses. Equine Vet J 1997;29:244–247.

16. Scott EA. Surgical repair of a dislocated superficial digital flexor tendon and fractured fibular tarsal bone in a horse. J Am Vet Med Assoc 1983;183:332–333.

17. Stashak TS. The femur-trochanteric bursitis. In Adams' Lameness in Horses, 4th ed. Lea and Febiger, Baltimore, 1987;747–748.

18. Tulleners EP, Reid CF. Osteomyelitis of the sustentaculum talus in a pony. J Am Vet Med Assoc 1981;178:290–291.

19. Welch RD, Auer JA, Watkins JP, et al. Surgical treatment of tarsal sheath effusion associated with an exostosis on the calcaneus of a horse. J Am Vet Med Assoc 1990;196:1992–1994.

20. Wilderjans H. New bone growth on the sustentaculum tali and medial aspect of the calcaneal bone surrounding the deep digital flexor tendon in a pony. Eq Vet Educ 1990;2:184–187.

OSTEOMYELITIS AND OSTEOLYTIC LESIONS OF THE CALCANEAL TUBER

The calcaneus is exposed at the plantar aspect of the hock and subject to injury from and by kicking. Penetrating trauma is also relatively common. Of 50 horses with radiographic calcaneal lesions, 29 had osteomyelitis, including 4 foals with septic apophysitis.[3] Infection and trauma tend to involve the attachments of the gastrocnemius tendon, SDFT, and calcaneal bursa.

Clinical Signs and Diagnosis

Lameness usually results at the time of the incident. Inflammation at the attachments of the gastrocnemius tendon and calcaneal bursitis can be extremely painful. Penetrating wounds with or without infection are obvious. All radiographic views are needed, but the 45° dorsomedial to plantarolateral oblique and flexed skyline views are especially useful if the horse is not too painful for the flexion (Figure 5.314).[3] Radiographic signs include soft tissue swelling, osseous lysis, fragments/sequestra, and new bone production more commonly associated with chronic conditions.

Ultrasound may reveal disruptions of the tendons or bursa. When drainage is present, there is a high probability of a sequestrum.[3] Penetrating wounds should be evaluated completely before septic tendinitis or bursitis becomes established. Contrast radiography under aseptic conditions may be advisable.

In 9 of 50 horses studied, chronic aseptic osseous lesions were seen on the medial, lateral, or caudolateral aspect of the calcaneus where the gastrocnemius and SDFT insert.[3] These radiographic signs were associated with persistent lameness.

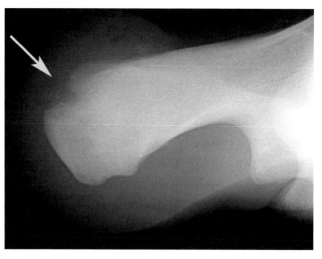

Figure 5.314. Skyline view of the calcaneus of a horse with osteomyelitis from a puncture wound (arrow).

Treatment

Septic wounds should be surgically debrided and drainage established for resolution of the infectious process. Bacterial culture and sensitivity is important in these cases, because the infection tends to be well established when treatment begins. In a series of 28 horses with calcaneal osteomyelitis, a statistical difference in results of surgical or medical therapy could not be demonstrated.[2] In another study, 9 of 14 horses worsened in spite of appropriate therapy,[3] demonstrating that this condition tends to persist. Horses with radiographic changes limited to soft tissue developed osseous lesions within an average of 9 weeks. Sound practice still dictates that septic necrotic tissue be removed because the septic processes tend to progress to the tendons or bursa.[3]

Non-infected bursitis still causes significant lameness. When medical therapy fails or if there are radiographic changes, arthroscopic exploration (bursoscopy) is indicated.[1] Bursal or osseous tissue is debrided where it has been disrupted. Local and systemic anti-inflammatory therapy is indicated.

Prognosis

The prognosis is guarded. Affected horses tend to be lame and may remain so for long periods of time, possibly due to the continued tension of weight-bearing at the attachments of the gastrocnemius and superficial flexor tendons and the compression beneath the superficial flexor on the bursal surface. The healing must be complete and congruent on the bursal surface or chronic bursitis will result.

Of 26 horses treated for calcaneal osteomyelitis, 6 became sound, although 18 survived.[2] Six horses returned for treatment, suffering from chronic osteomyelitis. Breeding soundness is a more certain goal. These relatively poor results were undoubtedly negatively influenced by the mean time of 2 months' duration of clinical signs before treatment.

Horses with aseptic bursitis also recover poorly.[1] The surface must be healed sufficiently to avert synovitis and chronic bursitis.

References

1. Bassage LH 2nd, Garcia-Lopez J, Currid EM. Osteolytic lesions of the tuber calcanei in two horses. J Am Vet Med Assoc 2000;217:710–716, 674.
2. MacDonald MH, Honnas CM, Meagher DM. Osteomyelitis of the calcaneus in horses: 28 cases (1972–1987). J Am Vet Med Assoc 1989;194:1317–1323.
3. Mattoon JS, O'Brien TR. Radiographic evaluation of the calcaneus in the horse: A retrospective study. Proc Am Assoc Eq Pract 1988;34:369–379.

SUBLUXATIONS AND LUXATIONS OF THE TARSAL JOINTS

Subluxations and luxations of all 4 tarsal joints have been reported in the literature, and avulsion fractures may occur concurrently.[1,4]

Etiology

A severe wrenching or twisting action that may occur from a sudden slip or fall is believed to be the cause in most cases.[1] Kicks from other horses and entrapment in fixed objects such as fences or cattle guards have also been implicated.[2,9] Even simply kicking a wall can result in a luxation.[5]

Clinical Signs and Diagnosis

The signs are usually quite obvious; an affected animal presents with a nonweight-bearing limb deformity associated with the tarsal joints. Usually the limb is freely moveable distal to the luxation. The exact location and extent of damage must be verified with radiographs. Luxation of the tarsocrural joint is the most severe, and the tibia is usually displaced distad and craniad, making it difficult or impossible to reduce (Figure 5.315). Talocalcaneal luxation is characterized by a separation between the affected joint.

Treatment

Reduction and immobilization with a full-limb cast suffices in many cases of subluxation, luxation, and simple fracture.[1,5,7] Early reduction is important because some luxations cannot be reduced. Flexion can facilitate reduction.[4] Suspending the dorsally recumbent horse from a hoist attached to the affected limb has worked, but the traction should be reduced so the joint surfaces are allowed to appose before fixation is applied. A luxation that is not severely displaced with a flat surface to buttress the proximal component is most amenable to simple cast immobilization. The cast should be applied as close to the stifle as possible to maximize immobilization of the tarsal area and maintained for at least 6 weeks. The congruity of the tarsocrural joint and buttress of the distal joint surfaces seem to aid in stabilization.[5]

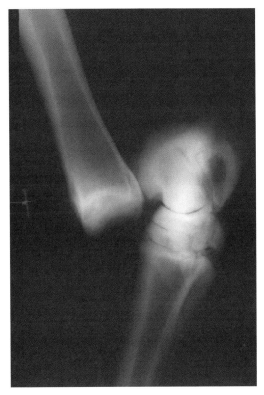

Figure 5.315. Lateromedial radiograph of a horse suffering a tarsocrural luxation. This type of luxation is extremely uncommon in horses but this horse survived.

The luxations associated with comminuted tarsal bone fracture or oblique weight-bearing surfaces require a combination of internal fixation and casting (Figure 5.316).[4,6,8] Some cases require an open approach and curettage or debridement to achieve reduction. When visible, curettage of the articular cartilage from the surfaces of the distal tarsal bones facilitates ankylosis. The tarsocrural joint has been successfully reduced.[3,7] However, it deserves special consideration of potential OA. The talocalcaneal luxation tends to be wedged apart by axial weight-bearing and requires internal fixation.

Prognosis

It is worthwhile to attempt reduction of any tarsal luxation in which stability could be expected. Complications such as excessive contamination or destruction of the tarsocrural joint surfaces are examples of important factors to be considered. The prognosis is reasonably good for simple luxation of the distal tarsal joints without fracture; however, the prognosis decreases from this point if fracture is present. Injuries restricted to the nonmoveable joints offer the most hope for a functional recovery (Figure 5.317). Successful reports include cast immobilization of distal tarsal[3] and tarsocrural[7] luxations reduced and placed in casts for 4 to 6 weeks. With internal fixation added, talocalcaneal[8] and unstable distal tarsal luxations[4,6] have been successfully treated.

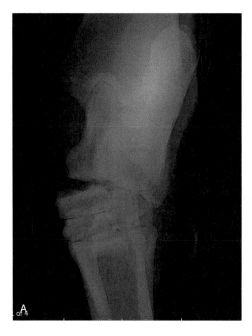
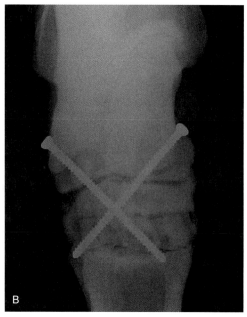

Figure 5.316. Pre- (A) and postoperative (B) dorsoplantar radiographs of a horse suffering a PIT joint luxation that was stabilized with cruciate screws and a full-limb cast. The horse did very well but after the cast was removed eventually broke one of the screws and the central tarsal bone. The screws should have been removed when the cast was removed.

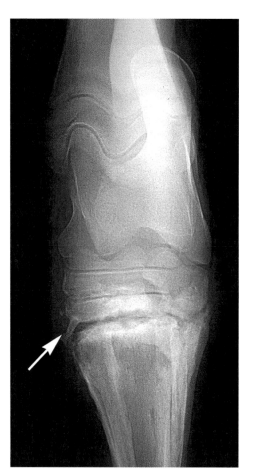

Figure 5.317. Dorsoplantar radiograph of a foal with luxation of the medial aspect of the TMT joint (arrow). A medial plate was used to stabilize the luxation and arthrodese the distal tarsal joints concurrently. (Courtesy of Dr. Gary Baxter.)

References

1. Fessler JF, Amstutz HE. Fracture repair. In Textbook of Large Animal Surgery. Oehme FW, Prier JE, eds. Williams and Wilkins Co., Baltimore, 1974.
2. Gross DR. Tarsal luxation and fracture in a pony. Mod Vet Pract 1964;45:68.
3. Laing JA, Caves SF, Rawlinson RJ. Successful treatment of a tarsocrural joint luxation in a pony. Aust Vet J 1992;69:200–201.
4. McIlwraith CW. Surgery of the hock, stifle, and shoulder horses, osteochondritis, injuries. Vet Clin N Am 1983;5:333–362.
5. Moll HD, Slone DE, Humburg JM, et al. Traumatic tarsal luxation repaired without internal fixation in three horses and three ponies. J Am Vet Med Assoc 1987;190:297–300.
6. Nixon A. Luxations of the hock. In Equine Fracture Repair. Nixon A, ed. WB Saunders, Philadelphia, 1996;270–271.
7. Reeves MJ, Trotter GW. Tarsocrural joint luxation in a horse. J Am Vet Med Assoc 1991;199:1051–1053.
8. Sullins KE. Diseases of the tarsus. In Equine Medicine and Surgery, Vol. II 5th ed. Colahan PT, Mayhew IG, Merritt AM, et al., eds. Mosby, St. Louis, 1999;1676.
9. Wheat JD, Rhoade EA. Luxation and fracture of the hock of the horse. J Am Vet Med Assoc 1964;145:341.

TALOCALCANEAL OSTEOARTHRITIS (TO)

Clinical Signs and Diagnosis

Twenty cases of TO have been reported in the literature.[1,3] Horses are reported to become acutely lame with no history of injury, although one had a history of being kicked. Some may have mild tarsocrural joint effusion and all are positive to hindlimb flexion. Response to IA anesthesia of the tarsocrural joint was variable but incomplete. Tibial/peroneal nerve anesthesia produced soundness in approximately 50% of the horses and improvement in the others.[1] Lateromedial radiographs demonstrated an irregular talocalcaneal joint space with subchondral sclerosis, osteolytic foci, and loss of joint space (Figure 5.318A). However, enhanced imaging such as MRI can be helpful to document the extent of these abnormalities (Figure 5.318B).

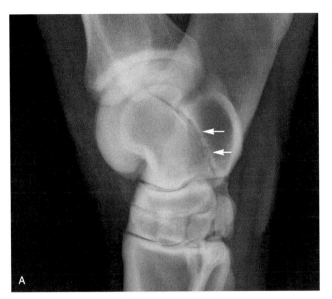 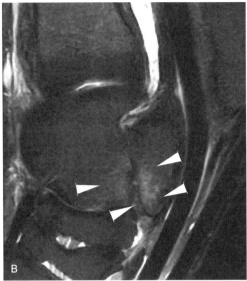

Figure 5.318. Lateral radiograph of the tarsus (A) with irregularity noted in the talocalcaneal joint (arrows) and sagittal MR image (B), demonstrating talocalcaneal degeneration as evidenced by the loss of joint space and bright signal signifying active inflammation in the subchondral bone (arrows). (Courtesy of Dr. Rich Redding [MRI] and Dr. Gary Baxter [radiograph]).

Treatment and Prognosis

In one study, all horses that were treated conservatively remained lame, and some were euthanatized. Six horses underwent surgical arthrodesis using 2 or 3 5.5-mm screws placed in a neutral fashion.[1] All of these horses improved significantly, but none became sound. One of the horses undergoing surgical arthrodesis developed contralateral TO 2 years later. One horse underwent partial tibial and deep peroneal neurectomy and another underwent surgical forage, but both remained lame.[1]

The section above on luxations of the tarsal joints described a horse that suffered a talocalcaneal luxation. The calcaneus was rotated away from the talus, opening the talocalcaneal articulation. Faced with no other choice, the talocalcaneal articulation was reduced as much as possible and stabilized with lag screw fixation, and became sound.[2] This anecdotal report together with the limited success of the surgical arthrodesis in the above reports suggests that horses with TO may be best treated surgically rather than conservatively.

References

1. Smith RKW, Dyson SJ, Schramme MC, et al. Osteoarthritis of the talocalcaneal joint in 18 horses. Equine Vet J 2005;37: 166–171(166).
2. Sullins KE. Diseases of the tarsus. In Equine Medicine and Surgery, Vol. II, 5th ed. Colahan PT, Mayhew IG, Merritt AM, et al., eds. Mosby, St. Louis, 1999;1676.
3. White NA, Turner TA. Hock lameness associated with degeneration of the talocalcaneal articulation: Report of two cases in horses. Vet Med 1980;75:678–681.

TARSOCRURAL COLLATERAL LIGAMENT DESMITIS/INSTABILITY/RUPTURE

Horses of all types are susceptible to collateral ligament (CL) injury. Affected horses comprise a diverse population of pleasure, dressage, eventing, and racehorses. One report included 9 Standardbred pacers.[1,4]

Etiology

The history varies, from observed incidents, to simply onset of lameness during training,[1] to unknown. The obvious injury is excessive strain in a valgus or varus direction, injuring the medial or lateral collateral ligament, respectively.

Because the long collateral ligaments seem to be more prone to injury, it appears that the injury occurs when the limb is extended, when those ligaments have been reported to be under the most tension.[5] The oblique angle of the trochlea causes lateral (outward) rotation of the talus during flexion.[5] In spite of relative loosening during flexion,[5] the long medial CL seems to be under more tension than the lateral. This possibly accounts for the more accidental injuries which predominately affect the long medial collateral ligament. The substance of the long medial CL is also less substantial than that of the long lateral CL.[5] The short medial CL was predominately affected in a report of one horse.[4]

Standardbred racehorses predominately injured the long lateral CL during training.[1] The long lateral CL spirals during flexion and straightens during extension as it takes the load from the short lateral CLs.[5] The authors of one study theorized that cyclic stress at racing speed was responsible,[1] which could be true. Seven of the 9 cases had histories of lameness in other limbs. Taking proportionately more weight on the hindlimb suffering the CL ligament injury could increase the forces on the CL, either from the shear forces[2] or varus tension.

Clinical Signs and Diagnosis

Horses present for hindlimb lameness localized to the tarsus relatively easily. The degree of lameness varies from subtle to nonweight-bearing; hindlimb flexion worsens the lameness. Physical exam findings usually include tarsal swelling characterized by edema and/or fibrosis localized over the medial or lateral collateral ligament region. A variable amount of tarsocrural effusion is often present but may be obscured by the periarticular edema, of which digital pressure often elicits a painful response from the horse. Local anesthesia is usually not required to isolate the problem.

Radiographs may only reveal soft tissue swelling. However, avulsion of fragments from origin or insertion of the affected collateral ligament on the adjacent tibial malleolus may be present.[4] Fragments may be intra- or extra-articular and buried within the substance of the ligament. Ultrasonography identifies the particular ligament involved and the degree of severity. However, horses with avulsion fractures seem to have short collateral ligament injury,[4] because the location of the fragments tends to be the dorsal limit of the ligamentous attachment. See the section on fractures of the tibial malleoli. Lateral collateral ligament calcification can also occur and was reported in a jumper, possibly related to sprain injury.[3] Scintigraphy is a further diagnostic aid in demonstrating the inflammation at the origin of the ligament and is useful when concurrent problems prevent a routine lameness exam.[1]

Treatment

NSAIDs are indicated for 10 to 14 days for acute injury. Cold therapy using ice water slurry in a plastic bag bandaged to the area for 20 minutes 3 to 4 times a day for 48 hours has proven beneficial. Support bandaging or splinting in the interim improves the response. Topical DMSO/furacin sweats or NSAIDs may help reduce the acute inflammation. If joint effusion is present, intra-articular sodium hyaluronate is indicated. The duration of stall rest is defined by monitoring the sonograms of the collateral ligament, but 30 to 90 days is the usual range. Horses with significant swelling or lameness should have a cast or bandage cast applied. Sleeve casts allowing continued weight-bearing and mobility of the fetlock usually suffice. Progressively decreasing the degree of immobilization from cast to bandage cast to bandage offers gradual increases in stress on the ligament. Perhaps the most important characteristics of this injury are that the instability and synovitis can subtly lead to OA, and return to work too early will result in re-injury. If the affected region continues to swell, more immobilization is indicated.

Radiographs or lack of response to IA therapy may signify co-existing intra-articular lesions. Although arthroscopic exploration is indicated, the risk of complete luxation of the joint during recovery from general anesthesia is real. The synovitis should be controlled until the collateral ligament has healed sufficiently to withstand normal forces or a cast should be used for recovery from anesthesia.

Although persisting synovitis is an indication for surgical evaluation, some prediction of the findings can be made. Fragments in either long CL are likely to be embedded in ligamentous tissue and inaccessible. Although affected less frequently, short CL injury is more exposed to the tarsocrural joint space because

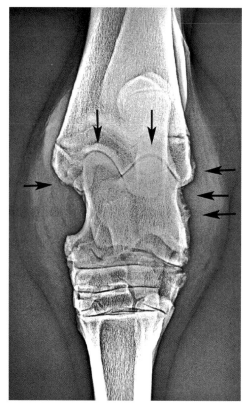

Figure 5.319. Collateral ligament desmitis and instability produces OA as shown in this Xeroradiograph. The TC joint space is narrowed and the subchondral bone has become sclerotic (vertical arrows), and enthesiopathy of most of the ligamentous attachments is present (horizontal arrows). This type of reaction is often accompanied by periarticular soft tissue thickening.

these ligaments attach on the cranial aspects of the respective malleolus. Concurrent radiographically inapparent articular cartilage damage must be considered.

Prognosis

In one study, 6 of 9 Standardbred racehorses returned to racing (3 at the previous level) following CL injuries. However, 2 reinjured the limb and 3 others required analgesics to train.[1] External coaptation was not used in the group of horses and ultrasound was not available.

To summarize, this condition can easily be taken too lightly. The subtle changes from the instability or joint damage sustained during the initial incident can produce OA before it is suspected (Figure 5.319). Immobilization and rest periods should err on the conservative side if CL injury of the tarsus is suspected.

References

1. Boero MJ, Kneller SK, Baker GJ, et al. Clinical, radiographic, and scintigraphic findings associated with enthesitis of the lateral collateral ligaments of the tarsocrural joint in standardbred racehorses. Equine Vet J 1988;Supplement 6:53–59.
2. Gabel AA. Lameness caused by inflammation in the distal hock. Vet Clin N Am 1980;2:101–124.

3. Moreau H, Denoix JM. Calcification of the medial collateral ligament of the hock in a jump horse. Pratique Veterinaire Equine 1994;26:219–220.
4. Rose PL, Moore I. Imaging diagnosis—avulsion of the medial collateral ligament of the tarsus in a horse. Vet Rad Ultra 2003;44:657–659.
5. Updike SJ. Functional anatomy of the equine tarsocrural collateral ligaments. Am J Vet Res 1984;45:867–874.

CURB

Curb is desmitis of the plantar ligament which originates on the plantar proximal aspect of the tuber calcis, courses laterally to the tarsal canal, and inserts on the distal part of the tuber calcis and the fourth tarsal and fourth metatarsal bones.[1,4] It is characterized by a thickening of the plantar distal aspect of the tarsus as viewed from the lateral side. Other structures that occupy the same area and may produce similar appearing swellings include the SDFT and subcutaneous thickening.[4]

Etiology

Plantar ligament desmitis results from excessive violent tension[8] or direct trauma. Sickle-hocked (curby hocks) or cow-hocked conformation impose exceptional stress on the plantar ligament and thus tend to produce curb. However, any horse can acquire curb from violent exertion, trauma from kicking walls or tailgates in trailers, and violent attempts to extend the hock. Rooney suggests that conditioning strengthens the tarsal ligaments.[8]

Foals with curby conformation are usually affected with wedging of the distal tarsal bones, which is described elsewhere in this chapter. However, the condition can persist into maturity and may be problematic in those individuals. Curby hocks were reported to be a factor that reduced starts in Standardbred race horses in one study.[5] The incidence of curby conformation in a series of 1,735 Dutch Warmblood horses was reported as 11.1%.[2]

Clinical Signs and Diagnosis

A curb is an enlargement on the plantar surface of the fibular tarsal bone. In the acute phase, there are signs of inflammation and lameness. The horse stands with the heel elevated when the limb is at rest, and heat and swelling can be palpated in the region.[6] Swelling usually does not diminish with exercise, and exercise may actually increase lameness in acute curb. In a severe case, in which trauma has been the inciting cause, periostitis on the plantar aspect of the fibular tarsal bone may result in new bone growth. If the inflammation is septic, extensive swelling and cellulitis may occur. In chronic cases, tissues surrounding the region often become infiltrated with scar tissue, and a permanent blemish results. Lameness may not be present, even though a considerable blemish is evident. Occasionally, the proximal end of the fourth metatarsal bone is large and causes false curb. Careful examination reveal that the swelling in this region is lateral to the plantar ligament and not on the ligament itself.

Although radiographs demonstrate only associated osseous involvement, confirmation of the ligamentous lesion is possible by ultrasonography[3,7]. It is important to differentiate the plantar ligament from other potentially more consequential sources of swelling such as proximal superficial digital flexor tendinitis or sepsis (Figure 3.53 in Chapter 3).[4]

Treatment

Treatment for acute injury to the plantar ligament includes rest and controlled exercise, application of cold packs for the first 48 hours following injury, and systemic administration of anti-inflammatory agents. Rest includes stall confinement for at least 6 weeks, and hand walking is often begun after 2 weeks and increased according to response. Although not reported, the application of shock wave therapy is a rational consideration. Follow-up ultrasound examination is generally done between 10 and 12 weeks to assess healing.

Prognosis

If the horse has good conformation, the prognosis is favorable, providing the initial acute inflammation is controlled. Poor conformation, however, serves as a continuing cause, and the prognosis is unfavorable. In most cases, some permanent blemish will remain after recovery, even though most horses will be serviceably sound, if conformation is good. Standardbred racehorses are often successful in spite of curby conformation.[6]

References

1. Adams OR. Lameness in Horses, 3rd ed. Lea and Febiger, Philadelphia, 1974.
2. Bos H, van der Mey GJW. Comparative study of the occurrence of some visible defects in Dutch Warmblood horses. Zuchtungskunde 1986;58:66–72.
3. Dik KJ. Ultrasonography of the equine tarsus. Vet Radiol Ultra 1993;34:36–43.
4. Dik KJ, Leitch M. Soft tissue injuries of the tarsus. Vet Clin NA Eq Pract 1995;11:235–247.
5. Dolvik NI, Klemetsdal G. Conformational traits of Norwegian cold-blooded trotters: Heritability and the relationship with performance. Acta Agriculturae Scandinavica Section A, Animal Science 1999;49:156–162.
6. Gill HE. Diagnosis and treatment of hock lameness. Proc Am Assoc Eq Pract 1973;19:257.
7. Rantanen NW, McKinnon AO. Equine diagnostic ultrasonography. Williams and Wilkins, Baltimore, 1998;536–537.
8. Rooney JR. An hypothesis of the pathogenesis of curb in horses. Can Vet J 1981;22:300–301.

LUXATION OF THE SUPERFICIAL DIGITAL FLEXOR TENDON (SDFT) FROM THE CALCANEUS

Occasionally, dislocation of the SDFT off the calcaneal tuber is seen in horses.[1] The dislocation occurs when one of the fascial attachments (usually medial retinaculum) of the SDFT to the calcaneus ruptures. Because of the severe swelling over the point of the hock, a misdiagnosis of capped hock or calcaneal bursitis can easily be made (Figures 5.320, 3.54). However, once the swelling decreases, dislocation is easily appreciated as a slippage of the SDFT off the point of the hock, usually laterally,[1,3] although medial dislocation has been reported.[4–6] One case of division of the SDFT

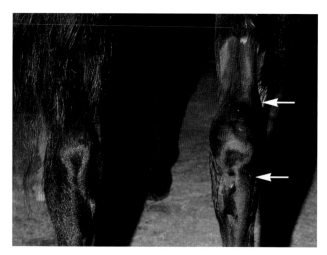

Figure 5.320. Caudal view of the tarsi in a horse with severe swelling within the right calcaneal bursa and evidence of lateral luxation of the right SDFT from the tuber calcanei (arrows). (Courtesy of Dr. Gary Baxter.)

and displacement in both directions has been described.[2] Initially, affected horses appear quite lame shortly after the injury, but with time the painful response diminishes and a partial loss of complete control of the hindlimb becomes apparent. Occasionally the condition can occur bilaterally.

Etiology

Dislocation of the SDFT has occurred as a racing injury,[3,6] simply bucking,[4] or trauma with accompanying fracture.[5]

Clinical Signs and Diagnosis

Shortly after the injury, the point of the hock is quite swollen, making it easy to misdiagnose it as a capped hock. The dislocation can be more easily appreciated as the swelling is reduced (Figure 5.320). In the acute stage, an obvious lameness is present. On palpation, the dislocation and relocation of the SDFT can be appreciated. The tendon often luxates when the tarsus is flexed. With time, the lameness diminishes. The horse will appear to have less control of its limb and a periodic displacement of the SDFT will occur. Although clinical signs alone can make the diagnosis, radiographs should be taken to rule out the possibility of a fracture. The severity of clinical signs varies with degree of mobility of the SDFT. Some horses only partially tear the attachments, and subluxation is the limit of dislocation.

Treatment

The degree of luxation and intended use of the horse dictates the treatment. When the tendon subluxates only mildly, stall rest for 3 to 6 months often returns the horse to work. If the tendon remains on the tuber calcis, horses often function in spite of the constant movement of the SDFT. Anecdotally, horses can be

pasture sound even if the SDFT remains completely luxated. If the luxation is severe or if an athlete is required, some prefer surgical repair. The timing of surgery is important because freshly torn tissues do not hold sutures well, and skin injury or infection may be present. However, the unaffected side of the fascia contracts, and complete reduction of the tendon becomes difficult after several days. It is very difficult to maintain reduction of the tendon in a bandage or cast in the preoperative period.

Several surgical techniques have been described. All involve debridement and repair of the torn fascia.[3-6] If the tendon does not reduce with the limb in extension, releasing incisions (without complete transection) are made in the bursal surface of the unaffected side until reduction can be maintained without undue tension.[6] One report describes a single case in which sutures were the only internal supporting device.[4] Supporting the suture line with a polypropylene mesh has also been described.[5-7] Strict asepsis must be maintained because infection resides in the nonabsorbable material. As much soft tissue as possible should be used to cover the implant. Support of the reduced flexor tendon with 2 screws placed on the unaffected side has also been described.[3]

All of these techniques were successful in the reported cases. In practical terms, the less that can be done successfully, the better. The screw technique is a long procedure during which the patients are rolled over. The mesh technique works well, but infection can be a problem in traumatized tissue. Every case has its own aspects to be addressed.

Most have immobilized the limb in a cast or sleeve cast for 30 to 45 day, after which the limb is supported in a Robert-Jones bandage followed by lesser amounts of support for a period of 30 days. Hand-walking exercise can be begun 7 days after the cast is removed and continued for the next 60 days. Free exercise is begun in a confined area about 4 months postoperatively. A recent report described complete immobilization for only 14 days and a bandage splint for another week.[4] Hand walking began 21 days after surgery.

Prognosis

The prognosis for breeding soundness or light pleasure riding is good. Realistically, too few cases have been treated surgically with long-term follow-up to make an objective prognosis about athletic ability, because every case is a bit different. One Thoroughbred racehorse recovered and raced 51 times, and another was retired for breeding.[3] An Arabian mare became sound in hand, but work was not described.[4] In another case, the horse did not return to previous performance.[6] Horses that have been operated may not retain perfect reduction of the tendon, but still return to work. In 5 cases treated at Colorado State University with the surgery described, 3 horses resumed to full performance 10 months after surgery. One horse was used as a mountain riding horse, another was used for ranch work, and the other horse was used for pleasure.[8] Complications associated with 2 of the 5 cases included 1 chronic infection and 1 repair breakdown. Horses can perform normal work with the altered appearance and slight movement of the tendon at the point of the hock.

References

1. Fessler JF, Amstutz HE. In Textbook of Large Animal Surgery. Oehme FW, Prier JE, eds. Williams and Wilkins Co., Baltimore, 1974;249.
2. Foerner JJ. Surgical treatment of selected musculoskeletal disorders of the rear limb. In Equine Surgery, 1st ed. Auer JA, ed. Saunders, Philadelphia, 1992;1055–1075.
3. Meagher DM, Aldrete AV. Lateral luxation of the superficial digital flexor tendon from the calcaneal tuber in two horses. J Am Vet Med Assoc 1989;195:495–498.
4. Reiners S, Jann HW, Gillis E. Repair of medial luxation of the superficial digital flexor tendon in the pelvic limb of a filly. Eq Pract 2000;22:18–19, 21.
5. Scott EA. Surgical repair of a dislocated superficial digital flexor tendon and fractured fibular tarsal bone in a horse. J Am Vet Med Assoc 1983;183:332–333.
6. Scott EA, Breuhaus B. Surgical repair of dislocated superficial digital flexor tendons in a horse. J Am Vet Med Assoc 1982;181:171.
7. Stashak TS. Luxation of the superficial digital flexor. In Adams' Lameness in Horses. 4th ed. Lea and Febiger, Baltimore, 1987; 718–220.
8. Stashak TS. Personal communication. 2001.

MEDIAL DISPLACEMENT OF THE DEEP DIGITAL FLEXOR TENDON

Medial displacement of the deep flexor from its position over the sustentaculum is a rarely diagnosed congenital anomaly. It produces no early clinical signs and is usually unobserved until the foal displays a tarsus/fetlock varus deformity due to a bowstring effect of the deep flexor tendon along the axial surface of the distal hindlimb. Closer inspection reveals the tendon to be even more misaligned than is usually seen with metatarsophalangeal varus deformity, and tracing its path proximally reveals the defect. The sustentacular defect is palpable and confirmed radiographically as compared to the contralateral hock. The applicable view is the flexed tangential projection.

Surgical correction is the only treatment option. The procedure consists of dissecting the tarsal sheath from the periosteal surface of the medial aspect of the sustentaculum and repositioning it in its correct position over the sustentaculum.[1] It must be supported in the position, and a cortical rib graft secured by bone screws has been used to form the shelf. Foerner confined the foal to a stall in a support bandage for a month before allowing normal exercise.[1] The author has operated the only other known case that had surgery. The procedure was performed in the same manner, and the foal was maintained in a sleeve cast early postoperatively. However, the tightening of the deep flexor tendon caused a plantar-to-dorsal bowstring hyperextension of the hock. The horse became breeding sound and the limb is straight. Given the same situation again, the author would transect the deep flexor in the distal portion of the muscle tissue to relieve the tension. A third case has been reported in a yearling.[2] That horse was lame but had no angular deformity; no treatment was applied. The degree of the displacement apparently varies.

References

1. Foerner JJ. Surgical treatment of selected musculoskeletal disorders of the rear limb. In Equine Surgery, 1st ed. Auer JA, ed. Saunders, Philadelphia, 1992;1055–1075.
2. Lepage OM, Leveille R, Breton L, et al. Congenital dislocation of the deep digital flexor tendon associated with hypoplasia of the sustentaculum tali in a thoroughbred colt. Vet Radiol Ultra 1995;36:384–386.

TARSAL SHEATH TENOSYNOVITIS (THOROUGHPIN)

The tarsal sheath is located on the medial aspect of the tarsus and begins 5 to 8 cm proximal to medial to the malleolus and extends distally to the proximal one-third of the metatarsus (Figure 5.321). It has a variable length (21 to 32 cm) and an estimated volume of 20 to 50 mL. It encloses the DDFT of the hindlimb as it courses over the sustentaculum tali on the medial aspect of the tarsus. Tenosynovitis or effusion of the tarsal sheath is often referred to as thoroughpin. Thoroughpin is a morphological description of the swelling. While some cases have idiopathic synovitis, potential causes for tarsal sheath tenosynovitis include damage to the DDFT, sustentaculum tali, or calcaneus, and infection from penetrating injuries or hematogenous spread.[1,3,5–7,9–11]

Etiology

Some horses have effusion within the tarsal sheath for what is thought to be no apparent reason. However, horses with effusion combined with lameness and/or a

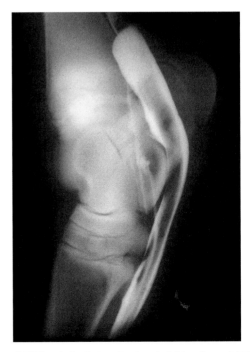

Figure 5.321. Iodinated contrast material has been injected into the tarsal sheath illustrating the proximal and distal limits of this synovial cavity of the medial aspect of the tarsus. (Courtesy of Dr. Gary Baxter.)

positive response to tarsal flexion most likely have an underlying cause. The most likely cause is previous trauma to the sustentaculum tali. The sustentaculum tali is very superficial on the medial aspect of the tarsus, and trauma such as kicks to this region can lead to open or closed fractures and other associated problems (Figure 5.322). Open fractures can predispose to infection within the sheath and closed fractures/trauma can lead to exostosis of the sustentaculum tali (Figure 5.313B). The exostosis, depending on the size, can cause signs of synovitis or actually damage the DDFT as it moves along the medial aspect of the tarsus. Damage to the DDFT within the tarsal sheath is also most likely trauma related but appears to be less common than damage to the sustentaculum tali. Penetrating injuries to the tarsal sheath may lead to infectious tenosynovitis similar to that of any synovial structure, and hematogenous infection within the sheath has been reported in one horse subsequent to bacterial peritonitis[1,7]. Osteomyelitis of the sustentaculum tali is a common finding in many of these horses.[6]

Clinical Signs

Horses with idiopathic tenosynovitis have effusion within the tarsal sheath but no apparent lameness or performance limitations. The effusion is typically located on the medial aspect of the tarsus and courses up and down the leg in the direction of the tarsal sheath. However, the effusion may also be visible and palpable from the lateral aspect of the tarsus (Figure 5.323). Horses with previous trauma to the sustentaculum tali (with or without DDFT abnormalities) often present for lameness and swelling of the medial aspect of the tarsus.

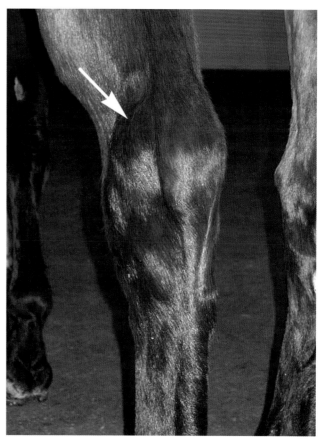

Figure 5.323. Thoroughpin can involve only the medial aspect of the tarsus, but may also project to the lateral side, as seen in this horse (arrow). (Courtesy of Dr. Gary Baxter.)

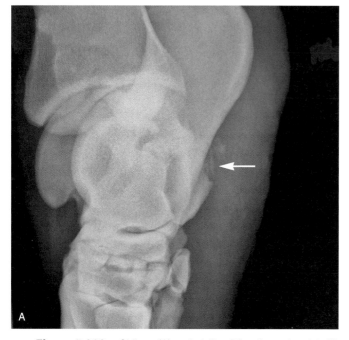
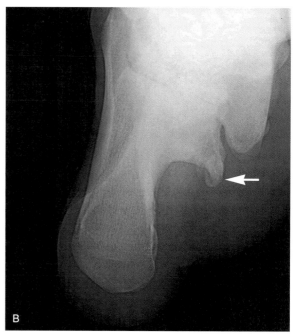

Figure 5.322. Oblique (A) and skyline (B) radiographs of 2 different horses with an open (A) and closed (B) fracture of the sustentaculum tali (arrows). (Courtesy of Dr. Gary Baxter.)

Most horses are grade 2 to 3 of 5 lame and positive to a tarsal flexion test. Intrasynovial anesthesia of the tendon sheath should improve the lameness in nearly all cases. Horses with infection of the tarsal sheath are usually nonweight-bearing, and are painful to digital pressure applied to the sheath. Effusion within the sheath may be difficult to determine in some horses, because diffuse swelling of the entire tarsus may be present.

Diagnosis

A presumptive diagnosis of tarsal sheath tenosynovitis can usually be made based on the clinical finding of effusion within the sheath. However, the findings of the lameness exam most likely determine whether the effusion is clinically significant. Abnormalities within the sheath should be suspected in horses that are lame, positive to tarsal flexion, or improve with intrasynovial anesthesia of the sheath. Radiographs of the tarsus, including a skyline view, should be performed in addition to ultrasonographic evaluation of the DDFT. The 45° dorsomedial-plantarolateral projection is also helpful (Figure 5.322A).[8,10]

Fractures, osteomyelitis, and proliferative exostosis of the sustentaculum tali are the most common radiographic abnormalities seen. Proliferative exostosis of the medial aspect of the calcaneus has also been reported to contribute to tenosynovitis in one horse.[12] Aspiration of synovial fluid from the sheath should be performed in horses with suspected sepsis or osteomyelitis of the sustentaculum tali to help document the presence of infection. Contrast radiography or a fistulogram may also be helpful to document synovial involvement of the tarsal sheath in horses with penetrating wounds. See Chapter 10 for further information on septic synovial structures.

Treatment

True idiopathic tenosynovitis without lameness can be treated with benign neglect or intrasynovial injections of anti-inflammatory medication such as corticosteroids and/or sodium hyaluronate (HA). Pressure bandaging the tarsus following intrasynovial treatment may help further reduce the effusion and prevent recurrence. Persistent idiopathic effusion may also be treated with intrasynovial atropine, but the lack of any predisposing cause should be documented before resorting to this treatment.

Horses with fractures, exostosis, or osteomyelitis of the sustentaculum tali are usually best treated surgically. This is especially true for open fractures and osteomyelitis with secondary infection of the sheath. There is some debate about whether horses with exostosis of the sustentaculum tali benefit from removal of the exostosis; however, these horses often do not respond or respond only temporarily to more conservative treatment[12]. In addition, concurrent damage to the DDFT is common with exostosis of the sustentaculum tali, and will most likely worsen if the exostosis is not removed.[4,10] Endoscopy of the sheath is the preferred technique,[2] although a small incision directly over the medial sustentaculum tali may also be used. The goal with either approach is to remove fracture fragments, exostosis, or infected bone from the sustentaculum tali. Endoscopy is usually essential to locate and debride damaged areas of the DDFT, similar to tendon injuries within the digital flexor tendon sheath. Horses with penetrating injuries or infection within the tarsal sheath are best treated with a combination of endoscopic lavage and debridement, parenteral and intrasynovial antimicrobials, and IV regional limb perfusion. Fibrin quickly accumulates, sequestering bacteria from antibiotics, and adhesions worsen the situation.

Deep digital flexor tenotomy (in the metatarsal region) or tenectomy within the tarsal canal was performed in 2 horses.[10] An extended heel shoe was necessary during convalescence, and both horses recovered to breeding soundness or were ridden lightly. The immediate effect of the procedure was relief of severe lameness and/or removal of necrotic tissue from the tendon sheath. Another report questions the necessity of tenotomy/tenectomy, which limits return to athletic soundness.[6]

Prognosis

The prognosis of horses with tarsal sheath tenosynovitis is variable, depending on the cause. Horses with idiopathic synovitis have a very good prognosis except for the cosmetic blemish. Horses with small fractures of the sustentaculum tali can do well, provided damage to the DDFT is minimal.

The overall prognosis for recovery from a septic tendon sheath is only fair. However, successful results can be accomplished if the debridement is complete and infection controlled.[3,12] The outlook is improved if no radiographic changes are present.[4] In one report of 10 horses treated for osteomyelitis of the sustentaculum tali, 9 were discharged from the hospital and 6 horses returned to their previous use.[6] Four of 5 horses treated endoscopically returned to their previous level of activity after surgery;[2] 4 of those had fragmentation of the sustentaculum tali. Six horses of a combined series of 17 horses were considered successfully treated.[4,9,10] A like number became breeding sound, while others were lost. The prognosis of horses with DDFT lesions within the tarsal sheath is unknown but most likely reflects the severity of the injury. The author has observed one horse that retained a mechanically abnormal gait that could not be changed with local analgesia.

References

1. Archer DC, Clegg PD, Edwards GB. Septic tenosynovitis of the tarsal sheath of an Arab gelding and suspected sepsis of the lateral digital flexor tendon subsequent to bacterial peritonitis. Vet Rec 2004;155:485–489.
2. Cauvin ER, Tapprest J, Munroe GA, et al. Endoscopic examination of the tarsal sheath of the lateral digital flexor tendon in horses. Equine Vet J 1999;31:219–227.
3. Dart AJ, Hodgson DR. Surgical management of osteomyelitis of the sustentaculum tali in a horse. Aust Vet J 1996;73:73–74.
4. Dik KJ, Merkens HW. Unilateral distension of the tarsal sheath in the horse: A report of 11 cases. Equine Vet J 1987;19:307–313.
5. Edwards GB. Changes in the sustentaculum tali associated with distension of the tarsal sheath (thoroughpin). Equine Vet J 1978;10:97–102.
6. Hand R, Watkins JP, Honnas CM, et al. Treatment of osteomyelitis of the sustentaculum tali and associated tenosynovitis in

horses: 10 cases (1992–1998). Proc Am Assoc Pract 1999; 45:158–159.

7. Lugo J, Gaughan EM. Septic arthritis, tenosynovitis, and infections of hoof structures. Vet Clin NA Eq Pract 2006; 22:363–388.

8. Mattoon JS, O'Briend TR. Radiographic evaluation of the calcaneus in the horse: A retrospective study. Proc Am Assoc Eq Pract 1988;34:369–379.

9. Peremans K, Verschooten F, Moor Ad, et al. Post-traumatic osteomyelitis of the sustentaculum tali in the horse: 4 cases. Vla Dierg Tijd 1988;57:410–417.

10. Santschi EM, Adams SB, Fessler JF, et al. Treatment of lesions of the sustentaculum of the calcaneus accompanied by tarsal sheath synovitis. Proceedings Am Assoc Equine Pract 1993;39: 249–250.

11. Tulleners EP, Reid CF. Osteomyelitis of the sustentaculum talus in a pony. J Am Vet Med Assoc 1981;178:290–291.

12. Welch RD, Auer JA, Watkins JP, et al. Surgical treatment of tarsal sheath effusion associated with an exostosis on the calcaneus of a horse. J Am Vet Med Assoc 1990;196:1992–1994.

RUPTURE OF THE PERONEUS TERTIUS

The peroneus tertius is a strong muscular band of tissue that lies between the long digital extensor and the tibialis cranialis muscle of the rear limb. It originates from the extensor fossa of the distal lateral femur and inserts distally as a tendinous band to the third metatarsal bone and laterally on the fourth metatarsal bone. It is an important part of the reciprocal apparatus, mechanically flexing the hock when the stifle joint is flexed. The muscle or tendon can rupture anywhere along its course and can result in an avulsion fracture at its origin in the extensor fossa. When this muscle is ruptured, the stifle flexes but the hock does not (Figure 5.324).[3]

In contrast, a congenital flexure deformity of the right hock in a foal resulted from an abnormally short peroneus tertius muscle, which rendered the foal unable to walk due to hyperflexion of the hock. Tension created by the short peroneus tertius limited the hock extension to 70°. The cause was thought to be the intrauterine positioning of the foal. After resection of the peroneus tertius, the foal was able to extend its hock another 30°, and 2 months later, hock flexion and extension appeared normal.[2]

Etiology

Rupture of the peroneus tertius is usually due to overextension of the hock joint. This may occur if the limb is entrapped and the horse struggles violently to free its limb. Rupture also may occur during the exertion of a fast start, when tremendous power is transferred to the limb, causing overextension, such as in jumping. It can also occur after a full-limb cast is applied to the hindlimb. The author has seen several in horses that barrel race.

Clinical Signs

Signs of rupture of the peroneus tertius are well defined. The stifle joint flexes as the limb advances and the hock joint is carried forward with very little flexion. That portion of the limb below the hock tends to hang limp, giving the appearance of being fractured as it is carried forward. When the foot is put down the horse has no trouble bearing weight and shows little pain. As the horse walks, however, it is noted that there is a dimpling in the Achilles tendon. If the limb is lifted from the ground, a dimpling can easily be produced in the Achilles tendon by extending the hock. It is noted that the hock can be extended without extending the stifle; this cannot be done in the normal limb (Figures 3.58 and 5.324). If the origin of the peroneus tertius fractures from the femur, femoropatellar effusion is a prominent feature, and the gait deficit is similar.

Diagnosis

The signs described above easily provide the diagnosis. If the injury appears to be proximal, radiographs are advised. However, ultrasound confirmation can be obtained.[1]

Treatment

Complete rest is the best treatment. The horse should be placed in a box stall and kept quiet for at least 4 to 6 weeks, and then limited exercise should be given for the next 2 months. Most cases heal and show normal limb action, and if properly conditioned, most horses can return to normal work. Surgical intervention is not recommended. Hand walking is advisable when exercise is first begun to help control the horse and prevent re-injury.

Prognosis

The prognosis is guarded to favorable. Healing usually occurs when the horse is properly rested by box stall confinement. If healing is not evident at the end of

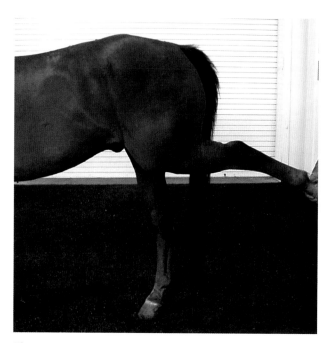

Figure 5.324. Rupture of the peroneus tertius disrupts the reciprocal apparatus allowing extension of the tarsus and fetlock with the stifle flexed. (Courtesy of Dr. Gary Baxter.)

4 to 6 weeks, the prognosis is unfavorable, because the tendon may not unite. Final appraisal should not be made for at least 3 months following the injury. The author has observed one horse that ruptured its peroneus tertius twice. It had returned to full work after the first incident before it happened again.

References

1. Leveille R, Lindsay WA, Biller DS. Ultrasonographic appearance of ruptured peroneus tertius in a horse. J Am Vet Med Assoc 1993;202:1981–1982.
2. Trout DR, Lohse CL. Anatomy and therapeutic resection of the peroneus tertius muscle in a foal. J Am Vet Med Assoc 1981;179:247.
3. Updike SJ. Anatomy of the tarsal tendons of the equine tibialis cranialis and peroneus tertius muscles. Am J Vet Res 1984;45:1379–1382.

GASTROCNEMIUS TENDINITIS/COMMON CALCANEAL TENDINITIS

Gastrocnemius tendinitis/common calcaneal tendinitis is uncommon but affects performance horses of all types. The condition is characterized by subtle to obvious lameness exacerbated by hindlimb flexion. The condition is somewhat similar to common calcaneal tendinitis,[5] but is more distal and affects the gastrocnemius individually.

Clinical Signs and Diagnosis

Some horses are perceived to have a reduced duration of weight-bearing during the caudal phase of the stride. Abaxial and generalized swelling of the tendinous insertion of the gastrocnemius may be evident, or the common calcaneal tendon may be enlarged (Figure 5.325). The firm swelling can be differentiated from thoroughpin and calcaneal bursitis by its location and lack of fluid distention. However, the superficial flexor bursa may be distended, resembling a capped hock in some horses.[4] Diagnostic anesthesia of the tibial and peroneal or only the tibial nerve improves the lameness.

Radiographs generally demonstrate no lesions, but chronic cases may have a calcification at the calcaneal attachment of the gastrocnemius tendon. Ultrasound reveals enlargement, focal or diffuse hypo- or anechoic regions, and loss of normal fiber alignment when viewed in the longitudinal plane.[4,6] Ultrasound of the unaffected contralateral tendon is advisable for reference.[4] Associated lesions are not common, but calcaneal bursitis[1,4] or superficial flexor tendon tendinitis[4] may exist concurrently.

Treatment

Therapy consists of rest with local and systemic anti-inflammatory therapy. The recovery can be quite prolonged. Return to work before the ultrasonographic lesion has healed is followed by reoccurrence of the lameness. Therapy that is begun in the more acute stages is more successful than for horses that have been lame for many weeks.[3] Even confined to a stall, this area is impossible to protect from normal weight-bearing.

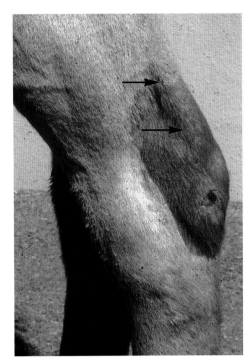

Figure 5.325. Firm enlargement of the common calcaneal tendon proximal to the tuber calcanei (arrows) may be associated with injury to the gastrocnemius tendon as it attaches to the point of the hock. (Courtesy of Dr. Gary Baxter.)

The author has surgically split the tendon of a show horse to accelerate healing that appeared to not be progressing. The horse became sound after approximately a year of rest and controlled exercise. One case of common calcaneal tendinitis became sound from rest and local anti-inflammatory therapy for 10 months.[5]

Prognosis

A series of horses that were lame up to 8 weeks were very slow to recuperate. Ultrasound monitoring continued to demonstrate the persisting or enlarging focal or generalized lesions. Horses that became sound again required 9 to 12 months.[2] Two horses that resumed work after 12 months again became lame, and others remained in slow advancing exercise for at least 8 months. Another group of horses that were diagnosed much earlier following onset of signs recovered much quicker and resumed flat racing or eventing.[3]

References

1. Dik KJ. Ultrasonography of the equine crus. Vet Radiol Ultra 1993;34:28–34.
2. Dyson SJ. Gastrocnemius tendinitis. Proc 15th Bain-Fallon Memorial Lectures 1993;15:63–70.
3. Dyson SJ. Personal communication. 2001.
4. Dyson SJ, Kidd L. Five cases of gastrocnemius tendinitis in the horse. Equine Vet J 1992;24:351–356.
5. Proudman CJ. Common calcaneal tendinitis in a horse. Eq Vet Educ 1992;4:277–279.
6. Reef VB. Equine Diagnostic Ultrasound. WB Saunders Co., Philadelphia, 1998.

RUPTURE OR STRAIN OF THE GASTROCNEMIUS/SUPERFICIAL DIGITAL FLEXOR (SDF) MUSCLE

The gastrocnemius muscle extends the tarsus by its insertion on the os calcis to support the stay apparatus and superficial digital flexor (SDF) muscle, which alone is not substantial enough to effect tarsal extension.[6] The origin of the lateral head of the gastrocnemius is closely associated with the SDF muscle and simultaneous injury often occurs.[5] The SDF muscle is responsible for the actual reciprocal action of flexing the digit when the tarsus and stifle are flexed, but it is insubstantial compared to the gastrocnemius and is aided by the more superficial additional parallel fibrous band. Loss of the gastrocnemius compromises tarsal extension along with the reciprocal apparatus. Complete gastrocnemius rupture significantly compromises tarsal extension. The clinical significance of partial disruption depends upon the size of the horse. Milder injury of the origin of the gastrocnemius muscles has been reported to cause persistent hindlimb lameness in performance horses.[8]

Etiology

It has been theorized that tension on the hindlimb during passive extension (e.g., trapping the hindlimb in extension beneath the horse) causes this injury.[5] Two of 3 affected adults were reported to have histories of falling.[2,5] The origin of the lameness may be unknown, but one horse with bilateral proximal gastrocnemius injury became cast in the stall.[8]

In neonates, the overriding strength of contraction of the biceps femoris and quadriceps muscles opposing the gastrocnemius has been theorized to be a factor with foals.[8] The injury is also associated with delivery of foals with flexure contractures, dystocia, and problems rising.[9] Lodging the hind feet against the mare's pelvis while traction is applied would overextend the stifles sufficiently to rupture the gastrocnemius, as well.[1,9]

Clinical Signs and Diagnosis

The tarsus of the affected limb is dropped so that there is a reduced angle to the joint and the os calcis is positioned closer to the ground than normal (Figure 11.50 and 5.326); bilaterally affected horses appear to

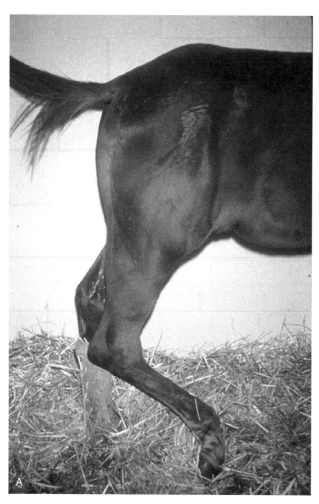 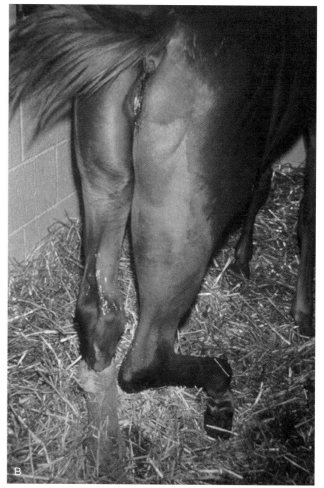

Figure 5.326. A. The ruptured gastrocnemius allows the tarsus to hyperflex (sink) with a flexed stifle demonstrating compromise or loss of the reciprocal apparatus.

B. There is extensive swelling in the affected gaskin from the soft tissue injury and the concurrent hemorrhage can be life-threatening.

squat or be unable to rise. The size of the horse affects the significance of partial rupture, which may progress to complete rupture.[5] Swelling caudal and lateral to the stifle is a consistent finding. Loss of the reciprocal apparatus as evidenced by extension of the hock with the stifle flexed and extension of the fetlock with the hock flexed is evident (Figure 5.326). Neonates often have concurrent musculoskeletal or metabolic conditions.[1,9] The trauma of the incident frequently causes hemorrhage due to tearing of the caudal femoral or possibly other vessels, which contributes to the swelling and may be fatal.[3,7] Abscessation at the site of rupture is not uncommon.[1,2,9]

Adult horses that are lame from proximal injury to the gastrocnemius have no external signs but demonstrate moderate lameness that is generally positive to hindlimb flexion. A characteristic lateral rotation of the calcaneus with medial rotation of the toe has been described.[8]

Radiographs are often normal, but avulsion of fragments from the distal femur have been observed,[1,9] as have calcifications of the caudal distal femur.[8] Scintigraphy was useful in isolating the gastrocnemius injuries on the caudodistal femurs of lame horses.[8] Ultrasound was used to successfully image the injury and defects of the lateral head of the gastrocnemius and superficial digital flexor muscles in foals.[9]

Partial disruptions in adults tend to involve the lateral head of the gastrocnemius and the SDF muscle,[2,4] whereas more foals had complete gastrocnemius rupture sparing the SDF muscle.[1,9]

Treatment

In adults, the goal is to support the limb with the hock extended to facilitate fibrosis at the rupture site. Surgical therapy is not a consideration. Methods used include a Robert-Jones bandage applied to the full limb and stall confinement.[5] A more rigid technique in a weanling consisted of a full-limb cast and a Thomas splint.[2] As the swelling diminished, the cast was replaced. The Thomas splint and cast were replaced with a Robert-Jones bandage after 21 days. Horses suffering from lameness due to proximal gastrocnemius injury generally respond to 6 to 12 months of rest.[8]

In neonates, treatment consists of supportive therapy and attempts to aid them in rising.

For a more distal injury, Valdez described the use of flexible carbon fiber for the repair of a ruptured gastrocnemius in a foal.[10] A transverse hole was drilled for the attachment of the carbon fiber distally. However, use of carbon fiber is not advisable.

Prognosis

In one study, 1 of 2 adults managed with Robert-Jones bandage and stall confinement for 90 days survived.[5] One improved, but reinjured the area and deteriorated. A less severely affected adult also recovered well with rest alone.[4] A weanling managed in a cast and Thomas splint was walking after 6 months and was normal in pasture after 17 months.[2] Adult horses with injuries to the gastrocnemius muscle appear to do well with prolonged rest.[8]

An older study of 9 neonates with rupture of the gastrocnemius muscle and hemorrhage reported that all were euthanatized due to the inability to rise and physical deterioration.[7] More successful results have been reported recently, and with unilateral milder disruption, complete recovery is possible.[1] Foals with more extensive injuries requiring prolonged intensive care may survive but may not reach athletic soundness.[1] In a recent series of 28 affected foals, 23 survived to discharge.[9] Foals without other concurrent conditions were more likely to become athletes. Thirteen of 16 that were of racing age at the time of the report were in training or had raced.

References

1. Jesty SA, Palmer JE, Parente EJ, et al. Rupture of the gastrocnemius muscle in six foals. J Am Vet Med Assoc 2005; 227:1965–1968.
2. Lescun TB, Hawkins JF, Siems JJ. Management of rupture of the gastrocnemius and superficial digital flexor muscles with a modified Thomas splint-cast combination in a horse. J Am Vet Med Assoc 1998;213:1457–1459.
3. Pascoe RR. Death due to rupture of the origin of the gastrocnemius muscle in a filly. Aust Vet J 1975;51:107.
4. Reeves MJ, Trotter GW. Reciprocal apparatus dysfunction as a cause of severe hind limb lameness in a horse. J Am Vet Med Assoc 1991;199:1047–1048.
5. Shoemaker RS, Martin, GS, Hillmann DJ, et al. Disruption of the caudal component of the reciprocal apparatus in two horses. School of Veterinary Medicine, Louisiana State University, Baton Rouge, Louisiana, 1988;1–11.
6. Sisson S, Grossman JD. Fasciae and Muscles of the Horse, 4th ed. WB Saunders, Philadelphia, 1953.
7. Sprinkle FP, Swerczek TW, Crowe MW. Gastrocnemius muscle rupture and hemorrhage in foals. Eq Pract 1985;7: 10–11,14–15,17.
8. Swor TM, Schneider RK, Ross MW, et al. Injury to the origin of the gastrocnemius muscle as a possible cause of lameness in four horses. J Am Vet Med Assoc 2001;219:215–219.
9. Tull TM, Woodie JB, Ruggles AJ, et al. Management and assessment of prognosis after gastrocnemius disruption in thoroughbred foals: 28 cases (1993–2007). Equine Vet J 2009;41: 541–546.
10. Valdez H, Coy CH, Swanson T. Flexible carbon fiber for repair of gastrocnemius and superficial digital flexor tendons in a heifer and gastrocnemius tendon in a foal. J Am Vet Med Assoc 1982; 181:154–157.

CAPPED HOCK/CALCANEAL BURSITIS

Swelling at the point of the hock (calcaneus) is usually attributable to damage to the subcutaneous calcaneal bursa (capped hock) or problems within the intertendinous calcaneal bursa located beneath the superficial digital flexor tendon (SDFT). The intertendinous calcaneal bursa may be further divided into the gastrocnemius calcaneal bursa and the intertendinous calcaneal bursa, but in most horses these 2 bursae communicate and should be considered as a single synovial structure.[6] The subcutaneous bursa at the tarsus is analogous to the bursa at the point of the olecranon but may communicate with the intertendinous bursa in about one-third of horses.[4] The intertendinous calcaneal bursa is a true synovial cavity analogous to the bicipital bursa and navicular bursa, and problems within this anatomic structure are much more problematic than those within the subcutaneous bursa. The calcaneal bursa extends approximately 7 cm distally and 9.6 cm

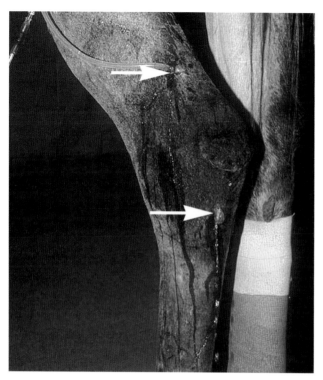

Figure 5.327. Lateral view of the calcaneal bursa with a drain placed to treat synovial infection. Note the proximal and distal extent of the calcaneal bursa (arrows) relative to the point of the hock. (Courtesy of Dr. Gary Baxter.)

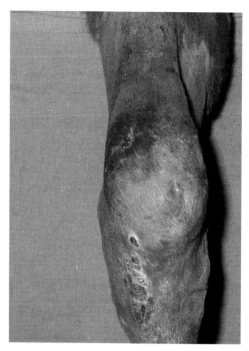

Figure 5.328. Caudal view of the calcaneus in a horse with synovial sepsis from a penetrating injury that occurred proximal to the tuber calcanei. The infection has resolved but the calcaneal bursa remains enlarged. (Courtesy of Dr. Gary Baxter.)

proximally relative to the tuber calcanei (point of the hock, Figure 5.327).[4] Therefore, it is very important to determine the location of the swelling over the point of the hock to best address treatment and prognosis. This is especially true for traumatic wounds in this location.

Etiology

Direct trauma to the point of the hock from a kick or the horse hitting a hard object such as a stall wall, fence, etc. is the most common cause of a capped hock.[8] These injuries may or may not be associated with a wound. True calcaneal bursitis may also be secondary to trauma such as that seen with luxation of the SDFT from the tuber calcanei and damage to the attachment of the gastrocnemius tendon to the tuber calcanei.[1,5] Nonseptic osteolytic lesions within the calcaneus at the insertion sites of the gastrocnemius tendon and the plantar ligament have also been reported to cause calcaneal bursitis.[1,3] However, penetrating wounds that enter the calcaneal bursa appear to be the most common cause for swelling and lameness referable to the calcaneal bursa.[7] These injuries are often small puncture wounds that do not seem to be important but subsequently result in infection within the bursa (Figure 5.328). Secondary osteomyelitis within the tuber calcanei is not uncommon. Wounds involving the subcutaneous bursa also occur but are usually not problematic.

Clinical Signs and Diagnosis

A capped hock (nonseptic) is usually characterized by a soft, fluctuant swelling located directly at the point of the hock (Figure 3.55). Subcutaneous edema in acute cases and thickening and fibrosis of surrounding tissues in chronic cases may make the diagnosis more difficult. Lameness may or may not be present depending on the time since injury but is usually minimal after a few days. In general, there are fewer signs of lameness for nonseptic injuries of the subcutaneous bursa than the calcaneal bursa.

Horses with nonseptic calcaneal bursitis can be a diagnostic challenge because fluid distention of the bursa is often not readily apparent. However, the area above and below the tuber calcanei is usually enlarged compared to the opposite calcaneus, and fluid distention is usually palpable either above or below the retinaculum on the medial or lateral aspects of the tuber calcanei. These horses are often painful to direct palpation of the bursa, lame at the trot, and very positive to tarsal flexion. Intrasynovial anesthesia directly into the calcaneal bursa is usually the best approach to confirm the location of the lameness.

Penetrating injuries/wounds at the point of the hock may involve the subcutaneous or intertendinous calcaneal bursae. The calcaneal bursa extends more proximally and distally to the tuber calcanei than the subcutaneous bursa and should be taken into account when evaluating these injuries. Small innocuous puncture wounds can cause subsequent infection within the bursa if not managed appropriately. These horses are often not very lame initially, but become nonweight-bearing with the development of synovial infection. The point of the hock is usually swollen and painful to palpation, and purulent exudate often exits the wound. The diagnosis of infection is similar to that of other sites of synovial infection and includes a combination of plain and contrast radiography, ultrasonography, aspiration of synovial fluid, and culture.

A definitive diagnosis of the cause of nonseptic calcaneal bursitis usually requires a combination of radiography and ultrasonography. However, endoscopy of the bursa is recommended as a diagnostic tool if other imaging results are negative. Scintigraphy and MRI also may be beneficial but usually are not necessary. The cause of nonseptic calcaneal bursitis may not be determined in all cases.

Treatment and Prognosis

Treatment of horses with a capped hock can vary depending on the severity. Small swellings may merely be a cosmetic concern and not require treatment. However, methods to prevent further trauma to the tuber calcanei are suggested to prevent the capped hock from worsening.[4] Larger swellings are treated in a manner similar to olecranon bursitis and carpal hygromas (Figure 5.329). Topical anti-inflammatories such as ice, DMSO, or topical diclofenac liposomal cream (Surpass) combined with bandaging may help in the acute stage. Other options include aseptic drainage and injection of corticosteroids or iodinated contrast agents.[4] Counterpressure with bandaging is recommended for at least 2 weeks but can be difficult in this high-motion area. A compressive sleeve-type bandage can be beneficial in these cases. Surgical drainage using Penrose drains or complete removal of the bursa are rarely recommended due to the problems with wound healing in this location.

Treatment of nonseptic calcaneal bursitis depends on the initiating cause, but is similar to other types of synovial inflammation. Acute bursitis without a defined

cause can be treated with intrasynovial triamcinolone and hyaluronan (HA) combined with a short period of rest. Known causes of calcaneal bursitis such as osteolytic lesions within the calcaneus should be debrided endoscopically.[1,3] In some chronic cases, endoscopy should be used as both a diagnostic and treatment tool for lesions within the gastrocnemius tendon, SDFT, and other soft tissue injuries within the bursa. Based on a very limited number of cases, horses with osteolytic lesions of the calcaneus and chronic wounds involving the bursa have a guarded prognosis for athletic activity.

The depth and involvement of the calcaneal bursa dictate the appropriate treatment of penetrating injuries to the tuber calcanei. Superficial wounds to the subcutaneous bursa usually resolve with routine wound care and have an excellent prognosis.[7] Wounds that involve the intertendinous calcaneal bursa are more problematic and should be treated aggressively in the acute stage to prevent synovial infection (Figure 5.328).[2] Horses with septic calcaneal bursitis should be treated with a combination of synovial lavage (endoscopy), local and parenteral antibiotics including IV regional perfusion, and NSAIDs.[2,3] Secondary osteomyelitis of the calcaneus should be debrided as part of the treatment protocol. In one study, 75% of horses with wounds involving the calcaneal bursa survived but only 44% of horses with secondary osteomyelitis of the tuber calcanei survived.[7] Horses with septic calcaneal bursitis tend to have a fair to guarded prognosis for athletic use because of the high motion required in this area during limb flexion. Further information on treating septic synovial cavities can be found in Chapter 10.

References

1. Bassage LH 2nd, Garcia-Lopez J, Currid EM. Osteolytic lesions of the tuber calcanei in two horses. J Am Vet Med Assoc 2000;217:710–716.
2. Baxter GM. Treatment of wounds involving synovial structures. Clinical Techniques in Equine Practice 2005;3:204–210.
3. Ingle-Fehr JE, Baxter GM. Endoscopy of the calcaneal bursa in horses. Vet Surg 1998;27:561–567.
4. McIlwraith CW. Diseases of bursae and other periarticular tissues. In Adams' Lameness in Horses, 5th ed. Stashak TS, ed. Lippincott Williams and Wilkins, Philadelphia, 2002;640–644.
5. Meagher DM, Aldrete AV. Lateral luxation of the superficial digital flexor tendon from the calcaneal tuber in two horses. J Am Vet Med Assoc 1989;195:495–498.
6. Post EM, Singer ER, Clegg PD. An anatomic study of the calcaneal bursae in the horse. Vet Surg 2007;36:3–9.
7. Post EM, Singer ER, Clegg PD, et al. Retrospective study of 24 cases of septic calcaneal bursitis in the horse. Equine Vet J 2003; 35:662–668.
8. Van Pelt RW, Riley WF Jr. Traumatic subcutaneous calcaneal bursitis (capped hock) in the horse. J Am Vet Med Assoc 1968;153:1176–1180.

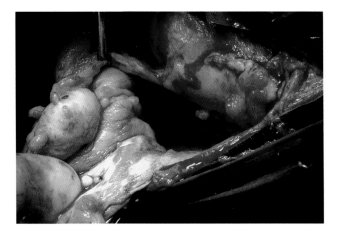

Figure 5.329. Surgery is being performed to remove the false bursa from a horse with an aseptic capped hock. The fibrous proliferative character of the lining makes it clear why medication will not resolve chronic lesions in this location.

STRINGHALT

Stringhalt is an involuntary hyperflexion of the hock when the horse moves, and the condition may affect one or both hindlimbs.[4,14] The extent of the motion may be minimal or so extensive that the fetlock contacts the abdomen. Atrophy of the distal muscles of the hindlimb has been described.[2] Two forms of the condition occur, and they are seemingly geographically predisposed.

Etiology

The condition is distributed worldwide, and one form affects isolated horses and is usually unilateral. It may follow an injury to the hindlimbs.[4,14] Spontaneous recovery is rare, but improvement may occur with rest.[4,14] The condition has been considered to involve the lateral digital extensor muscle tendon unit. Some cases are observed following trauma to this tendon, and adhesions of the tendon may form as it crosses the lateral surface of the hock joint. A series of 10 cases reported the development of stringhalt after dorsoproximal metatarsal injury to the extensor structures that healed by second intention. Most had suffered extensor tendon lacerations.[4] However, these 10 horses were only 19% of the total number of horses diagnosed with stringhalt during the same 5-year period.

Australian stringhalt has been restricted to Australia and New Zealand and commonly occurs in outbreak proportions, although sporadic incidence also occurs.[9] It is usually bilateral, and occurs more frequently in the late summer and fall of years with poor pasture. During those times, affected horses are exposed to exceptionally large amounts of certain toxic weeds including *Taraxacum officinael*, *Malva parviflora*, or *Hypochaeris radicata*, a dandelion.[3,5,12,13] The condition also has occurred under similar conditions in the Western Hemisphere in northern California, Washington, and southern Chile.[1,6,7] However, the Washington episode did not occur during a dry spell.

Although the plants mentioned are strongly associated with the condition, they have not been definitively linked as direct causes. Feeding trials using *H. radicata* failed to reproduce the condition, and *T. officinale* has been recommended for horse pastures. All exposed animals do not contract the disease.[7] An associated mycotoxin has been theorized to be present during the times at risk, while the plants themselves may not contribute directly to the situation. The incidence in Australia coincides with peak incidences of other plant-related mycotoxic diseases.[12]

The pathologic effect stems from axonopathy of the long peripheral nerves. The most noticeably affected are the recurrent laryngeal, peroneal, and tibial nerves, which account for laryngeal dysfunction and atrophy of the muscles of the gaskin.[2] The more distal portions of the axon may be affected earlier, which would tend to spare the nerve cell body and favor regeneration in the time required to cover the distance of degeneration.[15] The effect on the muscle is typical of neurogenic atrophy in that type II fibers are more affected. Many muscles are affected, most notably the cricoarytenoideus dorsalis, the long and lateral digital extensors, and the gastrocnemius.[15] The pathophysiology of the hyperflexion remains unknown. A plausible theory is that the action-debilitated extensors are overridden by the comparatively minimally affected flexors, biceps femoris, and semitendinosus.[15] However, the persistence of the flexion in severely affected horses remains unexplained.

Clinical Signs

The gait associated with typical Australian stringhalt has been graded.[9] Signs of the disease are quite variable; some horses show a very mild flexion of the hock during walking, whereas others show a marked jerking of the foot toward the abdomen. The dorsal surface of the fetlock may actually hit the abdominal wall in severe cases. Some horses show these signs at each step, whereas in others it is spasmodic. See the DVD for an illustration of stringhalt. In nearly all cases, the signs are exaggerated when the horse is backing. It is usually most noticeable after the horse has rested, but the signs may be intermittent and may disappear for variable periods of time. Any breed may be affected, and mild cases may not hinder the horse's use. Cold weather may cause an increase in signs, and signs usually decrease in intensity during warm weather. Most horses affected have a nervous disposition, which may play a part in the etiology. Laryngeal hemiparesis results from the effect on the recurrent laryngeal nerve.

Diagnosis

For either form of stringhalt, the alteration in gait is characteristic enough to make the diagnosis, but in some cases signs may be absent at the time of examination. The condition must be differentiated from fibrotic myopathy, which produces the opposite gait with a downward jerk. Intermittent upward fixation of the patella and shivering also should be ruled out. Horses affected with Australian stringhalt may exhibit other muscle involvement, including laryngeal paresis.

Treatment

The classic treatment for typical North American stringhalt has been removal of the tendon and a portion of the distal muscle of the lateral digital extensor (Figure 5.330). Spontaneous recovery of horses affected with this disease is uncommon.[4] In one study, 1 of 4 treated with rest and controlled exercise recovered, 2 improved, and 1 remained the same.[4] The author has had one case of acute-onset stringhalt in which a yearling recovered following treatment with therapeutic ultrasound. Following myotenectomy of the lateral digital flexor, 2 of 5 recovered completely and another improved significantly, but 1 remained intermittently affected and another had adhesions precluding complete myotenectomy and failed to improve.[4] In another case, a single horse affected with similar clinical signs responded to distal tarsal analgesia and subsequent steroid injection of those joints.[8] The hyperflexion was possibly the horse's response to the pain of distal tarsitis. Some benefit has been seen with treatment of acupuncture in a limited number of cases.

Surgical resection can be performed in a standing position, or in lateral recumbency on a surgical table. An incision approximately 8–10-cm long is made over the muscle of the lateral digital extensor just above the level of the point of the hock. The muscle belly cannot be identified until several layers of fascia have been severed. Pulling on the muscular portion reveals movement in the distal portion just before it attaches to the long digital extensor, where it is transected distally. Rarely, there are variations in the insertion of the

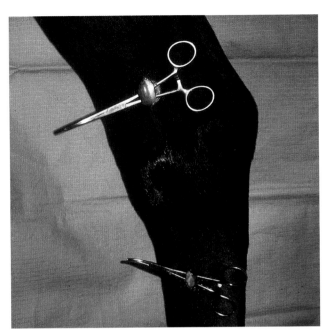

Figure 5.330. Lateral digital extensor myotenectomy, illustrating the proximal and distal incision sites to perform this procedure. (Courtesy of Dr. Gary Baxter.)

tendon, such as 2 tendons of insertion and insertion of the tendon on the proximal phalanx. Tension is then exerted on the proximal portion of the muscle until the tendon is pulled proximally. Considerable tension is sometimes required to break adhesions that are formed around the tendon where it crosses the hock joint, and further dissection of the proximal portion of the tendon may need to be performed to free it from adhesions and fascia. When the whole tendon is exposed, about 7 inches of it have been pulled through the upper incision. The tendon should then be transected, removing a 7- to 10-cm portion of the muscle belly with it.

Many cases show an almost immediate improvement, with complete recovery within 2 to 3 weeks. Other cases may take several months for any great improvement to occur, and still others may never show complete recovery. In cases that recur after several months or a year, an additional portion of the lateral digital extensor muscle may be removed.

There is little rationale for lateral digital extensor myotenectomy in horses suffering from Australian stringhalt, although some perform the procedure. The pathology is diffuse; the majority of horses recover spontaneously without treatment once they are removed from pasture. Recovery can often be protracted, lasting from several weeks to 1 year. The successful use of mephenesin in 1 case of stringhalt has been reported.[5] The drug was given in series of 3 injections both intravenously and intramuscularly. There was a relapse between the first and second series of injections. The drug merits further study on a significant number of cases. Other centrally-acting muscle relaxants, including phenytoin[10] and baclofen,[11] appear to be effective, but more experience is required with these agents before their efficacy is established.

Prognosis

For North American stringhalt, the prognosis is guarded to favorable. Most horses show some improvement after surgery, but the degree of improvement is not predictable. The prognosis is similar for Australian stringhalt. Many horses recover after removal from the pastures; however, some do not recover completely.

References

1. Araya O, Krause A, Solis de Ovando M. Outbreaks of stringhalt in southern Chile. Vet Rec 1998;142:462–463.
2. Cahill JI, Goulden BE. Stringhalt—current thoughts on aetiology and pathogenesis. Equine Vet J 1992;24:161–162.
3. Cahill JI, Goulden BE, Pearce HG. A review and some observations on stringhalt. NZ Vet 1985;33:101.
4. Crabill MR, Honnas CM, Taylor DS, et al. Stringhalt secondary to trauma to the dorsoproximal region of the metatarsus in horses: 10 cases (1986–1991). J Am Vet Med Assoc 1994;205:867–869.
5. Dixon RT, Stewart GA. Clinical and pharmacological observations in a case of equine stringhalt. Aust Vet J 1969;45: 127–130.
6. Galey FD, Hullinger PJ, McCaskill J. Outbreaks of stringhalt in northern california. Vet Hum Toxicol 1991;33:176–177.
7. Gay CC, Fransen S, Richards J, et al. Hypochoeris-associated stringhalt in North America. Equine Vet J 1993;25:456–457.
8. Hebert C, Jann HW. Intra-articular corticosteroid treatment for stringhalt in a Quarter horse: A case report. J Eq Vet Sci 1994;14:53–54.
9. Huntington PJ, Jeffcott LB, Friend SCE, et al. Australian stringhalt—epidemiological, clinical and neurological. Equine Vet J 1989;21:266–273.
10. Huntington PJ, Seneque S, Slocombe RF, et al. Use of phenytoin to treat horses with Australian stringhalt. Aust Vet J 1991;68:221–224.
11. Kannegieter NJ, Malik R. The use of baclofen in the treatment of stringhalt. Aust Equine Veterinarian 1992;10:90.
12. Pemberton DH, Caple IW. Australian stringhalt in horses. Vet Ann 1980;20:167.
13. Robertson-Smith RG, Jeffcott LB, Friend SCE, et al. An unusual incidence of neurological disease affecting horses during a drought. Aust Vet J 1985;62:6–12.
14. Seddon HO. Sudden case of stringhalt in a horse. Vet Rec 1963;75:35.
15. Slocombe RF, Huntington PJ, Friend SCE, et al. Pathological aspects of Australian stringhalt. Equine Vet J 1992;24: 174–183.

SHIVERING

Shivering is an uncommon problem characterized by involuntary flexion of the limbs and elevation of the tail. The course is often progressive and worsens over a long period of time. The hindlimbs and tail are more frequently affected, but sometimes the forelimbs may be involved.[1,2,4,6]

Etiology

The precise etiology of shivering is unknown; no documented lesions have been reported. Some have suggested that it is a peripheral nerve[5] or neuromuscular disorder subsequent to influenza, strangles, or other systemic diseases.[3] However, more recent evidence incriminates myopathy due to polysaccharide storage disease.[6] Draft horses are reported to be more frequently affected.[1] There are so many asymptomatic draft horses that have some degree of glycogen storage abnormality that it is difficult to positively attribute the signs of shivers to this myopathy.[7]

Clinical Signs and Diagnosis

In mild cases the signs may be difficult to detect, because they occur at irregular intervals, but in most cases the signs are characteristic.

Clinical signs consist of tension or trembling of the hindlimb with jerky tail movements,[4] progressing to sudden elevation and abduction of the hindlimb which is held suspended for several seconds.[1,8] Signs are exacerbated by backing the horse.[4] Fine body tremors may occur, but are possibly related to a more chronic debilitated state of the disease.[7] Horses may become progressively more debilitated and emaciated. Neurologic examination reveals no abnormalities. Stringhalt is the most important differential diagnosis.

Treatment

There is no curative treatment. Clinical signs have been reduced or controlled by feeding a high-fat, low-carbohydrate diet, and the effect is more profound when changes are made early in the progression of the disease.[9]

Prognosis

The prognosis is unfavorable because the signs usually increase in severity over time. Dietary management instituted early may control signs indefinitely, but relapse is always possible.

References

1. Baird JD, Firshman AM, Valberg SJ. Shivers (shivering) in the horse: A review. Proceedings Am Assoc Equine Pract 2006; 359–364.
2. Deen T. Shivering, a rare equine lameness. Eq Pract 1984;6: 19–21.
3. Mayhew IG. Large Animal Neurology. A Handbook for Veterinary Clinicians. Lea and Febiger, Philadelphia, 1989.
4. Neal FC, Ramsey FK. The nervous system. In Equine Medicine and Surgery, 2nd ed. American Veterinary Publications, Santa Barbara, 1972;486.
5. Neuman AJ. Well doc, what do you know? Draft Horse Journal 1990;27:34–35.
6. Palmer AC. Introduction to Animal Neurology, 2nd ed. Blackwell Scientific Publications, Oxford, 1976.
7. Valentine BA. Polysaccharide storage myopathy in draft and draft-related horses and ponies. Eq Pract 1999;21:16–19.
8. Valentine BA, deLahunta A, Divers TJ, et al. Clinical and pathologic findings in two draft horses with progressive muscle atrophy, neuromuscular weakness, and abnormal gait characteristic of shivers syndrome. J Am Vet Med Assoc 1999;215: 1661–1665.
9. Valentine BA, Divers TJ, Lavoie JP. Severe equine polysaccharide storage myopathy in draft horses: Clinical signs and response to dietary therapy. Proc Am Assoc Eq Pract 1996;42:294–296.

THE TIBIA: TYPES OF FRACTURES AND IMMOBILIZATION METHODS

Tibial fractures occur with roughly the same frequency as fractures of other proximal long bones, although regional differences are evident.[2,3] The more elastic bones in younger horses have less tendency to become severely comminuted, and open physes provide additional sites for fractures to occur. Younger horses are usually injured by a traumatic incident such as a kick, being stepped on by the mare, or pivoting at speed while running in pasture. Adult athletes may sustain stress fractures in addition to all types of trauma-induced injuries.

Complete or potentially complete diaphyseal fractures must be immobilized for transport to minimize soft tissue injury and eburnation of the bony fragments. In addition, tibial fractures can become open quite easily. See Chapter 7 for further information on first aid and methods of immobilization for tibial fractures.

There are several different types of tibial fractures, and a detailed discussion of each of these fracture types is below. Emphasis has been placed on treatment and prognosis because the cause, clinical signs, and methods of diagnosis are similar, regardless of the type of fracture.

The tibia is difficult to stabilize because the stifle is impossible to completely immobilize. Casts and splints simply add weight to the distal limb, causing further motion at the fracture site. A foal can be sedated and kept down, and can even be held, so further trauma is prevented.

Two devices are somewhat effective for immobilizing the stifle. The simpler is a temporary bandage splint with a lateral component that extends to the hip (Figure 7.32).[1,4,5] A Robert Jones bandage is applied to the limb and a lateral splint is affixed to the bandage with non-elastic tape. Alternatively, a 12-mm steel rod bent into a loop conforming to the caudolateral and caudomedial surfaces of the limb and extending to the tuber coxae can be used.[5] Sequential addition of thin layers of cotton wrapped tightly from the toe to the proximal tibia makes the eventual bandage extremely stiff.[5] A final layer of cast material further stiffens the bandage.[4]

The Thomas splint is more effective, but not as quickly applied (Figure 5.331). It consists of a frame with a ring that fits over the thigh and into the groin of the horse with cranial and caudal extensions reaching the foot to apply traction to the limb. Traction is applied to stabilize the entire limb. Hemicircumferential tape encircles one side of the limb and the opposite support bar to further immobilize the tibia without a tourniquet effect. The foot can be taped to the splint in foals, but weanlings and adults require wires through the hoof wall or bolts to a shoe for solid connection to the splint. The padded distal/medial hip ring is curved medially at the distal side to position tightly against the groin, and the lateral/proximal side of the ring contacts the hip closely.

Construction material depends upon the size of the horse. A heavy aluminum rod bent by hand suffices for foals. Weanlings or adults require hollow electric conduit or galvanized pipe, respectively. For splints constructed with hollow stock, the distal portion of the splint is comprised of threaded rod inserted into the tubes. Dual nuts are placed against the hollow tube to lock the splint in position. At the foot, foals' feet can be taped to the aluminum rod. In adults, threaded rod

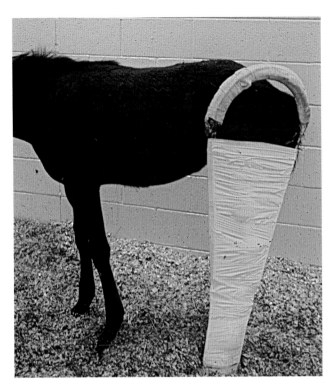

Figure 5.331.   A Thomas splint has been applied to a weanling with an open comminuted tibial fracture. The Thomas splint places the limb in traction and the tape supports the fracture in all directions. Bandages were changed as needed.

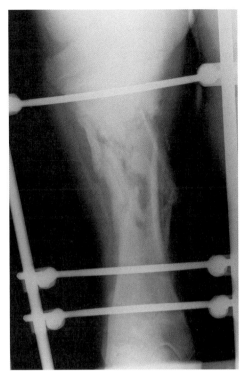

Figure 5.332.   Radiograph of an open comminuted midshaft tibial fracture in the weanling shown in Figure 5.331 that was managed in a Thomas splint and an external fixator. The fracture healed; however, the foal underwent subsequent surgery to correct forelimb tendon contracture and was never athletically sound.

is fixed to the dorsal and plantar portion of a plate holding wires or fixed to a shoe.

The length of the splint is adjusted to apply traction to the affected limb. In the middle of the splint, applying tape hemicircumferentially around the limb and the splint stabilizes the fracture without constricting the vascular supply; a bandage may be applied before the splint is taped if needed for a wound or padding. If this arrangement is not stable enough, a sleeve cast or external fixator can be added (Figure 5.332). As swelling subsides and muscles atrophy, the tension must be adjusted. For emergency use, the splint can be prepared in general sizes. For long-term application, general anesthesia is usually better; materials should be organized, and a farrier should be present.

If the tibia is fractured in the distal third of the diaphysis or more distally, a cast has some effect if it is applied as proximally as possible. Although the reciprocal apparatus may be disabled, application of a full-limb cast on the hindlimb of a standing horse is difficult. The distal portion of the cast is not needed to immobilize the tibia, and a sleeve cast ending at the distal metatarsus may suffice. Without the fetlock and foot included, the cast is lighter and easier to apply in the standing animal.

If these stabilization methods are not available, be sure that anything applied does not worsen the instability. Without the proper materials, leaving the affected limb alone may be a better choice.

References

1. Bramlage LR. First aid for the fracture patient. Proc Am Assoc Eq Pract 1982;28:97–105.
2. Crawford WH, Fretz PB. Long bone fractures in large animals. A retrospective study. Vet Surg 1985;14:295–302.
3. Haynes PF, Watters JW, McClure JR, et al. Incomplete tibial fractures in three horses. J Am Vet Med Assoc 1980; 177:1143–1145.
4. Janicek JC. How to provide limb stabilization for orthopedic emergencies. 2007:409–414.
5. Walmsley JP. First aid splinting for the equine fracture patient. Eq Vet Educ 1993;5:61–63.

TIBIAL TUBEROSITY/CREST FRACTURES

The physis of the tibial tuberosity is partially ossified at birth and forms a fibrocartilage union with the epiphysis during the second year of life. The irregular physis remains radiographically visible until 36 to 42 months of age,[6] and may be mistaken for a fracture. The terms tibial tuberosity and tibial crest are sometimes used interchangeably; however, tuberosity refers to the area of attachment of the quadriceps tendons and crest to the remainder of the cranial ridge on the tibia. The tibial tuberosity is relatively broad with regional insertions for the 3 patellar ligaments. Growth disturbance is not a factor with tibial crest fractures.

Lameness associated with naturally occurring variations in ossification of the tibial tuberosity has been reported (Figure 5.333).[3,8] Bilateral hindlimb lameness

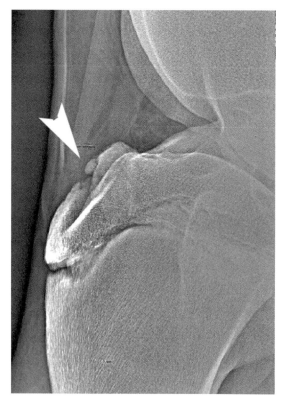

Figure 5.333. Lateromedial Xeroradiograph demonstrating an incompletely ossified tibial crest in a yearling Standardbred filly. The fragment (arrow) will become incorporated into the remainder of the tibial crest in time.

in a yearling Thoroughbred colt exacerbated by hindlimb flexion was associated with irregular ossification of the physis.[8] Radiographs revealed bilateral changes on the tibial tuberosities consisting of small osseous separations on the most cranial aspect of each. The physes were also considered wider than normal distally. Radiographs taken after 7 weeks of stall rest demonstrated that the cranial densities had ossified to become part of the remainder of the apophysis. A previously less-apparent lucency in the apophysis at the distal limit of the separate osseous density had become more radiolucent. A similar finding was reported in 8 Thoroughbred horses 1 to 3 years old.[3] Unilaterally affected horses were described to move away from the affected limb at the trot. Treatment consisted of rest up to 3 months.

Fractures are usually in the frontal plane and occur from direct trauma such as a kick or from hitting a jump, and are the second most common stifle injury in event horses.[1,4] Horses may occasionally avulse the fragment due to sudden quadriceps tension. Displacement is in the proximal and cranial direction and quadriceps integrity usually remains intact. However, if the middle patellar tendon is compromised, the stifle may be dropped, and the horse may not be willing or able to fix the limb in extension.[2] An open wound may be present from the initial trauma, which must be taken into consideration when planning internal fixation. Severity of lameness at the onset of the injury varies widely but is not related to eventual return to soundness.[1]

The lateromedial radiograph demonstrates the fracture, but the caudolateral-craniomedial oblique projection may provide additional information (Figure 5.334).[1] If an open physis complicates the radiographic diagnosis of a minimally displaced fracture, comparison to the

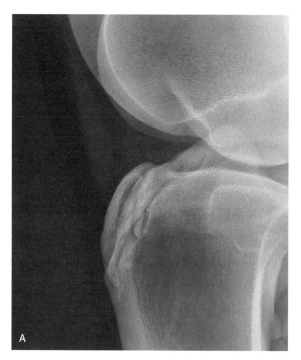
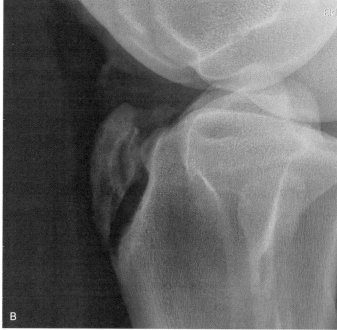

Figure 5.334. A. Lateromedial radiograph of a horse with a complete fracture of the tibial tuberosity. B. Caudolateral-craniomedial oblique projection of the same fracture, demonstrating improved characterization of the fracture by the additional radiographic projection.

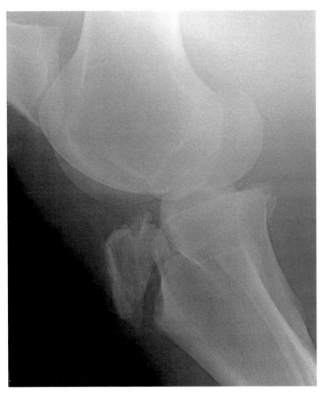

Figure 5.335. Lateromedial radiograph of a horse with a chronic, displaced, complete fracture of the tibial tuberosity that was repaired with a single locking plate. (Courtesy of Dr. Laurie Goodrich.)

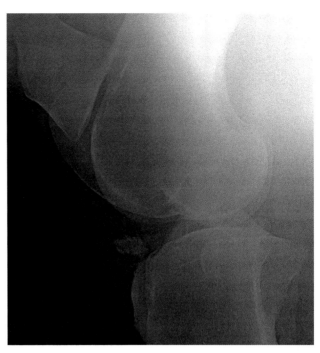

Figure 5.336. This small, chronic fracture of the lateral tibial tuberosity was removed because it was contributing to chronic drainage and lameness. (Courtesy of Dr. Gary Baxter.)

contralateral limb is useful, as is the horse's response to direct palpation. Most tibial tuberosity fractures are nonarticular; those with fracture lines at or caudal to the intercondylar eminence of the proximal tibia may be articular.[1]

Traction by the patellar ligaments tends to distract the fragment, which impairs healing (Figure 5.335). However, non- or minimally displaced fractures can heal following stall rest for several weeks.[1] Radiographic monitoring is done at 6-week intervals to document healing and detect delayed separation of the fracture.[10] These fractures take much longer to heal than usually expected, and complete radiographic union is not always required for soundness.[1] In a series of 17 horses with nonarticular fractures of the tibial tuberosity, 14 became sound and 12 returned to work in an average of 6.3 months.[1] The initial period of stall rest was 2 to 3 months followed by hand walking. All long-term radiographs demonstrated osteolysis of the fracture fragment and a fibrous union. Three horses with associated soft tissue injuries did not become sound. One horse with multiple ultrasonically confirmed ligamentous and meniscal injuries was not surprising, but 2 horses with seemingly isolated lateral patellar ligament desmitis also failed to become sound.[1] Perhaps more extensive imaging would have revealed other areas of involvement.

Ultrasound is a valuable adjunct to radiographs for detecting potentially limiting soft tissue injury[1] as well for identifying which patellar ligament insertions are

involved and potential articular involvement. Fractures not involving the insertion of the middle patellar ligament may be removed; these have usually been confined to the insertion of the lateral patellar ligament.[10] The area of the insertion of lateral patellar ligament to the tibial tuberosity protrudes prominently and is often involved. Removal of the bone fragment may facilitate a more efficient healing of the soft tissue to the parent bone, particularly if improvement does not occur with stall rest (Figure 5.336). Even structurally less significant fractures can take a very long time to heal and may cause lameness.

Unstable, displaced, or articular fractures require internal fixation (Figures 5.335 and 5.337). The fragment must be reduced and stabilized in a tension-band fashion which converts the quadriceps distraction to compression.[2,9] Tension-band wire,[5] headless screw fixation with cable tension band,[7] or lag-screws alone have been used successfully. Plate fixation improves the repair when the fragment is large and/or unstable[9,10] or when the fragment has undergone osteolysis, which occurs relatively rapidly (Figures 5.335 and 5.337).

Single-[10] or dual-plate fixation with proximal lag screws for rotational stability[9] have been reported. A single narrow dynamic compression plate placed cranially is sufficient; the patellar ligament insertion is broad enough to allow exposure of the bone for plate application. Locking compression plates provide additional stability, but locking screws must be applied perpendicularly to the plate.

In a series of 6 horses that had tibial tuberosity fractures repaired with cranially placed narrow dynamic compression plates, the mean time for return to their

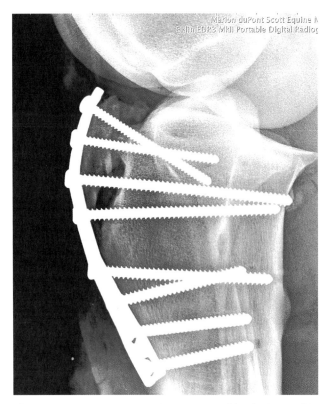

Figure 5.337. Radiograph of the proximal tibia of a horse with a tibial tuberosity fracture that did not respond to stall rest. After several weeks there was noticeable osteolysis of the fragment. A single plate has been applied to provide a tension band support for the distracting forces of the patellar tendon. The screws crossing the fracture line were placed in lag fashion. The fracture line was debrided, but bone resorption had occurred, preventing radiographic demonstration of bone contact. The fracture healed uneventfully.

previous level of activity was 28 months.[10] Two of 4 horses with fractures repaired with 2 plates and proximal lag screws were euthanatized after the fixation failed, and 2 other horses returned to their previous level of work after a few months.[9]

The recovery rate from surgically repaired tibial tuberosity fractures is generally good, provided stable fixation can be accomplished. Complicating factors include failure of the fixation, infection from the wound, and disruption of the cranial tibial articular surface. Occasionally chronic pain with exercise or focal loosening or infection may require removal of the implants.

References

1. Arnold CE, Schaer TP, Baird DL, et al. Conservative management of 17 horses with nonarticular fractures of the tibial tuberosity. Equine Vet J 2003;35:202–206.
2. Auer JA, Watkins JP. Diseases of the tibia. In Equine Medicine and Surgery, Vol. II, 5th ed. Colahan PT, Mayhew IG, Merritt AM, et al., eds. American Veterinary Publications, Santa Barbara, 1999;1696–1701.
3. Baker RH. Osteochondrosis of the tibial tuberosity of the horse. J Am Vet Med Assoc 1960;137:354–355.
4. Dyson SJ. Stifle trauma in the event horse. Eq Vet Educ 1994;6:234–240.
5. Gerring EL, Davies JV. Fracture of the tibial tuberosity in a polo pony. Equine Vet J 1982;14:158–159.
6. Getty GR. Sisson and Grossman's Anatomy of Domestic Animals, 5th ed. W.B. Saunders, Philadelphia, 1975.
7. Johnson NL, Galuppo LD. Use of a stainless steel cable and headless tapered compression screw for repair of a tibial crest fracture in a 10-year-old horse. Vet Comp Orth Traum 2004;17:247–252.
8. Kold SE. Traction apophysitis in a yearling colt resembling Osgood-Schlatter disease in man. Equine Vet J 1990;22:60–61.
9. Smith BL, Auer JA, Watkins JP. Surgical repair of tibial tuberosity avulsion fractures in four horses. Vet Surg 1990;19:117–121.
10. Wright IM, Montesso F, Kidd LJ. Surgical treatment of fractures of the tibial tuberosity in 6 adult horses. Equine Vet J 1995;27:96–102.

FRACTURES OF THE PROXIMAL TIBIAL PHYSIS

Fracture of the proximal tibial physis has been observed in foals up to 8 months of age.[1] The injury usually occurs from direct trauma (e.g., kick) while the limb is bearing weight[2] or from bending while having the limb somehow entrapped or stepped upon by the dam.[1] The forces apply pressure in a valgus direction, causing medial tension to separate the physeal cartilage. The physis opens until the lateral metaphyseal bone fractures, producing a Salter-Harris type II fracture.[3] The epiphysis and bone fragment becomes displaced laterally due to the ramp defect left in the proximal lateral metaphysis (Figure 5.338). The lateral metaphyseal component commonly occupies a third or less of the physeal surface. Uncommonly, the medial collateral ligament ruptures, which reduces the prognosis. The affected proximal limb assumes a stifle valgus position.[1,3]

Conservative management was used to successfully treat a non-displaced tibial fracture of the proximal physis in a foal[6] and 2 horses.[4] For displaced fractures, the preferred treatment is internal fixation.[1,3] Because the bone surfaces rapidly become eburnated and will not fit as well, repair should be performed as soon as possible. Surgical techniques reported include lag-screw fixation,[7] cross pinning,[8] medial plate application,[1,3,11] or bone plates and external fixation.[10]

Most surgeons approach the proximal tibia medially to place either a dynamic compression or T-plate. A screw that extends the entire length of the epiphysis is used so that the most possible screw threads engage the epiphysis for maximum holding power (Figure 5.339). If possible, the second screw engages the metaphyseal fragment. This technique does not adhere strictly to the principles of internal fixation in that the medial cortex of the tibia is the compression side of the bone. However, this fracture tends to maintain itself in reduction by friction if the epiphysis has an adequate contact area. Fractures in which the metaphyseal fragment occupies significantly more than the typical one-third of the physeal surface area are more difficult to maintain in reduction because the proximal fragment tends to slide off laterally (Figure 5.340). Cross-pin fixation has been reported for foals less than 50 kg.[5,8,9] Foals should bear more weight on the limb immediately and be walking well in 7 to 10 days.[3] Some fracture disease should be expected if this does not occur. The plate should be removed in 2 to 3 months. Angular deformity due to the medial physeal bridging is possible, but it usually corrects after the plate is removed.

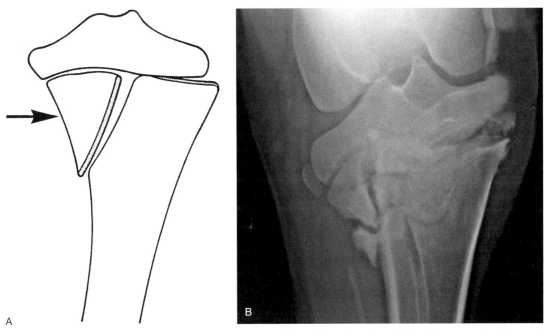

Figure 5.338. Line illustration (A) and caudocranial radiograph (B) of the stifle demonstrating a Salter-Harris type II fracture of the proximal tibial physis. The metaphyseal component is always lateral (arrow) and usually involves approximately one-third of the distance across the physis. (Image courtesy of Dr. Gary Baxter.)

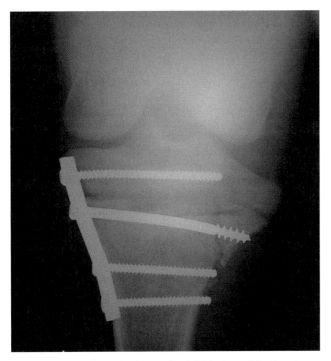

Figure 5.339. Repair of a proximal tibial physeal fracture in a foal using a medial plate. The first screw was placed as far as possible across the epiphysis and the 2nd screw engaged the metaphyseal component of the proximal fragment.

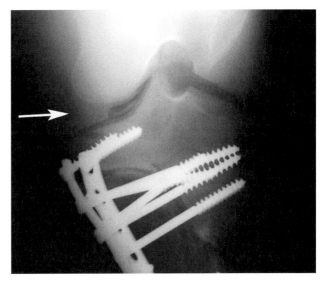

Figure 5.340. Valgus stressed craniocaudal radiograph of a repaired Salter-Harris type II fracture of the proximal tibia in a foal. The medial collateral ligament has ruptured as evidenced by the widened medial femorotibial joint space (arrow). The metaphyseal fragment in this fracture approximated 50% of the transverse measurement of the physis which permitted it to slide off more easily than most similar fractures; it was therefore repaired with 2 plates and 7 screws in the proximal fragment. Presumably more stress would have been applied on the medial aspect of the stifle to fracture such a large metaphyseal fragment.

The prognosis is generally favorable barring complications such as failure of the fixation, angular limb deformity, infection, or wound dehiscence.[1,3] The smaller the foal, the better the prognosis. The proximal physis is comparatively resilient and usually does not limit normal development. The prognosis for athletic activity following successful fixation is approximately 50%.[3]

References

1. Auer JA, Watkins JP. Diseases of the tibia. In Equine Medicine and Surgery, Vol II, 5th ed. Colahan PT, Mayhew IG, Merritt AM, Moore JN, eds. American Veterinary Publications, Santa Barbara, 1999;1696–1701.
2. Bramlage LR. Long bone fractures. Vet Clin North Am Large Anim Pract 1983;5:285–310.
3. Bramlage LR. The Tibia. In Equine Surgery, 2nd ed. Auer JA, Stick JA, eds. W.B. Saunders, Philadelphia, 1999;862–867.
4. Harrison LJ, May SA, Richardson JD, et al. Conservative treatment of an incomplete longbone fracture of a hindlimb of four horses. Vet Rec 1991;129:133–136.
5. Juswiak JS, Milton JL. Closed reduction and blind cross-pinning for repair of a proximal tibial fracture in a foal. J Am Vet Med Assoc 1985;187:743–745.
6. Turner AS. Fracture of specific bones. In Equine Medicine and Surgery, 3rd ed. Mansmann RA, McAllister ES, eds. American Veterinary Publications, Santa Barbara, 1982;1018.
7. Wagner PC, DeBowes RM, Grant BD, et al. Cancellous bone screws for repair of proximal growth plate fractures of the tibia in foals. J Am Vet Med Assoc 1984;184:688–691.
8. Watkins JP. Fractures of the tibia. In Equine fracture repair. Nixon AJ, ed. WB Saunders, Philadelphia, 1996;273–283.
9. Watkins JP, Auer JA, Taylor TS. Crosspin fixation of fractures of the proximal tibia in three foals. Vet Surg 1985;14:153–159.
10. White NA, Wheat JD. An expansion and compression technique for reducing and stabilizing proximal epiphyseal fractures of the tibia in foals. J Am Vet Med Assoc 1975;167:733–738.
11. White NA, Blackwell RB, Hoffman PE. Use of a bone plate for repair of proximal physeal fractures of the tibia in two foals. J Am Vet Med Assoc 1982;181:252–254.

FRACTURES OF THE DISTAL TIBIAL PHYSIS

Fractures of the distal tibial physis are less common than those of the proximal physis. These may be true physeal fractures[2] or the physis may be entered by a diaphyseal fracture.[1] One instance of bilateral non-displaced fractures extending down to the medial aspect of the physes was reported in a weanling Appaloosa; conservative therapy was successful.[4]

Treatment must achieve reduction and stability of the fracture; if the tarsocrural joint is involved, the articular surface is reconstructed. The distal tibial physis is comparatively thin and irregular, which complicates inserting an implant. External coaptation such as a cast applied as closely to the stifle as possible may be required to augment internal fixation. When the entire epiphysis is intact, Rush pins have been suggested.[3] Alternatively, Steinman pins placed in a cruciate fashion can be used.[5] If the fracture can be reduced and there is no articular involvement, a Thomas splint can be applied to immobilize the mid- to distal tibia in foals (Figure 5.331). Some fractures simply cannot be adequately reduced or immobilized, and euthanasia is indicated.

References

1. Auer JA, Watkins JP. Diseases of the tibia. In Equine Medicine and Surgery, Vol. II, 5th ed. Colahan PT, Mayhew IG, Merritt AM,

Moore JN, eds. American Veterinary Publications, Santa Barbara: 1999;1696–1701.
2. Embertson RM, Bramlage LR, Herring DS, et al. Physeal fractures in the horse. I. Classification and incidence. Vet Surg 1986;15 (3):223–229.
3. Foerner JJ. Surgical treatment of selected musculoskeletal disorders of the rear limb. In Equine Surgery, 1st ed. Auer JA, ed. Saunders, Philadelphia, 1992;1055–1075.
4. Frankeny RL, Johnson PJ, Messer NT, et al. Bilateral tibial metaphyseal stress fractures associated with physitis in a foal. J Am Vet Med Assoc 1994;205:76–78.
5. Stashak TS. The tibia. Fractures. Adams' Lameness in Horses, 4th ed. Lea and Febiger, Baltimore, 1987;726–728.

DIAPHYSEAL AND METAPHYSEAL TIBIAL FRACTURES

Most complete fractures of the tibial shaft have a spiral configuration and/or are comminuted.[5] The smaller the patient, the better the prognosis for successful treatment.[24]

The causes of these fractures include external trauma (e.g., kicking) or other stresses.[3,5,6,8,9,12,18,21,23] Fractures due to torsion combined with bending and axial compressions have been described.[18] Midshaft tibial fractures have resulted from falls during a race and have also occurred spontaneously.[23] The author has seen several cases in which the horse simply pivoted while running in pasture. Transverse fractures seem to be more common in foals, and adult horses often sustain highly comminuted fractures.

A recent *in vitro* study demonstrated that direct high velocity midshaft tibial trauma produced an oblique fracture or a fracture with butterfly fragment comminution opposite the point of cortical impact, which is where the apex of the triangle is located.[10] Small fragments occurred at the point of impact, and 98% had additional fissures.

Complete fracture of the tibia is characterized by the inability to bear weight on the affected limb, marked soft tissue swelling, angular deformity, and regional crepitation (Figure 5.341). Craniomedial overriding of the proximal fragment coupled with valgus angulation frequently results in an open fracture due to the lack of soft tissue covering the medial aspect of the tibia. The obvious instability, swelling, and pain make the diagnosis obvious. Radiographs are required to define the fracture configuration and formulate a treatment plan.

Incomplete or nondisplaced fractures of the tibia can be difficult to diagnose; acute lameness may abate with time (Figure 5.342). Visible or palpable swelling or pain is often absent, making localization difficult. Minimally displaced fractures may cause edema in the soft tissues overlying the thinly covered medial tibial cortex, but it can be subtle. The degree of lameness varies from severe to mild, depending upon degree of instability and duration.[12,13] Chronic fractures may begin to produce externally visible callus that appears as swelling.[12]

Radiographs in several oblique projections may be needed to demonstrate the fracture. Radiographic findings may include a fracture line, but intra-medullary or extra-cortical callus may be the only abnormality. Nuclear scintigraphy is an invaluable imaging technique for obscure tibial lesions (Figure 5.342).[13,17,19]

Conservative management has been used successfully for only non- or minimally displaced tibial fractures,

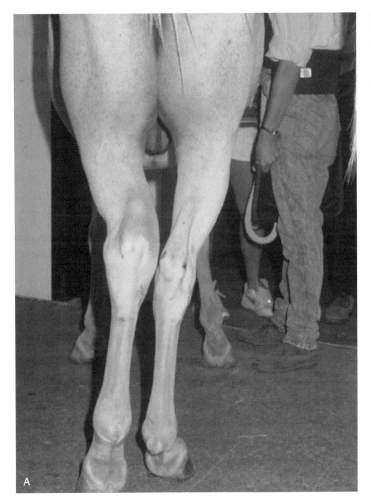

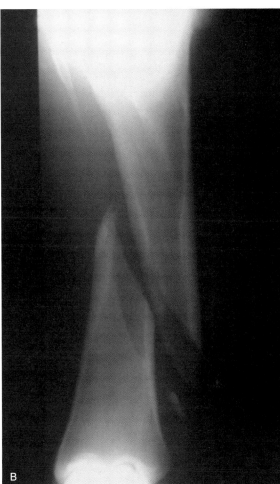

Figure 5.341. A. Caudal view of a horse with a left midshaft oblique tibial fracture. Note the valgus deviation at the point of fracture. B. Caudocranial radiograph of the fracture in the horse depicted in (A). This fracture is closed; however, the overriding proximal fragment is at risk of puncturing the thin soft tissue covering on the medial aspect of the tibia. (Courtesy of Dr. Ted Stashak.)

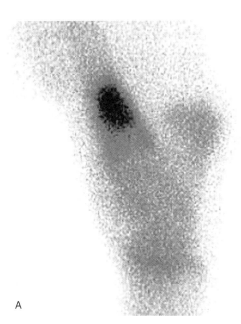

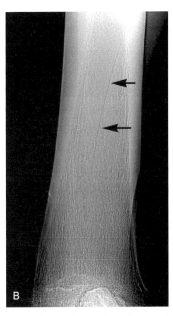

Figure 5.342. Lateral scintigram (A) and tibial radiograph (B) demonstrating an incomplete tibial fracture (arrows). (Courtesy of Dr. Gary Baxter.)

provided catastrophic separation does not occur during convalescence.[12,13] Stall confinement for 3 to 6 months with radiographic and/or scintigraphic monitoring is feasible.[12,13] Horses may remain significantly lame for several weeks or become sound at a walk. Most withhold pain control to cause the horses to take better care of themselves due to the possibility of progression to a complete fracture.[12] Although a high incidence of complete separation of minimally displaced tibial fractures has been reported,[12] 6 of 10 tibiae with fissure fractures recovered.[7] Horses with long (12- to 15-cm) spiral fissure lines generally did not remain stable and survive (Figure 5.343), whereas those with shorter (3- 7-cm) visible fissure lines survived.[7] The radiographically visible lengths of fissures tended to increase before finally healing. Additionally, nondisplaced fractures located on the compression or caudal side of the bone tended to become unstable (Figure 5.343).[7]

A bandage splint extending to the hip and putting the horse on a wire to prevent it from laying down has been recommended.[5] If the diagnosis is uncertain but believed to be a nondisplaced tibial fracture, the horse should be treated as described and radiographs taken in 10 days to establish a diagnosis.[5]

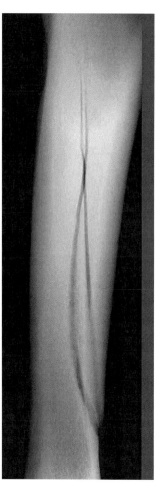

Figure 5.343. Lateral radiograph of a horse with a long spiral oblique tibial fracture that will most likely displace further if left untreated. (Courtesy of Dr. Gary Baxter.)

The decision to apply internal fixation on nondisplaced fractures can be difficult if the fracture appears to be stable. Persisting severe lameness is one sign that stability is not secure. From the above description, fractures traversing much of the length of the tibia should receive stronger consideration for internal fixation.[7]

The effective use of external coaptation for unstable tibial fractures is difficult. Distal fractures that self-abut to resist collapse are more amenable and can be treated with a cast and/or a Thomas splint (Figure 5.331).[21] However, external coaptation may be reconsidered when the fracture is too comminuted for internal fixation (Figure 5.332). Sleeve casts cause less leverage on the fracture than full-limb casts and may be applied with the horse standing when reduction of the fracture is not required. Thomas splints partially immobilize the stifle and provide traction to stabilize the fracture but are time consuming to prepare and usually must be custom built by a welder and a farrier.

Foals are more amenable to external coaptation, but are also more subject to fracture disease, which refers to problems affecting the entire patient as a result of lack of complete weight-bearing in the affected limb. Examples in foals include varus deformity of the contralateral limb and forelimb flexural deformities. Unless the external coaptation is effective and achieves a quick result, the fractured limb may ultimately be the best limb on an unsound horse after the limb heals. The most common complication in the adult is laminitis in the contralateral or other limbs. In general, athletic function should not be expected in horses with complete tibial fractures treated by external coaptation.

Internal fixation is the best option when applicable.[1,5,6,8,24] Success depends upon sufficient space proximal and distal to the fracture to place enough screws for adequate stability and interfragmentary compression along the fracture line. Bramlage has reported the successful treatment of a tibial fracture in an adult horse.[6] In the tibia, the tension surface is cranial and the compression surface is caudal.[11,20]

With the horse in dorsal recumbency and using a cranial approach, 2 plates should be placed, one craniolaterally and the other craniomedially at a 90° angle to each other. Plates should extend the entire length of the bone, but the 2 plates should not begin or end at the same points. The caudal cortex should have a buttress to prevent cycling of the plates.[4,24] Foals occasionally require less fixation for successful repair. When necessary, the fracture may be reconstructed using lag screws beside the plates to stabilize the fracture for plate application and provide better interfragmentary compression (Figure 5.344). Locking compression plates should provide more secure fixation than regular dynamic compression plates.

Interlocking nails have been developed to treat proximal equine long bone fractures.[14–16] Although promising in some respects, the torsional strength of the interlocking nail has not reached that of double-plating. Additionally, a specific fracture configuration is required.[2]

A cast should not be applied for recovery, because it will change the tension forces on the bone and result in additional stresses in the fracture.[6,20] A recovery pool is an advantage, but the horse should at least be assisted

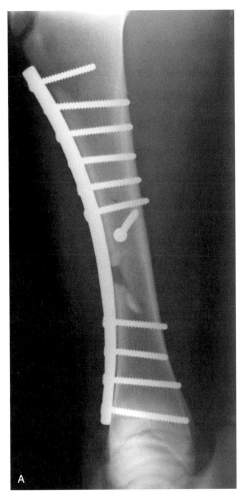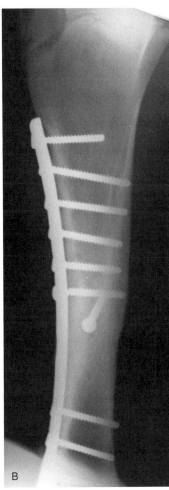

Figure 5.344. Lateromedial radiograph of a tibial fracture in a foal at the time of repair using a single plate placed on the cranial aspect of the tibia (A) and after the fracture has healed (B). The single screw was used to compress the fracture line. Note the solid caudal buttress on the caudal aspect of the tibia. (Courtesy of Dr. NA White.)

in its recovery from anesthesia. Euthanasia is advised for adult horses that have sustained irreparable severely comminuted fractures that cannot be stabilized.

In foals, half-pin[3] and full-transfixation pinning have been used successfully by the author. Successful experimental external fixation has been reported in foals.[22] The author believes this technique used alone can be successfully applied only to a transverse, mid-shaft fracture with no proximal or distal fracture lines in a patient weighing less than 125 kg. These conditions are rarely seen simultaneously in the clinical situation. Full-pin fixation is more stable than half-pin fixation. If external fixation is chosen, pin placements should be limited to the transverse plane and not placed in the cranial-caudal direction. In some cases, external fixation may be used to aid stability achieved with external coaptation such as a Thomas splint. The general success and lack of after care with internal fixation override consideration of external fixation alone in most situations, except where soft tissue loss has occurred.

The prognosis for a fractured tibia in an adult is guarded to poor. Non-displaced fractures may heal with stall rest, but complete separation remains a possibility for several weeks. The difficulty in successfully repairing a complete tibial fracture in an adult is reflected in the few reports in the literature. Each case is different with its own set of considerations.

In a series of 9 foals with tibial fractures repaired by internal fixation using plates and screws, 6 achieved excellent results and 2 others recovered.[24] However, the prognosis depends on the type of fracture sustained, its duration, and the treatment selected.

References

1. Auer JA, Watkins JP. Diseases of the tibia. In Equine Medicine and Surgery, Vol. II, 5th ed. Colahan PT, Mayhew IG, Merritt AM, et al., eds. American Veterinary Publications, Santa Barbara, 1999;1696–1701.
2. Auer JA, Watkins JP. Instrumentation and techniques in equine fracture fixation. Vet Clin North Am Equine Pract 1996; 12:283–302.
3. Bignozzi L, Gnudi M, Masetti L, et al. Half pin fixation in 2 cases of equine long bone fracture. Equine Vet J 1981;13: 64–66.
4. Bramlage LR. Long bone fractures. Vet Clin North Am Large Anim Pract 1983;5:285–310.
5. Bramlage LR. The tibia. In Equine surgery, 2nd ed. Auer JA, Stick JA, eds. W.B. Saunders, Philadelphia, 1999;862–867.
6. Bramlage LR, Hanes GE. Internal fixation of a tibial fracture in an adult horse. J Am Vet Med Assoc 1982;180: 1090–1094.
7. Derungs S, Fuerst A, Haas C, et al. Fissure fractures of the radius and tibia in 23 horses: A retrospective study. Eq Vet Educ 2001;13:313–318.
8. Dingwall JS, Duncan DB, Horney FD. Compression plating in large animal orthopedics. J Am Vet Med Assoc 1971;158: 1651–1657.

9. Fessler JF, Amstutz HE. Fracture repair. In Textbook of Large Animal Surgery. Oehme FW, Prier JE, eds. Williams and Wilkins Co., Baltimore, 1974.

10. Fürst AE, Oswald S, Jäggin S, et al. Fracture configurations of the equine radius and tibia after a simulated kick. Vet Comp Orth Traum 2008;21:49–58.

11. Hartman W, Schamhardt HC, Lammertink JL, et al. Bone strain in the equine tibia: An *in vivo* strain gauge analysis. Am J Vet Res 1984;45:880–884.

12. Haynes PF, Watters JW, McClure JR, et al. Incomplete tibial fractures in three horses. J Am Vet Med Assoc 1980; 177:1143–1145.

13. Johnson PJ, Allhands RV, Baker GJ, et al. Incomplete linear tibial fractures in two horses. J Am Vet Med Assoc 1988; 192:522–524.

14. McDuffee LA, Stover SM. An *in vitro* biomechanical investigation of an interlocking nail for fixation of diaphyseal tibial fractures in adult horses. Proceedings Am Coll Vet Surg 1993:390.

15. McDuffee LA, Stover SM, Bach JM, et al. An *in vitro* biomechanical investigation of an equine interlocking nail. Vet Surg 2000;29:38–47.

16. McDuffee LA, Stover SM, Taylor KT. *In vitro* cyclic biomechanical properties of an interlocking equine tibial nail. Vet Surg 2000;29:163–172.

17. Pilsworth RC, Webbon PM. The use of radionuclide bone scanning in the diagnosis of tibial 'stress' fractures in the horse: A review of five cases. Equine Vet J 1988;Supplement 6:60–65.

18. Rooney JR. The mechanics of humeral and tibial fractures of the horse. Cornell Vet 1965;55:599.

19. Ross MW. Bone scintigraphy: Lessons learned from 5,000 horses. Proceedings Am Assoc of Equine Pract 2005;51:6–20.

20. Schneider RK, Milne DW, Gabel AA, et al. Miltidirectional *in vivo* strain analysis of the equine radius and tibia during dynamic loading with and without a cast. Am J Vet Res 1982;43: 1541–1550.

21. Springstead BK. Fracture of the tibia in a horse. J Am Vet Med Assoc 1967;155:1370–1373.

22. Sullins KE, McIlwraith CW. Evaluation of 2 types of external skeletal fixation for repair of experimental tibial fractures in foals. Vet Surg 1987;16:255–264.

23. Vaughan LC, Mason BJE. A clinicopathologic study of racing accidents in horses. Adlard and Son, Ltd., Dorking, Surrey, 1975;70.

24. Young DR, Richardson DW, Nunamaker DM, et al. Use of dynamic compression plates for treatment of tibial diaphyseal fractures in foals: Nine cases (1980–1987). J Am Vet Med Assoc 1989;194:1755–1760.

TIBIAL STRESS FRACTURES

Remodeling due to cyclic fatigue of bone in horses that work at speed is thought to result in stress fractures.[10] Acute lameness may or may not abate with time, and visible or palpable swelling is often absent. Tibial stress fractures in racehorses tend to have particular patterns. Two-year-olds and occasionally 3-year-olds are predominately affected,[1,3,5,7] but variation occurs.[2] In a series of 61 Thoroughbreds, 70% had not raced.[3] Thoroughbreds may develop lesions in the proximal caudal to lateral aspect of the tibia[1,5] or mid-diaphyseal region,[3,6,12] similar to Standardbreds and racing Quarter horses.[4,7]

Scintigraphy or high detail imaging is often required to image the lesion (Figures 4.204, 5.342, and 9.150). When radiographically present, the beam usually must strike the fracture line exactly to see the lesion unless callus is present (Figure 5.342B). When present, the radiographic lesion is variable, depending upon the stage of development of the lesion; follow-up radiographs may be similar, improved, or appear to have worsened.[6]

Scintigraphic findings were quantitated in 42 tibiae with stress fractures in 35 horses.[12] Affected horses returned to racing in a mean of 10.6 months (range 5 to 42 months). No difference in return to racing with regard to severity of lameness or the scintigraphic lesion was found.[3,6,12] A series of 13 Standardbred race horses with tibial stress fractures were managed with 8 to 16 weeks of stall rest followed by 4 to 12 weeks of pasture turn-out before return to training.[7] Healing was determined by radiographic follow-up without repeating scintigraphy. Healing was evident as soon as 60 days after diagnosis. After a mean time of 9.5 months, 10 horses returned to racing, approximating other results.[3]

Determining the time of healing in such an obscure lesion is difficult. Racing at speed produces stresses that could cause catastrophic separation of incompletely healed stress fractures.[11]

Extracorporeal shock wave therapy (ESWT) has been applied to tibial stress fractures.[8] The number of horses treated is few, precluding any conclusions. Benefit has been observed after treating metacarpal stress fractures.[9] Importantly, the desensitization effect of ESWT may facilitate premature return to work with disastrous results. Complete healing should be documented before allowing complete return to work.

References

1. Mackey VS, Trout DR, Meagher DM, et al. Stress fractures of the humerus, radius, and tibia in horses. Clinical features and radiographic and/or scintigraphic appearance. Vet Rad 1987; 28:26–31.

2. Nelson A. Stress fractures of the hind limb in 2 Thoroughbreds. Eq Vet Educ 1994;6:245–248.

3. O'Sullivan CB, Lumsden JM. Stress fractures of the tibia and humerus in Thoroughbred racehorses: 99 cases (1992–2000). J Am Vet Med Assoc 2003;222:491–498.

4. Peloso JG, Watkins JP, Keele SR, et al. Bilateral stress fractures of the tibia in a racing American Quarter horse. J Am Vet Med Assoc 1993;203:801–803.

5. Pilsworth RC, Webbon PM. The use of radionuclide bone scanning in the diagnosis of tibial 'stress' fractures in the horse: A review of five cases. Equine Vet J 1988;Supplement 6:60–65.

6. Ramzan PHL, Newton JR, Shepherd MC, et al. The application of a scintigraphic grading system to equine tibial stress fractures: 42 cases. Equine Vet J 2003;35:382–388.

7. Ruggles AJ, Moore RM, Bertone AL, et al. Tibial stress fractures in racing Standardbreds: 13 cases (1989–1993). J Am Vet Med Assoc 1996;209:634–637.

8. Scheuch B, Whitcomb M, Galuppo L, et al. Clinical evaluation of high-energy extracorporeal shock waves on equine orthopedic injuries. Equine musculoskeletal high-energy shock wave therapy symposium 2001.

9. Scheuch B, Whitcomb M, Galuppo L, et al. Clinical evaluation of high-energy extracorporeal shock waves on equine orthopedic injuries. 20th Annual Meeting of the Association of Equine Sports Medicine (AESM) 2000.

10. Stover SM, Ardans AA, Read DH, et al. Patterns of stress factors associated with complete bone fractures in racehorses. Proc Am Assoc Eq Pract 1993;39:131–132.

11. Stover SM, Johnson BJ, Daft BM, et al. An association between complete and incomplete stress fractures of the humerus in racehorses. Equine Vet J 1992;24:260–263.

12. Valdés-Martínez A, Seiler G, Mai W, et al. Quantitative analysis of scintigraphic findings in tibial stress fractures in Thoroughbred racehorses. Am J Vet Res 2008;69:886–890.

ENOSTOSES OF THE TIBIA

Enostoses are intra-medullary osseous densities that are usually demonstrated radiographically after being

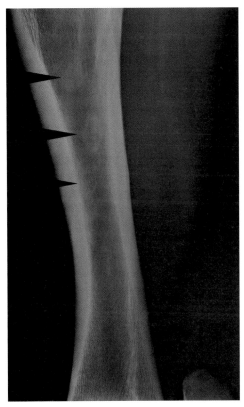

Figure 5.345. Lateral tibial radiograph with enostosis lesions visible within the medullary cavity (arrows). (Courtesy of Dr. PS Doyle.)

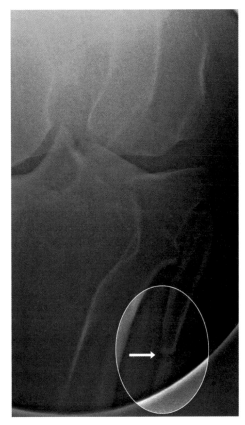

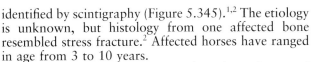

Figure 5.346. Craniocaudal radiograph of the proximal tibial region. The arrow indicates a fibrous union in the fibula that is typical of features commonly mistaken for fractures.

identified by scintigraphy (Figure 5.345).[1,2] The etiology is unknown, but histology from one affected bone resembled stress fracture.[2] Affected horses have ranged in age from 3 to 10 years.

The horses in which enostoses have been diagnosed were lame but not always in the limb where the lesion was discovered. The focal or multi-focal round or irregular scintigraphic lesions may coincide with lameness or they may be considered incidental findings. Some have been located close to the nutrient foramen.[1]

Five of 10 horses with enostoses were affected in the tibia; other sites included the radius, humerus, and metatarsus. Two of those 5 horses were believed to be lame from the enostosis lesion.[1]

Treatment consists of rest and systemic anti-inflammatory therapy. The tibia cannot benefit from any support or local anti-inflammatory measures.

The prognosis is generally good, provided the rest is allowed. Lameness resolves after 2–6 months. Follow-up scintigraphic examination in 3 horses (2, 6, and 9 months later, respectively) revealed normal radioisotope uptake in the affected areas.

References

1. Bassage LH, Ross MW. Enostosis-like lesions in the long bones of 10 horses: Scintigraphic and radiographic features. Equine Vet J 1998;30:35–42.

2. Ross MW. Bone scintigraphy: Lessons learned from 5,000 horses. Proceedings Am Assoc Equine Pract 2005;51:6–20.

FRACTURE OF THE FIBULA

Obscure hindlimb lameness has occasionally been diagnosed as fracture of the fibula.[3,5,6] Extensive radiologic studies have revealed that what often appears to be a fracture of the fibula is merely a defect in the union of the proximal and distal segments of the bone (Figure 5.346).[2,8,9] This defect in union of the bone can be demonstrated in a high percentage of horses. When radiographs are taken of the opposite fibula, the defect is usually there as well.[1]

That historical perspective notwithstanding, fracture of the fibula does occur.[7] A single case of a chronic, nonhealing proximal fibular fracture in a Standardbred racehorse was reported. The diagnosis was made based upon scintigraphic and radiographic findings, and scintigraphy also revealed a probable contralateral femoral neck stress fracture. The nonunion was treated by placement of an autogenous cancellous bone graft with the horse standing. The fracture ossified by 90 days after surgery, and the horse was training 11 months after surgery. The contralateral lameness persisted, and the horse was retired.

Histologically necrotic foci of fibrous tissue, islands of bone, and cartilage in the discontinuous part of the fibula have been observed. Associated with this were organic changes within the peroneal (fibular) and tibial nerves that the investigators thought may contribute to a mild disorder of locomotion of the hindlimb.[4]

References

1. Banks WC. Additional studies of fibular defects in horses. J Am Vet Med Assoc 1958;133:422.
2. Delahanty DD. Defects—not fractures—of the fibula in horses. J Am Vet Med Assoc 1958;133:258.
3. Editorial. A phenomenon in equine lameness. J Am Vet Med Assoc 1957;130.
4. Kaneko M, Kiryu K, Oikawa Ma, et al. Discontinuous condition in the fibulae in the light horse. Experimental Reports of Equine Health Laboratory 1975:1–11.
5. Lundvall RL. Fracture of the fibula in the horse. J Am Vet Med Assoc 1956;129:10.
6. Lusk ND, Rosborough JP. Fibular fracture in a filly. J Am Vet Med Assoc 1957;130:4.
7. O'Rielly JL, Bertone AL, Genovese RL. Treatment of a chronic comminuted fracture of the fibula in a horse. J Am Vet Med Assoc 1998;212:396–398.
8. Zeskov F. Fracture or congenital discontinuity of the fibula in the horse. Br Vet J 1958;114:145.
9. Zeskov F. A study of discontinuity of the fibula in the horse. Am J Vet Res 1959;78:852.

THE STIFLE

Kenneth E. Sullins (Femoropatellar Joint) and
Chris Kawcak (Femorotibial Joints)

FEMOROPATELLAR JOINT

The stifle is the largest and most complex joint in the horse; therefore, it is not surprising that injury to the stifle is an important cause of hindlimb lameness. The stifle consists of three synovial compartments: the femoropatellar joint and the medial and lateral femorotibial joints.

Vaughan recorded 63 cases of stifle problems of 835 horses (8%) that presented with hindlimb and spinal conditions.[30] In another report, stifle lameness occurred in 2% of 5,388 specified conditions of the musculoskeletal system.[1] Of a series of 553 horses with hindlimb lameness, 795 stifles were radiographed, demonstrating changes in 326 horses.[23] Femoropatellar and femorotibial lesions occurred at the similar rates of 27% and 32%, respectively, and there was an overall incidence of 32% with osteoarthritis (OA). Stifle problems are quite common in routine referral practice and are probably increasing due to the improved ability to make specific diagnoses.[12,15]

Clinical Signs

The evaluation of stifle lameness is made by visual observation, palpation of the joints, gait evaluation, and elimination of other types of lameness. The examiner should become acquainted with normal palpation and normal variations; asymmetry usually indicates a problem. Swelling may be impressive with acute injuries, which complicates the ability to make a precise anatomic diagnosis. Acutely painful horses usually do not fix the limb in extension when walking or standing. Bruising from external trauma is common from being kicked and in horses that jump over fences. Local and systemic anti-inflammatory therapy may be required to reduce the swelling before a complete diagnosis can be made.[8]

Distention of the femoropatellar joint is better observed when viewing the horse from the side, and may be obvious (Figure 5.347). On palpation, distention and thickening of the femoropatellar joint capsule may be detected between the patellar ligaments. Comparison with the opposite stifle should be made; both stifles can be palpated while standing behind most horses. Femoropatellar effusion, reflecting only a medial femorotibial (MFT) joint disease (if present at all), often is less than with primary femoropatellar joint involvement. Some normal horses retain mild femoropatellar effusion without a clinical problem being present. Femoropatellar effusion may be simple fluid distention or there may be thickening of the periarticular soft tissue. Such thickening may be edema or consist of fibrosis from chronic inflammation. With chronic lameness, atrophy of the gluteal and quadriceps muscles on

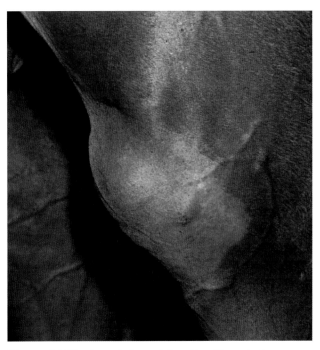

Figure 5.347. Lateral photo of the stifle with marked femoropatellar effusion. (Courtesy of Dr. Gary Baxter.)

the affected side may be apparent. This may be obvious, or careful comparison from the rear and side may be necessary. Hindlimb flexion induces a painful response in most cases.

Stifle pain causes typical hindlimb lameness. Viewed from the side, the cranial phase of the stride is shortened, and the foot is carried closer to the ground. The toe may drag when the horse advances the limb at a trot, and toe wear may be obvious. When viewed from the rear at a trot, asymmetry in the gluteal rise is observed. The duration of gluteal rise is shorter, resulting in an early limb unweighting. This is frequently referred to erroneously as the hip hike. What occurs is that the horse takes on less weight and spends less time on the affected limb, which results in a reduction in gluteal use; this is visualized as a hip roll. The degree of lameness varies according to the severity of the injury. Stifle lameness usually cannot be definitively distinguished from hock pain or other sites in the hindlimb.

Flexion of the hindlimb affects the digit, hock, stifle, and hip. Digital flexion is minimized if the limb is held loosely around the fetlock. However, the source of any increased pain following flexion must still be localized. The stifle flexion test can provide the examiner with some assuredness that the region is involved if the horse reacts in a painful manner to flexion and the test exacerbates the lameness. See Chapter 3 and the accompanying DVD for more information.

Lameness can be localized to the stifle with intrasynovial anesthesia. All 3 joints may be blocked at once (see Chapter 3). In some cases it may be desirable to block the 3 joints separately, which more accurately determines the site of the problem, for the possibility of surgical intervention or medication. In spite of the frequent femoropatellar-medial femorotibial communication, communication between the femoropatellar joint and lateral femorotibial joint is rare.[21] The femoropatellar joint in horses with OA occasionally communicates with both femorotibial joints.[21] None of the femorotibial joints communicate with their counterpart.

Diagnostic local analgesia in the stifle is usually performed after the remainder of the limb has been ruled out as a cause of the lameness. Without effusion, the MFT joint is the logical starting point if each joint is to be blocked separately, because the femoropatellar joint usually will visibly fill if there is a problem, and the lateral femorotibial joint is not the site of a problem as often. However, if clinical impression or previous diagnostic imaging incriminates the stifle, long-acting intrasynovial anesthesia may be the starting point of a lameness examination.

Diagnosis

A complete series of good quality radiographs is needed to evaluate the stifle joints and provide a definitive diagnosis. Digital radiography has made it possible to obtain good films in the field.[3] Routine survey views include caudocranial (CaCr) and lateromedial (LM) views. The 30° lateral craniomedial oblique separates the lateral from the medial trochlear ridge, if that is needed.[26] The articular surface and sagittal integrity of the patella are demonstrated best by a flexed cranioproximal-craniodistal tangential (skyline) view.[7,10,22] Many horses may have radiographically inapparent lesions or more extensive involvement than radiographs demonstrate.[5,15]

Ultrasonography is extremely helpful for evaluating the femoropatellar region. The character of the articular surfaces and subchondral bone,[4,6,17] joint capsule,[15] synovial fluid,[12,18] patellar ligaments,[17] and periarticular tissues[6,17] can be ultrasonographically demonstrated.[18–20] However, the articular surface of the patella is not readily accessible.[15]

Scintigraphy is quite useful for lesions in the stifle region.[15,16] Particularly with bilateral lameness, the need for ascending sequential local anesthesia may be obviated. Normal horses have patterns of uptake highlighting the patella and caudoproximal tibia.[9] However, osteochondrosis or subchondral cystic lesions may not have the increased vascularity required to sequester the radiopharmaceutical.[24]

Magnetic resonance imaging provides the most anatomic detail available for imaging the equine stifle (Figure 5.348).[11] Although many facilities are acquiring magnets, units capable of imaging a stifle are still very limited.

In clinical trials, computed tomography was accurate for imaging the trochlea and ridges, condyles, and proximal tibia.[27] Of most value was the detail in the caudal

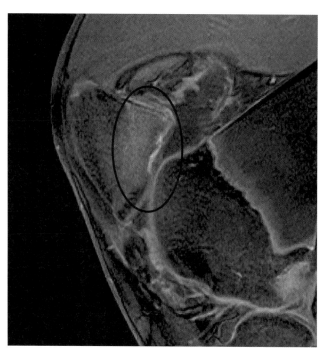

Figure 5.348. Sagittal MR image (contrast enhanced T1 sequence) demonstrating patellar subchondral contusion and articular surface disruption (black oval). There were no radiographic changes on the patella. (Courtesy of Dr. Carter Judy.)

portions of the joint,[27] including loose fragments, and the intercondylar fossa. When combined with contrast, computed tomography offers more potential to image intra-articular soft tissues than other techniques currently available.[2]

Arthroscopy has become the standard for femoropatellar exploration and surgical treatment because it provides access to the entire femoropatellar joint without significant risk of incisional complications and produces a better result.[29] Arthrotomy fails to provide sufficient visualization for exploration, and the large incision is at risk of dehiscence.[28] Arthroscopy is the definitive diagnostic tool for problems isolated to the femoropatellar joint but inapparent on any type of imaging.[13,14,25,26]

References

1. Anon R. British Equine Veterinary Association survey of equine diseases. 1962–1963. Vet Rec 1965;77:528.
2. Bergman EHJ, Puchalski SM, Van der Veen H, et al. Computed tomography and computed tomography arthrography of the equine stifle: Technique and preliminary results in 16 clinical cases. Proc Am Assoc Eq Prac 2007;46–55.
3. Bindeus T, Vrba S, Gabler C, et al. Comparison of computed radiography and conventional film-screen radiography of the equine stifle. Vet Radiol Ultra 2002;43:455–460.
4. Bourzac C, Alexander K, Rossier Y, et al. Comparison of radiography and ultrasonography for the diagnosis of osteochondritis dissecans in the equine femoropatellar joint. Equine Vet J 2009;41:686–692(687).
5. Dabareiner RM, Sullins KE, White NA. Progression of femoropatellar osteochondrosis in nine young horses. Clinical, radiographic and arthroscopic findings. Vet Surg 1993;22:515–523.
6. Dik KJ. Ultrasonography of the equine stifle. Eq Vet Educ 1995;7:154–160.

7. Dik KJ, Nemeth F. Traumatic patella fractures in the horse. Equine Vet J 1983;15:244–247.

8. Dyson S. Stifle trauma in the event horse. Eq Ath 1994;7:1, 9–14.

9. Dyson S, McNie K, Weekes J, et al. Scintigraphic evaluation of the stifle in normal horses and horses with forelimb lameness. Vet Rad Ultra 2007;48:378–382.

10. Dyson S, Wright I, Kold S, et al. Clinical and radiographic features, treatment and outcome in 15 horses with fracture of the medial aspect of the patella. Equine Vet J 1992;24:264–268.

11. Holcombe SJ, Bertone AL, Biller DS, et al. Magnetic resonance imaging of the equine stifle. Vet Rad Ultra 1995;36:119–125.

12. Martinelli MJ, Rantanen NW. Lameness originating from the equine stifle joint: A diagnostic challenge. Eq Vet Educ 2009;21:648–651(644).

13. McIlwraith CW. Inferences from referred clinical cases of osteochondritis dissecans. Equine Vet J 1993;Suppl. 16:27–30.

14. McIlwraith CW, Nixon AJ, Wright IM, et al. Arthroscopic surgery of the femoropatellar joint-osteochondritis dissecans. In Diagnostic and Surgical Arthroscopy in the Horse, 3rd ed. Elsevier, Philadelphia, 2005;197–246.

15. McLellan J, Plevin S, Hammock PD, et al. Comparison of radiography, scintigraphy and ultrasonography in the diagnosis of patellar chondromalacia in a horse, confirmed by arthroscopy. Eq Vet Educ 2009;21:642–647.

16. Myhre GD, Boucher N, Aiken L. Incidence and correlation of scintigraphic findings to referral lameness at a private hospital. Proc Am Assoc Eq Pract 1998;44:218–221.

17. Penninck DG, Nyland TG, O'Brien TR, et al. Ultrasonography of the equine stifle. Vet Rad 1990;31:293–298.

18. Rantanen NW, McKinnon AO. Equine diagnostic ultrasonography. Williams and Wilkins, Baltimore, 1998;500–511.

19. Reef VB. Equine diagnostic ultrasound. WB Saunders Co., Philadelphia, 1998;74–75.

20. Reef VB. Equine diagnostic ultrasound. WB Saunders Co., Philadelphia, 1998;160–164.

21. Reeves MJ, Trotter GW, Kainer RA. Anatomical and functional communications between the synovial sacs of the equine stifle joint. Equine Vet J 1991;23:215–218.

22. Richard E, Alexander K. Nonconventional radiographic projections in the equine orthopaedic examination. Eq Vet Educ 2007;19:551–559.

23. Samy MT, Hertsch R, Zeller R. Radiologic changes in the equine stifle joint. Eq Pract 1985;7:13–30.

24. Squire KRE, Fessler JF, Cantwell HD, et al. Enlarging bilateral femoral condylar bone cysts without scintigraphic uptake in a yearling foal. Vet Rad 1992;33:109–113.

25. Steinheimer DN, McIlwraith CW, Park RD, et al. Comparison of radiographic subchondral bone changes with arthroscopic findings in the equine femoropatellar and femorotibial joints: A retrospective study of 72 joints (50 horses). Vet Rad Ultra 1995;36:478–484.

26. Stick JA, Nickels FA. The stifle. In Equine Surgery, 2nd ed. Auer JA, Stick JA, eds. Saunders, Philadelphia, 1999;867–881.

27. Tietje S. Computed tomography of the stifle region in the horse: A comparison with radiographic/ultrasonographic and arthroscopic evaluation. Pferd 1997;13:647–658.

28. Trotter GW, McIlwraith CW, Norrdin RW. A comparison of two surgical approaches to the equine femoropatellar joint for the treatment of osteochondritis dissecans. Vet Surg 1983; 12:33–40.

29. Vatistas NJ, Wright IM, Dyson SJ. Comparison of arthroscopy and arthrotomy for the treatment of osteochondritic lesions in the femoropatellar joint of horses. Vet Rec 1995;137:629–632.

30. Vaughan JT. Analysis of lameness in the pelvic limb and selected cases. Proc Am Assoc Eq Pract 1965;11:223.

FEMOROPATELLAR OSTEOCHONDRITIS DISSECANS (OCD)

Femoropatellar OCD is a very common cause of stifle lameness rivaled in occurrence only by that in the tarsocrural joint.[11,13] In one study, Thoroughbreds were the most commonly affected of a series of 161 horses having surgery.[7] Seventy-eight percent were 2 years old and younger (most were yearlings), twice as many males as females were affected, and they were typically the better individuals in the herd.[21] Femoropatellar OCD affected the lateral trochlear ridge in 161 of 252 joints.[7] However, lesions may be located on the medial trochlear ridge, the trochlear groove, the articular surface of the patella, or in any combination.[7]

Clinical Signs

Femoropatellar OCD usually causes visible joint effusion (Figure 5.347) and variable hindlimb lameness. The lesion is a cartilage or osteochondral defect with separation, producing synovitis. Subtle effusion can be compared to the contralateral stifle, but at least half of affected horses have bilateral lesions.[7] Synovial fluid analysis is usually unremarkable. Uncommonly, horses with stifle lesions may also be affected in other joints; a complete physical exam noting effusion in other joints is indicated.[7,14]

The lameness may be so mild that joint effusion is the only presenting complaint; however, hindlimb flexion is usually positive in horses with clinically significant OCD. Others may be extremely lame, and some youngsters may have difficulty rising from recumbency. Chronic hindlimb lameness in foals may cause forelimb flexural deformities, which could be the actual presenting complaint. The severity of synovitis depends upon the lesion itself and the amount of inflammation caused by physical activity; the degree of synovitis was not always comparable to the size of lesions in one report.[2] Uncommonly, the lateral trochlear ridge defect can be so severe that the patella luxates laterally. Conversely, previously immobile OCD fragments may separate, causing sudden clinical signs in athletes.[6]

The usual age at presentation varies from weanling to 2- to 3-year-olds in training; more than half of a series 161 horses were 1 year of age or younger.[7] Training may be required to cause clinical signs; presumably the osteochondral defect becomes disrupted, causing synovitis. Horses presenting after training has begun generally have less severe lesions than weanlings or yearlings that present earlier, which is probably why the older group has an overall better outcome after surgery.[7,14] Some horses have radiographic evidence of OCD without clinical signs. The clinical significance of the lesion should be confirmed by intra-synovial analgesia, particularly among horses in active training or older horses with minimal femoropatellar effusion or radiographic change. Weanlings with femoropatellar OCD may present with joint effusion, lameness, and no radiographic changes.[4]

Diagnosis

Lateromedial radiographs usually demonstrate a flattened defect in the proximal portion of the lateral trochlear ridge of the femur where it articulates with the distal patella (Figure 5.349). Ossification within the defect is variable, and loose bodies may be present.[4,7,12] Less commonly, deeper ossification defects or subchondral cystic lesions occur (Figure 5.350) or the defect may be so large that the patella is unstable (Figure 5.351).[4,12,14] Caudolateral to craniomedial oblique films may provide more information about the severity of lateral trochlear ridge defects, which may extend over

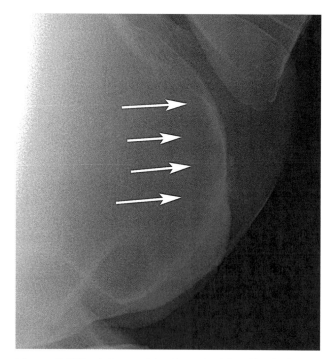

Figure 5.349. Lateromedial radiograph of the stifle of a horse with OCD of the lateral trochlear ridge. The arrows indicate the subchondral limits of the lesion, which could involve cartilage more extensively.

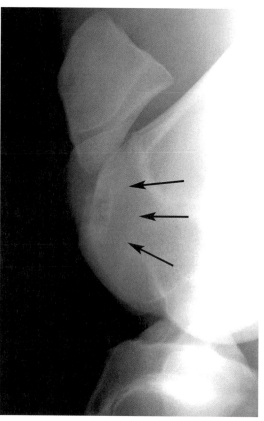

Figure 5.350. Lateromedial radiograph of the stifle of a horse with OCD of the lateral trochlear ridge. A subchondral cyst (arrows) has formed beneath the surface fragments.

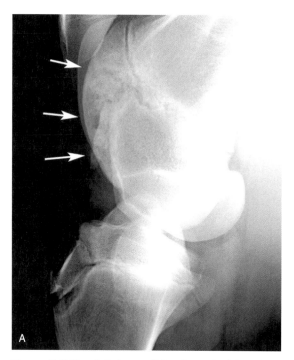

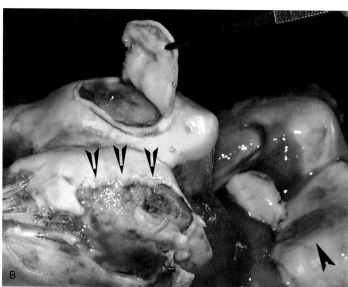

Figure 5.351. A. Lateromedial radiograph of the stifle of a horse with severe OCD. Most of the subchondral bone in the lateral trochlear ridge is affected (arrows). The patella had been luxating laterally. B. Necropsy photo of the same femoropatellar joint. The lateral trochlear ridge is hypoplastic and the lesion is broad (slotted arrows). A radiographically inapparent cartilage flap from the medial trochlear ridge is being held in the forceps. Additionally, the patellar cartilage is eburnated (single arrow).

the lateral side of the trochlear ridge. Patellar changes may be due to primary OCD or secondary to irritation from a severe lateral trochlear ridge lesion, but may not be discovered until surgery is performed. However, severe patellar lesions can be observed in the laterome-dial view.

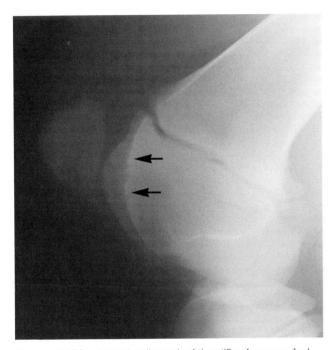

Figure 5.352. Lateral radiograph of the stifle of a young foal that demonstrates the normal irregularity of the subchondral bone along the proximal aspects of the trochlear ridges (arrows).

In one study, radiographically normal areas contained lesions detectable only by arthroscopy in 40% of 72 femoropatellar joints,[19] and more than half had lesions worse than anticipated from the radiographs.[4,19] Young foals have normally irregular contours of the proximal trochlear ridges (Figure 5.352 and 5.369, later in text).[1,9]

Ultrasound should be considered as an adjunct to radiographs.[2] The trochlear surfaces of the distal femur are readily imaged using ultrasound.[2,16] In addition, the lateromedial extent of defects and the trochlear groove can be imaged, whereas they may be obscured on radiographs. The sensitivity and specificity of detection of lateral trochlear ridge OCD is quite good.[2] The cartilage on the lateral trochlear ridge is reported to be thicker than that of the medial ridge.[17] Underscoring the value of exploratory arthroscopy, accuracy on the proximal medial trochlear ridge is not high for ultrasound or radiography.[2,16,19] Although numbers were low, lesions in the mid portion of the medial trochlear ridge were better detected by ultrasound than radiography in one study.[2] Synovial membrane proliferation and echolucent synovial effusion can be associated with the articular defects.[16] The majority of the patellar articular surface is not accessible for ultrasonic imaging.

In summary, a minority of horses with mild lateral trochlear ridge defects have no cartilage defect during surgery (Figure 5.353). Conversely, horses with more severe radiographic changes probably have cartilage defects there and possibly elsewhere in the same joint. When radiographic lesions are absent, lameness and synovial effusion dictate the clinical significance.

Figure 5.353. A. Lateromedial radiograph of a yearling with radiographic signs of lateral trochlear ridge OCD. Femoropatellar effusion was mild and the horse was affected with a clinically significant medial condylar subchondral cystic lesion in the same limb. B. While being operated for the SCL, the femoropatellar joint was evaluated arthroscopically. The cartilage contained an elevation but was intact (arrows), and no debridement was performed. As a 3-year-old, the horse was sound.

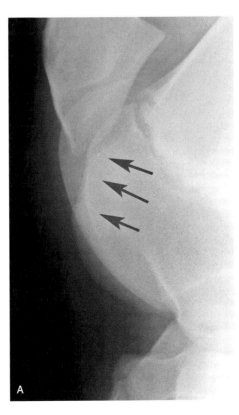

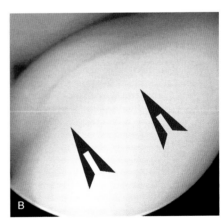

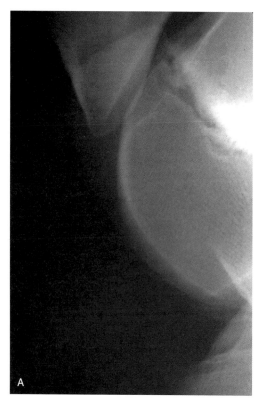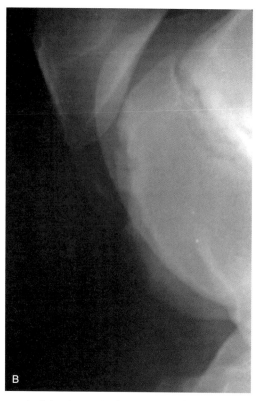

Figure 5.354. Lateromedial radiographs of the stifle of a weanling. A. Radiograph taken when foal presented with femoropatellar effusion and lameness. B. Radiograph taken 14 weeks later demonstrating extensive OCD of the lateral trochlear ridge. The unaffected bone of the lateral trochlear ridge has grown around the defective portion, revealing the lucency.

Treatment

Surgical debridement produces better results than conservative therapy when clinical signs are present in adults.[18,20] However, in one study, some lesions detected up to 8 months of age were found to resolve;[5] no worsening of the lesion should occur after 11 months of age. Stall confinement is recommended to protect the articular surface from disruption to facilitate healing.[15] Surgery is indicated if the clinical signs persist.

Intra-articular and systemic anti-inflammatory therapy to minimize the chance of degenerative change and improve healing is advisable.[20] Sodium hyaluronate is recommended for IA treatment and polysulfated glycosaminoglycan is most often used for systemic treatment. Intra-articular steroids are inadvisable where healing is needed,[3] and negative effects of steroids have been observed in immature equine joints.[8] The fluid is drained at the time of treatment so that resolution of the synovitis can be monitored. In one study, half of 23 affected foals that were diagnosed early with OCD and treated with stall rest eventually raced.[15] The successfully treated horses tended to have less severe lesions.

Sequential radiographs and clinical response to therapy are used to determine whether surgery is advisable. Surgery has been recommended for young horses with radiographic lesions greater than 2 cm in length or deeper than 5 mm or lesions with ossification in the defect and femoropatellar joint effusion.[14] However, the need to progress with the horse's conditioning schedule may dictate earlier surgical intervention.

Weanlings and short yearlings can present with effusion and lameness but no radiographic lesions (Figure 5.354).[4,15] Conservative therapy is indicated unless clinical signs persist. Subsequent radiographs may demonstrate healing or larger trochlear ridge ossification defects because the lesion has persisted while the surrounding trochlear ridge has ossified normally as the epiphysis has expanded.[4] Some believe that surgical lesions in foals and weanlings may progress, suggesting that surgery be delayed until the lesion has fully developed.[4] This consideration will have passed after a period of conservative therapy. Medical therapy in cases without radiographic changes is diagnostic as well because a permanent response indicates that there is no articular surface lesion.

Arthroscopic surgery is indicated when it is obvious that the lesion will not heal with conservative therapy and in horses beyond a year of age with clinical signs. Arthroscopy offers better visualization and access to the lesion without the inherent risk of post-operative dehiscence of the large incision.[14] A comparison of arthroscopy and arthrotomy for a series of horses affected with femoropatellar OCD revealed that arthroscopically treated horses returned to athletic activity at a higher rate and sooner and overcame the synovial effusion more often than horses treated by arthrotomy.[22] The most logical explanation for the functional difference after surgery is that the lesions were not debrided as completely or other lesions may not have been discovered.

The technique for arthroscopic debridement of femoropatellar OCD lesions has been well-described.[14,23] The author prefers to insert the arthroscope at the described level but medial to the middle patellar ligament (MidPL) to debride large lateral trochlear ridge lesions because there is more space for instrument access. To examine the suprapatellar pouch, the arthroscope must be moved to a more lateral instrument portal.

The objective of surgery is to remove all loose osteochondral tissue and debride the lesion to leave healthy subchondral bone to fill with fibrocartilage and resolve the synovitis (Figure 11.39 in Chapter 11). Aside from the usual lateral trochlear ridge lesion, the remainder of the joint and the articular surface of the patella should be evaluated. It is important to remove all the debris generated during the debridement process because it contributes to synovitis;[10] debris can be evacuated in the process of surgery using power-facilitated arthroscopic debridement.

Prognosis

The prognosis for athletic activity following arthroscopic surgery for femoropatellar OCD is generally good. Of a series of 134 horses, only 16% were unsuccessful for reasons related to the OCD.[7] Slightly fewer were successful when OCD in other joints underwent surgery concurrently. Increased lesion size had a significantly negative effect upon outcome. Defects less than 2 cm, between 2 cm and 4 cm, and greater than 4 cm had decreasing success rates of 78%, 63%, and 54%, respectively. The overall success rate of 64% was comparable to the starting rate of normal Thoroughbred horses in the same time period. Outcome could not be correlated to sex, function of the horse, lesion location, uni- vs. bilateral involvement, or presence of loose bodies.[7] Because of the bone-to-bone contact in horses with apposing lateral trochlear ridge and patellar lesions, the author extends the period of stall rest for those cases to 90 days.

References

1. Adams WM, Thilsted JP. Radiographic appearance of the equine stifle from birth to 6 months. Vet Rad 1985;26:126–132.
2. Bourzac C, Alexander K, Rossier Y, et al. Comparison of radiography and ultrasonography for the diagnosis of osteochondritis dissecans in the equine femoropatellar joint. Equine Vet J 2009;41:686–692.
3. Carter BG, Bertone AL, Weisbrode SE, et al. Influence of methylprednisolone acetate on osteochondral healing in exercised tarsocrural joints of horses. Am J Vet Res 1996;57:914–922.
4. Dabareiner RM, Sullins KE, White NA. Progression of femoropatellar osteochondrosis in nine young horses. Clinical, radiographic and arthroscopic findings. Vet Surg 1993;22:515–523.
5. Dik KJ, Enzerink E, Weeren PR. Radiographic development of osteochondral abnormalities, in the hock and stifle of Dutch warmblood foals, from age 1 to 11 months. Equine Vet J 1999: 9–15.
6. Dyson SJ. Stifle trauma in the event horse. Eq Vet Educ 1994;6:234–240.
7. Foland JW, McIlwraith CW, Trotter GW. Arthroscopic surgery for osteochondritis dissecans of the femoropatellar joint of the horse. Equine Vet J 1992;24:419–423.
8. Glade MJ, Krook L, Schryver HF, et al. Morphologic and biochemical changes in cartilage of foals treated with dexamethasone. Cornell Vet 1983;73:170–192.
9. Hertsch B. Ossification processes in the stifle of young horses. Zentralbl Veterinarmed 1980;27A:279–289.
10. Hurtig MB. Use of autogenous cartilage particles to create a model of naturally occurring degenerative joint disease in the horse. Equine Vet J 1988;Supplement 6:19–22.
11. Jeffcott LB, Kold SE. Stifle lameness in the horse: A survey of 86 referred cases. Equine Vet J 1982;14:31–39.
12. McIlwraith CW. Clinical aspects of osteochondrisis dissecans. Osteochondrosis dissecans of the femoropatellar joint. In Joint Disease in the Horse. McIllwraith CW, Trotter GW, eds. WB Saunders, Philadelphia, 1996;363–368.
13. McIlwraith CW. Inferences from referred clinical cases of osteochondritis dissecans. Equine Vet J 1993;Suppl. 16:27–30.
14. McIlwraith CW, Nixon AJ, Wright IM, et al. Arthroscopic surgery of the femoropatellar joint-osteochondritis dissecans. Diagnostic and surgical arthroscopy in the horse. 3rd ed. Elsevier, Philadelphia, 2005;197–246.
15. McIntosh SC, McIlwraith CW. Natural history of femoropatellar osteochondrosis in three crops of Thoroughbreds. Eq Vet J Supp 1993:54–61.
16. McLellan J, Plevin S, Hammock PD, et al. Comparison of radiography, scintigraphy and ultrasonography in the diagnosis of patellar chondromalacia in a horse, confirmed by arthroscopy. Eq Vet Educ 2009;21:642–647.
17. Rantanen NW, McKinnon AO. Equine diagnostic ultrasonography. Williams and Wilkins, Baltimore, 1998;500–511.
18. Steenhaut M, Verschooten F, Moor AD. Osteochondrosis dissecans of the stifle joint in the horse. Vla Dierg Tijd 1982;51:173–191.
19. Steinheimer DN, McIlwraith CW, Park RD, et al. Comparison of radiographic subchondral bone changes with arthroscopic findings in the equine femoropatellar and femorotibial joints: A retrospective study of 72 joints (50 horses). Vet Rad Ultra 1995;36:478–484.
20. Stromberg B, Rejno S. Osteochondrosis in the horse. I. A clinical and radiologic investigation of osteochondritis dissecans of the knee and hock joint. Acta Radiol Suppl (Stockh) 1978;358: 139–152.
21. van Weeren PR, Oldruitenborgh-Oosterbaan MMS, Barneveld A. The influence of birth weight, rate of weight gain and final achieved height and sex on the development of osteochondrotic lesions in a population of genetically predisposed Warmblood foals. Equine Vet J 1999:26–30.
22. Vatistas NJ, Wright IM, Dyson SJ. Comparison of arthroscopy and arthrotomy for the treatment of osteochondritic lesions in the femoropatellar joint of horses. Vet Rec 1995;137:629–632.
23. Vinardell T, David F, Morisset S. Arthroscopic surgical approach and intra-articular anatomy of the equine suprapatellar pouch. Vet Surg 2008;37:350–356.

INTRA-ARTICULAR FRACTURES OF THE FEMOROPATELLAR JOINT: FRACTURES OF THE FEMORAL TROCHLEA

Etiology and Diagnosis

Chip fractures have been reported in both trochlear ridges of the distal femur of 3 horses.[3] One horse sustained the injury by striking a jump (stone wall) and the other 2 occurred from punctures. Sepsis should be considered in these cases. All 3 horses underwent routine arthroscopic debridement and returned to normal work after 4 to 5 months.

Dyson has reported medial or lateral trochlear fragmentation in eventers after hitting jumps.[2] Without concurrent associated injury, fragment removal is usually curative. Separation of previously quiescent OCD fragments can also occur after direct trauma.[2]

Salter-Harris type IV fractures of the distal femur in young horses occur from direct trauma.[1,4] Lameness is severe and femoropatellar effusion is obvious. The fracture may involve one or both trochlear ridges. The tangential view in addition to the craniocaudal and lateromedial radiographic projections may be helpful (Figure 5.355).

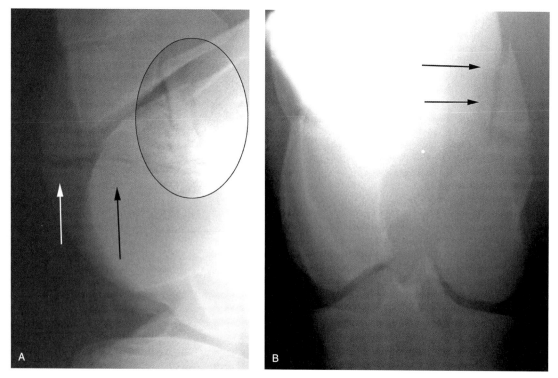

Figure 5.355. A. Lateromedial view of a Salter-Harris type IV fracture of the distal medial femur. Arrows, articular component; circle, metaphyseal component. B. Craniocaudal view of the same fracture. Arrows, metaphyseal fracture line.

Treatment and Prognosis

Acute fractures can generally be reduced, and fixation is performed using lag screws.[1] If necessary, screws can be placed distal to proximal through the articular surface; the screw heads are countersunk into the subchondral bone.[1] Although it is possible to accomplish the fixation arthroscopically in some cases, the spatial orientation can be challenging. Depending upon the case, it may be more efficient to use the direct approach. The prognosis is reasonable for normal activity. Though none of the reported cases reached training age, they were sound.[1]

References

1. DeBowes RM, Grant BD, Modranisky PD. Lag screw stabilization of Salter type IV femoral fracture in a young horse. J Am Vet Med Assoc 1983;182:1123–1125.
2. Dyson SJ. Stifle trauma in the event horse. Eq Vet Educ 1994;6:234–240.
3. Montesso F, Wright IM. Removal of chip fractures of the femoral trochlear ridges of three horses by arthroscopy. Vet Rec 1995;137:94–96.
4. Walmsley JP, Summerhays GES. Repair of a Salter-Harris type IV fracture of the distal femur of a yearling Thoroughbred by internal fixation. Eq Vet Educ 1990;2:177–179.

INTRA-ARTICULAR FRACTURES OF THE FEMOROPATELLAR JOINT: FRACTURE OF THE PATELLA

Patellar fractures occur infrequently in horses, but several configurations, including sagittal,[2,5,7,11] transverse,[10] comminuted,[13] basilar (proximal),[3,7,18] and distal fragmentation of the patella[12,17] have been described. Combinations of types of patellar fracture and associated fracture of the femur may occur.[7]

Etiology

Direct trauma to the patella while the stifle joint is in a semi-flexed position is commonly the cause. The patella is immobilized when the stifle is semi-flexed, making it more susceptible to direct trauma.[4] Horses that jump can strike jumps and sustain bilateral patellar fractures,[8,11] or the fractures can occur as a result of a kick. Sudden lateral slips may cause a separation of the medial fibrocartilage.[5] The prominence of the medial trochlear ridge may be a point of contact, causing a relative higher incidence of fractures toward the medial side of the patella.

Some horses suffer fragmentation of the distal patella when they return to work soon after undergoing a medial patellar ligament desmotomy (MPD); this is still probably due to the direct trauma of temporary patellar instability.[12,17] This condition is discussed in the next section.

Clinical Signs

Horses present with an acute onset of lameness and a significant painful swelling associated with the cranial aspect of the stifle. Femoropatellar effusion is usually profound, but significant soft tissue swelling may obscure palpation. Pain and sometimes crepitation is noted, and fragments may be palpable. Flexion of the stifle joint exacerbates the lameness and the painful

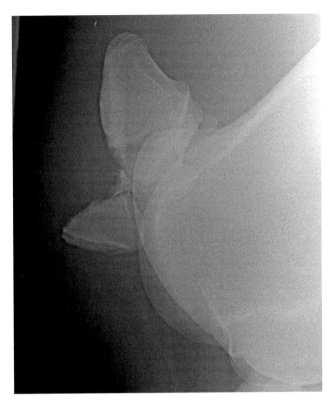

Figure 5.356. Lateromedial radiograph demonstrating a transverse fracture of the patella. (Courtesy of Dr. Gary Baxter.)

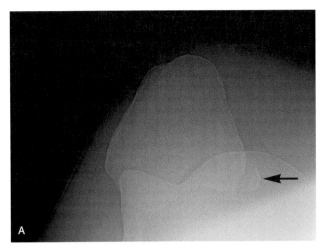

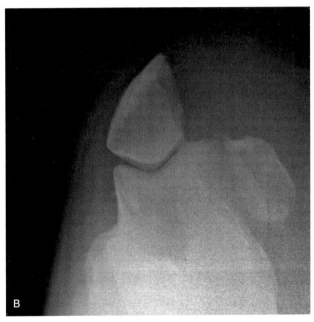

Figure 5.357. Cranioproximal to craniodistal (skyline) projections showing a typical medial patellar fracture fragment (arrow, A) and a large displaced sagittal fracture (B). Arthroscopic removal is indicated in (A). (Courtesy of Dr. Gary Baxter).

response. Weight-bearing may be difficult with compromise of the quadriceps or from pain, so the horse may stand with the limb partially flexed without locking the stifle. Clinical signs may diminish over a period of days to weeks of rest if smaller fragments do not affect the mechanics of the stifle.

Diagnosis

Radiographs are required to document the type and extent of the fracture. Routine lateromedial and caudocranial projections usually demonstrate transverse or comminuted fractures (Figure 5.356). The caudolateral-to-craniomedial oblique projection accentuates the apex (distal border) of the patella. Although swelling and pain may cause some resistance, flexed views are helpful or required to demonstrate some lesions. The flexed lateromedial projection may accentuate some transverse fractures, and sagittal fractures, particularly the relatively common small medial fragments, require a cranioproximal to craniodistal (skyline) projection (Figure 5.357). Placing the plate proximal to the stifle with the beam traveling distoproximad separates the patella more completely from the trochlea, making it more visible.[5,13] Ultrasound is useful for identifying small fracture fragments, patellar ligament disruption, or lesions that may not be radiographically visible, such as medial fibrocartilage separation.[16]

Treatment

Patellar fractures are often accompanied by severe soft tissue trauma involving the ligaments and joint capsule of the stifle joint.[6] Therefore, time and anti-inflammatory therapy may be required before treating the fracture. Nonarticular or small medial or basilar fragments may heal with rest and anti-inflammatory therapy.[7] Horses with relatively large incomplete apical fractures have become sound with extended confinement.[2,5] Some horses have returned to work with fibrous unions of the fracture.[5,13]

Horses with intra-articular fractures seldom remain sound when returned to work,[5,6,11] and stable fragments may displace when horses return to sustained work.[6] With adequate quadriceps stability, fragments approximating one-third of the patellar substance can be successfully removed.[3,6,11] If surgery must be delayed due to soft tissue injury or skin trauma, intra-articular sodium hyaluronate can be used to reduce the synovitis in the interim.

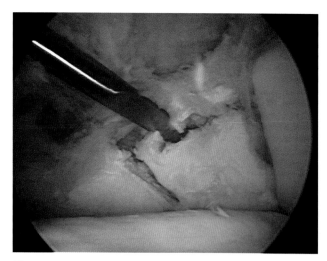

Figure 5.358. Arthroscopic view of a medial patellar fragment. The elevator is separating the patellar fragment from the soft tissue attachments.

Arthroscopy provides better visualization of the fractures, facilitating complete removal of fracture fragments and exploration of the remainder of the joint without the risk of incisional complications of an open approach (Figure 5.358).[11] The fragment can be dissected from the patellar tendon with a large elevator or a motorized soft tissue resector. If the fragment is large, it can be divided with an osteotome or reduced with motorized equipment.[11]

Internal fixation should be considered for distracted or displaced fractures with sizeable fragments. The patellar ligaments are the insertions of the quadriceps femoris and biceps femoris muscles. The goals of repair of larger articular fractures are integrity of the quadriceps mechanism and prevention of OA. Successful internal fixation of transverse distracted and longitudinally displaced fractures of the patella have been reported.[1,4,9,10,13] The longitudinal fracture is easier to reduce and stabilize,[1] and there is less chance of having it distract postoperatively. Transverse fractures require firm fixation because of the tendency of the proximal segment to become distracted by the pull of the quadriceps muscles,[4,10,13] although perfect anatomic reduction may not be required in every case.[4] Tension band support is a good option for transverse patellar fractures.[10]

Large extra-articular fractures can be removed, but it may not be necessary.[18] One consideration is whether the healing tissue between the fragments will be as strong as the new fibrous tissue from the soft tissue attachments if the fragment is removed. The inciting injury may cause sequestration or necrosis in the cranial aspect of the patella, requiring debridement.[14]

Prognosis

The ultimate outcome depends upon retaining quadriceps function and adequate congruent articular surface; instability or persistent synovitis will result in OA. Following conservative or surgical therapy, lameness may persist for an undetermined period while the synovitis resolves and any patellar ligament desmitis or enthesiopathy heals.[5,11,15,16]

In a combined series of 19 horses from which articular medial fragments were removed, 16 returned to full work.[6,11] Failures occurred primarily because of pre-existing OA, luxated patella during recovery from anesthesia, and one unexplained ensuing OA. These failures may point to the value of thorough pre-operative ultrasonographic evaluation or more prolonged postoperative stall rest.

Internal fixation provides the most ideal set of circumstances for a favorable outcome for displaced and distracted fractures. Recovery from anesthesia may be the most critical point in the postoperative period. Horses with severely comminuted fractures are likely to remain lame. Some of these may attain breeding soundness with prolonged stall rest. However, if the quadriceps function is compromised or if severe OA develops, euthanasia should be considered.

References

1. Aldrete AV, Meagher DM. Lag screw fixation of a patellar fracture in a horse. Vet Surg 1981;10:143–148.
2. Anderson BH, Turner, TA, Jonson GR. What is your diagnosis? Fracture of the patella in a horse. J Am Vet Med Assoc 1996;209:1847–1848.
3. Colbern GT, Moore JN. Surgical management of proximal articular fracture of the patella in a horse. J Am Vet Med Assoc 1984;185:543–545.
4. DeBowes RM, Grant BD, Chalman JA, et al. Fractured patella in a horse. Eq Pract 1980;2:49–53.
5. Dik KJ, Nemeth F. Traumatic patella fractures in the horse. Equine Vet J 1983;15:244–247.
6. Dyson S, Wright I, Kold S, et al. Clinical and radiographic features, treatment and outcome in 15 horses with fracture of the medial aspect of the patella. Equine Vet J 1992;24:264–268.
7. Dyson SJ. Stifle trauma in the event horse. Eq Vet Educ 1994;6:234–240.
8. Fessler JF, Amstutz HE. In Textbook of Large Animal Surgery. Oehme FW, Prier JE, eds. Williams and Wilkins Co., Baltimore, 1974;321.
9. Hance SR, Bramlage LR. Fractures of the femur and patella. In Equine Fracture Repair. Nixon AJ, ed. WB Saunders Co., Philadelphia, 1996;284–293.
10. Hunt RJ, Baxter GM, Zamos DT. Tension band wiring and lag screw fixation of a transverse, comminuted fracture of a patella in a horse. J Am Vet Med Assoc 1992;200:819–820.
11. Marble GP, Sullins KE. Arthroscopic removal of patellar fracture fragments in horses: Five cases (1989–1998). J Am Vet Med Assoc 2000;216:1799–1801.
12. McIlwraith CW. Osteochondral fragmentation of the distal aspect of the patella in horses. Equine Vet J 1990;22:157–163.
13. Pankowski RL, White KK. Fractures of the patella in horses. Compend Contin Educ Pract Vet 1985;7:S566-S570, S572-S573.
14. Parks AH, Wyn-Jones G. Traumatic injuries of the patella in five horses. Equine Vet J 1988;20:25–28.
15. Rantanen NW, McKinnon AO. Equine Diagnostic Ultrasonography. Williams and Wilkins, Baltimore, 1998;500–511.
16. Reef VB. Equine Diagnostic Ultrasound. WB Saunders Co., Philadelphia, 1998;160–164.
17. Riley CB, Yovich JV. Fracture of the apex of the patella after medial patellar desmotomy in a horse. Aust Vet J 1991;68: 37–39.
18. Wilderjans H, Boussauw B. Treatment of basilar patellar fracture in a horse by partial patellectomy. Eq Vet Educ 1995;7: 189–192.

FRAGMENTATION OF THE DISTAL PATELLA

Etiology

Fragmentation of the distal patella is an uncommon condition associated with previous medial patellar desmotomy (MPD);[3–8] however, not all cases have undergone MPD.[4] Malalignment of the patella has been reported shortly after MPD,[1,6] and radiographically evident fragmentation was experimentally reproduced in 11 of 12 horses undergoing MPD.[2] See the section on upward fixation of the patella, below, for more information. In addition, it is important to remember that fragmentation of the patella can occur from trauma or use-related injuries of the femoropatellar joint.

Clinical Signs

The clinical signs consist of variable uni- or bilateral hindlimb lameness and stiffness. Femoropatellar joint effusion is common and palpable thickening of the joint capsule is often present, particularly in horses that have had MPD.[4] Radiographic changes include bony fragmentation, spurring, subchondral roughening, and subchondral lysis of the distal aspect of the patella (Figure 5.359).[4,5,8] Cartilage fibrillation without radiographic change also has been reported.[2]

Treatment

All horses are treated with arthroscopic surgery. The lesions observed at arthroscopy vary from flaking, fissuring, undermining, or fragmentation of the articular cartilage, to fragmentation or lysis of the bone at the distal aspect of the patella. The subchondral bone is involved in all cases that had previous MPD. Fragments may be buried in the synovial membrane and tend to emanate from the more lateral portion of the distal patella.[4,7]

Prognosis

Eight of 12 horses that had a previous MPD became sound for their intended use. Of the 3 that did not have a previous patellar desmotomy, 2 performed their intended use well but 1 was unsatisfactory.[4] Three of 49 mixed population horses undergoing MPD remained lame.[1] One with patellar fragmentation did not become sound following arthroscopic debridement of the lesion,

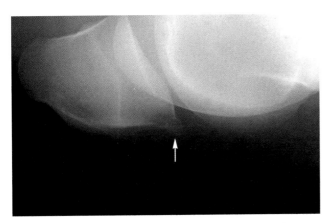

Figure 5.359. Flexed lateromedial radiograph of the stifle demonstrating fragmentation of the apex of the patella (arrow). (Courtesy of Dr. Gary Baxter.)

another had middle patellar ligament (MidPL) enthesiopathy, and another had no discernible reason for the persisting stifle lameness. One additional horse with documented patellar fragmentation was able to work with intra-articular medication. The patellar misalignment was reported to correct in 5 months[5] and was not reported 3 months after experimental MPD.[2]

References

1. Bathe AP, O'Hara LK. A retrospective study of the outcome of medial patellar desmotomy in 49 horses. Proceedings Am Assoc Equine Pract 2004;476–478.
2. Gibson KT, McIlwraith CW, Park RD, et al. Production of patellar lesions by medial patellar desmotomy in normal horses. Vet Surg 1989;18:466–471.
3. Grosenbaugh DA, Honnas CM. Arthroscopic treatment of patellar lesions resulting from medial patellar desmotomy in a horse. Eq Pract 1979;17:23–25.
4. McIlwraith CW. Osteochondral fragmentation of the distal aspect of the patella in horses. Equine Vet J 1990;22:157–163.
5. Riley CB, Yovich JV. Fracture of the apex of the patella after medial patellar desmotomy in a horse. Aust Vet J 1991; 68:37–39.
6. Squire KRE, Blevins WE, Frederick M, et al. Radiographic changes in an equine patella following medial patellar desmotomy. Vet Rad 1990;31:208–209.
7. Walmsley JP. Medial patellar desmotomy for upward fixation of the patella. Eq Vet Educ 1994;6:148–150.
8. Wright JD, Rose RJ. Fracture of the patella as a possible complication of medial patellar desmotomy. Aust Vet J 1989; 66:189–190.

UPWARD FIXATION OF THE PATELLA (UFP)

Upward fixation of the patella occurs when the medial patellar ligament (MPL) becomes caught over the medial trochlear ridge. If it becomes fixed in that position, the hindlimb cannot be flexed and the horse assumes a posture with the affected limb extended in a caudally abducted position with the fetlock flexed due to the reciprocal apparatus (Figure 5.360).

Etiology

Upward fixation of the patella generally has been considered to occur in horses that have exceptionally straight hindlimbs. Rooney considers most horses to have femorotibial angles approximating 135° and has stated that the problem occurs when the angle reaches 143° to 145°.[20] Although the exact angle of occurrence likely varies among horses, it is reasonable to say that a straight-legged horse has a greater chance of reaching its individual point of injury. Furthermore, hyperextension of the limb exacerbated by walking a horse downhill causes the upward fixation of the patella to occur more frequently.

Body type is strongly inherited, thus it is likely that the tendency for UFP could be congenital. Shetland ponies are particularly affected, and UFP predisposes them to coxofemoral luxation.[4]

The condition also appears when the medial patellar ligament becomes long enough to reach over the medial trochlear ridge in spite of normal conformation. Examples of this include loss of quadriceps muscle tone and traumatic hyperextension of the hindlimb. The ligaments may become stretched once upward fixation occurs, so recurrence is common.

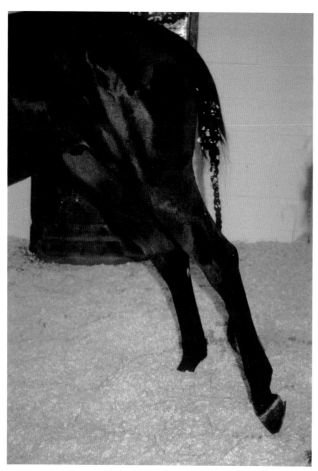

Figure 5.360. The horse has upward fixation of the patella. The limb is locked in extension and extended caudally and a bit laterally. The digit is also fixed in the flexed position.

The MPL is weaker than the other 2 patellar ligaments.[21] Furthermore, younger horses, when they begin training, often lack the muscle tone they will acquire as they work. Upward fixation also has been observed in horses abruptly taken out of training and confined to a stall.

A recent report of 76 horses affected with UFP cites hoof balance and angle as predisposing factors, along with reduced muscle tone from seasonally reduced work.[6] Higher medial hoof wall and elongated toes were reported to cause hyperextension of the stifle and outward rotation of the limb, contributing to UFP. Corrective trimming and shoeing alleviated UFP in half of the horses and reduced the incidence in an additional 20% (see Treatment, below).

Clinical Signs and Diagnosis

In acute upward fixation of the patella, the hindlimb is locked in extension, as described above. The condition may relieve itself, or it may remain locked for several hours or even days. In other cases, there is only a "catching" of the patella as the horse walks. Hyperextending the stifle by walking down an incline may cause a jerking gait from intermittent catching of

the MPL, and the horse may assume a crouched position, presumably to prevent stifle extension. Backing or moving in a tight circle also exacerbates the signs. When the MPL releases, the hindlimb usually jerks up quickly, mimicking stringhalt. UFP must be differentiated from stringhalt; see the accompanying DVD for a visual illustration.

Both hindlimbs usually are predisposed to the condition; however, truly unilateral cases often have a history of an inciting cause in the affected limb.

Palpation when the limb is locked in extension reveals tense patellar ligaments and that the patella is locked above the medial trochlear ridge of the femur. The horse drags the front of the hoof on the ground when it is forced to move forward with the limb locked. When the limb is in a normal position, the predisposition can be evaluated by forcing the patella upward and outward with the hand. If the limb can be manually locked in extension for 1 or more steps, it is predisposed to UFP; manual induction of UFP should not be possible in a normal horse. The examiner should take care not to be in the path of the limb when it releases.

Lameness usually is not severe or constant, but femoropatellar synovitis and distention may occur with repeated episodes. Coxofemoral strain may be associated with persistent UFP, as well.[4]

Radiographs of the stifle should be taken to eliminate conditions that predispose to UFP. Although uncommon, hypoplasia of the medial trochlear ridge, such as occurs with OCD, facilitates the displacement. Most affected horses do not have radiographic changes from intermittent UFP.[6]

Treatment

For a persistently fixed patella, a sideline may be applied to the affected limb so that as the limb is drawn forward, the patella is pushed medially to unhook the MPL, and downward, which often disengages the fixed patella. Backing the horse may also dislodge the patellar ligament. Personnel should take care to be out of the range of the "jerk" when the MPL releases.

Many horses respond to controlled conditioning to increase quadriceps strength and tone, which tightens the MPL.[17] However, if the horse's fitness level drops below optimal, the UFP recurs. Obviously, rest or confinement is contraindicated. Conditioning, including going up hills without coming back down the incline, which exacerbates the hyperextension of the stifle, strengthens and tones the quadriceps.

Dumoulin, et al. reported higher medial hoof walls and elongated toes along with reduced muscle tone from seasonally reduced work as predisposing factors in a series of 76 horses affected with UFP.[6] Shortening the toe and lowering the medial hoof wall sufficient to move break-over medial to the toe alleviated UFP in half of the horses and reduced the incidence in an additional 20%. Anecdotally, the author's master farrier shares that opinion.

If conditioning and/or shoeing fails to halt the incidence of upward fixation of the patella, the MPL can be tightened with scar tissue by creating a series of longitudinal incisions in the MPL. This substantially thickens the MPL and presumably causes a functional shortening and tightening of the MPL.[23] In one study, upward fixation of the patella was eliminated in all 7 reported cases. The advantage of this procedure compared to MPD is that the patella remains stable.

The author has performed this procedure in the standing horse as well. Once the area has been surgically prepared and local anesthesia has been administered, aseptic ultrasound is performed to delineate the areas to the incised. A #15 blade is held securely between the thumb and forefinger, protruding to the depth shown by ultrasound. The cranial and caudal limits of the MPL are easily palpable with the horse bearing weight. Once inserted, elevating the blade from the depth of its insertion extends the incision in the longitudinal plane of the ligament without extending the length of the skin incision. No transverse cutting of fibers should be done. The stab incisions are not sutured. A similar technique using a 14-gauge needle instead of a scalpel blade has been reported.[18]

A much older treatment that has been commonly used for horses with intermittent upward fixation and no palpable swelling of the femoropatellar joint capsule is the injection of counterirritants into the middle and medial patellar ligaments.[17] The injections are usually performed on the standing horse using mild sedation and nose twitch. Commonly used irritants contain 2% iodine; 1 to 2 ml is injected in 6 equally distributed sites along the medial patellar ligament. The description includes a similar amount in the MidPL. Most horses exhibit a slight stiffness and swelling for a few days after the injections. Daily mild exercise is recommended so there is minimal loss of muscle tone. While most horses respond well to this treatment, a few require re-treatment.

The commonly held opinion about the effectiveness of counterirritant injections into the medial patellar ligament is that the ligament tightens, thereby mimicking increased tone from conditioning. A study was performed in which the tissues were harvested and evaluated histologically.[3] The majority of the (severe) inflammatory reaction and all of the drug was found in the endotenon and peritenon. Apparently, the injection follows planes of least resistance. Within the dense collagen bundles, collagen fibers were disrupted without the same severe reaction, although there was fibrous tissue production and overall thickening. The mechanism of action, although still unproven, could lie in reduced expansile ability of the fibrous medial patellar ligament.

Ethanolamine oleate, a sclerosing agent, was compared to 2% iodine in almond oil for injection of medial and MidPL in experimental horses.[11] Although both induced inflammation, 2% iodine in almond oil caused more thickening and a more significant inflammatory reaction, which would be expected to lead to more functional shortening of the ligaments. None of the horses were lame after the injections. A report of 70 horses treated with weekly homeopathic anti-inflammatory injections 2 to 4 times related 82% success, with the remainder undergoing surgery.[5] Possibly the number and frequency of injections contributed to local fibrosis.

When nothing else helps or the UFP cannot be reduced, an MPD is performed using local anesthesia in the standing horse. In the past, MPD was performed on most horses with UFP and many others with undiagnosed hindlimb lameness. Complications from that procedure should deem it the treatment of last resort.[8,12,15,19,22,25] To perform the procedure in the standing horse, a 1-cm incision should be made along the medial limit of the middle patellar ligament near its tibial attachment. A curved mosquito hemostat is inserted and dissected axial to the medial patellar ligament. A Udall's teat bistoury, or other suitable blunt bistoury, is inserted along the path created with the blade directed distally. The tip of the bistoury is palpated subcutaneously in the same position caudal to the medial patellar ligament as the hemostat was just palpated. Once the medial patellar ligament has been transected, determination of remaining MPL vs. gracilis/sartorius aponeuroses can be difficult, although transection of some of those fibers may not be a problem (see below).[26] The horse should be kept in the stall, with hand walking gradually increasing over a period of 90 days. From that point a conservative conditioning program for regular work can begin.[25]

An alternative procedure performed with the horse under general anesthesia in dorsal recumbency has been described.[26] It is similar to the above procedure except the incision is continued into the aponeuroses of the gracilis and sartorius muscles until the limb can be fully extended and flexed without resistance or catching.

Failure of MPD to correct the problem has been reported.[6,10] The persisting tissue continues to displace over the medial trochlear ridge. An alternative procedure was suggested in which the accessory cartilage of the patella is transected proximal to the ligamentous tissue.[10] Wright's more extensive procedure may prevent this as well.[26] Accidental transection of the middle patellar ligament produces a catastrophic result.[26]

As early as 1979, fragmentation of the distal patella (FDP) following MPD was reported.[9] Gibson, et al. observed articular cartilage fibrillation or fragmentation in all horses 3 months after MPD.[8] The patellar lesions were located distolaterally or centrally. Horses were stall confined for 3 weeks followed by turn-out and exercised on a walker for 25 minutes 4 times weekly for the remainder of the study. All horses were lame in the operated limb 1, 2 and 3 months after MPD. Since then there have been several reports of distal patellar fibrillation, fragmentation, or subchondral lysis associated with varying degrees of lameness, femoropatellar synovitis, and periarticular change consisting of fibrosis or enthesiopathy at the origin or insertion of the MPL in horses having undergone MPD.[15,19,22,27] Onset of clinical signs was 10 days.[27]

A lateral shift in the patellar position[1] and increase in the patella-femoral angle[1,19] along with traction from the middle patellar ligament seems to explain the distal and lateral lesions that typically appear on the patella. Ultrasonographic evidence of middle patellar ligament desmitis was observed in experimental horses subjected to MPD and stall rested for 120 days, but no patellar fragmentation was detected.[14] Long-term middle patellar ligament desmitis and enthesiopathy were discovered in a horse presented for purchase with obvious previous MPD and patellar fragmentation,[13] and 2 of 9 horses with patellar ligament desmopathy had middle patellar ligament desmitis associated with previous MPD.[7] The latter horses did not regain soundness.

Although not in its original form, the MPL heals after MPD.[13] The femoropatellar angle reduced to normal after 5 months in one clinically affected horse.[19] An experimental study in normal horses demonstrated a trend toward normal, but the study was not as long.[1] Most accounts suggest that the risk of lameness subsides after a suitable convalescence; some (including this author) have recommended 90 days.[25] One experimental study that kept the horses stall-confined for 120 days revealed positional change in the patella and middle patellar ligament enthesiopathies, but neither lameness nor patellar fragmentation or femoropatellar synovitis were reported.[1]

The clinical significance of residual extra-articular changes has not been confirmed. Once initial inflammation resolves, it seems possible for horses to be sound despite soft tissue fibrosis or calcification. In one study, ultrasonically evident medial and middle patellar ligament desmitis occurred following injection with a counterirritant, but neither lameness nor femoropatellar effusion occurred,[11] and neither lameness nor femoropatellar effusion was reported in 8 horses with periarticular changes but without patellar lesions.[1] Middle patellar ligament enthesiopathy was the only radiographic finding in 1 horse that remained lame following MPD for clinically occurring UPF but further diagnostics were not performed.[2]

A 2-month-old foal with unilateral persistent UFP underwent MPD and became sound. Although femoropatellar effusion persisted, no radiographic changes were present at 6 months of age.[24] Although an encouraging report, longer follow-up to resolve the cause of the persisting joint effusion would have been useful.

Medial patellar desmotomy was performed on a series of 15 horses and 6 ponies of various disciplines.[16] All were rested or hand walked only for 47 days postoperatively. No recurrence of UFP was observed and 19 of 21 returned to their original work. One horse and 1 pony returned with lameness attributed to issues other than UFP or MPD. Postoperative radiographs were taken and revealed no changes in the ponies. However, 4 horses had fragmentation of the distal patella, and 8 horses had ossification at the tibial insertion.

In a retrospective study, 46 of 49 diversely occupied horses undergoing uni- or bilateral MPD over a 10-year period by multiple surgeons became sound.[2] Training was resumed after routine standing MPD and a 2- to 4-week convalescence. Of the 3 that remained lame, 1 had fragmentation of the patella for which surgery did not resolve the lameness, 1 had bone formation on the distal patella, and 1 had no detectable cause for the persisting stifle lameness. One additional racehorse developed fragmentation of the distal patella but raced with intra-articular medication. Four other horses required extended time and/or medical therapy to become sound. The authors' proposed explanation for this overall good result is that horses that are actually suffering from UFP have different stifle angles than normal horses that may prevent the more severe complications that have been described.

Prognosis

The prognosis is good for horses that respond to a conditioning program and maintain that fitness level. After conditioning and ensuring correct shoeing, the logical progression is counterirritant injection, medial patellar ligament splitting, and then medial patellar ligament desmotomy. The diagnosis should be confirmed before surgery is performed because more complications have appeared when MPD is performed on unaffected horses. The author recommends a 90-day convalescence following surgery. Regardless of the method of treatment, the critical factor is prevention of UFP without allowing synovitis to progress to OA.

References

1. Baccarin RYA, Martins EAN, Hagen SCF, et al. Patellar instability following experimental medial patellar desmotomy in horses. Vet Comp Orth Traum 2009;22:27–31.
2. Bathe AP, O'Hara LK. A retrospective study of the outcome of medial patellar desmotomy in 49 horses. Proceedings Am Assoc Equine Pract 2004;476–478.
3. Brown MP, Moon PD, Buergelt CD. The effects of injection of an iodine counterirritant into the patellar ligaments of ponies: Application to stifle lameness. J Eq Vet Sci 1984;4:82–87.
4. Clegg PD, Butson RJ. Treatment of a coxofemoral luxation secondary to upward fixation of the patella in a Shetland pony. Vet Rec 1996;138:134–137.
5. Dreismann GM. Conservative treatment of dorsomedial patella dislocation in the horse. Biol Tiermed 2003;20:59–61.
6. Dumoulin M, Pille F, Desmet P, et al. Upward fixation of the patella in the horse: A retrospective study. Vet Comp Orth Traum 2007;20:119–125.
7. Dyson SJ. Normal ultrasonographic anatomy and injury of the patellar ligaments in the horse. Equine Vet J 2002;34:258–264.
8. Gibson KT, McIlwraith CW, Park RD, et al. Production of patellar lesions by medial patellar desmotomy in normal horses. Vet Surg 1989;18:466–471.
9. Grosenbaugh DA, Honnas CM. Arthroscopic treatment of patellar lesions resulting from medial patellar desmotomy in a horse. Eq Pract 1979;17:23–25.
10. Hickman J, Walker RG. Upward retention of the patella in the horse. Vet Rec 1964;76:1198–1199.
11. Van Hoogmoed LM, Agnew DW, Whitcomb M, et al. Ultrasonographic and histologic evaluation of medial and middle patellar ligaments in exercised horses following injection with ethanolamine oleate and 2% iodine in almond oil. Am J Vet Res 2002;63:738–743.
12. Jansson N. Treatment for upward fixation of the patella in the horse by medial patellar desmotomy: Indications and complications. Eq Pract 1996;18:24–29.
13. Labens R, Busoni V, Peters F, et al. Ultrasonographic and radiographic diagnosis of patellar fragmentation secondary to bilateral medial patellar ligament desmotomy in a Warmblood gelding. Eq Vet Educ 2005;17:201–204.
14. Martins EAN, Silva LC, Baccarin RYA. Ultrasonographic changes of the equine stifle following experimental medial patellar desmotomy. Can Vet J 2006;47:471–474.
15. McIlwraith CW. Osteochondral fragmentation of the distal aspect of the patella in horses. Equine Vet J 1990;22:157–163.
16. Muller-Kirchenbauer D, Furst A, Geissbuhler U, et al. Clinical evaluation of the medial patellar desmotomy for treatment of proximal patella fixation in horses and ponies. Pferd 2001;17:208–216.
17. Norrie RD. Diseases of the rear leg. In Equine Medicine and Surgery. Mansmann RA, McAllister ES, eds. American Veterinary Publications, Santa Barbara, 1982;1137.
18. Reiners SR, May K, DiGrassie W, et al. How to perform a standing medial patellar ligament splitting. Proc Am Assoc Equine Pract 2005;51:481.
19. Riley CB, Yovich JV. Fracture of the apex of the patella after medial patellar desmotomy in a horse. Aust Vet J 1991;68:37–39.

20. Rooney JR. The abnormal rear leg. In The Lame Horse, 1st ed. AS Barnes and Co., Inc., Cranbury, N.J, 1973;175.
21. Sisson S. Equine syndesmology. In Anatomy of Domestic Animals. Getty GR, ed. WB Saunders, Philadelphia, 1975;366–367.
22. Squire KRE, Blevins WE, Frederick M, et al. Radiographic changes in an equine patella following medial patellar desmotomy. Vet Rad 1990;31:208–209.
23. Tnibar MA. Medial patellar ligament splitting for the treatment of upward fixation of the patella in 7 equids. Vet Surg 2002;31:462–467.
24. Toniato M, Torre F. Persistent acquired upward fixation of the patella in a Standardbred foal. Eq Vet Educ 2003;15:233–235.
25. Walmsley JP. Medial patellar desmotomy for upward fixation of the patella. Eq Vet Educ 1994;6:148–150.
26. Wright IM. Ligaments associated with joints. Vet Clin NA Eq Pract 1995;11:249–291.
27. Wright JD, Rose RJ. Fracture of the patella as a possible complication of medial patellar desmotomy. Aust Vet J 1989;66:189–190.

DESMITIS OF THE PATELLAR LIGAMENTS

Desmitis of patellar ligaments is an infrequently reported condition most often diagnosed in the middle patellar ligament (Figure 5.361).[1,4,5] Affected horses are usually athletes, mostly eventers, jumpers, or steeplechasers for which direct trauma from striking a jump is a risk factor.[1,2,4] Among eventers, frequency of patellar ligament injuries followed cruciate ligament and meniscal injuries.[2] Many cases are diagnosed after a prolonged lameness with no recognized inciting incident.[1] One report cited the incidence of MidPL combined with lateral (LPL) and LPL alone following MidPL injury.[1] Desmitis of the LPL may accompany fracture of the tibial tuberosity.[4]

Clinical Signs and Diagnosis

Lameness is variable and usually exacerbated by stifle flexion.[1] The desmitis may not be evident upon physical examination, and palpable swelling or eliciting pain from a specific point may require partial flexion of the stifle.[1] More extensive lesions or ruptured patellar ligaments are usually easy to locate. Intra-articular or regional local analgesia produced equivocal results.[1]

Middle patellar ligament lesions have been described as a linear lucency with fiber tearing or central hypoechoic regions similar to other desmopathies.[1,5] In addition to direct trauma, MPL injury may accompany palpable patellar instability.[1] Proximal and distal enthesiopathies reflect bony disruption in addition to the soft tissue lesion,[4] but their role in lameness if the inciting inflammation subsides is unclear.[5,6]

Lateral patellar ligament injury was observed simultaneously with MidPL injury and less commonly alone.[1] Tibial tuberosity fracture has been observed to be associated with simultaneous LPL desmopathy.[4]

The medial patellar ligament is affected less commonly by primary desmitis. Similar trauma seems to cause avulsion fracture of the medial aspect of the patella,[3] although the author has diagnosed one case of medial patellar ligament rupture which healed quickly with stall rest (Figure 5.362).

Upward fixation of the patella influences the medial patellar ligament. Extensive loss of density has been observed in animals with chronic intermittent upward fixation of the patella; after resolution, the tissue was healed yet thickened.[4] Generalized enlargement/fibrosis that is evident ultrasonographically also is evident after medial patellar ligament desmotomy.[4]

Scintigraphic evidence of patellar ligament inflammation may be present and appears to be related to the proximity to the most significant desmitis.[1]

Treatment

When the injury is confined to the soft tissue, therapy consists of rest and local and systemic anti-inflammatory therapy. Smaller enthesiopathies or fragments also may be treated conservatively with stall rest.

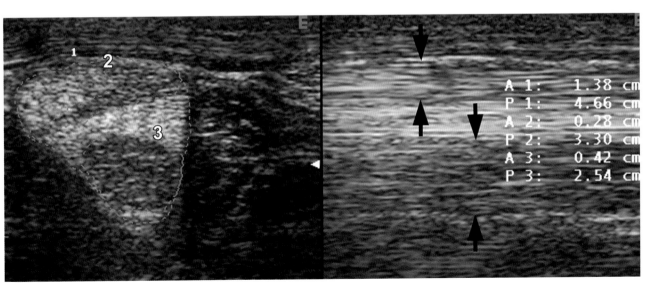

Figure 5.361. Ultrasound images of a middle patellar ligament injury. The cross-sectional view on the left demonstrates 2 areas of reduced fiber density (#2 and #3). The black arrows on the longitudinal view on the right outline the same areas at the same horizontal level as the image on the left. (Courtesy of Dr. Anne Desrochers.)

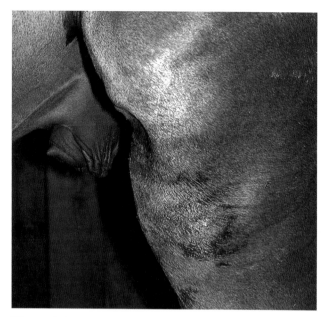

Figure 5.362. This horse developed a ruptured medial patellar ligament with an obvious palpable defect after hitting a jump. It healed completely and the horse became sound, although there were subtle radiographic changes on the distal patella.

Ultrasonographic monitoring of the healing process is advisable. Rest should be extended if medial patellar ligament laxity has occurred to prevent distal patellar changes.

Prognosis

Of a series of 9 patellar ligament injuries, none became completely sound for athletic performance, although working soundness was achieved in one.[1] These injuries might heal better with longer periods of restriction, or with desmoplasty with or without regenerative medicine intervention. Pain control should be used cautiously with continued training due to the potential for instability leading to OA.

The author suspects that ultrasonographic abnormalities in patellar ligaments detected after injury bear more pathophysiologic significance than those reported following MPD. Loss of tension following MPD could affect the ultrasonographic image. The improved outcomes reported for MPD in horses with a confirmed diagnosis compared to experimental MPD in normal horses suggest a difference.

References

1. Dyson SJ. Normal ultrasonographic anatomy and injury of the patellar ligaments in the horse. Equine Vet J 2002;34:258–264.
2. Dyson SJ. Stifle trauma in the event horse. Eq Vet Educ 1994;6:234–240.
3. Marble GP, Sullins KE. Arthroscopic removal of patellar fracture fragments in horses: Five cases (1989–1998). J Am Vet Med Assoc 2000;216:1799–1801.
4. Rantanen NW, McKinnon AO. Equine diagnostic ultrasonography. Williams and Wilkins, Baltimore, 1998;500–511.
5. Reef VB. Equine Diagnostic Ultrasound. WB Saunders Co., Philadelphia, 1998;160–164.
6. Wright I. Ligaments associated with joints. 1st Dubai International Equine Symposium 1996;241–272.

PATELLAR LUXATION/SUBLUXATION

Although patellar subluxation and luxation have been well documented in the literature, they are still considered to be uncommon.[4,5,8–12,15,17] The condition is usually recognized shortly after birth, but may be delayed in acquired cases. Acquired patellar luxation also occurs in older horses but even less commonly than congenitally.[12] Lateral,[2,4,6,10,12] medial,[1,7,14] distal,[13] unilateral, and bilateral luxations have been described, but lateral luxation is most common. Severity can range from a mild intermittent subluxation to a complete luxation that is difficult to manually replace.

Etiology

Hypoplasia of the trochlear ridges (primary bone deformity) and hypoplasia of the ligamentous support structures have been suggested as causes.[15,17] The medial patellar ligament is not as substantial as the other 2 patellar ligaments.

In ponies and miniature horses, lateral patellar luxation is considered heritable.[8] The lack of adequate trochlear groove and/or lateral trochlear ridge is a factor. Congenital trochlear inadequacy is not always bilateral, at least in the pony.[7] Lateral patellar luxation can also occur in association with defective development of the lateral trochlear ridge caused by OCD.[16] When the condition occurs in the mature horse, trauma is thought to be the cause. Partial tearing of the insertion of the quadriceps femoris muscles on the proximal patella has been cited as the cause for distal patellar luxation between the femoral trochlea.[13]

Clinical Signs and Diagnosis

Foals with bilateral lateral luxation may not be able to stand or may stand in a crouched position because the displaced patella causes the quadriceps muscle group to become a flexor rather than function as an extensor (Figure 5.363). Signs vary according to the frequency, position, and degree of displacement of the patella. Periods of normal ambulation occur if the displacement is intermittent. On palpation, there are varying degrees of patellar displacement and joint capsule distension. The intermittent patellar subluxations are usually readily replaced, whereas complete patellar luxation can be difficult to replace.

Persistent lateral subluxation of the patella presents much like a horse with upward fixation of the patella.[9] The limb is held in extension, causing the patella to be placed caudolaterad. When the limb is advanced, an awkward swinging toe-dragging gait occurs. Because some of these animals have a fairly normal gait, the condition may be missed until serious degenerative changes within the joint occur.[12]

In one case of distal patellar luxation, the limb was locked in flexion with the quadriceps femoris muscle stretched over the trochlea of the femur. This position was fixed and could not be altered by manipulation.[13]

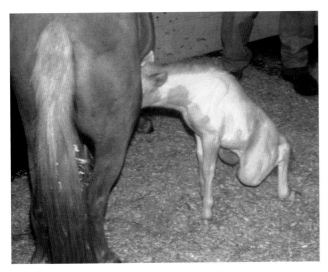

Figure 5.363. This foal has bilateral patellar luxation. The quadriceps muscles cannot extend the stifle without the pulley of the patella on the trochlea. (Courtesy of Dr. Cliff Honnas.)

General anesthesia was required to reduce the luxation, and the horse recovered uneventfully.

Radiographs should be taken to confirm the diagnosis and identify the amount of degenerative changes within the joint. The flexed cranioproximal-craniodistal tangential (skyline) view is particularly beneficial to assess the degree of displacement and the depth of the trochlea. In the neonate, the normal irregular borders of subchondral ossification in the proximal trochlea should not be confused with degenerative changes (Figure 5.352).

Treatment

In one reported case of bilateral congenital lateral patellar luxation in a miniature horse, the foal overcame the crouched stance and began to walk normally by 6 months of age, although the patellae remained luxated. Most are treated surgically to minimize permanent deformity of the soft tissues and the development of OA.

When a sufficient femoral trochlea is present, stabilization of the patella in the correct position by imbrication is performed. Release of the opposite soft tissue, including the contralateral patellar ligament, is often required to reduce tension on the repair.[4,9,12,14] Imbrication has commonly been accomplished using suture alone, but a recent case report in a pony employed screws in the femur to anchor the suture which was also placed through patellar drill paths and screws to anchor it and a nonabsorbable mesh for greater strength.[14]

Horses with hypoplasia of the lateral trochlear ridge resulting in an insufficient trochlear groove to stabilize the patella require reconstruction by sulcoplasty and/or tibial tuberosity transposition.[1,3,6,10] Significant misalignment of the patellar tendons also requires transposition of the tibial tuberosity.[1] When OCD is the cause of the hypoplastic trochlear ridge, the cartilage surface and underlying bone are usually insufficient to sustain correction.[16]

Prognosis

The outlook for soundness without surgical correction is poor,[12] although pasture soundness may be possible, at least in miniature horses. The outcome is better for horses undergoing stable correction before the soft tissues contract and OA occurs. For some reason, cases reported in the literature tend to be presented for treatment after weeks or months of clinical signs, which decreases the chance of successful stabilization.

In one study, a miniature horse requiring medial release, sulcoplasty, and tibial transposition became sound for its intended use.[1] In another study, 4 miniature foals undergoing imbrication alone to stabilize bilateral lateral patellar luxations survived to be functional, although 1 experienced a recurrence of unilateral lateral luxation.[4] Five horses were surgically treated by release of the lateral patellar ligament and imbrication of the medial joint capsule.[12] Three succumbed to wound dehiscence, infection, or failure of the repair. The stabilization was successful in 1 5-month-old Standardbred, but pre-existing OA limited the outcome. A yearling Trakehner-Thoroughbred was sound in light work 1 year postoperatively. The same procedure was successful for stabilizing a congenital bilateral lateral patellar luxation in a 6-week-old Shetland pony.[6]

Two full-sized horses and 1 miniature horse underwent sulcoplasty and medial imbrication of the joint capsules to stabilize lateral patellar luxations.[10] A 2-day-old Standardbred filly succumbed to incisional dehiscence and sepsis. A 3-month-old miniature horse and a 1-month-old Arabian filly recovered and were sound 2 years after surgery.

More recently, a newborn Shetland pony was diagnosed with the more uncommon medial patellar luxation.[7] Radiographs revealed unilateral patellar hypoplasia and essentially no trochlear groove in the distal femur. The foal underwent sulcoplasty and lateral imbrication and was sound 6 months postoperatively. Early recognition and correction would have contributed to success.

Although successful cases have been reported in horses, and it is true that miniature horses and ponies generally have fewer athletic expectations. From the above results it appears that horses have more difficulty sustaining the repair than ponies or miniature horses. Certainly horses have relatively longer, more flexible hindlimbs that probably place more tension on the repair. One report suggested minimal tension on the repairs when sulcoplasty was performed.[10] However, there are relatively few cases from which to draw conclusions regarding the best approach.[13]

References

1. Arighi M, Wilson JW. Surgical correction of medial luxation of the patella in a miniature horse. Can Vet J 1993;34:499–501.
2. Burba DJ, Collier MA. What is your diagnosis? Bilateral congenital patella luxation in horse. J Am Vet Med Assoc 1991;198:693–694.
3. Edinger H, Stanek C. Surgical correction of a congenital bilateral lateral stationary patellar luxation in a Shetland filly using trochleoplasty by wedge osteotomy. Pferd 1991;7:197–203.
4. Engelbert TA, Tate LP, Richardson DC, et al. Lateral patellar luxation in miniature horses. Vet Surg 1993;22:293–297.
5. Finocchio EJ, Guffy MM. Congenital ectopia in a foal. J Am Vet Med Assoc 1970;156:222.

6. Garlick MH, Thiemann AK. Treatment of luxating patellae. Vet Rec 1993;133:602–603.
7. Hart JCA, Jann HW, Moorman VJ. Surgical correction of a medial patellar luxation in a foal using a modified recession trochleoplasty technique. Eq Vet Educ 2009;21:307–311.
8. Hermans WA, Kersjes AW, van der Mey GJ, et al. Investigation into the heredity of congenital lateral patellar (sub)luxation in the Shetland pony. Vet Q 1987;9:1–8.
9. Jones RD, Henton JA, Cantrell GW, et al. Medial imbrication of the stifle to relieve lateral subluxation of the patella in a miniature horse. Eq Pract 1981;3:19–29.
10. Kobluk CN. Correction of patellar luxation by recession sulcoplasty in three foals. Vet Surg 1993;22:298–300.
11. Lafrance NA, Leaner DJ, O'Brien TR. Bilateral congenital lateral patellar luxation in a foal. Can Vet J 1971;12:119.
12. Leitch M, Kotlikoff M. Surgical repair of congenital lateral luxation of the patella in the foal and calf. Vet Surg 1980; 9:1–4.
13. McIlwraith CW, Warren RC. Distal luxation of the patella in a horse. J Am Vet Med Assoc 1982;181:67–69.
14. O'Meara B, Lischer CJ. Surgical management of a pony with a traumatic medial luxation of the patella. Eq Vet Educ 2009;21:458–463.
15. Rooney JR. Congenital lateral luxation of the patella in a horse. Cornell Vet 1971;61:670.
16. Stromberg B, Rejno S. Osteochondrosis in the horse. I. A clinical and radiologic investigation of osteochondritis dissecans of the knee and hock joint. Acta Radiol Suppl (Stockh) 1978; 358:139–152.
17. Van Pelt RW, Keahey KK, Dalley JB. Congenital bilateral extopia of the patella in the foal. Vet Med 1971;66:445.

SYNOVIAL OSTEOCHONDROMA IN THE HINDLIMB

Osteochondroma is a uni- or bilateral benign mass associated with cartilage growth centers. It is discussed as a distinct entity in Chapter 7. Young horses generally present with the problem, but they can remain clinically silent for long periods of time; therefore, older horses may also present.[3] In the hindlimb, osteochondroma has been reported in the femorotibial bursa on the proximal lateral tibia,[3] the plantar distal tibia within the tarsocrural joint,[2] within the tarsal canal on the fibular tarsal bone,[4] and on the calcaneus.[1]

Clinical Signs and Diagnosis

Synovial effusion with or without lameness is the usual presenting complaint. The location depends upon which synovial structure is affected. Often the mass can be palpated percutaneously. Radiographs usually demonstrate a focal semi-ossified variably sized mass associated with a growth plate or ossification center. The presenting signs and radiographic findings are often sufficient to make a presumptive diagnosis. Biopsy is usually better performed as excision. The radiographic appearance indicates that trauma is unlikely.

Treatment

In spite of the likelihood of it being a benign lesion, complete excision should be accomplished. If the horse is actively competing, palliation of the synovitis may be accomplished by local anti-inflammatory therapy. Routine postoperative bandaging and exercise restriction are tailored to the affected site. Intrasynovial anti-inflammatories such as sodium hyaluronate are advisable.

Prognosis

Although intrasynovial therapy is worthy of consideration, the prognosis for horses has been good following surgical excision. Each case is different, and the lesions are likely to occur in more difficult locations than have been observed in the past.

References

1. Chan CCH, Munroe GA, Callanan JJ. Congenital solitary osteochondroma affecting the tarsus in a filly foal. Eq Vet Educ 1996;8:153–156.
2. Kenzora KT, Von Matthiessen PW, Sheehan RM. A uniquely located solitary plantar tibial osteochondroma in a Thoroughbred racehorse. Eq Pract 1995;17:23–25.
3. Kirk MD. Radiographic and histologic appearance of synovial osteochondromatosis of the femorotibial bursae in a horse: A case history report. Vet Rad 1982;23:167–170.
4. Welch RD, Auer JA, Watkins JP, et al. Surgical treatment of tarsal sheath effusion associated with an exostosis on the calcaneus of a horse. J Am Vet Med Assoc 1990;196:1992–1994.

FEMOROTIBIAL JOINTS

The medial and lateral femorotibial joints are separate structures that usually lack communication except in cases of severe osteoarthritis and cruciate ligament damage and some cases of postoperative arthroscopy in which the septum separating the two structures is perforated. The medial femorotibial (MFT) joint usually communicates with the femoropatellar joint through a fenestration in the proximal aspect of the joint. This is important from the standpoint that disease in the MFT joint can manifest as femoropatellar joint effusion, sometimes leading to confusion about the true site of damage, since diagnostic anesthesia of one joint can influence the other. Consequently, heavy emphasis is placed on diagnostic imaging and sometimes arthroscopy to resolve the confusion.

Both the medial and lateral femorotibial joints are comprised of a femoral condyle and tibial plateau and a meniscus between the two. A soft tissue septum separates the two compartments, which continues caudally to surround the cranial and caudal cruciate ligaments, making them extrasynovial in this location. The same is true for the medial and lateral collateral ligaments.

Horses with lameness originating from the femorotibial joints can vary in severity. Some cases are subtle enough to create a training issue without the presence of noticeable lameness, whereas others are severe enough to lead to non-weight-bearing lameness. In more severe and chronic cases, horses typically stand with the limb abducted and there is usually noticeable atrophy of the hip and quadriceps musculature.

Whereas effusion in the lateral femorotibial (LFT) joint is difficult to palpate, effusion of the MFT joint is readily palpable, especially in the recess just cranial to the medial collateral ligament and proximal to the meniscus and tibial plateau (Figures 3.60 and 3.140). However, in more severe and chronic cases, significant soft tissue thickening can also occur in this area, often obscuring the ability to palpate effusion. This is referred to as a tibial buttress and is usually associated with advanced OA within the joint. The degree of effusion and swelling is usually graded as normal, mild, moderate, or severe, and any pain and thickening of the collateral ligament is noted.

There are no distinguishing characteristics to limb use in horses with stifle pain compared to those with pain at other sites in the hindlimb. All horses should be walked and trotted in a straight line. Subtle lameness is sometimes more noticeable in soft footing, especially when horses are jogged in a circle. Although most horses are more lame when the limb is on the inside of the circle, occasionally the lameness is worse when the limb is on the outside of the circle.

Horses with stifle pain is positive to full limb flexion. However, some information can be gained by attempting to isolate flexion to the stifle area. This is done by keeping the tarsal area as straight as possible and bringing the limb caudally from the tibia distally (Figure 3.77). A positive response to this flexion is not absolutely indicative of stifle pain, but it can give important information about the site of pain.

More severe cases of lameness attributable to the stifle are often obvious on clinical examination due to severe effusion, soft tissue swelling, pain on palpation, and severe response to flexion. However, diagnostic anesthesia is needed to confirm the site of pain in many horses. The approach to diagnostic anesthesia of the stifle can be complex. Some clinicians block all 3 joints of the stifle at once to expedite the process, rather than starting with one joint and then blocking the other joints. Consequently, if all 3 joints are blocked at once, the clinician may need to further isolate the joints later to determine which one(s) contribute to the lameness.

Regardless of how stifle pain is confirmed in affected horses, accurate imaging of the joints is difficult. Improvements in radiography, ultrasound, computed tomography, and magnetic resonance imaging help to characterize the disease processes, but the lack of visualization during arthroscopic surgery and a minimal number of postmortem studies have prevented investigators from truly correlating imaging results to gross damage. Unlike other species, the femorotibial joints in the horse are closely packed, preventing arthroscopic visualization of most of the joints. Consequently, the ability to truly characterize and repair damage in many parts of the femorotibial joints is limited.

SUBCHONDRAL CYSTIC LESIONS (SCL) OF THE STIFLE

This section focuses on the clinical signs, diagnosis, and treatment of SCL in the stifle. Although this occurs most commonly in the medial femoral condyle, it also can occur in the lateral femoral condyle and proximal tibia. See Chapter 11 for further discussion of SCLs as they relate to developmental orthopedic disease.

Etiology

Although SCL is usually attributed to developmental orthopedic disease,[19,21] some clinicians strongly believe and experimental evidence has shown that it can also occur after trauma to the subchondral bone.[30,39] Ray, et al.[30] have shown that creation of a lesion 3 mm deep and 5 mm in diameter into the subchondral bone created SCL in 5 of 6 horses. Furthermore, Von

Rechenberg, et al.[40] showed that the lining of the cysts contains significant inflammatory mediators that may be responsible for enlargement and persistence of the cyst. The tissues from postmortem cystic material had significant osteoclastic function on bone. Therefore, regardless of the cause of cyst formation, persistent enlargement of some lesions may be due to a vicious cycle of inflammation.

Clinical Signs

Horses with SCL of the stifle can present in several different ways. Historically, these lesions are found on survey films of yearlings in which no lameness is present. They can also be found in any age horse in which no lameness is apparent. However, most horses with stifle SCLs present at or near the time that training begins, when a mild to moderate degree of lameness is usually found. Effusion may or may not be present within the MFT and femoropatellar joints. When lameness is present the horse is usually positive to upper limb flexion that is isolated to the stifle joint.

Horses with SCL in the stifle commonly improve 50% or more with intra-articular analgesia of the joints. It is important to evaluate these horses within 15 minutes of performing the intra-articular analgesia and after 60 minutes to get a full appreciation for the improvement in lameness. In older horses that have been in training and competition, it is particularly important to perform intra-articular analgesia to prove the significance of an SCL because if a horse has been working well with the presence of a SCL, other factors may be involved in the lameness.

Imaging and Diagnosis

Radiography

Radiography is standard for accurate diagnosis (Figure 5.364). In a grading scheme for SCLs developed by Howard, et al., type 1 lesions are less than 10 mm in depth and typically dome-shaped; type 2 are greater than 10 mm in depth and either dome, conical, or spherical shaped; and grade 3 are flat or irregular bone surface.[16] Wallis, et al. modified the grading scheme to include type 2A, which are more than 10 mm deep and have a lollipop or mushroom shape with a narrow cloaca and a round cystic lucency; type 2B lesions are more than 10 mm deep with a large dome shape extending down to a large articular surface defect; type 3 are condylar flattening or small defects in the subchondral bone, usually noted in the contralateral limb to that of the clinically significant SCL, and type 4 are those that have a lucency in the condyle with or without an articular defect but no radiographic evidence of a cloaca in the subchondral bone plate (Figure 5.364).[41]

A grading scheme for characterizing pre-sale films in yearlings and 2-year-old Quarter horses has been developed that describes lesions in general.[8] In yearlings that do not show clinical signs, it is important to follow the progression of the lesions with radiographs over time to monitor the SCL, because some may resolve. Likewise, they should be monitored clinically because some may

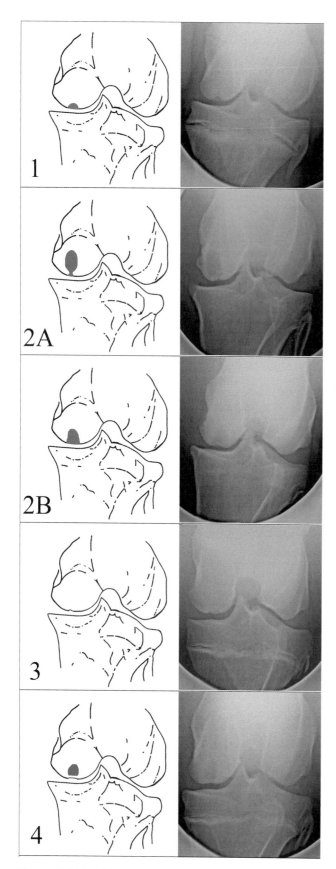

Figure 5.364. Grades of subchondral cystic lesions (SCLs). (Reprinted with permission from Wallis TW, et al. Equine Vet J 2008;40:461–467.)

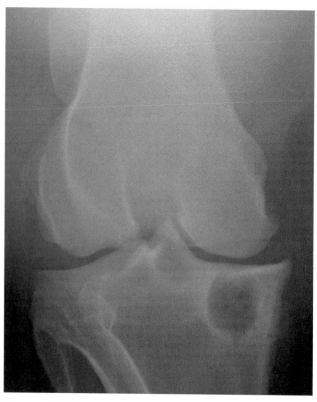

Figure 5.365. A caudal-cranial radiographic image of a proximal tibial subchondral cystic lesion with concurrent signs of osteoarthritis within the MFT joint.

worsen and begin to induce lameness. It is not uncommon in older horses to see radiographic signs of osteoarthritis (OA) such as periarticular osteophytes and joint space narrowing in addition to the cyst. It is also important to compare radiographs in both limbs because SCLs may be bilateral, especially if they are developmental in origin.

Subchondral cystic lesions are not uncommon in the proximal tibia (Figure 5.365).[38] In horses younger than 2 years of age, tibial SCLs have been shown to occur in the cranial aspect of the lateral condyle of the tibia, and in horses older than 2 years, it commonly occurs in the medial condyle of the tibia, either cranial or caudal. The author's colleagues have seen subchondral cystic lesions of both the medial femoral condyle and the tibia in a single horse. It is also typical in older horses to see OA changes concurrent with these lesions (Figure 5.365).

Nuclear Scintigraphy

The usefulness of nuclear scintigraphy in diagnosing SCL is questionable. It may be helpful for identifying the significance of SCL in the tibia,[38] but it has not been shown to demonstrate high specificity other than for identifying joint disease. Therefore, especially in older horses, it is difficult to rely on nuclear scintigraphy to determine the significance of an SCL because it cannot discern an SCL from generalized joint disease, such as OA.

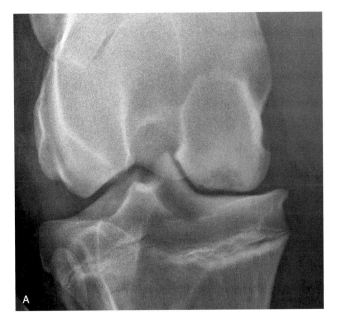

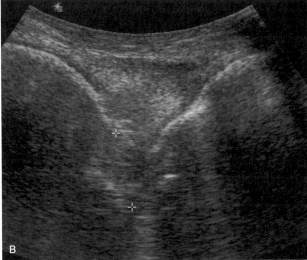

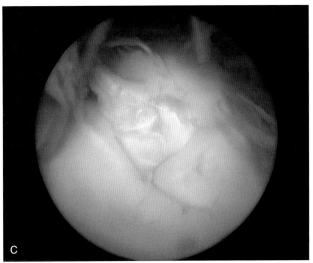

Figure 5.366. Radiograph (A), ultrasound (B), and intraoperative (C) images demonstrating an SCL that involved a large percentage of the articular surface. Note the joint space narrowing on the radiographic image (A), and the presence of the SCL as demonstrated by a defect in the subchondral bone on the ultrasonographic images (B). Thickening of the articular cartilage can be seen arthroscopically (C).

Ultrasonography

Ultrasonography helps to evaluate articular cartilage surface, joint effusion, debris, and changes that may occur in the meniscus and cruciate ligaments. Subchondral cystic lesions typically show an irregularity on the condylar surface and thickening of the articular cartilage (Figure 5.366). Because most cases of SCL are examined arthroscopically for treatment, the author does not routinely perform ultrasound of these cases unless there is concern about the integrity of the medial meniscus. However, if surgery is not an option at the owner's request, then ultrasound examination is recommended to obtain further information about the integrity of the surrounding articular cartilage and to later guide cyst injection. The femoral condyle becomes quite superficial beneath the skin when the limb is flexed, and the smooth, anechoic nature of the articular cartilage on the curved condyle can be easily appreciated super-ficial to the hyperechoic subchondral bone (Figure 5.366B). In cases of SCL, a defect is appreciated in the subchondral bone, the depths of which sometimes cannot be appreciated.[18] See Chapter 4 for further details on the use of ultrasonography to evaluate the MFT joint.

Treatment

Conservative therapy can be used in horses younger than 1 year old in which lameness may or may not be present. These horses may be treated with intra-articular medication. Corticosteroids in particular may have an effect on the cystic lining to prevent cyst enlargement. These horses should be confined to a small pen and radiographs re-evaluated every 4 to 6 weeks. If no change is present or if the cyst is enlarging, then surgical options should be considered. However, there are some horses of various ages that respond well to intra-articular and systemic medications, and in some instances may be maintained for competition. Cases that respond to medical management have SCLs that are either small, have a small articular component, or may show limited communication between the cyst and the joint surface. It is unknown whether the SCL is relatively stable in these cases, leading to adequate support of the articular surface. Rest has also been reported to be successful in treating some cases of SCL in the tibia[38].

Surgery is common to treat SCLs, because horses that suffer lameness from this problem can rarely perform with the existence of the cyst.[21] Several methods of surgical treatment have been used with varying degrees of success, including debridement of the cyst contents, injection of the cystic lining with corticosteroids, and grafting of the debrided cyst with various products.

Debridement of cystic contents has been shown to be effective in 56% to 77% of cases that undergo surgery. In these cases, the joint is arthroscopically explored and the contents of the cyst removed. It is important to remove the lining of the SCL because it contains inflammatory mediators.[40] Some have advocated drilling of the subchondral bone to facilitate access of blood supply to the cyst; however, Howard, et al, showed that in some of these cases, the drill holes lead to enlargement of the lesions.[16] Nevertheless, some advocate using microfracture on the cyst wall, especially when sclerosis is present.

A lateral approach is typically used during arthroscopic surgery; however, if the depths of the cyst are not visualized, then a cranial approach can be used. It is important to place the instrument portal directly over the site of the cyst to facilitate removal of all cystic contents. These horses are typically rested 6 to 12 months after surgery.

The prognosis generally is good for these lesions. Lewis has shown that 72% of horses had returned to intended use, although 14 of the 67 horses studied had occasional lameness that was managed medically.[20] Howard, et al. showed that although 74% were successful, that the prognosis was relatively lower for Quarter horses compared to other breeds.[16] Sandler, et al. showed that 77% of 150 Thoroughbreds intended for racing raced after debridement of the SCL. However, horses in which more than 15 mm of the surface of the joint was involved had a reduced prognosis compared to those with less than 15 mm.[33] Therefore, it appears that the depth of the cyst is of little importance in the prognosis but the percent of joint surface involved is important (Figure 5.366).

An osteochondritis dissecans (OCD) lesion may be present at the cyst opening and require debridement at the time of surgery.[16] Smith, et al. showed that horses older than 3 years had a dramatically lower chance of soundness and return to work than horses 3 years and younger.[36] This study also confirmed that the presence of articular cartilage lesions within the MFT joint remote to the site of the SCL negatively impacted the prognosis. In addition to age and other articular lesions, SCL enlargement[16] and damage to the menisci and/or meniscal ligament can further reduce prognosis.

Some have advocated bone grafting to facilitate repair and filling in the bony defect. However, the prognosis is really no different than debridement.[17] Others have advocated the use of some form of bone graft (cancellous bone graft, tricalcium phosphate or hydroxyapatite) with an overlay of fibrin, growth factors, and chondrocytes or stem cells to improve the prognosis.[22]

Subchondral cystic lesions of the tibia that occur laterally can be approached with an arthroscope and are typically beneath the cranial ligament of the lateral meniscus. They too can be debrided. However, in some lesions, especially those involving the medial tibial condyle of older horses, an extra-articular approach may be required for debridement.[38]

Some surgeons advocate intralesional steroid therapy for treating SCLs. Based on the work of von Rechenberg, et al., in which showed inflammatory mediators within the cyst lining, this treatment makes sense.[40] However, it is important to inject corticosteroids into the cystic lining and not just into the depths of the cyst. Cyst injection is best facilitated by an arthroscopic approach[41] so that concurrent articular cartilage lesions can be debrided if necessary. However, injection of the lesion can be done with ultrasound guidance of a needle into the cystic material. Triamcinolone acetonide (10 to 30 mg/cyst) or methylprednisolone acetate (40 to 80 mg/cyst) or both are typically injected into the SCL. These horses are rested post-operatively and re-radiographed after 2 months, at which time clinical signs often improve and the horses can be put into light work.

Wallis, et al. showed that this technique was successful in 67% of horses and 77% of cysts.[41] There was no significant influence of age, 90% of horses that had unilateral cysts were successful vs. 67% that were affected bilaterally, and the presence of osteophytes within the MFT joint reduced the success to 63% vs. 87% for those without.

Prognosis

Overall, 56% to 77% of horses returned to their intended use with surgery for SCL of the medial femoral condyle. The limited work in tibial cysts has shown that in younger than 2 years, 3 out of 4 returned to work. Older horses with tibial SCLs had reduced work. The prognosis was poor for those with lesions in the caudal aspect of the joint in which access was limited.

FRACTURES

Etiology

Intra-articular fractures of the stifle usually are due to acute trauma from internal forces; it is uncommon to see these problems in horses with outward signs of external trauma. They commonly occur with rotation and may involve an avulsion fracture, usually of the intercondylar eminence of the tibia. Intra-articular fractures of the femorotibial joints are rare compared to fractures in the femoropatellar joint and other joints in the horse.

Clinical Signs

Horses typically present with significant acute lameness, often with significant synovial effusion and joint capsule swelling. They may or may not be painful on palpation and they often show an outward rotation of the distal limb when standing. These are also very painful to flexion, both passively and with movement. Horses with tibial tuberosity fractures can be painful on palpation of the area, and are mentioned here because concurrent damage to the soft tissues of the femorotibial joints has been reported with this fracture.[1]

Diagnosis and Imaging

Radiographs typically demonstrate the presence of fractures. They can occur on the caudal aspect of the medial femoral condyle (Figure 5.367A),[9,13] caudal aspect of the medial tibial condyle, intercondylar eminence (Figure 5.367B),[24,43] Salter-Harris type III fracture of the lateral condyle,[12] Salter-Harris type IV fracture of the distal femoral physis,[12] origin of the long digital extensor muscle (Figure 5.368) or peroneus tertius muscle,[4,15] and as loose fragments within the lateral femorotibial joint.[37]

Peroneus tertius origin avulsion fractures usually induce flexion of the stifle with corresponding extension of the hock, and fragments are usually contained within the femoropatellar joint. Fragmentation of the origin of the long digital extensor muscle can induce lameness (Figure 5.368), although the author has seen these as incidental lesions on routine radiographs of yearlings. Fragments can be removed arthroscopically and the prognosis is good. Radiographs can confirm the diagnosis, and ultrasound is sometimes useful in identifying the exact location of the fragment. Fragments originating from the medial intercondylar eminence of the tibia are thought to be avulsion fractures from the insertion of the cranial cruciate ligament; however, some fragments in this location do not involve the ligament insertion. Walmsley demonstrated that the cranial cruciate ligament insertion was not involved in 7 of 12 horses

with medial intercondylar eminence fractures of the tibia. Ultrasound examination is valuable in assessing prognosis, which can be worsened by significant secondary damage to soft tissues of the joints.[1]

Treatment

Small intra-articular fragments can be excised and removed arthroscopically in most cases. It is important to explore the entire joint, both front and back, because fragments can migrate to the caudal aspect of the joint, and to determine if secondary damage to the soft tissues (such as the meniscus and the articular cartilage) are present. Proliferative lesions are found in the intercondylar area of the tibia and femur, which can be debrided if they are clinically significant. Specifically, fibrous proliferation of the soft tissues can be present in chronic cases, as can bony proliferation that may impinge on soft tissue structures with movement. Large fragments in the medial intercondylar eminence of the tibia that have a stable fibrous adhesion often can be left intact. If the fragment is large and involves a large portion of the intercondylar eminence, then lag screw fixation can be used to stabilize the area.

Fragment removal should be performed if there is no compromise to the weight-bearing aspect of the joint; however, internal fixation is recommended if the joint surface needs to be reconstructed and/or vital attachments retained.[43] For the condylar surface, a cannulated screw can be used to stabilize a fracture of the medial femoral condyle. Conservative therapy is sometimes best in horses with Salter-Harris fractures.[12]

Prognosis

Prognosis is often good for horses with small fragmentation in which minimal soft tissue debridement occurs and minimal secondary damage is present. The

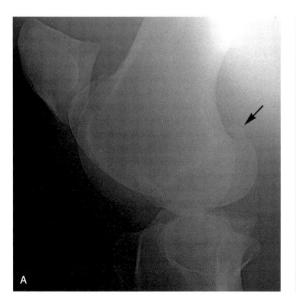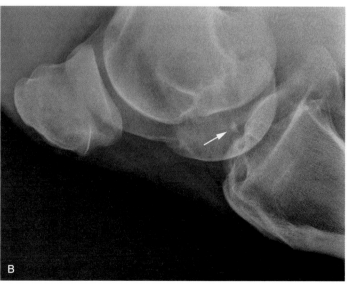

Figure 5.367. A. Standing lateral radiograph identifying a fracture of the caudal aspect of the medial femoral condyle (arrow). B. A flexed lateromedial radiographic image that demonstrates fragmentation of the intercondylar eminence of the tibia (arrow). The fragment was attached to the cranial cruciate ligament, but was loose during arthroscopic examination. (Courtesy of Dr. Gary Baxter.)

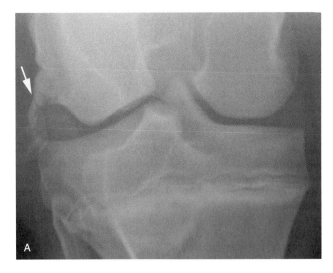

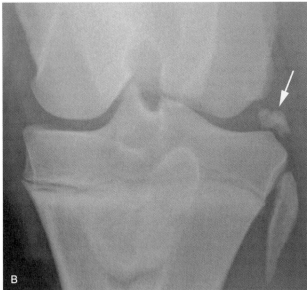

Figure 5.368. Caudal-cranial radiographic images of fragmentation of the origin of the long digital extensor tendon (arrows).

prognosis is reduced for horses with larger fracture fragments involving more of the articular surfaces and for those with significant soft tissue and articular cartilage damage.

FEMORAL CONDYLE LESIONS

Etiology

Femoral condyle lesions fall into 2 broad categories based on the age of the horse: septic or developmental lesions in foals and osteochondral disease in adults. In foals, Hance, et al. showed that 3 separate categories of femoral condyle lesions can occur.[13] Type I lesions are septic, and subchondral bone lysis is present in the face of septic arthritis and osteomyelitis. Type II lesions show osseous irregularity in less than 50% of the femoral condyle surface. Type III lesions show widespread irregularity and some have a thin osseous frag-

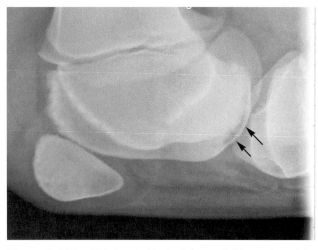

Figure 5.369. Subchondral lysis of the medial femoral condyle (arrows) was present on the lateromedial radiographic image of this foal's stifle. Arthroscopic examination revealed severe articular cartilage and subchondral bone degeneration.

ment. The authors of the study concluded that types II and III lesions may be some form of developmental orthopedic disease or vascular insult.

Osteochondral lesions of the femoral condyles in adult horses nearly always involve the medial femoral condyle. These lesions are usually considered to be traumatic in origin; however, there is growing concern that some of the lesions may be developmental in origin because abnormalities in condylar shape, such as dimpling or flattening, may predispose horses to this problem.

Clinical Signs and Diagnosis

Foals with types I and III lesions are typically severely lame, and those with type II lesions are usually moderately lame. However, all cause clinical signs that obviously point to a stifle problem. Radiographs typically reveal subchondral bone lucency indicative of the damage (Figure 5.369).

Medial femoral condyle osteochondral lesions are common in young Western performance athletes; however, they can occur in any type of horse. Adult horses with medial femoral condyle lesions may or may not have effusion, are usually positive to hindlimb flexion, and respond to intra-articular analgesia. Although these horses may not respond 100%, anything over 50% improvement is often considered significant.[20,34]

Radiographs are commonly negative in these horses, and ultrasound may or may not demonstrate articular cartilage lesions. Flattening and sclerosis of the medial femoral condyle are subtle radiographic abnormalities that may suggest osteochondral lesions.[34]

The key is that the lameness improves following IA anesthesia, often necessitating arthroscopic visualization to further characterize the lesions. As mentioned above, Contino has classified these changes in yearling and 2-year-old Quarter horses, but the significance of these changes is unknown at this time.[8] Magnetic resonance imaging has been advocated by some for characterizing these lesions; however, often the lesions are smaller than the resolution of the machine, and instead, any changes in subchondral bone can aid in the diagnosis.

Treatment

Arthroscopic surgery in foals should be preceded by obtaining a synovial fluid sample for culture and sensitivity. Debrided bone also may be submitted. Care should be taken during debridement because the normal subchondral bone of foals is soft and easily removed. Therefore, it is difficult to assess the extent of damage.

Arthroscopic findings in adults usually include focal or generalized articular cartilage lesions (Figure 5.370). Focal lesions are usually dimples, wrinkles, or folded pieces of articular cartilage which may or may not be detached from the subchondral bone (Figure 5.370).[34] Articular cartilage fibrillation, erosion, or subchondral bone lysis also can be involved.[20]

Walmsley has classified the types of articular cartilage lesions using human classification systems, and in particular uses the Outerbridge classification for reporting. The Outerbridge system grades the lesions on a scale of 1 to 4: grade 1 includes softening and swelling of the articular cartilage, grade 2 includes partial thickness defects with fissures on the surface that do not extend to the subchondral bone and/or do not exceed 1.5 cm in diameter, grade 3 includes fissuring to the subchondral bone and/or a lesion that exceeds 1.5 cm in diameter, and grade 4 includes those with exposed subchondral bone.

Schneider, et al. reported that 6 of 7 horses with focal disease returned to intended use, whereas only 1 of 4 with generalized condylar damage recovered.[34] Lewis stated that only 6 of 20 horses returned to intended use.[20] Walmsley, et al., found that in horses with Outerbridge grades 1 and 2, 78% returned to their intended use, compared to 63% of those with Outerbridge grades 3 and 4. In the study by Cohen, et al., 60% of horses improved, of which 46% became sound and 37% returned to intended use. In general, however, the severity of articular cartilage lesions was an inconsistent indicator of prognosis (Figure 5.370).[7]

There is no consensus on how best to treat these cases. In horses with fibrillation, the fibrillated tags of tissue should be debrided. For those with partial-thickness cracks and erosions, only superficial debridement should be performed. Some surgeons have proposed using radiofrequency probes to shrink the involved areas of cartilage disease to cause them to recede and theoretically alleviate loading on the area. This procedure is untested, and even in human medicine is contentious, because the radiofrequency procedure has been shown to cause chondrocyte death. Lesions with subchondral bone lysis can be lightly debrided and the bone area injected with corticosteroids in the hope of reducing the inflammatory components that may have an influence on the bone resorption. Some cases of full-thickness erosion have visible evidence of subchondral bone necrosis that require debridement. Some surgeons advocate the use of microfracture to augment healing;

however, in the medial femoral condyle this procedure could lead to the development of SCL.

It is currently unknown why medial femoral condyle lesions occur. Although some think that they may be developmental in nature, acute trauma and/or chronic competitive trauma cannot be ruled out. There is also concern that flattening or dimpling of the subchondral bone may predispose these horses to this injury. Contino showed that these lesions are common in young Quarter horses,[8] but there has been no correlation in clinical studies. Scott, et al. found that horses with flattening or mild lysis are likely to have articular cartilage lesions that require debridement.[35] Of those horses, 7 of 9 with focal lesions were sound postsurgery compared to 2 of 6 with generalized lesions. Care must be taken, however, because overly aggressive debridement and microfracture may lead to secondary SCL formation.

Prognosis

The prognosis for foals with type III lesions is guarded, even with surgical debridement; 11 of 20 horses in one study were euthanized due to poor prognosis.[13] As noted under the treatment section, the prognosis for medial femoral condyle lesions in adults depends on the severity of articular cartilage damage and must be estimated on a case-by-case basis.

COLLATERAL LIGAMENT INJURY

Etiology

Collateral ligament injury primarily occurs to the medial collateral ligament in the femorotibial joint, usually in adults. It is not uncommon to see that other structures are involved, including the meniscus and the cranial cruciate ligament.[5] These injuries are usually acute in nature, although chronic low-grade damage to the ligament may be seen in cases of chronic intra-articular disease.

Clinical Signs

Clinical signs are usually acute and severe, but minor injuries cause more subtle signs. Often there is swelling in the medial collateral ligament area and pain on palpation. The horses are usually very positive to flexion and worsen after manipulating the limb into a valgus position. This involves placing pressure over the lateral aspect of the femorotibial joints with one hand and pulling the limb laterally to stress the medial collateral ligament. Horses with complete rupture may show significant lateral movement of the distal limb and a palpable widening of the MFT joint space on the medial aspect of the stifle.

Diagnosis

Radiographic findings often are normal; however, the MFT joint may distract on a stressed caudocranial view (Figure 5.371). Signs of OA, such as an enthesiophyte, in the area of attachment in the medial collateral ligament are not uncommon in more chronic cases. Ultrasound is usually the primary method of diagnosis,

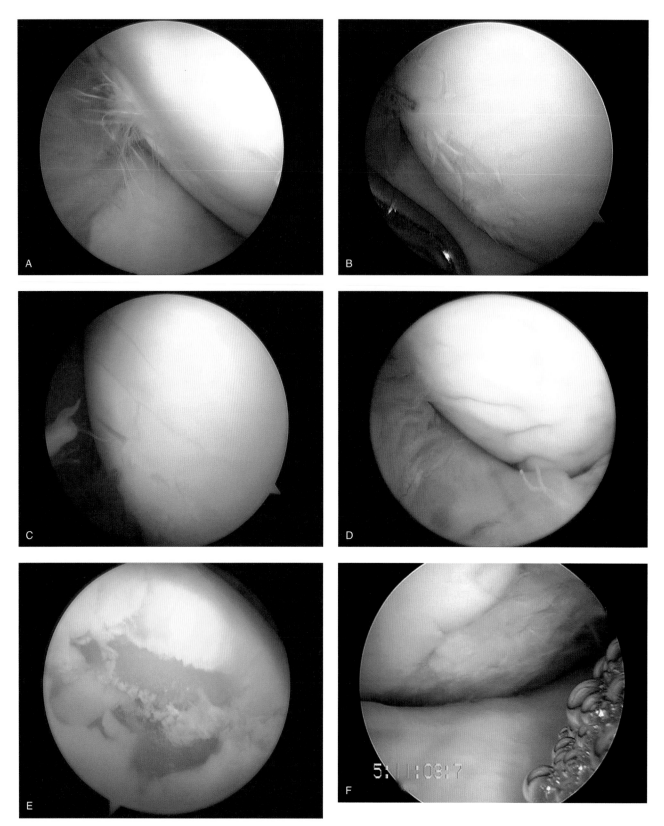

Figure 5.370. Various articular cartilage lesions that can be seen arthroscopically in adult horses. Small, focal area of cartilage fibrillation (A) or partial-thickness cracking can be seen (B). More extensive cracking, some of them full thickness, can also be present (C). More extensive cracks can also contain soft, thickened articular cartilage in between the cracks (D), and in some cases, dead, necrotic subchondral bone can be present (E). In advanced cases of OA, extensive articular cartilage erosion can be seen as well as fibrocartilage healing (F).

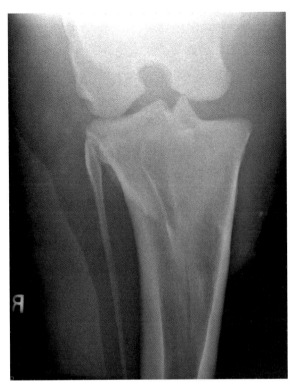

Figure 5.371. Caudal-cranial radiographic image of a stifle with a ruptured medial collateral ligament. Notice the widened joint space medially.

which often shows fibrin disorganization either in the body or the insertions of the ligament.

Treatment and Prognosis

Treatment is usually conservative in nature and may include rest, intra-articular medication, topical anti-inflammatory medication such as diclofenac acid, extra-corporeal shockwave therapy at both the body and the insertions of the ligament, or stem cell therapy into any hypoechoic region of the ligament. Surgical therapy has been advocated in some cases, although this is usually aimed at treating other problems within the joint such as fibrillation and tearing of the meniscus or the cranial cruciate ligament. The prognosis is often poor overall, except in horses with mild injuries to the ligament.

CRUCIATE LIGAMENT DISEASE

Etiology

Damage to the cranial cruciate ligament is usually acute in nature due to a traumatic event in which the limb is stressed in an abnormal direction, although the cause is rarely recognized. Other structures are usually involved, including the medial meniscus and the medial collateral ligament. Partial degeneration of the cranial cruciate ligament can occur in jumpers and racehorses. Horses with these lesions are less lame and tend to have a better prognosis with treatment.

The types of stresses that induce this problem are truly unknown. In an *ex vivo* study by Rich et al., in which mechanically induced tearing of the cranial cruciate ligament was assessed, 9 of 15 limbs failed in the ligament, 5 failed at the tibial insertion, and 2 failed at the femoral origin. This study suggested that there is no consistent change due to the type of injury that occurs.[31]

Clinical Signs

The degree of lameness is often associated with the degree of damage, and most horses present for an acute lameness, with significant effusion and response to flexion. However, in an attempt to mechanically assess the joint using the cranial drawer test, Prades, et al. found that only 1 of 10 horses was deemed to be unstable in the standing position and 6 of the 10 were deemed to be unstable under anesthesia.[29] A tibial thrust test in the caudal direction may worsen the lameness in some horses, but this is not considered specific for cranial cruciate ligament damage.

Diagnosis

Radiographs are usually unremarkable unless the origin of the ligament avulses from the intercondylar fossa,[11] a midbody tear shows dystrophic mineralization, or a medial tibial eminence fragment is present. However, the latter finding is not pathognomonic for cranial cruciate ligament damage because a fracture at the apex of the eminence may not involve the ligament. Ultrasound gives variable results because the cranial cruciate ligament area is difficult to image; however, a small section of the cranial cruciate ligament insertion on the tibia can be visualized with the limb flexed. MRI is available in limited locations, and probably demonstrates the best chances of acquiring an accurate diagnosis. High-field, short bore magnets can accommodate some horses for accurate imaging. Arthroscopic surgery can be used to explore the joint and assess the extent of damage, and is currently the best method to accurately diagnose cranial cruciate damage.[25,28]

Treatment

Osteochondral fragments from the tibial eminence can be removed and damaged tissues debrided arthroscopically. Microfracture may help stimulate endogenous repair of avulsed ligament from bone in the intercondylar space. Damaged tissue can be debrided, and although no repair technique has been successfully developed for the horse, partial tears can be augmented with platelet-rich plasma or mesenchymal stem cells injected into the tissues.[25] Other therapies to consider include intra-articular stem cell or IRAP therapy to use the growth factor properties that these 2 treatments are meant to induce. Overall, the prognosis depends on the extent of damage, but is often considered poor. However, some horses have returned to work.[20,25,29] Caudal cruciate ligament injuries have been reported and most of them involve longitudinal fraying and not true ligament rupture.[2,23,27,32]

MENISCAL INJURIES

Etiology

Meniscal lesions can be acute or chronic. Acute damage can occur with a bad step or an accident that leads to shifting or shear forces between the femur and tibia. Lesions are often seen in other structures such as cruciate ligaments and articular cartilage. Horses of any breed and use are susceptible to these lesions, especially those that jump. Chronic lesions often occur secondary to primary lesions in the opposing articular cartilage or instability due to damage in other structures. Western performance and sport horses have a high incidence of stifle lesions, and consequently are predisposed to secondary meniscal lesions. Both lateral and medial meniscal lesions occur, but damage to the medial meniscus is most common.

Clinical Signs

Meniscal injuries are acute or insidious in onset and usually affect the medial meniscus. Signs of medial meniscal injury can vary. In a study by Walmsley, 40% of cases presented acutely and 53% were insidious in onset.[46] The median lameness grade was 3 out of 10, 66% were positive to upper limb flexion, 47% had MFT joint and/or femoropatellar effusion, and 93% responded to intra-articular analgesia.[46] However, meniscal injury can be secondary to chronic OA or subchondral cystic lesions, and signs can include capsule thickening of the MFT joint and disuse atrophy of the surrounding musculature.

Diagnosis and Imaging

Radiographs can be normal in acute cases of primary meniscal damage. However, damage to the meniscus may lead to joint space narrowing so it is important that these images be reassessed because poor positioning can lead to false interpretation of the radiographs. In addition, radiographic abnormalities often accompany meniscal tearing in more chronic cases, as has been shown in several studies.[3,10,42] Mineralization of the meniscus (Figure 5.372) and osteophytes on the medial tibial plateau (Figure 5.373), and intercondylar eminence of the tibia are common in horses with more chronic lameness. In updated results from Walmsley,[45] 23% of horses with meniscal damage had new bone formation at the medial intercondylar eminence of the tibia, and this was associated with cranial cruciate injury in only 7% of cases.

Ultrasonographic findings can include characterization of an abnormal size, thickness, variability in echogenicity, location of the meniscus, prolapsing of the meniscus medially, and overt meniscal tearing.[3,6,10,14] It is important when assessing for a tear that the area is imaged in both weight-bearing and nonweight-bearing stances (Figures 5.374 and 5.375). Nonweight-bearing imaging often causes opening of the meniscus for better demonstration of the tear. For acute severe injuries, the cranial cruciate ligament and medial collateral ligament may also be involved but it is not uncommon to see isolated meniscal injuries. Despite its widespread use to diagnose meniscal lesions, it is difficult to validate ultra-

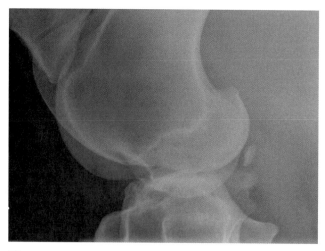

Figure 5.372. A lateromedial radiographic image demonstrating mineralization of the caudal aspect of the meniscus. Arthroscopic removal of this mineralization is rarely indicated because the OA is often advanced.

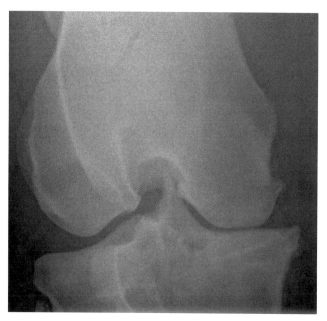

Figure 5.373. A caudal-cranial radiographic image showing osteophytes on the medial aspect of the tibia and the intercondylar eminence, which are common in many types of diseases involving the femorotibial joints.

sonographic findings since most of the meniscus is inaccessible at surgery, leading to potential false positive and/or negative findings.

Other diagnostic techniques include nuclear scintigraphy, which is highly sensitive but has poor specificity,[3] MRI, which is useful but limited in availability, and arthroscopy which is an important diagnostic tool that is readily available but unable to visualize much of the weight-bearing surface of the meniscus. Therefore, the lack of findings of a meniscal lesion with arthroscopy does not necessarily rule out the absence of a lesion.

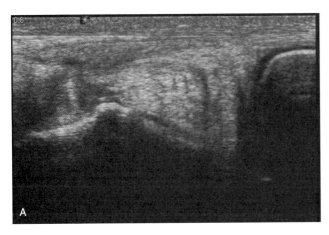

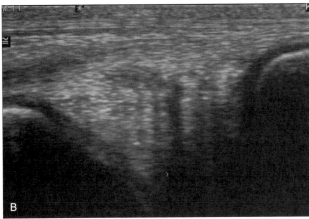

Figure 5.374. Ultrasonographic images of the medial meniscus in both weight-bearing (A) and nonweight-bearing positions (B). Notice how the meniscal tear becomes more apparent in the nonweight-bearing position.

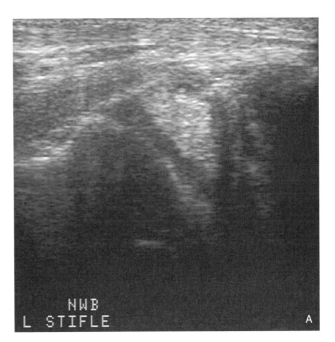

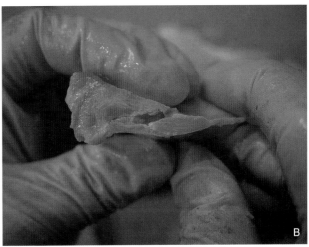

Figure 5.375. Ultrasonographic image (A) of a severe meniscal tear that correlated well with the gross appearance (B). (Courtesy of Dr. Laurie Goodrich.)

Treatment

Treatment usually involves arthroscopic surgery and debridement of the disrupted meniscal fibers that can be seen. In addition, it is common to test the looseness of the meniscus with a probe during surgery. The significance of this finding is unknown, but subjectively seems to be associated in some cases with damage and protrusion of the meniscus identified on ultrasound. In addition, manipulation of the meniscus permits better visualization of the tibia for evidence of secondary damage.

Walmsley developed a grading scale for meniscal injuries: grade I is characterized by axial tearing through the cranial ligament of the medial meniscus and into the meniscus, grade 2 is the same as grade I but with torn tissue and visible extent of the damage, and grade III is a severe tear that extends beneath the femoral condyle.[46]

In an updated review of cases, Walmsley found that of 126 cases of meniscal damage, 111 were medial and 25 lateral. 53% were grade I, 28% grade II and 17% grade III.[44] In that study, 76% had articular cartilage damage and 14% had damage to the cranial cruciate ligament. Of those with medial meniscal tearing, 45% were sound compared to 75% of those with lateral meniscal involvement. Sixty percent of horses with

grade I tearing were sound compared to 65% of those with grade II and 10% of those with grade III. Overall, 51% of the horses were sound with surgery.[44] Because most of the meniscus cannot be visualized arthroscopically, a tear or lesion in the body of the meniscus may be treated by extracapsular injection of stem cells or platelet-rich plasma (PRP) into the lesion(s). If the tear is visible arthroscopically, then various suturing and staple techniques are also available.[26] In general, suturing is preferred over stapling. The efficacies of these latter techniques to treat meniscal lesions are currently unknown.

Prognosis

As noted above, the prognosis for lesions of the medial meniscus is relatively guarded, but for the lateral meniscus can be quite good. In addition, horses with small lesions that can be debrided can do relatively well, although horses with significant tearing carry a poor prognosis. Great efforts are currently being made to provide augmentive therapies, such as stem cells, but at this time are limited in improving prognosis.

SYNOVITIS/CAPSULITIS/OA

Etiology

Horses that undergo chronic repetitive stress to the hindlimbs, such as young Western performance horses, are susceptible to synonovitis in the femorotibial joints, especially the medial compartment. This is similar to racehorses that develop synovitis in their metacarpophalangeal and carpal joints. A primary source of synovitis is usually not apparent in these horses. However, all of the diseases described in this section can lead to synovitis, and in some cases, ultimately, OA.

Clinical Signs and Diagnosis

Horses with synovitis of the femorotibial joints may not be lame, but have mild to moderate effusion in the MFT joint. These horses may show some response to flexion and a gait that can be described as stiff. Some horses can compete well with this finding, but they should be monitored closely. As mentioned previously, all diagnostic techniques can be negative in these cases, including arthroscopic surgery.

Horses with synovitis secondary to other primary lesions within the MFT joint usually have a history of a short response period to intra-articular medication. However, trainers and owners usually note that the horse either never fully regains its level of performance, or constant medication is needed. In these cases, additional diagnostics, including diagnostic arthroscopy, are often required to fully characterize the problem.

Horses with significant OA of the femorotibial joints are usually noticeably lame with loss of muscle mass and swelling of the MFT joint. Concurrent abnormaliltes such as OA, SCL of the medial femoral condyle, and medial meniscal damage are common (Figure 5.376). Although a history of predisposing injury and disease of the stifle are usually noted, some horses may develop this problem insidiously without a notable injury.

Treatment

Horses with synovitis usually respond well to intra-articular medication, topical anti-inflammatories, systemic medication, and extracorporeal shockwave therapy. These medications are described in depth in Chapter 8. Horses typically respond well to rest or a reduction in training, which are often recommended. However, failure to respond to medication or recurrence of lameness are often the key findings that lead to more intensive imaging and possibly diagnostic arthroscopy.

Treatment of OA of the femorotibial joints is the same as for other joints. However, arthrodesis is not an option, and clinicians are often forced to try several different treatment options. Exercise in the form of

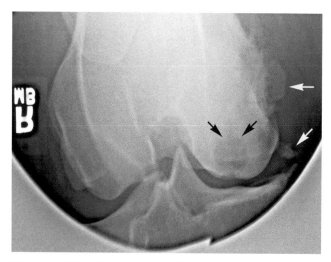

Figure 5.376. Caudal-cranial radiograph of the stifle of a 6-year-old Quarter horse mare with multiple radiographic abnormalities within the MFT joint (arrows). Concurrent medial meniscal injuries should also be suspected in these types of horses. (Courtesy of Dr. Gary Baxter.)

small paddock turn-out appears to help, although owners must ensure that another horse does not induce overstressing of the patient. Arthroscopic surgery can help to reduce the progression of OA by removing debris and fibrillated articular cartilage, but it must be stressed to the owners that this is not a cure and the disease process will most likely progress.

Prognosis

Horses with synovitis are easily managed medically as long as a primary disease process is not present. However, there is concern that chronic, persistent synovitis can lead to secondary damage to the articular cartilage, which may predispose to the onset of OA in the future. The prognosis for OA of the femorotibial joints depends on severity and appears no different than for other joints in the horse. However, severe OA can lead to significant lameness, making it difficult for the horse to stand, and secondary complications such as decubital ulcers.

References

1. Arnold CE, Schaer TP, Baird DL, et al. Conservative management of 17 horses with nonarticular fractures of the tibial tuberosity. Equine Vet J 2003;35:202–206.
2. Baker GJ, Moustafa MA, Boero MJ, et al. Caudal cruciate ligament function and injury in the horse. Vet Rec 1987;121:319–321.
3. Barr ED, Pinchbeck GL, Clegg PD, et al. Accuracy of diagnostic techniques used in investigation of stifle lameness in horses—40 cases. Equine Vet Educ 2006;18:326–331.
4. Blikslager AT, Bristol DG. Avulsion of the origin of the peroneus tertius tendon in a foal. J Am Vet Med Assoc 1994;204:1483–1485.
5. Bukowiecki CF, Sanders-Shamis M, Bramlage LR. Treatment of a ruptured medial collateral ligament of the stifle in a horse. J Am Vet Med Assoc 1988;193:687–690.
6. Cauvin ER, Munroe GA, Boyd JS, et al. Ultrasonographic examination of the femorotibial articulation in horses: imaging of the cranial and caudal aspects. Equine Vet J 1996;28:285–296.

7. Cohen JM, Richardson DW, McKnight AL, et al. Long-term outcome in 44 horses with stifle lameness after arthroscopic exploration and debridement. Vet Surg 2009;38:543–551.

8. Contino EK. The prevalence of radiographic changes in yearling and 2-year-old Quarter horses. Department of Clinical Sciences, Colorado State University, Fort Collins, 2009.

9. Dabareiner RM, Sullins KE. Fracture of the caudal medial femoral condyle in a horse. Equine Vet J 1993;25:75–77.

10. De Busscher V, Verwilghen D, Bolen G, et al. Meniscal damage diagnosed by ultrasonography in horses: A retrospective study of 74 femorotibial joint ultrasonographic examinations (2000-2005). J Equine Vet Sci 2006;26:453–461.

11. Edwards RB 3rd, Nixon AJ. Avulsion of the cranial cruciate ligament insertion in a horse. Equine Vet J 1996;28:334–336.

12. Hance SR, Bramlage LR, Schneider RK, et al. Retrospective study of 38 cases of femur fractures in horses less than one year of age. Equine Vet J 1992;24:357–363.

13. Hance SR, Schneider RK, Embertson RM, et al. Lesions of the caudal aspect of the femoral condyles in foals: 20 cases (1980–1990). J Am Vet Med Assoc 1993;202:637–646.

14. Hoegaerts M, Nicaise M, Van Bree H, et al. Cross-sectional anatomy and comparative ultrasonography of the equine medial femorotibial joint and its related structures. Equine Vet J 2005;37:520–529.

15. Holcombe SJ, Bertone AL. Avulsion fracture of the origin of the extensor digitorum longus muscle in a foal. J Am Vet Med Assoc 1994;204:1652–1654.

16. Howard RD, McIlwraith CW, Trotter GW. Arthroscopic surgery for subchondral cystic lesions of the medial femoral condyle in horses: 41 cases (1988–1991). J Am Vet Med Assoc 1995;206:842–850.

17. Jackson WA, Stick JA, Arnoczky SP, et al. The effect of compacted cancellous bone grafting on the healing of subchondral bone defects of the medial femoral condyle in horses. Vet Surg 2000;29:8–16.

18. Jacquet S, Audigie F, Denoix JM. Ultrasonographic diagnosis of subchondral bone cysts in the medial femoral condyle in horses. Tutorial article. Equine Vet Educ 2007;19:47–50.

19. Kold SE, Hickman J, Melsen F. An experimental study of the healing process of equine chondral and osteochondral defects. Equine Vet J 1986;18:18–24.

20. Lewis RD. A retrospective study of diagnostic and surgical arthroscopy of the equine femorotibial joint. Proceedings Am Assoc Equine Pract 1987;23.

21. McIlwraith CW. Subchondral bone cysts in the horse: aetiology, diagnosis and treatment options. Equine Veterinary Education 1998;10:313–317.

22. McIlwraith CW, Nixon AJ, Wright IM, et al. Diagnostic and surgical arthroscopy of the femoropatellar and femorotibial joints. Diagnostic and Surgical Arthroscopy in the Horse, 3rd ed. Mosby Elsevier, Edinburgh, 2005;197–268.

23. Moustafa MA, Boero MJ, Baker GJ. Arthroscopic examination of the femorotibial joints of horses. Vet Surg 1987;16:352–357.

24. Mueller PO, Allen D, Watson E, et al. Arthroscopic removal of a fragment from an intercondylar eminence fracture of the tibia in a two-year-old horse. J Am Vet Med Assoc 1994;204:1793–1795.

25. Nixon AJ. Anterior cruciate ligament—diagnostic techniques decision making repair. Equine Stifle Specialty Arthroscopy Course 2008.

26. Nixon AJ. Meniscal tears: Suture reconstruction rehabilitation outcomes. Equine Stifle Specialty Arthroscopy Course 2008.

27. Nixon AJ. PCL—definition and treatments. Equine Stifle Specialty Arthroscopy Course 2008.

28. Peroni JF, Stick JA. Evaluation of a cranial arthroscopic approach to the stifle joint for the treatment of femorotibial joint disease in horses: 23 cases (1998–1999). J Am Vet Med Assoc 2002;220:1046–1052.

29. Prades M, Grant BD, Turner TA, et al. Injuries to the cranial cruciate ligament and associated structures: summary of clinical, radiographic, arthroscopic and pathological findings from 10 horses. Equine Vet J 1989;21:354–357.

30. Ray CS, Baxter GM, McIlwraith CW. Development of subchondral cystic lesions after articular cartilage and subchondral bone damage in young horses. Equine Vet J 1996;28:225–232.

31. Rich FR, Glisson RR. *In vitro* mechanical properties and failure mode of the equine (pony) cranial cruciate ligament. Vet Surg 1994;23:257–265.

32. Rose PL, Graham JP, Moore I, et al. Imaging diagnosis—caudal cruciate ligament avulsion in a horse. Vet Radiol Ultrasound 2001;42:414–416.

33. Sandler EA, Bramlage LR, Embertson RM, et al. Correlation of lesion size with racing performance in Thoroughbreds after arthroscopic surgical treatment of subchondral cystic lesions of the medial femoral condyle: 15 cases (1989–2000). Proceedings Am Assoc Equine Pract 2002;48:255–256.

34. Schneider RK, Jenson P, Moore RM. Evaluation of cartilage lesions on the medial femoral condyle as a cause of lameness in horses: 11 cases (1988–1994). J Am Vet Med Assoc 1997;210:1649–1652.

35. Scott GS, Crawford WH, Colahan PT. Arthroscopic findings in horses with subtle radiographic evidence of osteochondral lesions of the medial femoral condyle: 15 cases (1995–2002). J Am Vet Med Assoc 2004;224:1821–1826.

36. Smith MA, Walmsley JP, Phillips TJ, et al. Effect of age at presentation on outcome following arthroscopic debridement of subchondral cystic lesions of the medial femoral condyle: 85 horses (1993–2003). Equine Vet J 2005;37:175–180.

37. Stick JA, Borg LA, Nickels FA, et al. Arthroscopic removal of an osteochondral fragment from the caudal pouch of the lateral femorotibial joint in a colt. J Am Vet Med Assoc 1992;200:1695–1697.

38. Textor JA, Nixon AJ, Lumsden J, et al. Subchondral cystic lesions of the proximal extremity of the tibia in horses: 12 cases (1983–2000). J Am Vet Med Assoc 2001;218:408–413.

39. Verschooten F, De Moor A. Subchondral cystic and related lesions affecting the equine pedal bone and stifle. Equine Vet J 1982;14:47–54.

40. von Rechenberg B, Guenther H, McIlwraith CW, et al. Fibrous tissue of subchondral cystic lesions in horses produce local mediators and neutral metalloproteinases and cause bone resorption *in vitro*. Vet Surg 2000;29:420–429.

41. Wallis TW, Goodrich LR, McIlwraith CW, et al. Arthroscopic injection of corticosteroids into the fibrous tissue of subchondral cystic lesions of the medial femoral condyle in horses: a retrospective study of 52 cases (2001–2006). Equine Vet J 2008;40:461–467.

42. Walmsley JP. Diagnosis and treatment of ligamentous and meniscal injuries in the equine stifle. Vet Clin North Am Equine Pract 2005;21:651–672.

43. Walmsley JP. Fracture of the intercondylar eminence of the tibia treated by arthroscopic internal fixation. Equine Vet J 1997;29:148–150.

44. Walmsley JP. Meniscal tears—approaches, debridement, rehabilitation outcomes. Equine Stifle Specialty Arthroscopy Course 2008.

45. Walmsley JP, Nixon AJ. Meniscal tears—diagnostic techniques and critical analysis of imaging techniques. Equine Stifle Specialty Arthroscopy Course 2008.

46. Walmsley JR, Phillips TJ, Townsend HG. Meniscal tears in horses: an evaluation of clinical signs and arthroscopic treatment of 80 cases. Equine Vet J 2003;35:402–406.

THE FEMUR AND COXOFEMORAL JOINT

Kenneth E. Sullins (Femur) and Gary M. Baxter
(Coxofemoral Joint)

THE FEMUR

Conditions of the femoral region that contribute to lameness are uncommon and can vary greatly in severity. For example, femoral fractures usually cause significant swelling in the region and severe nonweight-bearing lameness. In contrast, horses with fibrotic myopathy may not be lame but have a gait alteration due to fibrosis of the muscle. Careful palpation and physical examination of the femoral region is often very important in making a diagnosis because imaging of the femoral region can be difficult, especially in adult horses.

DIAPHYSEAL AND METAPHYSEAL FEMORAL FRACTURES

Fractures of the femur are relatively common in horses.[1,3,5,6,9,13] In young animals, fractures often involve the proximal or distal growth plate, and diaphyseal fractures are usually oblique and spiralling.[8] Adults often sustain irreparable comminuted fractures of the femoral shaft. Intra-articular fractures involving the stifle and coxofemoral joints are described in those respective sections.

Etiology

Foals frequently sustain femoral fractures during initial handling or during halter breaking. Occasionally a mare will step on a foal, or the foal may become trapped under a fence. In a study of 38 horses under 1 year of age, causes included a fall or severe adduction, external trauma, or being caught in a fence.[9] The author has diagnosed femoral condylar avulsion fractures in horses that had been cast with a sideline for castration without sedation.

Clinical Signs

The obvious sign is non-weight-bearing lameness. When viewed from the side, the affected limb may appear slightly shortened with the hock held higher than the opposite hindlimb; a dimpling of the musculature overlying the fracture may be observed. Obvious swelling may be present, especially in horses with diaphyseal fractures (Figure 5.377).

Diagnosis

Excessive movement of the distal limb is usually present on palpation. Moderate to severe swelling may be associated with the fracture site and crepitation may be apparent; a stethoscope may be helpful for detecting crepitation, although sounds may be muffled due to the massive musculature and swelling (e.g., hematoma) or

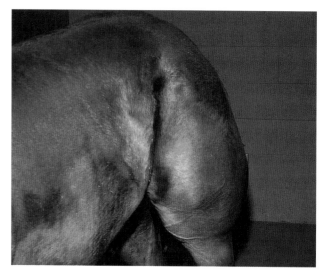

Figure 5.377. Cranial view of a yearling with severe swelling of the femoral and stifle region associated with a diaphyseal femoral fracture. The limb is also externally rotated.

just minimal with severe comminution. Because of overriding, the patella may feel loose and may be manipulated easily in a horizontal direction. Uncommonly, clinically significant or fatal hemorrhage results, and suspected vascular compromise should be investigated.[9,18]

Young horses that sustain proximal growth plate fractures (slipped capital epiphyses) can be difficult to diagnose, and they must be differentiated from coxofemoral luxations. Femoral neck fractures in older horses or ponies are similar. If the fracture overrides proximally, the hock on the affected limb is higher than the hock on the normal limb. These foals may bear weight, and swelling may not be readily apparent in the acute case. Palpation, and in some cases auscultation over the greater trochanter while the limb is being manipulated, may be helpful. If the horse is large enough, a rectal exam may reveal subtle crepitation when the limb is manipulated. Additionally, swelling may be palpated on the medial aspect of the thigh, particularly if the fracture is several days old. Fractures of the distal growth plate are usually more evident because of displacement, instability, or swelling in the stifle region (Figure 5.378).

Although physical exam findings may suffice to diagnose a femoral fracture, radiographs are important to make a definitive diagnosis and demonstrate the exact location and configuration of the fracture. Particularly in adults, a recumbent position facilitates quality radiographs of the proximal two-thirds of the femur. The most useful radiograph of the proximal two-thirds of

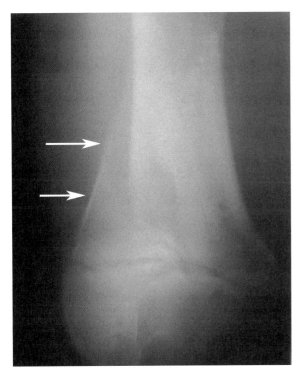

Figure 5.378. Lateral radiograph of a weanling with a type II distal femoral fracture (arrows) that was successfully treated with confinement.

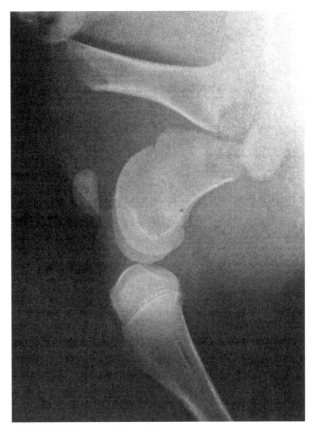

Figure 5.379. Lateromedial view of a closed oblique midshaft fracture of the femur. (Courtesy of Dr. Ted Stashak.)

the femur is taken medial to lateral with the horse in dorsal recumbency but tipped onto the injured limb. Adequate penetration is difficult for the cranial to caudal projection but the image may still be useful. A standing view of the proximal femur/coxofemoral region may suffice.[12] Digital radiography has significantly facilitated acquisition of quality images of this region, and standing oblique projections of the femoral shaft may demonstrate a lesion almost as well as in an anesthetized horse. The suspected gravity of the injury and the anticipated ability for the horse to recover from general anesthesia without further injury must be considered.

Ultrasound may demonstrate cortical disruption when radiographs are not possible or advisable.[7,17] Scintigraphy, particularly for less severe or more chronic injuries, also may localize femoral lesions not amenable to radiographic imaging.[19]

In a series of 38 foals with femoral fractures, 26 had fractures of the femoral diaphysis (Figure 5.379), and 18 involved two-thirds of the length of the diaphysis.[9] Twelve foals had distal physeal fractures with the most common configuration being Salter-Harris type II (Figure 5.378). A separate series of 25 foals sustained fractures of the capital femoral physis, neck, or greater trochanter (Figure 5.380).[10]

Treatment

Treatment of femoral shaft fractures depends on the age of the animal and the type and location of the fracture. Generally, euthanasia is indicated for adults that

have sustained femoral shaft fractures unless exceptional circumstances exist.

Diaphyseal fractures have been treated with stall rest in foals weighing up to approximately 200 kg;[13] however, misalignment and fracture disease are risks in young horses (Figure 5.381). Compression plating is the treatment of choice for foals that have sustained diaphyseal fractures when athletic soundness is desired. Fourteen of 15 foals in which diaphyseal fractures were plated were repaired using 2 plates, 1 lateral and 1 cranial.[9] However, single-plate application has been used occasionally.[1,9] A very stable repair can result when the fracture is midshaft and transverse.[22] More distal fractures can be repaired using angled blade plates or dynamic condylar screw plates.[2,9] The plates are not removed when there are no complications. Fractures without caudal cortical buttress remaining are at risk of an unstable repair and should be given a poor prognosis.[9]

Intramedullary pinning using the stacked pin technique or a single half-inch pin has been used successfully in young foals with femoral diaphyseal fractures.[20] However, problems with pin migration should be expected. One report in experimental fractures in donkeys (65 to 140 kg) reported some success.[21] However, the work was performed in adult donkeys. Creating controlled, relatively atraumatic fractures in what is really adult bone does not simulate clinical fractures in foals.

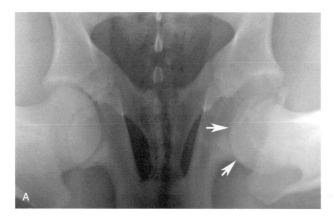

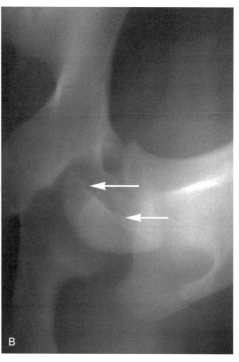

Figure 5.380. Recumbent radiographs of the pelvis of 2 different foals with capital physeal fractures (arrows) of the left proximal femur.

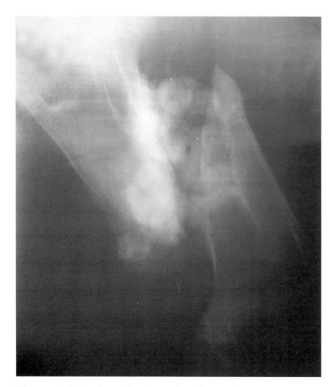

Figure 5.381. Lateral radiograph of the yearling in Figure 5.377, revealing a chronic diaphyseal fracture with a nonunion. Notice the proximal displacement and overriding of the fracture fragments that often occur without internal fixation.

Interlocking nails (ILN) have been investigated for repair of diaphyseal femoral fractures.[14,16] Three successfully managed transverse midshaft femoral fractures in neonates have been reported using the ILN alone, along with 4 of 6 successfully managed with an ILN-dynamic compression plate combination.[23] Double plate fixation has been reported to provide greater stiffness compared to ILN alone.[16]

Proximal growth plate fractures (slipped capital physeal fractures) are covered in the section on the coxofemoral joint. Most distal physeal fractures are Salter-Harris type II fractures. Minimally displaced distal physeal fractures may heal quite well with conservative therapy (Figure 5.378).[8] Unstable distal physeal fractures have little space for an adequate number of screws to be placed distal to the fracture and many are not treated.[9] Options for stabilizing distal physeal fractures include an angled blade plate,[9] condylar buttress plate,[15] a cobra-head and dynamic compression plate,[11] and cross-pins or Rush pins (Figure 5.382). Successful repair of a Salter-Harris type II fracture in a yearling Pony of America was reported using a condylar buttress plate.[15] A displaced Salter-Harris type IV fracture in a yearling was successfully treated using a lag-screw repair countersunk into the articular surface.[4]

Prognosis

The prognosis for fracture of the femur depends on the age of the horse, the location and type of fracture, and its intended use. Generally, femoral fractures in horses older than yearlings carry a very poor prognosis for a successful outcome. A much better prognosis can be expected in young animals with nondisplaced fractures or oblique midshaft fractures that are stabilized

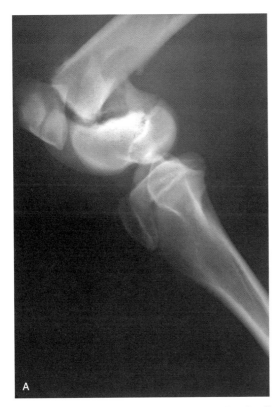 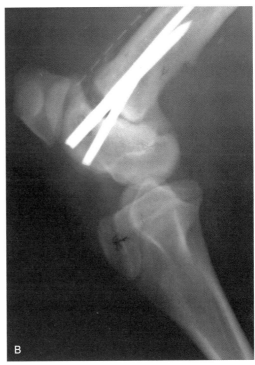

Figure 5.382. A. A Salter-Harris type II fracture involving the distal femur. B. The fracture was stabilized with Steinmann pins placed in cruciate fashion. The fracture healed successfully, and the pins were removed 3 months after surgery. (Courtesy of Dr. Ted Stashak.)

by internal fixation.[9] Nine of the 17 surgically repaired diaphyseal fractures healed.[1,9] Six of those were considered to have no sign of previous fracture.[9] The mean age for successfully treated foals was 2 months vs. 4 months for unsuccessfully treated foals.[9] Aside from size of the foals being an influence, development of a postoperative seroma was negatively associated with success.[9] Three of 4 foals with oblique mid-shaft femoral fractures treated by stall rest alone became sound for breeding, but fracture disease associated with prolonged nonweight-bearing presented problems during the healing period.[13]

In one report, only 1 of the 2 surgically repaired distal physeal fractures healed.[9] A minimally-displaced Salter-Harris type IV fracture treated conservatively in a yearling healed to racing status.[9] Aside from size of the foals being an influence, development of a postoperative seroma was negatively associated with success.[9]

References

1. Boulton CH, Dallman MJ. Equine femoral fracture repair: A case report. J Equine Vet Sci 1983;3:60–64.
2. Byron CR, Stick JA, Brown JA, et al. Use of a condylar screw plate for repair of a Salter-Harris type-III fracture of the femur in a 2-year-old horse. J Am Vet Med Assoc 2002;221:1292–1295.
3. Clayton-Jones DC. The repair of equine fractures. Vet Rec 1975;97:193.
4. DeBowes RM, Grant BD, Modranisky PD. Lag screw stabilization of Salter type IV femoral fracture in a young horse. J Am Vet Med Assoc 1983;182:1123–1125.
5. Denny HR. The surgical treatment of equine fractures. Vet Rec 1978;102:273–277.
6. Fessler JF, Amstutz HE. Fracture repair. In Textbook of Large Animal Surgery. Oehme FW, Prier JE, eds. Williams and Wilkins Co., Baltimore, 1974.
7. Geburek F, Rötting AK, Stadler PM. Comparison of the diagnostic value of ultrasonography and standing radiography for pelvic-femoral disorders in horses. Vet Surg 2009;38:310–317.
8. Hance SR, Bramlage LR. Fractures of the femur and patella. In Equine Fracture Repair. Nixon AJ, ed. WB Saunders Company, Philadelphia, 1996;284–293.
9. Hance SR, Bramlage LR, Schneider RK, et al. Retrospective study of 38 cases of femur fractures in horses less than one year of age. Equine Vet J 1992;24:357–363.
10. Hunt DA, Snyder JR, Morgan JP, et al. Femoral capital physeal fractures in 25 foals. Vet Surg 1990;19:41–49.
11. Kirker-Head CA, Fackelman GE. Use of the cobra head bone plate for distal long bone fractures in large animals. A report of four cases. Vet Surg 1989;18:227–234.
12. May SA, Patterson LJ, Peacock PJ, et al. Radiographic technique for the pelvis in the standing horse. Equine Vet J 1991;23:312–314.
13. McCann ME, Hunt RJ. Conservative management of femoral diaphyseal fractures in four foals. Cornell Vet 1993;83:125–132.
14. McClure SR, Watkins JP, Ashman RB. In vivo evaluation of intramedullary interlocking nail fixation of transverse femoral osteotomies in foals. Vet Surg 1998;27:29–36.
15. Orsini JA, Buonanno AM, Richardson DW, et al. Condylar buttress plate fixation of femoral fracture in a colt. J Am Vet Med Assoc 1990;197:1184–1186.
16. Radcliffe RM, Lopez MJ, Turner TA, et al. An in vitro biomechanical comparison of interlocking nail constructs and double plating for fixation of diaphyseal femur fractures in immature horses. Vet Surg 2001;30:179–190.
17. Reef VB. Equine Diagnostic Ultrasound. WB Saunders Co., Philadelphia, 1998.
18. Rose PL, Watkins JP, Auer JA. Femoral fracture repair complicated by vascular injury in a foal. J Am Vet Med Assoc 1984;185:795–797.
19. Steckel RR. The role of scintigraphy in the lameness evaluation. Vet Clin NA Eq Pract 1991;7:207–239.

20. Stick JA, Derksen FJ. Intramedullary pinning of a fractured femur in a foal. J Am Vet Med Assoc 1980;176:627–629.
21. Taneja AK, Singh J, Behl SM, et al. Repair techniques for femoral fractures in horses. Equine Pract 1986;8:35–40.
22. Turner AS, Milne DW, Hohn RB, et al. Surgical repair of fractured capital femoral epiphysis in three foals. J Am Vet Med Assoc 1979;175:1198–1202.
23. Watkins JP. Intramedullary interlocking nail fixation in equine fracture management. European Society of Veterinary Orthopaedics and Traumatology 2004;12:195–196.

FIBROTIC AND OSSIFYING MYOPATHY

Fibrotic and ossifying myopathy is a fibrosis with or without ossification of the muscle tissue in the crus that often results in adhesions between the semitendinosus, semimembranosus, gracilis, or biceps femoris muscles (Figure 5.383).[1] It is significant because the fibrosis and adhesions limit the action of the semitendinosus muscle, causing an abnormal gait characterized by a slapping down of the foot at the end of the cranial phase of the stride (Figure 5.384). If the semitendinosus is more affected, the slap is cranial to caudal. If the gracilis is more affected, the slap is from lateral to medial. The character of the gait of a semitendinosus-affected horse has been described in detail.[3] The affected hindlimb approaches the ground more vertically than normal and strikes it toe-first, making more of a slap than the normal heel-toe manner of landing. Some have reported a semi-flexed stance at rest with the toe touching the ground.[3,4] Rarely, the condition occurs in the forelimb.[1] The largest case series reported in the United States related a predisposition for occurrence in Quarter horse mares.[5]

A congenital form of fibrotic myopathy-type syndrome has been reported.[2] Foals are born with an altered gait characteristic of fibrotic myopathy in the hindlimb. On palpation, a tightening of the semitendinosus muscle was appreciated but no firm thickening of the muscle typical of fibrotic myopathy was palpated. Because no fibrous thickening of the muscle is present, congenital restrictive myopathy may be a more appropriate description of this entity.

Etiology

The cause of the fibrosis is always trauma, which takes several forms. Involved muscles may be injured during sliding stops in rodeo work, or from slipping and catching the hindlimb on the underside of a horse trailer, resisting a sideline, catching a foot in a halter, receiving intramuscular injections, or being kicked.[2] The lesions are usually unilateral, but a case of bilateral fibrotic myopathy resulting from a trailer accident was reported.[2] The author has diagnosed fibrotic myopathy in horses with histories of having been cast for castration without sedation. In some cases the exact cause of the injury is not known; cumulative injury must be considered in cases such as Western performance horses or those that involve any other repetitive situation. When the injury heals, the lack of muscle compliance and adhesions between the involved muscles contribute to the gait abnormality. Ossification is believed to be a more severe progression from the fibrosis.

The etiology of the congenital form is unknown, although parturient muscle trauma has been described to cause rupture of the gastrocnemius muscle.[6] It is conceivable that similar trauma could also affect the semitendinosus under different stresses at birth or shortly after.

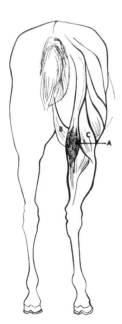

Figure 5.383. Drawing depicting the muscles in the fibrotic area in the gaskin of a horse affected with fibrotic myopathy. A. Semitendinosus. B. Semimembranosus. C. Biceps femoris.

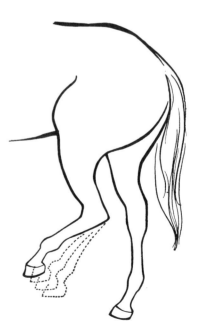

Figure 5.384. Characteristic action of the hindlimb of a horse affected with fibrotic myopathy. The limb jerks backward and downward (dotted outline of the affected foot) during the last 3 to 5 inches of the stride, resulting in slapping of the foot on the ground. If the gracilis muscle is affected, the swing of the hindlimb is lateral to medial instead.

Three cases of fibrotic myopathy accompanied by neurogenic atrophy of the affected muscles have been reported.[8] All 3 underwent necropsy, where peripheral nerve and muscle degeneration were discovered. One horse had a fracture of the greater trochanter and accompanying sciatic nerve impingement. No gross lesions were found in the other 2 horses.

Clinical Signs

The signs are due to lack compliance of the affected muscle(s) and adhesions between the semitendinosus muscle and the semimembranosus muscle medially, and between the semitendinosus and the biceps femoris muscle laterally (Figure 5.385). These adhesions partially inhibit the normal action of the muscles. See the DVD for examples of the gait abnormality. In the cranial phase of the stride, the foot of the affected hindlimb is suddenly pulled caudally 3 to 5 inches just before contacting the ground (Figure 5.384). The cranial phase of the stride is shortened, so consequently the caudal phase is lengthened. Usually the lameness is most noticeable when the horse walks. This abnormal gait, which is easily identified, may result from either fibrotic or ossifying myopathy. An area of firmness can often be palpated over the affected muscles on the caudal

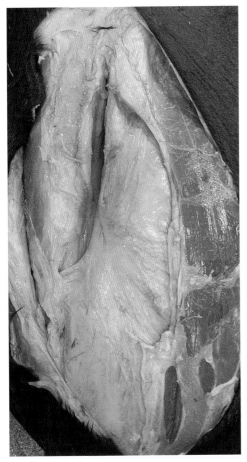

Figure 5.385. Cadaver dissection of the gaskin of a horse with fibrotic myopathy. The central pale mass is the fibrotic semitendinosus muscle.

surface of the affected limb at the level of the stifle joint and immediately above it (Figures 5.383 and 5.385). Occasionally, the lesion is deep and difficult to palpate or it may be in the medial gaskin affecting the gracilis muscle. If the gracilis is affected, the slap motion of the foot is in a more lateral to medial direction.

Diagnosis

The diagnosis is based upon the altered gait and palpation of a hardened area on the caudal or caudo-medial surface of the limb proximal to the level of the stifle joint. In making the diagnosis, stringhalt should also be considered. In stringhalt, the limb is pulled sharply toward the abdomen during the cranial phase of the stride, while in fibrotic myopathy the foot is pulled toward the ground in a caudal direction just before the foot contacts the ground. In fibrotic myopathy the limb is limited in the cranial phase of the stride by adhesions and by lack of elasticity in the affected area of the muscle belly, causing the limb to be pulled caudally before the full length of stride is reached.

Treatment

Three approaches for surgical correction of fibrotic myopathy have been described; each must be adjusted if more than the semitendinosus muscle is involved. Adams originally described complete removal of the affected fibrotic/calcified muscle tissue.[1] In a retrospective study of 18 horses undergoing this procedure, all of 11 horses available for follow-up had mild to complete persistence of the gait deficit.[7] Anecdotally, quadriceps rupture has been observed following resection of an extensive calcified mass. The failures were most likely due to recurrence of fibrosis in the defects created, but it is possible that there was more extensive involvement in some cases.

Bramlage described a semitendinosus tenotomy at the level of its insertion on the proximal medial tibia caudal to the saphenous vein.[2] The procedure is much less invasive and is expected to be effective if the problem is unaffected by other muscles. To perform the semitendinosus tenotomy,[2] the horse is positioned in lateral recumbency with the affected limb down. The tibial insertion of the semitendinosus tendon is palpated caudomedial to the proximal end of the tibia. An 8-cm incision is created over the tendon to expose it. The tendon is then isolated with a hemostat and transected. Hand-walking is started when the skin has healed, and normal exercise is allowed after 6 weeks.

Three of 4 (1 mature and 2 congenital) horses recovered completely; the fourth (a congenital) case underwent more distal transection of the calcaneal insertion of the semitendinosus tendon 2 months later, which provided sufficient improvement for race training. Of 2 additional cases in mature horses, 1 experienced complete recovery and 1 improved slowly but incompletely.[4] The author's experience with the tenotomy has been positive. Any incisional complications are unlikely to affect the outcome.

Magee and Vatistas reported a series of 39 horses that underwent a standing focal semitendinosus myotomy.[5] Average wound healing time was 4.7 weeks

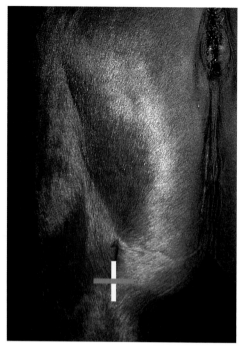

Figure 5.386. Caudal thigh region where the myotomy procedure is performed to correct fibrotic myopathy. The skin incision is made vertically (white line) and the fibrotic muscle is transected with a bistoury horizontally (red line).

overall. 83% of horses were able to perform at their pre-injury level. Nineteen were considered normal and 10 had some persistent restrictive gait. The incision is made directly over the affected semitendinosus muscle, which is transected using a blunt bistoury. The incisions are left open, partially closed, or completely closed, depending upon the surgeon's preference (Figure 5.386). No cases of involvement of muscles other than the semitendinosus were reported.

Prognosis

With partial myectomy, some relief is evident in all cases. After healing, some cases develop characteristic, but less pronounced, signs, although limb function is nearly normal and signs are not noticeable except in the walk. Occasionally, 3 to 7 days are needed for the maximum benefits of surgical correction to become evident. With the standing myotomy technique, 83% of horses were able to perform at their pre-injury level, although the restrictive gait pattern did not resolve in all horses.[5] The prognosis for successful surgery in horses affected by neurogenic atrophy of the muscles is poor. If the muscle mass appears abnormal, nerve conduction studies or electromyography are advisable.

References

1. Adams OR. Fibrotic myopathy in the hindlegs of horses. J Am Vet Med Assoc 1961;139:1089.
2. Bramlage LR, Reed SM, Embertson RM. Semitendinosus tenotomy for treatment of fibrotic myopathy in the horse. J Am Vet Med Assoc 1985;186:565–567.
3. Clayton HM. Cinematographic analysis of the gait of lame horses V: Fibrotic myopathy. Equine Veterinary Science 1988; 8:297–301.
4. Gomez-Villamandos R, Santisteban J, Ruiz I, et al. Tenotomy of the tibial insertion of the semitendinosus muscle of two horses with fibrotic myopathy. Vet Rec 1995;136:67–68.
5. Magee AA, Vatistas N. Standing semitendinosus myotomy for the treatment of fibrotic myopathy in 39 horses (1989–1997). Proc Am Assoc Equine Pract 1998;44:263–264.
6. Sprinkle FP, Swerczek TW, Crowe MW. Gastrocnemius muscle rupture and hemorrhage in foals. Equine Pract 1985;7:10–11, 14–15, 17.
7. Turner AS, Trotter GW. Fibrotic myopathy in the horse. J Am Vet Med Assoc 1984;184:335–338.
8. Valentine BA, Rousselle SD, Sams AE, et al. Denervation atrophy in three horses with fibrotic myopathy. J Am Vet Med Assoc 1994;205:332–336.

FEMORAL NERVE PARALYSIS (CRURAL PARALYSIS)

Paralysis of the femoral nerve affects the quadriceps femoris group of muscles. This muscle group is comprised of the rectus femoris muscle, vastus lateralis muscle, vastus medialis muscle, and vastus intermedius muscle. This large muscular mass covers the front and sides of the femur and inserts onto the patella to extend and fix the stifle.

Etiology

Femoral nerve paralysis may arise from trauma or unknown causes, and may be associated with rhabdomyolysis. Injury to the nerve may occur from overstretching the limb during exertion, kicking, slipping, or while the horse is tied in a recumbent position. It has also been reported as a complication of general anesthesia.[1]

Hemorrhagic neuritis has been described in 1 horse that was euthanatized due to femoral paralysis.[1] Unaffected horses had no such lesion at necropsy. The affected horse also had lesions of rhabdomyolysis, and the urinary system was affected by myoglobinuria. Postmortem studies with cadavers revealed that the femoral nerves were placed in tension by extending the hindlimbs behind the horse, whereas lifting the horse by the hindlimbs did not place tension on the femoral nerves.[1] The potential roles or interaction of femoral paralysis and rhabdomyolysis warrant further investigation.

Clinical Signs and Diagnosis

The horse assumes a crouched position with the fetlocks flexed and the toes on the ground and is unable to bear full weight on the affected limb. There is difficulty advancing the limb, but the affected horse can do so because the hock can be sufficiently flexed to pull the limb forward. After the condition has been present for some time, atrophy of the quadriceps muscles occurs, causing them to lose their normal softness and become more like tendinous structures. If rhabdomyolysis is present, the horse is more painful and less willing to attempt to stand.

The signs listed above are characteristic and are used for diagnosis. The condition should be differentiated from lateral (true) luxation of the patella, rupture of the quadriceps femoris muscles, avulsion of the tibial crest, and distal luxation of the patella. Any of these conditions could cause a similar syndrome; however, all are rare. Lateral luxation of the patella can be diagnosed by palpation of the displaced patella; rupture of the quadriceps femoris muscle also can be palpated. A radiographic examination can determine avulsion of the tibial crest where the patellar ligaments insert. Electromyography of the quadriceps femoris muscles 5 days after the first signs of femoral nerve paralysis provide a definitive diagnosis.

Treatment

No treatment is known. If the condition is due to injury of the femoral nerve, the animal should be stalled until improvement occurs. If rhabdomyolysis is present, intensive care and support is indicated, and repeated attempts to use the muscles should be discouraged.

Prognosis

The prognosis is guarded to unfavorable. In a report of 2 cases of post-anesthetic femoral paralysis, 1 had concurrent rhabdomyolysis and was euthanatized. The other responded to supportive therapy and was standing well 7 days after the onset.[1,2] The prognosis should be withheld until sufficient time has elapsed to determine whether any function will return.

References

1. Dyson S, Taylor P, Whitwell K. Femoral nerve paralysis after general anaesthesia. Equine Vet J 1988;20:376–380.
2. Mackay RCJ. Peripheral nerve injury. In Equine surgery, 3rd ed. Auer J, Stick J, eds. Elsevier, St. Louis, 2006;684–691.

CALCINOSIS CIRCUMSCRIPTA

Calcinosis circumscripta in the horse is a calcified mass commonly located on the lateral aspect of the gaskin adjacent to the stifle. The condition also has been observed over the carpus,[5] tarsus,[3] shoulder, and pectoral region.[7] A review of 18 reported cases of calcinosis circumscripta revealed that 16 were adjacent to the stifle and all were in young male horses.[4] In another report, the age at presentation ranged from 1 to 13 years.[7] The condition has not been reported in foals younger than 6 months of age.

Etiology

The etiology is unknown. The description of the lesion best fits that of dystrophic calcinosis characterized by calcinosis circumscripta. Tumor calcinosis implies a metabolic derangement in calcium/phosphorous metabolism leading to hyperphosphatemia and resulting accumulation of deposits of calcium phosphate.[9] Although few have investigated the serum chemistries of affected horses, hyperphosphatemia has not been a reported feature of the condition in horses.

Clinical Signs and Diagnosis

Because clinical signs of lameness seldom occur, horses may carry the lesion for years before presentation to a hospital. The masses are generally 3 to 12 cm in diameter. The skin is freely moveable over the density because it lies beneath the superficial and deep fascia. They are often attached to the joint capsule of the lateral femorotibial joint.

Once dissected free, the lesions are encapsulated in a tough, white, fibrous capsule.[4] The interior is comprised of loculations of finely granular, gritty, white, paste-like material.[3] Histologically, the granules are surrounded by a granulomatous inflammatory reaction.[3] Although it is difficult to make a broad comparison, the lesion in humans is believed to be secondary to collagen necrosis.[10]

Treatment

The only treatment is surgical excision. However, the lesions seldom cause a clinical problem. The location is one that tends to dehisce following surgery and must be taken seriously in that respect. One report in horses describes 3 of 4 cases that dehisced postoperatively and 1 horse was lost to septic arthritis.[4] If surgery is performed, a tension-relieving closure using mattress sutures and a sutured stent bandage is advised. A circumferential adherent surgical drape is helpful in preventing swelling.

Prognosis

The prognosis is good for soundness and future use. Clinical problems or lameness are uncommon. The prognosis after surgery is guarded, depending upon the size of the lesion due to potential for incisional complications.[1]

References

1. Bertoni G, Gnudi G, Pezzoli G. Two cases of calcinosis circumscripta in the horse. Annali della Facolta di Medicina Veterinaria, Universita di Parma 1993;13:201–210.
2. Dodd DC, Raker CW. Tumoral calcinosis (calcinosis circumscripta) in the horse. J Am Vet Med Assoc 1970;157:968–972.
3. Goulden BE. Tumoral calcinosis in the horse. NZ VetJ 1980;28:217–219.
4. Grant BD, Wagner PC. Unusual causes of carpitis. Mod Vet Pract 1980;61:131–134.
5. Hutchins DR. Tumoral calcinosis in the horse. Aust Vet J 1972;48:200–202.
6. Stone WC, Wilson DA, Dubielzig RR, et al. The pathologic mineralization of soft tissue: Calcinosis circumscripta in horses. Compend Contin Educ Pract Vet 1990;12:1643–1649.
7. Thomson SW, Sullivan DJ. Calcifying collagenolysis (tumoral calcinosis). Br J Radiol 1966;39:526–532.

TROCHANTERIC BURSITIS (TROCHANTERIC LAMENESS, WHIRLBONE LAMENESS)[8]

Trochanteric bursitis is an inflammation of the bursa beneath the tendon of the middle gluteus muscle as it passes over the greater trochanter of the femur. The tendon of the middle gluteus muscle also may be involved, as well as the cartilage over the trochanter. The deep portion of the gluteus medius muscle has a strong, flat tendon that passes over the convexity of the trochanter before it inserts into the crest (Figure 5.387). The trochanter is covered with cartilage and the trochanteric bursa is interposed between it and the tendon.

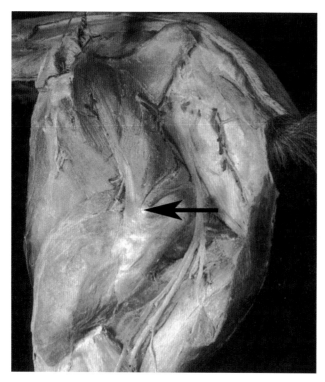

Figure 5.387. Cadaver specimen illustrating the location of the trochanteric bursa under the tendon of the middle gluteal muscle (arrow) at the cranial aspect of the greater trochanter. (Courtesy of Dr. Frank Nickels.)

Etiology

In many cases, there is a concurrent source of chronic lameness in the same limb, particularly distal tarsitis. Chronic forelimb lameness causes the horse to place more strain on the hindlimbs and may contribute.[2,6] Lameness may also be caused by bruising as a result of the horse falling on the affected side or by strain during racing or training.

Trochanteric bursitis occurs in horses racing on small tracks, where the turns are close together, and in horses working on their hindlimbs that are frequently exercised in soft, deep arenas. Short heels and long toes in the hind feet seem to predispose to this lameness. When the etiology is severe trauma, such as a direct kick, the cartilage or the bone of the trochanter may be fractured, causing persistent lameness. It also has been found following an attack of strangles.

Clinical Signs and Diagnosis

Pain may be evident when pressure is applied over the greater trochanter. Careful interpretation is required, because some horses naturally tend to shy away when pressure is applied over the hip joint. At rest, the limb may remain flexed; as the horse moves, weight may be placed on the inside of the foot so that the inside wall of the foot wears more than the outside wall. This can be best seen when observing the horse from behind—the foot is carried inward and the horse sets the foot down on a line between the forelimbs. The horse tends to travel "dog fashion" since the hindquarters move toward the sound side because the stride of the affected limb is shorter than that of the sound side. After the condition has been present for some time, atrophy of the gluteal muscles occurs.

The foregoing symptoms should be used in diagnosis. The condition is difficult to differentiate from inflammation of the coxofemoral joint. The lameness, which is not common, may be confused with spavin lameness. A lameness of unknown cause is sometimes ascribed to trochanteric bursitis. Injection of a local anesthetic into the bursa is helpful in differentiating the condition from coxofemoral joint osteoarthritis. Nuclear scintigraphy should identify the area as inflamed.

Treatment

It is important to address any associated source of lameness. Rest and anti-inflammatory treatment may be helpful in some cases. Injection of the bursa with corticoids appears to be the most effective method of treatment (Figure 5.387). Other reported treatments consist of injections of Lugol's solution of iodine into or around the bursa as a counterirritant. Hot packs applied to the affected area in the acute stages relieve some pain. Phenylbutazone therapy for 3 to 4 is weeks may be useful. Treatment is difficult when the cartilage or bone has been damaged with fracture or periostitis. Although surgery may be indicated in these cases, no reports could be found regarding the use of surgery.

Prognosis

The prognosis is guarded to unfavorable and may be associated with the prognosis of a second source of lameness. The horse may return to soundness if it responds to therapy within 4 to 6 weeks. However, if the injury is more severe, the lameness may remain indefinitely or may recur when the horse is put back into training.

References

1. Bertoni G, Gnudi G, Pezzoli G. Two cases of calcinosis circumscripta in the horse. Annali della Facolta di Medicina Veterinaria, Universita di Parma 1993;13:201–210.
2. Churchill EA. Lameness associated with the lower back and pelvis. Proc Am Assoc Equine Pract 1982;28:277–280.
3. Dodd DC, Raker CW. Tumoral calcinosis (calcinosis circumscripta) in the horse. J Am Vet Med Assoc 1970;157:968–972.
4. Goulden BE. Tumoral calcinosis in the horse. NZ VetJ 1980;28:217–219.
5. Grant BD, Wagner PC. Unusual causes of carpitis. Mod Vet Pract 1980;61:131–134.
6. Hawkins D. The thigh-trochanteric bursitis. In Diagnosis and Management of Lameness in the Horse. Dyson SJ, Ross MW, eds. WB. Saunders, Philadelphia, 2003;472–473.
7. Hutchins DR. Tumoral calcinosis in the horse. Aust Vet J 1972;48:200–202.
8. Stashak TS. The femur-trochanteric bursitis. In Adams' Lameness in Horses. 4th ed. Lea and Febiger, Baltimore, 1987;747–748.
9. Stone WC, Wilson DA, Dubielzig RR, et al. The pathologic mineralization of soft tissue: Calcinosis circumscripta in horses. Compend contin educ pract vet 1990;12:1643–1649.
10. Thomson SW, Sullivan DJ. Calcifying collagenolysis (tumoral calcinosis). Br J Radiol 1966;39:526–532.

RUPTURED QUADRICEPS MUSCLE

Ruptured quadriceps muscle is a rare condition that causes the horse to present with a dropped stifle.[1] A single case of unknown etiology was observed in a nursing foal. The patella was prominent due to the cranial position of the stifle without the quadriceps attachment.[2] Anecdotally, quadriceps rupture has been observed following extensive resection of a calcified and fibrotic mass causing a fibrotic myopathy.

References

1. Nicoletti JLM, Hussni CA, Thomassian A, et al. Rupture of the quadriceps femoris muscle in a horse. Ars Veterinaria 1989;5:117–119.
2. Stashak TS. Personal communication. 2001.

THE COXOFEMORAL JOINT

The femoral head and the acetabulum form a ball-and-socket type articulation that makes up the coxofemoral joint. The heavy musculature and extensive ligament network surrounding and within the joint make the hip joint inherently stable.[6] The transverse acetabular ligament, ligament of the head of the femur (round), and femoral accessory ligament help to stabilize the coxofemoral joint.[6,15] In addition, the acetabulum is surrounded by a fibrocartilaginous rim that increases the bony margin of the acetabulum.

The accessory ligament is the largest and strongest ligament and is unique to equids.[15] It arises from the fovea capitis of the femoral head, passes through the acetabular notch to the pubic groove, and becomes part of the prepubic tendon. The smaller ligament of the head of the femur (round) arises in the head of the femur adjacent to the accessory ligament and attaches to the pubic groove.[15] This ligament of the head of the femur can be seen and debrided arthroscopically but the accessory ligament is difficult to visualize.[23–25] The transverse ligament courses from the outer fibrocartilaginous rim medially across the acetabular notch.[15] See Chapter 1 for more information on the anatomy of the coxofemoral area.

In general, problems related to the coxofemoral joint appear to occur most commonly in foals, miniature horses, and ponies.[6,9,13,17,25] However, horses of any age may sustain damage to the coxofemoral joint from trauma. Most conditions are either developmental (osteochondrosis, osteochondritis dissecans, hip dysplasia), infectious (joint ill involving the coxofemoral joint or proximal femoral physis), or traumatic (tearing of the ligament of the head of the femur, rupture of the round ligament, capital physeal fractures, hip luxation, intra-articular acetabular fractures, and osteoarthritis) in origin.

Many of these conditions cause a moderate to severe lameness and the limb is often outwardly rotated when viewed from the rear (toe-out, hock-in conformation). In addition, the limb may appear straighter than the contralateral limb and the horse may lean away from the affected limb (Figure 5.388). External swelling of the coxofemoral joint is often difficult to detect, but visual enlargement over the greater trochanter may be evident (Figure 5.389). Pain can often be elicited with direct inward pressure of this area. Rectal palpation may reveal swelling along the axial aspect of the joint but can only be performed in larger horses and gives many false negative results. Crepitus with limb manipulation is not a common finding except with acetabular or more extensive pelvic fractures, hip luxations, or some cases of complete ligament rupture.

A definitive diagnosis of a hip problem can be challenging without additional diagnostics. Arthrocentesis of the joint with or without intra-articular (IA) anesthesia can be performed but is often difficult in large horses.[11,25] Transcutaneous ultrasound-guided arthrocentesis may be helpful in these cases.[5] In addition, it is often much easier to perform arthrocentesis of the hip in foals and ponies in lateral recumbency under anesthesia. In many cases of chronic hindlimb lameness, IA anesthesia is necessary to confirm that the hip is the site of the lameness. Rectal and transcutaneous ultrasound may be helpful to document capital physeal and acetabular fractures and hip luxations.[2,10] Nuclear scintigraphy has improved the potential to localize lameness to the hip region but does not provide a definitive diagnosis. In many cases, radiography of the coxofemoral region using a standing technique or under anesthesia is necessary to either rule in or rule out a problem in the coxofemoral joint.[19,20,34]

In general, the prognosis for horses with hip disease is guarded to poor for athletic use. However, this depends on the type of lesion, the extent of secondary OA, and whether the lesion is accessible for arthroscopic debridement.[23–25] Young horses with OCD lesions that can be debrided arthroscopically and foals with joint ill without secondary osteomyelitis appear to have the best prognosis. Horses with complete rupture of the ligament of the head of the femur or accessory ligament, complete joint luxation, and OA tend to do poorly, regardless of treatment.

OSTEOCHONDROSIS (OCD)/HIP DYSPLASIA OF THE COXOFEMORAL JOINT

Developmental lesions of the coxofemoral joint are rare in comparison to other joints in the horse. Malformation of the joint, hip dysplasia, osteochondritis dissecans, and subchondral cystic lesions (SCLs) have been described in the coxofemoral joint.[11,22,25,31,34]

Etiology

The cause of these developmental lesions is assumed to be the same as for other OCD-type lesions. It is unknown why there is a low prevalence of OCD-type lesions in the hip compared to other locations. Much of the coxofemoral joint is weight-bearing; therefore, the development of SCLs could be trauma-induced, similar to other weight-bearing joint surfaces.

Clinical Signs

Clinical signs of young horses with OCD of the hip may be similar to those of any hindlimb lameness. They may include a stilted hindlimb gait, low foot-flight arc, shortened cranial phase of the stride, and dragging of the hind feet.[22] In cases of bilateral disease, the hindlimbs

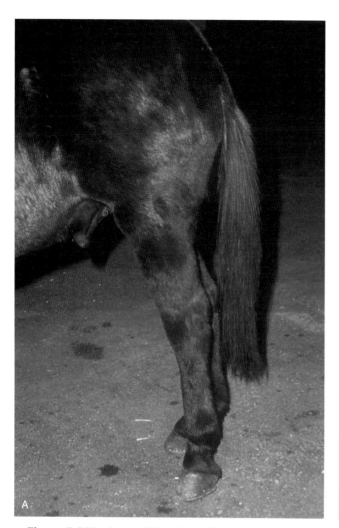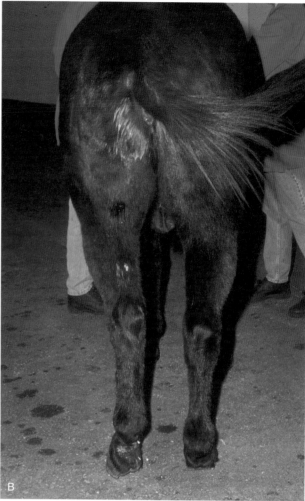

Figure 5.388. Lateral (A) and rear (B) views of an aged pony with the typical toe-out, hock-in stance characteristic of a hip/pelvic problem. The left hindlimb is straighter than the contralateral limb and from behind, the left point of the hock is higher than the right.

may be carried very straight and the weight shifted toward the forelimbs.[11,31,34] Physical abnormalities of the limb(s) or palpable pain may be difficult to document.

Diagnosis

Lameness in young horses may be localized to the hip by eliminating the remainder of the limb as the source of pain along with the characteristic stance of the limb. Physical examination findings may reveal pain on palpation and manipulation of the hip. Intra-articular anesthetic of the coxofemoral joint can be performed to aid diagnosis, but young horses do not tolerate the procedure very well. A definitive diagnosis is usually achieved via radiography. Better quality radiographs can generally be obtained under general anesthesia, although ventrodorsal and oblique radiographs of the pelvis can be performed in the standing horse.[19,20,25] Radiographic abnormalities consistent with OCD of the hip are similar to those of other locations and include SCLs, osteochondral fragments, abnormal contour of

the femoral head or acetabulum, and shallow and irregular acetabulum (Figure 5.390A).

Treatment

Depending on the severity of the OCD lesion, conservative or medical treatment is usually unsuccessful. However, palliative treatments aimed at cartilage and joint healing may be used in young horses with the hope of joint remodeling over time. Surgical debridement of the lesion is usually the treatment of choice, especially if osteochondritis dissecans lesions are present.[25] Arthroscopy of the coxofemoral joint is more easily performed in foals and weanlings, but can be accomplished in older horses with proper equipment.[12,23–25] Surgical debridement is also the treatment of choice for affected cartilage and subchondral bone. However, access to all areas of the coxofemoral joint is not possible. In severe cases of unilateral hip malformation or dysplasia (Figure 5.390A), a femoral head ostectomy may provide a salvage procedure for breeding soundness.[32] These procedures are performed infrequently in the horse.

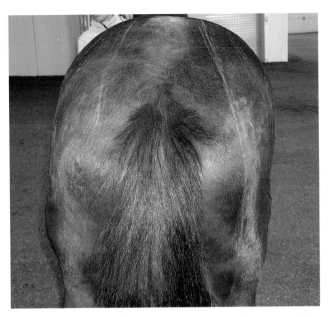

Figure 5.389. An older Quarter horse mare with grade 3 of 5 hindlimb lameness. Swelling over the left greater trochanter could be seen when compared to the opposite side, and pain was elicited with firm palpation. Radiographs revealed severe OA of the coxofemoral joint (Figure 5.394).

Prognosis

The coxofemoral joint is a major weight-bearing joint and articular abnormalities such as OCD often lead to OA. Young animals with small OCD lesions that can be debrided arthroscopically and have minimal evidence of OA may do well.[25] However, the prognosis for most horses with hip OCD should be considered guarded to poor for future athletic use.

INFECTIOUS ARTHRITIS/PHYSITIS OF THE COXOFEMORAL JOINT

Infection of the coxofemoral joint and the capital physis of the femur are part of the joint ill complex in foals.[18,26] Infections around the hip occur less frequently than at other sites in foals and can be very difficult to diagnose.

Etiology

Joint and physeal infections in foals are hematogenous in origin and bacteria usually gain access to the circulation through the umbilicus, gastrointestinal tract, or respiratory tract.[18,26,33] Affected foals usually have a history of failure of passive transfer. Bacteria localize in and around the physes and joints because of the specific low-flow circulation that is present in these areas. The syndrome may be classified according to the location of the lesion; S-type involves the synovium/joint, E-type involves the epiphysis, and P-type involves the physis.[18] Most infections are from Gram-negative bacteria. Infection of the proximal femoral physis may spread to the coxofemoral joint and surrounding tissues of the hip region.

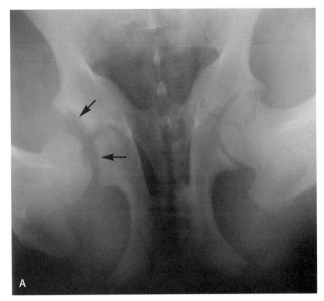

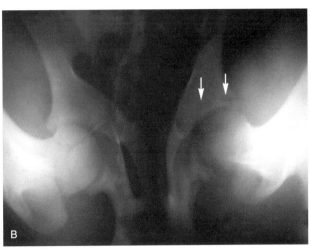

Figure 5.390. Ventrodorsal radiographs of the pelvis of 2 3-month-old fillies with a history of increasing lameness. A. Remodeling of the femoral head and acetabulum (arrows) consistent with a developmental abnormality. B. Lysis of the left acetabulum (arrows) consistent with infectious arthritis and osteomyelitis.

Clinical Signs

Infection of the coxofemoral joint can be a diagnostic challenge because joint effusion, heat, and pain are often not found on physical examination. Typically, these foals are less than 4 months of age and often present with a unilateral hindlimb lameness of unknown cause.[21] They may have a characteristic toe-out, stifle-out, hock-in appearance. Pain is often elicited with deep palpation over the greater trochanter and hip region. It can often be confused with trauma to the limb but the infection and therefore the lameness is often progressive, whereas a traumatic injury often improves with time. Any young foal with severe hindlimb lameness but no definable lesions in the lower limb should be suspected of having infection of the hip joint. In addition, infections of the capital physis can spread to the hip musculature and the foal may present with an abscess in the gluteal region.

Diagnosis

A complete blood count is often very helpful to help differentiate trauma from a potential hip infection. High white blood cell counts and fibrinogen concentrations help confirm the presence of an infection.[21] However, a definitive diagnosis of infectious arthritis is made by analyzing the synovial fluid of the hip joint following arthrocentesis. Synovial white blood cell counts of 30,000 cells/μL or more and total protein concentrations of 4.0 g/dL or more are consistent with infection. Physeal infections can be documented with radiographs of the hip region, where lysis around the capital physis, epiphysis, and occasionally the acetabulum is seen (Figure 5.390B).

Treatment

Treatment is similar as for any other joint/physis with a hematogenous infection. Broad-spectrum systemic antimicrobials, intra-articular antimicrobials, and joint lavage/drainage are all important. Arthroscopy can be performed in small horses and foals to help lavage and debride these lesions but cannula lavage alone can be very helpful.[12,23–25] Unfortunately, many of these infections are not diagnosed in the early stages and significant osteomyelitis is often present, worsening the prognosis (Figure 5.390B).

Prognosis

The prognosis is usually poor because the diagnosis is seldom made before significant joint abnormalities and osteomyelitis have occurred. However, foals with coxofemoral infectious arthritis without radiographic abnormalities should respond well to aggressive treatment and their prognosis for athletic use is similar to that of foals with joint ill at other locations.

PARTIAL TEAR/RUPTURE OF THE LIGAMENT OF THE HEAD OF THE FEMUR (ROUND LIGAMENT)

A partial tear or rupture of the ligament of the head of the femur (round ligament) of the coxofemoral joint is a relatively rare condition that can affect any age or breed of horse. Nevertheless, it appears to be more common in small breed horses (miniatures and ponies) and young horses.[25] The hip joint is usually very stable but occasionally a partial tear or complete rupture of ligament of the head of the femur can occur without a complete joint luxation. In these cases, the head of the femur may have greater range of motion within the joint, contributing to synovitis, joint effusion, and lameness.[11] Subsequent degenerative changes within the joint often lead to OA. Definitive diagnosis of a ruptured ligament of the head of the femur can be difficult.

Etiology

Trauma is the most common cause of either a partial tear or complete rupture of the ligament of the head of the femur. The same type of forces/stresses that cause luxation of the coxofemoral joint may also damage this ligament without resulting in a joint luxation.

Clinical Signs

Affected horses often have an acute onset of lameness and a history of trauma. Visible swelling over the hip is often difficult to detect but gluteal atrophy may be present if the condition is chronic. Horses often stand with a toe-out, stifle-out, and hock-in appearance of the affected hindlimb that is typical of problems in the coxofemoral region.[11] Unlike horses with a complete hip luxation, the limbs are the same length and the points of the hocks are at the same height.[11] Firm intermittent pressure applied over the greater trochanter usually elicits a painful response. Limb manipulation, flexion of the hip joint, and upper limb flexion tests may also be painful. Crepitation over the joint may be present because of the excessive motion of the femur, but can be difficult to document.[1]

Although the clinical signs often localize the problem to the hip region, intrasynovial anesthesia may be required to prove that the joint is affected. Aspiration of hemorrhagic synovial fluid during arthrocentesis is consistent with joint trauma. For information regarding the technique for intrasynovial anesthesia of the hip joint, see Chapter 3.

The clinical signs associated with partial tearing of the ligament of the head of the femur are not as clear as those seen with complete rupture of the ligament. The hock-in and stifle and toe-out appearance is generally not observed and these horses may present with a chronic hindlimb lameness. Varying degrees of gluteal muscle atrophy may occur in chronic cases but this is not a consistent finding. Limb manipulation, particularly hip abduction and flexion of the joint, may be present but less so than with complete ligament rupture. Intermittent firm pressure applied externally to the greater trochanter usually elicits a painful response.[1]

Diagnosis

A presumptive diagnosis of a complete rupture of the ligament of the head of the femur is based on a history of trauma combined with an acute lameness with clinical signs characteristic of a hip problem. However, several other hip-related injuries (capital physeal fractures, other ligamentous injuries, acetabular fractures) may present with similar histories and clinical signs. Hip luxations usually can be ruled out based on the physical findings of a shorter limb and a higher point of the hock on the affected limb.[11]

Radiography or ultrasound of the hip region is necessary to rule out other possible problems. Ventrodorsal and oblique radiographs of the hip can be performed with the horse under general anesthesia or standing. Radiographs of the hip may be normal with rupture of the ligament of the head of the femur, or an abnormal position of the femoral head within the acetabulum may be identified.[1] Subluxation of the coxofemoral joint may also be diagnosed with dynamic ultrasound (weight-bearing and nonweight-bearing views) of the hip region in standing horses.[2] An abnormal position of the femoral head seen on radiographs or with dynamic ultrasound together with hemarthrosis of the hip identified with arthrocentesis is highly suggestive of an acute ruptured round ligament. If the condition is chronic, radiographic signs consistent with OA are often present. These include osteophytes on the cranial and caudal rim of the acetabulum and at the capsular attachment on the femoral neck.[25]

Diagnostic approaches used to identify a partial tear of the accessory ligament may include scintigraphy, radiography, and arthroscopy. Although not diagnostic for a partial tear, scintigraphy may show a mild to moderate radionucleotide accumulation in the affected hip, particularly if secondary degenerative joint changes are present.[11,16,23,25] Radiography may identify changes associated with OA of the hip joint but is not specific for damage to the ligament of the head of the femur. Subluxation of the coxofemoral joint due to partial tearing of the ligament of the head of the femur was diagnosed in 2 horses with dynamic ultrasound, and should be considered in these cases.[2] Arthroscopy of the coxofemoral joint also may be used to diagnose and potentially treat (debridement) partial and complete ruptures of the ligament of the head of the femur.[23-25]

Treatment

There is no effective treatment for complete rupture of the ligament of the head of the femur of the hip joint. Affected horses often develop osteoarthritis and remain lame.[25] However, arthroscopy of the hip joint has been used successfully to debride partial tears of the round ligament and to perform a synovectomy.[23-25] Ligament tearing in small breeds of horses, particularly miniature horses, can be adequately debrided and a return to soundness is possible.[25]

Prognosis

The prognosis is poor for horses with complete rupture of round ligament, regardless of treatment. Secondary osteoarthritis of the hip joint appears to be a likely sequela. However, the response to debridement of partial tears in small-breed horses has been favorable in a limited number of cases.[25]

COXOFEMORAL LUXATION (DISLOCATION OF THE HIP JOINT)

Luxation of the coxofemoral joint is an uncommon condition in horses compared to cattle because of the numerous ligaments and heavy musculature surrounding the joint. The femoral accessory ligament and the round ligament both attach to the femoral head and provide the primary stability to the hip.[6] The fibrocartilaginous rim around the acetabulum further stabilizes the head of the femur within the joint. In horses, the ilium tends to fracture before the hip luxates.[11] Foals, miniature horses, and ponies are most frequently affected.[6,11,17,27,28] Coxofemoral luxation is unilateral and the head of the femur nearly always becomes craniodorsal to the acetabulum.[6]

Etiology

Both the accessory and the ligament of the head of the femur (round) must rupture for a luxation to occur.[11] Trauma is nearly always the cause. Violent overextension and falling on the point of the stifle with the femur in a vertical position occasionally produces fracture and/or luxation of the coxofemoral joint.[11] A tethered horse that catches its foot in a rope or a halter may dislocate the hip in the struggle to free itself.

Because the acetabulum is deep and the head of the femur is large, excessive trauma is usually necessary to dislocate this joint. Fractures of the dorsal rim often accompany the luxation because of the deep acetabulum in the horse.[11] Additionally, absence or partial tearing of the ligament of the head of the femur may predispose to subluxation and luxation with or without associated trauma.[1,2,11]

Coxofemoral luxations may be complicated by upward fixation of the patella.[4,9,11] The upward patellar fixation may potentially contribute to the luxation or occur as the result of. If it precedes the luxation, the secondary hip luxation is believed to occur as a result of the violent contraction of the quadriceps muscles trying to flex the limb while the stifle is locked in extension. The net result is that the head of the femur luxates out of the acetabulum rather than the stifle flexing.[11] The patella usually becomes unfixed at the time of the luxation. Alternatively, the patella becomes locked following the luxation because the craniodorsal position of the femur causes the limb to become much straighter, predisposing to upward fixation of the patella (Figure 5.391). Luxation of the hip also may occur secondary to wearing a full-limb hindlimb cast, especially in foals.[35]

Clinical Signs

A history of trauma resulting in a severe nonweight-bearing lameness is common. Some horses may toe-touch when walked because the affected limb is shorter than the opposite limb due to the craniodorsal position of the femur.[6] The limb may "dangle" somewhat because of shortening and the point of the hock on the affected side is higher than that of the opposite limb (Figure 5.388B). The toe and stifle turn outward and the point of the hock turns inward (Figure 5.388A). Affected horses generally have a limited cranial stride because of limb shortening and a more prominent greater trochanter of the femur. Soft tissue swelling may make this prominence difficult to see in the early stages. Crepitus with limb manipulation may be present as a result of the femur rubbing on the shaft of the ilium.[11] This may also occur with acetabular and pelvic fractures. Pushing the greater trochanter in a caudal to cranial direction may displace the femur further cranially than normal when a hip luxation is present.

Diagnosis

A presumptive diagnosis can often be made based on the history and clinical signs. Radiography confirms the diagnosis and also rules out other possible causes of the lameness such as pelvic fractures, acetabular fractures,

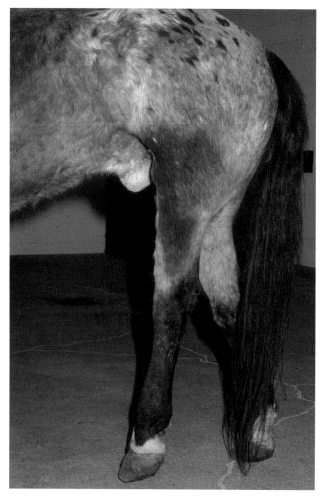

Figure 5.391. Horse with luxation of the hip and concurrent upward fixation of the patella. The craniodorsal positioning of the femoral head straightens the limb, contributing to upward fixation.

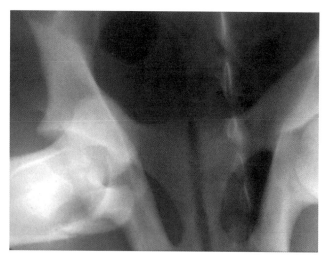

Figure 5.392. Ventrodorsal radiograph of the pelvis confirming luxation of the coxofemoral joint. The femoral head is outside the acetabulum and no other pelvic fractures can be identified.

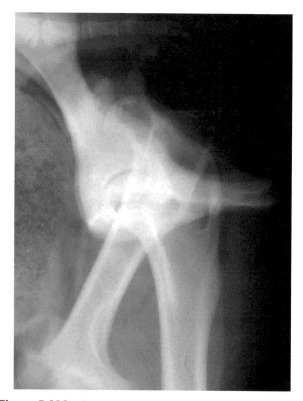

Figure 5.393. Lateral radiograph of the pelvis in a miniature horse which confirmed a craniodorsal luxation of the femoral head.

and capital physeal fractures (Figures 5.392 and 5.393).[19,20] Ultrasound is being used more frequently to examine the pelvic region and also may be able to confirm luxation of the femoral head.[10]

Treatment

In general, treatment of hip luxation is problematic, especially in adult horses. Many horses with this condition are euthanized because of the often unsuccessful treatment options and the poor prognosis. Closed reduction of the luxation is usually the best treatment option, but it can be very difficult to perform in adult horses and re-luxation is common. The likelihood of re-luxation after closed reduction increases if the dorsal rim of the acetabulum is fractured. If the luxation is chronic, the acetabulum may be filled with fibrin and granulation tissue, preventing a successful closed reduction. In a recent report of 17 cases of coxofemoral luxation, 35% had other orthopedic injuries and no form of closed or open reduction was successful.[17]

Horses with an acute luxation with no secondary fracture of the dorsal rim of the acetabulum are the best candidates for closed reduction. General anesthesia with or without muscle relaxation is required. The luxation may be reduced by manual traction and manipulation if good muscle relaxation is obtained.[11,17] Traction also can be applied by using a hoist with the horse placed in dorsal recumbency or with a calf jack if lateral recumbency is selected. Traction combined with external rotation and adduction of the limb followed by internal rotation as the traction is reduced completes the reduction. Reduction can be appreciated when the hip clicks or pops into place. Closed reduction is often difficult, and even when it is successful re-luxation may occur within a few days.[9,17] An Ehmer sling was used to prevent re-luxation after the second closed reduction in a pony and successfully improved the outcome.[4] However, this is only possible in foals or small-breed horses.

Several surgical approaches have been described for cases that re-luxate or those that cannot be corrected with closed reduction. However, these are most applicable for foals or small-breed horses. They include open reduction alone, transposition of the greater trochanter, femoral head and neck resection, toggle pinning, or augmentation of the lateral joint capsule with synthetic sutures attached to screws.[1,6,9,27,28] A combination of toggle pinning, synthetic capsular repair, and trochanteric transposition was used to successfully repair a hip luxation in an adult miniature horse.[9] Open surgical approaches should be performed soon after the luxation occurs; otherwise, contraction of the musculature will make reduction difficult. In addition, excision of the femoral head and neck and dorsal rim of the fractured acetabulum should be considered in smaller horses to aid in the development of a pseudoarthrosis.[8,11,32]

Prognosis

The prognosis is typically guarded to poor because successful closed reduction is not always possible. Conservative treatment is not an option and euthanasia is recommended. A minority of horses may return to complete soundness after the head of the femur is replaced, but this is the exception.[11] There is usually a better chance of maintaining permanent reduction if the femur stays in place for approximately 3 months.[11] Most horses can become sound enough for breeding purposes if the reduction can be maintained.[11] Surgical correction may be warranted if the horse is valuable and small, but is performed infrequently

OSTEOARTHRITIS (OA) OF THE COXOFEMORAL JOINT

Osteoarthritis of the coxofemoral joint is a sequel to all of the conditions described in this section. It can also occur from any type of soft tissue trauma to the hip region that does not necessarily result in a ligament injury or intra-articular fracture. Trauma to the joint capsule and surrounding musculature can contribute to the development of OA. It is seen most frequently in older animals and must be considered in any horse with chronic hindlimb lameness.

Etiology

Any hip-related traumatic injury can lead to OA. Reported causes of coxofemoral joint OA include idiopathic infection,[3] abnormal development of the coxofemoral joint,[31,34] joint ill, and trauma.

Clinical Signs

No clinical signs are specific for coxofemoral joint OA. However, hip OA should be suspected in older horses with chronic hindlimb lameness problems that have a history of trauma (Figure 5.389). Many of these horses have significant lameness (grade 3 to 4 on a scale of 5) and have a low arc of foot flight and a reduced cranial phase of stride. Horses with hip pain tend to move with the limb rotated externally and carry the limb abducted during advancement. Firm swelling over the greater trochanter and hip area may be present in chronic cases and the characteristic toe-out, hock-in stance may or may not be observed. In horses with bilateral disease, the hindlimbs are often carried very straight with a shift of weight onto the forelimbs.[11]

Diagnosis

A presumptive diagnosis of severe hip OA often can be made based on the history and clinical exam. Milder cases of OA can be a diagnostic challenge. Intra-articular anesthetic of the coxofemoral joint is the best method to localize the lameness to the hip. Nuclear scintigraphy may be helpful to localize the problem to the hip but is not very sensitive nor specific for coxofemoral joint OA. Radiographs are often necessary for a definitive diagnosis and usually reveal evidence of bone remodeling and osteophyte production in chronic cases (Figure 5.394). Good quality radiographs of both hips (to permit comparison between the 2) are necessary to diagnose mild to moderate hip OA.

Treatment

Treatment of hip OA is usually palliative because there is no cure. Horses with unilateral mild or

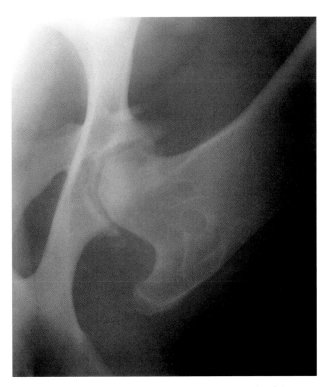

Figure 5.394. Ventrodorsal radiograph of the pelvis of the horse in Figure 5.389, demonstrating severe OA of the coxofemoral joint. The OA was reportedly secondary to trauma to the area from a previous fall.

moderate OA may benefit from coxofemoral joint arthroscopy to debride cartilage lesions and determine the inciting cause. Focal femoral head cartilage lesions have been debrided with good results in a limited number of cases.[25] Horses with hip OA usually respond well to oral nonsteroidal anti-inflammatory drugs and/or intra-articular treatment with hyaluronan and corticosteroids. Horses with mild or moderate hip OA may benefit from medications directed at joint healing such as IV hyaluronan, IM polysulfated glycosaminoglycans, and oral nutraceuticals. See Principles of Therapy for more information on treatment of OA.

Prognosis

There are no long-term reports on the prognosis of horses with coxofemoral joint OA. In general, any treatment is a temporary fix and the prognosis for athletic use in horses with severe OA is thought to be poor. However, many of these horses can be used for breeding or maintained as pets because they tend to do well at the walk. Horses with mild or moderate OA may respond well to treatment and may be used at a reduced performance level.

CAPITAL PHYSEAL FRACTURES OF THE FEMORAL HEAD

Fractures of the capital physis of the femoral neck occur commonly in foals under than 1 year of age.[7,13] They are usually a type I Salter-Harris physeal fracture but types II and III are also observed.[7,13] Another term that has been used to describe them is a "slipped capital physis" (Figure 5.380).

Etiology

Trauma such as violent falls, struggles, and kicks are the cause of these fractures. In particular, falling on the greater trochanter is thought to cause shearing forces across the physis, resulting in displacement between the epiphysis and metaphysis.

Clinical Signs

There is usually a history of trauma with an immediate severe lameness. However, some foals are still able to bear some weight but often stand with a toe-out, hock-in appearance. Swelling and pain over the hip, pelvic asymmetry, gluteal muscle atrophy, and crepitus with hip manipulation may be present. However, these signs were found inconsistently in a report of 25 foals with capital physeal fractures.[13]

Diagnosis

Because of the inconsistency of clinical signs, radiography of the hip is necessary for an accurate diagnosis. Separation of the epiphysis and metaphysis of the femoral neck confirms the diagnosis (Figure 5.380). However, other radiographic abnormalities are often found, such as comminution of the epiphysis, greater trochanter or acetabular fracture, or coxofemoral joint luxation/subluxation.[3] Concurrent radiographic findings often make potential surgical repair unlikely.

Treatment

Nonsurgical management of these fractures is not recommended because malunion, avascular necrosis, and secondary hip OA can lead to debilitating lameness.[13,36] However, surgical treatment is difficult and is not recommended in foals with concurrent radiographic abnormalities. Surgical treatments that have been used to repair capital physeal fractures include the use of cancellous or cortical bone screws, IM or Knowles pins, and an interfragmentary compression system.[13,14,30,36] Small foals with a type 1 or 2 physeal fracture are the best candidates for surgery.

Prognosis

Unfortunately, the majority of foals with this condition are euthanized because of the poor prognosis with nonsurgical treatment and the questionable results with surgery. If the epiphysis can be reduced and maintained until healing, athletic soundness can be achieved.

INTRA-ARTICULAR ACETABULAR FRACTURES

Acetabular fractures can occur independently or together with other fractures of the pelvis. They may be non-displaced but more frequently are comminuted and displaced. They appear to be more common in young horses and frequently result when the horse slips or splits (spread eagle).[11]

Etiology

Trauma is the cause in nearly all cases. Stress or fatigue fractures occur elsewhere in the pelvis such as the ilium, but are usually not confined to the acetabulum.[6]

Clinical Signs

Horses with acetabular fractures present with similar clinical signs as horses with pelvic fractures or hip disease. They usually have a significant unilateral lameness and may have gluteal muscle atrophy if the condition is chronic. Swelling, pain, and crepitus may be palpable over the greater trochanter, and there is often pelvic asymmetry if other pelvic fractures are present (Figure 5.395). A rectal examination may also reveal swelling axial to the coxofemoral joint but it may be difficult to detect with acetabulum fractures alone.

Diagnosis

Radiography or ultrasound is necessary to document an acetabular fracture and rule out other possible problems in the hip and pelvis (Figure 5.396).[6,10,20] Non-displaced acetabular fractures may be difficult to visualize with ultrasound. Concurrent fractures of the pelvis and hip are not uncommon.

Treatment

Conservative treatment with stall confinement is often the treatment of choice with acetabular fractures.

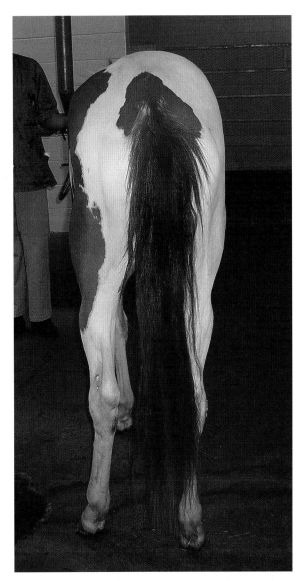

Figure 5.395. Young horse with asymmetry of the pelvis, muscle atrophy over the left hip, and a toe-out stance. The horse was lame at the walk and an acetabular fracture was present on radiographs.

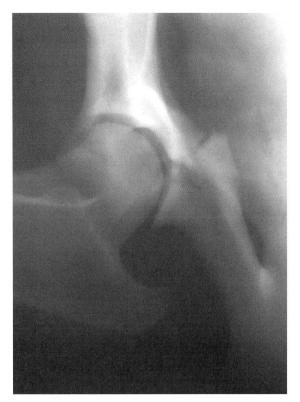

Figure 5.396. Ventrodorsal radiograph of the coxofemoral joint demonstrating a minimally displaced acetabular fracture. Intra-articular fragmentation was not identified and the horse was treated with stall confinement.

Euthanasia may be indicated with severely displaced fractures because there is no known surgical treatment. Small intra-articular fractures from the cranial and caudal perimeter of the acetabulum may be removed from the joint with the arthroscope to potentially improve the prognosis.[25] However, removal of large fragments appears to rarely be successful. Minimally displaced acetabular fractures heal very well with confinement and horses often can achieve their full athletic potential (Figure 5.396).

Prognosis

In general, horses with fractures of the acetabulum have a worse prognosis for soundness than those with fractures elsewhere in the pelvis.[6,28,29] However, most acetabular fractures respond better to conservative treatment than many other hip problems such as capital physeal fractures, luxation, and round ligament rupture. Approximately 20% of horses with articular fractures are capable of athletic performance.[29] However, this greatly depends on the fracture configuration and degree of displacement.

References

1. Adams OR. Lameness in Horses, 3rd ed. Lea and Febiger, Philadelphia, 1974;299–303.
2. Brenner S, Whitcomb MB. How to diagnose equine coxofemoral subluxation with dynamic ultrasonography. Proceedings Am Assoc Eq Pract 2007;53:433–437.
3. Clegg PD. Idiopathic infective arthritis of the coxofemoral joint in a mature horse. Vet Record 1995;137:460–464.
4. Clegg PD, Butson RJ. Treatment of a coxofemoral luxation secondary to upward fixation of the patella in a Shetland pony. Vet Record 1996;138:134–137.
5. David F, Rougier M, Alexander K, et al. Ultrasound-guided coxofemoral arthrocentesis in horses. Equine Vet J 2007;39: 79–83.
6. Ducharme NG. Pelvic fracture and coxofemoral luxation. In Equine Fracture Repair. Nixon AJ, ed. WB Saunders Co., Philadelphia, 1996;295–298.
7. Embertson RM, Bramlage LR, Herring DS, et al. Physeal fractures in the horse. I. Classification and incidence. Vet Surg 1986;15:223–229.
8. Field JR, McLaughlin R, Davies M. Surgical repair of coxofemoral luxation in a miniature horse. Can Vet J 1992;33: 404–405.
9. Garcia-Lopez JM, Boudrieau RJ, Provost PJ. Surgical repair of a coxofemoral joint luxation in a horse. J Am Vet Med Assoc 2001;219:1254–1258.

10. Goodrich LR, Werpy NM, Armentrout A. How to ultrasound the normal pelvis for aiding diagnosis of pelvic fractures using rectal and transcutaneous ultrasound examination. Proceedings Am Assoc Equine Pract 2006;52:609–612.
11. Hendrickson DA. The coxofemoral joint. In Adams' Lameness in Horses, 5th ed. Stashak TS, ed. Lippincott Williams and Wilkins, Philadelphia, 2002;1037–1043.
12. Honnas CM, Zamos DT, Ford TS. Arthroscopy of the coxofemoral joint of foals. Vet Surg 1993;22:115–121.
13. Hunt DA, Snyder JR, Morgan JP. Femoral capital physeal fractures in 25 foals. Vet Surg 1990;19:41–49.
14. Hunt DA, Snyder JR, Morgan JP. Evaluation of an interfragmentary compression system for the repair of equine femoral capital physeal fractures. Vet Surg 1990;19:107–116.
15. Kainer RA. Functional anatomy of the equine locomotor organs. In Adams' Lameness in Horses, 5th ed. Stashak TS, ed. Lippincott Williams and Wilkins, Philadelphia, 2002;1–72.
16. Lamb CR, Morris EA. Coxofemoral arthrosis in an aged mare. Equine Vet J 1987;19:350–352.
17. Malark JA, Nixon AJ, Haughland MA, et al. Equine coxofemoral luxations: 17 cases (1975–1990). Cornell Vet 1992;82:79–90.
18. Martens RJ, Auer JA, Carter GK. Equine pediatrics: septic arthritis and osteomyelitis. J Am Vet Med Assoc 1986;188:582–585.
19. May SA, Patterson LJ, Peacock PJ, et al. Radiographic technique for the pelvis in the standing horse. Equine Vet J 1991;23:312–314.
20. May SA. Standing and conventional pelvic radiography. In Current Techniques in Equine Surgery and Lameness. NA White, JN Moore, eds. WB Saunders Co., Philadelphia, 1998;584–586.
21. Newquist J, Baxter GM. Plasma fibrinogen as an indicator of physeal/epiphyseal osteomyelitis in foals: A retrospective study (2000–2007). J Am Vet Med Assoc 2009;235:415–419.
22. Nixon AJ, Adams RM, Teigland MB. Subchondral cystic lesions (osteochondrosis) of the femoral heads in a horse. J Am Vet Med Assoc 1988;192:301–362.
23. Nixon AJ. Coxofemoral joint arthroscopy. In Current Techniques in Equine Surgery and Lameness. White NA, Moore JN, eds. WB Saunders Co., Philadelphia, 1998;448–451.
24. Nixon AJ. Diagnostic and operative arthroscopy of the coxofemoral joint in horses. Vet Surg 1994;23:377–385.
25. Nixon AJ. Diagnostic and surgical arthroscopy of the coxofemoral (hip) joint. In Diagnostic and Surgical Arthroscopy in the Horse. McIlwraith CW, Nixon AJ, Wright IM, et al., eds. Mosby Elsevier, Philadelphia, 2005;337–246.
26. Paradis MR. Update on neonatal septicemia. Vet Clin of North Am Equine Pract 1994;10:109–135.
27. Platt D, Wright IM, Houlton JEF. Treatment of chronic coxofemoral luxation in a Shetland pony by excision arthroplasty of the femoral head: A case report. British Vet J 1990;146:374–379.
28. Richardson DW. The femur and pelvis. In Equine Surgery, 2nd ed. Auer JA, Stick J, eds. WB Saunders, Philadelphia, 1999;881–886.
29. Rutkowski JA, Richardson DW. A retrospective study of 100 pelvic fractures in horses. Equine Vet J 1989;21:256–259.
30. Smyth GB, Taylor EG. Stabilization of a proximal femoral physeal fracture in a filly by use of cancellous bone screws. J Am Vet Med Assoc 1992;201:895–898.
31. Speirs VC, Wrigley R. A case of bilateral hip dysplasia in a foal. Equine Vet J 1979;11:202–204.
32. Squire DRE, Fessler JF, Toombs JP, et al. Femoral head ostectomy in horses and cattle. Vet Surg 1991;20:453–458.
33. Steel CM, Hunt AR, Adams PL, et al. Factors associated with prognosis for survival and athletic use in foals with septic arthritis: 93 cases (1987–1994). J Am Vet Med Assoc 1999;215:973–977.
34. Talbot AM, Barrett EL, Driver AJ, et al. How to perform standing lateral oblique radiographs of the equine pelvis. Proceedings Am Assoc Eq Pract 2006;52:613.
35. Trent AM. Bilateral degenerative coxofemoral joint disease in a foal. J Am Vet Med Assoc 1985;186:284–287.
36. Trotter GW, Auer JA, Warwick A, et al. Coxofemoral luxation in two foals wearing hindlimb casts. J Am Vet Med Assoc 1986;189:56.
37. Turner AS, Milne DW, Hohn RB. Surgical repair of fractured capital femoral epiphysis in three foals. J Am Vet Med Assoc 1979;175:1198–1202.

Lameness Associated with the Axial Skeleton

THE AXIAL SKELETON

ROB VAN WESSUM

Back pain is increasingly recognized as contributing to or even causing equine lameness.[2,4,11,16,20] Previously back pain was generally considered to be a secondary problem, with the primary lameness of a limb causing changes in movement and affecting the spine. In recent years, more and more primary spine injuries have been acknowledged.[3,9,10,11,20] To understand the function of the vertebral column, its attached tissues, and their relationship to the physics of equine locomotion, some basic anatomical and biomechanical knowledge is necessary.

ANATOMY AND BIOMECHANICS OF THE VERTEBRAL COLUMN

There are approximately 260 joints between the vertebrae; the vertebrae and ribs, the sacrum and pelvis, and the head and the first cervical vertebra all contribute to mobility in the entire spine. In most of these joints, the total range of motion is limited in both direction and degree, but the overall effect of all of the joints within the spine creates a significant amount of motion in the entire spine.[5,12] Because of its connection to the limb, a major function of the spine and the attached muscles is the positioning of the limbs. Some of the muscles controlling limb position have their origin at the spine and their insertion on an extremity; other muscles with both origins and insertions on the spine regulate mobility in the spine itself.

Joints of the spine allow mobility dorsally, ventrally, and laterally, and some allow rotation. In particular areas of the spine, the vertebrae have specific ranges of motion within the three basic axes: lateroflexion, dorsi-

and ventroflexion, and rotation. Any specific change in the posture of the horse causes a change in the direction in 1 or more of these 3 planes. The cervical intervertebral joints allow a relatively large range of flexion dorsiventrally as well as laterally, while the intervertebral joint between the first and second cervical vertebra permits rotation. In the thoracic vertebrae the mobility is mainly lateral flexion, with some minor dorsi-ventral motion. In addition, the mobility of the costo-vertebral joints is necessary for breathing. In the lumbar spine the main mobility is in dorsi-ventral flexion with some rotation. In the sacral region there is a small amount of dorsi-ventral flexion, while in the tail there is considerable dorsi-ventral and lateral flexion but no rotation.[4,5]

The pattern of motion of the spine also is gait-specific. The support and the positioning of the spine are a specific function of each gait, enhancing the range of motion of the extremities by facilitating optimal positioning of the limb relative to the spine and the other limbs. The axial muscles can function as a stabilizer of the spine and hold certain portions of the spine during locomotion. The epaxial muscles are symmetrically arranged between the transverse and dorsal spinous processes. The spinalis muscle, semispinalis muscle, and multifidus muscle form the most axial and deepest epaxial muscle group. The multifidus muscle consists of a large number of separate muscle units, each covering only 2 to 6 vertebral segments along the entire vertebral column. The middle epaxial muscular layer, called the lateral system, extends from C1 to the pelvis and sacrum. The lateral part of this system is formed by the iliocostal muscle and the medial part by the longissimus muscle, which is very well developed in the lumbar region. The most superficial layer of epaxial muscles is formed by the splenius muscle in the cervical and cranial thoracic region.

Adams and Stashak's Lameness in Horses, 6e, edited by Gary M. Baxter
© 2011 Blackwell Publishing, Ltd.

Walk

In the walk, the main motion of the spine can be described as a "snake-like" motion. A sinusoidal pattern of motion is present in the spine with lateral flexion in the thoracic region, some rotation in the lumbar spine, and dorsi-ventral flexion in the cervical region, all contributing to support the walk.[6] Electromyographic evaluation has shown the action of the splenius muscles is to elevate the head and neck and facilitate forelimb protraction by the elongated brachiocephalicus muscle. The sternocephalicus muscle contributes to the stance phase of the front limb. The longissimus dorsi muscle acts during the stance phase of the hindlimb, whereas the rectus abdominus muscle is not active at all but limits vertical acceleration of the abdominal visceral mass. The multifidus lumborum muscle is active in the intermediate part of the stance phase of the ipsilateral limb and the obliquus externus abdominal muscle shows intermittent activity.[4]

Trot

At the trot there is only modest dorsi-ventral flexion in the thorax and the neck. The maximal thoracolumbar extension occurs in the mid stance phase due to the visceral inertia. The splenius muscle acts before and during the first part of the stance phase of each forelimb to limit lowering of the neck, and the sternocephalicus muscle controls neck elevation. The brachiocephalicus muscle acts to achieve protraction of the forelimb. The rectus abdominus muscle limits the passive thoracolumbar extension caused by the visceral mass inertia during the stance phase. The longissimus dorsi muscles act at the end of the stance phase and during the suspension phase to induce lumbosacral extension to facilitate hindlimb protrusion. In the trot, most muscles act to stabilize the spine, not to move it.[6,7]

Canter

There is more lumbar and sacral motion in the canter than in any other gait, with lumbar rotation and dorsi-ventral flexion in the lumbar, thoracic, and sacral spine.[8] In the neck, the splenius muscle is active during the trailing diagonal stance phase. It limits the neck to lower and causes neck extension during the leading stance phase, and the sternocephalicus muscle shows reciprocal activity. The brachiocephalicus muscle is mainly active during the stance phase. The longissimus dorsi muscles are active during the suspension phase and during the trailing hindlimb stance phase. The rectus abdominus muscles act reciprocally during the support phase of the non-leading diagonal to support the visceral mass and initiate thoracolumbar flexion. The sublumbar muscles, psoas major and minor, are active during the suspension phase and are part of the propulsion forces in the canter.[4]

Table 6.1 is an overview of the degrees of mobility and their relationship to the 3 gaits. It is easy to understand that this relationship can make a lameness examination more of a challenge. Some common symptoms are associated with specific parts of the spine, as shown in Table 6.2.

Table 6.1. Mobility of the spine.

| Gait | Axis | Part of the spine | | | |
		Cervical	Thoracic	Lumbar	Sacral
Walk	DV	++	+	+	+
	Lat	+	++	–	+
	Rot	+–	–	+	–
Trot	DV	+	+	–	–
	Lat	–	–	–	–
	Rot	–	–	–	–
Canter	DV	++	+	+++	++
	Lat	+–	+	–	–
	Rot	–	–	++	+

DV = dorso- and ventroflexion, Lat = lateroflexion, Rot = rotation, – = not present, + = minor mobility, ++ = major mobility, +++ = maximum mobility.
Reprinted with permission from van Wessum R. Evaluation of back pain by clinical examination. In Current Therapy in Equine Medicine, 6th ed. Robinson NE, Sprayberry KA, eds. Saunders, St. Louis, 2009, 469.

History

As in every examination, investigating the horse with back pain starts with the history.[15] Taking time for a good interview with the client is the first step to better comprehending the problem. Listening to the information provided by the client is a good start. Asking guiding questions such as whether there are time-related changes in the quality of the gaits or difficulties in keeping the correct lead can provide information about the gait in which the complaints are more evident. Common complaints from owners of horses with back problems include resistance to bending to one direction more than to another; not accepting the bridle; kicking and bucking (especially in one gait, most commonly the canter); poor quality canter, cross canter, or switching leads; or generalized stiffness.[1] The poor quality canter may be a no-sound, 4-beat canter, more "bunny-hop-like" with less separation between the subsequent footfalls of the hindlimbs.

Some complaints are specific to the discipline. Complaints indicative of back pain in dressage horses include difficulties in the walk and canter pirouettes, a poor quality or a lateral walk, and unsatisfactory collection and "coming under" (carriage of the hindquarters). In jumpers, common complaints are unsatisfactory bascule (balance above the fence), lack of propulsion and power, unwillingness to jump and/or turn, and landing in the wrong lead canter. The quality of the lope is a complaint in Western pleasure horses. In racing horses, back pain is often located in the lumbar region,

Table 6.2. Symptoms and locations.

Symptom	Location within spine			
	Cervical	Thoracic	Lumbar	Sacral
Gait abnormalities				
Lateral walk	Rare	Sometimes	Often	Often
Bunny hop canter	Rare	Sometimes	Often	Often
Cross cantering	Rare	Sometimes	Often	Often
Toe dragging behind	Rare	Rare	Often	Often
Narrow behind	Rare	Rare	Sometimes	Often
Wide behind	Rare	Sometimes	Often	Rare
Hip lowered	Rare	Rare	Sometimes	Often
Tail fixed to one side	Rare	Rare	Sometimes	Often
Head out on circles	Often	Rare	Rare	Rare
Front limb lameness	Sometimes	Sometimes	Rare	Rare
Reduced stride length, behind	Rare	Sometimes	Often	Often
Reduced stride length, front	Sometimes	Sometimes	Rare	Rare
Behavioral issues				
Downward transition difficult	Rare	Often	Often	Often
More complaints when ridden	Sometimes	Often	Often	Often
Refusal to accept the bit	Often	Sometimes	Sometimes	Sometimes
Refusal to jump	Sometimes	Often	Often	Often
Poor lateral bending	Sometimes	Sometimes	Often	Often
Poor collection	Sometimes	Rare	Often	Often
Resistance when tacked up	Rare	Often	Sometimes	Sometimes
Collapsing in hind limbs	Rare	Rare	Sometimes	Sometimes
Rearing	Rare	Rare	Sometimes	Rare
Poor engagement of hindquarters in trot	Rare	Often	Sometimes	Sometimes
Poor engagement hindquarters in canter	Rare	Rare	Often	Often
Bucking	Sometimes	Often	Often	Often

Reprinted with permission from van Wessum R. Evaluation of back pain by clinical examination. In Current Therapy in Equine Medicine, 6th ed. NE Robinson, KA Sprayberry, eds. Saunders, St. Louis, 2009, 471.

which can limit dorsi-ventral flexion, thus decreasing propulsion and reducing the efficiency of the canter and gallop, and ultimately leading to poor performance.

Other usual lameness issues also may be mentioned. Forelimb lameness can be a result of thoracic problems because the attachment of the scapula to the thoracic spine causes painful mobility in the thoracic vertebrae.[4,14,17] A reduced stride length of a hindlimb or lack of propulsion can be caused by pain in the lumbosacral region,[9,10,13,17] and a lowered hip can be a sign of back pain as well as an indication of hindlimb lameness.

Clinical Examination

Clinical examination of the horse is performed as with any lameness case, with more emphasis on observation of lateral bending in walking serpentines, and circles at the walk, trot and canter. The quality of the walk (4-beat) and canter (3-beat) can give essential information about location of a lesion within the spine due to the specific loads that are generated by these gaits to specific parts of the spine (Table 6.1).

In the walk and trot in hand on a straight line, observation of the gait and the position of the hindlimbs in relation to the front limbs and the position of the tail can assist in the assessing for the presence and location of back pain. For example, do the hindlimbs track the forelimbs and are the haunches more to one side? Because there is more mobility of the lumbosacral spine in the canter, lumbosacral pain is more obvious at this gait. By contrast, thoracic pain appears more as stiffness in the trot and resistance to going downhill, or in making downward transitions from canter to trot or trot to walk. More detailed signs and the locations they may identify are presented in Table 6.2.

Information gleaned from palpation of the back can be confusing. Most horses with any kind of back pain exhibit some muscle tension in the epaxial muscles. It is nearly impossible to differentiate between muscle tension caused by guarding spinal structures and primary muscle tension due to muscle problems. See the section on muscle diseases in Chapter 7.

Sensitivity to touch or pressure is another symptom that can be difficult to interpret. Some horses initially show a defensive reaction to every contact with their back, even when there is no pathological condition present. To make an initial differentiation, touch or apply pressure very gently and when the horse resists, maintain it and wait for the initial reaction to fade. In behavioral issues, when the pressure persists without correction or change, quite often the initial resistance will diminish. With pain, the same reaction will be shown over and over again.

Manual compression of the muscles in the withers area can give information about sensitivity of this region, which can indicate saddle fit issues (see the section on saddle fit in Chapter 10), as can spots of white hairs in this region. Bald spots or spots with damaged hairs are another indication of poor saddle fit as a cause for back pain and related muscle tension.

Specific Tests

Passive mobility tests should be performed to assess the mobility of the spine and the range of motion within every part of the spine.[19] Symmetry of range of motion is very important because muscle tension, which is a manifestation of pain, impedes symmetrical movement.[18] Gentle bending of the neck to the left and right, with one hand of the examiner on the head of the horse and the other fixing a specific cervical vertebra, provides information about the intervertebral mobility as well as the range of motion to the left and the right (Figure 6.1). A carrot or other palatable treat used to tempt the horse to move its head can indicate the willingness of the horse to bend its neck laterally and dorsoventrally.

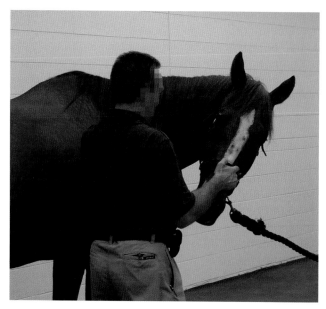

Figure 6.1. Flexion of the neck to the right. The left hand of the examiner is at C6 while the right hand gently asks for lateral motion.

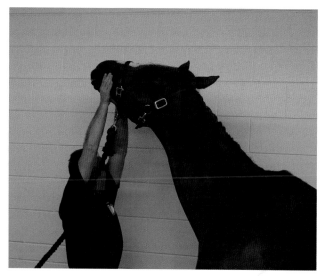

Figure 6.2. Extension of the neck. The examiner lifts the head of the horse, evaluating the extent of stretching of the neck and symmetry of the cervical vertebrae in a ventral aspect.

Lifting the head allows assessment of the amount of dorsiflexion as well as the symmetry of the muscles and location of anatomical landmarks on the ventral aspect of the neck (Figure 6.2).

In the thorax, a similar manipulation (pulling on the tail with one hand and placing the other arm as a fulcrum at an individual horizontal process of a specific vertebra) provides information about the range of motion and intervertebral mobility in the lateral plane (Figure 6.3). Palpation of the withers, dorsal processes of the thoracic vertebrae, and associated muscles indicate pain in this region that is very susceptible to discomfort caused by poor saddle fit. Triggering the

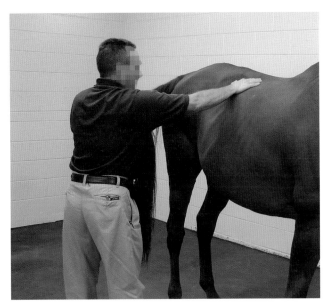

Figure 6.3. Lateroflexion of the caudal thoracic spine. The examiner pulls on the tail with the left hand to gain lateral excursion of the spine, while the right hand functions as a fulcrum on the transverse process of T17 so the mobility between T17 and the more caudal spine can be evaluated.

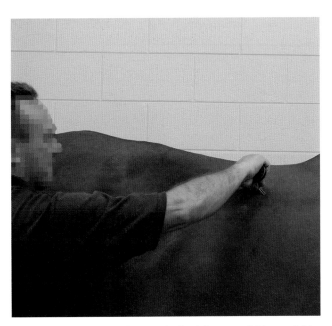

Figure 6.4. Moving a key on the back from cranial to caudal in a paramedian line checks for the reflectory movement of the horse with dorsoflexion and some lateroflexion.

dorsiflexion reflex by pressure with a pen in a paramedian motion from cranial to caudal (Figure 6.4) gives information about dorsal mobility in the thoracolumbar spine as well as symmetry in these reflexes. The same technique applied to the ventral aspect of the thorax and abdomen provides information about ventral mobility. An evasive reflex to these procedures is normal and absence of such reflexes can be neurological in

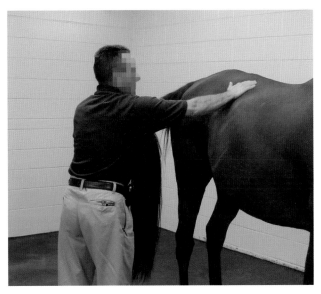

Figure 6.5. Lateroflexion of the lumbar spine, as in Figure 6.3, now with the hand as a fulcrum on the transverse process of L3.

origin (lack of skin sensation) or a consequence of pain that occurs when the spine is in motion.

Specific manipulation techniques in the lumbosacral region can yield information about the mobility of the spine. Lateroflexion of the lumbosacral spine and rotation of the lumbar spine can be tested by pulling intermittently on the tail base with one hand while fixing the spine at the tuber coxae with the other "fulcrum" hand (Figure 6.5). Information is obtained about the mobility of individual intervertebral regions by moving the fulcrum hand more cranially to the lateral process of each lumbar vertebra. Introducing a wavelike motion in the spine by gentle but powerful manipulation between tail base (pulling) and the tuber coxae facilitates evaluation of tension in all epaxial muscles. This wave can be observed to move over the spine to the head in a horse with relaxed muscles. Abruptly halted motion of this induced wave is a good indicator of higher muscle tension in that part of the spine.

Specific tests to localize pain include manual pressure on the individual dorsal processes of the thoracic and lumbar vertebrae (Figure 6.6) and on the tuber sacrale (Figure 6.7), as well as testing for sacroiliac pain by lateral manipulation of the pelvis. The latter provocation test introduces rotation and friction in the sacroiliac joints, so a positive response to the test is indicative for sacroiliac pain. The tests are executed with one hand on the tuber coxae and the other hand on the tuber ischium to manipulate the pelvis in cranial, ventral, dorsal, and caudal directions to cause friction and rotation in the sacroiliac and lumbosacral regions (Figures 6.8 and 6.9). Finally, an inspection of the entire spine can be performed by standing on a step stool to gain a higher position to evaluate the spine and potential deviations that have not been noticed previously.

PRIMARY VS. SECONDARY BACK PAIN

A common topic in equine back pain discussions is whether the back pain is primary, caused by a primary

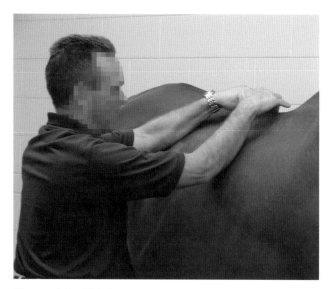

Figure 6.6. Digital pressure on the dorsal process of T16. Both index fingers are located on the dorsal process with strong downward pressure to place load on the intervertebral ligament, facet joints, and the intervertebral disc.

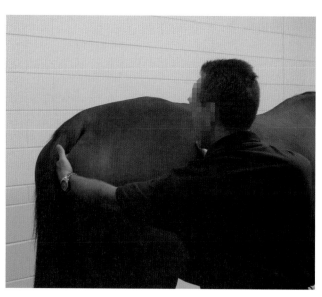

Figure 6.8. Provocation test for sacroiliac joint pain. The left hand of the examiner is on the right tuber ischium and the right hand is on the tuber coxae, making rocking motion in the cranial direction.

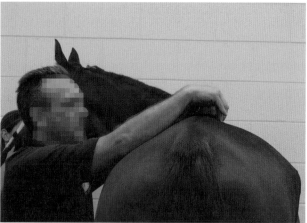

Figure 6.7. Digital pressure on the right tuber sacrale. Pressure is placed downward and slightly to the median so pressure is placed on the bone, dorsal sacral ligaments, and sacroiliac joint.

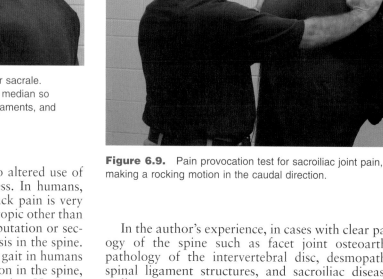

Figure 6.9. Pain provocation test for sacroiliac joint pain, making a rocking motion in the caudal direction.

lesion in the spine, or secondary, due to altered use of the spine that stems from limb lameness. In humans, contrary to the belief that secondary back pain is very common, there is little literature on this topic other than some papers on the influence of leg amputation or secondary back pain due to tumor metastasis in the spine. One can assume that specific changes in gait in humans can eventually lead to (over)compensation in the spine, resulting in secondary pathology in the spine. However this requires a considerable duration of time to occur because this phenomenon typically presents in people in their 50s. One could question whether secondary pathology of the spine has time to develop in horses, since most performance horses are much younger, between 4 and 16 years of age.

In the author's experience, in cases with clear pathology of the spine such as facet joint osteoarthritis, pathology of the intervertebral disc, desmopathy of spinal ligament structures, and sacroiliac disease, as well as cases with fractures of spinal structures, very often in the history there is an incident that indicates significant trauma to the spine, resulting in later symptoms of back pain. In the author's opinion, these are clear cases of primary back pain. When the pathology is located more in the soft tissues of the spine, with strain of spinal ligamentous structures or muscles, it is more difficult to assess whether this is primary or secondary back pain.

Complete physical examination is necessary to evaluate the complete condition of the horse and assess potential sources of coexisting limb lameness (primary or secondary). In the author's experience, when no clear pathology is found in the spinal structures and coexisting limb lameness is present, back pain is secondary. When the coexisting limb lameness is treated, the accompanying back pain diminishes or dissolves.

References

1. Bromiley MW. Physical therapy for the equine back. Vet Clin NA Equine Pract 1999:15:223–246.
2. Cauvin E. Assessment of back pain in horses. Equine Practice 1997;19:522–533.
3. Denoix JM. Ultrasonographic evaluation of back lesions. Vet Clin NA Equine Pract 1999;15:131–159.
4. Denoix JM, Audigie F. The neck and back. In Equine Locomotion. Back W, Clayton HM, eds. W.B. Saunders, London, 2001; 167–191.
5. Denoix JM. Spinal biomechanics and functional anatomy. Vet Clin NA Equine Pract 1999;15:27–60.
6. Faber M. Basic three-dimensional kinematics of the vertebral column of horses walking on a treadmill. In Kinematics of the equine back during locomotion. PhD Thesis, Utrecht, 2001.
7. Faber M. Basic three-dimensional kinematics of the vertebral column of horses trotting on a treadmill. In Kinematics of the equine back during locomotion. PhD Thesis, Utrecht, 2001.
8. Faber M. Basic three-dimensional kinematics of the vertebral column of horses cantering on a treadmill. In Kinematics of the equine back during locomotion. PhD Thesis, Utrecht, 2001.
9. Haussler KK, Stover SM. Stress fractures of the vertebral lamina and pelvis in Thoroughbred racehorses. Equine Vet J 1998; 30:374–381.
10. Haussler KK, Stover SM, Willits NH. Pathologic changes in the lumbosacral vertebrae and pelvis in Thoroughbred racehorses. Am J Vet Res 1999;60:143–163.
11. Haussler KK. Osseous Spinal Pathology. Vet Clin NA Equine Pract 1999:15:103–111.
12. Haussler KK. Anatomy of the thoracolumbar vertebral region. Vet Clin NA Equine Pract 1999;15:13–26.
13. Jeffcott LB. Diagnosis of back problems in the horse. Compendium Cont Ed 1981;3:134.
14. Jeffcott LB. Disorders of the thoracolumbar spine of the horse—A survey of 443 cases. Eq Vet J 1980;12:197.
15. Jeffcott LB. Guidelines for the diagnosis and treatment of back problems in horses. Proceedings Am Assoc Equine Pract 1980; 26:381.
16. Jeffcott LB. Historical perspective and clinical indications. Vet Clin NA Equine Pract 1999;15:1–12.
17. Jeffcott LB. Effects of induced back pain on gait and performance of trotting horses. Equine Vet J 1982;14:129.
18. Licka T, Peham C. An objective method for evaluating the flexibility of the back of standing horses. Equine Vet J 1998, 30:412–415.
19. Ridgeway K, Harman J. Equine back rehabilitation. Vet Clin NA Equine Pract 1999;15:263–280.
20. van Wessum R. Evaluation of back pain by clinical examination. In Current Therapy in Equine Medicine, 6th ed. Robinson NE, Sprayberry KA, eds. Saunders, St. Louis, 2009;469–473.

THE PELVIS

FRACTURES OF THE PELVIS

Fractures of the pelvis are rather uncommon, ranging from 0.9% to 4.4% of all equine lameness cases.[11] Most reports in the literature are from before 2000, and in the last few years no real new information about treatment of pelvic fractures has emerged. Therefore, the emphasis in this chapter is given to diagnosis and imaging modalities.

Diagnosis of pelvic fractures can be a challenge in practice. In most cases, therapy focuses on stall confinement and adjuvant therapy rather than invasive surgery.[12,19] However, for prognosis it is important for the veterinarian to have a confirmed diagnosis. Some pelvic fractures have a favorable prognosis for return to an athletic career; others only guarantee a breeding career. Some fractures are accompanied by severe pain and invalidation of the animal; therefore, euthanasia is a favorable option.

Etiology

Most pelvic fractures are traumatic fractures; common causes include falling, slipping, fighting, and accidents with cars or in trailers. The history of a sudden onset of the lameness is usually a clear indication of a traumatic event. Often the event is observed, but simply finding the horse very lame in the field is a common finding in the history.

However, ilial wing fractures are an example of common stress fractures caused by repetitive overloading of certain portions of the pelvis. These occur in young, immature Thoroughbred racehorses. The lameness is usually less severe with a more gradual onset than that of horses with a traumatic injury.[2–4,6,13,16,17,22]

Clinical Examination and Signs

Clinical examination of the horse with a suspected pelvic fracture starts with a complete inspection of the horse, emphasizing symmetry of the hindquarters. Important observations include muscle atrophy, position of the tuber sacrales, limb length, and pelvic height (height of the tuber coxae). The tuber coxae height is easier to determine when standing behind the horse and palpating both tuber coxae, left and right, to exactly determine their position. For accurate inspection, the horse should be taken out of its stall and made to stand completely square on a firm, level surface. This may be difficult when the horse is severely lame.

Particular attention should be paid to limb position; an abnormally straight limb may reflect luxation of the coxofemoral joint and secondary upward fixation of the patella. Toe-out, hock-in position is more often found with pelvic fractures. The muscles of the lumbar and pelvic regions should be assessed carefully to identify abnormal muscle tension and pain as well as swelling or hematoma. Firm manual or digital pressure on bony prominences such as the tuber sacrale, tuber coxae and tuber ischium should be applied to identify pain or defensive reactions. Keeping contact with the hand on these bony prominences when the horse is asked to walk can assist in detecting crepitation or abnormal (and asymmetrical) motion of the pelvic region. Auscultation during motion also can reveal crepitation.

Careful examination of the pelvic canal per rectum is indicated to asses the aorta and iliac arteries; psoas muscles; and the caudal aspect of the ilial shaft, pubis, and ischium. Some authors advocate rectal examination while the horse is rocked or even walked, but this can be dangerous for the horse (risk for rectal tear) and examiner (when horse acts up or falls). This author does not recommend such examination.

Most horses with pelvic fractures have a significant lameness, depending on the duration of the fracture. Most are lame at the walk, and gluteal muscle atrophy tends to occur more quickly in horses with pelvic fractures than with other severe lameness conditions of the hindlimb. Horses often stand with the affected limb outwardly rotated (toe-out, hock-in stance), and often lean away from the affected limb. Pelvic asymmetry, muscle atrophy, and pain and crepitus on manipulation of the pelvis are common clinical findings. The exceptions are horses with stress-type fractures or other types of non-displaced fractures.

Diagnosis

Diagnostic imaging involves radiography, ultrasonography, and scintigraphy. Particularly when the horse is reluctant to move and transportation to the clinic is difficult or dangerous, on-site imaging is needed to make decisions about first aid and follow-up examination. Standing radiography with mobile equipment is possible[5,14,17] but does not always give a final diagnosis. More complete radiography in dorsal recumbency under general anesthesia may be needed, with all of its associated risks during recovery.

Ultrasonography can be performed on site and is capable of imaging ilial wing fractures, ilial shaft fractures, and acetabular fractures with percutaneous probe placement. Transrectal ultrasonography can be used to diagnose acetabular and pubis fractures.[1,9,17,22] Due to the risks associated with radiography under general anesthesia and the potential for ultrasonography to confirm a tentative diagnosis of pelvic fracture, radiography has fallen out of favor as the first choice of imaging of horses suspected of having a pelvic fracture, in the author's opinion.[3,8] Ultrasonography has the advantage of not adding to the risks associated with transport when the horse must be taken to a facility for radiography. Most portable ultrasound equipment, in the hands of skilled clinicians, can confirm the diagnosis of pelvic fracture (PA Pease and MB Whitcomb, personal communications). When radiography is available at the location where the horse is presented for evaluation, it is still very useful, especially when the procedure can be performed in the standing horse.

On-site Management

Because of their traumatic origin, many of the pelvic fractures occur during a work-out, in competition, in a race, or in the pasture. With the more serious injuries, such as ilial shaft and acetabular fractures, the horse may be down or impossible to move. In these cases it is good practice to establish a preliminary diagnosis with a thorough clinical exam, which should at least include a rectal and/or vaginal exam. Crepitation and major swelling in the pelvic region at least can provide a severe suspicion for pelvic fractures, but not confirmation. Transportation to a clinical facility to perform more diagnostics can be contraindicated or at least undesirable. In the field, ultrasonography can be a perfect technique to confirm the diagnosis of a pelvic fracture and make transportation unnecessary.[1,9,17,22]

Treatment and Prognosis of Pelvis Fractures

Treatment for pelvic fractures is conservative, including with anti-inflammatory medication (NSAIDs).[3,11,18,19,21,23] Strict stall rest for at least 30 days is most important. Some clinicians advocate tying the horse in its stall for periods of up to 30 to 60 days to minimize the chance of a complete fracture when getting up. In general, any horse will lie down after some time, tied or untied. Therefore, tying the horse may increase the risk of other injuries associated with trying to lie down or getting up when tied. Furthermore, stress levels of horses that are tied up, or the public opinion about the possible stress this procedure can evoke in the horse, decrease the acceptability of this procedure.

Normal bone healing of pelvic fractures takes 2 to 3 months, so motion must at least be restricted during this period. Brief periods of hand-walking (with the horse under control) can assist in keeping muscle tension and development more progressive than when complete stall rest is prescribed. The use of hot walkers or treadmills must be avoided, because there is no permanent control with these types of rehabilitation equipment. Use of this equipment risks the chance of a brief moment of joy or fear, in which the horse can damage itself severely. Ultrasonographic examination can be a good technique to monitor healing and determine when to increase the workload.[1,22]

It is important to realize that complete healing of pelvic fractures (e.g., tuber coxae or tuber ischium fractures) and the adaptation of the adjacent structures to a changed anatomical conformation can take several months to a year. Sometimes it is possible after this period to give a final prognosis for the return to an athletic career. It is a good practice to communicate this at an early stage with the owner and/or trainer so they are aware that the final outcome after such a long period of treatment and rehabilitation may be unfulfilling.

SPECIFIC TYPES OF PELVIC FRACTURES

Ilial Wing Fractures

Ilial wing fractures are most commonly found in the young Thoroughbred racehorse, age 1 to 2.5 years, with an immature skeleton. Lameness is sudden in onset, and can vary in severity from 2 to 5 on a scale of 5, according to the AAEP grading scale. The horse has the tendency to plait with the hindlimbs or cross over the hindlimbs in a trot. The severity of the lameness diminishes or decreases in 24 to 48 hours. Profound muscle atrophy can occur within the first 2 weeks after injury, which can give the horse a very asymmetric appearance when the injury is unilateral. When a complete fracture is present, the ipsilateral tuber sacrale can be displaced. Manual pressure on the tuber sacrale (see Clinical Examination, above) can be painful, as when sacroiliac injuries are present (see the section on the sacroiliac region, below).

The major risk in these cases is when an initial incomplete fracture extends to a complete fracture. When this is the case bilaterally, the horse can become recumbent with the chance for adjacent severe neurological damage or a catastrophic injury during work-out or race. Therefore, correct diagnosis is important.[19,20,23]

Ultrasonography is the first choice for a diagnosis in a practical field situation.[1,9,17,22] With a 3.5–5 MHz transducer, nearly all commonly available ultrasound equipment will facilitate imaging of the ilial wing. Preparation of the imaging site is achieved by moisturizing the skin and coating it with alcohol. A better image can be obtained by clipping the coat before imaging. Following the contour of the ilial wing with the probe in a craniocaudal position and moving the probe from tuber sacrale out to the tuber coxae provides an outline figure of the ilial wing, and step-like changes can be observed at the fracture site (Figure 6.10).

Scintigraphy is very useful for evaluating incomplete stress fractures (Figure 6.11) as well as evaluating the adjacent structures of the tuber sacrales and sacroiliac joints for involvement. In most cases, scintigraphy is the most sensitive technique 5 to 10 days after initial injury.[7,8,14] Prognosis in most cases is good for a full recovery to an athletic career when no involvement of the sacroiliac joint(s) is present. When sacroiliac joint involvement is present and not diagnosed correctly, osteoarthritis of the sacroiliac joint(s) can be career limiting at a later stage. See the sacroiliac region section.

Tuber Coxae Fractures

Tuber coxae fractures are nearly always associated with trauma, such as running into a door post or fence, fighting, and kicking, and trailer accidents.[11] In cases of high-energy impact to the tuber coxae (e.g., high-speed collisions), adjacent structures in the sacroiliac region may be involved and require attention later. See the sacroiliac region section. Tuber coxae fractures are associated with moderate to severe lameness that decreases to mild lameness in 24 to 48 hours.

These fractures are fairly easy to recognize because the contour of the tuber coxae is changed (Figures 6.12 and 6.13). The fractured portion moves cranioventrally due to traction of the internal abdominal oblique muscle. The edges of the remainder of the tuber coxae are palpable through the skin. In rare cases the sharp edges of the ilium can penetrate the skin and cause a fresh laceration. In a later stage, sequestration can

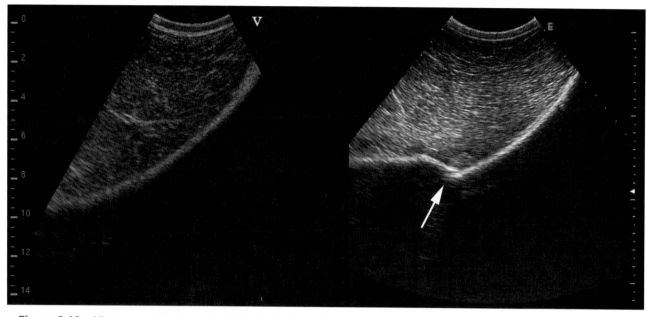

Figure 6.10. Ultrasonographic image of an ilial wing fracture. Left, the sonogram of a normal ilial wing. Right, an ilial wing fracture (arrow). (Courtesy of Dr. Mary Beth Withcomb.)

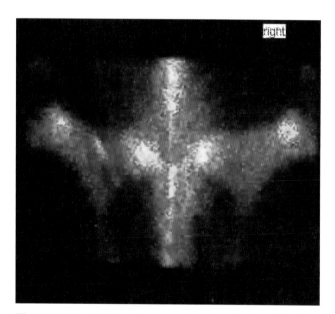

Figure 6.11. Scintigraphy image of a stress fracture of the left ilial wing. Increased radiopharmaceutical uptake (IRU) in the left ilial wing, as well as IRU at both tuber sacrales and the right tuber coxae, is indicative for trauma to these structures.

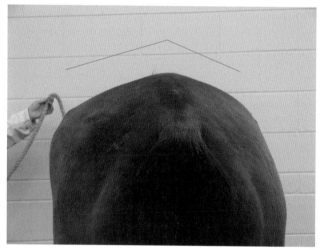

Figure 6.12. Fracture of a large part of the right tuber coxae. Note the shorter distance between the right tuber sacrale and tuber coxae compared with this distance on the left.

cause draining tracts or nonhealing wounds and the sequestrum must be removed.

Ultrasonographic examination is again the first choice for imaging, because it can show the irregular bone edge of the ilium and the displaced part of the tuber coxae (Figure 6.14).[1] Ultrasonography can identify a draining tract when present, and provide a guide to the sequestrum. Radiography in this region can be disappointing; however, sometimes a mediolateral oblique projection can show the fragmentation of the tuber coxae.[5,13,14,19] A recent study described a dorsome-dial-centrolateral 50° oblique radiographic view in the standing horse as being very helpful[5].

Scintigraphy is a very sensitive technique to show involvement of the tuber coxae,[8,14] but is unnecessary in most cases, at least in the initial diagnostic procedure. Later, when sacroiliac problems are suspected due to the initial trauma, scintigraphy is the first choice for imaging. The prognosis is favorable in most cases. A fibrotic and functional union between the dislocated fragment and the adjacent structures facilitate recovery to full athletic performance. In a recent study, up to 93% of the horses returned to athletic performance.[5] For higher level dressage, however, prognosis is less favorable due to the asymmetric position of the pelvic region. The horse appears to be asymmetrical and gives

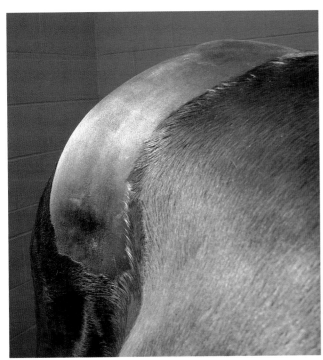
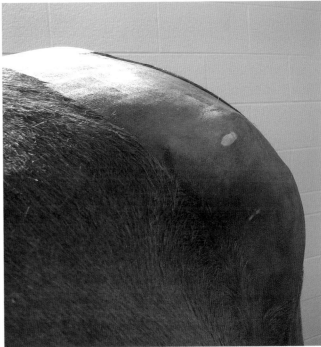

Figure 6.13. Images of the horse in Figure 6.12, right and left side views. Note the rounded aspect of the right tuber coxae and the atrophy of the quadriceps muscles.

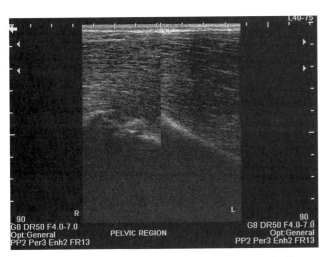

Figure 6.14. Ultrasound image of the same horse as in Figure 6.13. Note the disrupted contour of the iliac wing just medial to the normal position of the right tuber coxae.

the judge the impression that it cannot do certain exercises. Some minor gait asymmetry (altered motion pattern of the hindlimb(s) and slight change in stride length and path) can affect scores at the higher levels of dressage competitions, when judging is more strict and sensitive to small gait irregularities.

Fractures of the Pubis and Ischium

Isolated fractures to the pubis and ischium are rare. In cases of severe trauma to the pelvic region with high-energy impact (e.g., fall, car accident) fractures to these

structures can be complementary to fractures of other pelvic structures. When they are isolated fractures, they often cause unilateral hindlimb lameness combined with clear swelling of the thigh area. After a few days, the swelling can progress downward due to gravity and cause remarkable swelling around the stifle, femur, or hock.

This descending swelling can lead the examiner away from the initial injury and place suspicion at the stifle or hock as being the initial injury site[7]. With palpation it is often quite difficult to feel crepitation because of the muscle spasm that accompanies the injury. The injury is very painful, and muscle spasm is very common, sometimes leading to an asymmetric position of the tail or even the entire pelvic region. Sweating can be noticed, sometimes in localized patches, especially when nerve involvement is apparent.

Scintigraphy can be used to diagnose these type of fractures (Figure 6.15). Again, this technique is very sensitive, but should be done 1 to 2 weeks after the initial trauma. Ultrasonography can be used to identify displaced fragments of the tuber Ischium (Figure 6.16), often after scintigraphy has identified the region of interest. Prognosis for isolated fractures of the tuber ischium is favorable for a return to an athletic career. The exception is higher level dressage, as mentioned above in the tuber coxae fractures section, for the same reasons.

Ilial Shaft Fractures

Ilial shaft fractures are associated with nonweight-bearing lameness.[18] The horse is extremely painful, with sweating, and has severe muscle spasms. When the fracture ends of the ilial shaft damage the internal iliac

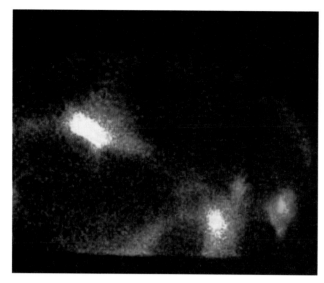

Figure 6.15. Lateral scintigraphy image of the hindquarters. Increased uptake is visible in the region of the tuber ischium.

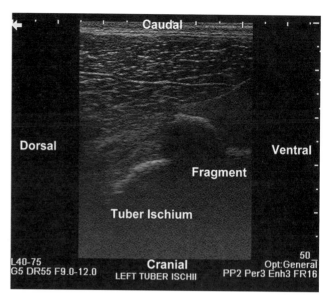

Figure 6.16. Ultrasound image of the tuber ischium of the horse in Figure 6.15. A large fragment that is avulsed from the tuber ischium is visible and is displaced ventrally. Note the attached muscle pulling it ventrally.

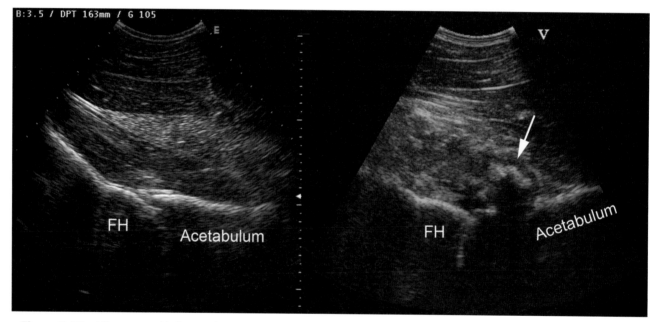

Figure 6.17. Ultrasonographic image of an acetabular fracture. At the left is a normal image, whereas a fracture of the acetabulum (arrow) can be seen on the right. FH = femoral head. (Courtesy of Dr. Mary Beth Whitcomb.)

artery, shock and exsanguination can occur. When the fracture is complete, the tuber coxae will be asymmetric and the affected limb will appear to be shorter. Rectal or vaginal examination reveals a possible hematoma and crepitation. Many of these fractures are multiple fractures that involve the pubis, ischium, and ilium. Prognosis is unfavorable and often euthanasia is performed.

Acetabular Fractures

Acetabular fractures are traumatic in origin (e.g., falling, slipping, trailering accidents) and very painful. In most cases the horse is nonweight-bearing lame and reluctant to move at all. Some horses are found nonweight-bearing standing in the pasture or paddock without any clear signs of the origin of the trauma. Crepitation can be found with a rectal or vaginal examination, especially when the horse is rocked a bit during the examination. Profound swelling can also be felt with the rectal or vaginal examination. Sometimes swelling is noticeable around the stifle and thigh area. Ultrasonography[1,22] (transcutaneously or transrectally) can assist in the diagnosis when there is a complete fracture (Figure 6.17). Radiography under anesthesia

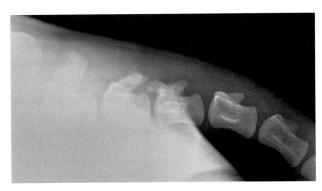

Figure 6.18. Radiograph of a horse with bone proliferation between the coccygeal vertebrae 1 and 2 at the dorsal aspect as the result of an avulsion fracture of the intervertebral ligament.

can confirm acetabular fractures, but adds the challenge of safe recovery afterward. Scintigraphy is the most sensitive technique, but should be performed at least 7 to 10 days after the initial cause; otherwise, the chance of false negative findings is great. Prognosis is unfavorable because of the chance of development of osteoarthritis of the coxofemoral joint, leading to permanent and progressing lameness.[17]

Fractures of the Sacrum and Coccygeal Vertebrae

Fractures of the sacral bone (primarily dorsal processes) or coccygeal vertebrae are rare but can cause lameness. When the proximal coccygeal vertebrae are involved, the normal locomotion pattern at the walk (the snake-like motion) and the canter can be influenced by pain in this region. Backing up (lowering the tail region) may be painful and the horse may be reluctant or completely refuse to back up. Often this is regarded by the owner as a dominancy problem more than a physical issue (many disciplines use backing as an obedience-test). Clinical examination can show enlargement of the soft tissues in the sacral or coccygeal region, and passive mobility can be painful. Radiography can be used to image the fracture site when coccygeal vertebrae are involved (Figure 6.18), as can a lateral image for sacral dorsal process fractures. Ultrasonography is also a good tool for imaging this region, but scintigraphy is the most sensitive.

Treatment can focus on anti-inflammatory therapy and reducing the workload. When nerves are involved, caudal epidural steroid administration has been used to treat this condition successfully.[12] Methylprednisolone acetate (200 mg) mixed with 10 to 20 ml of saline can be used to perform an epidural injection. Surgery may be indicated when fracture fragments are displaced or sequestration occurs. The prognosis is generally good for a return to athletic performance. Sometimes coccygeal fractures are a coincidental finding during a prepurchase examination, because they do not cause clinical symptoms.

References

1. Almanza A, Whitcomb MB. Ultrasonographic diagnosis of pelvic fractures in 28 horses. Proceedings Am Assoc Equine Pract 2003;50–54.
2. Bathe AP. 245 fractures in Thoroughbred racehorses: results of a 2-year prospective study, Proceedings Am Assoc Equine Pract 1994;40:174.
3. Brown K. Pelvic Fractures. In Current Therapy in Equine Medicine, 6th ed. Robinson E, Sprayberry KA, eds. Saunders, Philadelphia, 2008;488,491.
4. Carrier TK, Estberg L, Stover SM, et al. Association between long periods without high-speed workouts and risk of complete humeral or pelvic fracture in Thoroughbred racehorses: 54 cases (1991–1994). J Am Vet Med Assoc 1998;212:1582–1587.
5. Dabareiner RM, Cole CC. Fractures of the tuber coxae of the ilium in horses: 29 cases (1996–2007). J Am Vet Med Assoc 2009;243:1303–1307.
6. Ducharme NG. Pelvic fracture and coxofemoral luxation. Equine Fracture Repair. In Nixon AJ, ed. WB Saunders Co., Philadelphia, 1996;295–298.
7. Dyson SJ. Pelvic Injuries in the Non-Racehorse. In Diagnosis and Management of Lameness in the Horse. Ross MW, Dyson SJ, eds. Saunders, Philadelphia, 2003;491.
8. Geburek F, Rotting AK, Stadler PM. Comparison of the diagnostic value of ultrasonography and standing radiography for pelvic–femoral disorders in horses. Vet Surg 2009;38:307–310.
9. Geissbuhler U, Busato A, Ueltschi G. Abnormal bone scan findings of the equine ischial tuberosity and third trochanter. Vet Rad and Ultrasound 1998;39:572–577.
10. Goodrich LR, Werpy NM, Armentrout A. How to ultrasound the normal pelvis for aiding diagnosis of pelvic fractures using rectal and transcutaneous ultrasound examination. Proceedings Am Assoc Equine Pract 2006;609–612.
11. Haussler KK, Stover SM. Stress fractures of the vertebral lamina and pelvis in Thoroughbred racehorses. Equine Vet J 1998; 30:374–381.
12. Hendrickson DA. Fractures of the Pelvis. In Adam's Lameness in Horses, 5th ed. Stashak TS, ed. Lippincott Williams and Wilkins, Philadelphia, 2002;1045–1049.
13. Little C, Hilbert B. Pelvic fractures in horses: 19 cases (1974–1984). J Am Vet Med Assoc 1987;190:1203–1206.
14. May SA, Patterson LJ, Peacock PJ, et al. Radiographic technique for the pelvis in the standing horse. Equine Vet J 1991; 23:312–314.
15. Pilsworth RC, Holmes MA, Sheperd M. An improved method for the scintigraphic detection of acute bone damage to the equine pelvis by probe point counting. Vet Rec 1993;133:490–495.
16. Pilsworth RC, Sheperd M, Herinckx BMB, et al. Fracture of the wing of the ilium, adjacent to the sacroiliac joint, in Thoroughbred racehorses. Equine Vet J 1994;26:94–99.
17. Pilsworth RC. Diagnosis and management of pelvic fractures in the Thoroughbred racehorse. In Diagnosis and Management of Lameness in the Horse, Ross MW, Dyson SJ, eds. Saunders, Philadelphia, 2003;484,490.
18. Reef VB. Diagnosis of pelvic fractures in horses using ultrasonography. Vet Rad 1992;33:121.
19. Richardson DW. The femur and pelvis. In Equine Surgery, 2nd ed. Auer JA, Stick J, eds. WB Saunders, Philadelphia, 1999; 881–886.
20. Rutkowsi JA, Richardson DW. The diagnosis and treatment of pelvic fractures in horses. Proceedings Am Assoc Equine Pract 1987;33:701–705.
21. Rutkowski JA, Richardson DW. A retrospective study of 100 pelvic fractures in horses. Equine Vet J 1989;21:256–259.
22. Shepherd MC, Pilsworth RC, Hopes R, et al. Clinical signs, diagnosis, management and outcome of complete and incomplete fracture to the ilium: A review of 20 cases. Proceedings Am Assoc Equine Pract 1994;40:177–180.
23. Shepherd MC, Pilsworth RC. The use of ultrasound in the diagnosis of pelvic fractures. Equine Vet Educ 1994;6:223.
24. Stashak TS. Fractures of the pelvis. In Adams' Lameness in Horses, 4th ed. Stashak TS, ed. Lea and Feibiger, Philadelphia, 1987;752–753.

THROMBOSIS OF THE CAUDAL AORTA OR THE ILIAC ARTERIES

Etiology

Thrombus formation in arteries of the limbs can cause blood supply interruption. Specific locations for these thrombi are the caudal aorta, iliac arteries, femoral artery in the hindlimb, and very rarely the brachial artery in the front limb. Circulatory problems in the muscles (and later in all tissues) can cause pain, resulting in lameness. The etiology has been described as being caused by the migrating larva of *Strongylus vulgaris*, but it is not clear why only these locations are affected. It is more likely that any damage to the intima of the blood vessels can cause a thrombus to form.

Clinical Signs and Diagnosis

This lameness is specific in that it occurs after or during work, is sudden in onset, and can be very severe (grade 3 to 5 of 5), but can diminish or disappear within minutes to hours after ceasing work. Because of the severe pain, horses may sweat, show anxiety, and be very restless, which can make the condition look like azoturia or even colic. Blood chemistry and a clinical work-up for colic are negative.[3,4]

Clinical examination shows lower perfusion in the affected limb, lower temperature (thermography can be useful in these cases), and absence or lower pressure of arterial pulse. On the nonaffected limb, the veins can show clearly while they are indistinct on the affected limb. Ultrasonography can show lower blood flow in the blood vessels of the affected limb (using Doppler).[6] With transrectal ultrasonography it is sometimes possible to find the thrombus and measure its size,[8] but with a rectal examination one can determine the decrease or absence of arterial pulse or fremitus in the iliac arteries.

Treatment and Prognosis

Treatment is focused on medication: anticoagulants (Heparin 100 IU/kg sc SID, aspirin 5 to 10 mg/kg po SID, Phenprocoumon 0.08 to 0.16 mg/kg IV initial bolus, gradually reduced), nonsteroidal anti-inflammatory drugs, and antimicrobial drugs (Metronidazole 25 mg/kg PO BID and thiabendazole 4g/45 kg PO once weekly for 3 weeks or Ivermectin or Moxydectin) to act against *Strongylus vulgaris* larvae when they are expected to be the cause.[4]

Successful surgical removal of the thrombus has been performed with a thrombectomy catheter,[2] but this requires that the exact location of the thrombus be determined by ultrasonography or scintigraphy.[1,5,7] Prognosis for thrombosis of the aorta and the iliac arteries is guarded, especially when the underlying cause is not known.

References

1. Boswell J, Marr C, Cauvin E, et al. The use of scintigraphy in the diagnosis of aorto-iliac thrombosis in a horse. Equine Vet J 1999;31:537.
2. Brama PAJ, Rijkenhuizen ABM, van Swieten HA, et al. Thrombosis of the aorta and the caudal arteries in the horse: additional diagnostics and a new surgical treatment. Vet Quart 1996;18(2): S85–S89.
3. Dyson SJ, Worth L. Aortoiliacofemoral thrombosis. In Current Therapy in Equine Medicine, 4th ed. Robinson N, Wilson MR, eds. WB Saunders, Philadelphia, 1997.
4. Hendrickson, DA. Thrombosis of the caudal aorta or iliac artery. In Adam's Lameness in Horses, 5th ed. Stashak TS, ed. Lippincott Williams and Wilkins, Philadelphia 2002;1044–1045.
5. Malton R. Aortoiliacofemoral thrombosis: First pass radionuclide angiography. In Equine Scintigraphy. Dyson SJ, Pilsworth RC, Twardock AR, et al., eds. Equine Vet J, Newmarket, 2003; 249–250.
6. Reef V, Roby K, Richardson DA, et al. Use of ultrasonography for the detection of aortic-iliac thrombosis in horses. J Am Vet Med Assoc 1987;190:286.
7. Ross M, Maxson A, Stacey V, et al. First-pass radionuclide angiography in the diagnosis of aortoiliac thromboembolism in a horse. Vet Radiol Ultrasound 1997;38:226.
8. Warmerdam E. Ultrasonography of the femoral artery in six normal horses and three horses with thrombosis. Vet Radiol Ultrasound 1998;39:137.

DISEASES OF THE SACROILIAC REGION

Diseases of the sacroiliac region are recognized more and more as a cause for low-grade lameness or lack of performance.[2,3,20] Recent studies show that the sacroiliac joint may not always be involved, but the soft tissue structures adjacent to the joints in this region can be the cause of sacroiliac disease.[18,21,22]

The skeletal structures involved in sacroiliac diseases include the pelvic bones and spine, especially the sacroiliac joints where the ventral aspect of the ilium and ilial wing come into close contact with the sacral bone. At this junction there are 2 synovial joints, 1 at the ilial facet with a thin layer of fibrocartilage and 1 at the sacral facet with hyaline cartilage (Figure 6.19).[10,12,13]

At the ventral aspect of the sacroiliac joint, support is provided by several ligamentous structures, the capsule of the joint itself, and a package of small fibrous ligaments known as the ventral sacral ligaments.[13] On the top of the pelvic bones, ligamentous structures, called the dorsal sacral ligaments, originate from the tuber sacrale. These include a long ligamentous branch, called the long part, that adheres to the fibrous structures of the pelvis (the sacrosciatic ligament), and a shorter portion, called the short part, that adheres to the sacral bone and the coccygeal vertebrae and ligaments (Figures 6.20 to 6.22). From the ventral aspect of the ilial wing, the interosseus sacroiliac ligament supports the sacroiliac joint (Figure 6.23).[10,13]

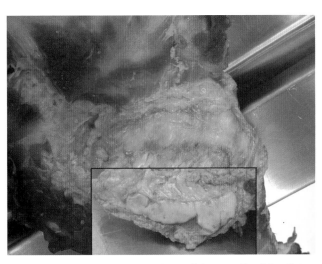

Figure 6.19. Anatomical specimen of the sacroiliac joint, ilial wing joint surface, and fibrocartilage. Insert: Sacral bone joint surface and hyaline cartilage.

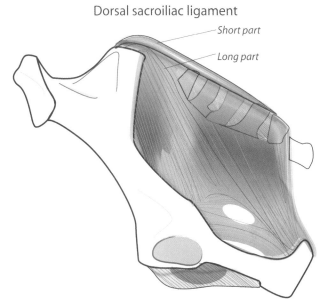

Dorsal sacroiliac ligament

Short part

Long part

Figure 6.20. Schematic drawing of the dorsal sacral ligament, including the short part and long part. (Drawing by Maggie Hoffman. Reprinted with permission from Sacroiliac Disease. In Current Therapy in Equine Medicine, 6th ed. Robinson NE, Sprayberry KA, eds. Elsevier, St. Louis, 2009; page 484.)

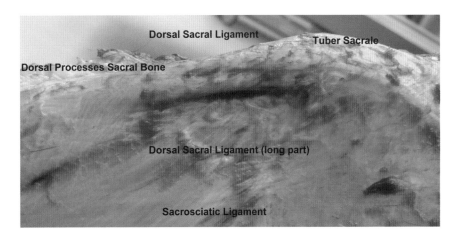

Dorsal Sacral Ligament

Tuber Sacrale

Dorsal Processes Sacral Bone

Dorsal Sacral Ligament (long part)

Sacrosciatic Ligament

Figure 6.21. Anatomical specimen of the dorsal sacral ligament, longitudinal view.

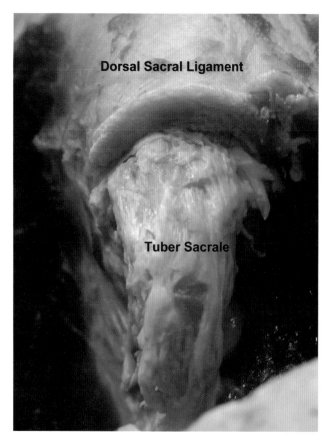

Figure 6.22. Anatomical specimen of the dorsal sacral ligament, cross-sectional view.

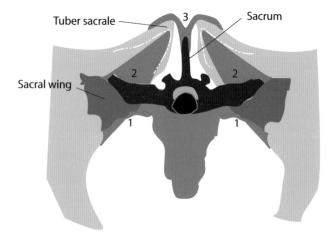

Figure 6.23. Schematic drawing of the sacroiliac joint region and the adjacent ligamentous structures, cranial aspect. 1 = ventral sacral ligaments, 2 = interosseus sacroiliac ligaments, 3 = dorsal sacral ligaments. (Drawing by Maggie Hofmann.)

ETIOLOGY

The muscles of the caudal spine and pelvis are major contributors to the stability of the sacroiliac region. On the dorsal aspect, the middle gluteal and superficial gluteal muscles and their fasciae support the sacroiliac region. On the caudal aspect are the semimembranosus and semitendinosus muscles, and at the ventral part of the pelvis are the psoas muscles, all of which are important contributors to stability. Under normal conditions, the muscles in this region maintain the mobility of the sacroiliac joints within their physical limits. However, when the muscles are not powerful enough to compete with the external forces that result from massive trauma due to falling, slipping, tipping over, etc., primary ligament damage and primary or secondary joint trauma can be sustained. Weakness in these muscles can be associated with sacroiliac injury. This weakness can have many causes, including fatigue from improper training techniques, overuse, and repetitive stress injuries that can occur in young horses not yet capable of the desired level of performance.[17]

The pelvic region is not a rigid structure, as was previously thought. Haussler, et al.[15] discovered that there is a small amount of deformation of the pelvic bone structures during the loading cycle in motion, and all of the involved structures (bone, ligamentous structures, and muscles) form a semiflexible complex to assist propulsion and transport this propulsion from the hindlimbs onto the spinal column.[11] These findings make it easier to understand the major impact of the dysfunction of the pelvis structures regarding locomotion and performance.

Three different types of injury occur in the sacroiliac region. In the author's experience, the most common seem to be those that cause damage to the dorsal sacral ligaments (the structure with the greatest span between tuber sacrale, sacral bone, and the sacrosciatic ligament, and the most potential motion between these structures). When trauma to the ligamentous structures of the sacroiliac region is more profound, the interosseus sacral ligaments and ventral sacral ligaments also can become damaged, with (sub)luxation of the sacroiliac joint(s) as a result. The last injury to the sacroiliac region occurs when damage to the sacroiliac joint is sustained with resultant osteoarthritis of the sacroiliac joint. In the author's experience, this only occurs in 5% to 10% of sacroiliac disease cases.[22]

CLINICAL SIGNS

Horses with sacroiliac pathology may come with a great diversity of owner/rider complaints, including reduced stride length in 1 or both hindlimbs, asymmetry of the hind end with 1 hip lowered, and sometimes obvious atrophy of the croup muscles. Owners report changes in both the rhythm and quality of the walk, with a more lateral walk seen especially during serpentines and circles, and a reduced stride length in 1 or both hindlimbs. There are no clear signs at the trot, perhaps just a little stiffness with slightly reduced propulsion and engagement. Downward transitions from canter to trot or from trot to walk can be of lower quality with a disturbance of the rhythm of the new gait in the first strides after the transition. Going downhill, even when the incline is small, can be difficult and a refusal to jump in hunting, cross country, or eventing can be a major complaint of the rider.[2,3]

The most remarkable signs of sacroiliac problems are usually shown when cantering. The pattern of the canter causes a very unilateral loading of the hindlimb and the sacroiliac region during the phase when the leading hindlimb (left hindlimb in left lead canter) carries the entire body load after the suspension phase. When sacroiliac lesions are present, the horse often alters its gait to relieve this unilateral loading by cantering more as a bunny hop in which there is less separation of footfalls of the hindlimbs. Horses with sacroiliac pathology also change leads or cross canter frequently. Due to this augmentation of signs in the canter, disciplines that are judged on the quality of the canter, for example, dressage and Western pleasure, or those that require a good quality canter for optimum performance, as in hunting, jumping, and racing, comprise a greater proportion of clients who bring their horses with sacroiliac pathology to the author's practice.

Racing horses with poor performance often have mild signs of sacroiliac disease, especially the young, immature Thoroughbred in which mild to moderate strain to the dorsal sacral ligaments is diagnosed frequently.[22] Sacroiliac disease is very common in Standardbred racehorses, again with desmopathy of the dorsal sacral ligaments as the most prominent diagnosis; however, in the author's experience, osteoarthritis of the sacroiliac joint(s) is diagnosed in this breed more often than in any other breed. Incomplete or complete rupture of the dorsal sacral ligaments and incongruence of the position of the tuber sacrales (as a sign for clinical subluxation of the sacroiliac joint) are seen, mostly in racehorses.

Behavioral issues such as kicking, rearing, striking, and bucking, as well as resisting going forward, are quite often associated with sacroiliac pathology. Riders frequently report that these behaviors occur when the horse is asked to canter, and it can be difficult to determine whether these are training/behavior issues or a reaction to pain.[2,3]

Some horses do not show evidence of sacroiliac disease until ridden under saddle. However, severe sacroiliac injury such as acute subluxation or even dislocation of one of the sacroiliac joints or rupture of the sacral ligaments can cause severe hindlimb lameness, even nonweight-bearing lameness.

DIAGNOSIS

Clinical examination of horses with suspected sacroiliac disease is the same as any other lameness examination. Emphasis is placed on observation of the gaits, in the walk, especially with serpentines, and at the canter in softer footing as well as eventually under saddle. Lateral walk (movement of the ipsilateral pair of legs at the same moment, like a camelid) in serpentines is a reliable sign of reduced mobility of the spine. When sacroiliac pain is present, especially when the dorsal sacral ligaments are involved, mobility of the tail can be reduced. Very often the tail is fixed in one position and does not move when the horse walks in a serpentine. Loss of the quality of the canter in one lead is a very strong sign for sacroiliac pain. This can be presented as less propulsion, less engagement, cross canter, no-sound 3-beat canter, or even a bunny hop canter. Asymmetry of the tuber sacrales can be observed; however, this is also found in clinically normal horses.[2,3,10,12,13]

With acute sacroiliac disease there is clear pain in the hindquarters or back. The horse can exhibit severe muscle spasm, clear asymmetry of the tuber sacrales, and favoring one hindlimb. Even nonweight-bearing lameness is sometimes found in cases of acute sacroiliac disease, as with subluxation.

The lameness is less pronounced in more chronic cases. Muscle atrophy of the affected side may be noticed with unilateral sacroiliac disease. Shorter stride length, mostly in the cranial phase, of the affected limb is a very common finding, as is lack of propulsion, less hindlimb engagement, and lack of collection (coming under).[22] The horse may appear stiff and rigid with lack of lateroflexion in the lumbosacral region. Asymmetric positioning of the tail is often observed, with a deviation of the tail in the direction of the affected ligament; this releases tension to the short part of the dorsal sacral ligament when the ligament is involved (Figure 6.20).[22]

In stance as well as in motion, the affected side often has a slight hip drop. This is different than with hindlimb lameness, in which the hip drop often is just evident in motion and less so in stance. Flexion tests of the hindlimbs may be positive; note that secondary overload of hindlimb structures may become more obvious in sacroiliac disease. In most cases with primary sacroiliac disease, the flexion tests are questionable or negative. However, standing on the affected limb when the contralateral limb is lifted and flexed can pronounce lameness of the affected side after the flexion test, resulting in more pronounced lameness on the contralateral side. During the flexion tests the horse may show reluctance to stand on the affected limb or lean over to the affected side, so the stance limb is in midposition, which reduces rotational forces to the pelvic structures.

Examination of the mobility of the spine can give specific information about reduced range of motion in the sacroiliac and lumbosacral region. Reflexes that induce dorsal and ventral flexion can be suppressed due to pain in the sacroiliac region. Passive lateral flexion is quite often reduced to the side of the location of the sacroiliac pain.

Provocation tests are useful to determine the location of the pain within the sacroiliac region. Manipulation of the tuber ischium forward with one hand and moving the tuber coxae of the same side upward and downward introduces ventroflexion and rotation in the sacroiliac joints. Pressure on the tuber sacrale identifies pain at the insertion of the dorsal sacral ligament.

Ultrasound examination provides more detailed information about the condition of the dorsal sacral ligaments.[7,16,18] Dorsal percutaneous ultrasonography using a linear probe with a higher frequency (10 to 15 MHz) is very useful for evaluating the dorsal sacral ligaments and their attachment to the tuber sacrale. Transverse views are used to identify the ligaments, check their size, and compare the left and right sides of these structures (Figure 6.24). Evaluation of the structures and the adjacent muscle tissue with Doppler ultrasonography can give valuable information about vascular activity in this area. Longitudinal views are better for evaluation of the alignment of the tissue and the contour of the tuber sacrale bone.

Ultrasonographic transrectal examination of the sacroiliac joints has been described to evaluate the bony edges of the joints[7] for bone proliferation (Figure 6.25).

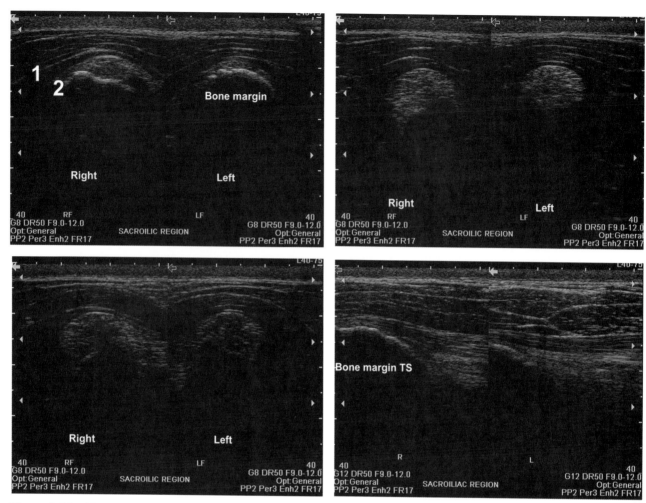

Figure 6.24. Ultrasonographic images. Right top view: Transverse view. 1 = short portion of the dorsal sacral ligament (DSL), 2 = long portion. Note the enlargement of the right DSL and the loss of echogenicity in the medial aspect when compared to the left. The bone margin on the right, however, is more smooth and normal than at the left, where the tuber sacrale is more irregular.

Left top view: Transverse view, more caudal than in right top view; the bone margin is no longer visible. Only ligament is visible, where it crosses the space between the tuber sacrale and the dorsal processes of the sacral bone. The right DSL is larger when compared to the left.

Right bottom view: Transverse view, more caudal than in left top view; the DSL starts to attach to the dorsal process of the sacral bone in the midline. Note again the increase in size of the right ligament. However, there is some loss of echogenicity in the body of both ligaments.

Left bottom view: Longitudinal view. In the right DSL there is loss of echogenicity and fiber pattern alignment; indicating desmitis of the DSL.

However, in the author's opinion there is little clinical relevancy for this technique, because necropsy findings show bone proliferation in this region in many horses without clinical symptoms. Radiographic techniques have been described for evaluation of the sacroiliac joint,[9] but they require general anesthesia and may not show a high correlation between radiological findings and clinical symptoms. Nuclear scintigraphy is the gold standard for showing clinically relevant involvement of the sacroiliac joint.[3,19,22]

Desmitis and enthesopathy (inflammation where ligaments attach to bone) are the most commonly diagnosed entities at the author's practice. Desmitis is seen as an enlargement of the dorsal sacral ligaments, usually combined with reduced echogenicity of the ligament in comparison to the contralateral one. The acute phase, often caused by a partial rupture of the ligament, is observed as an area with very low echogenicity. The vascular activity around the ligaments is clearly increased when compared to the healthy contralateral ligament. Quite often small avulsion fragments can be observed within the ligament.

More chronic desmitis and enthesopathy can be recognized as a higher echogenicity of the ligament, nearly comparable to the contralateral one, but enlarged and with an irregular and less clearly defined bone margin. This is more a repetitive stress injury than an acute trauma.

In cases with massive damage to the ligamentous structures, a more complete displacement of the sacral bone is visible with the ilial wings displaced dorsally and the sacral bone displaced ventrally. In this case,

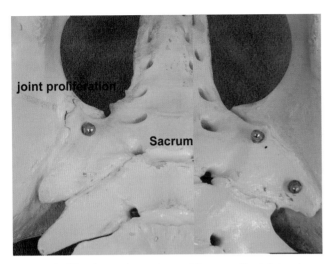

Figure 6.25. Anatomic specimen of the sacroiliac joint region. Note the visible bone proliferation at the ventral edge of the joints at the left view when compared with the right smooth joint margins.

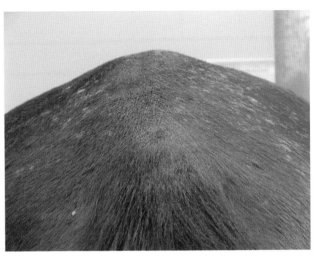

Figure 6.26. Caudal view of a horse with asymmetric tuber sacrales. Due to ligament damage, the right tuber sacrale is much higher than the left.

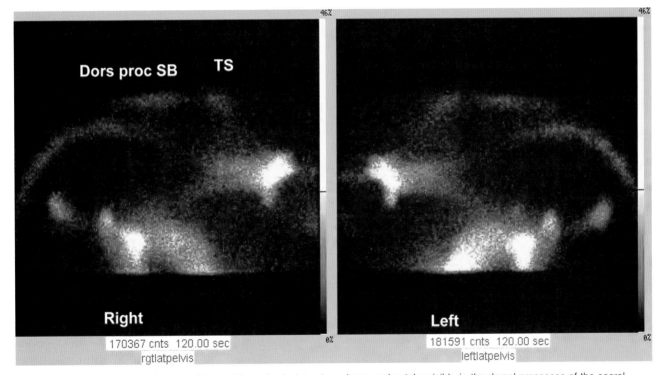

Figure 6.27. Scintigraphic images of the pelvic region in lateral view from left and right. Note the slightly higher uptake in the left tuber sacrale when compared to the right. There is also slightly increased uptake visible in the dorsal processes of the sacral bone. This can be a sign of enthesopathy of this structure or an indication of lower musculature size in this region.

one or both of the tuber sacrales are more pronounced (Figure 6.26). The latter condition is often called "hunter's bump."

In the case of significant displacement of the sacral bone, the incongruence in the articular surfaces of the sacroiliac joints leads to osteoarthritis. Osteoarthritis also can be a consequence of sacroiliac instability due to chronic desmitis of the dorsal sacral ligaments.

Scintigraphy facilitates evaluation of the sacroiliac joints as well as identification of enthesopathy of the tuber sacrale and the dorsal processes of the sacral bone.[3,19] Lateral (Figure 6.27), dorso-ventral, and oblique views of the sacroiliac region pinpoint increased bone metabolism of the tuber sacrale in the case of enthesopathy, and a more condensed higher bone metabolism in the ilial wing in the case of sacroiliac joint pathology (Figure 6.28). Lateral views taken in the first stage of uptake of radiopharmaceutical (soft tissue phase) can show increased uptake in the dorsal sacral ligaments as well as in the epaxial muscles.

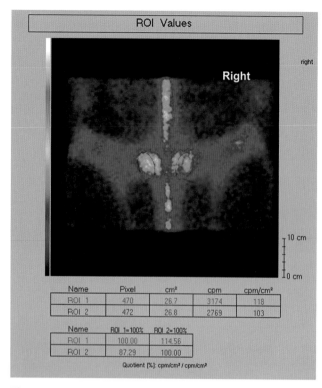

ROI Values

Right

Name	Pixel	cm²	cpm	cpm/cm²
ROI 1	470	26.7	3174	118
ROI 2	472	26.8	2769	103

Name	ROI 1=100%	ROI 2=100%
ROI 1	100.00	114.56
ROI 2	87.29	100.00

Quotient [%]: cpm/cm² / cpm/cm²

Figure 6.28. Scintigraphic image of the pelvic region with region of interest counts. The count on the left sacroiliac joint region is significantly higher (14% higher) than at the right joint region.

TREATMENT

In all cases of sacroiliac disease, a complete and intensive rehabilitation program is of paramount importance for the complete recovery of the horse.[2,3,14,21,22] When enthesopathy and desmitis are the most obvious diagnoses, an initial 2-month period of rest to immobilize the region is the first step of treatment. Uncontrolled motion in the pelvic region must be prevented and complete stall rest with no turn-out for the first 2 months of treatment is the only effective way to achieve immobilization of the pelvic region. During this period of stall rest, the horse is hand-walked on a straight, flat surface 2 to 3 times a day for 10 to 15 minutes. During this time oral medication with NSAIDs is needed to assist in the complete reduction of inflammation in the ligaments and bones. In the author's practice, phenylbutazone (1 g q 12 hours for a 500- to 600-kg horse) is the drug of choice.

After the initial 2 months of stall rest, 1 month of walking under saddle can begin. During this time, the horse is walked in serpentines and circles to increase lateroflexion and rotation in the lumbosacral and sacroiliac region. The rider should make the horse bend on the circles, and gradually reduce the circle to a smaller diameter, thus increasing lateroflexion.

In the fourth month of rehabilitation, the same exercises are done at the walk and also at the trot to increase speed and thus loading of the lumbosacral and sacroiliac region.

In the last 2 months of rehabilitation, the horse is ridden for longer periods, until achieving 1 to 1.5 hours of work daily. The canter is introduced with emphasis on brief episodes with many downward transitions to trot, creating more dorsal and ventral flexion in the lumbosacral and sacroiliac region. Short intervals of canter are extremely important to prevent fatigue of the muscles that support flexion and extension of the joints and their supporting ligaments to avoid mobility beyond their physical limits which may be diminished by the primary injury.

This rehabilitation program gradually introduces more mobility and develops better muscle support of the sacroiliac region. The exercises develop more muscle power in the epaxial muscles as well as in the muscles of the croup, which are of eminent importance in limiting the range of motion of the sacroiliac joints and their supportive ligamentous tissue.

When the sacroiliac joints are involved (in the author's practice this is only 10% to 15% of all cases and is almost always unilateral), injection of the joint with a corticosteroid may be needed. The author prefers triamcinolone over prednisolone, it causes less tissue irritation (AP Pease, personal communication).

A single injection of the affected joint with triamcinolone (20 to 30 mg) coupled with concurrent phenylbutazone and the rehabilitation program described above gives results that are quite similar to those described for treatment of enthesopathy and desmitis. In the author's experience, when scintigraphy findings lead to the diagnosis of sacroiliac joint disease, results of oral medication and a prolonged rehabilitation program without an injection are disappointing.

Injection directly into the sacroiliac joint is very difficult because the ilial wing makes access into the joint nearly impossible. However, depositing a corticosteroid very close to the joint can be effective in reducing inflammation within the joint. There are different techniques for depositing a corticosteroid close the joint.[1,4–6,8] At Michigan State University, a novel technique for injection of the sacroiliac joint (region) has been tested and shown to be preferable.[23] This approach is with a straight needle (15-gauge, 20 to 25 cm) with an insertion site 3 to 4 cm cranial and 1 to 2 cm paramedian to the contralateral tuber sacrale, through the interspinous ligament of L5 and L6, and aimed toward the ipsilateral tuber ischium (Figure 6.29). The medication is deposited when the tip of the needle makes contact with the ventral aspect of the ilial wing as ventral as possible. Landmarks for the location of the insertion site of the needle are the dorsal process of L5 and the tuber coxae. The insertion site of the needle is located on the contralateral side of the joint to be injected. The length between the cranial palpable tips of the dorsal processes of L5 and L6 is measured. Half of this length is the distance that the insertion site is lateral of the cranial tip of L5 on the contralateral side. This technique facilitates insertion of the needle at the correct location in horses of different sizes.[23]

In cases with severe damage to the dorsal sacral ligaments (disruption of the fiber pattern) as with partial or complete rupture of these ligaments, injection of platelet-rich plasma (PRP) into the damaged tissue has shown impressive results at the author's hospital. In

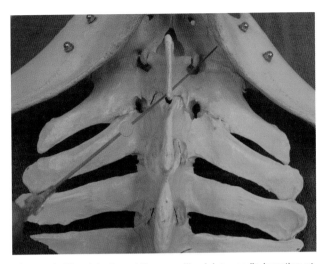

Figure 6.29. Injection of the sacroiliac joint: needle insertion at the left side 2 cm out of the median, through the intervertebral ligament between the dorsal processes of L5 and L6 into the right sacroiliac joint. The red dot indicates the location of needle insertion on the skin.

comparison to cases that were treated conservatively, the architectural structure of the ligament improved much faster and was more completely restored after treatment with PRP. However, no change of overall rehabilitation time (4 to 6 months) has been observed.[24]

PROGNOSIS

In nearly all of the past reports, prognosis for sacroiliac diseases has been rather guarded.[3,14,20] In the author's experience with more than 200 cases in the last 4 years involving desmopathy of the dorsal sacral ligaments and unilateral OA of the sacroiliac joint, more than 90% of the horses returned to work at their original level or higher. All of these cases were on a 6-month rehabilitation program with re-checks at 2-month intervals. The horses were evaluated clinically and ultrasonographically at every re-check and adjustments to the rehabilitation program were made based on the outcome of this evaluation.

For cases with partial or complete rupture and subluxation of the sacroiliac joint, prognosis seems to be favorable; however, at Michigan State University the author has seen fewer than 10 cases with this type of injury over the last 4 years. With enough time for initial healing of the ligamentous structures (2-plus months of stall rest with some hand walking) and 4 to 6 months for rehabilitation exercises, these horses were able to return to their original level of performance.

References

1. Denoix JM, Jacquet S. Ultrasound-guided injection of the sacroiliac area in horses. Eq Vet Educ 2008;4;203–207.
2. Dyson SJ. Pain associated with the sacroiliac joint region: a diagnostic challenge. Proceedings Am Assoc Equine Pract 2004;50:357–360.
3. Dyson SJ, Murray RC. Clinical features of pain associated with the sacroiliac region: A European perspective. Proceedings Am Assoc Equine Pract 2004;50:367–371.
4. Engeli E, Haussler KK, Erb HN. Development and validation of a periarticular injection technique of the sacroiliac joint in horses. Equine Vet J 2004;36:324–330.
5. Engeli E, Haussler KK, Erb HN. How to inject the sacroiliac joint region in horses. Proceedings Am Assoc Equine Pract 2002; 48:257–260.
6. Engeli E, Haussler KK. Review of sacroiliac injection techniques. Proceedings Am Assoc Equine Pract 2004;50:372–378.
7. Engeli E, Yeager AE, Haussler KK. Use and limitations of ultrasonography in sacroiliac disease. Proceedings Am Assoc Equine Pract 2004;50:385–391.
8. Florent D, Cousty M, Rossier Y. How to do ultrasound-guided injection of the sacroiliac region in horses. Proceedings Am Assoc Equine Pract 2007;53:430–432.
9. Gorgas D, Kircher P, Doherr MG, et al. Radiographic technique and anatomy of the equine sacroiliac region. Vet Radiol Ultrasound 2007;48:501–506.
10. Goff LM, Jeffcott LB, Jasiewicz J, et al. Structural and biomechanical aspects of equine sacroiliac joint function and their relationship to clinical disease. Equine Vet J 2008;176; 281–293.
11. Gomez Alvarez CB, L'Ami JJ, Moffat D, et al. Effect of chiropractic manipulations on the kinematics of back and limbs in horses with clinically diagnosed back problems. Equine Vet J 2008;40:153–159.
12. Haussler KK, Stover SM, Willits NH. Pathologic changes in the lumbosacral vertebrae and pelvis in Thoroughbred racehorses. Am J Vet Res 1999;60:143–163.
13. Haussler KK. Functional anatomy and pathophysiology of sacroiliac joint disease. Proceedings Am Assoc Equine Pract 2004; 50:361–366.
14. Haussler KK. Treatment options for sacroiliac joint disease. Proceedings Am Assoc Equine Pract 2004;50:392–395.
15. Haussler KK, McGilvray KC, Ayturk UM, et al. Sacroiliac joint motion and pelvic deformation in horses. Proceedings Am Assoc Equine Pract 2008;54:258–259.
16. Kersten AA, Edinger J. Ultrasonographic examination of the equine sacroiliac region. Equine Vet J 2004;602–608.
17. Pilsworth RC, Sheperd M, Herinckx BMB, et al. Fracture of the wing of the ilium, adjacent to the sacroiliac joint, in Thoroughbred racehorses. Equine Vet J 1994;26:94–99.
18. Tomlinson JE, Sage AM, Turner TA. Ultrasonographic abnormalities detected in the sacroiliac area in twenty cases of upper hindlimb lameness. Equine Vet J 2003;35:48–54.
19. Tucker RL, Schneider RK, Sondhof AH, et al. Bone scintigraphy in the diagnosis of sacroiliac injury in twelve horses. Equine Vet J 1998;30:390–395.
20. Tracy AT. Back problems in horses. Proceedings Am Assoc Equine Pract 2003;49:71–74.
21. van Wessum R. Sacroiliac disease. In Current Therapy in Equine Medicine, 6th ed. Robinson NE, Sprayberry KA, eds. Saunders Elsevier, St. Louis, 2008;483–487.
22. van Wessum R, Nickels F, Pease AP, et al. Clinical data on 206 equine back pain cases. In preparation.
23. van Wessum R, Johnston KA, Nickels F, et al. A novel technique for injection of the sacroiliac joint. In preparation.
24. van Wessum R, Johnston KA, Nickels F, et al. The use of PRP for the treatment of ligament and tendon pathology in 20 cases. In preparation.

THE THORACOLUMBAR SPINE

OVERRIDING/IMPINGEMENT OF DORSAL SPINOUS PROCESSES

Etiology

The impingement of the summits of the dorsal vertebral processes, also known as "kissing spines," is a relatively common diagnosis in horses with back pain.[10–12] The most common location for these lesions is in the thoracic spine (between T5 and T18), but impingement of the lumbar dorsal processes has also been reported.[11,19] Pathology may be caused by the repetitive, traumatic contact between the dorsal processes. Sclerosis of the cortical margins of the dorsal processes, narrowing or loss of the interspinous space, and osteolysis of the spinous processes are affirmative signs of bony pathology. When the supraspinous ligament or the interspinous ligaments are involved, enthesiophytes and avulsion fragments may be present at the summit (supraspinous ligament) or at the caudal or ventral aspect of the dorsal spinous process (interspinous ligament).[9]

When adjacent structures are damaged, they can lead to impingement of the spinous processes. A primary injury to the ventral and ventrolateral supportive structures of the annulus fibrosis of the intervertebral disc can cause asymmetrical narrowing or collapse of the intervertebral joint, which may tilt the dorsal vertebral processes towards each other.[31] In that case, the impingement may be a secondary finding at the initial radiological examination, underestimating the extent of the trauma. Spondylosis at the ventral aspect of the spine and narrowing or the loss of definition of the intervertebral disc space can be an additional radiological finding, pointing to the involvement of more spinal structures than just the spinous processes.

Clinical Signs

Impingement most often reduces the ventrodorsal mobility of the spine, but when pain is present, the lateral mobility may be limited due to reflectory muscle spasm, thus affecting performance.[10] Horses with impingement of spinous processes have a variety of symptoms, often related to the discipline in which they perform. Although show jumpers and hunters seem to be more affected, many horses that perform without clinical signs of back pain show radiological evidence of impingement. When impingement is present in the cranial part of the thoracic spine (T5 to T12 or T13), the horse may have a painful or violent response when putting the saddle on or when the rider mounts. Differentiating an injury from saddle fit issues can be a challenge.

Diagnosis

Palpation along the back may reveal irregularities in the size of the summits of the spinous processes of the thoracic or lumbar vertebrae. Deep digital palpation is necessary in most cases to reveal these changes. Examination should begin at the withers and work toward the sacrum. It is important to differentiate the resentment shown by some horses to this examination from distress resulting from other back conditions.[10] Clinical examination can show pain with localized digital pressure of the specific dorsal process or the supraspinous ligament.[12] Limitation of dorsoventral mobility as well as possible lateral reduction of motion is limited to the specific part of the spine.

Radiological examination can clearly identify bony changes as sclerosis and osteolysis.[27,39] Ultrasonographic examination is very useful to evaluate the contact and remodelling between 2 adjacent spinous processes, transverse thickening of the processes, and abnormal alignment. Concomitant lesions in the supraspinous ligament and enthesopathy on the summits of the spinous processes also can be imaged with ultrasonography.

Scintigraphy may help to identify evidence of active bone metabolism and remodeling of the spinous processes (Figure 6.30), as well as adjacent structures of the spine that can be involved (intervertebral disc, facet joint, vertebral body).[34] Localized increased activity may be observed or absent in completely sound and clinically asymptomatic horses, as well as in horses with clear symptoms of back pain caused by impingement of spinous processes.[15]

Infiltration with a local anaesthetic of a site that is suspect for pain caused by impingement can give more information about the likelihood of the observed impingement causing the symptoms.[13,14]

Treatment

Conservative therapies include rest, nonsteroidal anti-inflammatories, local injections of anti-inflammatory agents, acupuncture, and physiotherapy. Horses that are rested often improve during the rest period but become sore again shortly after reinstating exercise. Systemic therapy with NSAIDs helps horses with very minor lesions, but does not cure more severe lesions. Injections of corticosteroids between affected spinous processes, combined with nonsteroidal systemic therapy, can be quite helpful in reducing or removing pain.

Several surgical techniques have been described to remove an affected part of a dorsal process.[28] Newer techniques are less invasive and endoscopic resection of the spinous process and the interspinous ligament has been performed.[7]

Prognosis

The prognosis for impingement of spinous processes is guarded when the symptoms are primarily caused by this disease. In a study by Erichsen,[15] scintigraphic and radiological signs of impingement were found in com-

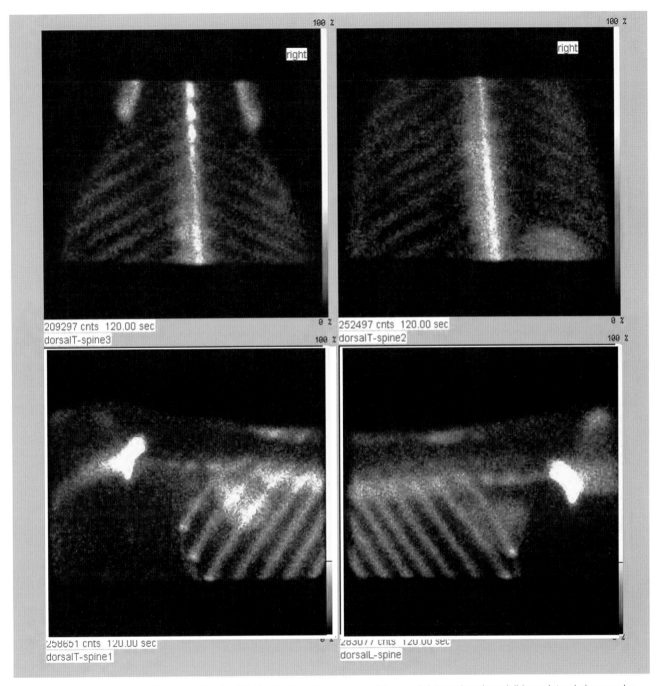

Figure 6.30. Scintigraphic image showing IRU in the dorsal processes of the caudal thoracic spine, visible on lateral views and a dorsal view. This horse was a 13-year-old show jumper with an international Grand Prix career that had no major clinical problems.

pletely sound horses. The most important factor in determining the prognosis for impingement of the spinous processes is the complete diagnosis. When ligamentous structures are involved (e.g., supraspinous ligament, intraspinous ligament, ventral longitudinal ligament) the prognosis for a quick recovery to the original workload is less favorable than when just osseous changes are seen on radiographs. When there are adjacent pathologic conditions in the intervertebral disc or the facet joints, prognosis is also less favorable.

For more severe cases, prognosis for a return to the original work level after months of rehabilitation seems to be better when resection is performed than when surgery is not performed.[7,28]

SUPRASPINOUS LIGAMENT INJURIES

Injuries of the supraspinous ligament are most common between T15 and L3.[12] They can be associated with localized thickening and pain.

Clinical Signs

Signs of desmopathy of the supraspinous ligament are similar to those of impingement of dorsal spinous processes. When only ligament pathology is present, signs can be mild and very difficult to detect. The increased size of the ligament (focal thickening) may be recognized by the owner, making this the primary complaint. In cases with more swelling in and around the ligament, the appearance of the shape of the spine can resemble kyphosis. In that case, radiography shows a normal configuration of the spine, but ultrasonography can show the soft tissue involvement and edema.

Diagnosis

Ultrasonography is the tool of choice to image these injuries.[17] Diagnosis of the pathology of the supraspinous ligament can be made with ultrasonographic examination. Radiography and scintigraphy can give additional information about the involvement of the spinous processes. Radiographic examination of desmopathy of the supraspinous ligament may show irregular bone margins of the summit of the dorsal spinal processes, avulsion fragments, and sclerosis. Scintigraphy may show increased uptake in the summits of the spinous processes (Figure 6.31). These findings are similar to those of impingement of the dorsal spinous processes, and quite often both pathologic conditions are found in the same horse.

A study of Henson et al. found ultrasonographic changes in the supraspinous ligament in clinically normal horses as well as in horses with signs of back pain.[12] They concluded that when ultrasonography alone does not confirm the diagnosis of desmitis of the supraspinous ligament, then local (infiltration) anesthesia should be performed as well.

Treatment

As with any ligamentous structure, treatment is focused on rest, medication, and rehabilitation. Controlled stretching of the ligament with a lower position of the head (i.e., in pasture, with hay on the ground, when ridden with a lower head and a longer neck) and a gradual increase in the workload is recommended.

Prognosis

When the ligament is the only affected structure and adequate time for a complete recovery before resuming the original work is allowed (4 to 6 months), the prognosis is usually favorable. When more structures are involved, as with impingement of dorsal spinous processes, facet joints, or intervertebral discs, the prognosis tends to be less favorable.

FRACTURES OF THE SPINOUS PROCESSES

Etiology

Fractures of the dorsal spinous processes occur mostly in the cranial thoracic spine (the withers region) when horses flip over, fall backwards, or run into objects with their withers (such as when the door is lower than the horse).[3,25] Sporadic fractures of the dorsal spinous processes in the lumbar spine can be caused by excessive trauma such as falling and turning at high speed, for instance in cross country riding, jumping, barrel racing, hunting, or traffic accidents. This places rotational force on the spine, which can cause fractures of the lumbar lateral spinous processes.[17]

Clinical Signs

Fractures of the withers have very clear symptoms, with swelling in this region and deformation of the normal contour of the withers. A significant dent can be observed in the normal curvature of the withers region, and the distal fragment will dislocate in most cases and end up lateral to the remaining spinous process, giving the withers a wider appearance. Fractures of the spinous processes of the more caudal thoracic spine and the lumbar spine are less pronounced in appearance. When the tips of the spinous processes are viewed from above, a clear change in the alignment may be visible, with the tip of the fractured spinous process out of line to the lateral side, possibly with some dislocation to the ventral side. A fracture of the lateral spinous process in the lumbar spine may be difficult to see when observing the horse due to the fact that they may not be dislocated.

In the acute stage, pain is present with generalized back stiffness, localized swelling, and muscle spasms in the epaxial muscles. In older cases, the change in the alignment of the withers or the caudal spine is the clear remains of the fracture, with few other clinical signs. When the mobility of the spine is evaluated, there may be slight alterations at the location of an older fracture, due to remodeling of the fragments and attached muscles.[18,29]

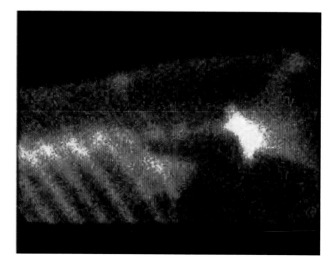

Figure 6.31. Scintigraphic image showing mild focal IRU at the summit of T18, indicative of desmitis of the supraspinous ligament. Radiography did not show any change, and ultrasonography showed mild desmitis with roughened bone margin of the summit of the spinous process of T18.

Diagnosis

Radiographic examination is the first diagnostic technique to image the spinous processes because the fragments, which are often dislocated, show clearly on the radiographs.[39] The summits of the thoracic spinous processes, especially in the withers region (T3 to T12), can vary in shape, show a variety in the pattern of accessory centers of ossification, and easily be misinterpreted as a fracture. Dislocation of the fragment is a very common finding in fractures of the spinous processes in the withers region, which helps to distinguish them from irregularities and delayed ossification. In the more caudal thoracic spine and lumbar spine, radiographic examination may be less useful because the muscle mass in these regions can make radiographic imaging incapable of identifying a nondisplaced fracture.

Ultrasonographic examination can give good additional information, especially to identify fractures of the lateral spinous processes in the lumbar spine.[8]

Scintigraphy can show increased radiopharmaceutical uptake after a fracture, but is not specific enough to identify the fractures. For lateral spinous process fractures, scintigraphy can be useful to identify the location of a possible fracture (Figure 6.32), but adjacent ultrasonography is needed to verify this.

Treatment

Treatment for fractured spinous processes is often not required, other than medication to deal with the associated pain of an acute fracture. Surgery is usually not required. Rest and controlled exercise for 1 to several months to keep the horse in good muscular condition usually is sufficient. The saddle should not be used when the withers region is involved.

Prognosis

Prognosis for most spinous process fractures is favorable. Sometimes after a fracture in the withers region

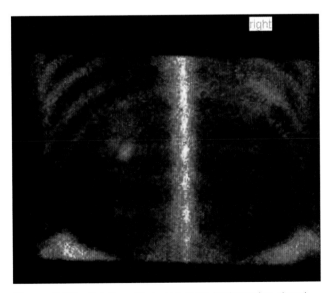

Figure 6.32. Scintigraphic image of the lumbar spine, dorsal view. Note the IRU in the left transverse spinous process of L2. This is indicative of a fracture of the transverse process.

it is difficult to make the saddle fit properly due to the changed shape of the withers. When the horse is judged on shape and conformation in its discipline (i.e., hand showing, breeding championships) the abnormal shape of the withers can influence the judging. Providing the client with a clear veterinary statement that the abnormality is caused by a traumatic event and not genetic, and that the horse is capable of competing, facilitates a successful show career.

VERTEBRAL FRACTURES

Etiology

Most vertebral fractures are traumatic in origin; however, pathological fractures can occur with processes affecting the vertebrae such as neoplasia, metastasis, and osteomyelitis.[35]

Stress fractures of the vertebra most likely occur more frequently than previously believed. In one study, 18 of 36 specimens had incomplete fractures and focal periosteal proliferation of the lamina stemming from vertebral stress fractures.[17] The fractures occurred most often near the junction of the cranial articular process and the spinous process.

Clinical Signs

Acute vertebral fractures are accompanied by severe pain. The horse is reluctant to move the affected part of the spine and shows increased muscle tension in the region of the fracture. Neurological symptoms are present when soft tissue swelling, hemorrhage, or fragments compress the spinal cord or root nerves. Unilateral root nerve compression can cause the horse to bend to the affected side when root nerve compression leads to irritability of the nerve and to the opposite side when the compression causes complete loss of neurotransmission.

Most stress fractures result in a lack of performance without clear-cut symptoms. Stiffness, lack of propulsion from behind, and mild back pain are common signs associated with laminar stress fractures in the young Thoroughbred racehorse. These are most often seen at the thoracolumbar junction and the lumbar vertebrae.[17,18]

Diagnosis

Radiography can image larger fragments; however, with the initial radiographic examination these fractures can be easily overlooked when there is little dislocation present. In addition, fractures with a longitudinal fracture line are nearly invisible on lateral views. Scintigraphy is a sensitive technique for vertebral fractures and is nearly the only way to determine active stress fractures.[34]

Treatment

Treatment is conservative in most cases of vertebral fracture without neurological symptoms. Stall rest with very controlled exercise and medication with NSAIDs and often muscle relaxants to reduce the pain and muscle spasms are sufficient. When neurological symptoms are present, treatment focuses more on reducing swelling around the spinal structures; medication with systemic corticosteroids and DMSO may be indicated.

Prognosis

The prognosis for nondisplaced vertebral fractures without neurological symptoms is favorable, as is the prognosis for most stress fractures. When neurological symptoms are present, the amount of time needed to reduce these symptoms with medication is a good indicator for future expectations. The longer it takes for the recovery of neurological functions, in general, the poorer the prognosis.

FACET JOINT ARTHRITIS AND VERTEBRAL FACET JOINT SYNDROME

Etiology

When facet joint osteoarthritis is present in the thoracolumbar spine, similar to this process in humans,[32,33] a complex of processes in and around the vertebral facet joints can lead to a painful condition known as facet joint syndrome. In the cervical spine, however, osteoarthritis of the facet joints seems to be less frequently related to facet joint syndrome than in the thoracolumbar spine, and the accompanying muscle spasms in the segmental muscles are absent. This gives the impression of an isolated joint disease with a reduced range of motion and pain in just the affected joint. However, compression of nerve roots due to proliferation of bone around the facet joints is a more common observation in the cervical spine than in the thoracolumbar spine.

The initiating incident in facet joint syndrome is damage to the facet joint, primarily to the joint capsule and the adjacent connective tissue, or else to the cartilage and/or subchondral bone. In the horse, this primary incident quite often is trauma, caused when the horse slips, falls, flips over, gets cast, or injures itself in any other way. Due to the rich innervation of the facet joint tissues, the inflammation reaction caused by the primary trauma starts a cascade of reactions that is more obvious than in the joints of the limbs.

One of the first reactions of the horse is stabilization of the spine by muscular contraction and spasm of the epaxial and subaxial muscles. This can occur in just the segment that is related to the injured vertebral facet joint, but a larger portion of the vertebral column may be involved. This muscle contraction can be short, last hours to days, or last weeks or even months. It is very likely that the prolonged contraction or spasm is very painful and partially immobilizes the spine, as is the situation in humans.[32,33]

As a consequence of this immobilization, the facet joint is more or less fixed in 1 position, which makes regaining later mobility a painful experience.[20] Due to the muscle spasm, no normal sequence of contraction-relaxation occurs in the muscle and the normal supportive function is less effective.[21] Consequently, when excessive force is applied to the spine again, repetitive injury to that facet joint can be the result.

Clinical Signs

Due to the contribution of the spine to the normal gait pattern in the horse, as described earlier in this chapter, horses that suffer from vertebral facet joint syndrome are often presented for lameness. In acute cases, the pain in and around the facet joints can be so severe that the horse does resists all movement, and stands with the hind feet parked out and the back lowered. This position closes the facet joints in the thoracic and lumbar spine, causing less tension in the joint capsules. The muscles of the back and hind end are contracted. This attitude can be difficult to differentiate from tying-up syndrome; however, with vertebral facet joint syndrome the serum levels of creatine kinase (CK) and aspartate aminotransferase (AST) are within normal limits or only slightly elevated.

With severe pain in the thoracic or lumbar spine, signs can be similar to those of colic, with restlessness, pawing, looking back, or standing with the hind legs parked far out, giving the impression of wanting to urinate. In those cases, the heart rate can be as high as 60 to 80 beats per minute, but an examination for colic reveals that the horse is within normal limits.

In more chronic cases, the locomotion of the horse can be altered and a stiff back noticed. At the trot, the propulsion of the hindlimbs can be reduced unilaterally or even bilaterally.[21,26] Due to the attachment of the front limbs with ligaments, tendons, and muscles to the thoracic vertebrae, motion of the front limbs also affects the position of the thoracic facet joints. At the trot, due to the diagonal gait, the thorax moves between the scapulae, with a maximum extent of motion in the dorsal processes of the withers of 1 to 3 cm to left and right. Pain in the facet joints of the thorax thus can lead to less mobility in the thoracic spine, and an altered gait pattern in the trot is best described as stiff or shortened.[21]

During the canter the thorax moves less, except in downward transitions (changing from canter to trot or trot to walk) when there is more loading of the facet joints, as well as in landing after a jump or going downhill. Therefore, when thoracic facet joints are involved, signs mentioned by the owner or rider can include stiffness, reluctance to go downhill or jump, and refusal or difficulty in extended trotting. Especially in jumping, a trainer or rider may note a preference of the horse to go left or right after a jump, and this is quite often thought to be related to an injury to the distal limb, but in fact is caused by facet joint problems.

Because lateral bending is a prominent mobility feature of the thoracic vertebrae, lateral bending of the horse may be reduced when thoracic vertebrae are involved with facet joint syndrome. This can be observed during circles and serpentines and in lateral exercises such as shoulder in, travers, and half pass of dressage; as well as in turns in barrel racing, polo, and eventing; or in between fences when jumping. Tightening the girth or putting the saddle on also can reveal an adverse reaction of the horse, because these actions can load the thoracic facet joints.

When lumbar facet joints are involved in facet joint syndrome, the most affected gait is the canter, because it is then that the dorsoventral flexion of the lumbar spine is most prominent. The lateral exercises—shoulder in, travers, and half pass—can show alterations when lumbar facet joints are involved because the rotation in the lumbosacral region makes an important contribution to these movements. In racing, dorsoventral flexion of the lumbar spine is a prominent contribution to the propulsion phase of the hindlimbs, so loss of performance may be caused by lumbar facet joint syndrome.

Diagnosis

The thoracic vertebrae can be viewed with radiography with the lungs facilitating radiographic imaging in the cranial part of the thorax. In most horses, the vertebral bodies of T1 through T15–T16 can be imaged adequately to evaluate the intervertebral disc spaces and vertebral body as well as the ventral aspect of the vertebrae.[33] In the more cranial part of the thorax it is difficult to get a clear image of the intervertebral disc space and the facet joints because of the superimposing structures of the scapulae. Depending on the conformation of the horse, the width of its thorax, musculature, and body condition, oblique lateral views can isolate the unilateral facet joints from T5–T7 to T18 (Figure 6.33). When pathology of the facet joints is present there are signs of sclerosis of the bone just around the facet joint, narrowing of the joint space, irregular shape of the joint space, and spur formation at the edges of

the joint space or complete ankylosis visible on the radiographs. Lumbar vertebrae are the most difficult to visualize with radiography. Especially well muscled horses of the bigger breeds often give disappointing images and it is difficult to differentiate their facet joints from the massive vertebral bodies of the lumbar spine. Oblique lateral views can sometimes facilitate imaging of the unilateral facet joints of the lumbar spine. Even under general anesthesia, the facet joints of the sacrum and the adjacent pelvic bones cannot be viewed accurately with radiography. However, the coccygeal vertebrae are easy to see with radiography.

Ultrasonography is a very useful tool for examining the facet joints of the vertebral column.[8] It can give information about ligamentous structures and muscle conditions (Figure 6.34), high muscle tension can be shown as increased muscle echogenicity, and fasciculations can be visualized in real-time ultrasonography. The supraspinous ligament, interspinous ligaments, and dorsal sacral ligaments can be examined with this as well. Paramedian longitudinal views of the facet joints can be used to determine the edges of these joints, which should normally be smooth and bilaterally symmetrical. Possible effusion of these joints, bony proliferations at the joint margins, as well as fractures and avulsion fragments and ankylosis of the facet joints (Figures 6.34 to 6.36) can be seen with ultrasound.

Doppler ultrasonography can provide valuable information about vascular activity around the facet joints

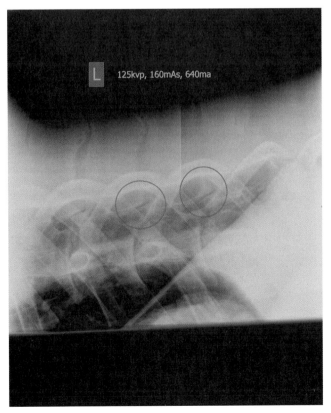
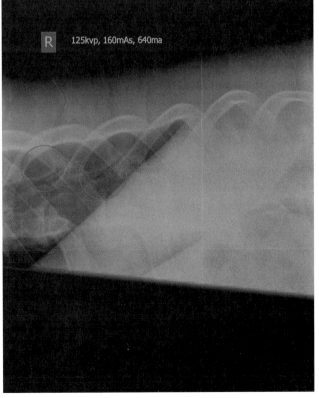

Figure 6.33. Radiographic image of the thoracic spine, (oblique lateral view) to expose the left facet joints (circles) at the left, and the right facet joints at the right. Note the more irregular joint space and some sclerosis in the right facet joints. This is indicative of osteoarthritis of the right thoracic facet joints.

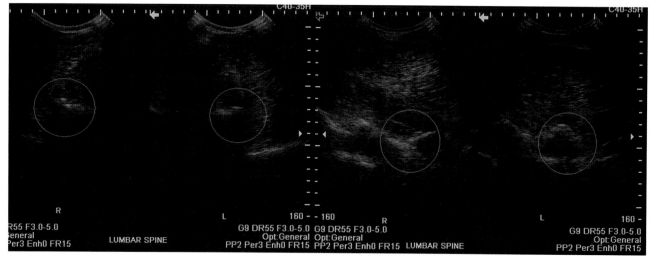

Figure 6.34. Ultrasonographic images of the lumbar spine. Transverse views (left images) of the left side and right side; the facet joint surfaces and the joint spaces are seen in the circles. Right side, 2 longitudinal paramedian views. The respective facet joints are seen in the circles; in the left circle is the joint space and both facets, and in the right circle the joint space is not visible.

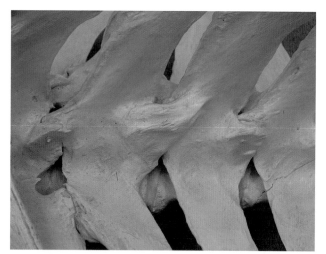

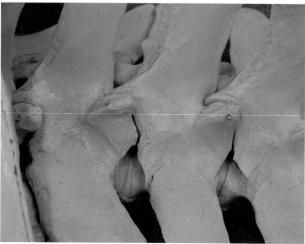

Figure 6.35. Anatomical specimen of the lumbar spine with the facet joints visible. In the lower image, the facet joints have smooth edges and appear to be normal. In the upper image the facet joints have more irregular edges when compared to the facet joints in the lower image. Complete ankylosis is present in one of the facet joints.

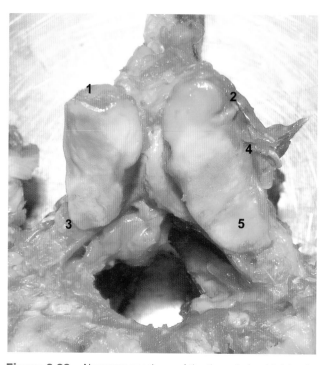

Figure 6.36. Necropsy specimen of the thoracic facet joints of T7. Note the asymmetry and difference in size from the left and right facet joint. 1 = erosion of cartilage and hemorrhage from the subchondral bone, 2 = fraying of the cartilage, 3 = compression damage of the cartilage, 4 and 5 = some ulceration of cartilage.

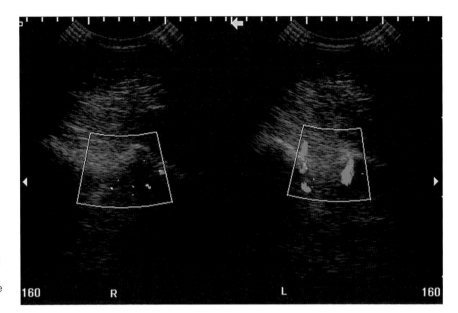

Figure 6.37. Ultrasonographic image of the lumbar facet joints. Doppler is used to identify higher blood flow around the facet joint at the left facet joint (right in the image).

(Figure 6.37). In cases of synovitis or osteoarthritis of a facet joint, increased vascular activity can be visualized around the facet joint, especially when the adjacent facet joints and the contralateral facet joint are compared. When muscles are evaluated with Doppler ultrasonography, vascular patterns within the muscles can provide information about myositis and muscle tension, in which cases increased and decreased vascular activity can be present, respectively.

Scintigraphy is a perfect modality for imaging the vertebral column. When the resolution of the gamma camera is adequate, it is possible to differentiate increased uptake of radiopharmaceutical in the vertebral body from that just dorsal in the facet joint. A recent study showed 61.5% of horses with back pain complaints had an increased uptake of radiopharmaceutical in 1 or more facet joints.[16] Comparison of images obtained from the left, right, and dorsal aspects can assist in determining the exact location of higher bone metabolism in a facet joint.

The final diagnosis of equine vertebral facet joint syndrome is often a summation of the results of 2 or 3 imaging techniques. When the results of Doppler ultrasonography and scintigraphy are combined, it may be possible to differentiate between synovitis with its increased vascular activity around the facet joint and osteoarthritis, which can have both increased uptake of radiopharmaceutical in the region of the facet joint and increased vascular activity.

The study by Gillen concluded a high predictive value for negative scintigraphy findings to exclude osteoarthritis of facet joints as the cause of back pain in horses.[16] They found a high predictive value for scintigraphy in the detection of radiographic lesions and back pain. Thus, scintigraphy is a valuable tool in the evaluation of thoracolumbar pain.[16]

Local anaesthesia is not a reliable tool for confirming facet joint pain. Anesthetic solution is deposited in muscle tissue rather than in the facet joint or its capsule, and diffuses rapidly within the muscle, affecting nerve sensation in the rami of the spinal nerves. Furthermore, the reflectory spasm that is caused by the facet joint arthritis takes several hours to relax, making it very difficult to adequately interpret the results of the block. In humans, anesthesia of a suspect facet joint is performed on a more regular basis, but people can communicate and tell the examiner when the main joint pain they were experiencing is diminished, even when a muscle spasm is still present.[32]

Treatment

Rehabilitation is a significant factor influencing the final outcome of facet joint arthritis and vertebral facet joint syndrome.[30] The primary goal is to break the vicious cycle of inflammation that triggers the nerves, which leads to muscle spasm, immobility of the spine, and repeated injury. Treatment can be aimed at multiple spots in this cycle but the best outcome can be expected with complex treatment plans that deal with as many aspects as possible.

Anti-inflammatory therapy is essential. NSAIDs, especially phenylbutazone (1 gm/500 kg BID), flunixin meglumine (0.5 mg/kg SID), naproxen (10 mg/kg SID), and meclofenamic acid (2 mg/kg SID) must be administered for a prolonged time, often up to 1 to 2 months. In that case, additional medication to prevent gastrointestinal side effects may be needed. The newer NSAID firocoxib may be a good choice for horses with gastrointestinal side effects that are on other NSAIDs, but it must be limited to a 3-week period of medication, according to the manufacturer. Some positive experience has been obtained in back pain cases with bisphosphonates, especially when osteolysis is present.[5]

More localized anti-inflammatory therapy is obtained by direct injections of a corticosteroid into or close to the facet joint. The author's drug of choice is triamcinolone (10 to 30 mg intra-articularly). The triggering facet joint must be established by scintigraphy that shows increased uptake of radiopharmaceutical in the area of the joint, possible radiographic changes, and/or ultrasonography that reveals increased vascular activity around the facet joint. With ultrasound guidance, a 20-gauge spinal needle is inserted into the dorsal aspect of the facet joint and 10 to 30 mg of the corticosteroid is injected into or close to the joint capsule. Because the medication is deposited in the joint capsule or in the adjacent multifidus muscle with an important proprioceptive function in intervertebral motion (the multifidus muscle stabilizes the spine and facilitates limb motion without deformation of the axial skeleton), the use of sarapin to reduce pain sensation is contraindicated.

Anti-inflammatory treatment should diminish muscle spasms, and quite often, muscle relaxation is observed within 2 to 3 days of facet joint injection. When only systemic medication is used, beneficial effects occur more slowly and muscle relaxation can take up to 2 to 3 weeks. Use of a muscle relaxant such as methocarbamol (15 to 25 mg/kg slow IV infusion) can be effective in reducing the muscle spasm but the supportive function of the spinal muscles may be diminished, so care must be taken to reduce the possibilities for injury to the spinal structures. No turn-out and a reduced workload is important in a horse that is on muscle relaxants; however, this may compromise an effective rehabilitation program.[30]

After reduction of inflammation and the adjacent muscle spasm, the next step in treatment is the design of a rehabilitation program aimed at gaining more mobility in the affected part of the spine as well as the development of better muscle support for that region. In the author's practice, rest is prescribed for 4 to 6 weeks. Pasture is ideal but if the horse is turned out with others, it must only be with pasture mates that will not force the patient to run. The more the horse walks, trots, and canters at its own pace, the better the mobility achieved. Grazing with the head down opens the facet joints in the thorax and lumbar region, thus counterbalancing the spasms in the dorsal epaxial muscles. In humans, one of the modern rehabilitation techniques with tendon and ligament injury is eccentric exercise. The stretching effect of the grazing position on the dorsal epaxial muscles as well as the tendons and ligaments around the spine may be a very important side effect of being out in pasture. When a patient cannot go out in pasture, mimicking this position by feeding small portions of feed and hay on the ground at multiple times during the day is a good alternative.

After the initial period of rest, a period of gradually increased work must be incorporated in the rehabilitation program. At first, just circling exercises at the walk and later at the trot facilitate more lateroflexion, thus providing stretch to the outside part of the spine and some compression and rotation to the inside part of the spine. By modulating the size of the circle and the direction of the circle in a 1- to 2-minute pattern, gradual mobilization of the entire spine can be achieved. In a later stage, some cantering can be introduced in circles as well as at the track or over terrain, together with more strenuous exercises to stimulate more powerful muscle contraction. In the author's clinic, a complete rehabilitation program can easily take 4 to 6 months, after which a large number of cases are fully serviceable at the original level of performance or even higher.

Prognosis

The prognosis for horses with thoracic or lumbar facet joint arthritis depends on a number of factors. The discipline in which the horse performs is very important. In the racing horse, thoracic facet joint arthritis has a better prognosis than facet joint arthritis of the lumbar facet joints, whereas the prognosis for thoracic facet joint arthritis for a barrel racer may be more performance limiting than lumbar facet joint arthritis. Three-day event horses and jumpers often have a more guarded prognosis than dressage horses. In the dressage discipline, rehabilitation of the core muscles of the trunk can assist in stabilizing the spine and prevent recurrent injury. Racing trotters seem to have the worst prognosis for full return to a racing career when diagnosed with facet joint arthritis or thoracolumbar pathology in general.

DISCOSPONDYLITIS

Etiology

Discospondylitis is an inflammatory condition involving the vertebral bodies adjacent to the symphysis between 2 vertebrae, and includes the intervertebral disc[31]. The most common cause is a septic process, in which the infection is caused by hematogenous spread. The primary site of infection should be identified. Blood flow through vertebral endplate venous channels is relatively slow and tortuous, which may promote localization of the infection in the vertebra and spread to adjacent discs.[37] Bacteria isolated from cases of equine adult discospondylitis include *Brucella abortus*, alpha-haemolytic *Streptococcus*,[1] coagulase negative *Staphylococcus*,[6] and *Staphylococcus aureus*.[36] *Rhodococcus equi* has been implicated in a foal.[4]

Traumatic discospondylitis has been documented in clinical cases and at postmortem examination.[31] Intervertebral disc lesions, including fissuration, calcification, and herniation, have been described ultrasonographically and at postmortem examination at the lumbosacral junction and the cervical spine.[9]

Clinical Signs

Signs of weight loss, back or neck pain, fever, stiffness, and ataxia may all be notable in discospondylitis. Atrophy of the epaxial muscle in the thoracolumbar region may be evident in some horses suffering from chronic discospondylitis in this region.[2] Some horses are so affected that they are reluctant to eat off the ground. Lateral neck flexion can be markedly obtunded as well, and the abdomen may be held rigid as though intra-abdominal pain were present.

When compression of the spinal cord or root nerves is present, neurological symptoms can be observed.[13]

Blood analysis may reveal a leucocytosis and elevated fibrinogen.

Diagnosis

Diagnosis of discospondylitis is based upon appropriate clinical signs and radiographical findings.[1] Radiographic features of discospondylitis include lysis and/or proliferation of the vertebral bodies adjacent to the affected disc. As the disease progresses, the intervertebral disc space may narrow and collapse, and a smooth bony bridge may unite the affected vertebrae.[37] Scintigraphy,[23] computed tomography,[35] and ultrasonography[36] have been used to facilitate the diagnosis of equine discospondylitis and vertebral osteomyelitis. Scintigraphy may be useful to determine whether multiple sites of bone involvement are present.[39]

Treatment and Prognosis

Successful treatment of discospondylitis usually involves long-term antimicrobial administration.[2,23,37] In specific cases surgical curettage of the lesion is an option when access to the lesion is possible.[36] If the causative organism is not isolated, as is usually the case, broad-spectrum antimicrobials should be administered. Intravenous antimicrobials often reach higher tissue concentrations than oral medication and are recommended at the onset of therapy. Antimicrobials allowing distribution and penetration into bone should be administered; therapeutic options may include fluoroquinolones, macrolides, cephalosporins, and potentiated sulphonamides.[2] The total duration of antimicrobial treatment can be 4 to 6 months, which can make the treatment very costly.

Although the prognosis for horses with discospondylitis has generally been considered guarded, favorable outcomes have been associated with early detection, nonseptic lesions, the absence of spinal cord compression, administration of long-term antimicrobial therapy, and surgical curettage.[1,23,36]

SPONDYLOSIS

Etiology

Spondylosis (deformans) is more common than discospondylitis. It involves the vertebral body only, without including the intervertebral disc.[31] It is a degenerative condition affecting the vertebral body on the ventral aspect in the thoracic spine and merely the lateral aspect in the lumbar spine. Spondylosis results in osteophytes, often seen in several adjacent vertebrae. The most common location for these osteophytes is the vertebral segment between T10 and T14.[13,14] Probably because of regional biomechanical influences, the osteophytes are located at the ventrolateral aspect of the vertebral bodies in the thoracic region. Pathogenesis of osteophyte formation involves mechanical stress at the attachment of the most peripheral fibers of the intervertebral disc and the ventral longitudinal ligament (enthesiophytes).

Postmortem results of acute cases showed hemorrhage and fraying of collagen fibers of the intervertebral disc, no deeper than the annulus fibrosis. The facet joints in these cases had been jammed together and there was evidence of fraying and erosion of cartilage and hemarthrosis.[31] The osteophytes resulted in reduced mobility of the spine at the site of the osteophytes (with the end stage of complete ankylosis), putting more of the motion load on the adjacent vertebrae which induces more active bone remodeling, often visible on scintigraphic examination.

Clinical Signs

In the more acute stage, when active bone remodeling is in progress, the horse can show severe back pain with generalized stiffness and reluctance to work. These cases seem to relate to the lay term of cold-back, in which saddling, mounting, or starting to ride initiates a violent reaction of the horse, including bucking, running away, and laying down. In older cases the condition is less painful but more limiting in the motion of the spine, giving the horse a more stiff appearance. In chronic cases, there is often loss of cartilage in the facet joints, and the dorsal spinous processes can come close or make contact, giving the horse the appearance of a hollow back or acquired lordosis. This condition seems to be more common in event horses, show jumpers, and hunters than in Thoroughbred and Standardbred racehorses. Working draft horses endure enormous forces on their spine when pulling heavy loads, and seem to be more predisposed for spondylosis.[31]

Diagnosis

Radiography and scintigraphy (Figures 6.38 and 6.39) are the main diagnostic tools to confirm spondylosis. Scintigraphy can show the amount of bone activity as an indicator for acuteness and activity.

Treatment

Medication with NSAIDs is the only option. No surgical techniques have been described in the horse to stabilize the spine.

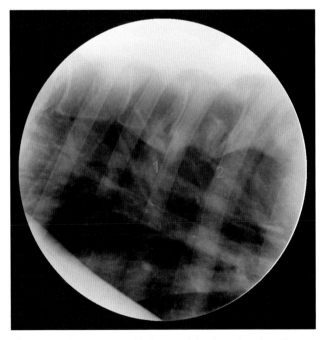

Figure 6.38. Radiographic image of the thoracic spine of a horse with severe spondylosis. There is proliferation of bone at the ventral aspect of the vertebral bodies. 1 = no complete contact between the proliferations, 2 = seemingly complete bridging of the intervertebral disk space.

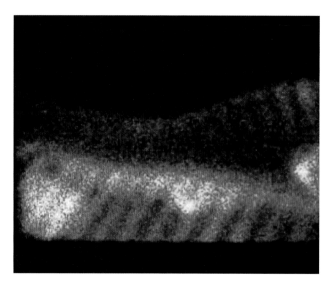

Figure 6.39. Scintigraphic image of a horse with IRU in the midthoracic spine, suggestive of spondylosis.

Prognosis

Prognosis for spondylosis to return to athletic career is guarded.

SCOLIOSIS, KYPHOSIS, AND LORDOSIS

These conditions can be congenital defects. The basic pathological defect of both scoliosis and lordosis is hypoplasia or aplasia of the articular facets of the intervertebral articulations, primarily in the thoracic spine.[38] Acquired lordosis can be seen in the older horse with osteoarthritis and ankylosis of the facet joints.[31]

Kyphosis in the lumbar spine seems to occur in Thoroughbreds (Figure 6.40). No data is available on the performance of horses with this condition.[31] With congenital deformities, it is likely that these conditions are not painful, but that they can limit athletic careers due to limitations in motion and propulsion. In the acquired cases, the initiating condition (osteoarthritis) can cause pain and clinical symptoms, as can localized pathology of the supraspinous ligament caused by focal kyphosis.

References

1. Adams SB, Steckel R, Blevins W. Diskospondylitis in five horses. J Am Vet Med Assoc 1985;186:270–272.
2. Alward AA, Pease AP, Jones SL. Thoracic discospondylitis with associated epaxial muscle atrophy in a Quarter Horse gelding. Eq Vet Educ 2007;3:67–71.
3. Cauvin E. Assessment of back pain in horses. Equine Practice 1997;19:522–533.
4. Chaffin MK, Honnas CM, Crabill MR, et al. *Cauda equina* syndrome, diskospondylitis, and a paravertebral abscess caused by *Rhodococcus equi* in a foal. J Am Vet Med Assoc 1995;206: 215–220.
5. Coudry V, Thibaud D, Riccio B, et al. Efficacy of tiludronate in the treatment of horses with signs of pain associated with osteoarthritic lesions of the thoracolumbar vertebral column. Am J Vet Res 2007;68(3):329–337.
6. Colbourne CM, Raidal SL, Yovich JV, et al. Cervical diskospondylitis in two horses. Aust Vet J 1997;75:477–479.
7. Desbrosse FG, Perrin R, Launois T, et al. Endoscopic resection of dorsal spinous processes and interspinous ligament in ten horses. Vet Surg 2007;36:149–155.
8. Denoix JM. Ultrasonographic evaluation of back lesions. Vet Clin North Am Equine Pract, 1999;15(1):131–159.
9. Denoix JM. Discovertebral pathology in horses. Eq Vet Educ 2007;3:72–73.
10. Denoix JM, Audige F, Robert C, et al. Alteration of locomotion in horses with vertebral lesions. Proc Conference Equine Sports Med Sci: The elite show jumper. Lidner A, ed. Arbeitsgruppe Pferd, Essen, 2000.
11. Denoix JM. Lesions of the vertebral column in poor performance horses. Proc World Eq Vet Assoc Symp Paris, 1999.
12. Denoix JM. Ligament injuries of the axial skeleton in the horse: Supraspinal and sacroiliac desmopathies. Dubai Int Eq Symp 1996.

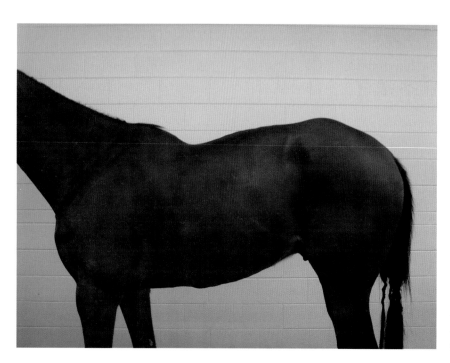

Figure 6.40. Seven-year-old Thoroughbred with marked kyphosis in the thoracolumbar spine. No clinical symptoms of back pain were present.

13. Denoix JM. Thoracolumbar malformations or injuries and neurological manifestations. Eq Vet Educ 2005;8:249–252.
14. Denoix JM, Audigié F, Coudry V. Review of diagnosis and treatment of lumbosacral pain in sport and race horses. Proceedings Am Assoc Equine Pract 2005;51:366–373.
15. Erichsen C, Eksel P, Roethlisberger HK, et al. Relationship between scintigraphic and radiographic evaluations of spinous processes in the thoracolumbar spine in riding horses without clinical signs of back problems. Eq Vet J 2004;36:458–465.
16. Gillen A, Dyson SJ, Murray R. Nuclear scintigraphic assessment of the thoracolumbar synovial intervertebral articulations. Eq Vet J 2009;41:1–7.
17. Haussler KK, Stover SM. Stress fractures of the vertebral lamina and pelvis in Thoroughbred racehorses. Equine Vet J, 1998; 30:374–381.
18. Haussler KK, Stover SM, Willits NH. Pathologic changes in the lumbosacral vertebrae and pelvis in Thoroughbred racehorses. Am J Vet Res 1999;60:143–163.
19. Haussler KK. Osseous spinal pathology. Vet Clin North Amer Equine Pract 1999;15(1):103–111.
20. Haussler KK. Chiropractic evaluation and management. Vet Clin North Am Equine Pract 1999;15(1):195–210.
21. Haussler KK, Bertram JE, Gellman K. *In vivo* segmental kinematics of the thoracolumbar spinal region in horses and effects of chiropractic manipulations. Proceedings Am Assoc Equine Pract 1999;45:327–329.
22. Henson FMD, Lamas L, Knezevic S, et al. Ultrasonographic evaluation of the supraspinous ligament in a series of ridden and unridden horses and horses with unrelated back pathology. BMC Vet Res 2007;1:3.
23. Hillyer MH, Innes JF, Patteson MW, et al. Diskospondylitis in an adult horse. Vet Record, 1996;139:519–521.
24. Hu AJ, Grant B, Grant J. Cervical vertebral osteomyelitis in a 4-month-old foal. Eq Vet Educ 2009;21:71–75.
25. Jeffcott LB. Disorders of the thoracolumbar spine of the horse—A survey of 443 cases. Eq Vet J 1980;12:197.
26. Jeffcott LB, et al. Effects of induced back pain on gait and performance of trotting horses. Eq Vet J 1982;14:129.
27. Johns S, Allen KA, Tyrrell LA. How to obtain digital radiographs of the thoracolumbar spine in the standing horse. Proceedings Am Assoc Equine Pract 2008;54:455–458.
28. Lauk H, Kreling I. Surgical treatment of kissing spines syndrome—50 cases. II. Results. Pferdeheilkunde 1998;14;123.
29. Licka T, Peham C. An objective method for evaluation of the flexibility of the back of standing horses. Equine Vet J 1998;30:412–415.
30. Ridgeway K, Harman J. Equine back rehabilitation. Vet Clin North Am Equine Pract 1999;15(1):263–280.
31. Rooney JR, Robertson JL. Equine Pathology. Wiley-Blackwell, Ames, 1996;218–223.
32. Schulte TL, Pietilä TA, Heidenreich J, et al. Injection therapy of lumbar facet syndrome: a prospective study. Acta Neurochir (Wien). 2006;148(11):1165–72.
33. Ständer M, März U, Steude U, et al. The facet syndrome: frequent cause of chronic backaches. Fortschr Med 2006;26;148(43):33–4.
34. Steckel RS, Kraus-Hansen AE, Fackelman GE, et al. Scintigraphic diagnosis of thoracolumbar spine disease in horses; a review of 50 cases. Proc Am Assoc Eq Pract 1991;37;583.
35. Stewart AJ, Salazar P, Waldridge BM, et al. Computed tomographic diagnosis of a pathological fracture due to rhodococcal osteomyelitis and spinal abscess in a foal. Eq Vet Educ 2007;6:231–235.
36. Sweers L, Carsten A. Imaging features of discospondylitis in two horses. Vet Rad Ultrasound 2006;47/2:159–164.
37. Thomas WB. Diskospondylitis and other vertebral infections. Vet Clin N Am Small Anim Pract 2000;30; 169–182.
38. Wong DM, Scarrat WK, Rohleder J. Hindlimb paresis associated with kyphosis, hemivertebrae and multiple thoracic vertebral malformations in a Quarter horse gelding. Eq Vet Educ 2005;8:249.
39. Weaver MP, Jeffcott LB, Nowak M. Radiology and scintigraphy. In The Veterinary Clinics of North America. Equine Practice. Back Problems. KK Haussler, ed. WB Saunders, Philadelphia, 1999;113–130.

THE NECK AND POLL

This section emphasizes the cervical disorders that directly cause or contribute to lameness. The developmental cervical disorders, most often causing neurological symptoms, are covered in Chapter 11.

As described in the first part of this chapter, the cervical spine has an important function in locomotion. Any dysfunction of the cervical spine can cause an altered gait pattern, often described as lameness. Sometimes the symptoms of the dysfunction of the cervical column are observed as altered behavior (head shaking, not connecting with the rider's hand, pulling, bucking, rearing, etc) but are presented to the veterinarian as lameness. Other cases are presented as lower limb-lameness or shoulder lameness. The following sections cover the common causes of cervical dysfunction and their symptoms, diagnosis, and treatment.

NUCHAL LIGAMENT

The Nuchal ligament connects the caudal aspect of the skull, dorsal processes of the cervical vertebrae, and withers region (the dorsal processes of the first thoracic vertebrae), and has an important function in supporting the entire neck. Elastic fibers in this structure store kinetic energy during locomotion and release the energy at specific phases of the locomotion when certain muscle groups move or activate parts of the cervical spine and the attached front limbs, thus contributing to an efficient gait. The head and neck function as a sling during propulsion and have a coordinating function in the specific pattern of the gait. For instance, the periodic sinusoid motion instigates activation patterns in the muscles of the neck and shoulder.[8]

Desmopathy at the origin of the nuchal ligament located at the base of the skull and the insertion to the dorsal processes of the cervical and cranial thoracic vertebrae is associated with pain and can alter this sinusoid pattern, thus altering the gait.[4,11] Tension in the nuchal ligament and its attachments is greater and symptoms of desmopathy can be more pronounced in specific positions, such as when the neck is more flexed, the head is more parallel to the vertical or even behind the vertical, or the head is in a higher or lower position.

Etiology

Etiology of desmopathy of the nuchal ligament is very often associated with trauma. Falling down or pulling backwards when tied, being caught in fences, and trailering accidents can put extreme force on the ligament and its attachments, causing trauma to the nuchal ligament and other structures in the neck and poll. Training methods such as tying the horse's head to the side or between the front limbs, as is sometimes practiced in preparation for Western pleasure, or hyperflexion or "Rollkur," as is practiced by some dressage trainers, can predispose horses in these disciplines for nuchal ligament pathology.

Clinical Signs

Symptoms of nuchal ligament pathology are diverse and very often more visible when the horse is worked. The horse may appear stiff, the neck does not move up and down as much as usual at the walk, and when worked on circles the head is out with no flexion of the neck according to the diameter of the circle.

When ridden or driven, the contact with the bit through the reins or lines can feel different to the rider/driver, with one side feeling more rigid or as if the horse is pulling on one side. Dental issues can have the same symptoms, so excluding dental problems helps to confirm or at least suspect neck problems. Particular head positions can cause pain, making the horse behave defensively or reluctant to perform certain exercises.

The neck is an important balancing tool for the horse during work, so in disciplines in which balance is of major importance for performance, such as jumping, dressage, and eventing, general lack of performance can be one of the more indistinctive signs.

Diagnosis

Desmopathy can be found at the attachment of the ligament to bone, which may cause enthesophytes that can be seen with radiographs. It also may be located in the ligament itself, in which case the altered fiber pattern is visible on ultrasonographic examination. Nuclear scintigraphy can show the increased bone turnover at the attachment sites (Figure 6.41). MRI and CT can give

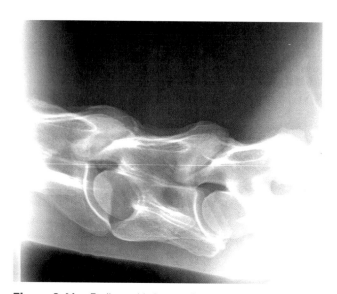

Figure 6.41. Radiographic image of the cervical spine with C5, C6, and C7 in view. There is mild enlargement of the facet joints between C5 and C6 and C6 and C7, with irregular joint spaces. This is indicative of mild to moderate osteoarthritis of the caudal cervical facet joints, and is a common finding in horses without clinical signs.

detailed information about the condition of the more cranial cervical vertebrae and the ligament. Newer MRI equipment (with smaller bore and larger aperture) facilitates imaging of the more caudal vertebrae, but in most cases imaging is limited to the level of the fourth or fifth cervical vertebra.

Treatment

Therapy for desmopathy of the nuchal ligament is similar to that of any desmopathy: rest and anti-inflammatory medication, as well as possible extracorporeal shock wave treatment. Biological treatments with stem cells, A-cell, and platelet-rich plasma are in the stage of experimental use and studies to be published in the near future on these therapy modalities will show their effectiveness in treatment of desmopathies in general and in the nuchal ligament in particular.

A specific structure in the poll, the nuchal bursa, which is present at the dorsal aspect at C1 in nearly all horses, and less frequent at C2, can be involved in pathology of the nuchal ligament. Bursitis is considered to be a rare condition. However, many veterinarians in the field of sports medicine diagnose bursitis of the nuchal ligament quite frequently. It is difficult to completely confirm this diagnosis on ultrasonographic examination alone. CT or MRI imaging, performed under general anesthesia, can give a more detailed image of the bursa(e) and its adjacent structures along with a more confirmed diagnosis. A common treatment modality for bursitis of the nuchal bursa is the ultrasound-guided injection of corticosteroids into the bursa. Calcifications in the bursa region are observed quite frequently in the author's clinic on routine radiographs of this region; however, in these cases the owner of the horse may not always remember any treatment or problem in this region.

Prognosis

When given enough time for complete recovery and rehabilitation, prognosis for nuchal ligament desmopathy is favorable.[4] The only exception may be the high-level dressage horses when the initial injury to the ligament has not been recognized and has developed into a more chronic phase or is considered to be a repetitive stress injury. In these cases, when the horse's head is in a very high and upright position, as needed for the highest grades of collection, strain to the ligament is the highest and the horse can show pain or defensive behavior such as rearing or shaking the head.

When calcifications are present due to mineralization of a hematoma or corticosteroid deposition, signs of altered behavior or performance are common and prognosis is guarded for complete recovery to the initial level of performance.

CERVICAL FACET JOINTS

Osteoarthritis of the cervical facet joints is very common in many horses, even without clinical signs.[4,10] Enlargement of the more caudal facet joints with irregularly shaped or narrowed joint spaces is common on cervical radiographs in horses of any breed at a slightly older age (older than 4 to 5 years) (Figure 6.41).

Etiology

Osteoarthritis of the cervical facet joints can be the result of osteochondrosis of the articular surfaces, as in any other joint affected by osteochondrosis. Trauma to the neck is often a cause for facet joint arthritis. The trauma may be the result of trailering accidents, falling or hanging in cross ties, running into objects with the neck, falling during exercise (racing, eventing, jumping), flipping backwards, etc. Instability of the neck due to malformation of vertebrae or joint surfaces predisposes the horse to facet joint arthritis, and it is often found in conjunction with several congenital or developmental cervical malformation syndromes.

Clinical Signs

Osteoarthritis of the cervical facet joints can cause a great diversity of symptoms. At first, pain can cause behavior similar to that described for nuchal ligament pathology.

When severe bone proliferation is present at or around the facet joints, mobility can be limited, thus limiting athletic performance. In dressage, the horse may be reluctant to bend the neck in a lateral direction, bring the head vertical in the collection position, or stretch down. A jumper can be difficult when asked for short turns or lack balance during the jump due to neck stiffness, while the barrel racer can be difficult to turn around the barrels.

Due in which several muscles originate at locations in the neck and have their insertion to the scapula (trapezius muscle, rhomboideus muscle) or humerus (brachiocephalicus muscle), contraction of these muscles can cause pain in the arthritic facet joints and thus alter the gait (e.g., shorter anterior stride, reduced protraction of the scapula) and mimic shoulder or even lower limb lameness.

Neurological symptoms can occur when bone proliferation of the arthritic joint structures protrudes into the spinal canal, with lower hindquarter activity as the most common sign. When the bony proliferation invades the intravertebral foramen, root nerves can be compressed.[9] The cervical nerves between C5 and C6, C6 and C7, and C7 and T1 (the sixth, seventh, and eighth cervical nerves) form the brachial plexus, so compression of these root nerves can be sensed as pain in the limb, and limb lameness may be observed.[10,13] When root nerve compression is present, a patchy spot of sweating may be noticed on one or both sides of the neck and/or thorax.

Diagnosis

At the clinical examination, cervical facet joint arthritis can be suspected when the range of motion in the neck is limited. With complete flexion to the side, the horse should be able to flex the neck laterally, touching the thoracic wall with its nose without rotation in C2 in both directions. A 20% to 30% limitation in the total range of motion in the lateral plane is found in many older horses without clinical symptoms and can be considered normal. Cervical facet joint arthritis is highly suspected with an asymmetric limitation of the range of motion. Range of motion in the dorsoventral plane can be tested by manually stretching the neck upward, while a carrot stretch between the front limbs can show the range of motion in the ventral direction. The dorsoventral range of motion tests are not as easy to interpret as the lateral plane, because they cannot be checked for symmetry, so there is no clear maximum range of motion to be defined. Palpation of the facet joints, left and right, can provide information about their size and shape, as well as pain when palpated.

When a particular joint is identified as highly suspected for causing the symptoms, ultrasound-guided intra-articular block of the facet joint can be used to verify the cause. This can best be seen when the horse is performing the work in which the symptoms are most obvious, for instance, so under saddle, at work, etc.

Radiography is the first imaging technique of choice.[1,6,7] Lateral views with a small degree of angle from the horizontal plane can be used to project the left or right facet joint without superimposing on top of the ipsilateral joint.

Ultrasonography can be used to image the facet joints as well, providing visual information about joint space size and shape and bone proliferation at the edges of the facet joint. Ultrasonography is also very helpful in treating cervical facet joint arthritis, because ultrasound-guided injection of the facet joint is not difficult.[2]

Nuclear scintigraphy (Figure 6.42) can be used to identify facet joints with an increased uptake of radio-

pharmaceutical as a sign of active inflammation to distinguish the older, consolidated proliferations, which are visible on radiographs, from signs of active arthritis/synovitis. This is useful in making decisions about the injection of corticosteroids.

MRI and CT imaging give much more detailed information about the size and shape of the facet joints and their potential compression effects on root nerves and the spinal cord, but are limited to the more cranial facet joints. These techniques also involve general anesthesia and carry higher costs.

Myelography is considered the gold standard for identifying possible involvement of root nerves and/or spinal cord compression; however, this technique is only 50% accurate at identifying the specific location of compression of the spinal cord when compared to necropsy findings (Pease AJ, personal communications). Electromyography can be used to identify changes in muscle signals in the segmental muscles in the neck and thorax to show decreased innervation of these muscles as a sign of root nerve compression.[14]

Treatment and Prognosis

As with any osteoarthritis, treatment for cervical facet joint osteoarthritis can include medication with NSAIDs. Intra-articular medication with corticosteroids, deposited in or close to the joint under ultrasound guidance, has been described as a useful treatment. Triamcinolone is the corticosteroid of choice because it does not cause as much irritation in the adjacent structures such as the ligamentous tissue and muscle as methylprednisolone acetate when not deposited in the joint itself.

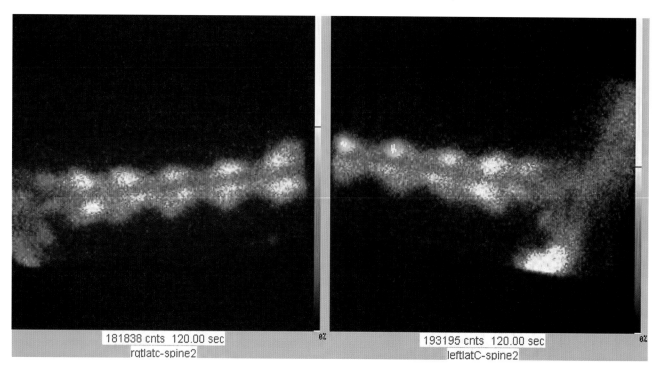

Figure 6.42. Scintigraphic images of the cervical spine. In the left image, IRU in C7 is visible at the right side of the neck in the arch and the body of C7; this is normal. In the right image, there is IRU visible in the arches of C4 and C5 on the left side of the neck, indicative for active facet joint osteoarthritis.

Osteoarthritis of facet joints, especially in the more caudal aspect of the cervical spine or cranial thoracic spine, may result in an associated enlargement of the joint capsule and subsequent pressure to the spinal cord or root nerves. Oral dexamethasone may be used to reduce this swelling and the signs of nerve compression.

DISCOSPONDYLITIS

As described in the section on the thoracolumbar spine, discospondylitis can occur in the cervical spine, most likely in the caudal cervical vertebrae. Signs of neck pain and front limb stiffness or lameness may be present. Diagnosis can be made with radiography and scintigraphy, and the prognosis is guarded.[3,4,13]

CERVICAL FRACTURES

As described earlier in this chapter, fractures of cervical vertebrae can occur, and in nearly all cases this is due to severe trauma. Fractures of facet joint surfaces are rather common, but laminar fractures and fractures of the body or the arch of the cervical vertebrae also have been described. Depending on the location and the extent of the fracture, hemorrhage and swelling can extend to the spinal cord and cause ataxia. Horses with

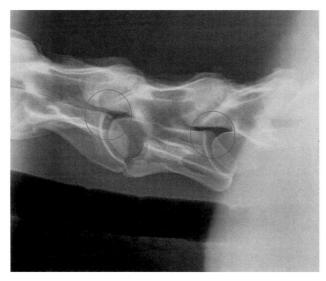

Figure 6.43. Radiographic image of the cervical spine. Note the change at the caudal aspect of the end plate of C5 and the small fragment (left circle) when compared to the clean appearance at C6 (right circle). This is most likely caused by trauma to the intervertebral ligament at the ventral base of the spinal canal, but also can be caused by local mineralization within the intervertebral disk. In the acute stage, swelling can cause neurologic symptoms related to compression of root nerves or the spinal cord.

an acute fracture show pain and are unable to move the cervical spine in the affected region. Radiography is the diagnostic tool of choice, and in most cases lateral views are sufficient to show the fracture. Ventrodorsal views can assist in determining the extent and location. In specific cases scintigraphy can give adjacent information from 7 to 10 days after the injury, when displacement of the fracture and recognition of the fracture line are difficult on the initial radiological examination. Ultrasonographic examination of the cervical spine is an option, but primarily shows fractured facet joints. It is difficult to make an interpretation of larger fractures through the body or arch of the vertebra.

When there is no damage to the spinal cord or the adjacent root nerves, and there is no displacement of the fragments, the prognosis can be moderate. Treatment includes stall rest or confinement in a small pen or paddock to reduce motion. However, callus formation can cause compression of the root nerves or the spinal cord in a later stage, and fractures of facet joint surfaces often result in facet joint arthritis. Trauma to ligamentous structures and the intervertebral disc may be not visible on initial radiographs (Figure 6.43), and can easily be overlooked or not recognized, but may result in discospondylitis, spondylitis, or osteoarthritis in a later stage.

References

1. Butler J, Colles C, Dyson SJ, et al. The spine. In Clinical Radiology of the Horse, 2nd ed. Blackwell Science, Oxford, 2000.
2. Chope K. How to perform sonographic examination and ultrasound-guided injection of the cervical vertebral facet joints in horses. Proceedings Am Assoc Equine Pract 2008;54:186–189.
3. Denoix JM. Discovertebral pathology in horses. Eq Vet Educ 2007;3:71–73.
4. Dyson SJ. Problems associated with the neck: Neck pain, stiffness or abnormal posture and forelimb gait abnormalities. In Current Therapy in Equine Medicine 4th ed. Robinson NE, Wilson MR, eds. WB Saunders, Philadelphia, 1997.
5. Hu, AJ, Grant B, Cannon J. Cervical vertebral osteomyelitis in a 4-month-old foal. Equine Vet Educ 2009;Feb:71–75.
6. Hudson NPH, Mayhew IG. Radiographic and myelographic assessment of the equine cervical vertebral column and spinal cord. Eq Vet Educ 2005;2:43–48.
7. Hughes KJ. Spinal radiography of the horse. Eq Vet Educ 2007;10:460–462.
8. Larson BE, Clayton HM, Elvin NG, et al. Modeling the inertial movement of the head and neck in the trotting horse—a pilot study. Poster. 2008.
9. Marks D. Cervical nerve root compression in a horse, treated by epidural injection of corticosteroids. J Equine Vet Sci 1999; 19:399.
10. Mayhew IG. The healthy spinal cord. Milne lecture, AAEP 1999.
11. Nowak M. Die insertiondesmopathie des nackenstrangurprungs beim pferd. Diagnostik; differentialdiagnostik. In Proc 7th Congress on Equine Medicine and Surgery, Geneva, 2001.
12. Olghowy TWJ. Vertebral body osteomyelitis due to Rhodococcus equi in two Arabian foals. J Am Vet Med 1994;26:79–82.
13. Ricardi G, Dyson SJ. Forelimb lameness associated with radiographic abnormalities of the cervical vertebrae. Eq Vet J 1993;25; 422.
14. Van Wessum R, Sloet MM, Clayton HM. Electromyography in the horse; a review. Vet Quart 1999;21:3–7.

Principles of Musculoskeletal Disease

JOINT INJURIES AND DISEASE AND OSTEOARTHRITIS

C. WAYNE MCILWRAITH

Arthritis may be defined simply as inflammation of a joint. It is a nonspecific term and does little to describe the nature of the various specific entities that affect equine joints. The role of inflammation also varies considerably among the different conditions. Such general terms are no longer appropriate in the management of equine joint conditions. Specific diagnoses must be made to effectively treat the horse and make accurate prognoses.

Knowledge of etiology, pathogenesis, diagnosis, and treatment of each of the different equine joint conditions has a separate textbook on equine joint disease.[67] To understand joint disease in the horse, a basic knowledge of the anatomy and physiology of joints, as well as their pathobiologic responses, is necessary.

ANATOMY AND PHYSIOLOGY OF JOINTS

Classification

Joints are most often classified according to their normal range of motion. Three groups are recognized: synarthroses (immovable joints), amphiarthroses (slightly movable joints), and diarthroses (movable joints), also known as synovial joints. Synovial joints have two major functions: (1) to enable movement and (2) to transfer load.[106] The entire structure is invested by a fibrous capsule. Diarthroses include most of the joints of the extremities. Because these are the joints that we are essentially concerned with in equine lameness, their anatomy and physiology are described in detail.

Adams and Stashak's Lameness in Horses, 6e, edited by Gary M. Baxter
© 2011 Blackwell Publishing, Ltd.

General Anatomy

The synovial or diarthrodial joint consists of the articulating surfaces of bone which are covered by articular cartilage and secured by a joint capsule and ligaments, and a cavity within these structures containing synovial fluid (Figure 7.1). The joint capsule is comprised of 2 parts: the fibrous layer, which is located externally and is continuous with the periosteum or perichondrium (and, ultimately, bone), and the synovial membrane, which lines the synovial cavity where articular cartilage is not present.

The fibrous portion of the joint capsule is comprised of dense fibrous connective tissue that provides some mechanical stability to the joint. The collateral ligaments are associated with the joint capsule. Intra-articular ligaments normally have a synovial membrane cover. Type I collagen predominates in the fibrous connective tissues of the joint.[106] It is vascular and has afferent pain fibers. Using immunohistochemistry with substance P as a more sensitive way of identifying the distribution of nociceptor fibers, it has been shown that sensory nerve fibers are present in the synovial membrane and subintimal layers as well as collateral ligaments, suspensory ligament, and distal sesamoid ligament attachments.[10]

The insertions of the fibrous capsule and articular ligaments into the adjacent bones demonstrate a zonal organization with a gradual transition of joint capsule and ligaments to mineralized fibrocartilage and then to bone. This enhances the ability of the insertions to distribute forces evenly and decrease the likelihood of pullout failure.[54]

Stability of the joint is provided by the bony configuration of the joint, the ligamentous and capsular support

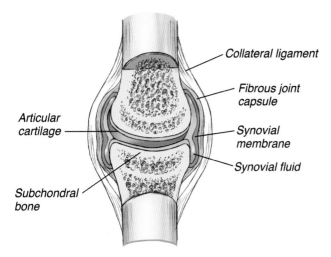

Figure 7.1.   Diagram of a typical synovial joint.

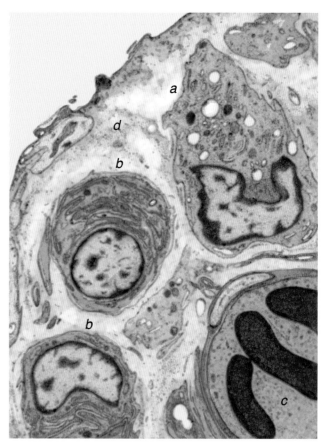

Figure 7.2.   Diagram of a portion of synovial membrane demonstrating synoviocytes (types A and B, a and b) within the intercellular stroma of the intima, capillary (c), and collagenous matrix of intima (d). Tissue deep to this is considered subintimal.

systems, and the musculotendinous units controlling the joint. In addition, there is a negative hydrostatic pressure within the synovial cavity of normal joints, and this is considered to impart a "suction" and stabilizing effect.[99]

It has also been demonstrated that only the periarticular soft tissues (capsule, ligaments, and synovial tissue) and bone have significant force-attenuating properties (these studies were done with longitudinally applied, external impulsive force on adult bovine interphalangeal joints).[82] Articular cartilage and synovial fluid have little effect in force attenuation. This emphasizes the importance of both soft tissues of the joint and bone in providing shock absorption.

Synovial Membrane Structure and Function

Equine synovial membrane (also called synovium) is smooth and glistening in some regions of the joint and is formed into numerous villi in other regions. These villi have specific locations and a diverse morphology. Although villi proliferate in association with trauma and other insults, they are present in the fetus and, therefore, at birth.

Histologically, the synovial membrane is a modified mesenchymal tissue and consists of 2 layers: the intima, an incomplete cellular lining layer that lies next to the joint cavity and overlies a deeper layer of connective tissue (fibrous, areolar, or adipose) termed the subsynovial layer, or the subintima. Generally, the synovial membrane is fibrous and flat in regions where it is subjected to increased pressure; it is areolar and may be folded where it must move freely and independently of the joint capsule. The areolar subintima consists of loose fibrous connective tissue that continues into the central core of the villi. Numerous blood vessels are present.

The synovial cells of the intima (synoviocytes) form an incomplete layer that is 1 to 4 cells thick, and no basement membrane can be detected (Figure 7.2).[65] The synoviocytes have been classified at the ultrastructural level into 2 principal types designated as types A and B. The type A cells resemble macrophages and type B cells

resemble fibroblasts. Intermediate cells are also observed. A concept has evolved in which type A and type B cells are not distinct, but rather merely cells whose differences in morphology reflect the functions they currently perform.[65]

Numerous blood vessels are present in the subintima and extend to within 5 to 10 microns from the intimal surface.[65] It appears that each joint has a dual nerve supply consisting of specific articular nerves that reach the joint capsule as independent articular branches of adjacent peripheral nerves, and by articular branches that are nonspecific and arise from related muscle nerves.[65]

The 3 principal functions of the synovial membrane are phagocytosis, regulation of protein and hyaluronan (HA) content of the synovial fluid, and regeneration.[65] Excessive phagocytic activity or disruption of lysosomal or cellular membranes releases enzymes into the environment (a typical feature of synovitis). The synovial membrane acts as an important permeability barrier which, in turn, controls synovial fluid composition. Most small molecules cross the synovial membrane by a process of free diffusion that is limited by the intercellular spaces in the synovial membrane rather than by blood vessel fenestrations.[99] In traumatic effusions, changes in protein content and composition have been

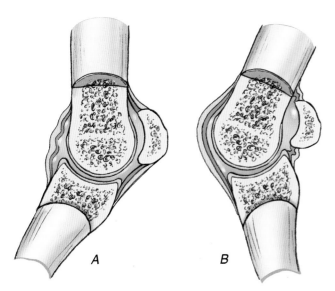

Figure 7.3. Diagram of a metacarpophalangeal joint demonstrating how redundant synovial membrane gathers at the dorsal aspect on extension (A) and at the palmar aspect on flexion (B).

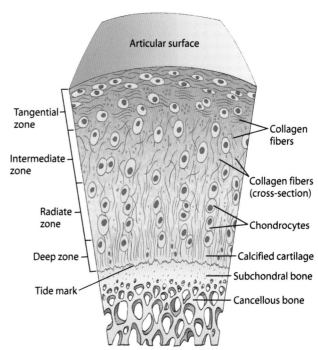

Figure 7.4. Diagram of adult articular cartilage showing the 4 layers and the arrangement of the chondrocytes and collagenous fibers.

associated with both increased vascular permeability and increased protein synthesis by the synoviocytes.

The ability of the synovial membrane to reform following synovectomy has been described in the horse[40,105] and reveals that 120 days after subtotal synovectomy, there is evidence of restoration and an intimal layer was present.[105] However, the synovium was devoid of villi and there was subintimal fibrosis.

Another important property of the joint capsule is its ability to allow complete range of motion. The example of a metacarpophalangeal (fetlock) joint, illustrated in Figure 7.3, shows that synovial membrane gathers at the dorsal aspect of the joint in extension and at the palmar aspect in flexion. This property of gathering is called "redundancy."[99] Inflammation and fibrosis impede this property and result in joint stiffness. Elasticity of the joint capsule is also important because of its role in shock absorption.[83]

Articular Cartilage Structure and Function

Grossly, normal articular cartilage appears milky and opaque in the thicker regions and translucent with a slight bluish tinge in the thinner regions. The surface is not smooth. Studies using the scanning electron microscope have demonstrated undulations and irregular depressions.[28] The articular cartilage of equine joints is generally of the hyaline type but fibrocartilage is also present at the junction of articular cartilage, synovial membrane, and periosteum (called the transition zone), and in menisci.[65]

Histologically, adult articular cartilage has been divided into 4 layers, and the chondrocytes have different appearances within these layers (Figure 7.4):

1. The tangential or superficial layer, containing flattened or ovoid chondrocytes and tangentially oriented collagenous fibrils

2. The intermediate or middle layer, containing larger chondrocytes that may be single or paired and randomly oriented collagenous fibrils
3. The radiate or deeper layer, containing chondrocytes arranged in vertical columns separated by collagenous fibrils that have an overall radial arrangement
4. The calcified cartilage layer, comprised of mineralized cartilage and chondrocytes in various stages of degeneration.

A basophilic-staining, undulating line of division between the radiate layer and the layer of calcified cartilage is termed the "tide mark" or "tide line." It delineates the elastic, nonmineralized layers of the articular cartilage from the layers of calcified cartilage that has little resilience. The extracellular matrix of the articular cartilage is a complex of collagen fibrils, proteoglycans, glycoproteins and water (Figures 7.5 and 7.6).[65]

Collagens

Type II collagen comprises 90% to 95% of the collagen in articular cartilage and forms fibrils and fibers intertwined throughout the matrix. Equine type II collagen has been characterized biochemically by cyanogen bromide-cleaved peptide profiles[109] and is secreted as a procollagen. The complete sequence of equine type II procollagen messenger RNA has been reported[86] and these authors also showed that chondrocytes harvested from juvenile horses exhibited more synthetic activity in culture with high steady state levels of messenger RNA for type II procollagen. These authors also showed that IL-1β and TNFα produced a dose-dependent decrease in the steady state mRNA levels for type II

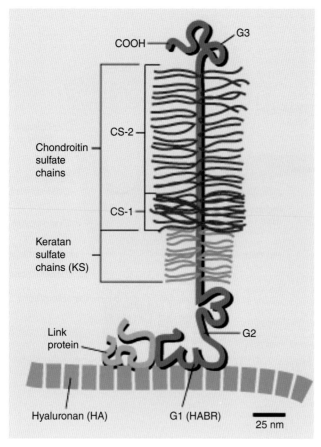

COOH — G3

CS-2

Chondroitin
sulfate
chains

CS-1

Keratan
sulfate
chains (KS)

G2

Link
protein

Hyaluronan (HA)   G1 (HABR)

25 nm

Figure 7.5. Diagram of a proteoglycan monomer formed by a protein core and glycosaminoglycan (chondroitin sulfate and keratin sulfate) side chains. Each proteoglycan core of the proteoglycan molecule is attached through a G-1 domain to an HA backbone through link protein to form aggregating proteoglycan (aggrecan). There are 2 other globular domains (G2 and G3).

collagen. Type II procollagen is expressed at very low levels in adult horses compared to younger ones. This may be relevant to naturally occurring changes of cartilage in the joints of older horses.

There are small amounts of type VI, IX, XI, XII, and XIV collagen, which help form and give stability to the type II fibril network.[76] The collagenous fibrils provide tensile strength to the articular cartilage in adult articular cartilage; this property chiefly resides in the superficial layers where the collagenous fibers are oriented parallel to the surface of the cartilage. In the middle layer of the cartilage the collagenous fibrils are randomly arranged and they become radially arranged in the deep layer. Tensile strength is not as critical in these deeper layers in normal cartilage, but if superficial erosion occurs, the collagen of these deeper layers is vulnerable to disruption. It has been shown that in immature cartilage the deeper layers also possess considerable tensile strength but this is lost with maturation.[93] The tensile properties automatically change with enzymatic degradation of hydroxy pyridinoline cross links, which emphasizes the importance of these cross links in providing cartilage stiffness, strength, and tension.[96]

Collagen fibers are also arranged concentrically around chondrocytes to form a capsule, called a chondron. Each chondron contains 1 or more chondrocytes, is invested by collagenous pericellular capsule, and is surrounded by a proteoglycan-rich territorial matrix.[80] Collagen type VI, fibronectin, and thrombospondin are present in this chondron capsule and help anchor the chondrocyte within the chondron and attach the chondron within the extracellular matrix.[76]

Proteoglycans

The proteoglycans (PG) (previously called mucopolysaccharides) are the other major solid component of the articular cartilage matrix. They occupy the spaces between the collagen fibrils. The basic PG molecule is a monomer formed by a protein core and glycosaminoglycan (GAG) side chains (Figure 7.5). Most of the proteoglycans (85%) form large aggregates by noncovalent attachment of the core protein of the proteoglycan to hyaluronan under the stabilization of a link protein (Figure 7.6). This aggregate is called aggregating proteoglycan or aggrecan.

The major glycosaminoglycans in adult articular cartilage are chondroitin-6-sulfate and keratan sulfate. Chondroitin-4-sulfate is an important constituent of immature articular cartilage, but its level decreases to a low percentage with cartilage maturity. The glycosaminoglycans consist of repeating units of disaccharides, which are important because of their polyanionic nature (carboxyl and sulfate radicals in chondroitin sulfate and sulfate radicals in keratan sulfate). The charges of the polyanionic GAG side chains both repel each other and attract a hydration shell. These properties, in turn, provide the articular cartilage with a physicochemical stiffness and affect cartilage permeability.[56] The aggrecan molecules are contained by the collagen network and hence the proteoglycans impart compressive stiffness.[46] It should be noted that enmeshment of the proteoglycans by the collagenous framework and specific interactions between the 2 components are necessary for the proteoglycans to function.[7]

The average proteoglycan unit in articular cartilage has a molecular weight of 3 million Daltons and contains 100 chondroitin sulfate side chains and 100 keratan sulfate side chains.[76] More than 100 of these proteoglycan monomers attach to a hyaluronan (HA) backbone to form the proteoglycan aggregate aggrecan, which has a molecular weight of more than 200 million Daltons (Figure 7.6). The proteoglycan monomer has been the subject of many studies. There are 2 globular domains (G1 and G2) at the HA-associated end followed by an extended glycosaminoglycan-containing region (E2), with a third globular domain (G3) at the other end. The N-terminal region of the aggrecan is attached to hyaluronan and the region that contains the majority of the glycosaminoglycans is an extended region lying between G2 and G3.

Other nonaggregating proteoglycans in articular cartilage include biglycan, decorin, and fibromodulin. Equine decorin has been characterized biochemically in the horse,[79] as have the gene sequences of biglycan and decorin.[86]

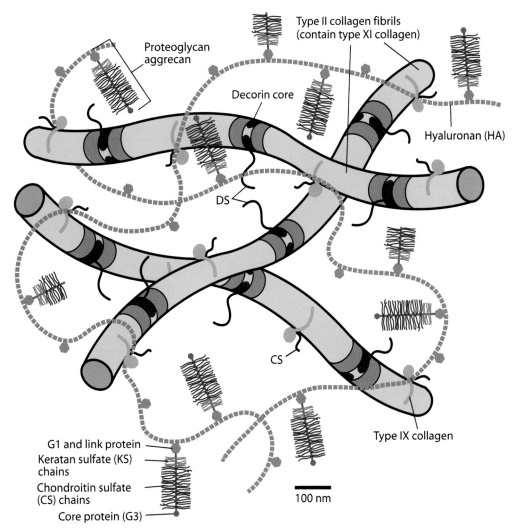

Figure 7.6. Diagram representing a portion of extra-cellular matrix showing organization of type II collagen fibers and multiple proteoglycan molecules that bind HA to form aggrecan entrapped within the collagen fibers. (Adapted from Poole AR. Cartilage in health and disease. In Arthritis and Allied Conditions. A Textbook of Rheumatology ATR. McCarty DJ, ed. Lea and Febiger, Philadelphia, 1993, pp. 279–333.)

Glycoproteins

Noncollagenous, nonproteoglycan glycoproteins constitute a small but significant portion of articular cartilage.[106] There are 3 fractions of equine link protein: LP1, LP2, and LP3.[23,79] Other glycoproteins of cartilage include chondronectin (thought to adhere chondrocytes to type II collagen surfaces), fibronectin (adheres cells to molecules and surfaces), cartilage oligomeric matrix protein (COMP), thrombospondin, and anchorin C-II, as well as cartilage-derived growth factor.

Cartilage Nutrition and Innervation

The articular cartilage is avascular, lacking both blood and lymph vessels. The deep layers of immature cartilage are penetrated extensively by vascular buds from the ossified portion of the epiphysis, which appear to play an important role in nutrition of the cartilage from the subchondral region.[65] Immature articular cartilage is an articular-epiphyseal complex with the deeper layers constituting a growth zone. In adults, the articular cartilage is separated from the subchondral vascular spaces by an end plate of bone (the subchondral plate), and nutrition of the articular cartilage occurs by diffusion from the synovial fluid. Chondrocytes function by anaerobic glycolysis. Under physiologic loads, cartilage can be compressed to 40% of its original height. The depth to which the diffusing nutritional gradient can extend is limited and was calculated to be a maximal cartilage thickness of 6 mm.[56] Because of this limit, necrosis secondarily occurs when retained thickened cartilage, as develops in some cases of OCD, exceeds diffusion limits.

There are no nerves in articular cartilage, and the bearing surface of the joint depends on nerve endings in the joint capsule, ligaments, muscle, and subchondral bone for appreciation of pain and proprioception.

Biomechanics

As indicated previously, articular cartilage is a tissue consisting of aggrecan that is stiff in compression, collagen that is stiff and strong in tension, and somewhat freely moving fluid carrying mobile ions (interstitial fluid). These components interact to provide the following mechanical and physical characteristics when young and healthy: (1) a permeable matrix that is stiff in compression, (2) a fibrous network capable of withstanding high tensile stresses, (3) a fluid that flows under load or deformation and aids in dissipating high stresses in the tissue, and (4) a high swelling pressure which results in a matrix swollen with water.[73] It has also been noted that an important function of aggrecan in cartilage is to retard the rate of stretch and alignment when a tensile load is suddenly applied, and that this mechanism may be useful in protecting the cartilage collagen network during physiologic situations.[96]

In an unloaded joint, the opposing articular surfaces are not completely congruent.[28] However, under physiologic loading, because the cartilage is soft, deformation causes an increase of contact area (reducing tissue stress levels) and increases joint conformity (which provides additional stability). The adaptation of the shape of loaded cartilage may also help to form and retain boundary lubrication (see below). As articular cartilage directly under load is compressed, the surrounding areas are subjected to transverse tensile strains. These forces tend to redistribute fluid away from the compressed area and into the stretched regions. As mentioned previously, the major contribution to the osmotic pressure provided by the proteoglycans is derived from negatively charged sulfate and carboxyl groups of the glycosaminoglycans and the associated cations (ionic or Gibbs-Donnan effect).[106] Water is attracted by the high charge density, and this osmotic pressure may contribute up to 50% of the compressive stiffness of the articular cartilage. The swelling pressure is balanced by the tensile stress of the collagen framework.

Mow and colleagues have described the extracellular matrix as a cohesive porous composite.[72] Their biphasic model for articular cartilage considers the tissue as an interacting mixture of 2 continua: a porous permeable elastic solid and interstitial fluid. Because of swelling pressure, the collagen network of the articular cartilage is under a tensile prestress even when unloaded. During compression, the concentration of the organic material and the charge density increase because the interstitial fluid is forced to flow from the matrix. A new equilibrium is reached when the charge density, collagen tension, and applied load are in balance (Figure 7.7). The deformation of this cartilage in association with fluid exudation is called creep. The compression time curve consists of the creep phase, controlled by fluid exudation, and the second phase, which is related to the collagen proteoglycan matrix component. During prolonged periods of stationary loading, fluid is slowly exuded and redistributed within the cartilage until an equilibrium position is reached. At this stage, the increased concentration of the fixed charge density is counterbalanced by the increased osmotic swelling pressure of the proteoglycan. When fluid motion ceases, the entire external load is borne by the solid extracellular matrix.

Intermittent pressures created by the interaction of the opposing articular surfaces pump fluid through the cartilage for nutrition and the removal of metabolic byproducts.[65] Expressed fluid from the articular cartilage resembles synovial fluid except for its low protein content and viscosity.[49] It has been shown that the concentration of fixed charges from glycosaminoglycans is the prime determinant of cartilage permeability.[56] Simple diffusion seems sufficient for nutrition of all but the deepest layers of articular cartilage, but joint movement probably facilitates the process.

Studies have shown that proteoglycans restrict solute movement within the tissue matrix. The proteoglycans restrict the diffusion of large, uncharged solutes but do not affect the diffusion of small, uncharged solutes. The molecular size and conformation of the solute is also an important factor. Removal of proteoglycans increases the influx of large molecules into the matrix, and this suggests that proteoglycan removal may also increase the efflux of large molecules out of the tissue matrix.[107] It has been suggested that the marked loss of aggrecan and newly synthesized proteoglycan monomer from the matrix in osteoarthritis is probably a direct result of the increased mobility of these macromolecules as the tissue matrix components continue to degrade.

It is also well accepted that mechanical forces modulate the metabolic activity of chondrocytes; however, the specific mechanisms of mechanical signal transduction in articular cartilage is still unknown. One proposed pathway is that chondrocytes may perceive changes in their mechanical environment through cellular deformation.[33] It is well established that the GAG content of habitually loaded areas of cartilage is greater than that of habitually unloaded areas. Work in sheep stifle joints has shown that different areas of articular cartilage subjected to differing mechanical stresses contain a phenotypically distinct chondrocyte population.[50] Chondrocyte phenotypes were identified by the relative biosynthesis of aggrecan, biglycan, and decorin.

Articular Cartilage Metabolism and Matrix Turnover

The chondrocytes synthesize all of the components of the cartilage matrix. At each stage of growth, development, and maturation, the relative rates of matrix synthesis and degradation are adjusted to achieve net growth, remodeling, or equilibrium. A unique interaction exists between chondrocytes and the surrounding matrix. This may be facilitated by a cilium from each chondrocyte that extends into the matrix and acts as a probe, sensing changes in the matrix composition such as a loss of proteoglycan or collagen or an increase or decrease in hyaluronan concentration. This information is relayed to the cell. Interaction between the pericellular and territorial matrix and the chondrocyte cell membrane also may include transmission of mechanical signals by changes in matrix tension or compression. Other investigators have provided support for the idea that forces perceived by chondrocytes dictate their shape and then stimulate alterations in cellular biochemistry and matrix metabolism.[36]

Collagen turnover times within normal articular cartilage have been estimated to be 120 years in the dog and 350 years in adult human articular cartilage.[106]

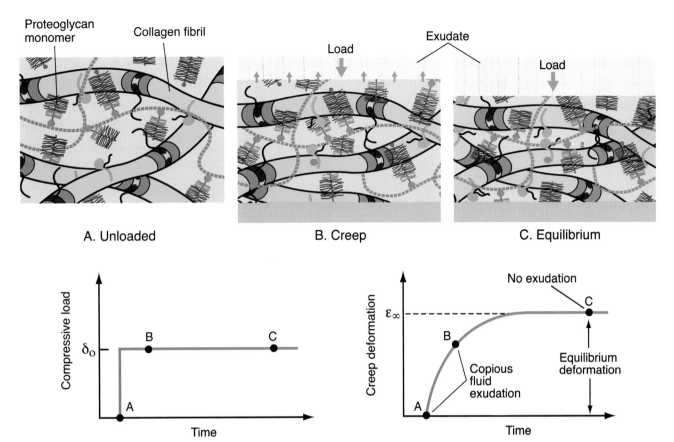

Figure 7.7. Deformation changes occurring over time during confined compression testing of articular cartilage. When a load is applied instantaneously to a confined piece of cartilage and held constant, compressive deformation increases with time (i.e., creep occurs) until an equilibrium position is obtained. The drawings at the top of the figure illustrate consolidation of the matrix under a constant load. The first phase component corresponds to the elastic spring of the biphasic model of cartilage behavior. The fluid is the second phase of the model and is exuded under load. The behavior of a non-viscoelastic material is shown by the graph on the lower left. The behavior of a viscoelastic material (articular cartilage) is shown by the graph on the lower right. The transient portion of the curve results from compression from a viscoelastic material as controlled by fluid exudation and equilibrium position by the elastic spring. (Adapted from Myers ER, Mow VC. Biomechanics of cartilage and its response to biomechanical stimuli. In Cartilage, Vol 1. Hall BK, ed. Academic Press, NY, 1983, p 324.)

However, collagen breakdown is an early event in OA and can be detected with biomarkers before it is apparent morphologically (see below).[66] On the other hand, the protein core of aggrecan is commonly cleaved, particularly the portion between the G1 and G2 domains. Cleavage here leaves a large C-terminal proteoglycan fragment which diffuses out of the tissue. The overall proteoglycan turnover time in adult rabbit and dog articular cartilage is about 300 days.

Dynamic load and the action of cytokines are thought to be involved in matrix turnover. The cytokines of principal interest at the moment are the interleukins and tumor necrosis factor-α (TNF-α). These factors act on chondrocyte receptors and influence the production and activation of metalloproteinases (MMPs), PGE$_2$, and aggrecanase. The activity of MMPs, in turn, is inhibited by tissue inhibitors of MMPs (TIMPs 1 and 2), and it has been shown that there is a slight excess of TIMP over metalloproteinase concentration in normal articular cartilage.[18] See the section on pathobiology for further information on the action of cytokines.

Not all cytokines cause degradation. There are a number of growth factors such as insulin-like growth factor 1 (IGF-1) and various members of the transforming growth factor (TGF) super family, which includes bone morphogenic proteins (BMPs), that are positively involved in articular cartilage synthesis.

Lubrication of Joints

The synovial joint contains 2 systems that require lubrication: a soft tissue system, involving the sliding of synovial membrane on itself or other tissues, and a cartilage-on-cartilage system. Lubrication of the synovial membrane is by boundary lubrication, and hyaluronan is the important component in the synovial fluid that performs this function.[65] The hyaluronan molecules stick to the surface of the synovial membrane and allow sliding of synovial membrane over the opposing surface. This function is important because a major part of the frictional resistance in joint movement is in the synovial membrane and fibrous joint capsule.[54]

Considerable investigations have clarified the lubrication of articular structures in synovial joints and the modes have been classified as fluid-filled or boundary. The operative lubrication modes depend on the normal and tangential forces on the articulating tissues, the relative rate of tangential motion between these surfaces, and the time and history of both loading and motion.[70] One type of fluid-mediated lubrication is hydrostatic. At the onset of loading and typically for a prolonged duration, the interstitial fluid within cartilage becomes pressurized and rises to the surface by a weeping mechanism. In boundary lubrication, the load is supported by surface-to-surface contact and the associated frictional properties are determined by lubricant surface molecules. This mode is thought to be important because the opposing cartilage surfaces make contact over approximately 10% of the total area, and this may be where most of the friction occurs.[70]

With increasing loading time and dissipation of hydrostatic pressure, lubricant-coated surfaces bear an increasingly high proportion of the load relative to pressurized film and consequently the friction coefficient is dominated by this mode of lubrication. Boundary lubrication is therefore important in reducing articulation-induced shear and wear. Boundary lubrication is mediated by synovial fluid.[97] Components of the synovial fluid involved in boundary lubrication include hyaluronan (HA),[78] proteoglycan 4 (PRG4),[101] and surface active phospholipids (SAPL)[98]. Maintenance of normal lubricating functions is considered critical to the health of articular cartilage.[94]

Subchondral Bone

The subchondral plate and epiphyseal bone beneath it form an integral part of the joint structure, providing structural support to the overlying articular cartilage. The subchondral plate consists of cortical bone that varies in thickness depending on the joint. With exercise, remodeling occurs and the amount of dense cortical bone can increase, at least in the carpus and fetlock, but there is marked variation between horses.[44]

The relationship between the mechanical properties and morphometry of the bones of horses has been explored.[116] In the third carpal bone, maximal subchondral bone stiffness occurs 10 mm palmar to the dorsal margin. There is also a significant negative correlation between subchondral stiffness and the porosity of the radial facet of the third carpal bone. Acquisition of such basic data is important in studying traumatic joint disease in the horse. Kawcak, et al. have shown microdamage in the subchondral bone (including microcracks and osteocyte death) as relatively early events in exercising horses.[44]

Cytokines and growth factors similar to those in articular cartilage are also present in bone. These include IGF-1, the TGFα family (including the bone morphogenic proteins 2 to 7), platelet-derived growth factor, and fibroblast growth factors. These peptides are produced by bone cells and are present in bone matrix. IL-1 and TNFα are also present in bone. Presumably, disease in subchondral bone would expose the articular cartilage to these cytokines. More details on the relationship

between articular cartilage and subchondral bone are presented in the section on pathobiology.

The innervation of the subchondral bone plate has been a subject of controversy. However, recent immunohistochemical techniques identifying substance P (a neuropeptide specifically located in sensory nerves and CNS elements) have helped study the innervation of the subchondral plate further.[75] Substance P immunoreactive neurofilaments have been identified in the subchondral bone of normal equine metacarpophalangeal joints. The nerves existed in the small cancellous spaces and diversion canals. Previous immunohistochemical studies of the subchondral plate of diseased human patellae revealed substance P fibers in the periosteum and subchondral plate of patellae affected with degenerative disease.[112] Another interesting finding in the human study was the observation of substance P fibers in erosion channels running through the subchondral plate to the deep surface of the articular cartilage, where nerve terminals were seen. Because the erosion channels were not seen in normal patellae, the presence of the substance P fibers in the erosion channels may represent a morphologic change explaining why degenerative patellae become painful.

PATHOBIOLOGY OF JOINTS AND THEIR REACTION TO INSULT AND INJURY

Traumatic Arthritis: Multiple Manifestations

In its broader sense, "traumatic arthritis" includes a diverse collection of pathologic and clinical states that develop after single or repetitive episodes of trauma, and may include one or all of the following:

1. Synovitis (inflammation of the synovial membrane)
2. Capsulitis (inflammation of the fibrous joint capsule)
3. Sprain (injury of specific ligaments associated with the joint)
4. Intra-articular fractures
5. Meniscal tears (femorotibial joints)
6. Osteoarthritis (when degradative changes have occurred in the articular cartilage)

Any of 1 through 5 above can potentially progress to osteoarthritis (OA). To facilitate the discussion of pathobiology it is convenient to divide articular trauma into three entities:

Type I: Traumatic synovitis and capsulitis without obvious disturbance of the cartilage or destruction of major supporting structures. This includes acute synovitis and most sprains.

Type II: Disruptive trauma with damage to the articular cartilage or complete rupture of a major supporting structure. This includes severe sprains, meniscal tears, and intra-articular fractures.

Type III: Post-traumatic osteoarthritis. Equine OA may be considered as a group of disorders characterized by a common end-stage in which progressive deterioration of the articular cartilage is accompanied by changes in the bone and soft tissues of the joint. It is inevitably the result of severe trauma to the joint or ineffective treatment of any of the predisposing conditions.

The joint is an organ and all of its tissues can be injured. Cyclic trauma to the synovial membrane and fibrous joint capsule results in synovitis and capsulitis, and is a common entity in the equine athlete. Direct trauma can occur to the articular cartilage and subchondral bone, whereas inflammatory mediators resulting from synovitis can cause biochemical damage. Intra-articular and extra-articular ligaments of the joint can be injured, as can the menisci in the stifle.

The reaction in the various joint-associated tissues should not be considered in isolation, as evidenced by the example of the carpus of a racehorse. Considerable damage may be inflicted directly to the articular cartilage and bone, resulting in cartilage ulceration and intra-articular fractures of the carpus that cause varying degrees of articular cartilage loss. However, cyclic fatigue damage to the collagen network could be an important step in the pathogenesis of a more insidious osteoarthritic entity, exposing chondrocytes to deleterious physical forces and inducing injury and metabolic changes.

Primary damage to the subchondral bone other than fracture also may occur (subchondral bone disease) and lead to secondary damage to the articular cartilage, either from loss of support or secondarily from release of cytokines. Subchondral sclerosis may also lead to further physical damage to the articular cartilage because of decreased shock absorption. Acute synovitis and capsulitis is a common problem in these same joints and may also contribute to the degenerative process by the release of deleterious mediators.[65]

Physiologic Trauma Leading to Osteoarthritis

Osteoarthritis is a disease that results from an interaction of a number of complex mechanical and biological processes and predominantly, but not solely, affects the diarthrodial joint. As noted above, the end result is progressive deterioration of the articular cartilage. While a definitive characteristic of OA is articular cartilage destruction, we have come to recognize the accompanying changes of synovitis and shown that it can be a primary disease process leading to OA. We also know that many of the mediators involved in early deterioration of the articular cartilage are present in increased amounts (or there are decreased amounts of their inhibitors), which represents an exaggerated normal metabolic process.

Athletic Activity Potentially Leading to a Pathologic Process

It is well accepted that equine athletes carry an increased risk for development of OA. It should be noted that intact articular cartilage possesses optimal load-bearing characteristics that adjust to the level of activity. Increasing weight-bearing activity in athletes and adolescents has been shown to improve the volume and thickness of articular cartilage[41] and increase cartilage glycosaminoglycan content in the human knee.[92] In the healthy human athlete, a positive linear dose-response relationship apparently exists for repetitive loading activities and articular cartilage function.[60] However, studies also indicate that the dose-response

curve reaches a threshold and activity beyond this threshold can result in maladjustment and injury of articular cartilage.[47]

High-impact joint loading above this threshold has been shown to decrease cartilage proteoglycan content, increase levels of degradative enzymes, and cause chondrocyte apoptosis.[1,52] If the integrity of the functional weight-bearing unit is lost, either through acute injury or chronic trauma in the high-impact athlete, a chondropenic response is initiated that can include loss of articular cartilage volume and stiffness, elevation of contact pressures, and development or progression of articular cartilage defects.[60] It has been proposed that concomitant histologic factors such as ligamentous instability, malalignment, meniscal injury, or deficiency can further support progression of the chondropenic cascade and without intervention, chondropenia leads to progressive deterioration of articular cartilage function and may ultimately progress to osteoarthritis.

Evidence has accumulated with regard to various inflammatory mediators having an impact on matrix homeostasis of articular chondrocytes by altering their metabolism.[57] The authors of a recent paper on inflammatory factors involved in human OA cited evidence that points to the pro-inflammatory cytokine interleukin-1β (IL-1β) as the most important factor responsible for the catabolism in OA.[57] However, the authors pointed out that new members of the IL-1 super family have recently been identified (ILF-5, ILF-10), some of which have been suggested to be of interest for arthritic disease, and that other pro-inflammatory cytokines such as tumor necrosis factor (TNF)-α-6 and other interleukins can be contributing factors. They also noted that the exact role and importance of each within the OA process is not yet clearly identified. In addition to cytokines, other inflammatory mediators that may play a major role in the OA process include nitric oxide (NO), eicosanoids (prostaglandins and leukotrienes), and a newly identified cell membrane receptor family, the proteases-activated receptors (PARs).

Discussion of mediators for equine traumatic joint disease and OA in this chapter focus on mediators that have been shown to be increased in equine joint disease and/or their inhibition can ameliorate progression of OA.

When considering a traumatically injured joint, 2 basic pathobiologic processes should be considered: inflammation of the synovial membrane and fibrous joint capsule (synovitis and capsulitis), and physical or biochemical damage to the articular cartilage and bone. Acute synovitis and capsulitis can cause significant clinical compromise and may also contribute to the degenerative process by releasing enzymes, inflammatory mediators, and cytokines.[66] These processes are outlined in Figures 7.8 and 7.9.

Synovitis and Capsulitis

Treatment of synovitis and capsulitis, particularly the acute form, is indicated to (1) alleviate the immediate compromising effects of inflammation, including pain and reduced function, (2) prevent the development of permanent fibrosis in the joint capsule, which in turn causes decreased motion and compromised shock

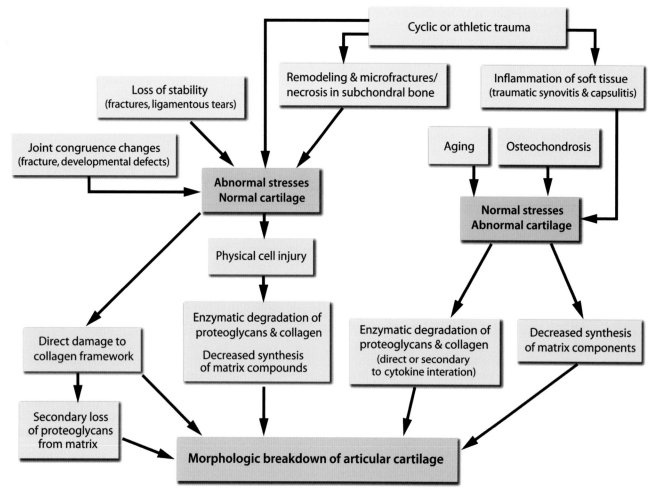

Figure 7.8. Possible pathways for degradation of articular cartilage secondary to joint trauma. (Redrawn from Figure 4, McIlwraith CW. Frank Milne Lecture: From Arthroscopy to Gene Therapy–30 Years of Looking in Joints. Proceedings Am Assoc Equine Pract 2005;51:65–113.)

absorption capabilities in that joint, and (3) prevent or minimize the development of OA.

Synovitis and capsulitis as primary entities in athletic horses are presumed to be associated with repeated trauma.[64] Severe injury to the fibrous joint capsule also can cause instability. The synovial membrane itself is mechanically weak and has no known biomechanical role but it is recognized that synovial injury may have pathophysiologic consequences in the joint.[24] Some injuries may affect diffusion across the synovial membrane and others have a primary effect on the metabolism of the chondrocyte.[24] Mechanically damaged synoviocytes may release degradative enzymes and cytokines, which alter the intra-articular environment and possibly affect articular cartilage. It has also been suggested that high intra-articular pressures in injured joints associated with effusion could be sufficient to impair the flow of blood through the synovial capillaries and potentially lead to reperfusion injury.[48] Flexion of a joint with sufficient synovial effusion could raise the intra-articular pressure to levels of impaired blood flow through the synovial capillaries.

In addition to direct injury that may occur to the synovial membrane, the reaction of the synovial mem-brane to articular cartilage damage or other mechanical destruction of intra-articular tissues is well recognized. The presence of cartilaginous wear particles increases the cellular production of prostaglandin E_2, cytokines, and the neutral metalloproteinases (collagenase, strome-lysin, and gelatinase).[24] It has also been shown that the proteoglycans released into synovial fluid cause synovitis.[6]

The ability of synovial membrane inflammation alone in the absence of trauma and/or instability to damage articular cartilage has previously been demon-strated in the horse.[62]

The Importance of Synovitis

Synovitis (and capsulitis) is important to the horse because it produces pain, the increased synovial effusion is uncomfortable and it eliminates the normal small negative pressure within the joint (therefore promoting micro-instability), and it produces products that are deleterious to joint health as a whole, and articular cartilage in particular. The mediators currently consid-ered to be of significance in equine joint disease include metalloproteinases and aggrecanases, prostaglandins,

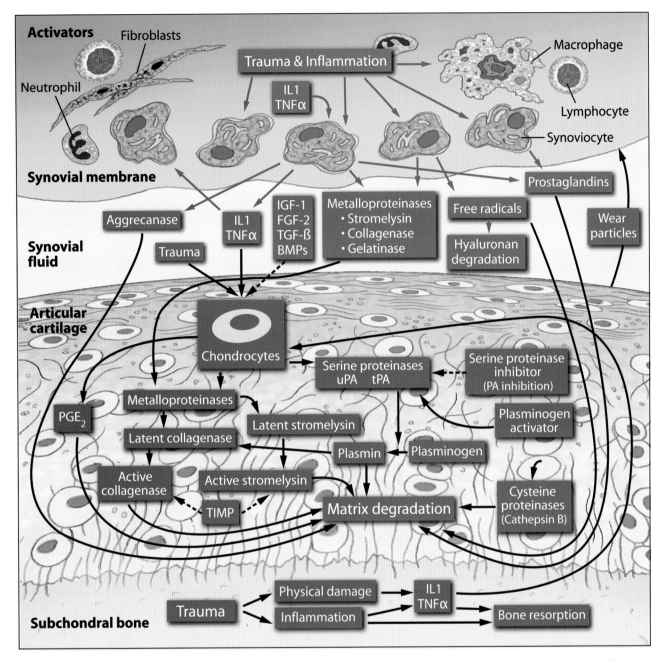

Figure 7.9. Factors involved in degradation of the articular matrix: interleukin-1, tumor necrosis factorα (TNFα), fibroblast growth factor-2 (FGF-2), PLA2, urokinase plasminogen activator (uPA), tissue plasminogen activator (tPA), plasminogen activator (PA), insulin-like growth factor-1 (IGF-1), transforming growth factor-β (TGF-β), and bone morphogenic protein (BMP). (Redrawn from Figure 5, McIlwraith CW. Frank Milne Lecture: From Arthroscopy to Gene Therapy—30 Years of Looking in Joints. Proceedings Am Assoc Equine Pract 2005;51:65–113.)

free radicals, cytokines, interleukin-1 (IL-1), and possibly tumor necrosis factor-alpha (TNFα) (Figure 7.9).

Matrix Metalloproteinases and Aggrecanases

Matrix metalloproteinases (MMPs) may be subdivided into collagenases, gelatinases, and stromelysins. Three collagenases have been identified and they are interstitial or tissue collagenase (also called MMP-1), PMN collagenase (or MMP-8), and collagenase 3 (also known as MMP-13). Based on evidence in both human and equine studies it appears that the primary collagenase involved in the degradation of type II collagen of articular cartilage is collagenase 3.[10,69] Caron, et al. found that MMP-13 is produced by equine chondrocytes and that MMP-13 expression was significantly stimulated by rhIL-1.[10]

Consideration of the breakdown of aggrecan initially focused on stromelysin (also called proteoglycanase or MMP-3), but now recognizes an initially undefined enzyme called "aggrecanase" (now known as aggrecanase-1 and -2 or ADAMTS-4 and -11). Stromelysin has a wide variety of substrates, including proteoglycans (aggrecan, decorin, fibromodulin, link protein) and type IV, V, VII, IX, and XI collagen. It also cleaves type II collagen in nonhelical sites.[115] In vitro study of IL-1-induced cartilage degeneration has revealed evidence of collagen degradation that could be attributed to stromelysin in addition to that attributed to collagenase.[21] Molecular cloning and cartilage gene expression of equine stromelysin 1 (MMP-3) has been described by Balkman and Nixon (1998).[2] Stromelysin cleaves the protein backbone of cartilage proteoglycans at the asparagine 341-phenylalanine 342 bond.[58] Cleavage due to aggrecanase, on the other hand, occurs at the GLU373-ALA373 site.[95] Based on preliminary work in the horse using markers that differentiate these 2 cleavage sites, it appears that aggrecanase is the principal enzyme degrading proteoglycan in equine joint disease.[51]

Equine MMPs 2 and 9 are 2 gelatinases that have been characterized in the horse.[11,12] It is known that the one-fourth and three-fourths fragments generated by cleavage by fibrin or collagens by collagenases can unwind and are then susceptible to further cleavage by MMP-2 and MMP-9. MMPs 2 and 9 are produced by a variety of equine cell types and these enzymes have been demonstrated in elevated levels in synovial fluids from horses with joint disease.[11,12]

The metalloproteinases are inhibited by 2 tissue inhibitors of metalloproteinase and these are known commonly as TIMP (TIMP-1 and TIMP-2).[74,100] TIMP is found in many connective tissues and may be the most important inhibitor found in articular cartilage. This current belief that the balance between MMPs and TIMP is important to prevent progression of articular cartilage degradation.

In summary, MMPs are considered to play a major role in articular cartilage degradation. They are secreted as latent proenzymes and activated extracellularly by serine proteinases. Plasmin may activate stromelysin, which in turn is an important activator of collagenase. Upregulation of these enzymes in synovial membrane and articular cartilage samples from traumatic equine joint disease has been demonstrated.[108] It is also known that the production of MMPs is upregulated by IL-1.

Prostaglandins

Prostaglandins (primarily E group) are produced in inflamed joints and can cause a decrease in the proteoglycan content of the cartilage matrix.[102] The presence of prostaglandin E_2 in synovial fluid from inflamed joints has been demonstrated in the horse.[103] In the author's laboratory PGE_2 measurements are used as an objective index of the level of synovitis.[27,42] Actions of PGE_2 in joints include vasodilation, enhancement of pain perception, proteoglycan depletion from cartilage (by both degradation and inhibition of synthesis), bone demineralization, and promotion of plasminogen activator secretion. PGE_2 is released from chondrocytes on stimulation of these cells by IL-1 and TNFα.

Oxygen-derived Free Radicals

Oxygen-derived free radicals, including superoxide anion, hydroxyl radicals, and hydrogen peroxide, may be released from injured joint tissues. Studies have demonstrated cleavage of hyaluronan by free radicals.[31,113] There is also evidence that superoxide can degrade the alpha chains of collagen based on the finding that superoxide treatment inhibits gelatin.[32] Proteoglycans may be cleaved by free radicals.[32] Increased free radicals in the synovial fluid of cases of equine joint disease have been demonstrated more recently.[20]

Nitric oxide has been recognized as an important physiologic mediator. It combines avidly with superoxide anion, and although this was originally thought to provide a protective function, it has been suggested that this reaction can generate further destructive species, including peroxynitrite anion and hydroxyl radicals.[81] A recent review has noted that the specific effect of a radical on a given cell function very much depends on experimental context. Specifically, the simultaneous presence of supraoxide, which leads to the formation of peroxynitrite (due to interaction of NO and supraoxide), a stronger and highly reactive radical, is likely to lead to cell and tissue damage.[53] However, NO has certain protective effects in cartilage and other tissues and inhibition of NO in vitro or in vivo can potentially lead to undesired exacerbation of inflammation and tissue destruction under certain conditions. Selective scavengers of peroxynitrite must be more promising candidates for the treatment of OA than specific inhibition of NO. The role of nitric oxide in joint disease needs, and is receiving, further attention.

Cytokines and Articular Cartilage Degradation

Cytokines are soluble peptides produced by one cell affecting the activity of other cell types. Studies of cytokines in joint tissues suggest that IL-1 and TNFα modulate the synthesis of metalloproteinases by both chondrocytes and synovial cells[16,17,114] and are therefore important mediators in joint disease. Because IL-1 and TNFα may be produced by synovial cells[17] they may therefore be of importance in the deleterious effects of synovitis on articular cartilage. It is thought that the normal turnover of the extracellular matrix of the articular cartilage is regulated by the chondrocytes under the control and influence of cytokines and mechanical stimuli. Articular cartilage degradation in association with disease represents an exacerbation of these normal processes. It is widely accepted that the cytokine interleukin-1 induces proteoglycan depletion in articular cartilage by either increasing the rate of degradation or decreasing synthesis in association with the release of proteinases and prostaglandins from chondrocytes (Figure 7.10). IL-1 produces its effects by binding with an IL-1 receptor on the cell. The presence of IL-1 in equine osteoarthritic joints was first reported by Morris, et al. (1990).[71] An equine IL-1 containing extract was produced by May in 1990.[35]

The significant role of equine IL-1 has been further consolidated, starting with the cDNA sequences for IL-1α and IL-1β being constructed.[34,35] After generation of these DNA sequences, the IL-1α and IL-1β recombinant proteins were purified. Prior to that, only human recombinant IL-1 protein was available. Using equine articular cartilage explants, significant proteoglycan release was induced by both rEq-IL-1α and rEq-IL-1β at concentrations greater than or equal to 0.01 ng/ml with 38% to 76% and 88% to 90% of total glycosaminoglycan released by 4 and 6 days, respectively.[102] Significant inhibition of proteoglycan synthesis (42% to 64%) was observed at IL-1 concentrations greater than or equal to 0.01 ng/ml at 2 and 4 days. Increased PGE_2 concentrations were observed at IL-1 concentrations greater than or equal to 1.0 ng/ml at 2 and 4 days. This work showed that the much lower concentrations of equine IL-1 could cause these effects compared with previously reported studies using human recombinant IL-1.[102]

The IL-1 system consists of the 2 agonist members IL-1α and IL-1β and these evoke signal production in response to binding IL-1R transmembrane receptors to induce downstream effects (Figure 7.10). The significant role of IL-1 in the pathogenesis of cartilage degradation in the horse was best demonstrated by the work of Frisbie, et al. (2002)[26] with interleukin-1 receptor antagonist (IL-1ra) using gene therapy. This study demonstrated that if IL-1 can be inhibited, articular cartilage degradation in experimental OA can essentially be stopped.

The role of TNFα in equine OA is less certain. Billinghurst, et al. (1995) first demonstrated induction of intra-articular TNF during acute inflammatory responses in equine arthritis.[5] It appears that IL-1 is the principal cytokine responsible for articular cartilage degradation and TNFα contributes more to clinical morbidity and pain. IL-1 and TNFα have been demonstrated using RT-PCR in the synovial membrane of inflamed equine joints,[108] and increased serum concentrations of soluble TNF receptors (S TNF-r) have been detected in human patients with RA and OA in comparison to healthy controls.[14] A mini review of the role of cytokines as inflammatory mediators in osteoarthritis concluded that it is generally accepted that IL-1 is the pivotal cytokine in early and late stages of OA, while TNFα is involved primarily in the onset of arthritis.[29] Both receptors of TNF have been identified in synovial tissue, with greater numbers seen in joints affected by RA in comparison to OA.[19]

The Pathways to Morphologic Breakdown of Articular Cartilage—the Critical Manifestation of OA

Trauma can cause an immediate physical defect or initiate a degradative process by direct damage to chondrocytes, causing release of enzymes as well as cytokine initiated release of metalloproteinases and PGE_2 from chondrocytes in response to IL-1. As outlined in Figure 7.8, any instability in a joint can lead to damage of normal cartilage. On the other hand, cartilage compromised by loss of glycosaminoglycans or collagen is vulnerable to normal forces.

As has been previously discussed, as cartilage is compressed, the collapse of the collagen network is countered by the resistance offered by the proteoglycan gel. The precise nature of the forces exerted through the network are complex and related both to mechanical entrapment and chemical bonding effects between the fibers and the proteoglycans.[7] The same author has addressed the general problem of abnormal softening in

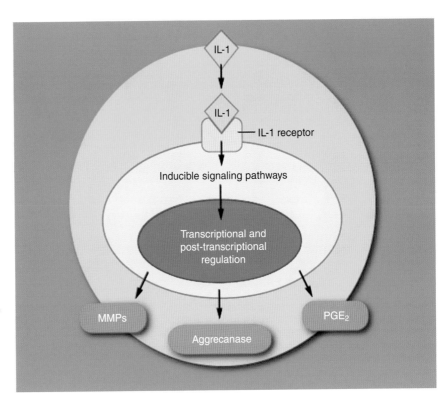

Figure 7.10. Diagram of IL-1 activation of MMPs, aggrecanase, and PGE2 release acting through IL-1 receptors on the cell membrane. (Redrawn from Figure 6, McIlwraith CW. Frank Milne Lecture: From Arthroscopy to Gene Therapy—30 Years of Looking in Joints. Proceedings AAEP 2005;51:65–113.)

articular cartilage with simultaneous micromechanical testing, interference-like microscopy, and transmission electron microscopy. A model has been developed in which this abnormal softening in articular cartilage is related to the presence of collagen fibers strongly aligned in a radial direction and this structure, having lost its 3-dimensional character, would have limited ability to contain the swelling proteoglycan aggregates remaining in the tissue and would therefore reflect a state of softening in articular cartilage.[7]

The most common reason for degradation of articular cartilage and the development of OA is generally synovitis and capsulitis. There is a progression, beginning with acute synovitis, when biochemical change can take place in the articular cartilage, but there is no morphologic change. With critical loss of matrical components, however, morphologic damage ensues, going through a cycle of chondromalacia with softening of the cartilage and swelling due to absorption of water, superficial fibrillation, fibrillation down to the middle zone of cartilage, followed by fibrillation progressing through the deeper layer of cartilage, which then allows for loss of articular cartilage components and full-thickness erosion. Figure 7.11 illustrates 4 stages of osteoarthritis in which the synovitis and capsulitis become more chronic. Close examination of articular cartilage shows change and the histologic equivalent of these macroscopic lesions is reflected as well.

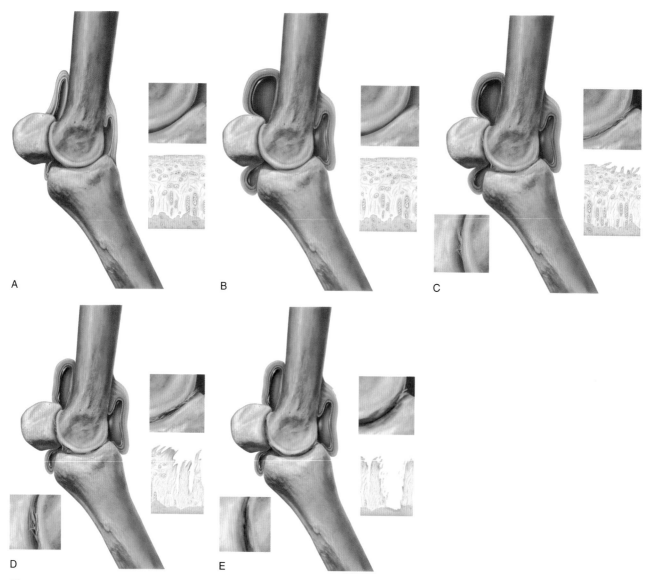

Figure 7.11. Diagrammatic series of development of osteoarthritis in a fetlock joint associated with cyclic trauma and traumatic synovitis and capsulitis. A. Diagram of a normal joint, as well as macroscopic and microscopic views of articular cartilage. B. Stage 1 acute synovitis without morphologic change in the articular cartilage. C. Stage 2 with synovitis persisting and early development of superficial fibrillation in the articular cartilage.

D. Stage 3 synovitis and capsulitis becoming chronic, and articular cartilage fibrillation down into the deep zone of articular cartilage. E. Stage 4 development of full-thickness erosions in the articular cartilage that are visible macroscopically and microscopically. Joint capsule change is chronic with fibrosis, but some degree of active synovitis is still present.

Articular Cartilage Repair

Healing refers to restoration of the structural integrity and function of the tissue after injury or disease, but repair usually has a more restricted meaning.[8] Repair refers to the replacement of damaged or lost cells and matrix with new cells and matrix, a process that does not necessarily restore the original structure or function of a tissue. Regeneration may be considered a special form of repair in which the cells replace lost or damaged tissue with a tissue identical to the original. It has been suggested that with the exception of bone fractures, most injuries and diseases of the musculoskeletal tissues do not stimulate regeneration of the original tissue.[8]

The limited potential of articular cartilage for regeneration and healing has been appreciated for more than 2 centuries. In 1743, Hunter stated, "From Hippocrates to the present age, it is universally allowed that ulcerated cartilage is a troublesome thing and that when once destroyed it is not repaired."[37] There is a limited response of cartilage to tissue damage and an inability of natural repair responses from adjacent tissues to produce tissue with the morphologic, biochemical, and biomechanical properties of articular cartilage.

The major limiting factor in the successful rehabilitation of any joint after injury or disease is the failure of osteochondral defects to heal.[61] Three mechanisms have been recognized as possible contributors to articular cartilage repair. Intrinsic repair (from within the cartilage) relies on the limited mitotic capability of the chondrocyte and a somewhat ineffective increase in collagen and proteoglycan production. Extrinsic repair comes from mesenchymal elements from the subchondral bone participating in the formation of new connective tissue that may undergo some metaplastic change to form cartilage elements. The third phenomenon, known as matrix flow, may contribute to equine articular cartilage repair by forming lips of cartilage from the perimeter of the lesion that migrate toward the center of the defect.[38,39]

The depth of the injury (full- or partial-thickness), size of defect, location and relation to weight-bearing or nonweight-bearing areas, and age of the animal influence the repair and remodeling of an injured joint surface.[9,13,68]

With a partial-thickness defect, some repair occurs with increased GAG synthesis and increased collagen synthesis.[68] However, the repair process is never completely effective. In humans, complete repair of chondromalacia of the patella has been reported to occur if matrical depletion and surface breakdown are minimal.[4] However, more recent work with arthroscopic debridement of partial-thickness defects in humans questions any actual regeneration.[96] In addition, superficial defects are not necessarily progressive and do not necessarily compromise joint function.

With full-thickness defects, the response from the adjacent articular cartilage varies little from that after superficial lesions and provides only the limited repair necessary to replace dead cells and damaged matrix at the margins of the wound. These defects heal by ingrowth of subchondral fibrous tissue that may or may not undergo metaplasia to fibrocartilage.[13,30,38,55,87,111]

Subchondral bone defects either heal with bone that grows up into the defect or fill in with fibrocartilaginous ingrowth.[111] Duplication of the tide mark in the calcified cartilage layer is rare, and adherence of the repair tissue to surrounding noninjured cartilage is often incomplete.[30,55]

A number of equine studies demonstrate that the size and location of articular defects significantly affect the degree of healing achieved. Convery, et al. first reported that large defects were less likely to heal.[30] A more recent study distinguished between large ($15~mm^2$) and small ($5~mm^2$) full-thickness lesions in weight-bearing and nonweight-bearing areas of the antebrachiocarpal (radiocarpal), middle carpal (intercarpal), and femoropatellar joints.[38] At 1 month, small defects were filled with poorly organized fibrovascular repair tissue; by 4 months, repair was limited to an increase in the amount of organization of this fibrous tissue, and by 5 months, small radiocarpal and femoropatellar lesions were hardly detectable because of combinations of matrix flow and extrinsic repair mechanisms. Large lesions showed good initial repair, but at 5 months, perilesional and intralesional subchondral clefts developed.

The repair tissue that forms after full-thickness injury to hyaline cartilage or as a natural repair process in joints with OA is primarily comprised of type I rather than type II collagen, at least at 4 months.[9,12] Identification of type II collagen is the critical biochemical factor distinguishing hyaline cartilage from repaired fibrous tissue and fibrocartilage. It is thought that the presence of an abnormal subchondral bone plate and the absence of a tide mark reforming may create a stiffness gradient and that shear stresses of the junction of the repair tissue and underlying bone develop. The propagation of such shear stresses would lead to the degradation of repair fibrocartilage and exposure of the bone. This mechanical failure has been observed experimentally and clinically in the horse.[38,63]

In a study looking at the long-term effectiveness of sternal cartilage grafting, the repair tissue in the nongrafted defects at 12 months consisted of fibrocartilaginous tissue with fibrous tissue in the surface layers, as was seen in control defects at 4 months. However, on biochemical analysis, the repair tissue of the non-grafted defects had a mean type II collagen percentage of 79%, compared with being non-detectable at 4 months.[109,110] On the other hand, the GAG content expressed as milligrams of total hexosamine per gram of dried tissue was 20.6 ± 1.85 mg/g, compared with 26.4 ± 3.1 mg/g at 4 months and 41.8 ± 4.3 mg/g DW in normal equine articular cartilage.[109,110]

The fibrocartilaginous repair seen in normal full-thickness defects is therefore biomechanically unsuitable as a replacement-bearing surface and has been shown to undergo mechanical failure with use. The lack of durability may be related to faulty biochemical composition of the old matrix and incomplete remodeling of the interface between old and repaired cartilage or to increased stress in the regenerated cartilage because of abnormal remodeling of the subchondral bone plate and calcified cartilage layer. Although recent work implies that it may be possible to reconstitute the normal collagen type in equine articular cartilage,[110] clearly there is continued deterioration of GAG content, and these are important components in the overall composition of the cartilage matrix.

The presence of a cartilage defect may not represent clinical compromise. In the equine carpus, loss of up to 30% of articular surface of an individual bone may not compromise the successful return of a horse to racing.[63] However, loss of 50% of the articular surface or severe loss of subchondral bone leads to a significantly worse prognosis.

The inadequate healing response may not necessarily apply to immature animals or to nonweight-bearing defects. An example is the young horse after surgery for osteochondritis dissecans (OCD) that shows impressive or at least functional healing responses. This may be related to increased chondrocytic capacity for mitosis and matrix synthesis and the presence of intracartilaginous vascularity. Complete restoration of the ultrastructure and surface configuration in a hinge-like gliding joint surface such as the femoropatellar joint may be unnecessary for clinical soundness, compared with the more severe loading on an osteochondral defect located on the weight-bearing portion of the medial condyle of the femur or the midcarpal joint.

It has been suggested that increasing age may affect the response of cartilage to injury in humans because the ability of the chondrocytes to synthesize and assemble matrix micromolecules could decline with age.[8] Buckwalter cites a study of transplanted chondrocytes, suggesting that older chondrocytes produce a more poorly organized matrix than do younger chondrocytes,[8] and other studies demonstrate that the proteoglycan synthesized by the chondrocytes changes with age.[3,85]

Much research is continuing to be done to develop better methods of cartilage repair and these have been reviewed elsewhere.[66]

PRIMARY DISEASE OF SUBCHONDRAL BONE

In addition to synovial mediated degradation of articular cartilage and direct mechanical damage, the subchondral bone can play a primary role in disease development (Figure 7.12).[77]

When considering possible pathways for mechanical destruction of articular cartilage in human OA it has been suggested that early subchondral bone sclerosis causes a reduction in the joint's shock-absorbing ability and thereby places cartilage at risk of shear-induced tensile failure of cartilage cross links, particularly under repetitive impulsive loading conditions.[84] Work in the author's laboratory[44] has demonstrated that when horses are subjected to athletic exercise on the treadmill, microdamage in the subchondral bone can develop early. On postmortem examination of racehorse joints (euthanized for catastrophic injuries in another limb), the range of microdamage includes not only microfractures, but also primary osteocyte death. It is thought that not only is the mechanical support of the articular cartilage lost when subchondral bone microdamage progresses to macrodamage, but that cytokine release from the bone also can potentially influence that state of the articular cartilage.[44,45,77] Figure 7.12 illustrates a specimen from a horse euthanized because of catastrophic injury in the other limb. An incidental finding

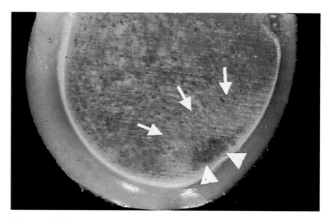

Figure 7.12. Postmortem sample of a distal metacarpus from the leg opposite to that suffering a catastrophic injury in a racehorse. Although there is intact articular cartilage, subchondral bone necrosis (arrowheads) and sclerosis (arrows) can be seen. (Norrdin RW, et al. Subchondral bone failure in an equine model of overload osteoarthrosis. Bone 1998;22:133–139, Figure 10.)

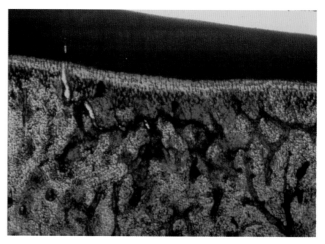

Figure 7.13. Histologic view of a section of articular cartilage and subchondral bone bulk-stained with basic fuchsin depicting microdamage with micro-crack formation in the subchondral bone. (Kawcak CE. In McIlwraith CW. Frank Milne Lecture: From Arthroscopy to Gene Therapy-30 Years of Looking in Joints. Proceedings AAEP 2005;51:65–113.)

at postmortem was the presence of subchondral bone necrosis, with a peripheral area of sclerosis and intact cartilage in the distal palmar area of the metacarpus. Figure 7.13 shows microdamage that can occur quite early in association with exercise.

Gross examination of MCP/MTP joints from racehorses revealed defects on the condylar surface that ranged from cartilage fibrillation and erosion to focal cartilage indentation and cavitation in subchondral bone. These lesions represented a spectrum of mechanically induced arthrosis in which microdamage is thought to play a role.[77] Lesions in the subchondral bone ranged from thickening of subchondral bone and underlying trabeculae, advancing sclerosis with increasing amounts of osteocyte necrosis, vascular channels with plugs of matrix debris, and osteoclastic remodeling. Apparent fragmentation lines in the subchondral bone suggested increased matrix fragility. Trabecular microfractures developed at a depth of a few millimeters, with increased vascularity with hemorrhage, fibrin, and fibroplasia seen in the marrow spaces at the more advanced stage. The articular cartilage in most of these instances was variously indented but remained largely viable, with degeneration and erosion limited to the superficial layers. Focally, breaks in the calcified layer appeared to lead to collagen and cartilage in-folding. In metacarpal condyles from experimental horses run on a treadmill,[45] change in the metacarpal condyles was milder. The significance of osteochondral injury in joint disease has also been well reviewed by Riggs.[90]

In addition to its role in contributing to OA, the presence of subchondral bone injury contributing to complete failure of the subchondral bone and fractures is important.[58] "Impact fracture" is a term that has been used recently to describe a pathologic fracture that shows up as an area of lucency in the bone.[15] Pathologic change in the distal condyles of the third metacarpal and third metatarsal bones of the horse as a pre-disposing factor for condylar fractures was first investigated in detail by Riggs, et al. (1999).[88,89,91] Recognition of this change potentially leading to fractures has led to investigations of imaging techniques to diagnose this at an early stage.[22]

References

1. Arokoski J, Kiviranta I, Jurvelin J, et al. Long-distance running causes site-dependent decrease of cartilage glycosaminoglycan content in the knee joint. Arth Rheum 1993;36:1451–1459.
2. Balkman CW, Nixon AJ. Molecular cloning and cartilage gene expression of equine stromelysin 1 (matrix metalloproteinase 3). Am J Vet Res 1998;59:30–36.
3. Bennett GA, Bauer W. Joint changes resulting from patellar displacement and their relation to degenerative joint disease. J Bone Joint Surg 1937;29:667–682.
4. Bentley G. Articular cartilage changes in chondromalacia patellae. J Bone Joint Surg [Br] 1985;67:769–774.
5. Billinghurst RC, Fretz PB, Gordon JR. Induction of intra-articular tumor necrosis factor during acute inflammatory responses in equine arthritis. Equine Vet J 1995;27:208–216.
6. Boniface RJ, Cain PR, Evans CH. Articular responses to purified cartilage proteoglycans. Arthritis Rheum 1988;31:258–266.
7. Broom ND. Abnormal softening in articular cartilage. Its relationship to the collagen framework. Arthritis Rheum 1982;25:1209.
8. Buckwalter JA, Mau DC. Cartilage repair in osteoarthritis. In Osteoarthritis. Diagnosis and Medical/Surgical Management, 2nd ed. Moskowitz RW, Howell DS, Goldberg VM, et al., eds. WB Saunders Co., Philadelphia, 1992;71–107.
9. Calandruccio RA, Gilmer S. Proliferation, regeneration and repair of articular cartilage of immature animals. J Bone Joint Surg [Am] 1962;44:431–455.
10. Caron JP, Tardif G, Martel-Pelletier J, et al. Modulation of matrix metalloproteinase 13 (collagenase III) gene expression in equine chondrocytes by equine interleukin-1 and corticosteroids. Am J Vet Res 1996; 57:1631–1634.
11. Clegg PD, Burke RM, Coughlan AR. Characterization of equine matrix metalloproteinase 2 and 9, and identification of the cellular sources of these enzymes in joints. Equine Vet J 1997a;29:335–342.
12. Clegg PD, Coughlan AR, Riggs CM, et al. Matrix metalloproteinases 2 and 9 in equine synovial fluids. Equine Vet J 1997b;29:343–348.
13. Convery FR, Akeson WH, Keown GH. Repair of large osteochondral defects—An experimental study in horses. Clin Orthop 1972;82:253.
14. Cope AP, Gibbons D, Brennan FM, et al. Increased levels of soluble tumor necrosis factor receptors in the sera and synovial fluid of patients with rheumatic diseases. Arth Rheum 1992;35:1160–1169.
15. Cullimore AM, Finney JW, Marmion WJ, et al. Severe lameness associated with impact fracture of the proximal phalanx in a filly. Equine Vet Educ 2009;21:247–251.
16. Dayer J-M, Beutler B, Serami A. Cachectin/tumor necrosis factor stimulates collagenase and prostaglandin E_2 production by human synovial cells and dermal fibroblasts. J Exp Med 1985;162:2163–2168.
17. Dayer J-M, de Rochemonteix B, Burrus B, et al. Human recombinant interleukin-1 stimulates collagenase and prostaglandin E_2 production by human synovial cells. J Clin Invest 1986;77:645–648.
18. Dean DD, Martel-Pelletier J, Pelletier JP, et al. Evidence for metalloproteinase and metalloproteinase inhibitor imbalance in human osteoarthritic cartilage. J Clin Invest 1989;84:678–685.
19. Deleuran BW, Chew CQ, Field M, et al. Localization of tumor necrosis factor receptors in the synovial tissue and cartilage-pannus junction in patients with rheumatoid arthritis. Arth Rheum 1992;35:1160–1169.
20. Dimock AN, Siciliano PD, McIlwraith CW. Evidence supporting an increased presence of reactive oxygen species in the diseased equine joint. Equine Vet J 2000;32:439–443.
21. Dodge GR, Poole AR. Immunohistochemical detection and immunochemical analysis of type II collagen degradation in human normal, rheumatoid, and osteoarthritic articular cartilage and in explants of bovine articular cartilage cultured with interleukin 1. J Clin Invest 1989;83:647–661.
22. Drum MG, Kawcak CE, Norrdin RW, et al. Comparison of gross and histopathologic findings with quantitative computed tomographic bone density in the distal third metacarpal bone of racehorses. Vet Radiol and Ultrasound 2007;48:518–527.
23. Dudhia J, Platt D. Complete primary sequence of equine cartilage link protein deduced from complementary DNA. Am J Vet Res 1995;56:959–965.
24. Evans CH, Mears DC, Stanitski CL. Ferrographic analysis of wear in human joints: Evaluation by comparison with arthroscopic examination of symptomatic knee joints. J Bone Joint Surg 1982;64B:572–578.
25. Flannery CR, Gordy JT, Lark MW, et al. Identification of a stromelysin cleavage site within the interglobular domain of human aggrecan: Evidence for proteolysis at this site in vivo. Proceedings 8th Ann Mtg Orthop Res Soc 84,1991.
26. Frisbie DD, Ghivizzani SC, Robbins PD, et al. Treatment of experimental equine osteoarthritis by an in vivo delivery of the equine-1 receptor antagonist gene. Gene Therapy 2002;9:12–20.
27. Frisbie DD, Kawcak CE, McIlwraith CW, et al. Effects of 6α-methylprednisolone acetate on an in vivo equine osteochondral fragment exercise model. Am J Vet Res 1998;59:1619–1628.
28. Gardner DL, McGillvray CD. Living articular cartilage is not smooth. Ann Rheum Dis 1971;30:3.
29. Goldring MB. The role of cytokines as inflammatory mediators in osteoarthritis: Lessons from animal models. Mini review. Overseas Publishers Assoc 1999;1–11.
30. Grant BD. Repair mechanisms of osteochondral defects in Equidae: A comparative study of untreated in x-irradiated defects. Proc Am Assoc Equine Pract 1975;21:95–114.
31. Greenwald R, Moy W. Effect of oxygen-derived free radicals on hyaluronic acid. Arth Rheum 1980;23:455–463.
32. Greenwald R, Moy W. Inhibition of collagen gelatin by actions of the superoxide radical. Arth Rheum 1979;22:251–259.
33. Guilak F, Ratcliffe A, Mow VC. Chondrocyte deformation and local tissue strain in articular cartilage: A confocal microscopy study. J Orthop Res 1995;13:410–421.
34. Howard RD, McIlwraith CW, Trotter GW, et al. Cloning of equine interleukin-1 alpha and equine interleukin-1 receptor antagonist and determination of their full length cDNA sequence. Am J Vet Res 1998b;57:704–711.
35. Howard RD, McIlwraith CW, Trotter GW, et al. Cloning of equine interleukin-1 alpha and equine interleukin-1 beta and determination of their full length cDNA sequences. Am J Vet Res 1998a;59:704–711.
36. Hung S-C, Nakamura K, Shiro R, et al. Effects of continuous distraction on cartilage in a moving joint: An investigation on adult rabbits. J Orthop Res 1997;15:381–390.

37. Hunter W. Of the structure and diseases of articulating cartilage. Clin Orthop and Rel Res 1995;317:3–6.

38. Hurtig MB, Fretz PB, Doige CE, et al. Effect of lesion size and location on equine articular cartilage repair. Can J Vet Res 1988;52:137–146.

39. Hurtig MB. Experimental use of small osteochondral grafts for resurfacing the equine third carpal bone. Equine Vet J 1988; S6:23–27.

40. Jones DL, Barber SM, Doige CE. Synovial fluid and clinical changes after arthroscopic partial synovectomy of the equine mile carpal joint. Vet Surg 1993;22:524–530.

41. Jones G, Bennell K, Cicuttini FM. Effect of physical activity on cartilage development in healthy kids. Br J Sports Med 2003; 37:382–383.

42. Kawcak CE, Frisbie DD, McIlwraith CW, et al. Effects of intravenous administration of sodium hyaluronate on carpal joints in exercising horses after arthroscopic surgery and osteochondral fragmentation. Am J Vet Res 1997;58:1132–1140.

43. Kawcak CE, Frisbie DD, Trotter GW, et al. Maintenance of equine articular cartilage explants in serum-free and serum-supplemented media compared with that in a commercially supplemented media. Am J Vet Res 1996;57:1261–1265.

44. Kawcak CE, McIlwraith CW, Norrdin RW, et al. Clinical effects of exercise on subchondral bone of carpal and metacarpophalangeal joints in horses. Am J Vet Res 2000;61:1252–1258.

45. Kawcak CE, McIlwraith CW, Norrdin RW, et al. The role of subchondral bone in joint disease: A review. Equine Vet J 2001;33:120–126.

46. Kempson GE, Muir H, Swanson SA, et al. Correlations between stiffness and the chemical constituents of cartilage on the human femoral head. Biochem Biophys Acta 1970;215:70.

47. Kiviranta I, Tammi M, Jervelin J, et al. Articular cartilage thickness and glycosaminoglycan distribution in the canine knee joint after strenuous exercise. Clin Orthop 1992;283:302–308.

48. Levick JR. Hypoxia and acidosis in chronic inflammatory arthritis: Relation to vascular supply and dynamic effusion pressure. J Rheumatol 1990;17:579–582.

49. Linn FC, Sokoloff L. Movement and composition of interstitial fluid of cartilage. Arthritis Rheum 1965;8:481–494.

50. Little CB, Ghosh P. Variation in proteoglycan metabolism by articular chondrocytes in different joint regions as determined by post-natal mechanical loading. Osteo and Cart 1997;5:49–62.

51. Little CB, McIlwraith CW. Unpublished data, 2004.

52. Lohmander LS, Roos H, Dahlberg L, et al. Temporal patterns of stromelysin, tissue inhibitor and proteoglycan fragments in synovial fluid after injury to the knee, cruciate ligament or meniscus. J Orthop Res 1994;12:21–28.

53. Lotz M. NO and other radicals in the pathogenesis of osteoarthritis. In Osteoarthritis, Inflammation and Degradation: A Continuum. Buckwalter JA, Lotz M, Stoltz J-F, eds. IOS Press, Amsterdam, 2007;182–191.

54. Mankin HJ, Radin E. Structure and function of joints. In Arthritis and Allied Conditions, 9th ed. McCarty DJ, ed. Lea and Febiger, Philadelphia, 1979;151–165.

55. Mankin HJ. The reactions of articular cartilage to injury in osteoarthritis. N Engl J Med 1974;191:1285–1292.

56. Maroudas A. Transport of solutes through cartilage: permeability to large molecules. J Anat 1976;122:335.

57. Martel-Pellieter P, Pellieter J-P. Inflammatory factors involved in osteoarthritis. In Osteoarthritis, Inflammation and Degradation: A Continuum. Buckwalter JA, Lotz M, Stoltz J-F, eds. IOS Press, Amsterdam, 2007;3–13.

58. Martinelli MJ. Subchondral bone and injury. Clinical commentary. Equine Vet Educ 2009;21:253–256.

59. May SA, Hooke RE, Lees P. The characterization of equine interleukin-1. Vet Immunol Immunopath 1990;24:169–174.

60. McAdams TR, Mandelbaum BR. Articular cartilage regeneration in the knee. Current Orthopedic Prac 2008;19:140–146.

61. McIlwraith CW, Vachon AM. Review of pathogenesis and treatment of degenerative joint disease. Equine Vet J 1988;S6:3–11.

62. McIlwraith CW, Van Sickle DC. Experimentally induced arthritis of the equine carpus: Histologic and histochemical changes in the articular cartilage. Am J Vet Res 1981;42:209–217.

63. McIlwraith CW, Yovich JV, Martin GS. Arthroscopic surgery for the treatment of osteochondral chip fractures in the equine carpus. J Am Vet Med Assoc 1987;191:531–540.

64. McIlwraith CW. Current concepts in equine degenerative joint disease. J Am Vet Med Assoc 1982;180:239.

65. McIlwraith CW. Diseases of joints, tendons and related structures. In Adams' Lameness in Horses, 5th ed. McIlwraith CW, ed. Lippincott, Williams and Wilkins, Philadelphia, 2002;457–644.

66. McIlwraith CW. Frank Milne Lecture: From Arthroscopy to Gene Therapy—30 years of Looking in Joints. Proceedings AAEP 2005;51:65–113.

67. McIlwraith CW. General pathobiology of the joint and response to injury. In Joint Disease in the Horse. McIlwraith CW, Trotter GW, eds. WB Saunders Co., Philadelphia, 1996.

68. Meachim G. The effect of scarification on articular cartilage in the rabbit. J Bone Joint Surg [Br] 1963;45:150–161.

69. Moldovan F, Pelletier JP, Hambor J, et al. Collagenase-3 (matrix metalloproteinase 13) is preferentially localized in the deep layer of human articular cartilage in situ. In vitro mimicking effect by transforming growth factor beta. Arth Rheum 1997;40:1653–1661.

70. Morel V, Berutto C, Quinn TM. Effects of damage in the articular surface on the cartilage response to injurious compression in vitro. Jour of Biomech 2005;39:924–930.

71. Morris EA, McDonald BS, Webb AC, et al. Identification of interleukin-1 in equine osteoarthritic joint effusion. Am J Vet Res 1990;51:59–64.

72. Mow VC, Holmes MH, Lai WM. Fluid transport of mechanical properties of articular cartilage: A review. J Biomechan 1984;17:377–394.

73. Myers ER, Mow VC. Biomechanics of cartilage and its response to biomechanical stimuli. In Cartilage. Hall BK, ed. Academic Press, New York, 1983;1:313–340.

74. Nagase H, Woessner JF Jr. Role of endogenous proteinases in the degradation of cartilage matrix. In Joint Cartilage Degradation: Basic and Clinical Aspects. Woessner JF Jr., Howell DS, eds. Marcel-Dekker Inc, New York, 1993;159–185.

75. Nixon AJ, Cummings JF. Substance P immunohistochemical study of the sensory innervation of normal subchondral bone in the equine metacarpophalangeal joint. Am J Vet Res 1994;55:28–34.

76. Nixon AJ. Articular cartilage surface structure and function. Equine Vet Educ 1991;3:72–75.

77. Norrdin RW, Kawcak CE, et al. Subchondral bone failure in an equine model of overload arthrosis. Bone 1998;22:133–139.

78. Ogston AG, Stanier J. The physiological function of hyaluronic acid in synovial fluid: Viscous, elastic and lubricant properties. J Phys 1953;119:244–252.

79. Platt D, Byrd JLE, Bayliss MT. Aging of equine articular cartilage: Structure and composition of aggrecan and decorin. Equine Vet J 1998;30:43–52.

80. Poole CA, Flint MH, Beaumont BW. Chondrons extracted from canine tibial cartilage: preliminary report on their isolation and structure. J Orthop Res 1988;6:408–419.

81. Price JS, Symons JA, Russell RGG. Cytokines: Inflammatory mediators of joint disease. Equine Vet J 1992;24:78–80.

82. Radin EL, Paul IL, Tolkoff MJ. Subchondral bone change in patients with early degenerative arthritis. Arthritis Rheum 1970;13:400.

83. Radin EL, Paul IL. Does cartilage compliance reduce skeletal impact loads? The relative force-attenuating properties of articular cartilage, synovial fluid, peri-articular soft tissues, and bone. Arthritis Rheum 1970;13:139.

84. Radin EL, Rose RN. The role of subchondral bone in the initiation and progression of cartilage damage. Clin Orthop Rel Res 1986;213:34–40.

85. Repo RB, Mitchell N. Collagen synthesis in mature articular cartilage of the rabbit. J Bone Joint Surg [Br] 1971;53:541–548.

86. Richardson DW, Dodge GR. Cloning of equine type II procollagen and the modulation of its expression in cultured equine articular chondrocytes. Matrix Biol 1997;16:59–64.

87. Riddle WE. Healing of articular cartilage in the horse. J Am Vet Med Assoc 1970;157:1471.

88. Riggs CM, Whitehouse CH, Boyd A. Structural variations of the distal condyles of the third metacarpal and third metatarsal bones of the horse. Equine Vet J 1999;31:130–139.

89. Riggs CM, Whitehouse CH, Boyd A. Pathology of the distal condyles of the third metacarpal and third metatarsal bones of the horse. Equine Vet J 1999;31:140–148.

90. Riggs CM. Osteochondral injury in joint disease in the athletic horse. Equine Vet Educ 2006;128–140.
91. Riggs CM. Multidisciplinary investigation of the aetiopathogenesis of parasagittal fractures of the distal metacarpal and third metatarsal bone–Review of the literature. Equine Vet J 1999;31:116–120.
92. Roos EM, Dahlberg L. Positive effects of moderate exercise on glycosaminoglycan content in knee cartilage. Arth Rheum 2005;52:3507–3514.
93. Roth V, Mow VC. The intrinsic tensile behavior of the matrix of bovine articular cartilage and its variation with age. J Bone Joint Surg 1980;62(A):1102.
94. Sah RL, McIlwraith CW, Pae KR, et al. Cartilage lubrication and diarthrodial joint biology. Proceedings 7th World Congress of ICRS, Warsaw, Poland 2007;121–122.
95. Sande JD, Neame PJ, Boynton RE, Flannery CR. Catabolism of aggrecan in cartilage explants. Identification of a major cleavage site within the interglobular domain. J Biochem 1991;266:8683–8685.
96. Schmid A, Schmid F. Ultrastructural studies after arthroscopical cartilage shaving. Arthroscopy 1987;3:137.
97. Schmidt TA, Sah RL. Effect of synovial fluid on boundary lubrication of articular cartilage. Osteo Cart 2007;15:335–347.
98. Schwarz IM, Hills BA. Surface-active phospholipids in the lubricating component of lubricin. J Rheumatol (Br) 1998;37:21–26.
99. Simkin PA. Synovial physiology. In McCarty DJ, ed. Arthritis and Allied Conditions, 9th ed. McCarty DJ, ed. Lea and Febiger, Philadelphia 1979;167–178.
100. Slether-Stevenson WG, Krutsch HC, Liotta LA. Tissue inhibitor of metalloproteinase (TIMP-2). A new member of the metalloproteinase family. J Biol Chem 1989;264:17374–17378.
101. Swann DA, Silver SH, Slayter HS, et al. The molecular structure and lubricating activity of lubricin isolated from bovine and human synovial fluid. Biochem J 1985;225:195–221.
102. Takafuji VA, McIlwraith CW, Howard RD. Effects of recombinant equine interleukin-1 alpha and interleukin-1 beta on proteoglycan metabolism and prostaglandin E_2 synthesis in equine articular cartilage explants. Am J Vet Res 2002;63:551–558.
103. Tamanini C, Seren C, Pezzoli G, et al. Concentrazione delle prostaglindiinne I1-E2 nel liquido synoviale di cavalla affetti da artropatie. Clinique Vet 1980;103:544–549.
104. Teitz CC, Chrisman OD. The effect of salicylate and chloroquine on prostaglandin-induced articular damage in the rabbit knee. Clin Orthop 1975;108:264–274.
105. Theoret CL, Barber SM, Moyana T, et al. Repair and function of synovium after arthroscopic synovectomy of the dorsal compartment of the equine antebrachiocarpal joint. Vet Surg 1996;25:142–153.
106. Todhunter RJ. Anatomy and physiology of synovial joints. In: Joint Disease in the Horse. McIlwraith CW, Trotter GW, eds. WB Saunders Co., Philadelphia, 1996; 1–48.
107. Torzilli PA, Arduino JM, Gregory JD, et al. Effect of proteoglycan removal on solute mobility in articular cartilage. J Biomechan 1997;30:895–902.
108. Trumble TN, Trotter GW, Oxford JRT, et al. Synovial fluid gelatinase concentrations and matrix metalloproteinase and cytokine expression in naturally occurring joint disease in horses. Am J Vet Res 2001;62:1467–1477.
109. Vachon AM, Keeley FW, McIlwraith CW, et al. Biochemical analysis of normal articular cartilage in horses. Am J Vet Res 1990;51:1905–1911.
110. Vachon AM, McIlwraith CW, Powers BE, et al. Morphologic and biochemical study of sternal cartilage autografts for resurfacing induced osteochondral defects in horses. Am J Vet Res 1992;53:1038–1047.
111. Vachon AM, McIlwraith CW, Trotter GW, et al. Morphologic study of induced osteochondral defects of the distal portion of the radial carpal bone in horses by use of glued periosteal autografts. Am J Vet Res 1991;52:317–327.
112. Wojtys TM, Beaman DN, Glover RA, et al. Innervation of the human knee joint by substance-P fibers. J Arthroscopy 1990;6:254–263.
113. Wong S, Halliwell B, Richmond R, et al. The role of superoxide and hydroxyl radicals in the degradation of hyaluronic acid induced by metal ions and by ascorbic acid. J Inorg Biochem 1981;14:127–134.
114. Wood DD, Ihrie EJ, Hamerman D. Release of interleukin-1 from human synovial tissue *in vitro*. Arth Rheum 1985;28:853–862.
115. Wu J-J, Lark M, Eyre DR. Sites of stromelysin cleavage in collagens type II, IX, X, and XI of cartilage. J Biol Chem 1991;266:5625–5628.
116. Young DR, Richardson DW, Markel MD, et al. Mechanical and morphometric analysis of the third carpal bone of Thoroughbreds. Am J Vet Res 1991;52:402–409.

BONE INJURIES AND DISEASE

Chris Kawcak and Gary M. Baxter

THE IMMATURE SKELETON

Longitudinal bone growth results from a series of events occurring at highly specialized regions at 1 or both ends of the bone. These regions are referred to as the physes, growth plates, or more correctly, the metaphyseal growth plates. The process occurring at the growth plate, endochondral ossification, is characterized by rapidly differentiating and maturing cartilage cells and the replacement of cartilage by bone. There are 2 types of growth plates: discoid and spherical.

The discoid growth plates are seen at the ends of long bones. Some bones have a physis at each end of the bone, whereas others, such as the third metacarpal/metatarsal bone and the proximal and middle phalanges, have only one. A discoid physis is located between the metaphysis (the flared end of the bone that contains spongy bone) and the epiphysis. An apophysis (which is a type of discoid physis) is an epiphysis that is subject to tensile rather than compressive forces, such as at the olecranon process, calcaneal tuber, and tibial tuberosity (Figure 7.14). The growth plate of an apophysis contains greater amounts of fibrocartilage than a true discoid physis, which is an adaptation to withstand tensile forces.[70]

Spherical physes are located in the small cuboidal bones of the foal's carpus and tarsus. These growth plates develop into bones by centrifugal expansion around a central cartilage core. They begin to ossify in the center and gradually assume the contours of the bone of an adult as bone development reaches the margins of the cartilage model.

See Chapter 11 for further information on the morphology and physiology of the physis.

Effect of External Trauma on the Physis

An epiphyseal or physeal injury is likely to occur when an excessive force is applied to a joint and its nearby physis. This is because the cartilaginous growth plate is weaker than the surrounding bone, ligamentous structures, and joint capsule. Physeal and epiphyseal injuries account for approximately 15% of all fractures in children and also occur commonly in foals. Injuries that would normally produce a ruptured ligament or joint dislocation in an adult may produce traumatic separation of the physis in a young animal. For example, trauma to the fetlock region usually causes fetlock luxations in adult horses, and a distal metacarpal/metatarsal physeal fractures in foals. Joint luxations are rare in young horses. See Chapter 11 for further information on physeal fractures in horses.

Developmental Orthopedic Diseases

Developmental orthopedic disease (DOD) complex is a group of abnormalities that occurs in foals and

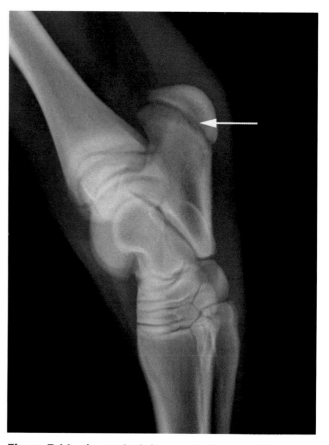

Figure 7.14. An apophysis is present at the point of the calcaneal tuber (arrow) in young horses and at the olecranon process and the tibial tuberosity.

young growing horses.[103] Other terms that are often used interchangeably with DOD include osteodystrophy or osteochondrosis, although this is considered erroneous. Most of the diseases included in the DOD complex can be attributed to alterations in bone growth or development (endochondral ossification), either at the metaphyseal or epiphyseal growth plates. These include physitis, angular limb deformities (ALDs), osteochondritis dissecans (OCD), subchondral cystic lesions, cuboidal bone collapse or incomplete ossification, juvenile arthritis, cervical vertebral malformations (CVM), and flexural deformities.[40,103] Clinical signs of these conditions are variable but are usually seen in young horses because this is an abnormality of developing bone. Signs include variable degrees of lameness, alteration in posture or positioning of the limb, crooked legs, joint effusion, limb enlargement, ataxia (CVM only), and possible fractures. Additionally, multiple DOD conditions may be present in the same animal.

Although the exact cause for DOD is not known, there are multiple risk factors that appear to predispose

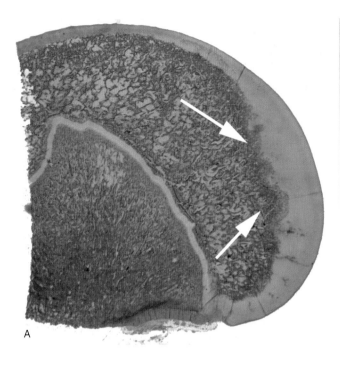

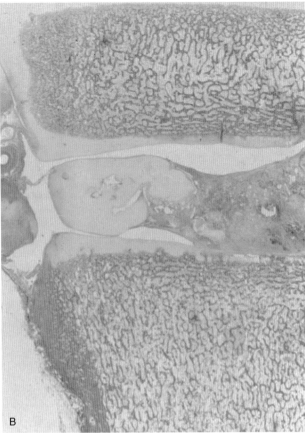

Figure 7.15. Histologic examples of abnormal bone formation typical of developmental orthopedic diseases. A. Retained articular cartilage in the subchondral bone area (arrows) that is typical of osteochondritis dissecans. B. Retained articular cartilage in the cuboidal bone of the tarsus leading to cuboidal bone malformation.

young horses to the development of these diseases. Many of the risk factors are manmade, such as management and breeding practices, and others have been extrapolated from research work in other species.[24,32,71] For instance, breeding for rapidly growing offspring that hopefully will perform better in the show ring, and feeding rations high in energy and protein appear to predispose these animals to DOD abnormalities, presumably by contributing to rapid bone growth.

Other risk factors include mineral imbalances such as copper deficiency or excess zinc, trauma, and genetic predilection.[77,99] Trace mineral deficiencies, particularly copper, have been incriminated in physitis and angular deformities in cattle,[84] and have been shown to cause clinical signs and joint pathology consistent with osteochondrosis in foals.[36,37] Copper is required for the enzyme lysyl oxidase, which itself is necessary for collagen cross linking. Therefore, defective collagen cross linking may impair the strength of bone collagen, essentially producing a "soft bone syndrome," particularly in the metaphyseal regions.[36] Excess zinc or alterations in the calcium/phosphorus ratios in the diet also may lead to clinical problems of DOD, but these are not as well defined in horses as copper deficiency.[77]

Trauma to the metaphyseal or epiphyseal growth plates can contribute to altered growth, subchondral bone damage, and avulsion of defective bone (Figure 7.15), all of which may also predispose to DOD conditions. Genetics most likely plays a role in the occurrence of these diseases, but its contribution is difficult to determine. However, in most cases the underlying cause of the DOD condition is multifactorial, usually obscure, and often never determined.[103] See Chapter 11 for further information on specific DOD conditions such as physitis and ALDs.

Incomplete Cuboidal Bone Ossification/Juvenile Spavin

Incomplete ossification of the cuboidal bones of the carpus or tarsus occurs most commonly in twins or premature or underdeveloped newborn foals. At birth, the cuboidal bones have not ossified sufficiently to withstand the forces of normal weight-bearing, predisposing to variable degrees of carpal or tarsal bone wedging or collapse (Figure 7.16). Incomplete ossification without collapse is not readily apparent clinically and is best diagnosed with radiography to document abnormal cuboidal bone appearance. Clinical signs associated with cuboidal bone collapse may be evident in the newborn foal as an angular limb deformity of the carpus or tarsus. Collapse of the tarsal bones is much more common than that of the carpal bones, and is often associated with a sickle or cow-hocked conformation of

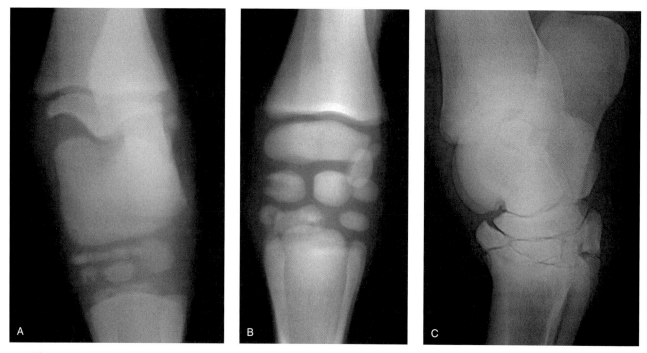

Figure 7.16. Radiographic images demonstrating incomplete ossification of the tarsal (A) and carpal (B) cuboidal bones in a premature foal. Without support, normal weight-bearing could lead to wedging and collapse of the tarsal bones (C).

the tarsus, or the tarsus looks like it has a curb. The degree of lameness is variable, and may not become clinically apparent until later in life.

Preventing cuboidal bone collapse in newborn foals with incomplete ossification involves minimizing compressive forces on the bones until they ossify. Confinement, sleeve casts, bandages, or bandages and splints may be used, depending on the severity. In a recent study, foals with only minor tarsal bone collapse were able to perform as intended, whereas foals with more severe tarsal bone collapse and fragmentation could not be used for their intended purposes (Figure 7.16C).[20] Additionally, incomplete ossification and mild collapse of the tarsal bones is thought to predispose to juvenile spavin in young horses. Horses with juvenile spavin have relatively severe signs of bone spavin at a young age with a history of minimal work (Figure 7.17). Inherent abnormalities of the central and third tarsal bones are thought to contribute to the development of osteoarthritis in the distal tarsal joints at such an early age. In young horses with obvious signs of juvenile spavin, surgical arthrodesis is often effective in salvaging the animal for athletic use.

Osteochondritis Dissecans (OCD)

Osteochondritis dissecans refers to cartilage or cartilage and bone (osteochondral) fragments or flaps that develop along the articular surfaces of joints in horses. These abnormalities are probably the most common manifestation of the DOD complex in horses. They usually occur along the non-weight bearing surfaces of the joint, and are especially common in the stifle, tarsus, and fetlock joints (Figure 7.18).[99] Horses with OCD lesions typically are only mildly lame but usually have

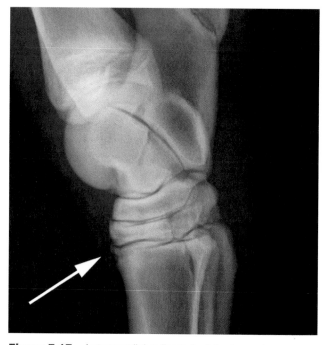

Figure 7.17. Lateromedial radiograph of the tarsus in a yearling colt with hindlimb lameness that improved with intra-articular anesthesia of the distal tarsal joints. Abnormal curvature to the third tarsal bone and osteophyte formation (arrow) are noted on the radiograph. Development of tarsal OA in young horses is often referred to as "juvenile spavin."

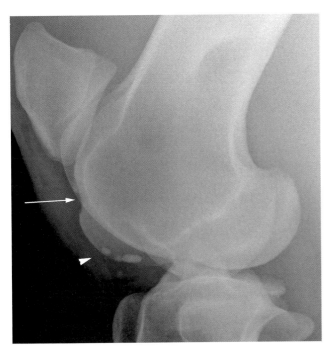

Figure 7.18. Lateromedial radiographic view demonstrating a typical lateral ridge OCD lesion of the distal femur (arrow) and the fragments that have migrated within the joint (arrowhead).

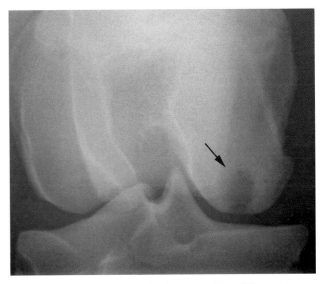

Figure 7.19. Caudal-cranial radiograph of the stifle reveals a subchondral cystic lesion within the medial femoral condyle (arrow) of this yearling Quarter horse filly.

joint effusion of the affected joint(s). These lesions are often bilateral and may or may not require arthroscopic surgery to remove the osteochondral fragment(s). The prognosis for performance of horses with OCD lesions is usually very good. More detailed discussion of OCD lesions can be found in Chapter 11.

Subchondral Cystic Lesions (SCLs)

Subchondral cystic lesions (bone cysts or osseous-cyst-like lesions) are commonly recognized pathologic entities of bones and joints in horses that may or may not cause lameness. They may be nonarticular or articular. However, most lesions that contribute to lameness involve the weight-bearing area of an articular surface. Nonarticular lesions (which may or may not be classified as subchondral cystic lesions) usually involve the metaphysis and can go undiagnosed because they may not cause clinical signs, and normal bone remodeling may resolve the defect. The most common age for diagnosis of SCLs, or at least the time when clinical signs develop, is usually 3 years or less.[5,34] However, horses demonstrate clinical signs related to SCLs over a wide age range, and the relationship between when the lesion develops and when the horse begins to show clinical signs is not known.[41] This relationship probably varies depending on the specific site of the SCL (the most common location is the medial femoral condyle), the age when the lesion develops, and the occupation of the horse. What causes or initiates the appearance of clinical signs in horses with articular SCLs remains unknown.

Subchondral cystic lesions have been reported at multiple locations in horses.[5,13] However, the most common sites that contribute to clinical problems appear to involve the stifle, fetlock, pastern, coffin, and elbow joints (Figure 7.19). Controversy exists as to whether these lesions are caused by a defect in endochondral ossification, intra-articular subchondral bone trauma, or a combination of both.[5,13,41] Joint trauma can lead to the development of SCLs, and this has been shown experimentally and has been seen clinically (Figure 7.20).[5] However, many of these lesions are seen in young horses and are bilateral, suggesting a developmental defect.

Subchondral cystic lesions have been described as resulting from an infolding of abnormal cartilage into the underlying bony spongiosa.[5] The infolded cartilage becomes necrotic and its matrix remains nonmineralized so that osteoclasts and blood vessels do not migrate into the defect to enable repair of the defective cartilage and bone. The cystic lining is made up of fibrous tissue with active fibroplasia and capillary proliferation present in the tissue adjacent to the bone. The cyst lining has been shown experimentally to contain significant inflammatory mediators that likely contribute to the formation and progression of the cyst.[97]

Treatment of SCLs involves the use of intra-articular medications (combined with systemic joint therapies), surgical debridement of the lesion, surgical debridement with bone graft, surgical debridement with augmentative therapies such as chondrocytes or stem cells, or intralesional injection with corticosteroids.[34,98] Because of the variable prognosis in horses with debridement of the lesion alone, some surgeons attempt additional treatment(s) of the bone defect. These include packing the entire defect with cancellous bone or packing the depth of the lesion with cancellous bone and filling the remaining bone defect with fibrin-laden chondrocytes containing growth factors. The goal of the latter treatment is to promote healing of both the bone and articular cartilage defects. Although nonsurgical treatment

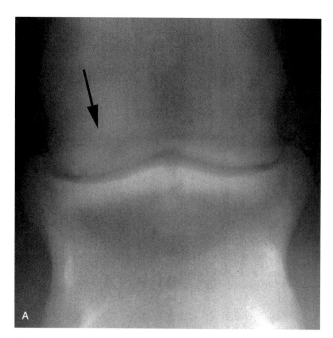

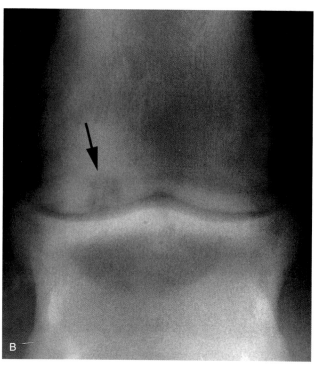

Figure 7.20. Dorsopalmar radiographs of the pastern in a 12-year-old Thoroughbred with a grade 4 out of 5 hindlimb lameness. Minimal radiographic abnormalities were visible on the initial radiograph (A, arrow). However, a subchondral cystic lesion with surrounding sclerosis was evident within the proximal phalanx on radiographs taken 6 months later (B, arrow).

has usually been recommended initially in most horses because of the variable success with surgical debridement of the lesions with or without the adjunctive treatments, the use of intralesional corticosteroid injections appears to give a more dependable prognosis.

Effects of Exercise on the Immature Skeleton

Beginning at birth, exercise can have a profound effect on the musculoskeletal system. There has been considerable interest in the effects of early exercise on foals in an attempt to strengthen the system to reduce the incidence of injuries later in life. In initial studies by van de Lest, et al., foals that were box-stall rested were more likely to have reduced development than foals that were turned out full time and those that were turned out intermittently along with box stall rest.[95] The author (CEK) has performed density studies in foals before and after exercise and found that prior to exercise, the subchondral bone pattern is blank, but at 6 months of age, the density pattern reflects the articulation between the joint surfaces (Figure 7.21).

In addition, in an attempt to strengthen musculoskeletal tissues later in life, a large study was performed in which foals that had additional exercise early in life were compared to those that were turned out. The goal was to provide galloping exercise in addition to normal pasture turn-out to a group of foals and compare tissue responses as yearlings and as 3-year-olds. The investigators found minimal effects on tendons and ligaments, but fairly significant effects on articular cartilage. Namely, exercised foals had significantly higher viable

chondrocyte content in their joints than pasture-reared foals, and they had fewer gross lesions in the carpi at 18 months of age.[21,45] However, there was no effect on articular cartilage changes in the palmar aspect of the parasagittal groove in the fetlock joints, a site of fracture and osteoarthritis (OA).[63] In the carpus, however, Wong, et al. showed that the incidence of gross lesions was significantly lower in the exercised group compared to the control group.[45] Subchondral bone formation was increased, but the overall bone content and density were no different between the groups. Overall, enforced galloping exercise did not produce negative effects and in fact provided benefit to the joints.

Clinically, lack of exercise seems to have a profound effect on bone. For instance, it is not uncommon for young foals to fracture their proximal sesamoid bones during normal pasture exercise after being confined, usually in a hospital setting (Figure 7.22). The stall confinement appears to prevent normal adaptation from occurring to the bones, especially the proximal sesamoid bones, and therefore creates a situation in which the bones cannot withstand normal exercise. Consequently, care must be taken in introducing foals to turn-out, especially if the mares sense competition with others in the pasture.

The proximal sesamoid bones seem to be the most sensitive to lack of exercise. For instance, cast application to a limb leads to radiographically apparent loss of bone density in the proximal sesamoid bones (Figure 7.23). The density of these bones is 30% to 40% lower with 6 weeks of casting. In other words, bones require a normal threshold of loading to maintain strength.

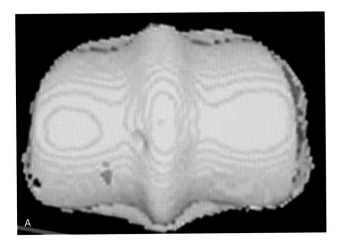

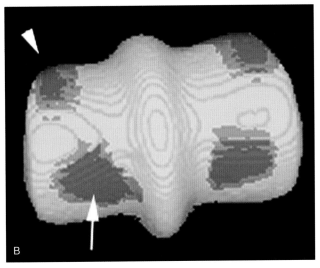

Figure 7.21. Three-dimensional computed tomographic images of the third metacarpal condyles, demonstrating the adaptation of bone to exercise in foals. In this example, subchondral bone density shortly after birth is homogeneous across the joint surface (A); however, after 6 months (B), the subchondral bone density increases in the areas that articulate with the proximal sesamoid bones (arrow) and the dorsal aspect of the first phalanx (arrowhead).

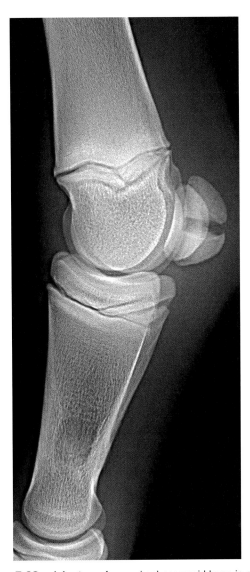

Figure 7.22. A fracture of a proximal sesamoid bone in a foal that was initially stall confined at birth.

LOCAL DISEASES OF BONE

Exercise-induced Bone Remodeling

Bone is very metabolically active under normal physiologic circumstances and in response to many types of injury. Its intricate micro- and macrostructural organization, combined with its high rate of metabolic activity, allow it to respond rapidly to many physical and biomechanical demands, especially in young animals.[50] Normal daily activity and exercise impose complex forces on the skeletal system that cause varying quantities of deformations of bone. Deformations within a bone are referred to as strains, and the local force intensities at these sites are the stresses, defined as a given force per unit area. The direction and magnitude of these stresses and strains depend on the geometry of the bone, the direction and magnitude of the load imposed on the bone, and the material properties of the bone.

Thus, joint surface geometry, limb conformation, and shoeing are so important to the causes and management of lameness.

Bone in any species can undergo remodeling or modeling. Equine bone remodels in response to the stresses placed on it according to Wolff's law, which in brief states that bone is laid down where it is needed and is resorbed where it is not needed. Examples of adaptive remodeling in equine bone include the cancellous portion of the proximal sesamoid bones becoming less porous (stiffer and stronger) when trained on dirt tracks compared to untrained horses,[104] and the shape of the metacarpus changing during training and racing to withstand the added forces applied to the bone.[64,67] Bone modeling occurs when the resorptive phase does not occur, and instead bone is laid down on top of normal trabecular structures. An example of this is the palmar aspect of the third metacarpal condyle and the radial facet of the third carpal bone becoming dense (Figure 7.24).[18,44]

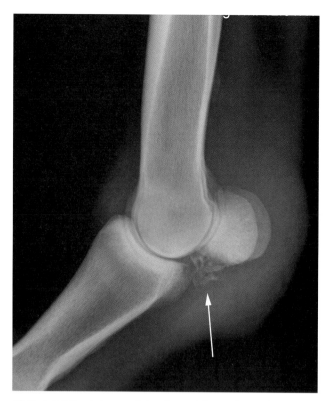

Figure 7.23. Lateromedial radiograph from a horse that was casted for 6 weeks. Notice the loss of bone density in the proximal sesamoid bones, as well as the formation of enthesiophytes distally (arrow).

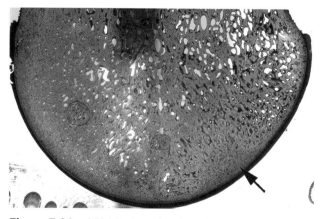

Figure 7.24. A histologic section through the palmar aspect of the third metacarpal condyle of a racehorse showing thickening of the subchondral bone (arrow) in the area that articulates with the proximal sesamoid bone. This area shows bone modeling in response to normal adaptation.

These are just a few examples of bone's response to exercise, which undoubtedly occurs in every bone during training and performance. Unfortunately, there is a fine line between what is considered to be normal adaptive training and over-training that may be pathologic to the bone (Figure 7.25). In addition, there is no objective means to characterize the threshold between normal and pathologic loading. The osteogenic response of bone to remodeling stimuli such as training or exer-

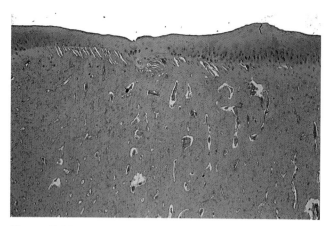

Figure 7.25. A histologic section through the palmar aspect of the third metacarpal condyles showing not only severe bone modeling, but also overlying articular cartilage damage. This example appears to represent a modeling response beyond the threshold of normal adaptation to exercise.

cise appears to be most dependent on the strain magnitude and strain rate. In other words, the greater the load, the faster the load is applied, and the more times bone is loaded (repetitions), the greater the remodeling response. Increased magnitude of loading may be achieved by exercising at higher speeds or on harder surfaces (or a combination of each).

Excessive repetitions of normal loads or excessively high loads are thought to contribute to the development of dorsal metacarpal disease or stress or fatigue fractures in racehorses.[64,66,90] Fatigue fractures indicate that the bone has not remodeled or gained enough strength to withstand the forces (loads) that are being applied to it.[66] In most cases, the exercise regimen should be altered to permit the bone to gain adequate strength to tolerate the higher loads. However, the clinical signs of fatigue fractures are vague, and often the horse shows no clinical signs until the fatigue fractures coalesce and cause a complete fracture. If an excessive load is applied to a bone as a single event, the ultimate stresses and strains that the tissue can tolerate are exceeded, and a complete fracture occurs. Single-event trauma is a cause of complete fractures in many horses and foals. However, fatigue or stress fractures predispose to complete fractures, especially in performance horses, presumably by decreasing the ultimate load that the bone can withstand before fracturing. This has been shown repeatedly at sites of injury in racehorses.[18,44] Examples include fatigue fractures of the cortical bone of the third metacarpus, tibia, pelvic structures, and humerus, as well as the subchondral bone of the carpal bones, proximal sesamoid bones, and third metacarpal condyles (Figure 7.26). In addition to fracture, stress-induced modeling can lead to pathologic sclerosis of subchondral bone, especially in the third carpal bone and third metacarpal condyles, that can lead to OA.

Fractures

When a fracture occurs there is usually a loss of structural continuity of the bone and its function is

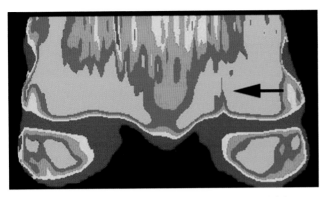

Figure 7.26. A computed tomographic image of the third metacarpal condyle of a Thoroughbred racehorse. Note the vertical demineralization in the area where condylar fractures typically occur (arrow).

impaired to varying degrees. The degree of altered function and the particular bone that is fractured often determine the type and severity of lameness. For example, a displaced fracture of the olecranon process or a fracture of one of the major load-bearing bones such as the radius or tibia usually produces severe lameness. Conversely, a so-called osteochondral or chip fracture of a carpal bone produces mild lameness that usually responds well to surgical removal, but if severe enough may predispose the horse to OA and cause a secondary lameness. Most acute fractures cause significant lameness regardless of their size and location. A fracture should always be considered as a possible cause of any nonweight-bearing lameness.

Fractures in horses are often due to single high-energy traumatic events that completely disrupt the bone (break the bone into at least 2 pieces). In contrast to most complete fractures, fatigue fractures are due to chronic trauma that weakens the bone, rather than a single traumatic event that fractures the bone.[90]

Specifically, chronic repetitive stress normally induces a bone-strengthening cascade in order to withstand these forces. This is a normal process in all athletes, especially the horse, and it creates normal patterns of bone enlargement or thickening, such as sclerosis, through the processes of bone modeling and remodeling. Specifically, repetitive stress can induce the response in 1 of 2 ways. Microdamage can result, stimulating remodeling events and leading to replacement of the damaged bone. Because osteoclastic function is more rapid than the osteoblastic response, this creates a window of vulnerability in which further high stresses can induce more damage within the relatively porous bone. The second form of bone strengthening in response to stress is through bone modeling, in which osteoid and mineral are added to existing bone to create either a dense sclerotic region (such as in subchondral bone) or geometric changes to bone architecture to maximize stress resistance (such as in cortical bone). This modeled bone is often more brittle than normal and in some instances can create pain and necrosis in these areas.

Fatigue fractures of the humerus, tibia, pelvis, and metacarpus/metatarsus (Figure 7.27) are commonly diagnosed in performance horses (primarily race-

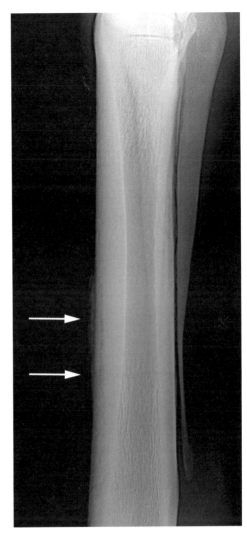

Figure 7.27. A radiograph of the third metacarpal bone from a 2-year-old racing Quarter Horse showing a fatigue fracture of the dorsal aspect of the bone (arrows).

horses).[90,91] Initially, these lesions cause variable degrees of lameness, but may contribute to complete fracture of the involved bone with continued use.[91] Diagnosis of incomplete fractures in racehorses is critical to prevent catastrophic bone failure, but can be difficult. These horses may not be overtly lame at the time of examination, but may have a history of not working correctly or being lame immediately after work. If lameness is present, then diagnostic analgesia can be performed, but the proximal location of many of these fractures often precludes its use. In addition, many subchondral bone lesions may not extend into the joint early in the disease process, making intra-articular analgesia of little use.[18] Nuclear scintigraphy can be very helpful in locating suspected fatigue fractures that are not apparent on radiographs. Care must be taken in overinterpretation though, because young, exercising horses typically show sites of intense remodeling, especially in the fetlock joints.

Treating incomplete fractures is much less complicated than treating complete fractures, and usually

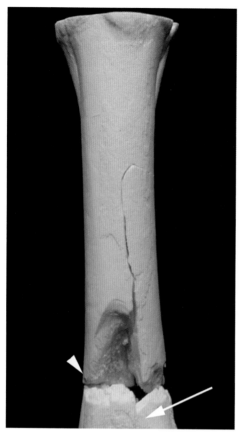

Figure 7.28. A severely comminuted, open, displaced fracture of the distal third metacarpus. Even though the condylar portion of this fracture is common and amenable to repair (arrow), the comminuted nature of the cortical portion of this fracture makes any repair futile, especially since the area was avascular from the degree of comminution (arrowhead).

Table 7.1. Contents of fracture first aid kit for horses.

Material	Purpose
Cotton, rolled and/or sheet	Padding under splint-cast combination or Robert-Jones bandage
Gauze, sterile and nonsterile	Applying dressing to wounds if present and Robert-Jones bandage
Razor or portable clippers	Removing hair from around wound
Antibiotic ointment	Topical dressing for open wounds
Support wrap (Vetrap, Elastikon, etc.)	Robert-Jones bandage or bandage under a splint-cast combination
White tape	Secure splints or boards to bandage
PVC splints (varying lengths)	Splint-cast combination
Fiberglass cast material	Splint-cast combination
Board splints (varying lengths) or aluminum rod	Splinting of radial and tibial fractures
Drugs (antibiotics, sedatives, NSAIDs)	Tranquilization, pain relief, and treatment of open fractures
"Leg saver" Kimzey splint (optional)	Immobilization of distal limb fractures

PVC = polyvinyl chloride, NSAIDs = nonsteroidal anti-inflammatory drugs

involves a period of inactivity combined with a change in training schedule. In contrast, complete fractures of long bones of horses are among the most difficult injuries to treat successfully and many horses are still euthanized because of the severity of the fracture (Figure 7.28). The prognosis of repairing complete fractures in horses depends on the specific bone affected, temperament of the horse, age and size of the horse, specific characteristics of the fracture, and expertise of the surgeon, to name just a few. However, proper stabilization of the fracture for transport to a surgical facility for repair is crucial to achieving a favorable outcome.

Fracture Stabilization for Transport/Fracture Immobilization at Specific Locations

Fractures are frequently diagnosed in horses and often require emergency first aid treatment (Table 7.1). Horses are not readily ambulatory on 3 limbs and often become very anxious when they are unable to place a fractured limb, which potentially can result in further injury. First aid measures should be directed toward minimizing further damage to the fractured limb and maintaining it in a position and condition that will facilitate repair.

The goals of first aid fracture management are to prevent damage to neural and vascular elements of the limb, prevent skin penetration of the fracture fragments or minimize further contamination of an existing wound, relieve anxiety of the animal by stabilizing the fractured limb, and minimize further damage to the fractured bone ends and surrounding soft tissue.[11,12] Most of these objectives can be accomplished by proper stabilization or splinting of the fracture. However, fractures of the upper forelimb and hindlimb in horses are nearly impossible to stabilize with external splints. Luckily, the bones in these locations are surrounded with large muscle groups, which inherently stabilize the fracture ends and make external coaptation less important.

Fracture immobilization serves several purposes. In horses, immobilization is more important to preserve limb vascularity than to prevent hemorrhage at the fracture site. Severe hemorrhage infrequently accompanies fractures in horses, but vascular thrombosis from continued stretching and direct trauma often lead to diminished vascularity of the distal limb. Limb immobilization also reduces the animal's anxiety, enabling the horse to regain control of the limb even though the limb cannot bear weight. Once stabilized, most horses will rest the limb instead of continually trying to place it in a normal stance, which causes further soft tissue and bone damage.

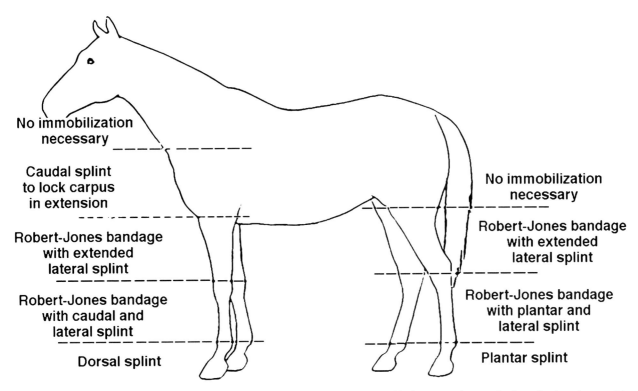

No immobilization
necessary

Caudal splint
to lock carpus
in extension

Robert-Jones bandage
with extended
lateral splint

Robert-Jones bandage
with caudal and
lateral splint

Dorsal splint

No immobilization
necessary

Robert-Jones bandage
with extended
lateral splint

Robert-Jones bandage
with plantar and
lateral splint

Plantar splint

Figure 7.29. Functional divisions of the horse's limbs that can be used as a guide for appropriate application of external support to immobilize fractures for transport.

Probably the most important purpose of immobilization is to prevent the development of an open fracture. Loss of intact skin coverage over a fracture is thought to predispose to infection, especially if internal fixation is performed. Equine skin is thin and readily penetrated by sharp bone fragments, and there is very little soft tissue support, such as muscle, below the carpus and tarsus. In general, fractures of the distal (phalanges) and upper (humerus, ulna, and femur) aspects of the horse's limbs rarely become open, suggesting that proper immobilization of fractures involving the metacarpus/metatarsus, radius, and tibia is the most critical aspect to preventing the development of an open fracture during transport. For the purposes of fracture immobilization, the fore- and hindlimbs in horses are divided into specific anatomical regions to help guide proper fracture splinting techniques (Figure 7.29).

PHALANGES AND DISTAL METACARPUS

The phalanges and distal metacarpus are probably the most common sites for fractures to occur in horses, and biomechanically they are dominated by the angle of the fetlock joint.[11,12] Therefore, proper splinting techniques should attempt to counteract the bending force at the fetlock. A cotton bandage combined with a dorsally placed polyvinylchloride (PVC) splint or a splint-cast combination with the limb maintained in a straight line from the carpus to the hoof appears to provide the optimal immobilization (Figure 7.30). Minimal padding (light bandage) should be used for the splint-cast combination, whereas a regular cotton bandage should be applied if a dorsal splint alone is used. Care must be taken not to apply too much padding, because fracture fragments can move within a large bulky bandage, and the bulk can sometimes make it difficult for the horse to ambulate efficiently.

To facilitate application of the splint and cast material, an assistant should hold the forelimb proximal to the carpus and let the limb hang. The PVC splint is applied to the dorsal aspect of the limb from the carpus to the hoof and secured with white tape. With the splint-cast, fiberglass cast material is applied over the entire distal limb to provide further stabilization. Alternatively, a Kimzey splint or the Farley compression boot may be used to stabilize fractures in this location. The disadvantages of these commercially available splints are that they are expensive to have on hand for only occasional use, and they cannot be easily modified to fit varying sized horses.

MIDFORELIMB (MID-METACARPUS TO DISTAL RADIUS)

Fractures in the midforelimb are stabilized best with a Robert-Jones type bandage combined with full-limb PVC splints applied caudally and laterally.[11,12] The bandage should be applied in several layers, with each layer of padding (cotton) no more than 1 inch in thickness and compressed with elastic or brown gauze to increase its stiffness. The bandage should contain only enough padding to help reduce swelling in the limb and protect the limb from the splint material. The splints should extend from the elbow to the ground at 90° to each other to help prevent movement of the fracture

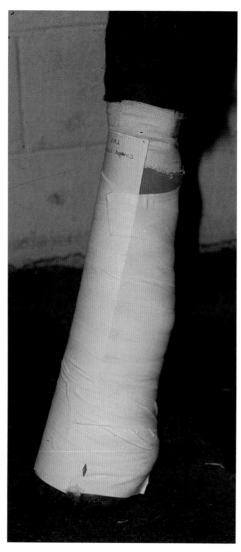

Figure 7.30. A bandage and PVC splint applied to the distal limb of a horse to immobilize a fractured phalanx. The splint was placed dorsally and secured with white nonelastic tape. (Courtesy of Dr. Chris Ray.)

during transport. The splints should be tightly secured to the bandage using nonelastic white tape. If PVC material is not available, any lightweight, rigid material such as wood, aluminum, or flat steel may be used effectively for splinting. Fractures in this location have the advantage of having portions of the forelimb above and below the fracture site, which can facilitate application of splints. However, because of the sparse soft tissue coverage of the metacarpal region, closed fractures in this location can easily become open if not adequately splinted. This is especially true for foals because their thin skin provides little resistance to bone penetration.

MIDDLE AND PROXIMAL RADIUS

Fractures in the middle and proximal radius cause the upper musculature of the forearm to abduct the distal limb.[11,12] This often results in adduction of the proximal fracture fragment and penetration of the skin on the medial side because of the lack of soft tissue coverage. Prevention of abduction of the distal limb is the goal when immobilizing fractures in this location. This is best achieved by applying a Robert-Jones bandage similar to that used with mid-forelimb fractures, but the lateral splint is extended up the lateral aspect of the shoulder, scapula, and chest, and taped securely to the proximal forelimb at the level of the axilla. A wide board (15 to 20 cm) or metal rod appears to work better than PVC for this lateral splint. The upper extension of the lateral splint should lie against the shoulder and scapula so that it prevents abduction of the distal limb during ambulation (Figure 7.31). A PVC splint that extends from the ground to the elbow should also be placed on the caudal aspect of the limb to provide additional stability for the fracture.

PROXIMAL TO THE ELBOW

The humerus and the ulna are well protected with muscles, which inherently stabilize and protect fractures of these bones. However, complete fractures of these bones disable the triceps muscle apparatus, making it impossible for the horse to fix the elbow in extension for weight-bearing. Restoring the triceps apparatus reduces the anxiety of affected animals and enables them to use the limb for balance during transport. A full-limb cotton bandage with a caudally applied PVC splint keeps the carpus extended and helps restore triceps muscle function. Some horses with ulna fractures bear considerable weight on the limb after splinting, but walking may be difficult. Not all fractures in these locations require stabilization because the risk of skin penetration is extremely low, and foals may not have the upper forelimb strength to move the limb with a splint in place.

PHALANGES AND DISTAL METATARSUS

Fractures in the distal hindlimb can be managed similarly to those in the forelimb except that the PVC splint is best placed on the plantar surface of the limb when using the splint-cast combination. Fiberglass cast material is applied over the splint and distal limb similar to the forelimb. Splints applied to the dorsal surface of the hindlimb over a bandage appear to be less useful than in the forelimb because they tend to break more readily. Additionally, the Kimzey splint or the Farley compression boot may be used to stabilize fractures in this location, similar to the forelimb.

MIDDLE AND PROXIMAL METATARSUS

A Robert-Jones bandage with PVC splints applied laterally and caudally using the calcaneus as a caudal extension of the metatarsus provide adequate support for fractures in this location.[11,12] The Robert-Jones bandage should be less extensive than in the forelimb because it is difficult to secure the splints to the limb if the bandage on the distal aspect of the metatarsus is too bulky.

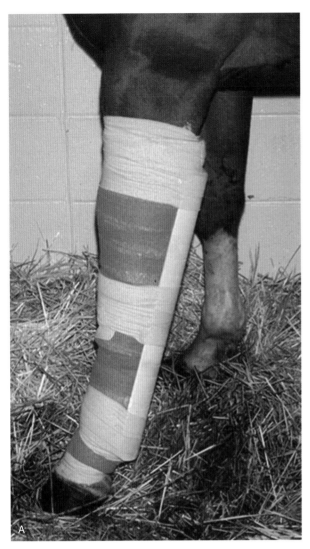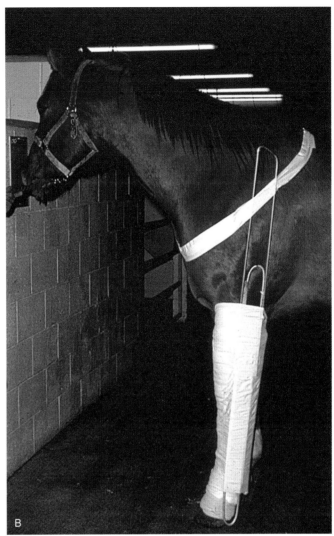

Figure 7.31.   A. A full-limb bandage with a caudal splint is placed and secured. B. A loop of aluminum rod has been shaped to extend from the ground up over the shoulder and scapula to help immobilize a radial fracture. (Courtesy of Dr. Chris Ray.)

TARSUS AND TIBIA

Fractures in the tarsus and tibia are particularly difficult to adequately stabilize because of the reciprocal apparatus and its effect on joint motion in the tarsus and stifle.[11,12] Fractures in this location tend to collapse when the stifle flexes, and the tarsus remains in a fixed position. The main principal for stabilization is similar to that of the radius, which primarily involves preventing abduction of the distal aspect of the limb. There is very little muscle coverage of the medial aspect of the tibia, and this is the site that is prone to becoming open. To prevent abduction, a single laterally placed splint that is bent to follow the angulation of the limb and extends proximally above the stifle joint works well. The splint is most effective if it is bent back on itself to mirror the hindlimb contour back to the ground, creating a double splint. The splint is applied over a full-limb Robert-Jones bandage, and is best made of lightweight metal such as aluminum that can be bent into the proper position, similar to the lateral support of a Schroeder-Thomas splint (Figure 7.32). An alternative to the metal splint is a wide board (15 to 20 cm) that extends from the ground to the ilium and is applied to the lateral aspect of the bandage.

Fracture Healing in Horses

Fracture healing can be considered a series of processes that occur in sequence but are often overlapping. The healing process can be divided into three distinct phases: inflammatory, reparative, and remodeling.[51] During this process the bone unites by 1 of 2 patterns: primary or direct healing and secondary or indirect healing. With primary bone healing, the bone ends heal directly by Haversian remodeling in contact and noncontact areas without the formation of a bone callus. Rigid fracture stabilization and correct anatomical reduction of the fracture are required for primary or direct bone healing to occur. With indirect or secondary bone healing, fibrous tissue or fibrocartilage is formed initially between the fracture fragments with subsequent replacement with new bone. Periosteal and endosteal callus is formed to unite the bone ends.[51]

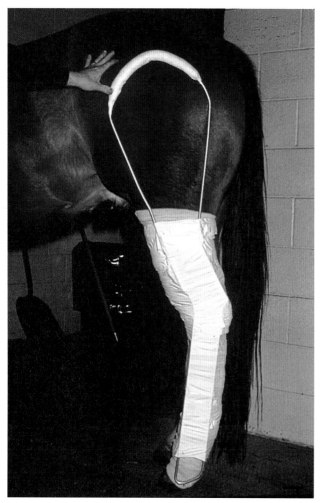

Figure 7.32. An aluminum rod has been shaped to extend from the ground up over the stifle and hip in this horse with a tibial fracture. Similar to radial fractures in the forelimb, the splint prevents abduction of the limb distal to the fracture, further stabilizing fractures of the tibia. A wide board may be used instead of the aluminum rod. (Courtesy of Dr. Chris Ray.)

INFLAMMATORY PHASE

The inflammatory phase occurs over the first 2 to 3 weeks after injury and is considered critical for the reparative phase of fracture healing that follows. During this phase the cellular mechanisms necessary for repair and the processes protecting the healing tissue from infection are activated. If the inflammatory response is impaired, tissue healing is compromised. Chemical messengers mediate the inflammatory reaction by causing vasodilation, migration of leukocytes, and chemotaxis of substances necessary for the repair process. In particular, bone morphogenetic proteins play an important role in the initiation of fracture repair.[73]

REPARATIVE PHASE

During the reparative phase, the pattern of fracture healing is highly susceptible to mechanical factors such as interfragmentary motion. With spontaneous fracture healing, periosteal and endosteal callus formation provides interfragmentary stabilization, and bone union occurs by intramembranous and endochondral ossification.[51] This process can take 2 to 12 months to be completed, depending on the method of fracture fixation, stability of the fracture, and size of the fracture gap (fracture displacement).

REMODELING PHASE

The remodeling phase occurs during and following the reparative phase. Avascular and necrotic regions of bone are replaced by Haversian remodeling.[51] Malalignment of fracture fragments may be corrected during this phase of healing by remodeling of the fracture site and functional adaptation, particularly in young animals. With weight-bearing and loading of the fracture, bone is removed from the convex surfaces and laid down on the concave surfaces. This process tends to realign the bone after malunion (Figure 7.33). However, fracture remodeling cannot correct torsional deformities associated with fracture healing. Theoretically, bone can heal completely and regain pre-fracture strength and function.

Fracture Fixation

In horses, more than any other domestic animal (except perhaps the racing greyhound), "successful" fracture healing must be carefully defined. For centuries, bone has been observed to heal by production of callus, but the end result was often angulation, rotation, or limb shortening. With intra-articular fractures, a certain amount of OA was often the end result. Fixation techniques used to achieve primary bone healing with intra-articular fractures have greatly decreased the morbidity associated with OA in these cases. In addition, improved techniques in internal fixation of long bone fractures have emphasized improving the implants to withstand massive functional forces and thus preventing failure due to mechanical overload. Such implants must also be strong enough to maintain their integrity until the bone has united, without breaking under fatigue. However, despite improvements in fracture fixation equipment, anesthetic protocols, and recovery methods, successful repair of some long bone fractures in horses remains very difficult.

Stress protection is a phenomenon that occurs when a bone that has been rigidly immobilized by a plate(s) undergoes certain histologic events, including loss of bone mass without a corresponding reduction in size (quantitative osteopenia).[94] Stress protection results in Haversian remodeling and has generated considerable interest in humans and small animals because of the potential for refracture of the bone following removal of the plate. Stress protection is almost an unknown occurrence in the horse, even in foals, because of the greater loads imparted on the implants compared to humans and other smaller animals.[94] Whereas research activity in humans and small animals has focused on the development of more flexible implants, in horses the emphasis has been in the reverse direction to provide stronger implants in an attempt to overcome the massive loading of the implants.

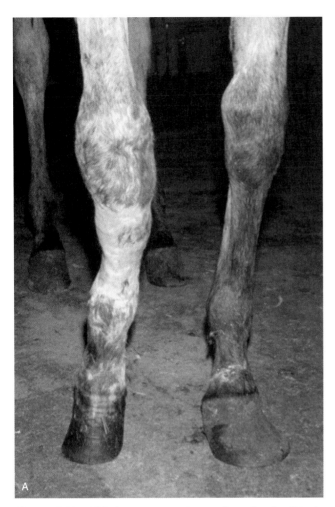 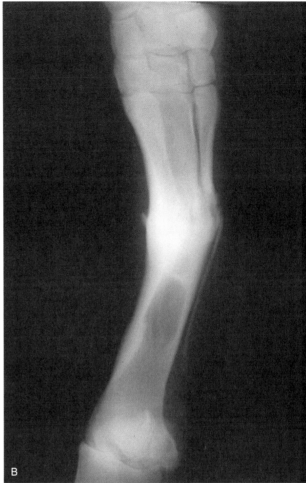

Figure 7.33. This horse presented several months after it had fractured the third metacarpus. The fracture had been treated by external splinting only. The fracture had healed but was mal-aligned both clinically (A) and radiographically (B). Considerable soft tissue swelling and fibrosis were also present in the metacarpal region, which is not uncommon following fracture healing.

Stress concentration is an important consideration in the horse. This is where biomechanical loads are concentrated in a small area of normal or weakened bone, potentially leading to complete bone failure.[94] It primarily occurs in the diaphysis of long bones but may also develop elsewhere along the bone. Examples of stress concentration include drill holes that are not filled with implants during internal fixation and vacant screw holes after implant removal (such as after metacarpal stress fracture repair).[64] Additionally, stress concentration occurs at the ends of bone plates, especially if they end in the mid-diaphyseal region of a bone, and at intramedullary pin hole sites following removal of external fixators. These locations are all areas where small areas of cortical bone are absent or have been weakened, and can fail if excessive loading of the bone occurs.

COMPRESSION FIXATION

Various methods of compression are widely accepted for treatment of fractures in humans and animals. Under stable conditions it is recognized that both can-cellous and cortical bones heal by primary bone union, without callus formation. Under these circumstances Schenk and Willenegger[80] showed that healing resulted by proliferation of new osteons growing parallel to the long axis of the bone, first through the necrotic bone ends, then across the fracture. This is termed "primary bone healing" and is the ultimate goal for repairing intra-articular fractures in horses or any species. With compression across the fracture, the mechanical stability with little or no motion between the fragments creates more favorable conditions for primary bone healing. Therefore, with internal fixation, the function of the implant (plate and/or screws) is to hold the bone fragments under compression with little to no movement until fracture union has occurred.[94]

Compression fixation of fractures is often the goal for fracture repair in horses. Intra-articular fractures, when rigidly compressed, usually heal rapidly without the development of secondary OA. Long bone fractures repaired with bone plates can heal without exuberant callus that would interfere with nearby soft tissue structures. However, compression fixation cannot be achieved in many cases due to the nature of the fracture and the temperament and size of the patient. In general, compression fixation and primary bone healing can be accomplished with most intra-articular fractures in horses, but is usually not achieved in long bone fractures. Most long bone fractures develop varying degrees of callus formation during the healing process, which in most cases is not a major problem. Specific methods for repair of certain fractures, particularly those amenable to lag screw fixation, are discussed in Chapter 5 (see discussions on particular bones or joints). Below are general principles regarding fracture fixation in horses.

LAG SCREW PRINCIPLE

Lag screw is a basic technique used routinely by carpenters and engineers that is also used to compress fractures. It is particularly suited for intra-articular fractures in horses where accurate anatomic alignment of the joint surface is essential to avoid secondary OA (Figure 7.34). Lag screws rarely are used alone to repair major long bone fractures in horses or even small foals, because they are simply not strong enough. They are ideally suited to repair condylar fractures of the distal

third metacarpus and metatarsus (Figure 7.34), slab fractures of the third carpal bone (Figure 7.35), sagittal fractures of the proximal phalanx, and some tarsal bone fractures. Additionally, lag screws can be used in conjunction with plates to repair comminuted fractures where fracture reconstruction is performed with screws and a so-called "neutralization plate" is applied or the lag screws are inserted through the plate holes. Varying sizes of cortical bone screws (3.5, 4.5, or 5.5 mm in diameter) can be used as lag screws. The 5.5-mm screw is being used more commonly in horses because of its increased strength and holding power compared to the 4.5-mm screw.

To achieve the lag screw principle, threads must gain purchase only in one bone fragment. For cortical screws this is achieved by overdrilling the fragment next to the screw head to such a size that the screw threads do not engage this portion of the bone. This hole is termed the glide hole (Figure 7.36). If this hole is not overdrilled, when the screw is tightened the gap between the fracture fragments is maintained and no compression is achieved. Therefore the screw should only achieve purchase in the "far" or transcortex, i.e., cortex away from the head.

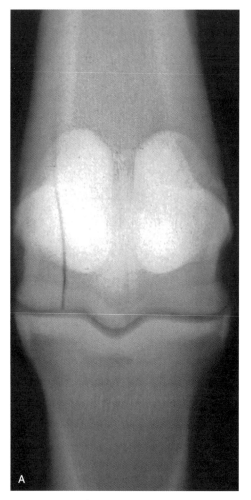
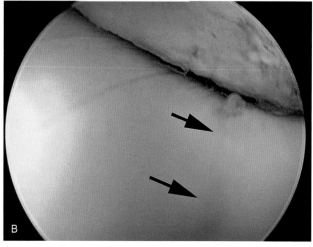

Figure 7.34.   A. A fracture of the lateral condyle of the distal third metacarpus that requires lag screw fixation to achieve precise alignment of the joint surface. B. An arthroscopic view showing compression of the fracture (arrows).

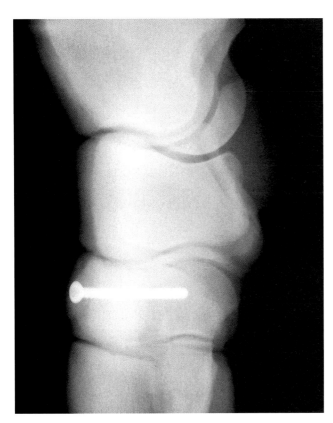

Figure 7.35. Lateral radiograph of the carpus in a racehorse following lag screw fixation of a third carpal bone slab fracture with a 3.5-mm cortical screw. Larger third carpal bone fractures in horses are often stabilized with 4.5-mm cortical screws.

In certain regions, particularly in the metaphysis of bones in foals, the bone may be too soft for cortical screws to gain purchase. Cancellous screws can be used to achieve compression between fragments in these locations. To increase the surface area of contact between the screw and bone, the ratio between the outer diameter and the core in cancellous screws is greater than that found in a cortical screw (Figure 7.37). A cancellous screw (6.5 mm in diameter) has a smooth shank near the head and a threaded portion near the tip (Figure 7.38). When employed as a lag screw the smooth shank must pass through one fragment and the threaded portion must gain purchase in the other to achieve compression.[94]

Cancellous screws have 2 lengths of thread at the tip, 16 mm and 32 mm (Figure 7.38). The longer threaded cancellous screws should be used whenever possible to achieve maximum holding power. Cancellous screws should be used with caution in dense cortical bone. However, if a cortical screw has been stripped, in some cases the only way to achieve compression is to use a cancellous screw in its place. During the healing process new bone forms around the smooth shank of the cancellous screw and, consequently, if screw removal is necessary, the cancellous thread must be able to cut its way through the bone. If the bone around the shank is too dense, breakage of the cancellous screw at the screw thread junction may occur. Therefore, whenever possible, cortical bone screws should be used in horses with the exception of young foals with very soft bone.

To exert the maximum amount of interfragmentary compression, lag screws should be inserted at right angles to the fracture plane. However, if the bone is under some axial load, the screws ideally should be inserted at right angles to the long axis of the bone. Therefore, the ideal direction to achieve maximum interfragmentary compression and resistance to axial

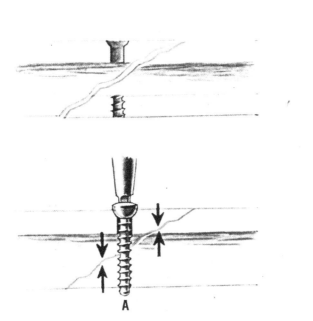
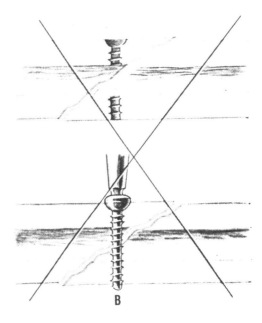

Figure 7.36. A. Correct execution of the lag screw principle. B. Incorrect execution of the lag screw principle. The cortex under the screw head was not overdrilled, and the gap between the bone fragments cannot close.

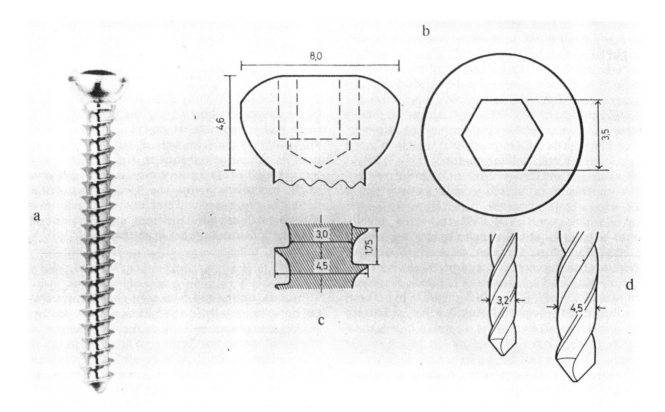

Figure 7.37. Design and dimensions of the Association for the Study of Internal Fixation (ASIF) 4.5-mm cortical screw. A. 4.5-mm cortical screw. B. Dimensions of the screw head. C. Dimensions of screw shaft and threads. D. Size of drill bits used to place the screw in lag or neutral fashion.

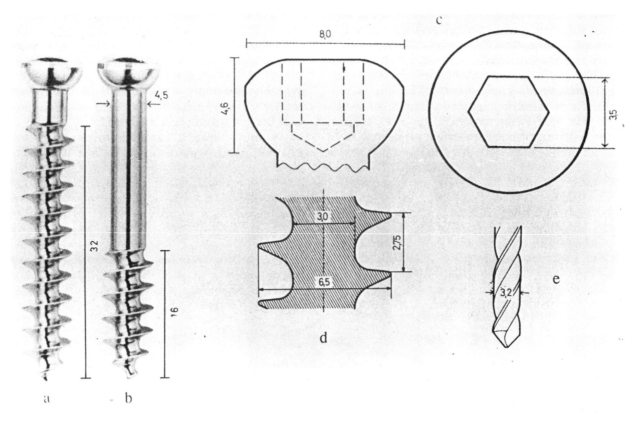

Figure 7.38. Design and dimensions of the ASIF cancellous bone screw. A. Fully threaded screw. B. Partially threaded screw. C. Dimensions of the screw head. D. Dimensions of screw shaft and threads. E. Size of drill bit used to place the screw.

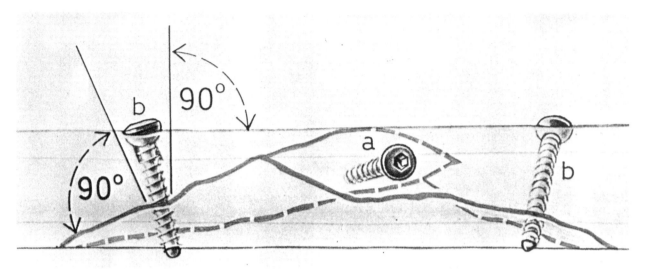

Figure 7.39. Ideal direction of screw placement for achieving maximum interfragmentary compression (A and B).

loading is a direction between these 2 extremes (Figure 7.39).[94] This is a somewhat hypothetical solution and is not always feasible in certain equine fractures. For example, in repair of a sagittal fracture of the proximal phalanx, insertion of the screws at right angles to the long axis of the bone usually achieves adequate compression and alignment of the joint surface. In general, 2 or more lag screws are used if possible to prevent rotation of the fragment. This is not always possible, especially for fractures involving the small carpal or tarsal bones.

Pre-tapped cortical screws are used primarily for lag screw fixation in horses. Self-tapping screws were originally thought to provide poor bone holding qualities compared to the pre-tapped screws.[94] Both 5.5-mm and 6.5-mm screws that were inserted pre-tapped into cadaver foal metacarpal/metatarsal bones had significantly greater holding power than the same size screws that were inserted self-tapped.[105] However, Schatzker, et al. and Andreas, et al. demonstrated in similar studies that self-tapping screws had the same holding power and pull-out strength as pre-tapped screws.[3,79,2] Use of self-tapping screws may be difficult in very dense cortical bone, and the screws may actually break. Self-tapping screws (4.5 mm) inserted into equine third metatarsal bones did not break, but could not be inserted continuously.[4] In addition, pre-tapped screws can be placed in the bone with greater precision, thereby producing better holding power.[78,79] In general, most cortical screws inserted into equine bone are pre-tapped.

Cannulated and bioabsorbable screws are also available for use in horses. Cannulated screws, available in a variety of sizes, are hollow, enabling screw placement over a guide pin that helps maintain fracture reduction and precise screw positioning during the lag screw procedure (Figure 7.40). They are used commonly in humans but less frequently in veterinary medicine. The concerns regarding using cannulated screws in horses are their questionable strength (because they are hollow) and the expense.[3,4,16] Cannulated 4.5-mm screws had significantly less pullout strength compared to standard

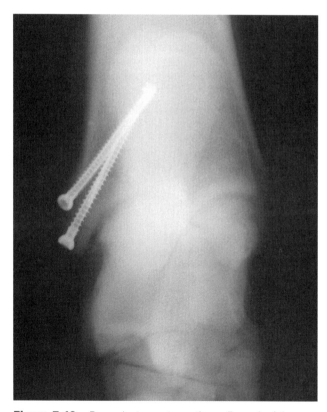

Figure 7.40. Dorsoplantar postoperative radiograph of the tarsus in a horse with a fracture of the medial malleolus of the tibia. The fracture was repaired using 2 4.5-mm cannulated screws.

4.5-mm cortical screws in an *in vitro* study suggesting that the interfragmentary compression achieved by these screws may be less than optimal and that screw failure is more likely to occur.[16]

Bioabsorbable screws are made of polylactic acid derivatives. Theoretically, they are not removed once they are placed. Bioabsorbable screws are used sparingly in horses because of the expense and their questionable strength, especially in shear.[25] However, one *in vitro* experimental study using equine third carpal slab fractures as a model suggested that they have biomechanical properties comparable to 4.5-mm cortical screws.[61]

A headless tapered variable pitch screw has also been advocated for use in horses.[14] The variable pitch nature of the screw allows for interfragmentary compression to occur without the presence of a screw head, which some surgeons feel can be a source of inflammation and irritation.

OTHER METHODS OF INTERNAL FIXATION

Many fractures in horses, especially those involving long bones, cannot be repaired with lag screws alone. Other methods of repairing long bone fractures include bone plating, tension band wiring (Figure 7.41), intramedullary (IM) pinning, IM interlocking nails, and the use of external fixators.[3,4] Bone plating provides the most rigid fixation of fractures but cannot be used in all cases because of the specific characteristics of the fracture and the expense. For those fractures amenable to bone plating, 1 (and many times 2) plate is used to provide adequate fixation (Figure 7.42). The plates (usually 4.5 mm in thickness) are best placed on the tension side of the bone and at right angles to each other when 2 plates are used. Either 4.5- or 5.5-mm cortical screws can be used to secure the plates to the bone, and

these should be placed as lag screws across the fracture if possible. Special purpose bone plates used occasionally in horses include the dynamic condylar screw (DCS) plate, dynamic hip screw (DHS) plate, angled blade plate (ABP), and the cobra head plate.[3,4]

Plate luting refers to placing polymethylmethacrylate, either under the plate or around the screw heads, to further increase the strength and stability of the fixation.[65,87] Improved bone-plate contact is achieved, and therefore luting is most beneficial in large horses to increase the overall strength of the implant.[87] However, locking plates have made the use of plate luting unnecessary. The locking plates are designed so that the screw heads fix into the plate with a screw mechanism and do not rely on friction between the plate and the bone for stability (Figure 7.43). Shearing of the screw heads is a common mode of failure, and this mechanism reduces the stress between the screw head and the plate, allowing for more stable fixation. This has been used routinely in equine fracture repair and arthrodesis, and lends itself well for use in minimally invasive percutaneous plate osteosynthesis.[39,47]

IM interlocking nails are relatively new in equine orthopedics and primarily have been used to repair humeral, femoral, and some metatarsal/metacarpal fractures.[4,56] The intramedullary nail is placed within the medullary cavity of the bone and transfixed to the bone above and below the fracture using bone screws.[56,57] This method is thought to create a more biomechani-

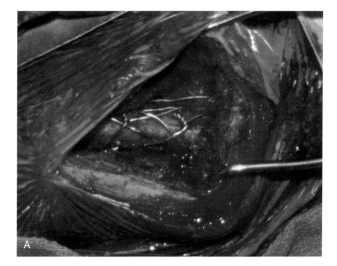

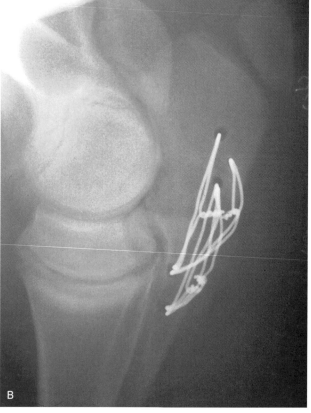

Figure 7.41. Intra-operative view (A) and postoperative lateral radiograph (B) of a fractured olecranon in a young foal that was repaired using tension band wires only. The foal did very well after surgery and the fracture healed without complications.

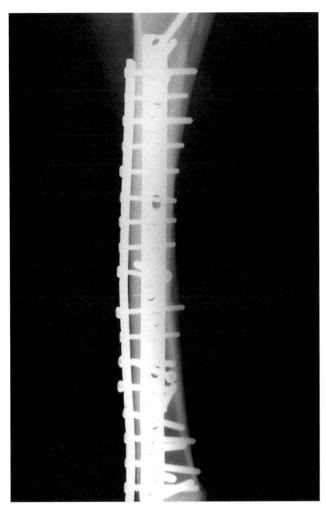

Figure 7.42. This midshaft radial fracture in an adult horse was repaired using 2 4.5 mm in diameter broad dynamic compression plates (DCP) placed at right angles to each other. All screws used in the repair were 4.5 mm in diameter; however 5.5-mm screws could have been used to provide further stability to the repair.

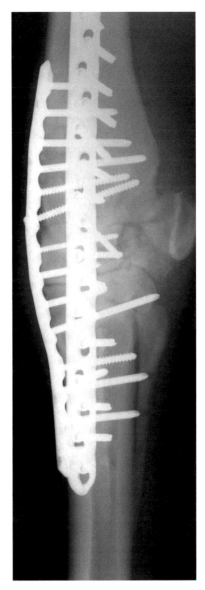

Figure 7.43. A pancarpal arthrodesis performed using 2 locking compression plates. (Courtesy of Dr. Laurie Goodrich.)

cally sound fixation by placing the implant within the bone, rather than applying bone plates to the external surface of the bone. The potential benefit of interlocking nails in equine orthopedics awaits further clinical use.

EXTERNAL FIXATION OF FRACTURES

External fixators or transfixation pin casts have become more widely used for fracture repair in horses over the last several years.[54,62] They are most useful to stabilize or prevent collapse of comminuted fractures of the distal limb where other forms of internal fixation cannot be used, and to treat open fractures where placement of implants would likely result in osteomyelitis.[52,69,75] The fixator pins (usually 0.25 inch or 6.35 mm in diameter for average adult horses) can be placed above and below the fracture, but in most cases pins are placed only above the fracture (Figure 7.44). Polymethylmethacrylate or stainless steel sidebars can be used as the construct of the fixator to connect the

pins if used above and below the fracture, or a fiberglass cast is applied to the limb to support the pins.[52,69,75] In most cases of phalangeal fractures, 2 to 3 pins are placed in the distal to middle aspect of the metatarsus/metacarpus and a half-limb fiberglass cast is applied to the limb to serve as the sidebars of the external fixator.[54,55] The transfixation cast permits the horse to ambulate on the limb without further displacement of the fracture during the healing process. Alternatively, a specially designed external fixator for horses (Nunamaker external fixator) that does not use a fiberglass cast may be used.[69]

Catastrophic failure of the bone through one of the external fixator pinholes is the most severe complication of this form of fixation. Other potential problems include infection around the pins, premature pin loosening, chronic pain associated with the pins, and prolonged fracture healing.

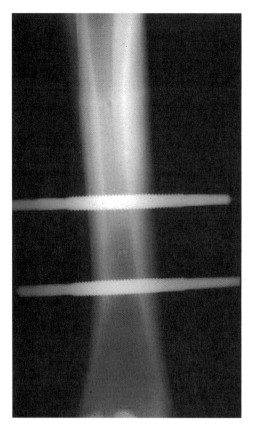

Figure 7.44. Two 0.25-inch (6.35-mm) in diameter threaded intramedullary (IM) pins were placed through the distal metatarsus and incorporated into a fiberglass cast (transfixation pin cast) to prevent collapse of a severely comminuted second phalanx fracture in this mare.

One method of reducing pin loosening is the development of a positive profile pin that is screwed into the bone. This allows greater fixation between the bone and pin, providing greater stabilization and less chance of loosening. Along with the development of a tapered sleeve,[68] the rigidity of external fixators has been improved.

Fractures as a Cause of Lameness

Consequences of fracture healing may lead to subsequent lameness. This has been termed fracture disease in humans and is seen under certain circumstances in horses. A major cause of disability in humans following fracture healing is stiffness of joints from disuse. This is rarely seen in horses and should not be confused with stiffening due to ankylosis of joints associated with the development of OA.[94] In fact, joint laxity, especially in young animals with fractures treated with casts, seems to occur more commonly than joint stiffness in horses. However, most fractures are accompanied by varying degrees of soft tissue (muscle, tendon, and ligament) damage that may be replaced with scar tissue (Figure 7.33). Subsequently, there is obliteration of normal tissue planes that may impair tendon function, produce stiffening of neighboring joints, and cause flexural deformities in growing animals.

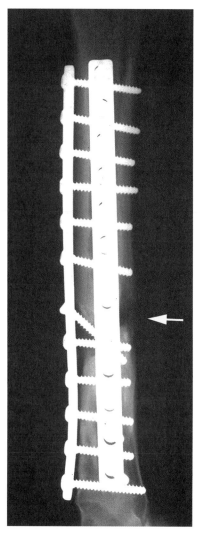

Figure 7.45. A radiograph of the third metacarpal fracture repaired with internal fixation. Note the lysis at the fracture line that is indicative of a nonunion (arrow).

A nonunion can occur due to infection, lack of vascularity, or relative instability (Figure 7.45). This instability leads to accumulation of fibrous tissue and fibrocartilage which, due to constant micromotion, cannot mineralize. A malunion of the fracture may also lead to athletic disability in some horses (Figure 7.33). In addition, implant-associated pain from bone plates or screws may cause chronic lameness or poor performance in athletic horses. In some cases, implants used for internal fixation of fractures must be removed in performance horses to prevent these problems.

Secondary problems related to casting can arise from fracture fixation. It is not uncommon to see significant loss of bone density, especially within the proximal sesamoid bones (Figure 7.23).[96] Tendon and muscle flaccidity and atrophy of surrounding muscles are also seen in horses with fractures treated with external immobilization such as casts. This usually is temporary and self corrects with time, but it may lead to permanent lameness. Other aspects of so-called fracture disease occur in the nonfractured limb, including angular limb deformities due to excessive axial loading on active growth plates in young horses, stretching of flexor tendons and associated muscles, and support limb laminitis due to excessive weight-bearing. Support limb laminitis with rotation of the distal phalanx is unique to the horse and is a potentially devastating complication of equine fracture repair.

Infection is a serious complication of fractures that can eventually lead to permanent lameness or a non-union of the fracture. Infection is most likely to occur with open fractures or those repaired with internal fixation.[6] Severe infections may necessitate euthanasia of the animal, whereas milder, more chronic infections may necessitate removal of the implants or necrotic bone to resolve the infection. Open, infected fractures that eventually heal are often accompanied by considerably more fibrosis with a greater chance of loss of function of surrounding structures than are closed, noninfected fractures. The limb may be permanently thickened due to scar tissue and callus formation, which may lead to impaired limb function.[94]

Bone Infections

Osteitis and osteomyelitis describe inflammation of bone involving the periosteum and connective tissues of the Haversian and Volkmann's canals as well as the medullary cavity.[42] If the process begins with or involves the periosteum and outer bone cortex, the terms osteitis or osteoperiostitis are used. If the infection involves the medullary cavity, the term osteomyelitis is used. The prognosis and treatments for osteitis and osteomyelitis are quite different, and it is important to make a distinction between the 2 categories of bone infection.[6]

Infectious Osteitis

Osteitis commonly occurs in the extremities of the horse (mostly metacarpal/metatarsal regions) because of the sparse soft tissue coverage in this location. It is usually the result of infection from a nearby septic process or from a break in the skin.[6,10] Osteitis is seen frequently when a horse is kicked without breaking the overlying skin, and may be similar to a bone bruise when no sequestrum develops. If the skin is broken, exposing the periosteum, the outer layers of cortical bone may eventually die, whereas the deeper cortical layers of bone survive due to the blood supply from endosteal vessels. For example, avulsion injuries with bone exposure of the dorsal aspect of the metacarpus/metatarsus frequently develop osteitis and sequestration.[7,10] Bacteria that gain entrance to the bone lodge in the superficial layers of the bone, resulting in a thin layer of dead bone (bone sequestrum) within the wound (Figure 7.46). Although granulation tissue may advance over the bone sequestrum, the rate of advancement is usually slow. Occasionally, granulation tissue advances under the sequestrum and extrudes it from the wound. The rate of healing of a wound can usually be accelerated by early removal of the sequestrum.

By definition, the 2 requirements for the formation of a sequestrum are avascularity and infection. Therefore, most surgeons believe that blunt trauma to the bone cortex does not cause sequestration in the

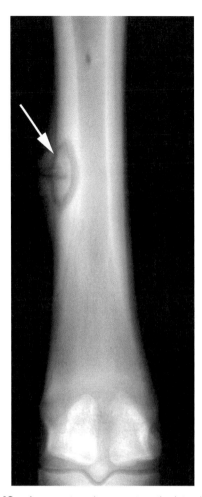

Figure 7.46. A sequestrum is present on the lateral aspect of the third metacarpal bone (arrow), secondary to trauma.

absence of infection.[6,7] Sequestration without skin penetration occurs in horses, although it is rare. In cases in which there is no break in the skin, the hematoma may become infected hematogenously, leading to sequestrum formation, fistulation, drainage, and a nonhealing wound. This appears to occur most commonly with injuries to the splint bones, but most have skin wounds that lead to secondary bacterial infection. Chronic persistent drainage from any wound in the horse suggests the presence of a bone sequestrum or foreign body. Without surgical removal of the sequestrum, drainage rarely subsides, or at the very least wound healing is substantially prolonged, because the pathogenic organisms reside within the necrotic bone, which is avascular, thereby resisting the animal's immune defenses.

The severity of lameness accompanying osteitis in horses is variable and inconsistent. In addition, the radiographic signs of osteitis depend on the length of time between the injury and examination. Initially, there may be soft tissue swelling with evidence of bone resorption seen radiographically. At 7 to 14 days following the injury, periosteal proliferation may be evident. Sequestrum formation may also be visible at that time as osteoclastic resorption occurs at the periphery of the damaged bone. Radiographic evidence of a sequestrum is usually not visible for a minimum 2 to 3 weeks after the injury.[10] At that time, the sequestrum and the sclerotic margin around the sequestrum, called the involucrum, are usually visible.[6]

Occasionally an osteitis may resolve spontaneously, especially if there is no infectious component or if the sequestrum is small and extruded from the wound. If bacteria and necrotic bone are present, the wound remains exudative indefinitely until the sequestrum is removed.[94] Wound debridement of unhealthy scar tissue and necrotic bone is usually required for healing to occur. Removal of bone sequestra is best performed with the animal under general anesthesia. However, thin cortical sequestra associated with avulsion injuries of the dorsal aspect of the cannon bone can often be removed in the standing, sedated horse. After the surrounding granulation and scar tissue have been excised, the area should be curetted until the bone appears to be healthy. Most wounds are either closed primarily or left to heal by second intention following debridement.

Parenteral antibiotics are of limited value when used alone to treat bone sequestra because of poor penetration of the antibiotics into the necrotic bone. Antibiotics are indicated if there are signs of cellulitis associated with the lesion, and following surgical debridement of the wound. Usually a wide variety of organisms (secondary pathogens) can be cultured from the wound and occasionally these bacteria are resistant to antibiotics that are of practical use in the horse. Culturing the sequestrum itself usually gives the most accurate diagnosis about the causative bacteria. The prognosis for horses with osteitis and sequestrum removal is usually excellent.

Osteomyelitis

Osteomyelitis is a more extensive inflammation of the bone than osteitis that begins within or extends into the medullary cavity. Osteomyelitis in horses can be divided into 3 categories based on the origin of the infection: hematogenous, traumatic, or iatrogenic.[6] Osteomyelitis from hematogenous origin occurs primarily in neonates and only rarely in adults. Traumatic osteomyelitis can occur in any age horse and is usually due to penetrating wounds or open fractures. Iatrogenic causes of osteomyelitis include surgery such as internal fixation of fractures or intra-articular injections of medications.

Hematogenous Infection

The localization of hematogenous osteomyelitis in the metaphyseal region can be explained by sluggish metaphyseal blood flow in which the blood vessels form terminal sinusoids. This permits the bacteria to localize in these areas and establish an infection (Figure 7.47). The infection in the bone spreads by way of Haversian and Volkmann's cavities, and prostaglandins are considered responsible for bone destruction.[94] Thrombosis of blood vessels also occurs as the infection spreads, producing death of the osteocytes in their lacunae.[6,94] The inflammatory process may increase pressure within the bone, further impairing blood supply. The end result is bone necrosis with possible sequestrum formation.

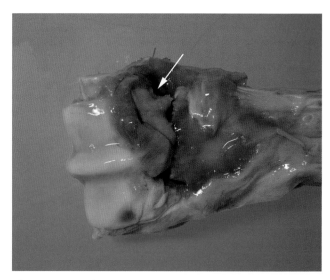

Figure 7.47. Gross image of a severely septic physis (arrow) that spread into the joint and led to a pathologic fracture of the limb.

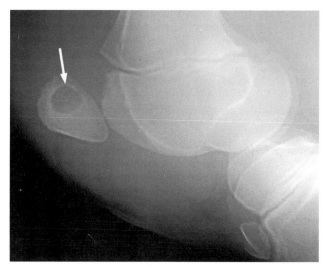

Figure 7.48. Lateral radiograph of the stifle in a foal with lameness and severe effusion of the femoropatellar joint. Lysis within the patella suggestive of hematogenous osteomyelitis was present (arrow). The caudal or ventral aspect of the patella directly below the lesion was removed using the arthroscope and the joint was lavaged.

Firth has classified hematogenous infections in foals into 3 categories depending on the location of the infection. S-type infections involve the synovial membrane of joints, P types involve the physis and usually the metaphysis, and E-type infections involve the epiphysis.[26] However, these infections are not completely isolated and foals may have multiple types of hematogenous infection at multiple sites (Figures 7.48 and 7.49). Bone infection due to *Salmonella spp.*, for example, typically involves multiple bones.[94]

Hematogenous osteomyelitis is frequently secondary to infections elsewhere in the animal's body, such as the umbilicus, gastrointestinal tract, or lungs.[6,26] Foals with

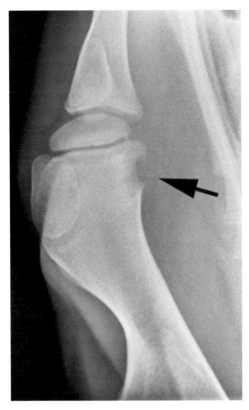

Figure 7.49. A radiographic view of a shoulder in a foal demonstrating a metaphyseal lytic lesion (arrow). This foal also had septic arthritis of the shoulder joint and bicipital bursa.

a compromised immune system due to failure of passive transfer or septicemia appear to be predisposed to hematogenous osteomyelitis. Many of these foals may have multiple body systems involved with signs referable to the infection in these regions, and therefore, a complete physical examination is essential. Some foals recover completely from the initial infection only to develop bone or joint infections several days later when they appear to be very healthy. The most common bacteria that cause hematogenous infections in foals are Gram-negative enterics such as *E. coli.*[6,26] Other causative organisms include *Staphylococcus spp., Streptococcus spp., Rhodococcus spp.,* and *Salmonella spp.*

TRAUMATIC OSTEOMYELITIS

An open fracture or a penetrating wound may lead to osteomyelitis in any age horse (Figures 7.50 and 7.51). There is usually some degree of trauma to the skin and surrounding soft tissues with these injuries, and the pathogenic organisms may directly enter the medullary cavity through the open wound. Bacteria associated with these types of infections include Gram-negative enterics, *Staphylococcus spp., Streptococcus spp.,* and anaerobes.[6,93] Infection spreads through the bone in a similar manner as for hematogenous osteomyelitis. Occasionally there is no overt break in the skin but the necrotic tissue provides a medium for bacterial proliferation and infection develops from a

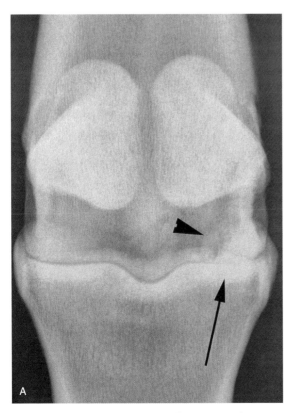
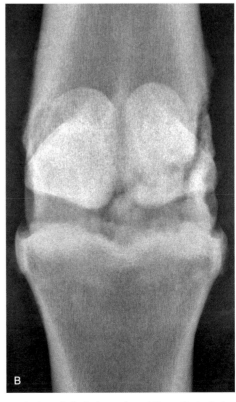

Figure 7.50. Radiographs of the fetlock joint from a mare that had a penetrating injury to the fetlock joint. The images were taken 2 weeks (A) and 6 weeks (B) after the injury. Note the severe lysis, ankylosis (arrow), and the pathologic fracture (arrowhead) in the joint secondary to long-standing sepsis.

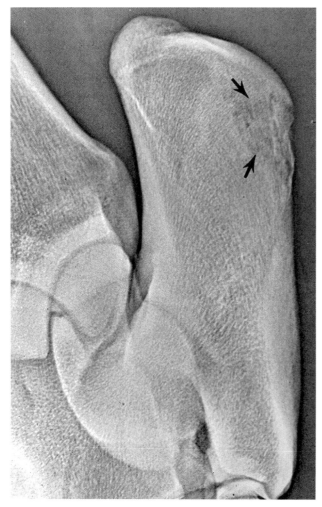

Figure 7.51. An oblique radiograph of the tarsus in a horse with a puncture wound and infection of the calcaneal bursa. Lysis within the proximal aspect of the calcaneus (black arrows) suggested concurrent osteitis or osteomyelitis of the bone.

hematogenous route. Avascularity is a major factor in the pathogenesis of osteomyelitis, and therefore, fractures with bone fragments isolated from a blood supply are at risk to develop infection.[6]

Treating an open fracture without providing absolute stability is usually futile unless the dead avascular fragments can be removed or reincorporated into the healing fracture where they can be revascularized.[94] Alternatively, some type of external fixator may be used to stabilize the fracture without disrupting the soft tissues around the fracture site.[54,69] In this manner, the potential for osteomyelitis is decreased because no implants are placed near the fracture, and the vascularity to the fracture is not further impaired.

IATROGENIC OSTEOMYELITIS

The cause of osteomyelitis following internal fixation of fractures is usually contamination of the wound from an open wound (open fracture). Regardless of the type of internal fixation used, infection following repair of open fractures is much more common than that follow-

ing repair of closed fractures. However, contamination of the fracture during the surgical procedure can and does occur, particularly if the procedure is prolonged (greater than 3 hours).[6] Usually the fracture hematoma and avascularity at the fracture site as well as the implantation of foreign material (pins, plates, screws, etc.) contribute to the development of osteomyelitis, because they provide favorable conditions for bacterial growth. Once bacteria become established where nutrients are available, proliferation occurs within a polysaccharide slime forming a biofilm-enclosed colony. This biofilm or bioslime is formed by bacterial extracapsular exopolysaccharide that binds to surfaces of the implants and helps maintain infection by protecting the bacteria from the host defenses. Therefore, osteomyelitis may develop despite prophylactic antibiotic coverage at the time of fracture repair, especially in open fractures. Highly resistant bacteria such as methicillin-resistant *Staphylococcus aureus* or Gram-negative enterics often cause these infections.[6]

CLINICAL SIGNS OF OSTEOMYELITIS

Hematogenous osteomyelitis may be missed in its early stages and often presents after the lameness has become unresponsive to medical therapy. Frequently the owner feels that the lameness was due to an injury such as a sprain or being stepped on by the mare. There is usually very severe lameness with cellulitis, similar to that seen with fractures. Pain is usually elicited with direct pressure and manipulation of the joint(s) adjacent to the infection, and a fever is commonly seen in foals. Clinical signs of traumatic or iatrogenic osteomyelitis are similar and include lameness, soft tissue swelling, retarded wound healing over the implants, drainage, and fistulation. Signs can be present as early as 7 to 10 days after injury or surgery or they may be delayed for 3 to 4 weeks.

RADIOGRAPHIC SIGNS OF OSTEOMYELITIS

Loss of bone density due to a reduction in the calcium salt content of the bone occurs gradually with osteomyelitis. Lytic changes in the bone are not visible until 30% to 50% of the bone mineral has been removed.[72] This is usually evident 10 to 14 days after the onset of infection (Figure 7.52). In more chronic cases, there are often sclerotic margins around the lytic regions due to new bone formation. Sequestrum formation with a surrounding envelope (called the involucrum) and endosteal and periosteal thickening may also be evident. Occasionally, osteomyelitis may penetrate into an adjacent joint, producing signs of a septic arthritis. With osteomyelitis following fracture repair, blurring of the cancellous trabeculation and a "moth-eaten" appearance at the fracture site are seen on radiographs.[94] Lysis along the screw threads or under the plate may become evident with time. Usually a piece of bone that is decalcified and surrounded by a lucent zone is a sign of sequestrum formation. A zone of bone destruction adjacent to the implants typically occurs under the plate and directly along the screw threads (Figure 7.53). In more chronic cases of osteomyelitis, zones of both bone production and destruction are visible radiographically.[6]

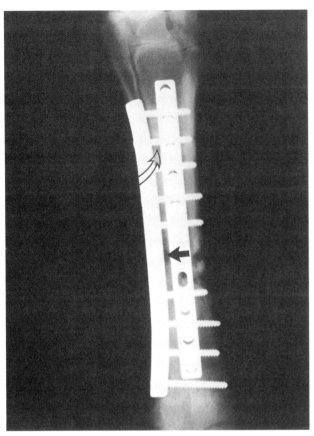

Figure 7.52. Osteomyelitis after internal fixation of a fractured third metacarpal bone. Lysis of the bone is occurring under the plate (solid arrow) and along one of the screw threads (open arrow).[6,76]

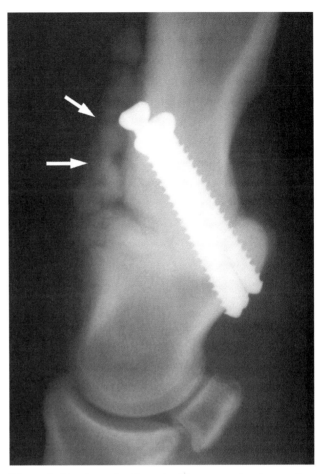

Figure 7.53. Lateral radiograph of the pastern in a horse with a chronic infection of the proximal interphalangeal joint that did not respond to systemic antimicrobials. The infection developed subsequent to a wound in the pastern region. Arthrodesis of the joint was performed following debridement of all damaged bone. Amikacin-impregnated PMMA beads were placed in the surgery site to help treat the infection (arrows). No recurrence of the infection occurred after surgery.

TREATMENT

The lameness in many foals with hematogenous osteomyelitis is frequently attributed to trauma, but is, in fact, the early stage of infection. Therefore, at the time of initial examination, the infection is often well advanced with obvious radiographic signs, making it difficult to treat medically.[6,76] However, if acute hematogenous osteomyelitis is suspected in foals despite having no radiographic signs, broad-spectrum bactericidal antimicrobials should be administered. The duration of antimicrobial use is largely empiric (usually a minimum of 3 weeks) and should be based on the clinical response of the animal. However, antimicrobials alone may be unsuccessful due to the ischemic nature of the disease and poor penetration of the antimicrobial into infected avascular bone. Antimicrobials are best used early in the course of the infection and at high doses. The antimicrobials used most commonly to treat horses and foals with osteomyelitis include penicillin, gentamicin, amikacin, ceftiofur, cefazolin, enrofloxacin, and vancomycin. Nonsteroidal anti-inflammatory drugs (NSAIDs) have been beneficial in treating acute osteomyelitis in humans and animals in conjunction with antimicrobials.[94]

If there is no response to medical therapy and/or the osteomyelitis is localized, then surgery in conjunction with medical therapy is recommended. If the lesion can be accessed through a joint, which is often seen with hematogenous infections, then arthroscopy should be used to remove the damaged bone (Figure 7.48). A sample of the bone should be obtained at surgery and submitted for culture and sensitivity testing. Debridement of infected fractures or open wounds should be performed to remove avascular bone and infected soft tissue, and to decrease bacterial numbers. Cancellous bone grafting is often used with infections of fractures to speed healing.

However, a major priority for treatment of osteomyelitis associated with fractures is to achieve stability of the fracture. Stability must be maintained not only for fracture healing but also to limit the spread of infection.[94] Loose implants should be removed and fracture stability achieved by other means such as replating, external fixators, interlocking nails, external immobilization, or a combination of these techniques. If it is impossible to stabilize the fracture either with internal fixation, external fixation, or both, euthanasia may be the only alternative because it is unlikely that the infection will resolve.

Other methods used to treat osteomyelitis include regional perfusion of antimicrobials directly into the medullary cavity of the bone or within the vascular system of the limb.[100–102] The goal is to obtain very high tissue concentrations of antibiotics to achieve better bacterial kill. A tourniquet should be placed above and below the site of infusion and maintained for a minimum of 20 to 30 minutes to achieve optimal results.[6,100] In addition, antimicrobial-impregnated polymethylmethacrylate (PMMA) may be placed locally into the wound to achieve high antibiotic concentrations in and around the fracture.[33,92] The antimicrobials are incorporated into the PMMA during mixing, and elute from the PMMA into the wound for several days to weeks after they are placed. The PMMA is usually molded into bead or cigar shapes and placed adjacent to the implants, fracture, or site of infection (Figure 7.53).[33] The use of antibiotic-impregnated PMMA is thought to greatly improve our ability to successfully treat iatrogenic osteomyelitis in horses, such as those associated with internal fixation.[33]

PROGNOSIS

The prognosis for foals with hematogenous osteomyelitis is variable but is usually poor if multiple sites are involved. However, the infection can usually be resolved if the site of osteomyelitis can be thoroughly debrided. The prognosis with traumatic osteomyelitis is also variable depending on the bone involved and the duration and severity of the infection. Traumatic osteomyelitis is usually less difficult to resolve than iatrogenic infections. Osteomyelitis following internal fixation of a fracture is one of the most difficult diseases to successfully resolve in horses.[6,33] Therefore, the prognosis for these animals is extremely guarded, particularly for adult horses.

Infectious Physitis

Hematogenous infections of the physes are not uncommon in foals and have similar predisposing factors as other bone and joint infections in foals. The physis is often the initial location of hematogenous bacteria and infection, which can subsequently spread to the neighboring epiphysis and joint (Figure 7.47). Multiple physes can be infected simultaneously, but this is uncommon. Clinical signs, radiographic findings, and treatment are similar to other bone infections.

Bone Cysts

True bone cysts that occur in other species (primarily aneurysmal and unicameral) have been reported to occur rarely in horses.[8,38,88] The most common site appears to be the mandible. Unicameral bone cysts are defined as solitary intraosseous cysts lined by thin connective tissue membranes.[38] Aneurysmal bone cysts are expansile lesions consisting of anastomosing cavernous spaces filled with unclotted blood and lined with fibrous walls of varying thickness.[49]

These cysts usually contain osteoid tissue or osseous components, without elastic laminae or muscle layers.[49] Aneurysmal and unicameral bone cysts are more characteristic of true cystic lesions because they do not involve an articular surface and are usually solitary, expansile, intraosseous lesions. The majority of these true bone cysts reported in dogs and people occur in the distal or proximal metaphyses of long bones.

The cause of aneurysmal and unicameral bone cysts in any species is uncertain. Unicameral cysts are thought to result from the encapsulation and alteration of a focus of intramedullary hemorrhage, supposedly from trauma. Alternatively, trauma results in a disturbance in endochondral ossification resulting in a cystic defect within the metaphysis.[15] Aneurysmal bone cysts are generally believed to develop secondary to a pre-existing lesion such as fibrous dysplasia, hematoma from trauma or bleeding disorders, or neoplasia.[88] An aneurysmal bone cyst of the distal metaphysis of the metatarsus in a horse was thought to be caused by trauma.[88]

Whether the pathogenesis of aneurysmal and unicameral bone cysts and subchondral cystic lesions are interrelated is controversial. Most of the evidence (including pathogenesis and clinical characteristics) suggest that subchondral cystic lesions, at least in horses, are a distinctly separate clinical entity from aneurysmal or unicameral bone cysts.[5] Additionally, aneurysmal and unicameral bone cysts can be difficult to differentiate from some bone tumors in horses (Figure 7.54).

Treatment of true bone cysts in horses usually involves surgical curettage of the lesion with or without autogenous cancellous bone grafting. Spontaneous resolution of the cyst may also occur, and some bone cysts in humans respond to intralesional steroid injections.[49] The prognosis for resolution of bone cysts in horses is usually good depending on the location of the cyst.

Bone Tumors

Primary bone neoplasia is rare in horses. The most common bone tumors that occur in horses include osteoma, ossifying fibroma, multilobular osteoma or osteochondrosarcoma, and osteosarcoma.[31] Although these tumors may develop at any location, the face and head (mandible, skull, and paranasal sinuses) appear to be the most common sites of occurrence. Osteomas are benign tumors that consist of well-differentiated bone that typically occur within the paranasal sinuses or on the skull. Ossifying fibromas are benign fibro-osseous lesions that usually involve the rostral aspect of the mandible, premaxilla, or paranasal sinuses (Figure 7.55).[31] Multilobular osteomas or osteochondrosarcomas are very rare in horses but usually involve the skull or paranasal sinus (Figure 7.56). These tumors are generally benign but locally aggressive, and can be removed surgically. Osteosarcomas are malignant tumors, arising from mesenchyme, in which neoplastic cells produce osteoid or bone. In horses, the skull, axial skeleton, ribs, and occasionally the limbs are commonly affected sites.

The clinical signs caused by these tumors depend on the location and specific type of neoplasia. The diagnosis of neoplasia is usually made based on its radiographic appearance and is confirmed by histopathology of biopsy or autopsy specimens. Treatment depends on

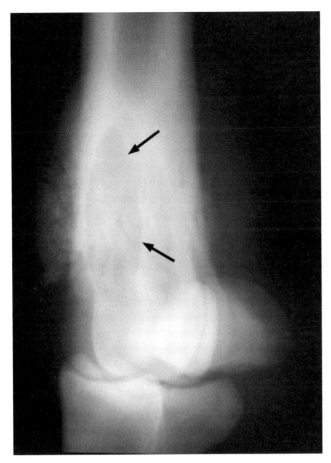

Figure 7.54. Oblique radiograph of the metatarsus in an adult horse with firm swelling of the metatarsus and mild lameness. Radiographs reveal a large lytic lesion within the bone with extensive periosteal new bone growth suggestive of neoplasia (arrows). The lesion was debrided and a biopsy suggested a possible osteosarcoma. However, this horse continued to do well with minimal progression of the lesion. Therefore, the lesion may be a true bone cyst and not a bone tumor.

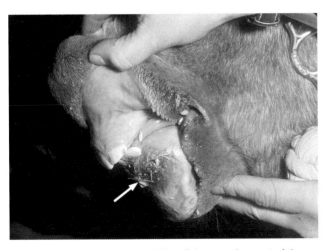

Figure 7.55. Large, firm swelling of the rostral aspect of the mandible in a young Quarter horse filly that was consistent with an ossifying fibroma (arrow). A rostral mandibulectomy was performed to completely remove the tumor.

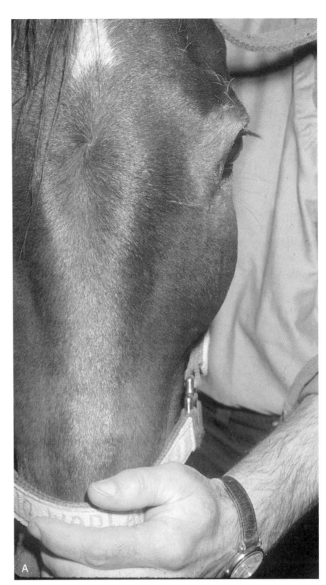

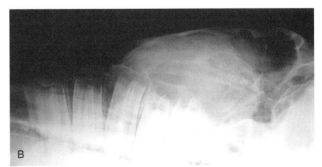

Figure 7.56. A. A large external swelling of the paranasal sinus region was evident on physical examination of this 3-year-old Quarter horse gelding. B. A lateral radiograph of the region revealed the presence of a large osseous mass within the maxillary sinuses. A biopsy of the mass suggested a diagnosis of multilobular osteochondroma.

the location of the tumor, involvement of the parent bone, and the specific type of osseous tumor present. In general, all tumors except osteosarcomas can potentially be removed successfully with minimal recurrence if complete tumor excision is achieved.[31] Unfortunately, complete tumor excision is not always possible.

Bone Contusion/Bruising/Periostitis

Bone contusions from direct or indirect trauma are known to occur in humans and contribute to orthopedic pain and lameness. The majority of joint pain in humans is thought to originate from bone and is typically seen as edema of the subchondral bone with magnetic resonance imaging (MRI). With the amount of trauma that horses seem to encounter, bone bruising probably occurs much more often than we currently recognize or are able to diagnose.

Diagnosing bone contusions and bruising in horses is very difficult and mostly subjective. This is especially true for bone pain originating in joints. Most bone contusions or bruises are diagnosed based on the history, clinical findings, and lack of radiographic abnormalities. However, MRI is now used routinely to diagnose bruising and edema within bone (Figure 7.57). With bone contusions, evidence of pain can usually be elicited with direct pressure over the affected site. In addition, bone pain usually causes more severe lameness than most soft tissue injuries, and pain is often elicited with manipulation of the affected bone or joint.

Radiographs are useful only to document the absence of fractures or other abnormalities within the affected bone or joint. Nuclear scintigraphy is useful to document abnormal bone metabolism of the affected site but cannot be used to definitively diagnose a bone bruise or contusion. Magnetic resonance imaging (MRI) or computed tomography (CT) are used in humans to help diagnose bone damage/contusion and are available for use in horses at referral hospitals.[52,59,86]

Treatment of bone contusions is similar to any type of acute musculoskeletal trauma, and includes inactivity, cold therapy, hydrotherapy, bandaging, and NSAIDs. Suspected bone contusions and bruising within joints also may be treated with intra-articular medications; however, they are somewhat limited in their effectiveness. Systemic bisphosphonate therapy has been advocated for treating bone bruising and edema.[43] The prognosis of horses with bone contusions is usually very good unless damage to the subchondral bone of a joint contributes to joint pathology and secondary OA (Figure 7.58).

SYSTEMIC DISEASES OF BONE

Osteoporosis

In osteoporosis, the bone mineral density (BMD) of the bone matrix is reduced. The bone becomes porous, light, and fragile and is prone to fracture. Osteoporosis in horses is an uncommon or at least an uncommonly recognized clinical problem. The term osteopenia is used if BMD is reduced but spontaneous fractures do not occur. Clinically, osteopenia is much more commonly recognized in horses than is osteoporosis.

Generalized Osteoporosis

The generalized osteoporosis seen in postmenopausal women has no counterpart in the aged horse. However, older mares may be more prone to long bone fractures during recovery from general anesthesia. Whether this may be due to declining estrogen levels associated with reproductive senescence is unknown. Osteoporosis is seen occasionally with undernutrition rather than actual deficiencies of calcium, phosphorus, or vitamin D. However, in most affected horses, osteoporosis is usually associated with a diet low in calcium, high in phosphorus, or low in vitamin D. Osteoporosis is asso-

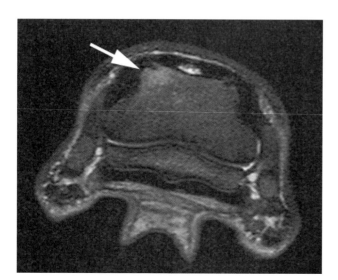

Figure 7.57. MR image of distal P2 of a horse that blocked in the distal limb and was moderately positive to digital flexion. Notice the area of bone edema in the distal aspect of P2 (arrow).

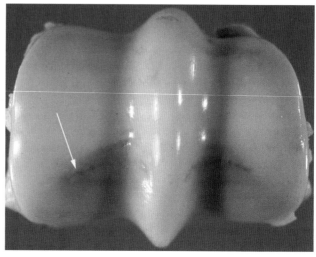

Figure 7.58. The distal aspect of the third metacarpal condyles typically shows subchondral bone bruising in racing Thoroughbred horses (arrow).

ciated with copper deficiency and chronic lead poisoning in lambs, but this has not been seen in foals.[9]

A condition first recognized in Thoroughbred foals may be a manifestation of generalized osteoporosis.[23] The condition is characterized by fractures of the proximal sesamoid bones and typically occurs when foals gallop to exhaustion while trying to keep up with their dams. Foals seem more prone to the condition if they are confined after birth. During this time of relative inactivity the bones are not subjected to the stresses required to strengthen them and are a potential weak link in the skeletal system (Figure 7.22). Some underlying metabolic problem or deficiency producing osteoporosis may exist, but is undefined at this time. Other lameness problems and unexplained fractures in horses may be attributed to generalized osteoporosis but their pathogenesis and cause are often unexplainable. The combination of age and pregnancy have also been shown to negatively influence bone strength,[30] with increased age and parity leading to significantly decreased bone strength.

Localized Osteopenia (Disuse Osteopenia)

Localized osteopenia is fairly common, especially in horses following rigid external immobilization of their limbs (casting). Disuse osteopenia also may occur in horses with severe or chronic lameness (Figure 7.59) or neuropathies such as radial nerve paralysis in which weight-bearing is reduced. With decreased weight-

bearing, there is increased resorption of bone and decreased bone formation. In one study, immobilization of the thoracic limb of a pony in a cast for 6 weeks caused a significant decrease in weight and specific gravity of the third metacarpal bone.[22] Histologically, the osteopenia was caused by atrophy of osteoblasts with failure of bone apposition.[22,94] However, external immobilization of the distal limb in horses has also been shown to have only a minor affect on articular cartilage with very little clinical significance.[74] If horses are brought back into work too quickly, distal sesamoidean ligaments can tear from the distal aspect of the proximal sesamoid bones, leading to significant lameness (Figure 7.23). Osteopenia is usually more severe in young animals due to the inherent rapid bone turnover compared with the adult horse. Bone cortices become thinner and more porotic. Fortunately, it rarely contributes to a clinical problem and is easily reversed when the external immobilization device is removed and the animal commences normal weight-bearing.

Localized osteopenia is essentially a radiographic diagnosis characterized by lack of cortical density and a more lucent appearance to the bones.[94] The sesamoid bones are often the first to manifest the problem radiographically (Figure 7.60). Loss of bone detected radiographically indicates a BMD loss of approximately 30%.

Further experiments have shown that treatment of osteopenia with 25-hydroxycholecalciferol has been beneficial.[22] Fortunately, localized osteopenia following immobilization rarely causes any problems. If the external support is suddenly removed, however, a pathologic fracture may result. To prevent this, the rigidity of the external support should be diminished gradually over time. For example, following cast removal a cotton bandage with a PVC splint incorporated into the bandage should be used to provide less stability than a cast but more support than a bandage alone.[94] Following removal of the splint, a lighter, less rigid bandage should be used until eventually no external support is applied to the limb. It may take several months before the bone regains normal density and strength following external immobilization. Occasionally, the original BMD is never reached.

Stress protection is another example of localized osteopenia seen in fractured bones that have been repaired with rigid internal fixation devices such as stainless steel bone plates.[94] Initially, rigid internal fixation enhances healing and permits mobility of neighboring joints. Over a period of months, however, the bone under these plates becomes porotic, producing a weakened bone with the possibility of a fatigue fracture when the plate is removed. Theoretically, plates should be removed as soon as healing has occurred. Plates with a lower modulus of elasticity have been designed to minimize stress protection, especially in humans and small animals. In horses, however, osteopenia generally does not occur to the same degree because a much larger animal places a greater force on the healing bone. Therefore, stress protection due to internal fixation is of minimal clinical significance in horses. In general, bone plates and other forms of internal fixation are not removed in horses unless they contribute to infection or cause lameness in performance horses.

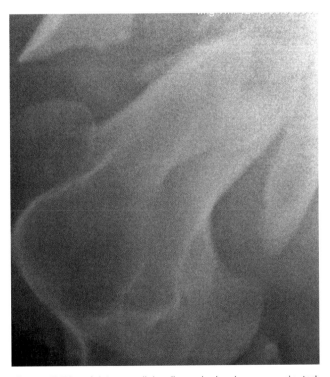

Figure 7.59. A lateromedial radiograph showing a comminuted fracture of the femur in a 23-year-old mare. This mare had severe lameness in the stifle of that limb since she was a yearling, and fractured it while getting up in her stall. It is likely that the bone was osteoporotic due to chronic, reduced weight-bearing from the lameness.

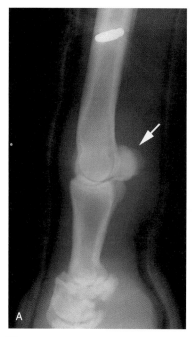 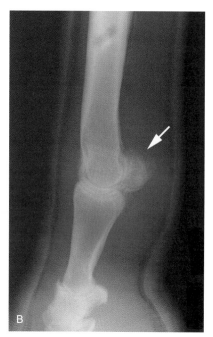 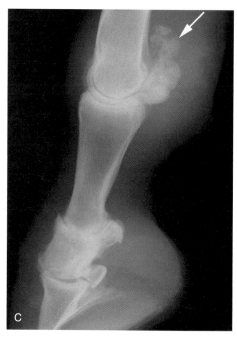

Figure 7.60. Radiographic images of a comminuted P2 fracture that was treated with a transfixation pin cast. A. At the initial pin placement. B. When the pins were removed 3 months later. C. Five months after pin removal. Note the progression of disuse osteoporosis of the sesamoid bones (arrows in A, B, and C) and distal limb with subsequent fracturing of the sesamoid bones (C, arrow).

Bone Fragility Disorder

Bone fragility disorder has been characterized recently by Anderson, et al.[1] These horses typically present with variable degrees of lameness that is difficult to regionalize on physical examination. The key diagnostic finding is that the horses have multiple sites of radioisotope uptake, mostly in the axial and proximal appendicular skeleton, and occasionally radiographic and ultrasonographic signs of bone remodeling at various sites. Rest appeared to help some horses in the report, but most were euthanized for humane reasons.[1]

Osteopetrosis

Osteopetrosis is a rare skeletal disease of horses characterized by an imbalance of bone apposition and resorption. It is an inherited disease of humans, rabbits, mice, and cattle, and it may be inherited in horses.[83] The underlying problem is a failure of bone resorption by osteoclasts. There is complete closure of the medullary canal at the mid-diaphysis of the bone because the canal has not been remodeled by osteoclasia during development from its embryologic state. The disease is also characterized by fractures due to a lack of a normal bone structure. Because there is no evidence of bone marrow in such bones, an anemia commonly accompanies this condition.

Osteopetrosis has been reported in a Peruvian Paso foal,[83] and it may be an inherited condition in this breed. In the case described by Singer and Whitenack,[83] metaphyseal diameters of long bones were wider than normal, and the cortices were abnormally thick with complete obliteration of the medullary canal. Trabecular bone was soft and could be crushed easily, and the bones were not as strong as normal bones in an animal of this age. Large calluses were formed at fracture sites, suggesting that such fractures had occurred *in utero*. Because of the inherited nature of the disease in other species, owners should be advised against future matings.[83]

Fluorosis

Fluorosis is occasionally seen in horses that ingest small but toxic amounts of fluorine in their diet or drinking water.[83] The source of the fluorine is usually contamination from nearby industries. Plants can become contaminated from industrial fumes and wells may become contaminated from an industrial effluent. In toxic amounts, the fluorine is deposited in bone, for which it has a great affinity. Osteomalacia, osteoporosis, and exostosis formation occur due to excessive mobilization of calcium and phosphorus to compensate for urinary excretion. The exostosis is usually first observed in the third metacarpal/metatarsal bones, commonly as hyperostotic lesions (Figure 7.61). There are also periosteal hyperostoses at tendon and ligament insertion sites.

Clinically, affected horses may be intermittently lame and show signs of generalized unthriftiness. The gait may be stiff and horses may stand with their feet abnormally placed and constantly shift their weight to relieve pain. Bones are more easily fractured, and there is usually a classic mottling of the teeth if the animal was exposed to fluorine during development of the teeth. Teeth are generally regarded as sensitive indicators of fluorosis.[81] The diagnosis is usually based on the clinical and radiographic signs and is confirmed by analysis of fluorine in bone and urine. The diagnosis should be confirmed by examining other animals exposed to a

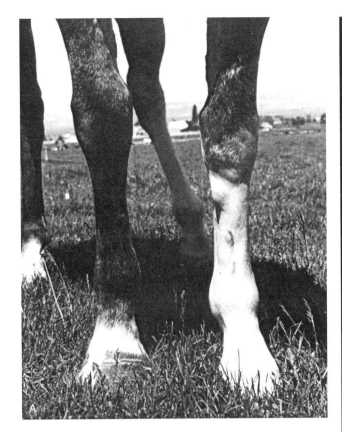
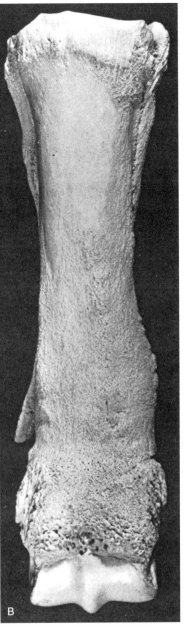

Figure 7.61. A. Enlargement of the metacarpi caused by fluorosis. B. Fluorosis of the third metacarpus with hyperostotic lesions. (Courtesy of JL Shupe.)

similar environment. The treatment is directed toward prevention as well as general symptomatic treatment of the affected horse.

Hereditary Multiple Exostosis (Multiple Cartilaginous Exostosis, Osteochondroma)

Hereditary multiple exostosis is an inherited skeletal disorder characterized by numerous abnormal projections from growing bones that result in an abnormal bone contour.[60,82] The condition affects most of the long bones as well as the ribs, scapula, and pelvis in horses and is used as a model for the condition in humans.[82] The characteristic swellings of hereditary multiple exostosis are usually present at birth, and the lesions are probably initiated during fetal osteogenesis. They are usually bilaterally symmetrical and consist of multiple firm, bony enlargements of various shapes and sizes that are firmly attached to bone.[82] Swellings on the limbs do not appear to enlarge as the animal matures, but others such as those located on the ribs and scapulae usually enlarge until maturity is reached (about 4 years of age) (Figure 7.62). Lameness, if present, is usually due to impingement of various tendons and muscle groups by the bony masses. Some horses may be presented for various joint and tendon sheath swellings.[46]

Grossly, the tumors adopt a variety of shapes, including conical, rounded, pedunculated, multilobulated, or spur-like. Histologically, such tumors appear as osteochondromas and do not appear to undergo malignant

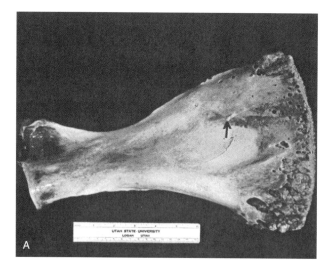

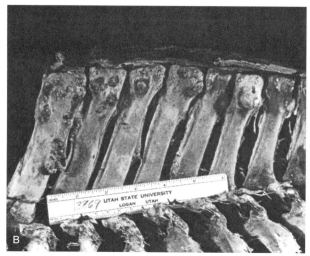

Figure 7.62. Hereditary multiple exostosis involving the scapula (A) and spinous processes of the thoracic vertebrae (B). (Courtesy of JL Shupe.)

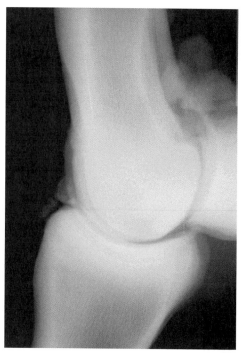

Figure 7.63. Lateral radiograph of a horse with multiple osteochondromas in both the dorsal and palmar aspects of the metacarpophalangeal joint.

transformation.[82] They usually have a small cartilage cap covering underlying spongy cancellous bone. There is no known treatment for this condition.

Solitary osteochondromas occur more commonly in horses, and usually develop on the caudomedial aspect of the distal radial metaphysis.[48,85] Solitary osteochondromas are not considered to be an inherited condition, like hereditary multiple exostosis. Horses with osteochondromas on the caudal aspect of the radius usually present for lameness and swelling of the carpal canal. The masses resemble hereditary multiple exostosis but the lesions are usually not symmetrical.[48,85] Radiographic examination usually reveals an osteocartilaginous exostosis protruding from the caudal aspect of the radius. Large exostoses may cause lameness by interfering with muscle movement such as the humeral head of the deep digital flexor muscle or pain from carpal canal effusion.[35,85] Carpal sheath effusion is usually due to the exostosis and generally does not resolve unless the bone is removed. Surgical removal of the lesion via tenoscopy of the carpal canal is now commonly performed.[85]

Solitary osteochondromas also may develop in joints associated with previous trauma or surgery. Small, dislodged pieces of cartilage may become trapped in the synovium, develop a blood supply, and grow to form osseous masses. These may or may not cause a clinical problem, but often lead to persistent synovial effusion. The dorsal aspect of the fetlock appears to be particularly susceptible to osteochondroma formation (Figure 7.63).

Tumoral Calcinosis (Calcinosis Circumscripta)

Tumoral calcinosis is the formation of calcified, granular, amorphous deposits in the subcutaneous tissues that induce a fibrosing granulomatous reaction.[89] The deposits usually occur in the subcutis near joints and tendon sheaths.[19,29] The condition occurs infrequently in the horse, although it may be more common than is actually recognized.[29] The etiology of the condition is unknown. Affected horses are usually presented for unsightly swellings that become progressively larger, and lameness is uncommon. The swellings are firm and painless, and the skin is usually intact and movable over the swellings. The most common location for tumoral calcinosis lesions is the lateral aspect of the stifle, lateral to the fibula, and beneath the aponeurosis of the biceps femoris and lateral crural fascia. Of 18 cases reported in the literature, lesions occurred over the lateral surface of the tibia close to the femorotibial joint in 16 horses.[29] Radiographically, the lesions are characterized by radio-opaque calcified deposits. On the cut surface of the lesions there is a honeycomb-like appearance with a calcareous, gritty deposit enclosed in a dense fibrous capsule.

The treatment for calcinosis circumscripta is surgical excision. This should be performed only in cases in which lameness can be directly attributed to the lesion. The lesion may be so firmly attached to the stifle joint capsule that it is impossible to dissect it free without opening the joint. Therefore, surgical excision of these lesions should be performed cautiously.

Osteodystrophia Fibrosa (Nutritional Secondary Hyperparathyroidism)

Osteodystrophia fibrosa or nutritional secondary hyperparathyroidism is a generalized bone disease caused primarily by a dietary calcium deficiency in the face of phosphorus excess.[17] It occurs in all equids, although the horse is more susceptible than its relatives.[42] It is most common in horses fed cereal and cereal byproducts such as bran (diets high in phosphorus and low in calcium), hence the name "bran disease." The addition to the diet of legume hay, which is high in calcium, usually prevents the disease.[17,58] The disease is also seen in horses grazing plants high in oxalates, which chelate the calcium and interfere with the absorption of calcium. Horses in Queensland, Australia, developed osteodystrophia fibrosa when grazed on tropical grasses.[94] A subclinical form of the disease may also occur but is difficult to diagnose because the clinical manifestations are subtle.

The underlying pathogenesis in osteodystrophia fibrosa is defective mineralization of bone. The diet high in phosphorus leads to increased absorption of phosphorus and elevation of serum phosphate levels. This tends to lower serum calcium and stimulate the parathyroid glands to increase secretion of parathyroid hormone. Parathyroid hormone increases activation of remodeling, leading to resorption of bone. With bone resorption there is a compensatory replacement with fibrous tissue,[27] which causes poorly mineralized bone that is eventually replaced with cellular connective tissue. Horses of both sexes and all ages are susceptible. Lactating mares and foals appear to be at increased risk to develop osteodystrophia fibrosa.

The classic form of osteodystrophia fibrosa is called "bighead" because of the predilection of the jaws and flat bones of the skull to respond to parathyroid hormone.[27] The classic clinical signs of the disease include a symmetrical enlargement of the mandible and facial bones. There is loss of lamina dura around the teeth due to osteoclastic resorption of alveolar margins and the teeth may eventually loosen. This can be identified radiographically and is one of the first signs of the disease. Swelling initially begins just above the facial crest and in the mandible, producing a reduction in intermandibular space. There may also be enough swelling of the palate, maxillae, and incisor bones to produce dyspnea.

The subclinical form of nutritional secondary hyperparathyroidism may cause a nebulous shifting limb lameness in horses that is difficult to localize with standard perineural anesthesia.[94] The condition may also contribute to unexplained fractures, especially in young horses. In such cases a dietary history is important in the diagnosis. Blood calcium and phosphorus levels are usually normal and the diagnosis is usually based on analysis of the diet and response to treatment with calcium supplementation.

Hypertrophic Osteopathy (Hypertrophic Pulmonary Osteoarthropathy)

Hypertrophic osteopathy is a progressive bilaterally symmetrical proliferation of subperiosteal bone and fibrous connective tissue on the appendicular and axial skeleton and facial bones.[94] It is relatively rare in the horse, and the pathogenesis is still unclear at present. Classically, the disease is associated with a space-occupying pulmonary lesion such as a neoplasm or chronic suppurative process such as a large abscess, tuberculosis, or a fractured rib with pleural adhesions.[53] The disease rarely occurs in horses with such thoracic lesions, but has been associated with a granular cell myoblastoma.[28] The term hypertrophic osteopathy is preferred because the disease also has been associated with intra-abdominal disorders without pulmonary involvement. Hypertrophic osteopathy has been reported in a mare with a dysgerminoma (a neoplasm of ovarian primordial germ cells) that had abdominal metastases but was free of thoracic lesions.[53]

The 2 most common mechanisms for the development of the disease are classified as neurogenic and humoral. The more popular neurogenic theory is based on the fact that an apparent stimulation of the vagus nerve produces an alteration of the vasculature and periosteum of bones by way of an unknown efferent pathway. Support for this theory is based on the fact that in dogs and humans, hypertrophic osteopathy lesions may regress following vagotomy. A humoral mechanism may also exist, because hypertrophic osteopathy has been shown to occur in people when urinary excretion of estrogen is increased. High levels of circulating estrogen have been reported in a mare with hypertrophic osteopathy, although the exact relationship between estrogen levels and hypertrophic osteopathy is purely speculative.[53]

The clinical signs of hypertrophic osteopathy are related to periosteal hyperostoses. There is symmetric enlargement of the long bones of the limb with all bones in the limb affected (Figure 7.64). There is pain and

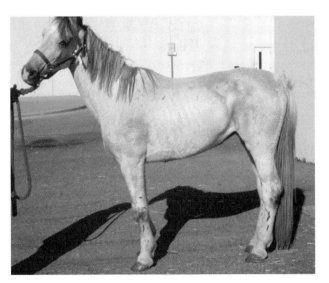

Figure 7.64. This horse had swellings of all 4 distal extremities associated with hypertrophic osteopathy.

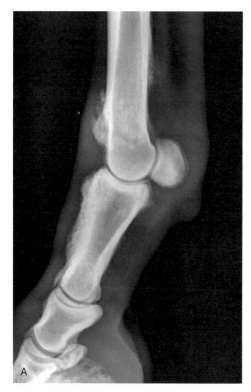
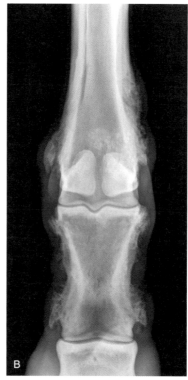

Figure 7.65. Lateral (A) and dorsopalmar (B) radiographs of the left front fetlock of a horse with hypertrophic osteopathy, showing irregular new bone growth. A definitive cause was never determined.

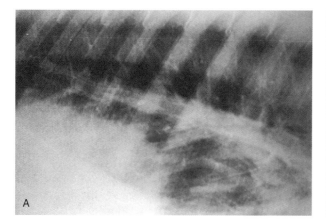
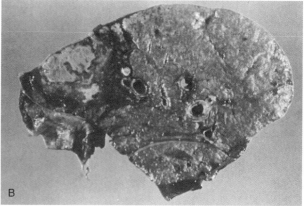

Figure 7.66. A. Radiograph of the thorax in a horse with hypertrophic osteopathy, revealing a large pulmonary abscess. B. Necropsy specimen of the lung showing the abscess. (Courtesy of Dr. N. Messer.)

edema of soft tissues and the horse may have a stiff gait and be reluctant to move. The joint surfaces are rarely involved; however, there may be decreased motion in affected joints as well as pain on manipulation. There may be signs referable to pulmonary abnormalities such as coughing and nasal discharge.

Radiographically, there is a generalized increase in soft tissue swelling and evidence of periostitis. Irregular new bone growth occurs, especially at the proximal and distal ends of the long bones (Figure 7.65).[94] The differential diagnosis should include fluorosis, but the gross appearance of the bones and absence of dental lesions, as well as blood and urine fluorine levels, can usually eliminate fluorosis as the cause. Lateral radio-

graphs of the chest or abdomen may help locate the causative lesion (Figure 7.66).

References

1. Anderson JD, Galuppo LD, Barr BC, et al. Clinical and scintigraphic findings in horses with a bone fragility disorder: 16 cases (1980–2006). J Am Vet Med Assoc 2008;232:1694–1699.
2. Andrea CR, Stover SM, Galuppo LD, et al. Comparison of insertion time and pullout strength between self-tapping and non-self-tapping AO 4.5-mm cortical bone screws in adult equine third metacarpal bone. Vet Surg 2002;31:189–194.
3. Auer JA. Surgical equipment and implants for fracture repair In Equine Fracture Repair, 1st ed. Nixon AJ, ed. W.B. Saunders Co., Philadelphia, 1996;52–62.

4. Auer JA, Watkins JP. Instrumentation and techniques in equine fracture fixation. Vet Clin North Am Equine Pract 1996; 12:283–302.

5. Baxter GM. Subchondral cystic lesions in horses. In Joint Disease in the Horse. McIlwraith CW, Trotter GW, eds. W.B. Saunders Co., Philadelphia, 1996;384–397.

6. Baxter GM. Treatment of orthopedic infections in horses. Vet Clin North Am Equine Pract 1996;12:303–336.

7. Belknap JK, Baxter GM, Nickels FA. Extensor tendon lacerations in horses: 50 cases (1982–1988). J Am Vet Med Assoc 1993;203:428–431.

8. Blackwell JC, Griffith AD, Crosby WJ. Surgical correction of an alveolar mandibular bone cyst. Equine Pract 1985;7: 70–73.

9. Blood DC, Henderson JA, Radostits OM. Veterinary Medicine. Lea and Febiger, Philadelphia, 1979.

10. Booth LC, Feeney DA. Superficial osteitis and sequestrum formation as a result of skin avulsion in the horse. Vet Surg 1982;11:2.

11. Bramlage LR. Current concepts of emergency first aid treatment and transportation of equine fracture patients. Comp Cont Educ Pract Vet 1983;5:S564-S574.

12. Bramlage LR. First aid and transportation of fracture patients. In Equine Fracture Repair. Nixon AJ, ed. W.B. Saunders Co., Philadelphia, 1996;36–42.

13. Bramlage LR. Osteochondrosis related bone cysts. Proceedings Am Assoc Equine Pract 1993;83–84.

14. Bueno AC, Galuppo LD, Taylor KT, et al. A biomechanical comparison of headless tapered variable pitch and AO cortical bone screws for fixation of a simulated slab fracture in equine third carpal bones. Vet Surg 2003;32:167–177.

15. Campanacci M, Capanna R, Picci P. Unicameral and aneurysmal bone cysts. Clin Orthop Relat Res 1986:25–36.

16. Colgan SA, Hecker AT, Kirker-Head CA, et al. A comparison of the Synthes 4.5-mm cannulated screw and the Synthes 4.5-mm standard cortex screw systems in equine bone. Vet Surg 1998;27:540–546.

17. David JB, Cohen ND, Nachreiner R. Equine secondary hyperparathyroidism. Comp Cont Educ Pract Vet 1997;19: 1380–1386.

18. Davidson EJ, Ross MW. Clinical recognition of stress-related bone injury in racehorses. Clin Tech Equine Pract 2003; 2:296–311.

19. Dodd DC, Raker CW. Tumoral calcinosis (calcinosis circumscripta) in the horse. J Am Vet Med Assoc 1970;157: 968–972.

20. Dutton DM, Watkins JP, Walker MA, et al. Incomplete ossification of the tarsal bones in foals: 22 cases (1988–1996). J Am Vet Med Assoc 1998;213:1590–1594.

21. Dykgraaf S, Firth EC, Rogers CW, et al. Effects of exercise on chondrocyte viability and subchondral bone sclerosis in the distal third metacarpal and metatarsal bones of young horses. Vet J 2008;178:53–61.

22. Eagle MT, Koch DB, Whalen JP. Mineral metabolism and immobilization osteopenia in ponies treated with 25-hydroxycholecalciferol. Cornell Vet 1982;72:372.

23. Ellis DR. Fractures of the proximal sesamoid bones in Thoroughbred foals. Equine Vet J 1979;11:48–52.

24. Farnum CE, Wilsman NJ. Ultrastructural histochemical evaluation of growth plate cartilage matrix from healthy and osteochondritic swine. Am J Vet Res 1986;47:1105–1115.

25. Field JR, Hearn TC, Arighi M. Investigation of bioabsorbable screw usage for long bone fracture repair in the horse: Interfragmentary compression and axial load response in equine cadaver long bone fractures. Vet Clin Orthop Trauma 1995;8:191–205.

26. Firth EC. Specific orthopedic infections. In Equine Surgery. Auer JA, ed. W.B. Saunders Co., Philadelphia, 1992;932.

27. Frank N, Hawkins JF, Couetil LL, et al. Primary hyperparathyroidism with osteodystrophia fibrosa of the facial bones in a pony. J Am Vet Med Assoc 1998;212:84–86.

28. Goodbary RF, Hage TJ. Hypertrophic pulmonary osteoarthropathy in a horse—a case report. J Am Vet Med Assoc 1960;137:602–605.

29. Goulden BE, O'Callaghan MW. Tumoral calcinosis in the horse. N Z Vet J 1980;28:217–219.

30. Hawkins DL, Stover SM. Pregnancy-associated changes in material properties of the third metacarpal cortical bone in mares. Am J Vet Res 1997;58:182–187.

31. Hawkins JF. Bone tumors and true cysts. In Current Techniques in Equine Surgery. White MR, Moore JN, eds. W.B. Saunders, Philadelphia, 1998;112–115.

32. Hill MA. Causes of degenerative joint disease (osteoarthrosis) and dyschondroplasia (osteochondrosis) in pigs. J Am Vet Med Assoc 1990;197:107–113.

33. Holcombe SJ, Schneider RK, Bramlage LR, et al. Use of antibiotic-impregnated polymethyl methacrylate in horses with open or infected fractures or joints: 19 cases (1987–1995). J Am Vet Med Assoc 1997;211:889–893.

34. Howard RD, McIlwraith CW, Trotter GW. Arthroscopic surgery for subchondral cystic lesions of the medial femoral condyle in horses: 41 cases (1988–1991). J Am Vet Med Assoc 1995;206:842–850.

35. Hunt DA, Snyder JR, Morgan JP, et al. Evaluation of an interfragmentary compression system for the repair of equine femoral capital physeal fractures. Vet Surg 1990;19:107–116.

36. Hurtig MB, Green SL, Dobson H, et al. Defective bone and cartilage in foals fed a low-copper diet. Proceedings Am Assoc Equine Pract 1990;637–643.

37. Hurtig MB, Green SL, Dobson H, et al. Correlation study of defective cartilage and bone growth in foals fed a low-copper diet. Equine Vet J Suppl 1993;66:66–74.

38. Jackman BR, Baxter GM. Treatment of a mandibular bone cyst by use of a corticocancellous bone graft in a horse. J Am Vet Med Assoc 1992;201:892–894.

39. James FM, Richardson DW. Minimally invasive plate fixation of lower limb injury in horses: 32 cases (1999–2003). Equine Vet J 2006;38:246–251.

40. Jeffcott LB. Osteochondrosis in the horse—searching for the key to pathogenesis. Equine Vet J 1991;23:331–338.

41. Jeffcott LB, Kold SE, Melsen F. Aspects of the pathology of stifle bone cysts in the horse. Equine Vet J 1983;15:304–311.

42. Jubb KV, Kennedy PC. Pathology of Domestic Animals. Academic Press, New York, 1970.

43. Kamm L, McIlwraith CW, Kawcak CE. A review of the efficacy of tiludronate in the horse. J Equine Vet Sci 2008;28: 209–214.

44. Kawcak CE, McIlwraith CW, Norrdin RW, et al. The role of subchondral bone in joint disease: a review. Equine Vet J 2001;33:120–126.

45. Kim W, Kawcak CE, McIlwraith CW, et al. Influence of early conditioning exercise on the development of gross cartilage defects and swelling behavior of cartilage extracellular matrix in the equine midcarpal joint. Am J Vet Res 2009;70: 589–598.

46. Lee HA, Grant BD, Galina AM. Solitary osteochondroma in a horse: A case report. J Eq Med Surg 1979;3:113.

47. Levine DG, Richardson DW. Clinical use of the locking compression plate (LCP) in horses: a retrospective study of 31 cases (2004–2006). Equine Vet J 2007;39:401–406.

48. Lundvall RL. Periosteal new bone formation of the radius as a cause of lameness in two horses. J Am Vet Med Assoc 1976;168:612–613.

49. Malghem J, Maldague B, Esselinckx W, et al. Spontaneous healing of aneurysmal bone cysts. A report of three cases. J Bone Joint Surg Br 1989;71:645–650.

50. Markel MD. Bone structure and the response of bone to stress. In Equine Fracture Repair, 1st ed. Nixon AJ, ed. W.B. Saunders Co., Philadelphia, 1996;3–9.

51. Markel MD. Fracture healing and its noninvasive assessment. In Equine Fracture Repair, 1st ed. Nixon AJ, ed. W.B. Saunders Co., Philadelphia, 1996;19–29.

52. Martinelli MJ, Baker GJ, Clarkson RB, et al. Magnetic resonance imaging of degenerative joint disease in a horse: a comparison to other diagnostic techniques. Equine Vet J 1996;28: 410–415.

53. Mauten DJ, Rendano VT Jr. Hypertrophic osteopathy in a mare with a dysgerminoma. J Equine Med Surg 1978;2:445.

54. McClure SR, Honnas CM, Watkins JP. Managing equine fractures with external skeletal fixation. Comp Cont Educ Pract Vet 1995;17:1054–1062.

55. McClure SR, Watkins JP, Ashman RB. *In vitro* comparison of the effect of parallel and divergent transfixation pins on breaking strength of equine third metacarpal bones. Am J Vet Res 1994;55:1327–1330.

56. McClure SR, Watkins JP, Ashman RB. *In vivo* evaluation of intramedullary interlocking nail fixation of transverse femoral osteotomies in foals. Vet Surg 1998;27:29–36.

57. McDuffee LA, Stover SM, Taylor KT, et al. An *in vitro* biomechanical investigation of an interlocking nail for fixation of diaphyseal tibial fractures in adult horses. Vet Surg 1994; 23:219–230.

58. McKenzie RA, Gartner RJ, Blaney BJ, et al. Control of nutritional secondary hyperparathyroidism in grazing horses with calcium plus phosphorus supplementation. Aust Vet J 1981;57:554–557.

59. Mehl ML, Tucker RL, Ragle CA, et al. The use of MRI in the diagnosis of equine limb disorders. Vet Clin North Am Equine Pract 1998;20:14–17.

60. Morgan JP, Carlson WD, Adams OR. Hereditary multiple exostosis in the horse. J Am Vet Med Assoc 1962;140:1320–1322.

61. Murray RC, Gaughan EM, Debowes RM, et al. Biomechanical comparison of the Herbert and AO cortical bone screws for compression of an equine third carpal bone dorsal plane slab osteotomy. Vet Surg 1998;27:49–55.

62. Nemeth F, Back W. The use of the walking cast to repair fractures in horses and ponies. Equine Vet J 1991;23:32–36.

63. Nugent GE, Law AW, Wong EG, et al. Site- and exercise-related variation in structure and function of cartilage from equine distal metacarpal condyle. Osteoarthritis Cartilage 2004;12:826–833.

64. Nunamaker DM. Metacarpal stress fractures. In Equine Fracture Repair, 1st ed. Nixon AJ, ed. W.B. Saunders Co., Philadelphia, 1996;195–199.

65. Nunamaker DM, Bowman KF, Richardson DW, et al. Plate luting: A preliminary report of its use in horses. Vet Surg 1986;15:289–293.

66. Nunamaker DM, Butterweck DM, Provost MT. Fatigue fractures in Thoroughbred racehorses: relationships with age, peak bone strain, and training. J Orthop Res 1990;8:604–611.

67. Nunamaker DM, Butterweck DM, Provost MT. Some geometric properties of the third metacarpal bone: a comparison between the Thoroughbred and Standardbred racehorse. J Biomech 1989;22:129–134.

68. Nunamaker DM, Nash RA. A tapered-sleeve transcortical pin external skeletal fixation device for use in horses: development, application, and experience. Vet Surg 2008;37:725–732.

69. Nunamaker DM, Richardson DW, Butterweck DM, et al. A new external skeletal fixation device that allows immediate full weight bearing. Vet Surg 1986;15:345–355.

70. Ogden JA. The development and growth of the musculoskeletal system. In The Scientific Basis of Orthopedics. Albright JA, Brand RA, eds. Appleton Century Crofts, New York, 1979.

71. Olsen SE, Reiland S. The nature of osteochondrosis in animals. Acta Radiol Suppl 1978;358:299.

72. Owen LN. The pathology of bone infection. In Bone in Clinical Orthopedics. Smith GS, ed. W.B. Saunders Co., Philadelphia, 1982.

73. Reddi AH. Initiation of fracture repair by bone morphogenetic proteins. Clin Orthop Relat Res 1998:S66–72.

74. Richardson DW, Clark CC. Effects of short-term cast immobilization on equine articular cartilage. Am J Vet Res 1993;54:449–453.

75. Richardson DW, Nunamaker DM, Sigafoos RD. Use of an external skeletal fixation device and bone graft for arthrodesis of the metacarpophalangeal joint in horses. J Am Vet Med Assoc 1986;191:316–321.

76. Rose RJ. Surgical treatment of osteomyelitis in the metacarpal and metatarsal bones of the horse. Vet Rec 1978;102:498–500.

77. Savage CJ. Etiopathogenesis of osteochondrosis. In Current Techniques in Equine Surgery and Lameness. White NA, Moore JN, eds. W.B. Saunders Co., Philadelphia, 1998;318–322.

78. Schatzker J. Concepts of Fracture Stabilization in Bone in Clinical Orthopedics. W.B. Saunders Co., Philadelphia, 1982.

79. Schatzker J, Sanderson R, Murnaghan JP. The holding power of orthopedic screws *in vivo*. Clin Orthop Relat Res 1975:115–126.

80. Schenk KR, Willenegger H. Zum histologischen bild der sogennanten primarheilung der knockenkompakta nch experimetellen osteomen am hund. Experimentia 1963;19:593.

81. Shupe JL. Flurosis. In Equine Medicine and Surgery, 4th ed. Colahan PT, et al., eds. American Veterinary Publications, Goleta, 1991;1293.

82. Shupe JL, Leone NC, Olson AE, et al. Hereditary multiple exostoses: Clinicopathologic features of a comparative study in horses and man. Am J Vet Res 1979;40:751–757.

83. Singer VL, Whitenacx DL. Osteopetrosis in a foal. Vet Clin North Am Equine Pract 1981;3:30.

84. Smart ME, Gudmundson J, Brockman RP, et al. Copper deficiency in calves in north central Manitoba. Can Vet J 1980;21:349–352.

85. Southwood LL, Stashak TS, Fehr JE, et al. Lateral approach for endoscopic removal of solitary osteochondromas from the distal radial metaphysis in three horses. J Am Vet Med Assoc 1997;210:1166–1168.

86. Spindler KP, Schils JP, Bergfeld JA, et al. Prospective study of osseous, articular, and meniscal lesions in recent anterior cruciate ligament tears by magnetic resonance imaging and arthroscopy. Am J Sports Med 1993;21:551–557.

87. Staller GS, Richardson DW, Nunamaker DM, et al. Contact area and static pressure profile at the plate-bone interface in the nonluted and luted bone plate. Vet Surg 1995;24:299–307.

88. Steiner JV, Rendano VT Jr. Aneurysmal bone cyst in the horse. Cornell Vet 1982;72:57–63.

89. Stone WC, Wilson DG, Dubiezig RR. The pathologic mineralization of soft tissue: Calcinosis circumscripta in horses. Comp Cont Educ Pract 1990;12:1643–1648.

90. Stover SM. Stress fractures. In Current Techniques in Equine Surgery and Lameness, 2nd ed. White NA, Moore JN, eds. W.B. Saunders Co., Philadelphia, 1998;451–459.

91. Stover SM, Johnson BJ, Daft BM, et al. An association between complete and incomplete stress fractures of the humerus in racehorses. Equine Vet J 1992;24:260–263.

92. Tobias KM, Schneider RK, Besser TE. Use of antimicrobial-impregnated polymethyl methacrylate. J Am Vet Med Assoc 1996;208:841–845.

93. Trotter GW. Osteomyelitis. In Equine Fracture Repair. Nixon AJ, ed. W.B. Saunders Co., Philadelphia, 1996;359–366.

94. Turner AS. Diseases of bone and related structures. In Adams' Lameness in Horses, 4th ed. Stashak TS, ed. Lea and Febiger, Philadelphia, 1987;293–338.

95. van de Lest CH, Brama PA, Van Weeren PR. The influence of exercise on the composition of developing equine joints. Biorheology 2002;39:183–191.

96. van Harreveld PD, Lillich JD, Kawcak CE, et al. Effects of immobilization followed by remobilization on mineral density, histomorphometric features, and formation of the bones of the metacarpophalangeal joint in horses. Am J Vet Res 2002;63:276–281.

97. von Rechenberg B, Guenther H, McIlwraith CW, et al. Fibrous tissue of subchondral cystic lesions in horses produce local mediators and neutral metalloproteinases and cause bone resorption *in vitro*. Vet Surg 2000;29:420–429.

98. Wallis TW, Goodrich LR, McIlwraith CW, et al. Arthroscopic injection of corticosteroids into the fibrous tissue of subchondral cystic lesions of the medial femoral condyle in horses: A retrospective study of 52 cases (2001–2006). Equine Vet J 2008;40:461–467.

99. Watkins JP. Osteochondrosis. In Equine Surgery, 1st ed. Auer JA, ed. W.B. Saunders Co., Philadelphia, 1992;971–984.

100. Whitehair KJ. Regional limb perfusion with antibiotics. American College of Veterinary Surgeons Veterinary Symposium 1995;59.

101. Whitehair KJ, Adams SB, Parker JE, et al. Regional limb perfusion with antibiotics in three horses. Vet Surg 1992;21:286–292.

102. Whitehair KJ, Blevins WE, Fessler JF, et al. Regional perfusion of the equine carpus for antibiotic delivery. Vet Surg 1992;21:279–285.

103. Williams MA, Pugh DC. Developmental orthopedic disease: Minimizing the incidence of a poorly understood disorder. Comp Cont Educ Pract Vet 1993;15:859–871.

104. Young DR, Nunamaker DM, Markel MD. Quantitative evaluation of the remodeling response of the proximal sesamoid bones to training-related stimuli in Thoroughbreds. Am J Vet Res 1991;52:1350–1356.

105. Yovich JV, Turner AS, Smith FW. Holding power of orthopedic screws: Comparison of self-tapped and pre-tapped screws in foal bone. Vet Surg 1986;15:55–59.

TENDON AND LIGAMENT INJURIES AND DISEASE

| Laurie R. Goodrich

ANATOMY

Tendons and ligaments are complex structures that exist in a hierarchical structure of subunits (Figure 7.67). Grossly, tendons are made up of many fascicles, which, during further macroscopic and microscopic examination, have decreasingly sized subunits, then fibers, and finally fibrils.

Structure

The anatomic structures of note are the paratenon, epitenon, endotenon, tendon fascicles, and tendon fiber/fibrils. Paratenon refers to the loose connective tissue and vessels which surround tendons. Epitenon is outside of tendon fascicles and is continuous with the endo-

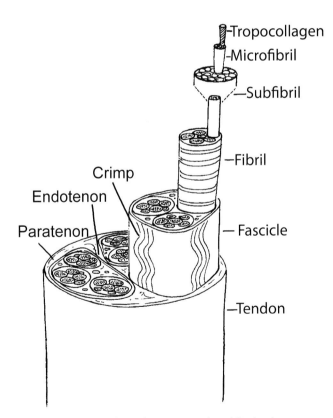

Figure 7.67. A schematic representation of the tendon hierarchy. The level of tendon fascicles can be viewed grossly, fibers may be seen microscopically, and individual collagen fibrils (tropocollagen) may be viewed via electron microscopy. (Modified from Davis CS, Smith RKW. Diagnosis and management of tendon and ligament disorders. In Equine Surgery. Auer JA, Stick JA, eds. Saunders, Philadelphia, 2006, 1087.)

tenon. Endotenon contains vascular and neural structures and separates cell populations. Furthermore, the endotenon may be a source for pluripotential cells. Tendon fascicles are the bundles of fibrocytes and tenocytes that are surrounded by endotenon. Tendon fibers/fibrils are made of long bundles of collagen filaments that are predominately type I collagen and have elastin and glycosaminoglycan in the extracellular matrix. Larger fibrils are stronger than smaller fibrils.[36]

Collagen fibrils have many triple helical collagen molecules that are arranged such that a characteristic banding pattern is seen on electron microscopy. Collagen molecules are secreted extracellularly through the pores of the tenocytes. Cross linking of these molecules results in fibril formation, and these fibrils fuse as horses age, leading to larger collagen fibrils.[19,22,36]

Under a light microscope, collagen fibers have a characteristic wavy pattern that is referred to as crimp (Figure 7.68). Crimp imparts elasticity to the tendon. A decrease in crimp occurs with aging along with a greater reduction in the central fibers.[29,36,42] When the tendon is stretched, the central fibers straighten primarily, and therefore a greater load is placed on these fibers relative to peripheral fibers. This may explain the more common occurrence of tendon lesions observed centrally (core lesions). Peripheral lesions are less clearly explained.

Cellular Components

Tenocytes are the primary cell types found within equine tendon; they are responsible for the formation and maintenance of tendon tissue.[36] Three types are described (Figure 7.69). Type I cells have thin, spindle-shaped nuclei, type II cells have rounded or oblong nuclei, and type III cells appear as cartilage-like cells with round nuclei and visible nucleoli.[36] Proportions vary with age of the horse, site, and whether a ligament or tendon. Type I cells are more frequently found in older horses, type II cells can be found in higher numbers in young horses and in ligaments, and type III cells are found in areas sustaining higher compressive loads.[36] It is logical to assume that Type II and III cells are metabolically active and maintain tendon extracellular matrix; however, Type I cells most likely do this to some extent as well.

Cellular numbers vary depending on age and location within the tendon. As maturity is reached, the numbers remain constant; however, areas of tendon become acellular and have changes consistent with chondroid metaplasia such as the center of the superficial digital flexor tendon (SDFT) or the deep digital flexor tendon (DDFT) in the metacarpophalangeal region.[36] These areas are often surrounded by type II

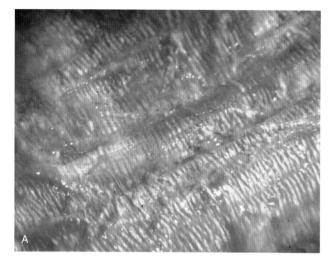

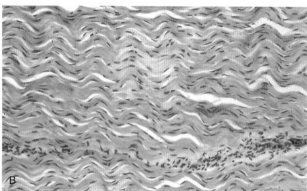

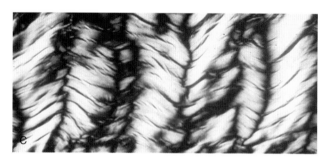

Figure 7.68. Gross (A) and hematoxylin- and eosin-stained microscopic section (B) and polarized light microscopy (C), revealing the classic crimp pattern formed by collagen fibers. (Courtesy of Dr. Roger Smith and Professor AE Goodship.)

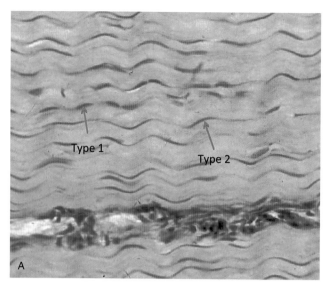

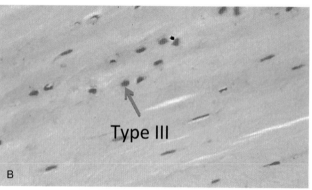

Figure 7.69. Type I, II (arrows in A), and III (arrow in B) cells found in the equine tendon. (Courtesy of Dr. Roger Smith.)

cells. Other cells found in tendon include synovial-like cells of the epitenon within the tendon sheaths and fibroblasts of the paratenon, epitenon, and endotenon. These probably have an integral role in tendon maintenance due to certain growth factors such as transforming growth factor-β (TGF-β) found in these areas.[10,20]

Tenocyte regulation has not been fully elucidated, but most likely it relies on mechanical and cytokine stimulation. Tenocytes have been shown to respond quickly to mechanical stimuli in cell culture.[2] However, tenocytes in culture also require growth factors to respond to mechanical load.[19] Recent research has discovered cellular communication through cytoplasmic extensions of tenocytes, which most likely result in a coordinated upregulation in response to mechanical stimuli.[26,36]

The growth factors most noted to have anabolic effects on tendons include TGF-β and insulin-like growth factor-I (IGF-I).[11,12] The concentration of these growth factors seems to be highest early in age, and decreases with maturity. Furthermore, it is believed they are deficient in healing tendon. Further research will elucidate the important growth factors that are essential to tendon health and healing.

Molecular Composition

Tendon and ligaments are highly hydrated and have a water content of approximately 65% (wet weight), which makes up the majority of the extracellular matrix. The remaining content consists of collagen (30% wet weight) and noncollagenous glycoproteins (5% wet weight). Type I collagen is the predominant collagen in tendon (greater than 95%) and the remaining is type III, which is present in endotenon and increases with age. Type II collagen, the main collagen found in cartilage, can only be found at tendon insertions and areas where tendon changes direction and takes on a fibro-cartilage-like character.[9] Collagen is synthesized outside of the cell as procollagen molecules. As the α-helical chains are produced and cleaved by procollagenases, they are cross linked to form a collagen fibril.[14]

Other non-collagenous glycoproteins include cartilage oligomeric matrix protein (COMP), proteoglycans and elastin, fibronectin, and thrombospondin.[36,45] COMP has recently been studied intensely due to its perceived importance in organization of the collagen fibril framework during tendon formation and growth.[14] Recent data have shown that COMP accelerated collagen fibril formation *in vitro*.[39] As collagen molecules form a fibril, COMP does not remain bound and is displaced from the fibril. As such, levels of COMP increase during growth, peak about 2 years of age in flexor tendons at the metacarpal level, and decrease once growth ceases and the animals age.[38] A correlation exists between tendon ultimate tensile strength and the level of COMP at maturity.[34]

Other noncollagenous proteins such as the small proteoglycans (decorin, fibromoedulin, lumican) can be found in the regions of tension; conversely, large proteoglycans (aggrecan and versican) are found in regions of compression where the tendon changes direction over a bony prominence (i.e., the DDFT at the level of the metacarpophalangeal joint).[14,16]

Collagen fibrils are bundled together into fibers that are separated by cellular cytoplasmic extensions of tenocytes (Figure 7.70).[26] Little is known about these cells; they may have different stages of activation. Various types of tenocytes have been described above; however, it is unknown how these cells function during growth, maturity, and aging.

Associated Structures

Blood Supply

Nutrients are supplied to the tendons and ligaments through diffusion and perfusion. Diffusion primarily occurs where a sheath encloses the structure with synovial fluid, playing an important role.[36] When blood is

delivered via perfusion, it originates from 3 separate sources, including the musculotendinous attachments proximally, the osseous insertion distally, and the intratendinous and extratendinous vessels.[25] The extratendinous blood supply comes from vessels within the paratenon (extrasynovially) or mesotenon (intrasynovially) attachments. An example of intrasynovial mesotenon is when vessels lie at the vinculum between the fetlock anular ligament and the SDFT.

Connective Tissue

Connective tissues associated with tendons include sheaths and retinaculi. The tendon sheath is comparable to the joint capsule with an outer fibrous sheath and an inner synovial membrane.[25] Sheaths of tendons are folded around the tendinous structures, most commonly in areas in which the tendon passes over joint structures, and bathes the tendon in synovial fluid. Annular ligaments, or retinacula, are tenacious fibrous bands that maintain tendons in the correct position (Figure 7.71).

Bursae are structures very similar to tendon sheaths except that they are located between tendinous structures and bone. Similar to tendinous bursae, they have a synovial membrane and rely on synovial fluid to provide nearly frictionless movement between the

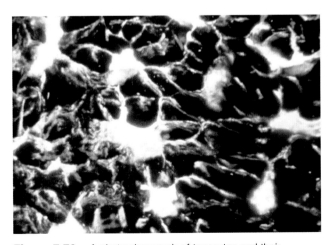

Figure 7.70. A photomicrograph of tenocytes and their extensions. The multiple connections allow the tenocytes to act in concert with mechanical influences. (From Davis CS, Smith RKW. Diagnosis and management of tendon and ligament disorders. In Equine Surgery. Auer JA, Stick JA, eds. Saunders, Philadelphia, 2006, 1087.)

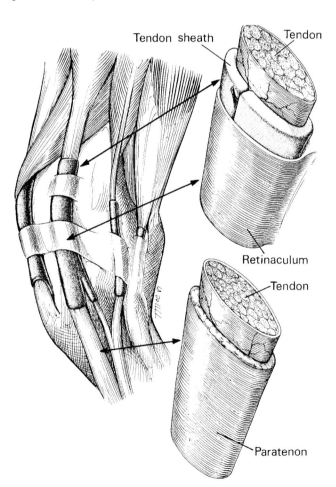

Figure 7.71. Diagram of tendons and their relationship to the retinaculum, endotenon, and tendon sheaths.

tendon and the bone. Bursae that are commonly dealt with in lameness primarily include the navicular bursa, calcaneal bursa, bicipital bursa, and the olecranon bursa.

FUNCTIONS OF TENDONS AND LIGAMENTS

The elaborate anatomical architecture of tendons and ligaments is designed to allow tendons to passively transfer force generated by muscle to bony attachments on the opposite side of a joint, or joints, to provide movement.[36] Conversely, ligaments resist distraction of 2 bony attachments such as the collateral ligaments and suspensory ligaments.[36] Because the tendon and ligaments are on the palmar aspect of the equine distal limb, they receive significant weight-bearing loads and therefore provide support to the metacarpophalangeal and metatarsophalangeal joints during weight-bearing and exercise and act as force transmitters during rapid and unexpected movement.[25]

Tendons should also be considered as elastic structures that store energy for efficient locomotion.[1,36] Structures such as the SDFT provide shock absorption through the elasticity of the tendon combined with the attachment of the musculotendinous portion to the caudal aspect of the radius by the accessory or superior check ligament. The undulating gait of a horse at speed has been compared to the motion of a pogo stick with the tendons providing the elasticity of the bounce.[44] The unique structural arrangement within tendons and ligaments allows the horse to exercise at high speeds while minimizing energy expenditure.[36]

BIOMECHANICAL PROPERTIES

Biomechanical characteristics of tendons are usually described by stress-strain curves. These curves reveal the force per unit area (stress) plotted against the percentage of elongation (strain) and can be used to calculate elastic modulus (Figure 7.72). The 4 areas that are important to a stress-strain curve of a tendon are:

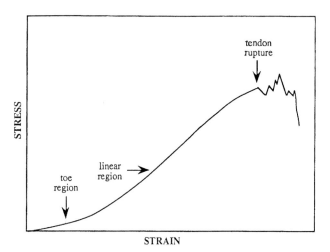

Figure 7.72. The stress strain curve for tendons. (From Goodship AE, Burch HL, Wilson AM. The pathobiology and repair of tendon and ligament injury. Vet Clin North Am Equine Pract 1994;10:335.)

1. The toe region, where stretch is nonlinear. This represents the area where the undulating pattern of collagen fibrils are eliminated; this is also the elastic phase.
2. Linear deformation, or midsection, where the elastic stiffness of the tendon is represented,
3. Yield region, in which irreversible lengthening of the tendon occurs and the plastic phase begins.
4. Rupture, in which the collagen cross links or fibrils sequentially rupture.

Initially, the tendon is highly compliant, but upon further extension, stiffness increases and viscoelastic (and permanent) changes occur.[25,40] It has been suggested that the second phase of the stress-strain curve for a tendon causes residual damage.[40] When the strain level is maintained between 3% and 5%, the normal linear stress-strain relationship is maintained; this is the typical strain that a tendon undergoes at a walk and trot. However, as strains reach 5% and 6%, the tendon is more viscoelastic, which results in permanent changes.[32] When the tendon reaches 10% to 12% strain (ultimate tensile strain), permanent, catastrophic changes such as rupture result. That said, maximum strains in Thoroughbreds at a gallop can reach 16%.[20,25] These are much greater than the strains most other species sustain at higher speeds and quite possibly explain why racing Thoroughbreds sustain a much greater incidence of disease affecting the SDFT.

The SDFT sustains loads of up to 1 metric ton at maximum weight-bearing.[36] Considering that the maximal cross section is approximately 1 cm^2 in cross-sectional area, it is little surprise that midmetacarpal tendon injury is so prevalent. Variability in ultimate tensile force exists within any population of horses, however, with up to a 2-fold difference reported between weak and strong tendons.[45]

The modulus of elasticity/stiffness is represented by the force required to extend the tendon by a unit length. The stronger the tendon, the stiffer it is.[36] Hysteresis refers to the phase between loading and unloading a tendon and importantly, results in loss of energy. It is estimated that approximately 5%[32] hysteresis occurs in equine tendon, increasing the temperature within the tendon core when repeated loads are applied to the tendon during exercise, and possibly causing flexor tendinitis (Figure 7.73).[43]

TYPES OF TENDON AND LIGAMENT INJURIES

Three types of injury may occur in tendons and ligaments: excessive strain, physical tearing, and percutaneous injury. Overstrain may result from overwhelming the resistive strength in an acute manner, and it is believed to be the most common reason for ligament and tendon injuries in the horse.[36] Strain-induced injuries are believed to occur after a phase of molecular degeneration or inflammation that is not clinically evident nor produces any reparative responses, but instead progressively weakens the structure.[36] Detection of asymptomatic lesions in postmortem studies of normal horses are consistent with this observation.[40] Furthermore, many strain-induced tendinopathies are bilateral.[14] Large studies analyzing epidemiologic data

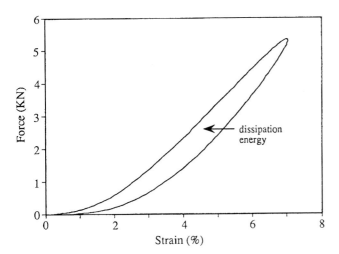

Figure 7.73. Loading of the SDFT, revealing the hysteresis loop. The area within the loop represents the energy lost during one loading and unloading cycle. (From Goodship AE, Burch HL, Wilson AM. The pathobiology and repair of tendon and ligament injury. Vet Clin North Am Equine Pract 1994;10:335.)

in both horses and humans have shown strong correlations between age and injury rate.[23] Experimental studies and postmortem analyses of normal tendons have indicated that increasing age and exercise may induce tendon matrix degeneration instead of adaptation in the adult horse.[14,37]

Tendinopathies often begin with degeneration. Minor changes in the structural integrity predispose an already high-risk structure to injury. When the structural integrity is overwhelmed, irreversible damage ensues.[14] Palmar structures, especially at the heel, sustain load increases during heel strike, quickly placing the SDFT and suspensory ligament (SL) at risk.[20] Conversely, load of the DDFT rises during stance.

Physical disruption occurs within the tendon matrix when structural strength is overcome. Various structural breakdowns may occur, including fibrillar stretching with breakage of cross links, fibrillar rupture, or in severe cases, separation of tendon tissue.[14] Once this occurs, the damage signals repair processes that are common throughout the body such as inflammation followed by repair mechanisms (see phases of healing).

The risk of strain-induced injury is increased by factors such as the horse's speed, track surface (the harder the track, the higher the risk of injury), the horse's weight, fatigue level, and shoeing. Increased heel elevation has been demonstrated to be protective for the DDFT, but it increases the extension of the MCP joint.[3] Although low heels have been viewed as protective of SDFT tendinitis, epidemiologic studies have correlated an increased risk of tendon and ligament injuries with a low heel and long toe conformation.[14]

Tearing of the tendon also occurs, although with much less frequency than tendon degeneration. The most common site is the DDFT of the forelimb, and occasionally the manica flexoria of the hindlimb. The mechanism of injury is not clear; however, it has been hypothesized that hyperextension of the fetlock canal combined with compression of the DDFT as it passes over the palmar aspect of the joint may predispose the

structure to injury.[14] The hindlimb manica tears may be a result of ongoing tenosynovitis that frequently occurs in the tendon sheath of the hindlimb combined with hyperextension in that region.

The third common mechanism for tendon and ligament injury is percutaneous trauma. The distal limbs have minimal soft tissue coverage and commonly sustain contusion. Injuries resulting from wire, kicks, blunt trauma, and overreaching contribute to most of the percutaneous injuries seen. The most serious include those to the palmar/plantar region of the limb and tendon lacerations that are from wire. Common locations of tendon lacerations are the mid-cannon area of the hindlimb and the pastern region (including the tendon sheath) of both the front and hindlimb. These injuries often result in moderate to severe adhesion formation and a poor return to athleticism.

EFFECT OF AGING AND EXERCISE ON TENDON INJURY

Recently, a number of controlled studies in young and adult horses have elucidated the effect of exercise on developing and mature tendons.[8,15,24] Subjects used in these studies had no evidence of previous tendinitis nor any evidence of tendinitis induced by the exercise protocols.

Histological analysis revealed that local differences occurred in collagen fiber diameter of older but not younger exercised horses.[30] In adult tendon, a reduction in crimp occurred with aging and exercise. Exercise also induced a greater number of smaller fibrils within the central region of the SDFT. This change did not correlate with new collagen formation, indicating that an adaptive response occurred rather than an elevation in collagen.

Molecular composition changes also occurred with exercise. A reduction in GAG content and loss of COMP occurred in the center of the tendon with long-term exercise.[5] This is in contrast to an increase in GAG and type III collagen found in the SDFT of exercising horses whose tendons were collected postmortem. Because damage to these tendons was thought to result from subclinical tendon degeneration, these molecular changes most likely reflect a response to injury (or a reparative response) rather than a degenerative change associated with age and/or exercise.

Similar to cartilage, a lack of load to tendon results in a deficit of COMP levels within the tendon. However, once adequate COMP has accumulated within tendons, loading does not appear to affect the COMP levels.[36] Clinically, this implies that a deficit of exercise in the developing tendon may likely result in a tendon prone to injury due to a poorer quality of matrix since COMP levels are directly correlated to tendon strength. In contrast, too much exercise may also result in tendon injury if the strain levels of the tendon are exceeded.[8]

Exercise studies suggest that as tendon ages, degenerative changes associated with exercise accelerate. Cellular activity decreases and most likely collagen turnover slows. Growth factors such as TGF-β also decrease, which may lead to a reduced ability of the tendon to undergo a reparative response. Furthermore, less adaptive changes may occur following maturity, as

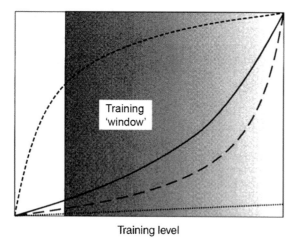

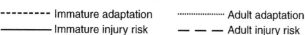

-------- Immature adaptation   ⋯⋯⋯⋯ Adult adaptation
————— Immature injury risk   — — — Adult injury risk

Figure 7.74. A representation of the adaptive and injury risk for growing (immature) and adult (older than 2 years of age) equine digital flexor tendons. (From Smith RKW. Pathophysiology of tendon injury. In Diagnosis and Management of Lameness in the Horse, Ross MW and Dyson SJ, eds. WB Saunders, Philadelphia, 2003, pg 624).

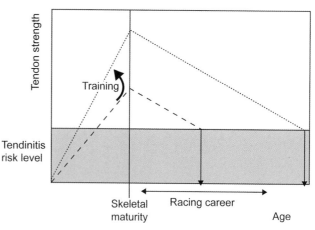

Figure 7.75. A diagram of an approach to tendinitis prevention. The dotted line represents a horse with strong tendons, in contrast to the dashed line, which represents a horse that has poor-quality tendons at skeletal maturity (approximately 2 years old). The horse with poor-quality tendons sustains tendinitis during its racing career due to cumulative fatigue damage to the tendon, whereas the horse with strong tendons, although sustaining the same degeneration, begins at a stronger point and does not suffer from tendinitis. Introduction of exercise throughout development improves tendon quality (arrow), potentially decreasing the incidence of tendinitis. (From Smith RKW. Pathophysiology of tendon injury. In Diagnosis and Management of Lameness in the Horse, Ross MW and Dyson SJ, eds. WB Saunders, Philadelphia, 2003, pg 624).

evidenced by epidemiological data in horses and humans that draw a strong correlation between age and exercise and the incidence of tendon injury.[36] Conversely, young, growing tendon appears to be much more adaptive and responsive to loading and exercise, especially during the early stages of growth.

Among the unknown factors are the level and amount of work necessary to initiate the response. The natural exercise intensity of foals at play may be ideal to allow strain rates that boost tendon matrix production. Figure 7.74 is a hypothesized schematic representation of adaptive responses to injury in mature and immature tendon. Figure 7.75 is a strategy for preventing tendinitis in the horse, focusing on tendinitis risk before and after skeletal maturity.

MECHANISMS OF TENDON DEGENERATION

Mechanisms of tendon degeneration may have several etiologies including mechanical, physical, vascular, and inflammatory. Mechanical influences such as overextension or direct low-grade repetitive forces cause fatigue and microdamage, leading to degeneration. This also predisposes the tendon to clinical tendinitis when an acute supra-maximal load is applied.

Hyperthermia during exercise is a physical influence that may predispose tendon to injury. Studies have determined that temperatures up to 45°C occur secondary to galloping.[43] These temperatures are high enough to damage most other tissue types; however, *in vitro* experiments have revealed that tenocytes may resist these increases.[7] Nevertheless, the hyperemia that occurs in tendon at high speeds may damage the tenocytes or even the extracellular matrix.

Vascular disturbances are also hypothesized to contribute to tendon damage. When tendon is maximally loaded, blood flow is limited or abolished due to the compressive forces generated.[36] This may lead to a relative hypoxic state of the tendon, predisposing the tissue to degeneration. Although certain areas of tendon have poor perfusion, there is histologic evidence of an adaptive state to ischemia because fewer cells exist in these areas (i.e., the dorsal surface of the DDFT in the area of the fetlock), and matrix components in ischemic areas have compression-resistant components. In addition, these areas may receive nutrition from synovial fluid components.

Despite a reduction in blood flow to certain areas of tendon such as the DDFT in the area of the fetlock, these regions seem to be resistant to degeneration except in the most severe cases of tendinitis. Furthermore, studies have shown that mechanically reducing oxidative metabolism does not lead to abnormal cell proliferation.[6] Therefore, tenocytes, and tendons and ligaments in general, may be resistant to hypoxia compared to other tissues in the body. Although resistance may exist, however, generation of toxic free radicals predisposes the tendon to degeneration. This mechanism of injury may occur as a result of reperfusion injury when perfusion is restored.

Finally, mechanical, vascular and hyperthermic environments may all lead to the release of proteolytic enzymes such as collagenase or aggrecanase that promote tendon degeneration. Elevations in these proteolytic enzymes result in a slowed matrix synthesis and an elevation in degradation, whereby overall degradation is high.[13,17,31]

In summary, tendon degeneration results from many factors that contribute to matrix and cellular abnormalities. Ultimately, the resident cell population cannot repair microdamage that is most likely due to deficient or absent growth factor stimuli (such as TGF-β) and cellular senescence within the tendon.[19] As loading continues and strain increases, failure of the fibrils occurs and results in tendon damage.

RESPONSE OF TENDONS AND LIGAMENTS TO INJURY: PHASES OF HEALING

When tendons and ligaments are damaged, the process of repair follows 3 stages of healing: the acute inflammatory phase, the subacute reparative phase, and the chronic remodeling phase. A subclinical phase of degeneration also exists; however, this phase is difficult to detect by clinical or ultrasonographic exam due to the minimal inflammatory reaction.

The initial inflammatory phase begins with an acute and substantial inflammatory response. The degree of inflammation depends on the severity of lesion and anti-inflammatory drugs that may be administered. This phase usually lasts 1 to 2 weeks and is characterized by intratendinous hemorrhage and edema, an increase in blood supply, leukocytes (initially neutrophils and then macrophages and monocytes), and proteolytic enzymes if unabated. Proteolytic enzyme release removes necrotic collagen; however, if the enzymes are not reduced with NSAID administration, their presence will result in expansion of the lesion within the inflammatory stage.

The subacute reparative phase peaks approximately 3 weeks following the initial injury.[36] This phase overlaps with the inflammatory phase and is marked by angiogenesis and the infiltration of fibroblasts in the damaged tissue. Fibroblasts originate from tendon, endotenon, and paratenon, and are also delivered from the vascular origin.[9] Scar tissue is formed from the fibroblasts, which are characterized by randomly arranged collagen that is initially type III. Similar to cartilage repair, the resulting scar tissue is weaker than the original tendon tissue, and therefore predisposed to re-injury at the original site of injury. When re-injury occurs, the inflammatory and reparative phases of healing are perpetuated, furthering the damage within the tendon.[36]

The poor healing response of tendon in areas of poor blood supply and paratenon may be explained by a lack of migration of fibroblasts. Adhesions are formed following tendon injury, and although detrimental, they allow healing factors to contribute to injured tissue. Therefore, although adhesions restrict movement of tendon, they allow tendon to form reparative tissue.[36]

The chronic remodeling phase consists of a slow conversion of type III collagen to type I collagen. This process occurs over several months, and the original tendon strength is never restored. Loading (exercise) that ensues in a controlled manner enhances conversion of type III to type I collagen. It improves the alignment of the collagen fibrils in the direction of force and results in better mechanical tendon strength.

Controlled exercise programs are integral to every successful tendon rehabilitation program. It is impor-

Table 7.2. A standard exercise program recommended following tendon injury. This protocol can be modified based upon ultrasound recheck examinations.

Exercise level	Week	Duration and nature of exercise
0	0–2	Box rest
1	3	10 minutes walking daily
1	4	15 minutes walking daily
1	5	20 minutes walking daily
1	6	25 minutes walking daily
1	7	30 minutes walking daily
1	8	35 minutes walking daily
1	9	40 minutes walking daily
1	10–12	45 minutes walking daily
Week 12: Repeat ultrasound examination		
2	13–16	40 minutes walking and 5 minutes trotting daily
2	17–20	35 minutes walking and 10 minutes trotting daily
2	21–24	30 minutes walking and 15 minutes trotting daily
Week 24: Repeat ultrasound examination		
3	25–28	25 minutes walking and 20 minutes trotting daily
3	29–32	20 minutes walking and 25 minutes trotting daily
Week 32: Repeat ultrasound examination		
4	33–40	45 minutes exercise daily, gradually increasing in amount
4	41–48	45 minutes exercise daily with fast work 3 times a week
Week 48: Repeat ultrasound examination		
5	48+	Return to full competition/race training

(Davis CS, Smith RKW. Equine Surgery. Auer JA, Stick JA, eds. Saunders, Philadelphia, 2006: 1110.)

tant to use ultrasound therapy and modify the exercise program based upon the quality of repair. Table 7.2 illustrates a standard rehabilitation program with ultrasound re-examination at specified times.

Re-injury is common following repair of tendons and ligaments; it has been reported to occur in 8% to 43% of racehorses.[16] Furthermore, the contralateral tendon or ligament also may become injured.[14] Although the strength of the remodeled tendon is improved 15 to 18 months following injury, the resulting elasticity is severely weakened, leading to elevated strains in the undamaged tendon. It is this tissue that often becomes damaged when re-injury occurs. Furthermore, if the SDFT is damaged and lengthened through the damage, the suspensory ligament may sustain microdamage and eventual injury due to increased strains.[23]

The basic goals of treatment programs are to initially minimize the acute inflammatory phase, thereby decreasing the ongoing damage of tendinous inflammation and edema. Next, the goals are to implement therapies that improve collagen type I and extracellular matrix production, thereby strengthening the tendon so that the structure can withstand the mechanical forces that it encountered before the initial injury. Finally, the adhesions that may form in the healing phases significantly reduce athletic function due to pain and lameness. Therefore, minimizing inflammation, enhancing regeneration, and controlling exercise optimize the chances of successful healing of tendons. For more detail on intralesional therapies, see Chapter 8.

MONITORING TENDON INJURY

Ultrasound examination remains the gold standard for monitoring tendinopathies. Clinical examination, while important, does not detect subtle changes and provides a poor objective assessment. Tendons and ligaments should be evaluated initially at the time of injury and then approximately 1 week following the injury due the frequent occurrence of expansion of the lesion in the first week. The prognosis for return to athleticism is determined by the appearance in the initial week.

The ultrasound exam is performed after clipping the hair and washing the limb to obtain the highest quality image. Transverse and linear images should be obtained and images should be recorded in a methodical fashion so that the images are accurately recorded. For example, during the examination, the limbs are divided into 7 subunits or, alternatively, the images are recorded as distance from the accessory carpal bones. Although one limb is almost always affected more severely than the others, ultrasound examinations should be done bilaterally due to the common occurrence of bilateral disease, especially in strain-induced tendon injury.

Ultrasound changes frequently associated with acute tendinopathy include enlargement, hypoechogenicity, alterations in tendon striated pattern viewed in the longitudinal images, and alterations in shape and margins (Figure 7.76).[14] Chronic tendinopathies are associated with enlargements or changes in echogenicity, and irregularities in striations observed on the longitudinal view.

BIOMARKERS FOR TENDON DISEASE

The field of biomarkers is of keen interest to many clinicians and researchers. Accurate detection of subclinical disease contributes to improved prevention of a common career-ending disease. Furthermore, early detection of disease enables more tailored rehabilitation programs and altered training regimens. Ultrasound remains the gold standard of detection,[18] permitting a more accurate reflection of cellular disease and sensitivity to subtle changes in the tissue state. Biomarkers that detect the stage of disease may also predict optimal treatment and rehabilitation protocols and evaluate their efficacy.

Markers that have been studied intensively include collagen synthesis (carboxy-terminal propeptide of type I collagen or PICP) and degradation (cross linked carboxyterminal telopeptide of type I collagen or ICTP) after tendon injury.[14,21] Significant elevations in PICP concentrations have been associated with tendinitis, whereas ICTP has been unchanged in control groups. These changes reflect the ability of serum concentrations of PICP to reveal disease of tendons and indicate that these markers are not necessary bone-specific.

COMP has also been intensively studied in tendon disease.[35] In one study, synovial fluid levels within tendon sheaths were significantly higher when tendons were damaged or sheaths were septic. However, serum levels were unaffected due to naturally high levels of COMP in blood. Although COMP appears to be a good marker in laboratory analysis of disease, it may not be an accurate marker for specific tendon disease.

COMMON CLINICAL CONDITIONS OF TENDONS AND LIGAMENTS

The most common tendon affected in tendinopathies is the SDFT. Although the lesion may be focal or generalized, it is usually centrally located in the tendon, just below the mid-metacarpal region of the limb. It can be focal or it may extend throughout the length of the tendon, giving rise to a palmar swelling of the metacarpal region (bowed tendon) (Figure 7.77). The section of the SDFT enclosed within the tendon sheath is affected much less often.

Desmitis of the accessory ligament of the DDFT can occur in association with superficial flexor tendinitis. Ponies have been observed to have a higher incidence of desmitis of the accessory ligament, while rarely experiencing superficial flexor tendinitis.[14] Lameness is usually much less severe than with superficial flexor tendinitis and swelling is often restricted to the proximal half of the metacarpus, immediately dorsal to the SDFT.

The suspensory ligament may sustain a desmitis along any section. Proximal suspensory desmitis (in both the front and hindlimb) is often restricted to that region, whereas midbody or branch lesions may occur concurrently or extend into each area. Branch lesions also may be found within the MCP joint and result in synovial effusion and lameness requiring arthroscopic debridement.[28] Synovial fluid may decrease the healing of these lesions, as well.[14] With severe suspensory desmitis, the limb may have a characteristic dropped fetlock either standing or at the walk due to decreased support of the fetlock.

The DDFT is more frequently associated with tendinitis within the digital tendon sheath, especially of the hindlimb (Figure 7.78).[33,41,46] These lesions may be a result of single excessive load cycles.[14] Two manifestations are typically observed with 1 lesion found within the substance of the tendon and the second found more

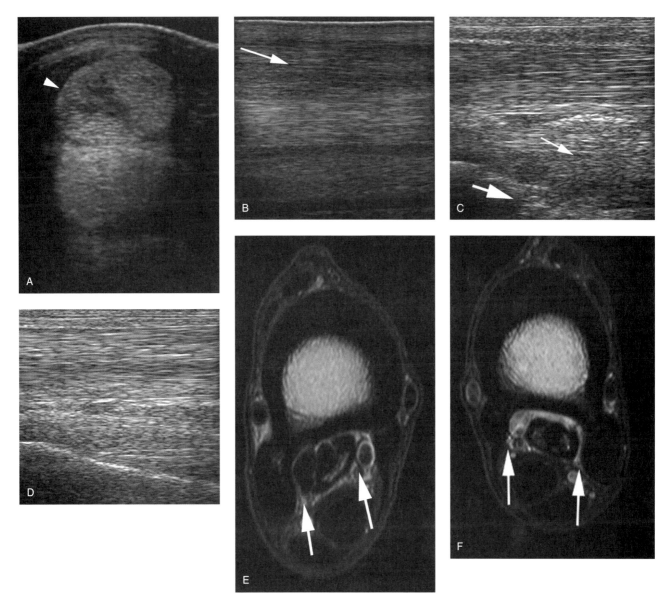

Figure 7.76. Examples of variations of tendon and ligament injuries detected on ultrasound or MRI examination. A. Enlargement and tearing of a SDFT (horizontal image). B. A longitudinal ultrasound image revealing tendon fiber disruption of the SDFT. C. Fiber and bone disruption (large arrow) of a proximal hind suspensory ligament (small arrow, ligament viewed longitudinally) in comparison to (D). D. A normal proximal hindlimb suspensory ligament. E. MRI examination of the disrupted and enlarged hind suspensory ligament (between arrows). F. MRI of the normal suspensory ligament of the contralateral limb. Note the space (white area) around the suspensory ligament, which is normal. (Images A and B courtesy of Dr. Natasha Werpy.)

in the periphery (medial and lateral borders) of the tendon, usually in the region of the MCP/MTP joint.[46] Invariably, these lesions result in synovial effusion of the digital sheath, with peripheral lesions being more difficult to detect with ultrasound.

Other tendon and ligaments may sustain strain-induced injury, although the frequency of strain to the palmar soft tissue structures of the metacarpus is much more common. Ligament injuries are much more common when the joint they support (and span) is inappropriately overloaded. When this occurs, desmitis and more seriously, subluxation or luxation, can result (Figure 7.79).

COMMON CLINICAL CHARACTERISTICS OF TENDON LACERATIONS

Complete loss of support of specific tendons leads to characteristic stances of the limb, which often helps the clinician determine which structure has been affected by the stance of the horse (Figure 7.80). When the SDFT is completely transected, the MCP/MTP joint is often hyperextended (dropped) when the limb is loaded but may be symmetrical to the contralateral limb in the standing horse. If the DDFT is lacerated alone or in addition to the SDFT, the toe will rise off of the ground when the limb is loaded. If the SL is completely

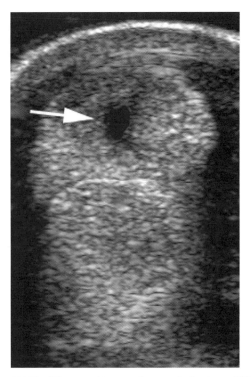

Figure 7.77. Ultrasound image of a core lesion in an SDFT. The arrow is pointing to the core lesion within the SDFT. (Courtesy of Dr. Natasha Werpy.)

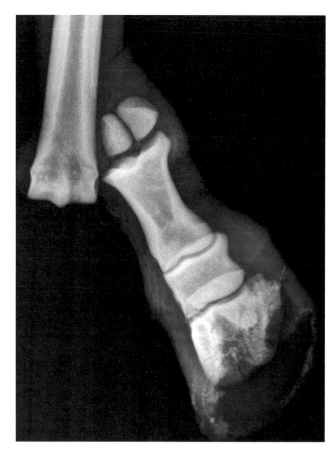

Figure 7.79. Radiograph of a complete fetlock luxation demonstrating failure of the collateral ligaments.

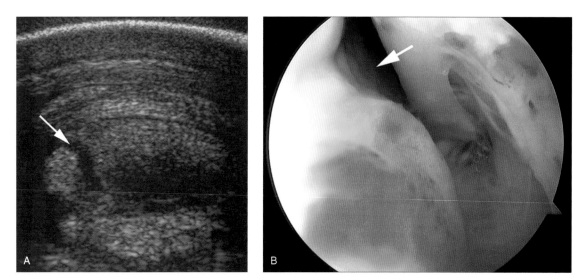

Figure 7.78. Ultrasound image of the DDFT with a linear tear located within the tendon sheath at the level of the fetlock (A) and the corresponding tenoscopic image (B). The arrow in both images points to the tear.

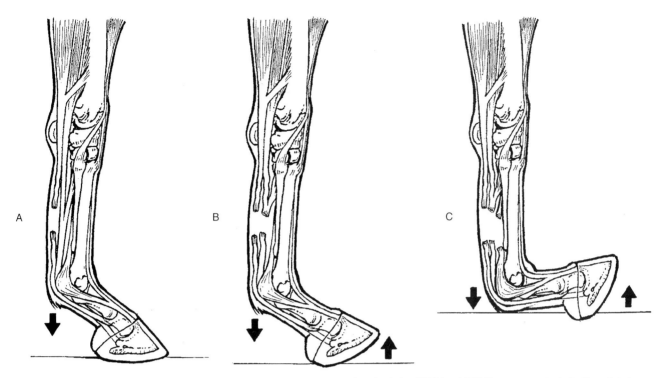

Figure 7.80. A. The amount of hyperextension of the metacarpophalangeal joint when the SDFT has been transected proximal to the joint. This amount of dropped fetlock also may be noted when there is a severe desmitis of the suspensory ligament. B. Hyperextension of the fetlock joint and elevation of the toe when both the SDFT and DDFT are transected. C. Complete loss of metacarpophalangeal joint support when both digital flexor tendons and the suspensory ligament have been disrupted. (From Davis CS, Smith RKW. Equine Surgery. Auer JA, Stick JA, eds. Saunders, Philadelphia, 2006, page 1098.)

transected in addition to the SDFT and the DDFT, there may be complete loss of the support of the MCP/MTP joint, resulting in complete contact of the joint to the ground. This often results in severe distress to the horse.

Lacerations to the extensor tendons frequently involve the metacarpal and metatarsal regions. Frequently the common and lateral extensor tendons are transected when lacerations to the front limb occur. These injuries usually do not cause severe lameness but interrupt the horse's ability to protract the limb and sufficiently place the foot flat on the ground in the cranial stride. This often leads to stumbling and distress if the limb is not splinted.[25] The prognosis for these injuries is usually favorable.[4,27] Lacerations to the proximal tarsus may involve the cranialis tibialis, long digital extensor tendon, or peroneus tertius tendon. More specific descriptions of tendon and ligament injuries are found in Chapter 5 based on the specific location of the injury.

References

1. Alexander RM. Energy-saving mechanisms in walking and running. J Exp Biol 1991;160:55–69:55–69.
2. Banes AJ, Tsuzaki M, Yamamoto J, et al. Mechanoreception at the cellular level: the detection, interpretation, and diversity of responses to mechanical signals. Biochem Cell Biol 1995; 73:349–365.
3. Barber SM. Arthrodesis of the distal intertarsal and tarsometatarsal joints in the horse. Vet Surg 1984;13:227–235.
4. Belknap JK, Baxter GM, Nickels FA. Extensor tendon lacerations in horses: 50 cases (1982–1988). J Am Vet Med Assoc 1993; 203:428–431.
5. Birch HL, Bailey AJ, Goodship AE. Macroscopic 'degeneration' of equine superficial digital flexor tendon is accompanied by a change in extracellular matrix composition. Equine Vet Journal 1998;30, 534–539.
6. Birch HL, Rutter GA, Goodship AE. Oxidative energy metabolism in equine tendon cells. Res Vet Sci 1997;62:93–97.
7. Birch HL, Wilson AM, Goodship AE. The effect of exercise-induced localised hyperthermia on tendon cell survival. J Exp Biol 1997;200:1703–1708.
8. Cherdchutham W, Becker C, Smith RK, et al. Age-related changes and effect of exercise on the molecular composition of immature equine superficial digital flexor tendons. Equine Vet J Suppl 1999;86–94.
9. Clegg PD, Strassburg S, Smith RK. Cell phenotypic variation in normal and damaged tendons. Int J Exp Pathol 2007;88: 227–235.
10. Dahlgren LA, Mohammed HO, Nixon AJ. Temporal expression of growth factors and matrix molecules in healing tendon lesions. J Orthop Res 2005;23:84–92.
11. Dahlgren LA, Mohammed HO, Nixon AJ. Expression of insulin-like growth factor binding proteins in healing tendon lesions. J Orthop Res 2006;24:183–192.
12. Dahlgren LA, van der Meulen MC, Bertram JE, et al. Insulin-like growth factor-I improves cellular and molecular aspects of healing in a collagenase-induced model of flexor tendinitis. J Orthop Res 2002;20:910–919.
13. Dalton S, Cawston TE, Riley GP, et al. Human shoulder tendon biopsy samples in organ culture produce procollagenase and tissue inhibitor of metalloproteinases. Ann Rheum Dis 1995;54: 571–577.
14. Davis CS, Smith RKW. Diagnosis and management of tendon and ligament disorders. In Equine Surgery. Auer JA, Stick JA, eds. Saunders, Philadelphia, 2006;1086–1110.
15. Dowling BA, Dart AJ. Mechanical and functional properties of the equine superficial digital flexor tendon. Vet J 2005;170: 184–192.
16. Dowling BA, Dart AJ, Hodgson DR, Smith RK. Superficial digital flexor tendinitis in the horse. Equine Vet J 2000;32:369–378.

17. Fortier LA, Smith RK. Regenerative medicine for tendinous and ligamentous injuries of sport horses. Vet Clin North Am Equine Pract 2008;24:191–201.
18. Genovese RL, Rantanen NW, Hauser ML, et al. Diagnostic ultrasonography of equine limbs. Vet Clin North Am (Equine Pract) 1986;2:145–226.
19. Goodman SA, May SA, Heinegard D, et al. Tenocyte response to cyclical strain and transforming growth factor beta is dependent upon age and site of origin. Biorheology 2004;41:613–628.
20. Goodship AE, Birch HL, Wilson AM. The pathobiology and repair of tendon and ligament injury. Vet Clin North Am (Equine Pract) 1994;10:323–349.
21. Jackson BF, Goodship AE, Eastell R, et al. Evaluation of serum concentrations of biochemical markers of bone metabolism and insulin-like growth factor I associated with treadmill exercise in young horses. Am J Vet Res 2003;64:1549–1556.
22. Kadler KE, Holmes DF, Graham H, et al. Tip-mediated fusion involving unipolar collagen fibrils accounts for rapid fibril elongation, the occurrence of fibrillar branched networks in skin and the paucity of collagen fibril ends in vertebrates. Matrix Biol 2000;19:359–365.
23. Kasashima Y, Takahashi T, Smith RK, et al. Prevalence of superficial digital flexor tendinitis and suspensory desmitis in Japanese Thoroughbred flat racehorses in 1999. Equine Vet J 2004;36: 346–350.
24. Lin YL, Brama PA, Kiers GH, et al. Functional adaptation through changes in regional biochemical characteristics during maturation of equine superficial digital flexor tendons. Am J Vet Res 2005;66:1623–1629.
25. McIlwraith CW. Diseases of joints, tendons, ligaments, and related structures. In Adams' Lameness in Horses. Stashak TS, ed. Lippincott Williams and Wilkins, Philadelphia, 2002; 459–644.
26. McNeilly CM, Banes AJ, Benjamin M, et al. Tendon cells *in vivo* form a three-dimensional network of cell processes linked by gap junctions. J Anat 1996;189:593–600.
27. Mespoulhes-Riviere C, Martens A, Bogaert L, et al. Factors affecting outcome of extensor tendon lacerations in the distal limb of horses. A retrospective study of 156 cases (1994–2003). Vet Comp Orthop Traumatol 2008;21:358–364.
28. Minshall GJ, Wright IM. Arthroscopic diagnosis and treatment of intra-articular insertional injuries of the suspensory ligament branches in 18 horses. Equine Vet J 2006;38:10–14.
29. Patterson-Kane JC, Firth EC, Goodship AE, et al. Age-related differences in collagen crimp patterns in the superficial digital flexor tendon core region of untrained horses. Aust Vet J 1997;75:39–44.
30. Patterson-Kane JC, Wilson AM, Firth EC, et al. Comparison of collagen fibril populations in the superficial digital flexor tendons of exercised and nonexercised Thoroughbreds. Equine Vet J 1997;29,121–125.
31. Rees SG, Flannery CR, Little CB, et al. Catabolism of aggrecan, decorin and biglycan in tendon. Biochem J 2000;350 Pt 1:181–8:181–188.
32. Riemersma DJ, van den Bogert AJ, Jansen MO, et al. Tendon strain in the forelimbs as a function of gait and ground characteristics and *in vitro* limb loading in ponies. Equine Vet J 1996;28:133–138.
33. Smith MR, Wright IM. Noninfected tenosynovitis of the digital flexor tendon sheath: a retrospective analysis of 76 cases. Equine Vet J 2006;38:134–141.
34. Smith RK, Gerard M, Dowling B, et al. Correlation of cartilage oligomeric matrix protein (COMP) levels in equine tendon with mechanical properties: a proposed role for COMP in determining function-specific mechanical characteristics of locomotor tendons. Equine Vet J Suppl 2002;241–244.
35. Smith RK, Heinegard D. Cartilage oligomeric matrix protein (COMP) levels in digital sheath synovial fluid and serum with tendon injury. Equine Vet J 2000;32:52–58.
36. Smith RKW. Pathophysiology of tendon injury. In Lameness in the Horse. Ross MW, Dyson SJ, eds. Saunders, Philadelphia, 2003;616–628.
37. Smith RKW, Webbon PM. The physiology of normal tendon and ligament. Proceedings, Dubai International Equine Symposium. 1996;55–81.
38. Smith RKW, Zunino L, Webbon PM, et al. The distribution of cartilage oligomeric matrix protein (COMP) in tendon and its variation with tendon site, age and load. Matrix Biology 1997;16,255–271.
39. Sodersten F, Ekman S, Eloranta ML, et al. Ultrastructural immunolocalization of cartilage oligomeric matrix protein (COMP) in relation to collagen fibrils in the equine tendon. Matrix Biol 2005;24:376–385.
40. Webbon PM. A postmortem study of equine digital flexor tendons. Equine Vet J 1977;9:61–67.
41. Wilderjans H, Boussauw B, Madder K, et al. Tenosynovitis of the digital flexor tendon sheath and annular ligament constriction syndrome caused by longitudinal tears in the deep digital flexor tendon: a clinical and surgical report of 17 cases in Warmblood horses. Equine Vet J 2003;35:270–275.
42. Wilmink J, Wilson AM, Goodship AE. Functional significance of the morphology and micromechanics of collagen fibres in relation to partial rupture of the superficial digital flexor tendon in racehorses. Research Vet Science 1992;53, 354–359.
43. Wilson AM, Goodship AE. Exercise-induced hyperthermia as a possible mechanism for tendon degeneration. J Biomech 1994;27:899–905.
44. Wilson AM, van den Bogert AJ, McGuigan MP. Skeletal muscle mechanics: from mechanisms to function. John Wiley and Sons, Chichester, England, 2000.
45. Woo SL. Mechanical properties of tendons and ligaments. I. Quasi-static and nonlinear viscoelastic properties. Biorheology 1982;19:385–396.
46. Wright IM, McMahon PJ. Tenosynovitis associated with longitudinal tears of the digital flexor tendons in horses: a report of 20 cases. Equine Vet J 1999;31:12–18.

MUSCLE INJURIES AND DISEASE

Stephanie J. Valberg

CLASSIFICATION OF MUSCLE DISORDERS

A muscle disorder is usually suspected because of altered muscle tone, weakness and/or exercise intolerance, muscle atrophy, muscle pain or swelling, or a gait abnormality not attributed to skeletal/tendon or ligamentous structures.

Altered Muscle Tone and Weakness

Increased muscle tone may result from sustained motor unit activity (e.g., ear ticks), dampened reflex inhibition by spinal interneurons (e.g., tetanus), persistent stimulation of nerve branches within a muscle belly (e.g., cramps), altered sarcolemmal ion channel function (e.g., myotonia and HYPP), or persistent contractures from increased myoplasmic calcium (e.g., exertional rhabdomyolysis). A full review of these disorders can be obtained elsewhere.[71]

Decreased muscle tone and weakness may be due to a decreased number of functional motor neurons (e.g., equine motor neuron disease), decreased neurotransmitter release at motor-end plates (e.g., botulism), marked loss of muscle mass (e.g., atrophy), altered depolarization of muscle/nerve membranes (hypokalemia), or impaired generation of adenosine triphosphate for muscle contracture (polysaccharide storage myopathy). When the few operative motor units fatigue, muscle fasciculations, shifting of weight, low head posture, prolonged recumbency, and difficulty rising may result. A full review of these disorders can be obtained elsewhere.[71]

Serum creatine kinase (CK) activity is usually normal or mildly elevated with most cases of altered muscle tone because little damage to muscle cell membranes occurs.

Muscle Atrophy

Gross muscle atrophy is the end result of a reduction in the diameter or cross-sectional area of muscle fibers. Denervation (neurogenic atrophy) results in fairly rapid atrophy because the normal low-level tonic neural stimulus that is necessary to maintain muscle fiber mass is absent. Complete denervation of a muscle results in more than a loss of 50% of muscle mass within 2 to 3 weeks.[17,33] Denervation can be focal (e.g., sweeney suprascapular nerve damage causes supraspinatus/infraspinatus atrophy) or generalized with slower progression (e.g., equine motor neuron disease).

Muscle biopsies of denervation atrophy are characterized by small, angular, slow-twitch type 1 and fast-twitch type 2 fibers with concave sides and pyknotic nuclear clumps. In some cases, hypertrophy of remaining motor units may occur and renervation is indicated by target fibers and fiber type grouping. Focal denerva-

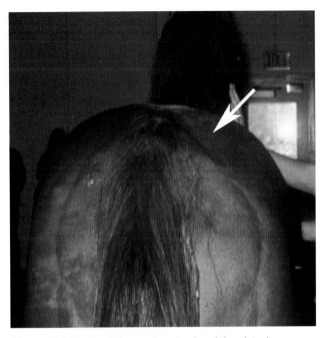

Figure 7.81. Focal denervation atrophy of the gluteal musculature (arrow) that was attributed to nerve root trauma. (Courtesy of Dr. Gary Baxter.)

tion atrophy may occur due to nerve trauma (Figure 7.81) or focal ventral spinal cord infection from equine protozoal myelitis. Degeneration of a peripheral nerve fiber progresses to the nearest node of Ranvier proximal to the site of injury. If the injury is mild, then most nerves can regenerate (at about 4 mm/day) and the original continuity to the muscle can be re-established. However, if the nerve injury is severe (e.g., transection), regrowth of the nerve to the muscle is delayed and may never occur. Furthermore, if concurrent muscle atrophy is severe, even if a functional connection is made, there may only be a limited number of fibers available for renervation. Generalized denervation atrophy occurs with diseases such as equine motor neuron disease and peripheral neuropathies.

Muscle atrophy can be myogenic in origin, resulting from disuse, malnutrition, hypovitaminosis E, cachexia, corticosteroid excess, severe rhabdomyolysis, type 2 polysaccharide storage myopathy (PSSM), and immune-mediated myositis (Figure 7.82). Disuse, malnutrition, cachexia, and corticosteroid excess are characterized by slow onset of atrophy over months of exclusively type 2 fast twitch muscle fibers and normal serum CK. Rhabdomyolysis and type 2 PSSM show marked elevations in serum CK activity and moderate onset of atrophy over a few weeks. In contrast, immune-mediated myositis shows rapid loss of 30% of muscle

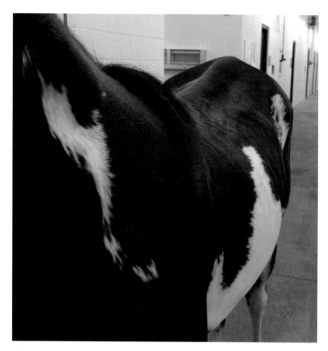

Figure 7.82. A young Paint horse with severe symmetrical epaxial and gluteal atrophy as a result of immune-mediated myositis.

mass over the topline within 48 hours (Figure 7.82), has lymphocytic infiltrates in biopsies of the atrophied muscle, and horses have elevated serum CK activity.[38] More information on immune-mediated myopathies can be obtained elsewhere.[71]

Muscle Pain, Swelling, Cramping, and Contracture

Trauma to skeletal muscle may damage the cellular architecture to a point at which regeneration of damaged myofiber segments is impossible and fibrosis results. This occurs with extensive physical trauma, prolonged compression, and ischemia. Muscles often initially appear swollen under these circumstances and as edema dissipates, atrophy appears. Muscle will regenerate over time unless muscle architecture is severely disrupted.

Many exertional causes of rhabdomyolysis result in segmental necrosis of muscle fibers with a preserved basement membrane. Segments of myofibers show segmental loss of cross-striations of contractile proteins, disruption of mitochondrial and sarcolemmal membranes, and vacuolar degeneration. Within 48 to 72 hours macrophages infiltrate and remove necrotic debris, which is followed by satellite cells migrating along the intact basement membrane to form regenerative myotubes within 3 to 4 days of injury. Regenerative fibers are basophilic with prominent central myonuclei, which eventually move to a normal peripheral location as myofilaments are produced and aligned. Mature muscle fibers form within a month of the original damage.[17]

Muscle pain with myonecrosis may or may not be present depending on whether painful contractures develop. Contractures are usually the result of a cellular energy deficit (PSSM) or sarcoplasmic reticulum ion channel defect (malignant hyperthermia, RER) that impair myofilament relaxation. Serum creatine kinase (CK) activity is elevated when muscle cell membranes are damaged and muscle biopsies show evidence of muscle fiber degeneration and potentially regeneration.

Gait Abnormalities

Horses with trauma or atrophy of individual muscle groups may show an asymmetric lameness. Those with generalized muscle soreness or myopathies affecting energy metabolism may show evidence of a mildly asymmetric gait, shifting lameness, poor performance under saddle, progressive stiffness, or inability to engage the hindquarters. Serum CK activities can range from normal to markedly elevated in such cases. Myopathies and skeletal/ligamentous causes of lameness often occur concurrently.

DIAGNOSIS OF SPECIFIC MUSCLE DISORDERS

Many times a complete examination of the musculoskeletal and neurologic systems is required to diagnose a myopathy. Myopathies can change the horse's movement to a point that lameness develops, and lameness can change muscle function to the point that soreness develops. Both possibilities should be considered. In addition, neurologic causes of muscle weakness, atrophy, and gait changes should also be fully evaluated. The topics below are key components of the examination of skeletal muscle.

History

A history of stiffness, muscle cramping, pain, muscle fasciculations, exercise intolerance, undiagnosed lameness, weakness, or muscle atrophy may all indicate a muscle disorder. Further characterization requires a detailed account of the horse's performance level, exercise schedule, previous lameness, diet, vaccination history, signs of respiratory disease, duration, severity and frequency of muscle problem, any factors that initiate the muscle problem, and all medications with which the horse is being treated.

Physical Examination

A detailed evaluation of the muscular system includes inspection of the horse for symmetry of muscle mass while standing with forelimbs and hindlimbs exactly square. Any evidence of fine tremors or fasciculations should be noted before palpating the animal. Horses originating in the Southwestern United States that have muscle pain and fasciculations should have their ears examined with an otoscope for ear ticks (*Otobes megnini*).[42]

The entire muscle mass of the horse should be palpated for heat, pain, swelling, or atrophy, comparing contralateral muscle groups. Firm, deep palpation of the lumbar, gluteal, and semimembranosus and semitendinosus muscles may reveal pain, cramps, or fibrosis. The triceps, pectoral, gluteal, and semitendinosus muscles should be tapped with a fist or percussion hammer and observed for a prolonged contracture suggestive of myotonia. Running a blunt instrument such as a needle cap or a pen over the lumbar and gluteal muscles should illicit extension followed by flexion in healthy horses. Guarding against movement may reflect abnormalities in the pelvic or thoracolumbar muscles, or pain associated with the thoracolumbar spine or sacroiliac joints.

The horse should be observed at a walk or trot for any gait abnormalities and flexion tests performed for lameness. In some cases it may be helpful to observe the horse under saddle and have the owner demonstrate the exact nature of the gait abnormality or performance problem.

Ancillary Diagnostic Tests

Muscle Enzymes

The best assessment of the extent of acute muscle damage is attained by measuring serum CK activity. CK is a relatively low molecular weight protein (80,000 Da) that is intimately involved in energy production within the cell cytoplasm. It is liberated within hours of muscle damage, or increased cell membrane permeability, into the extracellular fluid and usually peaks at 4 to 6 hours after muscle injury.[11] A 3- to 5-fold increase in serum CK from normal values is believed to represent necrosis of approximately 20 g of muscle tissue.[83] Limited elevations in CK (less than 1,000 U/L high range of normal value = 380 U/L) may accompany training or transport.[4] Extreme fatiguing exercise, (e.g., endurance rides or the cross-country phase of a 3-day event) may result in CK activities being increased to more than 1,000 U/L, but usually less than 5,000 U/L. Under these circumstances serum CK activities rapidly return to baseline (i.e., less than 350 IU/L in 24 to 48 hours). Recumbent animals also may have slightly elevated CK activities that are usually less than 3,000 U/L. In contrast, more substantial elevations (from several thousand to hundreds of thousands of U/L) in the activity of this enzyme may occur with rhabdomyolysis.[75]

Serum AST is a larger molecular weight protein that has high activity in skeletal and cardiac muscle as well as in liver, red blood cells, and other tissues. Elevations in AST are not specific for myonecrosis, and increases could be the result of hemolysis, muscle, liver, or other organ damage. AST activity rises more slowly in response to myonecrosis than does CK, often peaking between 12 and 24 hours after the insult. In addition, AST is cleared slowly by the reticuloendothelial system and may persist for 2 to 3 weeks after rhabdomyolysis.[10,11]

By comparing serial activities of CK and AST, information concerning the progression of myonecrosis or muscle cell membrane permeability may be derived. Elevations in both CK and AST reflect relatively recent or active myonecrosis; persistently elevated serum CK indicates that myonecrosis is likely to be continuing. Elevated AST activity accompanied by decreasing or normal CK activity indicates that myonecrosis has ceased. The degree of elevation of CK and AST does not necessarily reflect the severity of clinical signs.

Elevations in plasma/serum myoglobin concentrations indicate acute muscle damage. Myoglobin is a low molecular weight protein (16,500 mw) that leaks into plasma immediately after muscle damage and is rapidly cleared in the urine by the kidney. Approximately 200 g of muscle or more must be damaged before it is detectable in the urine in human patients.[10] Normal serum concentrations in resting horses have been determined by nephelometry (range 0 to 9 microgram/L), with measured concentrations with rhabdomyolysis ranging from 10,000 to 800,000 micrograms/L.[32,58,75]

Exercise Response Test

Diagnosing chronic exertional rhabdomyolysis may be difficult in horses that have normal serum AST and CK when examined and only historical evidence of exertional rhabdomyolysis. In such cases, an exercise challenge can be helpful in detecting subclinical exertional rhabdomyolysis. In addition, quantifying the extent of rhabdomyolysis during mild exercise is helpful in deciding how rapidly to put a horse back into training. Blood samples should be taken before exercise and about 4 to 6 hours after exercise to evaluate peak changes in CK. Serum CK activity measured immediately post-exercise does not reflect the amount of damage occurring during the exercise test. Small fluctuations in serum CK activity may occur with exercise due to enhanced muscle membrane permeability, particularly if exercise is prolonged or strenuous and the horse is untrained.[57]

A sub-maximal exercise test is often valuable for detecting rhabdomyolysis because it provides more consistent evidence of subclinical rhabdomyolysis than maximal exercise tests.[75,78] Fifteen minutes of trotting is often sufficient to produce subclinical muscle damage in horses prone to chronic exertional myopathies.[36] If signs of stiffness develop before this, exercise should be concluded. A normal response is less than a 3- to 4-fold increase from basal CK. In the author's experience, horses with type 1 PSSM and active RER are more likely to have a positive exercise response than horses with type 2 PSSM or well-managed type 1 PSSM.

Ultrasonography

Physical disruption of muscle fibers and fibrosis can be detected by diagnostic ultrasonography. The typical striated echogenic pattern[37,59] of skeletal muscle varies according to the muscle group, and careful comparisons must be made between similar sites in contralateral limbs, in both transverse and longitudinal images. The appearance of muscle is also sensitive to how the horse stands and whether the muscle is under tension, so it is important that the horse stand squarely and bear weight evenly. Muscle fascia appears as well defined, relatively echodense bands. Care must be taken in identifying large vessels and artifacts created by them.[72]

Relatively hypoechoic areas within muscle that lack the normal muscle fiber striation indicate acute injury. The jagged edge of the margin of the torn muscle may be increased in echogenicity. Tears in the muscle fascia may be identified. A loculated hematoma may fill the injured area and slowly be replaced by hypoechoic granulation tissue. As muscle fibers regenerate there is a progressive increase in echogenicity. Relatively hyperechoic regions may develop due to fibrous scarring. Hyperechoic regions causing shadowing artifacts reflect mineralization.[72]

Electromyography (EMG)

EMG is particularly useful for evaluating muscle atrophy, muscle fasciculations, and myotonia. Normal muscle shows a brief burst of electrical activity when the EMG needle is inserted and then quiescence unless motor units are recruited (motor unit action potentials) or the needle is very close to a motor end plate (miniature end plate potentials). Spontaneous electrical activity, fibrillation potentials, and positive sharp waves are seen in horses with denervation and myotonic discharges, or complex repetitive discharges are seen in horses with muscle conduction system abnormalities (e.g., myotonia, HYPP).

Muscle Biopsy

A number of specific equine myopathies have been identified through the routine examination of muscle biopsies from horses with evidence of muscle dysfunction. Muscle fiber sizes, shapes, and fiber type distribution; mitochondrial distribution; polysaccharide staining pattern; neuromuscular junctions; nerve branches; connective tissue; and blood vessels can be fully evaluated in frozen sections using a battery of tinctorial and histochemical stains.

Inflammation, muscle fiber necrosis, cellular infiltrates, and proliferation of connective tissue are evident in formalin and frozen sections. However, there are many pathologic alterations that cannot be detected in formalin-fixed tissue but can readily be seen in histochemical stains of fresh-frozen biopsy samples.[17] These include identification of muscle fiber types to differentiate between neurogenic and myogenic atrophy, characterization of vacuolar storage material, characterization of inclusion bodies, and mitochondrial density. In addition, frozen samples may be used for biochemical analysis of substrate concentrations and enzyme activities as well as DNA isolation.

Muscle biopsies are preferably collected from abnormal/diseased muscle. A 6-mm outer diameter percutaneous needle biopsy technique can be used to obtain small muscle samples through a 1.5-cm skin incision using a local anesthetic subcutaneously. If this technique is used, enough muscle should be obtained to form a 1.5-cm square sample at a minimum. These samples do not tolerate shipment to an outside laboratory well. The optimum biopsy for shipment of histopathologic tissues to a laboratory is collected using surgical or open techniques, performed under local anesthesia (Figure 7.83).

Semimembranosus samples are often selected for open biopsy in cases of exertional rhabdomyolysis. Care must be exercised to infiltrate only the subcutaneous tissues, not the muscle, with local anesthetic agent. The objective is to obtain approximately a 2-cm cube of tissue without crush artifact; hence, a suitably long skin incision is required. Subsequently, 2 parallel incisions 2 cm apart should be made longitudinal to the muscle fibers with a scalpel. The muscle should only be handled in one corner using forceps, and care should be taken not to crush the tissue. The muscle sample is then

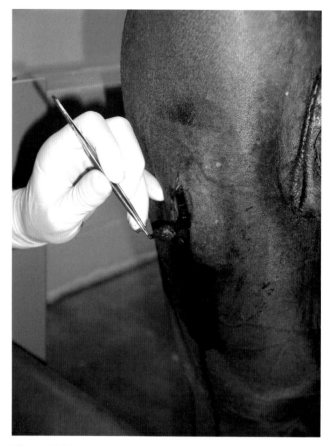

Figure 7.83. Muscle biopsy of the semimembranosus muscle. Note that the sample is gently handled at one end without crushing the tissue. Samples can be wrapped in saline-moistened gauze and shipped in a hard container on ice packs for frozen sections.

excised by transverse incisions 2 cm apart, and the tissue fixed appropriately.

Routine histopathologic samples can be placed in formalin. Fresh specimens are best shipped overnight in gauze slightly moistened with saline in a plastic jar on ice packs to specialized laboratories where they are frozen in isopentane (methylbutane) that is suspended in liquid nitrogen to minimize freeze artifact. Samples that potentially may be used for biochemical analysis should be immediately frozen in liquid nitrogen.

Genetic Testing

DNA tests are available for the diagnosis of hyperkalemic periodic paralysis, glycogen branching enzyme deficiency, type 1 polysaccharide storage myopathy, and malignant hyperthermia. Some laboratories prefer submission of a minimum of 20 mane or tail hairs pulled out with roots intact. Others analyze whole blood submitted in EDTA tubes.

MUSCLE DISEASES OF FOALS

Nutritional Myodegeneration

Foals with nutritional myodegeneration (NMD) may show clinical signs of dysphagia, muscle stiffness, trembling, firm muscles, difficulty rising, and myoglobin-uria.[73] If the myocardium is also involved, signs of dyspnea, a rapid irregular heartbeat, and sudden death may also be present. Aspiration pneumonia is a frequent complication. NMD is common in young, rapidly growing foals born to dams that consumed selenium-deficient diets during gestation. Selenium and vitamin E appear to be synergistic in preventing NMD. A diagnosis is based on finding moderate to marked elevated serum CK and AST activities combined with low whole blood selenium concentrations (less than 0.07 ppm) or serum vitamin E (less than 2 ppm). Hyperkalemia, hyperphosphatemia, hyponatremia, hypochloremia and hypocalcemia can occur with severe rhabdomyolysis when the normal distinction between extracellular and intracellular compartments is destroyed by massive tissue necrosis.[56] Selenium-dependent glutathione peroxidase formed in the red cells during erythropoiesis is another enzyme that can provide an index of body selenium status.

Treatment includes intramuscular injection of selenium at 0.055 to 0.067 mg/kg body weight and either injectable or oral vitamin E (0.5 to 1.5 IU/kg body weight). Supportive therapy may include administration of antibiotics to help combat secondary pneumonia, feeding via nasogastric tube if dysphagic, provision of adequate energy intake, and attention to the fluid and electrolyte balance.

Glycogen Branching Enzyme Deficiency

Glycogen branching enzyme deficiency (GBED) is a fatal autosomal recessive glycogen storage disorder in Quarter horse and Paint foals.[66,79] Foals may be weak at birth with contracted tendons, and stillbirths and abortions may be seen. Flexural deformities respond to conservative treatment; however, foals have low energy levels and may have periodic hypoglycemia and collapse. Death may be sudden when exercised on pasture, associated with ventilatory failure, or the result of euthanasia due to persistent recumbency. The longest an affected foal has lived is 18 weeks. Clinical signs are due to a lack of intracellular glucose stores for normal tissue metabolism. Persistent leukopenia, intermittent hypoglycemia, as well as moderate elevations in serum CK (1,000 to 15,000 U/L), AST, and gamma glutamyl transferase (GGT) activities are common laboratory findings.

A mutation in the glycogen branching enzyme gene (*GBE1*) results in an abnormally configured glycogen molecule in numerous tissues.[85] Approximately 8% of Quarter horses and Paint horses are carriers of the mutation and 3% of second and third trimester abortions submitted to 2 diagnostic laboratories were found to be homozygous for GBED.[84] Pleasure horses and working cow horses have the highest incidence of GBED carriers.[69] Many GBED cases likely are undiagnosed due to the similarity of clinical signs with many neonatal diseases and the current lack of awareness of available genetic testing for stillborn foals and aborted feti.

Routine postmortem examination usually reveals few abnormalities. Periodic acid Schiff's (PAS) staining of muscle, heart, and sometimes liver show notable lack of normal PAS staining for glycogen and a variable amount of abnormal PAS positive globular or crystalline intracellular inclusions. The most accurate diagnosis of GBED can be obtained through genetic testing where affected foals are homozygous and the dam/sire are heterozygous for the mutation. The Veterinary Genetics Laboratory at the University of California, Davis (www.vgl.ucdavis.edu) and Vet Gen in Michigan (www.vetgen.com) are licensed by the University of Minnesota to test for GBED. Mane or tail hairs with roots intact can be submitted. Diagnostic laboratories should be encouraged to screen aborted feti for GBED either through PAS staining of cardiac samples or via genetic testing. Testing also should be strongly advised for prepurchase evaluation of broodmares or stallions.

Hyperkalemic Periodic Paralysis

Hyperkalemic periodic paralysis (HYPP) is an autosomal dominant trait affecting Quarter horses, American Paint horses, Appaloosas, and Quarter horse cross-breeds worldwide.[65] A point mutation in the voltage-dependent skeletal muscle sodium channel alpha subunit occurs in about 4% of Quarter horses but this percentage is much higher in halter and pleasure horse performance types.[64, 69]

Clinical signs range from asymptomatic to intermittent muscle fasciculations and weakness, and are first identified from foals to 3 years of age. Homozygous horses are often more severely affected and may be identified at a younger age than heterozygotes.[14] A brief period of facial myotonia and prolapse of the third eyelid may be seen initially. Muscle fasciculations beginning on the flanks, neck, and shoulders may become more generalized. Whereas most horses remain standing during mild attacks, weakness with swaying, staggering, dogsitting, or recumbency may be seen, with severe attacks lasting 15 to 60 minutes or longer. Heart and respiratory rates may be elevated, but horses remain relatively bright and alert. Respiratory distress occurs in some horses as a result of upper respiratory muscle paralysis. Once episodes subside, horses regain their feet and appear normal with absent or minimal gait abnormalities. Young horses that are homozygous for the HyPP trait may have respiratory stridor and periodic obstruction of the upper respiratory tract that can be fatal.

Common factors that trigger episodes include sudden dietary changes or ingestion of diets high in potassium (less than 1.1%), such as those containing alfalfa hay, molasses, electrolyte supplements, and kelp-based supplements.[61] Fasting, anesthesia or heavy sedation, trailer rides, and stress also may precipitate clinical signs. The onset of signs, however, is often unpredictable. Exercise per se does not appear to stimulate clinical signs; serum CK shows no or minimal increases during episodic fasciculations and weakness.

Descendents from the "Impressive" stallion with episodic muscle tremors should be strongly suspected of having HyPP. Hyperkalemia (6 to 9 mEq/L), hemoconcentration, and hyponatremia are seen during clinical episodes, but a definitive diagnosis requires DNA testing of mane or tail hair. Electromyographic examination of affected horses between attacks reveals abnormal fibrillation potentials and complex repetitive discharges, with occasional myotonic potentials and trains of doublets between episodes.[54] Differential diagnoses for hyperkalemia include delay before serum centrifugation, hemolysis, chronic renal failure, and severe rhabdomyolysis.

Many horses recover spontaneously from HyPP episodes. Owners may abort early mild episodes using low-grade exercise or feeding grain or corn syrup to stimulate insulin-mediated movement of potassium across cell membranes. In severe cases, administration of calcium gluconate (0.2 to 0.4 mL/kg of a 23% solution diluted in 1 L of 5% dextrose) or IV dextrose (6 mL/kg of a 5% solution), alone or combined with sodium bicarbonate (1 to 2 mEq/kg), often provides immediate improvement.[65] With severe respiratory obstruction, a tracheotomy may be necessary. Acute death is common, especially in homozygous animals.

Prevention requires decreasing dietary potassium to 0.6 to 1.1% total potassium concentration and increasing renal losses of potassium.[60] High-potassium feeds such as alfalfa hay, first cutting hay, brome hay, sugar molasses, and beet molasses should be avoided. Optimally, later cuts of timothy or Bermuda grass hay; grains such as oats, corn, wheat, and barley; and beet pulp should be fed in small meals several times a day. Regular exercise and/or frequent access to a large paddock or yard are also beneficial. Pasture is ideal for horses with HyPP because the high water content of pasture grass makes it unlikely that horses will consume large amounts of potassium in a short period of time. Complete feeds for horses with HyPP are commercially available. For horses with recurrent episodes, even with dietary alterations, acetazolamide (2 to 4 mg/kg, PO, BID-TID) or hydrochlorothiazide (0.5 to 1 mg/kg, PO, BID) may be helpful.

Breed registries and other associations have restrictions on the use of these drugs during competitions. Some horses have both HyPP and PSSM, which may result in an episode of rhabdomyolysis during a hyperkalemic paralytic event with subsequent elevated serum CK activity and prolonged recumbency.

MUSCLE DISORDERS IN ADULT HORSES

Overuse and Muscle Strain

It is often difficult to assess the presence of muscle pain in horses because it is a subjective assessment and often coexists with a more easily recognized lameness. Frequently the lameness is treated without managing muscle soreness. In human athletes muscle stiffness and soreness are more easily recognized causes of decreased performance. In humans, muscle pain and stiffness are reported 24 to 48 hours after unaccustomed use of certain muscles; this is referred to as delayed onset muscular soreness (DOMS). Pain resolves spontaneously, assuming the muscles are not overworked again; however, continued overstress may result in ultrastructural damage to myofilaments and eventually histological evidence of myofiber necrosis. Gradual training involving the activity that provoked the original DOMS decreases the amount of soreness associated with that condition over time. The muscles most prone to strain in horses appear to be the back muscles (Standardbreds, dressage and jumping horses), semimembranosus/tendinosus muscles (reining, roping, cutting horses) and pectoral muscles (event horses after cross country jumping). Poor racing performance or poor jumping techniques as well as the horse twisting itself over jumps are common complaints in horses with sore backs.

Muscle Trauma

When muscle has been strained to the point of tearing through entire muscle fascicles, hemorrhage and inflammation can result in acute muscular pain and recognizable swelling in superficial muscles. The most common sites of injury in the forelimb include biceps brachii, brachiocephalicus, pectorals, and the musculotendinous junction of the superficial digital flexor.[72] In the hindlimb, semimembranosus and semitendinosus, adductor, gluteal, and gastrocnemius muscle injuries are common (Figure 7.84).[72] Whereas acute trauma is associated with swelling or herniation of a muscle belly through

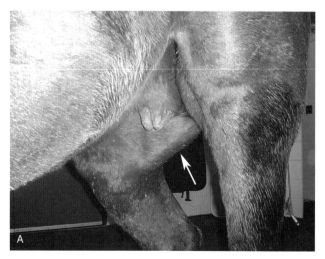
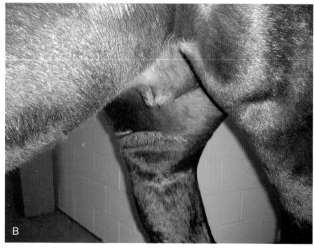

Figure 7.84.   A. Acute swelling of the right adductor muscles (arrow) in a mare that slipped in a muddy paddock. B) The same muscle 2 weeks later after cold therapy and treatment with a nonsteroidal anti-inflammatory.

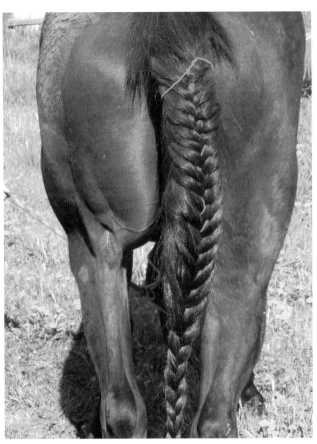

Figure 7.85. Severe atrophy, fibrosis, and contracture of the left hamstring region in a horse with previous trauma to the area. (Courtesy of Dr. Gary Baxter.)

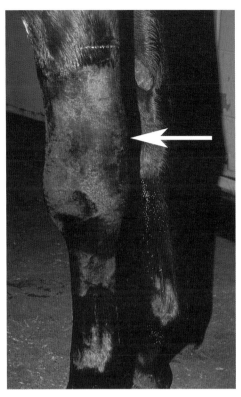

Figure 7.86. Trauma and associated swelling to the caudolateral antebrachium (arrow) that can cause ischemia of the enclosed structures, leading to signs suggestive of compartment syndrome. (Courtesy of Dr. Gary Baxter.)

the overlying fascia, chronic injury may be associated with loss of muscle bulk, fibrosis, mineralization, or rarely ossification (Figure 7.85).

Diagnosis

An acute muscle tear may produce a palpable defect, but this becomes filled with edema, hemorrhage, and eventually granulation tissue. Localization of deeper muscle injury is more challenging, because the clinical signs are more subtle.

Pain and limitations in movement should be evaluated in a full range of passive movement of the neck, limbs, and thoracolumbar region. The horse should be observed for gait abnormalities at both the walk and the trot. However, overt lameness may not be present if pain only occurs when the muscle contracts strongly or is stretched maximally. Serum muscle enzyme concentrations are usually in the normal range for focal muscle trauma.

Treatment

The choice of treatment depends upon the type of muscle injury and the stage of injury and repair. The goal is to relieve muscle spasm, decrease inflammation, restore circulation, minimize scarring, and maintain range of motion. Treatment modalities include cold

therapy, therapeutic ultrasound or laser therapy, transcutaneous electrical stimulation, massage, passive stretching combined with box rest, and a graduated, controlled exercise program. Relief of acute muscle spasm may require chiropractic manipulation. The extent of rest depends upon the degree of tearing and hemorrhage. Once initiated, the exercise program must be carefully moderated according to the site of the injury to avoid overstress in the early stages of repair but encourage a progressive increase in strength. Aqua treadmills can provide an excellent controlled means of building muscle strength.

Muscle Ischemia

Muscle ischemia is extremely painful and occurs with acute trauma, vascular occlusion, and the crush/compartment syndrome. Vascular occlusion may be a sequela to infarctive purpura hemorrhagica, disseminated intravascular coagulation, and iliac thrombosis.

Compartmental syndrome develops when high pressure within a closed fascial space reduces capillary blood perfusion below a level necessary for muscle tissue viability. Trauma to the caudolateral compartment of the antebrachium can cause ischemia of the enclosed lateral digital extensor, ulnaris lateralis, superficial and deep digital flexor, and flexor carpi ulnaris muscles, as well as the median artery, vein, and nerve (Figure 7.86).[68] Lameness is acute and severe in onset, with reluctance to bear weight on the limb associated with firm swelling on the caudolateral aspect of the antebrachium. Treatment of compartment syndrome is by fasciotomy. In one case, incising the superficial fascia over the ulnaris lateralis resulted in immediate separation of the fascia by 3 to 4 cm and rapid relief of clinical signs.[68]

In recumbent or anesthetized horses, the triceps muscle, gluteal muscles, longissimus dorsi, or extensors of the hindlimb may become ischemic because of compression, prolonged hypoperfusion, and subsequent reperfusion and edema. Hypotension during surgery in which mean arterial blood pressure is less than 60 mm Hg contributes to the development of this syndrome. Clinical signs are usually evident as soon as the horse tries to stand, but may be delayed for up to 2 hours. In severe cases the horse is unable to stand.

Triceps myopathy is often characterized by a dropped elbow stance typical of radial nerve paralysis. Involvement of the gluteal muscles may result in unwillingness to bear weight on the hindlimbs. Horses may appear distressed, with profuse sweating, tachycardia, and tachypnea. The degree of distress depends on the severity of the muscle damage. Affected muscles may feel very hard. There may be localized swelling. Neuropathy also may develop in the compressed muscles, resulting in temporary radial or peroneal nerve damage. Serum CK levels greater than 2,000 IU/L often occur within 4 hours after anesthesia as blood flow returns to the affected muscles.

Treatment of postanesthetic myopathy or neuropathy in horses is similar to that described in the section on acute exertional rhabdomyolysis. Bandaging and splinting of limbs with neuropraxia may help the horse stand and ambulate more easily, thus relieving much of the animal's anxiety. Horses that can stand on 3 legs have a good prognosis for recovery from myopathies or neuropathies and generally respond to treatment within 72 hours. Horses that are affected bilaterally and unable to stand have a very poor prognosis.

Muscle Cramping

Muscle cramping is a painful condition that arises from hyperactivity of motor units caused by repetitive firing of the peripheral and/or central nervous system. The origin of the cramp in most cases is believed to be the intramuscular portion of the motor nerve. Most muscle cramps are also accompanied by fasciculations in the same muscle and normal serum CK activity. In contrast, muscle contractures, such as those seen in exertional rhabdomyolysis, are painful muscle spasms that represent a state of muscle contracture unaccompanied by depolarization of the muscle membrane. Muscle cramps can be induced by forceful contraction of a shortened muscle, changes in the electrolyte composition of extracellular fluid, and ear tick infestations in horses.

Electrolyte Disturbances

Muscle cramping in endurance horses is most frequent in hot, humid weather when horses develop remarkable deficits in sodium, potassium, chloride magnesium, and calcium due to extensive sweating. Synchronous diaphragmatic flutter may be seen in association with cramping.[13] Mild muscle cramping is self-limiting, and the signs abate with rest or light exercise. Exhausted horses with metabolic derangements, however, require immediate treatment, including plasma volume expansion with oral or intravenous isotonic polyionic fluids and cooling (using water and fans).[12] Because most horses with this condition are alkalotic, administration of solutions containing sodium bicarbonate is contraindicated. Daily direct addition of 2 oz. of sodium chloride and 1 oz. of potassium chloride to the feed is recommended for horses with recurrent cramping in addition to electrolyte supplementation before and after endurance rides.

Muscles may also develop intensely painful spasms, particularly following trauma to the caudal thoracic and lumbar regions. Manipulation to release muscle spasm can produce relief of pain and rapid restoration of normal performance.[72]

Ear Ticks

Intermittent painful muscle cramps not associated with exercise have been described in horses with severe *Otobius megnini* infestations.[42] These horses show intermittent signs of severe muscle cramping of pectoral, triceps, abdominal, or semitendinosus/semimembranosus muscles lasting from minutes to a few hours, with severe pain that often resembles colic. Horses may fall over when stimulated. Between muscle cramps, horses appear to be normal. Percussion of triceps, pectoral, or semitendinosus muscles results in a typical myotonic cramp. Horses have serum CK activities ranging from 4,000 to 170,000 IU/L. Numerous ear ticks (*O. megnini*) can be identified in the external ear canal of affected horses. The spasms continue without treatment for ear ticks; however, local treatment of the ear ticks using pyrethrins and piperonal butoxide results in recovery within 12 to 36 hours. Acepromazine is helpful to relieve painful cramping.

Muscle Abscesses

Staphylococcus aureus, *Streptococcus equi*, and *Coynebacterium pseudotuberculosis* are common causes of skeletal muscle abscessation. Abscesses develop following penetrating injuries or local or hematogenous spread of infection. Ultrasonography and culture of aspirated fluid are the best means of diagnosis in superficial sites. Deeper abscesses may be diagnosed using fibrinogen, nucleated white blood cell count, and the synergistic hemolysin inhibition test for abscesses due to *C. pseudotuberculosis*.

Clostridial Myositis

Clostridial myositis most commonly occurs following penetrating wounds, parturition injuries, castration, and especially intramuscular injections.[55] Spores of *Clostridia* species involved are found in soil and feces, and may lie dormant in skeletal muscles. When tissue is traumatized by injection or injury (low oxidative potential and alkaline pH), organisms proliferate, elaborate exotoxins, and cause extensive necrosis of muscle and surrounding tissue. Death can occur quickly from toxemia with *C. sordelli*, *sporogenes*, and *chauvei* species. Cases of *C. perfringens* have a lower mortality rate and initially present with swelling and crepitus in an area in muscle, as well as moderate systemic signs of toxemia. Ultrasound is useful in identifying air bubbles in muscle exudate and clostridial species can be identified in aspirates by fluorescent antibody staining and anaerobic bacterial culture. Antibiotic therapy, wound fenestration, aggressive surgical debridement over the entire affected area, and supportive care are the hallmarks of successful treatment.[55] High doses of intravenous potassium penicillin are recommended every 2 to 4 hours until the horse is stable (1 to 5 days) combined with or followed by oral metronidazole. Supportive fluid therapy and anti-inflammatory agents for control of pain and swelling are recommended. Extensive skin sloughing over the affected area is common in surviving horses.

Exertional Rhabdomyolysis

Exertional rhabdomyolysis (ER) occurs in about 3% of exercising horses[15] and in a wide variety of breeds, including draft breeds, Warmbloods, Thoroughbreds, Standardbreds, Arabians, Morgans, Quarter horses, Appaloosas, American Paint horses, and many more. Terms such as tying-up, set fast, azoturia, and Monday morning disease have been used to describe this syndrome. It has become apparent that some horses develop exertional muscle damage as a result of nutritional or environmental factors. These sporadic cases of ER are usually amenable to treatment once the extrinsic cause of muscle damage is identified. Some horses, however, develop chronic ER, and many of these cases are due to an intrinsic and inherited dysfunction of muscle metabolism or muscle contraction.

Sporadic Exertional Rhabdomyolysis

Etiology

The most common extrinsic cause of sporadic ER is exercise that exceeds the horse's underlying state of training. Horses that are advanced too quickly in their training, those that are only ridden sporadically while being continually fed full rations, and horses performing strenuous exercise such as racing or endurance riding without sufficient conditioning commonly develop rhabdomyolysis. In addition, rhabdomyolysis may be more common in horses exercising during an outbreak of respiratory disease. Both equine herpes virus 1 and equine influenza virus have been implicated as causative agents.[26, 28]

Dietary imbalance: Horses consuming a high grain diet appear to be more likely to develop exertional rhabdomyolysis than horses fed a low grain or fat supplemented diet.[46,56,60] The grain itself may not be responsible for rhabdomyolysis; however, high starch intake may trigger rhabdomyolysis in horses with particular myopathies such as recurrent exertional rhabdomyolysis (RER) and PSSM.

Electrolyte depletion in horses can occur due to dietary deficiency and losses in sweat with strenuous exercise. Sodium, potassium, magnesium, and calcium play key roles in muscle fiber contractility. With severe acute electrolyte depletion such as that found following endurance exercise, serum electrolytes may be below normal ranges.[12] With chronic dietary depletion, however, serum concentrations may not reflect total body electrolyte imbalances.

Work by Harris, et al. established renal fractional excretions as a technique to evaluate electrolyte concentrations in horses with chronic ER.[27,30] Blood and urine samples are obtained concurrently and creatinine and electrolyte concentrations measured in both. Serum creatinine/urine creatinine multiplied by the reciprocal for urine and serum electrolyte concentrations ×100 provides the fractional excretion of a particular electrolyte. It can be difficult to obtain consistently representative renal fractional excretions of electrolytes in horses, however.[52] Hypokalemia has also been suggested to play a role in chronic ER, although it is not a common finding in horses consuming adequate quantities of forage.[7] Supplementation with good quality forage or 30 g of KCl/day (light salt) is recommended for horses with low renal fraction excretion of potassium.

Vitamin E and selenium: Another postulated cause of sporadic ER is the increased generation of free radicals from oxidative metabolism associated with exercise. It has not been shown whether horses that experience repeated episodes of ER may generate more free radicals than normal horses. Primary selenium deficiency has rarely been demonstrated as a cause of exertional rhabdomyolysis.[63] In fact, many racehorses with chronic ER have higher concentrations of selenium and vitamin E due to zealous dietary supplementation by the owner. Adequate values for blood selenium are greater than 0.07 mcg/ml.

Horses with low serum vitamin E may present with muscle soreness, muscle fasciculations, muscle weakness, and loss of muscle mass. In early stages this may be due to a reversible myopathic process. After years of deficiency, oxidative damage to motor nerves can result is generalized denervation typical of equine motor neuron disease.[19] Adequate values for serum vitamin E are above 2.0 mcg/ml.

Clinical Signs and Diagnosis

Classically, horses lose impulsion and develop a stiff, stilted gait, particularly involving the hindquarters. There is excessive sweating and a high respiratory rate due to pain. Horses may be unable to walk forward after resting due to firm, painful muscle contractures involving the back and hindquarters.

Gluteal, biceps femoris, semitendinosus, and semimembranosus muscles are usually symmetrically affected with less frequent involvement of the forelimbs. Severe cases of rhabdomyolysis show signs of colic, become recumbent, and develop occult myoglobinuria. Attempts to move more severely affected animals may result in extreme pain, obvious anxiety, and exacerbation of the condition. Exertional rhabdomyolysis may accompany the exhaustion syndrome in endurance horses with concurrent evidence of a rapid heart rate, dehydration, hyperthermia, synchronous diaphragmatic flutter, and collapse.[12] Muscle contractures are not always consistent in endurance horses with exhaustion.

Diagnosis is usually obvious based on the clinical signs, but measurement of serum muscle enzyme activities provides an assessment of the severity of muscle damage and confirms the diagnosis. The degree of elevation of muscle enzyme activity does not necessarily reflect the severity of clinical signs.

TREATMENT OF ACUTE RHABDOMYOLYSIS

If the attack occurs during exercise some distance from where the horse is normally stabled, the horse should not be made to walk home. If an attack occurs at a competition the horse should be treated there and should not be transported home over a long distance for at least 24 to 48 hours.

The objectives of treatment are to relieve anxiety and muscle pain, as well as correct fluid and acid base deficits (Table 7.3). Acepromazine is helpful in relieving anxiety and may increase muscle blood flow but should not be given to dehydrated horses due to hypotensive effects that produce recumbency. Alternatively, xylazine may provide short-term relief or in very painful horses, detomidine combined with butorphanol provides excellent sedation and analgesia. NSAIDs such as ketoprofen, phenylbutazone, or flunixine meglumine provide additional pain relief. Analgesic treatment is continued to effect, but most horses are relatively pain free within 18 to 24 hours. For horses with extreme pain and distress, a constant rate infusion of detomidine, lidocaine, or butorphanol can make the difference between adequate time for recovery and euthanasia.

Intravenous or intragastric dimethyl sulfoxide can be used as an anti-oxidant, anti-inflammatory, and osmotic diuretic in severely affected horses. Muscle relaxants such as methocarbamol seem to produce variable results, possibly depending on the dosage used. Dantrium sodium in severely affected horses may decrease muscle contractures and possibly prevent further activation of muscle necrosis. This can be repeated in 4 to 6 hours.

Severe rhabdomyolysis can lead to renal compromise due to the ischemic and the combined nephrotoxic effects of myoglobinuria, dehydration, and NSAIDs. The first priority in horses with hemoconcentration, or myoglobinuria, is to re-establish fluid balance and induce diuresis. In mild cases, administration of fluids via a nasogastric tube may be adequate, but generally fluids are better given intravenously. Balanced polyionic electrolyte solutions are best. If severe rhabdomyolysis is present, then isotonic saline or 2.5% dextrose in 0.45% saline may be necessary because horses often have hyponatremia, hypochloremia, and hyperkalemia.[56] If hypocalcaemia is present, then supplementing intravenous fluids with 100 to 200 ml of 24% calcium borogluconate is recommended, but serum calcium should not exceed a low normal range. Affected animals are usually alkalotic, making bicarbonate therapy inappropriate.

Chronic Exertional Rhabdomyolysis

Horses that have repeated episodes of exertional rhabdomyolysis from a young age, from the time of purchase, or when they are put back into training after

Table 7.3. Potential medications that can be used to treat acute rhabdomyolysis in the horse.

Category	Drug	Dose	Comment
Tranquilizer	Acepromazine	0.04–0.07 mg/kg IV	May be hypotensive; use caution if dehydrated
	Xylazine	0.4–0.8 mg/kg IV	
	Detomidine	0.02–0.04 mcg/kg IV	
	Butorphanol	0.01–0.04 mg/kg IV	Use with xylazine/detomidine
Anti-inflammatory	Phenylbutazone	2.2–4.4 mg/kg IV or oral	Use caution if dehydrated
	Flunixine meglumine	1.1 mg/kg IV or oral	Use caution if dehydrated
	Ketoprofen	2.2 mg/kg IV	Use caution if dehydrated
	DMSO	1–2 mg/kg IV or oral	Use as a solution diluted to less than 20%
Pain control: CRI	Lidocaine	1.3 mg/kg IV followed by 0.05 mg/kg/min IV	
	Detomidine	0.22 mcg/kg IV followed by 0.1 mcg/kg/min IV	
	Butorphanol	13 mcg/kg/hour	
Muscle relaxant	Methocarbamol	5–22 mg/kg IV slowly	
	Dantrolene	2–4 mg/kg oral QID	

a long period of rest may have an underlying intrinsic abnormality of muscle function. Many of the horses with intrinsic muscle defects have repeated episodes of rhabdomyolysis with minimal exercise, even when the dietary and training recommendations for sporadic ER are followed. Four specific intrinsic causes of exertional rhabdomyolysis have been identified to date: recurrent exertional rhabdomyolysis (RER),[35,78] type 1 polysaccharide storage myopathy (PSSM),[48,76] type 2 polysaccharide storage myopathy,[45,47] and malignant hyperthermia.[2,44] It is likely that there are other specific causes that have yet to be identified (idiopathic chronic exertional rhabdomyolysis).

In all of these intrinsic forms of chronic exertional rhabdomyolysis it appears that there are specific environmental stimuli that are necessary to trigger muscle necrosis in genetically susceptible animals. Horses cannot be cured of their susceptibility to this condition, but if the specific disease is identified changes in management can be implemented to minimize episodes of rhabdomyolysis.

Recurrent Exertional Rhabdomyolysis

Prevalence: About 5% to 10% of Thoroughbred racehorses develop exertional rhabdomyolysis during a racing season and 75% of these horses have more than 4 episodes in 4 months.[40] Approximately 6% of National Hunt Horses[70] and 13% of polo horses develop exertional rhabdomyolysis.[50] Horses with a nervous disposition, especially fillies, are highly predisposed. Research suggests that a subset of Thoroughbred horses with chronic ER have a specific form of exertional rhabdomyolysis, denoted as recurrent exertional rhabdomyolysis (RER).[35,36,78] RER appears to be an inherited, intermittent, stress-induced defect in the regulation of muscle contraction.[35,36] A breeding trial using Thoroughbred horses with RER confirmed that the characteristic abnormality in muscle contracture is inherited in an autosomal dominant fashion.[21] Recurrent episodes of rhabdomyolysis in Standardbreds and Arabian horses may be due to a similar abnormality but this has not been confirmed. A heritable basis for RER in Standardbreds was supported by equine lymphocyte antigen profiles in affected horses.[16]

Clinical signs: Horses with RER have intermittent elevations in serum CK activity. Episodes of muscle stiffness, sweating, and firm muscle contractures often occur in horses once they become fit and are frequently associated with excitement at the time of exercise. In Thoroughbreds, rhabdomyolysis occurs most frequently during training when horses are held to a slow gallop.[40] In Standardbreds, rhabdomyolysis often occurs 15 to 30 minutes into jogging.[74] Obvious clinical signs are rare after racing. A history of poor performance and elevated serum AST and CK may be the only presenting complaints in some horses. Older Thoroughbreds used as riding horses may have very intermittent episodes of rhabdomyolysis associated with lay-up of fit horses. Event horses often develop clinical signs after the steeplechase phase of a 3-day event, or in the "10 minute box," or less commonly during the cross country phase. Muscle stiffness and reluctance to collect may be present on a continual basis between episodes in some of these

older horses. Arabian horses often develop clinical signs with little exertion, frequently in association with excitement.

Etiology: RER is characterized by abnormal sensitivity of intact muscle bundles to contractures induced by the addition of caffeine or halothane to a muscle bath.[35] Elevated myoplasmic calcium concentration has been reported in muscle of horses with acute ER[39] and in myoblasts derived from Thoroughbreds with RER.[36]

There are physiological similarities between the contracture results of RER and contracture tests for malignant hyperthermia. Biochemical studies of isolated muscle cell membranes[86] and linkage analysis[20] do not support an identical biochemical basis for malignant hyperthermia and RER. Currently whole genome association analyses are under way to identify the genetic basis for RER in Thoroughbred horses. The increased halothane sensitivity of the muscles in RER horses may explain why many Thoroughbreds with RER develop rhabdomyolysis under halothane anesthesia.

Factors that trigger rhabdomyolysis in susceptible horses include gender, temperament, excitement, stress, dietary starch, exercise duration/intensity, season, and lameness. Females are most commonly afflicted with RER (67% female:33% male), particularly those that are 2 years of age and in race training.[40,49] Nervous horses are 5 times more likely to develop RER and horses with lameness are 4 times more likely to develop rhabdomyolysis. Susceptible horses receiving more than 5 kg of concentrate feed (oats, corn, molasses mix) are more likely to develop rhabdomyolysis than those receiving 2.5 kg of concentrate feed/day.[53] Dietary effects of high carbohydrates in recurrent exertional rhabdomyolysis may in part be related to the psychogenic effects of grain on excitability. Glycogen storage does not increase substantially in horses with RER.[78] Inclement weather has been cited as a trigger of exertional rhabdomyolysis and rhabdomyolysis is reported more commonly in the autumn and winter in the United Kingdom.[29]

A contribution of reproductive hormones to triggering ER has been postulated because the incidence of RER appears to be highest in mares.[25,31] Many owners report that episodes of rhabdomyolysis occur most commonly during estrus, but in one study of racehorses, no direct correlation was shown between progesterone fluctuations and serum CK activity.[25] It is likely that the estrus cycle is one of many factors that combine to trigger ER in susceptible horses. Many racetrack practitioners report that the incidence of ER declines when susceptible mares are treated with testosterone. Hypothyroidism and lactic acidosis have also been suggested as a cause of ER but never substantiated.

Diagnosis

Acute cases of ER are readily diagnosed by serum muscle enzymes. Identification of RER in a horse that presents with a history of poor performance unrelated to signs typical of tying up may be facilitated by a submaximal exercise test with pre- and 4-hour post serum CK activity assessed. This test is useful for horses with concurrent problems but is not adequate to screen for RER in asymptomatic horses.

Muscle biopsies from horses with RER that are in training have increased numbers of centrally located nuclei in mature muscle fibers. They may have evidence of varying stages of muscle degeneration and regeneration and they have normal to slightly increased subsarcolemmal muscle glycogen staining.[78] Histopathologic changes are often lacking in horses that have been laid up for a period of time prior to biopsy.

Polysaccharide Storage Myopathy (PSSM)

PREVALENCE

Recent research has shown that there are at least 2 forms of glycogen storage disorders in horses. Type 1 PSSM is due to an autosomal dominant gain of function mutation in the glycogen synthase gene (*GYS1*).[48] This mutation is found in at least 20 different breeds of horses in Europe and North America, including Quarter horses; American Paint horses; Appaloosa horses; Draft horse breeds including American Cream, Belgian, Percheron, Gypsy Vanner, Cob Normande, Trekpard, Haflinger, Morgan, Mustang, and Rocky Mountain horse; Tennessee walking horse breeds, mixed breed horse, Cobs, Hannoverians, Rheinlanders, and Warmblood horses of unspecified type.[46,47] The prevalence of PSSM due to the *GYS1* mutation ranges from 8% in Quarter horses and Paints[43,69] to 36% in Belgian Draft horses,[23] with no reported cases in the Thoroughbreds, Standardbreds, and Arabians tested.[46]

Type 2 PSSM refers to horses with excessive muscle glycogen storage that do not have the *GYS1* mutation. Type 2 PSSM appears to account for about 25% of PSSM cases in Quarter horse-related breeds and 80% of PSSM cases in many Warmblood breeds.[46,47] The acronyms EPSM and EPSSM have also been used for polysaccharide storage myopathy, although they do not indicate a specific genotype.[80, 81]

CLINICAL SIGNS

Horses with both forms of PSSM often have a calm and sedate demeanor. Clinical signs of muscle stiffness, reluctance to exercise, exercise intolerance, or overt muscle contractures and reluctance to move usually are apparent at the commencement of training.[24] Most horses have numerous episodes of ER, or a consistent history of poor performance; however, some mildly affected horses are asymptomatic or have only 1 or 2 episodes of ER per year. In Quarter horses, type 1 PSSM has the highest frequency in halter horses, followed by pleasure horses and working cow horses.[69] It is uncommon in racing Quarter horses. Serum CK activities are often elevated in untreated Quarter horses, even when horses are rested, and while clinical signs are active, CK will usually increase by 1,000 U/L or more 4 hours after 15 minutes of exercise at a trot.[78] Muscle atrophy, renal failure, and severe colic-like pain are less common presenting complaints. Both type 1 and type 2 PSSM occur in Quarter and Paint horse foals and weanlings without rhabdomyolysis necessarily being induced by exercise.

Draft horses with type 1 PSSM may be asymptomatic if not in work but may also show signs of a generalized decrease in muscle mass, overt muscle atrophy, weakness in the hindlimbs with difficulty rising, reluctance to back up, and gait abnormalities.[23,67,82] Exertional rhabdomyolysis can be a debilitating feature of type 1 PSSM in Draft breeds. Although shivers was suggested to be a sign of PSSM, recent studies show there is no causal relationship.[23] Draft horses with PSSM often have only a mild elevation in serum CK and AST. The prevalence of type 1 PSSM is so high in many Draft breeds that many homozygous affected horses can be identified (S. Valberg. personal observation). These homozygotes may have more severe clinical signs.

Warmbloods derived from Draft crosses may have type 1 PSSM. However, European Warmblood breeds are more frequently affected by type 2 PSSM.[47] One of the most common presenting complaints in Warmbloods with PSSM is a gait abnormality characterized by lack of impulsion and shifting, undiagnosed lameness.[34] Suspensory strains in hindlimbs seem to accompany type 2 PSSM, possibly due to the abnormal hindlimb gait and inability to engage the hindquarters under the body. Warmbloods with PSSM also present with sore muscles and intermittent exertional rhabdomyolysis.

DIAGNOSIS

Genetic testing for the *GYS1* mutation is performed on whole blood or hair root samples at Veterinary Diagnostic Laboratory at the University of Minnesota (http://www.vdl.umn.edu/vdl/ourservices/neuromuscular. html). The distinctive features of type 1 PSSM in muscle biopsy samples are numerous subsarcolemmal vacuoles and dense, crystalline periodic acid Schiff's (PAS)-positive, amylase-resistant inclusions in fast twitch fibers.[48,76] A false negative diagnosis of type 1 PSSM by muscle biopsy may occur if biopsy samples are small or if horses are less than 1 year of age.[18]

Type 2 PSSM must still be diagnosed by muscle biopsy at present.[45] Muscle biopsies from horses with type 2 PSSM have increased PAS staining for glycogen and aggregates of granular PAS-positive polysaccharide in the cytoplasm or under the sarcolemmal. The PAS-positive polysaccharide in type 2 PSSM is frequently but not always amylase sensitive. False positive diagnosis is possible for type 2 PSSM in highly trained horses that normally have higher muscle glycogen concentrations or in formalin fixed sections which show a greater deposition of subsarcolemmal glycogen in healthy horses. Other features that may be present with both forms of PSSM include muscle necrosis and macrophage infiltration of myofibers, regenerative fibers, and atrophied type 2 fibers.

ETIOLOGY

Muscle glycogen concentrations in horses with type 1 PSSM are 1.5 to 4 times normal.[6] Increased muscle glycogen concentrations in type 1 PSSM appear to be due to increased and unregulated glycogen synthase activity as a result of a gain of function mutation in the glycogen synthase 1 gene (*GYS1*).[48] Horses with PSSM show increased glycogen synthase activity both in the basal state and when stimulated by glucose 6 phosphate. Elevated insulin in the bloodstream can further enhance glycogen synthase activity. Abnormal amylase-resistant polysaccharide appears to result from production of a polysaccharide with a higher ratio of straight glucose chains, which are created by glycogen synthase, relative to branched chains, which are created by the less active glycogen branching enzyme.[6] Rhabdomyolysis in type 1 PSSM appears to result from a deficiency of energy within individual contracting muscle fibers.[5] The genetic defect combined with a high-starch diet appears to produce substrate limited muscle oxidative metabolism by both impairing production of acetyl CoA from glycogen as well as by preventing lipolysis and delivery of free fatty acids to skeletal muscle mediated by insulin release.[9] Clinical signs of muscle pain in horses with the *GYS1* mutation may be exacerbated by enhanced individual insulin sensitivity[6] as well as by meals that produce elevated blood glucose and insulin levels.[9,62] The etiology of type 2 PSSM is not known at present.

Malignant Hyperthermia

A genetic form of malignant hyperthermia (MH) due to an autosomal dominant mutation in the skeletal muscle ryanodine receptor (*RYR1*) has been identified in 1% or fewer of American Quarter horses.[3]

CLINICAL SIGNS

Horses with MH may develop classic signs under general anesthesia of excessive body temperature, rigor, metabolic acidosis, and death.[1] In addition, affected horses may show signs of exertional rhabdomyolysis and high body temperatures. Some MH affected horses have died suddenly after an episode of ER.[2] The MH defect can co-exist with the *GYS1* mutation for type 1 PSSM.[44] The combination of these 2 mutations makes signs of ER more severe and increases recurrence of high serum CK, and horses do not respond as well to changes in diet and exercise.[44]

DIAGNOSIS

Genetic testing is recommended in Quarter horses and Paint horses with difficult to manage forms of PSSM or a family history of post-anesthetic complications. Testing is available through the Veterinary Diagnostic Laboratory at the University of Minnesota. http://www.vdl.umn.edu/vdl/ourservices/neuromuscular. html.

Management of Chronic Forms of Exertional Rhabdomyolysis

EXPECTATIONS

Most horses with chronic forms of ER always have an underlying predilection for muscle soreness. However, with proper management most cases can have successful competitive careers. A few RER horses (speculatively homozygous fillies) are extremely difficult to manage and may be retired from racing. Most type 1 PSSM horses can be successful pleasure and trail horses but usually do not achieve success in upper-level dressage or fast-paced activities such as barrel racing. This limitation may not be true of type 2 PSSM horses.

Following clinical episodes, more than 80% of PSSM horses show notable improvement with adherence to both the diet and exercise recommendations provided below.[24] There is, however, a wide range in the severity of clinical signs shown by horses with PSSM; horses with severe or recurrent clinical signs require more stringent adherence to diet and exercise recommendations to regain muscle function. PSSM horse that also have the mutation for MH do not respond as well to diet and exercise recommendations and may continue to develop ER with the possibility of a fatal episode.[44]

REST

Stall rest appears to be counterproductive and predisposes RER and PSSM horses to further episodes of rhabdomyolysis. Providing daily turn-out with compatible companions can be very beneficial. It decreases anxiety in RER horses and enhances energy metabolism in PSSM horses. PSSM horses that are confined for days following an episode of rhabdomyolysis often have persistently elevated serum CK activity. In contrast, PSSM horses kept on pasture with little grain supplementation often show few clinical signs of rhabdomyolysis and have normal serum CK activity.[43]

ENVIRONMENT

If excitement is a triggering factor for RER, stressful environmental elements should be minimized. Many horses respond to a regular routine including feeding prior to other horses and training before other horses, especially if the horse becomes impatient while waiting. Other ways to decrease excitement include housing in an area of the barn where horses are not always walking past and next to calm companionable horses. The use of hot walkers, exercise machines, and swimming pools should be evaluated on an individual basis, because some horses develop rhabdomyolysis when using this type of equipment. Horses that develop rhabdomyolysis at specific events, such as horse shows, may must be reconditioned to decrease the stress level associated with such events.

Most PSSM horses are calm and not easily stressed. They do best when turned out on large pastures without lush grass where they move about on a daily basis. Grazing muzzles may be of benefit to PSSM horses for periods when grass is particularly lush.

EXERCISE

Regular daily exercise is important for managing all forms of ER. Thoroughbreds and Standardbreds with RER should avoid days off exercise. This prevents the elevations in serum CK activity that occur after a day of rest.[53] Following chronic episodes of ER in Thoroughbreds and Standardbreds, mild, calm, low-intensity daily exercise (less than 15 minutes) or preferably extensive daily turn-out is recommended until serum CK is less than 1,500 U/L. Thoroughbred racehorses often develop rhabdomyolysis when riders fight to keep horses at a slower speed (gallop exercise); therefore, this should be avoided.[40] Standardbreds often develop ER after 15 to 30 minutes of submaximal jogging and therefore interval training and reduction of jog miles to no more than 15 minutes per session is recommended.[75] For riding horses with RER, a prolonged warm-up with adequate stretching is recommended. Rest periods that allow horses to relax and stretch their muscles between 2- and 5-minute periods of collection under saddle may be of benefit. Event horses may require training that incorporates calm exposure to speed work to prevent rhabdomyolysis, as well as interval training at the speeds achieved during competitions.

Important principles to follow when starting exercise programs in PSSM horses include:

1. Providing adequate time for adaptation to a new diet prior to commencing exercise
2. Recognizing that the duration of exercise is more important than restricting the intensity of exercise
3. Ensuring the exercise is gradually introduced and consistently performed
4. Minimizing any days without some form of exercise.

If horses have experienced an episode of ER recently, 2 weeks of turn-out and diet change are often beneficial prior to recommencing exercise. Exercise should be very relaxed, and the horse should achieve a long, low frame without collection. For many horses this is most readily achieved in a round pen or on a lunge line. Successive daily addition of 2-minute intervals of walk and trot beginning with only 4 minutes of exercise and working up to 30 minutes after 3 weeks is recommended. Advancing the horse too quickly often results in poor adaptation or an episode of ER and repeated frustration for the owner.

Work under saddle after 3 weeks of ground work should be a gradually accelerating program that adds 2-minute intervals of collection or canter to the initial relaxed warm-up period at a walk and trot. Unless a horse shows an episode of overt ER during the initial first 4 weeks of exercise, re-evaluating serum CK activity is not helpful for the first month. This is because it is very common to have subclinical elevations in CK activity when exercise is re-introduced in PSSM horses, and a return to normal levels often requires 4 to 6 weeks of gradual exercise.[9,62] Keeping horses with PSSM fit seems to be the best prevention against further episodes of ER. This gradual approach aims to enhance the oxidative capacity of skeletal muscle, which in most Quarter horses is very low but can be increased with daily exercise. The objective of enhancing oxidative metabolism is to facilitate the metabolism of fat and blood borne fatty acids as energy substrates.

DIETARY MANAGEMENT

A nutritionally balanced diet with appropriate caloric intake and adequate vitamins and minerals is the core element of treating all forms of ER. Dietary recommendations are summarized in Table 7.4. Diets with a restricted amount of starch and sugar and supplemental calories supplied with fat are the basis for dietary management. In general, grass hay is preferable to alfalfa hay. For RER Thoroughbreds and Standardbreds, the challenge is supplying an adequate amount of calories in a highly palatable feed to meet daily energy demands. Controlled experimental studies using Thoroughbreds with RER show that serum CK activity is significantly lower when horses are fed a specially formulated high-fat, low-starch feed rather than an isocaloric amount of high-starch grain.[41,53] Given the close relationship between nervousness and RER, assuaging anxiety and excitability by reducing dietary starch and increasing

Table 7.4. Feeding recommendations for an average sized 1,000-lb horse with exertional rhabdomyolysis due to recurrent exertional rhabdomyolysis (RER) or polysaccharide storage myopathy (PSSM).

	RER			PSSM		
Exercise intensity	Light	Moderate	Intense	Light	Moderate	Intense
Caloric intake (megacalories/day)	20	25	33	18	23	30
% of daily digestible energy as NSC	15–20	15–20	15–20	Less than 10	Less than 10	Less than 10
% of daily digestible energy as fat	15	15–20	20–25	20	15–20	15–20
Selenium mg/day	2.2	2.8	3.1	2.2	2.8	3.1
Vitamin E† units	1,000	2,000	4,000	1,000	2,000	4,000
Daily amount (lbs) of 12% NSC, 10% fat concentrate*	5	7	10	4	6	8
Grass hay (lbs) with less than 12% NSC by weight	15–20	15–20	15–20	15–20	15–20	15–20
Sodium chloride (g)	34	34	41	34	34	41

† = natural vitamin is preferable to synthetic vitamin E due to better absorption, * = concentrate such as Re-Leve made by Kentucky Equine Research for horses with exertional myopathies.

dietary fat may decrease susceptibility by making these horses calmer prior to exercise. Some racehorse trainers prefer to supplement with a titrated amount of grain 3 days prior to a race if horses are on a low-starch, high-fat feed to increase the horse's energy during the race.

For PSSM horses, the challenge can be to provide adequate fat for energy metabolism while preventing excessive weight gain. If horses are overweight, reducing caloric intake by using a grazing muzzle, restricting hay to 1.5% of body weight, and providing a vitamin/mineral ration balancer is recommended. Adding excessive calories in the form of fat to an obese horse is inadvisable. Until horses are a normal weight, fat metabolism can be enhanced by riding horses after a 5- to 8-hour fast as a means to elevate plasma-free fatty acids.

Once a horse has achieved the desired body weight, feeds low in starch and sugar combined with dietary fat can be introduced. The starch and sugar content of the diet of PSSM horses must be managed more stringently than for RER horses (Table 7.4). Owners report that this type of diet improves clinical signs of muscle pain, stiffness, and exercise tolerance in Draft horses, Warmbloods, Quarter horses, and other breeds with PSSM when combined with the recommended exercise program. The addition of fat alone is not beneficial and an exercise program must be instituted for PSSM horses to show clinical improvement. Dietary change appears to have lesser impact on alleviating gait changes such as shivers.[34] Based on antecdotal experience, some authors recommend that more than 20% of daily caloric intake be supplied by fat (0.5 kg of fat). However, there are no controlled studies that support the "must feed every PSSM horse 1 pound of fat" (3 cups or more of oil) theory, and there are controlled studies to show PSSM horses can consume less fat and have normal CK activity.[9] In the author's experience, there is a great deal of variation in individual needs for fat supplementation and this should be balanced with the horse's weight.

A number of well balanced low-starch high-fat commercial diets are suitable for horses with RER and PSSM; however, the amount of starch and sugar can vary widely, as can the type of fat. Not all of these feeds are equally effective. At present, the NSC content of equine feed products is not listed on the feed tag, and consultation with the feed manufacturer is necessary to obtain this information. Nutritional support is available through most feed manufacturers in designing an appropriate diet. There are published peer reviewed studies to show the beneficial effect of one commercial diet on both RER and PSSM.[53,62]

MEDICATIONS

Low doses of acepromazine prior to exercise have been used in RER horses prone to excitement. A dose of 7 mg IV 20 minutes before exercise is reported to make horses more relaxed and manageable. Reserpine and fluphenazine, which have a longer duration of effect, are also used for this purpose. Horses given fluphenazine may occasionally exhibit bizarre behavior. Use of tranquillizers may only be necessary when horses

are in their initial phase of training and accommodation to a new environment because they obviously cannot compete on these medications.

Dantrolene sodium acts to decrease release of calcium from the calcium release channel in skeletal muscle and is used to treat malignant hyperthermia. Dantrolene given to horses with RER 90 minutes before exercise prevented abnormal elevations in CK following exercise.[51] A dose of 800 mg of dantrolene was given to Thoroughbred horses in the UK 1 hour prior to exercise and resulted in significantly lower postexercise CK activity than a placebo.[22] It must be given 60 to 90 minutes prior to exercise.

Phenytoin (1.4 to 2.7 mg/kg PO BID) acts on a number of ion channels within muscle and nerves, including sodium and calcium channels. Therapeutic levels vary, so oral doses are adjusted by monitoring serum levels to achieve 8 ug/ml and not to exceed 12 ug/ml.[8] Drowsiness and ataxia are evidence that the dose of phenytoin is too high and the dose should be decreased by half. Initial dosages start at 6 to 8 mg/kg orally twice a day for 3 to 5 days. If the horse still experiences rhabdomyolysis but is not drowsy, the dose can be increased by 1 mg/kg increments every 3 to 4 days.

Intramuscular injections of vitamin E and selenium are used in an attempt to prevent RER. Ensuring adequate oral intake may prevent the muscle soreness associated with IM injections.

HORMONE THERAPY

Some mares appear to exhibit signs of ER during estrus and it may well be beneficial in these horses to suppress estrus behavior using progesterone injections. Testosterone and anabolic steroids are used at racetracks to prevent signs of RER, but the efficacy has not been evaluated.

ELECTROLYTE SUPPLEMENTATION

Horses require daily dietary supplementation with sodium and chloride either in the form of loose salt (30 to 50 g/day) or a salt block. Additional electrolyte supplementation is indicated in hot, humid conditions. Some studies suggest that electrolyte imbalances, as reflected by low urinary fraction excretion of sodium or high dietary excretion of phosphorus, may contribute to ER, although others have not found a consistent abnormality.

OTHER DIETARY SUPPLEMENTS

A number of supplements are purported to decrease lactic acid build-up in skeletal muscle of ER horses. These include sodium bicarbonate, B vitamins, branched chain amino acids, and dimethylglycine. Because lactic acidosis is no longer implicated as a cause for ER, it is difficult to find a rationale for their use.

ADJUNCT THERAPIES

Massage, myofascial release, mesotherapy, stretching, and hot/cold therapy performed by experienced therapists may be of benefit in individual cases of ER.

Many but not all cases of exertional myopathies in horses are characterized by the development of muscle pain contractures, stiffness, and abnormal elevations in serum CK activity. Some disorders that affect muscle metabolism may result in exercise intolerance without inducing muscle necrosis. Two presently known metabolic disorders that are often characterized by normal serum CK activity include mitochondrial myopathy and type 2 PSSM.

MITOCHONDRIAL MYOPATHY

Mitochondrial myopathy is characterized by early onset of fatigue, normal serum CK activity, and development of lactic acidosis with as little as 10 minutes of trotting. A young Arabian filly with these signs was found to have a deficiency of complex 1, the first step in the mitochondrial respiratory chain.[77] Marked lactic acidosis, extremely low maximum oxygen consumption, and exercise intolerance occurred with light exercise. Histopathologic evaluation of muscle biopsies showed an abnormal increase in mitochondrial density which had an abnormal ultrastructural appearance. The horse has shown slowly progressive signs of muscle atrophy but has otherwise remained healthy at rest.

References

1. Aleman M, Brosnan RJ, Williams DC, et al. Malignant hyperthermia in a horse anesthetized with halothane. J Vet Intern Med 2005;19(3):363–6.
2. Aleman M, Nieto JE, Magdesian KG. Malignant hyperthermia associated with ryanodine receptor 1 (C7360G) mutation in Quarter horses. J Vet Intern Med 2009;23(2):329–34.
3. Aleman M, Riehl J, Aldridge BM, et al. Association of a mutation in the ryanodine receptor 1 gene with equine malignant hyperthermia. Muscle Nerve 2004;30(3):356–65.
4. Anderson MG. The influence of exercise on serum enzyme levels in the horse. Equine Vet J 1975;7(3):160–5.
5. Annandale EJ, Valberg SJ, Essen-Gustavsson B. Effects of submaximal exercise on adenine nucleotide concentrations in skeletal muscle fibers of horses with polysaccharide storage myopathy. Am J Vet Res 2005;66(5):839–45.
6. Annandale EJ, Valberg SJ, Mickelson JR, et al. Insulin sensitivity and skeletal muscle glucose transport in horses with equine polysaccharide storage myopathy. Neuromuscul Disord 2004; 14(10):666–74.
7. Bain FT, Merritt AM. Decreased erythrocyte potassium concentration associated with exercise-related myopathy in horses. J Am Vet Med Assoc 1990;196(8):1259–61.
8. Beech J, Fletcher JE, Tripolitis L, et al. Effects of phenytoin in two myotonic horses with hyperkalemic periodic paralysis. Muscle Nerve 1992;15(8):932–6.
9. Borgia L, Valberg SJ, McCue ME, et al. The effect of varying dietary starch and fat on metabolic response to exercise and plasma creatine kinase activity in Quarter horses with Polysaccharide Storage Myopathy. Am J Vet Res 2010;236(6):663.
10. Cardinet GH III, Fowler ME, Tyler WS. The effects of training, exercise, and tying-up on serum transaminase activities in horses. Am J Vet Res 1963;24:980–4.
11. Cardinet GH, Littrell JF, Freedland RA. Comparative investigations of serum creatine phosphokinase and glutamic-oxaloacetic transaminase activities in equine paralytic myoglobinuria. Res Vet Sci 1967;8(2):219–26.
12. Carlson GP. Medical problems associated with protracted heat and work stress in horses. Reno NV 1985;84–99.
13. Carlson GP. Synchronous diaphragmatic flutter. In Current Therapy in Equine Medicine, 2nd ed. Robinson NE, ed. WB Saunders, Philadelphia, 1987;485–6.
14. Carr EA, Spier SJ, Kortz GD, et al. Laryngeal and pharyngeal dysfunction in horses homozygous for hyperkalemic periodic paralysis. J Am Vet Med Assoc 1996;209(4):798–803.
15. Cole FL, Mellor DJ, Hodgson DR, et al. Prevalence and demographic characteristics of exertional rhabdomyolysis in horses in Australia. Vet Rec 2004;155(20):625–30.
16. Collinder E, Lindholm A, Rasmuson M. Genetic markers in Standardbred trotters susceptible to the rhabdomyolysis syndrome. Equine Vet J 1997;29(2):117–20.
17. Cumming WJK, Fulthorpe JJ, Hudgson P, et al. Color Atlas of Muscle Pathology, 1st ed. Mosby-Wolfe, London, UK, 1994.
18. De La Corte FD, Valberg SJ, MacLeay JM, et al. Developmental onset of polysaccharide storage myopathy in 4 Quarter horse foals. J Vet Intern Med 2002;16(5):581–7.
19. Divers TJ, Mohammed HO, Cummings JF, et al. Equine motor neuron disease: Findings in 28 horses and proposal of a pathophysiological mechanism for the disease. Equine Vet J 1994;26(5):409–15.
20. Dranchak PK, Valberg SJ, Onan GW, et al. Exclusion of linkage of the RYR1, CACNA1S, and ATP2A1 genes to recurrent exertional rhabdomyolysis in Thoroughbreds. Am J Vet Res 2006;67(8):1395–400.
21. Dranchak PK, Valberg SJ, Onan GW, et al. Inheritance of recurrent exertional rhabdomyolysis in Thoroughbreds. J Am Vet Med Assoc 2005;227(5):762–7.
22. Edwards JG, Newtont JR, Ramzan PH, et al. The efficacy of dantrolene sodium in controlling exertional rhabdomyolysis in the Thoroughbred racehorse. Equine Vet J 2003;35(7):707–11.
23. Firshman AM, Baird JD, Valberg SJ. Prevalences and clinical signs of polysaccharide storage myopathy and shivers in Belgian draft horses. J Am Vet Med Assoc 2005;227(12):1958–64.
24. Firshman AM, Valberg SJ, Bender JB, et al. Epidemiologic characteristics and management of polysaccharide storage myopathy in Quarter horses. Am J Vet Res 2003;64(10):1319–27.
25. Fraunfelder HC, Rossdale PD, Rickets SW. Changes in serum muscle enzyme levels associated with training schedules and stages of oestrus cycle in Thoroughbred racehorses. Equine Vet J 1986;18:371–4.
26. Freestone JF, Carlson GR. Muscle disorders in the horse: A retrospective study. Equine Vet J 1991;23(2):86–90.
27. Harris P, Colles C. The use of creatinine clearance ratios in the prevention of equine rhabdomyolysis: A report of four cases. Equine Vet J 1988;20(6):459–63.
28. Harris PA. An outbreak of the equine rhabdomyolysis syndrome in a racing yard. Vet Rec 1990;127(19):468–70.
29. Harris PA. The equine rhabdomyolysis syndrome in the United Kingdom: epidemiological and clinical descriptive information. Br Vet J 1991;147(4):373–84.
30. Harris PA, Snow DH. Role of electrolyte imbalances in the pathophysiology of the equine rhabdomyolysis syndrome. In Equine Exercise Physiology, 3rd ed. Persson S, Lindholm A, Jeffcott LB, eds. ICEEP Publications, Davis CA, 1991;435–42.
31. Harris PA, Snow DH, Greet TR, et al. Some factors influencing plasma AST/CK activities in Thoroughbred racehorses. Equine Vet J Suppl 1990;(9):66–71.
32. Holmgren N, Valberg S. Measurement of serum myoglobin concentrations in horses by immunodiffusion. Am J Vet Res 1992;53(6):957–60.
33. Hulland TJ. Muscle and tendons. In Pathology of Domestic Animals, 3rd ed. Jubb KVF, Kennedy PC, Palmer N, eds. Academic Press, Orlando, FL, 1985; 139–99.
34. Hunt LM, Valberg SJ, Steffenhagen K, et al. An epidemiological study of myopathies in Warmblood horses. Equine Vet J 2008;40(2):171–7.
35. Lentz LR, Valberg SJ, Balog EM, et al. Abnormal regulation of muscle contraction in horses with recurrent exertional rhabdomyolysis. Am J Vet Res 1999;60(8):992–9.
36. Lentz LR, Valberg SJ, Herold LV, et al. Myoplasmic calcium regulation in myotubes from horses with recurrent exertional rhabdomyolysis. Am J Vet Res 2002;63(12):1724–31.
37. Levaille R, Biller D. Muscle evaluation, foreign bodies and miscellaneous swellings. In: Equine Diagnostic Ultrasonography. McKinnon AO, Rantanen N, eds. Williams and Wilkins, Baltimore, 1998.
38. Lewis SS, Valberg SJ, Nielsen IL. Suspected immune-mediated myositis in horses. J Vet Intern Med 2007;21(3):495–503.
39. Lopez JR, Linares N, Cordovez G, et al. Elevated myoplasmic calcium in exercise-induced equine rhabdomyolysis. Pflugers Arch 1995;430(2):293–5.
40. MacLeay JM, Sorum SA, Valberg SJ, et al. Epidemiologic analysis of factors influencing exertional rhabdomyolysis in Thoroughbreds. Am J Vet Res 1999;60(12):1562–6.

41. MacLeay JM, Valberg SJ, Pagan JD, et al. Effect of ration and exercise on plasma creatine kinase activity and lactate concentration in Thoroughbred horses with recurrent exertional rhabdomyolysis. Am J Vet Res 2000;61(11):1390–5.

42. Madigan JE, Valberg SJ, Ragle C, et al. Muscle spasms associated with ear tick (*Otobius megnini*) infestations in five horses. J Am Vet Med Assoc 1995;207(1):74–6.

43. McCue ME, Valberg SJ. Estimated prevalence of polysaccharide storage myopathy among overtly healthy Quarter horses in the United States. Am J Vet Res 2007;231(5):746–50.

44. McCue ME, Valberg SJ, Jackson M, et al. Polysaccharide storage myopathy phenotype in Quarter horse-related breeds is modified by the presence of an RYR1 mutation. Neuromusc Disorders 2009;19:37–43.

45. McCue M, Armien A, Lucio M, et al. Comparative skeletal muscle histopathologic and ultrastructural features in two forms of polysaccharide storage myopathy in horses. Vet Pathol 2009;46:1281–1291.

46. McCue ME, Ribeiro WP, Valberg SJ. Prevalence of polysaccharide storage myopathy in horses with neuromuscular disorders. Equine Vet J Suppl 2006 August;(36):340–4.

47. McCue ME, Valberg SJ, Lucio M, et al. Glycogen synthase 1 (GYS1) mutation in diverse breeds with polysaccharide storage myopathy. J Vet Intern Med 2008.

48. McCue ME, Valberg SJ, Miller MB, et al. Glycogen synthase (GYS1) mutation causes a novel skeletal muscle glycogenosis. Genomics 2008;91(5):458–66.

49. McGowan CM, Fordham T, Christley RM. Incidence and risk factors for exertional rhabdomyolysis in Thoroughbred racehorses in the United Kingdom. Vet Rec 2002;151(21):623–6.

50. McGowan CM, Posner RE, Christley RM. Incidence of exertional rhabdomyolysis in polo horses in the USA and the United Kingdom in the 1999/2000 season. Vet Rec 2002;150(17):535–7.

51. McKenzie EC, Valberg SJ, Godden SM, et al. Effect of oral administration of dantrolene sodium on serum creatine kinase activity after exercise in horses with recurrent exertional rhabdomyolysis. Am J Vet Res 2004;65(1):74–9.

52. McKenzie EC, Valberg SJ, Godden SM, et al. Comparison of volumetric urine collection versus single-sample urine collection in horses consuming diets varying in cation-anion balance. Am J Vet Res 2003;64(3):284–91.

53. McKenzie EC, Valberg SJ, Godden SM, et al. Effect of dietary starch, fat, and bicarbonate content on exercise responses and serum creatine kinase activity in equine recurrent exertional rhabdomyolysis. J Vet Intern Med 2003;17(5):693–701.

54. Naylor JM, Robinson JA, Crichlow EC, et al. Inheritance of myotonic discharges in American Quarter horses and the relationship to hyperkalemic periodic paralysis. Can J Vet Res 1992;56(1):62–6.

55. Peek SF, Semrad SD, Perkins GA. Clostridial myonecrosis in horses (37 cases, 1985–2000). Equine Vet J 2003;35(1):86–92.

56. Perkins G, Valberg SJ, Madigan JM, et al. Electrolyte disturbances in foals with severe rhabdomyolysis. J Vet Intern Med 1998;12(3):173–7.

57. Poso AR, Soveri T, Oksanen HE. The effect of exercise on blood parameters in standardbred and Finnish-bred horses. Acta Vet Scand 1983;24(2):170–84.

58. Rasanen LA. Exercise-induced purine nucleotide degradation and changes in myocellular protein release. Equine Vet J Suppl 1995;18:235–8.

59. Reef V. Musculoskeletal ultrasonography. In Equine Diagnostic Ultrasonography. W.B. Saunders Co., Philadelphia, 1998; 39–186.

60. Reynolds AJ. Equine hyperkalemic periodic paralysis (HYPP): Overview and management strategies. http://www admani com/ AllianceEquine/TechBulletins/HYPP htm 2007.

61. Reynolds JA, Potter GD, Greene LW. Genetic-diet interactions in the hyperkalemic periodic paralysis syndrome in Quarter horses fed varying amounts of potassium: III. The relationship between plasma potassium concentration and HYPP Symptoms. J Equine Vet Sci 1998;18(11):731–5.

62. Ribeiro WP, Valberg SJ, Pagan JD, et al. The effect of varying dietary starch and fat content on serum creatine kinase activity and substrate availability in equine polysaccharide storage myopathy. J Vet Intern Med 2004;18(6):887–94.

63. Roneus B, Hakkarainen J. Vitamin E in serum and skeletal muscle tissue and blood glutathione peroxidase activity from horses with

64. the azoturia-tying-up syndrome. Acta Vet Scand 1985;26(3):425–7.

64. Rudolph JA, Spier SJ, Byrns G, et al. Periodic paralysis in Quarter horses: A sodium channel mutation disseminated by selective breeding. Nat Genet 1992;2(2):144–7.

65. Spier SJ, Carlson GP, Holliday TA, et al. Hyperkalemic periodic paralysis in horses. J Am Vet Med Assoc 1990;197(8):1009–17.

66. Sponseller BT, Valberg SJ, Ward TL, et al. Muscular weakness and recumbency in a Quarter horse colt due to glycogen branching enzyme deficiency. Equine Vet Educ 2003;14:182–8.

67. Sprayberry KA, Madigan J, Lecouteur RA, et al. Renal failure, laminitis, and colitis following severe rhabdomyolysis in a draft horse-cross with polysaccharide storage myopathy. Can Vet J 1998;39(8):500–3.

68. Sullins KE, Heath RB, Turner AS, et al. Possible antebrachial flexor compartment syndrome as a cause of lameness in two horses. Equine Vet J 1987;19(2):147–50.

69. Tryon RC, Penedo MC, McCue ME, et al. Allele frequencies of inherited disease genes in subpopulations of American Quarter horses. J Am Vet Med Assoc 2009;234(1):120–125.

70. Upjohn MM, Archer RM, Christley RM, et al. Incidence and risk factors associated with exertional rhabdomyolysis syndrome in National Hunt racehorses in Great Britain. Vet Rec 2005;156(24):763–6.

71. Valberg SJ. Diseases of muscle. In Large Animal Internal Medicine, 4rd ed. Smith BP, ed. Mosby Elsevier, St. Louis, 2009;1388–11418.

72. Valberg SJ, Dyson S. Skeletal muscle and lameness. In Lameness in the Horse, 1st ed. Ross M, Dyson S, eds. Saunders, Philadelphia, 2003;723–43.

73. Valberg SJ, Maas J. Diseases of muscles: Nutritional myodegeneration. In Large Animal Internal Medicine, 4th ed. Smith BP, ed. Mosby Elsevier, St. Louis, 2009;1405–8.

74. Valberg S, Haggendal J, Lindholm A. Blood chemistry and skeletal muscle metabolic responses to exercise in horses with recurrent exertional rhabdomyolysis. Equine Vet J 1993;25(1):17–22.

75. Valberg S, Jonsson L, Lindholm A, et al. Muscle histopathology and plasma aspartate aminotransferase, creatine kinase and myoglobin changes with exercise in horses with recurrent exertional rhabdomyolysis. Equine Vet J 1993;25(1):11–6.

76. Valberg SJ, Cardinet GH III, Carlson GP, et al. Polysaccharide storage myopathy associated with recurrent exertional rhabdomyolysis in horses. Neuromuscul Disord 1992;2(5–6):351–9.

77. Valberg SJ, Carlson GP, Cardinet GH, III et al. Skeletal muscle mitochondrial myopathy as a cause of exercise intolerance in a horse. Muscle Nerve 1994;17(3):305–12.

78. Valberg SJ, Mickelson JR, Gallant EM, et al. Exertional rhabdomyolysis in Quarter horses and Thoroughbreds: One syndrome, multiple aetiologies. Equine Vet J Suppl 1999;30:533–8.

79. Valberg SJ, Ward TL, Rush B, et al. Glycogen branching enzyme deficiency in Quarter horse foals. J Vet Intern Med 2001;15(6):572–80.

80. Valentine BA. Polysaccharide storage myopathy: a common metabolic disorder of horses. Vet Pathol 2002;39:630.

81. Valentine BA, Cooper BJ. Incidence of polysaccharide storage myopathy: necropsy study of 225 horses. Vet Pathol 2005;42(6):823–7.

82. Valentine BA, Habecker PL, Patterson JS, et al. Incidence of polysaccharide storage myopathy in draft horse-related breeds: A necropsy study of 37 horses and a mule. J Vet Diagn Invest 2001;13(1):63–8.

83. Volfinger L, Lassourd V, Michaux JM, et al. Kinetic evaluation of muscle damage during exercise by calculation of amount of creatine kinase released. Am J Physiol 1994;266(2 Pt 2):R434-R441.

84. Wagner ML, Valberg SJ, Ames EG, et al. Allele frequency and likely impact of the glycogen branching enzyme deficiency gene in Quarter horse and Paint horse populations. J Vet Intern Med 2006;20(5):1207–11.

85. Ward TL, Valberg SJ, Adelson DL, et al. Glycogen branching enzyme (GBE1) mutation causing equine glycogen storage disease IV. Mamm Genome 2004;15(7):570–7.

86. Ward TL, Valberg SJ, Gallant EM, et al. Calcium regulation by skeletal muscle membranes of horses with recurrent exertional rhabdomyolysis. Am J Vet Res 2000;61(3):242–7.

Principles of Therapy for Lameness

SYSTEMIC/PARENTERAL

LAURIE R. GOODRICH

Systemic/parenteral administration of medications to treat musculoskeletal diseases in the horse mainly encompasses oral nonsteroidal anti-inflammatory drugs (NSAIDs), oral nutraceuticals, intramuscular (IM) poly-sulfated glycosaminoglycans (PSGAGs), and intravenous (IV) hyaluronan (HA). Less commonly used systemic medications include oral HA, IV bisphosphonates, and a few other miscellaneous medications covered below. Excluding NSAIDs, there has been controversy regarding these drugs in the horse and whether they reach high enough concentrations at the intended area to be treated. Many (or most) of the drugs or nutraceuticals have been intended for systemic administration in humans, and levels high enough to be efficacious in the horse are often in question. NSAIDs and nutraceuticals are discussed in the oral/nutritional section later in this chapter.

PARENTERAL NSAIDS

The most commonly used intravenous NSAIDs are phenylbutazone and flunixin meglumine. Ketoprofen and carprofen are less commonly used intravenously. The NSAIDs mentioned above usually are used orally; however, in the acute case of inflammation when pain and swelling have not yet been addressed, the IV route of delivery is more effective and yields the desired pharmacological effect faster. Repeated IV injections are not recommended, however, due to perivasculitis that may develop in conjunction with constant IV use of NSAIDs. When NSAIDs are used consistently in horses, oral for-

mulations are recommended. For more information on specific NSAIDs, dosages, and indications, see the section on oral/nutritional therapy later in this chapter.

POLYSULFATED GLYCOSAMINOGLYCANS

Polysulfated glycosaminoglycans (PSGAGs) are a mixture of low molecular weight (approx 6 to 10,000 Daltons) glycosaminoglycans (GAG) that are very similar in structure to chondroitin sulfate, the major GAG in normal cartilage.[3] PSGAG administration has been associated with reducing the severity of clinical signs in both human and equine patients with arthritis.[17,28] Beneficial clinical effects are, at least in part, attributable to anti-inflammatory effects consisting of the inhibition of prostaglandin E_2 (PGE_2), cytokine release, and stimulatory effects on cartilage matrix components.[31] Modes of administration include intramuscular (IM) and intra-articular (IA) routes. Elevated risks have been identified with IA administration; therefore, many practitioners still prefer to administer PSGAGs intramuscularly.[3] The efficacy of IM administration may be lower compared to direct injection into the joint. Typically, when a favorable response to IM administration occurs, it is rapid.

The PSGAG Adequan® (Luitpold Pharmaceuticals, Inc., Shirley, NY) is produced from bovine trachea and lung, and is in a class of drugs that exhibits chondroprotective properties in cartilage. Pentosan polysulfate, also within the same class of drugs, is produced from a plant source and is not licensed in the United States but is widely used in the UK.

This section focuses on the use of IM PSGAG. IA use is covered in the section on intrasynovial therapy.

Adams and Stashak's Lameness in Horses, 6e, edited by
Gary M. Baxter
© 2011 Blackwell Publishing, Ltd.

Mechanism of Action

While there has been convincing evidence of the beneficial effects of PSGAGs on cartilage, the exact mechanism of action remains unknown. It has been theorized that PSGAGs form stable complexes with fibronectin and collagen fibers and are deposited in cartilage.[1] Studies have shown that PSGAGs inhibit a plethora of degradative enzymes that contribute to the osteoarthritic (OA) process, including lysosomal elastase, cathepsins, lysosomal hydrolases, serine proteinases, neutral metalloproteinases, plasminogen activators, and inducible nitric oxide expression.[16,32] An anti-inflammatory role based on the inhibitory effects on leukocyte migration and interleukin levels has also been suggested.[13,20] A biosynthetic role has been documented in terms of its stimulation of HA and collagen synthesis.[25,32,35] A recent study in rabbits revealed a reduction in mechanical stiffness of patellar cartilage 30 weeks after induced trauma.[10]

Adequan® was originally intended for IA use; however, alterations in the complement pathway that potentiated subinfective doses of *Staphylococcus aureus* resulted in IM administration becoming a more popular mode of administration. There is less clinical data for IM use of the drug, although anecdotal reports of efficacy abound.[22] Reports in the literature reveal that IM administration of a single 500-mg dose of Adequan® in horses resulted in therapeutic levels of the drug in antebrachiocarpal, metacarpophalangeal, tibiotarsal, and distal interphalangeal joints within 2 hours of injection.[18] In an earlier clinical study, however, IM administration of Adequan® every 4 days for 7 treatments in a full-thickness cartilage defect model in ponies was unable to significantly improve cartilage healing.[33] Furthermore, Fubini, et al. reported an inability of IM Adequan® to have a protective effect on methylprednisolone-injected joints in ponies.[14]

Despite a lack of scientific data to support IM administration of Adequan®, some clinicians believe that it has a beneficial effect on certain horses. In a survey of more than 400 equine practitioners, IM Adequan® was one of the most commonly administered medications (not in the steroid category) in horses.[11] The current dosing recommendations are 500 mg IM every 3 to 5 days for 5 to 7 treatments.

Clinical Indications

Indications for systemic administration of Adequan® include synovitis, cartilage degradation, osteoarthritis, and capsulitis. Theoretically, this drug should prevent or at least minimize progression of osteoarthritis if it reaches high enough levels in the joint. Many practitioners also use it to prevent joint inflammation/disease in sport horses in heavy work. Results seem to vary, but if effective, the results are usually seen in the first 2 to 3 months of treatment.

HYALURONAN

Hyaluronan (or hyaluronic acid, HA) is a large unbranched nonsulphated glycosaminoglycan composed of repeating units of D-glucouronic acid and N-acetyl glucosamine. It is an integral component of synovial fluid and articular cartilage. Intrasynovial injections are most likely the most efficacious route of administration; however the desire to treat multiple joints simultaneously has driven clinicians to use IV and oral preparations.

Mechanism of Action

HA actions in the synovial joint include increasing viscosity of synovial fluid, lubricating unloaded joints, restoring the rheologic properties of synovial fluid, and most importantly, inhibiting inflammation.[16,19,26] Many of these effects appear to depend on molecular size of the HA molecule administered, with molecular weights of .5 to 1×10^6 Da having the greatest ability of decreasing inflammation.[15]

Intravenous administration of HA is noninvasive and a route for treating multiple joints. The benefits are most likely due to the effects in the synovial membrane because plasma half-life is less than an hour and is no longer detectable after 3 hours.[23,27] The effects of IV administration may be due to the fact that the synovial membrane is highly vascularized, which may allow greater exposure to synoviocytes than IA administration. The anti-inflammatory effects may be due to the binding characteristics of HA to CD44 receptors present on several cell types within the synovial membrane, causing an inhibition of the expression of various cytokines.[30]

The only study to evaluate IV administration of HA in the horse used an osteochondral chip model and exercised horses following induction of the osteochondral fragment.[21] Horses treated with IV HA had reduced lameness, better synovial membrane scores, significantly lower total protein concentrations, and most importantly, reduced prostaglandins in joints compared to horses receiving saline. The study extended to 72 days following injection. Interestingly, HA did not have any effects on GAG content, synthetic rate, or morphologic scoring in articular cartilage, which lends credence to the theory that HA has mainly anti-inflammatory effects in joints. Currently, Legend® (Bayer Animal Health, Shawnee Mission, KS) is the only licensed HA product for IV administration. Another product, Polyglycan® (Arthrodynamic Technologies, Inc., Versailles, KY), is licensed as a medical device and is used by practitioners both intravenously and intrasynovially.[11] Clinical studies are currently under way to determine the clinical and biochemical effects of the IV administration on the osteochondral chip fragment model in horses (Frisbie DD, personal communication).

Clinical Indications

Indications for IV HA are similar to those for IM PSGAGs in that IV HA reduces inflammation in 1 or multiple joints or prevents an inflammatory process in sport horses that are in heavy use. Although IA administration is the most effective way to deliver this drug to the joints, IA and IV administration are often concurrent. IV HA is still probably more effective for controlling inflammation rather than being a disease-modifying drug for cartilage. Nevertheless, horses in which inflammation is controlled in many joints have a reduced risk of cartilage degeneration.

ISOXSUPRINE

Isoxsuprine has been suggested for treating navicular syndrome, sesamoiditis, and laminitis in horses. It is a β-adrenoreceptor antagonist with β-adrenoreceptor agonistic properties that causes vasodilation. Isoxsuprine also can decrease blood viscosity and platelet aggregation.[9] Several clinical studies have been performed to determine efficacy of dosages ranging from 0.6mg/kg to 1.2mg/kg orally twice daily. Results in several clinical trials were variable, with little control of shoeing and other concurrent treatments.[9,24,34] Despite reports of limited bioavailability, advocates of isoxsuprine recommend a trial dose of 0.6mg/kg twice a day for 30 days and continuation indefinitely if a treatment effect is realized.[24] In horses that do not respond to the twice daily 0.6mg/kg dose, a 0.9mg/kg or 1.2 mg/kg twice daily dose may be more favorable.[24] Poor responses most likely occur in cases with major radiological abnormalities.

BISPHOSPHONATES

Bisphosphonates have been used for decades to inhibit loss of bone mass in human patients with osteoporosis associated with age or steroid administration as well as rheumatoid arthritis.[4] Bisphosphonates inhibit osteoclast-mediated bone resorption, a property which clinicians believe plays a role in treating conditions in which reduction in bone turnover may have beneficial effects, such as OA and navicular bone edema/sclerosis.

Three studies in horses report the effects of the bisphosphonate tiludronate in clinical diseases such as navicular disease, vertebral pain related to OA of the thoracolumbar column, bone spavin, and bone loss due to cast immobilization.[5,6,8] All 3 studies reported reduced lameness, back soreness, and loss of bone with IV administration of the drug. More randomized controlled studies are needed to determine the efficacy as well as justify the current expense of this drug. Currently it is not licensed for use in horses in the US but veterinarians can obtain the drug with a letter of approval from the US Food and Drug Administration. Current pharmacokinetic studies suggest the drug be administered slowly at 1 mg/kg IV rather than at 0.1 mg/kg IV once daily for 10 days.[7] Flunixin meglumine is recommended concurrently because occasionally horses suffer from colic secondary to administration.

TETRACYCLINES

Tetracycline antibiotics have historically been used as treatments for rheumatoid arthritis and OA in humans. Clinical effects include improved joint pain and reduced cartilage erosion. Horses in which tetracyclines have been used empirically to treat Lyme disease while awaiting titer results have realized an improvement in lameness despite the fact that titers were negative.[12] Effects such as this have been attributed, at least in part, to the ability of tetracyclines to reduce matrix metalloproteinase (MMP) activity.[29] Ongoing studies will reveal the utility of low-dose tetracyclines or chemically modified tetracyclines in the horse that may reduce the catabolic effects of interleukin-1 and MMPs without an antimicrobial effect.[12]

ESTROGEN

Estrogen therapy has been used to treat upward fixation of the patella in horses.[36] The rationale is that estrogens can cause tendon and ligament relaxation; however, it is unclear whether horses with upward fixation have overly tense patellar ligaments and if estrogen has any effect on patellar ligaments and tendons. It is possible that estrogen affects muscle cell metabolism and muscle tone. There is anecdotal evidence that some horses may benefit from this type of therapy. There is a range of dosages, but generally they are 1 mg of estradiol cypionate/45 kg of body weight (i.e., 11 mg/500 kg) once weekly for 3 to 5 weeks.

ROBAXIN (METHOCARBAMOL)

Muscle relaxants are occasionally used to treat various pathologies of muscle disease in horses. Methocarbamol seems to produce variable results. However, it seems to benefit some horses that are prone to rhabdomyolysis or sore backs. The dose administered ranges from 6 to 22 mg/kg but usually is 10 mg/kg twice daily for 5 to 10 days.[2]

References

1. Andrews JL, Sutherland J, Ghosh P. Distribution and binding of glycosaminoglycan polysulfate to intervertebral disc, knee joint articular cartilage and meniscus. Arzneim Forsch 1985;35:144–148.
2. Black JB. The Western performance horse. In Diagnosis and Management of Lameness in the Horse. Ross MW, Dyson SJ, eds. Saunders, Philadelphia, 2003:1017–1020.
3. Caron JP. Intra-articular injections for joint disease in horses. Vet Clin North Am Equine Pract 2005;21:559–73.
4. Cohen SB. An update on bisphosphonates. Curr Rheumatol Rep 2004;6:59–65.
5. Coudry V, Thibaud D, Riccio B, et al. Efficacy of tiludronate in the treatment of horses with signs of pain associated with osteoarthritic lesions of the thoracolumbar vertebral column. Am J Vet Res 2007;68:329–337.
6. Delguste C, Amory H, Doucet M, et al. Pharmacological effects of tiludronate in horses after long-term immobilization. Bone 2007;41:414–421.
7. Delguste C, Amory H, Guyonnet J, et al. Comparative pharmacokinetics of two intravenous administration regimens of tiludronate in healthy adult horses and effects on the bone resorption marker CTX-1. J Vet Pharmacol Ther 2008;31:108–116.
8. Denoix JM, Thibaud D, Riccio B. Tiludronate as a new therapeutic agent in the treatment of navicular disease: A double-blind placebo-controlled clinical trial. Equine Vet J 2003;35:407–413.
9. Erkert RS, MacAllister CG. Isoxsuprine hydrochloride in the horse: A review. J Vet Pharmacol Ther 2002;25:81–87.
10. Ewers BJ, Haut RC. Polysulphated glycosaminoglycan treatments can mitigate decreases in stiffness of articular cartilage in a traumatized animal joint. J Orthop Res 2000;18:756–761.
11. Ferris DJ, Frisbie DD, McIlwraith CW. Current joint therapies in equine practice: A survey of veterinarians, 2009. Proceedings Am Assoc Equine Pract 2009.
12. Fortier LA. Systemic therapies for joint disease in horses. Vet Clin North Am Equine Pract 2005;21:547–557.

13. Francis DJ, Forrest MJ, et al. Retardation of articular cartilage degradation by glycosaminoglycan polysulfate, pentosan polysulfate, and DH-40J in the rat air pouch model. Arthritis Rheum 1989;32:608–616.

14. Fubini SL, Boatwright CE, Todhunter RJ, et al. Effect of intramuscularly administered polysulfated glycosaminoglycan on articular cartilage from equine joints injected with methylprednisolone acetate. Am J Vet Res 1993;54:1359–1365.

15. Ghosh P, Guidolin D. Potential mechanism of action of intra-articular hyaluronan therapy in osteoarthritis: Are the effects molecular weight dependent? Semin Arthritis Rheum 2002; 32:10–37.

16. Goodrich LR, Nixon AJ. Medical treatment of osteoarthritis in the horse—A review. Vet J 2006;171:51–69.

17. Hamm D, Jones EW. Intra-articular (IA) and intramuscular (IM) treatment of noninfectious equine arthritis (DJD) with polysulphated glycosaminoglycan (PSGAG). Eq Vet Science 1988; 8:456–459.

18. Haugland LM, Collier MA, DeBault LE, et al. 3H-PSGAG concentration in the synovial fluid of the equine antebrachiocarpal, metacarpophalangeal, coronopedal, and tibiotarsal joints following a 500 mg injection. J Equine Vet Sci 1995;15:274–278.

19. Howard RD, McIlwraith CW. Sodium hyaluronate in the treatment of equine joint disease. Compend Contin Educ Pract Vet 1993;15:473–481.

20. Jones IL, Sandstrom T. Enhanced breakdown of bovine articular cartilage proteoglycans by conditioned synovial medium *in vitro*. The effect of glycosaminoglycan polysulfate. Arzneim Forsch 1985;35:141–144.

21. Kawcak CE, Frisbie DD, Trotter GW, et al. Effects of intravenous administration of sodium hyaluronate on carpal joint in exercising horses after arthroscopic surgery and osteochondral fragmentation. Am J Vet Res 1997;58:1132–1140.

22. Kollias-Baker C. Therapeutics of musculoskeletal disease in the horse. Vet Clin North Am Equine Pract 1999;15:589–602.

23. Laurent UB, Fraser JR, Engstrom-Laurent A, et al. Catabolism of hyaluronan in the knee joint of the rabbit. Matrix 1992; 12:130–136.

24. Madison JB, Dyson SJ. Treatment and prognosis of horses with navicular disease. In Lameness in Horses. Ross M, Dyson SJ, eds. Saunders, Philadelphia, 2003:299–304.

25. Nishikawa H, Mori I, Umemoto J. Influences of sulfated glycosaminoglycans on biosynthesis of hyaluronic acid in rabbit knee synovial membrane. Arch Biochem Biophys 1985;240:146–153.

26. Pisko EJ, Turner RA, Soderstrom LP, et al. Inhibition of neutrophil phagocytosis and enzyme release by hyaluronic acid. Clin Exp Rheumatol 1983;1:41–44.

27. Popot MA, Bonnaire Y, Guechot J, et al. Hyaluronan in horses: Physiological production rate, plasma and synovial fluid concentrations in control conditions and following sodium hyaluronate administration. Equine Vet J 2004;36:482–487.

28. Raatikainen T, Vaananen K, Tamelander G. Effect of glycosaminoglycan polysulfate on chondromalacia patellae. Acta Ortho Scand 1990;61:443–448.

29. Smith GN Jr., Yu LP Jr., Brandt KD, et al. Oral administration of doxycycline reduces collagenase and gelatinase activities in extracts of human osteoarthritic cartilage. J Rheumatol 1998; 25:532–535.

30. Tamoto K, Tada M, Shimada S, et al. Effects of high-molecular-weight hyaluronates on the functions of guinea pig polymorphonuclear leukocytes. Semin Arthritis Rheum 1993;22:4–8.

31. Todhunter RJ, Lust G. Polysulfated glycosaminoglycan in the treatment of osteoarthritis. J Am Vet Med Assoc 1994; 204:1245–1251.

32. Trotter GT. Polysulfated glycosaminoglycan (Adequan). In Joint Disease in the Horse. McIlwraith CW, Trotter GT, eds. W.B. Saunders, Philadelphia, 1996:270–280.

33. Trotter GW, Yovich JV, McIlwraith CW, et al. Effects of intramuscular polysulfated glycosaminoglycan on chemical and physical defects in equine articular cartilage. Canadian Journal of Veterinary Research 1989;53, 224–230.

34. Turner AS, Tucker CM. The evaluation of isoxsuprine hydrochloride for the treatment of navicular disease: A double blind study. Equine Vet J 1989;21:338–341.

35. Vacha J, Pesakova V, Krajickova J, et al. Effect of glycosaminoglycan polysulphate on the metabolism of cartilage ribonucleic acid. Arzneim Forsch 1984;34:607–609.

36. Valentine BA. Mechanical lameness in the hindlimb. In Diagnosis and Management of Lameness in the Horse. Ross MW, Dyson SJ, eds. Saunders, Philadelphia, 2003:475–480.

TOPICAL/LOCAL

Laurie R. Goodrich

Topical and local therapies are commonly used to treat equine musculoskeletal diseases, both acutely when inflammation is most pronounced and chronically when ongoing inflammation results in soreness and/or lameness. Although NSAIDs are commonly used orally to control musculoskeletal inflammation, and intravenously in the acute stages of inflammation, clinicians often look for local modes of therapy to control associated edema and release of inflammatory mediators. The need for systemic NSAID therapy can be reduced and associated edema and tissue damage minimized with effective use of topical therapy.

TOPICAL NSAIDS

A topical formulation of diclofenac liposomal cream (DLC, Surpass®, Boehinger Ingelheim Vetmedica, Inc., St. Joseph, MO) is now approved for treatment of horses with osteoarthritis (OA).[12] The drug comes in a cream form, which is applied locally to areas of inflammation. Studies in horses revealed that when the drug was incorporated into liposomes, it readily penetrated skin and significantly attenuated carrageenan-induced local production of PGE_2.[8] Furthermore, minimal concentrations of diclofenac were detectable in plasma. In a recent study of 24 horses that had induced OA in the middle carpal joint via an osteochondral chip fragment model, application of 7.3 g of DLC twice daily (label dose) to the skin led to significant improvement in lameness, and significantly less carpal bone sclerosis and overall gross cartilage erosion compared to controls.[12] A study reporting the serum and urinary concentrations at 1×, 2×, and 4× the recommended dose applied over 10 days revealed slow absorption and elimination of the cream. This study is a useful resource to determine withdrawal times to prevent an inadvertent positive drug test.[1]

Clinical Use

Surpass® is used commonly in clinical practice. It can be used under a bandage and there are currently are no reported adverse effects. Although the dose is 7.3 g BID, some clinicians use this drug once daily or every other day for less acute inflammation. It is used for osteoarthritis, periostitis, tendinitis, and various musculoskeletal inflammatory conditions. Concurrent use of this product with systemic NSAIDs is common and seems to be very effective for a variety of inflammatory conditions.

TOPICAL FIRST AID (COLD THERAPY AND BANDAGING)

With acute inflammation associated with tendon injury or joint trauma (capsulitis, synovitis), initial cold therapy using ice boots, cold water hosing/

hydrotherapy, or medical devices that provide cold therapy and compression (Game Ready®, Alameda, CA) are useful therapies. Cold compression in the early stages of inflammation retard the inflammatory processes of exudation and diapedesis and reduce edema.[17] The use of cold therapy as a primary treatment for most acute joint or tendon injuries is commonly practiced and is extremely beneficial. Following an initial cooling out phase, usually 48 to 72 hours, warm hydrotherapy is often used to relieve pain and tension in tissues as well as stimulate the vasodilatory effect to aid with fluid resorption and the stimulation of phagocytic cells.[17]

Bandaging and pressure wraps are also commonly used to decrease edema formation and generalized swelling that results from inflammatory mediators released from the torn tendon or joint capsule. Bandage support also may assist healing as stimulation of mechanoreceptors occurs, and this may decrease pain sensation.[17] To date, there are no clinical studies that determine how long pressure bandages should be applied, nor the necessary thickness of the bandage. The general practice is to apply pressure wraps for as long as ongoing inflammation occurs, and then slowly discontinue their use to prevent swelling from recurring.

DIMETHYL SULFOXIDE (DMSO)

The chemical solvent DMSO has been used alone or mixed with corticosteroids to treat soft tissue swelling and inflammation resulting from acute trauma.[17] Its main benefit is considered to be reduction of edema.[22] DMSO also has been shown to possess superoxide dismutase activity and to inactivate superoxide radicals. Further, the drug enhances penetration of percutaneous steroid when mixed with DMSO, and when cortisone was dissolved in DMSO, the dilution of cortisone necessary to stabilize lysosomes was reduced from one-tenth to one-thousandth.[22] If applied under a bandage, DMSO should be used with caution because it may cause skin irritation. Some practitioners combine furacin, DMSO, and glycerin as a sweat to reduce inflammation and edema.

EXTRACORPOREAL SHOCK WAVE THERAPY

Extracorporeal shockwave therapy (ESWT) is used by veterinarians to treat many different musculoskeletal conditions in horses. Extracorporeal shock waves are acoustic waves generated outside the body, characterized by transient high peak pressures followed by negative pressure and that return to zero pressure. Pressures reached by current equipment range from 10 to 100 MPa with a rapid rise time of 30 to 120 ns and a short pulse duration (5 μs). Other variables include energy level, pulse frequency, and depth of penetration. Originally designed to treat bladder and ureteral stones (lithotripsy), ESWT has been used to treat select musculoskeletal conditions in the horse, including suspensory ligament desmitis, OA of the low-motion joints of the tarsus, and dorsal metacarpal disease.[14,15]

Shockwaves behave like sound waves in tissue. The energy of the waves is liberated into tissue as a function of the difference in acoustic impedance of the adjacent tissues. Tissues that have an air-fluid interface absorb the greatest amount of energy; conversely, tissues that have muscle-fat interfaces absorb small amounts of energy.[15] Tissues such as the lung should be avoided due to the potential for causing injury such as subcutaneous hemorrhage and pain. Large nerves and blood vessels also are generally avoided. A study performed by Verna, et al. used nonfocused shockwave therapy applied directly over the digital vascular bundle and did not detect any evidence of vascular abnormalities.[20]

The exact mechanism of action that extracorporeal shock wave therapy has on specific tissues has not been elucidated. Through its ability to cause cavitation, or the rupture of gas bubbles within the tissues, it is postulated that ESWT affects the tissues that are influenced by pressure, energy flow, and pulse frequency of the machine generating the waves.[15] Work in laboratory animals has demonstrated various dose-dependent effects, including microfracture of the cortical bone, medullary hemorrhage, subperiosteal hemorrhage, and stimulation of osteogenesis. Work in tendons has also demonstrated various dose-dependent effects, from hematoma formation and tendon cell damage, to increased glycosaminoglycan and protein syntheses.[6,7]

Analgesic properties attributed to ESWT have also long been recognized. Concerns over its use at racetracks has stimulated debate due to its abilities to reduce or eliminate pain from an injury that may become catastrophic if the horse continues to race. Two studies have been performed in the equine that have detected decreases in nerve conduction properties.[5,16] One of those studies observed significant disruption of the myelin sheath with no evidence of damage to Schwann cell bodies or axons following treatment with nonfocused ESWT.[5] Further, bone effects have also been documented in the horse in which both focused and radial shock waves resulted in an increase of microcracks on the dorsal surface of the third metacarpus and metatarsus.[13]

Several musculoskeletal conditions in horses have been treated with ESWT, including the bucked-shin complex, tibial stress fractures, proximal sesamoid bone fractures, incomplete proximal phalangeal fractures, subchondral bone pain, insertional desmopathies (most notably proximal ligament suspensory desmitis), impinging dorsal spinous processes, OA of the distal hock joints, navicular disease, and superficial digital flexor tendinitis.[6] Clinical trials have been performed in the horse; however, the units used varied as did energy levels, pulse frequency, depth of penetration, and number of treatments.

One of the most common clinical entities in which shockwave therapy has been used is proximal suspensory ligament desmitis. Data from clinical trials in Germany and the United States revealed a 70% to 80% success rate of return to work 6 months following focused or radial shockwave therapy.[6] Another popular use of shockwave therapy is in the treatment of navicular syndrome. In a German study, 80% of horses treated with shockwave therapy in the area between the heel bulbs improved in lameness.[4] This was in contrast to a 50% improvement in which the shockwaves were administered through the frog. Finally, clinical trials have been performed in horses with OA.[11] In a clinical model of induced OA in the middle carpal joint of horses, no disease modification was seen with ESWT; however, significant improvement in analgesia was observed in horses. Most likely, this effect is due to the nerve sheath alterations observed in other studies.[5]

Use of ESWT will most likely continue in equine practice. Large clinical trials are required to validate the appropriate uses and ideal settings, units, and specific diseases that will benefit from this treatment modality.

THERAPEUTIC ULTRASOUND, LASERS, AND ELECTROMAGNETICS

The use of therapeutic ultrasound, lasers, and electromagnetics is not uncommon in the horse industry. Horse owners who have done extensive investigation on the Internet, where anecdotal reports abound, frequently request equine clinicians' input on this therapy. Therapeutic ultrasounds emit unfocused sound waves that may have the potential to penetrate underlying tissues. The exact mechanism of action is unknown, but thermal energy purportedly is produced as the sound energy contacts the tissues. *In vitro* studies have reported alterations in blood flow, angiogenesis, collagen and protein synthesis, and osteogenesis. Clinical trials have shown conflicting results in treating tendon injuries. Therapeutic ultrasound did not improve muscle regeneration in injured tissue nor alleviate chronic heel pain in people.[3,9] One trial in horses reported improved healing characteristics 4 and 6 weeks following tendon injury.[18] Until more clinical trials become available, use of this treatment remains empirical.

Therapeutic laser therapy is based on light that is emitted from the instrument, a focused beam of photon energy. The power output of lasers used in physical therapy is in the milliwatt range (low). Mechanisms of action of therapeutic lasers are thought to include alterations in mitochondrial enzymes, and cytochromes within the electron transport chain and cellular calcium channels.[3] Cellular alterations may trigger mitosis and cellular proliferation which may have biomodulatory effects on circulation and analgesia. Only one study has been done in the horse, which showed no benefit in the treatment of wounds.[19] As with therapeutic ultrasound, more clinical studies are needed to determine if this therapy has a place in treating equine musculoskeletal conditions.

Magnetic and electromagnetic therapy remains a controversial subject. A great deal of anecdotal information is available, especially from equipment manufacturers. Ironically, this information is highly available to lay horsemen, despite a lack of technical information, understanding, and direction for its use. In general, an electromagnetic field is created by passing an electric current through a coil of insulated wire. When piezoelectrical properties of bone were discovered, evidence supported use of electromagnetic fields on bone healing.[3]

Limited studies are available in horses. Some benefit in fracture healing was observed after 2 hours of daily therapy.[2] Conversely, pulsed electromagnetic field therapy delayed tendon healing in experimentally created defects in the SDFT in horses.[21] However, in a rabbit study, beneficial effects were demonstrated in tendon healing.[10] As with therapeutic ultrasound and therapeutic laser therapy, magnetic therapy applications will most likely continue to be touted by the lay horseman until clinical trials are available to prove or disprove efficacy.

COUNTERIRRITATION

Topical blistering and pin firing have long been part of veterinary medicine, but fortunately, they are rarely practiced today due to the lack of clinical data as well as their inhumane ramifications. They are mentioned in this section only to acknowledge their common usage in the past. Topical blisters historically were made of iodine or mercuric iodide and were mainly used on splints, sore shins, or curbs. More severe blistering agents were made from cantharides or croton oil. The technique involved application to the skin and light exercise.

Firing most typically involves the use a pinpoint hot iron applied to the skin over the affected structure. Most commonly, firing is used for bucked shins and plantar ligament desmitis (curb) when the condition has not responded favorably to other conditions. The expectations that counterirritation may result in an improved fiber pattern with crimp and collagen are curious at best. Beyond enforced rest and low-grade exercise, the benefits of the treatment on underlying structures are most likely minimal. Occasionally, the technique continues to be used, but with the retirement of veterinarians who commonly used this technique it is seldom practiced.

References

1. Anderson D, Kollias-Baker C, Colahan P, et al. Urinary and serum concentrations of diclofenac after topical application to horses. Vet Ther 2005;6:57–66.
2. Auer JA, Burch GE, Hall P. Review of pulsing electromagnetic field therapy and its possible application to horses. Equine Vet J 1983;15:354–360.
3. Ball M. Therapeutic use of ultrasound, lasers, and electromagnetics. In Diagnosis and Management of Lameness in the Horse. Ross MW, Dyson SJ, eds. Saunders, Philadelphia, 2003: 811–814.
4. Blum N, Kreling K, Litzke LF. The use of extracorporeal shock-wave therapy in horses with navicular disease. Der Einsatz der Extrakorporalen Stosswellentherapie zur Behandlung des Podotrochlose-Syndroms. Pferdeheilkunde 2005;21:29–38.
5. Bolt DM, Burba DJ, Hubert JD, et al. Determination of functional and morphologic changes in palmar digital nerves after nonfocused extracorporeal shock wave treatment in horses. Am J Vet Res 2004;65:1714–1718.
6. Bonder D, Boening JK. Extracorporeal shock wave therapy. In Diagnosis and Management of Lameness in the Horse. Ross MW, Dyson SJ, eds. Saunders, Philadelphia, 2003:825–826.
7. Bosch G, Lin YL, Schie HTM, et al. Effect of extracorporeal shock wave therapy on the biochemical composition and metabolic activity of tenocytes in normal tendinous structures in ponies. Equine Vet J 2007;39:226–231.
8. Caldwell FJ, Mueller PO, Lynn RC, et al. Effect of topical application of diclofenac liposomal suspension on experimentally induced subcutaneous inflammation in horses. Am J Vet Res 2004;65:271–276.
9. Dyson M, Suckling J. Stimulation of tissue repair by ultrasound: a survey of the mechanisms involved. Physiotherapy 1978; 64:105–108.
10. Frank C, Schachar N, Dittrich D, et al. Electromagnetic stimulation of ligament healing in rabbits. Clin Orthop Relat Res 1983;263–272.
11. Frisbie DD, Kawcak CE, McIlwraith CW. Evaluation of the effect of extracorporeal shock wave treatment on experimentally induced osteoarthritis in middle carpal joints of horses. Am J Vet Res 2009;70:449–454.
12. Frisbie DD, McIlwraith CW, Kawcak CE, et al. Evaluation of topically administered diclofenac liposomal cream for treatment of horses with experimentally induced osteoarthritis. Am J Vet Res 2009;70:210–215.
13. Gomez TM, Radtke CL, Kalscheur VL, et al. Effect of focused and radial extracorporeal shock wave therapy on equine bone microdamage. Vet Surg 2004;33:49–55.
14. Loffeld S, Boening KJ, Weitkamp K, et al. Radial extracorporeal shock wave therapy for horses with chronic insertion desmopathy of the proximal suspensory ligament—a controlled study. Radiale extrakorporale Stosswellentherapie bei Pferden mit chronischer Insertionsdesmopathie am Fesseltroñgerursprung—eine kontrollierte Studie. Pferdeheilkunde 2002;18:147.
15. McClure SR, Merritt DK. Extracorporeal shock-wave therapy for equine musculoskeletal disorders. Compend Contin Educ Pract Vet 2003;25:68–70, 75.
16. McClure SR, Sonea IM, Evans RB, et al. Evaluation of analgesia resulting from extracorporeal shock wave therapy and radial pressure wave therapy in the limbs of horses and sheep. Am J Vet Res 2005;66:1702–1708.
17. McIlwraith CW. Diseases of joints, tendons, ligaments and related structures. In Adams' Lameness in Horses. Stashak TS, ed. Lippincott Williams and Wilkins, Philadelphia, 1998: 459–644.
18. Morcos MB, Aswad A. Histological studies of the effects of ultrasonic therapy on surgically split flexor tendons. Equine Vet J 1978;10:267–268.
19. Petersen SL, Botes C, Olivier A, et al. The effect of low level laser therapy (LLLT) on wound healing in horses. Equine Vet J 1999;31:228–231.
20. Verna M, Turner TA, Hayden DW. Short-term effects of nonfocused extracorporeal shockwave therapy on the palmar digital vasculature. Proceedings Am Assoc Equine Pract 2006.
21. Watkins JP, Auer JA, Gay S, et al. Healing of surgically created defects in the equine superficial digital flexor tendon: Collagen-type transformation and tissue morphologic reorganization. American Journal of Veterinary Research 1985;6, 2091–2096.
22. Wood DC, Wood J. Pharmacologic and biochemical considerations of dimethyl sulfoxide. Ann N Y Acad Sci 1975;243: 7–19.

INTRASYNOVIAL

Laurie R. Goodrich

Intrasynovial therapies are used to diminish the inflammatory response in synovium, cartilage, tendon (or tendon sheath), or meniscus. An effective therapy should halt progression of degradation of these structures and restore the normal intrasynovial environment, which will alleviate pain. Equine practitioners currently have several options available to treat intrasynovial inflammation. Intrasynovial therapies, specifically corticosteroids, are used frequently in horses to minimize or control pain associated with synovitis and osteoarthritis(OA).[10] New therapies are also beginning to be used intrasynovially as potential disease modifying agents of osteoarthritis (DMOAD); their reputed properties are prevention, retardation, or reversal of morphologic cartilaginous lesions of OA. While claims of these properties exist, evidence-based clinical studies about their true abilities to reverse OA are still in their infancy. The intrasynovial therapies covered in this section are the most commonly used treatments currently available for equine practitioners.

CORTICOSTEROIDS

Corticosteroids (CS) are the most potent anti-inflammatory drugs available to decrease the catabolic effects of joint disease. Historically, their use has been highly controversial due to the negative effects associated with overuse and high dosages used in the past.[46] Current clinical studies suggest judicious use of corticosteroids may be extremely beneficial and can result in long-lasting pain relief and control of inflammation.[19,38]

Mechanism of Action

Corticosteroids have powerful inhibitory effects on inflammation through stabilization of cellular lysosomal membranes, reduction of vascular permeability and leukocyte adherence to vessel walls (margination), inhibition of platelet aggregation, and leukocyte diapedesis. Furthermore, they inhibit prostanoids and nitric oxide, mediators integral to the progression of osteoarthritic lesions.[5,31] Corticosteroids are considered to be disease modifying through their actions on the abrogation of important mediators of inflammation, interleukin-1 (IL-1), and tumor necrosis factor-α (TNF-α). Degradative enzymes such as matrix metalloproteinases (MMPs) and other related proteinases are also decreased through the actions of corticosteroids which alter the progression of an inflamed joint toward osteoarthritic conditions.[15,33]

Detrimental Effects and Concerns Regarding Intra-articular Corticosteroids

The literature is replete with reports describing the deleterious effects of CS on cartilage. They include decreased chondrocyte size, loss of GAGs and decreased GAG synthesis, inhibition of proteoglycan synthesis, chondrocyte necrosis, and hypocellularity.[8,13,34,62] Particularly at high concentrations, CS inhibit production of important components of cartilage such as proteoglycans, collagen, and hyaluronic acid, and furthermore result in chondrocyte necrosis.[13,64] It is believed the high concentrations and extended exposure used in earlier studies resulted in the detrimental effects of CS on cartilage. As more realistic clinical models have emerged, such detrimental effects are noted less and more cartilage-sparing effects have been observed with use of low-dose corticosteroids.[38,54] The emerging stand by many clinicians seems to be that IA steroids can be extremely beneficial when used judiciously.

Post-injection flare associated with CS use in the horse is rare and usually self-limiting, but it is associated with some discomfort, necessitating NSAID therapy. The inflammation is believed to be caused by the microcrystalline characteristics of CS preparations, as well as the dose and particular ester that is injected, however; the incidence of post-injection flare has decreased with the advent of branched-chain esters.[66] More concerning is the potential for infection following CS injections. While the incidence is low, the occurrence of infection can be devastating and expensive to treat; therefore, strict adherence to aseptic technique is mandatory and the combination with an antimicrobial such as amikacin is commonly practiced.

It is important for practitioners to be aware that a delayed appearance of symptoms occurs due to the powerful ability of CS to inhibit inflammation. Symptoms associated with joint sepsis following steroid usage may take up to 10 days to become apparent. When faced with determining between a corticosteroid flare and joint sepsis, a synovial aspirate should be performed to detect a presence or absence of a leukocyte level and differential consistent with bacterial infection. Clinicians should bear in mind that CS can falsely lower WBC count post CS injection.

Laminitis has been associated with CS administration, and although rare, its occurrence subsequent to IA steroids can be devastating. In a study in which 205 horses were injected with triamcinolone at a dosage between 10 to 80 mg/treatment, only 2 of 205 horses developed laminitis and 1 of those cases was considered unrelated to the treatment because the laminitic event occurred several months following the treatment. This study reveals the low incidence of this complication.[47]

Clinical Choices

Despite decades of CS use to treat IA inflammation in the horse, the choice of formulation, dose, and frequency of administration remains somewhat empiric. Currently, the most commonly used formulations are

Table 8.1. Commonly used intra-articular corticosteroids.

Corticosteroid	Trade name	Manufacturer	Drug conc.(mg/ml)	Dose (mg)	Duration of action
Triamcinolone acetonide	Kenalog	Bristol-Myers Squibb	10	6–12	Medium
Methylprednisolone acetate	Depo Medrol	Pfizer	40 or 20	40–100	Long
Betamethasone acetate	Celestone Soluspan	Schering-Plough	6	3–18	Medium to long

triamcinolone acetonide, methyl-prednisolone acetate, and betamethasone acetate.[18] Less commonly used CS include isoflupredone acetate and flumethasone. In a recent survey of more than 400 equine practitioners, triamcinolone acetonide was found to be more commonly used in high-motion joints and methylprednisolone acetate in low-motion joints.[18]

Clinicians currently use lower dosages of CS than in the past because they seem to result in similar inhibition of inflammation with fewer detrimental effects on cartilage metabolism. Doses vary depending on the volume of synovial fluid in the joint, severity of inflammation, and the number of other joints requiring treatment. The formulations in Table 8.1 represent currently used CS and the associated dosages most commonly administered.

Triamcinolone Acetonide

The effects of low doses of triamcinolone on chondrocytes and extracellular matrix in both in vitro and in vivo studies have been impressive in terms of its ability to inhibit the degradative metalloproteinases with minimal negative effects on extracellular matrix of cartilage.[25,58] Frisbie, et al. showed that 12 mg of triamcinolone administered twice, 2 weeks apart, minimized the development of OA secondary to osteochondral chip fractures.[25] Interestingly, these effects were also noted in the contralateral joint. Furthermore, subchondral bone remodeling or fragility were not detected.[38] These studies suggest that a dose of 6 to 12 mg/joint should be adequate for anti-inflammatory effects. A study by Celeste, et al. revealed that 12 mg of TA administered at 3, 5, and 7 weeks in normal joints significantly altered cartilage metabolism both in injected and remote joints.[12] Although the joints in this study were not inflamed, clinicians should bear in mind that joints injected with triamcinolone as well as remote joints may change regulatory processes important in cartilage metabolism. The remote effects of triamcinolone have not been observed with other CS.

Methylprednisolone Acetate

Methylprednisolone acetate (MPA) has been studied extensively both in vitro and in vivo. Various beneficial and detrimental effects have been noted in cartilage, subchondral bone, and synovium.[11,16,58] Beneficial effects of MPA include reduction in the transcription of harmful molecules such as IL-1β, TNFα, MMPs, and others that directly cause matrix degeneration. Harmful effects include chondrocyte necrosis, inhibition of proteogly-

cans, and procollagen synthesis.[45,63] The dose of MPA seems to predict the fine balance between inhibition of inflammation with overall beneficial effects of the joint or destruction of matrix and disruption of normal cartilage metabolism. Ongoing studies will determine what level of MPA inhibits the destructive cascade of inflammation while preserving the normal joint environment.

Studies suggest that more physiological doses between 10 and 40 mg/joint inhibit inflammation and preserve normal joint environment.[16,50,64] Furthermore, results from Farquhar, et al. suggest the propensity for matrix changes tends to occur immediately following injection (softening), and thus horses should be prohibited from applying excessive loads for 6 days after injection.[16] In contrast, Murray, et al. found that microhardness of subchondral bone did not change with repeated injections of MPA and treadmill exercise; however, this study was done in normal joints.[51] Most notably, in a study by Frisbie, et al., horses that had osteochondral fragments induced in the middle carpal joints, had MPA injected at 100 mg, and underwent exercise on a treadmill revealed lower PGE$_2$ levels but also exhibited articular cartilage erosion and morphologic lesions associated with intra-articular MPA. In a survey of more than 400 practitioners regarding the use of corticosteroids, 75% revealed that they use MPA in low-motion joints, 36% use a dose of 20 to 40 mg, and 44% use 40 to 80 mg/joint injection.[18]

Betamethasone

Similar to MPA, betamethasone is considered an intermediate-to-long-acting glucocorticoid. A clinical study was performed by Foland, et al. in which osteochondral fragments were created in the middle carpal joint and 15.9 mg of betamethasone were administered to the joint at 2-week intervals followed by treadmill exercise. Although no statistically significant differences were seen between treated and control joints 56 days following treatment, there were trends toward decreased GAG staining in treated joints.[19] Although this study suggests mainly beneficial effects from betamethasone, practitioners should be aware that in vitro work still suggests potential detrimental effects as measured by suppressed proteoglycan synthesis at medium-to-low physiological doses.[21]

HYALURONAN

Hyaluronic acid (HA), or hyaluronan, is a large unbranched nonsulphated glycosaminoglycan comprised of repeating units of D-glucuronic acid and N-acetylglucosamine, and is secreted by the type B synoviocytes of the synovial membrane.[37,57] HA serves various important functions in the joint, such as providing viscoelasticity to the joint fluid and boundary lubrication of the intra-articular soft tissue. HA also may influence the composition of synovial fluid through steric hindrance of active plasma components and leukocytes from the joint cavity.[37] Furthermore, hyaluronan appears to modulate the chemotactic response within the synovial membrane by reducing cell migration and decreasing rates of diffusion and flow of solutes.[35]

HA is locally synthesized by chondrocytes and is the backbone of the proteoglycan aggregate in the extracellular matrix. The compressive stiffness in articular cartilage depends on the integrity of the matrix proteoglycans.[29]

Mechanism of Action

Although the exact mechanism of action is unclear, studies suggest that exogenously administered HA supplements or even replaces the actions of depleted or depolymerized endogenous HA in the synovial fluid, which restores viscoelasticity, steric hindrance, and lubrication of the articular soft tissues. *In vitro* studies suggest additional effects, including the ability to inhibit macrophage chemotaxis, reduce lymphocytic ability to proliferate and migrate, reduce the formation and release of prostaglandins from macrophages during phagocytosis, and scavenge oxygen-derived free radicals and degradative enzymes.[6,20,29,56] HA also possesses direct analgesic properties that seem to be partially attributable to reductions in the sensitivity of articular nerve endings.[10,30] Furthermore, it is suspected that exogenous injection of HA into osteoarthritic joints increases synthesis of high molecular weight HA by the synoviocytes.[37]

Many clinical studies in horses have supported HA administration in joint disease.[2,3,23,44,59,60] While the criteria for treatment success vary, the overall clinical impression is favorable. Inherent to clinical trials, duration of post-treatment observation periods is varied and short in some studies. Nevertheless, parallel clinical trials in humans also indicate symptomatic efficacy measured by improvement in pain, activity level, and function, especially following use of high-molecular weight products.[1]

Molecular Weight and Efficacy

The controversy continues regarding efficacy and molecular weight of high versus low molecular weight HA. Proponents of the visco-supplementation theory believe higher molecular weight products are more effective,[55] while others minimize the importance of size and suggest the activity of HA is mediated pharmacologically rather than physically.[4] More clinical studies are necessary to prove efficacy of higher or lower molecular weights of hyaluronic acid. Table 8.2 lists commonly used HA products and their molecular weights and current recommended dosages.

Clinicians who use HA should bear in mind that injections can be expensive due to the cost of the formulations; therefore, use in joints with advanced disease may yield less satisfying results compared to joints with incipient disease. This is consistent with human medicine, where people with less severe joint disease demonstrate greater improvement to intra-articular HA compared to those with more advanced radiographic changes.[67]

CORTICOSTEROID AND HA COMBINATIONS

The combination of HA and steroids to treat inflammation intrasynovially is commonplace.[9,14,42] Practitioners have recognized a beneficial effect of combination therapy for quite some time.[36] Synergistic

Table 8.2. Commonly used hyaluronan preparations.

Trade name	Concentration (mg/mL)	Manufacturer	Molecular weight (Daltons)[a]	How packaged	Current recommended dose (mg) per joint
Hylartin-V	10	Pharmacia and Upjohn	3.5×10^6	2-ml syringe	20
Hyvisc	11	Boehringer Ingelheim	2.1×10^6	2-ml vial	22
HY-50	17	Bexco Pharma		3-ml syringe	51
Equron	5	Solvay	$1.5–2 \times 10^6$	2-ml syringe	10
Equiflex	5	Chesapeake Biological	1×10^6	5-ml vial	10
Synacid	10	Schering-Plough	$0.15–0.20 \times 10^6$	5-ml vial	50
Hylovet	10	Fort Dodge/Vetrepharm	$4–7 \times 10$	2-ml syringe	20
Legend[b]	10	Bayer	3×10^5	4-ml vial	40 (IV)

[a] Manufacturer's reported molecular weight
[b] Marketed for IV and IA use

effects have been reported in human patients and similar effects have been seen *in vitro* in horses.[43,69] Many clinicians believe that the combination allows a smaller dose of corticosteroids to be administered with the HA, although further clinical studies are needed to determine the efficacy of combinations. The combination of HA and CS also is thought to provide a longer clinical effect than either injection alone, especially in high-motion joints.

INTRA-ARTICULAR POLYSULPHATED GLYCOSAMINOGLYCANS (PSGAGs)

PSGAGs are principally comprised of chondroitin sulfate, a glycosaminoglycan found in the aggregating proteoglycan of cartilage. It is a semisynthetic preparation from bovine trachea and is reported to have chondroprotective and anti-inflammatory properties as well as the ability to induce articular cartilage matrix synthesis and minimize matrix degradation.[65]

Mechanism of Action

The exact mechanism of action remains unclear. The drug most commonly is administered intramuscularly because intra-articular administration was initially associated with joint infections due to a reduction in complement activity in the joint. Intra-articular administration is now most commonly combined with 125 to 250 mg of amikacin to deter any infection, and this practice appears to be effective.

Many *in vitro* studies mimic the IA administration of PSGAGs because it is unlikely that concentrations injected intramuscularly can translate to similarly elevated concentrations in the joint fluid. *In vitro* studies and *in vivo* IA administration have revealed a significant ability of the drug to decrease lameness, modify OA through reducing bone remodeling, promote synthesis of endogenous HA, and inhibit mediators of inflammation, specifically PGE_2 production. Additionally, it has been found to reduce the levels of MMPs that rise in response to production of IL-1β.[10,27,29] Most recently, IA PSGAGs were compared to HA in an osteochondral chip fragment model and PSGAGs were demonstrated to reduce joint effusion and reduce synovial membrane vascularity and subintimal fibrosis compared with control horses when the drug was administered weekly for 3 weeks.[23] When compared to HA, neither PSGAGs nor HA had an effect on lameness. PSGAGs significantly reduced synovial membrane vascularity and subintimal fibrosis and HA significantly reduced fibrillation of the cartilage. It was concluded that in the osteochondral fragment model, both drugs had beneficial disease-modifying effects. Furthermore, in a study that compared PSGAGs to IA CS (MPA 40 mg), a regimen of weekly IA PSGAGs for 3 treatments gave significantly improved results (67%) compared to 1 treatment of CS (46%) in terms of returning horses to athleticism.[41]

Clinical Considerations

PSGAG is most likely more efficacious if administered intra-articularly, and this route of administration should be accompanied with amikacin due to the drug's ability to inhibit complement. Currently, the recommended frequency of IA administration is 3 to 5 injections weekly. It may be most efficacious in joints with known or suspected articular cartilage pathology.

POLYGLYCAN

Polyglycan®, which is not yet licensed for use as an IA medication, is a patented formulation comprised of hyaluronic acid, chondroitin sulfate, and N-acetyl-D-glucosamine, and has been used clinically in horses intra-articularly for viscosupplementation. This product is currently used extensively in equine practice; however, only one randomized blinded placebo controlled study has been performed to assess its efficacy. Frisbie, et al. compared Polyglycan® in an OA model of the middle carpal joints in which an osteochondral fragment was induced.[24] In horses in which Polyglycan® was administered intra-articularly at days 0, 7, 14, and 28, significant improvements were observed in lameness, bony proliferation, and degree of full-thickness articular cartilage erosions observed, grossly. Success with this IA medication will be further studied as the medication becomes more widely used in practice.

AUTOLOGOUS CONDITIONED SERUM (ACS)

ACS (also called interleukin receptor antagonist protein, IRAP) has been used extensively in practice to treat intrasynovial inflammation, especially in cases that are refractory to IA corticosteroids. Although clinical impressions have been favorable, this method of treatment is not widely used due to cost. IRAP, a substance that inhibits IL-1 activity, decreases the progression of joint disease and is believed to be present in high amounts in ACS.[26] Specifically, it has been reported that production of IL-4, IL-10, IRAP, and other growth factors are stimulated through incubation of whole blood with medical-grade glass beads exposed to chromium sulfate.[49]

A study by Frisbie, et al. in which ACS was injected into the middle carpal joints on days 14, 21, 28, and 35 following induction of OA through a chip fragment model revealed significant clinical improvement in lameness and reduced gross cartilage fibrillation and synovial membrane pathology. Elevated levels of IRAP were detected in the synovial fluid of the horses injected with ACS at 70 days post OA induction.[26] Clinical trials in humans with OA have also been encouraging, with people injected with ACS experiencing greater reduction in clinical signs and improved quality of life compared to those whose joints were injected with HA.[7,68] Use of this medication requires incubation of equine serum with beads coated with chromium sulfate to obtain the ACS solution. The ACS is usually administered intra-articularly weekly for 3 to 4 treatments, depending on the quantity of ACS obtained.

BONE- OR FAT-DERIVED MESENCHYMAL STEM CELL THERAPY

The use of bone-marrow or fat-derived mesenchymal stem cells (MSC) has grown in popularity in equine practice in the last decade. It is believed that these cells possess anti-inflammatory properties and may also contribute to healing of musculoskeletal tissues by becoming incorporated into the repair tissue.[52] Ferris, et al. recently reported on a retrospective study with a follow-up that included 40 horses that received IA injection of bone-marrow-derived mesenchymal stem cells which had been expanded to approximately 10 million to 20 million cells. Results from this study revealed a return to athleticism in 72% of all horses with IA injuries, ranging from mild to severe.[17] Although much more is known regarding the efficacy of MSCs in tendon injuries, early results suggest that these cells may also have a place in intrasynovial therapies. However, more randomized controlled clinical trials comparing efficacy to other treatments are needed.

MISCELLANEOUS

Other modes of therapy that control intrasynovial inflammation are currently being investigated. Gene therapy modalities engineered to overproduce beneficial cytokines such as insulin-like growth factor (IGF-I) and interleukin receptor antagonist protein (IRAP) are currently being developed.[22,28] Clinical trials will clarify the utility of these therapies.

Atropine is an anticholinergic drug that is occasionally used intrasynovially to reduce joint effusion. Its efficacy in a mouse model was proven by reducing induced joint effusion.[48] It has been used with some success in the horse; however, its use for reduction of joint effusion remains empirical. It is primarily used to reduce effusion in synovial cavities (mostly joints and tendon sheaths) that have not responded to other forms of therapy. The dose used is 7 mg IA, and if used for treatment of hygroma, should be combined with bandaging.[39] Horses should also be observed for colic following IA injection.

INTRASYNOVIAL THERAPY: PRACTICAL CONSIDERATIONS

Intrasynovial therapies are an integral part of the treatment of lameness in horses. Of course, success of the therapy depends on the correct synovial structure being medicated and that decision should be based on an accurate lameness examination and appropriate imaging. Furthermore, success of diminishing lameness also depends on the severity of the disease in the synovial structure being medicated as well as the efficacy of the medication being injected. For example, a recent study found a direct correlation between the success of intrabursal injections and the severity of the disease seen on MRI, with less severe disease having greater long-term success in treatment.[9] There are no accurate reports of how long a horse should be rested following corticosteroid injections; however, common practice is to combine the intrasynovial injection with at least 4 to 5 days of rest because the mechanical integrity of the cartilage has been shown to be compromised for several days following injection.[16] It is recommended that horses be returned to exercise slowly, over 1 to 2 weeks.

Sepsis may be a complication with any intrasynovial medication, so it is paramount for the clinician to be aware of any worsening of lameness following medica-tion of the structure. It should also be borne in mind that corticosteroid injections associated with sepsis may take several days to manifest due to their powerful inhibitory properties on inflammation. Although joint flares can also occur, a reaction to medication should be treated as a septic process until proven otherwise. Strict adherence to aseptic technique should also be practiced. A long accepted practice of aseptic prepping after clipping the hair over the injection site has been challenged recently by a study comparing aseptically prepared clipped and unclipped injection sites. The study found that areas could be adequately prepared without clipping.[32] Nevertheless, clipping the area of injection is still recommended by the author due to the devastating consequences of synovial infection. Furthermore, synovial injection should always be performed using sterile gloves and single-use syringes and needles and avoiding multiple-dose bottles or vials.

Occasionally, an intrasynovial structure is injected with medication and anesthetic as a combination of treatment and diagnostic aid. Recently a study found that the combination of TA and mepivacaine does not alter the potency or duration of TA's action.[40]

Finally, clinicians should realize that intrasynovial medications may diffuse between synovial structures. Two recent studies found that intrasynovial corticosteroids diffused between the coffin joint and navicular bursa[53] (when medication was injected into the coffin joint) and between the tarsal metatarsal joint and the distal intertarsal joint (when medication was injected into the tarsometatarsal joint).[61] This is often a desirable effect and further research will determine which synovial structures that approximate each other will adequately result in effective concentrations of drugs from the injected structure.

References

1. Aggarwal A, Sempowski IP. Hyaluronic acid injections for knee osteoarthritis. Systematic review of the literature. Can Fam Physician 2004;50:249–256.
2. Asheim A, Lindblad G. Intra-articular treatment of arthritis in race-horses with sodium hyaluronate. Acta Vet Scand 1976; 17:379–394.
3. Auer JA, Fackelman GE, Gingerich DA, et al. Effect of hyaluronic acid in naturally occurring and experimentally induced osteoarthritis. Am J Vet Res 1980;41:568–574.
4. Aviad AD, Houpt JB. The molecular weight of therapeutic hyaluronan (sodium hyaluronate): How significant is it? J Rheumatol 1994;21:297–301.
5. Axelrod L. Glucocorticoids. In Textbook of Rheumatology. Harris ED, Kelley WN, Ruddy S, et al., eds. WB Saunders, Philadelphia, 1993:779–796.
6. Balazs EA, Darzynkiewicz Z. The effect of hyaluronic acid on fibroblasts, mononuclear phagocytes, and lymphocytes. In Biology of Fibroblasts. Kulonen E, Pikkarainen JPKK, eds. Academic Press, New York, 1973:237.
7. Baltzer AW, Moser C, Jansen SA, et al. Autologous conditioned serum (Orthokine) is an effective treatment for knee osteoarthritis. Osteoarthritis Cartilage 2009;17:152–160.
8. Behrens F, Shepard N, Mitchell N. Alteration of rabbit articular cartilage by intra-articular injections of glucocorticoids. J Bone Joint Surg 1975;57:70–76.
9. Bell CD, Howard RD, Taylor DS, et al. Outcomes of podotrochlear (navicular) bursa injections for signs of foot pain in horses evaluated via magnetic resonance imaging: 23 cases (2005–2007). J Am Vet Med Assoc 2009;234:920–925.
10. Caron JP. Intra-articular injections for joint disease in horses. Vet Clin North Am Equine Pract 2005;21:559–73.

11. Caron JP, Tardif G, Martel-Pelletier J, et al. Modulation of matrix metalloprotease 13 (collagenase 3) gene expression in equine chondrocytes by interleukin 1 and corticosteroids. Am J Vet Res 1996;57:1631–1634.

12. Celeste C, Ionescu M, Robin PA, et al. Repeated intra-articular injections of triamcinolone acetonide alter cartilage matrix metabolism measured by biomarkers in synovial fluid. J Orthop Res 2005;23:602–610.

13. Chunekamrai S, Krook LP, Lust G, et al. Changes in articular cartilage after intra-articular injections of methylprednisolone acetate in horses. Am J Vet Res 1989;50:1733–1741.

14. Dabareiner RM, Carter GK, Honnas CM. Injection of corticosteroids, hyaluronate, and amikacin into the navicular bursa in horses with signs of navicular area pain unresponsive to other treatments: 25 cases (1999–2002). J Am Vet Med Assoc 2003;223:1469–1474.

15. Di Rosa M. Role in inflammation of glucocorticoid-induced phospholipase inhibitory proteins. Prog Biochem Pharmacol 1985;20:55–62.

16. Farquhar T, Todhunter RJ, Fubini SL, et al. Effect of methylprednisolone and mechanical loading on canine articular cartilage in explant culture. Osteoarthritis Cartilage 1996;4:55–62.

17. Ferris DJ, Frisbie DD, Kisiday JD, et al. Clinical follow-up of 40 orthopaedic cases treated with bone marrow derived stem cells intra-articularly. Manuscript in preparation 2009.

18. Ferris DJ, Frisbie DD, McIlwraith CW. Current joint therapies in equine practice: A survey of veterinarians, 2009. Proceedings Am Assoc Equine Pract 2009.

19. Foland JW, McIlwraith CW, Trotter GW, et al. Effect of betamethasone and exercise on equine carpal joints with osteochondral fragments. Vet Surg 1994;23:369–376.

20. Forrester JV, Balazs EA. Inhibition of leukocyte locomotion by hyaluronic acid. J Cell Sci 1981;48:315–330.

21. Frean SP, Cambridge H, Lees P. Effects of anti-arthritic drugs on proteoglycan synthesis by equine cartilage. J Vet Pharmacol Ther 2002;25:289–298.

22. Frisbie DD, Ghivizzani SC, Robbins PD, et al. Treatment of experimental equine osteoarthritis by *in vivo* delivery of the equine interleukin-1 receptor antagonist gene. Gene Ther 2002;9:12–20.

23. Frisbie DD, Kawcak CE, McIlwraith CW, et al. Evaluation of polysulfated glycosaminoglycan or sodium hyaluronan administered intra-articularly for treatment of horses with experimentally induced osteoarthritis. Am J Vet Res 2009;70:203–209.

24. Frisbie DD, Kawcak CE, McIlwraith CW, Werpy NM. Intra-articular treatment of osteoarthritis with polyglycan assessed using an equine experimental model. Proceedings Am Assoc Equine Pract 2009.

25. Frisbie DD, Kawcak CE, Trotter GW, et al. Effects of triamcinolone acetonide on an *in vivo* equine osteochondral fragment exercise model. Equine Vet J 1997;29:349–359.

26. Frisbie DD, Kawcak CE, Werpy NM, et al. Clinical, biochemical, and histologic effects of intra-articular administration of autologous conditioned serum in horses with experimentally induced osteoarthritis. Am J Vet Res 2007;68:290–296.

27. Gaustad G, Larsen S. Comparison of polysulphated glycosaminoglycan and sodium hyaluronate with placebo in treatment of traumatic arthritis in horses. Equine Vet J 1995;27:356–362.

28. Goodrich LR, Brower-Toland BD, Warnick L, et al. Direct adenovirus-mediated IGF-I gene transduction of synovium induces persisting synovial fluid IGF-I ligand elevations. Gene Ther 2006;13:1253–1262.

29. Goodrich LR, Nixon AJ. Medical treatment of osteoarthritis in the horse—A review. Vet J 2006;171:51–69.

30. Gotoh S, Onaya J-I, Abe M, et al. Effects of the molecular weight of hyaluronic acid and its action mechanisms on experimental joint pain in rats. Ann Rheum Dis 1993;52:817–822.

31. Gray RG, Tenenbaum J, Gottlieb NL. Local corticosteroid injection treatment in rheumatic disorders. Semin Arthritis Rheum 1981;10:231–254.

32. Hague BA, Honnas CM, Simpson RB, et al. Evaluation of skin bacterial flora before and after aseptic preparation of clipped and nonclipped arthrocentesis sites in horses. Vet Surg 1997;26:121–125.

33. Higgins AJ, Lees P. The acute inflammatory process, arachidonic acid metabolism and the mode of action of anti-inflammatory drugs. Equine Vet J 1984;16:163–175.

34. Higuchi M, Masuda T, Susuda K, et al. Ultrastructure of the articular cartilage after systemic administration of hydrocortisone in the rabbit: an electron microscopic study. Clin Orthop 1980;296–302.

35. Howard RD, McIlwraith CW. Sodium hyaluronate in the treatment of equine joint disease. Compend Contin Educ Pract Vet 1993;15:473–481.

36. Howard RD, McIlwraith CW. Sodium hyaluronate in the treatment of equine joint disease. Compend Contin Educ Pract Vet 1993;15:473–483.

37. Howard RD, McIlwraith CW. Hyaluronan and its use in the treatment of equine joint disease. In Joint Disease in the Horse. McIlwraith CW, Trotter GT, eds. WB Saunders, Philadelphia, 1996:257–269.

38. Kawcak CE, Norrdin RW, Frisbie DD, et al. Effects of osteochondral fragmentation and intra-articular triamcinolone acetonide treatment on subchondral bone in the equine carpus. Equine Vet J 1998;30:66–71.

39. Kawcak CE, Trotter GT. Other joint conditions. In Diagnosis and Management of Lameness in the Horse. Ross MW, Dyson SJ, eds. Saunders, Philadelphia, 2003:610–613.

40. Kay AT, Bolt DM, Ishihara A, et al. Anti-inflammatory and analgesic effects of intra-articular injection of triamcinolone acetonide, mepivacaine hydrochloride, or both on lipopolysaccharide-induced lameness in horses. Am J Vet Res 2008;69:1646–1654.

41. Kristiansen KK, Kold SE. Multivariable analysis of factors influencing outcome of 2 treatment protocols in 128 cases of horses responding positively to intra-articular analgesia of the distal interphalangeal joint. Equine Vet J 2007;39:150–156.

42. Labens R, Mellor DJ, Voute LC. Retrospective study of the effect of intra-articular treatment of osteoarthritis of the distal tarsal joints in 51 horses. Vet Rec 2007;161:611–616.

43. Leardini G, Mattara L, Franceschini M, et al. Intra-articular treatment of knee osteoarthritis. A comparative study between hyaluronic acid and 6-methyl prednisolone acetate. Clin Exp Rheumatol 1991;9:375–381.

44. Lynch TM, Caron JP, Arnoczky SP, et al. Influence of exogenous hyaluronan on synthesis of hyaluronan and collagenase by equine synoviocytes. Am J Vet Res 1998;59:888–892.

45. Macleod JN, Fubini SL, Gu DN, et al. Effect of synovitis and corticosteroids on transcription of cartilage matrix proteins. Am J Vet Res 1998;59:1021–1026.

46. McCarty OJ. Glucocorticoids. In Arthritis and Allied Conditions. McCarty OJ, ed. Lea and Febiger, Philadelphia, 1989:604–621.

47. McCluskey MJ, Kavenagh PB. Clinical use of triamcinolone acetonide in the horse (205 cases) and the incidence of glucocorticoid-induced laminitis associated with its use. Equine Veterinary Education 2004;16:86–89.

48. McDougall JJ, Elenko RD, Bray RC. Cholinergic vasoregulation in normal and adjuvant monoarthritic rat knee joints. J Auton Nerv Syst 1998;72:55–60.

49. Meijer H, Reinecke J, Becker C, et al. The production of anti-inflammatory cytokines in whole blood by physico-chemical induction. Inflamm Res 2003;52:404–407.

50. Murphy DJ, Todhunter RJ, Fubini SL, et al. The effects of methylprednisolone on normal and monocyte-conditioned medium-treated articular cartilage from dogs and horses. Vet Surg 2000;29:546–557.

51. Murray RC, Znaor N, Tanner KE, et al. The effect of intra-articular methylprednisolone acetate and exercise on equine carpal subchondral and cancellous bone microhardness. Equine Vet J 2002;34:306–310.

52. Pacini S, Spinabella S, Trombi L, et al. Suspension of bone marrow-derived undifferentiated mesenchymal stromal cells for repair of superficial digital flexor tendon in race horses. Tissue Eng 2007;13:2949–2955.

53. Pauwels FE, Schumacher J, Castro FA, et al. Evaluation of the diffusion of corticosteroids between the distal interphalangeal joint and navicular bursa in horses. Am J Vet Res 2008;69:611–616.

54. Pelletier JP, Martel-Pelletier J. Protective effects of corticosteroids on cartilage lesions and osteophyte formation in the Pond-Nuki model of osteoarthritis. Arthritis and Rheumatism 1989;32,181–193.

55. Peyron JG. A new approach to the treatment of osteoarthritis viscosupplementation. Osteoarthritis and Cartilage 1993;1, 85–87.

56. Pisko EJ, Turner RA, Soderstrom LP, et al. Inhibition of neutrophil phagocytosis and enzyme release by hyaluronic acid. Clin Exp Rheumatol 1983;1:41–44.

57. Prehm P. Hyaluronate is synthesized at plasma membranes. Biochem J 1984;220:597–600.
58. Richardson DW, Dodge GR. Dose-dependent effects of corticosteroids on the expression of matrix-related genes in normal and cytokine-treated articular chondrocytes. Inflamm Res 2003; 52:39–49.
59. Rose RJ. The intra-articular use of sodium hyaluronate for the treatment of osteo-arthrosis in the horse. New Zealand Vet J 1979;27:5–8.
60. Rydell N. Decreased granulation tissue reaction after installment of hyaluronic acid. Acta Orthopaedica Scandinavia 1970; 41:307–311.
61. Serena A, Schumacher J, Schramme MC, et al. Concentration of methylprednisolone in the centrodistal joint after administration of methylprednisolone acetate in the tarsometatarsal joint. Equine Vet J 2005;37:172–174.
62. Silberberg M, Silberberg R, Hasler M. Fine structure of articular cartilage in mice receiving cortisone acetate. Arch Pathol 1966;82:569–582.
63. Todhunter RJ, Fubini SL, Vernier-Singer M, et al. Acute synovitis and intra-articular methylprednisolone acetate in ponies. Osteoarthritis Cartilage 1998;6:94–105.
64. Todhunter RJ, Fubini SL, Wootton JA, et al. Effect of methylprednisolone acetate on proteoglycan and collagen metabolism of articular cartilage explants. J Rheumatol 1996;23: 1207–1213.
65. Todhunter RJ, Lust G. Polysulfated glycosaminoglycan in the treatment of osteoarthritis. J Am Vet Med Assoc 1994;204: 1245–1251.
66. Trotter GT. Intra-articular corticosteroids. In Joint Disease in the Horse. McIlwraith CW, Trotter GT, eds. W.B. Saunders, Philadelphia, 1996:237–256.
67. Wang CT, Lin J, Chang CJ, et al. Therapeutic effects of hyaluronic acid on osteoarthritis of the knee. A meta-analysis of randomized controlled trials. J Bone Joint Surg Am 2004;86-A: 538–545.
68. Wehling P, Moser C, Frisbie D, et al. Autologous conditioned serum in the treatment of orthopedic diseases: The orthokine therapy. BioDrugs 2007;21:323–332.
69. Yates AC, Stewart AA, Byron CR, et al. Effects of sodium hyaluronate and methylprednisolone acetate on proteoglycan metabolism in equine articular chondrocytes treated with interleukin-1. Am J Vet Res 2006;67:1980–1986.

INTRALESIONAL

| Laurie R. Goodrich

Therapies that are injected intralesionally are usually directed at healing tendon or ligament. They are most often intended to augment the healing processes locally by providing the necessary components of healing to the tissue being treated. Alternatively, they may act locally to reduce inflammation and/or signal the cellular and molecular components of the injured and surrounding tissue to begin the reparative processes. During repair, injured elastic fibers are replaced with modified fibrous scar tissue, resulting in repair that is suboptimal. The quality of repair varies greatly, depending on the severity of lesion, the inherent healing properties of the individual, the rehabilitation program, and the local environment of the lesion. Some injuries may repair and resolve with enough mature collagen that they return to normal size, with sufficient remodeling that results in parallel alignment of the fibers within the tissue. Other injuries form a scar, with a resulting increase in size of the tendon/ligament, poor or random fibrous tissue alignment, and peritendinous/ligament fibrosis.

Intralesional approaches are directed at maximizing the chances for a more physiologically functioning tendon. Rehabilitation and constant ultrasonographic monitoring must accompany any treatment. Treatments usually reduce the acute inflammatory response and hemorrhage in the acute phase and improve fiber alignment during the reparative phase. Ultimately, the goal is to maximize the chances for a tendon or ligament to repair with adequate strength and elasticity for a return to a similar level of performance with minimal risk for re-injury.

HYALURONAN (HA)

HA has been investigated for tendon injuries and adhesion prevention throughout the last 2 decades. Its use is predicated on its abilities to decrease inflammation and prevent adhesion formation through its mechanical characteristics.[24] Furthermore, it is thought to stabilize the fibrin clot early in wound healing, enhance the migration and replication of fibroblasts in the wound,[16] and improve fiber and biochemical characteristics of tendons.[44]

Multiple clinical trials have studied the effects of HA on tendon healing. Spurlock, et al. observed positive effects of Hylartin V (sodium hyaluronate) in a collagenase induced tendinitis model; improved weekly ultrasonographic evaluations were noted up to 42 days following treatment compared to saline.[37] Ten years later, Spurlock et al. reported that 60% of clinical cases in which horses with superficial flexor tendinitis (SDFT) received intralesional high molecular weight hyaluronan had ultrasonic resolution of lesions compared to 24% that had intralesional saline injections.[38] Gaughan et al., performed 2 separate clinical trials using the collagenase-induced tendinitis in the deep digital flexor tendon (DDFT),[17] DDF tendon sheath,[16] and SDFT.[15] Horses in which the DDF tendons were injected with hyaluronan had improved ultrasonographic appearance but no difference in histological outcome and morphometric evaluation at 6 weeks. Horses in which the DDF tendon sheaths were injected with HA revealed considerably fewer adhesions and improved appearance histologically, as measured by inflammatory cell infiltration, improved tendon structure, and less intratendinous hemorrhage compared to sheaths that were injected with methylcellulose. However, a significant difference in ultrasonographic appearance, lameness, or gross pathological or histological examination could not be detected in horses in which the SDFTs were injected with hyaluronan subsequent to collagenase-induced tendinitis. Most recently, Dyson, et al. reported no difference in outcome or re-injury rate in performance horses (race, National Hunt, dressage, and jumper horses) when horses were injected with intralesional HA, PSGAG, or nothing following diagnosis of superficial flexor tendinitis.[13] Collectively, studies performed in induced collagenase models suggest improvements in some healing characteristics; however, the benefits do not seem to be borne out in the few clinical trials available.

POLYSULFATED GLYCOSAMINOGLYCANS (PSGAG)

The use of PSGAGs intralesionally is based on the their known abilities to inhibit many of the enzymes associated with connective tissue degradation. *In vitro* studies have shown that PSGAGs are capable of inhibiting lysosomal elastase, cathepsins G and B, lysosomal hydrolases, keratin sulfate glycoanhydrolase, serine proteases, neutral metalloproteinases, b-glucuronidase, α-glucosidase, β-N-acetylglucosaminidase, and hyalurondase.[2,4,27] Additionally, PSGAGs have been reported to inhibit prostaglandin E synthesis, influx of leukocytes into inflammatory sites, and production of superoxide radicals and interleukin-1. They also possess a dose-related effect on fibroblast and tenocyte metabolism, causing elevated production of collagen, noncollagen proteins, and sulfated glycosaminoglycans.[4] In the horse, radioactive PSGAGs are distributed to serum, urine, articular cartilage, and synovial fluid following intramuscular (IM) administration.[20] Although no studies have been done to verify that IM administration of PSGAGs are found in tendon, a study performed in rabbits verified radioactive PSGAG in the SDFT, serum, and urine following IM administration.[40] No studies have reported the molecular and biochemical contributions of intralesional injections of PSGAGs into the ligament or tendon in the horse.

There are few clinical studies regarding the effects of intralesional PSGAGs in the horse. One report had a higher rate of horses (National Hunt and point-to-point) return to work with no difference in re-injury rate, compared to conservatively managed horses.[25] Another study reported improved results following treatment with PSGAGs but the results were based on subjective data.[12] Additionally, both of those studies used IM administration of PSGAGs. The only clinical study in horses in which SDFT were injected with intra-lesional PSGAGs (and intramuscular PSGAGs at the same time) found no difference in re-injury rate when horses were compared to patients injected with intral-esional HA or conservative management.[13]

MESENCHYMAL STEM CELL THERAPY

The use of mesenchymal stem cell (MSC) therapy in veterinary orthopedics has generated much enthusiasm in the last decade. Various uses have been described, including treatment of subchondral bone cysts, bone fracture repair, and cartilage repair.[23,29] However, by far the most frequent use of mesenchymal stem cells has been in the treatment of overstrain-induced injuries of tendons in horses.[32]

Although the mechanism of action in how these cells influence their trophic activity is still under intense investigation, many models of animal studies suggest that MSCs secrete bioactive molecules that: inhibit apoptosis and limit the field of damage or injury, inhibit fibrosis or scarring at sites of injury, stimulate angio-genesis and bring in a new blood supply, and stimulate the mitosis of tissue-specific and tissue-intrinsic progeni-tor cells.[5]

In racehorses, the re-injury rate in tendons sustaining SDF tendinitis is approximately 56%.[13] Due to the scar tissue formation, the primary need to restore functional-ity to tendons has encouraged development of regenera-tive strategies. Regenerative therapies require an exogenous cell source. Tendons and ligaments do not have a lack of cellular inflammation following injury; however, cells actually involved in the synthesis of new tissues are mostly locally derived. Transplantation of MSCs into various injured skeletal tissues has been shown to promote healing, and the use of autologous cells is beneficial because they do not incite an immune response from the host.[6,14,21] It is currently theorized that when transplanted MSCs are injected intrathecally, they either differentiate into cells capable of synthesiz-ing tendon matrix or they secrete important factors that induce adjacent cells to synthesize tendon matrix.[32]

Currently, there are 2 techniques for MSC transplan-tation using intrathecal injections. One uses a nonadi-pocyte-cell mixture from fat, and the second uses a cultured bone marrow aspirate. The fat-derived stem cells do not involve a culture step and therefore have the advantage of lower cost and speed of preparation (cells are returned to the practitioner within 48 hours). However, the cell mixture is believed to be heteroge-nous with regard to cell type. A recent small controlled study using nonadipocyte-cell mixtures from fat in a collagenase model of tendon injury reported some benefit in terms of crimp pattern.[30] Another study reported a return to athleticism in 14 out of 16 horses with SDF tendinitis, with no comment on re-injury rate.[11] However, larger scale clinical data are lacking.

The bone marrow derived MSC technique involves aspirating bone marrow from the sternum or tuber coxae, transferring it to a laboratory for culture and expansion, and then implanting the cell population (approximately 10 to 50×10^6) under ultrasound guid-ance.[18] The optimal time of injection is still unclear; however, cells will most likely maintain viability in an environment that is not associated with acute inflam-mation. Therefore, cells are injected 2 to 3 weeks fol-lowing the injury. Although success has been noted several weeks after the initial injury, many believe that the repair tissue maximally benefits when the cells are injected in the initial phase of healing, at least by 4 to 5 weeks following injury.

This technique has been widely used in the US, UK, Europe, and Australia. Long-term follow-up is encour-aging. More than 168 racehorses undergoing this regimen have been followed.[36] Of horses that returned to work, only 18% have suffered re-injury. This is in contrast to a 56% re-injury rate for horses receiving no intralesional therapy. No adverse effects were reported other than ultrasonographic evidence of needle tracks. Two smaller scale studies, one in research horses[33] and one in 11 racehorses,[31] also reported improved tendon repair. Although current data are encouraging in this area, large-scale clinical trials that compare untreated to treated horses are needed.

PLATELET-RICH PLASMA (PRP)

Platelet-rich plasma has been used to treat soft tissue and in bone healing and has been investigated for regen-eration of bone, cartilage, tendon, and ligament. Growth factors are released from platelet-α granules, including platelet-derived growth factor (PDGF), transforming growth factor-β (TGF-β), fibroblastic growth factor (FGF), vascular endothelial growth factor (VEGF), insu-lin-like growth factor-I (IGF-I), and epidermal growth factor (EGF). Many animal models have demonstrated positive effects of these growth factors—both alone and in concert with each other—in enhancing cellular migra-tion and proliferation, angiogenesis, and matrix deposi-tion in tendon and wound healing and repair.[1,3,34]

Current studies recently report benefits of PRP on equine ligament and tendon, both *in vitro* and *in vivo*.[26,35,42] *In vitro* studies support the belief that PRP supplies high levels of growth factors, which result in higher type I collagen, or cartilage oligomeric matrix protein (COMP), and reduced levels of inflammatory mediators such as matrix metalloproteinases (MMP) 3 and 13. A recent *in vivo* study reported improved repair of the SDFT when core lesions were induced mechani-cally.[35] When lesions that were injected with PRP were compared to lesions injected with saline, tendons had better mechanical characteristics as well as higher col-lagen, glycosaminoglycan, and cellularity. These find-ings correlate with the *in vitro* effects reported. Currently, the only clinical trial reported in the horse is by Waselau, et al., in which 9 Standardbred racehorses with midbody suspensory ligament tears were injected with 1 intrale-sional dose of PRP.[42] All of the horses returned to racing for a minimum of 2 years.

Optimal timing of injection, like that of mesenchy-mal stem cells, is still unclear; however, early in the healing process (2 to 4 weeks following injury) is most likely ideal so that the growth factors present in the PRP can contribute to the cellular environment and enhance matrix components integral to healthy repair tissue. Future clinical trials should further reveal the success rate of this treatment modality, now that this treatment is being used more frequently.

AUTOLOGOUS CONDITIONED SERUM (IRAP)

Autologous conditioned serum, also known as inter-leukin receptor antagonist protein (IRAP), is being used intralesionally in cases of tendinitis and desmitis. In addition to high levels of IRAP, preliminary work suggests that this product has high levels of other growth factors as well, which also may benefit tendon and ligament healing.[43] There are no studies evaluating this product in tendons and ligaments, but many practitioners feel that there is a benefit in these injuries. As with mesenchymal stem cell treatment and platelet-rich plasma, optimal timing is unclear, but most likely the maximal benefit is obtained 2 to 4 weeks following injury.

INSULIN-LIKE GROWTH FACTOR-I (IGF-I)

IGF-I protein is anabolic in tendon and cartilage and contributes to proliferation of tenocytes and matrix production.[7-10] Although the half-life of the protein is short, there seems to be a beneficial effect on tendon healing when injected into injured tendon in a collagenase model of tendinitis.[10] Recently, a gene therapeutic trial also revealed beneficial effects of tendon healing when IGF-I was overexpressed using gene therapy in mesenchymal stem cells.[33] Future clinical trials will reveal if this treatment can improve tendon and ligament repair tissue.

ACELLULAR URINARY BLADDER MATRIX (ACELL)

Acellular urinary bladder matrix (ACELL) was proposed to promote improved healing in tendinitis by supplying a matrix for tenoblasts and tenocytes to migrate and fill in the tendon defect.[28,41] Early reports of clinical results appeared promising.[28] However, when tested in a collagenase model, no beneficial effects were noted when compared to saline injection in horses.[41] With the advent of newer biologics such as mesenchymal stem cells and platelet-rich plasma, this treatment seems to have fallen out of favor.

CORTICOSTEROIDS

Perilesional corticosteroids are occasionally used in acute or chronic cases to treat tendinitis/desmitis. However, they are contraindicated, especially for long-term use, because they may delay collagen formation.[22] Nevertheless, some clinicians use a single perilesional dose of triamcinolone (6 to 9 mg) or methylprednisolone acetate (40 mg) perilesionally in horses with peripheral tendon lesions or suspensory ligament desmitis. Results from this therapy vary and probably should be reserved for tendon or ligaments in which minimal or no structural damage is seen ultrasono-graphically. Furthermore, if dexamethasone acetate is used, dystrophic mineralization has been noted following injection of this corticosteroid into soft tissues.

Numerous other uses have been described for local injection of corticosteroids in areas of inflammation, such as over splint bones, muscle/back soreness, and various soft tissue inflammatory conditions or trauma. The choice and amount of steroid seem to be empirical and clinician dependent; however, this does not seem to greatly impact the efficacy of the injections.

MISCELLANEOUS

Sarapin and/or 2% iodine in almond oil are other intralesional treatments that are occasionally used to treat proximal suspensory desmitis and/or upward fixation of the patella. The rationale behind iodine is unclear, although it is believed that the sclerosing action of this compound tightens loose ligaments (for upward fixation of the patella).[39] The theoretical mechanism of action for suspensory ligament desmitis is less clear. When iodine is used it is often combined with sarapin. Sarapin is an extract derived from the pitcher plant and is believed to have a numbing effect in chronic pain. The only study performed in the horse, however, could not detect analgesic effects of sarapin in a model of acute pain using heat.[19] Nonetheless, this therapy is commonly used to treat various forms of desmitis and muscle soreness with a widely believed suspicion that a temporary analgesic effect is produced. In addition to iodine, sarapin is often combined with corticosteroids to treat lameness conditions of the axial skeleton such as back and sacroiliac problems.

References

1. Akeda K, An HS, Pichika R, et al. Platelet-rich plasma (PRP) stimulates the extracellular matrix metabolism of porcine nucleus pulposus and anulus fibrosus cells cultured in alginate beads. Spine Phila Pa 1976;2006 20;31:959–966.
2. Andrews JL, Sutherland J, Ghosh P. Distribution and binding of glycosaminoglycan polysulfate to intervertebral disc, knee joint articular cartilage and meniscus. Arzneim Forsch 1985;35:144–148.
3. Anitua E, Andia I, Ardanza B, et al. Autologous platelets as a source of proteins for healing and tissue regeneration. Thromb Haemost 2004;91:4–15.
4. Burba DJ, Collier MA, Default LE, et al. *In vivo* study on uptake and distribution of intramuscular tritium-labeled polysulfated glycosaminoglycan in equine body fluid compartments and articular cartilage in an osteochondral defect model. Journal of Equine Veterinary Science 1993;13: 696–702.
5. Caplan AI. Why are MSCs therapeutic? New data: New insight. J Pathol 2009;217:318–324.
6. Caplan AI, Fink DJ, Goto T, et al. Mesenchymal stem cells and tissue repair. In The Anterior Cruciate Ligament: Current and Future Concepts. Jackson DW, et al., eds. Raven Press Ltd., New York, 1993;405–417.
7. Dahlgren LA, Mohammed HO, Nixon AJ. Temporal expression of growth factors and matrix molecules in healing tendon lesions. J Orthop Res 2005;23:84–92.
8. Dahlgren LA, Mohammed HO, Nixon AJ. Expression of insulin-like growth factor binding proteins in healing tendon lesions. J Orthop Res 2006;24:183–192.
9. Dahlgren LA, Nixon AJ. Cloning and expression of equine insulin-like growth factor binding proteins in normal equine tendon. Am J Vet Res 2005;66:300–306.
10. Dahlgren LA, van der Meulen MC, Bertram JE, et al. Insulin-like growth factor-I improves cellular and molecular aspects of healing in a collagenase-induced model of flexor tendinitis. J Orthop Res 2002;20:910–919.

11. Del Bue M, Ricco S, Ramoni R, et al. Equine adipose-tissue derived mesenchymal stem cells and platelet concentrates: their association *in vitro* and *in vivo*. Vet Res Commun 2008;32 Suppl S51-S55.

12. Dow SM, Wilson AM, Goodship AE. Treatment of acute superficial digital flexor tendon injury in horses with polysulphated glycosaminoglycan. Veterinary Record 1996;139:413–416.

13. Dyson SJ. Medical management of superficial digital flexor tendinitis : A comparative study in 219 horses (1992–2000). Equine Vet J 2004;36:415–419.

14. Ferrari G, Cusella-De Angelis G, Coletta M, et al. Muscle regeneration by bone marrow-derived myogenic progenitors. Science 1998;279:1528–1530.

15. Gaughan EM, Gift LJ, DeBowes RM, et al. The influence of sequential intratendinous sodium hyaluronate on tendon healing in horses. Veterinary and Comparative Orthopedics and Traumatology 1995;8, 40–45.

16. Gaughan EM, Nixon AJ, Krook LP, et al. Effects of sodium hyaluronate on tendon healing and adhesion formation in horses. Am J Vet Res 1991;52:764–773.

17. Gift LJ, Gaughan EM, DeBowes RM, et al. The influence of intratendinous sodium hyaluronate on tendon healing in horses. Veterinary and Comparative Orthopaedics and Traumatology 1992;5:151–157.

18. Goodrich LR, Frisbie DD, Kisiday JD. How to harvest bone marrow derived mesenchymal stem cells for expansion and injection. Proceedings Am Assoc Equine Pract 2008;54.

19. Harkins JD, Mundy GD, Stanley SD, et al. Lack of local anaesthetic efficacy of Sarapin in the abaxial sesamoid block model. J Vet Pharmacol Ther 1997;20:229–232.

20. Haugland LM, Collier MA, DeBault LE, et al. 3H-PSGAG concentration in the synovial fluid of the equine antebrachiocarpal, metacarpophalangeal, coronopedal, and tibiotarsal joints following a 500 mg injection. Journal of Equine Veterinary Science 1995;15:274–278.

21. Hildebrand KA, Jia F, Woo SL. Response of donor and recipient cells after transplantation of cells to the ligament and tendon. Microsc Res Tech 2002;58:34–38.

22. Jorgensen JS, Genovese RL. Superficial digital flexor tendinitis. In Diagnosis and Management of Lameness in the Horse. Ross MW, Dyson SJ, eds. Saunders, Philadelphia, 2003:628–639.

23. Kraus KH, Kirker-Head C. Mesenchymal stem cells and bone regeneration. Vet Surg 2006;35:232–242.

24. Madison JB. Acute and chronic tendinitis in horses. Compend Contin Educ Pract Vet 1995;17:853–856.

25. Marr CM, Love S, Boyd JS, et al. Factors affecting the clinical outcome of injuries to the superficial digital flexor tendon in National Hunt and point-to-point racehorses. Veterinary Record 1993;132:476–479.

26. McCarrel T, Fortier L. Temporal growth factor release from platelet-rich plasma, trehalose lyophilized platelets, and bone marrow aspirate and their effect on tendon and ligament gene expression. J Orthop Res 2009;27:1033–1042.

27. McIlwraith CW. General pathobiology of the joint and response to injury. In Joint Disease in the Horse. McIlwraith CW, Trotter GT, eds. W.B. Saunders, Philadelphia, 1996:40–70.

28. Mitchell RD. Treatment of tendon and ligament injuries with UBM powder. Management of Lameness Causes and Sport Horses: Muscle, Tendon, Joint and Bone disorders. Lindner, A. Conference on Equine Sports Medicine and Science, Cambridge, UK, 21–23 July 2006. Wageningen Academic Publishers, Wageningen, Netherlands.

29. Nixon AJ, Brower-Toland BD, Bent SJ, et al. Insulin like growth factor-I gene therapy applications for cartilage repair. Clin Orthop Relat Res 2000;S201-S213.

30. Nixon AJ, Dahlgren LA, Haupt JL, et al. Effect of adipose-derived nucleated cell fractions on tendon repair in horses with collagenase-induced tendinitis. Am J Vet Res 2008;69:928–937.

31. Pacini S, Spinabella S, Trombi L, et al. Suspension of bone marrow-derived undifferentiated mesenchymal stromal cells for repair of superficial digital flexor tendon in race horses. Tissue Eng 2007;13:2949–2955.

32. Richardson LE, Dudhia J, Clegg PD, et al. Stem cells in veterinary medicine-attempts at regenerating equine tendon after injury. Trends Biotechnol 2007;25:409–416.

33. Schnabel LV, Lynch ME, van der Meulen MC, et al. Mesenchymal stem cells and insulin-like growth factor-I gene-enhanced mesenchymal stem cells improve structural aspects of healing in equine flexor digitorum superficialis tendons. J Orthop Res 2009.

34. Schnabel LV, Sonea HO, Jacobson MS, et al. Effects of platelet rich plasma and acellular bone marrow on gene expression patterns and DNA content of equine suspensory ligament explant cultures. Equine Vet J 2008;40:260–265.

35. Smith JJ, Ross MW, Smith RK. Anabolic effects of acellular bone marrow, platelet rich plasma, and serum on equine suspensory ligament fibroblasts *in vitro*. Vet Comp Orthop Traumatol 2006;19:43–47.

36. Smith RK. Mesenchymal stem cell therapy for equine tendinopathy. Disabil Rehabil 2008;30:1752–1758.

37. Spurlock GH, Spurlock SL, Parker GA. Evaluation of hylartin V therapy for induced tendinitis in the horse. Equine Veterinary Science 1989;9,242–246.

38. Spurlock SL, Spurlock GH, Bernstad S, et al. Treatment of acute superficial flexor tendon injuries in performance horses with high molecular weight sodium hyaluronate. J Eq Vet Sci 1999; 19:338–344.

39. Valentine BA. Mechanical lameness in the hindlimb. In Diagnosis and Management of Lameness in the Horse. Ross MW, Dyson SJ, eds. Saunders, Philadelphia, 2003:475–480.

40. Walesby HA, Rosenbusch R, Booth LC, et al. Uptake and distribution of tritium-labeled polysulfated glycosaminoglycan in serum, urine, and superficial digital flexor tendon of rabbits after intramuscular administration. Am J Vet Res 2000;61:20–23.

41. Wallis TW, Baxter GM, Werpy NM, et al. Acellular urinary bladder matrix in a collagenase model of superficial digital flexor tendinitis in horses. Proceedings Am Assoc Equine Pract 2007;260–261.

42. Waselau M, Sutter WW, Genovese RL, et al. Intralesional injection of platelet-rich plasma followed by controlled exercise for treatment of midbody suspensory ligament desmitis in Standardbred racehorses. J Am Vet Med Assoc 2008;232: 1515–1520.

43. Wehling P, Moser C, Frisbie D, et al. Autologous conditioned serum in the treatment of orthopedic diseases: The orthokine therapy. BioDrugs 2007;21:323–332.

44. Yamamoto E, Hata D, Kobayashi A, et al. Effect of beta-aminopropionitrile and hyaluronic acid on repair of collagenase-induced injury of the rabbit Achilles tendon. J Comp Pathol 2002;126:161–170.

ORAL/NUTRITIONAL

Nicolas S. Ernst and Troy N. Trumble

Lameness is one of the most prevalent diseases that affects the equine industry. It is considered the most common and important performance-limiting problem in horses. This section discusses oral formulations used to treat the causes of lameness. Specifically, it focuses on oral formulations of nonsteroidal anti-inflammatory drugs (NSAIDs) and the most common compounds used in equine nutraceuticals.

NONSTEROIDAL ANTI-INFLAMMATORY DRUGS

Nonsteroidal anti-inflammatory drugs are a large group of drugs with differing degrees of analgesic, anti-inflammatory, and antipyretic properties (Table 8.3). In a recent survey by Merial of 1,400 horse owners and trainers, 96% of respondents stated that they use NSAIDs and 82% said they administer them without consulting a veterinarian,[89] demonstrating that owners and trainers are comfortable administering NSAIDs for treatment of musculoskeletal injuries. Oral formulations come in many varieties such as pills, paste, granules, and powder, allowing the consumer to choose which formulation is best for each individual. Some of these medications can also be administered systemically via intramuscular or intravenous injection (Table 8.3). NSAIDs have a wide range of side effects involving mainly the gastrointestinal, renal, and cardiovascular systems. These side effects can result from multiple doses and vary among the different drugs.[84]

In general, NSAIDs act by inhibiting cyclooxygenase (COX) enzymes that convert arachadonic acid into prostaglandins and thromboxanes. There are 2 well-known isoenzymes of the COX enzymes, COX-1 and COX-2, and recently, a third distinct isoenzyme, COX-3, has been identified.[141] In general, COX-1 is considered the housekeeping isoenzyme responsible for producing prostaglandins involved in normal physiological functions such as gastric and renal function and hemostasis.[88] The COX-2 isoenzyme is considered to be an important inducible mediator of inflammation in several organs and is primarily responsible for the inflammatory pathway.[88] However, the concept that COX-2 is purely involved in inflammation has changed since the COX-2 isoenzyme has been found to be constitutively formed in the brain, spinal cord, kidney, uterus, and some other regions.[118]

The variation in efficacy and toxicity of the different NSAIDs is closely related to inhibition of the different COX isoenzymes (Table 8.3). Some are more potent inhibitors of COX-1 than COX-2, some equally inhibit both, and others inhibit COX-2 more than COX-1.[88] In general, the anti-inflammatory and analgesic properties of NSAIDs are believed to be mainly due to inhibition of the inducible COX-2, whereas the adverse effects seem to be caused by inhibition of the constitutive COX-1.[84] This has led to the development of NSAIDs with a selective inhibition of COX-2, thereby decreasing the gastrointestinal and renal side effects.

Recommendations for NSAID usage should be formulated in attempt to minimize adverse effects when it is determined that an oral NSAID may be a beneficial treatment option. In general, oral NSAIDs should be used at the lowest effective dose and frequency as possible, for the shortest period of time. In addition, they

Table 8.3. Commonly used NSAIDs and their modes of action, formulations, and doses for equine musculoskeletal disorders.

Name of NSAID	Primary inhibitory action	Available formulations	Recommended dose
Phenylbutazone	Cox-1 and -2	Powder, tablets, paste, injectable solution	2.2–4.4 mg/kg SID or BID
Flunixin meglumine	Cox-1 and -2	Paste, granules, injectable solution	1.1 mg/kg SID
Acetylsalicylic acid	Cox-1 > Cox-2	Gel, powder, granules, paste, tablets	25–35 mg/kg SID or BID
Meclofenamic acid	Cox-1 and -2	Granules	2.2 mg/kg SID for 5–7 days
Naproxen	Cox-1 and -2	Granules, tablets, suspension	10 mg/kg SID or BID
Firocoxib	Cox-2	Paste, injectable solution	0.1 mg/kg SID, 0.09 mg/kg SID IV
Carprofen	Cox-2 > Cox-1	Tablets, injectable solution	0.7 mg/kg SID
Vedaprofen	Cox-2 > Cox-1	Gel, injectable solution	2 mg/kg loading dose followed by 1 mg/kg q 12 hours
Meloxicam	Cox-2 > Cox-1	Suspension, injectable solution	0.6 mg/kg SID for max of 14 days

should not be combined with other NSAIDs (oral or injectable), and special consideration should be used when treating susceptible breeds (ponies), foals, and systemically ill, dehydrated, or old horses. NSAIDs are commonly used in performance horses for recovery of minor injuries. However, most sport horse disciplines have rules about using NSAIDs before or during competitions. See each individual governing body for guidelines regarding appropriate therapeutic use of NSAIDs for that discipline.

Phenylbutazone (Butazolidin®, Butatron™, Bizolin®, Phenylbute™, Phenylzone®, Equiphen®, Butequine®, Superiorbute®, Equizone 100™)

Phenylbutazone (PBZ) is an inexpensive oral anti-inflammatory agent used for a wide range of musculoskeletal problems in horses.[92] Treatment with oral PBZ paste has been shown to control pain and improve function in horses with naturally occurring chronic osteoarthritis (OA).[31] PBZ is an acidic, lipophilic NSAID that is classified as an enolic acid and is metabolized in the liver and excreted in the urine. Following oral administration, PBZ is well absorbed in the stomach and small intestine.[82] The plasma half-life after oral administration has been reported to be between 6.2 and 6.7 hours.[64] However, absorption can be influenced by the drug's formulation and the route of administration.[3,64] For example, the paste formulation offers a greater rate and extent of absorption than tablet or powder formulations, and peak plasma concentrations and onset of action can be delayed by administration close to feeding.

Oral PBZ has been the most common drug used to treat many musculoskeletal conditions, including OA. However, studies have demonstrated that oral PBZ may have negative effects on cartilage and bone metabolism. A study in healthy horses receiving oral PBZ reported a decrease in bone activity (decrease in mineral apposition rate and a reduction in the magnitude of healing) compared to horses not receiving PBZ.[108] In another study, PBZ administered (4.4 mg/kg) orally twice daily for 14 days to healthy horses resulted in significant decreases in proteoglycan synthesis by suppressing chondrocyte metabolism in articular cartilage explants.[6] Recovery of chondrocyte metabolism took 2 weeks to normalize after cessation of treatment with PBZ. In contrast, no significant adverse effects were identified using systemic cartilage and bone biomarkers when PBZ (4.4 mg/kg) was administered orally twice daily for 3 days followed by a lower dose (2.2 mg/kg) for 7 days in healthy horses.[39]

Oral PBZ has been widely studied for its toxic effects on horses. It is considered relatively nontoxic at repeated doses of 2.2 mg/kg twice a day or less.[121] Clinical signs reported with PBZ toxicity in horses are anorexia, depression, loss of weight, abdominal edema, hypoproteinemia, leukopenia, anemia, and death within 4 to 7 days.[117] The gastrointestinal tract is the most commonly affected area following oral administration, causing ulcers (oral, esophageal, gastric, cecal, and right dorsal colon) and a protein-losing enteropathy.[117] Renal papillary necrosis has also been described and may be due to the inhibition of prostaglandins that maintain renal blood flow and/or direct toxic effect of the drug or its metabolites.[73]

Combination of oral PBZ with other NSAIDs enhances the analgesic properties of these drugs in performance horses.[63,105] Studies have shown a better clinical improvement in lameness when a combination of drugs is used than when PBZ is used alone. However, several toxic effects have been reported with this type of treatment in horses sensitive to NSAIDs.

In general, oral PBZ is an inexpensive NSAID that has potent pain relief, antipyretic, and anti-inflammatory properties. It provides pronounced analgesia and reduction in inflammation in many common lameness problems. In addition, it is usually very good at minimizing pain and inflammation associated with orthopedic surgical procedures when it is administered prior to surgery. However, caution should be used due to its narrow margin of safety and adverse effects. Special considerations or alternative therapies should be considered when horses require long-term administration. Often in severely affected orthopedic cases, horses can be safely maintained on 2.2 mg/kg/day for months when used in conjunction with gastroprotectants.

Flunixin Meglumine (Banamine®)

Oral flunixin meglumine can be used to treat musculoskeletal disorders in horses,[51] but because of its cost compared to PBZ, oral formulations are used infrequently. Flunixin meglumine is a derivative of nicotinic acid that exhibits analgesic, anti-inflammatory, and antipyretic activity. After oral administration the drug is rapidly absorbed with a peak in plasma levels within 30 minutes, and the plasma half-life is approximately 1.6 hours.[17] This rapid absorption may be important in minimizing potential ulcerogenicity.[17] The onset of action after oral administration occurs after 2 hours, with the greatest effect between 2 and 16 hours; some activity may persist for up to 30 hours.[51] Similar to phenylbutazone, recent feeding delays absorption.[136] Oral administration of flunixin is relatively safe. In one study, 3× the recommended dose given orally for 15 days failed to induce toxic effects.[51] However, oral administration of flunixin at 1.1 mg/kg/day for 30 days in foals resulted in oral and gastric ulceration.[125] In addition, high doses for long periods can cause gastrointestinal intolerance, hypoproteinemia, and hematological abnormalities.

In general, oral flunixin has been used mostly to treat musculoskeletal injuries associated with soft tissue structures such as muscle and tendons. However, there are no studies indicating that it is better or worse than other NSAIDs at controlling pain and inflammation associated with the musculoskeletal system. Combination of flunixin with other NSAIDs enhances the analgesic properties of these drugs in performance horses.[63,105]

Acetylsalicylic Acid (Aspirin)

Acetylsalicylic acid is the oldest of the NSAID group. Aspirin is a weak acid that reduces platelet aggregation and has analgesic, anti-inflammatory, and antipyretic properties. It is only available in oral forms and has a limited clinical use in the horse. It is best absorbed in the acidic environment of the upper gastrointestinal tract. In ponies, oral administration of salicylate demonstrated rapid absorption with a peak in plasma levels within an hour, with the highest concentrations of drug attained in the liver, heart, lungs, renal cortex, and plasma.[25] Aspirin affects platelet function at low dose rates, reducing clotting times and thrombus formation.[14] Aspirin has been reported to decrease platelet numbers and prolong bleeding time in horses with doses between 12 mg/kg to 24 mg/kg.[14,59,126] These effects can occur after a single dose and can last as long as 48 hours.[14,59] Therefore, caution should be used and close monitoring performed when using this drug on horses before surgery or with bleeding tendencies or anemia. Due to its effect on platelets, aspirin has been historically used for the treatment of navicular syndrome and chronic laminitis.[85] However, its therapeutic benefits for these diseases are not well defined.

Meclofenamic Acid (Arquel)

Meclofenamic acid (MA) is another oral NSAID used to treat lameness and chronic musculoskeletal conditions such as navicular disease, OA, and laminitis in horses.[22] Compared with other NSAIDs, MA has a slow onset of action of 36 to 96 hours for full effect.[22] It is not clear whether feeding time dramatically affects absorption because one study demonstrated that fasted and nonfasted ponies had similar oral absorption,[115] whereas another study demonstrated that plasma levels could be delayed by feeding.[120] The reported bioavailability after oral administration varies between 56% and 90%.[57,115] MA may prove to be useful for OA because high levels can be found in synovial fluid and articular cartilage.[22] High doses produced clinical signs of toxicity similar to those of PBZ (at a dose 13 to 18 mg/kg.[73,123]

Naproxen (Equiproxen, Naprosyn)

Naproxen is an NSAID with analgesic and antipyretic properties that has been used primarily to treat myositis and soft tissue problems.[123] In a study using an equine myositis model, oral naproxen was reported to be superior to oral PBZ, with faster relief of inflammatory swelling and associated lameness.[58] After oral administration the bioavailability of the drug is approximately 50% with peak plasma levels reached at 3 to 4 hours; the plasma half-life is approximately 4 hours.[123] Naproxen has a wide margin of safety. Oral administration of 4 × the recommended dose for 42 days did not cause signs of toxicity.[123] In another study, administration of the recommended dose of Naproxen for 14 days, followed by twice the dose for another 7 days, did not alter plasma protein concentrations.[116] Even though this drug has been marketed for soft tissue conditions, successful usage in the human field for treating joint pain may suggest that it can be used to treat inflammatory swelling and associated lameness.[58,85]

Firocoxib (Equioxx®)

Firocoxib is a new coxib-class of NSAID that reduces inflammation, pain, and fever, and decreases the risks of toxicities of other traditional NSAIDs. It has been approved by the FDA for controlling pain and inflammation associated with OA in horses. The bioavailability after oral administration in horses is 79%, with a time to peak concentration of 3.9 hours and elimination half-life of 30 hours.[69] It is metabolized in the liver and excreted in the urine. It is well distributed in the body, including synovial fluid, liver, fat, kidney, and muscle.

In a study of horses with chronic OA and navicular syndrome,[31] no significant differences in clinical improvement were found between horses treated for 14 days with firocoxib compared to PBZ treatment. However, a greater proportion of horses treated with firocoxib had improvement in scores for pain on manipulation or palpation, joint circumference, and range of motion compared to PBZ. Another study evaluated the efficacy of different doses of firocoxib in horses with chronic lameness using objective assessment with a force plate.[2] A dose of 0.1 mg/kg orally once a day was found to be most effective in reducing chronic lameness in horses.

Compared with other NSAIDs, firocoxib is relatively safe, with no clinical and biochemical signs of NSAID toxicity reported using the recommended dose.[35] Toxicity signs were reported when the drug was used at 3 to 5 × the recommended dose for 30 to 92 days. In several species, COX-2 has been associated with healing of gastric ulcers; therefore, firocoxib should be avoided or used with caution in horses that are known to have gastric ulcers.[8] The main downfall to firocoxib is that it is more expensive than PBZ. Therefore, the economic feasibility must be discussed with the client.

Carprofen (Zenecarp, Rimadyl®)

Carprofen is a propionic acid NSAID approved in Europe for oral use in horses. Its mechanism of action in horses is still unclear; however, it is described as being a more effective analgesic than anti-inflammatory agent.[87] Carprofen in horses was well tolerated when given at twice the oral dose for 14 consecutive days.[87] The benefit of using this NSAID in horses compared to other available NSAIDs requires further investigation.

Vedaprofen (Quadrisol®)

Vedaprofen is an arylpropionic acid NSAID with anti-inflammatory, anti-pyretic, and analgesic properties. Vedaprofen is approved in Europe for oral use in horses. It is recommended for musculoskeletal disorders and soft tissue lesions. Side effects of this drug are those associated with the use of NSAIDs in general. The main toxic effect is ulcer formation in the gastrointestinal tract, making it contraindicated for use in foals under 6 months of age.[130] Use of this NSAID in horses compared to other available NSAIDs requires further investigation.

Meloxicam (Metacam®)

Meloxicam is an NSAID of the oxicam class intended for the treatment of inflammatory orthopedic problems, including chronic musculoskeletal and soft tissue disorders. It is available for horses in Europe. Side effects seen with this drug are those routinely associated with the use of NSAIDs. Caution should be used and close monitoring performed when using this drug on horses treated concurrently with another NSAID, corticosteroid, or nephrotoxic medication.[132] Use of this NSAID in horses compared to other available NSAIDs requires further investigation.

NUTRACEUTICALS

In the absence of a cure for OA, management in horses has historically focused on symptom relief by using NSAIDs or intra-articular steroids. One of the main goals of orthopedic research has been the development of an ideal therapeutic agent that is capable of preventing, slowing, or reversing structural and pathological alterations and preventing further degradation while restoring function in osteoarthritic joints. Because NSAIDs and intra-articular steroids have not fulfilled these requirements and have been associated with several side effects, alternative therapies have been proposed to help alleviate the side effects or incomplete relief of symptoms of conventional therapies. Nutraceutical/supplement administration is one of the most commonly used alternative therapies in horses.

The nutraceutical term has undergone many different definitions over time, but is basically any substance that is a food, or part of a food, that can be administered orally to provide or stimulate production of raw materials or biochemical pathways required for normal bodily functions. Although these substances are neither nutrients nor pharmaceuticals, they are generally used in an attempt to lower the dose of other drugs that are more problematic and provide medical benefits that prevent or treat disease. Included in this broad category of products are nutrients, dietary supplements, functional foods, and phytochemicals (including herbs).

In general, the FDA does not recognize nutraceuticals as foods or drugs. However, based on the definition of nutraceuticals, the FDA perceives veterinary nutraceuticals as unapproved drugs even though they are not labeled or marketed as drugs. The FDA does not regulate these products unless they become unsafe or are associated with labels that claim a drug use. The Center for Veterinary Medicine (CVM) has allowed products to be marketed as nutraceuticals provided that they do not claim to treat, cure, or mitigate disease. Ultimately, there is no requirement to prove safety or efficacy of a nutraceutical for its intended use.[10]

In 1994, the Dietary Supplement Health Education Act (DSHEA) was enacted to define and place some restrictions on human supplements. The DSHEA allows manufacturers to make claims with regard to health, structure or function, and nutrient content of a nutraceutical, and requires that the manufacturer ensure that its product is safe before marketing.[127] In general, the manufacturer must identify each dietary ingredient contained in the product and adhere to state licensing requirements.[86] However, neither the DSHEA nor FDA have set up a system to monitor manufacturers. There is no requirement for manufacturers to guarantee high quality and batch-to-batch consistency, and product safety is completely up to each individual manufacturer.[127] In 2001, the National Animal Supplement

Council (NASC), a nonprofit trade organization, was founded by animal supplement industry stakeholders to try to improve and standardize the industry.[129] As part of this goal, the NASC developed the concept of a "Quality Seal Program." The idea was that the presence of the seal on a product indicates to the consumer that the company is reputable and has undergone some form of quality control. To have a seal placed on their product, the company must demonstrate compliance in four main areas to NASC investigators: a quality control manual that demonstrates standard operating procedures are in place, an adverse event reporting system to evaluate the ingredients within each product, proper labeling guidelines, inclusion of any warning and caution statements recommended by the FDA's CVM for particular ingredients.

According to a study by Packaged Facts, the total retail sales of pet supplements and nutraceuticals in 2007 was $1.2 billion and is expected to reach $1.7 billion by 2012.[133] Equine-related supplements and nutraceuticals accounted for the majority of the market (51%) in 2007, which translates into a $600 million equine market/year. Nutraceuticals are often used by many owners or trainers independent of their veterinarians. Products have become widely available (there are more than 100 products) in many formulations including capsules, tablets, and powder, and they are incorporated within packaged feed. When using or recommending these products, documentation validating the contents, purity, and quality control procedures should be requested from the manufacturer to examine and understand the quality, efficacy, tolerance, and safety of each individual nutraceutical.[127,138]

Several of the products in the equine market have considerable variability in purity, formulation, and consistency between batches. Although these products are marketed with "guaranteed analysis," only a small number consistently meet the label claims.[1,74,75,103,128] In fact, truth-in-labeling problems have been documented, in which ingredients listed on the package were not present at the claimed concentration or purity. The products that have the most inconsistency in concentrations compared to the label claims tend to be those that state that they are a "complex," "formula," or "blend" of ingredients with no weight of each component listed.[128] In general, products should be avoided if they do not have information on the quality, make exaggerated claims, or rely on testimonials.[127] The presence of lot numbers and expiration dates generally offers some evidence of accuracy in labeling, but does not guarantee it.[10]

Many manufacturers with similar products attempt to compete in the market based with claims based on research conducted by another company, even though there is no proof of comparable efficacy. Because these products are oral, it is also important to ensure that there is adequate evidence of absorption in the species of interest, or else the product is essentially useless.[127] As with many medications, each particular individual may respond in an adverse fashion to various ingredients within the product. This could be a reaction to the main ingredients, contaminants, or inert ingredients that are added to help disperse or dilute the product.[10] Possible interactions with traditional therapies (NSAIDs) should also be taken into account because the nutraceutical could potentially render the traditional therapy useless. Unfortunately, to date little to no information exists about these products, which is important to consider when discussing safety of the product with a horse owner or trainer. Most of the information is anecdotal and is based on the lack of any major adverse reactions after treatment.[127]

One should not, and cannot, assume that these products will not cause harm. Just because there is a lack of published adverse reactions to a nutraceutical does not mean that one should extrapolate that the product is safe. In fact, most manufacturers will not spend the money to prove safety, so the lack of side effects does not mean that a product is safe.[127] Unfortunately, even when safety data is present on a particular product, the variability in concentrations of the ingredients within and between batches can make this data inaccurate. It is also worth noting that these products have only been around for a little over a decade, so there is no data regarding the effects of long-term administration.

The remainder of this section discusses the known scientific effects of the most common compounds contained in equine nutraceuticals that are currently available. A basic knowledge of the pathophysiology of joint disease is assumed and can be reviewed in Chapter 7.

Glucosamine (GLN)

Glucosamine is an aminosaccharide essential for normal growth and repair of articular cartilage.[102,124] Glucosamine compounds have been used as nutraceuticals in horses due to their possible role in stimulating chondrocyte metabolism and reducing inflammation in the articular cartilage.

Exogenous glucosamine can be produced synthetically or derived from marine exoskeletons or beef carcasses. There are 3 commercially available forms of exogenous GLN: hydrochloride (HCl), sulfate, and N-acetyl-D-glucosamine. Several reports have demonstrated differences among the available GLN forms. For instance, in vitro studies have demonstrated that GLN HCl and GLN sulfate appear to inhibit cartilage degeneration more consistently than N-acteyl-D-glucosamine.[36,37,113] The GLN sulfate form has been postulated to be more efficacious because serum and/or synovial fluid concentrations of sulfate increase after GLN sulfate administration.[49,53,90,114]

Oral bioavailability of GLN HCl in the horse has been reported to range from 2.5% to 6.1% and has been attributed to a large volume of distribution, poor absorption from the gastrointestinal tract, and extensive tissue uptake.[32,71] Radiolabeling studies have shown that there is good distribution of GLN to articular cartilage with levels exceeding those in the plasma, and multiple dosing results in accumulation of GLN in the cartilage.[112] However, GLN delivery to the articular cartilage does not necessarily mean that it becomes incorporated into articular cartilage. In fact, after oral dosing in the horse, it has been shown that synovial fluid levels of GLN are less than 10% of those in the serum at the same time.[71] This indicates that GLN does not diffuse readily into the synovial fluid from the plasma, suggesting that the effects of GLN may lie in

its effect on nonarticular tissues.[71] The presence or absence of joint disease can influence the concentration of GLN in the joint. In one study, the presence of synovial inflammation induced by E. coli lipopolysaccharide in carpal joints led to significantly higher synovial GLN concentrations compared to levels attained in healthy joints following oral administration of GLN HCl.[91]

Exogenous GLN has been shown in vitro to have no detrimental effects on normal articular cartilage explants[26] or on chondrocyte metabolism after long-term exposure.[56] Many in vitro studies have generally found that GLN induces the production of new cartilage while protecting cartilage that is already present.[4,26,27,29,60] GLN stimulates synthesis of proteoglycans (PG) and collagen while inhibiting PG degradation. This may occur partly via down-regulation of matrix metalloproteinases (MMP) and aggrecanases.[97,110] The anti-inflammatory effects are likely prostaglandin-independent and may be due to enhanced production of HA by synoviocytes.[37,54,70,100,113] In addition, GLN may protect against some of the negative effects of steroids on cartilage, as demonstrated in an in vitro equine chondrocyte pellet model in which GLN had a protective effect against the inhibition of proteoglycan production caused by methylprednisolone.[12]

Few equine in vivo studies have used only GLN. Oral administration of GLN in young horses in training showed no significant treatment effect on serum biomarker concentrations of bone and cartilage metabolism.[15,38] High levels of GLN used for in vitro experiments that were effective have never been achieved in experimental models in humans and animals.[135] Therefore, extrapolating the results from in vitro studies to the in vivo setting must be done with caution. The most consistent information that can be extrapolated from human studies is that it appears to take 4 to 8 weeks before GLN begins to act, and that GLN would likely give the best results when used preventatively—when minor lesions are present prior to the advancement of the disease process.[96]

The quality of products that contain GLN has been questioned. One study compared the measured amount of GLN in commercially available equine oral supplements to levels listed on each product's label.[99] The study concluded that of the 23 products considered, 9 (39.1%) contained less GLN than claimed by the manufacturer and 4 (17.4%) contained less than 30% of the listed amount. In another study examining 5 GLN equine products, the actual composition of GLN varied between 63.6% and 112.2% of the label claim.[103] A large variation in the average recommended daily maintenance dose of GLN was also found in the product labels, ranging from 1,800 to 12,000 mg GLN orally/day for an average sized mature horse. This variability should be considered when evaluating the efficacy of these products.[99]

Chondroitin Sulfate (CS)

CS is a long chain polysaccharide that is a normal constituent of aggrecan, and it constitutes about 80% of all glycosaminoglycans in articular cartilage. It is also an important component of the extracellular matrix of bone, ligaments, and tendons. Within the cartilage it plays an important role in creating osmotic pressure due to its polyanionic charge. CS is often derived from shark and bovine cartilage and it is rather expensive to synthesize and extract. The species or tissue of origin of CS can determine differences in the concentrations, pharmacokinetics profile, molecular composition and weight, metabolic fate, and therapeutic results.[65,142] Therefore, it cannot be assumed that all CS products have the same clinical effect.

CS is orally absorbed in horses; however, the molecular weight and source can have a direct influence on its permeability across the gastrointestinal tract and its bioavailability.[32,33] Studies in other species have shown that the gastrointestinal mucosa contains a variety of GAG-degrading enzymes, suggesting that CS is not absorbed as an intact molecule due to a potential enzymatic degradation.[76,77] It has been proposed that the liver can further modify the final CS molecule prior to reaching circulation.[44,76,77] Reports using radiolabeled CS have demonstrated that it achieves high concentrations in plasma, articular cartilage, and synovial fluid.[21]

Exogenous CS has been shown *in vitro* to have no detrimental effects on normal articular cartilage explants[26] and to increase the synthesis, or decrease the turnover, of proteoglycans/GAGs. *In vitro* studies have also demonstrated a profound anti-inflammatory effect on several tissues involved with joint metabolism. This may be due in part to exogenous CS stimulating hyaluronan synthesis in synoviocytes along with improved composition (viscosity) of HA.[20,104,109] In addition, anti-inflammatory effects may stem from a down-regulation of PGE_2 as well as from NO production.[16,100] CS has also been shown to inhibit MMP and aggrecanase expression/activity in a dose-dependent manner.[100,109,119]

In a synovitis model in horses, CS was found to be markedly less effective than polysulfated glycosaminoglycans (PSGAG) administered intramuscularly (Adequan®, Luitpold Pharmaceuticals, Inc., Shirley, NY) for relief of lameness, stride length, and carpal flexion.[139] In another study using the same model, there was evidence that CS had therapeutic value irrespective of the route of administration (oral or intramuscularly) by improving joint function and reducing lameness scores.[30] However, the time of onset of clinical improvement was slower with oral administration of CS. In a human study, response to treatment with oral CS appeared later (at 60 days), was greater at the end of the 3 months' treatment, and lasted up to 3 months after the treatment,[93] suggesting that response may take time but may also last beyond the last administration. In a study examining 5 CS equine products, the actual composition of chondroitin sulfate ranged from 22.5% to 155.7% of the label claim.[103]

Glucosamine and Chondroitin Sulfate (GLN-CS)

Many equine nutraceuticals contain a combination of GLN and CS. Synergistic effects have been suggested in a rabbit instability model in which the combination was more efficacious in delaying cartilage lesions than with either agent alone.[79] It has also been shown that the combination improves collagen synthesis in tenocytes and ligament cells, and it may be important for use in accessory joint structures.[78]

In vitro studies demonstrated no detrimental effects of GLN-CS on cartilage metabolism.[26] *In vitro* studies have also suggested that the combination inhibits proteolytic activity, potentially via retardation of the molecular and biochemical events associated with pro-inflammatory cytokines, including decreased PGE_2 and NO levels, while also preventing GAG degradation.[16,26,100] These studies suggest that the GLN would be best for potentially inhibiting OA progression, whereas CS may be best for controlling symptomatic action of OA.

Oral administration of GLN-CS at doses greater than those recommended in horses is associated with a good safety profile, with no alterations in hematological or clotting profiles.[68] In an induced synovitis model in horses, a GLN-CS product showed no clinical detectable benefits.[137] However, there was a significant treatment effect for both the oral and intramuscular administration in another study.[30] In studies of clinical cases treated with this compound, horses showed improved lameness, flexion, and stride length, while navicular horses showed significant improvement in soundness compared to placebo controls.[45,46] GLN-CS was also evaluated in horses with tarsal OA using gait analysis, demonstrating significant improvement in the left-to-right symmetry of peak vertical ground reaction forces and impulses, as well as tarsal range of motion and joint energy generation during stance.[19]

Hyaluronic Acid

Hyaluronic acid (HA) is a natural component of articular cartilage synthesized by synoviocytes, fibroblasts, and chondrocytes. It is responsible for the viscoelastic and lubricating properties of synovial fluid and plays an important physiologic role in nutrition of the articular cartilage.[52] HA has been increasingly used in horses as a therapy for OA via intra-articular and intravenous administration. Many oral formulations of HA have become available for horses. There are several anecdotal reports about the use of these products in horses, but scientific evidence of oral absorption, bioavailability, distribution, and controlled evaluation of the efficacy of oral HA products in the horse is lacking. One controlled double-blinded study using yearling Thoroughbreds that had arthroscopic surgery to remove osteochondritis dessicans (OCD) lesions from the tarsus demonstrated that the mean effusion score for the treated horses (100 mg orally once daily) was significantly lower than for the placebo group.[9]

Methylsulfonylmethane

Methylsulfonylmethane (MSM) is a normal oxidative metabolite product of industrial-grade dimethyl sulfoxide (DMSO) that is an odorless and tasteless organic form of sulphur. It is naturally found in small amounts in fruit, alfalfa, and corn, and is very soluble in water.[106,131] It can be found as a product by itself or in combination with GLN and/or CS. It has been used as a nutraceutical because of its analgesic, anti-inflammatory, and antioxidant properties.[67,101,134] There is little known about the pharmacokinetics of MSM. Similar to DMSO, MSM has been suggested for the management of musculoskeletal pain as well as OA. It has been suggested that MSM may relieve muscle discomfort by decreasing the nerve impulses via cholinesterase inhibition and subsequently reducing muscle spasm.[34]

Very little is known about oral administration of MSM safety and toxicity. In a study in rats, MSM given for more than 90 days did not cause any adverse effects nor increase mortality.[50] Few studies have been published to support the use of MSM for managing OA in horses. Horses receiving oral MSM and vitamins demonstrated that MSM could exert some protective effect on oxidative and inflammatory exercise-induced injury related to jumping.[83] In another uncontrolled, nonpeer-reviewed study, MSM was associated with improved performance in Standardbred racehorses in training.[107]

Avocado and Soybean Unsaponifiable Extracts (ASU)

The unsaponifiable portions of avocado and soybean oils are extracted via hydrolysis to make up fractions of one-third avocado oil and two-thirds soybean oil. It appears that this mixture has synergistic properties; however, the active ingredient is still unknown.[81] *In vitro* studies have suggested that ASU extracts may have a positive effect on both the inflammatory cascade and structural components of the cartilage matrix. Studies have demonstrated that the extracts reduce MMPs, cytokines, nitric oxide, and prostaglandin E2, while increasing growth factors and aggrecan production.[11,47,135] One controlled study that used horses with induced OA in the middle carpal joint failed to demonstrate any significant clinical effects.[61] However, the study demonstrated that ASU displays disease modifying capabilities because of a significant decrease in intimal hyperplasia and histologic cartilage disease score along with an increase in articular cartilage GAG synthesis in joints with OA. ASU has been combined with GLN-CS in some products, which may help to decrease some of the symptomatic signs.

Fatty Acids

Polyunsaturated fatty acids (PUFAs) are essential fatty acids that are found in fish and plants. Essential fatty acids are components of cell membranes, involved in lipid transport, and serve as precursors to the eicosanoid hormone family, which regulates inflammatory processes.[42] The 2 principle essential fatty acids are linoleic acid and α-linolenic acid. In the body they are desaturated and elongated to produce analogs of arachadonic acid (N-6 fatty acid) called eicosapentaenoic acid (EPA omega-3 fatty acids) and docosahexaenoic acid (DHA omega-3 fatty acids).

In horses, it was reported that the source of essential fatty acids affects the concentration of EPA and DHA in serum.[98] When horses received fish oil in the diet, there was an increase in the concentration of EPA and DHA in their serum, compared to horses that received corn oil. The anti-inflammatory effects of fatty acids have been attributed to stabilization of cell membranes, inhibition of the formation of inflammatory mediators, and protection against oxidation.[13,23,43] Studies have demonstrated that N-3 fatty acid supplementation can reduce or inhibit the inflammatory and matrix degradative response elicited by chondrocytes during OA progression.[23,24] An *in vitro* study using an LPS challenge model in equine synovial explants demonstrated that pretreatment with α-linolenic acid significantly decreased prostaglandin E2 production induced by lipopolysaccharide (LPS), reducing the inflammatory response.[95] However, the clinical usefulness in the treatment of joint disease is still not entirely clear due to the uncertainty of which components of the oils might be effective.

Cetyl myristoleate (CM) is another fatty acid that is used in equine nutraceuticals. It is an ester, omega-5 fatty acid that may act by inhibiting the 5-lipo-oxygenase pathway,[55] which is responsible for the metabolism of leukotrienes (potent inflammatory mediators from the arachadonic acid cascade). CM has been shown to confer protection against adjuvant-induced arthritis in rats.[28] Humans with knee OA that were administered CM showed improvements in knee flexion and function.[48] One equine product demonstrated lower lameness scores compared to placebo horses in a double-blinded OA clinical trial.[62] However, there are no published reports on safety, absorption, and metabolism of CM in horses.

Collagen Hydrolysate

Collagen hydrolysate (CH) is a food ingredient that has been used in humans to improve joint comfort and function.[94] CH is derived from bovine or porcine skin and bones. Orally administered CH has been shown to be absorbed intestinally and to accumulate in cartilage.[144] In contrast with other nutraceuticals, no direct analgesic and anti-inflammatory effects have been found after using CH.[7] The theory behind CH is that it provides amino acids specific to the collagen network, playing an important role in the structure and function of cartilage by directly stimulating chondrocytes to synthesize collagenous matrix. Several studies in humans have indicated that the use of CH in people with OA is safe and provides improvement in some measures of joint pain and function.[5,7] There are no published reports on the safety, absorption, metabolism, or clinical use of CH in the horse.

Vitamins, Minerals, and Trace Elements

Many vitamins, minerals, and trace elements are included in many equine nutraceutical products in an attempt to supply elements that are necessary for the maintenance of normal cartilage metabolism as well as provide protection against reactive oxygen species.[127]

Vitamin C has been shown to stimulate collagen and aggrecan synthesis.[18,40,111] In addition, vitamin C is a free-radical scavenger that potentially provides anti-arthritic effects by protecting chondrocytes from damage by pro-oxidants.[80] α-tocopherol (vitamin E) may have anti-inflammatory effects in the joint, in part by protecting chondrocytes from damage by reactive oxygen species.[66,80,143] In addition, vitamin E can enhance chondrocyte growth and increase the synthesis of proteoglycan.[41,122] Beta-carotene (provitamin A), selenium, zinc, manganese, niacinamide, and bioflavanoids all have potential anti-oxidant effects.[72,80]

Herbs

Many equine nutraceuticals contain herbal ingredients. Many plants, parts of plants, or plant-derived substances have anecdotally been suggested to have antioxidant and/or anti-inflammatory properties.[140] Some pharmaceuticals have "natural" plants as one or more of their components. Although some of these may have clinical merit, there are numerous products available and none have been proven effective in the horse.[140] Nutraceuticals that contain herbal supplements should be carefully evaluated to avoid potential toxicity or drug interactions and to determine whether there is any research regarding their effects on the joint as well as potential side effects.[140]

References

1. Adebowale A, Cox D, Liang Z, et al. Analysis of glucosamine and chondroitin sulfate content in marketed products and the caco-2 permeability of chondroitin sulfate raw materials J Am Nutraceut Assoc 2000;3:37–44.
2. Back W, MacAllister CG, van Heel MC, et al. The use of force plate measurements to titrate the dosage of a new cox-2 inhibitor in lame horses. Equine Vet J 2009;41:309–312.
3. Baggot JD. Bioavailability and bioequivalence of veterinary drug dosage forms, with particular reference to horses: An overview. J Vet Pharmacol Ther 1992;15:160–173.
4. Bassleer C, Rovati L, Franchimont P. Stimulation of proteoglycan production by glucosamine sulfate in chondrocytes isolated from human osteoarthritic articular cartilage in vitro. Osteoarthritis Cartilage 1998;6:427–434.
5. Bello AE, Oesser S. Collagen hydrolysate for the treatment of osteoarthritis and other joint disorders: A review of the literature. Curr Med Res Opin 2006;22:2221–2232.
6. Beluche LA, Bertone AL, Anderson DE, et al. Effects of oral administration of phenylbutazone to horses on in vitro articular cartilage metabolism. Am J Vet Res 2001;62:1916–1921.
7. Benito-Ruiz P, Camacho-Zambrano MM, Carrillo-Arcentales JN, et al. A randomized controlled trial on the efficacy and safety of a food ingredient, collagen hydrolysate, for improving joint comfort. Int J Food Sci Nutr 2009;1–15.
8. Bergh MS, Budsberg SC. The coxib NSAIDs: Potential clinical and pharmacologic importance in veterinary medicine. J Vet Intern Med 2005;19:633–643.
9. Bergin BJ, Pierce SW, Bramlage LR, et al. Oral hyaluronan gel reduces post operative tarsocrural effusion in the yearling Thoroughbred. Equine Vet J 2006;38:375–378.
10. Boothe DM. Balancing fact and fiction of novel ingredients: definitions, regulations and evaluation. Vet Clin North Am Small Anim Pract 2004;34:7–38.
11. Boumediene K, Felisaz N, Bogdanowicz P, et al. Avocado/soya unsaponifiables enhance the expression of transforming growth factor beta-1 and beta-2 in cultured articular chondrocytes. Arthritis Rheum 1999;42:148–156.
12. Byron CR, Benson BM, Stewart AA, et al. Effects of methylprednisolone acetate and glucosamine on proteoglycan production by equine chondrocytes in vitro. Am J Vet Res 2008;69:1123–1128.
13. Calder PC. Omega-3 polyunsaturated fatty acids, inflammation and immunity. World Rev Nutr Diet 2001;88:109–116.
14. Cambridge H, Lees P, Hooke RE, et al. Antithrombotic actions of aspirin in the horse. Equine Vet J 1991;23:123–127.
15. Caron JP, Peters TL, Hauptman JG, et al. Serum concentrations of keratan sulfate, osteocalcin, and pyridinoline crosslinks after oral administration of glucosamine to Standardbred horses during race training. Am J Vet Res 2002;63:1106–1110.
16. Chan PS, Caron JP, Rossa GJ, et al. Glucosamine and chondroitin sulfate regulate gene expression and synthesis of nitric oxide and prostaglandin E(2) in articular cartilage explants. Osteoarthritis Cartilage 2005;13:387–394.
17. Chay S, Wood WE, Nugent T, et al. The pharmacology of nonsteroidal anti-inflammatory drugs in the horse: flunixin meglumine (Benamine®). Equine Pract 1982;4:16–23.
18. Clark AG, Rohrbaugh AL, Otterness I, et al. The effects of ascorbic acid on cartilage metabolism in guinea pig articular cartilage explants. Matrix Biol 2002;21:175–184.
19. Clayton HM, Almeida PE, Prades M, et al. Double-blind study of the effects of an oral supplement intended to support joint health in horses with tarsal degenerative joint disease. Proceedings Am Assoc Equine Pract 2002;48:314–317.
20. Conte A, de Bernardi M, Palmieri L, et al. Metabolic fate of exogenous chondroitin sulfate in man. Arzneimittelforschung 1991;41:768–772.
21. Conte A, Volpi N, Palmieri L, et al. Biochemical and pharmacokinetic aspects of oral treatment with chondroitin sulfate. Arzneimittelforschung 1995;45:918–925.
22. Cotter GH, Riley WF, Beck CC, et al. Arquel (Cl-1583). A new nonsteroidal anti-inflammatory drug for horses. Proceedings Am Assoc Equine Pract 1973;19:81–90.
23. Curtis CL, Harwood JL, Dent CM, et al. Biological basis for the benefit of nutraceutical supplementation in arthritis. Drug Discov Today 2004;9:165–172.
24. Curtis CL, Hughes CE, Flannery CR, et al. N-3 fatty acids specifically modulate catabolic factors involved in articular cartilage degradation. J Biol Chem 2000;275:721–724.
25. Davis LE, Westfall BA. Species differences in biotransformation and excretion of salicylate. Am J Vet Res 1972;33:1253–1262.
26. Dechant JE, Baxter GM, Frisbie DD, et al. Effects of glucosamine hydrochloride and chondroitin sulphate, alone and in combination, on normal and interleukin-1 conditioned equine articular cartilage explant metabolism. Equine Vet J 2005;37:227–231.
27. Derfoul A, Miyoshi AD, Tuan RS. Glucosamine promotes chondrogenic phenotype in both chondrocytes and mesenchymal stem cells and inhibits IL-1 beta induced MMP-13 expression and matrix degradation. In Transactions of the 51st Annual Meeting of the Orthopaedic Research Society 2005:1477.
28. Diehl HW, May EL. Cetyl myristoleate isolated from Swiss albino mice: An apparent protective agent against adjuvant arthritis in rats. J Pharm Sci 1994;83:296–299.
29. Dodge GR, Jimenez SA. Glucosamine sulfate modulates the levels of aggrecan and matrix metalloproteinase-3 synthesized by cultured human osteoarthritis articular chondrocytes. Osteoarthritis Cartilage 2003;11:424–432.
30. Dorna V, Guerrero RC. Effects of oral and intramuscular use of chondroitin sulfate in induced equine aseptic arthritis. J Equine Vet Sci 1998;18:548–555.
31. Doucet MY, Bertone AL, Hendrickson D, et al. Comparison of efficacy and safety of paste formulations of firocoxib and phenylbutazone in horses with naturally occurring osteoarthritis. J Am Vet Med Assoc 2008;232:91–97.
32. Du J, White N, Eddington ND. The bioavailability and pharmacokinetics of glucosamine hydrochloride and chondroitin sulfate after oral and intravenous single dose administration in the horse. Biopharm Drug Dispos 2004;25:109–116.
33. Eddington ND, Du J, White N. Evidence of the oral absorption of chondroitin sulfate as determined by total disaccharide content after oral and intravenous administration to horses. Proceedings Am Assoc Equine Pract 2001;47:326–328.
34. Evans MS, Reid KH, Sharp JB Jr. Dimethylsulfoxide (DMSO) blocks conduction in peripheral nerve C fibers: a possible mechanism of analgesia. Neurosci Lett 1993;150:145–148.
35. FDA-CVM. Freedom of information summary. EQUIOXX oral paste-0.82% firocoxib (w/w). NADA Rockville, Md: FDA, 2005;141–253.
36. Fenton JI, Chlebek-Brown KA, Peters TL, et al. The effects of glucosamine derivatives on equine articular cartilage degradation in explant culture. Osteoarthritis Cartilage 2000;8:444–451.
37. Fenton JI, Chlebek-Brown KA, Peters TL, et al. Glucosamine HCl reduces equine articular cartilage degradation in explant culture. Osteoarthritis Cartilage 2000;8:258–265.
38. Fenton JI, Orth MW, Chlebek-Brown KA, et al. Effect of lunging and glucosamine supplementation on serum markers of bone and joint metabolism in yearling Quarter horses. Can J Vet Res 1999;63:288–291.
39. Fradette ME, Celeste C, Richard H, et al. Effects of continuous oral administration of phenylbutazone on biomarkers of cartilage and bone metabolism in horses. Am J Vet Res 2007;68:128–133.

40. Gaby AR. Natural treatments for osteoarthritis. Altern Med Rev 1999;4:330–341.

41. Gerstenfeld LC, Kelly CM, Von Deck M, et al. Effect of 1,25-dihydroxyvitamin D3 on induction of chondrocyte maturation in culture: Extracellular matrix gene expression and morphology. Endocrinology 1990;126:1599–1609.

42. Goggs R, Vaughan-Thomas A, Clegg PD, et al. Nutraceutical therapies for degenerative joint diseases: a critical review. Crit Rev Food Sci Nutr 2005;45:145–164.

43. Grimm H, Mayer K, Mayser P, et al. Regulatory potential of n-3 fatty acids in immunological and inflammatory processes. Br J Nutr 2002;87 Suppl 1:S59–67.

44. Gustafson S, Bjorkman T. Circulating hyaluronan, chondroitin sulphate and dextran sulphate bind to a liver receptor that does not recognize heparin. Glycoconj J 1997;14:561–568.

45. Hanson RR, Brawner WR, Blaik MA, et al. Oral treatment with a nutraceutical (Cosequin) for ameliorating signs of navicular syndrome in horses. Vet Ther 2001;2:148–159.

46. Hanson RR, Smalley LR, Huff GK, et al. Oral treatment with a glucosamine-chondroitin sulfate compound for degenerative joint disease in horses: 25 cases. Equine Pract 1997;19:16–22.

47. Henrotin YE, Sanchez C, Deberg MA, et al. Avocado/soybean unsaponifiables increase aggrecan synthesis and reduce catabolic and proinflammatory mediator production by human osteoarthritic chondrocytes. J Rheumatol 2003;30:1825–1834.

48. Hesslink R Jr., Armstrong D 3rd, Nagendran MV, et al. Cetylated fatty acids improve knee function in patients with osteoarthritis. J Rheumatol 2002;29:1708–1712.

49. Hoffer LJ, Kaplan LN, Hamadeh MJ, et al. Sulfate could mediate the therapeutic effect of glucosamine sulfate. Metabolism 2001;50:767–770.

50. Horvath K, Noker PE, Somfai-Relle S, et al. Toxicity of methylsulfonylmethane in rats. Food Chem Toxicol 2002;40:1459–1462.

51. Houdeshell JW, Hennessey PW. A new non-steroidal, anti-inflammatory analgesic for horses. J Equine Med Surg 1977;1:57–63.

52. Howard RD, McIlwraith CW. Hyaluronan and its use in the treatment of equine joint disease In Joint Disease in the Horse, 1st ed. McIlwraith CW, Trotter GW, eds. WB Saunders, Philadelphia, 1996;257–269.

53. Humphries DE, Silbert CK, Silbert JE. Glycosaminoglycan production by bovine aortic endothelial cells cultured in sulfate-depleted medium. J Biol Chem 1986;261:9122–9127.

54. Hungerford D, Navarro R, Hammad T. Use of nutraceuticals in the management of osteoarthritis. J Am Nutraceut Assoc 2000;3:23–27.

55. Iguchi K, Okumura N, Usui S, et al. Myristoleic acid, a cytotoxic component in the extract from Serenoa repens, induces apoptosis and necrosis in human prostatic LNCaP cells. Prostate 2001;47:59–65.

56. Ilic MZ, Martinac B, Handley CJ. Effects of long-term exposure to glucosamine and mannosamine on aggrecan degradation in articular cartilage. Osteoarthritis Cartilage 2003;11:613–622.

57. Johansson IM, Kallings P, Hammarlund-Udenaes M. Studies of meclofenamic acid and two metabolites in horses—pharmacokinetics and effects on exercise tolerance. J Vet Pharmacol Ther 1991;14:235–242.

58. Jones EW, Hamm D. Comparative efficacy of phenylbutazone and naproxen in induced equine myositis. J Equine Med Surg 1978;2:341–347.

59. Judson DG, Barton M. Effect of aspirin on haemostasis in the horse. Res Vet Sci 1981;30:241–242.

60. Karzel K, Lee KJ. Effect of hexosamine derivatives on mesenchymal metabolic processes of in vitro cultured fetal bone explants. Z Rheumatol 1982;41:212–218.

61. Kawcak CE, Frisbie DD, McIlwraith CW, et al. Evaluation of avocado and soybean unsaponifiable extracts for treatment of horses with experimentally induced osteoarthritis. Am J Vet Res 2007;68:598–604.

62. Keegan K, Hughes F, Lane T, et al. Effects of an oral nutraceutical on clinical aspects of joint disease in a blinded, controlled clinical trial: 39 horses. Proceedings Am Assoc Equine Pract 2007;53:252–255.

63. Keegan KG, Messer NT, Reed SK, et al. Effectiveness of administration of phenylbutazone alone or concurrent administration of phenylbutazone and flunixin meglumine to alleviate lameness in horses. Am J Vet Res 2008;69:167–173.

64. Keller H, Hashem A. The concentration changes of different phenylbutazone formulations in horse plasma. Dtsch Tierarztl Wochenschr 1996;103:224–230.

65. Kelly GS. The role of glucosamine sulfate and chondroitin sulfates in the treatment of degenerative joint disease. Altern Med Rev 1998;3:27–39.

66. Kheir-Eldin AA, Hamdy MA, Motawi TK, et al. Biochemical changes in arthritic rats under the influence of vitamin E. Agents Actions 1992;36:300–305.

67. Kim LS, Axelrod LJ, Howard P, et al. Efficacy of methylsulfonylmethane (MSM) in osteoarthritis pain of the knee: a pilot clinical trial. Osteoarthritis Cartilage 2006;14:286–294.

68. Kirker-Head CA, Kirker-Head RP. Safety of an oral chondroprotective agent in horses. Vet Ther 2001;2:345–353.

69. Kvaternick V, Pollmeier M, Fischer J, et al. Pharmacokinetics and metabolism of orally administered firocoxib, a novel second generation coxib, in horses. J Vet Pharmacol Ther 2007;30:208–217.

70. Largo R, Alvarez-Soria MA, Diez-Ortego I, et al. Glucosamine inhibits IL-1beta-induced NFκB activation in human osteoarthritic chondrocytes. Osteoarthritis Cartilage 2003;11:290–298.

71. Laverty S, Sandy JD, Celeste C, et al. Synovial fluid levels and serum pharmacokinetics in a large animal model following treatment with oral glucosamine at clinically relevant doses. Arthritis Rheum 2005;52:181–191.

72. Leach RM, Muenster AM, Wien EM. Studies on the role of manganese in bone formation. II. Effect upon chondroitin sulfate synthesis in chick epiphyseal cartilage. Arch Biochem Biophys 1969;133:22–28.

73. Lees P, Higgins AJ. Clinical pharmacology and therapeutic uses of non-steroidal anti-inflammatory drugs in the horse. Equine Vet J 1985;17:83–96.

74. Liang Z, Bonneville C, Senez T, et al. Development and validation of a photometric titration method for the quantitation of sodium chondroitin sulfate (bovine) in Cosequin DS chewable tablet. J Pharm Biomed Anal 2002;28:245–249.

75. Liang Z, Leslie J, Adebowale A, et al. Determination of the nutraceutical, glucosamine hydrochloride, in raw materials, dosage forms and plasma using pre-column derivatization with ultraviolet HPLC. J Pharm Biomed Anal 1999;20:807–814.

76. Liau YH, Galicki N, Horowitz MI. Degradation of chondroitin 4-sulfate by rat stomach exoglycosidases, sulfohydrolase and hyaluronidase-like enzymes. Digestion 1981;21:117–124.

77. Liau YH, Horowitz MI. Desulfation and depolymerization of chondroitin 4-sulfate and its degradation products by rat stomach, liver and small intestine. Proc Soc Exp Biol Med 1974;146:1037–1043.

78. Lippiello L, Prudhomme A. Advantageous use of glucosamine combined with S-Adenosylmethionine in veterinary medicine: Preservation of articular cartilage in joint disorders. Intern J Appl Res Vet Med 2005;3:6–12.

79. Lippiello L, Woodward J, Karpman R, et al. In vivo chondroprotection and metabolic synergy of glucosamine and chondroitin sulfate. Clin Orthop Relat Res 2000;229–240.

80. Machlin LJ, Bendich A. Free radical tissue damage: protective role of antioxidant nutrients. FASEB J 1987;1:441–445.

81. Maheu E, Mazieres B, Valat JP, et al. Symptomatic efficacy of avocado/soybean unsaponifiables in the treatment of osteoarthritis of the knee and hip: a prospective, randomized, double-blind, placebo-controlled, multicenter clinical trial with a six-month treatment period and a two-month follow-up demonstrating a persistent effect. Arthritis Rheum 1998;41:81–91.

82. Maitho TE, Lees P, Taylor JB. Absorption and pharmacokinetics of phenylbutazone in Welsh Mountain ponies. J Vet Pharmacol Ther 1986;9:26–39.

83. Maranon G, Munoz-Escassi B, Manley W, et al. The effect of methyl sulphonyl methane supplementation on biomarkers of oxidative stress in sport horses following jumping exercise. Acta Vet Scand 2008;50:45.

84. May SA, Lees P. Nonsteroidal anti-inflammatory drugs In Joint Disease in the Horse, 1st ed. McIlwraith CW, Trotter GW, eds. W.B. Saunders, Philadelphia, 1996;223–236.

85. McIlwraith CW. Medications for joint disease: Nonsteroidal anti-inflammatory drugs. In Adams' Lameness in Horses, 5th ed. Stashak TS, ed. Lippincott Williams and Wilkins. Philadelphia, 2002;494–498.

86. McIlwraith CW. Licensed medications, "generic" medications, compounding, and nutraceuticals—what has been scientifically

validated, where do we encounter scientific mistruth, and where are we legally? Proceedings Am Assoc Equine Pract 2004; 50:459–475.

87. McKellar QA, Bogan JA, von Fellenberg RL, et al. Pharmacokinetic, biochemical and tolerance studies on carprofen in the horse. Equine Vet J 1991;23:280–284.

88. Meade EA, Smith WL, DeWitt DL. Differential inhibition of prostaglandin endoperoxide synthase (cyclooxygenase) isozymes by aspirin and other non-steroidal anti-inflammatory drugs. J Biol Chem 1993;268:6610–6614.

89. Merial. Horse Owner Survey Shows NSAID Use Trends. www.thehorse.com. April 30, 2009.

90. Meulyzer M, Vachon P, Beaudry F, et al. Comparison of pharmacokinetics of glucosamine and synovial fluid levels following administration of glucosamine sulphate or glucosamine hydrochloride. Osteoarthritis Cartilage 2008;16:973–979.

91. Meulyzer M, Vachon P, Beaudry F, et al. Joint inflammation increases glucosamine levels attained in synovial fluid following oral administration of glucosamine hydrochloride. Osteoarthritis Cartilage 2009;17:228–234.

92. Moore RM, Walesby HA. Pharmacotherapy of joint and tendon disease. In: Equine Sports Medicine and Surgery: Basic and Clinical Sciences of the Athletic Horse, 1st ed. Hinchcliff KW, Kaneps AJ, Geor RJ, eds. Elsevier Limited, Philadelphia, 2004;486–514.

93. Morreale P, Manopulo R, Galati M, et al. Comparison of the anti-inflammatory efficacy of chondroitin sulfate and diclofenac sodium in patients with knee osteoarthritis. J Rheumatol 1996;23:1385–1391.

94. Moskowitz RW. Role of collagen hydrolysate in bone and joint disease. Semin Arthritis Rheum 2000;30:87–99.

95. Munsterman AS, Bertone AL, Zachos TA, et al. Effects of the omega-3 fatty acid, alpha-linolenic acid, on lipopolysaccharide-challenged synovial explants from horses. Am J Vet Res 2005;66:1503–1508.

96. Neil KM, Caron JP, Orth MW. The role of glucosamine and chondroitin sulfate in treatment for and prevention of osteoarthritis in animals. J Am Vet Med Assoc 2005;226: 1079–1088.

97. Neil KM, Orth MW, Coussens PM, et al. Effects of glucosamine and chondroitin sulfate on mediators of osteoarthritis in cultured equine chondrocytes stimulated by use of recombinant equine interleukin-1beta. Am J Vet Res 2005;66:1861–1869.

98. O'Connor CI, Lawrence LM, Hayes SH. Dietary fish oil supplementation affects serum fatty acid concentrations in horses. J Anim Sci 2007;85:2183–2189.

99. Oke S, Aghazadeh-Habashi A, Weese JS, et al. Evaluation of glucosamine levels in commercial equine oral supplements for joints. Equine Vet J 2006;38:93–95.

100. Orth MW, Peters TL, Hawkins JN. Inhibition of articular cartilage degradation by glucosamine-HCl and chondroitin sulphate. Equine Vet J Suppl 2002;34:224–229.

101. Parcell S. Sulfur in human nutrition and applications in medicine. Altern Med Rev 2002;7:22–44.

102. Platt D. Articular cartilage homeostasis and the role of growth factors and cytokines in regulating matrix composition. In: Joint Disease in the Horse, 1st ed. McIlwraith CW, Trotter GW, eds. WB Saunders, Philadelphia, 1996;29–39.

103. Ramey DW, Eddington N, Thonar E. An analysis of glucosamine and chondroitin sulfate content in oral joint supplement products. J Equine Vet Sci 2002;22:125–127.

104. Redini F, Moczar E, Poupon MF. Effects of glycosaminoglycans and extracellular matrix components on metastatic rat rhabdomyosarcoma tumor and myoblast cell proliferation. Clin Exp Metastasis 1990;8:491–502.

105. Reed SK, Messer NT, Tessman RK, et al. Effects of phenylbutazone alone or in combination with flunixin meglumine on blood protein concentrations in horses. Am J Vet Res 2006;67:398–402.

106. Richmond VL. Incorporation of methylsulfonylmethane sulfur into guinea pig serum proteins. Life Sci 1986;39:263–268.

107. Riegel RJ. The correlation of training times, thermographic and serum chemistry levels to provide evidence as to the effectiveness of the use of oral Alavis MSM (Methylsulfonylmethane) upon the musculature of the racing Standardbred. www.sheld.com/pdf/msm_race_horse.pdf_August 20, 2009.

108. Rohde C, Anderson DE, Bertone AL, et al. Effects of phenylbutazone on bone activity and formation in horses. Am J Vet Res 2000;61:537–543.

109. Ronca F, Palmieri L, Panicucci P, et al. Anti-inflammatory activity of chondroitin sulfate. Osteoarthritis Cartilage 1998;6 Suppl A:14–21.

110. Sandy JD, Gamett D, Thompson V, et al. Chondrocyte-mediated catabolism of aggrecan: aggrecanase-dependent cleavage induced by interleukin-1 or retinoic acid can be inhibited by glucosamine. Biochem J 1998;335:59–66.

111. Schwartz ER, Adamy L. Effect of ascorbic acid on arylsulfatase activities and sulfated proteoglycan metabolism in chondrocyte cultures. J Clin Invest 1977;60:96–106.

112. Setnikar I, Giacchetti C, Zanolo G. Pharmacokinetics of glucosamine in the dog and in man. Arzneimittelforschung 1986;36:729–735.

113. Shikhman AR, Kuhn K, Alaaeddine N, et al. N-acetylglucosamine prevents IL-1 beta-mediated activation of human chondrocytes. J Immunol 2001;166:5155–5160.

114. Silbert JE, Sugumaran G, Cogburn JN. Sulphation of proteochondroitin and 4-methylumbelliferyl beta-D-xyloside-chondroitin formed by mouse mastocytoma cells cultured in sulphate-deficient medium. Biochem J 1993;296:119–126.

115. Snow DH, Baxter P, Whiting B. The pharmacokinetics of meclofenamic acid in the horse. J Vet Pharmacol Ther 1981; 4:147–156.

116. Snow DH, Douglas TA, Thompson H, et al. Effect of non-steroidal anti-inflammatory agents on plasma protein concentration of ponies. Vet Res Comm 1983;7:205–206.

117. Snow DH, Douglas TA, Thompson H, et al. Phenylbutazone toxicosis in equidae: A biochemical and pathophysiological study. Am J Vet Res 1981;42:1754–1759.

118. Steinmeyer J. Pharmacological basis for the therapy of pain and inflammation with nonsteroidal anti-inflammatory drugs. Arthritis Res 2000;2:379–385.

119. Sugimoto K, Takahashi M, Yamamoto Y, et al. Identification of aggrecanase activity in medium of cartilage culture. J Biochem 1999;126:449–455.

120. Sullivan M, Snow DH. Factors affecting absorption of non-steroidal anti-inflammatory agents in the horse. Vet Rec 1982;110:554–558.

121. Taylor JB, Walland A, Lees P, et al. Biochemical and haematological effects of a revised dosage schedule of phenylbutazone in horses. Vet Rec 1983;112:599–602.

122. Tiku ML, Shah R, Allison GT. Evidence linking chondrocyte lipid peroxidation to cartilage matrix protein degradation. Possible role in cartilage aging and the pathogenesis of osteoarthritis. J Biol Chem 2000;275:20069–20076.

123. Tobin T. Pharmacology review: The non-steroidal anti-inflammatory drugs. II. Equiproxen, meclofenamic acid, flunixin and others. J Equine Med Surg 1979;3:298–302.

124. Todhunter RJ. Anatomy and physiology of synovial joints. In Joint Disease in the Horse, 1st ed. McIlwraith CW, Trotter GW, eds. WB Saunders, Philadelphia, 1996;1–28.

125. Traub-Dargatz JL, Bertone JJ, Gould DH, et al. Chronic flunixin meglumine therapy in foals. Am J Vet Res 1988;49:7–12.

126. Trujillo O, Rios A, Maldonado R, et al. Effect of oral administration of acetylsalicylic acid on haemostasis in the horse. Equine Vet J 1981;13:205–206.

127. Trumble TN. The use of nutraceuticals for osteoarthritis in horses. Vet Clin North Am Equine Pract 2005;21:575–597.

128. Unknown. Joint health supplements for pets (dogs and cats) and horses with glucosamine, chondroitin. MSM available at www.ConsumerLab.com_August 20, 2009.

129. Unknown. National Animal Supplement Council. http://nasc.cc/index.php; August 20, 2009.

130. Unknown. Vedaprofen. Summary report. European Agency for the Evaluation of Medicinal Products Veterinary Medicines Evaluation Unit. Committee for Veterinary Medicinal products. http://www.emea.europa.eu/pdfs/vet/mrls/014496en.pdf; July 10,2009.

131. Unknown. Natural medicines in the clinical management of osteoarthritis. http://www.naturaldatabase.com; April 2, 2009.

132. Unknown. Metacam. Scientific discussion. European Agency for the Evaluation of Medicinal Products Veterinary Medicines Evaluation Unit. Committee for veterinary medicinal products. www.emea.europa.eu/vetdocs/PDFs/EPAR/metacam/032397 en6.pdf; July 10, 2009.

133. Unknown. Pet supplements and nutraceutical treats in the U.S., 2nd ed. Packaged Facts. http://www.packagedfacts.com/pet-supplments-market-c1641/; August 20, 2009.

134. Usha PR, Naidu MU. Randomized, double-blind, parallel, placebo-controlled study of oral glucosamine, methylsulfonylmethane and their combination in osteoarthritis. Clin Drug Investig 2004;24:353–363.

135. Verbruggen G. Chondroprotective drugs in degenerative joint diseases. Rheumatology (Oxford) 2006;45:129–138.

136. Welsh JC, Lees P, Stodulski G, et al. Influence of feeding schedule on the absorption of orally administered flunixin in the horse. Equine Vet J Suppl 1992:62–65.

137. White G, Sanders T, Sites T, et al. Efficacy of systemically administered anti-arthritic drugs in an induced equine carpitis model. Proceedings Am Assoc Equine Pract 1996;42:135–138.

138. White GW, Bertone J, Stenbom R, et al. Luitpold animal health roundtable discussion on compounding for the equine veterinary profession. J Equine Veterinary Science 2003;23:517–536.

139. White GW, Stites T, Jones EW, et al. Efficacy of intramuscular chondroitin sulfate and compounded acetyl-d-glucosamine in a positive controlled study of equine carpitis. Proceedings Am Assoc Equine Pract 2004;50:264–269.

140. Williams CA, Lamprecht ED. Some commonly fed herbs and other functional foods in equine nutrition: A review. Vet J 2008;178:21–31.

141. Willoughby DA, Moore AR, Colville-Nash PR. COX-1, COX-2, and COX-3 and the future treatment of chronic inflammatory disease. Lancet 2000;355:646–648.

142. Yamanashi S, Toyoda H, Furuya N, et al. Metabolic study on chondroitin sulfates in rabbits. Yakugaku Zasshi 1991;111:73–76.

143. Yoshikawa T, Tanaka H, Kondo M. Effect of vitamin E on adjuvant arthritis in rats. Biochem Med 1983;29:227–234.

144. Zeijdner EE. Digestibility of collagen hydrolysate during passage through a dynamic gastric and small intestinal model (TIM-1). TNO Nutrition and Food Research Report June 24, 2002.

THERAPEUTIC TRIMMING AND SHOEING

Andrew Parks

INTRODUCTION

The terms "corrective shoeing" and "therapeutic shoeing" are frequently used interchangeably, and to make the differentiation yet more confusing, they mean different things to different people. Literally, corrective implies changing a situation to prevent something harmful, whereas therapeutic suggests a measure designed to heal a pathological process. For the purposes of this discussion, they will be considered synonymous and the term therapeutic shoeing will be used.

Most horses requiring therapeutic shoeing present with either lameness, including poor performance, or undesirable foot/distal limb conformation/balance as the primary problem.

Ideally, therapeutic shoeing would follow a logical sequence of thought. An accurate understanding of foot function would determine 1 of 2 things: how foot conformation or imbalance has predisposed to or caused a disease process to occur in the foot, and/or how a disease process in the foot has altered foot function. From this it should be possible to deduce what principles need to be employed to counteract the causes or effects of the problem, and devise a practical strategy to implement those principles.

There are obvious limitations at all these steps. While sometimes a diagnosis can be definitive, there are other occasions when the most specific diagnosis a clinician can make is heel pain. Although significantly improved over the last 10 to 20 years, our understanding of foot function is still quite incomplete, and therefore, the clinician must often pick the most rational explanation.

Most disease processes of the distal limb are traumatic in origin; more specifically, they are the result of repetitive stress resulting from normal athletic activity. The stresses on the distal limb vary with the phase of the stride.[18] The impact phase of the stride is separated into 2 overlapping collisions. The primary collision occurs as the foot contacts the ground and is associated with high accelerations but low mass. The secondary impact phase of the stride occurs as the mass of the body collides with the foot that is then firmly planted on the ground, but by this phase of the stride the shock waves are diminishing. During the support phase of the stride the accelerations have ceased, but the overall load increases to a maximum at approximately mid-stride, after which the load diminishes.[18] The break-over phase of the stride is also associated with accelerations as the foot rotates. The distal limb has sophisticated mechanisms to dampen shockwaves and spread out the duration of loading and unloading, but extreme exercise, or changes to the foot or ground surface that enhance the accelerations within the distal limb or shorten the duration of loading, increase the likelihood of injury. Both shock waves and large loads associated with weight-bearing are potentially injurious. In addition, attaching steel shoes with nails is known to increase the magnitude and frequency of impact shock waves.[2,6] Therefore, once the principle abnormality is determined, the goals of therapeutic shoeing are almost always designed to strategically address the way structures in the distal limb are stressed to prevent, palliate, or heal injury to the structures that are at risk or diseased. Consequently, it is important to consider the way the structures of the distal limb are stressed during weight-bearing and locomotion.

The hoof capsule normally endures stress under tension or compression, depending on circumstances. These stresses may be longitudinal, radial, or circumferential, and likely a complex combination of these. Ligaments and tendons are built primarily to resist tensile forces; cartilage best resists compression; and bones can withstand compression, tension, bending, or torsion to different degrees. The stresses associated with bending and torsional forces are much more dangerous to the bones of the distal limb than are those of compression, in which the bones are primarily loaded. Therefore, injury prevention is aimed at normalizing the stresses in the distal limb, and treatment is designed to protect a structure from stress as it heals.

The definition of ideal conformation is elusive. However, deviation from an optimal conformation is likely to lower the threshold at which injury related to the stresses of locomotion and weight-bearing is likely to occur. The hoof capsule, as part of the integument, differs from the musculoskeletal structures of the distal limb because it constantly grows and wears away, and because it has remarkable viscoelastic properties. In response to prolonged application of abnormal stresses, the hoof capsule becomes distorted, and prolonged altered load-bearing changes both wear and growth patterns.

EXAMINATION OF THE LIMB FOR THERAPEUTIC SHOEING

Examination of the horse and its limbs should identify both predisposing factors and disease. When the disease process is identified, a specific strategy may be formulated that includes a combination of therapeutic shoeing, medication, and/or surgery. Frequently, the clinician is expected to develop a strategy to treat a lameness originating from the digit that cannot be ascribed to a particular structure or process, compensate for a conformational abnormality, correct an apparent imbalance in the foot, or a combination of the above. This necessitates careful examination of the morphology of the foot, the relationship between the foot and the rest of the limb, and the way the foot interacts with the ground. Radiography is a useful adjunct to assess the relationship between the phalanges and the relationship between the phalanges and the hoof capsule.

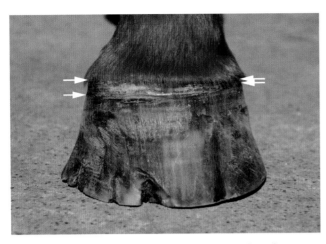

Figure 8.1. Photograph of a horse with growth rings that diverge markedly from medial to lateral (arrows). This horse has medial distal displacement of the distal phalanx.

Examination of the hoof capsule morphology indicates where the wall is unduly stressed, though care must be taken not to overemphasize any one characteristic, but rather correlate all findings. The hoof capsule should be examined from all sides with the foot on the ground, and from the solar perspective with the foot off the ground. With the foot on the ground the following findings suggest too much stress in the wall in one portion of the foot: compression of growth ring (Figure 8.1), flares at the quarter or toe, underruning of the heels, and proximal and/or abaxial displacement of the coronary band. With the foot held up, the ground surface should be examined for approximate mediolateral symmetry, including position of the heels and irregularities in the outline of the capsule. Additionally, the ground surface should be evaluated for appropriate width in relation to length, and position of the widest point of the foot in relation to the center of the ground surface (See Chapter 12).

The phases of the stride are best observed at a walk. The normal pattern of landing at a walk or trot is either lateral heel/quarter first or both heels simultaneously. Toe-first landing and medial-first landing are both indicative of an abnormality in gait when a horse is moving in a straight line. Excessive lateral landing, especially if seen at the trot, is also considered abnormal.

Lateral and dorsopalmar radiographs are required to assess conformation and balance of the distal limb. For lateral radiographs, the center of the x-ray beam should be centered approximately 1.5 cm above the ground surface of the foot and midway between the toe and heels. In a foot with good conformation and balance, the dorsal wall is parallel to the dorsal surface of the distal phalanx, the sole depth is appropriate for the size of horse (optimally greater than 15 mm),[12] the center of rotation of the distal interphalangeal joint is slightly palmar to the center of the weight-bearing surface of the foot, and the average angle that the solar margin of the distal phalanx makes with the ground is 6°.[15]

Dorsopalmar radiographs must be taken with the metacarpus vertical and aligned with the median plane of the foot, which may not be the same as the median plane of the more proximal limb or the trunk. Both feet should be weight-bearing because elevating the contralateral limb induces collateromotion and rotation within the digit.[5] There should be no forced rotation in the limb. The most important observations are the angle of the articular surface of the distal phalanx to the ground and the symmetry of the articulations. The height of the coronet should be correlated with the position of the distal phalanx, and any flares identified.

THE TRIM

The foundation for any corrective shoeing is the trim. If the trim is not appropriate, whatever shoe is used will be less than optimal. The ideal shape of the foot and basic technique of trimming is well described in Chapter 12. In short, there are just 3 basic variables that can be altered: depth of sole, angle of the dorsal wall, and mediolateral symmetry. The length of the wall at the toe is predicated on the depth of the sole; the wall is either level or slightly longer than the adjacent sole. The length of the heels is then predicated on the length of toe and the angle of the foot-pastern axis. Distortions in the hoof capsule may necessitate additional measures. Likewise, application of techniques described below may require variation from the basic pattern.

SHOEING

There are only so many basic principles that can be implemented to improve the function of the equine foot, and these include increasing shock absorption, moving the center of pressure, easing movement about the distal joints in the limb, altering the distribution of force, and altering the motion of the limb during the flight phase of the stride (Table 8.4). However, there is a wide range of tools that can be applied to achieve these principles, and the combinations thereof are almost infinite. Some of these modifications to the shoe are covered in Chapter 12. Unfortunately, all too often the focus is on the method rather than underlying principles.

Shock Absorption

High-frequency, high-energy shock waves are generated during the impact phase of the stride, and to a lesser extent during the break-over phase. They occur in all planes, and the magnitude and frequency of these waves are affected by the structure of the distal limb, the presence of shoes and pads, and the nature of the ground surface.[2,14] Numerous manipulations of the foot influence—potentially influence—the magnitude of shockwaves, including the application of a shoe, the method of shoe attachment, the material of the shoe, pads interposed between the shoe and hoof, traction devices on the shoe, and the surface of the ground.

Usually, it appears that most interventions that involve shoeing increase the shock waves associated with impact. Therefore, the natural damping mechanisms within the digit almost always function better in a healthy horse if it is barefooted. However, conditions of the working environment frequently necessitate shoeing. Most research has compared attachment of a steel shoe with nails to the barefoot condition and the

Table 8.4. Principles for therapeutic trimming and shoeing.

Modification	Goal of modification	Examples of how to achieve goal
Move the center of pressure	Move the ground reaction force in relation to the center of the foot/center of rotation of the distal interphalangeal joint to move the load of weight-bearing from one side of the foot to the other	Wedges, extensions; alter width of web unevenly, either medial vs. lateral or dorsal vs. palmar
Shock absorption	Dampen vibrations associated with deceleration and acceleration	Aluminum shoes instead of steel, synthetic polymer shoes, viscoelastic pads
Ease movement about the distal interphalangeal joint	Shorten arm of extensor moment about the distal interphalangeal joint at break-over	Roll the toe, rocker the toe, square the toe, set the shoe back
Change distribution of force	Increase ground contact of part or all of sole, bars, and frog to reduce load on wall	Heart-bar shoes, custom pad (e.g. heart-bar pad), pour-in pads
Motion of limb during flight	Prevent interference or improve esthetics of gait	Forging: Speed up break-over of forelimb and retard break-over of hindlimb Brushing in hindlimbs: Widen gait by squaring toe, adding traction or trailer to lateral branch, ± lowering medial wall

horse exercised on a firm, flat surface. Under these circumstances, the steel shoe reduces the natural damping mechanisms and reduces—but does not abolish—foot expansion.[4,6] Research also shows that aluminum and synthetic shoes may impede the natural damping mechanisms less than steel.[1,2]

The effect of rim pads inserted between the shoe and ground surface of the foot vary, depending on the material they are made from. Rigid pads and those that become compressed with use are unlikely to be of much benefit, but pads that undergo viscoelastic compression and relaxation with the phases of the stride may offer significant benefit. Unfortunately, there is virtually no information about commercially available pads to know which are likely to provide the greatest benefit. Similarly, there is a wide range of synthetic shoes available, some of which dampen impact vibrations, whereas others do not show a detectable improvement.[1,2]

The nature of the ground surface is also important in the interaction between the shoe and the ground in both damping impact shock waves and loading and unloading the osseous and tendinous structures of the limb.[14,18] Usually, the surface is dictated by the nature of the work. Numerous devices such as calks, toe grabs, and modifications to the shoe profile (such as rims) are used to increase traction. Wide-web flat shoes or half-round shoes may decrease traction. Too much traction increases the horizontal impact vibrations, and too little predisposes to slipping and potential ligamentous injury. There are few data to assist a clinician in the choice of these devices to optimize traction, except to implicate the use of toe grabs in causing musculoskeletal injuries in racehorses.[8,10] Therefore, their application is largely based on individual experience. It is wise to err on the side of caution and use creases or low rims if possible, and if calks or grabs are needed, to use the lowest, broadest devices applicable.

Weight-bearing and the Center of Pressure

The center of pressure determines the relative load bearing by the medial and lateral and dorsal and palmar halves of the foot, which in turn determines the loads and subsequent compressive and tensile stresses on the different structures of the foot. At rest, the center of pressure is at or near the center of the ground surface of the foot. The center of pressure changes during the course of the stride; it can be most simply described as moving rapidly from the point of contact to the point at or near the middle of the ground surface of the foot for the majority of the stride, until break-over, when it moves toward the toe.

The center of pressure can be moved in numerous ways. The simplest that works on all surfaces is to increase the relative length of one side of the foot to the other, which moves the center of pressure to the elevated side.[21] Increasing the length of the heel or toe moves the center of pressure toward or away from the center of rotation of the distal interphalangeal joint (Figure 8.2). In doing so, it shortens or lengthens the arm of the extensor moment about the distal interphalangeal joint.

Other manipulations to move the center of pressure without altering the relative lengths of one side of the foot are based on increasing or decreasing the resistance of the foot to descend into the surface of a yielding substrate. Extension of the shoe outside of the normal perimeter of the foot increases the length of the lever arm on that side. This increases the leverage that the substrate can exert about the center of rotation; for example, an egg-bar shoe moves the center of pressure away from the toe.[13] A similar effect can be achieved by altering the width of the shoe at any point about the perimeter in relation to the rest of the shoe. A decrease in the width of the web increases the descent of the shoe

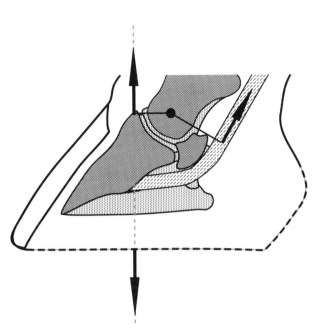

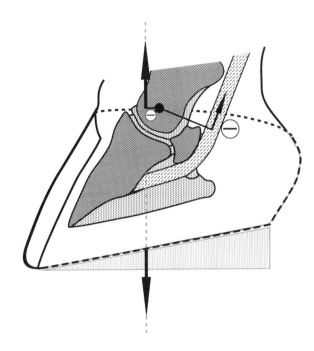

Figure 8.2. Schematic illustration demonstrating effect of heel wedge on moments about the distal interphalangeal joint. Elevating the heel shortens the moment arm of the extensor moment. As the flexor moment arm remains approximately the same, the force in the deep digital flexor tendon is decreased. The center of pressure remains approximately in the center of the foot. (Vectors represented by arrows are for illustrative purposes and do not represent real values.)

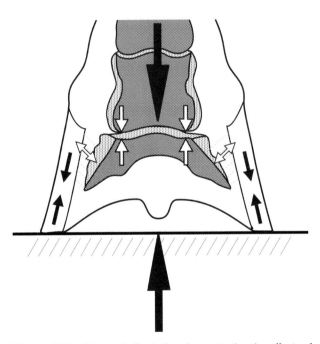

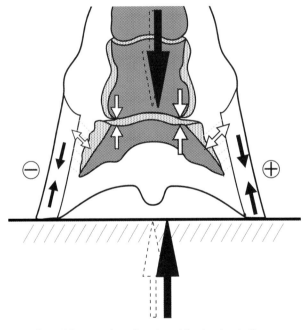

Figure 8.3. Schematic illustration demonstrating the effects of moving the center of pressure in the frontal plane on the structures in the foot. As more weight is borne by one side of the foot, the bones and joints become more compressed, the tension in the collateral ligament is reduced, and the tension in the lamellae is increased. These changes are reversed in the opposite side of the foot. (Vectors represented by arrows are for illustrative purposes and do not represent real values.)

into the substrate at that point; an increase in web width decreases it. Moving the center of pressure in this manner to one side of the foot decreases the stress in the ipsilateral collateral ligament and the contralateral lamellae and articular surfaces (Figure 8.3). Moving the center of pressure toward the heels reduces tensile stress in the deep digital flexor tendon, compressive stress on the navicular bone, and tensile stress in the dorsal lamellae (Figure 8.4).

Each of these manipulations has a concurrent side effect. The manner in which horses place their foot on the ground suggests that proprioceptive feedback, rather

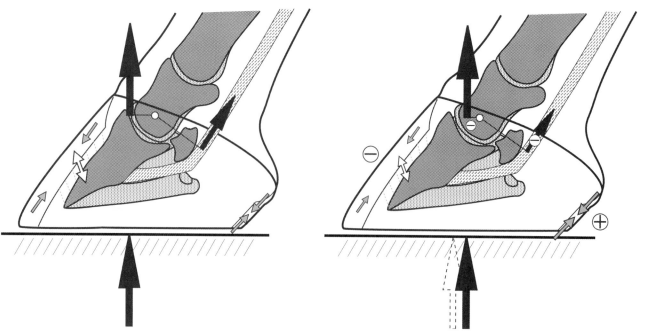

Figure 8.4. Schematic illustration demonstrating the effect of moving the center of pressure in a palmar direction. The arm of the extensor moment becomes shorter, and because the arm of the flexor moment remains approximately the same, the force in the deep digital flexor tendon is decreased. (Vectors represented by arrows are for illustrative purposes and do not represent real values.)

than the ground surface of the hoof, controls the position of the distal phalanx. Therefore, extending the effective border of the hoof distally at any point around its circumference increases the tendency that the foot will land on the lengthened wall first. Extensions on the medial side of the foot of a horse should be used with caution because of the risk of interference. Similarly, toe extensions should be used with caution because they increase the propensity of a horse to trip. Lateral extensions may be used without such obvious side effects but are likely to alter flight of the foot as the limb is protracted due to increased air resistance, the magnitude and significance of which have not been determined. Changing the width of the web of one branch of the shoe causes the foot to become asymmetrically weighted, changing the inertia that must be overcome as the foot accelerates away from the ground at break-over and decelerates at impact. The significance of this effect has not been investigated.

Ease of Movement

Clinicians have long thought that making the break-over point more palmar improves the function of the foot and relieves mild lameness, particularly that associated with palmar heel pain. However, several studies have examined the effect of changing break-over in this manner and have been unable to demonstrate a decrease in the duration of the break-over or a change in the flight of the foot.[7,11] Additionally, it does not change the peak moment about the distal interphalangeal joint or the peak force on the navicular bone, even though it decreases the length of the moment arm of the ground reaction force about that the distal interphalangeal joint at break-over (Figure 8.5).[7]

The most likely explanation for the improvement seen by clinicians is that the foot breaks over (unrolls) more smoothly, thereby decreasing the abruptness in changes in stress in the underlying tissues.[19] To a lesser extent the medial and lateral abaxial branches of the shoe can be beveled to improve the ease of motion as a horse is turning. While this has not been explicitly studied, it is known that a turning horse loads the side of the hoof on the inside of the turn. Therefore, it is rational to anticipate that rolling or beveling the abaxial margins of the shoe smoothes out the changes in stress in the underlying tissues on the ipsilateral side of the foot.

Distribution of Force

The main rationale for distributing part of the load of weight-bearing over more of the sole and frog is to reduce load bearing by the lamellae and wall, which assumes that most of the load is normally born by the wall. This is frequently done by recruiting the entire ground surface in horses with laminitis. In those with underrun heels, reducing weight-bearing by the heels is attempted by increasing weight-bearing by the frog, bars, and angles of the sole.

However successful these manipulations appear clinically, the mechanical effectiveness of this manipulation is uncertain because the role of the sole and wall in weight-bearing is poorly understood. It has been clearly demonstrated that when a horse that has been at pasture barefoot stands on a firm surface, it bears weight in a "4-point" pattern;[9] that is, on its heels and at the toe-quarter junctions. If the same horse is housed on concrete, the wear of the ground surface of its foot causes it to bear weight around more of the perimeter of its

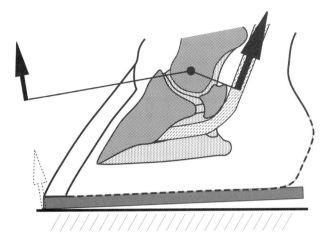

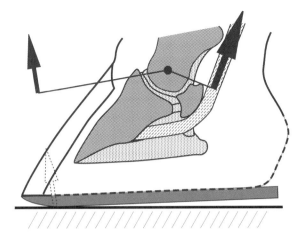

Figure 8.5. Schematic illustration demonstrating the effect of moving the point of break-over in a palmar direction. At the moment the heel leaves the ground, the arm of the extensor moment is shorter in shoes with rolled toes compared to shoes without rolled toes. (Vectors represented by arrows are for illustrative purposes and do not represent real values.)

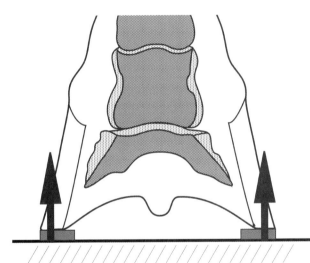

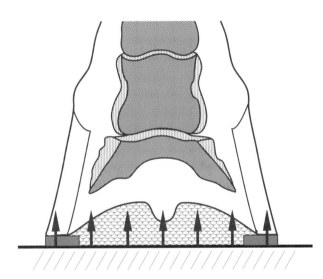

Figure 8.6. Schematic illustration demonstrating the effect of distribution of pressure. It is unknown how the redistribution of force on the ground surface of the foot affects the transmission of load to the distal phalanx. (Vectors represented by arrows are for illustrative purposes and do not represent real values.)

foot and frog. If the same horse is made to stand on sand, the weight is distributed over a much greater area, which is no longer distributed around the periphery of the foot, but over the sole in a band running from quarter to quarter.[9]

What is much less clear is how the weight is transmitted from the hoof capsule to the distal phalanx. Intuitively, it would seem that when a horse is bearing weight on a flat, firm surface and only the wall is in contact with the ground, all of the load is transferred through the wall to the distal phalanx through the lamellae and that the sole has little role in weight-bearing.

What then is the manner of load transmission when the horse is standing on a deformable surface such as sand or turf? Intuition might suggest that now weight is directly transmitted from the sole to the distal phalanx. However, evidence from finite element analysis suggests that this is not the case.[17] Rather, evidence suggests that the load is transmitted through the sole to the wall, and presumably then to the lamellae. This model also suggests that expansion of the foot is caused by the wall at the quarters spreading, which causes the sole to spread and flatten. In doing so, the sole descends more than the distal phalanx. The implication behind the latter observation is that completely filling the space between the branches of the shoe, as with pour-in pads, may decrease the sole from descending, limiting expansion of the wall, and hence decreasing one of the hoof's mechanisms for dissipating shock waves.

The distribution of force on the ground surface of the foot can be changed by increasing the area of contact with the ground during the stride, so that the force on the ground surface of the foot is more broadly distributed (Figure 8.6). This may be achieved by increasing the ground surface area of the web of the shoe so that it has greater contact with the ground and the foot. Alternatively, a variety of materials, such as polyurethane or silicone putty, may be placed inside the contour of the shoe to either partially or completely fill the space between the branches of the shoe, the ground surface of the foot, and the ground. A similar result may be achieved by using a heel plate in conjunction with a composite (Figure 8.7). A symmetrical increase in distribution of load about the center of pressure across the ground surface of the foot is unlikely to alter the center of pressure, but any asymmetrical redistribution of load bearing is likely to cause the center of pressure to shift. Additionally, there is a risk that making the ground surface of the foot completely flat reduces traction excessively, depending on the surface, and hence predisposing to ligamentous injuries related to slippage.

Clinical experience indicates that the lameness of some horses can be dramatically improved by distribution of weight across the sole while in others it is made worse, and in yet others it seems to make little difference. The failures only serve to emphasize that our knowledge is insufficient to accurately apply scientific principles to the use of redistributing weight-bearing across the ground surface in a predicable manner. That said, the successes encourage further exploration to determine when and why it is successful.

Motion of Limb During Flight

The flight phase is the least investigated of the phases of the stride with respect to the effects of shoeing. Therefore, most modifications to change it are based on reasoned arguments, with all their flaws, and experience. The way the foot lands influences the position of the foot during the stance phase, and the position of the foot during the stance phase influences the way the foot leaves the ground. Thus, the patterns of the stance and flight phases are at least in part intertwined. Redirection of the path of flight of the foot is primarily directed at preventing interference injuries, but might also be directed at improving the appearance of flight path for esthetic reasons. Any manipulation of the foot to change to flight path that causes the structures to move outside of their normal plane of motion or increases their range of motion potentially predisposes these structures to injury.

Interference between 2 limbs is a potential cause of injury. It may occur between 2 forelimbs, 2 hindlimbs, 2 ipsilateral limbs, and in pacers between diagonal limbs. Interference is more common in shod horses and it is thought that conformation, imbalance, and fatigue are the main precipitating factors. In nonracehorses, the most common causes are forging and brushing between the hindlimbs.

Given the likely etiology of interference, the best starting point is to ensure the foot is balanced and use the lightest, appropriately sized shoe compatible with the level of work. Although the general strategy to avoid interference that occurs between ipsilateral limbs is to speed up break-over of the forelimb and slow down break-over of the hindlimb, this practice is not well supported by scientific evidence. Changing the point of break-over on a forelimb does not change the kinematics of break-over. Furthermore, while lengthening the

toe and therefore moving the point of break-over dorsally in the hindlimb does prolong break-over, the limb compensates during protraction to impact the ground at the same time as it would with a shorter toe.[3,11]

The general principle in treating interference between contralateral limbs is to widen the gait. This is generally achieved by a combination of squaring the toe, increasing traction laterally, and using a lateral trailer on the hind foot, with or without lowering the medial side of the foot. Again, evidence to substantiate these modifications of the shoe to achieve these goals is lacking, but they are longstanding traditional approaches. When these approaches do not work, and interference persists, then the limb that is interfered with is protected with boots, and the shoe on the interfering limb may be safed.

PROTECTION AND SUPPORT

Protection and support are goals of therapeutic shoeing, and they deserve separate consideration since there is some overlap in their implementation. The term protection in relation to shoeing is usually used to indicate reduction or prevention of pressure on part of the ground surface of the foot. Therefore, protection is usually provided by eliminating pressure in a given area by redistributing the force associated with weight bearing on the distal surface of the foot or placing a shielding device superficial to the area. This may involve using a wider web shoe, a strategically placed bar, or a treatment plate across the entire ground surface of the foot.

The use of the term support is more ambiguous. Support can be used in relation to maintaining an anatomical relationship; for example, after the deep digital flexor tendon has been severed, a heel extension may be used to maintain the foot flat on the ground. Alternatively, a structure can be considered supported when the stress in it is reduced; for example, in the case of a strained deep digital flexor tendon, elevating or extending the heels decreases the stress in the tendon. In these examples, one action meets both definitions of support; however, this is not always the case. It is common to hear that a modification to the shoe supports the heels, usually by extending or elevating them. In reality, extending or elevating the heels maintains the alignment of the foot pastern axis and supports the deep digital flexor tendon, but increases the load on the heels, thereby increasing the likelihood that they will deform and decrease their growth. Most actions that provide support involve movement of the center of pressure.

CLINICAL APPLICATIONS OF PRINCIPLES

The specific diseases of the equine digit are covered in detail elsewhere in the text, but it is useful to briefly examine how the above principles might be applied to several common conditions. Because navicular syndrome is generally considered to be progressive, prolonged rest for a working horse is not usually an option. Therefore, therapeutic measures are primarily directed at palliation, and therapeutic shoeing is pivotal.

Moving the point of break-over in a palmar direction by aggressively rolling the toe smoothes out break-over. Increasing the ground contact in the palmar half of the

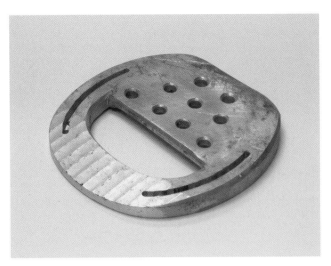

Figure 8.7. Shoe with a heel plate welded between the palmar aspect of the branches. (Courtesy of James Gilchrist.)

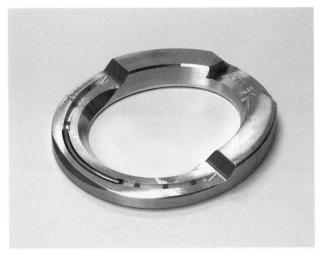

Figure 8.8. KB navicular shoe, a variant of the Tennessee navicular shoe. (Manufactured by G.E. Forge and Tool, Inc., 959 Highland Way Grover Beach, CA 93433.)

foot, such as with a straight bar, heel plate (Figure 8.7), or egg-bar shoe, decreases the descent of the heel into a yielding substrate, and thereby acts as a mild wedge. Therefore, these measure move the center of pressure in a palmar direction to decrease the tension in the deep digital flexor tendon at rest and in the support phase of the stride.

To move the center of pressure in a palmar direction more aggressively, the heels may be raised by one of several means including a graduated shoe or a wedge pad. The compromise made in moving the center of pressure in a palmar direction is that the palmar hoof capsule will bear more load and will be more likely to become deformed. Therefore, the center of pressure should be moved as little as possible to produce the desired result.

There are several shoe designs in which the palmar half of the shoe is flat, but the design of the shoe incorporates a break-over point at or just dorsal to the mid point of the foot; for example, the Tennessee navicular shoe (Figure 8.8). Presumably, this shoe acts as a flat shoe for the landing and support phases of the stride, but as a wedge during break-over. It appears to mitigate some of the disadvantages of heel elevation.

Finally, impact vibrations can be potentially dampened by switching from a steel shoe to an aluminum or synthetic shoe, or by incorporating a viscoelastic pad.

Strains and rupture of the deep digital flexor tendon share features with navicular disease in that they are likely caused by repetitive excessive strain; therefore, similar measures should benefit both. However, the goal of treatment of a deep digital flexor tendon injury is to promote repair. The horse is rested, and reducing tension on the tendon at rest or in the support phase of the stride becomes the primary goal of shoeing. Consequently, the center of pressure is moved in a palmar direction more aggressively, usually by extending the shoe in a palmar direction and by elevating the heels, often using a custom forged patten shoe (Figure 8.9). Prolonged used of this type of shoe causes marked distortion of the hoof capsule by decreasing heel growth,

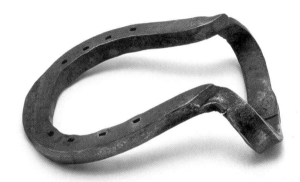

Figure 8.9. Patten shoe used to elevate and extend the heels in horses with severe deep digital flexor tendon injury.

causing the heels to underrun and contract, increasing growth at the toe and causing the dorsal wall to assume a marked convex shape. Therefore, the degree of elevation must be reduced as rapidly as is compatible with healing of the tendon.

Laminitis is a complex disease that has many clinical manifestations. The goals of shoeing are to minimize additional injury and control pain in the early chronic stages of the disease, and in later stages of the disease to encourage realignment of the hoof wall with the distal phalanx and normal hoof wall growth. Because the lamellae are stressed under tension, which contributes to the pain, the center of pressure should be moved to the opposite side of the foot. In a horse with rotation, this is commonly accomplished with heel extension or elevation to decrease stress in the dorsal lamellae. Additionally, because it is preferable to reduce weight on all the lamellae as much as possible, part of or the entire ground surface of the foot between the branches of the shoe may be recruited to bear weight (this is apparently used to good effect when standing an acutely laminitic horse on sand). However, caution must be taken to ensure that the shoe or packing material/pad do not put pressure on the sole where the solar margin of the distal phalanx has displaced distally. If the horse has sunk unilaterally, then the center of pressure should be moved to the contralateral side of the foot. This has been attempted by setting a shoe, either metal or wood, wide to act as an extension on the contralateral side of the foot. In horses that have complete loss of lamellar integrity and have distal displacement of the distal phalanx, there is little advantage to moving the center of pressure.

In addition, spreading the load across the sole is problematic because in unloading the wall it loads the sole where the distal phalanx has displaced. Generally, once the distal phalanx has become more stable and the sole thickened, horses with this type of displacement can be shod. Then a seated out wide-web shoe is used to protect the sole adjacent to the wall and a composite such as silicone putty is used to recruit weight-bearing by the sole, bars, and frog. While this outline suggests logical approaches to protect the affected lamellae as they heal, more documented experience is needed.

Pedal osteitis is a syndrome associated with a flattened sole, bruising of the solar dermis, and osteopenia of the solar margin of the distal phalanx. Therefore, the principal goal of treatment is to protect the affected areas by limiting their contact with the ground. Wide-web shoes that have been seated out protect that area immediately adjacent to the wall, the principally affected area, and therefore are the most common shoe modification used. Pads that elevate the ground surface of the foot may also decrease the likelihood of ground contact. However, pads that cover the ground surface of the foot are of mixed benefit because while they may dissipate the energy of contact, they may actually increase the likelihood of contact; this particularly applies to pads of the pour-in variety. Therefore, the use of a pad must be decided on a case-by-case basis and careful choice of material.

Osteoarthritis of the interphalangeal joints is progressive, and pain can be exacerbated by concussion and extreme motion within the joint. Therefore, the goals of treatment should be to decrease concussion associated with impact and loading and decrease the abruptness in changes of stress associated with locomotion. This can be accomplished by using aluminum or synthetic polymer shoes instead of steel shoes, using viscoelastic rim pads, and ensuring that the shoe has limited traction to decrease the jarring associated with deceleration. Moving the break-over in a palmar direction and beveling the abaxial margins of the shoe minimize strain on the joint capsule and collateral ligaments. These may be achieved with a roller motion shoe (Figure 8.10), but other shoes, such as half-round shoes, can be modified to provide similar all-around benefits.

Ideal distal limb conformation is poorly defined and depends on the nature of athletic activity a horse performs. Nevertheless, some generalizations can be made about the various forms it takes. Most are related to mediolateral angulation within limb, rotation within the limb, and changes in relative length and angle of the pastern. If one of these is present, without clinical lameness, hoof wall distortion, or changes in foot flight, it is usually unadvisable to perform anything other than routine trimming and shoeing because almost all measures will have an unintended consequence. For example,

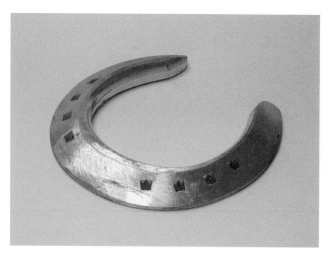

Figure 8.10. Colleoni rolling shoe, a form of roller motion shoe (Colleoni S.R.L., VIA Boscaccio N. 40, Cassano Magnago-VA 21012, Italy.)

it has been proposed that if the foot is lateral to the median plane of the metacarpus, a medial extension should be placed on the foot to bring the center of pressure under the metacarpus. The potential benefit is that the metacarpophalangeal joint is more evenly loaded.[20] Unfortunately, this also loads the medial structures of the foot that are under compression and the lateral structures that are under tension. At a minimum, the compression of the medial hoof capsule causes decreased hoof wall growth and flaring of the capsule at the quarters.

Similarly, it has been proposed that when the foot is further dorsal in relation to the metacarpus than "normal," the shoe is extended farther in a palmar direction to bring the center of pressure closer to the axis of the metacarpus to decrease the strain on the tendons.[16] However, the tendon that receives the greatest benefit is the deep digital flexor tendon, whereas the tendons most affected by the length/low angle of the pastern are the superficial flexor tendon and the suspensory apparatus. This strategy also places greater load on the heels, increasing the likelihood that they will deform. Nevertheless, it can be envisaged that there are occasions when these compromises are necessary. Indeed, in foals, both strategies are used. Abaxial extensions are used to treat angular and rotational deformities and palmar extensions to treat flexor tendon laxity. In part, these techniques are successful in foals because they are only needed temporarily and the growth plates have not fused.

In brief, the treatment of imbalance restores the shape of the hoof capsule, its relationship to the skeletal structures of the limb, and the pattern of landing. Because imbalance takes so many forms, there is no universal recipe, but there are some general guidelines. Imbalance of the hoof capsule is best treated by trimming rather than shoeing if possible. Imbalance may be a more general problem, i.e., when it affects the symmetry of the whole foot, either medial vs. lateral or dorsal vs. palmar. Alternatively, it may be a local phenomenon, such as occurs when there is proximal displacement of the coronary band immediately proximal to the ground surface of the heel buttress associated with a quarter crack.

The trimming is best guided by examining the hoof capsule for evidence of areas with increased stress, such as flares and compression of growth rings (Figure 8.1). If possible, the length of the wall should be trimmed in these areas. If there is not enough wall below the preferred plane of the sole to trim to correct it—for example, when the wall has moved proximally in relation to the distal phalanx or correction of a local imbalance leaves an uneven ground surface—then it is best to leave the hoof unshod. This encourages migration of the wall into a more normal position.

Graduated shoes, pads, and attachment of shoes with composites can also be used to correct imbalance. However, placement of a shoe may also limit or prevent movement of the hoof capsule that contributes to restoring the desired shape of the foot. There are occasions when indicators of imbalance suggest conflicting actions; then it is advisable to go with the preponderance of the evidence and be prepared to use trial and error.

SUMMARY

The science of farriery is far from fully developed. It is important that clinicians understand the limited amount of experimental evidence that is available to support different trimming and shoeing techniques. For experiments to have value, they must be performed under very specific constraints. Extrapolation beyond these constraints increases the variability of expected results, and therefore, an apparently rational approach is not always successful. Consequently, a willingness to use trial and error greatly increase a clinician's chances of success; it also builds the clinician's body of knowledge. It is natural for any veterinarian or farrier to prefer a given technique based on experience because practice improves success, and it is difficult, if not impossible, to be adept at all techniques available. The goal should always be to find the simplest solution that meets the objectives. Finally, it is important to remember that whenever a change is made to a shoe, there is an unintended, though potentially anticipated, consequence.

References

1. Back W, van Schie MH, Poll JN. Synthetic shoes attenuate hoof impact in the trotting Warmblood horse. Equine Comp Ex Physiol 2006;3:143–151.
2. Benoit P, Barrey E, Tegnault JC, et al. Comparison of the damping effect of different shoeing by the measurement of hoof acceleration. Acta Anat 1993;146:109–113.
3. Clayton HM. The effect of an acute angulation of the hind hooves on diagonal synchrony of trotting horses. Equine Vet J Suppl 1990;9:91–94.
4. Colles CM. The relationship of frog pressure to heel expansion. Equine Vet J 1989;21:13–16.
5. Denoix J-M. Functional anatomy of the equine interphalangeal joints. Proc Am Assoc Equine Pract 1999;45:174–177.
6. Dyhre-Poulsen P, Smedegaard HH, Roed J, et al. Equine hoof function investigated by pressure transducers inside the hoof and accelerometers mounted on the first phalanx. Equine Vet J 1994;26:362–366.
7. Eliashar E, McGuigan MP, Rogers KA, et al. A comparison of three horseshoeing styles on the kinetics of break-over in sound horses. Equine Vet J 2002;34:184–190.
8. Hernandez JA, Scollay MC, Hawkins DL, et al. Evaluation of horseshoe characteristics and high-speed exercise history as possible risk factors for catastrophic musculoskeletal injury in Thoroughbred racehorses. Am J Vet Res 2005;66: 1314–1320.
9. Hood DM, Taylor D, Wagner IP. Effects of ground surface deformability, trimming, and shoeing on quasistatic hoof loading patterns in horses. Am J Vet Res 2001;62:895–900.
10. Kane AJ, Stover SM, Gardner IA, et al. Horseshoe characteristics as possible risk factors for fatal musculoskeletal injury of thoroughbred racehorses. Am J Vet Res 1996;57:1147–1152.
11. Ramey D. Do rolled or squared toes affect rate of break-over in horses? Equine Vet Education 2007;19:447–448.
12. Redden RF. Clinical and radiographic examination of the equine foot. Proc Am Assoc Equine Pract 2003:49:169–185.
13. Rogers CW, Back W. Wedge and eggbar shoes change the pressure distribution under the hoof of the forelimb in the square standing horse. J Equine Vet Sci 2003;23:306–309
14. Setterbo JJ, Garcia TC, Campbell IP, et al. Hoof accelerations and ground reaction forces of Thoroughbred racehorses measured on dirt, synthetic, and turf track surfaces. Am J Vet Res 2009;70:1220–1229.
15. Smith SS, Dyson SJ. Proc Am Assoc Eq Pract 2004; 50:328–331.
16. Snow VE, Birdsall DP. Specific parameters used to evaluate hoof balance and support. Proc Am Assoc Equine Pract 1990;35:299–311.
17. Thomason JJ. The hoof as a smart structure: Is it smarter than us? In Equine Podiatry. Floyd AE, Mansmann RA, eds. WB Saunders, Philadelphia, 2007, pp 46–56.
18. Thomason JJ, Peterson L. Biomechanical and mechanical investigations of the hoof-track interface in racing horses. Vet Clin N Am Equine Pract 2008;24:53–77.
19. van Heel MCV, van Weeren PR, Back W. Shoeing sound Warmblood horses with a rolled toe optimizes hoof-unrollment and lowers peak loading during break-over. Equine Vet J 2006;38:258–262.
20. Williams G, Deacon M. Hoof capsule deviations. In No Foot, No Horse. Kennilworth Press Ltd, Addington. 1999, pp 65–80.
21. Wilson AM, Seelig TJ, Shield RA, et al. The effect of foot imbalance on point of force application in the horse. Equine Vet J 1998;30:540–545.

SURGICAL

C. Wayne McIlwraith

INTRODUCTION

Surgical techniques for joint problems have grown increasingly sophisticated in the last 30 years. The 2 greatest advances in equine orthopedics in that period have been internal fixation of fractures and arthroscopic surgery, and the fruits of these developments are particularly evident in the management of joint injuries. Fracture fixation techniques evolved from the Swiss Association of Internal Fixation (ASIF), which were introduced to the United States by Dr. Jacques Jenny at the University of Pennsylvania in the mid-1960s. These techniques led to considerable improvement in the reduction and fixation of fractures, and they help decrease the degree of pathologic change where the fracture enters the joint surface. At the same time, arthroscopic surgery replaced arthrotomy as a means of assessing fractures before and after treatment. It also became a means by which reduction (in the case of internal fixation) is achieved in most instances.

As these techniques were evolving, the development of osteoarthritis (OA) after certain fractures or joint injuries and the subsequent effect of OA on the prognosis and athletic outcome was increasingly being recognized. Both diagnostic and surgical uses of arthroscopic surgery are now well documented.[25] Joints can be examined with greater accuracy than was previously possible. In addition to most pathologic change, new conditions are also being recognized with the technology. All types of surgical manipulations can be performed through stab incisions under arthroscopic visualization. These procedures are less traumatic and less painful, and provide immense cosmetic and functional advantages.

INDICATIONS FOR SURGICAL TREATMENT

The primary indication for surgical treatment of articular injury or disease in the equine athlete is normalization of the interior of the joint and the prevention of OA.[5,24] Once articular cartilage degeneration is well established, surgical treatment cannot reverse the loss. Surgery for salvage for nonathletic procedures might include the re-establishment of pain-free weight-bearing and the prevention of structural collapse in severely injured joints.[4]

Damage to a joint is resolved by negating or reversing the effect of one of the common causes for joint damage and inflammation, including direct trauma, such as from a single overloading blow from an external force that may result in a fracture, or stress trauma, which is the more common cause of articular damage during athletic exercise. Repeated submaximal loads result in the accumulation of damage, and failure at these damage sites can result in a stress fracture, gross subchondral microdamage, complete fracture, or a more insidious failure, as well as persistent inflammation that causes biochemical and molecular degradation of articular cartilage.

Most articular fractures resulting from athletic activity are the results of stress accumulation, and not a single acute overload.[19,31] In addition, athletic activity can lead to primary damage to the articular cartilage and ulceration of the articular surface as well as inflammation of the synovial membrane (synovitis). Synovitis, in turn, may result in pain on use as well as eventual enzymatic degeneration in the joint if the synovitis is left untreated. Developmental abnormalities can damage the joint; the best example is osteochondrosis leading to osteochondritis dessicans (OCD). Infections may be an indication for surgical intervention. There is also a category of unknowns in the treatment of equine patients, in which the history or cause is not discernible.

The surgical treatments for neutralization of these pathologic insults to the joint include:[24]

1. Fragment removal, when an isolated fragment of bone, cartilage, or soft tissue exists within the joint and interferes with normal joint motion or function
2. Debridement of a surface defect to stabilize the defect and eliminate joint irritation
3. Internal fixation and joint reconstruction to establish normal joint anatomy in fractures that pass through an articulation and cause large articular surface defects
4. Lavage and decontamination of the joint to eliminate infectious debris and metabolic byproducts in diseases such as infectious arthritis
5. Soft tissue debulking and debridement where overuse trauma causes proliferation of the soft tissue structures and creation of an intra-articular mass that may affect joint function, such as synovial pad fibrotic proliferation (villonodular synovitis) as seen in the dorsal compartment of the MCP joint
6. Arthrodesis of a joint when the trauma or degeneration has damaged the joint to the extent that normal joint function cannot be re-established, or in the case of the MCP joint, when stability of the lower limb is required.

If elimination of joint inflammation cannot be accomplished and pain-free weight-bearing restored, then surgical fusion of a joint (arthrodesis) to eliminate the motion that initiates the pain cycle is another method of circumventing the pain.

Diagnostic examination is also an important part of surgical treatment when a problem does not respond to medication. Arthroscopy can diagnose structural damage to one of the soft tissue structures, such as an intra-articular ligament, and often leads to diagnosis of an osteochondral problem that was not obvious with conventional imaging techniques. In most instances, the normal physiologic response of the joint to the pathologic insult neutralizes routine insults.

Surgical treatment is aimed at improving the quality or speed of the natural recovery mechanism. Chronic inflammation within joints causes permanent damage to that joint.[24,26] Progressive degeneration of articular cartilage can often be stopped or decreased by timely surgical intervention. The improvements in the articular treatment of joint injuries and technology have greatly enhanced our capabilities and willingness to invade a joint for surgical treatment, leading to better end results of the natural healing process.

SURGICAL TECHNIQUE OPTIONS

Arthroscopy has replaced arthrotomy in nearly every joint in the horse because of its reduced morbidity and, with experience, better visualization and increased versatility of the joint treatment.[25] In addition, techniques for endoscopic exploration of nearly every tendon sheath and bursa within the horse have replaced most open approaches to these synovial cavities. Diagnostic examination, fragment removal, and surface debridement are all improved with the ability to manipulate the arthroscope for closer, more varied, and more complete visualization of these synovial structures.

Soft tissue debridement and debulking can be performed to reduce soft tissue inflammation. Control of internal fixation of fractures that do not require gross manipulation, such as third carpal slab fractures, is easily accomplished via arthroscopic control. More recently, arthroscopy has replaced arthrotomy for major reduction and manipulation such as in the case of displaced metacarpal condylar fractures or midbody sesamoid fractures (although not all surgeons practice arthroscopy to treat the latter). Arthrodesis remains the exception; open arthrotomy is required for articular cartilage removal and monitoring of fixation, although minimally invasive approaches are being developed for specific joints.

The lavage that accompanies arthroscopy and endoscopy is critical for removing particulate matter and biologic debris, such as with synovitis and OA. Motorized resection of fibrin under arthroscopic visualization has replaced more radical drainage techniques in the treatment of infective arthritis/synovitis. Further information on diagnostic arthroscopy is available in Chapter 4.

While there are many benefits of arthroscopy, it is technically demanding and there is a need for training as well as time on the learning curve. Critical recommendations during arthroscopy are:

1. Avoid the use of a sharp trochar.
2. Only use instruments if they can be seen clearly.
3. Never cut tissues blindly; always have tissues under direct visualization.
4. Take care with power instruments, particularly when suction is applied, because this can rapidly result in joint evacuation and compromised visibility.[1]

Hemarthrosis is an intra-operative problem in equine arthroscopy. It is uncommon and less likely when the horse is in dorsal recumbency. Tourniquets are sometimes necessary when the horse is in lateral recumbency. Hemorrhage is minimized with joint distention, particularly in debridement of subchondral defects. Obstruction of the view by synovial villi can be associated with inadequate distention or excessive fluid movement.[25] Extrasynovial extravasation of fluid is associated with time in surgery and excessive intra-articular pressure during manipulation of instruments. Iatrogenic damage to articular cartilage, as well as intrasynovial instrument breakage, are risks that can be obviated by careful technique.

Postoperative complications of equine arthroscopy include infection, which can be minimized by good aseptic technique, and postoperative synovitis and capsulitis, which usually resolve after surgery but may persist in the tarsocrural joint after OCD surgery. Failure to remove fragments is a problem that is minimized by intra-operative radiographs. Postoperative capsulitis and enthesitis are minimized by case selection and careful avoidance of trauma to the fibrous joint capsule. Postoperative pain is usually quite transient.

OSTEOCHONDRAL FRAGMENTATION AND REMOVAL

Pathobiologic Principles

Fragmentation in equine joints is derived from 2 main sources: traumatic injury and OCD. The most common instances of traumatically induced osteochondral chip fragmentation are in the carpal and fetlock joints.

Although chip fractures have been frequently considered to be acute injuries, it is now well accepted that they are secondary complications that affect joint margins previously altered by OA[31] or the result of microdamage associated with cyclic trauma.[22,30] Fragmentation can arise from at least 2 different pathogenic conditions: (1) fragmentation of the original tissue of the joint margin (with this lesion starting as a progressive disease induced by the repetitive trauma of training and racing, with eventual damage of articular cartilage and subchondral bone), or (2) within the base of periarticular osteophytes forming in OA. Experience with arthroscopic surgery of carpal fragmentation supports both of these roles in various instances. Fresh fracture lines through an articular surface that otherwise appears grossly normal simply represent the acute final failure of an area of subchondral bone disease.

Fragmentation of the osteochondral articular surfaces has direct physical effects because of the loss of a smooth congruent articular surface, as well as the release of cartilage and bone debris, which may lead to synovitis. Sufficiently severe compromise of the articular surface leads to instability, as does tearing of fibrous joint capsule and ligaments. Synovial membrane in turn has the potential to respond directly to mechanical trauma, indirectly to injury elsewhere in the joint, or both. Direct damage to synoviocytes within the synovial membrane liberates mediators that can lead to articular cartilage degeneration (see Chapter 7). Damage to articular cartilage also releases wear particles and, possibly, other soluble breakdown products. These materials in turn can activate the synovial membrane to result in increased production of harmful mediators and cytokines.[10]

It is important to recognize the chronic effects that result in the loss of motion after joint surgery. Arthrofibrosis is minimized by the use of skilled arthroscopic techniques,[11] However, it may still be a complication because inflammation arising from injury can lead to collagen deposition and cross-linking, not only within individual injured tissues but also between periarticular tissues, which normally glide on one another. Physical therapy and anti-inflammatory medications can help minimize swelling and stiffness postoperatively. Direct damage to chondrocytes can lead to release of mediators that can cause breakdown in the extra-cellular matrix of the cartilage.

Osteochondral Fragmentation

Osteochondral chip fractures of the equine carpus are common in racehorses (580 of 591 horses in one series).[20] Arthroscopic surgery for the removal of these osteochondral fragments is indicated for the immediate relief of clinical signs, as well as to prevent further development of OA. Arthroscopic surgery to remove osteochondral fragment involves a triangulation technique using two portals that remain consistent for all locations of fractures in these joints (Figure 8.11). Priority of portal is given for the instrument, as this is straight, whereas the wide angle lens can be positioned almost anywhere to see the fragment.

Arthroscopic surgery is always the ideal option for removal of osteochondral fragmentation. This is particularly so in the middle carpal joint, where failure to remove fragments from the distal radial carpal bone, for instance, is quickly accompanied by secondary OA. Fragments in the antebrachiocarpal joint tend to be

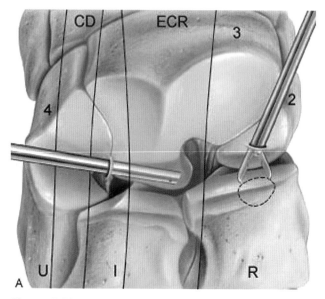

Figure 8.11. Diagram of positioning of arthroscope and instrument used during operations involving fragmentation of the distal radial carpal bone. (Reproduced with permission from McIlwraith CW, et al. Diagnostic and Surgical Arthroscopy in the Horse, 3rd ed., 2005, Figure 4.29).

more forgiving, but arthroscopic surgery is certainly the preferred option.

Fragmentation is more severe when visualized at arthroscopy than on the radiographs (Figures 8.12 and 8.13). When horses in one study were separated into 4 categories of articular damage, the performances of the 2 most severely affected groups were significantly inferior. The success rate with grade I damage was 71.1% (less than 5 mm articular cartilage loss peripheral to the fragment), 75% with grade II damage (up to 30% of the articular surface involved), 53.2% with grade III damage (greater than 50% articular cartilage loss) and 54% with grade IV (significant loss of subchondral bone.[20]

Osteochondral Fragmentation in the Fetlock Joint

Proximodorsal osteochondral fracture fragments of the first phalanx are the most common of the fetlock joint. In most instances, the fragment is considered to be the result of trauma (compression of the dorsoproximal portion of the proximal phalanx against the distal part of the third metacarpal bone when extreme extension of the fetlock joint occurs during racing or fast training).[7,17] Nonracehorses sometimes manifest with fragments that are rounded and more chronic. All fragments, if accompanied by clinical signs, are indications for surgery (Figure 8.14). The damage that is evident arthroscopically is always more extensive than what is seen in radiographs. Consequently, many referred cases have persistent evidence of synovitis and capsulitis despite medical therapy and relatively minor fragmentation or with only a radiographic defect off the proximal phalanx. Good results are obtained with surgery.[18]

Osteochondral fractures of the proximal sesamoid bone amenable to removal occur at the apical, abaxial, and basal margins. Arthroscopic techniques for the removal of these fragments have been developed.[25] Previous dogma proposed limitations of fragment removal based on the size of the fragment and degree of attachment in the suspensory ligament and distal sesamoidean ligaments. However, current follow-up on the author's cases that have been treated arthroscopically suggest that the limitation should be redefined.

The technique for an apical sesamoid fragment removal is illustrated in Figure 8.15. Abaxial fragments are removed using a similar approach. These can be depicted radiographically and are confirmed arthroscopically (Figure 8.16). The results of apical, abaxial, and basal sesamoid fragments have been documented.[35–37] Basal sesamoid fragments are candidates for arthroscopic removal when no other pathologic changes are present in the fetlock joint (at least on radiographs). Their removal does not comprise the distal sesamoidean ligament attachments, and racing success has been achieved with quite large fragments (Figure 8.17). The exact size limitations have been defined.[35]

Axial osteochondral fragments of the proximal palmar or plantar aspect of the proximal phalanx (type I osteochondral fragments of the palmar-plantar aspect of the fetlock joint)[12,14] were initially reported as chip fractures.[3] Although some authors have suggested they are a manifestation of osteochondrosis, pathologic

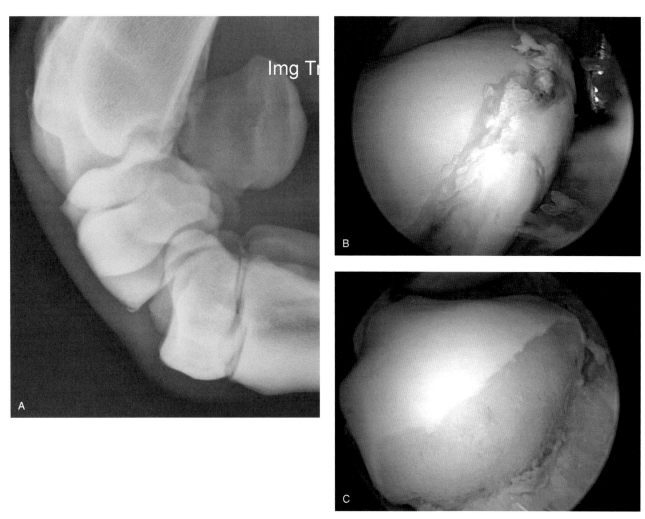

Figure 8.12. Radiograph (A) and arthroscopic view of a fresh fragment on distal aspect of the radial carpal bone before (B) and after (C) removal and debridement.

examination supports the concept of a traumatic etiology.[29] To be considered a surgical candidate, the patient must have demonstrable lameness referable to the fetlock. The fracture is visualized with optimal definition of the lesion using a special oblique view; it is useful for the tube to be at a 30° angle distad.[25] Nonsurgical treatment usually lowers the horse's performance.[2] Arthroscopic surgery is the standard technique for removal.[25]

Synovial Pad Fibrotic Proliferation (Villonodular Synovitis)

Synovial pad fibrotic proliferation was initially designated as villonodular synovitis and later described as chronic proliferative synovitis.[39,41] It involves a proliferative response from the synovial pad in the proximal dorsal aspect of the MCP joint. The term synovial pad fibrotic proliferation is now preferred.[8] Repetitive trauma during fast exercise can result in irritation and enlargement of the synovial pad and development of clinical signs of lameness, as well as chronic joint effusion that often resolves temporarily with rest and intra-articular medication. Persistence of the problem leads to the diagnosis. Concavity of the distal dorsal aspect of MCIII is suggestive of synovial pad proliferation. Ultrasound is the method of choice to further define this proliferation. The condition is most common in the racehorse, but has been seen in other horses not subject to fast athletic exercise. Arthroscopic removal of the synovial pad is the recommended treatment, and follow-up of 55 horses after arthroscopy indicated that 43 (85%) that had surgery returned to racing with 34 (68%) racing at an equivalent or better level than before surgery.[8]

Arthroscopically Assisted Repair of Fractures with Lag Screw Fixation

The use of the arthroscope allows verification of articular alignment as well as compression of carpal bone slab fractures and lateral condylar fractures of the distal MCIII and MTIII, as well as complete diagnostic examination of the joint.[32,33] With correct technique, even displaced condylar fractures can be accurately reduced and repaired without a large surgical exposure.

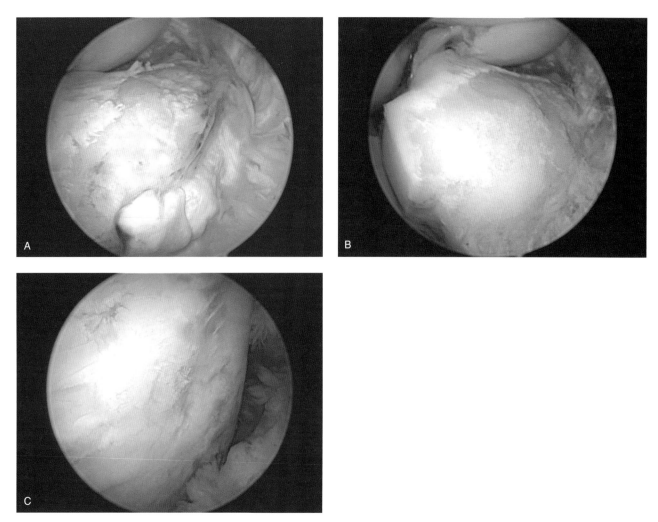

Figure 8.13. Fragment removal and a severe lesion of the distal radial carpal bone. Arthroscopic view of fragment before (A) and after (B) debridement. Kissing lesion (C) on the opposing third carpal bone.

Figure 8.18 illustrates reduction of a displaced condylar fracture under arthroscopic visualization. Good results have been reported.[32,33,43]

Osteochondral Fragmentation in the Femoropatellar and Tarsocrural Joints

Intra-articular chip fragments in the tarsocrural joint occur, although they are relatively uncommon. The most common location is the proximal aspect of the medial trochlear ridge in association with traumatic injury.[25] In these cases the fragments may be removed arthroscopically using an approach through the plantar pouch. The most common fracture associated with tarsocrural joints are lateral malleolar fractures.[42] Only a small portion of the lateral malleolus is intra-articular, with most of the fragmented bone enclosed within the joint capsule and collateral ligament, but arthroscopic removal (albeit an advanced technique) is possible.[25]

Osteochondral fragmentation of the distal aspect of the patella has been described and is commonly associated with medial patellar desmotomy.[16,21] Successful treatment with surgery has been evaluated. Fracture fragments also occur off the lateral and medial aspects of the patella (usually associated with direct trauma). There is usually severe lameness referable to the stifle as well as swelling, including femoropatellar effusion. A skyline radiograph of the femoropatellar joint best defines the lesion (Figure 8.19). These fractures are also removed with arthroscopic surgery.

Osteochondritis Dissecans (OCD)

Cases of OCD can be treated conservatively and with surgery. For many years, the author recommended arthroscopic surgery for all cases of OCD in the femoropatellar joint, particularly if an athletic career was planned; however the study by McIntosh and McIlwraith (1993)[27] showed that with conservative management (stall or pen confinement for 60 days) quite a number of femoropatellar OCD cases can heal. Generally these are defects that are less than 2 cm long and less than 5 mm deep with no obvious mineralization or fragmentation on the flap on radiographs.

It has also been noted by Dik, et al. (1999)[9] that it is possible for radiographic OCD in the femoropatellar

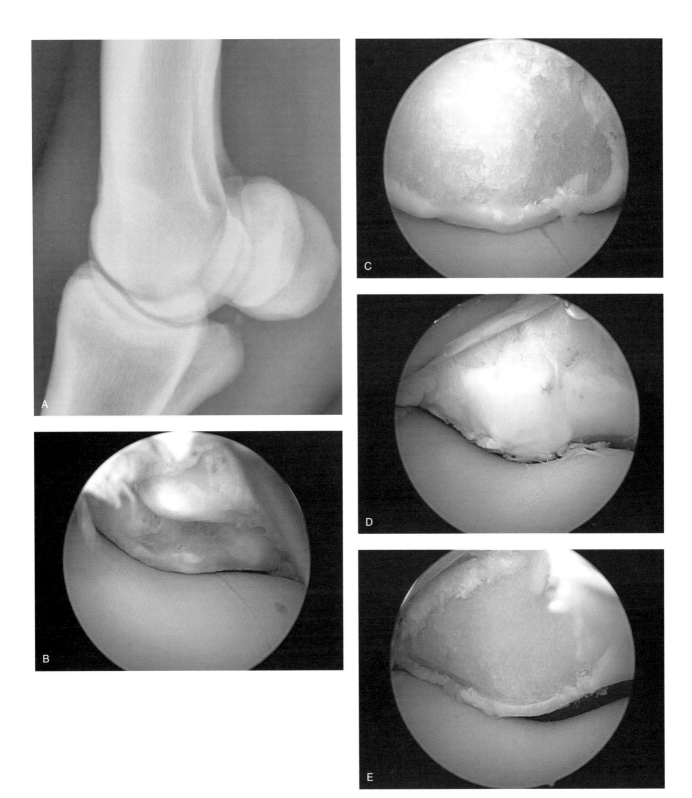

Figure 8.14. Radiographic (A) and arthroscopic views (B through E) of proximal phalanx fragmentation on both the medial and lateral eminences. The small fragment off the lateral eminence can be seen superimposed over the larger fragmentation off the medial eminence (A). The arthroscopic views show the lateral eminence fragment before (B) and after (C) removal. The arthroscopic views are the larger proximal medial P1 fragment shown before (D) and after (E) removal and debridement of the defect.

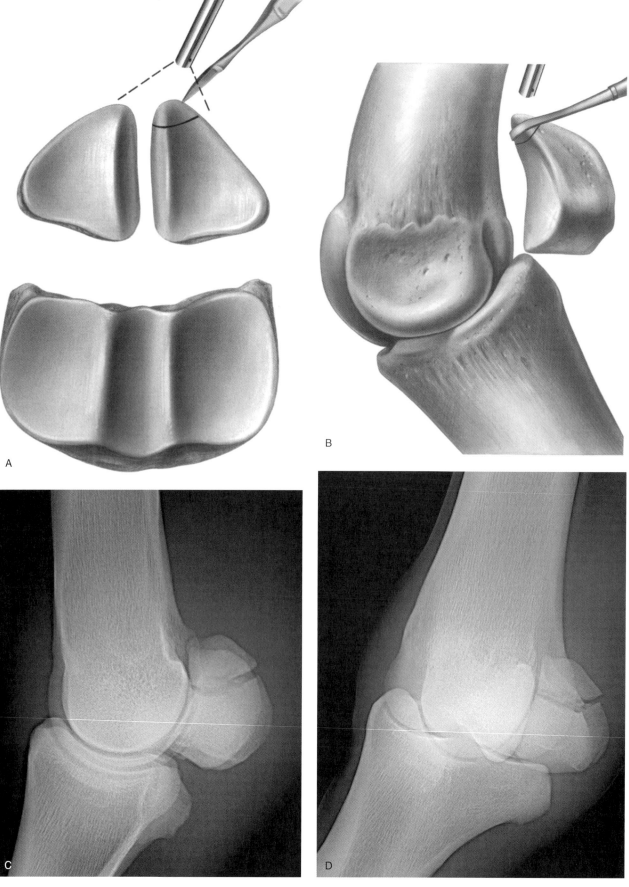

Figure 8.15. Diagram of position of arthroscope and instrument to dissect apical fragments of the sesamoid bone from the suspensory and sesamoidean ligaments using an ipsilateral approach. A. Dorsal view. B. Lateral view. C and D. Radiographs of a large apical sesamoid fragment. E and F. Arthroscopic views of a fracture and dissection of fragment from the suspensory ligament attachments.

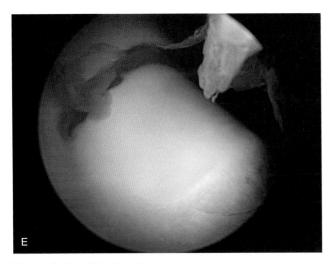

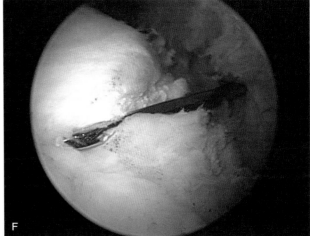

Figure 8.15. (*Continued*)

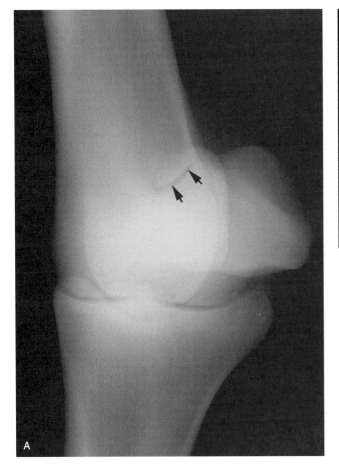

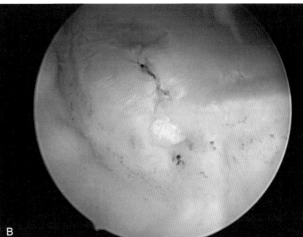

Figure 8.16. Radiographic (A) and arthroscopic view (B) of an abaxial fracture fragment (arrow) of the proximal sesamoid bone. (Reproduced with permission from McIlwraith, CW, et al. Diagnostic and Surgical Arthroscopy in the Horse, 3rd ed., 2005, Figure 5.56.)

joint to heal up to age 8 months. In a longitudinal study of Dutch Warmblood foals radiographed at 1 month old and subsequently at 4-week intervals, the mid-region of the lateral femoral trochlear ridge became radiographically abnormal from 3 to 4 months of age. Subsequent progression of radiographic abnormalities was usually followed by regression and resolution, whereby at 5 months 20% of the stifles were abnormal radiographically, but at 11 months this percentage had decreased to 3%.

When clinical signs persist or horses are older than 8 months of age, arthroscopic surgery is indicated. The

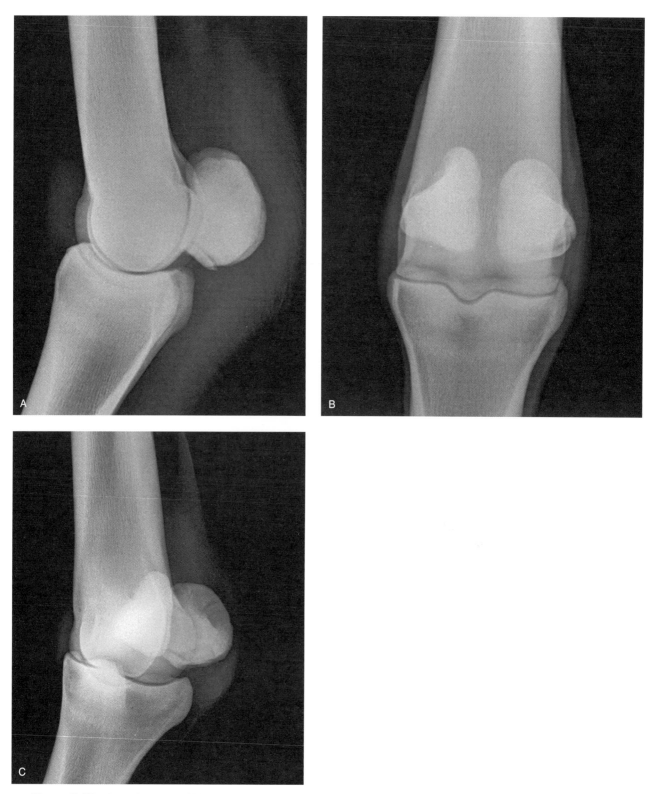

Figure 8.17. Lateral to medial (A), dorsopalmar (B), and DPMLO (C) radiographic views of basal fragmentation of the medial sesamoid bone. Despite the extent of this fragmentation, the horse was able to come back and race successfully.

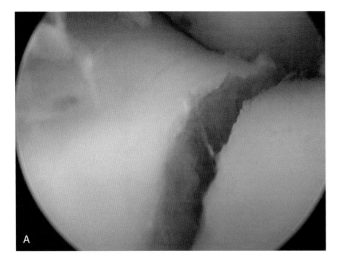

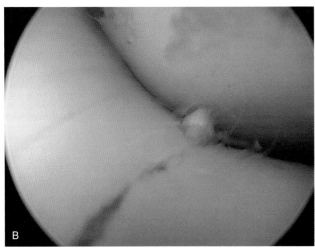

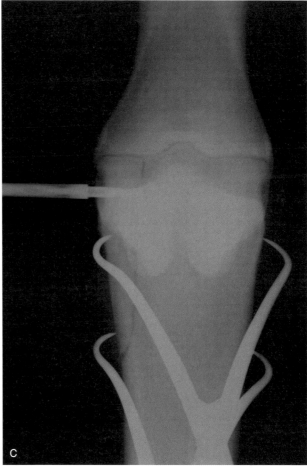

Figure 8.18. The use of large (AO/ASIF) reduction forceps to reduce displaced condylar fracture. Arthroscopic view before reduction (A) and after reduction (B). C. Radiographic view with reduction forceps reducing the fracture and the distal hole being drilled. Dorsal (D) and palmar (E) arthroscopic views following reduction and compression. F. Post-operative radiograph. (Reproduced with permission from McIlwraith CW, et al. Diagnostic and Surgical Arthroscopy in the Horse, 3rd ed., 2005, Figure 5.70.)

techniques have been previously described[25] and positive results also reported.[13]

When clinical signs as well as a radiographic OCD lesion are present in the tarsocrural joint, arthroscopic surgery is indicated because conservative management has not been shown to resolve any of these problems once clinical signs are present. The technique and results of arthroscopic surgery for OCD in the 4 locations where it occurs (distal intermediate ridge of tibia [DIRT], lateral trochlear ridge of talus [LTR], medial malleolus of tibia, and medial trochlear ridge of tibia, in descending order of frequency) has been reported.[23,25] Dik, et al. also reported that resolution of radiographic lesions can occur in the tarsocrural joint.[9] At 1 month of age the appearance of the intermediate ridge of the distal tibia was frequently abnormal (grades 1 to 3 of 4 in 67%). Abnormal appearances of the distal aspect of the lateral trochlear ridge of the talus were less common (grades 1 to 3 of 4 in 25%). Only 18% of the DIRT (and 3% of LTR) lesions were still abnormal at these sites at age 11 months. For both predilection sites

on the hock, normal and abnormal appearances were permanent from age 5 months.

Management of OCD in the fetlock joints is discussed in Chapter 11.

Arthroscopic Treatment of Osteoarthritis

There is considerable controversy over the value of arthroscopic treatment of OA in humans.[6,28,34] As recently reviewed by Sipalsky, et al. (2007)[34], there is only a single level one study and the design has flaws. This study concluded that arthroscopic lavage or arthroscopic debridement was no better than those after placebo procedure.[28] However, the author is aware of considerable benefit being gained from lavage with distention breaking down adhesions within the joint, removal of debris and focal debridement of fibrillated lesions in humans. In a recent study 69 knees in 61 patients were treated with an arthroscopic regimen including joint insufflation, lysis of adhesions, anterior interval release, contouring of cartilage defects to a

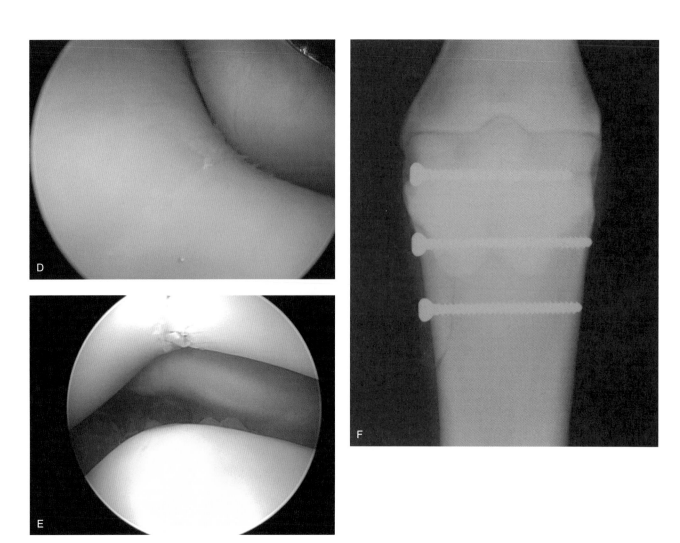

Figure 8.18. (*Continued*)

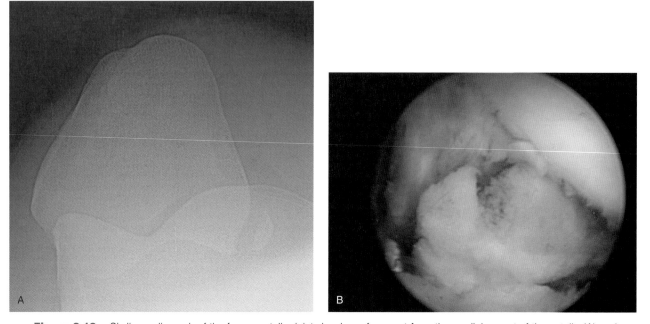

Figure 8.19. Skyline radiograph of the femoropatellar joint showing a fragment from the medial aspect of the patella (A) and arthroscopic view after separation from the soft tissue but prior to removal (B).

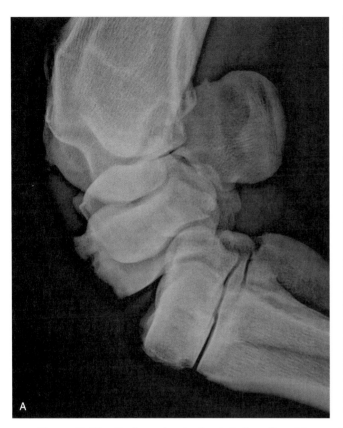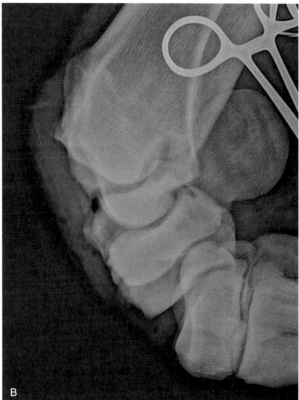

Figure 8.20. Radiographs of osteophyte formation of the proximal intermediate and radial carpal bones before (A) and after (B) removal.

stable rim, shaping of meniscal tears to a stable rim, synovectomy, removal of loose bodies, and removal of osteophytes that affected terminal extension.[38] Inclusion criteria included severe OA and a minimum of 2 years' follow-up. Nine knees failed, with survivorship of 83% at 3 years. At an average follow-up of 31 months the average Lysholm score improved 25 points, the average Tegner score was 4, and average patient satisfaction was 8 (scale of 10). The conclusion was that this regimen could improve function and activity levels with moderate to severe OA. Of 69 patients, 60 (87%) had satisfactory results, but 11 needed a second procedure, which resulted in a net 71% satisfactory result after one surgery.

Similar rationale has been applied to symptomatic and selective debridement of problems in equine joints. Although there is controversy regarding the value of removing fibrillated cartilage and the use of radiofrequency probes is to be discouraged, selective removal of loose cartilage as well as loose bodies and debris has achieved improvement in clinical results. Debridement of articular defects is limited to removal of loose tissue, loose separated cartilage and bone, and calcified cartilage when the defect appears to be full-thickness. Partial-thickness defects (if there is no detached tissue) are left alone.

The removal of spurs or osteophytes is often a difficult decision. The author considers it appropriate if they have fractured off or if their interposition into the joint makes them likely candidates for later

fracture. Figure 8.20 illustrates a case in which the osteophytes were removed. Most spurs that are visible radiographically are not candidates for removal. In most instances the experienced surgeon can predict whether removal of a spur is appropriate by examining the radiographs.

The author only uses microfracture if there is a defect completely surrounded by articular cartilage to protect the repair tissue created. Defects in the femoropatellar and femorotibial joints are the best candidates because of the greater thickness of articular cartilage. Microfracture is avoided in the center of the weight-bearing area of the medial femoral condyle in most instances to avoid the possibility of secondary subchondral cystic lesion development. Recent work suggests that the use of new grafting techniques such as autologous cartilage fragments could be beneficial, but the availability of appropriate staples (as has been demonstrated in experimental work)[15] is necessary.

References

1. Allum R. Complications of arthroscopy of the knee. J Bone Joint Surg (Br) 2002;84B:937–945.
2. Barclay WP, Foerner JJ, Philips TN. Lameness attributable to osteochondral fragmentation of the plantar aspect of the proximal phalanx in horses: 19 cases (1981–1985). J Am Vet Med Assoc 1987;191:855–857.
3. Birkeland R. Chip fractures of the first phalanx in the metatarsophalangeal joint of the horse. Acta Radiol Suppl 1972; 29:73–77.

4. Bramlage LR. Arthrodesis of the fetlock joint. In Equine Medicine and Surgery, 3rd ed. Mansmann RA, McAllister GS, eds. American Veterinary Publications, Santa Barbara, 1982;1064.

5. Buckwalter JA. Mechanical injuries of articular cartilage. In: Biology and Biomechanics of the Traumatized Synovial Joint: The Knee as a Model. Finerman GAM, Noyes FR, eds. American Academy of Orthopedic Surgeons, Rosemont, Illinois, 1992;83–96.

6. Calvert GT, Wright RW. The use of arthroscopy in the athlete with knee osteoarthritis. Clin Sports Med 2005;24:113–152.

7. Copelan R, Bramlage LR. Surgery of the fetlock joint. Vet Clin North Am 1983;2:221–231.

8. Dabareiner RM, White NA, et al. Metacarpophalangeal joint and synovial pad fibrotic fibrillation in 63 horses. Vet Surg 1996;5:199–206.

9. Dik KJ, Enzerink E, van Weeran PR. Radiographic development of osteochondral abnormalities in the hock and stifle of Dutch Warmblood foals from age 1 to 11 months. Equine Vet J Suppl 1999;31:9–15.

10. Evans CH, Mears DC, Cosgrove JL. Release of neutral proteinases from mononuclear phagocytes and synovial cells in response to cartilaginous wear particles *in vitro*. Biochem Biophys Acta 1981;677:287–294.

11. Finerman GAM, Noyes FR, eds. Biology and Biomechanics of the Traumatized Synovial joint: The Knee as a Model. American Academy of Orthopedic Surgeons, Rosemont, Illinois, 1992;1265–1274.

12. Foerner JJ, Barclay WP, Philips TN, et al. Osteochondral fragments of the palmar/plantar aspect of the fetlock joint. Proceedings Am Assoc Equine Pract 1987;33:739–744.

13. Foland JW, McIlwraith CW, Trotter GW. Arthroscopic surgery for osteochondritis dissecans of the femoropatellar joint. Equine Vet J 1992;22:419–423.

14. Fortier LA, Foerner JJ, Nixon AJ. Arthroscopic removal of axial osteochondral fragments of the palmar/plantar proximal aspect of the proximal phalanx in horses: 119 cases (1988–1992). J Am Vet Med Assoc 1995;206:71–74.

15. Frisbie DD, Lu Y, Kawcak CE, et al. *In vivo* evaluation of autologous cartilage fragment loaded scaffolds implanted into equine articular cartilage defects (a one-step procedure). Am J Sports Med 2009;37:71S-80.

16. Gibson KT, McIlwraith CW, Park RD, et al. Production of patellar lesions by medial patellar desmotomy in normal horses. Vet Surg 1989;18:466–471.

17. Haynes PF. Diseases of the metatarsophalangeal joint and metacarpus. Vet Clin North Am Large Anim Pract 1980;2:33–85.

18. Kawcak CE, McIlwraith CW. Proximodorsal first phalanx osteochondral chip fragments in 320 horses. Equine Vet J 1994; 26:392–396.

19. Kawcak CE, McIlwraith CW, Norrdin RW, et al. The role of subchondral bone in joint disease: A review. Equine Vet J 2001;33:120–126.

20. McIlwraith CW, Yovich JV, Martin GS. Arthroscopic surgery for the treatment of osteochondral chip fractures in the equine carpus. J Am Vet Med Assoc 1987;191:531–540.

21. McIlwraith CW. Osteochondral fragmentation of the distal aspect of the patella in the horse. Equine Vet J 1990a;22: 157–163.

22. McIlwraith CW, Voorhees M. Management of osteochondritis dissecans of the dorsal aspect of the distal metacarpus and metatarsus. Proceedings Am Assoc Equine Pract 1990b;35:547–550.

23. McIlwraith CW, Foerner JJ, Davis DM. Osteochondritis dissecans of the tarsocrural joint: Results of treatment with arthroscopic surgery. Equine Vet J 1991;23:155–162.

24. McIlwraith CW, Bramlage LR. Surgical treatment of joint injury. In Joint Disease in the Horse, 2nd ed. McIlwraith CW, Trotter GW, eds. WB Saunders Co, Philadelphia, 1996;292–317.

25. McIlwraith CW, Nixon AJ, Wright IM, et al. In Diagnostic and Surgical Arthroscopy of the Horse, 3rd ed. Mosby Elsevier, Edinborough, 2005a.

26. McIlwraith CW. Frank Milne Lecture: From Arthroscopy to Gene Therapy—30 Years of Looking in Joints. Proceedings Am Assoc Equine Pract 2005b;51:65–113.

27. McIntosh SC, McIlwraith CW. Natural history of femoropatellar osteochondrosis in three crops of Thoroughbreds. Equine Vet J Suppl 1993;16:54–61.

28. Moseley JB, O'Malley K, Petersen NJ, et al. A controlled trial of arthroscopic surgery for osteoarthritis of the knee. N Engl J Med 2002;347:81–88.

29. Nixon AJ, Pool RR. Histologic appearance of axial osteochondral fragments from the proximoplantar/proximopalmar aspect of the proximal phalanx in horses. J Am Vet Med Assoc 1995;207:1076–1080.

30. Norrdin RW, Kawcak CE, McIlwraith CW. Subchondral bone failure in an equine model of overload arthrosis. Bone 1998;22:133–139.

31. Pool RR, Meagher DM. Pathologic findings and pathogenesis of racetrack injuries. Vet Clin North Am Equine Pract 1990;6:1–30.

32. Richardson DW. Technique for arthroscopic repair of third carpal bone slab fractures in the horse. J Am Vet Med Assoc 1986;188:288–291.

33. Richardson DW. Arthroscopically assisted repair of articular fractures. Clin Equine Pract 2001;1:211–217.

34. Sipalksy P, Ryzwicz M, Peterson B, et al. Arthroscopic treatment of osteoarthritis of the knee. Are there any evidence-based indications? Clin Orthop 2007;455:105–112.

35. Southwood LL, Trotter GW, McIlwraith CW. Arthroscopic removal of abaxial fracture fragments of the proximal sesamoid bones in horses: 47 cases (1989–1997). J Am Vet Med Assoc 1998;213:1016–1021.

36. Southwood LL, McIlwraith CW. Arthroscopic removal of fracture fragment involving a portion of the base of the proximal sesamoid bone in horses: 26 cases (1984–1997). J Am Vet Med Assoc 2000;217:236–240.

37. Southwood LL, McIlwraith CW, Trotter GW, et al. Arthroscopic removal of apical fractures of the proximal sesamoid bone in horses: 98 cases (1989–1999). Proceedings Am Assoc Equine Pract 2000;46:100–101.

38. Steadman JR, Remappa AJ, Maxwell RB, et al. An arthroscopic treatment regime for osteoarthritis of the knee. Arthroscopy 2007;23:948–955.

39. van Veenendaal JC, Moffatt RE. Tissue masses in the fetlock joint of horses. Aust Vet J 1980;56:533–566.

40. Walmsley JP. Vertical tears of the cranial horn of the meniscus and its cranial ligament in the equine femorotibial joint: 7 cases and their treatment by arthroscopic surgery. Equine Vet J 1995;27:20–25.

41. White NA, Sullins KE, Spurlock SL, et al. Diagnosis and treatment of metacarpophalangeal synovial pad proliferation in the horse. Vet Surg 1988;17:46.

42. Wright IM. Fractures of the lateral malleolus of tibia in 16 horses. Equine Vet J 1992;24:424–429.

43. Zekas LJ, Bramlage LR, et al. Results of treatment of 145 fractures in the third metacarpal/metatarsal condyles in 155 horses (1986–1994). Equine Vet J 1999;31:309–313.

ACUPUNCTURE TREATMENT OF LAMENESS AND BACK PAIN

Kevin K. Haussler

INTRODUCTION

Acupuncture is the stimulation of specific anatomical landmarks with the goal of providing pain relief or normalizing physiologic function. The exact location of equine acupuncture points has been debated and clear consensus on anatomic locations and naming systems is lacking.[11] Numerous studies have proposed unique anatomical or physical characteristics of acupuncture points, such as sites of palpable indentation or tenderness, decreased electrical resistance, increased free nerve endings, motor points, or neurovascular bundles. A Western perspective of acupuncture points is that most sites correspond to underlying nerves that produce specific local, autonomic, and central neurophysiologic effects.[15] Acupuncture has many reported effects via neurophysiologic, humoral, and bioelectric mechanisms. Needle insertion into the skin produces local tissue effects and afferent sensory stimulation of central neural pathways.

The most commonly reported mechanisms of action for acupuncture-induced analgesia include stimulation of endogenous opioids and peripheral electrical stimulation of large sensory afferent nerves that modulate nociceptive input in the dorsal horn of the spinal cord (i.e., gate control theory of pain) via release of neurotransmitters and neuromodulators.[14,22] However, there is no consistent relationship between the level of analgesia and plasma or cerebrospinal fluid concentrations of β-endorphins or cortisol. Neurologic connections between acupuncture points on the trunk and sympathetic pathways in the thoracolumbar spinal cord also provide possibilities of influencing internal organ function by stimulating paraspinal acupuncture points.[11] Recent neuroimaging studies using functional MRI to measure brain activity have revealed that acupuncture stimulation modulates the human central nervous system, including cerebral limbic/paralimbic and somatosensory cortex.[23]

De qi is a characteristic needling sensation as perceived by the patient and the sensation of needle grasp as perceived by the acupuncturist. During needle grasp, the acupuncturist feels pulling and increased resistance to further movement of the inserted needle, which is considered to be due to mechanical coupling between the needle and connective tissue.[5] A large number of acupuncture points have been reported to occur along intermuscular or intramuscular connective tissue planes. Evaluation of connective tissue responses to acupuncture stimulation has revealed quantitative differences between acupuncture and nonacupuncture points, which may provide a valid anatomical and physiological explanation for acupuncture meridians. Mechanical coupling between the acupuncture needle and connective tissue produces mechanical, neurologic, and chemical extracellular signaling, which may explain some of the local and remote as well as long-term effects of acupuncture.[4] This may provide one explanation why inserting a needle anywhere in the body can produce measurable physiological responses.[10] Further research is needed to fully explain the physiologic effects of acupuncture.

TECHNIQUES OF STIMULATION

Numerous forms of stimulation have been applied to acupuncture points. Different pain-controlling mechanism can be evoked by changing the type or intensity of acupuncture stimulation.[15] The most common methods of acupuncture stimulation include the insertion of solid needles (i.e., dry needling), electroacupuncture, and aquapuncture. Dry needle acupuncture uses disposable, 25- to 34-gauge, filiform, solid needles of varying lengths. Dry needle insertion causes immediate changes in neural or segmental interactions and local inflammatory responses.[15] Prolonged stimulation can induce humoral responses and activation of the opiate system, which creates generalized analgesia.

Electroacupuncture is the application of electrical stimulation to inserted needles, with the goal of providing more intense or focused neurologic stimulation and muscle relaxation (Figure 8.21). Electroacupuncture and dry needle acupuncture both provide cutaneous analgesia in horses, compared to controls.[14] However, electroacupuncture is more effective than needle acupuncture for activating the release of β-endorphins into

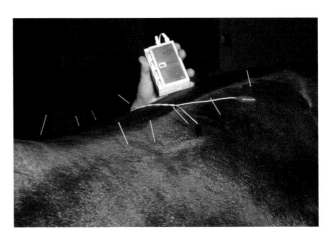

Figure 8.21. Electroacupuncture of the longissimus muscle near the thoracolumbar junction in a horse with back pain and muscle hypertonicity. (Courtesy of Dr. Gary Baxter.)

the cerebrospinal fluid. Electroacupuncture produces effects according to the polarity, frequency, intensity, and duration of electrical stimulation, as well as the number and pairing of needles stimulated.[22] Low-frequency (less than 20 Hz), high-amplitude stimulation causes visible muscle contractions and produces generalized analgesia with slow, prolonged, and cumulative effects that are mediated by endorphins.[15] High-frequency (80 to 100 Hz), low-amplitude stimulation activates low-threshold skin and muscle receptors and produces nonopiate derived analgesia that has a rapid onset and decline, is localized segmentally, and is not cumulative.

In a randomized control trial, 4 different electroacupuncture protocols were evaluated for antinociceptive effects on thermal stimulation of the pastern region.[22] Local acupuncture points and high-frequency (80 to 120 Hz) stimulation was more effective in blocking limb pain than the use of distant acupuncture points and low frequency (20 Hz) stimulation.

Aquapuncture uses a 20- to 25-gauge, hypodermic needle to mechanically stimulate acupuncture points, followed by injection of various solutions in an effort to produce longer-lasting or combined pharmacological effects. Some of the more commonly injected substances include saline, vitamin B_{12}, and 2% iodine in peanut oil. Other substances include corticosteroids, Sarapin, Traumeel (a homeopathic remedy), vitamin B_1, 25% magnesium sulfate, 2% procaine, and 15% dextrose.[19] Injected volumes at each site vary from 0.5 to 5 ml (and up to 30 ml)/site, depending on the injected substance and desired response. Some practitioners believe that treatment effects last longer with injected substances, compared to dry needling. Other practitioners prefer dry needling with solid acupuncture needles due to the increased risk of breaking off hypodermic needles under the skin due to skin or fascial movement.

Additional forms of acupuncture stimulation include acupressure (i.e., digital pressure), implantation of gold beads or surgical staples for long-term stimulation, and laser stimulation, which uses low-level laser generation to stimulate superficial acupuncture points. Laser acupuncture provides the benefit of having no physical puncturing of the skin, but the initial cost of equipment is expensive. Anecdotal evidence experienced by the author suggests that low-level laser stimulation is effective for producing a temporary reduction in acute or severe back pain when affected horses do not tolerate acupuncture needle placement or forms of manual therapy. Dry needling, laser stimulation, and injection of saline into acupuncture points appear to be equally effective for treating horses with chronic back pain.[6]

GENERAL INDICATIONS FOR TREATMENT

Acupuncture case selection is often based on thorough physical examination and elimination of conditions that are judged to respond more effectively to conventional therapies.[9] Because of the lack of proven effective medical or surgical approaches for the treatment of chronic back pain in horses, acupuncture is often considered as a first treatment of choice.[9] If clinical signs of back pain persist after a few acupuncture treatments, then additional diagnostics and re-examina-tion is indicated in an attempt to better localize and identify the source of pain and to prescribe a targeted treatment or a combination of therapies. Acupuncture is generally not sufficient by itself to manage overt lameness, unless the lameness is judged to be caused by muscle hypertonicity.[8] Acupuncture may be used in cases that have an incomplete or lack of response to traditional medical and surgical approaches or compensatory lameness associated with primary joint or limb pain.[9] The use of acupuncture or the combination of acupuncture with conventional care is believed to produce beneficial and lasting effects and provides an opportunity to expand a veterinarian's diagnostic and therapeutic armamentarium. Acupuncture combined with diagnostic joint blocks and intra-articular therapy is thought to provide a more comprehensive diagnostic and treatment approach to chronic lameness.[7,8]

Contraindications for acupuncture include acute injuries, fractures, severe cardiac disease, extremely nervous or exhausted patients, acute infections, and neoplasia. Patients with organic disease or overt musculoskeletal pathology need a complete diagnostic work-up and consideration of appropriate Western treatments with documented efficacy and safety for the condition of interest.

LAMENESS

Acupuncture is reportedly useful for treating myofascial pain, osteoarthritis, stifle or hock pain, tendinitis, laminitis, and navicular disease, but there is a lack of controlled studies to validate efficacy.[17] Most evidence is in the form of clinical experience, case reports, and case series.[13] Numerous equine acupuncture case series on lameness are reported in the Chinese literature; however, poor scientific quality and lack of controls makes the evidence difficult to interpret.[18] A review of several case series on non-specific shoulder lameness, fetlock injuries, and laminitis report overall success rates ranging from 87% to 94% after 1 to 5 treatments, applied every 1 to 4 weeks.[18] However, the lack of details about case selection, diagnostic findings, objective outcome parameters, and nonuniform point selection and type of stimulation reduces the strength of the studies.

Only a few randomized, controlled trials have evaluated the effectiveness of acupuncture for limb pain or lameness. Cutaneous nociceptive thresholds to mechanical and heat stimuli during control and electroacupuncture trials in 23 horses showed significant cutaneous analgesia within 5 areas of the trunk, but not in the head or limbs.[1] Electroacupuncture has demonstrated variable effectiveness for reducing pain associated with either experimentally induced or naturally occurring lameness.[16,22] In a randomized controlled trial, electroacupuncture was used to treat horses with chronic laminitis (n = 10) and navicular disease (n = 10).[16] The degree of lameness was assessed by changes in subjective lameness scores, stride lengths, and ground reaction forces. Although 7 out of 10 horses with chronic laminitis improved clinically during the trial, there were no statistically significant differences between treatment and control groups. Six out of 10 horses with navicular disease improved, but there were no significant differ-

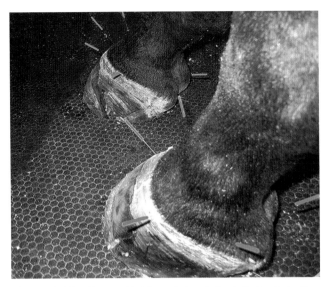

Figure 8.22. Horse with bilateral chronic laminitis treated with acupuncture needles placed around the coronary band at *Ting* acupuncture points. (Courtesy of Dr. Tim Holt.)

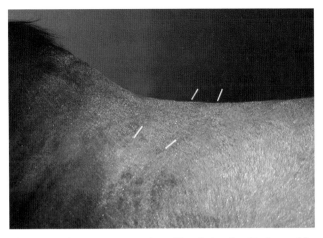

Figure 8.23. Horse presenting with pain localized to the saddle region treated with acupuncture needles placed along the dorsal midline adjacent to the spinous processes and within the epaxial musculature. (Courtesy of Dr. Tim Holt.)

ences between treatment and control groups. Reasons for failing to demonstrate efficacy of acupuncture treatment include small sample size and inappropriate point selection, frequency, or intensity of stimulation.

Electroacupuncture has also been evaluated in an experimentally-induced lameness model using an instrumented shoe to apply transient localized sole pressure.[21] Electroacupuncture was able to partially reduce lameness scores, compared to bupivacaine or saline controls. Inconsistent changes in stride kinematics were noted, but there was no change in overall stride lengths. In another study using instrumented shoes to induce lameness in 6 horses, there was inconsistent evidence to suggest that pain, as measured by increased heart rates, was reduced after needle puncture to induce bleeding (hemoacupuncture) around the coronary band and dry needle placement between the heel bulbs.[2] For empirical treatment of laminitis, acupuncture points around the coronary band (*Ting* points) reportedly reduce local pain, and proximal thoracic limb points are used to address the sustained laminitic posture and subsequent muscle hypertonicity and pain associated with chronic laminitis (Figure 8.22).

CHRONIC BACK PAIN

The majority of the equine acupuncture literature addressing musculoskeletal issues is focused on treatment of chronic back pain (Figure 8.23). In one review of acupuncture treatment for back pain, 11 different types of acupuncture stimulation have been described; however, some methods are quite unconventional and not used in Western acupuncture.[19] In acupuncture case series for treating back pain, success rates range from 66% to 100%; however, many studies have small sample sizes and all studies lack objective outcome parameters.[18,19] In a case series of 200 horses treated with acupuncture, 73% had primary back problems or back problems combined with pelvic limb lameness.[9] Of

the horses that received treatment for primary back pain, 58% (84 of 146) received acupuncture treatment alone. Another case series of 25 horses with back pain and poor performance reported that all horses returned to their previous level of competition following a combination of acupuncture treatment, changing saddle pads, and addressing poor saddle fit.[3] In a large case series (n = 350) reported over several successive studies, horses presenting with a chief compliant of poor performance, presumably due to primary back pain, were treated with different forms of acupuncture stimulation, and pain alleviation varied from 53% to 87%.[6] Out of the 350 horses, 75% were able to perform at an acceptable level after acupuncture treatment. Unfortunately, there were no control groups in these studies so the natural course of back pain resolution or true effectiveness of acupuncture treatment could not be determined.[6]

In a randomized controlled study, both dry needle acupuncture and electroacupuncture of the trunk significantly increased cutaneous analgesia measured by thermal stimulation, compared to sham needle placement.[14] Another randomized, controlled study reported that electroacupuncture produced significant decreases in thoracolumbar pain scores after 3 treatments, which remained reduced 14 days after the last treatment, compared to oral phenylbutazone and control (i.e., oral saline) groups.[20] A third randomized, double-blind, controlled trial evaluated the effectiveness of electroacupuncture on chronic back pain using pressure algometry to assess mechanical nociceptive thresholds.[12] A series of electroacupuncture treatments over 15 days combined with rest was significantly more effective for increasing mechanical nociceptive thresholds (i.e., reducing pain) than sham electroacupuncture and rest.

ADVERSE EFFECTS

Adverse effects associated with acupuncture use in horses are largely unreported. Bleeding at the site of needle insertion is common and may actually be used as a treatment technique (i.e., hemoacupuncture) for certain conditions. In one equine study, approximately 20% of horses experience increased signs of back pain the day after saline aquapuncture treatment, which was alleviated by prescribed exercise.[6] Bent or retained needles are most commonly due to the use of excessive force to insert needles through thick skin, muscle spasms, or patient movement. Close patient monitoring is indicated, and repeat acupuncture treatment sessions may need to be revised by changing point selection or the method or intensity of stimulation. Equine acupuncture is considered a safe treatment modality for practitioners experienced in addressing pain associated with lameness or back problems.

References

1. Bossut DF, Page EH, Stromberg MW. Production of cutaneous analgesia by electroacupuncture in horses: Variations dependent on sex of subject and locus of stimulation. Am J Vet Res 1984;45:620–625.
2. Hackett GE, Spitzfaden DM, May KJ, et al. Acupuncture: Is it effective for alleviating pain in horses? Proc Am Assoc Equine Practitioners 1997;43:333–335.
3. Harman JC. The effects of acupuncture on the performance of horses. The Equine Athlete 1993;6:22–25.
4. Langevin HM, Bouffard NA, Badger GJ, et al. Dynamic fibroblast cytoskeletal response to subcutaneous tissue stretch *ex vivo* and *in vivo*. Am J Physiol Cell Physiol 2005;288:C747–756.
5. Langevin HM, Yandow JA. Relationship of acupuncture points and meridians to connective tissue planes. Anat Rec 2002;269:257–65.
6. Martin BB Jr., Klide AM. Acupuncture for treatment of chronic back pain in horses. In Veterinary Acupuncture: Ancient Art to Modern Medicine. Schoen AM, ed. Mosby, Inc., St. Louis, 2001:467–473.
7. McCormick WH. Oriental channel diagnosis in foot lameness of the equine forelimb. J Equine Vet Sci 1997;17:315–321.
8. McCormick WH. Understanding the use of acupuncture in treating equine lameness and musculoskeletal pain. In Diagnosis and Management of Lameness in the Horse. Ross MW, Dyson SJ, eds. Saunders, St. Louis, 2003:798–803.
9. Merriam JG. Acupuncture in the treatment of back pain and hind leg pain in sport horses. Proc Amer Assoc Equine Practitioners 1997;43:325–326.
10. Moffet HH. Sham acupuncture may be as efficacious as true acupuncture: a systematic review of clinical trials. J Altern Complement Med 2009;15:213–216.
11. Robinson NG. The need for consistency and comparability of transpositional acupuncture points across species. Am J Traditional Chinese Vet Med 2006;1:14–21.
12. Rungsri PK, Trinarong C, Rojanasthien S, et al. The effectiveness of electro-acupuncture on pain threshold in sport horses with back pain. Am J Traditional Chinese Vet Med 2009;4:22–26.
13. Schoen AM. Equine acupuncture for lameness diagnosis and treatment. In Diagnosis and Management of Lameness in the Horse. Ross MW, Dyson SJ, eds. Saunders, St. Louis, 2003: 792–798.
14. Skarda RT, Tejwani GA, Muir WW. Cutaneous analgesia, hemodynamic and respiratory effects, and beta-endorphin concentration in spinal fluid and plasma of horses after acupuncture and electroacupuncture. Am J Vet Res 2002;63:1435–1442.
15. Steiss JE. Neurophysiological basis of acupuncture. In Veterinary Acupuncture: Ancient Art to Modern Medicine. Schoen AM, ed. Mosby Publications, St. Louis, 2001:24–46.
16. Steiss JE, White NA, Bowen JM. Electroacupuncture in the treatment of chronic lameness in horses and ponies: A controlled clinical trial. Can J Vet Res 1989;53:239–243.
17. Sutherland EC. Integration of acupuncture and manipulation into a standard lameness examination and treatment approach. Proc Amer Assoc Equine Practitioners 1997;43:319–321.
18. Xie H. Treating equine lameness with acupuncture. Compendium 2001;23:838–841, 852.
19. Xie H, Asquith RL, Kivipelto J. A review of the use of acupuncture for treatment of equine back pain. J Equine Vet Sci 1996; 16:285–290.
20. Xie H, Colahan P, Ott EA. Evaluation of electroacupuncture treatment of horses with signs of chronic thoracolumbar pain. J Am Vet Med Assoc 2005;227:281–286.
21. Xie H, Ott EA, Colahan P. Influence of acupuncture on experimental lameness in horses. Proc Amer Assoc Equine Pract 2001; 47:347–357.
22. Xie H, Ott EA, Harkins JD, et al. Influence of electro-acupuncture on pain threshold in horses and its mode of action. J Equine Vet Sci 2001;21:591–600.
23. Yoo SS, Kerr CE, Park M, et al. Neural activities in human somatosensory cortical areas evoked by acupuncture stimulation. Complement Ther Med 2007;15:247–254.

MANUAL THERAPY TECHNIQUES

| Kevin K. Haussler

INTRODUCTION

Manual therapy is application of the hands to the body with a therapeutic intent.[11] Chiropractic, osteopathy, physical therapy, massage therapy, and touch therapies are all considered forms of manual therapy techniques that have been developed for treatment of musculoskeletal disorders in humans and transferred for use in horses. Each technique has unique origins and different proposed biomechanical or physiological effects; however, all forms of manual therapy are characterized by applying variable gradations of manual force and degrees of soft tissue or articular displacement. The goal of all manual therapies is to influence reparative or healing processes within the neuromusculoskeletal system.

Therapeutic effects may be generalized to the entire body by inducing relaxation or altering behavior, regional effects may include alterations in pain perception or neuromuscular control, or effects may be localized to specific tissues and cellular responses.[11] The challenge is in selecting the most appropriate and effective form of manual therapy to produce the desired physiological effect within an individual patient, such as increasing joint range of motion, reducing pain, or promoting general body relaxation. Anecdotally, all forms of manual therapy have reported levels of effectiveness in humans and horses. Unfortunately, most claims are not supported by high levels of evidence such as randomized controlled trials or systematic reviews of the literature.

THERAPEUTIC TOUCH

The physical act of touching someone can induce physiologic responses and is often considered therapeutic.[3] In horses, touch therapies have been primarily developed and promoted by Linda Tellington-Jones in a collection of techniques named the Tellington Touch Equine Awareness Method (TTEAM) or Tellington TTouch.[20] Anecdotally, therapeutic touch is thought to improve behavior, performance, and well-being of horses, and enhance the relationship between horse and rider, but no controlled studies support these claims. Similar touch therapy techniques have been used in foals at birth to assess the effects of touch or imprint-training on behavioral reactions during selected handling procedures.[18] Conditioned foals are reported to be significantly less resistant to touching the front and hind limbs and picking up the hind feet at 3 months of age. More controlled studies are needed to determine the effectiveness of touch theories in managing behavioral or musculoskeletal issues in horses.

MASSAGE THERAPY

Massage therapy is the manipulation of the skin and underlying soft tissues either manually (e.g., by rubbing, kneading, or tapping) or with an instrument or machine (e.g., mechanical vibration). Massage techniques include many named methods such as Swedish massage, sports massage, trigger point therapy, cross-fiber friction massage, lymphatic drainage, and acupressure. Clinically, massage and soft tissue mobilization are thought to increase blood flow, promote relaxation, relax muscles, increase tissue extensibility, reduce pain, and speed return to normal function.[2] In horses, massage therapy has been shown to be effective at reducing stress-related behavior and pain thresholds within the thoracolumbar spine.[12,19] A noncontrolled, clinical trial using 8 horses measured increased stride lengths at the walk and trot compared pre and postmassage, but changes were not significant due to a small sample size.[24] More high-quality, scientific evidence is needed to support the use of massage therapy in horses.[15]

PASSIVE STRETCHING EXERCISES

Passive stretching consists of applying forces to a limb or body segment to lengthen muscles or connective tissues beyond their normal resting lengths, with the intent of increasing joint range of motion and flexibility (Figure 8.24).[1] The amplitude of motion and length of time that an individual stretch is held is gradually increased over time, according to patient tolerance and ability. Stretching exercises are thought to increase joint range of motion, enhance flexibility, improve coordination and motor control, increase blood flow to muscles,

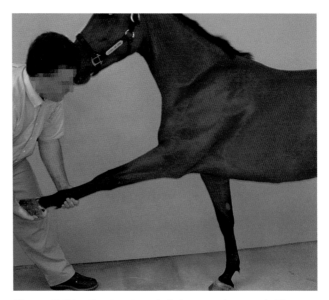

Figure 8.24. Passive thoracic limb protraction stretch. The thoracic limb is fully extended and held at the end range of motion to promote elongation of soft tissues and increase joint range of motion.

and help to prevent injuries. In horses, passive stretching of the limbs and axial skeleton have anecdotal effects of increasing stride length and joint range of motion and improving overall comfort.[5] In a noncontrolled study, passive thoracic limb stretching lowered wither height due to possible relaxation of the fibromuscular thoracic girdle.[6] However, a randomized controlled trial in riding school horses evaluating the effect of 2 different 8-week passive stretching programs reported no significant changes in stride length at the trot but did measure decreased joint range of motion within the shoulder, stifle, and hock articulations, instead of the expected increased joint range of motion.[16] The authors concluded that daily stretching may be too intensive in normal horses and may actually cause negative biomechanical effects.

MOBILIZATION

Mobilization is manually-induced movement of articulations or soft tissues for therapeutic purposes. Soft tissue mobilization focuses on restoring movement to the skin, connective tissue, ligaments, tendons, and muscles with the goal of modulating pain, reducing inflammation, improving tissue repair, increasing extensibility, and improving function.[2] Joint mobilization is characterized as nonimpulsive, repetitive joint movements induced within the passive range of joint motion with the goals of restoring normal and symmetric joint range of motion, stretching connective tissues, and restoring normal joint end-feel.[17] Manipulation is a manual procedure that involves a directed impulse that moves a joint or vertebral segment beyond its physiological range of motion, but does not exceed the anatomical limit of the articulation. Therefore, the primary biomechanical difference between joint mobilization and manipulation is the presence of a high-speed thrust or impulse. Spinal manipulation involves the application of controlled impulses to articular structures within the axial skeleton with the intent of reducing pain and muscle hypertonicity and increasing joint range of motion (Figure 8.25).

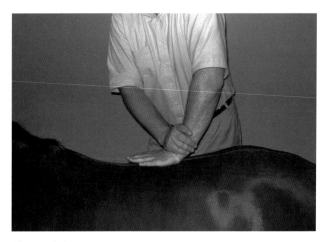

Figure 8.25. Thoracolumbar spinal extension mobilization. A gentle rhythmic force is applied over the dorsal spinous processes of the thoracolumbar junction in an effort to assess regional spinal flexibility and local pain or muscle hypertonicity.

Manual techniques used by physical therapists consist primarily of soft tissue and joint mobilization to assess the quality and quantity of joint range of motion and as a primary means of treating musculoskeletal disorders. Subjective assessment of the ease of joint motion, joint stability, and joint end-feel provide insights into the biomechanical and neurologic features of an articulation. Few formal studies support the use of limb or spinal mobilization techniques in horses.[10] Most mobilization studies in horses involve a period of induced joint immobilization by a fixture or cast followed by allowing the horse to spontaneously weight bear and ambulate on the affected limb, without evaluation of specific soft tissue or joint mobilization techniques.[21]

JOINT MOBILIZATION AND MANIPULATION

The chiropractic and osteopathic professions have many overlapping philosophies, techniques, and potential mechanisms of action related to joint mobilization and manipulation. Manual osteopathic techniques use a combination of mobilization and manipulation methods to address impaired or altered function of the musculoskeletal system (i.e., somatic dysfunction). From an osteopathic perspective, somatic dysfunction relates to impaired or altered function of skeletal, articular, myofascial, and related vascular, lymphatic, and neural elements.[13] Human osteopathic techniques also include highly controversial methods associated with mobilizing cranial bones and abdominal viscera, which have questionable application to horses.[22] Equine osteopathic evaluation and treatment procedures have been described in textbooks and case reports, but no formal hypothesis-driven research exists.[14, 22]

Chiropractic treatment is characterized primarily as the application of high-velocity, low-amplitude (HVLA) thrusts to induce therapeutic effects within articular structures, muscle function, and neurological reflexes. From a chiropractic perspective, the basic elements of joint or spinal dysfunction include altered articular neurophysiology, biochemical alterations, pathological changes within the joint capsule, and articular degeneration. Recent equine chiropractic research has focused on assessing the clinical effects of spinal manipulation on pain relief, improving flexibility, reducing muscle hypertonicity, and restoring spinal motion symmetry. Obvious criticism has been directed at the physical ability to even induce movement in the horse's back. Pilot work has demonstrated that manually applied forces associated with chiropractic techniques are able to produce substantial segmental spinal motion within the thoracolumbar region of horses.[8]

Two randomized controlled clinical trials using pressure algometry to assess mechanical nociceptive thresholds (MNTs) in the thoracolumbar region of horses have demonstrated that both manual and instrument-assisted spinal manipulation can reduce spinal nociception (or increase MNT values).[9,19] Additional studies have assessed the effects of equine chiropractic techniques on increasing passive spinal mobility (i.e., flexibility) and reducing longissimus muscle tone.[10,23] The effect of manipulation on asymmetrical spinal movement patterns in horses with documented back pain suggest that chiropractic treatment elicits minor but

Table 8.5. Types of manual therapy, proposed mechanisms of action, and possible clinical applications.

Manual therapies	Mechanisms of action	Clinical applications
Touch therapies	Psychological: Calming Behavioral deconditioning Novel cutaneous stimulation Mechanoreceptive stimulation	Behavioral issues Anxiety or nervousness Poor proprioception or body awareness Pain
Therapeutic massage	Psychological: Relaxation Mechanical: Soft tissues Neurophysiological: Pain	Anxiety or nervousness Soft tissue restriction Muscle hypertonicity Pain
Passive stretching exercises	Mechanical: Articular and soft tissues Neuromotor learning	Soft tissue restriction Muscle hypertonicity Joint stiffness Pain
Mobilization		
Soft tissue	Mechanical: Soft tissues	Soft tissue restriction Muscle hypertonicity Pain
Articular	Mechanical: Articular and soft tissues	Restricted joint motion Joint effusion Pain
Manipulation	Mechanical: Articular and soft tissues Neurophysiological: Pain Mechanoreceptive stimulation	Restricted joint motion Joint motion asymmetry Muscle hypertonicity Pain

significant changes in thoracolumbar and pelvic kinematics and that some of these changes are likely to be beneficial.[4,7]

Manual therapy is believed to produce physiological effects within local tissues, on sensory and motor components of the nervous system, and at a psychological or behavioral level.[11] It is likely that specific manual therapy techniques are inherently more effective than others in addressing each of these local, regional, or systemic components (Table 8.5). The question is choosing the most appropriate form of manual therapy or combination of techniques that will be efficacious for an individual patient with specific musculoskeletal disabilities.

CONTRAINDICATIONS

Contraindications for mobilization and manipulation are often based on clinical judgment and are related to the technique applied and skill or experience of the practitioner.[17] Few absolute contraindications exist for touch therapies, massage, and joint mobilization, if the techniques are applied appropriately. Manual therapy is generally contraindicated in the presence of fractures, acute inflammatory or infectious joint disease, osteomyelitis, joint ankylosis, bleeding disorders, progressive neurological signs, and primary or metastatic tumors.[17] Acute episodes of osteoarthritis, impinged dorsal spinous processes, and severe articular instability, such as joint subluxation or luxation, are also often contraindications for manipulation. All horses with neurologic diseases should be evaluated fully to assess the potential risks or benefits of joint mobilization or manipulation. Serious diseases requiring immediate medical or surgical care must be ruled out and treated by conventional veterinary medicine before any routine manual therapy is initiated.

References

1. Blignault K. Stretch Exercises For Your Horse. J.A. Allen, London, 2003.
2. Bromiley MW. Massage Techniques for Horse and Rider. The Crowood Press Ltd., Wiltshire, England, 2002.
3. Coppa D. The internal process of therapeutic touch. J Holist Nurs 2008;26:17–24.
4. Faber MJ, van Weeren PR, Schepers M, Barneveld A. Long-term follow-up of manipulative treatment in a horse with back problems. J Vet Med A Physiol Pathol Clin Med 2003;50:241–245.
5. Frick A. Fitness in motion: Keeping your equine's zone at peak performance. The Lyons Press, Guilford, CT, 2007.
6. Giovagnoli G, Plebani G, Daubon JC. Withers height variations after muscle stretching. Proceedings of the Conference on Equine Sports Medicine and Science. Oslo, Norway, 2004:172–176.
7. Gómez Alvarez CB, L'Ami JJ, Moffat D, et al. Effect of chiropractic manipulations on the kinematics of back and limbs in horses with clinically diagnosed back problems. Equine Veterinary Journal 2008;40:153–159.
8. Haussler KK, Bertram JEA, Gellman K. In-vivo segmental kinematics of the thoracolumbar spinal region in horses and effects of chiropractic manipulations. Proc Amer Assoc Equine Practitioners 1999;45:327–329.

9. Haussler KK, Erb HN. Pressure algometry: Objective assessment of back pain and effects of chiropractic treatment. Proc Amer Assoc Equine Practitioners 2003;49:66–70.

10. Haussler KK, Hill AE, Puttlitz CM, et al. Effects of vertebral mobilization and manipulation on kinematics of the thoracolumbar region. Am J Vet Res 2007;68:508–516.

11. Lederman E. Fundamentals of Manual Therapy: Physiology, Neurology and Psychology. Churchill Livingstone, St. Louis, MO, 1997:1–4.

12. McBride SD, Hemmings A, Robinson K. A preliminary study on the effect of massage to reduce stress in the horse. J Equine Vet Sci 2004;24:76–82.

13. Parsons J, Marcer N. The osteopathic lesion or somatic dysfunction. In Osteopathy: Models for Diagnosis, Treatment and Practice. Churchill Livingstone, Philadelphia, 2006:17–39.

14. Pusey A, Colles C, Brooks J. Osteopathic treatment of horses—a retrospective study. Br Osteo J 1995;16:30–32.

15. Ramey DW, Tiidus PM. Massage therapy in horses: assessing its effectiveness from empirical data in humans and animals. Compendium 2002;24:418–423.

16. Rose NS, Northrop AJ, Brigden CV, et al. Effects of a stretching regime on stride length and range of motion in equine trot. Vet J 2009;181:53–5.

17. Scaringe J, Kawaoka C. Mobilization techniques. In Principles and Practice of Chiropractic, 3rd ed. Haldeman S, ed. McGraw-Hill, New York, 2005:767–785.

18. Spier SJ, Berger Pusterla J, Villarroel A, et al. Outcome of tactile conditioning of neonates, or "imprint training" on selected handling measures in foals. Vet J 2004;168:252–8.

19. Sullivan KA, Hill AE, Haussler KK. The effects of chiropractic, massage and phenylbutazone on spinal mechanical nociceptive thresholds in horses without clinical signs. Equine Veterinary Journal 2008;40:14–20.

20. Tellington-Jones L, Lieberman B. The Ultimate Horse Behavior and Training Book. Trafalgar Square Books, North Pomfret, VT, 2006.

21. van Harreveld PD, Lillich JD, Kawcak CE, et al. Clinical evaluation of the effects of immobilization followed by remobilization and exercise on the metacarpophalangeal joint in horses. Am J Vet Res 2002;63:282–288.

22. Verschooten F. Osteopathy in locomotion problems of the horse: A critical evaluation. Vlaams Diergeneeskd Tijdschr 1992;61:116–120.

23. Wakeling JM, Barnett K, Price S, et al. Effects of manipulative therapy on the longissimus dorsi in the equine back. Equine and Comparative Exercise Physiology 2006;3:153–160.

24. Wilson J. The effects of sports massage on athletic performance and general function. Massage Therapy J 2002:90–100.

REHABILITATION/PHYSICAL THERAPY

Narelle C. Stubbs

INTRODUCTION

Rehabilitation and physical therapy (PT) play an important role in performance enhancement, injury prevention, and restoration of full function during recovery from injury. The principles of rehabilitation and PT are based on a combination of evidence-based medicine, clinical reports, and comparative human sports sciences. Veterinary medicine continues to follow the principles of human sports medicine and rehabilitation to encompass many professional fields, including PT. Rehabilitation encompasses broad-based concepts with a focus on tissue healing, biomechanics, and neuromotor control. These concepts relate to morphology, conformation, training, environmental conditions, type of competition, age, performance limitations, exercise effects on the neuromuscular and skeletal systems, and interaction between horse and rider. The sciences underlying rehabilitation/PT include biomechanics, motor control, and exercise physiology.[3,10,34,45]

The word rehabilitation comes from the Latin "rehabilitare," meaning to make fit again. Rehabilitation/PT techniques are individually tailored to each patient rather than prescriptive for a given lesion or pathoanatomical diagnosis, taking into account the whole horse, short- and long-term goals, type of equitation, and overall prognoses. Each individual patient protocol is designed to complement medical management and facilitate the process of recovery by promoting tissue healing, assisting the normal physiological processes, and restoring the patient to its former capacity following an illness or injury. This includes manual therapies, electrotherapy, functional retraining, and therapeutic exercise-based treatments, along with education and ongoing owner-managed procedures. These are the founding principles of the physiotherapy or PT profession as described by the World Confederation for Physical Therapy (WCPT).[72] PT in all species is concerned with identifying and maximizing quality of movement potential within the spheres of promotion, prevention, treatment/intervention, rehabilitation, and more recently, sports medicine and performance enhancement.

Rehabilitation in veterinary medicine involves the veterinarian as the primary pathoanatomical diagnostician, a thorough objective functional assessment of the patient, and consultation with other health professionals.[45] Using knowledge and skills unique to these professions, the movement potential of the patient is assessed, with all information and confounding factors incorporated to establish an accurate functional diagnosis, problem list, management plan, and goals. Clinically, it is imperative that during the rehabilitation process valid and reliable objective measures are taken to determine accurate outcome measures. It is the author's opinion and one that is advocated in all modern sports medicine literature that rehabilitation should begin as soon as possible after the injury occurs, alongside therapeutic pharmacological measures such as anti-inflammatory and other painkilling agents.[19] This might also begin before or immediately after surgery; therefore, the rehabilitative process is managed by a multi-disciplinary team.

There is still a great need for further research on the effects of PT in horses to complement the considerable research in pathology and the high prevalence of injuries in athletic horses.[3,17,64] Although peer-reviewed research is limited in equine rehabilitation,[11,12,30,60,70,79,81] many animal models have been used for human rehabilitation research, with many findings able to be related to current concepts in equine rehabilitation. A recent textbook, Animal Physiotherapy: Assessment, Treatment and Rehabilitation of Animals, laid the foundations of animal physiotherapy; it is a good reference with respect to evidence-based rehabilitation.[45] Furthermore, 4 recent journal publications have reviewed the principles and practice of equine PT, including the science behind the profession,[47] manual therapy,[22,28] and therapeutic exercises,[52] all of which highlight the potential input of equine rehabilitation. Other useful texts are Physical Therapy and Massage for the Horse" which complements both evidence-based and clinical practice,[14] and Equine Injury, Therapy and Rehabilitation, third edition, (2007) by Mary Bromiley, one of the founding physical therapists and authors in this field.[7] Many other clinical and evidence-based articles, text chapters, and textbooks exist[32,57], some of which are listed in the references below. The profile of rehabilitation and performance enhancement has been heightened by the official use of PT and other allied health professionals during international level equestrian competitions, highlighting how equestrian sports are rapidly catching up to other international competitive sports.

Readers are directed toward the many evidence-based human therapeutic texts to extend the scope of evidence-based techniques that may be enlisted to rehabilitate joint and soft-tissue disorders and lesions. These include manual therapies, soft tissue mobilization/massage[6], myofascial pain and dysfunction[65], electrotherapy and physical agents,[48,80] and integrative therapeutic approaches relating to mechanical passive constraints of locomotion and neuromotor control, including facilitation and strengthening techniques.[42,44,50]

It is beyond the scope of this section to cover all aspects of equine rehabilitation. The aim is to present some fundamental evidence-based concepts of PT/rehabilitation focusing on manual therapies, electrotherapy, and exercise-based treatments.

CLINICAL AND CLIENT DEMAND FOR REHABILITATION/PT

The clinical need for rehabilitation interventions is verified by the amount of waste and loss of performance in equine sports due to musculoskeletal injuries.[17,4,53,75] Statistics indicate that diseases of the musculoskeletal system are the predominant cause of loss of use and death in sport horses.[1,8,16,31,54] For example, as described elsewhere in the text, it is well established that flexor tendon and suspensory ligament injuries are the most frequently reported injuries in sport horses, resulting from the horse performing at high speed and over jumps.[13,39,43,49,61–63]

Gibson, et al. (2002) highlighted the importance of veterinary management, rehabilitation, and PT in the sport horse in relation to these injuries. The report emphasized the frequency of soft tissue injury in elite horses at the 2000 Sydney Olympics (n = 70): dressage (8), show jumping (15), and eventing (n = 47).[21] Many of the dressage horses were able to continue competing despite a suspensory desmitis, yet others withdrew. The most common lesion in show jumpers (n = 10) was suspensory desmitis; interestingly 4 medalists were among this group. The authors suggest that show jumpers can continue to successfully compete with good management, despite chronic low-grade injury. As expected in eventing, tendon and ligament lesions occur with greater frequency; all but 2 horses that presented (n = 45) had a soft tissue lesion, and 10 horses had multiple lesions. Many did not complete due to retirement (n = 10), elimination (n = 3) on course, or withdrawal before the third inspection (n = 6). Twenty horses passed the veterinary inspection and completed the event, adhering to the veterinary rules of the Fédération Equestre Internationale (FEI)[18] with respect to nonpharmaceutical treatments, again highlighting the importance of careful management and use of rehabilitation and PT techniques.

Equine back pain is a condition in which rehabilitation strategies are widely recognized as being of great clinical use. As discussed elsewhere in the text, back problems are considered to be a major cause of alterations in gait and performance. Within the literature there is variability with respect to prevalence of back pain in horses; Haussler, et al. (1999) highlighted the prevalence and underdiagnosis of lesions in the caudal thoracolumbar and pelvic regions in Thoroughbred racehorses as a potential contributor to poor performance and lameness.[29] McGowan, et al. (2007)[46] also reported on osseous pathology in a group of 22 Thoroughbred racehorses euthanized for reasons unrelated to back pain at the Hong Kong Jockey Club, with similar results. In a recent owner survey of 11,363 registered dressage horse owners in the United Kingdom, Murray et al. (2009)[51] reported that 40% (n = 644) had a back problem, although the majority of these had not been diagnosed by a veterinary surgeon (80%). Complementary therapies were used as a treatment in 63%. Veterinary care was combined with other treatments including saddle fit and change of training regimes but without complementary therapy in 3%, and only veterinary care in 2.5%. This reflects the demand for multidisciplinary treatment strategies and long-term

management for chronic and recurrent back pain in horses, as is the case in humans.

In a study by Turner (2003), 5,352 medical records (1997 to 2002) were evaluated. The occurrence of diagnosed back problems was 2.2% (118) in the lameness case load, and 102 (82%) in the back pain case load.[73] The treatment was administration of systemic anti-inflammatories, and/or local anti-inflammatory injection, along with a variable combination of acupuncture, chiropractic techniques, massage therapy, electro-stimulation, magnetic therapy, therapeutic ultrasound, extracorporeal shockwave therapy, and training (exercise) management. Follow-up information was available on 112 horses, with 90% returning to work; however, 15 of those horses did not return to their previous level and were retired or used for other activities. Of the 86 horses that returned to their previous level of work, 52 (60%) did not require further therapy; however, the remaining 34 (40%) horses continued to receive some therapy. The need for therapy was based on the owner's and trainer's impressions of the horse's behavior.

MANUAL THERAPY

Manual therapy techniques are suitable for many conditions following a veterinary pathoanatomical diagnosis, when possible. These techniques encompass the application of very specific passive and/or active assisted movements by the therapist to the horse to manage and/or alter pain and dysfunction of the articular, neural, and muscle systems.[17] Manual therapy techniques are based on a wide range of methods and theories related to the intervertebral and peripheral joint complexes, myofascia, and the neuromuscular system.

It is beyond the scope of this section to describe each technique. Passive accessory and physiological joint mobilization techniques are specific to PT and osteopathy and have been clinically reported to be successfully adapted to treat the horse. Some technique examples used in human manual therapy include Maitland, Mulligan, Karltenborn, McKenzie, and muscle energy techniques. Numerous myofascial and neuromuscular mobilization techniques also can be used, some of which include massage (friction, effleurage, petrissage, tapôtement, vibrations, and shaking), trigger point therapy, direct and indirect myofascial release, positional release, reflex inhibition techniques, craniosacral therapy, adverse neural tension techniques, and stretching.

To effectively establish a treatment protocol and apply these techniques, an accurate functional assessment of the musculoskeletal and neuromuscular systems is vital, identifying the primary and secondary condition(s) that may be responsible for and/or attributed to pain and loss of function. The assessment procedure, where applicable, includes a full static and dynamic examination as described elsewhere in the text, followed by palpatory evaluation including specific manual testing and provocation tests. Examination procedures determine the regions of altered range of motion, quality of movement, muscle function, and tissue irritability that may be related to pain, pathology, altered motor control, and/or dysfunction.[25,26,56]

Joint Mobilization

Degenerative joint disease or osteoarthritis is an example of a common dysfunction and cause of lameness and loss of performance in the horse in which manual therapy can be successfully applied, as is the case in humans. Many manual therapy techniques such as passive mobilizations can be applied to the articular system, including the vertebral column and peripheral joints, with complementary soft tissue techniques applied to the associated neuromuscular and fascial tissues in this condition. These repeated movement techniques have reported effects on the intra-articular, periarticular (joint capsule and ligament), and extra-articular structures (muscle, fascia, and neural tissue), and thus affect the passive and active constraints of the joint complex and primarily assist in pain modulation.[22,25,28,56]

There is a vast amount of scientific evidence in the human literature to support manual therapy techniques and the possible biomechanical and neurophysiological mechanisms behind the effects, with many studies using animal models.[2,38,66,67] The neurophysiological mechanisms that explain the pain-relieving effects are now supported by scientific evidence, both in the vertebral column and in peripheral joints. Evidence has shown that manual therapy produces an initial treatment-specific hypoalgesic and sympathetic-excitatory effect locally in the treatment area beyond placebo or control conditions, and then a nonopioid-mediated hypoalgesia systemically.[55,66,77,78,82]

Passive mobilizations are applied at different amplitudes, velocities, and directions determined by the assessment procedure and biomechanics of the joint complex.[23] It is the author's experience (which is in agreement with that described by Goff [2009][17]) that manual passive assessment and treatment techniques directed at a joint, soft tissue, or neural structure are well tolerated by the horse due to the rhythmic motion being applied at a comfortable speed. This may include a high-velocity thrust technique which is described elsewhere within this chapter. Similar techniques have been widely reported in humans.[37]

Two very effective mobilization techniques often used to restore joint motion and reduce pain in the horse are described by Goff (2009):[22] (1) passive physiological mobilizations, whereby the forces being directed reproduce passive physiological or coupled joint motion around the 3 axes of motion of the affected joint complex, as occurs with voluntary motion, and (2) passive accessory movements, in which the motion produced is a translation that accompanies rotations, which cannot be voluntarily performed by the horse. Figure 8.26 is

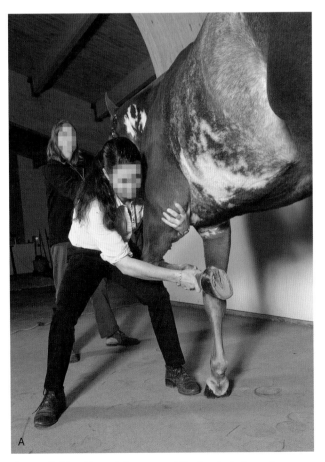 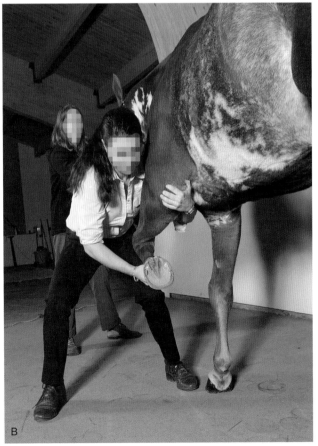

Figure 8.26. Manual therapy mobilization technique. A combination of passive physiological and passive accessory mobilization techniques is applied to the carpus to increase the available range of motion into flexion. The carpus is flexed, the radius is stabilized, and medial (A) and lateral motion (B) are applied to the end of range via the third metacarpus.

an example of the application of a combination of these techniques applied to the carpus.

It is the author's experience and opinion that these techniques are highly applicable in mid- and end of range of motion positions (as seen in figure 8.26), which is commonly the practice in human PT, rather than treatment taking place only in the neutral standing posture. Clinically this is particularly effective in relation to inter-segmental motion in the spine. The practitioner is able to use combined mobilization with movement techniques as described below, or with an assistant to maintain the desired postures. Direct dorsoventral and lateral passive accessory glides can then be performed manually over the dorsal spinous processes, ribs, vertebral bodies (cervical spine) and transverse processes (lumbar spine), in the end-of-range functional positions.

Soft-tissue Mobilization

The aim of many manual therapy techniques directed at the myofascia, tendons, and ligaments is to normalize tissue irritability, muscle tone, extensibility, length, contractility, strength, and coordination, and ultimately improve motor control. Addressing these impairments in an attempt to regain function and optimize performance is a key feature of the rehabilitation process.

As discussed elsewhere in the text, muscular dysfunctions are often seen occurring secondarily to underlying bone pathology in horses with limb and/or back pain; however, dysfunction and/or atrophy may also be due to pathology of actual muscles such as a generalized muscle disorder, or muscle damage attributed to a poorly fitting saddle.[20,27,59,74] Valentine (2008)[75] investigated the pathological findings in equine muscle (excluding polysaccharide storage myopathy) in 229 equids. Sixty-five percent (n = 129) suffered muscle lesions, (13.1%, n = 30) generalized muscle atrophy, and (6.1%, n = 14) denervation atrophy. Clinical signs of myopathies have been shown to improve with dietary management along with a regulated exercise routine as part of rehabilitation.[36]

Following soft-tissue trauma or pathology, dynamic stretching regimes can be implemented to regain and maintain full range of motion during the healing process. As a preventative measure, this also applies to any horse that is on a restricted exercise regime or confined to the stable for other reasons to help avoid the detrimental effects of immobilization.[52]

Passive stretching techniques are much more difficult in the horse because the horse is never entirely passive with respect to muscle tonicity, because it is usually standing during treatment. Therefore, the stretching procedure is dynamic and never completely passive, even when stretching limbs.

However, an osteopathic technique that is reported in the clinical literature suggests that a form of gentle stretching ("positional release") in the treatment of chronic myofascial restrictions can be performed under sedation or anesthesia. This technique has been reported to have some success.[58] The technique is often used after all other avenues have been exhausted due to the anesthetic risk. Therefore, tissue mobilization with movement may be a more apt title for many forms of

stretching techniques in the horse. These techniques are performed rhythmically or in a sustained manner depending on the desired response and effect on the tissues. Examples of these techniques are described below in the section on mobilization with movement exercises.

If there is a primary lesion of a soft-tissue structure such as muscle, ligament or tendon, stretches or active mobilizations with movement exercises in conjunction with other therapies may be appropriate to avoid excessive scar formation and disorientation of the fiber alignment in the subacute and chronic phases of healing. With respect to rehabilitation of distal tendon and ligament lesions, it has been widely reported in the human literature that dynamic motor-control-based exercises, including eccentric loading exercises, accelerate healing and tensile strength, especially in relation to Achilles tendon lesions.[41] This type of rehabilitation strategy is beginning to be more commonly implemented where appropriate in horses. In these cases the horse undergoes "active rest" and begins a walking program along with other forms of therapy, once the lesion is determined to be stabilized. It is the author's suggestion to also include unmounted exercises to increase the dynamic core muscle strength as described below.[69] Fibrotic myopathy is an example of a chronic condition in which repeated sustained positioning of a limb may be warranted in combination with other forms of therapy. In this case, the affected limb is manually moved to the available range of motion to stress the desired soft tissue structures.

Mobilization with Movement Techniques/Exercises

Indirect mobilization with movement techniques/exercises in conjunction with direct manual therapy techniques are also very effective clinically, especially in relation to functional motor control. Altered motor control (neuromuscular function) may be a result of the underlying lesion in the spine and/or peripheral joint disease, with pain and inflammation causing reflex inhibition of motor neurons, which in turn causes weakness and atrophy of associated muscles.[83] This is widely reported in the human literature, indicating that motor control is a vital component of the management of musculoskeletal conditions, especially related to spinal disorders and dysfunction.[33] McGowan, et al. (2007)[46] reported that there is a relationship between muscle function and pathology via ultrasonography and necropsy analysis, whereby significant atrophy of the multifidus muscles was evident at the level and side of the thoracolumbar lesion in 22 racehorses. This has been widely reported in the human literature.[33] This is also an area of veterinary medicine in which rehabilitation/PT techniques may be of great use.

Many of these mobilization techniques/exercises use neuromuscular reflexive responses along with muscular facilitation and inhibition. They use similar theoretical principles to those used in human manual therapy, including muscle energy techniques to gain motion that is limited by restrictions of neuromuscular structures, as well as restore or normalize motor control. In people, the patient is asked to contract and relax specific muscles in a given range of motion, and often resistance is applied to the body part. These techniques promote muscle relaxation by activating the Golgi tendon reflex.[15] The techniques implement the principles of reciprocal inhibition and post-isometric relaxation. Reciprocal inhibition uses the body's antagonist-inhibition reflex to induce relaxation of a muscle.

A simplified example in people: if there is a loss of elbow flexion range of motion due to triceps muscle hypertonicity, the elbow is placed into end-range of flexion, biceps (agonist) are then contracted, which induces the triceps (antagonist) into relaxation. The joint is then moved farther into maximal flexion and the technique is repeated, with incremental restoration of range of motion. Conversely, other techniques use the antagonist-inhibition reflex to incrementally restore range of motion, whereby a muscle is stretched immediately following its isometric contraction due to the neuromuscular apparatus becoming briefly refractory, or its inability to respond to further excitation.

It is the author's opinion that many of these applied techniques/exercises are very useful in the majority of rehabilitation cases to maintain and improve mobility, strength, and dynamic stability. This is especially true in those cases involving regions where the affected joint complexes are inaccessible due to the horse's morphology.

As described elsewhere in the text, the horse alters its posture reflexively in response to digital pressure on various regions of the axial skeleton, both into dorsoventral flexion-extension and into coupled lateral bending/rotation and dorsoventral motion. For example, this can be seen when there is a reduction of dorsoventral motion into flexion and/or lateral bending of the cervicothoracic and thoracolumbar-lumbopelvic regions due to pain, muscle spasm, and/or joint pathology or dysfunction. The intention is not only to increase the joint mobility but to activate and strengthen the muscles required to move the horse's body to the desired position.

A simple example of these exercises is seen in Figure 8.27, where the therapist applies a slow, constant pressure to the ventral midline and dorsal sacral region simultaneously, facilitating end-of-range of motion via a dorsoventral flexion response of the cervicothoracic and thoracolumbar spine and the pelvis. In this example, activation of the horse's core muscles, serratus ventralis and hypaxial muscles (pectoral, abdominal, and iliopsoas complexes), produces the desired posture in

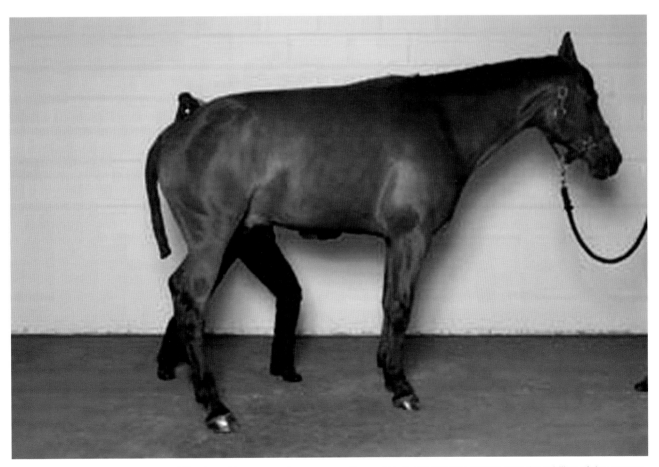

Figure 8.27. Manual therapy mobilization with movement technique. A combined rounding response into end-of-dorsoventral flexion range of motion of the thoracolumbar spine and pelvis. This is performed by manual finger pressure to the ventral midline with one hand and dorsally directly over the midline of the sacrum with the other hand. Depending on the size of the horse, this may need to be performed by 2 people.

combination with relaxation and lengthening of the opposing epaxial muscles. This posture is maintained for 3 to 5 seconds and repeated multiple times as reported by Stubbs and Clayton (2008) to incrementally restore range of motion and strengthen the core muscles.[72] Indirect techniques can also be used to mobilize other inaccessible regions such as the cervicothoracic junction, whereby a muscle reflex/response occurs on deep palpation (constant index and thumb pressure) of the distal third of the brachiocephalicus muscle, producing flexion in this region. The brachiocephalicus response is shown in Figure 8.28. This can also be coupled with ventral pressure to the sternum to mobilize the joint complexes into an increasing range of upper thoracic flexion.

Many combinations of mobilization, core strengthening, and stability/balancing exercises have been described in the literature.[22,52,69] These often use a food incentive or bait (such as a carrot) to encourage the horse to move into the desired posture. Baited exercises encourage the horse to move into end-of-range postures of the cervicothoracic and lumbopelvic regions spine; for example, into flexion with movement of the chin to chest, between carpi and fetlocks; or coupled lateral/ rotation bending and flexion, with movement of the chin to girth, flank, and hock (Figure 8.29). The aim of

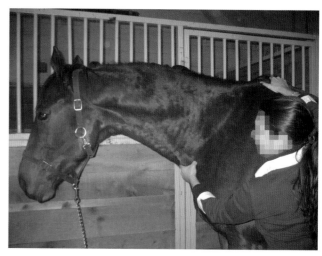

Figure 8.28. Mobilization with movement technique. The brachiocephalic response results in flexion of the mid-lower cervical spine, including the cervicothoracic region. Gradual digital pressure is applied by the forefinger and thumb (pincer) to the distal third of the brachiocephalicus muscle. Pressure is maintained and gradually increased until the desired posture is attained, then held for 3 to 5 seconds.

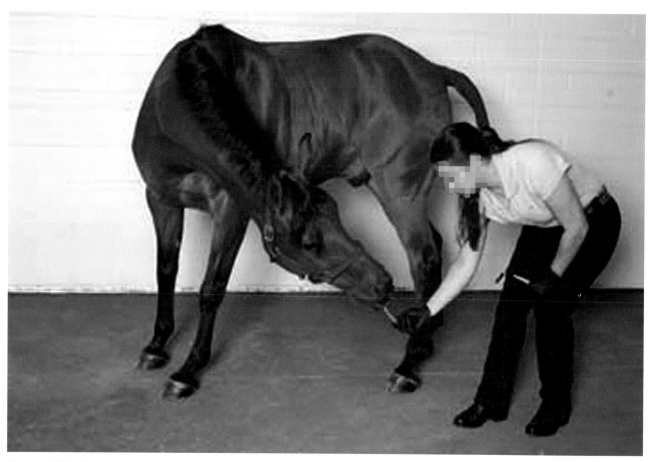

Figure 8.29. Baited mobilization with movement exercises; lateral bending coupled with flexion and rotation. The horse's functional end-of-range posture is attained by the horse's chin following the carrot toward its hock/fetlock. The position is held for 3 to 5 seconds to increase the activity of the core muscles of the thoracic sling, trunk, and pelvic sling, as seen in the photograph.

these exercises is not only to mobilize both the axial and distal skeletons but also to facilitate core muscle activity (thoracic sling, hypaxial/epaxial, and pelvic musculature), improve neuromuscular control, and strengthen over time.[69] This is a key concept in human rehabilitation and sports medicine.

ELECTRO-PHYSICAL AGENTS: TREATMENT MODALITIES

It is beyond the scope of this section to define and describe all forms of electromodalities and biophysical agents that alter and/or accelerate tissue healing and minimize the effects of disuse atrophy, immobilization, and denervation. The reader is advised to consult texts that are specifically aimed at evidence-based practices in the field of PT, electromodalities. and physical agents.[5,48,80]

It is well established in the human literature that cryotherapy is an effective method of modulating pain and inflammation in the acute phase of healing following injury (first 48 hours) if the tissue temperature is reduced to a therapeutic threshold of 10°C to 19°C at depths of 1 to 4 cm.[48] Hocutt, et al. (1982) reported that in human ankle ligament sprains, if ice is applied immediately after the injury, vs. 36 hours post-trauma, there is a more rapid return to full activity (13.2 days compared with 33.3).[35]

In the horse, considerable research has been associated with cryotherapy in distal limb pathology. Cryotherapy, when applied to the distal limbs, has been shown to markedly reduce the severity of acute laminitis due to the reduction of enzymatic mediators.[76] The most effective form of cryotherapy in the equine limb is ice water immersion,[40] which is common practice in many forms of equestrian sports post-exercise, such as eventing. Horses can stand immersed in the ice below the carpi for extended periods of time due to perfusion relying on the foot's anastomosis pumping mechanism. Further research is lacking; therefore, it is suggested that elsewhere in the horse, wet ice applications (wet towel with crushed ice) are best applied for up to 20 minutes every 2 to 4 hours to avoid tissue damage and cold-induced vasodilation (hunting response). Tissue damage has been shown to occur in humans if the temperature goes below 10°C.

Superficial heat therapy (e.g., hot packs and hot water hosing) may be less useful in the horse. A study by Kaneps (2000) showed that subcutaneous and deep tissue temperatures never reached the therapeutic threshold of 41°C; however, this study only observed the metacarpal region.[40]

Therapeutic ultrasound is another modality commonly used in people to heat tissue (3 to 5 cm depth) and increase fluid motion around cell membranes,[80] but sufficient evidence of clinical efficacy is still lacking.[52] The optimal methods of application in the horse are also uncertain, with no peer-reviewed studies to date. Factors to consider are the horse's coat (which must be shaved to apply therapeutic ultrasound), thickness of the skin, fascia, and amount of subcutaneous fat, all of which alter penetration and absorption of the vibration currents.

Electrotherapy introduces electrical currents to the body to gain therapeutic effects. This modality uses various types and frequencies of current, depending on the desired effect. In humans, transcutaneous electrical nerve stimulation (TENS) has been well documented to provide temporary pain relief by release of endogenous endorphins and opioids centrally, and/or stimulate inhibitory interneurons at the spinal level.[80] Although there is no evidence that TENS is effective in horses, it is the author's experience that it is well-tolerated and a clinically useful modality to complement other treatment strategies.

Neuromuscular electrical stimulation (NMES) is a useful electromodality in cases of muscle atrophy due to disuse, immobility, and or nerve damage in humans. When a patient is unable to voluntarily contract the muscle, NMES can be applied to generate 80% to 90% of the maximal voluntary contraction, assisting in maintaining neuromuscular control and muscle development.[52] The literature regarding this modality in denervated muscle is still conflicting, with some evidence of a delay in denervation atrophy.[80] Again, to date there are no studies in the horse; however, it is the author's opinion that if NMES is tolerated by the individual horse, it is a useful adjunct to assess and treat muscle dysfunction and/or atrophy in such cases as suprascapular and radial nerve lesions.

MOTOR CONTROL: EXERCISE-BASED TREATMENT TECHNIQUES

Normalizing and/or altering motor control, in addition to managing pain and dysfunction, is directly related to and mediated by proprioceptive and mechanoreceptive afferent feedback from joints, tendons, ligaments, fascia, and skin, which modulate efferent neuromuscular control. Therefore, a vital facet of musculoskeletal and neurological rehabilitation and performance enhancement is related to motor control and motor-skill retraining. This ensures that the appropriate neuromuscular pathways are stimulated and strengthened over time, allowing the horse to return to maximal sport-specific function.

Sensory integration techniques involve tactile stimulation during exercise and are reported to be clinically helpful in the horse.[11,12,22,24,52,60] The goal of these techniques is to stimulate the afferent proprioceptive/mechanoreceptive input that modulates and coordinates motor function. These techniques are potentially very effective due to the horse's heightened skin-mechanoreceptive system in conjunction with the underlying cutaneous trunci myofascial attachments to the skin. For example, the horse has the ability to feel the smallest tactile stimulus such as a fly, and respond by altering its muscle activity (i.e., fasciculation of cutaneous trunci). Tactile stimulants or cues can be applied to the skin over targeted regions, including the limbs or specific muscles, to alter mechanoreceptive/proprioception feedback and thus potentially alter motor control.

There is a vast amount of evidence in the human literature that supports these techniques with respect to enhancing motor control and performance. This also appears to be the case in the horse, as is evidenced in 2 recent studies that showed that the application of a very light tactile stimulus (55 grams) to the coronet band (Figure 8.30) altered the kinetics and kinematics of gait, including increasing the peak hoof height during the swing phase.[11,12] It is thought that the effect of a light

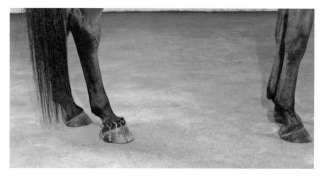

Figure 8.30. Sensory integration technique. A lightweight (55-gram) tactile stimulation device is placed around the coronary band of a horse and worn during exercise to increase the peak height of the swing phase of gait.

tactile device is different from that of weighted boots, hence, the stimulus applied is very specific to the desired outcome and training effect.[12,81]

A body wrap is another form of sensory integration used during training. This involves wrapping materials such as bandages, Vetwrap, and Thera-Band around the horse's hindquarter, abdomen, and/or chest.[22,24,52,71] It is the author's opinion that Thera-Band is the best choice because it appears to increase the horse's body awareness (i.e., kinesthesia) and its ability to use its core muscles. The benefit of the body wrap is that it can be used on horses performing exercises both in-hand and ridden.

The functional proprioceptive taping technique is another extremely clinically effective sensory stimulation method that is widely used in human rehabilitation, sports medicine, and athletic performance. In the veterinary literature, Ramon, et al. (2004) reported that rigid mechanical athletic taping of the fetlock does not alter the kinematics of the forelimb during stance, but it does limit flexion of the fetlock during the swing phase.[60] However, there was a decrease in the peak vertical force, which may be due to an increased proprioceptive effect. The authors concluded that the

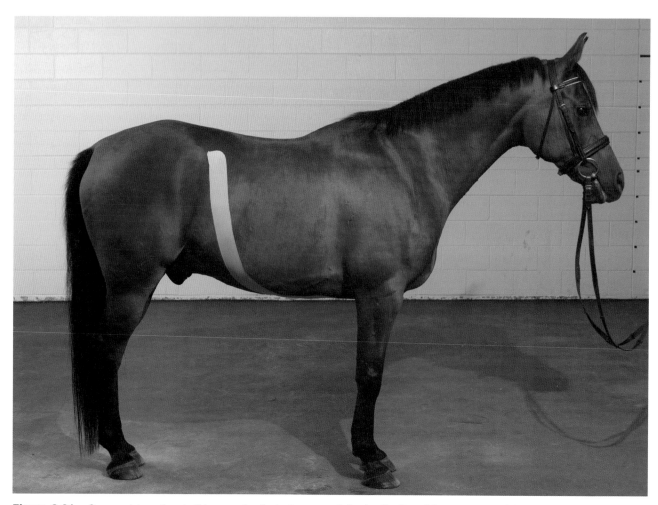

Figure 8.31. Sensory integration. In this example of a taping technique of the abdominal complex, Kinesio Tape™ is applied to stretch from the transverse processes of the lumbar vertebrae, following the line of the transverse abdominus, internal oblique, and rectus abdominus muscles. The tape finishes on the ventral aspect of the sternum and pectoral muscle complex.

reduced peak vertical forces may be helpful in preventing or reducing injury and potentially could be applied for tendinous or ligamentous rehabilitation in equine patients.

These effects also may differ if using a non-mechanical but functional taping technique, as is commonly used in human athletes and has been widely researched. Kinesio Tex™ tape is elastic, hypo-allergenic, and semi-waterproof, and allows the horse to sweat due to a porous weave. Theoretically, tape is stretched and placed along the length of a muscle that the practitioner wishes to facilitate. This is achieved through tension that increases the kinesthetic awareness across the fibers of the muscle where an inhibitory effect is desired. The horse can perform specific exercises with the tape attached, including individual sport-specific activities under saddle, which is an advantage with respect to alteration of neuromotor function over time. The author has successfully used taping techniques in the regions of the core dynamic stability musculature, specifically the biceps femoris and the abdominal complex (Figure 8.31).

These techniques may be combined with many forms of in-hand and ridden exercises that are widely described in the clinical literature.[22,24,52,68,71] The exercise protocol should be individually tailored by the therapist, with a skilled handler/trainer required to perform these exercises on a daily basis. The exercise protocol should follow the principles of conditioning,[9] with constant re-assessment of the horse's motion to ensure that compensatory strategies are minimal and the desired effects evident. The program should be gradually increased with consideration given to exercise time, gaits, transitions, direction, surfaces, and gradients/slopes. The horse should be constantly monitored for excessive fatigue.

Training aids that may be used include long-lining; the Pessoa lunging system; and various combinations of equipment to alter gait, including poles, cavaletti, obstacles, balancing boards, a variety of surfaces (asphalt, turf, gravel, sand, water), swimming pools, and treadmills/aqua-treadmills. These aids alter the horse's motor control and provide neuromuscular and/or cardiovascular training effects over time.

CONCLUSION

Although there is currently relatively limited scientific evidence regarding rehabilitation strategies and PT in equine veterinary medicine, their use is rapidly expanding. Research and documented clinical experiences are still needed to complement the adaptation of the scientific-based principles presented in this section. Nevertheless, it is the author's opinion and clinical experience that rehabilitation/PT strategies can be successfully incorporated in conjunction with traditional veterinary medicine. A team approach with the necessary clinical reasoning skills is vital in choosing the appropriate rehabilitation strategy and PT technique, and monitoring the patient's progress. Constant reassessment and, where possible, objective measures to validate the outcome of the interventions, are indicated for successful treatment strategies involving PT and rehabilitative techniques.

References

1. AGRIA 90–94-Femà6rsskrift AGRIA, Stockholm (Insurance Statistics 1990–1994), 1995. In: Wallin L, Strandberg EJ, et al. Estimates of longevity and causes of culling and death in Swedish Warmblood and coldblood horses. Livest Prod Sci 2000; 63:275–289.
2. Babbage CS, Coppieters MW, McGowan CM. Strain and excursion of the sciatic nerve in the dog: Biomechanical considerations in the development of a clinical test for increased neural mechano sensitivity. Vet J 2007;174:330–336.
3. Back W, Clayton HM. Equine Locomotion, 2nd ed. WB Saunders, 2010; in press.
4. Barr ED, Pinchbeck PD, Clegg PD, et al. Post mortem evaluation of palmar osteochondral disease (traumatic osteochondrosis) of the metacarpo/metatarsophalangeal joint in Thoroughbred racehorses. Equine Vet J 2009;41:366–371.
5. Baxter DG, McDonough SM. Principles of electrotherapy in veterinary physiotherapy. In Animal Physiotherapy: Assessment, Treatment, and Rehabilitation of Animals. McGowan C, Goff L, Stubbs N, eds. Blackwell Publishing, Ames, IA, 2007; 177–186.
6. Boyling JD, Jull GA. Grieve's Modern Manuel Therapy: The Vertebral Column, 3rd ed. Churchill Livingstone, Elsevier, Philadelphia, 2004.
7. Bromiley M. Equine Injury, Therapy and Rehabilitation, 3rd ed. Blackwell Publishing, Ames, IA, 2007.
8. Clausen M, Preisinger R, Kalm E. Analyse von krankenheitsdaten in der Deutschen Warmblutzucht. Züchtungskunde 1990;62: 167–178.
9. Clayton HM. Conditioning Sport Horses. Sport Horse Publications, Mason, MI, 1991.
10. Clayton HM. The Dynamic Horse. Sport Horse Publications, Mason, MI, 2004.
11. Clayton HM, White AD, Kaiser LJ, et al. Short-term habituation of equine limb kinematics to tactile stimulation of the coronet. Vet Comp Orthop Traumatol 2008;3:211–214.
12. Clayton HM, White AD, Kaiser LJ, et al. Hind limb response to tactile stimulation of the pastern and coronet. Equine Vet J 2010; in press.
13. Colbourn CM, Yovich JV. Suspensory ligament injuries in racing horses: Ultrasonographic diagnosis and long-term follow up. Aust Equine Vet J 1994;12:119–128.
14. Denoix JM, Pailloux JP. Physical Therapy and Massage for the Horse, 2nd ed. Trafalgar Square Publishing, North Promfret, VT, 2001.
15. DiGiovanna EL, Schiowitz S, Dowling DJ. An Osteopathic Approach to Diagnosis and Treatment, 3rd ed. Lippincott Williams and Wilkins, Philadelphia, 2005.
16. Egenvall A, Lonnell C, Roepstrorff L. Analysis of morbidity and mortality data in riding school horses, with special regard to locomotor problems. Prev Vet Med 2009;88:193–204.
17. Ely ER, Avella CS, Price JS, et al. Descriptive epidemiology of fracture, tendon and suspensory ligament injury in National Hunt racehorses in training. Equine Vet J 2009;41:372–378.
18. FéDération Equestre Internationale. www.fei.org. Accessed Jan. 8, 2010.
19. Frontera WR. Rehabilitation of Sports Injuries: Scientific Basis. Blackwell Science, Malden, MA, 2003.
20. Gellman K. An integrated approach to diagnosing and treating back pain in horses. Proceedings Conf Equine Sports Med and Sci 1998;119.
21. Gibson KT, Snyder JR, Spier SJ. Ultrasonographic diagnosis of soft tissue injuries in horses competing at the Sydney 2000 Olympic Games. Equine Vet Ed 2002;14:149–156.
22. Goff LM. Manual therapy for the horse—A contemporary perspective. J Equine Vet Sci 2009;29:799–808.
23. Goff L, Stubbs N. Applied animal biomechanics. In Animal Physiotherapy: Assessment, Treatment and Rehabilitation of Animals. McGowan C, Goff L, Stubbs N. eds. Blackwell Publishing, Ames, IA, 2007;32–55.
24. Goff L, Stubbs N. Equine treatment and rehabilitation. In Animal Physiotherapy: Assessment, Treatment and Rehabilitation of Animals. McGowan C, Goff L, Stubbs N, eds. Blackwell Publishing, Ames, IA, 2007;238–251.
25. Goff L, Jull G. Manual therapy. In Animal Physiotherapy: Assessment, Treatment and Rehabilitation of Animals. McGowan C, Goff L, Stubbs N, eds. Blackwell Publishing, Ames, IA, 2007;164–176.

26. Goff L, Cook T. Physiotherapy assessment for animals. In Animal Physiotherapy: Assessment, Treatment and Rehabilitation of Animals. McGowan C, Goff L, Stubbs N, eds. Blackwell Publishing, Ames, IA, 2007.

27. Harman J. Tack and saddle fit. Vet Clin N Am Equine Prac 1999;15:247–261.

28. Haussler KK. Review of Manual Therapy Techniques in Equine Practice. J Equine Vet Sci 2009;29:849–869.

29. Haussler KK, Stover SM, Willits NH. Pathologic changes in the lumbosacral vertebrae and pelvis in Thoroughbred racehorses. Am J Vet Res 1999;60:143–153.

30. Haussler KK, Hill AE, Puttlitz CM, et al. Effects of vertebral mobilization and manipulation on kinematics of the thoracolumbar region. Am J Vet Res 2007;68(5):508–516.

31. Heisele C. Schadenfälle in der Langfristigen Pferdelebensversicherung unter berucksichtigung der tierärztlichen Mitwirkung in der Pferdelebensversicherung. Thesis, University of München. München, Germany: 1995.

32. Henson FMD. Equine Back Pathology: Diagnosis and Treatment. Blackwell Publishing, Ames, IA, 2009.

33. Hides J, Gilmore C, Stanton W, et al. Multifidus size and symmetry among chronic LBP and healthy asymptomatic subjects. Manual Ther 2008;13:43–49.

34. Hinchcliff KW, Geor RJ, Kaneps AJ. Equine Exercise Physiology: The Science of Exercise in the Athletic Horse. Saunders Elsevier, Philadelphia, 2008.

35. Hocutt JE, Jaffe R, Rylander CR, et al. Cryotherapy in ankle sprains. Am J Sports Med 1982;10:316–319.

36. Hunt LM, Valberg SJ, Steffenhagen K, et al. An epidemiological study of myopathies in Warmblood horses. Equine Vet J 2008;40:171–177.

37. Hurwitz E, Aker P, Adams A, et al. Manipulation and mobilization of the cervical spine: a systematic review of the literature. Spine 1996;21:1746–1759.

38. Indahl A, Kaigle A, Reikeras O, et al. Sacroiliac joint involvement in activation of the porcine spinal and gluteal musculature. J Spinal Dis 1999;12:325–330.

39. Jeffcott LB, Rossdale PD, Freestone J, et al. An assessment of wastage in Thoroughbred racing from conception to 4 years of age. Equine Vet J 1982;14:185–198.

40. Kaneps AJ. Tissue temperature response to hot and cold therapy in the metacarpal region of a horse. Proc Amer Assoc Equine Practitioners 2000;46:208–213.

41. Kingma JJ, de Knikker R, Wittink HM, et al. Eccentric overload training in patients with chronic Achilles tendinopathy: a systematic review. Br J Sports Med 2007;41:e3.

42. Lee D, Vleeming A. An integrated therapeutic approach to the treatment of pelvic girdle pain. In Movement, Stability and Lumbopelvic Pain, 2nd ed. Vleeming A, Mooney V, Stoeckart R, eds. Churchill Livingstone, Elsevier, Philadelphia, 2007; 622–638.

43. Marr CM, Love S, Boyd JS, et al. Factors affecting the clinical outcome of injuries to the superficial digital flexor tendon in National Hunt and point-to-point racehorses. Vet Rec 1993; 132:476–479.

44. McGill SM. The painful and unstable lumbar spine: a foundation and approach for restabilization. In Movement, Stability and Lumbopelvic Pain, 2nd ed. Vleeming A, Mooney V, Stoeckart R, eds. Churchill Livingstone, Elsevier, Philadelphia, 2007; 529–545.

45. McGowan C, Goff L, Stubbs N. Animal Physiotherapy: Assessment, Treatment and Rehabilitation of Animals. Blackwell Publishing, Ames, IA, 2007.

46. McGowan CM, Hodges PW, Jeffcott LB. Epaxial musculature and its relationship with back pain in the horse. In RIRDC Horse Projects, completed in 2006–07, and Horse Research in Progress, June 2007. Rural Industries Research and Development Corporation, 2007;37.

47. McGowan CM, Stubbs NC, Jull GA. Equine physiotherapy: a comparative view of the science underlying the profession. Equine Vet J 2007;39:90–94.

48. Michlovitz SL, Thermal Agents in Rehabilitation, 3rd ed. FA Davis, Philadelphia, 1996.

49. Mohammed HO, Hill T, Lowe J. Risk factors associated with injuries in Thoroughbred horses. Equine Vet J 1991;23:445–448.

50. Mooney V. Effective Rehabilitation of Lumbar and Pelvic Girdle Pain. In Movement, Stability and Lumbopelvic Pain, 2nd ed. Vleeming A, Mooney V, Stoeckart R, eds. Churchill Livingstone, Elsevier, Philadelphia, 2007;573–588.

51. Murray RC, Walters JM, Snart H, et al. Identification of risk factors for lameness in the dressage horse. Vet J 2009; in press.

52. Paulekas R, Haussler KK. Principles and practice of therapeutic exercise for horses. J Equine Vet Sci 2009;29:870–893.

53. Pelso JM, Mundy GD, Cohen ND. Prevalence of and factors associated with musculoskeletal racing injuries of Thoroughbreds. J Am Vet Med Assoc 1994;204:620–626.

54. Pennell JC, Egenvall A, Bonnett BN, et al. Specific causes of morbidity among Swedish horses insured for veterinary care between 1997 and 2000. Vet Rec 2005;157:470–477.

55. Perry J, Green A. An investigation into the effects of a unilaterally applied lumbar mobilization technique on peripheral sympathetic nervous system activity in the lower limbs. Man Ther 2008;13:492–499.

56. Petty NJ, Moore AP. Neuromusculoskeletal Examination and Assessment: A Handbook for Therapists, 2nd ed. Churchill Livingstone, Elsevier, Philadelphia, 2001.

57. Porter M. Equine rehabilitation therapy for joint disease. Vet Clin N Am Equine Prac 2005;21:599–607.

58. Pusey A, Brooks J, Jenks A. Osteopathy and the Treatment of Horses. Wiley-Blackwell, John Wiley and Sons Ltd., Ames IA, 2010.

59. Quiroz-Rothe M, Novales M, Aguilare-Tejero E, et al. Polysaccharide storage myopathy in the M. longissimus lumborum of show jumpers and dressage horses with back pain. Equine Vet J 2002;34:171–176.

60. Ramon T, Prades M, Armengou L, et al. Effects of athletic taping of the fetlock on distal limb mechanics. Equine Vet J 2004;36(8):764–768.

61. Reef VB. Musculoskeletal ultrasonography. In Equine Diagnostic Ultrasound. Reef VB, ed. W.B. Saunders, Philadelphia, 1998;39–186.

62. Rooney JR, Genovese RL. A survey and analysis of bowed tendon in Thoroughbred racehorses. Equine Vet Sci 1981;5:49–53.

63. Rossdale PD, Hopes R, Wingfield Digby NJ, et al. Epidemiological study of wastage among racehorses, 1982 and 1983. Vet Rec 1985;116:66–69.

64. Scott M. Musculoskeletal injuries in nonracing quarter horses. Vet Clin Equine Prac 2008;24:133–152.

65. Simons DG, Travell JG, Simons LS. Travell and Simons' Myofascial Pain and Dysfunction: The Trigger Point Manual, 2nd ed. Lippincott Williams and Wilkins, Philadelphia, 1999.

66. Sluka KA, Skyba DA, Radhakrishnan R, et al. Joint mobilization reduces hyperalgesia associated with chronic muscle and joint inflammation in rats. J Pain 2006;7:602–607.

67. Somers DL, Clemente FR. Transcutaneous electrical nerve stimulation for the management of neuropathic pain: The effects of frequency and electrode position on prevention of allodynia in a rat model of complex regional pain syndrome type II. Phys Ther 2006;86:698–709.

68. Steiner B, Bryant J. A Gymnastic Riding System Using Mind, Body and Spirit. Progressive Training for the Horse and Rider. Trafalgar Square Publishing, Hong Kong, 2003.

69. Stubbs NC, Clayton HM. Activate Your Horse's Core: Unmounted Exercises for Dynamic Mobility, Strength, and Balance. Sport Horse Publications, Mason, MI, 2008.

70. Sullivan KA, Hill AE, Haussler KK. The effects of chiropractic, massage and phenylbutazone on spinal mechanical nociceptive thresholds in horses without clinical signs. Equine Vet J 2008;40:14–20.

71. Tellington-Jones L, Bruns U, Isenbugel VMDE. An Introduction to the Tellington-Jones Equine Awareness Method: The T.E.A.M. Approach to Problem-Free Training. Breakthrough Publications, New York, 1988.

72. The World Confederation for Physical Therapy. http://www.wcpt.org/. Accessed Jan. 8, 2010.

73. Turner T. Back problems in horses. Proceedings Am Assoc Equine Practitioners, 2003.

74. Valberg S. Spinal muscle pathology. Vet Clin N Am Equine Prac 1999;15:87–96.

75. Valentine BA. Pathologic findings in equine muscle (excluding polysaccharide storage): A necropsy study. J Vet Diagn Invest 2008;20:572–579.

76. Van Eps AW, Pollitt CC. Equine laminitis: Cryotherapy reduces the severity of the acute lesion. Equine Vet J 2004;36:255–260.

77. Vicenzino B, Collins D, Benson H, et al. An investigation of the interrelationship between manipulative therapy-induced hypoalgesia and sympathoexcitation. J Manipulative Physiol Ther 1998;21:448–453.

78. Vicenzino B, Paungmali A, Buratowski S, et al. Specific manipulative therapy treatment for chronic lateral epicondylagia produces uniquely characteristic hypoalgesia. Man Ther 2001;6: 205–212.

79. Wakeling JM, Barnett K, Price S, et al. Effects of manipulative therapy on the longissimus dorsi in the equine back. Equine and Comparative Exercise Physiology 2006;3:153–160.

80. Watson T. Electrotherapy: Evidence-based Practice (Physiotherapy Essentials), 12th ed. Churchill Livingstone, Elsevier, Philadelphia, 2008.

81. Wennerstrand J, Johnston C, Rhodi M, et al. The effect of weighted boots on the movement of the back in the asymptomatic riding horse. Equine and Comparative Exercise Physiology 2006;3:13–18.

82. Wright A. Hypoalgesia post-manipulative therapy: A review of the potential neurophysiological mechanisms. Man Ther 1995;1:11–16.

83. Young A. Current issues in arthrogenous inhibition. Ann Rheum Dis 1993;52:829–834.

Occupation-related Lameness Conditions

THE THOROUGHBRED RACEHORSE

ROBERT J. HUNT AND FOSTER NORTHROP

The incidence and impact of lameness in Thoroughbred racehorses is significant. Essentially all horses participating in training and racing are vulnerable to injury with resultant lameness. In one review, 37 of 40 juvenile horses became lame during training.[43] Failure to train due to lameness had a significant detrimental economic impact in this study. Monetary considerations coupled with the recent increased public awareness focused on the welfare of horses in general has resulted in a new era of philosophy in lameness management in the Thoroughbred racehorse. As a result, there is marked emphasis on injury prevention, early recognition of lameness, and early proactive intervention prior to the onset of serious lameness. It is important to be able to differentiate potential life-threatening disorders from those that are transient or pose minimal threat to the horse's well being while continuing to compete.

The focus of this discussion predominately pertains to lameness of musculoskeletal origin. Several etiologic factors have been incriminated in racing and training injuries. Variables include genetics, racing surface, number of starts, age of the horse, pre-existing disease, conformation, and trauma. Monotonic injuries causing lameness result from single acute incidents in which tissue is momentarily loaded beyond its ultimate strength. Most injuries, however, are cumulative and result from fatigue associated with cyclical or repetitive overuse of a structure. This applies to all tissue types. The degree of damage and resultant lameness covers the spectrum from almost imperceptible to catastrophic failure. Most conditions are manageable with appropri-

ate intervention, and the goal is to prevent potentially serious injuries from becoming catastrophic.

RISK FACTORS FOR INJURY

Emphasis has been given to the identification of risk factors for development of musculoskeletal injury with special attention to fatal injuries.[14,32,37,38,40,51] As noted, the occurrence of lameness is extremely high. Fortunately, the incidence of catastrophic breakdown in racehorses is very low; approximately 1 to 2 catastrophic events occur per every 1,000 starts.[40]

Several postmortem studies have categorized injuries that result in destruction of the horse. These studies have elucidated not only training factors that appear to predispose racehorses to specific injuries, but also apparent geographic differences. For example, the incidence of soft tissue injuries incurred during racing differs among various racetracks in the United States. One Australian study of fatal injuries in Thoroughbred racehorses found that most were euthanized after a catastrophic injury to a forelimb; however, there was no statistically significant difference between forelimb affected.[6] Conversely, there was a predisposition for right forelimb injury in the United Kingdom.[38] In the United States, horses were more likely to sustain fracture of the left forelimb during racing and right forelimb during training.[25] Fractures of the proximal sesamoid bones were the most common injury in the United States, but Australian studies showed that fracture of the front or rear cannon bone was most common during racing, followed by accompanying fractures of the proximal sesamoids and proximal phalanx.[5,6]

Training and racing schedules have been scrutinized.[1,10–12,15–18,23] The risk of catastrophic injury and

Adams and Stashak's Lameness in Horses, 6e, edited by Gary M. Baxter
© 2011 Blackwell Publishing, Ltd.

forced lay-up in fit California Thoroughbred racehorses was significantly increased following 2 months of high-speed exercise with distance accumulation.[17] Two-year-olds exceeding 0.76 furlongs/day, 3-year-olds exceeding 0.85 furlongs/day, and 4-year-olds exceeding 0.95 furlongs/day were at higher risk of sustaining injury than those working shorter distances. In another study, the racing injury rates were inversely proportional to the success of the individual trainer.[52] The incidence of tibial and pelvic stress fractures rises with increasing distances cantered during a 30-day training period but not over a 60-day period.[35,50]

Track conditions also correlate with injury.[8,9,41] Fracture rates in Japan increased as dirt tracks became muddier and decreased as turf surfaces became softer.[34] The differences between synthetic surfaces, dirt, and turf courses are still under investigation, and to date there is no uniform consensus on superiority, although track base uniformity and surface maintenance are necessities for safety.

Individual conformation has been recognized clinically to affect locomotion and long-term soundness.[29,31] Some traits have been shown to influence the onset of clinical abnormalities. For example, horses with offset knees have an increased incidence of stress-related disorders of the knees and an increased risk of fetlock problems.[29] Other flaws that likely predispose a horse to injury include back-in-the-knee conformation and carpal or fetlock varus deviation.

DIAGNOSIS OF LAMENESS

History and physical evaluation, economics, and personal preferences help determine the appropriate diagnostic steps for every horse. Knowledge of the exercise and racing schedule, including when fast work has taken place, intensity level of training, and past performance is important. It is also important to be aware of recent lay-up, convalescence, and previous surgery.

The physical evaluation is straightforward and basic, but it must be thorough. It is especially helpful if the veterinarian is familiar with the patient. The general health of the horse must be considered, including appetite, hair coat, general disposition, and the presence of any current medical conditions as well as treatment thereof. Recognition of previous lameness in the specific patient coupled with results from current diagnostic procedures may raise the level of suspicion for a recurrent injury.

Racetrack practitioners who are familiar with their patients have a number of advantages, including the ability to perform multiple examinations either in-hand or on the racetrack in the horse's routine work environment. A disadvantage of known history is the potential for bias in diagnoses. Another disadvantage for the racetrack practitioner is potential obstacles in the working environment, where there is often excessive commotion that may preclude a thorough locomotor examination. Special scheduling may be required to accomplish a complete examination. The behavior of a fit racehorse likewise limits the time allowed for the evaluation, in addition to presenting an inherent safety hazard. Many racehorses become rank and difficult to handle after only a few jogging sessions, and may hide

a subtle lameness due to excitement. Diagnosis of a new injury may be challenging if there are pre-existing healed injuries that are not clinically active.

Lameness may be displayed in a broad spectrum of clinical signs, ranging from behavioral changes, reluctance to train, and poor performance, to mild or overt gait alterations. It is common for horses to display changes in temperament, such as aggressive or passive behavior, prior to displaying actual lameness. Horses may become track sour or display changes during training such as lugging in or out or running off. Other manifestations include reduced appetite, poor hair coat, soft palate displacement, or tying-up.

Lameness associated with pain is the manifestation of an avoidance response. The character of lameness is largely determined by the location or source of an injury, although it is difficult to differentiate exact foci of pain or specific disorders based on gait alone. Generalities of gait combined with the rest of the clinical picture often aid in lesion localization, but there are no absolutes based solely on gait.

Gait alterations associated with mechanical limitations may be challenging to distinguish from lameness associated with pain. An example of characteristic gait patterns is a delay in contact of the foot with the ground (drift) caused by a foot bruise or developing abscess in a front foot; a similar problem in a hind foot produces a stringhalt appearance. Abduction of a limb prior to ground contact is often observed with a fracture of the lateral wing of the coffin bone, incomplete lateral condylar fracture, and fracture of the lateral aspect of the carpus. Changes in advancement of a limb and stride length occur with many lameness conditions and vary with location and severity. Horses with a humeral stress fracture or other proximal limb injury do not advance the limb fully in the cranial phase of the stride. Tibial stress fractures often display a limited contact or support phase of the stride, which results in a jerking lift-off of the limb in addition to a limited cranial phase of the stride.

Diagnosis of lameness should be confirmed by isolating the source of lameness. Ancillary diagnostic anesthesia may be employed to localize the pain if necessary and feasible. Diagnostic nerve blocks may be difficult to perform for 2 reasons: the fractious behavior of some horses and potential regulatory hurdles if the horse is scheduled to compete. Caution is imperative in the racehorse if the possibility of anesthetizing a potential fracture exists. The results of local anesthesia are sometimes open to interpretation, due to the effectiveness of the block and the time frame required for anesthesia to develop. Results may also be confused because excitement of the horse can obscure the lameness independent of the regional anesthesia.

Further ancillary diagnostic techniques include imaging modalities such as radiographs, ultrasound, nuclear scintigraphy, MRI, and computed tomography. It is routine for race track practitioners to be equipped with portable digital radiographic and ultrasonographic equipment.[4] Instant stall side diagnosis of fracture or other injury has become standard.

Nuclear scintigraphy has had a tremendous impact on understanding bone disease in the racehorse and the management of many of these conditions. Because it provides a reflection of the physiologic status of tissue, pathology may be detected and therefore addressed earlier than with plain radiography. For example, detection of stress-related bone injuries may be observed before catastrophic failure occurs.

COMMON CONDITIONS

An almost endless number of clinical problems resulting in lameness regularly confront the race track practitioner. Certain problems occur routinely and become standard and expected, while other conditions are uncommon and may be overlooked because of their relative infrequence. As more information is gained with advancement of studies, our knowledge base and future management of these conditions may be subject to change.

Foot

The foot of the racehorse is the single most common region affected by lameness. It is standard belief that the hoof of the North American Thoroughbred is inferior to that of the European Thoroughbred due to less mass. The front feet of the average racehorse undergo conformational changes as it progresses through its training and racing career. It is common to develop a long toe and underslung heel with the axis of the foot becoming reoriented in a broken back fashion. Improper shoeing is often implicated; however, these changes are also the result of the mechanical forces on the foot associated with training. These conformational changes combined with the trauma to which the foot is subjected contribute to many lameness conditions in the foot.

The most frequent problem is bruising in the subsolar region, heels, or frog. Treatment for bruising is to rest and protect the region, remove the offending load responsible for the bruising, and prevent abscessation. Generally little training is missed as a result of a foot bruise because most are self-limiting problems; however, abscessation may occur if sepsis occurs. Abscessation is treated with plain hot water soaks and a softening hoof pack (Animalintex) until the horn is pliant enough to allow eruption of the abscess. Most resolve uneventfully and carry a good prognosis if managed with proper hygiene and rest.

Quarter cracks occur less commonly but often enough to be a particular nuisance. They almost always occur in horses that have shearing of the heels, thin walls, an unbalanced foot, and often underslung heels. The side with the crack is taller than the unaffected side. An integral component of management involves balancing the foot in addition to stabilizing the wall. Without balancing the foot, repair of the crack is futile and it will recur. A support shoe such as a Z-bar shoe or a three-quarter shoe with a Z bar is helpful at lessening the shearing forces of the involved wall while healing occurs. Direct repair of the crack by lacing and/or patching is often necessary to stabilize the hoof wall. The crack must be free of sepsis and if there is sensitive tissue involved, a drain must be placed beneath the crack. Many horses are able to continue training while undergoing treatment for quarter cracks, while others must be convalesced to allow hoof regrowth and con-

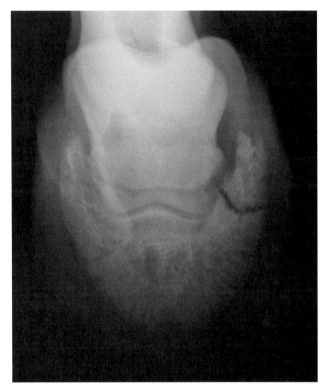

Figure 9.1. 45° degree dorsoproximal palmarodistal radiograph illustrating a wing fracture of the third phalanx.

ditioning. The farther palmar the crack, the more difficult it is to manage.

Six types of coffin bone fractures are described in the literature and occur in racehorses, but the most common are articular or nonarticular fractures of the lateral wing of the left forelimb and medial wing of the right (Figure 9.1).[24,44] These may be recognized with nuclear scintigraphy prior to the appearance of radiographic changes, suggesting a stress-related bone injury basis for development.[44] Fractures may not be apparent on radiographs until 7 to 10 days after they occur. Conventional management includes rest with a bar shoe with or without clips for 8 to 12 weeks. If lameness is evident it is common to perform palmar digital neurectomy. There is a good prognosis for return to racing, even though there is commonly evidence of osteoarthritis (OA) or a step defect once healing is completed.

Fetlock

The fetlock joints of the front- and hindlimbs are plagued with multiple problems that contribute to lameness, and they are the most commonly affected articular structure in the racehorse. One report indicates that up to 56% of the total days lost in training as 2-year-olds are attributed to fetlock injuries.[3] Most are associated with some form of cumulative stress-related disease which may involve bone, cartilage, or soft tissue. Synovitis and capsulitis of 2-year-old training horses are common and often self limiting so long as training is reduced and tissue is allowed to heal.[30]

The predominant clinical sign is joint effusion with or without heat. Lameness is mild if present but there is usually resentment to flexion of the joint. Radiographs are unremarkable, whereas ultrasonography confirms increased joint fluid and mild thickening or proliferation of the synovium. Treatment includes local therapy with ice, hydrotherapy, poultice, and bandaging. Joint injection with chondroprotective agents and corticosteroids is common. Systemic nonsteroidal anti-inflammatory drugs (NSAIDs) are also frequently administered.

Common areas of cartilage and osteochondral trauma involve the dorsal rim of the proximal phalanx (P1), usually medially or medially and laterally. This is believed to occur from the repetitive trauma and wear of the rim against the distal metacarpus, and is the most common area for development of chip fracture in the fetlock.[48] Usually there is joint effusion, warmth, and varying degrees of pain on flexion, along with focally sensitive palpation on the area of the rim that is involved. Lameness is usually only transient if present at all, unless advanced changes have occurred in the joint. Most commonly there is a reduction in performance rather than an overt lameness. The prognosis is good with arthroscopic removal of dorsal P1 chips in racehorses as long as appropriate convalescence is allowed.[13] Recuperation time averages 3 months or longer. Reports indicate that there is no difference in prognosis with different sizes of fragments, but larger fragments usually induce more cartilage damage and wear on the distal metacarpus, especially if they are longstanding.

Dorsal frontal fractures of proximal P1 occur relatively frequently. These fractures are usually insidious and chronic problems because many have a callus by the time they are recognized, and they affect the hindlimbs more commonly. There is no specific gait characteristic associated with this injury, but affected horses are often described as having an upper limb lameness. Frequently this injury is confused with tibial stress fractures. Diagnosis is often made with nuclear scintigraphy and confirmed by radiographs. Unless extreme displacement occurs, which is infrequent, the treatment is rest for 90 to 120 days or less. There is a good prognosis for return to racing.

The proximal sesamoid bones and other components of the suspensory apparatus are subject to tremendous tensile forces and fatigue, especially when under full load at high velocity. Several fracture types occur in the proximal sesamoid bones but apical fractures predominate. Other fracture types include midbody, basilar, abaxial, and comminuted fractures, but all occur less frequently than fractures of the apex (Figure 9.2).

Apical fractures are articular; therefore, joint effusion is usually observed if the fracture is displaced. There is pain on flexion and on focal pressure of the involved sesamoid. Diagnosis is confirmed radiographically and there is a good prognosis for return to racing with forelimb involvement (67%) with an even better prognosis for return to racing for hindlimbs (83%).[46] The medial sesamoid of the front fetlock carries the worst prognosis; only 47% return to race. A major determinant in the prognosis is the integrity and degree of damage of the suspensory ligament.

Abaxial, transverse midbody, and basilar fractures occur less commonly and carry a guarded prognosis for future racing, with or without surgery. Surgical removal of abaxial fragments is routinely performed but likely has little benefit unless the fragment is significantly displaced. Generally, if marked displacement has occurred there is excessive suspensory damage and there is a poor prognosis for racing. Midbody fractures may be managed with conservative or surgical treatment with lag screw fixation or circumferential wiring.[22] Contrary to literature reports, there is a guarded prognosis for future racing. Degenerative joint changes often accompany these injuries and worsen the prognosis. With conservative management, horses usually become sound and are useful for breeding or light athletic use.

Stress-related bone disease of the distal third metacarpus or metatarsus is an extremely common cause of lameness in juvenile horses and is also seen in older horses. The most common clinical manifestation is a variable severity of lameness, usually seen when cooling after a work out or on the following day.

Nuclear scintigraphy shows intense focal uptake of radioisotope of the involved condyle. Radiographs generally have some degree of resorption of subchondral bone.[27] At this stage, conservative therapy yields a good prognosis. If continued training is allowed, resorption will progress to a fracture line. In this instance, lameness is usually eminent and once present surgical intervention is necessary if there is any distraction at the fracture site (Figure 9.3). If initial radiographs only show subchondral resorption it is imperative to perform follow-up radiographs in 3 to 4 weeks to assess for development of a fracture line once resorption is complete. The front fetlocks develop fractures of the lateral condyle more frequently than medial, while the hind fetlocks sustain medial and lateral fractures in approximately equal numbers. There is a tendency for lateral condylar fractures to remain in a relatively simple configuration and exit the metacarpus laterally, whereas the medial fractures tend to spiral proximally and may exit medially and laterally. Prognosis is directly correlated with the extent of articular injury.

Cannon

The third metacarpal bone is commonly subject to stress-related bone injury. The most common manifestation is dorsal cortical disease which ranges from mild bucked shins to dorsal cortical fracture.[33] Numerous configurations of bone reaction and resorption are recognized, including periosteal reaction, dorsal cortical thickening, vertical resorption lines in the dorsal cortex, and saucer fractures (Figure 9.4).

Diagnosis is based on clinical findings of palpable sensitivity of the dorsal cortex while holding the limb in a nonweight-bearing frame. Local anesthesia is occasionally necessary to isolate the lameness. Radiographs eventually detect periosteal new bone proliferation or bone resorption but these changes may not be evident for several weeks. Treatment is based on the severity of the disease and degree of lameness, but the most common and effective treatment is reducing the intensity of training or rest. Ancillary treatments include topical blistering, pin firing, shock wave therapy, needle periosteal scraping, osteostixis, and cortical screw placement.[7] Generally there is a good prognosis for future racing.

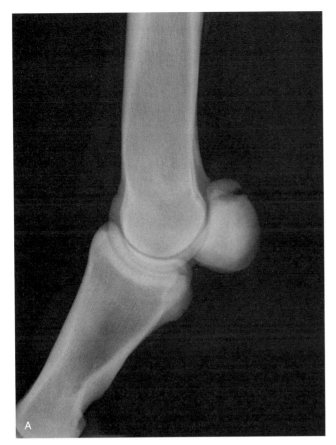 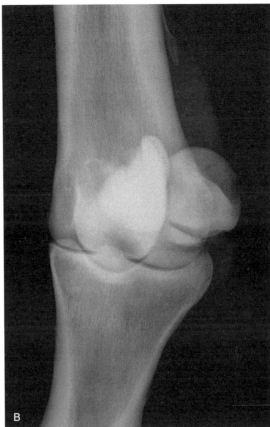

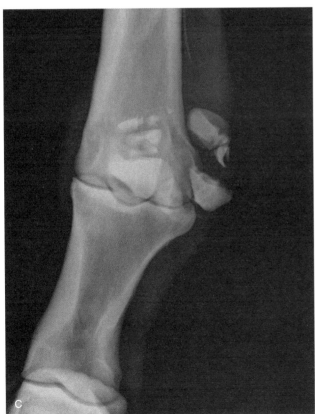

Figure 9.2. A. Lateromedial radiographic view of the metacarpophalangeal joint, showing a displaced apical sesamoid fracture. B. Lateromedial radiographic view of the metatarsophalangeal joint, showing a wedge-shaped basilar fracture fragment of a proximal sesamoid bone. C. Dorsolateral palmaromedial oblique radiographic view of the metacarpophalangeal joint illustrating a suspensory ligament breakdown injury where comminuted fractures of both proximal sesamoid bones have occurred.

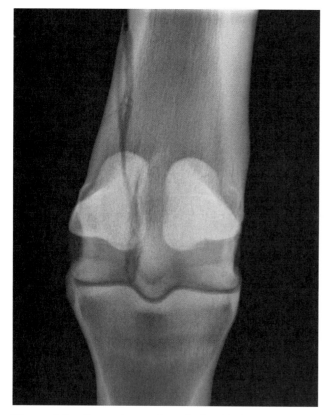

Figure 9.3. Dorsopalmar radiograph of a right front fetlock showing a displaced comminuted lateral condylar fracture of the third metacarpus.

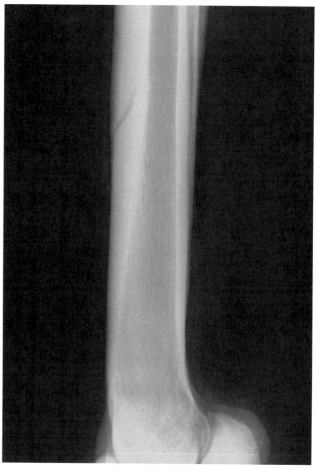

Figure 9.4. Lateromedial radiograph showing a dorsal cortical fracture of the third metacarpal bone.

Proximal palmar cortical fractures develop at the origin of the suspensory ligament and may be a source of significant lameness. Two common types of bone injury occur in this region. The first is a circular resorptive region in which there is usually an avulsion of the suspensory ligament. The other type consists of palmar cortical vertical fractures, which typically do not involve the suspensory ligament. Diagnosis may be made with a combination of local anesthesia, nuclear scintigraphy, radiographs, and ultrasound. Both injuries have a favorable prognosis with conservative management and monitoring to assess healing. A convalescence period of 3 to 5 months is usually sufficient for training to restart.

Knee

Carpal lameness is extremely common in Thoroughbred racehorses of all ages, especially so in juveniles. The carpus is a complex joint which is susceptible to a multitude of injuries associated with training and racing. Stress-related injury is involved in most of the bone, cartilage, and other soft tissue injuries of the carpus.

Common conditions include synovitis and/or capsulitis, cartilage wear and erosion, and stress-related bone injury of the third carpal bone. Numerous chip fractures of the radial carpal and middle carpal joints also occur (Figure 9.5).[36]

Clinical signs of carpal lameness vary depending on the disease process, but generally the horse tracks in a base-wide manner to facilitate lateral placement of the knee. The middle carpal joint is far more frequently affected than the proximal joint. Young horses with synovitis of the middle carpal joint display minimal lameness. The joint is often warm and there may be a change in behavior or performance. Radiographs are normal and the condition is self-limiting with a reduction in training. Joint injection is frequently performed using a corticosteroid in conjunction with a chondroprotective agent. If the condition persists or recurs after treatment, a rest period of 30 to 60 days is indicated.

Third carpal disease is very common in juvenile thoroughbreds, and is considered to be an integral component in the development of third carpal slab or sagittal fracture. Radiographs including a skyline projection of the third carpal bone should be performed and are diagnostic for third carpal disease. Common radiographic changes are sclerosis, bone resorption beginning at the radial facet, and slab and sagittal fractures (Figure 9.6).[19] Prognosis is correlated with the amount of displacement of the fracture and degree of damage to the articular cartilage.[28]

Other fracture configurations of the middle carpal joint include chip fracture of the distal radial carpal bone, the proximal third carpal bone, and the distal intermediate carpal bone. Prognosis for return to racing

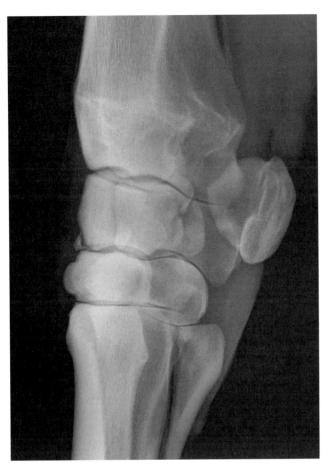

Figure 9.5. Dorsolateral palmaromedial oblique radiographic view of the carpus showing a chip fracture of the distal radial carpal bone.

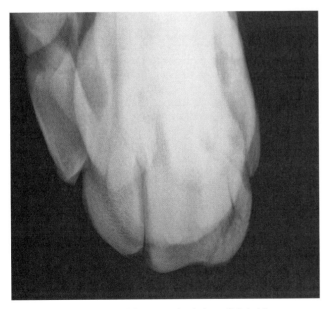

Figure 9.6. 30° flexed dorsoproximal dorsodistal oblique radiograph showing a slab fracture of the third carpal bone with frontal and sagittal components.

soundness depends on the extent of damage to the articular cartilage and amount of exposed subchondral bone at the load-bearing surface. Poor prognostic signs include extensive cartilage damage or a void on a load-bearing surface. Free fragments in the palmar aspect of the joint are also considered a poor prognostic indicator.[21]

The radial carpal joint is less frequently involved than the middle carpal joint, but pathology affecting this joint occurs routinely. Bone and cartilage injury usually manifests on the distal lateral radius, which often develops large (0.5 to 1.0 cm), partially or completely displaced fragments. In many cases the proximal intermediate carpal bone has a kissing lesion associated with this fragment or a chip fracture itself. Fragments of the distal medial radius and proximal radial carpal bone also commonly occur. Although there is a good prognosis associated with removal of fragments in the radial carpal joint, the incidence of future recurrent injury is high and the horse is predisposed to development of OA.

Hock

Tarsal lameness is a common clinical diagnosis. Affected horses travel with a characteristic gait in which the involved hindlimb hits the ground in a stabbing manner and may not readily change leads during high-speed exercise. Routine treatment consists of injecting the lower tarsal joints with corticosteroids and chondroprotective agents. Radiographs are often normal and have little correlation with tarsal lameness. Exceptions include overt pathology such as fracture of the third or central tarsal bones, or tarsal crushing or wedging.[26,49] Overt radiographic changes carry a declining prognosis. Reports suggest a poor prognosis for return to racing with slab fractures of the third and central tarsal bones; however, clinical experience indicates that the prognosis is favorable as long as healing occurs with preservation of normal articular margins and normal shape of cuboidal bones.

Stifle

Lameness in the stifle is commonly diagnosed by clinical evaluation. It is largely believed to be associated with strain and subsequent injury, primarily of the soft tissue structures of the medial femorotibial joint with occasional involvement of the femoropatellar joint. Manifestations of this lameness include the following gait disturbances: the horse travels wide behind, often does not push off the affected limb normally, and has an unsteady appearance of the hind leg. The medial femorotibial compartment usually has joint effusion but radiographs are typically normal. Intra-articular anesthesia is not typically performed but does improve the lameness if used as a diagnostic aid. Treatment with intra-articular placement of corticosteroids and chondroprotective agents improves the lameness. If the gait worsens following initial improvement, often a tibial stress fracture is implicated.

Upward fixation of the patella is usually seen in 2-year-olds but may be seen in older horses as well. Most horses with upward fixation of the patella respond favorably to treatment with systemic intramuscular administration of 3.0 ml of 30 mg/ml mephentermine hemisulfate (90 mg/horse) for 3 consecutive days. Treatment options for refractory cases include internal blister of the patellar ligaments, hormonal therapy, or medial patellar desmotomy. Prognosis for racing is good after resolution of the fixation.

Tibial and Humeral Stress Fractures

Tibial and humeral stress fractures are now recognized as a component of the stress-related bone injury complex.[35] Tibial stress fractures are most commonly seen in 2-year-old horses in training; however, these fractures may be seen occasionally in mature horses. They may be unilateral or bilateral. One limb is generally more severely affected in bilateral cases. These fractures often improve with anesthesia of the stifle, which may confuse accurate diagnosis. History commonly includes a recent episode of tying up. Lameness ranges in severity from very mild to nonweight-bearing and is usually transient in nature.

Diagnosis is confirmed by nuclear scintigraphy; however, caution is issued because in an acute tibial stress fracture, uptake of radioisotope may not be sufficient for diagnosis. Therefore, repeat scintigraphy may be necessary. Radiographs, when positive, may likewise confirm the diagnosis with characteristic signs of endosteal and periosteal callus, cortical thickening, and occasionally a fracture line (Figure 9.7). Treatment is conservative and convalescent time is commensurate with the degree of lameness. In general, a 90-day period is necessary before returning to exercise. Prognosis for return to training and racing is good.

Humeral stress fractures are diagnosed predominantly with nuclear scintigraphy. These injuries are seen in horses that have raced and are actively racing, as well as in horses that are just beginning to gallop after returning to work following convalescence. They occur on the caudal aspect of the distal humerus or on the cranial or caudal aspect of the proximal humerus. Radiographically, a callus is often recognized, indicating chronicity, especially in the distal humeral fractures. Prognosis is good for future racing with a period of convalescence similar to that for other stress-related bone injuries (90 to 120 days).

Pelvis

The pelvic and sacral regions are plagued with a number of soft tissue and bone injuries, which are usually stress induced. All types of pelvic fractures described in the literature may occur as a result of some form of acute trauma.[45] Stress fractures of the wing of the ilium and sacroiliac injury are the most common sites of bone injury in this area.[42] Prognosis for most injuries in this region is favorable with rest as long as the fracture is not displaced.

Soft tissue injuries are recognized in the hip area and are believed to occur during propulsion at fast work. Synthetic surfaces with increased traction have been incriminated in development of this condition; however, there is no current evidence to support this theory. Treatment consists of rest, and the prognosis is good for full recovery.

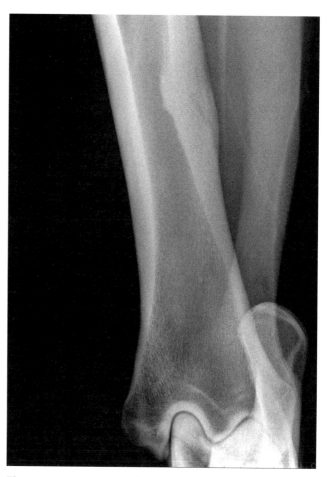

Figure 9.7. Craniocaudal radiograph showing a stress fracture response in the tibial diaphysis.

Tendons and Ligaments

Tendon and ligament injuries in racing Thoroughbreds occur predominantly from intrinsic sources, although extrinsic trauma or injury occasionally occurs. The etiology is multifactorial, but cumulative excessive strain rates in addition to the gradual demise of structural stability incurred with degenerative aging changes which are accelerated by exercise are the primary components.[47] Repetitive loading of a compromised tendon (one that has sustained subclinical, microscopic damage) may be responsible for the often progressive nature of these injuries.[39] Incidence of tendon injury is high and in one study was reported to be responsible for up to 46% of all racetrack injuries,[2] although in clinical experience the rate is not this high.

The forelimb superficial digital flexor tendon (SDFT) is frequently injured (Figure 9.8). The suspensory ligament, including the origin of the suspensory and medial or lateral branches of the front and hindlimbs, is commonly affected, as are the distal sesamoidean ligaments. The SDFT develops several characteristic lesions in different locations. A common site is the core area in the mid metacarpal region.[39] Central core lesions may be due to unequal strains on fibrils within the tendon. It has been suggested that strain levels on central core fibrils are greater than on peripheral fibers.[2] The second

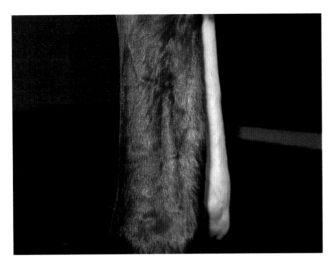

Figure 9.8. Typical bowed tendon appearance associated with superficial digital flexor tendinitis.

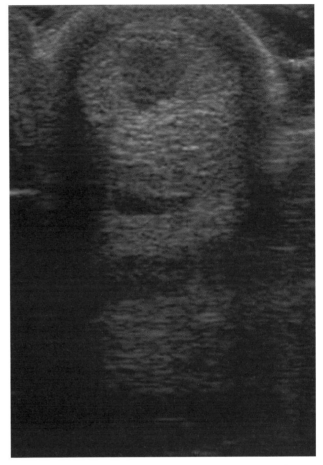

Figure 9.9. Ultrasound image of the flexor tendons showing a core lesion of the superficial digital flexor tendon.

most common lesion of the SDFT recognized clinically involves tearing of the peripheral fibers located on the lateral aspect of the tendon.

Physical evaluation often reveals warmth, mild to moderate edema, and pain upon palpation of an affected area. Horses may exhibit palmar metacarpal swelling without SDFT swelling, usually with very low-grade involvement of the tendon.[20] Lameness may be nonexistent, subtle, and transient, or overt. Ultrasound examination is the gold standard to gauge the tendon injury. Caution must be used in interpretation, especially in the acute phase, in which fluid accumulation between fibers may resemble a tear. The follow-up sonogram several weeks later is critical for accurate determination of the degree of tendon injury. Tears are recognized as hypoechoic areas within the tendon, range dramatically in diameter and length, and may be partial or complete. Complete tears appear as anechoic areas and partial tears appear as hypoechoic, or echogenicity is mixed (Figure 9.9). Affected tendons and ligaments may have a larger cross-sectional diameter than unaffected, contralateral structures, and periodically this is the only visible indicator of the problem on ultrasound.[20] More refined imaging may be obtained via MRI, and most likely will influence the future management of tendon injuries.

Treatment varies according to the degree of injury. Severe injuries may require complete rest coupled with systemic NSAIDs, hydrotherapy, sweating, and gradual return to work, whereas minimal lesions may only need a reduction in training. Serial ultrasonographic examinations help determine the rate of healing and ability to return to full training. Very large defects may benefit from surgical intervention in the form of tendon splitting to allow fluid drainage.

The prognosis for return to racing is guarded following tendon injuries. The more severe the tear, the worse the prognosis. Tendons undergo repair in phases, and the final result is remodeled, mature scar tissue.[39] Frequently, healed areas contain cicatrical tissue that does not have the elasticity of an uninjured tendon and

therefore there is a possibility for repetitive injury. The majority of tendon injuries tend to recur in racehorses, regardless of the treatments employed. Recurrence may be at the original site but is often in a region distinct from the original injury.

References

1. Anthenill LA, Stover SM, Gardner IA, et al. Risk factors for proximal sesamoid bone fractures associated with exercise history and horseshoe characteristics in Thoroughbred racehorses. Am J Vet Res 2007;68:760–769.
2. Arnoczky SP. Role of mechanobiology in the pathogenesis of tendinopathy: Lessons learned from horses and humans. Proc Am Assoc Equine Pract 2008;54:470–474.
3. Bailey CJ, Rose RJ, Reid SW, et al. Causes of wastage in 2-year-old Thoroughbreds in training: A longitudinal study. Proc Am Assoc Equine Pract 1997;43:425–426.
4. Blevins WE, Widmer WR. Radiology in racetrack practice. Vet Clin North Am Equine Pract 1990;6:31–61.
5. Boden LA, Anderson GA, Charles JA, et al. Risk of fatality and causes of death of Thoroughbred horses associated with racing in Victoria, Australia. Equine Vet J 2006;38:312–318.
6. Boden LA, Charles JA, Slocombe RF, et al. Post-mortem study of Thoroughbred fatalities in Victoria, Australia between 2001 and 2004. Proc Am Assoc Equine Pract 2005;51:303–305.
7. Cervantes C, Madison JB, Ackerman N, et al. Surgical treatment of dorsal cortical fractures of the third metacarpal bone in Thoroughbred racehorses: 53 cases (1985–1989). J Am Vet Med Assoc 1992;200:1997–2000.

8. Cheney JA, Shen CK, Wheat JD. Relationship of racetrack surface to lameness in the Thoroughbred racehorse. Am J Vet Res 1978;34:1285–1289.

9. Clanton C, Kobluk C, Robinson RA, et al. Monitoring surface conditions of a Thoroughbred racetrack. J Am Vet Med Assoc 1991;198:613–620.

10. Cogger N, Perkins N, Hodgson DR, et al. Risk factors for musculoskeletal injuries in 2-year-old Thoroughbred racehorses. Prev Vet Med 2006;74:36–43.

11. Cohen ND, Berry SM, Peloso JG, et al. Thoroughbred racehorses that sustain injury accumulate less high speed exercise compared to horses without injury in Kentucky. Proc Am Assoc Equine Pract 2000;46:51–53.

12. Cohen ND, Mundy GD, Peloso JG, et al. Results of physical inspection before races and race-related characteristics and their association with musculoskeletal injuries in Thoroughbreds during races. J Am Vet Med Assoc 1999;215:654–661.

13. Colon JL, Bramlage LF, Hance SR, et al. Qualitative and quantitative documentation of the racing performance of 461 Thoroughbred racehorses after arthroscopic removal of dorso-proximal first phalanx osteochondral fractures (1986–1995). Equine Vet J 2000;32:475–481.

14. Cruz AM, Poljak Z, Filejski C, et al. Epidemiologic characteristics of catastrophic musculoskeletal injuries in Thoroughbred racehorses. Am J Vet Res 2007;68:1370–1375.

15. Estberg L, Gardner IA, Stover SM, et al. A case-crossover study of intensive racing and training schedules and risk of catastrophic musculoskeletal injury and lay-up in California Thoroughbred racehorses. Prev Vet Med 1998;33:159–170.

16. Estberg L, Gardner IA, Stover SM, et al. Intensive exercise schedules and risk of catastrophic musculoskeletal injury and lay-up in California Thoroughbred racehorses. Proc Am Assoc Equine Pract 1997;43:269–270.

17. Estberg L, Stover SM, Gardner IA, et al. High-speed exercise history and catastrophic racing fracture in Thoroughbreds. Am J Vet Res 1996;57:1549–1555.

18. Estberg L, Stover SM, Gardner IA, et al. Relationship between race start characteristics and risk of catastrophic injury in Thoroughbreds: 78 cases (1992). J Am Vet Med Assoc 1998; 212:544–549.

19. Fischer AT, Stover SM. Sagittal fractures of the third carpal bone in horses: 12 cases (1977–1985). J Am Vet Med Assoc 1987; 191:106–108.

20. Genovese R, Longo K, Berthold B, et al. Quantitative sonographic assessment in the clinical management of superficial digital flexor injuries in Thoroughbred racehorses. Proc Am Assoc Equine Pract 1997;43:285–290.

21. Getman LM, Southwood LL, Richardson DW. Palmar carpal osteochondral fragments in racehorses: 31 cases (1994–2004). J Am Vet Med Assoc 2006;228:1551–1558.

22. Henninger RW, Bramlage LR, Schneider RK, et al. Lag screw and cancellous bone graft fixation of transverse proximal sesamoid bone fractures in horses: 25 cases (1983–1989). J Am Vet Med Assoc 1991;199:606–612.

23. Hernandez J, Hawkins DL, Scollay MC. Race-start characteristics and risk of catastrophic musculoskeletal injury in Thoroughbred racehorses. J Am Vet Med Assoc 2001;218: 83–86.

24. Honnas CM, O'Brien TR, Linford RL. Distal phalanx fractures in horses: A survey of 274 horses with radiographic assessment of healing in 36 horses. Vet Radiol 1998;29:98–107.

25. Johnson BJ, Stover SM, Daft BM, et al. Causes of death in racehorses over a 2-year period. Equine Vet J 1994;26: 327–330.

26. Kane AJ, McIlwraith CW, Park RD, et al. Radiographic changes in Thoroughbred yearlings. Part 2: Associations with racing performance. Equine Vet J 2003;35:366–374.

27. Kawcak CE, Bramlage LR, Embertson RM. Diagnosis and management of incomplete fracture of the distal palmar aspect of the third metacarpal bone in five horses. J Am Vet Med Assoc 1995;206:335–337.

28. Kraus BM, Ross MW, Boston RC. Surgical and nonsurgical management of sagittal slab fractures of the third carpal bone in

racehorses: 32 cases (1991–2001). J Am Vet Med Assoc 2005;226:945–950.

29. McIlwraith CW, Anderson TA, Douay P, et al. Role of conformation in musculoskeletal problems in the racing Thoroughbred and racing Quarter horse. Proc Am Assoc Equine Pract 2003; 49:59–61.

30. McIlwraith CW, Frisbie DD, Kawcak CE. Current treatments for traumatic synovitis, capsulitis and osteoarthritis. Proc Am Assoc Equine Pract 2001;47:180–206.

31. Morgan JW, Leibsle SR, Gotchey MH, et al. The forelimb conformation of Thoroughbred racing prospects and racing performance from 2 to 4 years of age. Proc Am Assoc Equine Pract 2005;51:299–300.

32. Mundy GD. Review of risk factors associated with racing injuries. Proc Am Assoc Equine Pract 1997;43:204–210.

33. Nunamaker DM. On bucked shins. Proc Am Assoc Equine Pract 2002;48:76–89.

34. Oikawa M, Kusunose R. Fractures sustained by racehorses in Japan during flat racing with special reference to track condition and racing time. Vet J 2005;170:369–374.

35. O'Sullivan CB, Lumsden JM. Stress fractures of the tibia and humerus in Thoroughbred racehorses: 99 cases (1992–2000). J Am Vet Med Assoc 2003;222:491–498.

36. Palmer SE. Prevalence of carpal fractures in Thoroughbred and Standardbred racehorses. J Am Vet Med Assoc 1986;188: 1171–1173.

37. Parkin TD. Epidemiology of racetrack injuries in racehorses. Vet Clin North Am Equine Pract 2008;24:1–19.

38. Parkin TD, Clegg PD, French NP, et al. High-level risk factors for fatal distal limb fracture in racing Thoroughbreds in the UK. Equine Vet J 2004;36:513–519.

39. Patterson-Kane JC, Firth EC. The pathobiology of exercise-induced superficial digital flexor tendon injury in Thoroughbred racehorses. Vet J 2009;181:79–89.

40. Peloso JG, Mundy GD, Cohen ND. Prevalence of, and factors associated with, musculoskeletal racing injuries of Thoroughbreds. J Am Vet Med Assoc 1994;204:620–625.

41. Peterson ML, McIlwraith CW. Effect of track maintenance on mechanical properties of a dirt racetrack: a preliminary study. Equine Vet J 2008;40:602–605.

42. Pilsworth RC, Shepherd MC, Herincks et al. Fracture of the wing of the ilium, adjacent to the sacroiliac joint, in Thoroughbred racehorses. Equine Vet J 1994;26:94–99.

43. Preston SA, Trumble TN, Zimmel DN, et al. Lameness, athletic performance, and financial returns in yearling Thoroughbreds bought for the purpose of resale for profit. J Am Vet Med Assoc 2008;232:85–90.

44. Rabuffo TS, Ross MW. Fractures of the distal phalanx in 72 racehorses: 1990–2001. Proc Am Assoc Equine Pract 2002;48:375–377.

45. Rutkowski JA, Richardson DW. A retrospective study of 100 pelvic fractures in horses. Equine Vet J 1989;21:256–259.

46. Schnabel LV, Bramlage LR, Mohammed HO, et al. Racing performance after arthroscopic removal of apical sesamoid fracture fragments in Thoroughbred horses age > or =2 years: 84 cases (1989–2002). Equine Vet J 2006;38:446–451.

47. Smith RK. Aetiopathogenesis of fatigue injuries to tendons. Proc Euro Soc Vet Ortho Trauma 2000;10:109.

48. Stashak TS. Lameness. In Adams's Lameness in Horses, 4th ed. TS Stashak, ed. Lea and Febiger, Philadelphia. 1987;568–573.

49. Tulamo RM, Bramlage LF, Gabel AA. Fractures of the central and third tarsal bones in horses. J Am Med Assoc 1983; 182:1234–1238.

50. Verheyen KLP, Newton RJ, Price JS, et al. A case-control study of factors associated with pelvic and tibial stress fractures in Thoroughbred racehorses in training in the UK. Prev Vet Med 2006;74:21–35.

51. Verheyen KLP, Wood JLN. Descriptive epidemiology of fractures occurring in British Thoroughbred racehorses in training. Equine Vet J 2004;36:167–173.

52. Wilson JH, Shaw KS, King V. Thoroughbred racing injury rates are inversely associated with trainer success. Proc Am Assoc Equine Pract 1997;43:229–230.

THE STANDARDBRED RACEHORSE

Kimberly Johnston and Frank A. Nickels

DESCRIPTION OF THE SPORT

The name Standardbred was first used in 1879. It originated with registration of horses capable of trotting 1 mile within a standard time of 2 minutes, thirty seconds. Today the Standardbred is a distinct breed with foals eligible for registration if both sire and dam are registered Standardbreds, regardless of racing performance. American Standardbreds currently race much faster than the original standard; most pacers complete a mile in less than 1 minute, 50 seconds, and trotters are only a few seconds slower than pacers. Racing is on an oval track, usually a mile in length, and horses pull lightweight carts with a single driver. In the United States racing is counterclockwise and commences from a moving start with horses at their post position behind a vehicle with a collapsible partition. Standardbreds race at either the trot, a 2-beat diagonal gait with the contralateral limbs (left front- and right hindlimb) advanced together, or the pace, in which the ipsilateral limbs (left front- and left hindlimb) move in unison. In the United States, pacers outnumber trotters 4:1, while in Europe and Australia, races are held at the trot only. A horse may have the ability to perform both gaits but Standardbreds tend to race at only one gait for their entire career. In general, pacers seem to tolerate lameness better than trotters due to the perpetual swinging motion of the pace.

The racy body type of the Standardbred is clearly indicative of the task for which it was bred. The Standardbred resembles the Thoroughbred; however, it is longer and does not stand as tall, averaging between 14.2 and 16 hands. Adequate body length is essential for a long stride and to allow free movement of the limbs without interference.

Conformation plays a pivotal role in the success of the racehorse and many conformational faults predispose to interference or lameness problems. Toeing out is undesirable in the front limbs, especially when accompanied by a base-narrow stance. This conformation affects the flight of the hoof and can cause interference. Toeing in causes less interference but results in an inefficient gait and increases the strain on the medial side of the limb, leading to carpal pain and the development of splints. Horses that are offset or back at the knees are at risk of carpal chips and slab factures. Sickle hocks used to be common in pacers and were even selected for, but this sharp angulation of the hindlimb predisposes to curb and hock arthritis. In contrast, many trotters are cow hocked, but unless severe, this conformation may be advantageous because it allows a passing gait in which the imprint of the hindlimb falls outside the imprint of the forelimb, providing a longer stride.

Standardbreds are broken to harness as yearlings and train for 7 to 9 months before racing as 2-year-olds. Horses are jogged at a slow trot/pace for several miles daily to gain fitness and stamina. Jogging is done "the wrong way" (clockwise) around the track and a few times a week horses are turned to work "the right way" for short bursts of speed training. During peak season, Standardbreds may race as often as once a week. This pounding on hard tracks for many miles and the fact that Standardbreds race and train in different directions makes them prone to repetitive stress and maladaptive bone injuries (Figure 9.10).

LAMENESS EXAM

Lameness is a leading cause of poor performance that plagues nearly every Standardbred racehorse at some point during its career. A high percentage of hindlimb lameness problems are encountered as a result of the Standardbreds' symmetrical gaits and having to pull a draft load.

At the exam, the history should include the age, stage of training, and whether the horse is a trotter or pacer. Owners should be asked if the horse is lame or simply not performing well? Young Standardbreds experience a subset of problems not commonly seen in the mature horse, and examination of unproven 2- and 3-year-olds with poor performance must be sufficient to rule out the cardiovascular or respiratory systems as the cause.

Lame horses should be examined for signs of localized inflammation (heat, swelling, or pain) and the owners asked about the duration of the problem. Specific questioning directs attention toward (or away from) various parts of the musculoskeletal system and helps establish a list of differential diagnoses. It is important to ask about the size of the track that the horse races on and whether lameness is worse in turns or on the straightaway. Most harness races are a mile long, but track lengths vary. On smaller tracks, horses must negotiate more turns and the turn diameter is less. Lameness from the medial side of the limb is more evident in the turns, whereas lameness from foot pain, splints, and curbs worsens with distance and is obvious at the end of a race. A change of racing venue may prove successful for horses with chronic lameness issues. A trotter with stifle arthritis, for example, may perform better on a 1-mile track where it only negotiates 2 turns.

It should be noted whether the horse breaks stride. Hock pain causes horses to get rough coming into or out of the turns, but they usually maintain the gait, whereas fetlock and stifle lameness often cause horses to break in the turns. Horses break for many reasons other than lameness, including excitement, immaturity, and incoordination. Interference is a major cause of breaking, and shoeing or tack changes may correct the problem. The bute test can be helpful to differentiate lameness from interference: A horse is prescribed a modest course of phenylbutazone and then

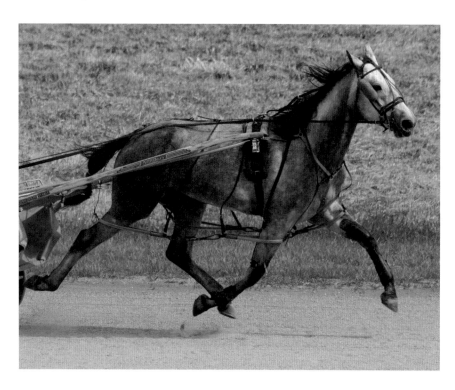

Figure 9.10. Although the pace is a natural gait, horses often wear hobbles to help maintain the gait while racing. This equipment commonly causes hairless areas on the legs, making a Standardbred pacer readily identifiable.

re-examined. It is believed that lameness improves with nonsteroidal anti-inflammatory medication (NSAID); however, interference remains unchanged. Neurologic disease also must be considered in any horse with unresolved gait abnormalities.

Several terms unique to Standardbred racing provide information about a horse's performance. Bearing in means a horse drifts toward the infield, whereas bearing out refers to a horse that drifts toward the outside rail. Drivers may comment that a horse is on a line, indicating that they must pull harder on one rein to keep the horse from bearing in or out. Horses drift away from a source of pain, so a horse on the right line is likely to have right front lameness. In rear limb problems, the hindquarters may move closer to one shaft of the sulky and the horse is then described as being on a shaft (Figure 9.11). There are exceptions; therefore, this information must only be used as a guide. Horses with right front medial heel pain, for instance, are commonly on the left line during a race because they try to avoid loading the inside of the limb (Figure 9.11).

Interference may mimic lameness if horses alter their stride to avoid hitting another limb, and it results in bruising and lacerations that cause lameness. Alterations in gait can also cause horses to overload other limbs and develop compensatory lameness, which is so common in the Standardbred that veterinarians must always consider the possibility that new problems have arisen. Both primary and secondary lameness issues must be addressed to achieve soundness. Trotters tend to develop diagonal lameness problems, whereas pacers may develop ipsilateral or contralateral issues. Tack changes such as the addition of hobbles, boots, or a head pole often indicate high-speed lameness and should be assessed.

Finally, the clinician must know the horse's history, including racing performance, prior lameness, treat-

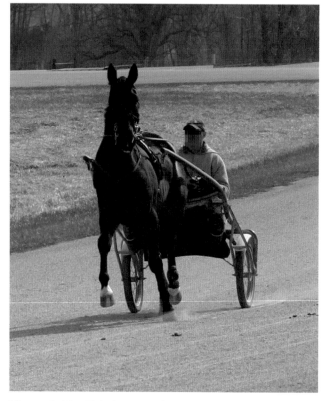

Figure 9.11. This 2-year-old Standardbred pacer demonstrates being on a shaft. The colt's hindquarters are positioned closer to the right shaft of the sulky. This colt is also on the left line and its head is turned to the left as the driver pulls harder on the rein in an attempt to keep the horse straight. This combination of findings suggests a left hindlimb lameness.

ments, and response to those treatments. Detailed record keeping is imperative, since many owners and trainers prefer jumping straight to treatment rather than pursuing extensive diagnostic tests. Without a complete diagnosis, response to treatment becomes the barometer of clinical accuracy. Standardbred trainers may try to treat problems on their own, resulting in conflicting clinical findings. It is not uncommon to be presented with a horse that has "had all his joints done" (meaning intra-articular injections) but is still not performing well. Careful inquiry may reveal that an area has been overlooked or the veterinarian may need to shift the focus to soft tissue structures rather than just injecting the horse again. It is also important to remain aware of the potential for joint infection following intra-articular injections. Onset of clinical signs can be delayed as long as 2 weeks if steroids are used.

A visual assessment of symmetry and general conditioning is made, and followed by palpation of the limbs and back in search of areas with pain or inflammation. False positive results may be encountered if the horse was recently fired or blistered. The entire horse should be examined, even if a problem is quickly recognized, because other subtle or compensatory conditions also may be identified.

An acceptable venue to watch a horse in hand can be difficult to find at the racetrack, and Standardbreds are not always amenable to jogging on a lead, making observation of the horse in the shed row typical. Unsound trotters sometimes prefer to pace at slow speeds; however, the pace is a forgiving gait and front limb lameness may be difficult to detect. Most horses, including pacers, will finally trot in hand after several attempts. Correlation between lameness seen in hand and that at racing speed is often poor, so observation of horses in harness on the track is routine.

Flexion tests are part of most exams, although their value is dubious. The carpus can be flexed exclusively and this manipulation is generally useful. In the hindlimb, an effort should be made to flex the fetlock separately from the upper limb, because problems are relatively common in this joint.

A few points regarding the use of diagnostic analgesia in the Standardbred deserve mention. Foot pain is so commonplace that blocking of a front limb should always begin with anesthesia of the palmar digital nerves to establish the significance of heel pain in the overall picture. The abaxial sesamoidean block is avoided because it can desensitize the foot, pastern, and parts of the fetlock. Inadvertent anesthesia of fetlock pain could be mistaken for lameness of the foot, with dire consequences if a fracture is present. Hindlimb foot pain is infrequent, so digital anesthesia is rarely warranted. However, low plantar anesthesia should be used to rule out the distal limb for all but the most obvious cases of hindlimb lameness. Observation of the horse on the track before and after diagnostic analgesia can be useful; however, there is risk of further injury, so the driver should be instructed to only drive the horse as far as is necessary to assess the effectiveness of the block and to avoid abrupt stops or turns. Propagation of incomplete fractures or catastrophic breakdown is possible following desensitization of a limb. Finally, the veterinarian must remember to abide by local juris-

dictions regarding the use of local anesthetics close to race day.

SPECIFIC LAMENESS CONDITIONS

Foot

Standardbreds race on compacted limestone tracks and are shod frequently, predisposing them to foot pain. It is not uncommon for a horse to be foot sore for several days after a race. Corns are particularly prevalent in the Standardbred and should be among the top differentials when presented with a sorefooted horse. The long-toe, low-heel hoof conformation seen in many Standardbreds, along with the repetitive concussion sustained from jogging on hard tracks, predisposes them to corns. Horses that are shod tight or have the heel of the shoe turned in to prevent it from being pulled off if they overreach are likely to develop corns from the focal pressure placed on the caudal angle of the bars.

Fracture of the distal phalanx is a relatively frequent cause of foot pain and should be considered in severely lame Standardbreds that have no localizing signs. Acute lameness is seen after a race, often in the winter months.

Distention of the distal interphalangeal joint is a nonspecific sign that may be noted in conjunction with foot soreness. Effusion is palpable as a soft dome 1 cm above the coronet, and placement of a needle into the joint reveals increased fluid pressure. Radiographic signs of coffin joint arthritis may not be present because synovitis can be a reflection of inflammation in nearby structures, including the podotrochlear apparatus. Response to intra-articular medication is generally favorable but often must be repeated, especially if an accurate diagnosis is never made.

Pastern

The pastern region is often overlooked in the Standardbred. Most practitioners are not familiar with the intricate anatomy of this area, so soft tissue injuries are likely underdiagnosed.

Injury to the distal sesamoidean ligaments, collateral ligaments, and flexor tendons in the pastern can all result in lameness and even joint instability, causing ringbone months or even years later.

Fetlock

Synovial or joint capsule inflammation is common and develops as the amount training increases. The condition can be secondary to altered gait from another lameness issue and it is frequently seen in horses with sore heels as a result of toe-first landing. Heat and effusion are present along with a positive response to joint manipulation, but overt lameness is not typical. Fibrosis and mineralization of the synovial pad can occur with chronicity.

Osteochondral fragments are frequently encountered in the fetlock, most commonly originating in the dorsomedial proximal margin of the first phalanx.[3] Concurrent thickening of the synovial pad is frequently observed because the 2 sites make contact during maximal extension of the joint. Small fragments may not be a significant problem, but larger fragments close to the articular surface result in lameness and can produce score lines on the metacarpal condyle. Frequent injection may keep horses going, but fragment removal is the treatment of choice to prevent joint deterioration.

Disease of the metatarsophalangeal joint is common in the Standardbred; therefore, the fetlock should be carefully evaluated in horses with hindlimb lameness. Fragments from the plantar eminence of the proximal phalanx are common. Not all fragments cause lameness, and when they do it is mild. The complaint more often involves an inability to go straight or breaks at high speed. Most fragments are found medially in the left hindlimb, and horses with an outwardly rotated hindlimb axis are predisposed.[3]

Demonstration of the lesion requires oblique views angled 30° to 45° distad to prevent overlap of the proximal sesamoid bones on the plantar aspect of the first phalanx. Problematic fragments can often be managed using intra-articular therapy until the end of the racing season without risk of further injury to the joint. Arthroscopic removal of axial fragments is then indicated. Abaxial fragments are not articular and surgical removal should not be attempted.

Fractures of the first phalanx occur and are generally straightforward; however, special mention should be made of incomplete sagittal fractures because they are common in the Standardbred and can represent a diagnostic challenge. Marked lameness after a race subsides quickly but recurs with return to work. Heat, swelling, and joint distention may be absent or minimal. This scenario, coupled with a positive response to fetlock flexion, should arouse suspicion. Radiographs prior to diagnostic anesthesia are warranted because propagation of the fracture has been reported. Short fractures may not be radiographically visible until bone resorption occurs 3 to 6 weeks following fracture.

Diagnosis is facilitated by observation of linear lucency in the proximal sagittal groove on the AP view and dorsal periosteal remodeling, which is best seen on the lateral to medial projection. Sclerosis near the mid-sagittal groove often precedes fracture and nuclear scintigraphy is likely to demonstrate the lesion much earlier. Until an accurate diagnosis can be made, these cases should be managed conservatively in a stall to prevent catastrophic injury. Short fractures may be treated with confinement alone, whereas longer, propagating, or nonhealing fractures benefit from internal fixation. Healing occurs in 4 to 6 months and the prognosis for racing is good, provided significant degenerative changes do not occur.[6]

Cyclic fatigue occurs in the Standardbred when bone adapts to the miles of low-speed jogging one way of the track and is then unable to endure the intense loads encountered during speed work in the opposite direction. Common sites of stress remodeling in the fetlock include the distal plantarolateral aspect of the metatarsal condyle, distal palmaromedial aspect of the metacarpal condyle, proximal sesamoid bones, and the proximal aspect of the first phalanx.[1]

Physical findings are minimal and affected horses have a variable response to fetlock flexion. Subtle high-speed lameness or frequent breaks in the turns are typical. Minimal improvement is seen with intrasynovial anesthesia, except in the most severe cases, because intact cartilage prevents desensitization of the subchondral bone. Nuclear scintigraphy is a valuable tool to reveal identifiable patterns of uptake for this disease entity. Radiographic findings offer insight for prognosis, because changes are nearly undetectable initially, then progress to sclerosis and flattening of the palmar/plantar condyle. A skyline view of the palmar aspect of the condyle is obtained by holding the limb in flexion as the X-ray beam is aimed dorsodistal to palmaroproximal through the fetlock joint (Figures 9.12 and 9.13). A characteristic "gull wing" pattern of sclerosis on the condyle provides the diagnosis. Exercise must be reduced to allow the adaptive process to equilibrate and microdamage to heal.

Arthritis is probably the most common condition of the fetlock. Joint distention, most notable in the palmar/plantar recess, is characteristic along with variable lameness exacerbated by flexion. Range of motion may be reduced due to joint capsule thickening and fibrosis. Some horses subsist surprisingly well and lameness does not become a prominent feature until the disease is advanced. A subclinical condition often becomes apparent after hard training or racing under adverse conditions. Diagnosis is based on the presence of degenerative changes on radiographs, and treatment is primarily palliative.

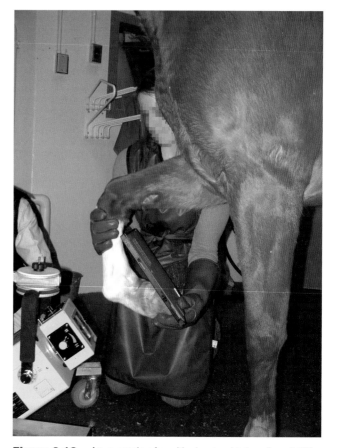

Figure 9.12.   An example of positioning to obtain a flexed 45° dorsodistal to palmaroproximal oblique (skyline) radiograph of the metacarpal condyle.

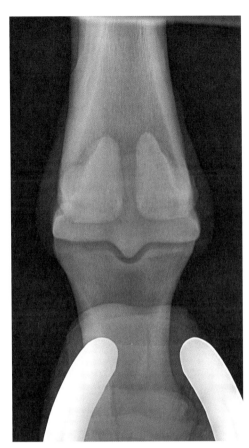

Figure 9.13. This radiograph of the metacarpus was obtained using the position described in Figure 9.12. This view is useful to demonstrate small fissures or sclerosis of the palmar aspect of the condyle, neither of which are present in this case.

Proximal Sesamoid Bones

Sesamoiditis is believed to result from minor tearing of the suspensory attachment to the proximal sesamoid bones, causing inflammation. Diagnosis is based on radiographic changes, including the presence of prominent vascular channels and patchy sclerosis within the bones. Many believe that the condition predisposes horses to sesamoid fracture but in a serial radiographic investigation of 71 young Standardbreds, horses that developed proximal sesamoid bone fractures did not have radiographic signs consistent with sesamoiditis.[4] Rest and NSAIDs are the mainstays of treatment, but prognosis for chronic cases is poor.

Fractures of the sesamoid bone are associated with trauma and generally occur in areas of attachment of the suspensory ligaments. It is believed that the suspensory ligament responds to conditioning faster than the sesamoid bone, predisposing the bone to failure during overloading. Horses present with lameness, joint swelling, and thickening of the branch of the suspensory ligament attached to the fracture. Pain is elicited with digital pressure over the bone. Treatment and prognosis vary depending on the type of fracture and extent of concurrent soft-tissue injuries. Surgical removal of apical and abaxial fragments is indicated in acute cases.

Metacarpus/Metatarsus

Standardbreds are not prone to the bucked shin complex seen in other racing breeds, although the problem is occasionally seen in forelimbs of 2-year-old pacers during late summer. Bruising of the hind shins may occur in trotters that interfere, with the front foot hitting the dorsal surface of the metatarsus.

Injury to soft tissue structures in this region is common. The majority of cases result from repetitive stress injury, although acute trauma and even tendon rupture can be seen in Standardbreds that race without adequate leg protection.

Tendon injuries are relatively easy to diagnose in the Standardbred; swelling and pain prompt ultrasonographic evaluation. Injury to the superficial digital flexor tendon (SDFT) is most common and the severity dictates the course of treatment. Horses with injury within the tendon sheath often develop constriction by the palmar annular ligament and may require transection of this ligament prior to racing. Prognosis for SDFT injury appears better in the Standardbred than other racing breeds.

Proximal metacarpal pain is regularly encountered in the Standardbred and differentials must include proximal suspensory desmitis (PSD), injury to the inferior check ligament, and sagittal fracture of the cannon bone, with PSD being most likely. Horses with PSD usually have a head nod that is pronounced when the limb is on the outside of a circle. Affected horses can move in a manner that mimics carpal pain, and lameness may be exacerbated by both fetlock and carpal flexion. In the hindlimb, swelling is minimal and horses can be positive to any or all hindlimb manipulations, including the Churchill test, making diagnostic anesthesia critical. Diagnosis is confirmed with ultrasound but radiographs should also be obtained to look for bone abnormalities at the ligament's origin, proximal sesamoid bones, and the splint bones, which are frequent in racing Standardbreds.

Branch desmitis is more common in the Standardbred than the general equine population and it is frequently seen in horses that train on tracks with tight turns or excessive banking. Single branch disease is related to hoof imbalance or poor conformation, whereas biaxial injury results from hyperextension of the fetlock joint. Lameness is not a prominent feature and many Standardbreds continue to race and train, accumulating damage and propagating injury toward the suspensory body. Injury is easily recognized by the visible swelling at the back of the fetlock and palpation of the enlarged branch(es).

Carpus

Carpal pain represents a significant cause of lameness in the Standardbred. A recent study revealed its presence in one-third of the population and found it to be the top reason for horses to require a layoff longer than 1 month.[13] Lameness results in a distinctive gait characterized by abduction of the limb and a shortened cranial phase of the stride from a reluctance to flex the carpus. Affected horses often stand in the stall with the knee(s) slightly flexed to reduce tension on the dorsal joint capsule. Heat and swelling are invariably present and often recognized by trainers.

Synovitis and capsulitis are frequently encountered in the young Standardbred. Sensitivity to palpation, pain on flexion, and reduced range of motion are typical. Treatment is aimed at returning the joint to normal as quickly as possible; NSAIDs and ice are helpful in the acute stage. Walking should follow to regain joint mobility and limit fibrosis. In some cases, intra-articular hyaluronan (HA) or steroids are needed to control the inflammatory process. Suppression of synovitis is important to prevent the products of inflammation from compromising the articular cartilage and causing arthritis.

Osteochondral fractures in the carpus are a direct result of race training. In the Standardbred, fragments are mainly seen in the middle carpal joint and are almost exclusively located dorsomedially, coming from either the distal radial carpal bone or the proximal third carpal bone.[10] Sudden onset of carpal swelling with lameness is typical. Flexion exacerbates the lameness, and digital pressure along the dorsal aspect of each bone while the joint is flexed may help localize the source of pain. A complete radiographic study of the carpus should be performed to document any chips as well as subchondral sclerosis. Remodeling occurs in both limbs simultaneously; therefore, the contralateral carpus should also be radiographed to look for concurrent disease. In the racehorse, most chips are clinically important and arthroscopic removal is the treatment of choice.

The third carpal bone is prone to maladaptive stress remodeling that causes pain and fractures. Evaluation of Standardbreds in training revealed middle carpal joint lameness in 30% of horses, with severity directly related to the degree of third carpal bone sclerosis.[6] Increased bone density and loss of vascular channels cause ischemic necrosis and predispose to further injury (Figure 9.14). Lucency of C3 is also associated with

lameness, and lesions in bone and cartilage are usually identified at surgery.[15] Etiopathogenesis is similar to that seen in the fetlock and requires similar management.

Incidence of carpal slab fractures is highest in 2-year-olds, with frontal plane fractures of the radial facet of the third carpal bone the most common configuration.[10] Distribution is nearly equal between the right and left limbs. Horses are lame and resentful of flexion, often leaning back or rearing to avoid it. Diagnosis is confirmed using radiography; the tangential view (skyline) of the third carpal bone is the most valuable. Fractures heal with conservative management, but surgery limits the severity of joint deterioration and provides the best chance to return to racing. Up to 77% of Standardbreds return to racing following slab fracture but earnings may be decreased.[14]

Hock

The hock is among the most frequently recognized sites of hindlimb lameness, and pain in the distal joints is common. Young Standardbreds with uneven gaits or those subjected to miles of jogging quickly develop tarsitis. Affected horses exhibit a shortened stride and may stab the toe laterally as they land, causing uneven wear to the shoe. Disease is most frequent in the tarsometatarsal joint but can occur solely in the distal intertarsal joint; therefore, these joints should be blocked (and treated) separately. Nuclear scintigraphy of the Standardbred with distal tarsitis reveals increased radiopharmaceutical uptake (IRU) in the dorsolateral region of the joints, in contrast to a medial location seen in most other sport horses.[2] Radiographic findings correlate poorly with disease severity. They are frequently negative in 2- and 3-year-olds despite a response to diagnostic anesthesia. Intra-articular use of HA and corticosteroids is beneficial, and older horses may require regular injections to remain competitive. Flat shoes with square toes ease break-over and removal of all shoe additives (toe grabs, etc.) helps to reduce shear strain.

Distention of the tarsocrural joint is usually associated with osteochondrosis (OCD). This condition is prevalent in the Standardbred, and the distal intermediate ridge of the tibia is the most frequent location. Fragment removal by arthroscopy is the favored treatment in young animals.

Fractures of the central or third tarsal bone are occasionally seen in the racing Standardbred. Lameness can be severe but other external signs are often limited and do not specifically incriminate the distal tarsus. Both conservative treatment and internal fixation have provided a fair prognosis for return to racing but arthritis remains an inevitable sequellae.[12,26]

Curbs frequently develop in 2-year-olds as speed training begins. In addition to swelling in the long plantar ligament, injury to the digital flexor tendons, collateral ligaments, and numerous other structures in this region can lead to the appearance of curb.[11] Causes include poor conformation (sickle hocks), kicking walls, or excessive training. Cryotherapy (freeze firing) is often employed for persistently painful curbs.

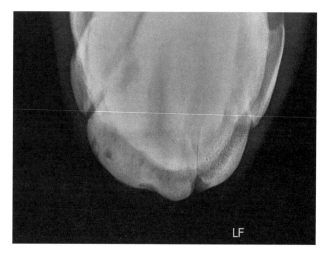

Figure 9.14. A flexed 35° dorsoproximal to dorsodistal (skyline) view of the distal row of carpal bones in a 3-year-old Standardbred filly with grade 2 of 5 right forelimb lameness. Note the generalized sclerosis of the third carpal bone along with focal lucent areas in the radial facet, indicative of bone necrosis.

Stifle

The stifle is frequently implicated as a source of lameness in the Standardbred, but a thorough work-up is rarely performed at the track and the true incidence of lameness attributable to this region is unknown. Usually, lameness blocks out lower in the limb. Horses with stifle lameness tend to carry the affected limb wide and land on the toe. Trotters may develop a bunny-hop gait, particularly if affected bilaterally.

Standardbreds with so-called loose stifles frequently have quadriceps muscle soreness that makes them resemble horses with intermittent upward fixation of the patella. They develop an abnormal cranial phase of the stride as the patella momentarily "catches" before the limb is brought to the ground. Generally, this is a fitness issue that is cured by trotting up and down hills or work in deep footing to hasten conditioning. Nevertheless, many veterinarians advocate internal blisters over the medial patellar ligament to induce scarring and decrease laxity. Medial patellar desmotomy should be reserved for cases of true upward fixation because fragmentation of the distal end of the patella has been reported following this procedure in normal horses.[8]

Stifle swelling should be a red flag whenever it is found. Marked femoropatellar effusion with minor lameness is characteristic of OCD and should prompt radiographic investigation. The postoperative prognosis is favorable in the Standardbred, as long as lesions are not extensive. Medial femorotibial effusion is a more subtle but ominous sign, often indicating advanced arthritis or injury to the intra-articular support structures of the stifle. These injuries usually end a racing career.

Upper Limb Stress Fractures

Racehorses can experience stress-related bone disease in the proximal appendicular skeleton, including the radius, humerus, tibia, and pelvis.[7,12] A high index of suspicion enhances the ability to diagnose these stress fractures, and a combination of nuclear scintigraphy and radiography is often needed. Tibial stress fractures are the most common and are usually seen in 2-year-olds. Lameness is noted after speed work and abates quickly with rest. Palpation is unrewarding but response to upper limb flexion may be dramatic. The fracture location is unique for the Standardbred, with the majority in the mid-diaphysis of the tibia, whereas fractures in Thoroughbreds are usually in the proximal caudal or caudolateral cortex.[12] Bilateral fractures can be seen, even in horses with unilateral lameness (Figures 9.15 and 9.16). Horses with scintigraphic evidence of stress remodeling should be treated conservatively, even if fracture is not radiographically visible. The prognosis is good for return to racing following appropriate rest.

Sacroiliac Pain

Sacroiliac pain is very common in the Standardbred and may present as poor performance rather than lameness. Drivers sometimes describe a horse's reluctance to take hold of the bit and think the problem is related to the teeth. Injury occurs during slips and falls and damage

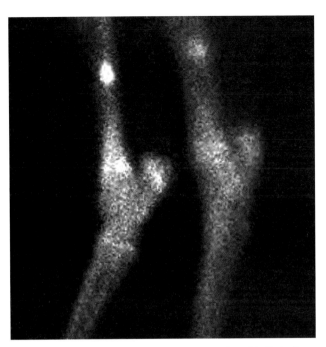

Figure 9.15. A lateral scintigraphic image of the hindlimbs in a 2-year-old Standardbred filly with obscure right hindlimb lameness. Note the focal intense radiopharmaceutical uptake in the middiaphysis of each tibia.

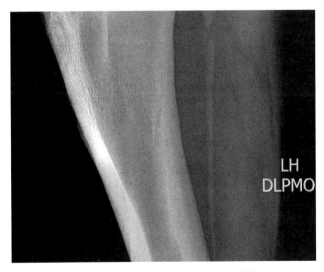

Figure 9.16. A dorsolateral to palmaromedial oblique radiograph of the tibia from the same horse as in Figure 9.15. Endosteal sclerosis and callus formation along the caudolateral cortex in the middiaphysis indicate the presence of a stress fracture. The horse was rested for 6 months and made a full recovery.

to either the ligaments supporting the pelvis or to the sacroiliac joint results in a similar clinical picture. Treatment includes rest and NSAIDs followed by a controlled exercise program with specific exercises to strengthen muscles of the back and croup. See Chapter 6 for more information on sacroiliac disease.

References

1. Davidson E. Clinical recognition of stress-related bone injury in racehorses. Clinical Techniques in Equine Practice 2003;2: 296–311.
2. Ehrlich PJ, Dohoo IR, O'Callaghan MW. Results of bone scintigraphy in racing Standardbred horses: 64 cases (1992–1994). J Am Vet Med Assoc 1999;215:982–991.
3. Grondahl AM. The incidence of bony fragments and osteochondrosis in the metacarpo- and metatarsophalangeal joints of Standardbred trotters: A radiographic study. J Equine Vet Science 1992;12:81–85.
4. Hardy J, Marcoux M, Breton L. Clinical relevance of radiographic findings in proximal sesamoid bones of two-year-old Standardbreds in their first year of race training. J Am Vet Med Assoc 1991;198:2089–2094.
5. Holcombe SJ, Schneider RK, Bramlage et al. Lag screw fixation of noncomminuted sagittal fractures of the proximal phalanx in racehorses: 59 cases (1973–1991). J Am Vet Med Assoc 1995; 206:1195–9.
6. Hopper BJ, Steel C, Richardson JL, et al. Radiographic evaluation of sclerosis of the third carpal bone associated with exercise and the development of lameness in Standardbred racehorses. Equine Vet J 2004;36:441–6.
7. Kraus BM, Ross MW, Boswell RP. Stress remodeling and stress fracture of the humerus in four Standardbred racehorses. Vet Radiol Ultrasound 2005;46:524–528.
8. McIlwraith CW. Fragmentation of distal patella—a complication of medial patellar desmotomy. Proceedings Am Assoc Equine Pract 1988;44:660–661.
9. Murphey ED, Schneider RK, Adams SB. Long-term outcome of horses with a slab fracture of the central or third tarsal bone treated conservatively: 25 cases (1976–1993). J Am Vet Med Assoc 2000;216:1949–54.
10. Palmer SE. Prevalence of carpal fractures in Thoroughbred and Standardbred racehorses. J Am Vet Med Assoc 1986;188: 1171–3.
11. Ross MW. Curb: A collection of plantar tarsal soft tissue injuries. Proceedings Am Assoc Equine Pract 2002;48:337–344.
12. Ruggles AJ, Moore RM, Bertone AL, et al. Tibial stress fractures in racing standardbreds: 13 cases (1989–1993). J Am Vet Med Assoc 1996;209:634–7.
13. Steel CM, Hopper BJ, Richardson JL, et al. Clinical findings, diagnosis, prevalence and predisposing factors for lameness localized to the middle carpal joint in young Standardbred racehorses. Equine Vet J 2006;38:152–7.
14. Stephens PR, Richardson DW, Spencer PA. Slab fractures of the third carpal bone in Standardbreds and Thoroughbreds: 155 cases (1977–1984). J Am Vet Med Assoc 1988;193:353–8.
15. Uhlhorn H, Carlsten J. Retrospective study of subchondral sclerosis and lucency in the third carpal bone of Standardbred trotters. Equine Vet J 1999;31:500–5.
16. Winberg FG, Pettersson H. Outcome and racing performance after internal fixation of third and central tarsal bone slab fractures in horses. A review of 20 cases. Acta Vet Scand 1999;40:173–80.

THE RACING QUARTER HORSE

Nancy L. Goodman

INTRODUCTION

Racing Quarter horses have specific lameness problems associated with their vocation—sprint racing, attaining speeds in excess of 50 mph in less than 21 seconds at a distance of one-quarter mile. The breed originated in colonial Virginia in the 1600s when imported English Thoroughbreds were crossed with "native" breeds of Spanish descent to produce a compact, heavily muscled horse that excelled at running short distances. They were known as Quarter Pathers or Quarter Milers, named after the quarter mile distance at which they excelled. The first race records are from Enrico County, Virginia, in 1674, where match races were run down village streets and in small, level fields.

Nearly everyone in the industry has dreamed of winning the All American Futurity, held annually on Labor Day at Ruidoso Downs in Ruidoso, New Mexico. The race features a $2 million dollar purse, with $1 million going to the winner. Los Alamitos Racetrack in Southern California, the only predominantly Quarter horse track, offers at least five races during the year with high dollar purses; the Los Al $2 Million Dollar Futurity is the richest. The Champion of Champions, held at the end of the racing year, is the most prestigious race for older horses, representing winners of the top races nationwide during the year.

The sport emphasizes 2-year-old racing, futurities, which require qualifying heats. The horses with the ten fastest times compete in a final race 2 weeks later. Horses must be nominated to futurities, and periodic payments are made to maintain eligibility. The same applies to derbies, which are held for 3-year-olds, but the purse money is less than for futurities. Yearling sale prices are driven by precocious, nicely conformed, and well-bred individuals with the potential to compete in these lucrative futurities and then derbies (Figure 9.17).

The American Quarter Horse Association (AQHA) studbook has remained open to the breeding of Thoroughbreds ever since the American Quarter horse breed was formally established. Breeding to Thoroughbreds is a useful outcross to expand an otherwise small gene pool and maintain the classic quarter mile distance of 440 yards, because some Quarter horses run their best at even shorter distances of 300 to 350 yards. Unlike Thoroughbreds, artificial insemination is the norm for breeding and embryo transfer is popular.

CONFORMATION RELATING TO LAMENESS

Conformational factors that have been associated with lameness in the forelimb are relatively large body mass, poor carpal conformation (back at the knee and bench-kneed), short upright pasterns, and poor hoof

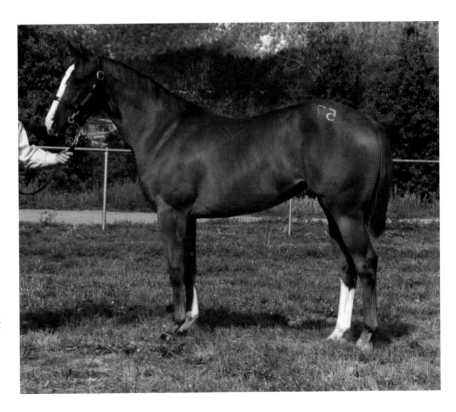

Figure 9.17. Precocious individuals with popular bloodlines are sought after at yearling sales. This horse (pictured as a sale yearling) won the All American Futurity the following year. (Courtesy of The American Quarter Horse Racing Journal.)

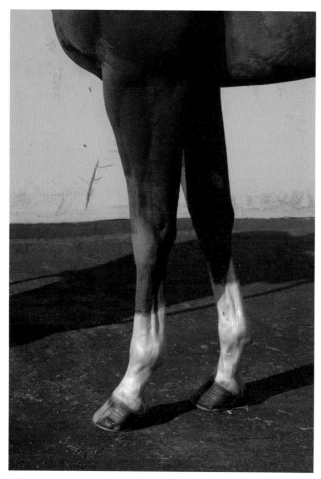

Figure 9.18. Back-in-the-knee conformation on a horse immediately prior to arthroscopic surgery for carpal chip fragmentation. (Courtesy of Dr. CW McIlwraith.)

conformation (Figure 9.18). In a scientific study, the most significant finding was that for every inch increase in toe length, the odds of sustaining a carpal chip fracture increased by a factor of 40.33.[13] Major hind-end conformational defects (e.g., sickle hocks, cow hocks, too straight in the stifles) are undesirable in the Quarter horse racing breed because breaking sharply from the starting gate is necessary to be competitive and any serious hind-end lameness may limit the individual's usefulness.

TRAINING THE RACING QUARTER HORSE

Horses are usually started under saddle in the latter part of the yearling year to prepare for racing as 2-year-olds. They are not allowed to race before March of their 2-year-old year and they are restricted from racing 440 yards until later in the year.[1] In California the horses are required to be truly 24 months of age before their first race. The early races are very short (220 yards) and their training schedule is light compared with the racing Thoroughbred. Most of the 2-year-old Quarter horses are very precocious, big bodied, and naturally fast. They can perform well with a low level of fitness, which is

possibly a risk factor for injury. Once they are fit, they gallop fewer days than Thoroughbreds and many older racehorses spend much of their time on a mechanical horse walker at the barn.

SHOEING

The most serious shoeing considerations in the Quarter horse are probably the same as in the Thoroughbred: long toe, low, excessively sloping heels, and medial to lateral hoof imbalance. Most racehorses are shod close to or on race day; consequently, corrective shoeing is not employed as often as needed in many cases because of the risk of sore feet on race day. Horses race in aluminum shoes and various types of pads are employed for foot-sore horses, including rim pads, wedge pads, full plastic pads, and even full aluminum pads with an assortment of hoof packing. Toe grabs are controversial, especially in Quarter horse racing. They have been associated with catastrophic injury in the racing Thoroughbred and racing regulators restrict their use in some states. There is very little published data regarding toe grabs in Quarter horse racing and one study found underrun heels as a more significant risk factor for catastrophic injury than toe grab length.[2] Historically, Quarter horse racehorses have used up to 8-mm (high) toe grabs to prevent stumbling and slipping from the starting gate but the norm now is 2- to 4-mm toe grabs, with higher ones used only rarely.

Races can be won or lost at the break in Quarter horse racing due to the short distance. The action of the front hooves pointing into the racing surface at the first jump out of the gate is different than that of Thoroughbreds, as is the fact that they actually pull with their front legs as well as push from the hindquarters (Figure 9.19). Some leading trainers feel that the use of higher toe grabs may be necessary for a few individuals after the horses have stumbled or fallen out of the starting gate while wearing a low toe grab. A 2-year survey in California found no adverse effect of toe grabs on the rate of catastrophic injury in racing Quarter horses, with a similar distribution of injury to the control population.[9] Further studies specific to Quarter horse racing and toe grabs correlated to injury rates are necessary, as is investigation into racing surfaces and the condition of the racetrack itself.

LAMENESS RELATED TO TRACK SURFACE

Quarter horses race on varying track surfaces around the country; however, trainers prefer a firmer surface because a loose or sandy surface poses problems with breaking at speed from the starting gate and gaining enough traction for sprinting at high speeds. A different set of injuries is associated with racing on a sandier track, particularly tendinitis of the superficial flexor tendon. Hind-end lameness, muscle pulls, back soreness, and suspensory ligament injuries also are more prevalent. Although firmer tracks are preferred, they may lead to a higher incidence of joint and bone injury due to greater concussive forces. There are currently no statistics for Quarter horse injuries associated with synthetic tracks.

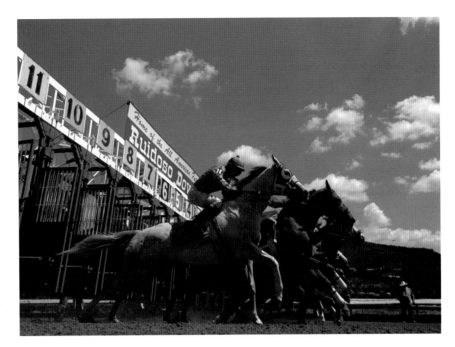

Figure 9.19. Quarter horses break from the starting gate at Ruidoso Downs. Notice the action of the front hooves pointing into the racing surface. (Courtesy of The American Quarter Horse Racing Journal.)

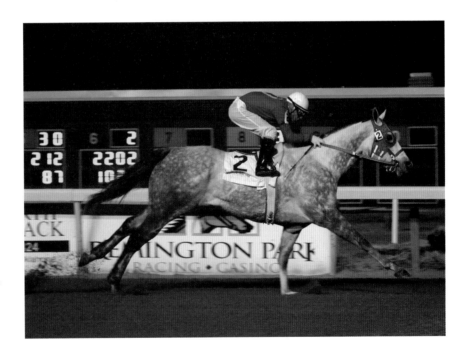

Figure 9.20. A champion 870-yard Quarter horse winning a stakes race at Remington Park. This is a good example of hyperextension of the carpus and metacarpophalangeal joints commonly seen in racehorses. (Courtesy of Dustin Orona Photography/Remington Park.)

LAMENESS EXAMINATION

There is no set procedure for lameness examination, but a systematic approach is essential to assure that it is complete. It is important to be efficient because many trainers like to examine every horse before it is entered to race. Soundness is imperative for optimum racing performance in the Quarter horse breed because the races are so short and they are won or lost by photo finishes on a regular basis. Lame horses may be fractious in the starting gate, and those with hind-end lameness may be slow to break from the gate. Quarter horses require a great deal of lameness monitoring to remain at the top of their game. Intra-articular therapy is frequently employed due to the high incidence of joint injury and inflammation associated with speed and concussive forces. Hyperextension of the carpus and metacarpophalangeal joints are common in racehorses and can contribute to lameness (Figure 9.20).

It is very useful to watch the horse walk out of the stall and down the shed row, and this is a good time to obtain a history from the trainer or barn foreman. A sore carpus may be noted immediately by a characteristic wide placement of the leg while walking. Observations such as "The horse gets hotter than usual at the track in the morning," or "He is digging a hole in the stall and standing in it," are useful parts of the history. Observing the horse walk and jog on a hard level surface may accentuate the lameness and aid in diagnosis. Hoof testers should always be used to define lameness pertaining to the foot. Joint flexion and palpation are particularly useful due to the high incidence of joint problems in the Quarter horse racehorse.

In addition to a conventional lameness examination, the author pays particular attention to certain examinations in the racing Quarter horse. This includes flexing the carpus with the leg in a raised position so that the radius is horizontal, and looking for an immediate withdrawal response of the neck and shoulder muscles as a response to pain, as well as directly palpating the carpal joints by placing the thumbs along the individual dorsal borders of the carpal bones while the fingers apply pressure behind the joint to further localize the lameness. The coffin joint is palpated for heat and excessive joint effusion and the digital pulse should always be checked because it is frequently elevated in horses with acute foot problems. A positive Churchill test may indicate hock soreness and is quickly performed while palpating the distal limb. The medial femorotibial joint is the most common area of soreness in the stifle and may or may not have effusion. The history of a poor performance (especially leaving the gate) usually initiates a more complete examination of the hindlimb.

Diagnostic blocks are used when necessary to localize the lameness. See Chapter 3.

SPECIFIC LAMENESS CONDITIONS

The lameness conditions discussed below are the most relevant for the Quarter horse racing breed. Most of the topics are covered extensively in other chapters; therefore, this section is meant as a review of Quarter horse injuries and differences from those of the Thoroughbred.

Arthrosis of the Distal Interphalangeal (DIP) Joint and Problems Associated with the Foot

Coffin joint synovitis is a significant cause of lameness in the Quarter horse.[6] The breed is well known for having undersized feet in relation to the body size, and this, coupled with the tendency for racehorses to develop long toes and excessively sloping heels, probably leads to greater stresses to the foot than in other breeds. They also tend to have short upright pasterns and they race at high speeds on firm track surfaces. Bilateral forelimb lameness is seen, and it can be accentuated by jogging on a hard surface. The stride is shortened with a transfer of weight to the hindlimbs. Horses typically respond to hoof testers over the central third of the frog (as in navicular syndrome). An increased digital pulse is usually evident and DIP joint effusion may be palpated above the coronet in many cases. Younger horses (2- and 3-year-olds) with synovitis show a greater degree of localizing inflammatory signs than older horses with chronic osteoarthritis (OA).[12]

Osteoarthritis of the DIP joint is occasionally evidenced by the presence of osteophytes involving the distal aspect of the middle phalanx or the extensor process of the distal phalanx. Generalized suspensory soreness as well as soreness in the area of the bicipital

bursa is often palpated secondary to inflammation of the DIP joint. Back pain may also be associated with the presence of sore feet and can be detrimental to racing performance due to the horse's reluctance to break sharply and extend its stride.[12] These secondary clinical signs usually disappear after resolution of the foot soreness.

Intra-articular anesthesia may be used to localize the lameness. The author uses intra-articular anesthesia in combination with intra-articular medication when necessary to confirm the diagnosis. Radiographs are frequently normal but may show some degree of pedal osteitis, and rarely, navicular syndrome changes.

Anti-inflammatory medications and corrective shoeing are often used to treat the condition. The shoeing is in accordance with individual needs, most commonly backing up the shoe as much as possible and protecting the sole. A wide variety of pads are used, including rim pads, full pads, and aluminum pads with various sole packings. Wedge pads or shoes may be used to correct the low heel conformation but care must be taken because the heel pain is often exacerbated. Some horses are trained in bar shoes until they are ready to race. NSAIDs (usually phenylbutazone) are useful and the feet are iced twice daily during the acute stage.

Intra-articular corticosteroids are effective in relieving the lameness. Betamethasone esters (Celestone Soluspan™) or triamcinolone acetonide (Vetalog™), with or without HA, are preferred by the author, especially if frequent joint injection is necessary. In the author's experience, frequent use of methylprednisolone acetate (Depo-Medrol™) in the coffin joint produces severe cases of OA over time.

Other differential diagnoses of the foot include bruises, abscesses, grabbed quarters, quarter cracks, and laminitis. See Chapter 5.

The Metacarpophalangeal (MCP) Joint

The MCP joint is another frequent site of lameness in Quarter horses. The most common conditions are synovitis/capsulitis, osteochondral chip fractures, osteochondritis dissecans (OCD), OA, and fractures of the proximal sesamoid bones.

Heat and synovial effusion are the first signs of synovitis, along with a varying degree of lameness. The condition is often bilateral and radiographic examination is negative. In the author's opinion, capsulitis does not occur as frequently as in the Thoroughbred because Quarter horses in training gallop less than Thoroughbreds do; therefore, much less stress is placed on the soft tissue structures of the fetlock joint.

Symptomatic treatment includes the use of ice, leg sweats or poultice, and NSAIDS. Intravenous HA (Legend™) or IM PSGAG (Adequan™) are often used as systemic treatments. Intra-articular therapy is very effective in these cases, with a good response from corticosteroids with or without HA. If the condition does not resolve with intra-articular therapy or if it recurs after a brief period of time, the training program should be altered or the risk of further joint damage is likely, with OA as the end result.

Many 2-year-olds are entered in multiple futurities, so training revolves around these races. Trainers try to

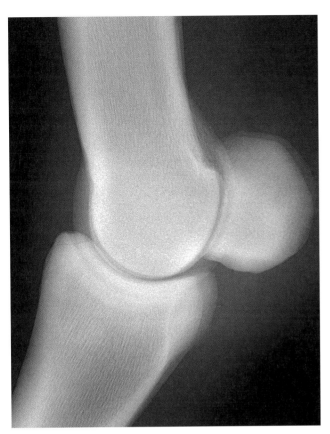

Figure 9.21. Radiograph showing a large P1 osteochondral chip fracture with a large frontal component. (Courtesy of Dr. CW McIlwraith.)

keep horses on schedule for their race dates without sustaining injuries that jeopardize their careers or require extended lay-up periods.

Intra-articular chip fractures of the dorsal aspect of the proximal phalanx are commonly seen in the forelimb of racing Quarter horses (but less than carpal chip fragments). These fractures are considered to be traumatic hyperextension injuries. They occur primarily on the medial aspect, but may also occur laterally.[7] In some cases, they are quite large, especially compared to the fragments that occur in the Thoroughbred, with a long frontal component (Figure 9.21). Horses usually exhibit lameness and synovial effusion, and are positive to flexion of the fetlock joint.

Osteochondritis dissecans (OCD) of the sagittal ridge of the metacarpus and metatarsus is usually noticed when the horse is in early training or still at the farm. It may be seen in either the MCP or metatarsophalangeal joints (more commonly, the latter). The joint is radiographed due to synovial effusion, and varying degrees of lameness may be noted. The defects are recognized on the sagittal ridge, along with fragmentation and loose bodies.

Osteoarthritis may be seen in association with proximal phalanx chip fractures, especially in older horses, and is manifested as wear lines and erosions on the distal metacarpophalangeal articular surface.[7] Defects of the palmar surface of the distal metacarpus are far

less common than in the Thoroughbred, but they do occur in older Quarter horses and the prognosis is similarly poor.

Fractures of the proximal sesamoid bones (apical, abaxial, mid-body, basilar, and comminuted) are relatively common in the Quarter horse, despite such fractures being considered fatigue-related injuries by other authors. Although most often associated with Thoroughbred racing, biaxial and comminuted sesamoid fractures occur in the Quarter horse, resulting in disruption of the suspensory apparatus.

Dorsal Metacarpal Disease

Bucked shins and stress fractures of the dorsal metacarpus are mainly problems of 2-year-old racehorses but are occasionally seen in 3-year-olds. Dorsal metacarpal disease (DMD) is basically a bone-remodeling phenomenon of the dorsal metacarpus along the lines of stress, resulting in various degrees of periostitis and osteoporosis.[14] The incidence is less now that trainers understand this bone remodeling process as it relates to exercise. Stress fractures are most often seen in the 2-year-old year, in contrast to those in Thoroughbreds, which often sustain stress fractures from 3 to 5 years of age.[14] Many of the fractures are longitudinal and cannot be seen to exit the cortex. They may be present bilaterally and the dorsolateral cortex is the most common location, as in the Thoroughbred. Surgery is not indicated with longitudinal fractures because they heal well with rest. Saucer fractures are generally treated with lag screw fixation.

The treatments for DMD are variable, depending on the owner, trainer, and the horse's racing schedule. Extracorporeal shock wave is a popular treatment, but some of the older methods of electrical hyfercation, pin firing, and periosteal scraping are still employed. They are all used with varying degrees of rest, depending on the level of disease.

Proximal Suspensory Desmitis

Proximal suspensory desmitis is usually seen as an acute lameness the day after a workout or race, with profound lameness (4 on a scale of 5). Often it is the fastest horse in the trainer's barn that suffers from this injury. In the acute stage, the horse may walk on the toe without dropping the heel down to contact the ground. Peri-neural anesthesia of the lateral branch of the palmar nerve may be necessary to localize the lameness without blocking the middle carpal joint of the carpus. Radiographs should be taken and an ultrasound examination should be performed. This condition responds well to shock wave treatment and altering the training schedule as necessary.

Tendinitis of the Superficial Flexor Tendon

Superficial flexor tendinitis may be seen in the racing Quarter horse but tends to be related to racetrack surface. The incidence increases with sandier tracks and the condition is more prevalent in horses that race at the 870-yard distance. Diagnosis and treatment are the same as for the racing Thoroughbred.

Arthrosis of the Carpus

Carpal synovitis is the most frequent condition seen in the young racing Quarter horse. Back-in-the-knee conformation is common, and this predisposes to carpal injury during hyperextension of the joint while running. Many 2-year-olds have a large body mass for their age and reach very fast speeds without much prior conditioning. The condition is characterized by heat and synovial effusion of the affected joints with the absence of radiographic changes. Lameness may be present but is generally not severe. Carpal flexion and palpation are used to localize the affected joints. The treatment is the same as for synovitis of the MCP joint.

Osteochondral Chip Fractures of the Carpus

The incidence of osteochondral chip fractures of the carpus is very high in racing Quarter horses. Multiple chip fractures are often seen and many times they are bilateral. The distal radial carpal bone is the most common site for chip fracture, followed by the proximal intermediate carpal bone. It is not uncommon to have distal radial carpal fragments in both middle carpal joints and proximal intermediate carpal bone fragmentation in both antebrachiocarpal joints in the same horse (Figure 9.22).[11]

The diagnosis is generally made by physical examination and digital radiography. The lameness is fairly obvious; most horses have a characteristic wide placement or circumduction of the involved limb at the walk. Most cases are sensitive to flexion of the carpus and palpation of the dorsal surface of the carpal bones. Heat and synovial effusion are often present.

Arthroscopic surgery is the treatment of choice, although some less valuable claiming horses are injected with corticosteroids and raced. Distal radial carpal chips are particularly associated with progressive cartilage damage and OA if the horse continues to race without removal of the chip fracture. Many Quarter horses have multiple surgeries during their racing careers due to the high incidence of osteochondral chip fragmentation.

Other important injuries include the more severe fractures (slab fractures and comminuted fractures), many of which are amenable to surgery. Whenever significant lameness is evident in the carpus, a thorough radiographic examination including skyline views of the carpus is necessary to ensure that degenerative lesions, incomplete sagittal fractures, and any nondisplaced fractures may be seen before a catastrophic injury occurs. All of the reported third carpal bone fractures can be seen in the Quarter horse, with a higher percentage of large frontal slab fractures involving both the radial and intermediate facets (Figure 9.23). The slab is often displaced in these cases, with the distal margin of the radial carpal bone collapsing into the proximal fracture site (Figure 9.24). Lag screw fixation is necessary for proper healing and to prevent further collapse of the joint.

Fractures involving both rows of carpal bones may be seen with some injuries. These can be challenging surgical cases due to the severe damage to the carpal bones and associated joint instability, requiring partial or pan-arthrodesis and the use of multiple bone plates. Most of these injuries can be managed successfully by using aggressive internal fixation techniques to produce pasture-sound breeding animals. Prompt surgical intervention is necessary due to the high risk of laminitis in the contralateral limb.[8]

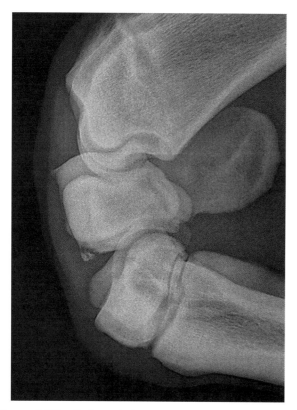

Figure 9.22. Radiograph demonstrating osteochondral chip fragments off the proximal intermediate and distal radial carpal bones (a common combination in the racing Quarter horse). (Courtesy of Dr. CW McIlwraith.)

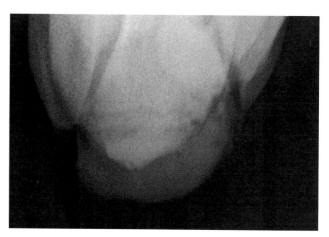

Figure 9.23. Skyline view of the third carpal bone with a slab fracture involving both radial and intermediate facets. (Courtesy of Dr. CW McIlwraith.)

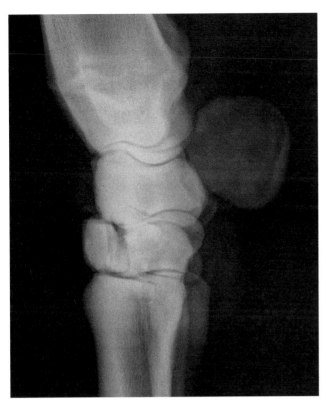

Figure 9.24. Radiograph of a collapsing slab fracture of the third carpal bone with the distal margin of the radial carpal bone collapsing into the proximal fracture site. (Courtesy of Dr. CW McIlwraith.)

Hock Lameness

Lameness associated with the distal tarsal joints, as well as other hind end lameness, is associated with a failure to break sharply from the starting gate. Upper hindlimb flexion tests may be equivocal, but a positive Churchill test along with the history of a poor performance may indicate tarsitis, although a negative test does not rule out the problem. The condition is generally bilateral and the horse may track close behind or cross midline when observed from behind.

Horses that wear patches behind to protect from scalping or horses with laceration marks seen on the medial aspect of the hock are highly suspect for hock soreness. Radiographs are negative in many instances, or subtle changes may be seen. Intra-articular corticosteroids are effective at relieving the lameness and/or improving performance. Even though the tarsometatarsal and centrodistal joints are low-motion joints, maintaining articular cartilage is important because these joints rarely fuse on their own. Betamethasone esters (Celestone Soluspan™) and triamcinolone acetate (Vetalog™) have been shown to have fewer deleterious affects on cartilage than methylprednisolone acetate (Depo-Medrol™).[4,5] If methylprednisolone acetate is used, low doses should be considered (20 to 40 mg).

Stifle Lameness

The most common site of stifle pain is the medial femorotibial joint, which is also the case in racing Thoroughbreds. This can be another cause of poor performance. The horse may be positive to upper hindlimb flexion or palpation but most often intra-articular anesthesia is required to localize the lameness. It is not always clear whether the condition is synovitis or early OA. Radiographs are useful to assess the joint and rule out certain conditions. More recently, ultrasound examination has become useful to pick up soft tissue conditions.[3]

Most stifle lameness responds well to intra-articular therapy; however, if lameness persists, diagnostic arthroscopy is necessary to make a definitive diagnosis. Lameness conditions involving the femoropatellar joint are often accompanied by the presence of joint effusion but in recent years most OCD lesions are operated on before the horse starts racing. Upward fixation of the patella may be an issue in immature horses in early training and subchondral cystic lesions of the medial femoral condyle are a rare but painful condition in the racehorse.

Tibial Stress Fractures

Stress fractures involving the tibia are seen in young horses around the time of their second qualifying work or first race. Diagnosis of the condition has become more common with the advances in imaging techniques and the access to nuclear scintigraphy. The lameness is unilateral and quite severe; the left hind leg is predominantly affected. This may be due to the fact that the horse pulls up quickly from high speed before entering a left-hand turn on the racetrack. If a tibial stress fracture is suspected, nuclear scintigraphy is the best way to demonstrate the injury. Alternatively, digital radiographs taken 1 week to 10 days after injury may show a lesion on the tibia. The horse is usually rested for at least 90 days before resuming training.

Miscellaneous Major Fractures

Proximal sesamoid fractures are the greatest cause of catastrophic injury in the racing Quarter horse. A retrospective study of racing fatalities found that carpal bone and vertebral body fractures were more common in Quarter horses than Thoroughbred racehorses. Sprinting vs. distance racing may play a role in a different distribution of skeletal injuries, but the greatest cause of death for both breeds was found to be fetlock injury.[15]

Fractures involving the back (predominantly lumbar vertebral body) and the distal metacarpus often result in a fall of horse and rider.[10] Falls due to lumbar vertebral fracture have been associated with serious injury to the jockey.

References

1. American Quarter Horse Association Handbook of Rules and Regulations, 2008;111:70.
2. Balch OK, Helman RG, Collier MA. Underrun heels and toe-grab length as possible risk factors for musculoskeletal injuries in Oklahoma racehorses. Proc Am Assoc Equine Pract 2004;47: 334–338.
3. Denoix J-M. Ultrasonographic examination in the diagnosis of joint disease. In Joint Disease in the Horse. McIlwraith CW, Trotter GW, eds. WB Saunders, Philadelphia, 1996;165–202.

4. Frisbie DD, Kawcak CE, Trotter GW, et al. Effects of triamcinolone acetonide on an *in vivo* equine osteochondral fragment exercise model. Equine Vet J 1997;29:349–359.

5. Frisbie DD, Kawcak CE, Baxter GM, et al. Effects of 6-α-methylprednisolone acetate on an *in vivo* equine osteochondral fragment exercise model. Am J Vet Res 1998; 59:1619–1628.

6. Goodman NL. Lameness diagnosis and treatment in the Quarter horse. Vet Clin North Am (Equine Pract) 1990;6:85–108.

7. Kawcak CE, McIlwraith CW. Proximal dorsal first phalanx osteochondral chip fragmentation in 336 horses. Equine Vet J 1994;26:392–396.

8. Lewis RD. Carpal arthrodesis—Indications and Techniques. Proc Am Assoc Equine Pract 2001;7:480–483.

9. Martinelli MJ, Overly LR, McIlwraith CW. Survey of horseshoe characteristics and their relationship to catastrophic injuries in a population of racing Quarter horses. Proc Am Assoc Equine Pract 2009;55:226–228.

10. Martinelli MJ, Overly LR, McIlwraith CW. Observations related to catastrophic injuries in racing Quarter horses from 2005 to 2008. Proc Am Assoc Equine Pract 2009;55:187–189.

11. McIlwraith CW, Yovich JB, Martin GS. Arthroscopic surgery for the treatment of osteochondral chip fractures in the equine carpus. J Am Vet Med Assoc 1987;191:531–540.

12. McIlwraith CW, Goodman NL. Conditions of the interphalangeal joints. Vet Clin North Am (Equine Pract) 1989;5:161.

13. McIlwraith CW, Anderson TM, Sanschi EM. Conformation and musculoskeletal problems in the racehorse. Clinical Tech Equine Pract 2003;2:339–347.

14. Nunamaker DM. The bucked shin complex. Proc Am Assoc Equine Pract 1986;32:457.

15. Sarrafian TL, Case JT, Kinde H, et al. Fatal musculoskeletal injuries of Quarter horse racehorses in California. Proc Am Assoc Equine Pract 2009;55:1909–191.

THE ENDURANCE HORSE

Todd C. Holbrook

THE SPORT

The sport of equine endurance has grown substantially since the American Endurance Ride Conference (AERC) was established as the national governing body for long distance riding in 1972. Under current rules, the AERC recognizes endurance competitions that cover distances of at least 50 miles per day, up to a maximum distance of 150 miles in 3 days. Pioneer rides may be up to 5 days in duration; in that case, 1 day must be 55 miles and the remaining are 50 miles.[2]

The sport originated in the United States, where the Western States Trail Ride 100-mile competition (also known as the Tevis Cup) has been held in the Sierra mountain range since 1955. Endurance events covering a minimal distance of 80 km were recognized as an international sport by the Federation Equestre Internationale (FEI) in 1978. The sport has subsequently undergone tremendous growth internationally. In 2010, a new world record was set in a 100-mile (160-km) endurance competition in Abu Dhabi, United Arab Emirates. The winning time was 6 hours, 21 minutes, 12 seconds, at a speed of 25.18 km/hour.[3] The trend of faster speeds associated with less technically demanding competitions in international events in comparison to national events is well recognized.

Typically, AERC rides are comprised of both limited distance competitions (25 to 35 miles), and AERC-recognized endurance competitions, ranging from 50 to 100 miles. Over the past 3 ride seasons (2005 to 2008) in the United States, the AERC recognized an average of 278 yearly rides in which 22,317 horses competed each year.[2] While completion rates typically vary with ride conditions and level of competition, the average completion rate over the past 3 AERC seasons has been 85.8% ± 0.2% to 0.5%.[2] Completion rates for international competitions are not typically this high. In a recent review of 120- and 160-km FEI competitions from 8 world regions from 2005 to 2007, completion rates varied from approximately 40% to 75%. Furthermore, a notable inverse relationship has developed between mean competition speeds and completion rates in 160-km races over the last 20 years (personal communication, David Marlin 2009). In both national and international venues, the primary reason for elimination from endurance competition is lameness.

ATHLETES AND EXERCISE CONDITIONS

The suitability of pure Arabians and Arabian crosses is well recognized for long distance aerobic exercise. However, most endurance rides are open to horses of other breeds, with the exception of breed sanctioned competitions (i.e., Arabian Horse Association).

Frequently, suitable athletes compete from the age of eligibility for 8 to 12 years. It is not uncommon for some horses to compete well into their 20s. The current minimum age limit is 5 years for AERC and novice levels of FEI competition.[2,4] FEI competitions are categorized by course difficulty: horses must be 6 years old to enter 1* and 2* rides, 7 years old to enter 3* rides, and 8 years old to enter 4* rides.[4]

Although most competitive horses in the sport are of Arabian influence, their individual conformation can vary widely. Those with a long competitive career usually have few striking conformational flaws; however many horses with less-than-perfect foot conformation (e.g., toed in or out, high/low heel, contracted heels, etc.) or limb conformation (e.g., post legged, sickle hocked, etc.) can be competitive in the sport. Coupled with the magnitude of distance covered, the environmental conditions in terms of both topographical terrain variation as well as heat and humidity extremes create exercise conditions that are among the most challenging of any equine sport. Lameness, followed by metabolic disturbances, are the 2 most common reasons for elimination during competition.

VETERINARY CONTROL

Endurance is one of the most stringently controlled equine sports in terms of veterinary oversight during competition. Horses are initially examined prior to the ride to determine suitability to enter competition. The examination includes a basic physical and lameness examination. At the pre-ride inspection, joint or tendon sheath effusion and abrasions or scars are entered on the ride card horse diagram, similar to markings on a Coggin's form (Figure 9.25).[2]

The ride is divided into segments or phases. An examination determines fitness to continue at the end of each phase at a veterinary check point or "vet gate." Short rides may only have 1 vet gate, whereas 160-km competitions may have as many as 7. Physical examination parameters evaluated and recorded on the ride card at each vet gate include temperature, pulse and respiratory rate (TPR), mucous membrane character, capillary refill time, jugular vein refill, skin turgor, gastrointestinal sounds, back and withers sensitivity, rubs or sores from the bit or tack, muscle tone, anal tone, gait, impulsion, and overall impression. Criteria are recorded on a ride card using a scale of A to D, with A considered normal (Figure 9.25).[2]

Horses must meet a pulse criterion that is set prior to competition (usually 64 beats/minute within 30 minutes of entering the vet gate). A cardiac recovery index is determined in conjunction with the lameness examination by assessing the heart rate before and 1 minute after initiating an 80-meter trot (40 meters out and back). After the trot-out, if the horse's heart rate increases by 4 or more beats, metabolic criteria coupled with other physical exam findings are scrutinized in more depth to determine fitness to continue competition. Horses with synchronous diaphragmatic flutter

RIDE NAME_____ DATE_____ DISTANCE_____

Rider Name _____ Weight Division _____

Junior Rider _____ Sponsor's Name (Juniors) _____

Horse Name _____ Age_____ Breed_____ Color_____

RIDER #

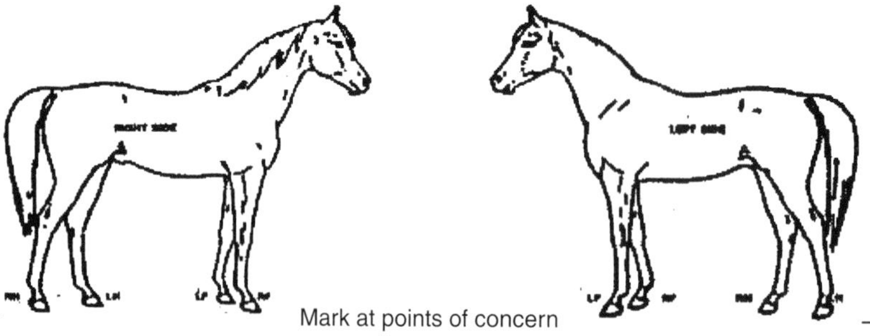

_____   Mark at points of concern   _____
_____   (can use contrasting color at final)   _____

Pre-Ride (First) Examination				Post-Ride (Final) Examination		
P_____				P_____		
R_____				R_____		Heart Rate
T_____				T_____		Recovery Index
Parameter	A,B,C,D	Comments		Parameter	A,B,C,D	Comments
Mucous Membranes				Mucous Membranes		
Capillary Refill				Capillary Refill		
Jugular Refill				Jugular Refill		
Gut Sounds				Gut Sounds		
Skin Tenting				Skin Tenting		
Anal Tone				Anal Tone		
Muscle Tone				Muscle Tone		
Back Withers				Back Withers		
Tack Galls				Tack Galls		
Wounds				Wounds		
Gait				Gait		
Impulsion				Impulsion		
Attitude				Attitude		
Overall Impression				Overall Impression		
Signature of Examiner_____				Signature of Examiner_____		
Reason of elimination_____ Signature_____						

A. file: RideCard 4/04 1.0

Figure 9.25. A. Front of a typical AERC ride card. B. Back of a typical AERC ride card.

coupled with evidence of significant metabolic distress are eliminated from competition. Those eliminated from competition by the control veterinary staff are typically referred to a treatment veterinarian for further evaluation and treatment on site.

Lameness is evaluated on the American Association of Equine Practitioners (AAEP) scale of 1 to 5. See Table 3.2 in Chapter 3. Competitors may not enter or proceed in the ride on a horse with lameness of grade 3 or higher. Typically the footing for lameness examination areas is well planned and controlled at international ride venues, whereas at regional AERC rides the footing and terrain

may be quite variable at the vet gates (Figure 9.26). Occasionally, when level topography is unavailable and the footing is inconsistent the lameness examination can be more challenging.

Maximum ride times are typically 12 and 24 hours for 50- and 100-mile competitions, respectively. In most rides the top 10 finishers are evaluated 1 hour after completion to determine best condition (BC). In contrast to examinations during competition, the BC exam often includes limb palpation and mild flexion. Similar to the routine exams during competition, horses are evaluated for lameness at a trot. In addition, during the

RIDER #_____   NAME_____

CHECK	#1	#2	#3	#4	#5	#6
ARRIVAL TIME						
PR TIME						
PULSE						
OUT TIME						
Mucous Membranes						
Capillary Refill						
Jugular Refill						
Gut Sounds						
Skin Tenting						
Anal Tone						
Muscle Tone						
Back Withers						
Tack Galls						
Wounds						
Gait						
Impulsion						
Attitude						
Overall Impression						
COMMENTS						
Heart Rate Recovery						
#1						
#2						
Examiner						

Figure 9.25. (*Continued*) B.

BC lameness examination, horses are also frequently evaluated in a circle in both directions.

Performance-enhancing medications are not allowed during endurance competitions and both the FEI and AERC governing bodies use random drug testing for prohibited substances.

THE LAMENESS EXAMINATION

It is not uncommon for an individual to perform several hundred lameness exams during any given ride, depending on entries, ride distance, and number of ride veterinarians. This provides a great training ground for students and new graduates as well as an enjoyable working environment for practitioners who are sports medicine enthusiasts.

As indicated above, lameness examinations during competition are typically limited to observation from a distance, with the exception of the foot evaluation. While limb palpation and joint flexion are used during the BC exam, this depth of examination during competition is typically reserved for horses that are eliminated to direct further diagnostics and treatment. If a soft tissue injury is suspected in horses with only a grade 1 or 2 lameness at a vet gate, the flexor surfaces are frequently palpated when considering elimination. Consistent examination of the foot also is important in these horses because removing a rock lodged in the frog sulcus or replacing a lost, displaced, or bent shoe may resolve or improve the lameness and allow the horse to continue (Figure 9.27). Thus, riders have the option to re-present for lameness evaluation after farriery.

Horses with grade 3 or greater lameness are eliminated from further competition and referred to the treatment veterinarian. Elimination of horses with grade 1 to 2 lameness is at the discretion of the control veterinarian and depends on the suspected underlying cause. Most horses with undetermined causes of lameness of this grade are allowed to continue, whereas elimination of horses with consistent sensitivity over the suspensory or flexor tendons is prudent. Prior to elimination at FEI and AERC national championship rides, it is common for a panel of 3 veterinary judges to observe the trot-out and vote with the majority consensus taken.

COMMON CAUSES OF LAMENESS

Lameness is by far the most common indication for elimination from endurance competition. Based on AERC post ride statistical reports, of 21,933 starts

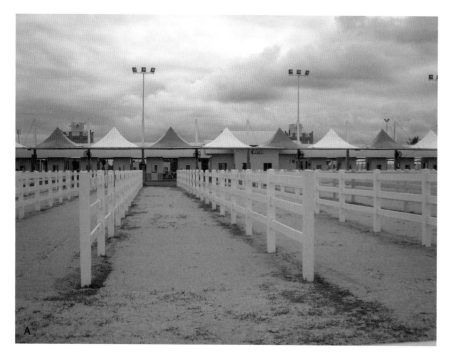

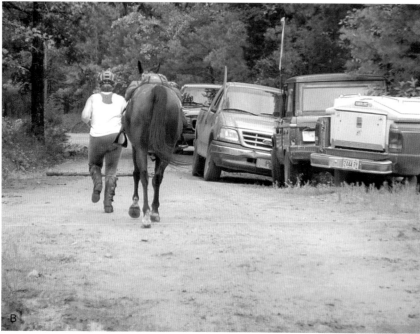

Figure 9.26. A. Veterinary gate trot-out area for the FEI World Endurance Championships in Terengganu, Malaysia in 2008. B. Veterinary gate trot-out area at an AERC ride near Poteau, OK.

during the 2007–2008 ride season, 1,410 horses were eliminated for lameness, accounting for 44% of all eliminations. Of these, the majority were unlocalized front limb (45.9%) and hindlimb (23.4%) lameness conditions. Keep in mind that diagnoses at the vet gate are based on brief examination only, usually without even the benefit of hoof testers, and definitely without the use of diagnostic nerve blocks. Considering the defined causes of lameness, hindlimb muscle comprised 9.4% of all lameness problems, followed by front suspensory (4.9%), front foot (4.4%), front tendon (3.3%), front muscle (2.5%), front joint (2.1%), hind tendon (1.1%), hind foot (0.78%), other front ligament (0.71%), other hind ligament (0.64%), hind joint (0.57%), and hind suspensory (0.28%).

Many causes of lameness in endurance athletes are transient, leading to elimination from competition on ride day, but resolving after rest with or without the benefit of anti-inflammatory treatment. Often, the exact cause of lameness in these situations is not specifically determined. Recurrent problems or significant acute soft tissue or orthopedic injuries are more likely to result in a full diagnostic and therapeutic approach similar to that performed for any other sport horse.

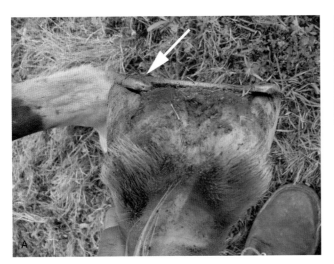 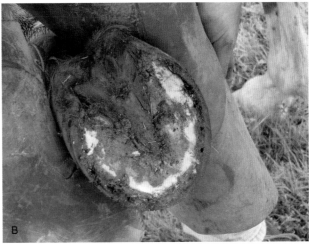

Figure 9.27. A. 50-mile endurance horse with grade 3 lameness of the left front limb. Note the displacement of the medial branch of the shoe and the compression of the heel (arrow).

B. Medial heel bruise that was evident after shoe removal. The medial heel was floated and the shoe straightened and replaced. Subsequently, the horse was sound enough to continue competition.

Muscle Disorders

Certain occupational conditions are common in the sport of endurance, including exertional rhabdomyolysis and other muscle disorders primarily of the hindlimbs, back, and neck. Data regarding the prevalence of exertional rhabdomyolysis in endurance horses is limited. Of 21,933 starts in the AERC 2007–2008 ride season, 2.19% were eliminated for rhabdomyolysis. Myopathy that may or may not be associated with overt signs of tying up is likely much more common. As indicated above, AERC post ride statistical data suggest that hindlimb myopathy is the most common cause of defined lameness in endurance horses. Subclinical myopathy may also predispose to the development of compensatory lameness.

In a recent study of 36 elite horses competing in a 160-km FEI 3-star competition, 22 horses that successfully completed had abnormally high mean creatine kinase (CK) activity (22,473 ± 41,192 IU/L) compared to pre-ride concentrations (702 ± 720 IU/L). Although there was no difference in CK activity between finishers and nonfinishers, 2 horses eliminated for lameness had the highest CK values (240,000 to 400,000 IU/L).[6]

Exertional rhabdomyolysis usually develops early in the ride (fewer than 15 miles), is often associated with anxiety, and may be influenced by cold weather and inadequate warm-up. Myopathy also develops late in the ride (more than 50 miles) and is associated with exhaustion or abrupt changes in footing (i.e., muddy hill work). Most commonly, the gluteals and lumbar epaxial muscles are affected. The gluteal and/or lower lumbar epaxial muscles may be affected asymmetrically, resulting in pronounced unilateral swelling or firmness in a specific area (e.g., middle gluteals). The most common gait abnormality is a shortened anterior stride phase at a walk. Further exercise is contraindicated with significant rhabdomyolysis, and aggressive treatment is warranted in most affected horses.

The primary goal of treatment is fluid diuresis until gross pigmenturia is resolved. Analgesics may be necessary in some horses. Doses of flunixin meglumine and other toxic NSAIDs should be minimized in the face of dehydration. Portable biochemistry analyzers are commonly used by treatment veterinarians, at even small local endurance rides. Field evaluation of serum electrolytes, muscle enzymes, and renal parameters in these patients helps to guide therapy.

Although the efficacy of dantrolene in the treatment of acute rhabdomyolysis in horses has not been well studied, its role in preventing recurrent episodes is established. In treadmill studies, dantrolene sodium (4 mg/kg PO) reduced biochemical evidence of muscle damage in Thoroughbreds with recurrent exertional rhabdomyolysis.[5] In addition, dantrolene reduced recurrent episodes of rhabdomyolysis in racing Thoroughbreds.[1] Although dantrolene cannot be used during competition due to medication rules, it is commonly used as an effective preventative in the training of elite Arabian endurance horses with recurrent myopathy.

Muscle spasms or cramps and muscle strains are also quite common in the sport. The gluteal muscles are commonly affected, but other muscle groups, including the gracilis, lumbar, triceps, biceps, forearm, and pectoral muscles, may be involved. Occasionally horses with muscle spasms are acutely painful; they may collapse and show signs similar to those of acute colic. These individuals usually benefit from prompt analgesic treatment. Most often an α-2 agonist (e.g., detomidine, xylazine) with or without a narcotic (butorphanol) is more effective and safer compared to high doses of NSAIDs, considering the likelihood of significant concurrent dehydration. Massage therapy, stretching or walking, and topical heat may help treat muscle cramps. On-site serum biochemical analysis in these patients is prudent because it may reveal electrolyte imbalances, necessitating correction.

Muscle pain affecting the back and skin sensitivity of the saddle and girth regions are common in endurance horses. It is likely both are related to rider imbalance and poor saddle fit, and compensatory back pain may develop secondary to hock lameness. In the neck region, sensitivity of the strap muscles in front of the shoulder (brachiocephalicus m.) is very common and likely develops as a consequence of forelimb lameness (usually in the feet or ankles), or fatigue.

More rarely, frank muscle tears may cause acute lameness. Occasionally, local hematomas may form. Rest and NSAIDs (post-rehydration) usually lead to full recovery.

Suspensory Desmitis

Forelimb suspensory desmitis (SD) is common in endurance horses, affecting both the proximal area and branches. Hindlimb suspensory desmitis is less common, but likely has a similar pathogenesis and the treatment options are identical. SD usually develops when local footing consists of deep sand, soft soil, or mud. Hence, in areas such the United Arab Emirates, suspensory desmitis is the most common cause of lameness in endurance horses. The diagnosis is suspected based on palpation of the limb and is confirmed by ultrasonography (Figure 9.28). The author's impression is that medial/lateral hoof imbalance predisposes endurance horses to suspensory branch desmitis. With branch lesions, usually only one branch is affected; therefore, notable swelling may be evident on palpation compared to the opposite branch or leg. In contrast, lesions of the proximal suspensory and body may be less obviously swollen, and diagnosis is usually based on sensitivity to palpation and ultrasound. Subtle, recurrent lameness associated with proximal SD may require diagnostic nerve blocks followed by ultrasonography for confirmation.

After an acute injury, the character of the ultrasonographic lesion severity may worsen over time, so serial examinations to follow lesion progression are recommended. Response to topical ice therapy can be dramatic and is warranted for the first 24 hours post injury. This should be followed by intermittent ice or cold water therapy and bandage support. After rehydration, NSAID treatment for the first 5 to 10 days post-injury is typical. The prognosis for return to function is good in horses with mild desmitis. Those with minimal to no ultrasonographic changes may only need 3 to 4 weeks of stall rest and hand walking before gradually returning to work under saddle, with an additional 4 to 6 weeks of walk/light trot intervals prior to returning to training work. With significant lesion size, long-term rest (minimum 6 to 8 months) is prudent. Horses with significant desmitis are best managed with a well controlled exercise program in which the intensity and duration of work is gradually increased over 6 to 12 months. This is often guided by improvement in lameness, and ligament healing based on serial ultrasonographic evaluations.

Foot Lameness

Foot conditions are common causes of lameness in endurance horses. If time permitted more routine use of the hoof tester at the vet gate examination during endurance events, the AERC post ride statistic results mentioned above would likely be quite different. Often evaluation of the digital pulse and comparison of its pre and post trot quality can be informative. Common conditions include foot bruising, corns, dislodged or sprung shoes, and heel bulb trauma from overreaching or other sources of injury.

Endurance horses are also subject to acute laminitis which may be related to repetitive concussive laminar trauma or associated with systemic exertional disease syndromes (e.g., heat stress, exhaustion, rhabdomyolysis, and renal failure). Severe laminitis may necessitate euthanasia. Aggressive medical treatment for acute laminitis is indicated in any endurance horse with prodromal signs thereof (shifting weight, forelimb lameness while turning, bounding digital pulses, etc). Early treatment is important because consistent clinical prognostic indicators are unclear. It is quite common for certain horses to develop horizontal hoof cracks as the hoof grows out

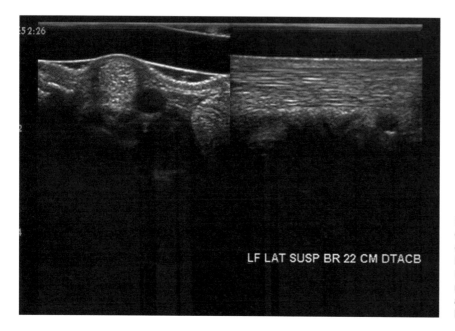

LF LAT SUSP BR 22 CM DTACB

Figure 9.28. Ultrasonographic image of the lateral suspensory branch from an endurance horse that developed grade 3 lameness after 83 miles of competition. Enlargement and fiber disruption were minimal, and the horse returned to work after several weeks of rest. (Courtesy of Dr. Patty Doyle.)

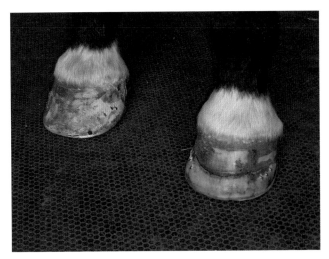

Figure 9.29. Typical horizontal hoof cracks common in competing endurance horses. (Courtesy of Wendy Bejarano.)

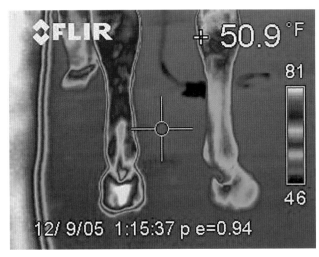

Figure 9.30. Thermographic image of an endurance horse with flexor tendinitis of the left forelimb. (Courtesy of Dr. Ken Marcella.)

that serve as a timeline of when laminitis may have occurred at previous competitive rides. (Figure 9.29). The majority of these horses complete the ride and do not develop lameness; thus, it is unclear whether this truly represents a laminitic event. Very rarely subsolar hematoma formation can cause acute lameness that can mimic acute traumatic laminitis in endurance horses.

Tendinitis

Superficial digital flexor tendinitis (SDFT) is a common cause of lameness in endurance horses, especially in the forelimb. While tendinitis occurs less commonly in the hindlimb, it appears to be more prevalent in the sport of endurance compared to other disciplines. Deep digital flexor tendinitis occurs less commonly than SDFT, but appears to have a predilection for the hindlimb in endurance horses. Clinical diagnosis is based on palpation and confirmed by ultrasonography. Thermography can be used to confirm regional hyperthermia associated with acute soft tissue injuries (Figure 9.30). Similar to other soft tissue injuries, early ice therapy and NSAIDs after rehydration are warranted. Rest duration, rehabilitation, and prognosis depend on lesion severity and location.

Other Causes of Lameness

Acute joint sprain is not uncommon and is often influenced by the condition of the trail footing. Although the fetlock appears to be more commonly affected, slipping on trail can potentially result in soft tissue injury of any other joint. Interference injury, especially of the medial fetlock of the hindlimb, is common, and occasionally lameness can result (Figure 9.31).

Splints can cause acute lameness and are likely more common during training, especially in horses with less than ideal forelimb conformation. This condition typically responds well to conservative treatment and rest. Recurrent lameness is uncommon unless there is impingement on the suspensory apparatus that causes chronic desmitis.

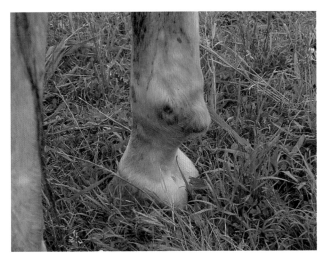

Figure 9.31. Interference lesion at the medial aspect of the right hind fetlock.

Chronic osteoarthritis affecting the metacarpophalangeal and hock joints is not uncommon. Prognosis with significant degenerative disease is guarded with the exception of distal tarsitis, which may respond well to intra-articular corticosteroids, enabling continued work.

References

1. Edwards JG, Newton JR, Ramzan PH, et al. The efficacy of dantrolene sodium in controlling exertional rhabdomyolysis in the Thoroughbred racehorse. Equine Vet J 2003;35:707–711.
2. www.aerc.org/.
3. www.endurance.net/international/UAE/2010PresidentsCup/.
4. www.fei.org/Disciplines/Endurance/Rules/Pages/Regulations.aspx.
5. McKenzie EC, Valberg SJ, Godden SM, et al. Effect of oral administration of dantrolene sodium on serum creatine kinase activity after exercise in horses with exertional rhabdomyolysis. Am J Vet Res 2004;65:74–79.
6. Schott HC 2nd, Marlin DJ, Geor RJ, et al. Changes in selected physiologic and laboratory measurements in elite horses competing in a 160-km endurance ride. Equine Vet J Suppl 2006; 36:37–42.

SHOW/PLEASURE HORSES

Ellis G. Farstvedt

PLEASURE HORSE/SHOW HORSE SPORT

Western Pleasure showing is a popular sport among Quarter horse enthusiasts. The American Quarter Horse Association (AQHA) maintains the integrity of this breed.[2] In 2008 the AQHA recorded nearly 850,000 total show entries with nearly 3,000 approved shows, and total World Show prize money was reported at $2.7 million.[3] The specific number of Western Pleasure entries was not reported; however, that is one of the most popular classes.[1] The AQHA has established comprehensive rules that safeguard the welfare of the horse while providing a level playing field for showing.[2] It is recommended that veterinarians working within this discipline be familiar with these regulations prior to administering treatments.

According to the AQHA, Western Pleasure horses should have a free-flowing stride of reasonable length in keeping with its conformation.[2] They should have a balanced, flowing motion while exhibiting the correct gaits in proper cadence.[2] Head carriage should be at the level of the withers or slightly above and should extend past vertical in the frontal plane.

The 3 standard gaits are the walk, jog, and lope. The lope can appear unusual to veterinarians because this show gait does not reflect the average motion of a Quarter horse that is not trained in this discipline. It is the most difficult of the 3 gaits required for the Western Pleasure horse.[1] During the lope the hindlimbs are driven up under the horse, thereby allowing the epaxial and hindlimb muscles to elevate the front end of the horse, resulting in forelimb advancement with minimal to no carpal flexion. This movement produces the flat knee gait that is characteristic of the Western Pleasure horse, and it is awarded accordingly by judges. The walk and jog more similarly reflect gaits of the average Quarter horse but are typically at a slower cadence with a flat knee. Maximum show credits "should be given to the flowing, balanced and willing horse that gives the appearance of being fit and a pleasure to ride," according to the AQHA Official Handbook of Rules and Regulations.[2]

The most critical component for a veterinarian handling orthopedic problems in the show horse is communication and establishing oneself as part of a team that usually includes an owner, trainer, and farrier. Many times the orthopedic veterinarian is just a part of the medical team, which may also include general practice veterinarians, acupuncturists, chiropractors, naturopaths, etc. One of the greatest challenges facing veterinarians in this discipline is trying to determine whether the horse is a poor athlete, being ridden poorly, or has an orthopedic problem. Spending time with an accomplished trainer in the field and obtaining some knowledge of this industry helps the veterinarian immensely in becoming familiar with its standards. The orthopedic problems that occur in the pleasure horse

are similar to those of other disciplines. There is limited statistical information regarding frequency of specific injuries, but the author's clinical experience suggests that problems occur most frequently in the front feet, followed by pain originating in the tarsus, suspensory ligaments, stifles, and back.

To be successful in the pleasure horse arena, the horses must be quiet and calm while being shown. To accomplish this without the use of illegal substances, many horses are exercised for prolonged time periods before entering the show pen. This activity tends to result in fatigue-related injuries and diseases such as synovitis, myositis, tendinitis, and desmitis.

MUSCULOSKELETAL PROBLEMS IN THE FORELIMB

Typical foot care in the pleasure horse consists of applying wedged aluminum shoes to the front hooves and flat steel shoes to the rear hooves. The front shoes may consist of aluminum egg bars, wedged aluminum shoes, or various assortments of wedged pads in combination with shoes (Figures 9.32 and 9.33). The wedged conformation in the front feet provides relief in the break-over phase of the stride, translating to less carpal movement (flat knee), which is desirable in this show discipline. Coffin joint synovitis is a common finding in

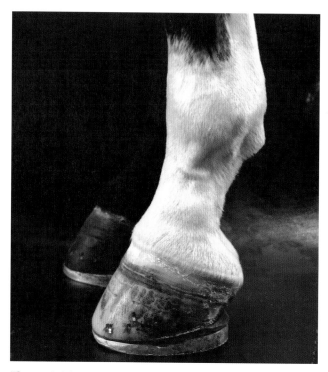

Figure 9.32. Example of a wedge pad and wedged shoe to create alignment of the foot pastern axis.

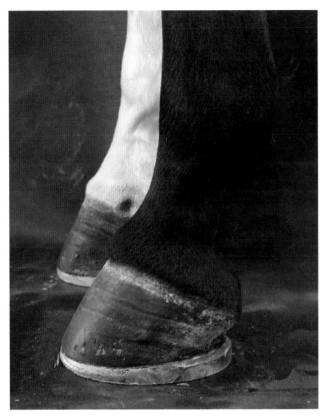

Figure 9.33. Example of wedged front shoes typically seen in the Western Pleasure show horse.

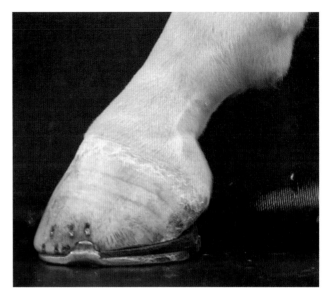

Figure 9.34. The use of a wedged shoe in the hindlimb to treat tarsal pain.

these horses; it typically manifests as forelimb lameness with coffin joint effusion. Diagnostic anesthesia isolates the lameness to the foot, and radiographic changes are uncommon.

In observing these horses at shows, it is clear that a majority of horses land toe-first or flat footed in the front feet. Clinical experience suggests that toe-first landing has a strong correlation to suspensory desmitis. The theory is that gradual tensile forces applied to the suspensory ligament through heel-first landing and transition to full weight-bearing are lost when a horse lands toe first. With toe-first landing, the suspensory ligament bears a minimal load until the instant of weight-bearing when the heels contact the ground and the flexor structures of the metacarpus experience instant maximum load. The suspensory ligament seems to be the most affected structure in the palmar metacarpus, possibly because of its origin and insertion in bone and lack of a muscle belly to absorb tensile forces.

These horses typically present with mild to moderate forelimb lameness with some degree of pain palpable in the proximal palmar metacarpus. At times they show lameness with the affected limb on the outside of a circle, but this finding is inconsistent because many of these horses also have foot pain that is exacerbated with the limb on the inside of the circle. Some patients exhibit a positive response to phalangeal and/or carpal flexion. Holding firm pressure over the proximal suspensory region for 30 to 45 seconds and trotting them off occasionally exacerbates the lameness.

Proper progression of diagnostic anesthesia is required to definitively identify the area of pain. The author prefers to anesthetize the foot with palmar digital nerve blocks and/or abaxial nerve blocks, followed by a low 4-point block. After that, the deep branch of the lateral palmar nerve is blocked. Palpable pain in the proximal suspensory region should be absent if the deep branch of the lateral palmar nerve is anesthetized properly. This progression of blocks isolates the region of interest to the proximal palmar metacarpus. It is important to review the anatomical structures anesthetized with this block. Imaging of this region is commonly performed with ultrasound. MRI imaging of this region is a valuable modality as well because of the limited sensitivity of ultrasound.

MUSCULOSKELETAL PROBLEMS OF THE HINDLIMB

The most common hindlimb problem in pleasure horses appears to involve the tarsus. Among most trainers, the tarsus is arguably the most common overall performance-limiting lameness in this discipline. Often these horses present with generalized poor performance. The horses commonly do not exhibit clinical baseline lameness and not all of them exhibit a response to tarsal flexion. When observed under saddle, these horses tend to have a subtle decreased anterior stride phase or axial stabbing when the affected limb is placed on the inside of the circle. Some horses with tarsal pain respond favorably to heel wedges placed on the hind feet (Figure 9.34).

As with other disciplines that require hard work from the hindquarters there are other areas that require attention, particularly the rear feet and suspensory ligaments. Problems in these areas are often mistaken for tarsal pain; therefore, a thorough lameness evaluation with diagnostic anesthesia and appropriate imaging is recommended.

A negative solar angle of the distal phalanx tends to be a common problem in the hind feet. These horses typically present with lameness, are phalangeal flexion positive, and usually block with a plantar digital nerve block. Occasionally the digital tendon sheath is concurrently effusive and painful to palpation, which may warrant further investigation and/or treatment. The dorsal hoof wall typically has a bullnosed appearance with a short heel. A lateral radiograph shows the position of the distal phalanx within the hoof capsule and helps guide corrective trimming and shoeing.

The author likes to leave approximately 1 to 1.2 cm of toe sole depth when performing the trim and correct the remaining angle deficit with a heel wedge if needed. If the horn tissue of the heels is solid and healthy, the author takes minimal to no depth in that area. However, if the tissue is unstable or crushed, the author recommends trimming to solid horn, after which the foot frequently requires a heel wedge to correct the solar angle of the distal phalanx (Figure 9.35). The aim is to obtain at least 3° elevation with the first trim and usually settle with about 4° to 5° after a couple of shoeing intervals. Typically, the author tends to get a good clinical result if the hind distal phalanx can be elevated at least 3°. See chapters 3 and 12 for further information on this topic.

Hindlimb suspensory pain occurs in this discipline. The author's approach for diagnosis is similar to that outlined for the forelimb, with the proper progression of diagnostic anesthesia and imaging. Concomitant disease in the tarsometatarsal joint makes diagnosis a challenge at times because of the lack of specificity with diagnostic anesthesia in this location. MRI imaging of hindlimb suspensory ligament disease is very valuable in determining the definitive diagnosis as well as location and severity of disease. Identifying lesions by ultrasonography is a challenge in this region and has less sensitivity than MRI imaging.

The stifles and hindlimb pastern joints also are affected. Lameness in these areas is diagnosed with routine examination and diagnostic anesthesia. The disease processes are typical of the general horse population.

MUSCULOSKELETAL PROBLEMS OF THE AXIAL SKELETON

Problems in the axial skeleton typically involve pain in the caudal lumbar muscles or sacroiliac region. The horse usually presents with complaints of back pain or not collecting in the hindquarters. Firm downward pressure on the tuber sacrale typically elicits a painful response evidenced by muscle fasciculations in the caudal lumbar epaxial muscles and/or a sitting posture. Caudal lumbar epaxial muscle soreness is palpated with a flat palm and firm pressure. A painful response is typically seen with tensing of the muscles and resistance to motion of that area. Acupuncture examinations are useful to show specific areas of reactivity that can be treated. Chiropractic examination and manipulation can help identify problem areas and may provide treatment.

GENERAL TREATMENT RECOMMENDATIONS

Problems in pleasure horses are treated similarly to those in other disciplines; however, veterinarians must be familiar with drug use regulations put forth by the AQHA which are updated and amended frequently. Some medications are allowed under a threshold and others have zero tolerance; therefore, dosage and frequency of administration are important. One challenge facing veterinarians at shows is recommending whether to continue or discontinue showing. The ultimate decision rests with the owner and/or trainer. Predicting future events in a horse's health or soundness is impossible, yet the veterinarian can provide sound medical information based on the exam and/or diagnostics that can help with these decisions. Communication with all parties involved is essential because some continue to show horses with minor injuries or soreness, and others elect not to do so.

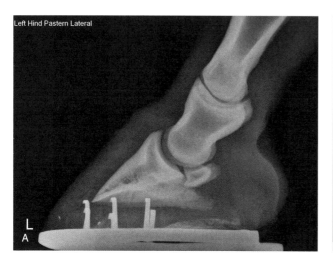
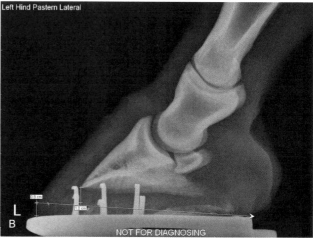

Figure 9.35.   A. Lateral radiograph of a hind foot illustrating a negative solar plane angle of the third phalanx. B. Determining the depth at which to safely trim the toe for correction of the negative solar angle.

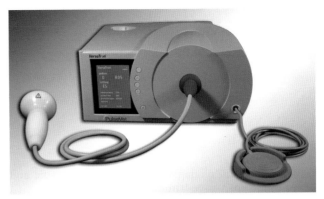

Figure 9.37. Versa Tron shockwave used to treat soft tissue injuries. (Courtesy of Pulse Veterinary Technologies LLC, Alpharetta, GA.)

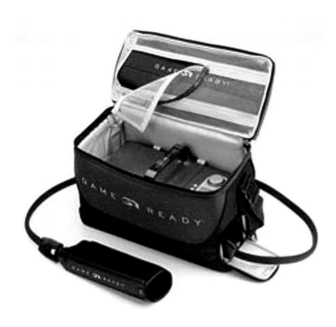

Figure 9.36. Game Ready™ Equine used to apply cold compression therapy to acute injuries. (Courtesy of Game Ready™, Alameda, CA, 2009.)

Acute synovitis (e.g., minimal radiographic changes) and tenosynovitis cases are usually medicated intrasynovially with 6 to 10 mg/joint triamcinolone acetonide (Kenalog or Vetalog) in combination with 20 mg of sodium hyaluronate (Hylartin V). The author tries not to exceed a 20-mg total body dose of triamcinolone, but has given total doses up to 40 mg without complications. For low-motion joints with radiographic evidence of osteoarthritis, the author typically gives 40 to 80 mg/joint methyl prednisolone acetate (Depo Medrol). Other intra-articular medications that are used commonly, depending on the case, include intra-articular Adequan and interleukin-1 receptor antagonist protein (IRAP) therapy (Arthrex Vet Systems). Horses can be ridden 24 hours after treatment, but results tend to be better if they are rested at least 2 days.

Acute tendinitis and desmitis diseases are typically treated with cold compression therapy at 36° to 40°F for 30 minutes with intermittent compression (Game Ready Equine™; Figure 9.36). The author then applies a cooling mud poultice for 12 hours. Shockwave therapy is used for pain management and to aid in healing, typically at a power setting of E4 and a dose range of 1,000 to 1,500 pulses (Figure 9.37). The use of shockwave therapy and the dose administered depends on the case and the stage of injury and/or healing.

Pain in various regions such as the epaxial, gluteal, neck, and shoulder muscle groups can be treated with a multitude of therapies. Muscle relaxant medications such as dantrolene sodium (Dantrium) or methocarbamol (Robaxin) and/or NSAIDs can be used in accordance with AQHA regulations. Shockwave therapy also alleviates pain and decreases muscle tension. Many other treatments have value as well, including electrical stimulation acupuncture, local injections, chiropractic manipulation, massage therapy, mesotherapy, and electromagnetic pulse therapy.

The competing Western Pleasure show horse can and will present with multiple performance-limiting problems—riding issues, training problems, medical conditions, or orthopedic conditions. Sorting through all of these potential sources for a performance problem can be difficult, and the veterinarian often works with several individuals to determine whether musculoskeletal problems exist. The majority of orthopedic cases can be diagnosed with thorough examination, proper diagnostic anesthesia, and appropriate imaging. Treatments before and during the shows must be in accordance with regulations governing the particular discipline.

References

1. Noble JK. Lameness in the Western Performance Horse. Proceedings Am Assoc Equine Pract 2001;47:12.
2. Official Handbook of Rules and Regulations, American Quarter Horse Association 2008;9:208–210.
3. www.aqha.com/association/pdf/showstats08.pdf.

THE WESTERN PERFORMANCE HORSE

Robin M. Dabareiner

INTRODUCTION

Western working stock horses are highly talented and bred to be extremely athletic. Its genetic instinct to control a cow, plus overall athletic ability, produces the near-perfect scenario for training- and competition-related injuries with subsequent pathologies. The role of attending veterinarians is to diagnose injuries accurately and initiate appropriate therapy as soon as possible, thereby minimizing recovery time. A thorough understanding of the nature of the horse's competition is necessary for advising the trainer and owner in the proper management of each athlete.

TEAM ROPING HORSES

Description of Event

Team roping is a timed event that begins with a horned steer weighing approximately 200 to 300 kg that is contained in a chute at the end of the arena. The heading box is to the left of the steer and the heeling box is to the left of the chute. The first member of the team, the header, asks for the steer to be released from the chute and the steer is allowed a head start, termed the score. The team is assessed a 10-second penalty if the header leaves the heading box before the steer crosses the score line. When cued by the rider, the heading horse leaves the roping box and chases the steer at maximum speed, much like a racehorse leaving the starting gate. As the header approaches the steer, it "rates off" or slows slightly as it reaches the steer's hip to allow the rider to rope the steer's horns. After the steer is roped, the rider wraps the rope around the saddle horn (dally), and the heading horse drops its hindquarters to slow the steer's momentum. The heading horse is then turned 90° to the left and pulls the steer across the arena, maintaining a constant reduced speed that allows the rider of the heeler to get into position to rope the hindlimbs of the steer. After the heeler's rider ropes the hind feet and slack is drawn out of the heel rope, the rope is dallied around the saddle horn and the heel horse is signaled to drop its hindquarters and come to an abrupt stop. The heading horse turns 180° to face the heeler, which signals the end of the run, at which point time is taken. A good time for the completed run is 7 to 8 seconds; the world record is 3.7 seconds.

Musculoskeletal Injuries

A recent study that identified the prevalence of specific musculoskeletal injuries sustained by horses used for team roping also showed differences between horses used specifically for heading vs. heeling. Horses used for heading were significantly older (12 years vs. 9 years) and heavier (545 kg vs. 500 kg) and at greater risk of lameness than horses used for heeling.[1] All were Quarter horses and all that presented for poor or change in performance were lame.

The type of performance change reported by the owners differed between horses used for heading or heeling. The primary owner complaint in horses used for heading was that the horse stopped pulling the steer after it was roped, followed by the horse acting nervous in the heading box, and the horse failing to slow down (rate) after reaching the steer to allow the roper to throw his rope. The primary owner complaint in horses used for heeling was that the horse quit stopping after the steer's feet were roped or the horse would nicker when asked to stop.

The right forelimb was most frequently affected by lameness in horses used for heading, whereas the left forelimb was most frequently affected in horses used for heeling. Horses used for heading had significantly more bilateral forelimb lameness, and those used for heeling had significantly more bilateral hindlimb lameness.

As the heading horse sets the steer and initiates the 90° turn to the left, the right front limb is placed cranially and laterally to decelerate and brace against its forward motion and the weight of the steer, placing a tremendous amount of weight and strain on the structures of the right forelimb. These actions and forces may explain the frequency of right forelimb problems in horses used for heading. As the heading horse turns the steer to the left, the heel horse changes directions and makes a quick left turn to position itself to the inside of the steer's left hip so the roper can throw his rope, which may account for the left forelimb involvement. The horse then stops abruptly which could place stresses on the hindlimbs (Figure 9.38).

The most common musculoskeletal problems diagnosed in horses used for heading were:

1. Pain in the navicular area only
2. Navicular area pain with distal tarsal joint osteoarthritis (OA)
3. Soft tissue injury in the pastern region of the right forelimb
4. Carpal joint OA

Heeling horses were most commonly affected by:

1. Navicular area pain
2. OA of the metacarpophalangeal joint
3. Distal tarsal joint OA
4. OA of the left forelimb proximal interphalangeal joint.

The joints of the majority of horses were treated with intra-articular medications; the distal interphalangeal joint was most frequently treated.

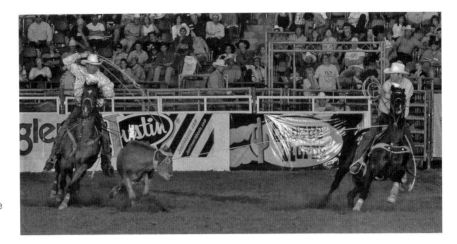

Figure 9.38. A team roping run just after the steer has been roped and the head horse and rider turned 90° degrees so the heeler can rope the heels. Note the right front limb on the heading horse and left front limb on the heeling horse.

TIE-DOWN AND BREAKAWAY ROPING

Description of Event

Tie-down roping, previously called calf-roping, is another timed roping event; however, it involves only 1 horse and rider and 1 calf without horns. Similar to team roping, the rider backs his horse into the roping box located to the right of the calf, which is confined in the chute. The calf is given a head start, the score, which varies depending on the length of the arena and the level of the roping event (professional calf ropers have a longer score compared to amateur ropers). A 10-second penalty is assessed if the horse and rider leave the roping box before the calf reaches the predetermined score line. The horse and rider chase the calf and the rider ropes it around the neck. The rider dismounts as the rope comes tight and must grab the calf's flank and put him on his side on the ground. The roper than ties 3 legs together with a pigging string that he carries during the run. The rider gets back on his horse and the calf must stay tied 6 seconds or he is disqualified. As the rider dismounts, the horse comes to a sudden stop (Figure 9.39) and backs up to take excess slack out of the rope. This allows the roper to catch and flank the calf. The calf roping horse constantly works the rope or keeps it tight throughout the entire run, placing a tremendous amount of pressure on the hindlimbs. A good tie-down roping time is 8 to 9 seconds.

Breakaway roping is similar to tie-down roping except the ropers are women or children and the rider does not dismount and tie the calf. The roper ropes the calf around the neck with a breakaway rope—a normal rope equipped with a breakaway device that releases the calf as soon as the rope becomes tight. Horse and rider chase the calf, the calf is roped around the neck, and the horse stops quickly, allowing the rope to come tight, at which point the breakaway rope opens. Time is stopped when the rope breaks free. A good time is 3 to 4 seconds for the run.

Musculoskeletal Injuries

The stop is critical and demanding in these horses. The horses are running at top speed and then must come to a complete stop very quickly. Hindlimb lameness

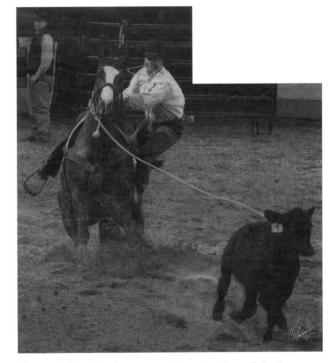

Figure 9.39. Tie-down roper after roping the calf. As the roper dismounts, the horse comes to a quick stop and backs up to take the slack out of the rope, allowing the roper to tie the calf.

issues are very common. The most common musculoskeletal injuries seen by the author are:

1. Distal tarsal joint OA
2. Medial femorotibial joint pain or arthritis
3. Hindlimb suspensory ligament desmitis and hindlimb flexor tendinitis
4. Hindlimb fetlock OA
5. Hindlimb pastern joint OA
6. Forelimb foot pain

BARREL RACING

Description of Event

Barrel-racing is a timed arena. The pattern consists of 3 barrels (55-gallon steel drums) in a cloverleaf

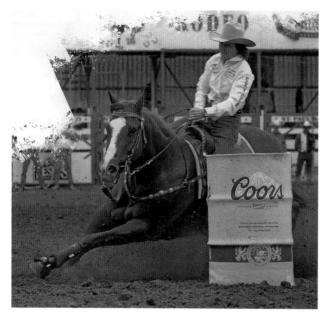

Figure 9.40. Barrel horse and rider turning a barrel.

pattern. The distance covered for the pattern varies with arena size, but generally the distance from the starting line to the first barrel is 14 to 18 meters. The distance between the first and second barrel is 21 to 27 meters and between the second and third is 27 to 32 meters. The horse and rider start at the alleyway or entrance into the arena, run at full speed to the first barrel (the contestant chooses to take the right or left barrel first), then slow down (rate) and complete a 360° degree turn around the first barrel. The horse and rider then speed up and run toward the second barrel and turn 360° degrees around it (Figure 9.40), repeat the process with the third barrel, and then sprint to the finish line. The fastest time to complete the pattern varies with arena size, but a good run for a large arena pattern is 15 to 16 seconds. If a rider gets too close to a barrel and tips it over, a 5-second penalty is assessed. If the horse and rider fail to negotiate the pattern correctly, they are disqualified.

Although the event is called barrel racing, it is important for the veterinarian to realize that these horses do not sustain the same type of injuries encountered by flat racing horses. The barrel horse does not run at top speed over long distances like flat and steeplechase racehorses; thus, injuries generally associated with speed and fatigue (such as superficial flexor tendinitis or metacarpophalangeal and carpal chip fractures) are usually not common in barrel-racing horses.

A recent study evaluated musculoskeletal injuries sustained by more than 100 horses used solely for barrel racing.[2] The median age was 9 years and the horses weighed an average of 509 kg. Sixty percent were examined due to an owner complaint of lameness and 40% because of a change in the horse's performance. The most common performance problem reported by owners was that the horse refused to turn correctly around the first (usually right) barrel or ran past it and down the arena. Other complaints included a decrease

in the horse's speed, failure to enter the arena, and failure to take the correct lead around the barrel.

Musculoskeletal Injuries

The right forelimb was most frequently affected by lameness (48%), followed by the left forelimb (43%), left hindlimb (26%), and right hindlimb (21%). Bilateral forelimb lameness (26%) was more common than bilateral hindlimb lameness (5%). The majority of horses that had a performance problem related to the first (right) barrel had right forelimb lameness.

The most common musculoskeletal problems diagnosed in horses used for barrel racing were forelimb foot pain only (33%), distal tarsal joint OA only (14%), suspensory ligament desmitis (13%), forelimb foot pain with distal tarsal joint OA (10%), and bruised feet (9%). Eighty-one of 118 (69%) horses had the affected joint(s) treated with intra-articular medications.

The majority of barrel horses begin the cloverleaf pattern by going to the right barrel. The horse runs at full speed, then slows to turn 360° around this first barrel. The first barrel is the hardest to turn because at this point in the pattern, the horse is at maximum speed. As the horse turns to the right, the inside right forelimb may be under great strain. As the horse approaches the 2 left turns (second and third barrels), its speed is slower than it was for the initial approach to the first barrel, which may account for slightly less left forelimb lameness. Perhaps these horses refuse to turn sharply to the right because they have subtle right forelimb lameness and are trying to avoid a painful stimulus. This has been previously suggested by other veterinarians who work on barrel racing horses.

REINING HORSES

Description of Event

Reining horses are judged individually as they complete 1 of 11 specified patterns (Figure 9.41). One or more judges score each horse between 0 and infinity, with 70 denoting an average score. Each horse automatically begins the pattern with a 70. The judge can either add or deduct up to 1.5 points on each maneuver in half-point increments based on the quality of the maneuver. Penalties are also allocated for minor deviations from the pattern; major deviations result in a zero score for the go. As the judges watch the execution of the pattern, individual scribes keep track of each judge's maneuver scores as well as penalty marks on a score sheet. Scores are tabulated and announced at the end of each run.

The judge's sheets with individual maneuver scores, penalties, and total scores are then posted for the benefit of the exhibitors following each class. In scoring, credit is given for smoothness, finesse, attitude, quickness, and authority when performing the various maneuvers. Controlled speed in the pattern raises the level of difficulty and makes the reining horse more exciting and pleasing to watch. An increased level of difficulty is rewarded with higher scores if the maneuvers are performed correctly.

Reining Pattern

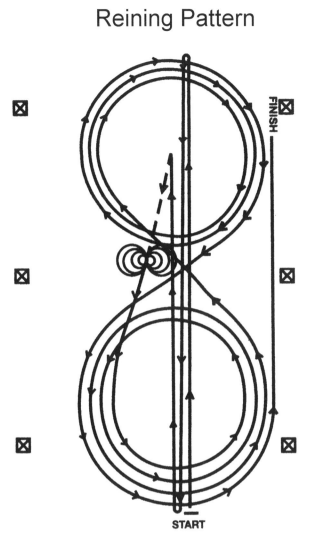

Figure 9.41. Reining horse pattern.

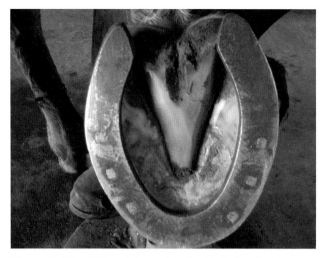

Figure 9.42. Sliding plate used on the hindlimbs of reining horses so that they will slide after a stop. (Courtesy of Jeff Ridley.)

the hind feet (Figure 9.42). These are usually made from .75-inch to 1.25-inch × .25-inch flat steel. The extended heels add support and balance to the stop and the extended heels rarely extend past the heel bulbs so that they do not cut the opposite leg during the turnaround. Most seasoned horses wear a 1-inch sliding plate throughout the shoe with equal length branches, which provides good support and adequate traction.

Many reining horses are plagued with hindlimb tendon and ligament injuries, of which hindlimb proximal suspensory desmitis is most common. This is likely due to the extensive sliding stop that they are asked to perform.

CUTTING HORSES

Description of Event

Cutting horses were born of necessity on the open grass plains of West Texas. They provided big ranches without barbed wire fences with the only means of working vast cattle herds. The task of the horse was quite simple, at least by definition. Guided by his rider, the cutting horse would enter a herd of cattle quietly and deliberately. A single cow was cut, or separated, from the herd. The cow's natural instinct is to return to the safety of the herd. The cutting horse, through breeding and training, controlled the calf with a series of moves and counter moves. The speed, agility, balance, and quickness of the cutting horse kept the cow from the herd, where other cowboys would hold the cut. The horse and rider would re-enter the herd again and again, cutting cattle out until the work was done.

Training of today's cutting horse begins early in its 2-year-old year. The horse is taught to mirror the movements of the cow as it moves around the perimeter of the large circular arena. The finished cutting horse must perform the necessary moves to keep the cow in proper position away from the herd without any hand cues from the rider. It relies on instinct alone to read the movement of the cow. Reining the horse is permitted

Musculoskeletal Injuries

The precision maneuvers performed at top speeds by reining horses require implementation of good preventative and balanced shoeing principles. These horses start from a standstill, gallop at top speed, and come to a 30-foot sliding stop. They perform turnarounds in which their body whirls around the inside hind foot as the forelimbs reach and cross over in a precise and smooth motion.

These horses are often plagued with distal limb bone bruises, fractured splints, and coronary band injuries from the turnaround spins. The high speed and lateral movements also lead to unilateral hoof impaction and forces that can cause high quarter cracks and blow out cracks.

Half-round shoes are often used on the front feet to ease break-over in all directions, especially with all of the lateral movement that these horses are required to perform. However, some trainers feel that the web of the half round is not wide enough for support and prefer the rounded edges of polo or rim shoes on the front feet. The sliding stops require a sliding plate on

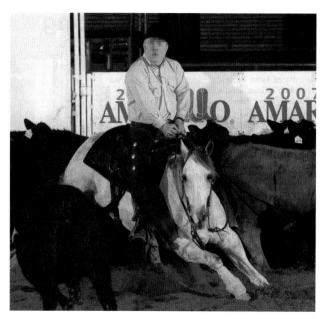

Figure 9.43. Twisting and rotation of the body as the cutting horse mirrors the movement of the cow.

only to make the cut of a single cow from the herd. After the cut is successfully made, the reins are placed in a relaxed position on the horse's neck and only leg cues are permitted from the rider during the actual working time. The instinctive ability of the working cow horse to contain the individual cow provides the excitement of competition in cutting.

Musculoskeletal Injuries

Due to the twisting and quick side-to-side movements (Figure 9.43), these horses are plagued with numerous hindlimb, pelvis, and thoracolumbar problems. Cutting horses usually have more hindlimb musculoskeletal injuries than forelimb problems. Distal tarsal joint pain and OA is the most common reason for decreased performance in cutting horses. Many have a decrease or change in performance prior to showing lameness. Common complaints from owners of horses with distal tarsal joint pain are that the horse will not hold the ground or a cow, the horse is late in making a turn on the cow, or it refuses to get low to the ground.

Cutting horses with distal tarsal joint pain are often found to be sore in the lumbar region of the back when palpated. Radiographic abnormalities may not be apparent in young cutting horses with distal tarsal joint inflammation. Treatment options consist of short periods of rest combined with NSAIDS and often IV sodium hyaluronate. Most trainers and owners prefer to keep the horse in work and elect for intra-articular medication of both the distal intertarsal and tarsometatarsal joints with a combination of corticosteroids and sodium hyaluronate.

Traumatic or developmental stifle problems also commonly cause hindlimb lameness. Horses with traumatic stifle injuries usually present with mild increased joint effusion within the medial femorotibial (MFT)

joints. Radiographs are usually normal and no detectable soft tissue injuries. In these mild cases, rest and anti-inflammatory medications or medicating the MFT joint(s) with a short-acting steroid such as triamcinolone acetonide and hyaluronic acid will often reduce the inflammation and allow the horse to continue training. In horses with evidence of soft tissue injuries or radiographic changes, longer periods of rest are usually required. Hindlimb proximal suspensory desmitis also occurs in cutting horses. Mild cases with minimal sonographic changes respond well to 6 to 8 weeks of stall rest with local injection of hyaluronic acid and corticosteroids. Horses with chronic, severe lesions require additional therapies and have a guarded prognosis for returning to athletic function.

Young cutting horses with hindlimb lameness may suffer concurrently with thoracolumbar myositis. These horses are painful on palpation of the back. They are often agitated when saddled or mounted and unwilling to stop or perform. Therapy is aimed at reducing the local inflammation and preventing muscle spasms. Rest is indicated but rarely is an option due to the horse's performance schedule. Systemic use of muscle relaxants such as methocarbamol (10 mg/kg PO BID for 10 days) may be beneficial in mild cases. Others may respond to a single injection of triamcinolone acetonide (12 to 16 mg, IM) in addition to the muscle relaxants.

Specific localized pain may be treated successfully by injecting anti-inflammatories directly into affected tissues. The combination of methylprednisolone acetate (200 to 400 mg) and Sarapin (50 ml) locally infiltrated aseptically with 2- to 3.5-inch needles is the author's treatment of choice. The injections are placed into areas of palpable pain by local infiltration.

Other management considerations are important to the recovery. Horses with low, underrun heels in the hind feet should be shod to encourage additional heel support and raise the heels. Typically, a 2° to 3° lift is indicated in the stock horse. Evaluation of the saddle fit, type of pad, and specific pressure points when ridden should be considered.

Other modalities such as pulse electromagnetic field and ultrasound therapy have been very useful in keeping these horses in competition. Long warm-up periods by ponying the horse at a walk and trot for 30 to 45 minutes without the rider is always indicated. The trainer must be cautioned to avoid overwork and severe fatigue at all times.

Strain and subluxation of the sacroiliac joint are not uncommon in the working stock horse. Unlike other types of horses that incur sacroiliac desmitis as a result of slipping or falling, the stock horse often incurs this type of injury from the twisting and rotation of the back and pelvis during work. This rotation is complicated by the weight of the tack and rider, who is attempting to maintain balance and remain stationary on top of the horse during sudden hard stops, turns, and bursts of speed.

Many of the symptoms observed with thoracolumbar myositis are also common with sacroiliac desmitis. A painful reaction to digital palpation of muscles in this region is common because of the bridging effect. The muscles undergo bridging during contraction to provide stability to the traumatized sacroiliac joint. This constant state of contraction leads to muscle fatigue, spasms, and pain. Unlike thoracolumbar myositis, observable pelvic limb lameness is often associated with unilateral sacroiliac strain and subluxation.

Clinical signs are extremely variable but include stiffness and alteration of gait, either bilaterally or unilaterally. Often the horse will show a right hindlimb lameness when the left hindlimb undergoes an upper limb flexion test or vice versa. Infiltration of local anesthetic into the suspected area of trauma may help in diagnosis, but seldom is 100% improvement achieved.

Therapy is similar to previously described treatments for thoracolumbar myositis. Deep intramuscular injections of methylprednisolone (400 mg) and Sarapin (50 ml) into the region of the sacroiliac joint have been very effective. Disposable needles at least 4 inches long are necessary to reach the affected area. Strict aseptic technique must be rigidly followed. Concurrent systemic therapy with NSAIDs is beneficial in sacroiliac desmitis. All classes of significantly lame horses with sacroiliac instability and subluxation must have rest. Two to 6 months out of training is often necessary, with strict stall confinement for the first 30 to 45 days.

The most common forelimb injuries are sore feet from repeated concussion and navicular area pain. The cornerstone of treatment is appropriate and consistent shoeing. An effort should be made to enhance break-over of the foot and provide adequate heel support. Proximal suspensory desmitis is another common forelimb injury. Because these horses must have a quiet demeanor while performing, most are ridden excessively prior to competition, which increases the risk of these fatigue type injuries. The horses usually have a lameness severity of grade 1 or 2 out of 5 and may or may not be painful to palpation of the proximal suspensory ligament. After radiographs and ultrasound determine the severity of the lesion, the horses are treated with NSAIDS, local cold therapy, and occasionally local injection into the lesion with corticosteroids or sodium hyaluronate. Most are stalled for 60 days with daily hand-walking, then reassessed via ultrasound to determine when they can return to work. Many cutting horses overuse the forelimbs if hindlimb pain is present.

References

1. Dabareiner RM, Cohen ND, Carter GK, et al. Lameness and poor performance in horses used for team roping: 118 cases (2000–2002). J Am Vet Med Assoc 2005;226:1694–1699.
2. Dabareiner RM, Cohen ND, Carter GK, et al. Lameness and poor performance in horses used for barrel racing in Texas. J Am Vet Med Assoc 2005;227:1646–1650.
3. Hill C, Klimesh R. Maximum Hoof Power. Macmillan Publishing Co., New York, 1994.

JUMPING/EVENTING/DRESSAGE HORSES

Omar Maher and Jack R. Snyder

INTRODUCTION AND HORSES USED FOR THESE DISCIPLINES

Jumping, dressage, and 3-day eventing constitute the 3 Olympic equestrian disciplines, which were first included in 1912. Their modern form developed mostly from military institutes and in recent decades became a civilian sport. All 3 disciplines have become increasingly popular and widespread and are practiced at various levels of performance. The United States Equestrian Federation (USEF) assures the governance of the sports in the United States and the Federation Equestre Internationale (FEI) does so at the international level.

Many breeds are used for these disciplines, especially at lower levels. As the level increases, particular breeds, better suited for the disciplines become predominant. The degree of specialization, adoption of specific training methods, structure of the competitions, selection of horses bred for the competitions, and level of competition predispose these horses to specific occupation related injuries.

Dressage

Dressage is a challenge that combines balance, obedience, suppleness, and hindlimb engagement. The objective is to have the horse move as asked, giving the impression that he is doing it willingly and generously. The horse must move upon the slightest command from the rider with rhythm, looseness and suppleness, and energy while remaining straight and on contact with the bit.

Grace, power, athleticism, and balance are needed along with the compatibility for complete obedience. High-level dressage horses are almost exclusively Warmbloods, with a few Thoroughbred crosses and a few purebred Spanish horses.

A study comparing gait and conformation of several Warmblood and Spanish horse breeds (3 years old), including Hanoverians, Westphalias, Oldenburgs and Selle Francais, and Spanish saddle horses concluded that the German Warmbloods, and particularly Hanoverians, were the most adapted for competitive modern dressage.[1] This is confirmed in the show ring, where Hanoverians are the most represented breed at the elite level.

Jumping/Hunting

Show jumping combines the athletic effort of jumping with speed. It requires balance, power, and agility, as well as caution to avoid hitting the rails. The objective is to jump a course obstacle with set distances between them, without knocking rails or refusal of the horse, in the minimal amount of time. The level of horse-rider coordination is extremely important, especially as the courses become more technical (e.g., turns and distances between obstacles) and the jumps become higher.

Show-hunting is specific to North America, and although it requires jumping fences without knocking down rails, more important is the elegance of the horse and rider's jumping style (Figure 9.44). The horses must travel elegantly, always in balance, with barely noticeable command from the rider. The horses are expected

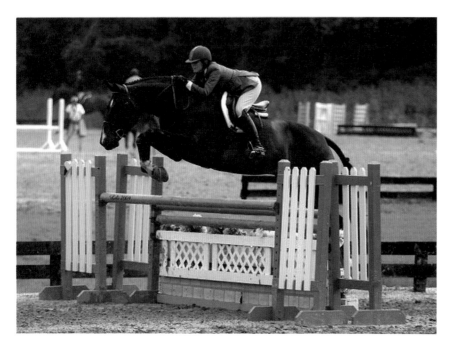

Figure 9.44. A show hunter. Manners, way of going, and style of jumping are being judged. (Courtesy of Dr. Eric Swinebroad.)

to jump fluidly with ease, style, and scope. Competitions are scored subjectively on these parameters.

Thoroughbreds, Warmbloods, American Quarter horses, and their crosses are commonly used as hunters and jumpers. Several breeds of ponies are often used by children. The appearance of the horse, its proportions, and the jumping styles are important, especially for the hunters, because they are judged subjectively. Many European Warmblood breeds (Selle Francais, Hanoverians, Dutch Warmbloods, etc.) have been selected for many decades with the help of government run programs (i.e., haras nationaux in France), using objective data and rigorous selection programs to produce competitive show jumpers; these horses dominate the show circuits.

Eventing

Eventing consists of the consecutive combination of dressage, cross-country (previously named speed and endurance), and jumping. Horses must show proficiency in each discipline; cross-country being the most important (Figure 9.45). Horses must display some of the qualities needed for dressage and jumping, with added emphasis on speed and endurance. Competitions, especially at higher levels, are extremely demanding on the horse's physique and are relatively dangerous for both the horse and rider.

Eventing is often a second career for these horses. This is partially due to their relatively lower financial value. Horses that are less successful at racing and jumping are sometimes selected because of the need for proficiency in the various tests. Most of the elite event horses are Thoroughbreds or Thoroughbred crosses because they have the endurance and speed needed for the cross-country phase. Australian, New Zealand, and Irish Thoroughbreds are particularly appreciated at the elite level because of their larger frame.

STRUCTURE OF TRAINING AND COMPETITION

The training of horses used for dressage or jumping starts much later than it does for racehorses. Horses are usually broken at 3 or 4 years of age, and their prime performance years are often at the age of 10 to 12.

Dressage

Training of the dressage horse follows a pyramid scale. At the bottom of the pyramid is rhythm and regularity (takt), which should remain consistent through the different exercises and their combination. Relaxation, or looseness, (losgelassenheit) is the second level; the goal is for the horse to be relaxed, loose at the pole, chewing at the bit, swinging its neck and tail along the strides, and making smooth transitions between gaits. The third level is contact (anlehnung) at the bit; it should result from the horse's forward motion rather than pulling by the rider's hand. Impulsion (schwung), the fourth level, is created by storing the energy of engagement. Straightness (geraderichtung) and collection (versammlung) are the last 2 levels. Straightness is when the spine is parallel to the straight line or long side of the dressage arena, known as the manege. Relative straightness in dressage terms means that a horse is going straight when the inside hindleg follows the track of the inside foreleg. Collection is the horse's ability to move its center of gravity more backward by taking more weight on its back end, lowering it, and lightening its forehand. This requires energy and muscular strength and allows the performance of more advanced exercises such as piaffe and passage.

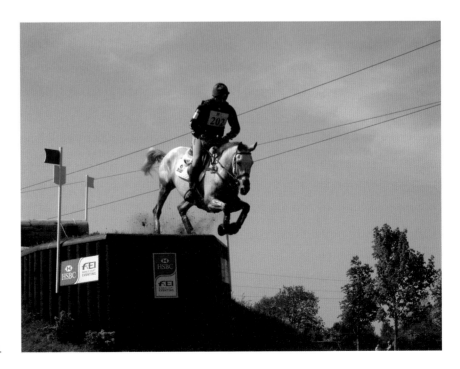

Figure 9.45. A cross-country obstacle.

Competition usually starts at the age of 5. Horses can reach medium levels by age 7 to 8 and for some, Grand Prix level by age 8 or 9. Under FEI rules, no dressage horse can show under the age of 6, and lower level competitions require mostly balance and freedom of movement; as the level of competition rises, so do the demands on lateral work and collection. Under the USEF governance, competitions are progressively ranked, beginning with training continuing with first level through fifth level. The fifth level corresponds to international competition. The progressive levels in Europe are L, M, and S, and S corresponds to international competitions.

International competitions, which fall under FEI governance, are classified (from lowest to highest) as Prix St. Georges, Intermediate I, Intermediate II, Grand Prix, and Grand Prix Special. Shows are also classified by order of competitiveness and difficulty, CDI* (concours de dressage international) to CDI***. Competitions are judged by 1 to 5 judges who score each movement/figure, awarding scores from 0 to 10. The scores of each figure are added and converted into a percentage.

The training and competition surfaces are usually well cushioned, usually artificial. The surfaces at the show grounds are very consistent and close to ideal, and therefore rarely blamed for contributing to lameness.

Dressage horses do not perform speed work or high-impact work, which shields them from acute traumatic orthopedic injuries. However, their training involves repetition of similar exercises, which makes them more prone to chronic accumulative stresses resulting in subclinical injuries. These injuries may lead to ultimate or periodic decreased performance, unwillingness to perform some tasks, and sometimes chronic lameness.

The combination of the collected and lateral work (Figure 9.46), placement of the saddle relatively far back, and a rider that sits almost exclusively places unique strains on dressage horses. This is accentuated by the fact that they have relatively long careers. Many compete until 15 to 20 years of age. Most horses are at their peak between 8 and 14 years then compete at lower levels with less experienced riders.

Jumping

Young jumper prospects are often free jumped before being broken (between the ages of 2 and 3). In some breeding programs, weanlings are free jumped and a first selection is made at 6 months, based on jumping style. One study found that superior jumping style could indeed be detected at such an age, although with some variability.[31] Foals' jumping technique was found to improve with training, and those with early training performed better than untrained foals at age 4. However, the difference did not carry over when horses reached 5 years of age, rendering the early training unnecessary[32].

After the horses are broken, training of the hunter jumper involves basic flat training, similar to basic dressage training, emphasizing collection and engagement. After a few months of training on the flat, they are brought over fences. The fences are raised as the training continues. The horses are also trained to jump combinations of fences and to jump fences at different

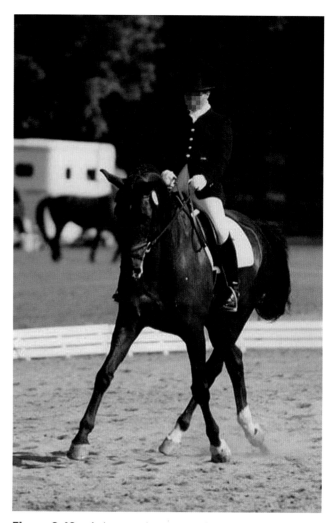

Figure 9.46. A dressage horse executing a half pass.

angles, different speeds, and from different distances. They are also taught to modulate their stride length and speed while approaching the fences.

Hunters are trained to jump in a relaxed, seemingly effortless fashion, with the jump a smooth continuation of the previous strides (i.e., the horse jumps in stride). Completions are scored subjectively on the style and cadence of the horse and rider. The height of the jumps starts at 0.75 m (2.5 feet) and increases with the levels but does not usually exceed 1.2 m (4 feet). It is not uncommon to ride hunters for an extended period just before the competitions to "take the edge off."

Less attention is given to the style of moving and jumping of jumpers. The competitions are scored objectively based on fallen rails, possible refusals, and time of completion of the course. The rail height varies between 0.90 m and 1.5 m, depending on the level of USEF competition, although it can be raised even higher in puissance. The maximum height in FEI competitions is 1.7 meters.

There are multitudes of classes and levels depending on the rider's status (amateur vs. professional) and age (adult vs. junior) as well as the horse's age, experience, and quality (e.g., young horse classes). As the level rises,

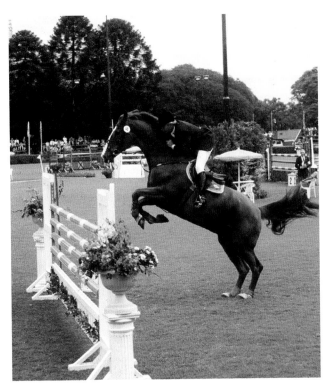

Figure 9.47. A show jumper. Note the hyperextension of the hind fetlocks.

so do the height of jumps and the technicality of the courses.

The competition season is exceptionally long for hunters and jumpers (10 months). Horses show several weeks every month and sometimes travel long distances between shows.

There are key events at each of the higher levels, and the horses are conditioned and prepped for a few main events a year. At each show, hunters tend to be ridden in several classes every day for up to 4 days of the show week. Jumpers are typically only ridden in 1 or 2 classes during the week.

The longevity of jumpers' and hunters' careers and the particular strains from the jumping (Figure 9.47) contribute to the development of occupational injuries.

Eventing

Event horses begin their dressage and jumping training at the age of 4. Some have had prior careers as racehorses. Cross country training includes familiarizing the horse with the cross country obstacles, but more importantly it emphasizes the horse's fitness. Horses begin competing at lower levels around the age of 5 and can reach the international level by age 7 or 8.

Competitions begin at the lower levels with 1-day events, during which all 3 tests are conducted. The levels for the USEF-regulated competitions are, in order of increasing difficulty, pre-novice, novice, training, preliminary, intermediate, and advanced. International competitions are sanctioned by the FEI and are divided between CIC (Concours International

Combine) and the more advanced CCI (Concours Complet International), which is characterized by more jumps and faster rates. CIC competitions are further rated with 1 to 3 stars, increasing with the level of difficulty.

The top level of international competition is the 3-day event, or Concours Complet International (CCI). It is conducted over 3 to 4 days: 1 or 2 days of dressage, 1 day of cross country, and 1 day of stadium jumping. Cross-country, in the classic form of the competition, is divided in 4 phases: trotting warm up (phase A), steeplechase (phase B), cool down (phase C), and the proper cross-country course with 30 to 45 fixed obstacles (phase D). There is significant veterinary involvement before and during each phase of the competition due to the strain on the horse's body.

In 2002, a new format of the CCI competition eliminated phases A, B, and C in an attempt to lessen the strain on the horses. However, it is still being debated whether or not changing the format had a real effect on the horses. Since the modification, the differences between CCI and CIC are the number of jumps, distances, and levels of difficulty.

CCI competitions are rated with 1 star (lowest) to 4 stars (highest). Each year there are very few CCI**** competitions worldwide. The CCI**** events include the Olympic games, FEI World Equestrian Games, Burghley horse trials (UK), Badminton horse trials (UK), Australian international 3-day event in Adelaide, Rolex Kentucky 3-day (USA), Luhmuhlen horse trials (Germany), and the Stars de Pau (France). Horses usually compete in only 1 or 2 CCI****/year. Horses competing at this level usually use 1-day events and lower level competitions for training and as fitness indicators.

Overall, fences for the jumping and cross-country phase are 1 meter to 1.30 meters in height, and 1.40 meters to 2 meters in spread (Figure 9.48). The cross-country distance varies from 2,500 meters or 7 200 meters. The length and required speed for these competitions, especially at high levels, pushes the horses close to their metabolic and musculoskeletal limits.

TRAINING SURFACES AND SHOEING

Training surfaces vary considerably among the 3 disciplines. Dressage training and competition arenas are relatively standard, usually made of artificial material, and provide great cushion. Three-day event horses are at the other end of the spectrum, tackling surfaces from hard ground to wet mud. Jumpers also compete on a variety of surfaces; however, they are meant to be somewhat controlled, varying from sandy rings to grass fields.

Deep, soft footing predisposes the horses to a multitude of soft tissue lesions related to fatigue, including suspensory desmitis, superficial digital flexor tendinitis, inferior check ligament desmitis, and gluteal myositis. Hard surfaces predispose to impact injury, such as foot soreness, as well as joint trauma, bone bruising, and axial skeleton pain. Competition on grass fields promotes the use of studs, which are placed on one or both branches of the front limbs or both front and hindlimbs. The use of only one stud per foot offsets the lateral

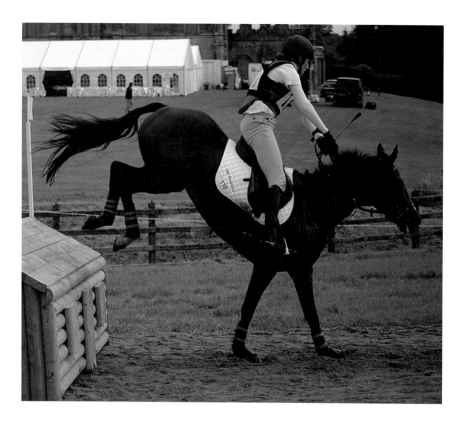

Figure 9.48. An event horse landing after a cross-country jump. Note the hyperextension of the front fetlocks. (Courtesy of Dr. Eric Swinebroad.)

medial balance and results in abnormal torque and forces. The use of studs on both branches is less problematic from a lateral-medial point of view, but might exacerbate hyperextension of the forelimbs by preventing the normal minimal sliding of the front feet upon landing from a jump.

Typically, a horse is shod at least a week before any significant competitions, which allows correction and sufficient rest in case of a shoe set too tight or a nail issue. An added constraint on the competition horses from a shoeing standpoint is that the constant traveling to shows requires using numerous farriers. As a result, the farriers lack familiarity with a particular horse's feet, so subtle fine tuning is lost.

LAMENESS DIAGNOSIS

The lameness evaluation of performance horses should be preceded by gaining good knowledge of the medical/orthopedic history; current and past performances; and any changes in training, riders, or shoeing.

Horses are evaluated at the walk, on straight line, and on short circles, then at the trot and canter, ideally on hard and soft surfaces. It can be extremely helpful to evaluate some horses under saddle. Palpation of the horse's joints, tendons, and back is performed as are limb flexion tests, and finally the cervical range of motion is evaluated. Hoof testers are then applied. Many elite barns have horses evaluated on a weekly basis to detect any small changes so that problems can be addressed early and the workload adjusted accordingly.

Depending on the severity of the gait abnormality, and bearing in mind the regulations and timing con-

straints from upcoming shows (FEI vs. USEF for the detection limits of traces of local anesthesia agents), local regional blocks may be performed. Nerve blocks are complemented by synovial blocks as needed to improve specificity. This process might take several days because it is often necessary to let a block wear off before trying a more specific one. This is especially true when trying to gain more information about foot lameness (e.g., after a positive palmar digital nerve block, using intrasynovial distal interphalangeal [DIP] joint, navicular bursa, and digital flexor tendon sheath [DFTS] blocks). This is also the case when differentiating hindlimb proximal suspensory ligament desmitis from lower hock joint pain.

The results of the blocks are evaluated on the horse while ridden or on hand. Having a rider is especially helpful for some types of mild lameness that are better felt than seen, or when the lameness is best seen under saddle. It has been shown that some lameness can be unconsciously well hidden by riders, and some exacerbated by such riders.[22]

The veterinarian's experience with a particular discipline plays a major role in the detection of such subtleties. This is especially true with dressage horses, because the veterinarian evaluates the trainer and rider to determine if they could be causing a particular gait irregularity or are unable to guide the horse properly to perform a certain task. Having an experienced rider available to help evaluate such a horse can prove to be invaluable.

If this approach is not successful, other diagnostic methods such as nuclear scintigraphy can be used. If the lameness is localized with nerve blocks, the entire array of imaging modalities could be used, starting with radiographs and ultrasound, and if necessary, cross sectional imaging modalities such as magnetic resonance imaging (MRI), computed tomography (CT), and contrast enhanced computer tomography (CECT).

COMMON LAMENESS PROBLEMS

Considering all 3 disciplines, combined, the most common sources of lameness are:

1. Foot problems including heel pain, solar pain, deep digital flexor tendon (DDFT) tendinitis within the foot, DIP joint synovitis/arthritis, collateral ligament desmitis of the DIP joint, and injuries to the navicular bone and associated ligaments
2. Lower hock pain
3. Suspensory desmitis (fore and hindlimbs, origin and branches)
4. Axial skeletal problems including cervical, thoracolumbo-sacral, and sacroiliac pain
5. Superficial digital flexor tendon (SDFT) and inferior check ligament injuries
6. Fetlock osteoarthritis (OA)
7. Stifle injuries

There are marked variations between disciplines as well as within disciplines between high- and low-level horses.[26]

Both high- and low-level dressage horses are significantly more prone to proximal suspensory desmitis than those in other disciplines. Those competing at lower levels are more prone to navicular bone and associated ligamentous (impar sesamoidean and suspensory ligament of the navicular bone) injuries. Elite dressage horses are more likely to suffer from distal hock OA than their low-level counterparts. High-level show-jumpers are more prone to DDFT injuries within the DFTS. Those at lower levels are more prone to navicular bone and associated ligament injuries. Both have a relatively high incidence of distal hock OA.

High-level event horses and high level jumpers are significantly more likely than others to suffer SDFT injuries. This is likely related to the significantly increased strain of the SDFT that accompanies speed, fatigue,[4] and height of the fences being jumped.[24]

DIAGNOSIS AND MANAGEMENT OF MOST COMMON LAMENESS COMPLAINTS

Foot Pain

Foot pain is the single most common cause of lameness in performance horses. Assessment of foot pain starts with the observation of its conformation. Low-heel, long-toe conformations, underrun heels, and lateromedial imbalances predispose horses to soreness. Evaluation of the symmetry of the collateral ligaments of the DIP joint and the presence of DIP joint effusion are better done by palpation. Hoof testers are applied carefully over the heels and sole and across the frog and the heels.

Most foot lameness responds to palmar digital nerve blocks, although such blocks are not completely specific to the foot, since they have been shown to diffuse and block out lesions in the pastern area, even when per-

formed most accurately.[35,27] A positive palmar digital nerve block should be interpreted as the lameness originating somewhere in the foot or pastern area. A positive DIP joint block helps localize the lameness to the coffin joint and the rest of the foot, including the navicular apparatus and the sole, but excluding the heels.[9,33,35]

A positive navicular bursa block localizes the origin of the lameness to the navicular apparatus or the sole.[34] A positive DFTS block, if interpreted within 10 minutes, should limit the origin of the lameness to the contents of the sheath, with DDFT lesions being most common,[16] but injuries of the distal sesamoidean ligaments also occur.

Heel and Sole Pain

Heel pain and solar pain are more common in event horses and jumpers than in dressage horses. This is probably partially due to the type of surfaces they work on. Proper farriery guided with radiographs is often sufficient to help correct these problems.

Full pads are often helpful for solar pain. Pour-on fillers are also very popular, but care must be taken not to over fill the shoe or under the plates, which causes undue pressure on the sole. Full plates are commonly used on hunter-jumpers and dressage horses but are unpopular with event horses because the plates can promote shoe loosening.

Heel pain and corns can be managed fairly well using onion shoes (open shoes with wide flares at the heels). Occasionally, in some of the more severe cases of under-run heels, loading the frog with dental impression material taped to the foot and going without a shoe for 4 to 6 weeks may help to promote some heel growth in a more vertical direction.

Sheared heels affect mostly jumpers and often start insidiously. The medial heel is often displaced proximally. Floating the affected heel and improving break-over by setting the shoe back and adjusting the lateral medial balance usually resolve the problem, although this process can take 6 months to a year. Addition of a hoof supplement rich in biotin seems to speed up hoof growth and improve hoof wall quality, but is most often already being used.[21,29]

Navicular Syndrome, DIP Joint, DDFT Lesions

Navicular bone and associated ligament injuries, DDFT lesions within the foot, DIP joint synovitis/arthritis, and DIP collateral desmitis can be difficult to pick apart using only diagnostic analgesia. Usually navicular bone and associated ligaments injuries (impar ligament and suspensory ligament of the navicular bone) will block out to a PD nerve block, but they will also do so to a DIP joint block and a navicular bursa block. Horses with DDFT lesions block only partially to a PD nerve block and to a DFTS block if located in the distal tendon sheath; will block well to a PD nerve block, the navicular bursa block, or a DIP joint block if located within the navicular bursa; and to a PD block and DIP joint block if the lesion is located at the level of the insertion.

Horses with DIP joint arthritis/synovitis usually display effusion of the DIP joint and block well to a PD nerve block and a DIP joint block. DIP collateral desmitis rarely displays palpable asymmetry, tends to block only partially to the PD block and a DIP joint block, and often requires a pastern ring block or a basi-sesamoid nerve block to resolve totally.

Navicular bone injuries such as subchondral bone cysts, fragmentation of the distal border, increased size of vascular channels, and enthesiopathy of the attachment of the suspensory ligament of the navicular bone are common and can be diagnosed easily with radiography. Physiologic affectation that does not yet appear on a radiograph may be detected using nuclear scintigraphy or cross-sectional imaging such as CT or MRI. Bone bruising or edema is best seen on MRI STIR sequences.

Affections of the impar ligament and distal aspect of the DDFT may be identified using transfurcal ultrasonography, although image quality is not always ideal, and there is a chance of missing subtle lesions as well as other lesions within the foot.

Effusion within the navicular bursa and some lesions of the DDFT proximal to the navicular bone can be seen with ultrasonography between the heel bulbs. This is enhanced when a microconvex probe is used because of the smaller footprint, which allows for a better contact. Injuries of the suspensory ligament of the navicular bone are harder to evaluate using ultrasonography.

Only 50% of the injuries to the collateral ligament of the coffin joints can be seen using ultrasonography. A small percentage has typical radiographic changes with osteolysis at the site of insertion onto the third phalanx. Initial management usually entails rest and corrective shoeing, and attempting to adjust the hoof pastern angles and lateral/medial balance. Bar shoes or onion shoes support the heels and help decrease the sinking of the heels during the caudal phase of the stance on soft ground, theoretically diminishing pressure on the navicular apparatus and coffin joint. Asymmetric shoes with a wider bar on the site of the injury are often used for suspect collateral desmitis, as are pads or fillers. Onion shoes with an open plate over the frog are becoming increasingly popular.

DIP joint and navicular bursa injections with corticosteroids and hyaluronic acid or glycosaminoglycans are often part of the initial treatment. Alternatively, biologics such as IRAP (interleukin 1 receptor antagonist protein)[12] are becoming increasingly popular, because they are sometimes effective in cases in which steroids have failed. IRAP also can be used near shows without the worry of possible testing.

When the initial management fails or is not sustained, cross sectional imaging such as MRI or CECT is warranted. Both are very valuable for foot injuries. In the author's experience, both MRI on anesthetized horses and CECT are equally sensitive for most soft tissue and structural bony lesions; however, MRI on standing horses has been less sensitive and more susceptible to motion artifact. MRI detects physiologic bony lesions (bone bruising or bone edema) on STIR. CECT is much faster and, more importantly, can be used to guide needles to perform intralesional therapeutic injections.

Once a definitive diagnosis is made, the most appropriate treatment is indicated. Bone injuries such as navicular bone edema or bruising or pedal osteitis may be treated with rest, anti-inflammatories, and possibly bisphosphonates (tiludronic acid or zoledronic acid). Collateral ligaments and DDFT lesions may be treated using extra corporeal shock wave therapy (ESWT) or intralesional injections. Intralesional injections are performed with ultrasound or CT guidance. See Chapters 5 and 8 for further information on these therapeutic options.

Lower Hock OA

Lower hock joint OA is extremely common in sport horses. The most common complaints include lameness, lack of engagement, loss of stride length, and poor impulsion. Complaints in jumpers and event horses often include loss of scope of jumping and the inability to stay centered while jumping. Dressage riders complain about the inability to perform advanced figures such as piaffe or passage that require significant collection. The affectation is usually bilateral. Spavin flexion tests are usually positive. Radiographs may show various degrees of bone spurring, sclerosis, and joint space thinning with little correlation to the degree of lameness.

In most cases intra-articular blocks of the tarsometatarsal (TMT) and distal intertarsal (DIT) joints significantly improve the lameness. Tibial and peroneal nerve blocks are sometimes necessary. Usually, these joints are medicated with corticosteroids and hyaluronic acid or glycosaminoglycan as a therapeutic trial without blocking. Using a shoe with a small lateral plantar extension is thought to normalize the landing pattern of the foot and is often used in conjunction with joint injections.

The use of corticosteroid is often limited by the show schedule and regulations. For example, methylprednisolone must be used at least 60 days before an FEI-regulated show and 15 days prior to a USEF-regulated show. Such treatment is often repeated at regular intervals to avoid losing performance and weeks of showing and to help prevent the development of secondary issues. Horses also are often treated with systemic injections of maintenance therapy such as glycosaminoglycans or hyaluronic acid.

In some cases that are refractory to steroids, biologics such as IRAP have been used with unexpected success. In advanced cases, fusion of the lower hock joints may be performed chemically (using ethyl alcohol[36] or monoiodoacetate[3,7,30]) or surgically. In these cases the horses usually perform at lower classes.

When hock injections seem to improve the lameness but only for short periods, the possibility of other injuries in the close proximity of the TMT and DIT joints, such as proximal suspensory ligament desmitis, should be considered.

Suspensory Desmitis

Proximal suspensory desmitis (PSD) is the single most common soft tissue lesion, especially in dressage horses and hunter-jumpers. In the hindlimbs, PSD is likely due to the increased load placed by collection work in dressage and by jumping in hunter-jumpers and eventers. In the forelimbs, it is often seen with overzealous movers and is related to the marked metacarpophalangeal hyperextension upon landing from jumps. Suspensory branch lesions are most common on the forelimbs in event horses and high-level show jumpers.[13]

PSD most often appears insidiously in the hindlimbs, and lameness or loss of performance seems to subside temporarily with brief periods of rest. The condition is often bilateral, which further delays recognition of the problem. Initially, there is often a more acute lameness in the forelimbs. Lameness is often more obvious on the circle with the leg on the outside. Palpation can reveal sensitivity at the site on forelimbs but interpretation can be difficult. Flexion tests, especially the carpal flexion test and the spavin test, may be positive, which can mislead the diagnostician.

Diagnosis is made with diagnostic analgesia: either direct infiltration of the ligament origin or specific nerve blocks. Sometimes no obvious lameness is present, and it may be helpful to use an experienced rider and potentially bilateral nerve blocks and re-evaluation of the horse's freedom of movement and ability to perform particular tasks better. This is especially true for dressage horses. Analgesia of the lateral palmar nerve at the level of medial aspect of the accessory carpal bone in the forelimb[5] and perineural injection of the deep branch of the lateral plantar nerve in the hindlimb[20] are gaining popularity because they are easy to perform and appear to decrease the incidence of unintentional analgesia of the carpometacarpal and TMT joints. Differentiation of distal hock pain and suspensor desmitis can be difficult, especially in the hindlimbs. A tibial nerve block can help differentiate between the two because it theoretically blocks the proximal suspensory but not the lower hock joints. Furthermore, it does not interfere with potential ultrasound evaluation. Such blocks may be performed on horses in hand or ridden if the lameness is most obvious then or only felt.

Ultrasonography is the most common method for diagnosing PSD and evaluating possible enlargement, loss of fiber pattern, and core lesions. Ultrasound evaluation can be challenging, especially when evaluating hindlimb suspensory ligaments, because the lesions are often subtle and there is significant variation in the muscle fibers of the suspensory ligament that could appear as lesions to even experienced ultrasonographers. The transducer should be applied from medial plantar and the ligament should be evaluated on cross sectional and longitudinal planes. Comparisons with the opposite limb should be performed if there are any doubts about potential muscle fibers.

Radiographs may show bony remodeling at the level of the proximal palmar or plantar cortex, and avulsion fractures in more severe cases. Nuclear scintigraphy is also useful for detecting increased radiopharmaceutical uptake at the level of the insertion, indicating a bony component to the lameness. In questionable cases, cross sectional imaging MRI and CECT are extremely useful, not only to confirm lesions, but also to rule out other causes of lameness responding to local analgesia of the site.

Treatment of PSD includes rest, controlled exercise, and therapeutic shoeing (shoe with wide toe and thin branches to load more of the DDFT), which is often sufficient for treating forelimb PSD, but rarely resolves hindlimb desmitis. Adding ESWT and intralesional injections (of scaffold, source of growth factors, or source of stem cells) is necessary when dealing with hindlimb desmitis, and has significantly improved the prognosis. Ligament splitting is performed when a fresh core lesion is present and in chronic cases.[18]

Fasciotomy and neurectomy of the deep branch of the lateral plantar nerve and neurectomy alone[2] have shown extremely promising results in horses with chronic hindlimb PSD, because these horses are believed to have a neuropathy[39] accompanying the compartmental syndrome created by the enlargement of the ligament. Both fasciotomy and neurectomy are believed to reduce the compartmental compression: directly with the fasciotomy and indirectly by the neurectomy because it causes atrophy of the muscular fibers[28] within the ligament, resulting in a reduction of cross sectional area.

Suspensory branch injuries often have an acute onset. Enlargement, heat, and pain to palpation are usually features of the early stages. Definitive diagnosis is made using ultrasonography; periligamentous fibrous tissue, core lesions, or enthesiopathy at the insertion on the proximal sesamoid bones can be seen. Rest and controlled exercise programs usually result in improvement and prevent re-injury. Large core lesions may be treated with splitting or intralesional injections. Enthesopathies respond well to ESWT. In some cases, the branch lesions communicate with the fetlock joints, creating some degree of synovitis and requiring intra-articular medication of the joint; in some cases arthroscopic debridement of the branch lesions is required.[25]

Axial Skeleton Pain

Cervical Pain

Cervical facet OA is an increasingly recognized condition that affects horses in several disciplines, but more commonly in event horses and jumpers. A wide range of clinical signs can be linked to this condition, including decreased jumping quality, resistance to sharp turns and advanced dressage figures involving exaggerated latero-flexion such as canter pirouette, resistance to work in a frame, resistance to the bit, abnormal head carriage, forelimb lameness, neck stiffness, and in the most advanced cases neurological proprioceptive deficits.

Range of motion (lateroflexion, ventroflexion, and extension) should be evaluated with minute attention to any range limitations, hesitation, or slowness. Some horses compensate and avoid maximal flexion by turning their heads at the level of the atlanto-axial joint. Radiographs of the cervical column can be difficult to interpret because many horses have evidence of some degree of OA of the last 2 inter-cervical facets (C5–C6 and C6–C7).[8] Nuclear scintigraphy confirms the suspicion or reveals the affected sites when evaluating a horse for poor performance or forelimb lameness that does not block out to the most commonly performed blocks.

Ultrasound can help to evaluate the articular facets and identify osteophytes and effusion, but is most often used to guide needles for therapeutic joint injections.

Horses with cervical pain associated with cervical facet OA can respond to physical therapy and osteopathic and chiropractic work. The vast majority respond to intra-articular injections of corticosteroids using ultrasound guidance. Depending on the show schedule, the authors usually use 40 to 80 mg of methylprednisolone in the left and right cervical facet articulations of C4–5, C5–6, and C6–7. Horses are usually rested for 1 week before returning to full work. Peak effects of the injections are reached after 2 to 3 weeks.

Back Pain

Back pain is common in performance horses and can manifest clinically through various performance limitations. Riders and trainers most often recognize it when it is accompanied by sensitivity to palpation, grooming, and saddling; reactivity to tightening the girth and to the rider's weight; and bucking. Horses with chronic back pain often lose some of their epaxial muscle mass. Significant information about the back pain can be gleaned by evaluating reported behavior, performing back palpation and manipulation (inducing lateroflexion, dorsiflexion, and extension at various levels), and observing the horse while ridden and lunging at the canter on soft ground (to evaluate the amplitude of the dorsiflexion).

Treatment of back pain includes treating the initiating cause if it can be identified, the primary lesion, and associated muscle spasm and pain. Chiropractic work, physical therapy, acupuncture, and training modification complement the medical management. The most common causes for back pain are discussed below.

Hindlimb lameness that causes compensatory muscle spasm in the thoracolumbar area. Treating the lameness usually results in the resolution of the back pain within a few weeks. Treating the muscle spasm and pain speeds up the return to optimal performance and may be needed depending on the timing of shows.

Suboptimally fit saddle that creates pressure points or restricts the horse's movement. Horses must be comfortable in their tack to perform optimally. Ideally, the saddle should be fitted to the individual horse. Adjustments should be made when the horse is in a state of fitness. The fitting should be evaluated at rest but most importantly during work when the muscles are tighter and more voluminous to ensure that the saddle is not constrictive. The saddle should have a good area of contact with the horse and should not create pressure points. A veterinarian or saddle fitter experienced in the particular discipline should perform the evaluation and recommend or make the adjustments because the saddle movement varies with the discipline. Some saddle companies provide pads with pressure sensors to help evaluate the fit, and thermography also can be used for this purpose.

Rider. Evaluating the rider as a potential cause of back pain is always a delicate task and requires the veterinarian to be very knowledgeable about the particular discipline. Horses with back issues that regularly recur after treatment often have lower level riders that sit crookedly or are heavy (relative to the horse) and are unbalanced.

Primary muscle strain and/or spasm. Primary muscle strain is usually acute, most common in jumpers and eventers, and presents with significant pain, swelling, and spasm. It usually is appreciated shortly after a significant workout. Treatment includes anti-inflammatory therapy (icing and NSAIDS or a systemic dose of corticosteroids depending on the severity), rest, and muscle relaxants.

More insidious and more frequent muscle spasms require finer back palpation to be identified. Treatments are various and include NSAIDS, muscle relaxants (methocarbamol) and epaxial muscle injections of trigger points or mesotherapy. Epaxial muscle injection can be performed with 80 ml of sarapin, 10 ml of DMSO, and a dose of corticosteroid (200 mg of methyl prednisolone and/or 40 mg of isoflupredone), injected with a 1.5-inch, 21-gauge needle. The injection should follow 3 parallel lines on either side of the dorsal spinous processes, spaced an inch apart, from the mid thoracic level, caudally to the sacroiliac area. Afterward, the horse is ideally given 2 days of rest and 2 weeks of lunge work before resuming training.

Kissing spine. Kissing spines or dorsal spinous processes impingement is one of the most common causes of primary back pain. The pain is chronic and diagnosis is made with radiography (evidence of overriding spinous processes, with areas of bony sclerosis and bony lysis) or nuclear scintigraphy. The supraspinous ligament also may be affected and should be evaluated with ultrasound.

Interpretation of radiographs, nuclear scintigraphy, and ultrasound of the supraspinous ligament should be performed with caution because many horses with no clinical signs of back pain have abnormalities.[17,11] Using local anesthetics around suspected areas may be useful, but should be performed cautiously because it also increases the amplitude of movement of normal horses.[19]

Treatment of impinging spinous processes involves injections of corticosteroids and sarapin in and around the affected interspinous spaces, muscle relaxants, NSAIDS, and bisphosphonates. Shock wave therapy is efficacious in some cases. Ancillary therapies (acupuncture, chiropractic work, etc.) and adaptation of the training aimed at encouraging dorsiflexion complement the treatment. Refractory cases can be treated surgically (partial resection of the spinous processes).

Intervertebral facet OA. Intervertebral thoracolumbar facet OA is suspected when horses have recurring back spasm and pain. Diagnosis can be made with nuclear scintigraphy, radiographs, or ultrasound. Facets are best evaluated on lateral oblique (horizontal 20° ventral-dorsal oblique) views taken from left to right and from right to left.[14] Using local anesthesia and re-evaluation helps confirm the diagnosis.[15] Treatment consists of intra-articular or periarticular injections of corticosteroids under ultrasound guidance and/or bisphosphonates added to the basic treatment of the associated muscle spasm.

Sacroiliac Pain

Sacroiliac pain is relatively common, more so in jumpers and eventers than in dressage horses. The disease is usually bilateral but one limb is often more affected than the other. The severity varies widely: most severely affected horses stand parked out and resent bearing weight on the most affected limb. A common complaint is that it is difficult for the farrier to shoe the horse). Mild to moderate lameness is often present and the horses tend to bunny hop at the canter. Affected horses are often sore to palpation/pressure over the tuber sacrale.

Diagnosis can be reached by using local analgesia around the joint. This should be done with extreme caution and never bilaterally due to the risk of anesthetizing the sciatic nerve, which will affect the horse's ability to walk and potentially stand. Nuclear scintigraphy using motion correction software can be diagnostic but is somewhat insensitive. Ultrasound evaluation of the dorsal sacroiliac ligament (transcutaneously) and the sacroiliac joint itself (transrectally) can provide supportive information.

Therapeutic trials using periarticular injections of corticosteroids are used most often to confirm the diagnosis. The injections are carried out blindly or with ultrasound assistance, using 8- to 10-inch spinal needles.[6,10] The authors' preference is to use a blind craniomedial approach, penetrating the skin just cranial to the opposite tuber sacrale and sliding against the inner surface of the ilium, or a caudal ultrasound-guided approach. Treatment includes periods of rest for the most severe cases (4 to 6 months), and periarticular injections using corticosteroids and potentially sarapin for the least affected cases.

SDFT and Inferior Check Ligament Injuries

SDFT Injuries

SDFT injuries are most common in event horses, somewhat common in jumpers (especially at the higher levels), and rare in dressage horses. They almost exclusively affect the forelimbs. Presentations range from subclinical progressive tendinitis and peritendinitis (most common in eventers, and associated with cyclic repetitive loading and damage) to acute severe tendinitis with large core lesions (most common in eventers and high-level jumpers) that are usually related to one misstep on deeper footing. They are especially associated with the use of studs within shoes.

Diagnosis is easily made by palpation. Ultrasonography further characterizes the injury and allows follow-up. Treatment in the acute stage is aimed at minimizing inflammation, using icing and NSAIDS to minimize edema and further fiber disruption. In extremely painful horses, placing the limb in a cast or a supportive boot seems to increase the comfort level. Supportive bandaging and local anti-inflammatory ointments such as DMSO or Diclofenac cream, alternated with icing, are helpful for the first few days.

After a few days, ultrasonographic examination is repeated. Large core lesions are treated using transcutaneous splitting. Treatment after that consists of rest and controlled exercise for 3 to 12 months, depending on the extent of the injury, using ultrasonography to monitor progress, and gradually increasing the workload. The use of intralesional injection is becoming routine for such lesions, using a source of stem cells (bone marrow, bone marrow concentrate, FAD-derived mesenchymal cells, cultured stem cells), a source of growth factors (platelet-rich plasma or bone marrow supernatant), a scaffold (porcine bladder submucosa;

Acell), or a combination thereof. Such injections are believed to improve the quality and speed of healing, and decrease the rate of re-injury. The use of therapeutic ultrasound is also popular, especially to treat peritendinitis.

Inferior Check Ligament Desmitis

Inferior check ligament desmitis mostly affects jumpers and eventers in their mid-teens and younger dressage horses, almost exclusively on the forelimbs. Lameness presents acutely with swelling and heat at the site. Ultrasonography confirms the diagnosis and treatments involves mostly rest and controlled exercise for 4 to 6 months. Intralesional injections of the inferior check ligament have not been rewarding in the authors' experience.

Some cases are complicated by adhesions to the DDFT that are identified during a dynamic ultrasound examination (holding the leg and performing ultrasound in the area as fetlock flexion and extension are induced). Such complications are managed by surgical separation and 3 to 4 repeated injections of corticosteroids between the DDFT and the check ligament, 2 weeks apart.

Metacarpophalangeal and Metatarsophalangeal (MCP/MTP) Joint Injuries

Synovitis and OA of the fetlock joints are fairly common in older jumping and event horses. Lameness is localized by a positive intra-articular analgesia or a low 4- or 6-point nerve block. Fragmentation of the proximodorsal aspect of the first phalanx is not uncommon and is better treated surgically, removing the fragment arthroscopically. Synovitis, with no evidence of radiographically or ultrasonographically visible pathology, responds usually well to intra-articular injections of corticosteroids and hyaluronan or glycosaminoglycan. Alternatively, series of IRAP injections may be used. If the response to intra-articular therapy is incomplete or transient, advanced imaging (such as MRI) or exploratory arthroscopy is warranted. Cartilage damage may be curetted. Severe bone bruising visible on MRI STIR sequences should be addressed and probably treated with bisphosphonates and rest to help prevent the development of subchondral bone cystic lesions.

Stifle Injuries

Osteochondrosis and Subchondral Cystic Lesions

Osteochondrosis of the trochlear ridges of the femur and of the patella along with subchondral bone cyst of the medial condyle of the femur are relatively frequent developmental disorders in Warmbloods. Radiographic surveys of yearlings and during prepurchase examination are highly recommended. Osteochondrosis lesions are treated surgically with debridement under arthroscopy and the prognosis is relatively good if the lesions are not too sizable.

Subchondral cystic lesions are treated with surgical debridement or injections of corticosteroids under the lining of the cyst,[40] but the prognosis is not as good for a long career, especially if the horse is older.[37] In the authors' experience, preoperative treatment with a bisphosphonate reduces the risk of postoperative enlargement of the cyst when debridement is elected.

Intermittent Upward Fixation of the Patella

Intermittent upward fixation of the patella especially affects larger, young horses and horses after a period of rest. The diagnosis is easy to make in the most severe cases, but necessitates a finer observation in the milder cases that only "catch" their patella. The best way to observe mild cases is during a transition from canter to trot, or when they are being asked to back up.

Milder cases respond well to blistering of the medial and middle patellar ligament to induce scarring and thickening (injection of 0.5 ml of 2% iodine in almond oil at 3 levels in each ligament). More tenacious cases may be treated by ligament splitting.[38] Medial patellar desmotomy is reserved for the most severe cases because it has been associated with complications such as patellar fragmentation.[23]

Synovitis and OA

Synovitis and OA can affect 1 or a combination of the 3 synovial compartments within the stifle. Ideally, each should be blocked separately during lameness examination. Radiographs and especially ultrasonography are necessary to evaluate the menisci. Osteophytes at the level of the medial tibial condyle are relatively common. If no soft tissue injuries are identified, intra-articular injections with a combination of corticosteroids and hyaluronan or glycosaminoglycan are warranted in each of the affected compartments. Alternatively, IRAP may be used. If the injections do not provide soundness or if they only do so for a short period, diagnostic exploratory arthroscopy is warranted.

Meniscal injuries are diagnosed after identifying one of the femorotibial joints as the source of lameness by using ultrasonography or during exploratory arthroscopy. Debridement of meniscal tears is warranted unless they are amenable to being sutured, and a period of 3 to 4 months of rest should ensue.[41]

Patellar Fractures

Patellar fractures are mostly seen in event horses and some jumpers. They are associated with moderate to severe lameness and effusion of the femoropatellar joint. Skyline radiographic views of the patella are necessary to fully evaluate the fracture. Most of the fractures are amenable to arthroscopic debridement and the majority of affected horses return to full work.

References

1. Barrey E, Desliens F, Poirel D, et al. Early evaluation of dressage ability in different breeds. Equine Vet J Suppl 2002:319–324.
2. Bathe A. Surgical treatment for tendinitis and suspensory. WEVA 2008;303–305.
3. Bohanon TC, Schneider RK, and Weisbrode SE. Fusion of the distal intertarsal and tarsometatarsal joints in the horse using intra-articular sodium monoiodoacetate. Equine Vet J 1991;23: 289–295.
4. Butcher MT, Hermanson JW, Ducharme NG, et al. Superficial digital flexor tendon lesions in racehorses as a sequela to muscle fatigue: a preliminary study. Equine Vet J 2007;39:540–545.
5. Castro FA, Schumacher JS, Pauwels F, et al. A new approach for perineural injection of the lateral palmar nerve in the horse. Vet Surg 2005;34:539–542.
6. Cousty M, Rossier Y, and David F. Ultrasound-guided periarticular injections of the sacroiliac region in horses: A cadaveric study. Equine Vet J 2008;40:160–166.
7. Dowling BA, Dart AJ, and Matthews SM. Chemical arthrodesis of the distal tarsal joints using sodium monoiodoacetate in 104 horses. Aust Vet J 2004;82:38–42.
8. Down SS and Henson FM. Radiographic retrospective study of the caudal cervical articular process joints in the horse. Equine Vet J 2009;41:518–524.
9. Dyson SJ and Kidd L. A comparison of responses to analgesia of the navicular bursa and intra-articular analgesia of the distal interphalangeal joint in 59 horses. Equine Vet J 1993;25: 93–98.
10. Engeli E, Haussler KK, and Erb HN. Development and validation of a periarticular injection technique of the sacroiliac joint in horses. Equine Vet J 2004;36:324–330.
11. Erichsen C, Eksell P, Holm KR, et al. Relationship between scintigraphic and radiographic evaluations of spinous processes in the thoracolumbar spine in riding horses without clinical signs of back problems. Equine Vet J 2004;36:458–465.
12. Frisbie DD, Kawcak CE, Werpy NM, et al. Clinical, biochemical, and histologic effects of intra-articular administration of autologous conditioned serum in horses with experimentally induced osteoarthritis. Am J Vet Res 2007;68:290–296.
13. Gibson KT, Spier SJ. Ultrasonographic diagnosis of soft tissue injuries in horses competing at the Sydney 2000 Olympic Games. Equine Veterinary Education 2002;192.
14. Gillen A, Dyson S, Murray R. Nuclear scintigraphic assessment of the thoracolumbar synovial intervertebral articulations. Equine Vet J 2009;41:534–540.
15. Girodroux M, Dyson S, Murray R. Osteoarthritis of the thoracolumbar synovial intervertebral articulations: Clinical and radiographic features in 77 horses with poor performance and back pain. Equine Vet J 2009;41:130–138.
16. Harper J, Schumacher J, Degraves F, et al. Effects of analgesia of the digital flexor tendon sheath on pain originating in the sole, distal interphalangeal joint or navicular bursa of horses. Equine Vet J 2007;39:535–539.
17. Henson FM, Lamas L, Knezevic S, et al. Ultrasonographic evaluation of the supraspinous ligament in a series of ridden and unridden horses and horses with unrelated back pathology. BMC Vet Res 2007;3:3.
18. Hewes CA, White NA. Outcome of desmoplasty and fasciotomy for desmitis involving the origin of the suspensory ligament in horses: 27 cases (1995–2004). J Am Vet Med Assoc 2006;229: 407–412.
19. Holm KR, Wennerstrand J, Lagerquist U, et al. Effect of local analgesia on movement of the equine back. Equine Vet J 2006;38:65–69.
20. Hughes TK, Eliashar E, Smith RK. In vitro evaluation of a single injection technique for diagnostic analgesia of the proximal suspensory ligament of the equine pelvic limb. Vet Surg 2007; 36:760–764.
21. Josseck H, Zenker W, Geyer H. Hoof horn abnormalities in Lipizzaner horses and the effect of dietary biotin on macroscopic aspects of hoof horn quality. Equine Vet J 1995;27: 175–182.
22. Licka T, Kapaun M, Peham C. Influence of rider on lameness in trotting horses. Equine Vet J 2004;36:734–736.
23. McIlwraith CW. Osteochondral fragmentation of the distal aspect of the patella in horses. Equine Vet J 1990;22:157–163.
24. Meershoek LS, Schamhardt HC, Roepstorff L, et al. Forelimb tendon loading during jump landings and the influence of fence height. Equine Vet J Suppl 2001:6–10.
25. Minshall GJ, Wright IM. Arthroscopic diagnosis and treatment of intra-articular insertional injuries of the suspensory ligament branches in 18 horses. Equine Vet J 2006;38:10–14.
26. Murray RC, Dyson SJ, Tranquille C, et al. Association of type of sport and performance level with anatomical site of orthopaedic injury diagnosis. Equine Vet J Suppl 2006:411–416.
27. Nagy A, Bodo G, Dyson SJ, et al. Diffusion of contrast medium after perineural injection of the palmar nerves: An in vivo and in vitro study. Equine Vet J 2009;41:379–383.

28. Pauwels FE, Schumacher J, Mayhew IG, et al. Neurectomy of the deep branch of the lateral plantar nerve can cause neurogenic atrophy of the muscle fibres in the proximal part of the suspensory ligament (M. interosseous III). Equine Vet J 2009;41: 508–510.

29. Reilly JD, Cottrell DF, Martin RJ, et al. Effect of supplementary dietary biotin on hoof growth and hoof growth rate in ponies: A controlled trial. Equine Vet J Suppl 1998:51–57.

30. Sammut EB, Kannegieter NJ. Use of sodium monoiodoacetate to fuse the distal hock joints in horses. Aust Vet J 1995;72:25–28.

31. Santamaria S, Bobbert ME, Back W, et al. Evaluation of consistency of jumping technique in horses between the ages of 6 months and 4 years. Am J Vet Res 2004;65:945–950.

32. Santamaria S, Bobbert MF, Back W, et al. Effect of early training on the jumping technique of horses. Am J Vet Res 2005;66: 418–424.

33. Sardari K, Kazemi H, Mohri M. Effects of analgesia of the distal interphalangeal joint and navicular bursa on experimental lameness caused by solar pain in horses. J Vet Med A Physiol Pathol Clin Med 2002;49:478–481.

34. Schumacher J, de Graves F, Schramme M, et al. A comparison of the effects of local analgesic solution in the navicular bursa of horses with lameness caused by solar toe or solar heel pain. Equine Vet J 2001;33:386–389.

35. Schumacher J, Steiger R, de Graves F, et al. Effects of analgesia of the distal interphalangeal joint or palmar digital nerves on lameness caused by solar pain in horses. Vet Surg 2000;29: 54–58.

36. Shoemaker RW, Allen AL, Richardson CE, et al. Use of intraarticular administration of ethyl alcohol for arthrodesis of the tarsometatarsal joint in healthy horses. Am J Vet Res 2006;67:850–857.

37. Smith MA, Walmsley JP, Phillips TJ, et al. Effect of age at presentation on outcome following arthroscopic debridement of subchondral cystic lesions of the medial femoral condyle: 85 horses (1993–2003). Equine Vet J 2005;37:175–180.

38. Tnibar MA. Medial patellar ligament splitting for the treatment of upward fixation of the patella in 7 equids. Vet Surg 2002;31:462–467.

39. Toth F, Schumacher J, Schramme M, et al. Compressive damage to the deep branch of the lateral plantar nerve associated with lameness caused by proximal suspensory desmitis. Vet Surg 2008;37:328–335.

40. Wallis TW, Goodrich LR, McIlwraith CW, et al. Arthroscopic injection of corticosteroids into the fibrous tissue of subchondral cystic lesions of the medial femoral condyle in horses: A retrospective study of 52 cases (2001–2006). Equine Vet J 2008;40:461–467.

41. Walmsley JR, Phillips TJ, Townsend HG. Meniscal tears in horses: An evaluation of clinical signs and arthroscopic treatment of 80 cases. Equine Vet J 2003;35:402–406.

THE DRAFT HORSE

Jan F. Hawkins

INTRODUCTION

Evaluating lame draft horses presents unique challenges due to of their large size, which complicates handling, routine farriery, and the lameness evaluation. Fortunately, most draft horses are docile and amenable to restraint. Draft horses are rarely exercised at speeds greater than a trot. This can delay the onset of obvious signs of lameness because of the lower amount of athletic demand required. This section reviews the anamnesis, physical and lameness examination findings, diagnostic tests, common lameness disorders, and treatments for lameness in the draft horse.

ANAMNESIS

Knowing the type of athletic demand placed on the horse is useful in determining the most likely cause of lameness. Common uses for draft horses include pulling, farm labor, showing in a hitch (either alone or with other horses), dressage, or use as a broodmare. Young horses (under 2 years of age) presenting with lameness should be evaluated for metabolic bone diseases such as osteochondrosis and subchondral bone cysts.

LAMENESS EXAMINATION

All draft horses should have a complete physical examination because some cases presented for lameness evaluation may have systemic disease (e.g., endocarditis). The lameness examination should begin with a visual examination of the limbs and trunk. Next, the limbs, neck, back, and pelvis should be carefully palpated for evidence of asymmetry and focal pain or swelling. Chronic forelimb lameness can contribute to foot asymmetry and muscle atrophy of the shoulder muscles. Chronic hindlimb lameness can result in gluteal muscle atrophy.

Palpation of the lower extremities is complicated by the presence of long hair (feathers) in the fetlock and pastern regions. Palpation is also hampered because of the thick nature of the skin covering the distal extremity. Picking up the foot for applying a hoof tester can be challenging because not all draft horses willingly allow the examiner to pick up the foot. If necessary, the horse can be placed in stocks and a hobble placed around the pastern of the affected limb. A rope is secured to the hobble and the foot hoisted. Hoof tester application is often not helpful because the soles and hoof walls are typically thick and hard. Nonetheless, hoof testers should be applied to fully evaluate the hoof capsule, sole, and frog.

Lameness should be evaluated at the walk and trot. Horses should be evaluated on a straight line and while trotted in a circle. If possible, competition hitch horses should be evaluated while pulling a cart or wagon.

Flexion tests and diagnostic anesthesia are performed as in light breed horses. Diagnostic nerve blocks are more difficult because of the thick skin of the distal extremity. The thick skin may limit diffusion of local anesthetic; therefore, sometimes greater amounts of anesthetic solution are needed and observation times should be longer to allow for greater diffusion. Higher kVp and mAs are required for radiography due to the increased size and thickness of the foot and distal extremity. Ultrasonography of the lower limb (below the hock or carpus) is complicated by the thick skin and dense hair on the distal extremity, making careful skin preparation necessary.

COMMON CAUSES OF LAMENESS

Lameness of the Foot

The most common cause of lameness in the draft horse involves the foot due to poor hoof wall quality, improper or no trimming, and inadequate hoof hygiene (Figure 9.49). Tie stalls and confinement in wet, manure-contaminated stalls can be risk factors for disorders such as subsolar abscessation and proliferative pododermatitis (canker). It is difficult for owners to regularly pick up and examine the foot, and many farriers are reluctant to provide routine hoof care for draft horses because of the physical demands of holding up a large draft horse.

Farriery can be greatly aided with shoeing stocks. Some owners possess shoeing stocks and perform routine farriery on their own. Feet also can be hoisted with the help of a rope secured to a hobble placed around the pastern. Shoes for draft horses are not

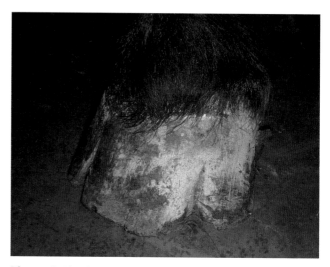

Figure 9.49. Hoof care can be more difficult in draft horses, predisposing to foot problems, including hoof cracks.

readily available because most are custom made, thus adding to the expense of routine hoof care.

Most draft horses not used for athletic use or pulling are frequently left unshod. Those left unshod and not trimmed regularly by a farrier are prone to overgrown hoof walls. Overgrown hoof walls are prone to hoof cracks, which can involve the sensitive laminae, and poor hoof care in general can contribute to chronic foot soreness and lameness (Figure 9.49).

Subsolar Abscessation

Subsolar abscessation is common in draft horses. Risk factors include inadequate hoof care and poor stall hygiene.[8,12,13,28] Hoof testers should be applied to the sole, hoof wall, and frog in an attempt to localize focal areas of pain. In some instances purulent discharge can be expressed with the hoof testers. Feet also should be carefully evaluated for foreign body penetration. Insensitivity to hoof testers does not preclude a diagnosis of subsolar abscessation. Draft horses believed to have subsolar abscessation should have a palmar digital or abaxial sesamoid block performed to confirm the diagnosis and aid in trimming of the foot and sole exploration for an abscess. If necessary, affected horses should be restrained in shoeing stocks or sedated for examination to facilitate foot examination. Inability to find an abnormal region of the sole following hoof trimming does not rule out a diagnosis of subsolar abscessation. Soaking the foot can help soften the sole and aid identification and drainage of subsolar abscessation.

Affected horses should be treated with NSAIDs as needed to facilitate patient comfort. Most abscesses resolve promptly with adequate drainage and do not require antimicrobials. It is important to remove the undermined sections of the sole involved in the abscess to ensure adequate drainage. The author recommends placing a foot bandage initially. Once cornification begins, a shoe with a treatment plate can be substituted for the bandage. The shoe can be removed following complete cornification of the sole defect, if desired, and the horse returned to use. The prognosis for routine subsolar abscessation is good.

It is a rare case (less than 5%) in which extensive subsolar abscessation leads to the development of septic osteitis of the distal phalanx in draft horses. Radiography is required to determine the amount of the distal phalanx involved. Debridement of the third phalanx is accomplished with the horse standing, and is combined with perineural anesthesia of the digital nerves.

To access the distal phalanx, a portion of the sole overlying the abnormal area must be removed and all abnormal bone should be curetted. The defect is packed with sterile gauze and a sterile bandage is placed on the foot. For large sole defects, a shoe with a treatment or hospital plate should be considered to protect the sole and facilitate foot hygiene. The prognosis for septic osteitis of the distal phalanx is fair to good as long as 25% or less of the distal phalanx is involved.[3,10]

Infectious Pododermatitis

Infectious pododermatitis (canker) is commonly diagnosed in stalls with inadequate hygeine.[18,30] Various treatments have been described for managing infectious pododermatitis, including topical application of caustic agents such as formalin and hydrochloric acid, topical sulfa drugs and metronidazole, cryosurgery, and limited and aggressive surgical debridement. The combination of limited surgical debridement and topical application of metronidazole results in the best outcome.

Surgical debridement can be performed under general anesthesia or while standing. Debridement under anesthesia is preferred because of improved visualization, lack of patient movement, and superior hemostasis. Standing surgical debridement is facilitated with intravenous sedation (detomidine hydrochloride and butorphanol tartrate) and perineural anesthesia of the palmar digital nerves. A hobble is secured around the pastern and the leg is hoisted and secured with a rope held by an assistant or attached to stocks. A tourniquet is essential to control hemorrhage and improve visualization. All visible portions of abnormal frog and sole are resected with a sharp hoof knife or scalpel blade. Following debridement, a paste of metronidazole tablets (equivalent to a systemic dose, 15 to 30 mg/kg) is applied to the debrided foot. A sterile bandage is then placed on the foot. A treatment plate aids postoperative management.

Topical application of metronidazole is performed at least once daily until the debrided area of the sole and frog are completely cornified, which may take 6 to 8 weeks. Aftercare is time consuming and must be performed daily until the defect has completely cornified. Owners must understand the absolute requirement for good foot hygiene following treatment. If the horse is placed back into the same hygienic conditions, the condition will most likely recur. The prognosis following treatment is fair to good.

Sidebone

Ossification of the collateral cartilage occurs to some degree in all draft horses. Fortunately, lameness related to sidebone is rare. Sidebone can be indicative of chronic foot lameness, even though it is not the primary cause for lameness. All suspected cases of sidebone should be confirmed with diagnostic anesthesia to rule out other more common disorders of the foot.

Radiographic findings compatible with sidebone include complete to incomplete ossification of the collateral cartilages.[22,23] Separate centers of ossification are not unusual and should not be confused with a fracture of the collateral cartilage. Bone phase nuclear scintigraphy can be useful in determining the significance of collateral cartilage ossification to lameness.[23] Corrective farriery is the treatment of choice for management of sidebone. The foot should be balanced medial to lateral and a long-toe, low-heel conformation should be avoided. Corrective shoeing should include a rolled toe with quarter clips to stabilize the foot, or a bar shoe with clips can be considered. The prognosis for sidebone in confirmed cases is favorable. Nonresponsive horses can be considered for palmar digital neurectomy.

Distal Phalanx Osteitis

Nonseptic osteitis (pedal osteitis) of the distal phalanx is not unusual. Contributing factors include heavy body weight, poor hoof care, thin soles, broken hoof walls, and exercise on hard surfaces. Horses with distal phalanx osteitis typically present with a history of bilateral forelimb lameness. Other historical findings include lameness on hard surfaces (e.g., gravel, pavement, dry ground). Most horses with distal phalanx osteitis have increased sensitivity to hoof testers across the toes, quarters, and sometimes the heels. When trotted in hand, affected horses have clinical signs of bilateral forelimb lameness, which may be worse when trotted in a circle. Approximately 50% of horses improve following a palmar digital nerve block, and the remaining 50% improve following a midpastern ring block or an abaxial sesamoid nerve block. The author prefers a midpastern ring block because it is more specific for the foot and pastern.

Radiographic findings associated with pedal osteitis include lucency along the margins of the distal phalanx and proliferative new bone formation along the margin of the distal phalanx, which can extend up the hoof wall. Treatment includes NSAIDs and corrective farriery, which should include the placement of a wide-web shoe with a rolled toe. The inside of the shoe should be filled with shock-absorbing material such as dental impression material. This type of material is very important in managing the lameness because it protects and supports the sole to minimize compression and concussion to the distal phalanx. Cases that do not respond to corrective farriery and sole support may be considered for a palmar digital neurectomy.

Hoof Cracks

Hoof cracks involving the insensitive and sensitive laminae are common in draft horses. This is in part due to the difficulty in keeping the feet trimmed, but may also be secondary to previous coronary band trauma. More than 75% of hoof wall cracks in draft horses involve the insensitive laminae, and these cracks can be managed with corrective shoeing and proper trimming of the hoof wall. Grooving the hoof wall at the most proximal aspect of the crack can be useful in preventing crack propagation toward the coronary band. If desired, insensitive hoof wall cracks can be managed with hoof wall staples and epoxy/acrylic repair, with a good prognosis.

Cracks involving the sensitive laminae result in lameness and require stabilization. Acceptable methods of stabilization include staples, acrylic repair, and a bar shoe with clips on each side of the crack.[19,20] If epoxy/acrylic repair is chosen, it is very important that the crack be completely cornified prior to repair to reduce the risk of abscessation. Hoof wall cracks associated with coronary band defects may require surgical reconstruction of the coronary band defect to prevent continued cracks. The prognosis is good. The most common complication is infection associated with hoof crack repair.

Laminitis

Laminitis, although not diagnostically challenging, is difficult to manage in draft horses because of their heavy body weight. Common causes of laminitis in

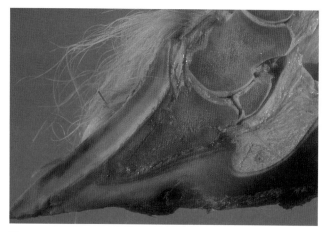

Figure 9.50. Cross-section of a Clydesdale's foot demonstrating the long toe and concavity of the dorsal hoof wall that may predispose these horses to laminitis.

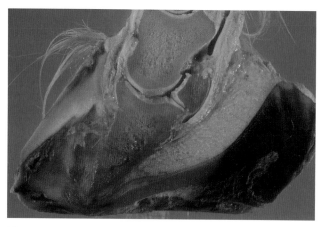

Figure 9.51. Cross-section of a Clydesdale's foot with severe chronic laminitis. Significant movement of the distal phalanx is often present at the initial evaluation of draft horses, and preventing further movement can be challenging.

draft horses include grain overload, following gastrointestinal disease (e.g., diarrhea, post abdominal surgery), retained placenta, and contralateral weight-bearing lameness. These horses are also commonly shod with long toes and exercised on hard ground, which also may predispose them to laminitis (Figure 9.50). Laminitis can involve rotation, distal displacement of the distal phalanx (sinking), or a combination of rotation and distal displacement of the third phalanx.[1] The author has found no universally successful method for managing laminitis in draft horses. Laminitis is difficult to stabilize so that no further rotation nor distal displacement occurs (Figure 9.51). The risk factor that most likely explains this is the large body weight.

The cornerstone of management is corrective shoeing, and working with a farrier is crucial to a successful outcome. The author prefers the application of wedge shoes with sole/frog support to relieve the pull of the deep digital flexor tendon and to support the sole and frog. Because of draft horses' large foot size, custom

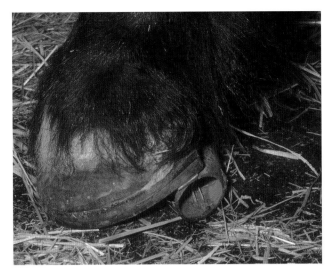

Figure 9.52. A custom made patten-type shoe has been applied to this Percheron draft horse to treat laminitis.

made shoes are required (Figure 9.52). Some draft horses respond well to application of heart-bar shoes with added sole and frog support. Draft horses with distal phalanx rotation greater than 15° are candidates for deep digital flexor tenotomy.[7] This should not be considered as a salvage procedure but as a useful tool in the management of laminitis. It can make a significant improvement, along with corrective farriery, in derotating the distal phalanx. Regardless of the treatment chosen, the prognosis for laminitis in draft horses is guarded to poor and is considered to be worse than for light breed horses.

Osteoarthritis of the Distal and Proximal Interphalangeal Joints

OA of the distal (low ringbone) and proximal interphalangeal (high ringbone) joints is not unusual. The greatest risk factor is a combination of large body size and work-related activities that pull and twist the lower limb. Radiographic evidence of ringbone is not unusual and may not be responsible for signs of lameness. The radiographic findings are similar to those found in other breeds of horses. Mild cases of ringbone can be managed successfully with conservative management consisting of corrective shoeing, NSAIDs, and intra-articular injection.

Moderate to severe cases of high ringbone that do not respond to conservative management should be considered for pastern arthrodesis. In draft horses, pastern arthrodesis should include at least 2 lag screws and locking plate application to ensure a strong enough construct to avoid cyclic fatigue.[15,16] Pastern arthrodesis is performed less commonly in draft horses than light breed horses, primarily because of the cost as well as anesthetic concerns related to their large body size. Most owners typically opt for retirement from exercise or use these horses for breeding. The prognosis for ringbone in draft horses is favorable in mild to moderately affected horses. Severely affected horses can only be successfully managed with pastern arthrodesis, with a fair to good prognosis.

Osteoarthritis of the distal interphalangeal joint in mildly to moderately affected horses can be managed with a combination of corrective farriery and intra-articular injections.[6] Surgical arthrodesis for severely affected horses may be considered, but most owners reject this for financial reasons.[2,25] Palmar digital neurectomy also can be considered. The prognosis for distal interphalangeal OA is lower than for proximal interphalangeal joint OA.

Suprascapular Nerve Injury

Suprascapular nerve injury, or shoulder sweeny, is caused by direct trauma to the suprascapular nerve. This condition is not uncommon in draft horses because of repetitive injury to the suprascapular nerve from ill-fitting collars. Clinical signs of shoulder sweeny include muscle atrophy of the supraspinatus and infraspinatus muscles, subluxation of the shoulder joint, and lameness. Nevertheless, all affected horses should have radiographs of the shoulder to rule out traumatic injury, including fracture, of the supraglenoid tubercle or proximal humerus. The clinical signs of this type of fracture and shoulder sweeny can be similar. Horses with clinical signs of suprascapular nerve injury but no radiographic abnormalities should be treated conservatively for at least 60 days before deciding on surgical decompression of the suprascapular nerve.

Conservative management consists of stall rest and NSAID therapy if needed.[5] Acute cases of shoulder sweeny can be administered corticosteroids and NSAIDs to decrease perineural inflammation. If following 60 days of conservative management no improvement in clinical signs has been observed, surgical decompression of the suprascapular nerve can be considered. The surgical technique has been described previously and is not detailed here.[24] The surgical success rate has been reported as favorable. However, muscle atrophy can persist in some cases, even though subluxation of the shoulder joint and mechanical lameness resolves. The prognosis for conservatively treated horses is fair to good, whereas the prognosis for horses treated with surgery is guarded. Horses that return to use should be monitored carefully for proper fitting of the collar to prevent recurrent suprascapular nerve injury.

Osteoarthritis of the Lower Hock Joints

OA of the tarsometatarsal or distal intertarsal joints (bone spavin) is a common cause of hindlimb lameness in competitive draft horses, especially in show horse hitches. Intra-articular anesthesia of the lower hock joints is indicated to confirm the diagnosis. The author recommends that lidocaine or mepivacaine be injected into both the tarsometatarsal and distal intertarsal joints. It is not unusual for affected horses which appear lame in only one limb during baseline evaluation and then switch to contralateral limb lameness following successful intra-articular anesthesia of the originally injected limb. Radiography is not required but is helpful to determine the amount of radiographic change present and establish a baseline for future examinations.

Mildly affected horses can be managed with corrective farriery and NSAID therapy. Corrective farriery can include a square or rolled toe shoe with a 2° to 3° heel elevation. The toe of the hoof should be trimmed short to aid break-over. Moderately affected horses also should be treated with intra-articular injections of corticosteroids. The author prefers methylprednisolone acetate for injection into the DIT and TMT joints. Ethyl alcohol also can be used for intra-articular injection to facilitate bony fusion of the lower hock joints.[27] Ethyl alcohol also is neurolytic, and injected horses frequently are more comfortable following intra-articular injection. Those that do not respond to intra-articular injections can be considered for surgical fusion of the lower hock joints. The author prefers to combine intra-articular drilling with the diode laser.[33]

The prognosis for conservatively treated horses is fair to good, with the majority responding satisfactorily. In the author's experience, fewer than 5% of horses diagnosed with OA of the lower hock joints require surgery. The prognosis following surgery is good, with most horses improving.

Stringhalt

Stringhalt is caused by hyperactivity of the lateral digital extensor (LDE) muscle. Causes include trauma to the LDE tendon, peripheral neuropathy, ingestion of toxic plants, and idiopathic causes.[4,14,29] The classical clinical sign for stringhalt is hyperflexion of the hindlimb with the limb being quickly moved toward the abdomen while walking or trotting. The diagnosis is made by clinical signs alone. The only conservative treatment for stringhalt is administration of phenytoin (15 mg/kg, PO, every 24 hours, for 14 days).[14] Phenytoin has been

used to improve the gait abnormality associated with Australian stringhalt.

Horses with traumatic injury to the lateral digital extensor tendon or musculotendinous junction are best treated with lateral digital extensor myotendonectomy. The author prefers to remove the lateral digital extensor tendon along with a 5 to 6 cm of the distal aspect of the LDE muscle belly, thus completely removing the musculotendinous junction. The inclusion of the musculotendinous junction seems to lessen the chance for adhesions between the stump of the resected tendon and extensor tendon sheath, which may contribute to recurrence. The prognosis following surgery is fair to good.

Shivers

Shivers affects draft horses along with other breeds, including Warmbloods.[9,32] Shivers is an unusual problem because the horse typically only does it once it begins to walk or trot. Affected horses pick up their leg quickly, toward the abdomen, and tend to shake the limb before setting it down. It can be confused with stringhalt and upward fixation of the patella. Accompanying the flexion of the hindlimb, the tail head may elevate. The abnormal gait can be exacerbated with lack of exercise, low ambient temperatures, and increased horse anxiety. The condition can be difficult for the farrier to deal with because the unexpected flexion of the limb makes limb restraint difficult. The condition can be unilateral or bilateral and can be progressive. For some horses, the progressive nature of the condition can make it difficult to stand, especially when the condition is bilateral. Clinical signs also can involve the forelimbs.

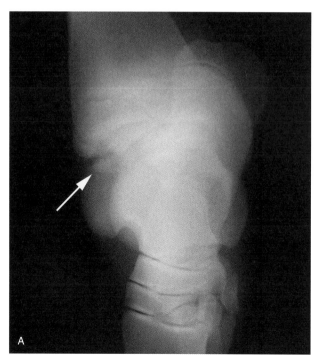 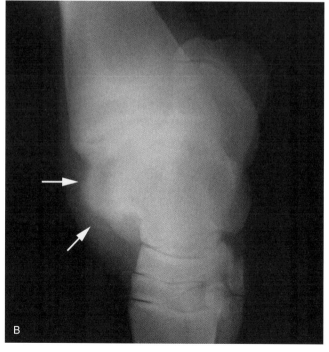

Figure 9.53. Fragmentation or osteochondral defects associated with OCD tend to be very large in draft horses and occur at more than one location within the joint. (A) A large OCD lesion of the distal intermediate ridge (arrow) and (B) an extensive subchondral defect involving most of the lateral trochlear ridge (arrows). The horse in (A) also had a large lesion of the lateral trochlear ridge in the same joint.

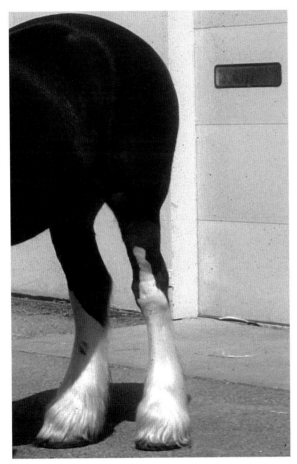

Figure 9.54. Tarsocrural joint effusion is a common finding in draft horses and may persist even if the OCD lesions are removed.

The cause of shivers is unknown, but equine polysaccharide storage myopathy (EPSSM) has been incriminated. A muscle biopsy may be obtained and submitted for evidence of EPSSM. Affected horses can be improved with a high-fat, low-carbohydrate diet. No other treatment for shivers has been shown to be consistently effective, and most owners learn to live with the disorder.

DISEASES OF YOUNG DRAFT HORSES

Septic Arthritis

Septic arthritis in draft horse foals is not uncommon and is usually associated with septic omphalophlebitis secondary to a patent urachus. The most commonly affected joints are the hock and stifle, and osteomyelitis is not an uncommon sequelae. The diagnosis and treatment for septic arthritis in draft horse foals is the same as for light breed horses.[26] The prognosis for draft horse foals is similar to that for light breed horses, although the expectations for athletic demand are less.

Osteochondritis Dissecans (OCD)

OCD in draft horses mimics the condition in light breed horses except that the size of the OCD lesion in draft horses is usually larger. The most commonly affected joints are the hock and stifle.[21] Large osteochondral fragmentation of the distal intermediate ridge of the tibia and the lateral trochlear ridge is not uncommon (Figure 9.53). Likewise, for the stifle, large lesions involving the lateral trochlear ridge of the femur are not unusual. Standard arthroscopic techniques for the hock and stifle are used. The prognosis following arthroscopic debridement is favorable in most instances due to the lower athletic demand placed on draft horses. However, despite arthroscopic debridement, some horses persist with joint effusion which may require intra-articular injections (Figure 9.54).

References

1. Baxter GM. Equine laminitis caused by distal displacement of the distal phalanx: 12 cases (1976–1985). J Am Vet Med Assoc 1986;189:326–329.
2. Busschers E, Richardson DW. Arthroscopically assisted arthrodesis of the distal interphalangeal joint with transarticular screws inserted through a dorsal hoof wall approach in a horse. J Am Vet Med Assoc 2006;228:909–913.
3. Cauvin ER, Munroe GA. Septic osteitis of the distal phalanx: Findings and surgical treatment in 18 cases. Equine Vet J 1998;30:512–519.
4. Crabill MR, Honnas CM, Taylor TS, et al. Stringhalt secondary to trauma to the dorsoproximal region of the metatarsus in horses: 10 cases (1986–1991). J Am Vet Med Assoc 1994;205:867–869.
5. Dutton DM, Honnas CM, Watkins JP. Nonsurgical treatment of suprascapular nerve injury in horses: 8 cases (1988–1998). J Am Vet Med Assoc 1999;214:1657–1659.
6. Dyson SJ. Lameness due to pain associated with the distal interphalangeal joint: 45 cases. Equine Vet J 1991;23:128–135.
7. Eastman TG, Honnas CM, Hague BA, et al. Deep digital flexor tenotomy as a treatment for chronic laminitis in horses: 35 cases (1988–1997). J Am Vet Med Assoc 1999;214:517–519.
8. Fessler JF. Hoof injuries. Vet Clin North Am Eq Prac 1989;5:643–664.
9. Firshman AM, Baird JD, Valbert SJ. Prevalences and clinical signs of polysaccharide storage myopathy and shivers in Belgian draft horses. J Am Vet Med Assoc 2005;227:1958–1964.
10. Gaughan EM, Rendano VT, Ducharme NG. Surgical treatment of septic pedal osteitis in horses: Nine cases (1980–1987). J Am Vet Med Assoc 1989;195:1131–1134.
11. Honnas CM. Standing surgical procedures of the foot. Vet Clin North Am Eq Prac 1991;7:695–722.
12. Honnas CM, Peloso JG, Carter GK, et al. Managing two infectious diseases of the horse's foot. Vet Med 1994;9:891–896.
13. Honnas CM, Peloso JG, Carter GK, et al. Diagnosing and treating septic conditions of the equine foot. Vet Med 1994;11:1060–1071.
14. Huntington PJ, Seneque S, Slocombe RF, et al. Use of phenytoin to treat horses with Australian stringhalt. Aust Vet J 1991;68:221–224.
15. Jones P, Delco M, Beard W, et al. A limited surgical approach for pastern arthrodesis in horse with severe osteoarthritis. Vet Comp Orthop Traumatol 2009;22:303–308.
16. Knox PM, Watkins JP. Proximal interphalangeal joint arthrodesis using a combination plate-screw technique in 53 horses (1994–2003). Equine Vet J 2006;38:538–542.
17. Martin CA, Kerr CL, Pearce SG, et al. Outcome of epidural catheterization for delivery of analgesics in horses: 43 cases (1998–2001). J Am Vet Med Assoc 2003;222:1394–1398.
18. Mishra PN, Bose VS, Rao AT, et al. Cryotherapy for canker in a horse. Vet Rec 1998;142:284.
19. Moyer W. Hoof wall defects: Chronic hoof wall separations and hoof wall cracks. Vet Clin North Am Equine Pract 2003;19:463–477.
20. Pardoe CH, Wilson AM. In vitro mechanical properties of different equine hoof wall crack fixation techniques. Equine Vet J 1999;31:506–509.

21. Riley CB, Scott WM, Caron JP, et al. Osteochondritis dessicans and subchondral cystic lesions in draft horses: A retrospective study. Can Vet J 1998;39:627–633.

22. Ruohoniemi M, Tulamo R-M, Hackzell M. Radiographic evaluation of ossification of the collateral cartilage of the third phalanx in Finnhorses. Equine Vet J 1993;25:453–455.

23. Ruohoniemi M, Makela O, Eskonen T. Clinical significance of ossification of the cartilages of the front feet based on nuclear bone scintigraphy, radiography, and lameness examinations in 21 Finnhorses. Equine Vet J 2004;36:143–148.

24. Schneider JE, Adams OR, Easley KJ, et al. Scapular notch resection for suprascapular nerve decompression in 12 horses. J Am Vet Med Assoc 1985;187:1019–1020.

25. Schneider RK, Bramlage LR, Hardy J. Arthrodesis of the distal interphalangeal joint in two horses using three parallel 5.5-mm cortical screws. Vet Surg 1993;22:122–128.

26. Schneider RK, Bramlage LR, Mecklenburg LM et al. Open drainage, intra-articular and systemic antibiotics in the treatment of septic arthritis/tenosynovitis in horses. Equine Vet J 1992;24:443–449.

27. Shoemaker RW, Allen AL, Richardson CE, et al. Use of intra-articular administration of ethyl alcohol for arthrodesis of the tarsometatarsal joint in healthy horses. Am J Vet Res 2006;67:850–857.

28. Steckel RR, Fessler JF. Surgical management of severe hoof wounds in the horse: A retrospective study of 30 cases. Comp Contin Educ Prac Vet 1983;5:S435–S443.

29. Torre F. Clinical diagnosis and results of surgical treatment of 13 cases of acquired bilateral stringhalt (1991–2003). Equine Vet J 2005;37:181–183.

30. Wilson DG, Calderwood Mays MB, Colahan PT. Treatment of canker in horses. J Am Vet Med Assoc 1989;194:1721–1723.

31. Witte S, Thorpe PE, Hunt RJ, et al. A lag-screw technique for bridging of the medial aspect of the distal tibial physis in horses. J Am Vet Med Assoc 2004;225:1581–1583.

32. Valentine BA, de Lahunta A, Divers TJ, et al. Clinical and pathologic findings in two draft horses with progressive muscle atrophy, neuromuscular weakness, and abnormal gait characteristics of shivers syndrome. J Am Vet Med Assoc 1999;215:1661–1665.

33. Zubrod CJ, Schneider RK, Hague BA, et al. Comparison of three methods for arthrodesis of the distal intertarsal and tarsometatarsal joints in horses. Vet Surg 2005;34:372–382.

Miscellaneous Musculoskeletal Conditions

GUIDELINES FOR PREPURCHASE EXAMINATION

TERRY D. SWANSON

PURPOSE OF THE EXAM

The purpose of the prepurchase examination is to evaluate the health and serviceability of a horse for a potential buyer. This information is then used to establish a prognosis for the buyer relative to the intended use of the horse. The veterinarian must be capable of performing a thorough physical exam including soundness of limbs, wind, and sight, and have an understanding of the intended use.

This process is an important function in the marketing of horses. The value of the exam is significant for the inexperienced horseman as well as the seasoned, veteran horseman. Historical documentation of horses being evaluated for purchase dates back to 400 BC. Xenophon, a Greek horseman, described an evaluation of a horse for purchase. The work has been documented and translated to English.[3] Much more recently, Beeman has described an excellent detailed examination of a horse for purchase.[1]

This discussion focuses on the evaluation of the musculoskeletal system for purchase.

BEFORE THE EXAM

Prior to the exam, the veterinarian should review the process and goals of the exam with the buyer, providing specific details for the inexperienced buyer. It is best to have both the buyer and/or buyer's agent and the seller and/or the seller's agent present for the examination. In reality, this may not be possible. In that case, extra effort must be made to ensure that all parties receive

accurate reporting of the examination. It is reasonable to expect that the buyer has determined the horse to be suitable for the intended use and the price for the horse has been established. While the findings of the exam could affect the price or value of the horse, the examination should not be primary in the negotiation of the price.

In some cases the process can take on a negative tone because the veterinarian is challenged with finding and identifying any health problems associated with the horse that has been selected for purchase. It is helpful for the novice buyer to have the counsel of a professional horseman when evaluating the examination results. As biological individuals, all horses have some abnormalities that require notation and evaluation.

The choice of veterinarian to conduct the exam should be discussed by both parties. To avoid potential conflict of interest, the veterinarian must be neutral in the transaction. In other words, he/she should not be the regular veterinarian for the horse or for the seller nor in a position to benefit from the sale of the horse. In many cases the best veterinarian to perform the exam is professionally involved with the horse or seller, and sometimes there may not be another qualified veterinarian in the area to do the exam. In some situations the veterinarian works directly for both the buyer and seller on a regular basis. The veterinarian's involvement with the specific discipline also can make them uniquely qualified to conduct a prepurchase exam.

On some occasions the best choice is the veterinarian with the potential conflict of interest, and in those cases all parties must understand some key points. First, the veterinarian must declare that he/she is working only for and in the best interest of the buyer at this time. Second, the buyer must understand the potential

Adams and Stashak's Lameness in Horses, 6e, edited by
Gary M. Baxter
© 2011 Blackwell Publishing, Ltd.

conflict of interest but believe that the veterinarian will function professionally. Third, the seller must understand that all of the veterinary information regarding this horse must be brought forward by the veterinarian and disclosed to the buyer. The veterinarian cannot be selective regarding the horse's veterinary history. In clinical practice, the exam results can be professional and creditable if these guidelines are followed.

The location for the examination requires adequate space to move the horse at the walk, trot, and canter. The surface should be firm and smooth with the option for a second, softer arena-like surface. It is helpful to observe the horse performing under saddle; however, that is not always an option. Close proximity to a veterinary facility with diagnostic equipment is also very helpful. If there is a compromise in the exam due to the facilities, this should be noted for the buyer, who should then have the option to arrange for a more suitable environment.

PHYSICAL EXAM

In theory, the same examination is performed for all horses without regard for the price or the respective discipline. However, each exam has its own area of emphasis. For the youth or inexperienced rider, the horse's attitude and respect for the rider becomes especially important. For cutting and reining horses, rear leg soundness, particularly in the stifle, is important. Horses that jump fences must be comfortable in their hocks for pushing off and on their front feet for landing. Those that run at speed and stop or turn must be comfortable on their front feet, and horses that do consistent, repetitive maneuvers, such as dressage horses, should have their soft tissue structures, including the tendons and suspensory ligaments, examined. Horses that perform in endurance events, such as higher level eventing horses, should have their orthopedic systems carefully examined because they are subject to stress.

The horse should be observed at rest in the stall or paddock, coming out of the stall, and standing at rest. The horse may exhibit vices while in the stall such as cribbing or stall weaving. In hand, the horse should be observed from 360° in a walk-around exam. The veterinarian should note posturing (particularly foot placement), attitude, character of respiration, muscle symmetry, and body conformation. Conformation should be regarded as 2 components; first the body's form as related to its potential athletic use, and second as the body's form as it relates to specific breed characteristics or style. The veterinarian is qualified to evaluate conformation for function and soundness and should not offer an opinion regarding breed conformation unless he is uniquely qualified and is asked to do so. The exam continues with hands-on evaluation of the horse's body. The head is evaluated for symmetry. The neck is evaluated for muscle symmetry and any sign of cervical vertebrae or muscle pain. The neck is moved to demonstrate left and right flexion as well as dorsal extension and ventral flexion.

The left front leg is examined, palpated from the withers to the foot, while observing for pain response and muscle symmetry with the right front leg. All joints are examined for evidence of enlargement, excessive synovial effusion, pain, and range of motion. Tendons and ligaments are palpated both weighted and unweighted, and any enlargement or pain is noted. Any bone enlargements or sensitivity also should be noted. The foot is carefully evaluated on shape, wall angle and consistency, and frog size and consistency, and compared to the opposite foot. Hoof tester evaluation is performed after the horse has been examined in motion.

The left rear leg is palpated and evaluated, as it is with the front leg. Each joint is palpated for increased synovial fluid and ligament changes. The flexor tendons and suspensory ligament are carefully palpated, both weight-bearing and nonweight-bearing. Any bony enlargements or sensitivity should be noted. The rear leg is evaluated for resistance to flexion when it is picked up for evaluation; shivers should be considered if there is unusual resistance. The same procedures are performed on the right front and right rear legs.

As the exam proceeds, any abnormalities are noted in the report for further consideration. These facts and their relevance to the entire context of the exam are evaluated at the end of the exam. In some cases there may be a point anywhere in the exam that a condition or combination of conditions is serious enough to warrant stopping the exam.

Next, the back and pelvis are evaluated. For many horses this is best done after the legs are examined, giving the horse time to relax and become comfortable with the process. The dorsal limits of the spinous processes are palpated along with the associated ligament; any deviations, pain, or swelling are noted. The skin and hair of the back is felt for pain, edema, or trauma. The muscles are then evaluated with a deep or firmer palpation from the withers to the croup, applying pressure in the direction that the hair lay.

Next, careful and detailed manipulation of the spinal column is performed, stimulating extension, flexion, and both right and left lateral flexions. Any resistance or pain is noted. The lumbosacral joint is evaluated for range of motion by applying downward pressure on each tuber coxae individually to assess the range of motion and any evidence of pain or muscle bunching. The pelvis and its associated musculature are examined for symmetry. This is best done from behind the horse, providing he is safe. The area of the tuber sacrale is evaluated for symmetry and evidence of pain. The tuber coxae are palpated for pain and symmetry along with symmetry of the gluteal muscles. The area of each tuber ischii is also evaluated for evidence of injury.

In some breeds the tail function must be evaluated for evidence of surgery or previous injections to limit tail function. Gentle anal stimulation of a normal horse will cause the horse to raise its tail. From the side view the tail should rise well above the horizontal plane with an arched profile. Caution is important with this test until it is certain the horse will tolerate anal simulation; this is no more risky than taking the temperature.

Flexion tests are performed on all 4 legs. The carpal and digit joints are flexed for 1 minute and the horse is trotted off in a straight line and then turned in the direction of the flexed leg. A preview trot is performed prior to the flexion. Any changes in gait are noted. For the rear leg, the stifle, hock, or whole leg and the digit are flexed. The digit is flexed for 1 minute while the upper joints are flexed for 1.5 minutes. Again, gait changes are noted. In some cases the veterinarian may feel it is necessary to do other stress tests based on the observations during the exam. These may include shoulder range of motion, rear leg abduction, and adduction tests.

Next, the feet are examined with hoof testers, and if there are pads the shoes must be removed. If there are considerations for not removing the shoes and pads, the buyer must be told of this compromise. The foot is squeezed from side to side, each heel to the opposite toe quarter, frog from the lateral sulci to the opposite wall and the medial sulci to the opposite wall, each bar to the respective hoof wall, and the perimeter of the sole as well as the central sole area. Abnormal or degree of pain response is noted.

The other body systems must be evaluated: cardiovascular, respiratory with consideration of the upper airway, ophthalmic, digestive tract including dental age, and reproductive systems if indicated. Neurological issues should surface during the physical and in-motion exam and if needed, further diagnostics or referrals are performed.

At this point a review of the exam information is discussed with the buyer. If there are no concerns this could be the end of the examination. Often, further diagnostics are indicated and performed.

OTHER DIAGNOSTIC PROCEDURES

It is the veterinarian's responsibility to suggest any further diagnostics that are deemed important to fully assess the health status of the horse. This includes radiographs, ultrasound, upper airway endoscopy, gastroscopy, rectal exam, blood work (Coggin's test, blood chemistry, and complete blood count), and testing for medications. Any procedures that carry potential physical risk to the horse require permission from the seller to proceed.

Radiographs of specific areas noted in the examination are offered to the buyer. For some disciplines, radiographs of the front feet and hocks are routine in a prepurchase exam. Unsoundness associated with the navicular area of the feet and the lower joints of the hock are common in some disciplines such as hunters and jumpers and others that require consistent and regular work. For these horses it is routine to radiograph the front feet and the hocks to establish the current radiographic status as well as provide a base line for future evaluations. The stifle is often included in the above group. In many cases previous radiographs of the horse can be evaluated in light of the current exam before deciding to take new radiographs.

An ultrasound exam of the lower leg is considered for tendon and ligament injuries, new or older. Magnetic resonance imagining (MRI) is helpful for some cases with a history of lower leg/foot injuries or specific lameness at the time of the exam. The MRI provides valuable information for the prognosis that cannot be determined by radiographs or ultrasound. This is especially true with horses that have extraordinary talent for their discipline but show a degree of lameness at the time of the prepurchase exam. Diagnostic blocks are occasionally used with the permission of the seller to localize lameness. This can provide important information to

the buyer or seller. The individual who is responsible for additional diagnostics must be designated prior to the procedure.

In some cases the decision to purchase the horse will be postponed due to certain findings, for instance, to allow time for healing in cases with mild lameness. A follow-up exam is scheduled for a time in the near future.

REPORTING THE RESULTS OF THE EXAM

The summary of the findings and the prognosis are reported to the buyer. The American Association of Equine Practitioners has established a form for reporting the findings of the prepurchase exam.[2] This information should be written down and discussed so everyone has the same report about the examination findings (Box 10.1). The prognosis is reported relative to the

---

Box 10.1. Guidelines for Reporting Prepurchase Examinations.[2]

The American Association of Equine Practitioners (AAEP) recognizes that for practical reasons, not all examinations permit or require veterinarians to adhere to each of the following guidelines.

1. All reports should be included in the medical record.
2. The report should contain:
   a. A description of the horse with sufficient specificity to fully identify it.
   b. The time, date, and place of the examination.
3. The veterinarian should list all abnormal or undesirable findings discovered during the examination and give his or her qualified opinions as to the functional effect of these findings.
4. The veterinarian should make no determination and express no opinions as to the suitability of the animal for the purpose intended. This issue is a business judgment that is solely the responsibility of the buyer that he or she should make on the basis of a variety of factors, only one of which is the report provided by the veterinarian.
5. The veterinarian should record and retain in the medical record a description of all the procedures performed in connection with the purchase examination, but the examination procedures need not be listed in detail in the report.
6. The veterinarian should qualify any finding and opinions expressed to the buyer with specific references to tests that were recommended but not performed on the horse (X-rays, endoscopy, blood, drug, EKG, rectal, nerve blocks, laboratory studies, etc.) at the request of the person for whom the examination was performed.
7. The veterinarian should record and retain the name and address of parties involved with the examination (buyer, seller, agent, witness, etc.).
8. A copy of the report and copies of all documents relevant to the examination should be retained by the veterinarian for a period of years not less than the statute of limitations applicable for the state in which the service was rendered.

task the horse is to perform. The prognosis can be expressed in percentages. This is helpful especially for the nonhorse individual or inexperienced horseman who is buying the horse. For example, a horse with minor problems could have an 80% chance of fulfilling the use as previously stated. Another case with a more serious problem could have a 50% chance of performing the intended use. This system provides the buyer with a relative risk factor, rather than simply broad terms such as fair or good. It is inappropriate for the veterinarian to use terms such as pass and fail. The acceptance or rejection of the horse is the buyer's decision, based on the findings of the veterinary examination. In addition, most horses have potential use; therefore, it is unfair to brand one as "failed."

The information from the examination is the property of the buyer and cannot be released to another party without his/her permission. The veterinarian must respect this level of confidentiality. If the horse is not purchased by the buyer it is reasonable to ask the buyer to release the details to the seller for personal use as a courtesy for allowing the detailed evaluation of the horse.

In summary, the prepurchase exam is performed to provide the buyer with all available information regarding the health of the horse in question. The veterinarian's responsibility is to examine the horse and report the findings to the buyer as a prognosis for the horse to be serviceable with respect to the intended use.

References

1. Beeman GM, Soule SG, Swanson TD. History and philosophy of the medical examination of horses for purchase. Veterinary Clinics of North America Equine Practice 1992;8:257–267.
2. www.aaep.org/purchase_exams.htm.
3. Morgan MH, translator. Zenophon: The Art of Horsemanship,: JA Allen and Company Limited, Great Britain. 1962;13–19.

THE POORLY PERFORMING HORSE

Robin M. Dabareiner

INTRODUCTION

One of the most challenging aspects facing the equine clinician is the poorly performing horse. These horses present to the veterinarian with an owner complaint of a recent change or decrease in performance and/or behavior rather than lameness. Many have a musculoskeletal problem that is not perceived by the owner or trainer. Most horses perform in an arena or grassy area, and many subtle lameness problems are not apparent on soft ground.

It is important to initially evaluate the poorly performing horse on a hard (concrete) surface in hand to accentuate a subtle musculoskeletal problem. After the initial standing musculoskeletal exam, which includes jogging the horse in hand on a hard surface and performing both lower limb and upper limb flexion tests, the next step is to observe the horse being ridden. It is crucial for the veterinarian to understand the horse's specific discipline and know which type of gait or movements are typical of the breed. For example, a Quarter horse hunter has different movements and a shorter length of stride than a larger Warmblood hunter. The veterinarian must also be able to assess the rider's ability. For instance, some horses appear clumsy and stiff when ridden by a novice rider. On the other hand, many experienced riders can mask a gait deficit or lameness problem in a poorly performing horse. It is helpful for the client to bring a videotape showing the horse performing its event normally and then another tape demonstrating the performance or behavior problem. One of the initial challenges facing the veterinarian is to determine if the perceived performance problem is secondary to a painful stimuli or simply a behavior problem exhibited by the horse. This section describes common performance problems associated with specific equine activities.

HISTORY AND SIGNALMENT

The history and horse signalment can provide valuable insight into the potential performance problem and can help differentiate between behavioral and pain-related issues. If possible, the veterinarian should determine the answers to the following questions:

1. Has anything changed recently in the horse's training schedule? For example, if the level of training has recently increased, the horse may object to the recent change because of lack of physical ability or it is suffering from physical or mental fatigue. Mental fatigue is more common in younger horses that advance too quickly in training.
2. Has there been a recent traumatic event? If the horse fell, was injured by another horse, had a trailer accident, etc., a chronic low-grade musculoskeletal problem may cause a painful stimulus.
3. Has there been a change in tack? The horse may object to a poor saddle or pad fit, or perhaps the new bit or mouth piece is too harsh for this particular horse's mouth.
4. Has there been a change in the day-to-day management of the horse? For example, some horses get too high and quit working properly if the diet is switched to a higher protein feed or from grass to alfalfa hay. Is the horse allowed turn-out activity? Has its location in the barn or order in which it is fed changed? Minor management changes can have a major impact on some horses, especially those that are high strung or have dominant personalities.
5. Is the performance problem consistent? Does it happen every time the horse performs or only on occasion? The owner should try to determine exactly when the problem occurs to see if it is related to a specific reason. For example, perhaps the horse only performs badly when it is in heat. Other horses object to a small arena or a loud announcer at the event.
6. Does the problem occur with a more advanced or different rider? The problem may be caused by a timid or inexperienced rider.
7. Has the horse had any recent illness? A low-grade respiratory problem may cause a decrease in the horse's performance.
8. Does the problem exist if the horse is medicated with nonsteroidal anti-inflammatory drugs (NSAIDs)? This may provide a clue about whether the decreased performance is behavioral or related to pain. A single dose usually is not sufficient. The author advises the client to give 2.2 mg/kg phenylbutazone orally once daily for a minimum of 7 to 10 days. The timing of the drug administration is important. The author recommends giving 2 grams of phenylbutazone orally or IV 1 hour before riding the horse.

COMPLAINTS OF POOR PERFORMANCE

A thorough knowledge of the horse's activity is important to determine the possible cause of decreasing performance. The following are common owner complaints of poor or decreased performance for several specific equine occupations.

Team Roping Horses

Performance problems differ between horses used primarily for heading or heeling the steer. The most common performance problems exhibited by a heading horse are:

1. The horse lunges across the arena when pulling the steer for the heeler to rope. This is often associated with a hindlimb musculoskeletal problem such as distal tarsal joint pain.

2. The horse acts up in the roping box—it looks away from the steer, rears, or spins as the steer is released from the chute to be roped. This gives the roper a poor head start and makes roping the steer very difficult. This may be related to a painful stimulus or it could be behavioral if the horse is tired and has had too many steers roped on him.
3. The horse's speed has decreased and the horse refuses to run hard to the steer. This is often associated with painful front feet.

The most common owner complaints for heeling horses are:

1. The horse nickers when it stops after the heels are roped or the horse refuses stay down in the stop and bounces up out of the stop. This is often associated with hindlimb pain.
2. The horse does not stop square to the steer, but rather stops at an angle. Again, this is usually associated with hindlimb pain such as distal tarsal joint pain.
3. The horse does not make a good turn into the steer after the header catches the horns and turns 90° for the heeler to get into position to rope the heels. This is often associated with left forelimb pain because this limb is loaded excessively at this point in the run.[2]

Tie-down and Breakaway Horses

These horses are big stoppers and must work the rope after the calf is roped. In other words, the horse comes to a sudden stop and backs up to keep tension on the rope, allowing the roper to catch and tie the calf. Common performance complaints include:

1. The horse does not stay in the stop or quits working the rope. This may be associated with hindlimb pain.
2. The horse drifts to one side after it stops and backs up at an angle instead of straight away from the calf. If the horse drifts to the right, the author usually looks for a left hindlimb musculoskeletal problem, and vice versa.
3. The horse does not run hard to catch the calf. This is associated with forelimb foot pain.

Barrel Racing Horses

The barrel horse runs a clover leaf pattern around 3 barrels. The majority of barrel horses run to the right as they approach the first barrel. The most common performance complaint about a barrel racer is that it runs past the first (right) barrel or takes a very wide turn around it. This is commonly associated with a right forelimb musculoskeletal problem. If the problem is with the second or third barrel (which is a left turn), then the author looks closely for a left forelimb or hindlimb musculoskeletal problem.

Another common complaint is that the horse's speed has recently decreased. The average barrel horse is quite consistent in its time for a specific arena size. A recent drop in speed may be related to pain or associated with a subclinical episode of exercise-induced pulmonary hemorrhage. The latter is very common in barrel racing horses and often goes undetected unless the horse has a major bleed and blood is noticed in the nasal passages.

If a musculoskeletal and lameness exam does not reveal any problems, the author recommends an endoscopic evaluation of the upper respiratory tract and a transtracheal or bronchiolar lavage to look for hemosiderin and degenerative neutrophils. This lavage should be performed within a day or 2 of a barrel racing performance.

Many barrel horses with decreased performance may be sound when jogged in a straight line or a 20- to 30-foot circle. If the handler jogs the horse in a small circle, 10 feet or less, which simulates a turn around the barrel, many subtle lamenesses will be easier to detect.

Cutting Horses

Training typically starts very early for cutting horses to prepare them for futurity classes in their 3-year-old year. Many of these horses suffer from over training, muscle fatigue, and musculoskeletal injuries induced by excessive training at a very young age. One common performance problem is that the horse does not stay down when stopping and changing directions to mirror the cow's movements. Often this is associated with hindlimb pain such as distal tarsal joint or medial femorotibial joint pain. Another common complaint is that the horse moves in one direction but not the other. For example, it cuts to the right to follow the cow but has difficulty moving to the left. The author looks for musculoskeletal problems on the side that the horse does not want to turn. Secondary thoracolumbar myositis is very common in horses used for cutting, and sacroiliac joint pain and desmitis are common and hinder performance.

Horses that Jump (Hunters, Jumpers, and Eventing Horses)

Riders report the following types of problems in horses that jump:

1. Refusal to jump. Possible causes include forelimb foot pain and lack of confidence from the horse or rider.
2. Knocking down rails of the jump. This may be a rider error in which the horse is not set up correctly to jump, or it may be pain related.
3. Inability to jump straight, or drifting to one side over the jumps. This is usually pain related, and the horse drifts to the hindlimb side that is painful.
4. Refusal to take the correct lead. This can be a rider problem or pain related. For example, if the horse refuses to take the left lead, it may be experiencing left forelimb pain.
5. The horse breaks into a canter instead of remaining in an extended trot. This usually reflects hindlimb pain.
6. Switching leads in the hindlimbs at the canter. This usually indicates a hindlimb musculoskeletal problem.

Dressage Horses

Dressage horses have problems similar to those of jumping horses, especially with incorrect leads. More specific to dressage horses are the performance problems that only occur when the horse is collected and not on a long or free rein. This may reflect cervical or upper forelimb muscular pain or hindlimb lameness.

Endurance Horses

Endurance horses train and compete over variable terrain including deep sand, rocky mountains, gravel roads, rivers and creeks, and hilly areas. The type of terrain that the horse trains and races on contributes to the specific injury sustained. Rocky and gravel areas cause bruised feet or traumatic laminitis, which is common in these horses. The long distance races and fatigue, especially in sandy terrain, put these horses at risk for superficial flexor tendinitis and suspensory ligament desmitis in any limb, although this is more common in the forelimbs. Exertional myopathy and gluteal myalgia also are common due to the long distances traveled in training and racing.[4]

Racehorses

Both Thoroughbred and racing Quarter horses have similar fatigue types of injuries. Carpal and fetlock chip fractures are very common. The middle carpal joint is more commonly affected in Thoroughbreds and the radiocarpal joint is most commonly affected in Quarter horses. Both also suffer from superficial flexor tendinitis and suspensory ligament desmitis. Osteoarthritis of the distal tarsal joints is common and seen in horses that leave the starting gate poorly.[1]

Issues Reported for all Horses

Other performance issues reported for all horses include bucking, cold-backed behavior, and agitation as the girth of the saddle is tightened. These horses should be checked for sternum pain (especially if the horse resents tightening of the girth or cinch), spinous process or rib bruising, and thoracolumbar myositis. Rearing is usually behavioral and seldom the result of a painful stimulus.

High-dose NSAIDS are helpful in trying to determine whether the poor performance is related to pain or behavior. The author gives 4 grams of phenylbutazone IV (for an average adult horse) and 2 hours later asks the rider to ride the horse. If the poor performance still occurs at this point, the owner is instructed to continue with 2.2 mg/kg phenylbutazone for 7 to 10 days, and then the horse is re-evaluated. If the performance does not improve, then it may be a rider or behavioral issue. Long-term sedatives such as reserpine (2.5 to 3 mg IM, every 30 days) may help with a behavioral problem, especially in high-strung or nervous horses.

NON-MUSCULOSKELETAL CAUSES OF POOR PERFORMANCE

There are many other reasons for a horse to experience a sudden decrease in performance, and all may need to be investigated. These include:

1. Neurologic disease. A subtle neurologic problem can have a dramatic effect on performance. A complete neurologic evaluation including diagnostics is indicated to rule out equine protozoa myelitis (EPM), cervical stenotic myelopathy, or cervical osteoarthritis.

2. Polysaccharide storage myopathy (PSSM) or recurrent exertional rhabdomyolysis (RER). Diagnostics include an exercise tolerance test by taking a resting AST/CK prior to exercise and then trotting the horse for 20 minutes and retesting the AST/CK 5 hours after the exercise. An elevation of these enzymes rules in disease. Hereditary testing for Quarter horses for type 1 PSSM can be accomplished by sending blood and tail hairs to the University of Minnesota (http://www.vdl.umn.edu/vdl/ourservices/neuromuscular.html). Alternatively, a muscle biopsy of the semimembranosus muscle can be submitted to the same laboratory. See Chapter 7 for further information on this subject.

3. Atrial fibrillation. An echocardiogram and cardiac ultrasound detect this problem, which can cause a decrease in performance.

4. Myocarditis. This can be detected by evaluating the cardiac Troponin I cardiac enzyme level. Heparinized blood is submitted and values should be less than 0.04 ng/ml, but may vary with reference levels at different labs.

5. Inflammatory airway disease. Diagnostics include a rebreathing exam, thoracic ultrasound, chest radiographs, and bronchoalveolar lavage.

6. Upper respiratory problems such as dorsal displacement of the soft palate, epiglottic entrapment, arytenoid pathology, cicatrix formation (especially if the horse is located in the southeastern states), and laryngeal hemiplegia. These should be ruled out, ideally with an endoscopic exam performed with the horse on a treadmill.

7. Subtle musculoskeletal problems. As a last resort, a full body nuclear scintigraphic examination may be beneficial in detecting problems that cannot be identified by other means.

The poorly performing horse can be a diagnostic and time-consuming challenge. Many horses just grow tired or bored with their job. In some challenging cases, the author has found it useful to have the owner change the horse's job for 3 to 6 months. For example, instead of running barrels, have the horse learn to rope steers and at a later date return to barrel racing. If the horse and rider are having problems, simply sending the horse to a professional trainer may be beneficial. Other horses simply need to find a different job or drop a level in training.[2]

References

1. Cohen ND, Dresser BT, Peloso JG, et al. Frequency of musculoskeletal injuries and risk factors associated with injuries incurred in Quarter horses during races. J Am Vet Med Assoc 1999; 215:662–669.
2. Dabareiner RM, Cohen ND, Carter GK, et al. Lameness and poor performance in horses used for team roping: 118 cases (2000–2003). J Am Vet Med Assoc 2005;226:1694–1699.
3. Dabareiner RM, Cohen ND, Carter GK, et al. Musculoskeletal problems associated with lameness and poor performance among horses used for barrel racing: 118 cases (2000–2003). J Am Vet Med Assoc 2005;227:1646–1650.
4. Misheff MM. Lameness in endurance horses. In Diagnosis and Management of Lameness in the Horse. Ross MW, Dyson SJ, eds. Saunders, Philadelphia, 2003;996–1002.

HEADSHAKING AND BIT-RELATED PROBLEMS

Dwight G. Bennett

A headshaker is a horse that displays uncontrollable, persistent or intermittent, sudden, and apparently involuntary bouts of head tossing with spontaneous and frequently repetitive intermittent vertical, horizontal, or rotary movements of the head and neck. Headshakers may also press their heads or rub the sides of their faces against the ground or other objects and strike at their faces or noses with their forefeet. Seasonality with worsening of clinical signs on exposure to bright light in the summer is a common feature of this syndrome.[13,16,17,21]

Some headshakers show only intermittent and mild clinical signs with facial muscle twitching and are still rideable.[25] However, others range from those showing more severe signs while still being rideable, albeit with some difficulty, to those that are unrideable and uncontrollable to the point of being dangerous with bizarre behavior patterns.[8,25]

It is important to realize that the condition is a clinical sign and not a diagnosis. It may be caused by environmental problems, medical problems, traumatic injury, inappropriate bitting or inappropriate riding techniques, or a compulsive disorder.[11] Rather than being a vice or a behavioral or reactive state, in the majority of cases headshaking is due to pain, irritation or discomfort.[4,18,29] In a survey of 31 head shaking horses, 100% of the owners considered the animal to be a good, reliable horse except for the headshaking problem and only 13% of the horses had another vice.[17]

Although headshaking has been identified for nearly 200 years and is easily clinically recognizable, a causative factor can be found in only a few exceptional cases.[3,4,15,16,20,28,29] In a distressingly high percentage of cases, treatments and/or interventions are of limited success.

ETIOLOGY

Some headshaking is a normal reaction to harassment by flies.[4,11] Because the use of insect repellents has uniformly failed to alleviate repetitive headshaking in horses, it seems unlikely that insect aggravation is a component of the problem.[17] Numerous medical disorders have been associated with headshaking, including dental, oral, ear, eye, neck, back, and respiratory problems.[5,8,11] Specific conditions that have been associated with headshaking include otitis, spinose ear ticks (*Otobius megnini*), ear mites,[6] foreign bodies and tumors in the ears,[7] fracture of the petrous temporal bone,[2,8] reactive or inflammatory airway disease,[19] equine protozoal myeloencephalitis,[24] pharyngitis, guttural pouch mycosis,[7] dentiguous cysts in the temporal region, and calcification of the ligamentum nuchae.[7]

However, the presence of an associated disease or condition in a horse may be an incidental finding, with no role in the etiology of its headshaking.[21] In few, if any, cases does the successful treatment of any of the above diseases resolve the headshaking.

The pressure of a bit in a horse's mouth, especially with an improperly fitting or severe bit or hard hands on the part of the rider, can lead to pain and head tossing.[1,2] When a horse has a sore mouth, the use of any bit, even the mildest possible bit with the reins in the hands of a skilled and gentle rider, can still lead to head tossing.[1] Many authorities consider the mechanical and physiological effects of the bit to be a primary initiating cause of headshaking.[1,4–11,15]

Because the horse is an obligate nasal breather, using a bit to force a horse into excessive vertical neck flexion, as is required in many riding disciplines, can interfere with breathing.[11] As a result, some horses toss their heads in an attempt to breath more freely.[4,8,11] Headshaking exhibited by a horse being held back at the start of an exercise gallop may be due to frustration.[4] Headshaking is rarely seen in racehorses, which run with their necks outstretched, which causes minimal resistance to air flow.[3]

The continued use of inappropriate bits, inappropriate riding techniques, or excessive flexion can result in behavioral conditioning to the point that the mere presence of a rider on the back or a bit in the mouth may lead to anxiety with consequential headshaking in conditioned horses.[11] The headshaking syndrome, when bit-induced, seems to be a manifestation of trigeminal neuralgia.[10] The trigeminal nerve, in its mandibular, maxillary, and ophthalmic branches, contains sensory fibers from most parts of the head.[27,30] The trigeminal pain can be transmitted directly to the brain from any branch of the trigeminal nerve in direct contact with the bit.[10] Or the oral branches of the trigeminal nerve may send signals to other trigeminal branches, resulting in referred pain in areas of the face, such as the eyes, ears, or upper forehead that have no direct contact with the bit.[10]

Whether or not related to bitting, all modern theories regarding the etiology of idiopathic headshaking have the trigeminal nerve in common.[5,11,12,16,17,20,25,26,30] Neuropathic pain, presumably with sensations that are unfamiliar and different from usual pain experiences, seems to be a major component of the syndrome.[12,17,26] Less of a stimulus of the trigeminal nerve may be required to evoke a response in headshakers than in normal horses.[12]

Trigeminal neuralgia, a well-recognized syndrome in humans,[27] is characterized by episodes of sharp, shooting pain following the course of one of the branches of the nerve, and is caused by compression, trauma, chemical irritation, or infection damaging one of the branches.[26,27] It is recognized that sensory trigger zones in the horse's face, nose, nasal cavity, and throat initiate headshaking comparable to the mechanisms in human trigeminal neuralgia.[26,27,29,30] Obviously, excessive bit pressure can lead to compression and trauma to the horse's mandibular and maxillary branches of the trigeminal nerve. The violent flicks or nods of the head appear suddenly and spontaneously, suggesting that sharp, shooting pain sensations could be the cause.[26] The rubbing of the face and muzzle might be a response to pain sensations that are similar but less sharp and sudden.[26]

The caudal nasal branch of the trigeminal nerve (originally called the posterior ethmoidal nerve) is more proximal than the infraorbital nerve and is most likely to be affected in headshaking horses because local anesthesia of this nerve results in an 80% to 100% reduction of clinical signs in most headshakers.[25,26] Infraorbital anesthesia almost never results in improvement.[25,26]

Some authors have questioned whether schooling, riding, and the bit have a role in the etiology of headshaking since the percentage of horses that exhibit headshaking only when ridden is small.[14,17,25] However, others have observed that many, if not most, horses with this problem shake their heads only during exercise.[5,8] Exercise may lower the threshold for trigeminal nerve stimulation.[17,18]

In a survey of 254 headshaking horses in the UK, all of the horses were reported to headshake at exercise, and 40.5% also did so at rest.[21] Most of the horses in the survey were more than 5 years old at the time of onset of headshaking, and nearly 20% were more than 10 years old.[21] Therefore, it seems likely that most of these horses had been bridled prior to the onset of headshaking. Many owners associated the onset of the problem with initial training for riding, reluctance to be bridled, and sensitivity of the muzzle, supporting the suggestion that one of the main causes of headshaking is neuralgia associated with bitting.[21]

While it certainly seems to be a common cause, bitting is not the only stimulus leading to trigeminal neuralgia in headshaking horses. The stimulation of ophthalmic and nasal trigeminal pain receptors also may lead to headshaking.

Headshaking is frequently a seasonal problem with an increased incidence in the summer.[8,13,16,17,21] So-called photic headshakers exhibit increased headshaking when exposed to bright light, such as when they are outside on sunny, summer days, and decreased headshaking when in a darkened, indoor environment.[11] Many headshaking horses exhibit conscious efforts to avoid light when outside during daylight hours.[16]

Most of 254 headshaking horses in the survey cited became worse on bright, sunny, summer days.[21] In another survey, light was a stimulus for headshaking in about 60% of the cases.[17] The headshaking shown by horses sensitive to light was the same as that in headshaking horses in which light was not a stimulus; therefore, light seems to be simply another means of altering the threshold for neuropathically mediated trigeminal nerve pain.[17]

Optic stimulation by light may lead to referred sensation not only in the parts innervated by the ophthalmic division of the trigeminal nerve, but in parts of the nose innervated by other branches of the trigeminal nerve.[16] The role of light may operate in the same fashion in the horse as in the photic sneeze in humans, which occurs upon sudden exposure to bright light and stimulates a tingling sensation in the sensory branches of the trigeminal nerve. The same sensation that results in sneezing in humans many lead to stimulation of the muzzle area of the horse, leading to nasal rubbing, snorting, and sudden flipping of the nose.[16] Some sort of nasal irritation seemed to afflict 80% of the 254 horses in the UK survey because they rubbed their noses on the ground or on nearby objects.[21]

There also appears to be a trigger zone for headshaking in the caudal nasal cavity of horses, which responds to fast-flowing air and particulate matter reaching the caudal areas. In one investigation, application of a nasal occlusal mask, which slowed airflow into the nasal cavities, resulted in a 90% to 100% reduction in clinical signs in most headshakers.[26] When the mask was removed, the signs returned.[26] Additional support for the caudal nasal trigger zone is the fact that local anesthesia of the caudal nasal nerve temporarily resolved headshaking.[26]

In addition to the above stimuli, headshaking may be a response to anything that frustrates a horse.[8] For example, a horse confined for lengthy periods in a small stall may nod its head from frustration and boredom.[4]

A major concern with headshaking in horses is that the condition may become a compulsive disorder with no direct nerve stimulus required to initiate the behavior. The neural malfunction may be central or peripheral, and pain thresholds and perceptions can be permanently affected.[17]

It is difficult to be certain whether compulsive headshaking in a horse is due to recurrent pain, such as in human trigeminal neuralgia, or has simply become a habitual behavior.

Some horses, often called head shy, have become conditioned to fear the approach of human hands and shake their heads only when people reach for their heads, with or without an object such as a bridle in their hands.[11] A horse with no medical abnormalities that shakes its head regardless of the presence of flies, a bit in its mouth, a rider on its back, hands reaching toward its head, or other environmental factors that might induce headshaking may have developed a compulsive disorder.[11]

CLINICAL SIGNS

The most common clinical signs are shaking the head in a vertical (much less commonly horizontal) plane, acting as if an insect is flying up a nostril, snorting excessively, or rubbing the muzzle on objects. A worsening of clinical signs with exposure to sunlight and improvement of clinical signs at night also are common.[13] Headshakers may also snort or sneeze excessively, flip their upper lips, strike their faces with their forelimbs, or have an anxious expression with the cutaneous muscles tense and the sclera showing.[11]

Once the signs of headshaking have begun during exercise, they generally become progressively worse to the extent that the horse becomes very distressed if it is kept working, and its behavior seems almost maniacal.[18] In these circumstances the horse is a danger to both itself and its rider.

DIAGNOSIS

A precise diagnosis can be reached in only a minority of cases of headshaking.[3,15,29,30] Even if an abnormality is detected, it is not always possible to establish its significance with respect to headshaking.[18] In the majority of cases, no major reason for head tossing can be found. While perhaps indicated to rule out related problems, thorough physical examination, even when it includes ophthalmologic, otoscopic, endoscopic, neurologic, and radiographic examination, plus complete blood count and blood chemistry profile, generally fails to reveal the cause of headshaking in horses.[16,20]

Headshaking should be addressed without delay before it becomes a compulsive habit that is nearly impossible to break.[11,15] Because of the likelihood that a reaction to biting causes the headshaking, it is worthwhile to establish whether the problem persists when the horse is lunged, with or without a bit in his mouth, and whether the headshaking is affected by riding the horse with a different bit or a bitless bridle.[18]

Trial treatments to help diagnose the cause of headshaking include floating teeth; removing wolf teeth; using a decongestant, corticosteroid, or local anesthetic nasal spray; medicating with sedatives or tranquilizers; blocking the trigeminal (caudal nasal) nerve (Figures 10.1 and 10.2); and treating any skin diseases.[6]

TREATMENT AND PREVENTION

As indicated, treatment is complicated by the fact that in most cases, a specific cause is never found.[18] Treatments with antihistamines, NSAIDs, corticosteroids, antimicrobials, fly control, chiropractic, and acupuncture have had limited success.[13,18]

Cyproheptadine, an anticholinergic serotonin antagonist and histamine blocking agent used to treat human migraine headaches and hypersensitivity reactions such as rhinitis, has been reported to be successful in treating some cases of headshaking.[13,16,17] However, in other reports, cyproheptadine alone has been ineffective.[25,26]

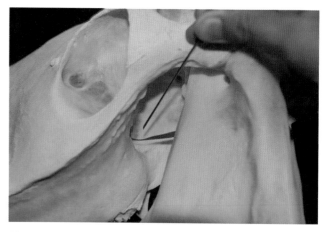

Figure 10.2. A 3.5 inch, 18 g needle in the proper position to block the caudal nasal branch of the trigeminal nerve (shown in red).

A combination of carbamazepine, an anti-convulsive and anti-epileptic drug used to treat trigeminal neuralgia in humans,[27] and cyproheptadine resulted in an 80% to 100% improvement in 80% of cases of equine headshaking.[25] However, carbamazepine alone was just as effective as the combination.[25,26] The positive response to carbamazepine, combined with clinical features, is consistent with involvement of the trigeminal nerve, particularly the more proximal branches such as the caudal nasal branch nerve.[25] Bilateral infraorbital neurectomy has not been successful in resolving headshaking.[20]

Serotonin reuptake inhibitors have been effective in the treatment of compulsive disorders in dogs.[22] Fluoxetine (Prozac) is the most commonly used such drug in dogs,[22] and at 0.25 to 0.5 mg/kg/day per os is probably the most economical medication that can benefit a horse with compulsive disorder.[11]

The use of a nose net or nose mesh to reduce turbulent air flow in the caudal nasal passages was reported

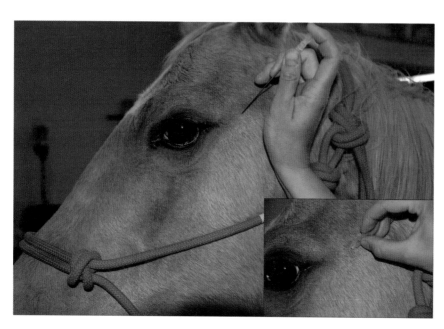

Figure 10.1. Proper location and direction for inserting the needle to block the caudal nasal branch of the trigeminal nerve.

by more than 25% of users to be completely successful in resolving headshaking.[3] In another survey, approximately 75% of owners reported some overall improvement with various types of nose net, 60% reported 50% or greater improvement, and 30% reported 70% or greater improvement.[23]

Photic headshaker horses stopped headshaking when they were blindfolded, had their eyes covered with light-filtering masks or gray lenses, or were turned out into night darkness.[16]

To the extent possible, any stressors in the horse's environment should be eliminated.[11] A horse that is confined for lengthy periods in a small stall may become frustrated and bored.[4] Horses are gregarious animals that are uncomfortable when isolated from other horses. It may help to keep the horse on pasture for a minimum of several hours a day with compatible horses.[11] In fact, turning the horse out onto pasture for several months may help if all other treatments fail.[7]

It generally takes considerable patience to resolve headshaking.[15]

Identifying and Dealing with Bitting Problems

In addition to headshaking, common signs of bitting problems include pulling on the bit; ear pinning; gaping of the mouth; failure to travel straight (sometimes mistaken for lameness); difficulty in guiding or stopping; excessive salivation; and sores, cuts, or bleeding from the mouth.[15]

A horse that is sore on one side of its mouth may lean on the bit on the tender side.[15] Oral discomfort causes horses to focus on pain rather than performance. An affected horse may fail to respond to the bit cues, evade the action of the bit, or ignore the bit completely.[15]

Clients that inquire about a headshaking horse or one that has any other performance problems should always be asked about the type of bit used (Figures 10.3 and 10.4), and the tongue, lips, lower interdental space, palate, chin, and nose examined carefully for subtle signs of injury.[15]

A horse may take a number of actions to evade a bit.[15] If it suffers discomfort every time the bit is inserted, it may resist being bridled by raising its head and clenching its teeth. When a horse is said to take the bit in his teeth, it is actually extending its nose, getting ahead of the bit, and retracting the corners of its lips.[15] The bit ends up resting against the lower second premolars, where contact with the mouth is painless. When a horse is said to spit out the bit, it is tucking its chin against its chest, getting behind the bit to avoid the bit's pressure.[15] The horse may brace its lower lip outside on the shank of a curb bit, thus taking the pressure off the tongue and gums. It can also turn the bit in its mouth with its tongue, sometimes called scissoring, thereby avoiding its pressure.[15] A horse may continually nod or toss its head in an attempt to position the bit in its mouth so that it will be more comfortable.[15]

Measures to prevent bitting problems include ensuring that bits are clean and free of defects and that they fit properly, and that the headstall and all accessories are adjusted properly.[15] A standing martingale (tie-down) should be adjusted with enough slack so that the

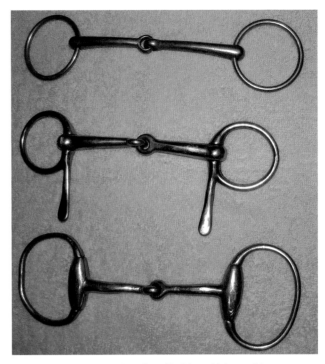

Figure 10.3. Examples of snaffle bits, which provide no leverage to the hands on the reins, and are considered the mildest of bits.

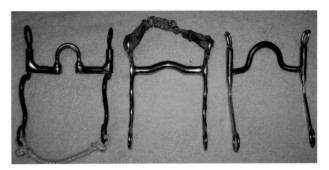

Figure 10.4. Examples of leverage (curb) bits, which are considered to be relatively severe bits because they provide a mechanical advantage. The forces on the horse's mouth exerted by a curb bit increase with the length of the shanks of the bit and with the ratio of the length of the shanks (below the mouthpiece) to the length of the cheeks (above the mouthpiece).

horse can stand comfortably and use its head and neck effectively for balance during performance. A running martingale should not be used with a shanked bit.[15] A horse should never be tied with the bridle reins and should never be punished by jerking on the reins. It should become a habit to check the horse's mouth for signs of tenderness or injury whenever the bit is inserted.[15]

If the history indicates that headshaking may have developed from inappropriate use of bits, retraining may be necessary.[11] An experienced trainer should address the rider's technique.[11] Bit- or rider-related headshaking can be prevented by experienced trainers encouraging beginning riders to learn how to use the

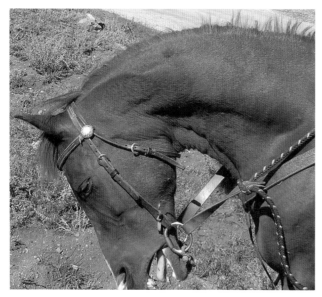

Figure 10.5. Even the mildest of bits, such as this egg-butt snaffle, can become severe if used with excessive rein pressure (hard hands).

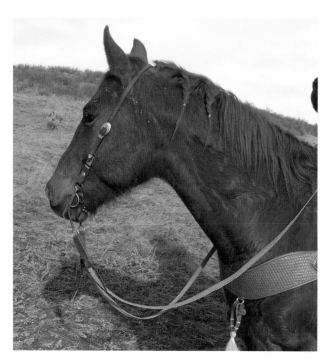

Figure 10.6. This potentially severe curb bit with a harsh, twisted wire mouthpiece does not damage the horse's mouth because the rider has soft hands and rides with a slack rein.

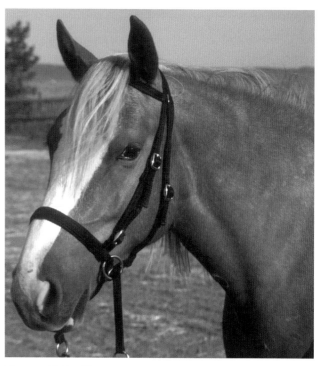

Figure 10.7. The cross-under bitless bridle developed by Dr. Robert Cook is perhaps the gentlest of all headgear with which to communicate with the horse.

bit lightly (Figures 10.5 and 10.6).[11,15] A change of bridling and riding tactics, allowing the horse to assume a head position that is natural and comfortable, and adjusting the position of the bit in the mouth may be necessary.[15] Attaching the bit to the reins with light rubber bands may be effective in preventing beginning riders from injuring horses' mouths.

It is frequently advisable to change the problem horse to a milder bit or, even better, to a bitless bridle. The cross-under bitless bridle (Figure 10.7) developed by Cook is very gentle and can be effective in treating or preventing headshaking and other problems.[1,9,15]

For horses that have developed a strong fear of the bit or of human hands as a result of abuse, many weeks of counterconditioning may be required to resolve the problem.[11] Attempts should be made to determine whether the horse responds adversely to excessively rapid movement of the hand, movement toward a specific location on its head, the presence of a bridle in the hand, and silence or the sound of a human voice.[11] It is important to identify how the hand can approach the head without the horse showing anxiety, and then these motions should be repeated while offering highly palatable food (e.g., sweet feed, apples, carrots) in the other hand.[11] Placing a bridle with a gentle bit on the horse while gently grooming it on the withers may help to reduce its fear.[11]

PROGNOSIS

Even when considerable time has been spent investigating and attempting to treat a headshaker, the results are often disappointing.[4] However, with careful observation, correction of bitting and riding problems, counterconditioning when indicated, and judicious use of drugs, many cases can be improved if not resolved.

References

1. Bennett DG. Bits, bridles and accessories In Equine Dentistry, 2nd ed. Baker GJ, Easley J, eds. Saunders Elsevier, London, New York, 2007;9–22.

2. Blythe LL, Watrous BJ, Pearson EJ, et al. Otitis media/interna in the horse—A cause of head shaking and skull fractures. Proceedings Am Assoc Equine Pract 1991;36:517–528.
3. Casey RA. Clinical problems associated with intensive management of performance horses. In The Welfare of Horses. Waran N, ed. Kluwer Academic Publishers, Boston, 2002;19–44.
4. Cook WR. Headshaking in horses. Part 1. Equine Pract 1979;1(5):9–17.
5. Cook WR. Headshaking in horses. Part 2. History and management tests. Equine Pract 1979;1(6):36–39.
6. Cook WR. Headshaking in horses. Part 3: Diagnostic tests. Equine Pract 1980;2(1):31–40.
7. Cook WR. Headshaking in horses. Part 4. Special diagnostic procedures. Equine Practice 1980;2(2):7–15.
8. Cook WR. Headshaking in horses: An afterword. Compendium Equine 1992;14(10):1368–1371,1376.
9. Cook WR. Use of the bit in the horse. Vet Rec 1998;142(8):200.
10. Cook WR. Bit-induced fear. Part 2: Bits and diseases they can cause. Vet Times 2007;37(15):22–23,25.
11. Crowell-Davis SL. Head shaking. Compendium Contin Educ 2008;3(9):466–470,474.
12. Dacre KJ, Madigan JE, Walsh V, et al. Measurement of somatosensory evoked potentials of the trigeminal nerve in the horse for investigation of headshaking (abstract). J Vet Internal Med 2007;21:667.
13. Feige K, Eser MW. Photic headshaking and cyproheptadine therapy. Pferdeheilkunde 1998;14(5):361–368.
14. Lane JG, Mair T. Observations on headshaking in the horse. Equine Vet J 1987;19(4):331–336.
15. Lynch B, Bennett DG. Bits and Bridles: Power Tools for Thinking Riders. Equi Media, Austin, TX. 2000.
16. Madigan JE, Kortz G, Murphy C, et al. Photic headshaking in the horse: 7 cases. Equine Vet J 1995;27(4):306–311.
17. Madigan JE, Bell SA. Owner survey of headshaking in horses. J Am Vet Med Assoc 2001;219(3):334–337.
18. Mair TS, Lane G. Headshaking in horses. In Practice 1990; 12(5):183–186.
19. Mair TS. Obstructive pulmonary disease in 18 horses at summer pasture. Vet Rec 1996;138(4):89–91.
20. Mair TS. Assessment of bilateral infra-orbital nerve blockade and bilateral infra-orbital neurectomy in the investigation and treatment of idiopathic headshaking. Equine Vet J 1999; 31(3):262–264.
21. Mills DS, Cook S, Taylor K, et al. Analysis of the variations in clinical signs shown by 254 cases of equine headshaking. Vet Rec 2002;150:236–240.
22. Mills D, Luescher A. Veterinary and pharmacologic approaches to abnormal repetitive behaviour. In Stereotypic Animal Behaviour: Fundamentals and Applications to Welfare, 2nd ed. Mason G, Rushen J, eds. CABI, Wallingford, UK, 2006; 286–316.
23. Mills DS, Taylor K. Field study of the efficacy of three types of nose net for the treatment of headshaking in horses. Vet Rec 2003;152(2):41–44.
24. Moore LA, Johnson PJ, Messer NT, et al. Management of headshaking in three horses by treatment of protozoal myeloencephalitis. Vet Rec 1997;141(11):264–267.
25. Newton SA, Knottenbelt DC, Eldridge PR. Headshaking in horses: Possible aetiopathogenesis suggested by the results of diagnostic tests and several treatment regimes used in 20 cases. Equine Vet J 2000;32(3):208–216.
26. Newton SA. Idiopathic headshaking in horses. Equine Vet Education 2005;17(2):83–9.
27. Ropper AH, Brown RH. Adams and Victor's Principles of Neurology, 8th ed. McGraw-Hill, New York, 2005.
28. Schule E, Herling A. Headshaking—A review. Pferdeheilkunde 2006;22(3):281–295.
29. Schwarz B. Idiopathic headshaking in horses—Thoughts on potential etiology and therapeutic approaches. Praktische Tierarzt 2008;89(3):208–213.
30. Taylor KD, Cook S, Mills DS. A case-controlled study investigating health, management and behavioural features of horses commonly described as headshakers. Ippologia 2001;12(3):29–37.

STANCE AND GAIT ABNORMALITIES CAUSED BY NEUROLOGICAL DISEASE

Lutz S. Goehring

PREVALENCE OF NEUROLOGICAL DISEASE IN HORSES

Neurological disease in horses is relatively rare, particularly when compared to horses that present with problems such as recurrent airway obstruction or lameness. The most common neurological presentation is a horse with gait abnormalities caused by a compressive, cervical spinal cord lesion or (in the U.S.) infection with *Sarcocystis neurona*, the cause of equine protozoal myelitis. An in-depth review of equine neurology can be obtained from a number of excellent text books.[1,3,4,7]

It is usually easy for a professional to recognize moderate to profound neurological gait abnormalities. Distinguishing minor gait changes caused by neurological defects from lameness or behavioral abnormalities, may be more of a challenge, however. Furthermore, all of these can contribute to an abnormal gait, and neurological and musculoskeletal conditions may co-exist independently or share a common pathophysiological background, confounding the diagnosis. Osteochondrosis is a perfect example of gait problems resulting from both musculoskeletal and neurological causes. It leads to limb lameness through joint problems, and facet joint osteochondrosis of the cervical vertebrae can lead to compression of the cervical spinal cord. See the section on cervical vertebral stenosis in Chapter 11 for more information on this topic.

From a neuro-anatomical standpoint, neurological gait abnormalities can be caused by diseases that affect the central and/or peripheral nervous system, either rostral or caudal of the foramen magnum. Lesions in the spinal cord, its segmental spinal nerves, and neuromuscular junctions cause most neurological gait abnormalities in horses.

NEUROLOGICAL GAIT

The first question veterinarians should ask themselves when a horse presents with suspected neurological gait abnormalities is, "Is what we observe caused by neurological disease?" To make a certain diagnosis of neurological disease, it is important to take a history and conduct physical and neurological exams each and every time. Furthermore, a neurological examination should always be completed, regardless of the presentation. This includes determining the patient's level of consciousness; conducting cranial nerve function testing; briefly examining both eyes; and observing eating, drinking, and, ideally, defecation/urination prior to a gait evaluation.[7]

A neurological gait can be described in terms of 3 distinct abnormalities: ataxia, dysmetria, and weakness. The neurological gait that is observed may be the result of a single abnormality or a combination of 2 or all 3 abnormalities. Each limb must be observed and evaluated for the presence of these findings, and graded using a predetermined scale.[4]

Ataxia

Ataxia is derived from the Greek word for indiscipline or lack of order. An ataxic gait is irregular and lacks predictability; it is best described as being "irregularly irregular." Ataxia results from an absent or decreased perception of proprioceptive information ascending to the cerebellum from the peripheral sensors, Golgi (tendon) organs in all limbs, and neck (and vestibular organ), and as a result the animal can no longer correctly perceive its position, posture, or equilibrium.

Ataxia is noticed in a horse if 1 of the following 3 components of the nervous system is affected: the vestibular organ, vestibular nerve, or nucleus; the cerebellum; or the spinal cord. Vestibular ataxia is usually associated with a head tilt and asymmetrical ataxia. Horses with one-sided vestibular ataxia show a head tilt toward the side of the lesion, and also tend to circle toward that side. A nystagmus may be present.

Cerebellar ataxia is characterized by a symmetrical ataxia and hypermetria, but without loss of strength. It is routinely accompanied by an intention tremor of the head and a base-wide stance.

Spinal ataxia is the most frequently encountered form of ataxia in the horse. Its cause is a disruption of ascending flow of proprioceptive information toward the cerebellum. As a result, descending information cannot appropriately streamline or fine tune muscle tone and motor function in the periphery. This results in ataxia and irregularly irregular placement of the limbs that are caudal to the spinal cord lesion(s).

Dysmetria

Dysmetria collectively describes a state of rigidity, spasticity, or exuberant limb flexion. It is associated with upper motor neuron (UMN) disease and affects the cerebellum or the descending UMN tracts in the spinal cord. These tracts have two major functions: some are involved in the initiation of movement, whereas others have an inhibitory effect on a peripheral reflex loop (e.g., a patellar reflex). Dysmetria is caused by a reduced inhibition of the peripheral reflex loop, and the uninhibited reflex is observed. A hypermetric gait is characterized by an increased range of movement and excessive joint flexion; hypometric gait is typified by limb stiffness and reduced joint flexion, particularly of the tarsal and carpal joints. This is often described as a tin soldier gait.

Weakness or Paresis

Paresis is the decreased ability to initiate gait, maintain posture, or resist gravity. Paralysis is the inability to do all three. Paresis can be further divided into UMN and lower motor neuron (LMN) paresis. UMN paresis, or flexor weakness, presents with a delay in initiating movement, followed by longer and, typically, lower stride. LMN paresis is usually observed as an antigravity or extensor weakness, presenting as short-strided gait, trembling due to muscle fatigue (muscle fasciculations), bunny-hopping during canter, and lowered neck carriage while standing. Muscle atrophy is more pronounced and often more localized in LMN than UMN paresis; both forms may take 2 to 3 weeks after damage before becoming noticeable. Toe dragging and abnormal hoof wear can be seen with either form of paresis. Severe weakness in all 4 limbs, but no ataxia or dysmetria, indicates diffusely affected neuro-muscular units and is by definition a LMN weakness.

EXPECTED FINDINGS FROM A NEUROLOGICAL EXAM

Consciousness and Body Position

The normal horse is quiet or bright, alert, and responsive (QAR or BAR). It pays attention to its surroundings, it recognizes visitors, and finds water and food. A horse stands on all 4 limbs placed vertically underneath the body. The exception to this is a standing horse with a locked stifle. In a QAR or BAR horse, the poll of the head should be above the level of the withers. The recumbent horse usually is found in a sternal position or in a flat lateral position. Minimal disturbance is usually necessary for arousal and getting up. A horse extends its forelimbs first, followed by an abrupt extension and lift-off with both hindlimbs.

An abnormal horse is either stuporous or (semi) comatose; wanders in circles within its confined space; may appear blind, agitated, or violent, or it has a seizure. All clinical signs relate to a problem rostral to the foramen magnum. An abnormal stance can be wide based (sawhorse stance) or narrow based (horse-on-a-ball or goat-on-a-rock stance). The sawhorse stance is typical for a horse with a cerebellar lesion, whereas the horse-on-a-ball stance is seen with diseases collectively affecting the LMN. Whenever a horse places limbs randomly, once it comes to a standstill (hence, an asymmetrical limb placement), this may be a sign for a lack of proprioception.

A conscious horse that cannot rise from recumbency is probably affected by profound weakness, which can be UMN or diffuse LMN weakness. Whether the horse can lift its neck from the ground, maintain a sternal position, or sits like a dog is a critical observation in determining where the lesion of the problem is located—the cranial or caudal neck, thoracolumbar spinal cord, multifocal, or diffusely involving gray and white matter of the spinal cord.

Horses with a head tilt and vestibular ataxia often stand slightly wide based, and the body may be concavely bent toward the side of the lesion. If recumbent, horses with a head tilt are more comfortable while lying on the affected side.

Head and Body Symmetry

The normal horse shows symmetry in the head position and the posture of the neck, limbs, and trunk. Symmetry also extends to facial expression and the carriage of the tail. A headtilt (a sign of central or peripheral vestibular damage), a dropped ear, and paralysis of facial muscles (facial nerve paralysis) are examples of head asymmetry. Regional muscle atrophy or complete unilateral atrophy is more likely a sign of UMN paresis. Defined muscle atrophy of a single muscle belly is best explained by peripheral nerve damage. However, generalized, symmetrical muscle atrophy without signs of ataxia or dysmetria is the result of diffuse LMN disease if it is a neurological disease to begin with.

Manipulations in the Standing Horse

The normal horse is able to extend and flex its head and neck dorsally and ventrally. The horse's muzzle should touch its ribs during lateral flexion of the head and neck toward the chest.

A severely ataxic horse resists extending its head and neck dorsally and to the sides. Some horses with cervical vertebral stenotic myelopathy (CVS or CVSM) may be reluctant or resent lateral flexion due to pain in the vertebral facets.

Both sides of the horse's neck and back musculature, from front to back, should be probed with a blunt instrument such as the handle of a neurology hammer or a ball-point pen. Mild stimulation of the chest and abdomen elicits a cutaneous trunci muscle response, but not in all horses. A 2-pinch technique with forceps elicits this local reflex first, and a pain response may be noticed with a deeper pinch. The dorsal processes of the thoracic and lumbar vertebrae must be palpated and percussed. No pain response or crepitus should be observed or palpated. With both hands placed over the withers, the horse is pushed away and pulled toward the examiner. A normal horse quickly contracts the extensor or anti-gravity muscles in the forelimbs to maintain a solid stance. An abnormal horse can easily be pushed away or pulled toward the examiner because of LMN weakness or a lack of proprioception.

Hopping should be done by picking up one forelimb at a time; however, caution is advised in the obviously severely affected horse. The examiner faces the same direction as the horse, holds the lifted forelimb at the pasterns, and pushes the horse away with her/his shoulder. The normal horse will hop one jump at a time with a nice lift-off and landing. The abnormal horse will have a delayed lift-off and a short, rigid jump followed by a clumsy landing. Hopping tests several aspects of the nervous system: muscular strength, proprioception, and dysmetria.

Stimulating the axial musculature of the back usually elicits a ventro-dorsal movement of the vertebral column, lordosis followed by kyphosis. The abnormal horse shows scoliosis or it appears stiff in the back. A normal horse has at least some degree of a tail tone, and a perineal reflex. A completely flaccid tail is a sign of LMN weakness. A tail should not continuously be held off the body; this can be a clinical sign of tetanus or tetany.

The (standing) tail-pull is probably the most important test of a neurological examination in the standing horse (Figure 10.8). It helps to distinguish between UMN and LMN weakness. The square, standing horse is gradually pulled at its tail laterally until the examiner notices a contraction of the quadriceps muscle. The horse will be pulled fairly easily toward the examiner due to lower motor weakness if there is lumbar lower motor neuron dysfunction.

A normal horse walks with a regular 4-beat movement. Limb placement should be graceful and regular, and a solid surface allows the examiner to listen to hoof placement. The hindlimbs follow the forelimbs, and the hindlimbs typically overreach the imprints of the forelimbs. Key abnormalities in the neurological horse are revealed in unpredictable limb placement, a shortened stride length, toe dragging, pacing, and generalized rigidity or stiffness resulting in a truncal sway. All of these signs can result from ataxia, weakness, or dysmetria. These may be mild and unobservable during a routine exam when walking the horse on a flat, hard surface.

In such cases the signs can be exacerbated by circling or spinning the horse, backing it up for several steps, and walking it, with and without head elevation, up and down a slope. A horse with a neurologically affected gait may exhibit circumduction (an exaggerated movement of the outer hindlimb) or pivoting (planting a forefoot and turning around without lifting it) during spinning. During backing, the limbs of a normal horse should move diagonally, with simultaneous placement of the contralateral fore- and hindlimbs. During uphill and downhill walking, a normal horse places its limbs solidly and securely, without knuckling in the fetlocks or carpal/tarsal joints. Insecure placement of limbs is a sign of ataxia. Particularly when walking downhill, simultaneous elevation of the head exacerbates insecurity with limb placement.

Neurologically abnormal horses also should be examined during a trot, and, if not too severely affected, during canter. A good test for proprioception is to trot a horse and bring it to a sudden stop. A smooth collection of all limbs underneath the body will be observed in a normal horse.

PITFALLS OF NEUROLOGICAL EXAMINATION

The clinical presentations discussed above suggest neurological damage that affects the gait. However, the signs also can arise from illnesses or problems unrelated to the nervous system. These should be considered when making the diagnosis, and possible explanations for suspect neurological findings are listed in Table 10.1.

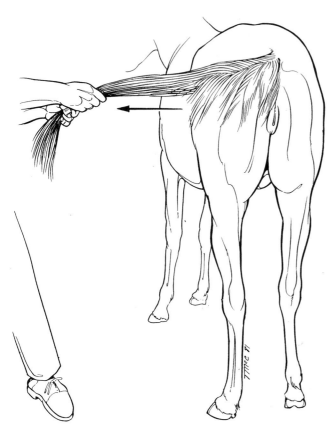

Figure 10.8. Tail-pull (arrow) in a standing horse tests the strength of the quadriceps muscle and the reflex activity of the femoral nerve as a part of the lower motor neuron system. A gradually increasing pull on the tail toward the examiner should result in a quadriceps muscle contraction, and the hindquarter of the horse should not move significantly. For example, a horse with a cervical spinal cord lesion showing a grade 3 out of 4 ataxia of the hindlimbs still has a strong response to the standing tail pull. Pulling on this horse's tail during a walk will show incoordination or ataxia.

Table 10.1. Alternative explanations for presentations with a suspected neurological presentation.

Clinical finding	Alternative, non-nervous system associated explanations
Generalized muscle atrophy	Starvation, emaciation, (intestinal) nutrient absorption disorder, paraneoplastic syndrome, chronic myopathies
Regional muscle atrophy	Lameness-associated disuse
Low head-neck carriage	Nuchal ligament desmitis or rupture, exhaustion, emaciation/starvation, fever, use of sedatives
Ataxia	Fever, sedation
Stiffness, short-strided	Lameness, myopathy
Hind limb hypermetria	Laminitis, Chorioptes spp. infestation, fibrotic myopathy
Recumbency	Exhaustion, colic, rhabdomyolysis, pain, laminitis

NEUROLOGICAL SYNDROMES AFFECTING THE GAIT

Cervical Vertebral Stenotic Myelopathy (CVSM)

CVSM is probably the most frequent cause of neurological gait abnormalities in performance horses. CVSM is described in detail in Chapter 11.

Botulism

Botulism is a feed-borne intoxication associated with *Clostridium botulinum* toxin. If several horses are on a property, botulism usually manifests as a herd outbreak.

Botulism toxins block the acetylcholine (ACh) release at presynaptic neuromuscular junctions, postganglionic parasympathetic nerve endings, and peripheral ganglia. Posture and gait deficits are noted initially, with muscle fasciculations and a short-strided gait, and are followed by recumbency. Stance is characterized by "goat-on-a-rock" stance. Hallmark findings of botulism are generalized weakness resulting in an abnormal gait and recumbency, and cranial (motor) nerve dysfunction. Excellent reviews of botulism are available in other texts.[3,12]

Equine Motor Neuron Disease (EMND)

EMND is a rare, slowly progressive disease that usually affects only a single animal in a herd. Although its etiology is unknown, lack of antioxidants, particularly vitamin E, has been implicated in its development. EMND causes lower motor neuron destruction of the spinal cord, leading to signs of symmetrical neurogenic muscle atrophy and weakness, without ataxia. Stance is characterized by "goat-on-a-rock" stance. Horses with EMND are described as having a loss of muscle mass in combination with a good appetite, and cranial nerves are not involved.[2,8]

Equine Protozoal Myeloencephalitis (EPM)

EPM is a disease of the Americas, most commonly caused by a protozoan organism, *Sarcocystis neurona*. The geographical restriction of *S. neurona* is linked to the restriction of its definitive host, the American opossum (*Didelphis virginiana*). *S. neurona* oocysts are produced in the opossums' gastrointestinal tract. After horses ingest the oocysts through contaminated feed, sporulation occurs and asexual replication of *S. neurona* merozoites may follow. In a small but poorly defined number of horses the protozoan enters the central nervous system, where replication can be prolonged and progressive, leading to multifocal disease of the brain and spinal cord. The most common presentation of EPM is asymmetrical gait, with a gradual worsening over weeks to months. Cranial nerve abnormalities are also common. EPM is well reviewed in several textbooks.[4,9,10]

West Nile Virus, Eastern/Western/Venezuelan Encephalitis Viruses

The implementation of a good vaccination program against West Nile virus and Eastern, Western, and Venezuelan encephalitis viruses means that disease should only be expected in poorly or nonvaccinated horses. Hallmark clinical findings of these viruses are active muscle fasciculations, tremors, and hyperesthesia. Cortex or general brain involvement appears to be more common with Eastern, Western, and Venezuelan encephalitis viruses, whereas the spinal cord and basal ganglia are frequent targets of West Nile virus.[5]

Equine Herpesvirus Type 1-associated Myeloencephalopathy (EHM)

EHM is a rare syndrome that can follow infection with equine herpesvirus type 1. It causes multifocal ischemic damage, primarily to the spinal cord, usually in adult horses of the tall breeds. Only horses that develop a cell-associated viremia during infection are at risk of EHM. The clinical presentation varies with the number of ischemic infarcts. A low to moderate number of infarcts results in asymmetrical ataxia and both upper and lower motor weakness; a high number leads to a coalescing disease with profound weakness, which often results in paralysis.[5,11]

Ryegrass Staggers

The clinical signs of ryegrass staggers present shortly after ingestion of a preformed toxin from an endophyte closely associated with perennial ryegrass (*Lolium perenne*), although a few other grasses are associated with a similar syndrome. The endophyte (*Neotyphodium lolii*) is in a symbiotic, lifelong relationship with the grass, and may produce significant amounts of the toxin, lolitrem B, under growth-related and environmental conditions. The syndrome has a regional occurrence, reflecting its close association with perennial ryegrass feeding. Lolitrem B affects the cerebellum and the inhibitory (inter) neurons in the spinal cord. The clinical signs are very typical: tremors, base wide stance, (micro)nystagmus, and a staggering, hypermetric gait. The signs worsen with exercise and persist as long as there is further toxin intake. Once toxin-free feed is provided, there is usually a fast recovery and return to full function.[6]

Stringhalt and Shivers

Although recognized as neuropathies, the etiology and location of a neurological lesion for both stringhalt and shivers remains poorly understood. A hyperreflexia seems to be involved in both syndromes. In stringhalt, this is a hyperreflexia of the lateral digital extensor muscle of the hindlimbs, typically hyperflexing 1 or both hindlimbs during a walk. Shivers is a hyperreflexia of the flexor muscles of the pelvic limbs, which becomes most noticeable when the horse is backed. Shivers is more common in draft and Warmblood breeds.[4] The affected hindlimb, often in combination with the tail base, shows jerky movements that are due to cyclic contraction followed by relaxation of the involved musculature.

Stringhalt is differentiated as a plant-associated form involving a toxin, in which case several horses sharing pasture may become affected simultaneously, and a sporadic, single-animal form. A peripheral axonopathy may be found in combination with a neurogenic myopathy with the plant-associated form of stringhalt. Involvement of the Golgi tendon organ is suspected with the sporadic form. This may also be true for Shivers; however, proprioceptive or UMN pathways in the CNS may also be affected.

References

1. De Lahunta A, Glass E. Veterinary Neuroanatomy and Clinical Neurology, 3rd ed. Saunders Elsevier, St. Louis, 2009.
2. Divers TJ, Mohammed HO, Cummings JF, et al. Equine motor neuron disease: Findings in 28 horses and proposal of a pathophysiological mechanism for the disease. Equine Vet J 1995;26:409–415.
3. Furr M. Clostridial neurotoxins: Botulism and tetanus. In Equine Neurology. Furr M, Reed S, eds. Blackwell Publishing, Ames, 2008;221–229.
4. Furr M, Reed S. Equine Neurology. Blackwell Publishing, Ames, 2008.
5. Goehring L. Viral diseases of the nervous system. In Equine Neurology. Furr M, Reed S, eds. Blackwell Publishing, Ames, 2008;169–186.
6. Goehring LS, van Maanen C, Sloet van Oldruitenborgh-Oosterbaan MM. Neurological syndromes among horses in the Netherlands. A 5-year retrospective survey (1999–2004). Vet Q 2005;27:11–20.
7. Mayhew IG: Large Animal Neurology, 2nd ed. Wiley-Blackwell, Ames, 2008.
8. McGorum BC, Mayhew IG, Amory H, et al. Horses on pasture may be affected by equine motor neuron disease. Equine Vet J 2006;38:47–51.
9. Reed S, Bayly W, Sellon D. Equine Internal Medicine, 2nd ed. Saunders Elsevier, St. Louis, 2004.
10. Sellon D, Dubey J. Equine protozoal myeloencephalitis. In Equine Infectious Diseases. Sellon DC, Long MT, eds. Saunders Elsevier, St. Louis, 2007;453–464.
11. Slater JD. Equine herpesviruses. In Equine Infectious Diseases. Sellon DC, Long MT, eds. Saunders Elsevier, St. Louis, 2007;134–153.
12. Whitlock R. Botulism (Shaker Foals; Forage Poisoning). In Large Animal Internal Medicine, 4th ed. Smith B, ed. Mosby Elsevier, St. Louis, 2009;1096–1101.

EVALUATION OF PROPER SADDLE FIT

Kevin K. Haussler

INTRODUCTION

Proper saddle fit and use is a critical component of optimum athletic performance and the prevention of back pain or discomfort in horses. Unfortunately, it is not always clear what is meant by "good saddle fit," and objective parameters for assessing saddle fit and function during dynamic activities are lacking and often difficult. Saddles are often fit for the seat of the rider; however, the correct width or length of the saddle for a particular horse, adequate padding, and stirrup attachment or positioning, which influence a rider's leg positioning and balance on the horse, are often overlooked.[6] Considerable interactions between the rider, saddle, and horse's back influence the rider's comfort and effectiveness in the saddle and the movement patterns of the horse's back and saddle.[5] Poorly fitting or improperly used saddles and saddle pads often contribute to back pain and poor performance. It is imperative to understand the basic principles of assessing proper saddle fit and the effects of proper vs. poorly fitting saddles on both the rider and the horse.

CLINICAL SIGNS OF POOR SADDLE FIT

Signs of asymmetric rider positioning in the saddle include uneven wear patterns on the seat from asymmetric rider contact with the seat bones (tuber ischii) or asymmetrical leather wear over the stirrup irons or stitching under the rider's legs. Horses with back pain related to poor saddle fit may display adverse or abnormal behavioral signs such as ear pinning, teeth grinding, head tossing, tail swishing, unwillingness to stand still during saddle or saddle pad placement, or biting or kicking while being saddled or while tightening the girth.[3] Asymmetric sweat patterns on the horse or saddle pad, asymmetric dirt patterns on the saddle pad, regional hair loss in areas of saddle contact, local edema, or open sores are all acute signs of poor saddle fit. Chronic signs of poorly fitting saddles include white hairs or granulomas and muscle atrophy in the saddle region.

Ill-fitting saddles can cause horses to hollow their backs (i.e., induced lordosis) and resent mounting. Affected horses often have reduced spinal mobility and are slow to warm up or relax during initial riding, but may be completely normal during lunging or work in the round pen due to unweighted exercise. Regular bucking or rearing, resistance to work that worsens with time, difficulty with collection or maintaining impulsion, and resentment or ignoring training aids also may be indicative of poor saddle fit issues related to ridden exercise. Reduced protraction of the thoracic limb (i.e., shortened stride), stumbling or tripping, or obvious lameness can be produced by poorly fitting saddles. Upper pelvic limb lameness and lack of impulsion also may be exacerbated by increased saddle pressure.[4]

SADDLE EXAMINATION

To evaluate proper saddle fit, the saddle is assessed for manufacturer defects or signs of wear and the rider-saddle and saddle-horse interfaces are evaluated during static and dynamic examinations. The ideal saddle provides uniform contact and pressure across all regions of the back during both static and dynamic assessments. There should be no elevated or depressed areas that predispose to increased pressure and no left-right or craniocaudal asymmetries. The most common saddle fitting faults include bridging, increased pressure over the withers at the front of the saddle, high overall pressure, or asymmetric or localized pressure points.[7]

Examination of the saddle begins with assessing saddle construction and wear. The seat is evaluated for asymmetric wear, which often indicates that the rider is uneven in the saddle. Uneven flaps or stirrup bar placement are manufacturing defects and an affected saddle should be returned for replacement. Worn or dried out leather straps must be replaced due to safety concerns.

Because the tree forms the foundation of the saddle, any saddle with a broken or asymmetric tree must be repaired or discarded. Saddles with broken trees have reduced stability and support, allowing the saddle to deform and causing localized increased pressure. Broken and twisted trees are evaluated visually by inspecting the symmetry. Excessive flexibility is assessed by applying craniocaudal forces to the bars or by applying lateral compressive forces to the head of the tree. The ventral surface of the panels is inspected for adequate flocking, left-right angular symmetry, and craniocaudal symmetry in the flocking. Horses with asymmetric withers often affect the symmetry of the cranial portion of the panels. The caudal edge of the panels should be wide and flat to maximize comfort for the horse, rather than narrow or pointed, which can cause localized pressure at the back edge of the saddle. In Western saddles, the fleece along the ventral surface should be palpated carefully with a flat hand to identify any protruding screws, nails, or plant burrs that can produce localized pressure or wounds. The width of the gullet should be 2 to 3 fingers wide along the entire length to allow positioning and movement of the dorsal spinous processes.[4]

STATIC EXAMINATION OF SADDLE FIT

The static examination of saddle fit on the horse's back is accomplished by visual inspection and palpation of the saddle-horse interface in the standing horse. A useful analogy for assessing saddle fit and proper saddle pad use is that the saddle should fit the horse's back like a well-made shoe and the saddle pad functions like a sock.

In a well fitting saddle, the addition of a thin saddle pad should result in optimal saddle and saddle pad function and should not produce increased pressure or back pain. However, a proper fitting saddle used with an excessive number or increased thickness of saddle pads will likely produce localized pressure and back problems. In poor fitting saddles, the addition of a thin pad will likely not improve saddle fit. Likewise, the use of several saddle pads to compensate for a poor fitting saddle (such as a poor fitting shoe with several socks) will likely exaggerate saddle pressure and produce back pain. That said, wide fitting saddles may benefit from the use of several pads as a temporary solution to mismatched saddle-horse sizes.

The static examination of saddle fit begins with the owner placing the saddle on the horse's back. The saddle is initially evaluated without any pads or girth to limit influence by other confounding variables. The owner is instructed to place and position the saddle on the horse's back in the usual manner. This provides an opportunity to qualitatively assess the horse's response and behavior to saddle placement and to evaluate saddle fit and positioning. Horses that pin their ears or attempt to bite or kick with saddle placement likely have or have had issues with poor fitting saddles and secondary back pain. As noted above, the tree provides the framework for the saddle and acts to transfer the rider's weight to the back of the horse. Therefore, the length, width, angles, and twist (or shape) of the tree ideally must match the contour and symmetry of the individual horse's back. The flare at the front of the tree should fit over the withers and allow free scapular movements. The width and angle of the tree must match the lateral slope of the withers.

In English saddles, the cranial edge of the saddle should rest at the caudal edge of the scapula. In Western saddles, the saddle normally covers the dorsal aspect of the scapulae, but the skirt should flare cranially to allow caudal rotation of the scapula during thoracic limb protraction. New saddles often have very stiff and inflexible skirts that may occasionally rub on the dorsal scapula cranially or lumbar region caudally. The length of the saddle should be proportionate to the length of the horse's back and the size of the rider. Saddles that are too short localize pressure and likely cause back pain. Saddles that are too long tend to bridge across the horse's back and localize pressure at the withers and caudal saddle, with little or no contact in the middle of the saddle where most of the rider's weight is located. Saddle bridging is a common problem in lordotic horses; this can be temporarily managed by placing additional padding or shims to fill in the non-contact areas at the center of the saddle to provide uniform saddle contact. Proper skirt length in Western saddles should provide 4 to 6 inches of clearance in front of the tuber coxae. Long skirts can cause friction rubs on the cranial aspect of the tuber coxae and restrict lateral bending of the trunk.

Stability of the saddle on the horse's back can be estimated by applying cranial-to-caudal, side-to-side, and diagonal rocking motions to the saddle. Properly fitting saddles are very stable and allow no displacement of the saddle. Wide saddles or the use of too many saddle pads causes instability and excessive displacement of the saddle during these induced movements.

In properly fitting and positioned saddles, the pommel and cantle of most saddles are horizontally level and the deepest portion of the seat should be located near the center of the seat. Saddles that slope downward in the front cause the rider's weight to be shifted over the withers. In contrast, caudally sloping seats cause the rider's weight to be shifted caudally, away from the horse's center of gravity. The position of the girth or cinch should correspond to the narrowest portion of the chest; otherwise, the saddle tends to constantly slide forward or backward, producing back pain and altering performance.

Properly fitting saddles should have 2 to 3 fingers-width (4 to 6 cm) of vertical clearance between the pommel gullet and the dorsal withers (Figure 10.9). Narrow saddles tend to sit higher and produce a taller saddle-wither gap, whereas wide saddles come close to resting on the dorsal spinous processes due to lack of lateral contact and support over the withers (Figure 10.10). Gliding a flat hand under the front edge of a well fitting saddle and over the withers should provide a sensation of a smooth, uniform, soft contact bilaterally (Figure 10.11). The angle of the head of the tree should coincide with the lateral slope of the withers. Asymmetric trees or scapulae can produce left-right differences in saddle contact over the lateral wither region.

Gliding a flat hand under the panels or skirt of a well fitting saddle should also provide a smooth, uniform contact bilaterally, which closely follows the contour of the horse's back. The flocking in English saddles should be symmetric, of uniform firmness, and evenly distributed with no prominences or depressions. Overstuffed panels form round, firm cylinders that do not readily conform to the shape of the horse's back. Underflocked panels are flat and provide no cushion. The panels at the back edge of an English saddle should be flat and in contact with the horse's back. Some saddles have pronounced upward curving panels that cause a substantial reduction in the surface area over which to distribute a rider's weight. The gullet can be visualized

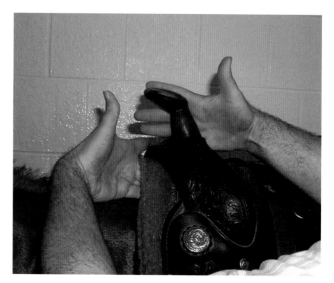

Figure 10.9. Proper spacing between the saddle and dorsal aspect of the withers, with a saddle pad in place.

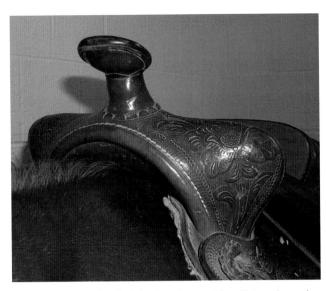

Figure 10.10. Poorly fitting Western saddle with too close of contact between the pommel gullet and the dorsal aspect of the withers.

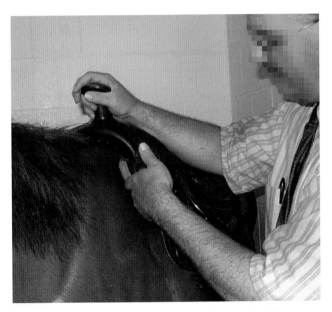

Figure 10.11. Evaluation of smooth, uniform contact between the front portion of the panel and the underlying dorsal aspect of the scapula. The contact pressure should be symmetrical from left to right.

from behind the horse and should provide ample clearance for the dorsal spinous processes.

STATIC EXAMINATION OF SADDLE PADS

Static evaluation of the combined saddle and saddle pad fit is accomplished by repeating the above examination with the saddle pad in place. If more than 1 saddle pad is typically used by a rider, then pads or blankets are sequentially added or exchanged during the exami-

nation to assess the influence of select saddle pads or saddle pad combinations on proper saddle fit. The size, shape, thickness, and material of the saddle pad should correspond to the intended use of the horse. Saddle pads should also be selected for specific temperature, moisture absorption, friction reduction, shock absorption or cushion, and uniform pressure distribution characteristics.

Saddle pads for a short-term dressage test have different requirements than do saddle pads used for racing or during extended ridden activities (e.g., a 100-mile endurance ride). One method for indirectly assessing saddle fit and pressure is to ask the rider to ride the horse in a clean, white saddle pad prior to saddle fit assessment. Properly fitting saddles produce symmetric and uniform dirt or sweat patterns on the saddle pad in the shape of a butterfly. Regions of increased dirt and lack of dirt are noted bilaterally, which can help determine where the saddle fit should be examined more closely.

The size and shape of the saddle and saddle pad should be compared. Half pads or pads that are too small can cause increased localized pressure along their margins, especially if the edges are not tapered. Again, like wearing socks in a well-fitting shoe, it is important to have no foreign objects, wrinkles, or step defects in the saddle pads, which can cause discomfort and localized pressure. Saddle pads should always be pulled up into the gullet of the saddle in an effort to reduce friction and pressure over the dorsal withers. Saddle pads should also be evaluated for excessive wear, cleanliness, and moisture.

DYNAMIC EXAMINATION OF SADDLE FIT

Dynamic examination of saddle fit and saddle pad use involves assessing both horse and saddle movement during unridden and ridden exercise. The horse initially should be assessed for pain reactions or abnormal behavior in response to saddle placement and tightening of the girth. Saddle movement and the influence of saddle fit and saddle pads can then be assessed during locomotion in hand, on the lunge, or in a round pen.

Proper saddle fit should allow fluid movements of the thoracic limb without restricting any flexion-extension or lateral bending motion of the thoracolumbar spine. Proper saddle fit provides seamless interactions between the rider and the horse during dynamic activities and intended use. Poorly fitting saddles often cause horses to guard their back due to pain or muscle hypertonicity.[3] Scapula or spinal movement asymmetries can produce obvious 1-sided or uneven saddle movement or saddle pad migration.

Evaluation of uniform sweat or dirt patterns on the saddle pad after both unridden and ridden exercise can provide insight into saddle fit and pressure distribution underneath the saddle. Recent research has used pressure-sensitive mats to obtain pressure distribution patterns and areas of peak pressures under both normally and abnormally fitting saddles.[1,2,6]

The effects of saddle pad thickness and weight distribution of the rider in the saddle also can be quantified and monitored over time. Evaluation and knowledge of saddle and saddle pad construction and fit, as well as rider-saddle-horse interactions is important in assessing causes of poor performance and back pain in horses.

References

1. de Cocq P, van Weeren PR, Back W. Saddle pressure measuring: Validity, reliability and power to discriminate between different saddle-fits. Vet J 2006;172:265–273.
2. Fruehwirth B, Peham C, Scheidl M, Schobesberger H. Evaluation of pressure distribution under an English saddle at walk, trot and canter. Equine Veterinary Journal 2004;36:754–757.
3. Harman J. The Horse's Pain-free Back and Saddle-Fit Book. Trafalgar Square Publishing, North Pomfret, VT, 2004.
4. Harman JC. Measurement of the pressure exerted by saddles on the horse's back using a computerized pressure measuring device. Pferdeheilkunde 1997;13:129–134.
5. Jeffcott LB, Holmes MA, Townsend HG. Validity of saddle pressure measurements using force-sensing array technology—preliminary studies. Vet J 1999;158:113–119.
6. Meschan EM, Peham C, Schobesberger H, et al. The influence of the width of the saddle tree on the forces and the pressure distribution under the saddle. Vet J 2007;173:578–584.
7. Pullin JG, Collier MA, Durham CM, et al. Use of force sensing array technology in the development of a new equine saddle pad: Static and dynamic evaluations and technical considerations. J Equine Vet Sci 1996;16:207–216.

PREVENTION AND TREATMENT OF MUSCULOSKELETAL INFECTIONS

Jeremy Hubert

At the very least, orthopedic infections are often severely debilitating condition to horses, and often they are life threatening. Attempts to minimize the likelihood of infection and to treat orthopedic infections aggressively and appropriately are important to ensure a satisfactory outcome and to return to normal athletic function.

PREVENTION OF ORTHOPEDIC INFECTIONS

Prevention of infection falls into two areas: management of traumatic wounds and peri-operative protocols to minimize surgical site infection (SSI) with strategies to minimize contamination of exposed tissue during a surgical procedure.

Preventing Infection in Traumatic Wounds

Lameness resulting from a traumatic injury is common and the sequelae of infection can result in a devastating outcome. The initial management of such injuries often determines the outcome. Limb wounds require a thorough examination to determine the structures involved and the degree of injury. Prior to invasive palpation, wounds should be clipped and cleaned in an aseptic manner. A sterile lubricant may be applied to the wound to prevent hair from getting into the wound while being clipped.

Povidone-iodine or chlorhexidine-based scrubs remove most debris from the area, minimizing further contamination.[50] Copious lavage with a similar povidone-iodine (0.1%) or chlorhexidine (0.05%) solution under moderate pressure (10 to 15 psi) removes bacteria but does not drive them into the damaged tissue; this is accomplished with a 60-cc syringe and a 19-gauge needle.[52]

Debridement can be done with a scalpel, removing superficial tissue until all notably contaminated or denuded tissue has been removed. Exposed bone usually needs superficial debridement as well. Debridement has been shown to be important in the management of traumatic wounds. Tissue that is contaminated beyond 10^5 microorganisms/gram of tissue is likely to become infected (Figure 10.12).[16,40] Contamination with soil can result in a 25-fold greater infection rate,[38] and specific soil factors can result in as few as 100 microorganisms/gram causing infection.[39]

Once debrided, the wound can be explored with a sterile instrument such as a probe or with sterile gloved hands (Figure 10.13). It is necessary to assess which structures are involved, especially in wounds that are located near synovial cavities. If synovial cavities are suspected to be involved it may be necessary to perform radiographic and ultrasonographic studies of the area

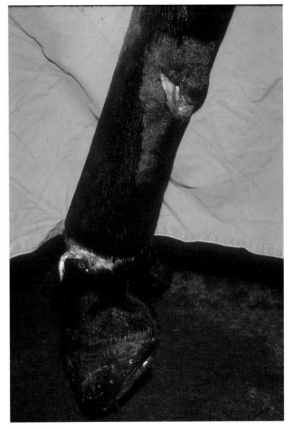

Figure 10.12. This traumatic wound was associated with an open comminuted fracture of the fourth metatarsus. Wound debridement and lavage are important to prevent osteomyelitis in these horses. (Courtesy of Dr. Gary Baxter.)

before any further attempts are made to determine whether the synovial structure is involved. This is because introduction of a needle may result in gas gaining entry into the cavity, which potentially complicates a radiographic diagnosis.

Other pertinent findings for a traumatic wound are the exposure of bone and the involvement of ligaments or tendons. Manipulating the joint, including stressing it, may be necessary to determine if ligaments are damaged. Discrete palpation determines whether bone has been exposed or if tendons are lacerated.

Topical antibiotics can help prevent infections and are indicated in wounds that are acute and clean or have been effectively cleaned and debrided to create a new, clean wound. Triple antibiotic ointments containing bacitracin, polymixin B, and neomycin are effective, with a wide spectrum of activity. Other useful creams

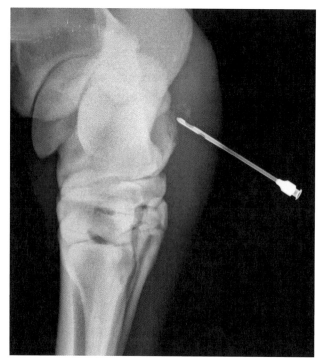

Figure 10.13. This relatively minor wound on the medial aspect of the tarsus was associated with fractures of the sustentaculum tali, and a probe went directly to the bone and entered the tarsal sheath. (Courtesy of Dr. Gary Baxter.)

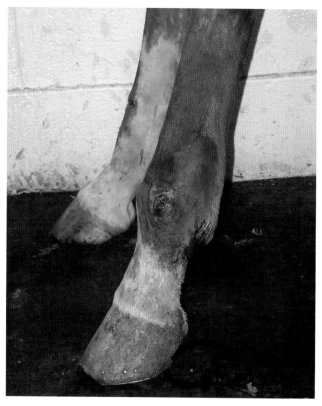

Figure 10.14. This wound on the dorsal aspect of the fetlock healed by second intention and trapped infection within the fetlock joint. Chronic synovial infections such as these are more difficult to resolve than acute injuries. (Courtesy of Dr. Gary Baxter.)

or ointments include silver sulfadiazine, povidone-iodine, and gentamicin ointments. Application of powder forms of antibiotics such as cefazolin are also effective in preventing wound infection.[51] For superficial wounds or some deeper wounds that are not complicated by the involvement of a synovial structure, systemic antibiotics alone for 5 days are usually sufficient. Organisms involved in superficial wounds can vary but often involve streptococci, staphylococci, enterobacteriaceae and *Pseudomonas* species.[55] Commonly used antibiotics are penicillins given intra-muscularly (IM) or oral doxycycline or trimethoprim-sulfas. More involved wounds may require an intravenous (IV) route of administration using a combination of aminoglycosides and penicillins or cepahlosporins to ensure adequate broad-spectrum coverage.

Acute wounds involving synovial structures, including joints, bursae, and tendon sheaths, often directly introduce bacteria and other contaminants into the synovial space. The clinician's primary concern is removing the bacteria from the space before infection can be established. Early recognition and treatment of a synovial penetrating wound is imperative to reduce the risk of developing septic arthritis. One study reported that horses treated within 24 hours had a lower risk of developing septic arthritis compared with those treated after 24 hours. Essentially, the quicker or earlier these cases are addressed, the better (Figure 10.14).[2,12] Therapies for preventing infection in a synovial cavity include parenteral broad-spectrum antimicrobials, some form of synovial lavage, drainage or endoscopic exploration, intrasynovial antimicrobials, wound debride-

ment with or without closure, and regional perfusion of antimicrobials when possible. These treatments are addressed later in this chapter.

Surgical Site Infection and Peri-operative Protocols

Preparation of a surgical site is important to minimize the likelihood of an SSI occurring. SSIs are classified into 3 categories: superficial incisional, deep incisional, and organ/space. Superficial infections occur within 30 days of the procedure and involve only the skin and/or subcutaneous tissues. A deep incisional infection involves infections up to 1 year after the procedure if implants are left in place. This also includes internal fixation fracture repairs when they involve deeper tissues planes. Organ/space infections involve any other structure apart from the incision that is involved in the procedure, including synovial structures or body cavities.[55]

Most elective procedures are considered to be clean, and aseptic techniques are employed to prevent infection from occurring. However, several risk factors can influence the development of SSIs (Table 10.2). Microbe-related factors relate to the numbers of microorganisms, their virulence, and the host tissue's ability to defend against these microbes.[55] The number of bacteria that result in an infection may well depend upon the host's immune status as well as the presence of foreign material. Certain structures appear to be more vulnerable

Table 10.2. Risk factors for surgical site infections.

Origin of factor	Specific risk factor
Microbe-related factors	Numbers of organisms Virulence of organisms Immune status of host Presence of contaminating materials

Host-related factors	Systemic condition of host:
	    Shock
	    Nutritional status: obesity or malnutrition
	    Presence of remote infections

Other factors	Patient and surgeon preparation Duration of surgical procedure Degree of surgical skill and tissue trauma Method of incising skin Use of implants

than others; synovial spaces are particularly vulnerable, because as few as 100 colony-forming units of *S. aureus* may cause infection in a joint,[15] compared to 10^5 organisms/gram of tissue causing infection in soft tissue wounds.[16,40]

The ability of the organism to establish infection depends upon its virulence and a myriad of bacteriologic factors. The presence of foreign material or implants in a wound is likely to potentiate infection as the bacteria adhere to these materials and maintain their presence by forming biofilm. The biofilm is an extensive fibrous matrix that ensures bacterial colony adherence and resists local host defenses and antimicrobials.[14,55] Bacterial adherence to bone has been reduced experimentally by adding hyperimmune plasma to the implant or surgical site.[1] This technique is not yet widely used clinically as an intraoperative lavage to prevent infection.

Host-related risk factors for SSI are related to the animal's systemic condition. Shock, malnutrition, obesity, and remote infections have all been shown to increase SSI. Other factors that must be considered for SSI are the duration of the procedure, degree of surgical skill (e.g., minimal hemorrhage, minimal tissue trauma, dead space formation), and methods used to incise the skin (stainless steel scalpel vs. electrosurgery or lasers). Latent thermal energy can result in tissue necrosis and increase the chance of infection at the incision site.[27]

SSI prevention relies on 3 main components: reducing bacterial numbers at the surgical site, promoting clearance at the site, and administering prophylactic antimicrobials. Routine protocols and correct surgical procedures should be strictly adhered to as best as possible, even for relatively benign procedures done under field circumstances, to minimize the first 2 components. This includes correct patient and surgeon preparation.

Prophylactic antibiotic use, the third component, is essential for procedures that carry an increased risk of SSI. Serum concentrations should peak prior to the initiation of the procedure and should remain at levels of 4 to 8 times the minimum inhibitory concentration for the expected bacteria. In horses, the most common

organisms in orthopedic infections include enterobacteriaceae, staphylococci, streptococci, and *Pseudomonas* species.[29,49]

Timing of antibiotic administration is important. Generally accepted protocols include administering IM drugs 1 hour before and IV drugs 30 minutes before the procedure commences. This permits tissue concentrations to peak at the time of incision. In human surgery, a second dose can be given during the surgery if a procedure lasts more than 3 hours and it is deemed necessary, and depending upon the antimicrobials used.[6,31,32] Antibiotics are continued after the surgery is completed. For clean procedures there is no evidence for continuing beyond 24 hours,[6] but for clean contaminated procedures the decision is left to the surgeon's discretion, usually 3 to 5 days.

Penicillins and aminoglycosides are commonly used antimicrobials for treating equine orthopedic SSI. Penicillin is generally effective against β-hemolytic streptococci and β-lactamase negative staphylococci and most anaerobes. Metronidazole can be added if there is concern about anaerobic coverage because *Bacteroides* species are often not covered using this regime. Cephalosporins are often used as part of a routine prophylaxis replacing penicillins; the advantage is a wider spectrum of activity. Gentamicin is commonly used in combination with penicillins or a cephalosporin. It is effective against Gram-negative species, pseudomonas, and staphylococcus, but it is not very effective against streptococcal species.

Routes of administration vary depending upon the structures involved and the classification of the procedure, i.e., whether it is clean, clean contaminated, contaminated, or dirty. For routine prophylaxis, antibiotics are systemically administered as described above. However, there are several other strategies that can be employed to minimize SSI or treat established infections when there are concerns about cost and ensuring that adequate tissue levels are established at remote sites such as the distal limb. These strategies include intraarticular (IA) antibiotic therapies, intraosseous regional perfusion, IV regional perfusion, and application of antibiotic-impregnated materials into wounds. These strategies are discussed below.

TREATMENT OF SEPTIC CONDITIONS

Systemic antibiotics are initiated for any infected wound, regardless of the structures, to provide a broad spectrum of activity against the previously mentioned suspected microbes. These antibiotics are maintained until sensitivity of the cultured organism is obtained. Most commonly, a combination of penicillin (22,000 IU/kg every 6 hours IV, every 12 hours IM) and gentamicin (6.6 mg/kg every 24 hours IV) is used initially. At this stage, the parenteral therapy can be altered accordingly.

Other antibiotics that are less commonly used include metronidazole, enrofloxacin, chloramphenicol, and vancomycin. Enrofloxacin is relatively commonly used when indicated; it is broad spectrum and often effective when aminoglycosides are ineffective. However, there is concern that articular cartilage damage may occur with its use in foals and younger horses.[17] Chloramphenicol also has a wide spectrum of activity and has good tissue penetration. The concern associated with this drug is the risk to human health due to the possibility of aplastic anemia in exposed people.[7] Vancomycin has been used successfully in cases of methicillin-resistant staphylococcal infections.[33]

For wounds that are obviously infected but do not appear to involve bone or synovial structures, principles similar to preventing infection of a wound are followed. The wound can be cleaned and then debrided. Once the extent and nature of the wound has been established, a decision can be made to allow for secondary intentional healing or to close the wound primarily. In general, infected wounds are chronic and primary closure usually is not attempted. Instead, once adequate cleaning and debridement of the wound have been performed, the wound should be bandaged with an appropriate dressing. Dressings that are indicated for heavily infected wounds include activated charcoal, gauze, hypertonic saline, and iodine-based dressings,[51] which continue to facilitate debridement and have antimicrobial effects. Topical antibiotics also may be applied, but IV regional perfusions may be more effective.

Wounds that are infected more deeply that may involve bone usually require more extensive debridement and further diagnostics. Radiographic studies may be required to appreciate the extent of an infected wound that involves bone or is an osteomyelitic lesion (Figure 10.15). Radiographs are very specific yet not

extremely sensitive; classically 30% to 50% of bone demineralization must occur before bone lysis is visible radiographically.

Other modalities such as scintigraphic examination, CT, and MRI can assist in the diagnosis. MR and scintigraphy are the modalities of choice for suspected cases of human osteomyelitis and septic arthritis.[18] Ultrasonography also can be effective in helping to diagnose osteomyelitis. The imaging of fluid pockets in and around bone assist in determination.[37]

If osteomyelitis is suspected, aggressive debridement is warranted. The infected bone should be exposed, curetted, and effectively removed. If the lesion is the result of an implant that has become infected, then the implant should be removed. The establishment of a biofilm around the implant makes it difficult for any antibiotic strategy to be effective. Regional perfusion by IV or intraosseous techniques is indicated, as is use of antibiotic-impregnated materials such as PMMA or sponges. In some cases, when the osteomyelitis is closely associated with a joint, such as in some cases of septic physitis, it may be prudent to treat the joint with IA antibiotics as well. Research has shown that IA administration of antibiotics provide adequate concentrations in the subchondral bone.[56]

Often the practitioner is presented with a chronically infected wound that reveals exposed bone. The bone may not appear infected but is dry, not bleeding, and has no obvious covering of granulation tissue. It is likely that the periosteum and underlying cortical bone has died and will form a sequestrum over time (Figure 10.16). This bone can be vigorously debrided back to bleeding bone to allow the formation of granulation tissue.

Chronic synovial cavity infections must be addressed in a manner similar to that of synovial wounds, with prevention of infection as the goal. Systemic antibiotics, arthroscopic debridement and lavage, arthrotomy or joint drains, and regional IV or intraosseous perfusion are all required to effectively resolve the infection. Most synovial wounds except those that are very acute benefit from arthroscopic debridement and lavage. As the infection develops, a considerable amount of fibrin collects in the joint. This renders through and through needle lavage ineffective because the needle is frequently blocked and arthroscopic removal of fibrin and debris is necessary. After flushing a severely and chronically infected joint, performing an arthrotomy to facilitate further drainage is sometimes effective. Larger holes allow fibrin to be evacuated, and further standing flushes with cannulas can be performed easily in the standing horse. Regional perfusions and IA antibiotics are indicated in conjunction with arthroscopic debridement.

SPECIFIC TREATMENT STRATEGIES

Lavage and Drainage for Synovial Cavities

Through and Through Needle Lavage

A simple, quick way to lavage a synovial cavity is to place large-bore needles into the joint at multiple sites and lavage a solution such as normal saline solution through the joint, alternating the ingress needle (Figure

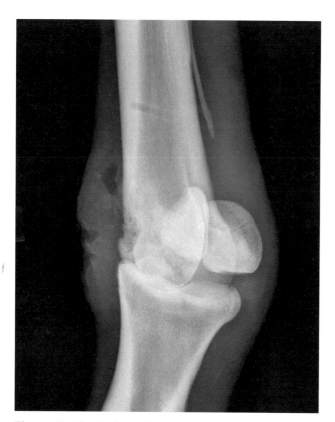

Figure 10.15. Radiographic evidence of osteomyelitis of the lateral condyle of the distal third metacarpal bone. There is significant soft tissue swelling, gas pockets, and bone lysis. Note the hole drilled in MCIII where intraosseous perfusion had been performed.

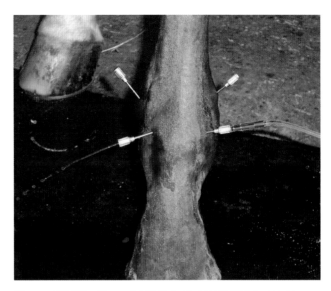

Figure 10.17. Through and through needle joint lavage is performed using hypodermic needles. The ingress needles are alternated during the lavage and all synovial pouches are lavaged if possible.

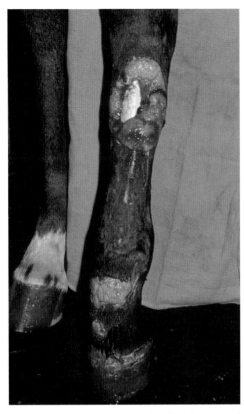

Figure 10.16. Avulsion injuries on the dorsal aspect of the metacarpus/metatarsus often have exposed bone that may develop into a surface sequestrum. (Courtesy of Dr. Gary Baxter.)

10.17).[4] The horse must remain sedated and the area desensitized to facilitate the procedure. Fourteen-gauge needles are placed into the cavity at appropriate locations and a fluid line is attached under a pressure system. The volume of fluid flushed through is important. At least 1 liter should be used for smaller joints such as the fetlock. This method is not effective in older infections because clots of fibrin block the needles. An additional shortcoming of this procedure is that any further damage to the joint cannot be assessed. Therefore, this method of joint lavage is probably best suited for acute simple punctures of joints.[41]

Arthroscopic/Endoscopic Lavage

Infected synovial cavities are best cleaned and debrided through arthroscopic/endoscopic visualization and lavage. Foreign material, fibrin, and bone fragmentation if present can be seen and removed and the joint itself can be debrided accordingly. A more accurate prognosis can be provided as well.[58] Lesions to the cartilage, tendons, and bone can be identified and treated appropriately. Partial synovectomy can be performed to aid in debridement of the joint by allowing better visualization of the entire space. Most joints, bursae, and tendon sheaths are accessible for an arthroscopic lavage, and this is the preferential treatment for any synovial injury that is more than 24 hours old.[3] Wounds that have large puncture holes are not suitable, however, because this precludes adequate distension of the joint for arthroscopic lavage.

Arthrotomy and Passive Drainage

After arthroscopic lavage or a through and through lavage, an arthrotomy may be performed to enlarge the arthroscopic portals to allow for continued passive drainage. One clinical study showed good results using open wound drainage;[47] however, a recent study shows this may not be necessary.[58] Yet some clinicians may choose to do so for some chronic synovial wounds. The arthrotomies can be used for further flushing and are allowed to close by second intention.

A variation to this technique is to place an ingress system within the synovial cavity with a smaller egress arthrotomy. This permits repeated lavage and instillation of antimicrobials into the cavity with continued passive drainage. This technique is commonly used for tendon sheath infections. Soft fenestrated drains, such as a Jackson Pratt drain (Jackson Pratt Hubless, American Hospital Supply, Chicago), are placed within a cavity with the drain distad and sutured in place. This same system can be used for constant infusion systems of antimicrobials.[26] A balloon reservoir is attached to the system, allowing a constant infusion.[21] One concern of this system is the potential for development of a superimposed infection if the system is not kept very clean with sterile bandaging and skin preparations.

Regional Antimicrobial Delivery Systems

Intrasynovial Antimicrobials

The administration of intrasynovial antibiotics is a cost-effective way to attain high concentrations of drugs (above minimum inhibitory concentration [MIC] values) in synovial fluid for at least 24 hours. Antimicrobials commonly are injected into a synovial cavity on a daily basis or they can be deposited after a synovial lavage. They are not administered alone, but rather in combination with parenteral antibiotics. They also can be delivered to the joint using a constant infusion system.[21] Initial studies using a single dose of 150 mg of gentamicin provided concentrations above the MIC for common pathogens for 24 hours.[23] A 150-mg dose of ceftiofur also has been shown to provide adequate concentrations for more than 24 hours.[28]

Amikacin has recently become one of the most widely used intrasynovial antibiotics; it has also been shown to be effective against a broader spectrum of bacteria than gentamicin and has concentrations above MIC values for common pathogens for up to 34 hours.[48] A dose of 250 to 500 mg is commonly administered. None of these antibiotics appear to have any ill effects on the joint, although there is some mild transitory inflammation in normal joints. Other antibiotics that have been used are cefazolin, timentin, methicillin, and imipenem-cilastatin.[3,46]

Regional Limb Perfusions

Regional limb perfusions have become the accepted method of providing increased tissue concentrations of antibiotics for the treatment of synovial and osseous infection, as well as for preventing the establishment of infection. The 2 main methods of delivery are IV or intraosseous. Both involve the application of a tourni-quet proximal to the affected site (distal as well if the infected tissue is relatively proximal on a limb), and the antibiotic is infused distal to the tourniquet. The infusate diffuses into the surrounding tissues. Several studies have shown that antimicrobial concentrations reach up to 100 times the MIC values for common pathogens.[8,30,35,42,45,56] Concentrations of amikacin in synovial fluid using regional perfusion have been compared to those of an isolated limb infusion system that administers an infusate with an extracorporeal system.[10] Both techniques reached adequate concentrations of amikacin greater than 10 times the MIC for most common pathogens, illustrating that retrograde IV perfusion is an acceptable technique.

The technique is simple to perform and can be done under field conditions in the standing sedated horse or under general anesthesia. A pneumatic tourniquet is preferentially used; however, an esmarch bandage applied tightly to the distal limb suffices (Figure 10.18).[10] A recent study compared a pneumatic tourniquet to wide and narrow rubber tubing tourniquets and showed that the highest concentrations of intrasynovial antimicrobials were obtained with the pneumatic tourniquet at 420 mm Hg. Wide rubber tourniquets were acceptable, but narrow rubber ones were not.[22]

The preferred pressure to be applied when a pneumatic tourniquet is used is unknown; however, com-

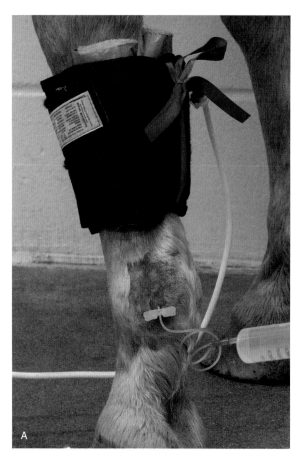

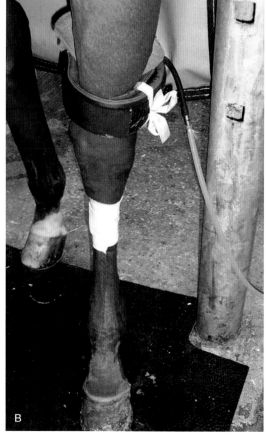

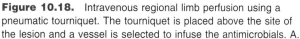

Figure 10.18.   Intravenous regional limb perfusion using a pneumatic tourniquet. The tourniquet is placed above the site of the lesion and a vessel is selected to infuse the antimicrobials. A. The palmar vein. B. The saphenous vein. Rolls of gauze can be applied over the vessels for extra pressure; these can be seen under the tourniquet in figures A and B.

monly applied pressures are in the range of 300 to 500 mm Hg.[5] To assist in applying pressure to the digital vessels in the standing horse, gauze rolls can be applied against these vessels under the tourniquet. A local nerve block also can be applied prior to injecting the vein to assist in the procedure. For regional IV perfusion, a 20- to 25-gauge butterfly catheter is used, the vein accessed, and the solution slowly infused. To the author's knowledge, the exact time needed for infusion has not been studied. Periods from 1 to 15 minutes have been recommended.[3,24] The tourniquet is left in place for 30 minutes.[34] The exact timeline for leaving the tourniquet in place is still relatively controversial. One study using a contrast medium showed maximal dye uptake in the soft tissues at 30 minutes.[20]

For intraosseous perfusion, a hole is drilled in the cortical bone of the third metacarpal bone for distal limb treatments. A 3.2-mm to 5.5-mm cannulated bone screw with a Luer lock head is placed in the drilled and tapped hole. Alternatively, the end of a catheter extension set fits securely into the drilled hole.

Factors that may favor osseous perfusion vs. IV include a lack of easy venous access due to cellulitis and edema, and the presence of osteomyelitis. Intraosseous perfusion is initially more invasive, but if the procedure is expected to be repeated over a significant period of time, it may be indicated. A recent study evaluated the perfusion of tissue with technetium Tc 99 and quantitatively evaluated the radio-isotope uptake.[25] The results of the 2 methods were similar, except there was a significant increase in uptake of the isotope in the distal MCIII with intraosseous perfusion. This leads to the assumption that osteomyelitic lesions may respond better to intraosseous perfusion. The volume of the perfusate is generally 30 to 60 mL. In a study of perfusion of the tarsus in horses, concentrations of amikacin were higher when a perfusate of 60 ml was used compared to 30 ml.[45] A smaller volume (30 ml) is recommended in foals.[19]

A variety of antibiotics have been used in regional perfusions. The most common are amikacin and gentamicin; also used are penicillin, ampicillin, cepahlosporins, enrofloxacin, and vancomycin. Doses vary considerably but in most clinical situations 500 mg of amikacin or gentamicin is used.[9] Doses of more than 250 mg of amikacin have been recommended.[35] In this same study, 1.5 mg/kg of enrofloxacin was recommended for orthopedic infections susceptible to enrofloxacin. Care must be taken when using enrofloxacin due to cartilage concerns as well as vasculitis of the perfused areas. Penicillins have been used at a dose of 10×10^6 units, and timentin (1 g) and ampicillin (9 g) have been used.[34,57] More recently, vancomycin has been studied for use in both IV and osseous perfusion. Intraosseous use of 300 mg vancomycin appeared to have better results in terms of greater concentrations in the lower limb synovial fluid concentrations, compared to IV use.[42]

Antibiotic-impregnated Materials

Antibiotics can be effectively delivered by slow release from impregnated materials. These products are left *in situ* to release the drug over an extended period of time, resulting in high local tissue concentrations. Commonly used materials include polymethylmethacrylate (PMMA), collagen, plaster of Paris, hydroxyapatite, polylactide-polyglycolide, and other bone cements.

PMMA is widely used, and there are a variety of commercially available brands, including Surgical Simplex P™ (Howmedica, Rutherford, NJ) and Palacos™ (Richards Medical, Philadelphia, PA). PMMA is nonbiodegradable and has been used when incorporated with a variety of antibiotics in horses. Most commonly are gentamicin, amikacin, and cephalosporins (ceftiofur); also used are timentin, tobramycin, amoxicillin, metronidazole, enrofloxacin, imipenem, and vancomycin.[13,36,44,46,54] The cement can be placed strategically around implants to prevent infection or as beads in areas of infection. Often the beads are incorporated in a strand of nonabsorbable material for ease of later removal, although they are commonly left in place unless they become a source of clinical concern themselves. The beads can be made prior to use and sterilized or made at the time of surgery. Gas sterilization is preferential because steam causes drug loss.[13] Commercial molds are available to place beads on a string.

Elution rates of incorporated antibiotics are highly variable and depend upon a number of factors. The drug used, ratio of drug to cement, environment in which it is placed, and size of the bead effect elution rates. For example, smaller spherical beads result in more rapid elution rates compared to cylindrical beads, because the higher the surface area, the greater the elution.[11] In general, a drug:cement ratio of 1:10 or 1:20 is used when preparing antibiotic-incorporated PMMA. The more drug that is used, the less stable the compound, which is detrimental if antibiotic-impregnated PMMA is being used to provide mechanical support to a construct such as a fracture repair with an implant.

Elution rates have been studied for 3 antibiotics impregnated into PMMA and hydroxyapatite (HA).[11] In this study 10-mm × 17-mm cylinders of material were prepared and placed in phosphate buffered saline to measure elution rates. All antibiotics eluted the greatest amount of drug in the first 24 hours. There was a greater elution of drug when it was added to the cement in a liquid form, compared to a powdered form. The rate of elution was proportional to the amount of drug, and drugs eluted quicker from HA than from PMMA. In this environment ceftiofur eluted the quickest, with the concentrations dropping below MIC by day 7. With amikacin and gentamicin, concentrations eluted remained above MIC for more than 30 days.

Based on the most common pathogens encountered in equine orthopedic infection, 0.5 to 1 gram of amikacin added to 10 grams of PMMA and made into smaller cylinders provides the ideal vehicle for drug elution in most clinical scenarios.

Plaster of Paris (POP) is a much cheaper alternative to PMMA and is biodegradable. A recent study used 20 g of calcium sulfate hemihydrate (POP) with 5 ml (500 mg) of gentamicin and 3 ml of phosphate buffered saline.[43] This provided 60 7-mm spherical beads on a PDS chain made with a commercial mold. Elution occurred rapidly; 80% of the drug was eluted in the first 48 hours. Based upon this finding, if POP is used it should be replaced relatively often in cases of sustained infection. Other materials are not commonly used in clinical situations. Gentamicin-impregnated bovine collagen sponges are commercially available outside the US and used in horses. Seven of 8 horses in which the sponges were an adjunctive treatment for synovial sepsis responded well.[53]

References

1. Bauer SM, Santschi EM, Fialkowski J, et al. Quantification of *Staphylococcus aureus* adhesion to equine bone surfaces passivated with Plasmalyte and hyperimmune plasma. Vet Surg 2004;33:376–381.
2. Baxter G. Retrospective study of lower limb wounds involving tendons, tendon sheaths, or joints in horses. Proceedings of American Association of Equine Practitioners 1987;715–728.
3. Baxter G. Treatment of wounds involving synovial structures. Clinical techniques in Equine Practice 2005;3:204–214.
4. Baxter GM. Instrumentation and techniques for treating orthopedic infections in horses. Vet Clin North Am Equine Pract 1996;12:303–335.
5. Blass C, Moore B. The tourniquet in surgery: A review. Veterinary Surgery 1984;13:111–114.
6. Bratzler DW, Houck PM. Antimicrobial prophylaxis for surgery: An advisory statement from the National Surgical Infection Prevention Project. Clin Infect Dis 2004;38:1706–1715.
7. Brumbaugh GW, Martens RJ, Knight HD, et al. Pharmacokinetics of chloramphenicol in the neonatal horse. J Vet Pharmacol Ther 1983;6:219–227.
8. Butt TD, Bailey JV, Dowling PM, et al. Comparison of 2 techniques for regional antibiotic delivery to the equine forelimb: Intraosseous perfusion vs. intravenous perfusion. Can Vet J 2001;42:617–622.
9. Cruz AM, Rubio-Martinez L, Dowling T. New antimicrobials, systemic distribution, and local methods of antimicrobial delivery in horses. Vet Clin North Am Equine Pract 2006;22:297–322.
10. Errico JA, Trumble TN, Bueno AC, et al. Comparison of two indirect techniques for local delivery of a high dose of an antimicrobial in the distal portion of forelimbs of horses. Am J Vet Res 2008;69:334–342.
11. Ethell MT, Bennett RA, Brown MP, et al. *In vitro* elution of gentamicin, amikacin, and ceftiofur from polymethylmethacrylate and hydroxyapatite cement. Vet Surg 2000;29:375–382.
12. Gibson KT, McIlwraith CW, Turner AS, et al. Open joint injuries in horses: 58 cases (1980–1986). J Am Vet Med Assoc 1989;194:398–404.
13. Goodrich LR. Osteomyelitis in horses. Vet Clin North Am Equine Pract 2006;22:389–417.
14. Gristina AG, Costerton JW. Bacterial adherence to biomaterials and tissue. The significance of its role in clinical sepsis. J Bone Joint Surg Am 1985;67:264–273.
15. Gustafson SB, McIlwraith CW, Jones RL. Comparison of the effect of polysulfated glycosaminoglycan, corticosteroids, and sodium hyaluronate in the potentiation of a subinfective dose of *Staphylococcus aureus* in the midcarpal joint of horses. Am J Vet Res 1989;50:2014–2017.
16. Hackett RP, Dimock BA, Bentinck-Smith J. Quantitative bacteriology of experimentally incised skin wounds in horses. Equine Vet J 1983;15:37–39.
17. Hughes K, Hodgson J, Hodgson D. Use of fluoroquinolone antimicrobial agents in equine practice. Equine Veterinary Education 2002;14:240–243.
18. Jaramillo D, Treves ST, Kasser JR, et al. Osteomyelitis and septic arthritis in children: Appropriate use of imaging to guide treatment. AJR Am J Roentgenol 1995;165:399–403.
19. Kettner NU, Parker JE, Watrous BJ. Intraosseous regional perfusion for treatment of septic physitis in a two-week-old foal. J Am Vet Med Assoc 2003;222:346–350.
20. Keys GJ, Berry DB, Pleasant RS, et al. Vascular distribution of contrast medium during intraosseous regional perfusion of the distal portion of the equine forelimb. Am J Vet Res 2006;67:1445–1452.
21. Lescun TB, Adams SB, Wu CC, et al. Continuous infusion of gentamicin into the tarsocrural joint of horses. Am J Vet Res 2000;61:407–412.
22. Levine DG, Epstein KL, Neelis DA, et al. Effect of topical application of 1% diclofenac sodium liposomal cream on inflammation in healthy horses undergoing intravenous regional limb perfusion with amikacin sulfate. Am J Vet Res 2009;70:1323–1325.
23. Lloyd KC, Stover SM, Pascoe JR, et al. Synovial fluid pH, cytologic characteristics, and gentamicin concentration after intraarticular administration of the drug in an experimental model of infectious arthritis in horses. Am J Vet Res 1990;51:1363–1369.
24. Lugo J, Gaughan EM. Septic arthritis, tenosynovitis, and infections of hoof structures. Vet Clin North Am Equine Pract 2006;22:363–388.
25. Mattson SE, Pearce SG, Boure LP, et al. Comparison of intraosseous and intravenous infusion of technetium Tc 99m pertechnate in the distal portion of forelimbs in standing horses by use of scintigraphic imaging. Am J Vet Res 2005;66:1267–1272.
26. Meagher DT, Latimer FG, Sutter WW, et al. Evaluation of a balloon constant rate infusion system for treatment of septic arthritis, septic tenosynovitis, and contaminated synovial wounds: 23 cases (2002–2005). J Am Vet Med Assoc 2006;228:1930–1934.
27. Middleton WG, Tees DA, Ostrowski M. Comparative gross and histological effects of the CO2 laser, Nd-YAG laser, scalpel, Shaw scalpel and cutting cautery on skin in rats. J Otolaryngol 1993;22:167–170.
28. Mills ML, Rush BR, St. Jean G, et al. Determination of synovial fluid and serum concentrations, and morphologic effects of intraarticular ceftiofur sodium in horses. Vet Surg 2000;29:398–406.
29. Moore RM, Schneider RK, Kowalski J, et al. Antimicrobial susceptibility of bacterial isolates from 233 horses with musculoskeletal infection during 1979–1989. Equine Vet J 1992;24:450–456.
30. Murphey ED, Santschi EM, Papich MG. Regional intravenous perfusion of the distal limb of horses with amikacin sulfate. J Vet Pharmacol Ther 1999;22:68–71.
31. Nichols RL. Preventing surgical site infections: A surgeon's perspective. Emerg Infect Dis 2001;7:220–224.
32. Nichols RL. Surgical wound infection. Am J Med 1991;91:54S–64S.
33. Orsini JA, Snooks-Parsons C, Stine L, et al. Vancomycin for the treatment of methicillin-resistant staphylococcal and enterococcal infections in 15 horses. Can J Vet Res 2005;69:278–286.
34. Palmar S, Hogan P. How to perform regional limb perfusion in the horse. Proceedings American Equine Practitioners, 1999;45:124–127.
35. Parra-Sanchez A, Lugo J, Boothe DM, et al. Pharmacokinetics and pharmacodynamics of enrofloxacin and a low dose of amikacin administered via regional intravenous limb perfusion in standing horses. Am J Vet Res 2006;67:1687–1695.
36. Ramos JR, Howard RD, Pleasant RS, et al. Elution of metronidazole and gentamicin from polymethylmethacrylate beads. Vet Surg 2003;32:251–261.
37. Reef V, Reimer J, Reid C. Ultrasonographic findings in horses with osteomyelitis. Proceedings American Association of Equine Practitioners. San Francisco, CA, 1991;37:381–391.
38. Robson MC. Wound infection. A failure of wound healing caused by an imbalance of bacteria. Surg Clin North Am 1997;77:637–650.
39. Rodeheaver G, Pettry D, Turnbull V, et al. Identification of the wound infection-potentiating factors in soil. Am J Surg 1974;128:8–14.
40. Roettinger W, Edgerton MT, Kurtz LD, et al. Role of inoculation site as a determinant of infection in soft tissue wounds. Am J Surg 1973;126:354–358.
41. Ross M. Clinical management of synovial infection. Proceedings of the American College of Veterinary Surgery, 1995;45.
42. Rubio-Martinez LM, Lopez-Sanroman J, Cruz AM, et al. Evaluation of safety and pharmacokinetics of vancomycin after intraosseous regional limb perfusion and comparison of results with those obtained after intravenous regional limb perfusion in horses. Am J Vet Res 2006;67:1701–1707.
43. Santschi EM, McGarvey L. *In vitro* elution of gentamicin from plaster of Paris beads. Vet Surg 2003;32:128–133.
44. Sayegh A, Moore R. Polymethylmethacrylate beads for treating orthopedic infections. Compendium of Continuing Education 2003;25:788.

45. Scheuch BC, Van Hoogmoed LM, Wilson WD, et al. Comparison of intraosseous or intravenous infusion for delivery of amikacin sulfate to the tibiotarsal joint of horses. Am J Vet Res 2002;63: 374–380.

46. Schneider RK. Synovial and Osseous Infections. In Equine Surgery, 3rd ed. Auer JA, Stick J, eds. Saunders Elsevier, St. Louis, 2006;1121–1129.

47. Schneider RK, Bramlage LR, Mecklenburg LM, et al. Open drainage, intra-articular and systemic antibiotics in the treatment of septic arthritis/tenosynovitis in horses. Equine Vet J 1992;24: 443–449.

48. Sedrish S, Moore R, Barker S. Pharmacokinetics of single dose intra-articular administration of amikacin in the radiocarpal joint of normal horses. Veterinary Surgery 1996;25:437–441.

49. Snyder JR, Pascoe JR, Hirsh DC. Antimicrobial susceptibility of microorganisms isolated from equine orthopedic patients. Vet Surg 1987;16:197–201.

50. Southwood LL, Baxter GM. Instrument sterilization, skin preparation, and wound management. Vet Clin North Am Equine Pract 1996;12:173–194.

51. Stashak T, Farstvedt E. Update on Wound Dressings: Indications and Best Use. In Equine Wound Management, 2nd ed. Stashak T, Theoret C, eds. Wiley-Blackwell, Ames, 2008;109–136.

52. Stevenson TR, Thacker JG, Rodeheaver GT, et al. Cleansing the traumatic wound by high pressure syringe irrigation. JACEP 1976;5:17–21.

53. Summerhays GE. Treatment of traumatically induced synovial sepsis in horses with gentamicin-impregnated collagen sponges. Vet Rec 2000;147:184–188.

54. Tobias KM, Schneider RK, Besser TE. Use of antimicrobial-impregnated polymethylmethacrylate. J Am Vet Med Assoc 1996;208:841–845.

55. Waguespack R, Moore R, Burba D. Surgical Site Infection and the Use of Antimicrobials. In Equine Surgery, 3rd ed. Auer JA, Stick J, eds. Saunders Elsevier, St. Louis, 2006;70–87.

56. Werner LA, Hardy J, Bertone AL. Bone gentamicin concentration after intra-articular injection or regional intravenous perfusion in the horse. Vet Surg 2003;32:559–565.

57. Whitehair KJ, Adams SB, Parker JE, et al. Regional limb perfusion with antibiotics in three horses. Vet Surg 1992; 21:286–292.

58. Wright IM, Smith MR, Humphrey DJ, et al. Endoscopic surgery in the treatment of contaminated and infected synovial cavities. Equine Vet J 2003;35:613–619.

Lameness in the Young Horse

THE PHYSIS/PHYSEAL FRACTURES

GARY M. BAXTER

THE PHYSIS

Growth and Development of the Musculoskeletal System

Longitudinal bone growth results from a series of events occurring at highly specialized regions at 1 or both ends of the bone. These regions are referred to as the physes, growth plates, or more correctly, the metaphyseal growth plates. The process occurring at the growth plate, endochondral ossification, is characterized by rapidly differentiating and maturing cartilage cells and the replacement of cartilage by bone.[20]

There are 2 types of growth plates: discoid and spherical.[1] The discoid growth plates are located at the ends of long bones. Some bones have a physis at each end of the bone, whereas others, such as the third metacarpal/metatarsal bone and the proximal and middle phalanges, have only one. A discoid physis is located between the metaphysis (the flared end of the bone that contains spongy bone) and the epiphysis. An apophysis (which is a type of discoid physis) is an epiphysis that is subject to tensile rather than compressive forces, such as at the olecranon process, calcaneal tuber, and tibial tuberosity. The growth plate of an apophysis contains greater amounts of fibrocartilage than a true discoid physis, which is an adaptation to withstand tensile forces (Figure 11.1).[12]

Spherical physes are located in the small cuboidal bones of the foal's carpus and tarsus. These growth plates develop into bones by centrifugal expansion around a central cartilage core.[1] The cartilage core begins to ossify in the center and gradually assumes the contours of the bone of an adult as bone development reaches the margins of the cartilage model (Figure 11.2).

Ossification of cartilage at 1 or both ends of long bones occurs early in life, forming the epiphyses. These

articular-epiphyseal complexes form in a manner similar to ossification of the cartilage models of the small cuboidal bones. The cellular events consist of vesiculation and chondrocyte death with calcification of matrix, invasion of vessels, and partial resorption and ossification.[12] Eventually, a subchondral bone plate forms, which is best imagined as a mini growth plate. This articular-epiphyseal growth plate contributes to the size of the epiphyses but very little to the length of the bone.

Morphology of the Physis (Growth Plate)

The metaphyseal growth plate or physis has a characteristic cellular architecture from birth to maturity. The cartilage cells of the growth plate can be divided into a number of zones, which vary in height and cell number, histological appearance, and cellular function. They are arranged in longitudinal columns, with cellular division occurring on the epiphyseal side of the cartilage, while simultaneous ossification progresses from the metaphysis to the diaphysis. There is a primary ossification center on the metaphyseal/diaphyseal side of the physis and a secondary ossification center within the epiphysis that contributes to radial growth of the epiphysis (Figure 11.3).[20,21]

Resting/Reserve Zone

The zone nearest the epiphysis is one of growth, where cell division is initiated. The chondrocytes are highly metabolic and are similar to those found in articular cartilage. These cells divide primarily in a longitudinal direction, and appear as small flattened chondrocytes, providing elongation to the columns of cells.[1] Epiphyseal vessels (arterioles and capillaries) are closely associated with early cellular events and may provide undifferentiated cells that can add to the pool of chondrocytes that later go on to divide.

Resting chondrocytes are also elaborated peripherally, forming a cartilaginous ring. This specialized

Adams and Stashak's Lameness in Horses, 6e, edited by Gary M. Baxter

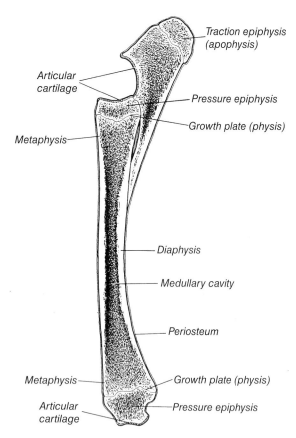

Figure 11.1. Sagittal section of the radius and ulna of a foal.

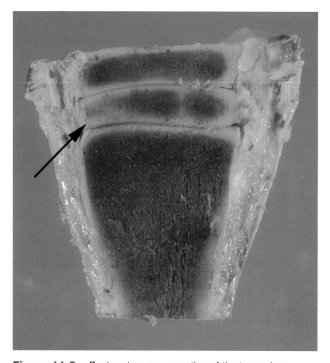

Figure 11.2. Postmortem cross section of the tarsus in a premature foal demonstrating bone surrounded by nonossified cartilage (arrow) within the cuboidal bones. These bones ossify by centrifugal expansion around a central cartilage core.

region of the perichondrium is called the zone of Ranvier and remains in contact with the metaphyseal growth plate.[22] It continues to grow on the epiphyseal side of the physis but is resorbed on the diaphyseal side. Continual bone resorption and bone formation is one of the hallmarks of bone growth and serves to keep bones the correct proportions in length and width.[22] For example, lack of bone resorption from the inner surface (endosteal side)combined with bone apposition from the periosteum would produce a bone that is too thick with an inadequate marrow cavity.

Proliferative Zone

The zone of growth or proliferation is where chondrocytes divide rapidly to form columns of isogenous groups.[20] This zone can be quite large, compared to other areas of the growth plate (Figure 11.3). Chondrocytes farther down the cell columns synthesize and secrete extracellular matrix (predominantly of type II collagen), aggrecan, and other proteoglycan aggregates.[20] Collagen that is randomly orientated in the resting zone becomes more longitudinally oriented between the columns of proliferating cells.

Hypertrophy Zone

After the cells are elaborated through cell division, they eventually hypertrophy due to increased metabolic activity. At this stage, they are no longer capable of dividing. Rates of longitudinal and radial growth depend on the increase in chondrocyte volume rather than on cell proliferation and matrix synthesis.[20] Collagen cross-linking occurs in the hypertrophy zone if copper-containing lysyl oxidase is present. The zone of hypertrophy is the structurally weak link of the physis and is usually where physeal fractures occur and trauma damages the physis.[1,13]

Zone of Calcification/Ossification

The zone of calcification is where the matrix between the cells gradually becomes mineralized due to deposition of hydroxyapatite crystals (Figure 11.3). This is thought to be initiated by cell-derived matrix vesicles and it depends on several factors such as the availability of calcium and phosphate ions, cobalt and collagen, the pH, and the enzyme alkaline phosphatase.[20]

The zone of ossification is sometimes called the zone of angiogenesis because the terminal ends of the capillary sprouts impinge on the hypertrophic chondrocytes. Here osteogenic buds, which consist of capillary sprouts and osteoprogenitor cells, invade the columns of calcifying cartilage.[10,20] Osteoblasts elaborate osteoid matrix, the organic part of bone, on the columns of calcified cartilage. This forms longitudinally orientated bony spicules (inside is a cartilaginous core) in the region called the primary spongiosa. Eventually the bone of the primary spongiosa is replaced by secondary spongiosa, which lacks remnants of the cartilage core.[22] As the bone elongates, bone at the diaphyseal end is removed by osteoclasts at the same rate that new bone is being formed on the epiphyseal side of the metaphysis. Thus, there is a continuous sequence of events, with cell divi-

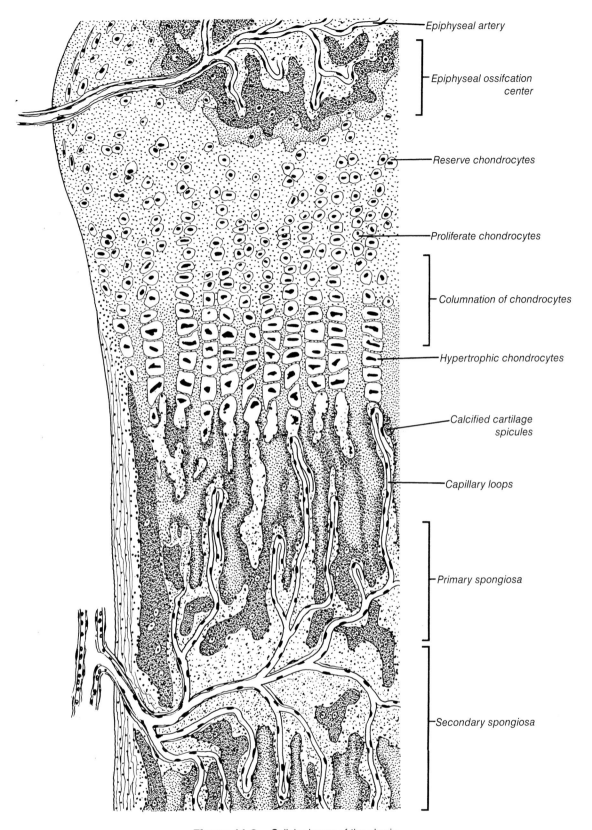

Figure 11.3. Cellular layers of the physis.

Epiphyseal artery

Epiphyseal ossifcation center

Reserve chondrocytes

Proliferate chondrocytes

Columnation of chondrocytes

Hypertrophic chondrocytes

Calcified cartilage spicules

Capillary loops

Primary spongiosa

Secondary spongiosa

sion at one end, bone formation, and bone destruction, which is an important process that contributes to the final shape of the bone (Figure 11.3).[22]

Vascularity of the Physis

The blood supply to the growth plate originates from the epiphyseal, metaphyseal, and perichondral circulations.[1,12] Transphyseal vessels (those crossing the growth plate) are present in large epiphyses and may serve as a route for spread of infection from the metaphysis to the epiphysis. The metaphyseal circulation forms a series of loops that penetrate the longitudinal septa, enlarging as they return toward the diaphysis and forming a sinusoid. This produces a sluggish pattern of blood flow within the physis that predisposes this region to bacterial localization and osteomyelitis.[22]

The integrity of the blood vessels within the zone of Ranvier is important for continued appositional growth at the periphery of the epiphyseal growth plate. Disruption of the blood supply of the perichondral region can potentially cause ischemia to the physis, contributing to asynchronous growth and a subsequent angular limb deformity (ALD). In addition, lack of blood supply, particularly to the ossification zone, can prevent proper bone formation and potentially contribute to disruption of bone growth or osteochondrosis.[2,14,25]

Biomechanical Aspects of the Physis

Although the exact mechanism is not completely understood, tension and compression (within a physiologic range) on the physis are essential for continued orderly bone development and growth.[22] Each growth plate has a biologic range of both tension and compression within which it will respond. Within this range increasing tension or compression will accelerate physeal growth while decreasing tension, or compression will decrease physeal growth.

Beyond the physiologic limits of tension or compression, physeal growth may be significantly decreased or even stopped; this is referred to as the Heuter-Volkmann law of physeal growth.[8,22] This law has an important practical application in the management of foals with ALDs. If we assume that a foal with an ALD of the carpus (carpus valgus) exerts an asymmetric load on the distal radial physis, then the physis will stimulate growth on the concave side of the physis and slow growth on the convex side of the physis, serving to straighten the limb without intervention. However, unrestrained exercise may cause physeal compression that is greater than the physiologic range and therefore prevent autocorrection of the ALD. In addition, foals with physitis or physeal dysplasia may have weaker metaphyseal bone than normal, which may be more susceptible to trauma.[1]

Cessation of Physeal Growth

As bone growth ceases, the physis becomes progressively thinner, and finally the epiphysis and metaphysis fuse.[12,13] The cartilaginous growth plate is replaced with trabecular bone, making it incapable of correcting an ALD. The timing of the physeal closure depends on the specific bone. Some close early in life and others remain open for several years. Functional (remaining growth potential) physeal closure occurs well before radiographic closure, and this difference has important bearing on the timing of surgery used to correct ALDs.[22] In general, the further distal on the limb the physis is located, the sooner it will become functionally inactive. For instance, the distal metacarpal/metatarsal physes close sooner than the distal radial or distal tibial physes, making correction of ALDs of the fetlock and pastern more important early in life than those of the carpus or tarsus. In addition, any injury to the physis such as excessive pressure, direct trauma, traction, circulatory loss, or shearing forces can lead to premature cessation of growth or asynchronous growth.[1,24]

External Trauma to the Physis

When excessive force is applied to a joint and its nearby physis, an epiphyseal or physeal injury is likely to occur because the cartilaginous growth plate is weaker than the surrounding bone, ligamentous structures, and joint capsule. Physeal and epiphyseal injuries account for approximately 15% of all fractures in children, and they are also common in foals.[3,4,15,18] Injuries that would normally produce a ruptured ligament or joint dislocation in an adult may produce traumatic separation of the physis in a young animal. For example, trauma to the fetlock region usually causes a fetlock luxation in an adult horse, and a distal metacarpal/metatarsal physeal fracture in a foal.[22] Joint luxations appear to be rare in young horses.

CLASSIFICATION OF PHYSEAL INJURIES/FRACTURES

The most widely accepted classification of growth plate injuries is based on Salter's system, which separates the injuries into 6 specific types.[18] Such a system has been applied to domestic animals including horses, although at times somewhat artificially (Figure 11.4).[3] One of the main purposes of the classification system in horses is to permit equine clinicians to communicate effectively when describing such injuries. Some information from children is applicable to foals, but in most cases the prognosis and method of treatment are different because of the dissimilarity in fracture repair between foals and children.[4,18,19]

Physeal fractures are relatively common in foals (accounting for approximately 20% of fractures) and may be considered more serious than diaphyseal fractures because of the risk of disturbed limb growth and articular involvement.[3,4,15] Type I and II physeal fractures are most common in horses. Frequent locations of physeal fractures include the distal metacarpus/metatarsus, distal and proximal radius, proximal humerus, proximal tibia, and distal and proximal femur (Figures 11.5 and 11.6). These fractures tend to heal quickly but usually reduce the growth potential remaining in the physis. Although the prognosis can be very good, one study indicated that only 25% of foals with physeal fractures achieved complete soundness.[4,15]

Type I

In a type I injury there is complete separation of the physis without fracture through the bone; the germinal

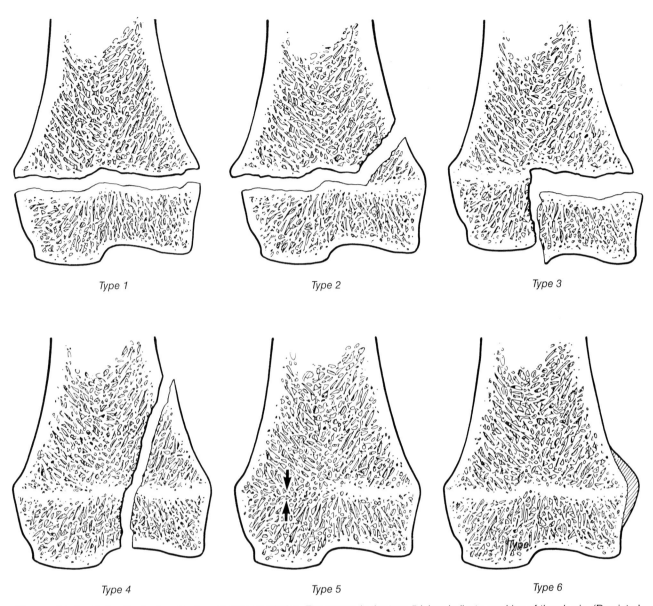

Type 1   *Type 2*   *Type 3*

Type 4   *Type 5*   *Type 6*

Figure 11.4. Salter-Harris classification of physeal injuries. The arrows in the type 5 injury indicate crushing of the physis. (Reprinted from Salter RB, Harris WR. Injuries involving the epiphyseal plate. J Bone Joint Surg 1963;45:587.)

cells of the growth plate remain with the epiphysis (Figure 11.4, type I). This fracture is usually due to shearing forces across the physis, as occurs in foals with proximal femoral physeal fractures (slipped capital femoral epiphysis).[1,22] This may also be seen in the proximal radial physis or proximal humeral physis with external trauma. The treatment and prognosis for this injury in foals varies and depends on the location and characteristics of the fracture. See Chapter 5 for additional information on physeal fractures in specific locations.

Type II

Type II is the most common type of physeal injury in foals as well as in virtually all domestic animals (Figure 11.4, type II).[22] The fracture line extends along the physis for a variable distance and then breaks out through a portion of the metaphysis, producing a triangular shaped metaphyseal fragment (Figures 11.5 and 11.6). Similar to nearly all physeal injuries, the germinal cells remain within the physis. This type of injury is usually the result of shearing and bending forces. The distal third metacarpal/metatarsal physis commonly incurs this injury when the mare steps on the foal. The periosteum is torn on the convex side of the angulation but is intact on the concave side. Thus, the intact periosteal hinge is always on the side of the metaphyseal fragment.[18] A similar injury also occurs in the proximal tibial physis in slightly older foals. Closed reduction with casting may be possible in foals with metacarpal/metatarsal type II physeal injuries but internal fixation is usually mandatory for type II proximal tibial fractures.

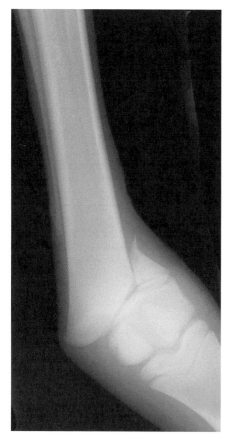

Figure 11.5. Dorsoplantar radiograph of the distal metatarsus of a weanling with a type II physeal fracture. The fracture was repaired with internal fixation.

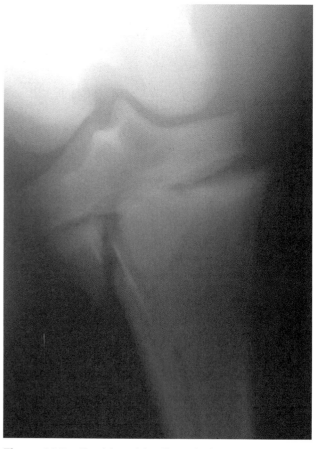

Figure 11.6. Caudal-cranial radiograph of a foal with a type II fracture of the proximal tibial physis. These fractures should be repaired surgically to prevent malalignment of the limb.

Type III

The type III fracture is intra-articular and extends from the joint surface to the deep zone of the growth plate and then along the physis to its periphery (Figure 11.4, type III).[18,19] This type of injury is uncommon in foals and is usually caused by an intra-articular shearing force or is secondary to infectious physitis (Figure 11.7). Open reduction and internal fixation are usually necessary to reconstruct the joint surface to prevent the development of secondary osteoarthritis (OA).

Type IV

Type IV fractures are intra-articular and extend from the joint surface through the epiphysis, across the entire thickness of the physeal plate, and through a portion of the metaphysis (Figure 11.4, type IV). This type of fracture is rare in foals. Open reduction and internal fixation are necessary not only to restore a normal joint surface but also to obtain perfect apposition of the physeal plate. It has been observed in children that unless the fractured surfaces of the physeal plate are kept perfectly reduced, fracture healing occurs across the plate and renders further longitudinal growth impossible.[18,19]

Type V

Type V fracture is also an uncommon injury in foals. It results from a severe crushing force applied through the epiphysis to one region of the physeal plate (Figure 11.4, type V). It may be associated with the distal third metacarpal/metatarsal physes in cases of severe varus deformity of the fetlock or the distal radial physis with severe carpal valgus. Excessive trauma to one part of the physis may be responsible for the severity of these deformities, although this is difficult to document.

Type VI

In a type VI injury, a periosteal bridge develops between the metaphysis and epiphysis (Figure 11.4, type VI, and Figure 11.8A). The new bone restrains growth on the affected side of the physis and has the same effect as a transphyseal staple or screws and wire. This type of injury may occur due to excessive trauma during placement or removal of staples or screws and wire, secondary to local infectious periostitis, or spontaneously from external trauma.[1,22] Removal of the periosteal bridge to help restore further growth in combination with transphyseal bridging on the opposite side of the physis is necessary to correct the problem

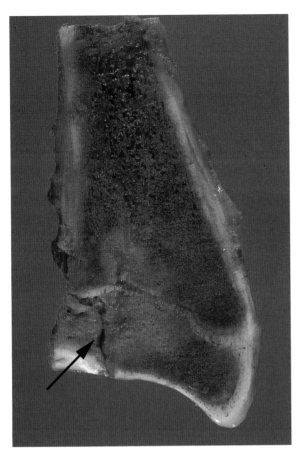

Figure 11.7. Postmortem cross section of the distal tibia physis with a pathologic type III physeal fracture (arrow) secondary to infectious physitis.

(Figure 11.8). This approach has been reported to successfully resolve type VI lesions of the distal radial physis in 2 yearling horses.[5]

DEVELOPMENTAL ORTHOPEDIC DISEASES

The developmental orthopedic disease (DOD) complex is a comprehensive group of growth disturbances that occurs in foals and growing horses.[20,24] These include physitis/physeal dysplasia, angular limb deformities (ALD), osteochondritis dissecans (OCD), subchondral cystic lesions (SCL), incomplete ossification or collapse of the cuboidal bones, juvenile arthritis, cervical vertebral malformations (CVM), and flexural deformities.[11,20,21]

These developmental conditions, with the exception of flexural deformities, are attributed to alterations in bone growth or development (endochondral ossification) at the metaphyseal or articular-epiphyseal growth plates. Clinical signs of these conditions vary depending on the specific disease and location, but are unique to growing horses. In one survey of Thoroughbreds, 11% of young horses needed treatment for DOD conditions, and ALD and physeal dysplasia constituted 73% of treated cases.[11] Signs include variable degrees of lameness, alterations in posture or positioning of the limb, crooked legs, joint effusion, limb enlargement, and ataxia (CVM only). Although uncommon, multiple DOD conditions may develop in the same animal.

Osteochondrosis, which is believed to have a similar pathogenesis as DOD, is a focal disturbance of endochondral ossification with a multifactorial etiology, with no single factor accounting for all aspects of the disease.[25] The most commonly cited etiologic factors are heredity, rapid growth, anatomic conformation, trauma, and dietary imbalances; however, only heredity and anatomic conformation are well supported by the scientific literature.[21,23,25] Formation of fragile cartilage, failure of chondrocyte differentiation, subchondral bone necrosis, and failure of blood supply to the growth cartilage all have been proposed as the initial step in the pathogenesis.[25] High-circulating insulin levels from high-energy feeding has also been suggested to contribute to altered matrix metabolism and faulty mineralization.[9]

Although the exact cause for DOD is unknown, several risk factors predispose young horses to develop these diseases. The major risk factors appear to be nutritional imbalances, trauma, and genetic predisposition.[21] Nutritional imbalances include energy and phosphorus excesses; calcium, phosphorus, and copper deficiencies; or any combination of these.[21] Feeding rations high in energy appears to predispose young animals to DOD abnormalities, presumably by contributing to rapid bone growth. However, in a recent study, weanling horses fed a high-starch diet had no increase in OCD lesions compared to those fed a medium-starch diet.[16] Trace mineral deficiencies, particularly copper, have been shown to cause clinical signs and joint pathology consistent with osteochondrosis in foals.[7]

Defective collagen crosslinking from a deficiency in lysyl oxidase may impair the strength of bone collagen, essentially producing a soft bone syndrome, particularly in the metaphyseal regions.[7,20] However, Cu supplementation of mares and foals had no significant effect on the frequency or severity of articular cartilage lesions in foals at 160 days of age.[6,17] The importance of Cu deficiency in the pathogenesis of OCD is currently thought to be overemphasized.[6] In addition, trace mineral supplementation to yearling horses had no effect on growth and development, and no skeletal abnormalities were detected.[16]

Trauma to the metaphyseal or epiphyseal growth plates may also contribute to altered growth, subchondral bone damage, avulsion of defective bone, and disruption of the physeal vasculature, all of which may predispose to DOD conditions. Weight, limb conformation, and excessive exercise may be contributing factors.[21,23] Genetics most likely plays a role in the occurrence of these diseases, but its contribution is difficult to determine.

Osteochondrosis is most likely a polygenic trait with a complex method of inheritance.[26] A genetic predisposition has been demonstrated in dogs, pigs, and horses.[21] However, in most cases, the underlying cause of the DOD condition is multifactorial, usually obscure, and often never determined.[1,24] Factors that may have contributed to the disease process are often long gone by the time a veterinarian is asked to evaluate the horse. In addition, the timing at which risk factors may exert their effects on bone growth and development is

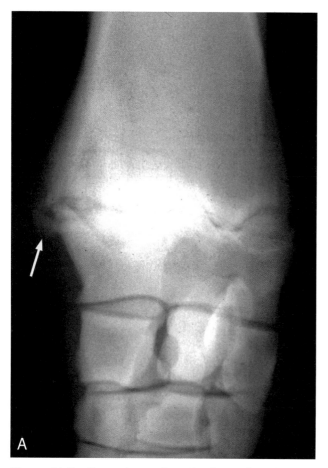

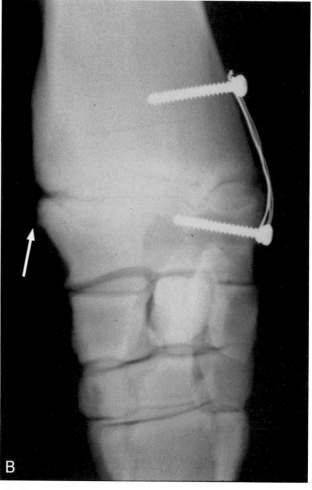

Figure 11.8. Dorsopalmar radiographs of a yearling with a carpal varus deformity. A. Type VI physeal injury with bone bridging the medial aspect of the physis (arrow).

B. Surgical removal of the exostosis (arrow) with transphyseal bridging on the lateral aspect of the physis to correct the deformity.

currently unknown. Discussions of each specific DOD condition seen in growing horses is presented in this chapter.

References

1. Baxter GM, Turner AS. Diseases of bone and related structures. In Adams' Lameness in Horses, 5th ed. Stashak TS, ed., Lippincott Williams and Wilkins, Philadelphia, 2002, pp 401–457.
2. Carlson CS, Cullins LD, Meuten DJ. Osteochondrosis of the articular-epiphyseal cartilage complex in young horses: Evidence for a defect in cartilage canal blood supply. Vet Pathol 1995; 32:641–647.
3. Embertson RM, Bramlage LR, Herring DS, et al. Physeal fractures in the horse: I. Classification and incidence. Vet Surg 1986;15:223–229.
4. Embertson RM, Bramlage LR, Gabel AA. Physeal fractures in the horse. II. Management and outcome. Vet Surg 1986;15:230–236.
5. Gaughan EM. Partial physiolysis with temporary transphyseal bridging for correction of physeal dysplasia and angular limb deformity in two yearling horses. Vet Clin Orthop Trauma 1996;9:101–105.
6. Gee EK, Firth EC, Morel PC, et al. Articular/epiphyseal osteochondrosis in Thoroughbred foals at 5 months of age: Influences of growth of the foal and prenatal copper supplementation of the dam. N Z Vet J 2005;52:448–456.
7. Hurtig MB, et al. Correlation study of defective cartilage and bone growth in foals fed a low-copper diet. Equine Vet J 1993;16(suppl):66–73.
8. Hueter C, Volkman R. Previous opinions concerning the reasons for the shape of bones. In The Law of Bone Remodeling. Wolf J, ed. Verlag, Berlin, 1982, pp 76–83.
9. Jeffcott LB, Henson FM. Studies on growth cartilage in the horse and their application to aetiopathogenesis of dyschondroplasia (osteochondrosis). Vet J 1998;156:177–192.
10. Mackie EJ, Ahmed YA, Tatarczuch L, et al. Endochondral ossification: How cartilage is converted into bone in the developing skeleton. Int J Biochem Cell Biol 2008;40:46–62.
11. O'Donohue DD, Smith FH, Strickland KL. The incidence of abnormal limb development in the Irish Thoroughbred from birth to 18 months. Equine Vet J 1992;24:305–309.
12. Ogden JA. The development and growth of the musculoskeletal system. In The Scientific Basis of Orthopedics. Albright JA, Brand RA, eds. Appleton Century Crofts, New York, 1979.
13. Olsen SE. Morphology and physiology of the growth cartilage under normal and pathologic conditions. In Bone in Clinical Orthopedics. Sumner-Smith G, ed. WB Saunders Co., Philadelphia, 1982.
14. Olstad K, Ytrehus B, Ekman S, et al. Early lesions of osteochondrosis in the distal tibia of foals. J Orthop Res 2007;25: 1094–1105.
15. Orsini JA, Kreuder C. Musculoskeletal disorders of the neonate. Vet Clin NA Equine Pract 1994;10:137–166.

16. Ott EA, Asquith RL. Trace mineral supplementation of yearling horses. J Anim Sci 1995;73:466–471.
17. Pearce SG, Firth EC, Grace ND, et al. Effect of copper supplementation on the evidence of developmental orthopedic disease in pasture-fed New Zealand Thoroughbreds. Equine Vet J 1998;30:211–218.
18. Salter RB. Birth and Pediatric Fractures in Fracture Treatment and Healing. Heppenstall BR, ed. WB Saunders Co., Philadelphia, 1980.
19. Salter RB. Textbook of Disorders and Injuries of the Musculoskeletal System. Williams and Wilkins Co., Baltimore, 1970, p 33.
20. Savage CJ. Etiopathogenesis of osteochondrosis. In Current Techniques in Equine Surgery and Lameness. White NA, Moore JN, eds. WB Saunders, Philadelphia, 1998, pp 318–322.
21. Savage CJ, Lewis LD. The role of nutrition in musculoskeletal development and disease. In Adams' Lameness in Horses, 5th ed. Stashak TS, ed. Lippincott Williams and Wilkins, Philadelphia, 2002, pp 377–399.
22. Turner AS. Diseases of bone and related structures. In Adams' Lameness in Horses, 4th ed. Stashak TS, ed., Lea and Febiger, Philadelphia1987, pp 293–338.
23. Van Weeren PR. Osteochondrosis. In Equine Surgery, 3rd ed. Auer JA, Stick JA, eds. Elsevier, Philadelphia, 2006, pp 1166–1178.
24. Williams MA, Pugh DC. Developmental orthopedic disease: Minimizing the incidence of a poorly understood disorder. Comp Cont Educ Pract Vet 1993;15:859–871.
25. Ytrehus B, Carlson CS, Ekman S. Etiology and pathogenesis of osteochondrosis. Vet Pathol. 2007;44:429–48.

EPIPHYSITIS/PHYSITIS/PHYSEAL DYSPLASIA

Gary M. Baxter

Physitis or epiphysitis is an important generalized bone disease of young growing horses characterized by enlargement of the growth plates of certain long bones (Figure 11.9).[1,3] It usually occurs in young, rapidly growing horses such as foals and weanlings, with a peak incidence between 4 to 8 months of age.[7] However, yearlings and even 2-year-old horses may also develop the condition. It may affect a single or multiple growth plates but is often bilaterally symmetrical.

Physeal dysplasia may be a more appropriate term because the condition is thought to be characterized by a disruption of endochondral ossification within the physeal growth cartilage.[3] However, in one study, physeal cartilage abnormalities and compromise of endochondral ossification were not frequently seen in Thoroughbred foals with visible bony enlargements of the distal metacarpus/metatarsus.[4] This study questions the clinical significance of these physeal swellings and suggests that they may be physiological swellings associated with normal bone remodeling.[4]

ETIOLOGY

Although the exact etiology of physitis is unknown, it is most likely multifactorial and may differ from case to case.[1,3] For instance, in foals with multiple limb involvement, a nutritional problem affecting the entire animal seems most plausible. In contrast, physitis involving a single site is likely due to trauma or excessive compression of the affected physis.[1] Secondary ALDs tend to occur more frequently with trauma-induced physitis than from other causes. Foals with severe lameness in 1 limb may develop physitis and an ALD in the contralateral limb because of excessive

weight-bearing.[2] However, in many cases physitis appears to have a mechanical as well as a nutritional component. Affected animals are frequently heavily muscled, overweight, and being overfed for rapid growth.[1] Regions of disturbed ossification within the physis from any number of these factors are susceptible to trauma, and may predispose the underlying subchondral bone to microfractures.[7] These microfractures could lead to clinical signs of inflammation, and potentially stimulate bone production and remodeling that is often seen radiographically in horses with physitis.[1,7]

The term physitis is often referred to as physeal compression, which further emphasizes the mechanical component of physitis.[6] When compression is applied to a physis, an increased thickening of the physis occurs due to retardation of provisional calcification and increased survival of chondrocytes.[1,6] This is an auto-correction phenomenon in which the animal corrects any minor angulation of the limb axis. However, if the compression is beyond the physiologic limits of the physis, complete arrest of endochondral ossification may occur. The end result is asynchronous physeal growth and the development of an ALD together with physitis. This is most commonly seen at the distal radial physis in horses with carpal varus (Figure 11.10).

CLINICAL SIGNS

The clinical appearance of a horse with physitis is characterized by enlarged physes, primarily of the distal aspects of the radius, tibia, and third metacarpal/metatarsal bones (Figures 11.9 to 11.11). The metaphyseal flaring results in an hourglass shape of the bones and the enlargement is often painful to deep palpation, with increased heat detected.

Physitis of the distal aspect of the cannon bones often involves all 4 limbs (Figure 11.11), whereas the distal aspect of the radius and tibia are usually not involved concurrently.[1] In addition, foals with metacarpal/metatarsal physitis are usually younger than foals with physitis in other locations. This may be related to the activity of the physes with respect to bone growth at varying ages. These metacarpal/metatarsal swellings also may have no clinical significance and be a normal part of bone growth and remodeling.[4] Lameness varies from slight stiffness in the gait to overt pain and a reluctance to stand.[3,7] Severely affected animals may have concurrent angular limb (Figures 11.10 and 11.11) or flexural deformities due to disturbed physeal bone growth and chronic pain, respectively.[7]

DIAGNOSIS

The most common radiographic abnormality observed with physitis is paraphyseal bone production,

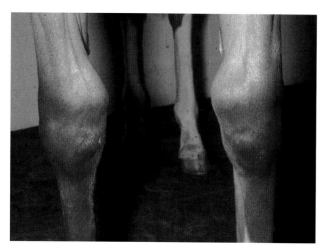

Figure 11.9. Typical swellings on the medial aspects of the distal radial physes associated with physitis.

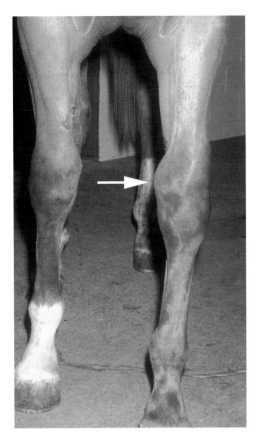

Figure 11.10. Physitis of the medial aspect of the distal radius (arrow) in a 12-month-old colt, which occurred after being kicked in the area. A carpal varus deformity developed after the trauma.

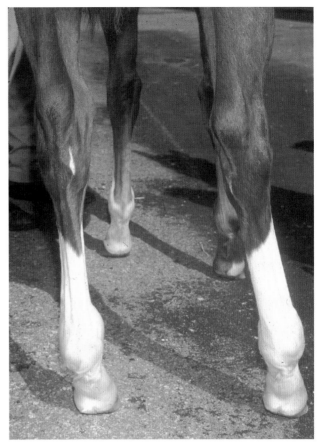

Figure 11.11. A 4-month-old Paint colt with severe physitis of all 4 distal cannon bones. Large swellings of the distal metatarsal physes and varus deformities of both hind fetlocks were present.

often termed physeal lipping or metaphyseal flaring (Figure 11.12).[3] Increased radiolucency or widening of the physis, asymmetry of the metaphysis, wedging of the epiphysis, metaphyseal sclerosis adjacent to the physis, and asymmetry of cortical thickness due to altered stress on the limb are less commonly observed.[1,7] Concurrent angular limb deformities or osteochondrosis lesions also may be present.

TREATMENT

One of the first steps in treating physitis, especially if it involves multiple locations, is to evaluate the feed ration. Often a geographic nutritional deficiency may exist, especially when multiple animals are affected. The ration should be altered accordingly and many times it is advised to reduce the animal's body weight or growth rate. However, retardation of growth rate by feeding poor-quality hay is considered irresponsible by many.[5] The recommended approach is a carefully formulated diet that specifically restricts starch and protein while supplying National Research Council (NRC) minimum requirements of other essential nutrients.[5] In general, affected horses should be fed less grain and fewer protein supplements, and the quantity of alfalfa hay should be reduced or replaced with good-quality grass hay.[1] With nursing foals, the milk production of the

mare should be decreased if possible. Specific balanced rations for growing horses to minimize the development of physitis and other DOD diseases have been developed and also should be considered.

Nonsteroidal anti-inflammatory drugs (NSAIDs) are indicated in most cases to decrease physeal inflammation and improve the animal's stiff gait. NSAIDs help diminish pain and may prevent the development of flexural deformities. These drugs may be required for 2 to 3 weeks at low doses (once-daily or every-other-day oral phenylbutazone or firocoxib works well) to completely resolve the inflammation. Further trauma to the physis should be prevented by minimizing exercise (with confinement) and correcting predisposing causes such as ALDs. With concurrent physitis and ALDs, the greatest degree of physeal abnormalities usually corresponds to the direction in which the limb is deviated. For example, weanlings with significant physitis of the medial aspect of the distal radial physis often develop carpal varus (Figure 11.10). This suggests that the physitis has contributed to arrested growth on the medial aspect of the physis. Auto correction of these deviations is unlikely and growth retardation procedures on the opposite side of the physis are often necessary to correct the ALD.

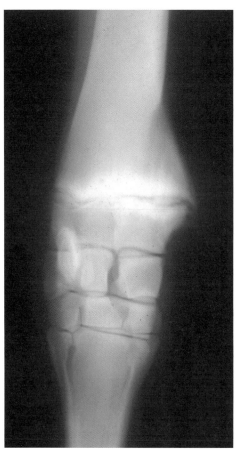

Figure 11.12. Dorsopalmar radiograph of the carpus illustrating the paraphyseal lipping of the physis that is often seen in horses with physitis.

PROGNOSIS

Fortunately, mild cases of physitis are often self-limiting and resolve when skeletal maturity is reached and growth of the affected physis ceases. Many cases may be normal aspects of bone remodeling and the foals simply grow out of the problem.[4] More severe cases of physitis that have concurrent orthopedic abnormalities, especially varus deformities, may cause residual problems severe enough to limit future athletic soundness.

References

1. Baxter GM, Turner AS. Diseases of bone and related structures. In Adams' Lameness in Horses, 5th ed. Stashak TS, ed. Lippincott Williams and Wilkins, Philadelphia. 2002;401–457.
2. Baxter GM, Morrison S. Complications of unilateral weight bearing. Vet Clin NA Eq Pract 2009;24:621–642.
3. Bramlage LR. Physitis in foals. Proc Am Assoc Equine Pract 1993;39:57–62.
4. Gee EK, Firth EC, Morel PC, et al. Enlargements of the distal third metacarpus and metatarsus in Thoroughbred foals at pasture from birth to 160 days of age. N Z Vet J 2005;53: 438–447.
5. Kronfield DS, Meachum TN, Donoghue S. Dietary aspects of developmental orthopaedic disease in young horses. Vet Clin NA Equine Pract 1990;6:451–465.
6. Turner AS. Diseases of bone and related structures. In Adams' Lameness in Horses, 4th ed. Stashak TS, ed. Lea and Febiger, Philadelphia, 1987, pp 293–338.
7. Watkins JP. Osteochondrosis. In Equine Surgery, 1st ed. Auer JA, ed. W.B. Saunders Co., Philadelphia, 1992, pp 971–984.
8. Williams MA, Pugh DC. Developmental orthopedic disease: Minimizing the incidence of a poorly understood disorder. Comp Cont Educ Pract Vet 1993;15:859–871.

INCOMPLETE CUBOIDAL BONE OSSIFICATION/ JUVENILE SPAVIN

Gary M. Baxter

Incomplete ossification of the cuboidal bones of the carpus or tarsus occurs most commonly in premature, twin, or underdeveloped newborn foals.[2,8] At birth, the cuboidal bones have not ossified sufficiently to withstand the forces of normal weight-bearing, predisposing to variable degrees of carpal or tarsal bone wedging or collapse.[6] In one study of foals with tarsal valgus deformities, 56% had concurrent incomplete ossification of the tarsal cuboidal bones.[5] Incomplete ossification without collapse is not readily apparent clinically in young foals and may go unrecognized until the horse has matured. These horses often develop OA of the distal tarsal joints at an early age and become lame when put into work.[3,4] This condition has been termed juvenile arthritis or spavin.

ETIOLOGY

Cuboidal bone ossification normally occurs during the last 2 to 3 weeks of gestation.[8] Foals born prematurely or immature may simply have a delay in the normal ossification of the cuboidal bones (Figure 11.2). Others foals with incomplete ossification may have similar congenital or developmental abnormalities that are associated with ALDs and OCD. For example, juvenile arthritis is thought to occur because of a defect in endochondral ossification of the cuboidal bones, similar to OCD. The articular-epiphyseal physes are affected with OCD and the spherical physes of the tarsal cuboidal bones with juvenile arthritis.

CLINICAL SIGNS

Clinical signs associated with cuboidal bone collapse may be evident in the newborn foal as an ALD of the carpus or tarsus. Concurrent laxity of soft tissue structures is often present.[7] The limb can usually be straightened manually but often bows inward or outward during weight-bearing. It is usually bilaterally symmetrical, and both the carpi and tarsi may be affected. Collapse or crushing of the tarsal bones occurs more commonly than that of the carpal bones (Figure 11.13).[5,6] Tarsal collapse is often associated with a sickle or cow-hocked conformation because the tarsus is often deviated cranially (reduced angle to the hock).[1] The tarsus may appear like it has a curb. There is usually no lameness initially but lameness is inevitable if the cuboidal bone collapse went unrecognized and was not clinically apparent until later in life (Figure 11.13).

Incomplete ossification and mild collapse of the tarsal bones is also thought to predispose to juvenile spavin in young horses (Figure 11.14).[2-4] These horses tend to develop hind lameness and moderate to severe

radiographic signs of distal tarsal osteoarthritis at a young age without a history of exercise.[3] Incongruencies or minor malformations of the central and third tarsal bones are thought to contribute to the development of osteoarthritis at such an early age (Figure 11.14B).[4] For unknown reasons, the distal intertarsal joint appears to be affected most commonly in horses with juvenile arthritis (Figure 11.14A).

DIAGNOSIS

The diagnosis is based on the history, characteristic limb conformation, and radiographs indicating incomplete ossification of the cuboidal bones. Radiographically, incomplete ossification is observed as wide joint spaces with small, rounded cuboidal bones, with or without compression or crushing.[7] In the tarsus, the collapse is usually located on the cranial aspect of the distal tarsus, contributing to the cranial deviation of the limb.[2,6] The lesions in the tarsus have been described as incomplete ossification with less than 30% collapse of the affected bones (type I) and more than 30% collapse with pinching or fragmentation of the affected bones (type II).[6] Type II lesions are more common and are associated with a worse outcome than type I lesions (Figure 11.13).[6] In addition, a skeletal ossification index has been proposed to classify osseous immaturity in the carpal bones, but it is not used clinically by the author.[1]

Milder forms of incomplete ossification may not become clinically apparent until later in life. However, young horses (under 2 years of age) with hindlimb lameness localized to the distal tarsus should be suspected of having malformation/incongruency of the tarsal cuboidal bones (Figure 11.14).[4] Some of these horses also may have a tarsal valgus or sickle-hock tarsal conformation. The diagnosis is confirmed by radiographs, which may indicate mild cuboidal bone collapse, wedging, or malformation, and signs of OA.[3,4]

TREATMENT

Treatment depends on the age of the foal, severity of the incomplete ossification, and the limbs affected. If diagnosed early, the goal of treatment is to prevent cuboidal bone collapse in newborn foals. This usually involves minimizing compressive (weight-bearing) forces on the bones until they have time to ossify completely. Confinement, sleeve casts, bandages alone, bandage-casts, or bandages and splints may be used, depending on the severity.[2,7,8] However, bilateral sleeve casts or bandages can be difficult to manage in newborn foals and the foals may have difficulty getting up and

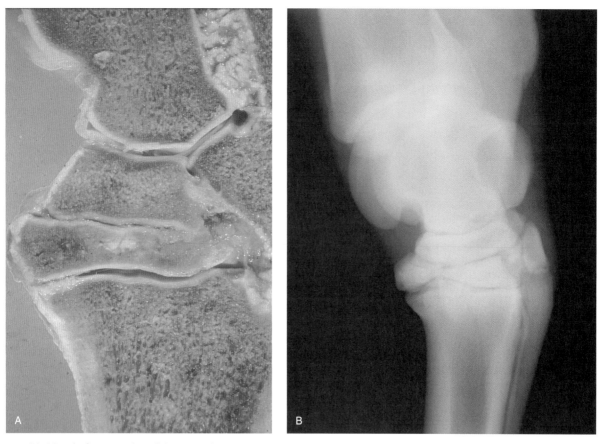

Figure 11.13. A. Cross section of the tarsus in a young horse with partial collapse of the third tarsal bone. B. Lateral radiograph of a yearling with complete collapse of the cuboidal bones.

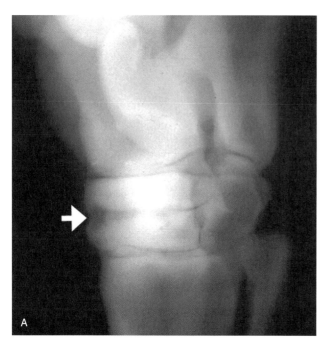
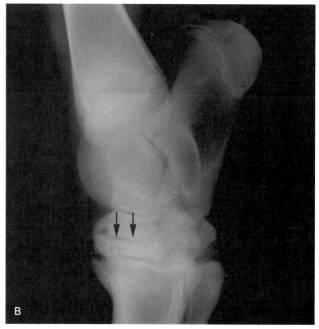

Figure 11.14. A. DMPLO radiograph of the tarsus in a 2-year-old Paint horse with hindlimb lameness. Subchondral bone lysis of the distal intertarsal joint (arrow) can be seen. B. Lateral radiograph of a 2-year-old demonstrating an undulating distal intertarsal joint surface with narrowing of the third tarsal bone (black arrows) and severe osteophyte formation consistent with distal tarsal OA.

down. The most important treatment is confinement. The decision whether to use external coaptation is made on a case-by-case basis. If cuboidal bone collapse has already occurred, any form of treatment is unlikely to be of benefit and abnormalities within the joints are inevitable.

PROGNOSIS

Foals that can be managed successfully to prevent cuboidal bone collapse can do well. Foals with only minor tarsal bone collapse (type I) were able to perform as intended, whereas foals with more severe tarsal bone collapse and fragmentation (type II) could not be used for their intended purposes.[6] No study has looked at the prognosis of foals with carpal bone collapse but it is logical to assume that these foals have a more guarded prognosis than those with tarsal bone collapse.

References

1. Adams R, Poulos P. A skeletal ossification index for neonatal foals. Vet Radiol 1988;29:217–220.
2. Baxter GM, Turner AS. Diseases of bone and related structures. In Adams' Lameness in Horses, 5th ed. Stashak TS, ed. Lippincott Williams and Wilkins, Philadelphia. 2002;401–457.
3. Baxter GM, Dechant JE, Southwood LL. Diagnosis of distal tarsal osteoarthritis in horses. Compendium Contin Educ Pract Vet 2003;25:138–147.
4. Bramlage LR. Traumatic and developmental lesions of the tarsus. In Proceedings Am Assoc Eq Pract 2006;52:1–4.
5. Dutton DM, Watkins JP, Honnas CM, et al. Treatment response and athletic outcome of foals with tarsal valgus deformities: 39 cases (1988–1997). J Am Vet Med Assoc 1999;215:1481–1484.
6. Dutton DM, Watkins JP, Walker MA, et al. Incomplete ossification of the tarsal bones in foals: 22 cases (1988–1996). J Am Vet Med Assoc 1998;213:1590–1594.
7. Orsini JA, Kreuder C. Musculoskeletal disorders of the neonate. Vet Clin NA Equine Pract 1994;10:137–166.
8. Trumble TN. Orthopedic disorders in neonatal foals. Vet Clin NA Equine Pract 2005;21:357–385.

ANGULAR LIMB DEFORMITIES (ALDS)

| Gary M. Baxter

Valgus and varus are terms used to describe ALDs in foals. Valgus and varus indicate a shift outward or inward of the distal limb from midline (distal to the site of origin).[4] Typically the deviation (valgus vs. varus) is further characterized by the joint of origin of the angulation. For instance, carpal valgus refers to a deformity in which the carpus is the site of the lesion, and the limb distal to this joint (third metacarpal bone and phalanges) is deviated away from the midline of the body (Figure 11.15). A carpal varus indicates the third metacarpal bone and fetlock are deviated toward the midline distal to the carpus (Figure 11.10).

Carpal valgus is the most common ALD seen in foals, followed by fetlock varus, carpal varus, and tarsal valgus.[2,3,9,12,15] Tarsal varus is rare, as are deviations of other parts of the limbs.[3,7,13] Foals with ALDs due to asynchronous physeal growth typically are not lame and have few physical examination abnormalities other than crooked legs. If lameness is present, physeal trauma, fracture, or collapse of the cuboidal bones should be suspected as the cause of the limb deformity (Figure 11.16).[4]

ETIOLOGY

Causes of ALDs in foals include laxity of periarticular supporting tissues, incomplete ossification of the tarsal or carpal cuboidal bones, direct trauma to the physis as with concussion or fractures, traumatic luxation or fracture of the carpal bones (Figure 11.16), and asynchronous longitudinal growth of the metaphysis and epiphysis (Figures 11.11 and 11.15).[3,4,15,21] By far the most common reason for ALDs in foals is asynchronous metaphyseal growth. For often unexplained reasons, one side of the growth plate grows faster than the other, resulting in a deviation of the normal limb axis.[12] Trauma across the growth plate is believed to be one of the main underlying causes of asynchronous growth.[12] Trauma may retard calcification of the matured and dying chondrocytes, resulting in thickening of the physeal plate with an increasing number of chondrocytes at the hypertrophied cell layer.[4] If compression is excessive, chondrocytes may undergo necrosis and the physis may prematurely close or growth is slowed. Any factor that causes asymmetric loading across a growth plate can lead to this sequence of events, resulting in an ALD.[4,9] Such factors include joint laxity, hypoplasia of the cuboidal bones, poor foot trimming, heavy muscling, excessively active foals, or lameness in the opposite limb.[3,4,12] Other proposed causes of ALD include malpositioning *in utero*, *in utero* chemical insults such as locoweed, and hormonal or nutritional imbalances.[4,14,17,21]

CLINICAL SIGNS

Laxity of Periarticular Support Tissues

Foals with ligamentous laxity are often termed windswept because their limbs are very flaccid and tend to deviate in the same direction. The carpus or tarsus is usually affected, and 1 limb has a valgus deviation and the other has a varus deformity (Figure 11.17). Usually the limbs can be manually straightened, indicating a soft tissue problem and not a deviation of the bony column. Affected foals are usually within 2 weeks of birth, may be premature, and usually are not lame. At the walk, the affected joint may deviate inward or outward when weight is placed on the limb (hence the term spaghetti legs) due to the weakness of the supporting soft tissue.

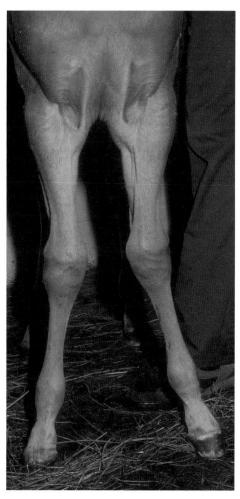

Figure 11.15. Young filly with bilateral carpal valgus.

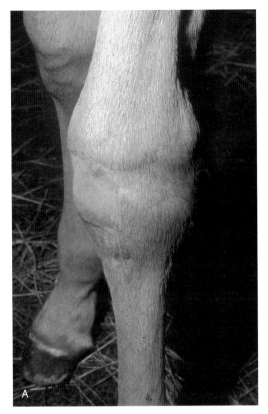

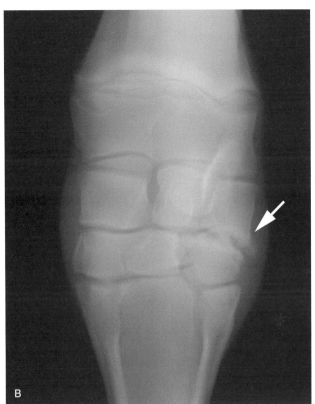

Figure 11.16.   Young horse with a traumatic injury to the carpus, contributing to a carpal valgus. A. Physical examination of the carpus revealed effusion of the middle carpal joint and pain on flexion. B. Dorsopalmar radiograph of the carpus, which revealed a fracture of the ulna carpal bone (arrow) and collapse of the lateral aspect of the middle carpal joint.

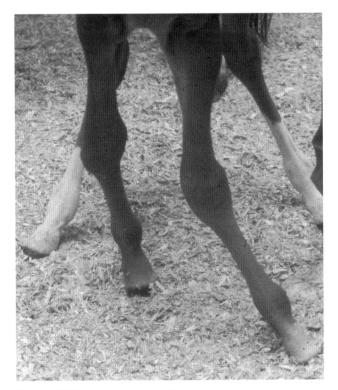

Figure 11.17.   Newborn foal with a windswept appearance to the carpi due to ligamentous laxity.

Delayed Ossification of the Tarsal or Carpal Cuboidal Bones

Affected foals are usually born premature or dysmature and may have concurrent ligamentous laxity.[17] The limbs are often straight at birth and then begin to deviate within a few days or weeks due to collapsing of the cuboidal bones (Figure 11.13). Valgus deviation of the carpus and tarsus occurs most commonly.

Physeal or Articular Trauma/Fracture

The majority of foals with physeal or articular trauma/fracture have no history of limb deformities until after a traumatic incident. They may have a single limb involved, are usually lame, and often have joint effusion (Figure 11.16). Lameness and pain on manipulation of the affected joint are the most important clinical findings to suggest trauma as the cause of the ALD.

Asynchronous Longitudinal Growth

Foals with asynchronous physeal growth appear clinically normal except for their crooked legs. No palpable abnormalities should be present and the limbs cannot be straightened manually. Varying degrees of outward rotation of the limb often accompany foals with carpal valgus (Figure 11.15).[4,21] Multiple types of ALD may be present in the same foal, especially if it has

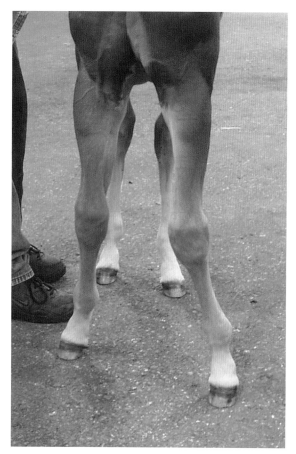

Figure 11.18. Foal with a combination of carpal valgus and fetlock varus. Straightening the carpal valgus would probably make the fetlock varus worse and must be considered when developing a treatment plan.

not been treated. Carpal valgus and fetlock varus may occur concurrently, and the treatment of one deformity most likely affects the other (Figure 11.18).

DIAGNOSIS

Foals with ALD of almost any joint can usually be diagnosed by visual exam. To avoid confusion with rotation of the limb, it can be helpful to elevate the limb and look down the limb from above, noting the relationship of the bone above to the bone below the joint of origin. Palpation and radiographs usually are necessary to determine the exact cause of the deformity. Most foals with limb deformities have no lameness or palpable abnormalities, and the only evidence of limb deviation is on dorsopalmar/plantar or craniocaudal radiographs.

Radiographs provide the most conclusive evidence about the location and potential cause of the ALD. In the case of asynchronous growth across the distal radial physis, the deviation arise from the distal metaphyseal region rather than within the carpus (Figure 11.19). This can be verified by drawing lines along the long axes of the bones, bisecting the radius and the third metacarpal bone.[4,17,21] The lines bisect in what has been

called the pivot point, which is considered to be the location of the limb deformity. Wedging of the epiphysis on the concave side of the deviation, abnormal contour of the cuboidal bones, and displacement of the splint bones often accompany limb deviations of the carpus and tarsus but usually resolve when the limb straightens (Figure 11.19).[4,15] Epiphyseal wedging is especially prominent with varus deformities of the fetlock (Figure 11.20), and collapse of the lateral aspect of the third carpal bone is common with carpal valgus deformities (Figure 11.19). However, severe abnormalities such as physeal or cuboidal bone fractures or crushing of the carpal or tarsal bones in conjunction with an ALD are a major concern and may contribute to permanent lameness problems, even if the deviation is corrected.

TREATMENT

Treatment depends on the cause, location, and severity of the ALD, as well as the age of the foal. In general, varus deformities appear to be more problematic for future soundness than valgus deformities. Varus deformities of the fetlock (pigeon-toed) are thought to contribute to pastern and fetlock lameness problems, whereas mild carpal valgus was found to be protective for carpal injuries in racing Thoroughbreds.[1] Most foals have a mild degree of carpal valgus conformation (approximately 5°) that tends to decrease as they grow older.[10,19] Foals tend to grow into the mild carpal valgus as the chest expands during growth.[10,21] If the limb is completely straight as a foal, a carpal varus may develop as the chest expands during growth. In contrast, fetlock varus deviations tend to worsen with age up to 6 months.[19] Therefore, mild carpal valgus deformities should not be treated, whereas minor varus deformities of the fetlock probably should be addressed because of the potential to worsen with age (Figure 11.11).

Conservative Treatment of Asynchronous Physeal Growth

Conservative treatment of asynchronous physeal growth usually involves a combination of time, exercise restriction, and foot care in foals with mild to moderate ALDs. Under normal circumstances, most foals auto correct their deformity because the bone grows faster on the concave side and slower on the convex side (Wolff's law).[8,11,21] This only occurs under physiologic loads, so the goal of confinement is to minimize overloading of the physis. Overactivity may cause or perpetuate physeal trauma and excessive loading, possibly preventing the limb(s) from auto correcting. Restricting the foal's exercise by confining the mare and foal to a stall and run or small paddock/pasture is usually adequate. Confinement is usually continued until the limb has straightened.

Foot trimming (or balancing) also may minimize compressive forces on the physis. In foals with varus deformities, the hoof does not wear as much on the medial side and becomes compressed on the lateral side. The opposite occurs with valgus deformities. The goal of trimming is to remove the hoof wall that is over-

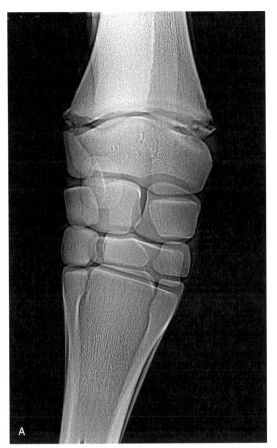 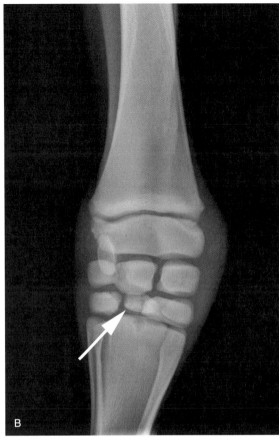

Figure 11.19. Dorsopalmar radiographs of two foals with mild carpal valgus without abnormalities of the carpal bones (A) and with wedging of the lateral aspect of the third carpal bone (arrow) (B).

grown (trim the hoof on the side that the leg goes; inside hoof for varus deformities and outside hoof for valgus deformities) to make the foot flat or balanced.[17,21] This should be done with only a rasp to avoid excessive trimming. Glue-on shoes (Dalric, Advanced Equine Products, Versailles, KY) with lateral or medial extensions also may be helpful to minimize asymmetrical loading of the physis and pull the limb inward or outward. Frequent re-evaluations (e.g., every 2 weeks) with or without radiographic examination should be performed to monitor the progress of conservative therapy.

Confinement and minor foot trimming can correct many foals with mild to moderate ALDs, and should always be considered as the initial therapy if possible. However, aggressive and prolonged trimming may lead to concurrent angular deformities elsewhere in the limb that may worsen the overall condition of the foal. For example, a secondary varus deformity of the fetlock may develop in some foals with carpal valgus treated conservatively.[3] Conservative management is usually not recommended or successful with a severe deformity of any physis in any age foal. The asymmetrical loading of the physis is usually beyond the physiologic limits in these cases, making auto-correction unlikely.[11,21] In addition, a severe ALD has a greater likelihood of causing permanent damage to the tarsal or carpal cuboidal bones if not corrected early in life.

Surgical Treatment of Asynchronous Physeal Growth

Surgical treatment of foals with ALDs is directed toward accelerating growth on the concave side or slowing growth on the convex side.[2,3,9,12,21] Hemi-circumferential transection of the periosteum and periosteal stripping (HCTP+PS) is used to stimulate growth, and various forms of transphyseal bridging (TPB) are used to retard growth.

Recently, physeal growth has been reported to occur by stimulation of the physis with fan-shaped stab incisions and placement of needles directly into the physis.[6] These techniques were reported as another method to treat ALDs and as an alternative to HCTP+PS.[6] The exact mechanism contributing to physeal growth stimulation is unknown but is thought to be a mechanical release of the periosteal restraint of growth.[2,3] However, there is controversy regarding the true benefit of HCTP+PS. A controlled model of ALD demonstrated no benefit of HCTP+PS compared with controls treated with confinement and hoof trimming.[18] In addition, practices in which foals can be examined consistently have found that most correct on their own, with only changes to the exercise regimen.[20] These studies and observations have questioned whether HCTP+PS is a necessary surgical procedure in foals with ALDs.

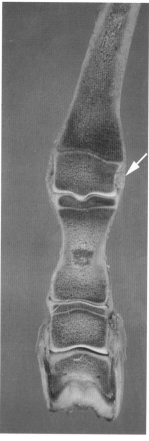

Figure 11.20. Cross section of a fetlock varus deformity in a young foal with collapse of the medial aspect of the epiphysis (arrow).

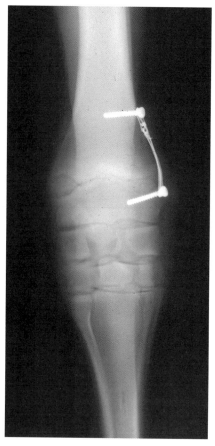

Figure 11.21. Dorsopalmar radiograph of a 4-month-old foal that had transphyseal bridging performed to correct a carpal valgus ALD. The limb has straightened and it is time to remove the implants.

However, many veterinarians remain convinced that it is beneficial because foals with ALDs treated conservatively improve after HCTP+PS is performed.[3,6,12]

Transphyseal bridging is effective and is currently the most reliable surgical technique to correct limb deformities. However, the advantages of HCTP+PS over TPB techniques are that the procedure is easy to perform, has minimal complications, is less expensive than TPB procedures, and the limb does not overcorrect. In addition, the majority of horses can perform well after surgery, although racing performance has been shown to be reduced if HCTP+PS is performed at 2 or more anatomic locations.[16] Despite these benefits, HCTP+PS appears to be most useful for mild to moderate cases of ALD that have not responded to conservative treatment. Foals with severe ALD at any location are best treated with TPB.

Retardation of endochondral ossification on the convex side of the deformity can be accomplished with various TPB procedures.[5,7,12,13,15,22] The bridges may consist of staples,[5,12] screws and wires,[3,15] a small plate spanning the growth plate,[12] or a transphyseal lag or positional screw placed across one side of the physis[13,22] (Figures 11.21 and 11.22). A positional screw is currently recommended to avoid screw breakage and difficulties in screw removal. The transphyseal screw technique is especially useful in the tarsus because of

the ease of screw placement (the epiphysis is narrow and angled), but can also be used primarily in the fetlock (Figure 11.22).[13,22]

The implants create a static compression across one side of the physis so that bone growth is retarded.[11,21] Slowed growth on one side of the physis and continued growth on the opposite equalizes the relative length of the medial and lateral aspects of the distal metaphysis, thereby straightening the limb. Once the limb is straight, the implants must be removed or the limb will over correct. Limb growth usually returns to normal following implant removal. However, continued growth retardation has been seen following removal of the transphyseal screw, and this should be considered when deciding when and where to use this technique. The advantages of the TPB procedures are that severe deformities can be corrected quickly and most surgeons feel that the results are more reliable than HCTP+PS. The disadvantages include that the procedure is more difficult to perform, there are more wound healing complications, a second surgical procedure is needed to remove the implants, and the limb can over-correct if the owners fail to monitor the limb or the implants damage the physis. For these reasons, most surgeons utilize TPB in severe deformities that will not correct with HCTP+PS alone or in older foals/weanlings where the growth potential of the physis may be limited.

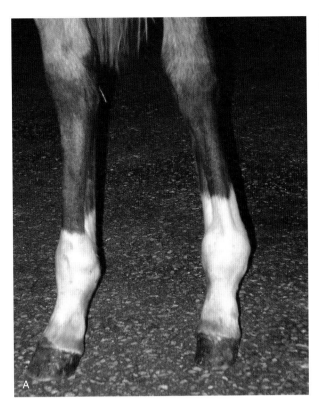
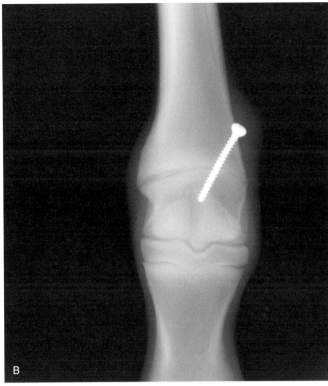

Figure 11.22.   A 3-month-old foal with varus deformity of the left hind fetlock (A) that had a positional transphyseal screw placed to correct the deformity (B). The screw was removed once the limb was straight.

The maximal growth potential in the distal physis is reduced by 2 months for the metacarpus/metatarsus, 4 months for the tibia, and 6 months for the radius.[3] In most cases, ALDs of the fetlock or phalanges should be treated surgically within 45 to 60 days of age, or sooner if they are worsening.[3,21] Hunt recommends that HCTP+PS be performed by 1 to 2 months and TPB by 3 to 4 months to achieve correction of ALDs at the fetlock.[12] However, some minor limb deviations of the fetlock may be corrected with TPB after 4 to 6 months of age. The distal radial and tibial physes close at a later age and therefore conservative therapy can be continued longer (up to 4 to 5 months). However, if the deformity is severe (more than 15°) or if limb deviation worsens with time, then surgery should be performed earlier.

In most cases of carpal and tarsal deformities, surgery is indicated if the limbs have not corrected by 4 to 5 months of age.[12,13,22] Carpal valgus deformities of less than 10° in foals less than 4 to 5 months of age may benefit from HCTP+PS alone.[2,3,12]

The HCTP+PS technique should be performed by 45 days of age to correct fetlock deformities, and in one study was most beneficial for tarsal valgus deformities if performed by 60 days of age.[7] TPB techniques are usually recommended for carpal deformities greater than 10°, especially in foals older than 4 to 5 months, and for most fetlock deformities in foals older than 2 months of age. The transphyseal screw is the recommended TPB technique for the tarsus because it is much easier to place than staples or screws and wires. The mean age of foals in 2 different studies with fetlock, tarsal, or carpal deformities that were treated with transphyseal screws was 94, 220, and 377 days, respectively.[13,22] These average ages were greater than what is currently recommended for TPB techniques but several older horses were treated in these studies, which contributed to the greater mean ages. Depending on the severity of the deformity and to ensure correction, the upper age limit for using TPB techniques should be approximately 6 months for the tarsus and carpus and 3 months for the fetlock. However, horses older than these upper limits have been treated successfully with TPB techniques, depending on the severity. TPB can be performed successfully up to 14 to 16 months of age in the carpus, up to 12 months of age in the tarsus, and up to 7 months of age in the fetlock.[12,22]

Many veterinarians' philosophy about managing foals with ALDs appears to have changed over the last several years. Mild carpal valgus is considered normal and there is less desire to obtain perfectly straight front limbs at an early age. Furthermore, more foals are being treated conservatively and for longer periods of time before surgery is performed. It also appears that correction of ALDs can be accomplished with TPB techniques in foals and weanlings older than what has been previously thought. All of these findings have led to a more conservative approach to manage foals with ALDs, relying more on normal bone remodeling and growth for correction. However, severe deformities at any location and varus deformities should still be considered problematic, less responsive to conservative treatment, and often an indication for surgical intervention.

PROGNOSIS

Foals with mild and moderate ALDs of any region usually have an excellent prognosis for correction and future athletic soundness. In general, varus deformities appear to be more problematic for future soundness than valgus deformities. Varus deformities of the fetlock (pigeon-toed) are thought to contribute to pastern and fetlock lameness problems, whereas mild carpal valgus may be protective for carpal injuries. Severe ALDs have the potential to cause asymmetrical loading of the carpal and tarsal cuboidal bones, contributing to collapse, articular cartilage damage, and future lameness. Early correction of severe ALDs usually helps prevent these problems and improves the long-term prognosis in affected foals.

References

1. Anderson TA, McIlwraith CW, Douay P. The role of conformation in musculoskeletal problems in racing Thoroughbreds. Equine Vet J 2004;36:571–575.
2. Auer JA, Martens RJ. Periosteal transection and periosteal stripping for correction of angular limb deformities in foals. Am J Vet Res 1982;43:1530.
3. Auer JA. Angular limb deformities. In Equine Surgery, 3rd ed. Auer JA, Stick JA, eds. Elsevier, Philadelphia, 2006, pp 1130–1149.
4. Baxter GM, Turner AS. Diseases of bone and related structures. In Adams' Lameness in Horses, 5th ed. Stashak TS, ed. Lippincott Williams and Wilkins, Philadelphia. 2002;401–457.
5. Caston SS, Reinertson EL, Kersh KK. How to make, place and remove transphyseal staples. Proceedings Am Assoc Eq Pract 2007;53:415–419.
6. Colles CM. How to aid the correction of angular limb deformities in foals using physeal stimulation. Proceedings Am Assoc Eq Pract 2008;54:60–63.
7. Dutton DM, Watkins JP, Honnas CM, et al. Treatment response and athletic outcome of foals with tarsal valgus deformities: 39 cases (1988–1997) J Am Vet Med Assoc 1999;215:1481–1484.
8. Frost HM. Structural adaptations to mechanical usage: a proposed three way rule for bone remodeling. Vet Comp Orthopaed Traumatol 1988;2:80–85.
9. Gaughan EM. Angular limb deformities in horses. Comp Cont Educ Pract Vet 1998;20:944–946.
10. Greet TRC. Managing flexural and angular limb deformities: The Newmarket perspective. Proceedings Am Assoc Eq Pract 2000;46:130–136.
11. Hueter C, Volkman R. Previous opinions concerning the reasons for the shape of bones. In The Law of Bone Remodeling. Wolf J, ed. Verlag, Berlin, 1982, pp 76–83.
12. Hunt RJ. Angular limb deviations. In Current Techniques in Equine Surgery and Lameness. White NA, Moore JN, eds. W.B. Saunders, Philadelphia, 1998, pp 323–326.
13. Kay AT, Hunt RJ, Thorpe PE, et al. Single screw transphyseal bridging for correction of forelimb angular limb deviation. Proceedings Am Assoc Eq Pract 2005;51:306–308.
14. McIlwraith CW, James LF. Limb deformities in foals associated with ingestion of locoweed by mares. J Am Vet Med Assoc 1982;181:255–258.
15. Mitton LA, Bertone AL. Angular limb deformities in foals. J Am Vet Med Assoc 1994;204:717–720.
16. Mitton LA, Bramlage LR, Embertson RM. Racing performance after hemicircumferential transaction for angular limb deformities in Thoroughbreds: 199 cases(1987–1989). J Am Vet Med Assoc 1995;207:746–750.
17. Orsini JA, Kreuder C. Musculoskeletal disorders of the neonate. Vet Clin NA Equine Pract 1994;10:137–166.
18. Read EK, Read MR, Townsend HG, et al. Effect of hemi-circumferential periosteal transaction and elevation in foals with experimentally induced angular limb deformities. J Am Vet Med Assoc 2002;221:536–540.
19. Santschi EM, Leibsle SR, Morehead JP, et al. Carpal and fetlock conformation of the juvenile Thoroughbred from birth to yearling auction age. Equine Vet J 2006;38:604–609.
20. Slone DE, Roberts CT, Hughes FE. Restricted exercise and transphyseal bridging for correction of angular limb deformities. Proceedings Am Assoc Eq Pract 2000;46:126–127.
21. Trumble TN. Orthopedic disorders in neonatal foals. Vet Clin NA Equine Pract 2005;21:357–385.
22. Witte S, Thorpe PE, Hunt RJ, et al. A lag-screw technique for bridging of the medial aspect of the distal tibial physis in horses. J Am Vet Med Assoc 2004;225:1581–1583.

FLEXURAL DEFORMITIES

| Gary M. Baxter

Flexural deformities or contracted tendons of limbs of young horses are classified as congenital (apparent at or near the time of birth) or acquired (develop during the growth period).[1,20] Limb deformities secondary to trauma also may be considered as acquired flexural deformities.[10] The term contracted tendons is often used synonymously with flexural deformities but the potential for contraction of dense tendinous tissue is limited and the primary defect is usually not in the tendon itself.[20] In many instances the effective functional length of the musculotendinous unit(s) is less than what is necessary for normal limb alignment. The term contracted tendons may be an effective means of describing the condition but other possible incompletely understood mechanisms most likely contribute to their development.[9] In addition, these abnormalities are most accurately discussed relative to the joint(s) around which the deformity is centered rather than the probable affected tendons and ligaments because more than 1 structure often is involved.

CONGENITAL FLEXURAL DEFORMITIES

Etiology

Several factors have been incriminated as causes of congenital flexural deformities in neonates. This condition primarily has been attributed to uterine malpositioning or overcrowding but more complex influences have been implicated, such as genetic factors, equine goiter, and teratogenic insults from toxic and infectious agents during the embryonic stage of pregnancy.[9,19,20] Arthrogryposis, as a cause of congenital flexural deformities, has been well documented in calves but is less well defined in horses.[20]

Clinical Signs

Congenital flexural deformities may affect 1 or more limbs but usually involve the carpus (most common) and fetlock (Figure 11.23). Congenital flexural deformities of the pastern, tarsus, and distal interphalangeal

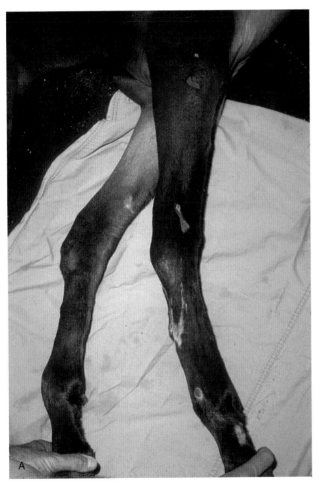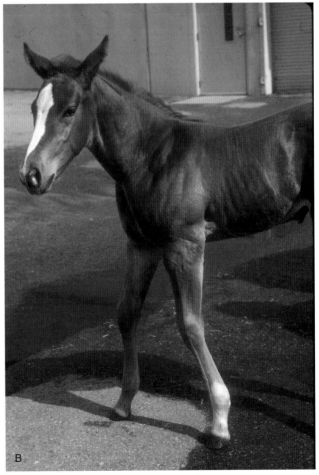

Figure 11.23.   A. Congenital flexural deformities of both carpi and front fetlocks. Neither limb could be straightened manually and the foal had difficulty walking with splinting. B. More typical flexural deformities of both carpi that cause the carpus to knuckle forward.

(DIP) joint occur, but much less frequently.[9,20] With fetlock flexural deformities the foals may be able to stand but knuckle over at the fetlock. In severe instances, the foals walk on the dorsal surface of the fetlock. Generally, both the superficial and deep digital flexor muscle tendon units are shortened and the carpus and/or fetlock cannot be straightened. Involvement of the deep digital flexor tendon (DDFT) alone may manifest as a flexural deformity of the DIP joint. Individual tendon involvement is difficult to define in severe cases and contracture of the carpal fascia and palmar ligaments may be the primary component. This contributes to an arthrogryposis-like position of the carpus with minimal flexion or extension capabilities (Figure 11.23A).

Rupture of the common digital extensor (CDE) tendon may occur concurrently with carpal or fetlock flexural deformities (Figure 11.24).[20,29] Occasionally, flexural deformities may not be noted despite evidence of a ruptured extensor tendon. The extensor tendon rupture may occur secondary to flexor tendon contracture or it may predispose to the flexural deformity. Affected foals may have other associated birth defects including prognathism, underdeveloped pectoral muscles, and incomplete ossification of the carpal/tarsal bones.[20]

Diagnosis

The diagnosis is usually based on the history of being born with the problem and physical examination of the foal. Affected limb(s) cannot be straightened manually and the foal may have difficulty standing. Radiographs

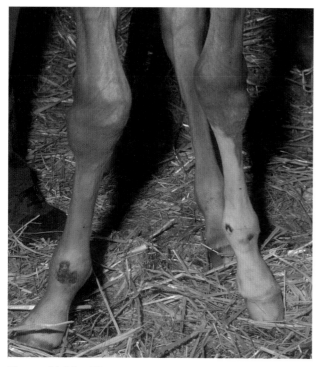

Figure 11.24. Bilateral symmetrical fluid swellings of the lateral aspects of both carpi in neonatal foals are characteristic of rupture of the common digital extensor tendons.

or ultrasound can be performed but are usually not necessary for the diagnosis. Concurrent extensor tendon rupture is characterized by the presence of bilaterally symmetrical swellings over the dorsolateral aspect of both carpi (Figure 11.24).[29] It may or may not be possible to palpate the enlarged ends of the ruptured tendon. Commonly, the ruptured CDE tendon is not recognized and the problem is diagnosed as a flexor tendon contracture.

Treatment

Treatment of congenital flexural deformities should be initiated soon after recognition of the problem, with the severity of the deformity dictating how quickly and aggressively treatment should proceed.[9] Medical treatment usually consists of NSAIDs and IV oxytetracycline, and is often combined with bandaging and splinting. Foals with minor congenital flexural deformities (particularly of the carpus) may improve spontaneously and do not require treatment (Figure 11.23B). In addition, most fetlock flexural deformities usually respond well to bandaging and splinting.[1,9,20]

Splints may be made from PVC pipe tubing and may be bent with heat to whatever conformation is desired. Fiberglass cast material molded over a padded bandage also works well. Splinting increases tensional forces to the flexor units during weight-bearing, which induces flexor relaxation through the inverse myotactic reflex (stretching the musculotendinous unit leads to relaxation).[20] All splinting devices require strategic placement of padding, constant evaluation, and changing of the splints to prevent complications. It is often easiest to apply bandages and splints with the foal sedated and positioned in lateral recumbency.

Concurrent rupture of the extensor tendon usually responds spontaneously with stall rest but bandaging and splinting may be needed to prevent knuckling over at the fetlock.[20,29] Exercise is usually restricted initially because the foals often have difficulty walking, but exercise may actually increase strength and tone in the flexor muscles.[9] Distal interphalangeal joint deformities may respond to glue-on toe extensions that stretch the DDFT and also prevent excessive wear of the toe. However, these should be used with caution because they may produce excessive tension on the laminae.[9]

Oxytetracycline remains a common treatment for foals with congenital flexural deformities.[1,2,9,16,20] Clinically, it appears to be more effective on congenital than acquired flexural deformities, but can be used for both types. The use of oxytetracycline was first described in 1985 by Lokai and again in 1992 by the same author.[15,16] All foals in the latter study (n = 123) were treated either once or twice with 3 grams of oxytetracycline intravenously (undiluted) and no external splinting was used. A 94% overall success rate was reported with the forelimbs responding better (98%) than the hindlimbs (75%).[16] Two controlled studies have documented changes in metacarpophalangeal (MCP) joint angles following treatment with oxytetracycline.[13,17] A significant decrease in mean MCP joint angles at rest was observed in foals 24 hours after treatment, and these angles returned to pretreatment value by 96 hours.[17] In another study, maximum MCP joint angles that occurred during the stance phase of the stride at a walk and range of joint motion were significantly increased in treated foals compared to controls.[13]

Currently, 2 to 3 grams of oxytetracycline diluted in a small amount of saline IV is recommended for the average sized foal. A dose of 44 mg/kg IV was used in 1 experimental study with good effects and no alterations in blood chemistry values.[17] One or 2 repeat treatments may be given but the risk of renal problems should be considered with multiple dosing or overdosing.[9,28] The author usually combines splinting with IV oxytetracycline treatment, especially in moderate to severe cases of congenital flexural deformities.

Oxytetracycline's mechanism of action has been hypothesized to result from chelation of calcium in muscle or to decrease the expression of the contractile protein α-smooth muscle actin.[11,16] A recent study found that myofibroblasts made up most of the cells in the distal check ligament and the DDFT in normal foals, supporting this rationale.[11] Oxytetracycline was also found to inhibit normal collagen organization in equine myofibroblasts through a matrix metalloproteinase-1 mechanism.[5] However it works, oxytetracycline appears to be an effective method to obtain a short-term moderate decrease in MCP joint angle in newborn foals.

Surgical treatment of congenital tendon contractures is usually the last resort and often unnecessary. Flexor tendon tenotomies and carpal (inferior) or radial (superior) check ligament desmotomies have been used successfully but are not commonly indicated.[9,20] Transection of the superior check ligament may benefit some foals that are chronically over at the knees because the carpus becomes more hyperextended following transection.[3] Transection of the palmar carpal ligament in the palmar carpal joint capsule has been used to treat foals with severe carpal flexural deformities.[26] Tenotomy of the ulnaris lateralis and flexor carpi ulnaris 2 cm proximal to the accessory carpal bone has been used to treat less severe carpal flexural deformities with a very favorable outcome.[1,8] Arthrodesis of the fetlock joint has also been used to correct severe flexural deformities of the fetlock in a donkey and miniature horse, and may be used as a salvage procedure in some cases.[1,27]

ACQUIRED FLEXURAL DEFORMITIES

Acquired flexural deformities can be unilateral or bilateral and usually affect the DIP joint (club foot) or MCP joint (dorsal knuckling of the fetlock). Acquired flexural deformities are grouped within the DOD complex because the potential causes and risk factors (nutritional imbalances, trauma, and genetics) are similar. Flexural deformities tend to occur in fast-growing horses or in those following a growth spurt, and often animals that are overfed. However, both overfeeding and imbalanced rations have been implicated as causes.[20]

Other types of DOD conditions such as physitis and OCD are seen concurrently in these animals and may actually contribute to the development of flexural deformities (Figure 11.25). For example, foals with OCD of the shoulder often have a concurrent club foot in the same leg, presumably from unweighting of the foot related to the lameness and pain. Flexural deformities

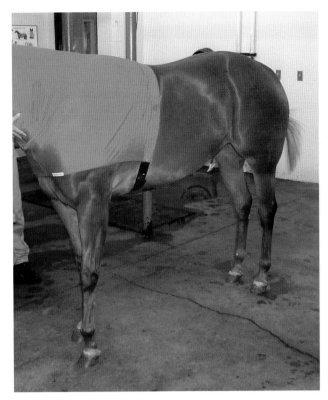

Figure 11.25. This yearling Quarter horse filly had flexural deformities of both front fetlocks and subchondral cystic lesions in both stifles.

of the DIP joint typically occur in foals and weanlings, and flexural deformities at the MCP joint are more typical of 1- to 2-year-old animals (Figures 11.26 and 11.27).[18,23,24,26] However, the relationship between age and the type of flexural deformity is not absolute.

Etiology

The cause(s) of acquired flexural deformities is/are thought to be similar to that of other DOD conditions (see above). However, unlike other DOD conditions, pain in the limb for any reason may initiate a flexion withdrawal reflex causing flexor muscle contraction and an altered position of the joint.[20] Chronic unweighting of the leg also may contribute to foot contracture, high heels, and the development of a club foot. Lack of exercise has been suggested to prevent proper stretching of the tendons and ligaments, contributing to limb contracture.[20] Severe trauma to a flexor tendon or its associated muscles is also known to cause tendon contracture due to fibrous tissue deposited during the reparative process.[10] The author has seen flexural deformities of both the DIP and MCP joints develop subsequent to trauma to the elbow region.

The mechanism by which the suggested risk factors produce flexural deformities is still uncertain. Suggested hypotheses include the failure of tendons and ligaments to develop at the same rate as bone lengthening and a discrepancy between bone growth and the capacity for lengthening of the check ligaments.[10,20] Flexor muscles

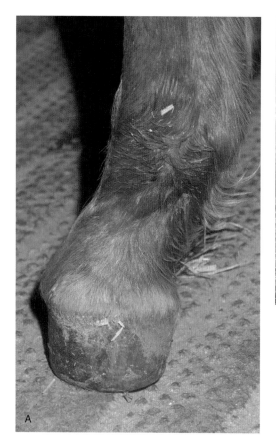
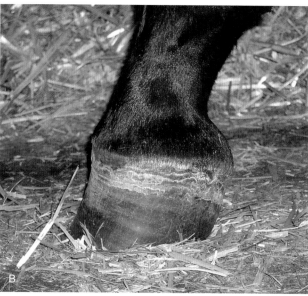

Figure 11.26. Weanling Quarter horses with typical club foot appearances. The dorsal hoof wall was vertical to the ground (A) with a concavity of the hoof wall (B). The deformities were corrected in both with an inferior check ligament desmotomy.

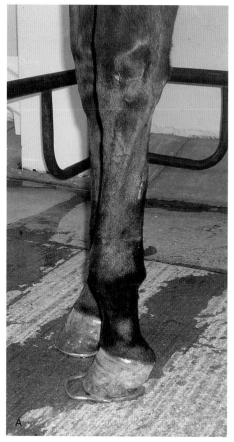
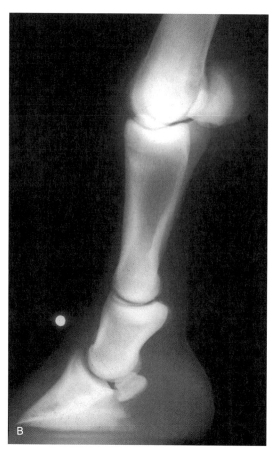

Figure 11.27. Visual (A) and radiographic (B) appearance of a yearling Quarter horse with a flexural deformity of the left front fetlock. The deformity did not respond to a previous inferior check ligament desmotomy.

are stronger than extensor muscles, and the foal consequently develops a flexural deformity. These theories are not entirely compatible with our knowledge of bone growth since the majority of bone growth occurs early in life (first few months) and many flexural deformities develop later than that time period.

Clinical Signs

Flexural deformity of the DIP joint or so-called DDFT contracture results in a raised heel and a "club foot" (Figure 11.26). The heel may be completely off the ground in severe cases (walking on the toe, Figure 11.28) but usually the heels maintain contact with the ground and grow excessively long (Figure 11.26). Most foals should not be lame and a pronounced lameness should cause wariness of other problems in the limb. Dishing or concavity of the dorsal hoof wall may occur in chronic cases (Figure 11.26B), and tearing of the dorsal laminae may lead to seedy toe and toe abscesses.

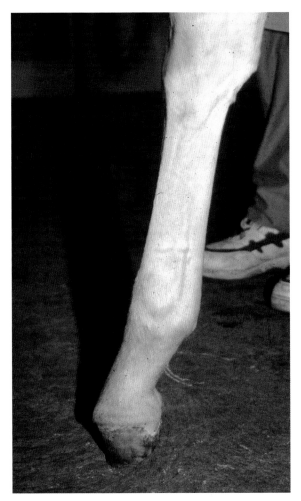

Figure 11.28. Young foal with a flexural deformity of the DIP joint, in which the hoof wall is beyond vertical and the heels are completely off the ground. Surgical treatment is recommended for these types of deformities. An inferior check ligament desmotomy was performed in this foal.

The severity of the deformity may be subdivided into stages I and II based on the visual position of the dorsal hoof wall.[18,20] Stage I contracture is when the dorsal hoof wall does not go beyond vertical and stage II is when the dorsal surface of the hoof passes beyond vertical. The more severe the deformity, the more shortening of the musculotendinous unit, and the more aggressive treatment should be. With severe contracture, pathologic changes may develop in the joint capsule and other tissues of the coffin joint, making permanent correction less likely.[10,20]

Flexural deformity of the MCP joint has been classically referred to as contracture of the superficial digital flexor tendon (SDFT). It is characterized by dorsal knuckling of the fetlock with the hoof itself remaining in normal alignment (Figure 11.27). The term SDFT contracture is a gross oversimplification because the SDFT, DDFT, both the SDFT and DDFT, and the suspensory ligament in chronic cases may the involved with the deformity. Early in the condition, the fetlock and pastern may begin to appear more upright with the fetlock angle approaching 180° measured from the dorsal surface (the normal angle is approximately 140°).[1] In more severe cases, the fetlock knuckles forward with every step and the horse may stand with a dorsal fetlock angle of more than 180° (Figure 11.29). As with flexural deformities of the DIP joint, when the deformity goes beyond vertical (constant dorsal knuckling of the fetlock), more aggressive treatment is usually required. In chronic cases, the suspensory ligament becomes involved, fibrosis of the joint capsule may occur, and osteoarthritic changes may develop in the fetlock joint.[20]

Diagnosis

A tentative diagnosis of flexural deformities of the DIP or MCP joints usually can be made based on the characteristic foot and limb conformation. Flexural deformities of the DIP joint only involve the DDFT. Determining which soft tissue structure(s) is involved with deformities of the MCP joint is more difficult.

The DDFT, SDFT, and the suspensory ligament may all contribute to an MCP deformity.[1] Careful palpation of the limbs in both the standing and flexed positions may suggest that the DDFT or SDFT is more taut on palpation. Forcing the fetlock into extension while palpating the tendons in the standing horse can be very helpful. This is very subjective but is the best clinical method to determine which structure may be more involved. However, if this cannot be determined, it is probably best to assume that both the DDFT and SDFT are involved to avoid failure in treatment. It is also the author's opinion that younger horses with MCP joint deformities usually have primary DDFT involvement, whereas older horses often have both SDFT and DDFT involvement (Figure 11.30). This decision is very important when selecting surgical treatment.

Radiographs can be used to confirm the diagnosis and assess any changes in the joints involved. Lateral to medial and 60° dorsopalmar views of the foot should be performed in foals with DIP joint deformities and at least 2 views of the phalanges/fetlock for MCP deformities. The degree of DIP joint subluxation, angle of the

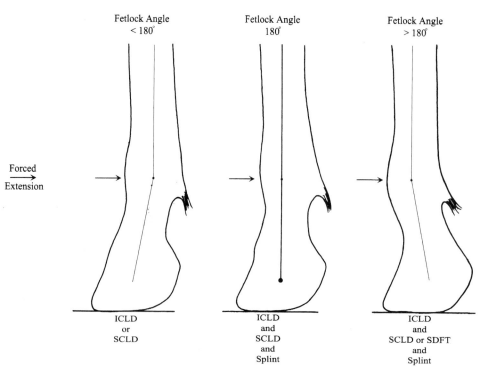

Fetlock Angle
< 180°

Fetlock Angle
180°

Fetlock Angle
> 180°

Forced
Extension

ICLD
or
SCLD

ICLD
and
SCLD
and
Splint

ICLD
and
SCLD or SDFT
and
Splint

Figure 11.29. Treatment guidelines based on the angle of the fetlock for horses with flexural deformities of the fetlock joint. (Reprinted with permission from Adams SB, Santschi EM. Management of congenital and acquired flexural limb deformities. Proc Am Assoc Eq Pract 2000;46:117–125.)

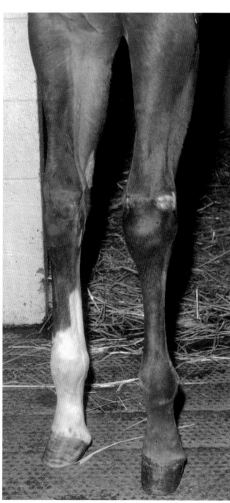

Figure 11.30. This 6-month-old Quarter horse filly with flexural deformities of both front fetlocks responded well to bilateral inferior check ligament desmotomies.

dorsal hoof wall, and abnormalities at the apex of the distal phalanx should be observed. Varying degrees of osteolysis in the distal part of the distal phalanx is not uncommon, and the foals with the most pronounced clinical signs usually display the most prominent radiologic changes (Figure 11.31).[4] Radiographs of the phalanges/fetlock in horses with MCP deformities usually reveal dorsal knuckling of the fetlock with no other bony abnormalities (Figure 11.27).

Treatment

Nonsurgical Treatment

Nonsurgical treatment may consist of changes in diet and exercise, corrective trimming and shoeing, splinting for MCP deformities, IV oxytetracycline, and the use of NSAIDs if pain is considered to be a contributing factor.[1,2,20] Mild deformities or those in the early stages of the disease are the most appropriate candidates for conservative treatment. Foals with DIP joint deformities that cannot touch the heel to the ground or MCP joint deformities that constantly knuckle forward at the fetlock are not candidates for nonsurgical treatment (Figures 11.28 and 11.29). Animals with flexural deformities of the DIP joint should have the heels trimmed to increase tension on the palmar flexor tendons (primarily the DDFT). Trimming of the heel combined with a toe extension or elevation also may be used. Extension of the toe may be accomplished with a steel shoe, glue-on shoe, or acrylic applied to the bottom of the foot, depending on the age of the foal.

It is generally recommended to raise the heels with corrective shoeing to treat horses with MCP joint deformities. This is thought to relax the DDFT and cause the fetlock to drop.[20,23] However, each case should be evaluated individually by placing wedges under the

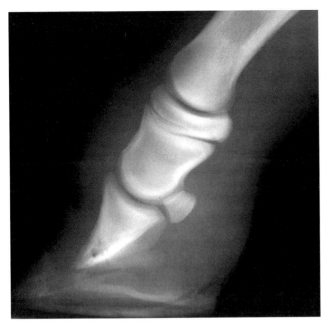

Figure 11.31. Lateral radiograph of a foal with a club foot. Remodeling and lysis of the distal aspect of the distal phalanx was present and the foal had a concurrent abscess in the toe.

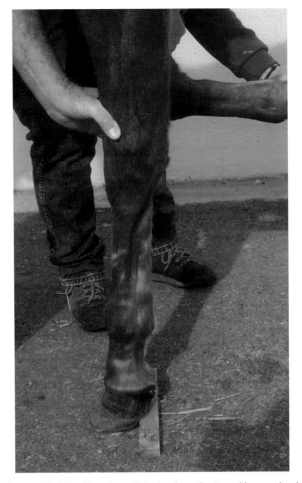

Figure 11.32. Elevation of the heel vs. the toe with a wedge in horses with flexural deformities of the fetlock can help guide both surgical and conservative treatment. In most horses, heel elevation causes the fetlock to drop and improves the angle of the fetlock.

foot to either elevate the heel or elevate the toe to observe which scenario improves the angle of the fetlock (Figure 11.32). Whether heel elevation reduces strain on the SDFT and suspensory ligament is debatable, but most clinical cases respond best to heel elevation in contrast to lowering the heels.[1,20] Heel elevation (2 to 3 cm) combined with a 1- to 2-cm toe extension also has been advocated.[1] Corrective shoeing is often combined with splinting of the MCP joint to prevent dorsal knuckling of the fetlock. The PVC splint is applied to the palmar aspect of the distal limb to pull the fetlock in a palmar direction. Conforming the PVC splint (using heat) to the palmar aspect of the limb may improve the effectiveness of the splinting.[1]

Corrective trimming and shoeing, and splinting if used, may contribute to lameness in some horses by increasing tension on the palmar soft tissues. In addition, horses must bear full weight on the limb(s) to achieve the maximum benefit of nonsurgical treatment. Therefore, low doses of oral NSAIDs are recommended for 1 to 2 weeks to help stretch the musculotendinous unit. Oxytetracycline IV can be used as an adjunct treatment similar to that in foals with congenital flexural deformities, but appears to be less effective in older animals.

Surgical Treatment

The decision for surgical treatment of DIP and MCP joint flexural deformities depends on the severity of the deformity, age of the horse, and response to conservative treatment. Surgical intervention is the only alternative in cases that do not respond to conservative methods.

Surgical options for foals with deformities of the DIP joint include an inferior check ligament desmotomy or

DDFT tenotomy at the level of the pastern or mid-metacarpus.[1,2,12,22,24] Foals treated at a younger age (younger than 6 to 8 months) with an inferior check ligament desmotomy have an improved prognosis for normal hoof conformation and for athletic performance.[22,26]

Surgical options for horses with deformities of the MCP joint include an inferior check ligament desmotomy, a superior check ligament desmotomy, both inferior and superior check ligament desmotomies, and SDFT tenotomy in the mid-metacarpus.[1,2,14,23] There is scarce information regarding the prognosis of horses with MCP flexural deformities following surgery. However, in the author's experience lack of response to surgery and recurrence of the flexural deformity is much more common with MCP joint deformities than with DIP joint deformities.

The majority of DIP deformities can be corrected with an inferior check ligament desmotomy. This includes all type I and many type II deformities if the surgery is performed at a young age (younger than 6 to 8 months) and if combined with corrective shoeing such as a toe extension and/or toe elevation.[20,26] An inferior

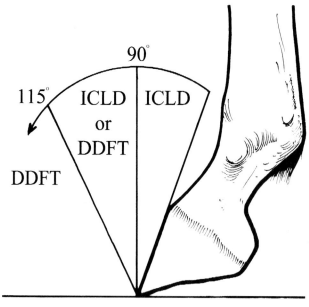

Figure 11.33. Treatment guidelines for foals with flexural deformities of the DIP joint based on the angle of the dorsal hoof wall relative to the ground. (Reprinted with permission from Adams SB, Santschi EM. Management of congenital and acquired flexural limb deformities. Proc Am Assoc Eq Pract 2000;46:117–125.)

check ligament desmotomy is recommended in foals with hoof-ground angles of 90° or less and in most foals with deformities between 90° and 115° (Figure 11.33).[1] An inferior check ligament desmotomy is highly recommended in foals that have not responded to conservative therapy, with hoof deformities approaching or beyond vertical, with osteolysis of the distal phalanx, that cannot touch the heel to the ground, and older than 1 year of age.

The surgery can be performed with the traditional open approach in the proximal metacarpus or with ultrasound guidance through a 1- to 2-cm incision.[12,18,20,22,24] Trimming the heel and using a shoe with a toe extension or toe elevation is recommended following surgery in most cases (especially older horses) to achieve a normal hoof conformation as quickly as possible. Normal limb alignment may be obtained almost immediately following surgery, but relaxation may progress for 7 to 10 days postoperatively.[20] Normal hoof conformation should be achieved within 2 weeks of surgery in most cases. Several studies have documented that the majority of foals treated with an inferior check ligament desmotomy develop a normal hoof conformation and can be used for their intended purpose.[18,22,24,26] Experimental studies also have documented that transection of the inferior check ligament causes minimal changes in locomotion, joint angles, or strains to the palmar soft tissue structures in normal horses.[6,7] The surgery itself should have minimal effects on future performance.

Tenotomy of the DDFT is usually reserved for older horses (older than 1 year) with severe deformities of the DIP joint. A DDFT tenotomy is recommended if the hoof-ground angle is more than 115° (Figure 11.33).[1] Foals with deformities between 90° and 115° may respond to an inferior check ligament desmotomy and this should be attempted initially. However, the response to surgery is less predictable in these cases.[1,20] The DDFT tenotomy may be performed in the mid-metacarpus or the palmar aspect of the pastern. Greater release of the DDFT and correction of the DIP joint deformity can usually be obtained with transection in the pastern, but the wider separation of the tendon ends is more of a concern with later function. Fewer complications and a better functional outcome are usually achieved with DDFT tenotomy in the mid-metacarpus compared to the pastern region.[1] Tenotomy of the DDFT should be considered a salvage procedure; however, many of these horses can be used for light riding.[1,2]

The results of surgical treatment of MCP joint deformities are less predictable than those of deformities of the DIP joint. The recommended surgery also is less defined and is often based on the clinical experience of the veterinarian and the physical examination findings of the horse. In one report of 15 cases of MCP joint flexural deformities, mild deformities were treated nonsurgically, moderate deformities were treated with an inferior check ligament desmotomy, and severe deformities were treated with both inferior and superior check ligament desmotomies.[20] In a more recent report of using tenoscopy to transect the superior check ligament, both desmotomies also were performed on horses with MCP flexural deformities.[14]

Often the decision of which desmotomy (or both) to perform is based on which tendon feels more taut on palpation. If the SDFT is most taut, then a superior check ligament desmotomy may be appropriate, or a SDFT tenotomy if the deformity is severe. If the DDFT is most taut, then an inferior check ligament desmotomy is indicated. However, this approach is very subjective and little information is available regarding its appropriateness. The author has found that younger horses (younger than 1 year) with MCP joint deformities respond better to inferior check ligament desmotomy alone than older horses. A combination of inferior and superior check ligament desmotomy is usually recommended by the author in yearlings or 2-year-olds with MCP joint flexural deformities. However, successful results have been reported with inferior check ligament desmotomy alone by some authors.[20,23] A tenoscopic approach is currently recommended for superior check ligament desmotomy to minimize the complications seen with the open approach.[14,21]

Surgical guidelines have been recommended based on the angle of the MCP joint (Figure 11.29).[1] Mild deformities have a fetlock joint angle of less than 180° degrees, and an inferior or superior check ligament desmotomy is recommended. Moderate deformities are those with a fetlock angle of 180° (straight upright), and both inferior and superior check ligament desmotomies are recommended. Severe deformities have a fetlock angle of more than 180 degrees (knuckled forward), and an inferior check ligament desmotomy combined with a superior check ligament desmotomy or SDFT tenotomy is recommended (Figure 11.29). Splinting is recommended after surgery for both moderate and severe MCP joint deformities.

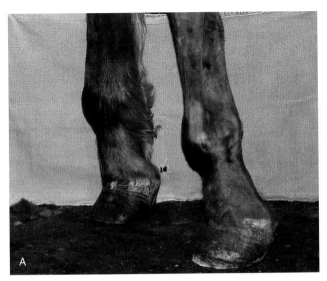
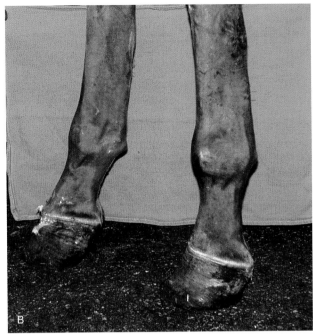

Figure 11.34. Before (A) and after (B) images of a 2-year-old with severe flexural deformities of the front fetlocks that had the SDFT transected in the midmetacarpal region. This horse had been treated previously with an inferior check ligament desmotomy.

Horses with severe MCP deformities have a poor prognosis and often do not improve with either or both check ligament desmotomy surgeries.[23] Transection of the SDFT in the mid-metacarpus in the standing, sedated horse is often the quickest, least expensive, and most beneficial procedure in these cases (Figure 11.34). However, a SDFT tenotomy combined with an inferior check ligament desmotomy has been recommended in these cases (Figure 11.29).[1] Suspensory ligament/branch desmotomy also may be considered when the MCP joint deformity is refractory to other surgical treatments, but is often unsuccessful due to fibrosis and scarring of the soft tissues around the fetlock that often accompany chronic cases.[20]

Prognosis

In general, the prognosis is much better for foals with DIP joint flexural deformities than older horses with MCP joint deformities. Most reports indicate that young (under 5 to 6 months) horses with a DIP joint deformity treated surgically have a better prognosis for future athletic use than older horses.[22,26] In addition, foals treated surgically with an inferior check desmotomy had an improved prognosis for racing than those treated conservatively.[22] In one report, 33 of 40 horses treated with an inferior check desmotomy were used for their intended purpose.[24] In contrast, the response to surgery is often unpredictable in horses with MCP joint deformities, and these horses often have a guarded to poor prognosis for soundness. In one report, horses with mild and moderate MCP joint deformities returned to useful work but none of the horses with a severe flexural deformity became athletes.[23] Similar to DIP joint deformities, it is the author's opinion that MCP joint deformities respond much better to either nonsurgical or surgical treatments in younger horses. The sooner treatment can be initiated in either type of deformity, the better the prognosis for correction and future athletic use.

References

1. Adams SB, Santschi EM. Management of Congenital and Acquired Flexural Limb Deformities. Proceedings Am Assoc Eq Pract 2000;46:117–125.
2. Adams SB, Santschi EM. Management of flexural limb deformities in young horses. Equine Pract 1999;21:9–14.
3. Alexander GR, Gibson KT, Day RE, et al. Effects of superior check desmotomy on flexor tendon and suspensory ligament strain in equine cadaver limbs. Vet Surg 2001;30:522–527.
4. Arnbjerg J. Changes in the distal phalanx in foals with deep digital flexor tendon contraction. Vet Radiol 1988;29:65–69.
5. Arnoczky SP, Lavagnino M, Gardner KL, et al. *In vitro* effects of oxytetracycline on matrix metalloproteinase-1 mRNA expression and on collagen gel contraction by cultured myofibroblasts obtained from the accessory ligament of foals. Am J Vet Res 2004;65:491–496.
6. Becker CK, Sabelberg HHCM, Buchner HHF, et al. Long-term consequences of experimental desmotomy of the accessory ligament of the deep digital flexor tendon in adult horses. Am J Vet Res 1998;59:347–351.
7. Becker CK, Sabelberg CM, Buchner HF, et al. Effects of experimental desmotomy on material properties and histomorphologic and ultrasonographic features of the accessory ligament of the deep digital flexor tendon in clinically normal horses. Am J Vet Res 1998;59:352–358.
8. Charmin RE, Vasey JR. Surgical treatment of carpal flexural deformity in 72 horses. Aust Vet J 2008;86:195–199.
9. Embertson RM. Congenital abnormalities of tendons and ligaments. Vet Clin North Am Equine Pract 1994;10:351–364.
10. Greet TRC. Managing flexural and angular limb deformities: The Newmarket perspective. Proceedings Am Assoc Eq Pract 2000; 46:130–136.
11. Hartzel DK, Arnoczky SP, Kilfoyle SJ, et al. Myofibroblasts in the accessory ligament (distal check ligament) and the deep digital flexor tendon in foals. Am J Vet Res 2001;62:823–827.

12. Jansson N, Sonnichsen HV. Acquired flexural deformity of the distal interphalangeal joint in horses: Treatment by desmotomy of the accessory ligament of the deep digital flexor tendon. A retrospective study. J Equine Vet Sci 1995;15:353–356.

13. Kasper CA, Clayton HM, Wright AK, et al. Effects of high doses of oxytetracycline on metacarpophalangeal joint kinematics in neonatal foals. J Am Vet Med Assoc 1995;207:71–73.

14. Kretzschmar BH, Desjardins MR. Clinical evaluation of 49 tenoscopically assisted superior check ligament desmotomies in 27 horses. Proceedings Am Assoc Eq Pract 2001;47:484–487.

15. Lokai MD, Meyer RJ. Preliminary observations in oxytetracycline treatment of congenital flexural deformities in foals. Mod Vet Pract 1985;66:237–239.

16. Lokai MD. Case selection for medical management of congenital flexural deformities in foals. Equine Pract 1992;14:23–25.

17. Madison JB, Garber JL, Rice B, et al. Effect of oxytetracycline on metacarpophalangeal and distal interphalangeal joint angles in newborn foals. J Am Vet Med Assoc 1994;204:246–254.

18. McIlwraith CW, Fessler JF. Evaluation of inferior check ligament desmotomy for treatment of acquired flexor tendon contracture in the horse. J Am Vet Med Assoc 1978;294:293–298.

19. McIlwraith CW, James LF. Limb deformities in foals associated with ingestion of locoweed by mares. J Am Vet Med Assoc 1982;181:255–258.

20. McIlwraith CW. Diseases of joints, tendons, ligaments and related structures. In Adams' Lameness in Horses 5th ed. Stashak TS, ed. Lippincott Williams and Wilkins, Philadelphia. 2002;459–644.

21. Southwood LL, Stashak TS, Kainer RA, et al. Desmotomy of the accessory ligament of the superficial digital flexor tendon in the horse with use of a tenoscopic approach to the carpal sheath. Vet Surg 1999;28:99–105.

22. Stick JA, Nickels FA, Williams MA. Long-term effects of desmotomy of the accessory ligament of the deep digital flexor muscle in Standardbreds: 23 cases (1979–1989). J Am Vet Med Assoc 1992;15:1131–1142.

23. Wagner PC, Shires MG, Watrous BJ, et al. Management of acquired flexural deformity of the metacarpophalangeal joint in Equidae. J Am Vet Med Assoc 1985;187:915–918.

24. Wagner PC, Grant BD, Kaneps AJ, et al. Long-term results of desmotomy of the accessory ligament of the deep digital flexor tendon (distal check ligament) in horses. J Am Vet Med Assoc 1985;187:1351–1356.

25. Wagner von Matthiessen PC. Case selection and management of flexural limb deformities in horses: Congenital flexural limb deformities, part II. Equine Pract 1994;16:7–11.

26. White NA. Ultrasound-guided transection of the accessory ligament of the deep digital flexor muscle (distal check ligament desmotomy) in horses. Vet Surg 1995;24:373–378.

27. Whitehair KJ, Adams SB, Toombs JP, et al. Arthrodesis for congenital flexural deformity in the metacarpophalangeal and metatarsophalangeal joints. Vet Surg 1992;22:228–233.

28. Wright AK, Petrie L, Papich MG, et al. The effect of high dose oxytetracycline on renal parameters in neonatal foals: Recommended dose for treatment of flexural limb deformities. Proc Am Assoc Equine Pract 1993;38:297–298.

29. Yovich JV Stashak TS, McIlwraith CW. Rupture of the common digital extensor tendon in foals. Comp Cont Educ Pract Vet 1984;6:S373.

OSTEOCHONDROSIS

C. Wayne McIlwraith

INTRODUCTION

Osteochondritis dissecans (OCD) is arguably the most important entity within the developmental orthopedic disease complex. It is a frequent cause of lameness in young athletic horses and is the most frequent condition of the complex requiring surgical intervention. OCD has been classically considered as a manifestation of osteochondrosis.[12] Rejno and Stromberg[19] described the first stages of osteochondrosis as a disturbance of cellular differentiation in the growing cartilage, and the second as involving the process of basal forces within the joint, giving rise to fissures in the damaged cartilage. The terms osteochondrosis, osteochondritis dissecans, and osteochondrosis dissecans have been regularly used as synonyms, but this is misleading. Poulos[17] distinguished them as follows: osteochondrosis is the disease, osteochondritis is the inflammatory response to the disease, and OCD is the condition in which a flap can be demonstrated. This is a simple but fairly appropriate representation.

Subchondral bone cysts (SBC) or subchondral cystic lesions (SCLs) were also proposed by Rejno and Stromberg[22] as a manifestation of osteochondrosis. The author considers that SCLs showing up clinically in the first 2 years of life are indeed manifestations of osteochondrosis. However, they represent quite a different disease than OCD. Examination of the lining of enucleated SCLs in the medial femoral condyle showed that they produce increased levels of PGE_2, neutral metalloproteinases, and nitric oxide (NO), and that there was enhanced osteoclastic resorption activity attributable to the tissue.[23] *In situ* hybridization of sections of fibrous tissue of SCLs showed that mRNA of IL-1β was upregulated at the periphery of the cystic lesion and IL-6 was upregulated in the fibrin tissue of the center.[24] Other work showed that SCLs could be produced after 5-mm in diameter, 3-mm deep defects were created in the subchondral bone plate at the central weight-bearing of the medial femoral condyle,[18] leading to an alternative pathogenesis for clinical cases in older horses.

Therefore, the discussion of osteochondrosis is limited to OCD and SCLs, because these are the important clinical manifestations. Osteochondrosis also can occur in the physis, but it is uncommon, and rare for it to cause a clinical problem. Figure 11.35 illustrates the proposed pathways of osteochondrosis leading to both OCD and SCLs.

OSTEOCHONDRITIS DISSECANS (OCD)

Disease Manifestation

Three categories of OCD lesions are recognized:

1. Those showing clinical and radiographic signs
2. Those showing clinical without radiographic (but arthroscopic) signs
3. Those showing radiographic, but no clinical signs.

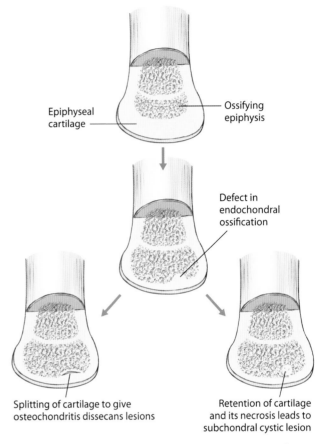

Epiphyseal cartilage

Ossifying epiphysis

Defect in endochondral ossification

Splitting of cartilage to give osteochondritis dissecans lesions

Retention of cartilage and its necrosis leads to subchondral cystic lesion

Figure 11.35. The proposed pathways of osteochondrosis leading to both OCD and SCLs.

Data from the first 2 categories of disease have been tabulated from the most commonly selected joints from the author's surgical case reports.[11] The relative incidence of clinical signs vs. radiographic lesions also has been documented in the femoropatellar joint by McIntosh and McIlwraith.[14] The third category of radiographic lesions has become increasingly important because of the common use of pre-sale radiographs of yearlings.[6,7]

The condition affects the articular (joint) cartilage, and often involves the subchondral bone beneath the cartilage surface (Figure 11.36A). Generally, a dissecting lesion develops that involves cartilage, or cartilage and bone, and the defection plane ultimately reaches the joint surface. It is theorized that clinical signs develop when the joint surface is reached by the dissecting lesions. Sometimes the OCD fragments can detach and become a loose body, or joint mouse. In most instances, however, the fragments remain loosely attached to the bone of origin, but the debris that is released into the joint from the flap results in synovitis or joint

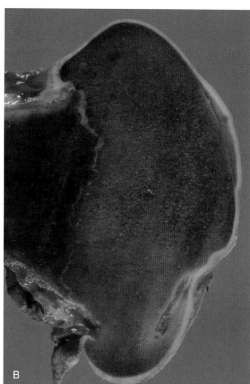

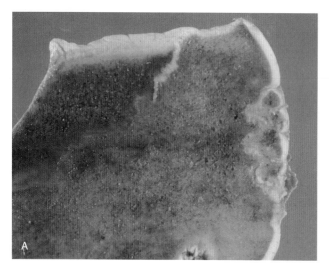

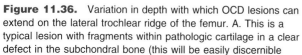

Figure 11.36. Variation in depth with which OCD lesions can extend on the lateral trochlear ridge of the femur. A. This is a typical lesion with fragments within pathologic cartilage in a clear defect in the subchondral bone (this will be easily discernible radiographically). B. Less commonly (and usually on the medial trochlear ridge of the femur), there can be elevated cartilage, which has normal fragments with normal bone contour and no evidence of an endochondral ossification defect.

inflammation and the clinical signs of pain and lameness that are seen with the disease.

In some instances there is no defect in the sub-chondral bone, but merely separation of cartilage (normal thickness) from a normal subchondral bone contour (Figure 11.36B). These manifestations not only lead to questioning of the classical defects in the endochondral ossification concept, but also provide diagnostic challenges because there is no defect seen on radiographs.

OCD can affect a number of joints, but the most commonly involved are the femoropatellar, tarsocrural, and fetlock joints. Shoulder joints also are affected, but are less frequently. Each of these entities is discussed separately.

Osteochondritis Dissecans of the Femoropatellar Joint

The femoropatellar joint is one of the principal joints affected with OCD. Although stifle OCD can be diagnosed in almost any breed, it seems to be more common in Thoroughbreds than in other breeds (Table 11.1).[4] Approximately 60% of affected horses are 1 year of age or younger when the condition becomes symptomatic, and younger animals that develop clinical signs often have more severe damage within the joint (Table 11.2).[4] However, incidental radiographic lesions are sometimes identified in older horses in which no clinical signs have ever been observed.

Table 11.1. Breed distribution of 161 horses presented for femoropatellar OCD.

Breed	Number	Percentage
Thoroughbred	82	50.9
Quarter horse	39	24.2
Arabian	16	9.9
Warmblood	9	5.6
Crossbred	5	3.1
Paint horse	3	1.9
Appaloosa	3	1.9
Other	4	2.5

(Foland et al. 1992)

Clinical and Radiographic Signs

Animals usually present with a sudden onset of joint swelling and lameness. A recent increase in the level of exercise is sometimes part of the history. Lameness may be very mild, with a stiff action and shortened stride

Table 11.2. Age distribution of 161 horses presented for femoropatellar OCD.

Age (year)	Number	Percentage
<1	22	13.7
1	68	42.2
2	36	22.4
3	21	13
>4	14	8.7

(Foland et al. 1992)

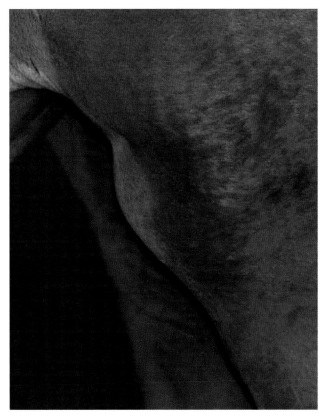

Figure 11.37. Synovial effusion typical of femoropatellar OCD.

observed, rather than the horse having a prominent lameness. Some more severely affected horses have a bunny hop action behind, and severe cases can sometimes be confused with a neurologic problem due to an inability to flex the stifle and may appear to be circumducting. Joint distention, however, is the most consistent sign seen with OCD of the stifle (Figure 11.37). Careful palpation of the joint may identify free bodies or the surface irregularity associated with the damage within the joint. Bilateral involvement is common in the femoropatellar joint, so both joints should be examined

carefully. Flexion of the limb usually exacerbates the lameness, and anesthetic placed into the joint improves or eliminates the lameness. However, intra-articular anesthesia is usually not necessary to confirm a diagnosis.

Lateral to medial radiographs provide the most useful information regarding specific lesion location and size (Figure 11.38). The most commonly identified defect is a variably sized irregularity or flattening of the lateral trochlear ridge of the femur. The area of the ridge that comes in contact with the distal aspect of the patella is most commonly involved. Partial mineralization of the tissue within the defect or fragment formation is often seen, and free bodies are also occasionally identified. It is rare to see OCD primarily affecting the patella, but secondary radiographic changes in the patella resulting from the trochlear ridge damage are often seen at arthroscopy. The medial ridge of the femur is less commonly involved.

Generally, the extent of damage to the joint identified at surgery is more extensive than would be predicted from radiographs.[21] Although other joints may be involved concurrently, this is uncommon. In one study of 161 horses with stifle OCD, 5 also had OCD affecting the rear fetlocks, 4 had hock OCD, and 1 had OCD of a shoulder joint.[4]

Treatment

It is generally accepted that surgical debridement of the lesions using arthroscopic surgery is the treatment of choice.[4,13] However, smaller lesions in younger horses may respond to rest and resolve radiographically.[14] It has also been shown in a study taking radiographs once a month for the first year of life in a group of Warmblood foals that femoropatellar OCD lesions can resolve.[3] They can develop into obvious lesions radiographically, but then completely heal. In the case of the femoropatellar joint, healing is completed (if they are going to heal) by 8 months of age. These are generally lesions that are not causing severe clinical signs. If lameness and swelling are prominent and the horse is older than 8 months, arthroscopic surgery is indicated.

As for all joint surgery, the joint is thoroughly explored, and suspicious lesions are probed. Loose or detached tissue is elevated and removed (Figure 11.39) and loose bodies are removed. The defect site is then debrided down to healthy tissue. Care must be taken to not be overly aggressive with bone debridement in young animals that have soft subchondral bone. Salvage and reattachment of OCD cartilage flaps in the stifle have been reported.[16] While not common, an OCD cartilage flap that is relatively smooth and is not detached on its entire perimeter can be elevated and the underlying necrotic cartilage and marrow fibrosis debrided. The flap can then be replaced and secured with polydioxaone (PDS) pins (OrthoSorb, Ethicon, Johnson and Johnson) or PLLA tacks (Chondral Darts, Arthrex, Naples, FL).

PROGNOSIS

In one study of 252 stifle joints in 161 horses with follow-up information available for 134 horses, 64%

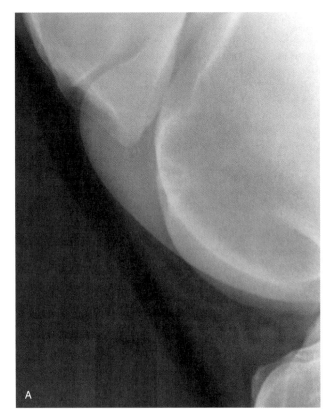

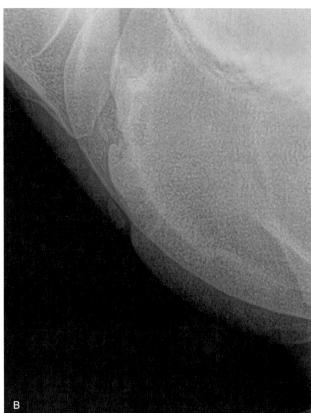

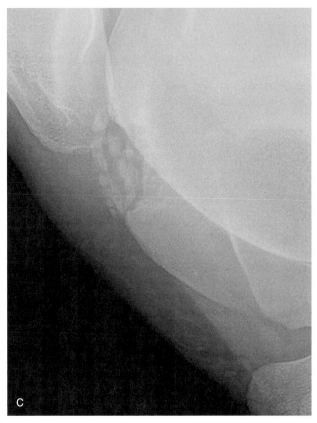

Figure 11.38. Radiographs of 3 cases of OCD of the lateral trochlear ridge of the femur in the femoropatellar joint. A. A small defect in the lateral trochlear ridge without obvious fragmentation within the defect (treated conservatively). B. A fragment within a defect. C. Multiple fragments in a more severe lesion.

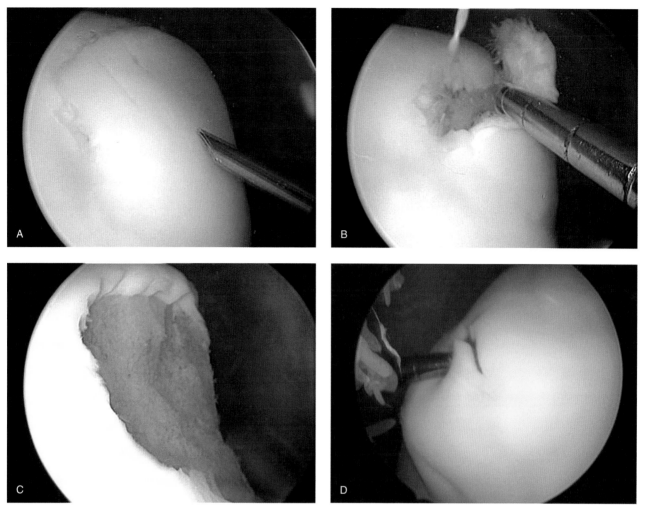

Figure 11.39. Arthroscopic views of OCD of the lateral trochlear ridge of the femur prior to probing (A), during elevation of the OCD flap (B), and after debridement of osteochondritic tissue (C). D. A lesion on the medial trochlear ridge of the femur manifesting as elevated cartilage of normal thickness without a subchondral defect beneath.

returned to their previous use, 7% were in training, 16% were unsuccessful, and 13% were unsuccessful due to reasons unrelated to the stifle.[4] The success rate was higher in horses with smaller lesions and in older horses. However, the age factor was considered to be due to the fact that the most severe lesions were generally identified in the younger horses.

Osteochondritis Dissecans of the Tarsocrural (Hock) Joint

Tarsal OCD most commonly involves the intermediate ridge of the tibia.[10] However, lesions can also develop on the trochlear ridges (the lateral ridge is much more common than medial ridge) and the medial malleolus of the tibia.

Clinical and Radiographic Signs

The most common clinical sign of hock OCD is effusion of the tarsocrural joint. Lameness also can be seen but it is uncommon and rarely prominent. Racehorses usually present as 2-year-olds, but nonracehorses usually present as yearlings prior to beginning training.

On radiographs, lesions, in order of incidence, can occur on the distal intermediate ridge of the tibia (DIRT) (Figure 11.40), followed by the lateral trochlear ridge of the talus (Figure 11.41), and then the medial malleolus of the tibia (Table 11.3). Lesions are identified as defects alone or defects containing fragmentation. The radiographic appearance often underestimates the extent of damage identified at surgery, particularly for lateral trochlear ridge lesions. The hock is also a joint in which radiographically silent lesions (those identified at surgery and in which no abnormality was seen on radiographs) occur more commonly than in other joints.[10]

Treatment

Although lameness is usually minimal with hock OCD, surgery is the recommended treatment. Lameness may only be a problem at racing speeds, or at upper

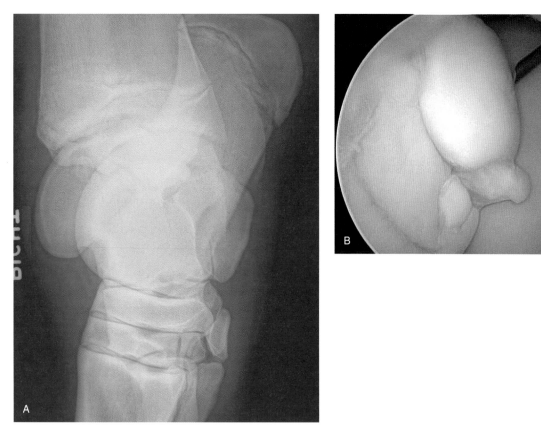

Figure 11.40. Radiographic view (A) and arthroscopic view (B) of OCD of the distal intermediate ridge of the tibia (DIRT) in the tarsocrural joint.

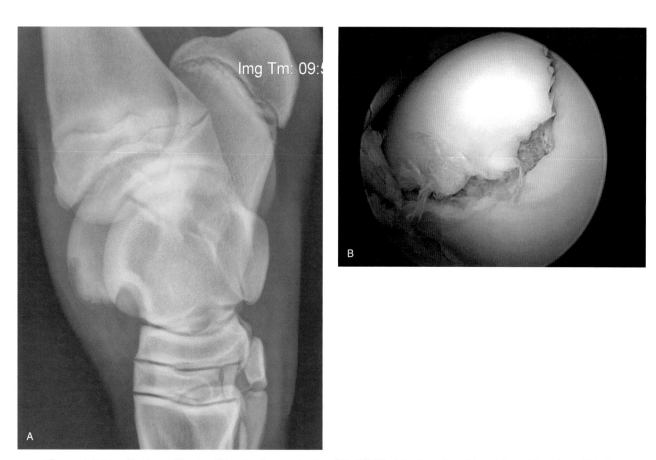

Figure 11.41. Radiographic view (A) and arthroscopic view (B) of OCD of the lateral trochlear ridge of the talus within the tarsocrural joint.

Table 11.3. Location of OCD lesions in 318 tarsocrural joints.

Number of joints	Location
244	Intermediate ridge (dorsal aspect) of distal tibia
37	Lateral trochlear ridge of talus
12	Medial malleolus (dorsal aspect) of tibia
11	Intermediate ridge of tibia plus lateral trochlear ridge of talus
4	Intermediate ridge plus medial malleolus of tibia
3	Intermediate ridge plus medial trochlear ridge of talus
3	Medial trochlear ridge of talus
3	Lateral trochlear ridge of talus plus medial malleolus of tibia
1	Lateral and medial trochlear ridge of talus
318	Total

(McIlwraith et al. 1991)

levels of performance, and this cannot be determined during a clinical examination. Resolution of the effusion cannot be expected without removal of the abnormal tissue. However, not all horses need surgery. Those with small lesions, minimal effusion, no lameness, and a potential career as a pleasure horse or light use horse may not require surgery. Sequential radiographs of Dutch Warmblood tarsocrural joints showed development (and resolution in most cases) of lesions of the DIRT and lateral trochlear ridge of the talus over the first 5 months of life.[3] Surgery should be considered early enough in the course of the disease (but after 5 months of age) so that the joint capsule is not unduly stretched, which makes resolution of the joint effusion less likely. Arthroscopic surgery with removal of fragments and debridement of defective tissue is recommended.

Prognosis

In a study involving 183 horses, 76% raced successfully or performed at their intended use after surgery.[10] Only 11% were unsuccessful because of a persistent hock problem. If degenerative changes were identified at surgery in the cartilage remote from the OCD lesion (wear lines on the medial trochlear ridge of the talus), the prognosis was less favorable. Complete resolution of effusion was inferior for lesions involving the lateral trochlear ridge and medial malleolus compared to the intermediate ridge of the tibia; however, this seemed to have no effect on subsequent performance (but can be a cosmetic issue for show horse owners). Further studies have confirmed the success rate with arthroscopic surgery.[1,8]

Osteochondritis Dissecans of the Fetlock Joint

The most common manifestation of OCD in the fetlock joint is fragmentation and irregularity that occurs on the dorsal aspect of the sagittal ridge and the condyles of the metacarpus or metatarsus (cannon bone). A second manifestation involving the fetlock is fragmentation of the dorsal aspect of the proximal phalanx. A third manifestation that has been considered by some to be osteochondrosis related is plantar/palmar fragments of the proximal phalanx. However, the consensus now is that these are avulsion fragments.

Osteochondritis Dissecans of the Dorsal Aspect of the Distal Metacarpus/Metatarsus

CLINICAL AND RADIOGRAPHIC SIGNS

Joint swelling (effusion) is the most common clinical sign, with lameness variable in both appearance and severity. Fetlock flexion tests are usually positive. It is not unusual for all 4 fetlocks to be involved, and bilateral forelimb or hindlimb involvement is quite common.

The diagnosis is confirmed on radiographs, and clinically silent lesions (no effusion or baseline lameness) are often identified along with the lesions causing clinical signs. Lameness can sometimes be induced by flexion in these clinically silent joints. A variety of radiographic presentations are seen with fetlock OCD. Some joints show only flattening or a defect in the sagittal ridge (type I OCD), others have a fragment in place within the area of flattening (type II OCD), and others have flattening with or without a fragment in place, but also have free or loose bodies within the joint (type III OCD).[13,26]

Treatment

A conservative approach is initially recommended for type I lesions. Many of these cases have resolution of clinical signs, as well as improvement or disappearance of radiographic signs;[9] however, surgery is eventually necessary in a small number of these cases. Surgical debridement is recommended for type II and III lesions, where fragmentation or loose bodies are present.[9]

Prognosis

The prognosis is quite favorable for type I lesions, but more guarded for type II and type III lesions. In one study involving 42 horses, the success rate was approximately 60%.[9] Horses with other signs of articular cartilage erosion or wear lines within the joint had a less favorable prognosis. If the lesion extended onto the condyle of the metacarpus/metatarsus from the sagittal ridge, the prognosis was also less favorable. It was determined that clinical signs would persist in approximately 25% of cases.

OCD Fragments of Proximal Dorsal Aspect of Proximal Phalanx

Joint swelling (effusion) is the most common clinical sign, with lameness variable in both appearance and severity. Quite often these fragments are identified on

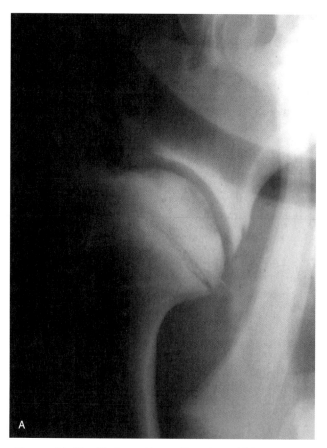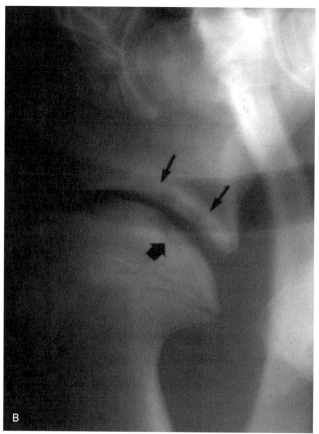

Figure 11.42. Radiographic manifestations of OCD of the shoulder. A. This defect in the humeral head is the only lesion. B. Defects in the humeral head (large black arrow) and glenoid of the scapula (2 black arrows).

survey radiographs and are presented for removal. The fragments are usually rounded in appearance and are off the proximal medial eminence of the proximal phalanx. Arthroscopically they show a typical OCD appearance with separated cartilage and defective cartilage underneath.

Osteochondritis Dissecans of the Shoulder Joint

OCD involving the shoulder joint is the most debilitating form of OCD affecting horses. Generally, large areas of the joint surfaces are involved, and secondary joint disease is common. However, it is unusual to have free or loose bodies develop. OCD of the shoulder is less common than for the other joints described, and seems to affect Quarter horses and Thoroughbreds with a similar incidence.

Clinical and Radiographic Signs

Most horses with shoulder OCD present at 1 year of age or younger, with a history of forelimb lameness of variable severity. Many of these horses have prominent lameness, and if lameness has been present for many weeks, shoulder muscle atrophy is also seen. Because of the altered gait and use of the limb, many cases develop an upright or club-footed appearance to the foot, and the foot may appear smaller on the affected limb. Deep pressure over the shoulder joint often causes discomfort, and forced flexion/extension of the limb sometimes accentuates the lameness that is seen. Intra-articular anesthesia improves or eliminates the lameness.

On radiographs, the most common sign is flattening or indentation of the humeral head (Figure 11.42). Often, defects or cystic type lesions are also identified in the glenoid cavity of the scapula. Productive remodeling changes are commonly identified along the caudal border of the glenoid cavity.[2]

Treatment

Conservative treatment is never associated with a successful outcome, and inadequate numbers of horses having surgery have been accumulated to accurately identify the prognosis with surgery. However, there is little doubt that surgery dramatically improves the clinical signs in most affected cases.[2,15] If extensive degenerative arthritic change is present on radiographs at the time of the initial examination, the prognosis for an athletic career is unfavorable, and surgery should only be considered for relative improvement in the degree of lameness. However, for more localized lesions, the prognosis is favorable for a successful outcome.

The shoulder is probably the most difficult joint on which to perform arthroscopic surgery, due to the depth of the joint below the muscles in the area—and there is

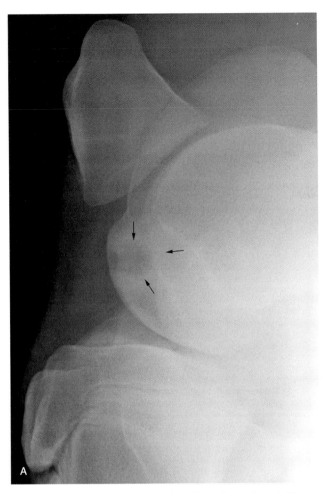
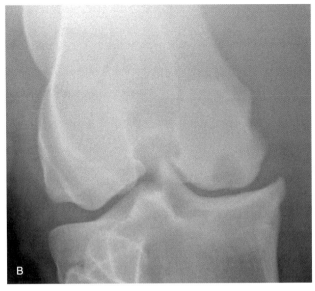

Figure 11.43.   (A) Flexed lateral-medial radiograph and (B) caudal-cranial radiograph of subchondral cystic lesions (arrows in A) of the medial femoral condyle of the femur.

a learning curve.[13] Surgery is easier on younger animals due to their relative muscle mass. Problems encountered in the shoulder are inaccessibility of lesions due to their location within the joint and extravasation or leakage of fluid outside the joint, which impairs visibility within the joint.

Prognosis

A large series of cases having surgery has not yet been reported, although preliminary results from 80 cases compiled at Colorado State University suggest that the overall prognosis is approximately 50%. The prognosis seems to be less favorable if lesions are present on both the humeral head and the glenoid cavity. In unsuccessful cases, further deterioration of the joint surfaces on subsequent radiographs is common.

SUBCHONDRAL CYSTIC LESIONS

Subchondral cystic lesions (SCLs) have been mentioned previously as a manifestation of osteochondrosis, at least in young horses. The most common location for clinically significant SCLs is within the medial condyle

of the femur in the medial femorotibial joint (Figure 11.43). Other areas of importance are the distal metacarpus or metatarsus in the fetlock joint, the distal proximal phalanx in the proximal interphalangeal joint, as well as shoulder, elbow, carpus, distal phalanx, and talus.

Lesions in the medial femorotibial joint have been treated with curettage,[5,20] but more recently they have been treated with intralesional injection of triamcinolone acetonide.[25] This technique was developed based on work previously cited by von Rechenberg, et al.,[23] in which the lining of SCLs produced increased levels of PGE_2, MMPs, and NO, as well as enhanced osteoclastic resorption activity. Recently published results have shown a 90% success rate with unilateral SCLs and 67% success rate with bilateral SCLs. Most other instances of SCLs have been treated with debridement because intralesional therapy is more difficult, but an increasing number of cases are being treated with intralesional injection under arthroscopic visualization.

It is important to note that most SCLs occur on central weight-bearing areas and this is considered to be a factor in them being more commonly clinically problematical. See chapters 5 and 7 for more information about SCLs at different anatomic locations.

References

1. Beard WL, Bramlage LR, Schneider RK, et al. Postoperative racing performance in Standardbreds and Thoroughbreds with osteochondrosis of the tarsocrural joint: 109 cases (1984–2000). J Am Vet Med Assoc 1994;204;1655–1659.
2. Bertone AL, McIlwraith CW, Powers BE, et al. Arthroscopic surgery for the treatment of osteochondrosis in the equine shoulder joint. Vet Surg 1987;16:303–311.
3. Dik KJ, Enzerink E, van Weeren PR. Radiographic development of osteochondral abnormalities in the hock and stifle of Dutch Warmblood foals, from age 1 to 11 months. Equine Vet J (Suppl 1) 1999;31;9–15.
4. Foland JW, McIlwraith CW, Trotter GW. Osteochondritis dissecans in the femoropatellar joint: Results of treatment with arthroscopic surgery. Equine Vet J 1992;24:419–423.
5. Howard RD, McIlwraith CW, Trotter GW. Arthroscopic surgery for subchondral cystic lesions of the medial femoral condyle in horses: 41 cases (1988–1991). J Am Vet Med Assoc 1995;206: 842–850.
6. Kane AJ, Park RD, McIlwraith CW, et al. Radiographic changes in Thoroughbred yearlings. Part I: Prevalence at the time of the yearling sales. Equine Vet J 2003a;15:354–365.
7. Kane AJ, McIlwraith CW, Park RD, et al. Radiographic changes in Thoroughbred yearlings. Part II: Associations with racing performance. Equine Vet J 2003b;35:366–375.
8. Laws EG, Richardson DW, Ross MW, et al. Racing performance in Standardbreds following conservative and surgical treatment for tarsocrural osteochondrosis. Equine Vet J 1993;25: 199–202.
9. McIlwraith CW, Vorhees M. Management of osteochondritis dissecans of the dorsal aspect of the distal metacarpus and metatarsus. Proceedings American Association of Equine Practitioners 1990;35:547–550.
10. McIlwraith CW, Foerner JJ, Davis DM. Osteochondritis dissecans of the tarsocrural joint: Results of treatment with arthroscopic surgery. Equine Vet J 1991;23;155–162.
11. McIlwraith CW. Inferences from referred clinical cases of osteochondritis dissecans. Equine Vet J 1993a;16:27–30.
12. McIlwraith CW. What is developmental orthopedic disease, osteochondrosis, osteochondritis, metabolic bone disease? Proceedings American Association Equine Practitioners 1993b; 39:35–44.
13. McIlwraith CW, Nixon AJ, Wright IM, et al. In: Diagnostic and Surgical Arthroscopy of the Horse, 3rd ed. Mosby Elsevier, Edinborough, 2005.
14. McIntosh SC, McIlwraith CW. Natural history of femoropatellar osteochondrosis in three crops of Thoroughbreds. Equine Vet J Suppl 1993;16:54–61.
15. Nixon AJ. Diagnostic and surgical arthroscopy of the equine shoulder joint. Vet Surg 1987;16:44–52.
16. Nixon AJ, Fortier LA, Goodrich LR, et al. Arthroscopic reattachment of select (OCD) lesions using resorbable polydioxaone pins. Equine Vet J 2004;36:376–383.
17. Poulos P. Radiologic manifestations of developmental problems. In AQHA Developmental Orthopedic Disease Symposium. McIlwraith CW, ed. Amarillo, TX, 1986, pp 1–2.
18. Ray CS, Baxter GM, McIlwraith CW, et al. Development of subchondral cystic lesions following articular cartilage and subchondral bone damage in young horses. Equine Vet J 1996;28:225–232.
19. Rejno S, Stromberg B. Osteochondrosis in the horse. II. Pathology. Acta Radiol Suppl 1978;358:153–178.
20. Smith MA, Walmsley JP, Phillips TJ, et al. Effective age at presentation on outcome following arthroscopic debridement of subchondral cystic lesions of the medial femoral condyle: 85 horses (1993–2003). Equine Vet J 2005;37:175–180.
21. Steinheimer DN, McIlwraith CW, Park RD, et al. Comparison of radiographic subchondral bone changes with arthroscopic findings in the equine femoropatellar and femorotibial joints: A retrospective study of 72 joints (50 horses). Vet Radiol 1995;36: 478–484.
22. Stromberg C, Rejno S. Osteochondrosis in the horse: A clinical and radiological investigation of osteochondritis dissecans of the knee and hock joint. Acta Radiol Suppl 1978;358:139–152.
23. von Rechenberg B, Guenther H, McIlwraith CW, et al. Fibrous tissue of subchondral cystic lesions produces local mediators and neutral metalloproteinases and cause bone absorption *in vitro*. Vet Surg 2000;29:420–429.
24. von Rechenberg B, Leutenegger C, Zlinsky K, et al. Upregulation of mRNA of interleukin-1 and -6 in subchondral cystic lesions of 4 horses. Equine Vet J 2001;33:143–149.
25. Wallis TW, Goodrich LR, McIlwraith CW, et al. Arthroscopic injection of corticosteroids into the fibrous tissue of subchondral lesions of the medial femoral condyle of horses: A retrospective study of 52 cases (2001–2006). Equine Vet J 2008;40:461–467.
26. Yovich JV, McIlwraith CW, Stashak TS. Osteochondritis dissecans of the sagittal ridge of the third metacarpal and metatarsal bones in horses. J Am Vet Med Assoc 1985;186:1186–1191.

LAMENESS IN FOALS

Robert J. Hunt

Lameness in foals is common and may be recognized shortly after birth or at any time during development. This chapter focuses on foals up to approximately 6 months of age.

By nature of their physical makeup, behavior, and environment, foals are particularly vulnerable to events resulting in lameness. There are multiple causes of lameness, including infectious and noninfectious etiologies. Because of the often rapid clinical progression of lameness with potentially life-threatening consequences, timely recognition along with accurate diagnosis and treatment are critical for a favorable outcome.

DIAGNOSIS

To make a diagnosis in a foal, it is important to know its age, sex, breed, and intended use, as well as husbandry information such as housing and level of hygiene, turn-out schedules, terrain and environment, behavior of the mare and foal, and concentration of horses. Medical histories of the lame foal and others in the herd must be obtained, along with information about the mare's general condition, presence of any medical or reproductive problems during pregnancy or parturition, as well as possible insufficient immunoglobulin transfer to the foal. The presence or absence of any febrile episodes and any alterations in the hemogram are important, and evidence of any infectious disease on the premises and equine traffic on the farm should also be noted.

The physical evaluation and locomotor assessment are the primary means of isolating lameness. It is important to evaluate the entire foal for its overall condition and development and compare it to the other foals on the premises. Any illness and or physical conformation abnormalities are also relevant to correct diagnosis and treatment and should be noted.

Palpation should begin on a sound limb to avoid confusion between behavior and pain responses. Thorough evaluation of the limb should begin at the foot, proceed proximally to the shoulder or pelvis, and include the vertebral column. Inspection of the foot includes evaluation for changes in shape and integrity, presence of cracks or separation in the wall or sole, or swelling at the coronary band. The foot temperature and digital pulse amplitude should be compared to that of the contralateral foot. Compression of the foot to assess for pain may be made with the hand and fingers on young foals rather than hoof testers. Care should be taken to evaluate the entire coronary band and all solar surfaces by applying pressure. Compression of the walls between the medial and lateral heels should also be performed routinely.

Moving proximally, any areas of swelling in the limb should be closely evaluated for character and consistency. Inspect for possible joint involvement, temperature alteration relative to surrounding areas, and pain on palpation and/or manipulation.

Isolation of the lame limb and the specific origin of pain may be challenging if subtle, but in general foals readily display locomotor evidence of the location of pain. Most foals attempt to avoid the painful component of the gait and usually display more exaggerated lameness reactions than adults. Observation of the young foal at rest and unrestrained in the company of the mare may be useful in detecting mild gait alterations or postural changes. Special attention should be given to the stance of the foal, particularly any trends in abnormal posture. Young, untrained foals may require gait evaluation while unrestrained and following the mare. The gait should be assessed at a slow walk in a straight line and in turns in both directions. Placement of the foot as well as limb and body carriage during ambulation is important in localizing lameness. Although there are some common findings with certain conditions (see below), there are no absolutes regarding gait characteristics and location of lameness in foals.

NONINFECTIOUS CAUSES OF LAMENESS

Virtually all components of the musculoskeletal system are susceptible to injury and lameness. Intrinsic and external sources of trauma commonly result in structural compromise to tissue of the musculoskeletal system. Other conditions resulting in lameness include those associated with DOD and disorders of vascular or neurogenic origin. Several disorders specific to foals occur routinely and are worth mention.

Foot Injuries

Fractures of the coffin bone wing are extremely common on Thoroughbred breeding operations and are recognized predominantly between 2 weeks and 5 months of age.[30] These fractures almost always involve the lateral wing but occasionally are biaxial or bilateral; seldom is only the medial wing involved. Although factors such as hard or soft surfaces or application of external hoof acrylics are incriminated, no single factor has been substantiated as causative.

Many fractures are discovered as incidental findings and never have an apparent lameness. Gait alteration displayed as abduction of the limb during the contact phase to load the medial aspect of the foot is sometimes seen. There is usually a palpable increase in the intensity of the digital pulse but only a mild increase in the temperature of the foot. The most consistent clinical finding is an increase in reaction to medial-to-lateral compression of the hoof wall at the quarters and heels (Figure 11.44). Palmar digital anesthesia of the involved side will eliminate the lameness. The diagnosis is confirmed

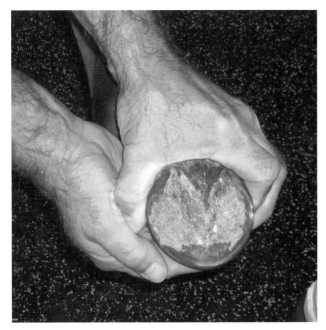

Figure 11.44. Manipulation of the foot to locate the focus of pain in a lameness examination in a foal.

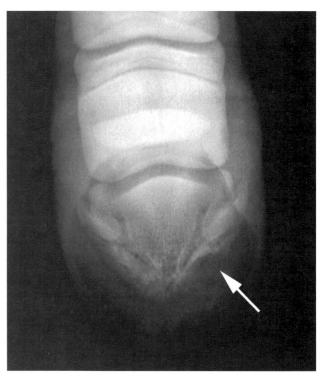

Figure 11.46. 45° Dorsoproximal palmarodistal radiograph showing septic osteitis of the third phalanx. There is a radiolucent area on the medial aspect of the solar margin (arrow).

Treatment for wing fractures of the coffin bone is conservative and consists of confinement to a small area on soft, uniform bedding for 2 to 3 weeks or until the horse is comfortable enough for paddock turn-out.[30] Rigid coaptation of the foot with a shoe, cuff, or cast material as well as surgical removal of the fragment are contraindicated. The prognosis for future soundness is good; rarely are there any long-term ramifications or gait deficits. Differentials include other types of coffin bone fractures, foot abscessation or bruising, septic osteitis, and a septic coffin or pastern joint.

Subsolar abscess with or without involvement of the coffin bone is common. It is discussed here because it is generally associated with trauma rather than hematogenous. Lameness may be recognized as early as 3 to 5 days of age or older. In the young foal the hind feet are most commonly involved and the abscess likely begins with bruising and subsolar hematoma beneath the soft keratinized sole that is present during the first few days of life. It is common for the abscess to involve a large portion of the subsolar tissue or dissect proximally up the dorsal hoof wall, or involve the coffin bone (Figure 11.46) with possible sequestration. Subsolar abscessation generally causes a severe nonweight-bearing or minimally weight-bearing gait.

Treatment includes draining purulent material and protecting the foot. Surgical curettage is indicated when the coffin bone is involved.[22] Regional perfusion with antimicrobials is frequently performed and clinically appears to be beneficial. Broad-spectrum systemic antimicrobials are routinely administered once drainage is established, or in refractory cases, or if surgical curettage is necessary.

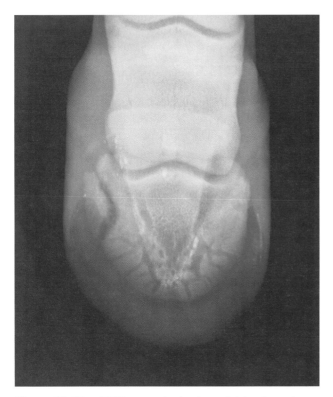

Figure 11.45. 45° Dorsoproximal palmarodistal radiograph showing a type VII fracture of the coffin bone.

radiographically using the 45° dorsal-ventral proximal-lateral to distal-medial oblique projections, although fractures may be seen on the lateral to medial, horizontal dorsal-palmar, and 45° dorsal-ventral projections (Figure 11.45).

It is not uncommon for the coffin joint to become secondarily involved through extension. In this case joint lavage is indicated in addition to the above treatments. Generally with joint involvement subsequent to hoof abscess, there is a guarded to poor prognosis because this is often associated with an aggressive and rapidly spreading infection.

Proximal Sesamoid Bone

Fracture of the proximal sesamoid bones is another common lameness condition on commercial breeding farms. These are most commonly seen in foals younger than 6 to 8 weeks of age; they are often associated with overexertion from running.[7] Essentially all configurations of proximal sesamoid bone fracture described in the literature occur in foals, but the most common types are apical and basilar fractures with a smaller number having midbody or comminuted fractures (Figure 11.47). It is common for the fractures to be unilateral and involve only one sesamoid, or to be bilateral and uniaxial, although sometimes they are biaxial.

The degree of lameness varies from mild and perceptible only on turns to nonweight-bearing. Gross instability of the suspensory apparatus resulting in a dropped fetlock only occurs with biaxial fractures of the body with extreme distraction. Depending on the fracture configuration, there may be a soft tissue profile over the involved sesamoid. There is often joint distension, especially with the basilar sesamoid fractures. Fetlock flexion and direct manual pressure applied over the involved sesamoid usually elicits pain.[7] The diagnosis is confirmed by radiographs and may be facilitated by ultrasound evaluation.

Treatment for proximal sesamoid bone fractures in foals is conservative and consists of confinement to a stall-sized area for 4 to 8 weeks, followed by a graduated turn-out schedule. The prognosis for future athleticism is good, but the sesamoid commonly heals in an elongated manner, which is often criticized if the horse is sold at public auction.

Only in rare instances is external coaptation with a cast or splint indicated. These devices are usually contraindicated for fear of promoting laxity of the flexor tendons. Likewise, surgical repair is usually futile and applies to salvage cases with total compromise of the suspensory apparatus which have marked distraction of the fracture fragments and dropping of the fetlock. The logical surgical technique is circumferential wiring or suturing of the fractured sesamoid bones. External coaptation and intensive rehabilitation to allow gradual loading of the limb is necessary. The sesamoid bones remodel in a distorted and deformed configuration and an athletic and sale future is unlikely. Alternatively, surgical arthrodesis of the fetlock may be performed to achieve comfort; however, this is considered only for salvage and not for athletic use.

Carpus and Tarsus

Lameness associated with the carpus is usually from trauma or sepsis. Trauma may be associated with compression injury, and dysmature neonates may be predisposed. Chip fracture also may occur as a result of trauma and is often accompanied by soft tissue trauma. There are almost always outward physical signs of carpal involvement, such as pain on manipulation and palpation, heat, joint effusion, and swelling of periarticular tissue. Most carpal injuries involving cartilage, bone, and intra-articular soft tissue carry a guarded prognosis, and management depends on the type of injury. Displaced fragments that are unstable require removal and have a poor prognosis.

Tarsal lameness may be associated with wedging or crushing of the cuboidal bones as a result of dysmaturity (Figure 11.48).[5,6] Accompanying clinical features include a boxy appearance of the distal tarsus when viewed from the front, and a curby or sickle hock appearance when viewed from the side. Radiographs should be performed on all dysmature foals to establish a baseline of the degree of mineralization of the cuboidal bones. Premature and dysmature foals are conventionally confined to a stall until 6 to 8 weeks of age, or until acceptable mineralization has occurred to minimize wedging or crushing. Tarsal wedging or crushing usually does not cause lameness in the neonate. Gait abnormalities are recognized only after periods of exertion following turn-out with other foals, or after athletic activity begins. If frank lameness is present in the neonate with a lack of mineralization of cuboidal bones, septic osteomyelitis must be ruled out.

Common injuries of the tarsocrural joint result in fracture of the distal lateral trochlear ridge of the talus and malleolar trauma with or without fracture. Marked synovial effusion is associated with these injuries, and the diagnosis is confirmed radiographically. If there is displacement of the fragment, surgical removal is the treatment of choice and the prognosis is favorable.

Soft tissue injury is common. A decubital wound of the lateral aspect of the tarsus overlying the lateral digital extensor tendon is the most frequently observed condition. This injury often occurs in young foals less than 2 to 3 weeks of age that have spent significant time in lateral recumbency as neonates, but it may be recognized in clinically normal foals as well. The condition causes mild lameness unless secondary sepsis extends into deeper bony structures or the tendon sheath, in which case lameness may be severe. Once the tissue opens and begins draining, the lameness resolves. There is a good prognosis with proper conservative wound management and good hygiene. These wounds should be allowed to heal by second intention, which may take weeks to months.

Elbow and Shoulder

Lameness of the elbow may be associated with trauma or infection. The presenting appearance may range from a subtle shortening of the gait to the classic dropped elbow recognized with olecranon fracture and disruption of the triceps apparatus (Figure 11.49).

Lameness involving the shoulder region of the foal is common and may be of septic or traumatic origin. It is not unusual to have 2 foals present simultaneously with shoulder injuries from colliding with one another while running head on. They may also undergo collision with a tree or sustain a kick injury. Most collision injuries resulting in nerve paralysis involve the radial nerve or

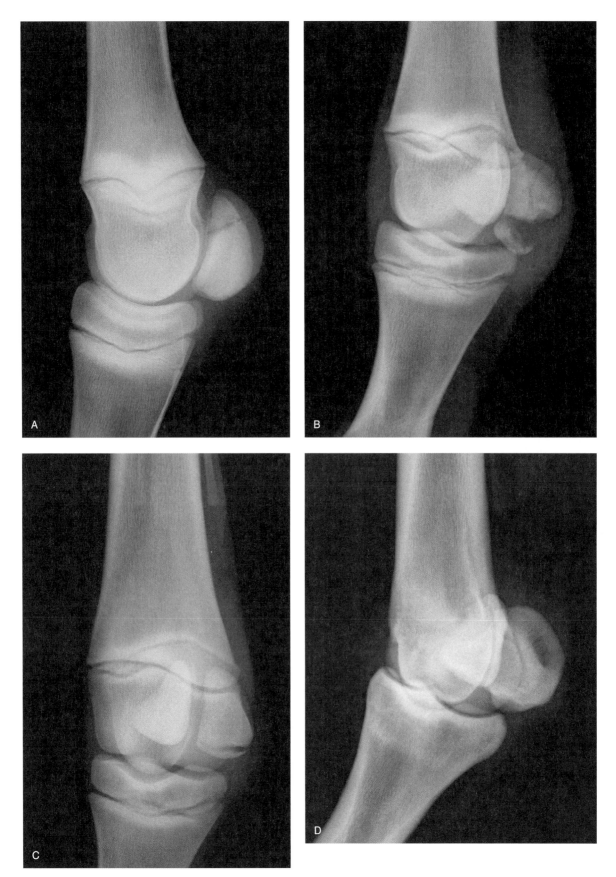

Figure 11.47. A. Lateromedial radiographic view of a nondisplaced apical sesamoid fracture. B. Dorsomedial to palmarolateral radiographic view of a displaced basilar sesamoid fracture. C. Dorsomedial to palmarolateral radiographic view of a mildly displaced medial basilar sesamoid fracture in a foal at time of injury. D. Radiograph of the same foal shown in C at 16 months of age after healing.

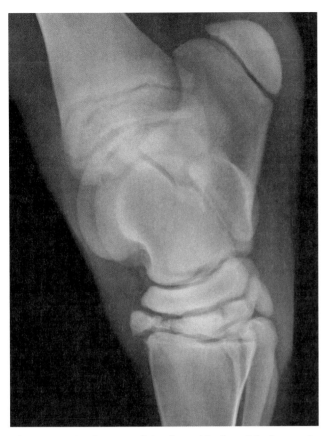

Figure 11.48. Lateromedial radiographic view of the tarsus of a foal showing collapse of the third tarsal bone.

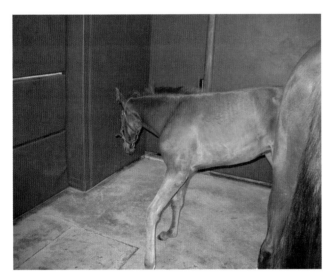

Figure 11.49. Typical dropped elbow appearance seen in fractures of the humerus and olecranon. Notice that the limb is also abducted and held in slight flexion.

brachial plexus, whereas kick injuries commonly cause fracture of the supraglenoid tubercle or other portions of the scapula.

Differentiating between nerve injury and fracture can be accomplished with physical exam and radiographs. With nerve injury, the foals are not painful on palpation

and manipulation, the shoulder is dramatically dropped, and the limb may be physically placed and maintained in normal position while applying pressure to the dorsal aspect of the carpus. There is usually less swelling over the point of the shoulder with nerve injury than with fracture. Radiographs are normal with nerve injury; however, they may be confusing to interpret because of the physes. Likewise, if a supraglenoid tubercle physeal fracture is initially nondisplaced, it may go undetected. Follow-up radiographs in several days to weeks may be necessary for an accurate diagnosis.

Prognosis for nerve injury is guarded, depending on the extent of injury. Foals with neuropraxia improve in a matter of hours to days, although it may take weeks to return to normal. There is often some degree of muscle atrophy that gradually improves. Ruptured and avulsed nerves do not improve and these cases may undergo prolonged treatment attempts before the involved limb develops severe contraction or there is breakdown of the contralateral limb. The prognosis for supraglenoid tubercle fracture is good for survival, pasture soundness, and light use, but poor for athletic use. Surgical removal of the fragmented tubercle and open reduction with internal fixation has been performed, but there is little difference between aggressive and conservative management in the long-term outcome regarding athletic potential of these animals.

Stifle

Lameness of the stifle in foals is usually septic in nature; traumatic injuries and developmental orthopedic disease of the stifle in foals occur less frequently. The proximal tibial physis is subject to fracture in a predictable configuration, which produces a Salter-Harris type II fracture. There is frequently accompanying soft tissue trauma that precludes athletic soundness after reduction and surgical repair, but these animals are most often sound for breeding as adults. Other traumatic injuries of the stifle are usually severe and result in intra-articular soft tissue injury involving the cruciate ligaments, collateral ligaments and menisci, or severe bone injury, necessitating destruction.

Pelvis

Injuries of the pelvic region are common and may be difficult to diagnose with great specificity because they may involve bone, cartilage, muscle, tendon and ligament, nerves, and blood vessels. There is no age limitation on pelvic injuries, which may occur as early as a few days or at any time later; however, most traumatic and septic causes of pelvic lameness occur prior to 4 months of age. Traumatic injuries of the pelvis and coxofemoral joint may result from rearing, twisting, and falling over, with torsional load causing the injury. Tuber coxae injuries are typically associated with external trauma such as a kick from another horse or striking the area during a fall or against a gate post or other fixed object. Injuries of the tuber ischii may occur from falling backwards or accelerating backwards and directly striking or landing on this bony prominence.

The gait and degree of lameness depends on the structures involved and their location. Fractures of the pelvis almost always involve both sides, with one side more extensively damaged than the other. Displaced pelvic fractures are generally nonweight-bearing lame during ambulation on the side with the most damage. When standing, however, foals generally bear weight on both limbs and may electively stand on the primary fracture side. Generally the tail is set away from the most severely affected side. If the injury is caudal to the coxofemoral joint, the caudal phase of the stride is prolonged and there is resentment during the cranial phase, whereas the opposite is true for injuries of the tuber coxae. Injuries to the superficial bony prominences such as the tuber coxae, tuber ischii, or greater trochanter of the femur as well as injury to the coxofemoral joint display a pain response on digital palpation. Deeper injuries of the pelvic floor or pubic symphysis may be more difficult to detect on physical palpation.

Radiographs are necessary to confirm the presence of a fracture and ultrasound may facilitate identification of other injured tissue. Nuclear scintigraphy is occasionally used to evaluate pelvic injuries and can effectively identify regions of injury, but does not allow identification of specific fracture types. Injuries of the physes and accompanying soft tissue are more effectively identified by magnetic resonance imaging.

Treatment for pelvic injury includes stall rest, and the duration depends upon the severity of the injury.[16] Once full weight-bearing returns, controlled exercise in the form of hand walking is beneficial for rehabilitation. The prognosis for pelvic injury depends upon severity. In general, the prognosis is favorable, but severe displacement accompanied by marked soft tissue trauma or significant involvement of the coxofemoral joint carries a poor prognosis. The main differentials for pelvic trauma are septic arthritis, osteomyelitis, septic physitis, and pelvic abscess.

Less severe lameness of the hip region is associated with tearing of the fascia of the lateral aspect of the biceps femoris or the vastus lateralis muscle. These injuries produce a transient lameness that manifests as a shortened gait at a walk. A palpable 3- to 5-cm deficit, oriented obliquely and parallel to the muscle fibers, is present and an associated hematoma may be observed. Treatment is rest and confinement for 1 to 2 weeks to allow any hemorrhage to stop. These tears should not be drained or opened for fear of sepsis. Rarely, if ever, do any long-term residual effects of these tears manifest, and future athletic potential should not be affected.

Physeal Fractures

Physeal fractures are common due to the relatively weak physeal bone compared with the diaphyseal bone. Diagnosis of physeal injuries is made on clinical and radiographic findings. Clinical signs vary depending on the degree of instability; they include lameness of varying degrees, pain on palpation, swelling, and occasionally angular deviation of the limb distal to the fracture. The primary differential for a stable physeal fracture is infectious physitis. Fracture of pressure physes (those that contribute to longitudinal bone growth) have been categorized and defined using the Salter-Harris classification scheme,[3,8] covered earlier in the chapter. Surgical repair is necessary in foals with displaced, unstable physeal fractures. If adequate reduction and stabilization are achieved, the prognosis for future soundness is good.

Long Bone Fractures

Long bone fractures usually result from external trauma such as a kick or having the limb pinned beneath an object while rolling. Rearing and misloading a limb may result in fracture of the tibia, femur, or pelvis. Physical evaluation may be diagnostic in foals with lameness of traumatic origin because unstable fractures or severe soft tissue injuries cause obvious, immediate clinical signs. If a fracture is suspected, radiographs are necessary to confirm the diagnosis and determine the severity of the injury. The prognosis for a foal after fracture depends on the anatomical location of the fracture; the complexity, orientation, and degree of soft tissue injury around the fracture; and whether the fracture is open. Secondary problems associated with contralateral limb overload from prolonged lameness or from immobilization often dictate the degree of long-term soundness.

Although mechanical laminitis is not as common as in adult horses, it occurs in foals. More common problems include excessive laxity of the metacarpophalangeal or metatarsophalangeal joint, varus deviation, or deformity of the foot, such as underslung or crushed heels and overgrowth of the toe. Contracture or excessive laxity of the fractured limb associated with disuse may prevent future soundness. See chapters 5 and 7 for additional information on long bone fractures.

Developmental Orthopedic Disease

Lameness may be associated with developmental orthopedic disease (DOD) in foals.[4,24] In a group of 378 foals evaluated radiographically at 6 months of age, 47% were affected by DOD and 36% by osteochondrosis.[14] Although osteochondrosis does not typically manifest until the late weanling and yearling period, it is occasionally recognized clinically as a cause of lameness in foals less than 6 months of age. See earlier sections of this chapter for specific DOD conditions.

Perinatal and Congenital Conditions

Foals may be born with musculoskeletal conditions that result in lameness or they may develop them shortly after birth. These conditions are relatively infrequent but worthy of mention because historically they have either been misdiagnosed or erroneously given a poor prognosis. As a result, foals that might have matured and had normal athletic potential have been humanely destroyed. Lameness may be directly caused by these conditions or it may be secondary to their occurrence.

Two such conditions of the neonate are flexural limb deformities and excessive laxity of flexor tendons, both of which are relatively common and may result in secondary lameness. Flexural limb deformity may produce mechanical limitations on ambulation or it may cause pain associated with attempts to correct the deformity. The most common cause of lameness from

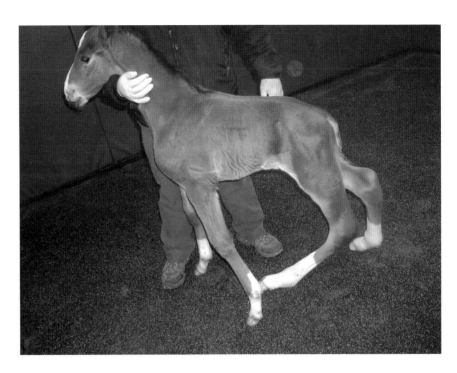

Figure 11.50. Excessive flexion of the hock in a foal with rupture of the left gastrocnemius muscle.

flexural deformity is excessive trauma to the sole of the foot at the toe region, which causes bruising and abscessation.

Flexor tendon laxity causes lameness from decubital sores, bruising, and abscessation in the heel bulbs of the hind feet. These may be prevented by lightly bandaging the heel bulbs for protection and preventing luxation of the distal limb by applying extended heels.

Certain structures in the neonate and young foal are prone to rupture, including that of the common and lateral digital extensor tendons of the forelimb, which usually occurs within 72 hours of birth. Foals with mild flexural deformities may be predisposed to develop these problems. In these contracted individuals, the condition may develop at 2 to 3 weeks of age. The predominant clinical sign is knuckling forward on the ankle and carpus and initially failure to advance the limb. This pathology is frequently mistaken for flexural limb deformity.

The 2 conditions may be differentiated with physical evaluation. Lateral and common digital extensor tendon rupture may be recognized by the presence of a characteristic swelling over the dorsal lateral surface of the carpus at the musculotendinous junction where the rupture occurs. The limb also may readily be placed in a normal position, whereas this is not possible in foals with flexural deformity.

Treatment is aimed at protecting the limb from excoriation of the dorsum of the fetlock with bandaging until the foal acclimates to walking. Continuous splinting or casting is not usually necessary but may be applied intermittently to facilitate use of the limb. Surgery is not necessary nor advisable because the tendons generally heal uneventfully over several weeks.

Ruptured gastrocnemius muscle is recognized in neonates following both normal deliveries and dystocias, but larger foals appear to be predisposed to this condition.[13] Rupture may be partial or total. With partial rupture there is moderate flexion of the tarsus but the foal can still bear weight on the limb. With a complete tear the foal is unable to extend the limb, which will collapse with weight-bearing and the excessive flexion of the hock with the stifle in a fixed position, resulting in a typical, crouched position on the affected side (Figure 11.50). Prognosis for future soundness is good with conservative treatment, providing the foal is not compromised with other concomitant disease processes.[13,27] Splinting is usually required and bandages must be changed frequently to prevent focal pressure necrosis, adequately support the limb, and support ambulation while healing occurs.

INFECTIOUS CAUSES OF LAMENESS

Lameness in foals caused by infectious agents is extremely common, so much so that it is a safe to assume that all lameness in foals is septic in origin until proven otherwise. Foals may be affected shortly after birth or up to 4 months of age, although such lameness may sporadically occur in older foals; approximately half the foals are affected by 60 days of age.[21] It is perplexing that foals appear to be plagued with these conditions more than other species with similar housing and hygiene practices.

The most common infectious conditions causing lameness include the complex of osteomyelitis, septic arthritis, septic physitis, and/or septic tenosynovitis.[9,17–19,25,28] Although there are numerous pathways by which these conditions may occur, such as external injury, the most common is believed to be hematogenous spread from a primary source.[10] Such sources include the urachus or urachal remnants, gastrointestinal tract, respiratory tract, or a distant site in the musculoskeletal system.[12,21] It is commonly thought that there is a propensity for bacterial colonization in the extensive vascular plexus comprised of venous sinusoids; metaphyseal loops; and epiphyseal, metaphyseal, and physeal vessels in growing long bones. The slow and sluggish blood flow and relative vascular stasis in this region allow bacteria to proliferate at or close to the cartilage interface.[3,9] Cartilage matrix degradation and proteoglycan loss may occur within 2 days, and loss of collagen within 9 days after inoculation by bacteria.[2,3,20] The chance of infection is increased in high-risk individuals such as a foal with failure of passive transfer or exposure of a naïve immune system to an aggressive pathogen.

Hematogenous osteomyelitis and septic arthritis have been classified into 5 types based on the structure involved and location.[9,29] Infectious synovitis, or S-type, most commonly affects younger (under 2 weeks) foals and involves only the synovial structure. Epiphyseal type (E-type) involves the joint and adjacent epiphysis. Involvement of subchondral bone results in eventual radiographic changes, although these may not be evident for a week or more. P-type involves the physis and is seen in foals 1 week to 4 months of age. Lesions are seen radiographically as lytic changes in the physis, metaphysis, or epiphysis. T-type involves the tarsal or carpal cuboidal bones and may result in collapse of these structures. These most commonly occur in neonates that suffer from dysmaturity, although normal foals may be affected. I-type involves periarticular soft tissue abscess infecting a physis or joint and often involves the hip or stifle, or more commonly the distal metacarpus or metatarsus. Foals older than 6 to 8 weeks are most often involved. The clinical appearance of the involved region is diffuse pitting edema, with eventual abscess development and drainage.

The common presenting complaint of osteomyelitis and/or septic arthritis is acute onset of lameness, and there is often a pyrexic episode at presentation or in the recent past. The degree of lameness varies from mild to nonweight-bearing and largely depends on the severity of the infection and structures involved. The foal may be noted in recumbent positions more often than normal. With joint involvement there is synovial distension as opposed to the diffuse swelling typically seen with osteomyelitis. The region is usually warm to hot and is painful on manipulation. Occasionally, the area may be cold if the swelling is excessive enough to create vascular compromise, or there may be vascular thrombosis associated with the sepsis.

Hemogram is often normal on presentation because of the localized and acute nature of the infection. When hemogram alterations occur, there is an elevation in the white blood cell count, with or without a left shift and an increase in fibrinogen of 500 mg/dl to 800 mg/dl or higher. Plasma fibrinogen concentration of more than 900 mg/dl may be useful as an indicator of physeal or epiphyseal osteomyelitis, and values may reach 1,500 mg/dl.[23]

If joint involvement is suspected, diagnosis is confirmed through arthrocentesis, joint fluid analysis, and culture and sensitivity. Unfortunately, culture results are often negative because of the bacteriostatic properties of synovial fluid and previously administered antimicrobials.[2,21] Fluid analysis typically reveals more than 20,000 white blood cells and an elevation in total protein. Diagnosis may be more challenging without articular involvement; however, ultrasound evaluation coupled with aspiration and analysis of any fluid pockets may facilitate accurate diagnosis.[12] Radiographs are helpful in establishing a diagnosis, prognosis, and treatment plan. Initial radiographs are often normal but begin to show areas of lysis within a few days of onset. Aspiration of a lytic area may be performed with a needle; however, if this technique is not productive, a sample may be acquired via passage of a drill into the lesion and shavings from the drill may be cultured.[12,17] This portal may also be used for therapy by instillation of antimicrobial agents through a needle or through a cannulated bone screw placed in the hole.

Treatment of septic arthritis includes systemic broad-spectrum antimicrobials while waiting on culture results. Pain control, protection against gastric ulceration, and overall support for the foal regarding hydration and nutritional intake are important, especially in young foals. In cases with joint involvement, local treatment by joint lavage using sterile polyionic fluids is important; alternatively, constant rate infusion therapy with antimicrobials has recently proven beneficial.[1,15] Joint lavage is not necessary if the lesion is isolated to bone. Regional perfusion has proven beneficial, as has intraosseous antimicrobial administration.[12]

Anecdotally, the use of chondroprotective agents parenterally, orally, and intra-articularly is believed to be beneficial in restoring and maintaining joint health, especially in systemically ill foals. Hyperbaric therapy for treatment of osteomyelitis has likewise gained favor for the benefits of revascularization of ischemic tissue and increasing the effectiveness of antimicrobial therapy. In debilitated or cachectic foals, the common clinical impression is that immediately following hyperbaric treatment, the animal is usually brighter and has an improved appetite.

With early diagnosis and appropriate treatment, the prognosis for the survival of foals with septic osteomyelitis is favorable;[12,21] however, with a delay in therapy the prognosis is guarded to grave. Younger foals (under 30 days) that display involvement of bone have a worsened prognosis because of a high incidence of multisystem disease.[21,26] Multiple sites of involvement have a significant detrimental impact on survival as well as future athletic potential.

References

1. Adams SB, Lescun TB. How to treat septic joints with constant intra-articular infusion of gentacmicin or amikacin. Proc Am Assoc Equine Pract 2000;46:188–192.
2. Bertone AL. Infectious arthritis in adult horses. Proc Am Coll Vet Intern Med 1991;9:409–412.
3. Bohanon TC. Developmental musculoskeletal disease. In The Horse: Diseases and Clinical Management, vol. 2. Kobluk CN, Ames TR, Geor RJ, eds. WB Saunders, Philadelphia, 1995, pp 815–858.
4. Douglas J. The pathogenesis and clinical manifestations of equine osteochondrosis. Vet Med 1992;87:826.
5. Dutton DM, Watkins JP, Honnas CM, et al. Treatment response and athletic outcome of foals with tarsal valgus deformities: 39 cases (1988–1997). J Am Vet Med Assoc 1999;215: 1481–1484.
6. Dutton DM, Watkins JP, Walker MA, et al. Incomplete ossification of the tarsal bones in foals: 22 cases (1988–1996). J Am Vet Med Assoc 1998;213:1590–1594.
7. Ellis DR. Fractures of the proximal sesamoid bones in thoroughbred foals. Equine Vet J 1979;11:48–52.

8. Embertson RM, Bramlage LR, Herring DS, et al. Physeal fractures in the horse: Classification and incidence. Vet Surg 1986;15:223.

9. Firth EC. Infectious arthritis in foals. In Current Practice of Equine Surgery. White NA, Moore JN, eds. JB Lippincott Co., Philadelphia, 1990, pp 577–85.

10. Hance SR. Hematogenous infections of the musculoskeletal system in foals. Proc Am Assoc Equine Pract 1998;44:159–166.

11. Hance SR, Bramlage LR, Schneider RK, et al. Retrospective study of 38 cases of femur fractures in horses less than one year of age. Equine Vet J 1992;24:357–363.

12. Hanson R. Septic joints in foals. Proceedings of the North American Veterinary Conference pp. 110–112. Reprinted with permission from the NAVC Conference, 2006.

13. Jesty SA, Palmer JE, Parente EJ, et al. Rupture of the gastrocnemius muscle in six foals. J Am Vet Med Assoc 2005;227:1965–1968.

14. Lepeule J, Bareille N, Robert C, et al. Association of growth, feeding practices and exercise conditions with the prevalence of developmental orthopaedic disease in limbs of French foals at weaning. Prev Vet Med 2009;89:167–177.

15. Lescun TB, Vasey RJ, Ward MP, et al. Treatment with continuous intrasynovial antimcrobial infusion for septic synovitis in horses: 31 cases (2000–2003). J Am Vet Med Assoc 2006;228:1922–1929.

16. Little C, Hilbert B. Pelvic fractures in horses: 19 cases (1974–1984). J Am Vet Med Assoc 1987;190:1203–1206.

17. Madison JB. Infectious orthopedic disease in foals. In Current Therapy in Equine Medicine, 4th ed. Robinson NE, ed. WB Saunders, Philadelphia, 1997, pp 619–23.

18. Madison JB, Sommer M, Spencer PA. Relations among synovial membrane histopathologic findings, synovial fluid cytologic findings, and bacterial culture results in horses with suspected infectious arthritis: 64 cases (1979–1987). J Am Vet Med Assoc 1991;198:1655–1661.

19. Martens RJ, Auer JA. Haematogenous septic arthritis and osteomyelitis in the foal. Proc Am Assoc Equine Pract 1980;26:47–63.

20. McIlwraith CW. Treatment of septic arthritis. Vet Clinics North Am Large Animal Pract 1983;5:363.

21. Neil KM, Axon JE, Begg AP, et al. A retrospective study of 108 foals with septic osteomyelitis: 1995–2001. Proc Am Assoc Equine Pract 2006;52:567–569.

22. Neil KM, Axon JE, Todhunter PG, et al. Septic osteitis of the distal phalanx in foals: 22 cases (1995–2002). J Am Vet Med Assoc 2007;230:1683–1690.

23. Newquist JM, Baxter GM. Evaluation of plasma fibrinogen concentration as an indicator of physeal or epiphyseal osteomyelitis in foals: 17 cases (2002–2007). J Am Vet Med Assoc 2009;235:415–419.

24. Pool RR. Pathologic manifestations of osteochondrosis. In AQHA Developmental Orthopedic Disease Symposium, April 1986, Amarillo, TX. McIlwraith CW, ed. American Quarter Horse Association. pp. 3–7.

25. Schneider RK, Bramlage LR, Moore RM, et al. A retrospective study of 192 horses affected with septic arthritis/tenosynovitis. Equine Vet J 1992;24:436.

26. Steele CM, Hunt AR, Adams PLE, et al. Factors associated with prognosis for survival and athletic use in foals with septic arthritis (1987–1994). J Am Vet Med Assoc 1999;215:973–977.

27. Tull TM, Woodie JB, Ruggles AJ, et al. Management and assessment of prognosis after gastrocnemius disruption in Thoroughbred foals: 28 cases (1993). Equine Vet J 2009;41:541–546.

28. Vatistas NJ, Wilson WD, Pascoe JR, et al. Septic arthritis in foals: Bacterial isolates, antimicrobial susceptibility, and factors influencing survival. Proc Am Assoc Equine Pract 1993;39:259.

29. Wagner PC, Watrous BJ, Darien BJ. Septic arthritis and osteomyelitis. In Current Therapy in Equine Medicine, 3rd ed. Robinson NE, ed. WB Saunders, Philadelphia, 1992, pp 455–462.

30. Yovich JV, Stashak TS, DeBowes RM, et al. Fractures of the distal phalanx of the forelimb in eight foals. J Am Vet Med Assoc 1986;189:550–554.

CERVICAL STENOTIC MYELOPATHY (WOBBLER SYNDROME)

Bonnie R. Rush

Cervical stenotic myelopathy (CSM) is a common cause of symmetric spinal ataxia in young horses. Neurologic gait deficits result from compression of the spinal cord by malformed cervical vertebrae. Pathologic lesions suggest that CSM is a manifestation of developmental orthopedic disease. Heritability has not been established, although genetic predisposition appears likely in specific breeds. The most important differential diagnoses for horses with symmetric spinal ataxia include protozoal myeloencephalitis, degenerative myeloencephalopathy, neuropathic equine herpesvirus-1, and spinal cord trauma.

SIGNALMENT

CSM has been reported in most light and draft breeds. Thoroughbreds, Tennessee Walking horses, and Warmblood breeds appear particularly predisposed.[8] Levine, et al. identified geldings and intact male horses to be more frequently affected than female horses (odds ratio 2.0 and 2.4).[8] Most horses with CSM are 6 months to 3 years of age at presentation, and are often rapidly growing horses.[21] Nonetheless, age (4 years or older) does not preclude the diagnosis; spinal cord compression due to vertebral malformation is routinely diagnosed in adult and aged horses.[7] Spinal cord compression is usually the result of osteoarthritic enlargement of the articular processes in the latter group.[7,21]

CLINICAL SIGNS

The onset of neurologic gait deficits is often reported as a progression of ataxia over several weeks, followed by stabilization (plateau) of clinical signs. Owners may report a traumatic incident with the onset of neurologic signs. The traumatic incident may be the result of mild neurologic deficits, with the injury exacerbating the clinical signs of spinal cord compression. Asymmetric ataxia and paresis may be observed in horses with dorsolateral compression of the spinal cord by proliferative articular processes and periarticular soft tissue structures.[5,18]

Neurologic examination is performed to assess symmetry and severity of weakness, ataxia, and spasticity. Gait analysis is performed at the walk, and neurologic deficits are accentuated by circling, elevation of the head, and maneuvering over obstacles and inclines.[23] Proprioceptive deficits manifest as circumduction of the hindlimbs, posting (pivoting on the inside hindlimb during circling), and truncal sway. Neurologic deficits are graded on a scale of 0 to 5. Grade 0 denotes a normal examination with no deficits detected. Grade 1 describes mild neurologic deficits, which are primarily detected by a trained clinician. Grade 2 indicates deficits that can be detected by most horse owners. Grade 3 deficits are prominent and are detected by all observers. Horses with grade 4 deficits may fall during the examination, but return to standing without assistance. A horse with grade 5 deficits is recumbent and unable to rise.

In most cases of CSM, pelvic limb ataxia is more pronounced than forelimb deficits; upper motor neuron tracts to the pelvic limbs are superficial and vulnerable to external compression.[21] Moderate to severely affected horses have lacerations on the heel bulbs (wobbler heels) and medial aspect of the forelimbs from overreaching and interference. Stumbling and toe dragging indicate weakness. The hooves of horses with prolonged clinical signs of CSM are chipped, worn, or squared at the toe. At rest, affected horses may have a base-wide stance and demonstrate delayed responses to proprioceptive positioning. When prompted to back, affected horses may stand base wide, lean backward, drag their hindlimbs, or step on a hind foot with a forelimb. Neck musculature may appear disproportionately thin compared to the rest of the body, and articular processes of the fifth and sixth cervical vertebrae may be prominant.[18]

Occasionally, weakness and stumbling are more pronounced in the forelimbs. This is observed in horses with stenosis of the caudal cervical vertebrae (C6-C7, C7-T1) due to compression of the cervical intumescence. Alternatively, osteoarthritis of the caudal cervical vertebrae may produce cervical pain and forelimb lameness due to peripheral nerve compression without producing clinical signs of spinal cord compression.[16] Affected horses travel with a short cranial phase of the stride and a low foot arc of their forelimb, and may stand or travel with their head and neck extended. Horses with osteoarthritis of the articular processes of the caudal vertebrae may demonstrate increased rate and depth of respiration with cervical manipulation due to pain.

ETIOLOGY

The breed predilection pattern of cervical stenotic myelopathy suggests that heritability plays a role in disease development. However, definitive evidence of a genetic component has been elusive.[21] Development of CSM is likely multifactorial with genetic predisposition and environmental influences (particularly diet) contributing to bony malformation and spinal cord compression.[6,21] Developmental orthopedic disease of the appendicular skeleton, such as physitis, osteochondrosis, and flexural limb deformities, occurs more often in horses with CSM, and CSM appears to be a manifestation of developmental orthopedic disease.[21]

Spinal cord compression can be dynamic or static in horses with CSM.[5,10,21] Dynamic compression occurs due to vertebral instability and causes intermittent spinal cord compression during ventroflexion of the neck; spinal cord compression is relieved when the neck is in the neutral position. Pathologic changes most commonly observed in horses with dynamic compression are instability between adjacent vertebrae, malformation of the caudal vertebral epiphysis (caudal epiphyseal flare), and malformation of the articular processes.[10,14] The intervertebral sites most commonly affected by dynamic compression are C3-C4 and C4-C5.[22]

Static compression results in continuous spinal cord impingement regardless of cervical position and occurs predominantly in the caudal cervical region, C5-C6 and C6-C7.[14] Static spinal cord compression is exacerbated by thickening of the dorsal lamina, hypertrophy of the ligamentum flavum, and osteoarthritis of the articular processes. Static and dynamic spinal cord compression are both associated with narrowing of the vertebral canal from C3-C6, regardless of the site of spinal cord compression, indicating that generalized vertebral canal stenosis is an important factor in the pathophysiology of CSM.[5,18]

Histopathologic examination of the spinal cord identifies myelin degeneration (ventral and lateral funiculi), malacia, focal neuronal loss, and fibrosis at the sites of spinal cord compression. Wallerian degeneration occurs in ascending white matter tracts cranial to the affected site and in descending tracts distal to the site of spinal cord compression.[21]

DIAGNOSIS

Radiographic examination and cerebrospinal fluid (CSF) analysis are indicated in horses with symmetric tetraparesis and ataxia to differentiate CSM from other spinal cord disorders. The most important differential diagnoses for horses with symmetric tetraparesis and ataxia include protozoal myeloencephalitis, degenerative myeloencephalopathy, neuropathic equine herpesvirus-1, and spinal cord trauma. Cytologic findings in the cerebrospinal fluid usually are unremarkable. When CSF analysis is abnormal, alterations are consistent with acute spinal cord compression, such as mild xanthochromia or increased protein concentration.

Survey radiographs of the cervical spine are obtained in standing, sedated horses. Cervical radiographs are evaluated by subjective assessment of vertebral malformation[5,10] and objective determination of vertebral canal diameter.[4,18] The 5 categories of cervical vertebral malformation that are subjectively assessed in horses with CSM are osteoarthritis of the articular processes, subluxation between adjacent vertebrae, flare of the caudal physis of the vertebral body, abnormal ossification patterns, and caudal extension of the dorsal laminae (Figure 11.51).[10,17] Osteoarthritis of the articular processes of the caudal cervical vertebrae is the most common malformation observed in affected horses,[14] but it is also common in horses without CSM. Osteoarthritis is prominent in aged-onset CSM. In some cases collapse of the intervertebral space is observed (Figure 11.52). In young horses subluxation between adjacent vertebrae and caudal epiphyseal flare are more

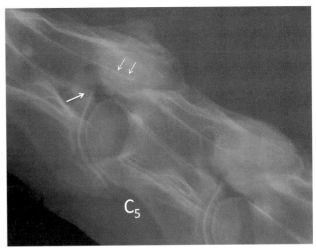

Figure 11.51. Radiograph of the C4-C5 articulation demonstrating caudal epiphyseal flare (arrow), subluxation between C4-C5 vertebra, osteoarthritis of the articular processes, and caudal extension of the dorsal laminae (double arrow).

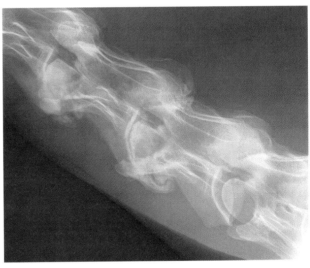

Figure 11.52. Radiograph of C4 and C5 from an aged mare with progressive spinal ataxia and cervical pain demonstrating osteoarthritis of the articular facets and degeneration and collapse of the intervertebral space.

discriminating findings than osteoarthritis of the articular processes.[10]

Two techniques have been described to objectively measure vertebral canal diameter: the sagittal ratio[17] and the intervertebral ratio.[4] Both measures eliminate error caused by magnification given that the vertebral canal and vertebral body are in the same anatomic plane. The sagittal ratio is obtained by dividing the minimum sagittal diameter of the vertebral canal by the width of the corresponding vertebral body.[17] The minimum sagittal diameter is measured from the dorsal aspect of the vertebral body to the ventral border of the dorsal laminae at the cranial aspect of the vertebra, and the vertebral body width is measured perpendicular to the vertebral canal at the widest point of the cranial

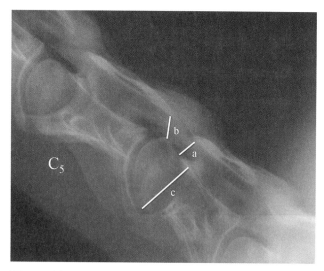

Figure 11.53. Radiograph of the C5-C6 vertebra demonstrating measurement of the sagittal ratio (a×c = 31%) and the intervertebral ratio (b×c = 35%), both of which are far below reference values.

aspect of the vertebral body (Figure 11.53). The sagittal ratio should exceed 52% from C4 through C6 and 56% at C7 in horses weighing more than 320 kg. Sensitivity and specificity of the sagittal ratio for identification of CSM-affected horses is approximately 89% for vertebral sites C4 through C7.[17]

Intervertebral ratios are obtained by determining the minimum distance from the craniodorsal aspect of the vertebral body to the caudal aspect of the vertebral arch of the immediately rostral vertebrae (Figure 11.53).[4,5] This value is divided by the width of the vertebral body. Reference ranges were determined using 8 affected horses; an intervertebral ratio equal to or less than 0.485 correctly classified each horse with CSM.[4]

Accurate determination of these objective measures requires a precise, lateral radiograph of the cervical vertebrae. Oblique views yield indistinct margins of the ventral aspect of the vertebral canal, resulting in erroneous values for vertebral canal diameter and vertebral body width. Survey radiographic examination of the cervical vertebrae determines the likelihood of spinal cord compression; qualitative and both quantitative techniques should be evaluated during assessment of cervical radiographs.

Myelographic examination provides a definitive diagnosis of CSM and identifies sites of spinal cord compression and classifies lesions as static or dynamic.[5,11] Myelographic examination is performed under general anesthesia in lateral recumbency.[11] The landmarks for cisternal puncture at the atlanto-occipital site are the cranial border of the wings of the atlas, the caudal border of the occipital protuberance, and the dorsal midline. The poll region is aseptically prepared and the head flexed at a 90° angle with the cervical vertebral column. The spinal needle (3.5-inch, 18-gauge) is introduced and directed toward the lower jaw. The spinal needle is advanced until the dura mater is penetrated, which often produces a popping sensation. Clear cerebrospinal fluid should drip rapidly or flow from the hub

with successful placement of the spinal needle. An equal volume (20 to 40 ml) of cerebrospinal fluid is removed prior to injection of contrast agent. Twenty to 40 ml of contrast medium produces sufficient positive-contrast opacity to identify spinal cord compression in adult horses. The bevel of the spinal needle is directed caudally and contrast medium is injected at a constant rate over 5 minutes. The head and neck are elevated under a wedged platform for 5 minutes at 30° to 45° to facilitate caudal flow of contrast medium. Iohexol (350 mg iodine/ml) is the most popular nonionic, water-soluble contrast media used for equine myelographic studies.[5,11]

It is difficult for investigators to agree on myelographic criteria for definitive diagnosis of CSM. In many cases, the site of compression (or lack thereof) is obvious and all recommended criteria would produce the same result. However, there is a population of horses for which myelographic interpretation is more difficult.[5,11,22] Early descriptions of equine myelography recommended a 50% or greater decrease in the sagittal diameter of the dorsal contrast column, paired with obliteration of the ventral contrast columns.[14] The decrease in the sagittal diameter of the contrast column is determined by comparing the value at the intervertebral space to a midvertebral site cranial or caudal to the suspected intervertebral space. The 50% reduction should be interpreted conservatively, given the propensity for false positive diagnosis; a 70% reduction may be more reliable. Some investigators prefer to use a diagnostic criterion of less than 2 mm of dorsal contrast column (or smaller) to reduce the occurrence of false positive results on myelographic studies; however, this criterion increases the risk of false negative diagnosis. Most recently, a 20% reduction in dural diameter (height of the dural sac) at a given intervertebral junction, compared to the dural diameter at the level of the mid-vertebral body, has been suggested as the most reliable indication of spinal cord compression specifically at C6-C7.[22] At mid-cervical sites, this criterion has low sensitivity and high specificity. A reliable decision criterion for mid-cervical myelographic examination has been difficult to identify.[22]

A complete myelographic examination should include neutral and stressed (flexed and extended) views of the cervical vertebrae.[11,22] Horses with dynamic spinal cord compression show narrowing of the dorsal and ventral contrast columns during ventroflexion of the neck (Figure 11.54), whereas spinal cord compression is not apparent with the neck in the neutral position. Static vertebral canal stenosis is characterized by constant spinal cord compression regardless of cervical position. In some cases of static compression, ventroflexion of the neck stretches the ligamentum flavum and relieves spinal cord compression, whereas hyperextension exacerbates compression. In horses with obvious sites of spinal cord compression on neutral myelographic views, excessive flexion and extension of the neck should be avoided to prevent exacerbation of spinal cord injury.

Horses should be monitored for 24 hours after the myelographic procedure for depression, fever, seizure, and worsening of neurologic status, which may result from spinal cord trauma during hyperflexion, iatrogenic puncture of the spinal cord, or chemical meningitis. Administration of phenylbutazone (4.4 mg/kg PO every

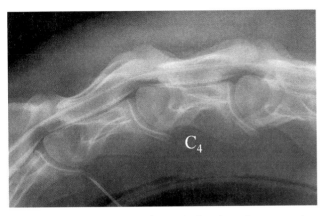

Figure 11.54. Myelogram demonstrating dynamic compression of the C3-C4 and C4-C5 articulations during ventroflexion of the cervical spine.

24 hours) 1 day before through 1 day after myelographic examination attenuates fever and depression associated with chemical meningitis.

Standing myelography via lumbosacral injection of nonionic contrast agent (0.20 ml/kg) can provide diagnostic images in just over half of the subjects without serious complication.[16] The justifications for recommending standing myelography are the economic value of the patient and ease of obtaining films.

TREATMENT AND PROGNOSIS

Conservative management of CSM-affected horses consists of administration of anti-inflammatory therapy (glucocorticoids and nonsteroidal anti-inflammatory drugs) and exercise restriction. Anti-inflammatory therapy alone may reduce the edema associated with spinal cord compression; however, full recovery is unlikely without dietary or surgical intervention.[19]

The most successful conservative treatment option for CSM-affected foals under 1 year of age is the paced diet program.[2] This dietary program consists of restricted energy and protein (65% to 75% of National Research Council recommendations) but maintains a balanced vitamin and mineral intake. Vitamins A and E are provided at 3 times NRC recommendations, and selenium is supplemented to 0.3 ppm. Roughage is provided by pasture or low-quality grass hay (6% to 9% crude protein). Solitary stall confinement is recommended to minimize repetitive spinal cord compression from dynamic instability. After 6 to 9 months of dietary restriction, horses appear markedly thin; however, cervical radiographs (bony malformation and objective measures) and neurologic status are often improved (Figure 11.55). Dietary-restricted horses appear osteopenic radiographically; cautious return to full feed and exercise is recommended over 6 to 8 weeks.

Horses with cervical pain and forelimb lameness due to cervical vertebral osteoarthritis may benefit from intra-articular administration of corticosteroids or chondroprotective agents.[3,8] Arthrocentesis of cervical vertebral articulations is performed with ultrasound guidance using a 6-inch, 18-gauge, spinal needle in the standing, sedated, or recumbent horse.[1] The cranial facet of the caudal vertebrae will appear superficial to the caudal facet of the cranial vertebrae. The articular space is accessed at the cranioventral opening of the articular facet, which is angled approximately 60° from the ultrasound beam.[11] The needle should be introduced 5 cm cranial to the facet and inserted at a 30° angle to the skin surface. Joint penetration may be confirmed by aspiration of synovial fluid. If the neck is extended, the transverse process of the cranial vertebrae may obscure the path to the articulation. Intra-articular triamcinolone (6 mg/joint) or methylprednisolone (100 mg/joint) have produced a positive clinical response in approximately 50% of horses with arthrosis of the articular

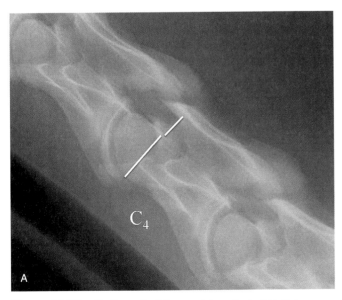
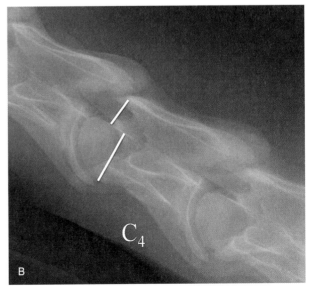

Figure 11.55. Radiograph of the cranial cervical spine in a young Quarter horse filly with CSM (A) before and (B) after institution of the paced diet. The sagittal ratio at C3-C4 articulation was 47.9% (19.1 mm × 39.8 mm) prior to and 53.5% (23.5 mm × 43.9 mm) after 8 months of dietary and exercise restriction. Grade II spinal ataxia had resolved.

processes.[3] The goal of intra-articular anti-inflammatory therapy should be to improve cervical mobility, reduce cervical pain, and/or eliminate forelimb lameness. It is unlikely that intra-articular therapy will significantly improve clinical signs of spinal ataxia.

Surgical intervention is the most widely reported treatment for CSM, and is indicated to stop repetitive trauma to the spinal cord.[13,19,23] The goals of surgical intervention are to stabilize cervical vertebrae and decompress the spinal cord. Ventral stabilization (interbody fusion) provides intervertebral stability for horses with dynamic spinal cord compression. Affected vertebrae are fused in the extended position to provide immediate relief of spinal cord compression and prevent repetitive spinal cord trauma.

Dorsal laminectomy (subtotal Funkquist type-B) is performed to decompress static lesions by removing portions of the dorsal lamina, ligamentum flavum, and joint capsule at the compressed site.[13] This procedure provides immediate decompression of the spinal cord; however, fatal postoperative complications may occur.[13,19] Ventral stabilization in horses with static compression causes remodeling and atrophy of the articular processes, resulting in delayed decompression of the spinal cord over a period of weeks to months.[19] Decompression is immediate with dorsal laminectomy; however, because of its relative safety, ventral stabilization using a threaded basket is the technique of choice for both dynamic and static compressive lesions.

Ventral stabilization improves the neurologic status in just over half of horses with CSM, with some horses returning to athletic function.[19,23] An improvement in 1 to 2 neurologic grades out of 5 is expected. The most important patient factor for determining the postoperative prognosis is the duration of clinical signs before surgical intervention; horses that have had clinical signs for less than 1 month before surgery are more likely to return to athletic function than are horses that have had clinical signs for longer than 3 months.[19] In addition, the number of compressive sites, severity of the compression, and severity of post-operative complications contribute to the long-term prognosis. Subtotal laminectomy and ventral stabilization for static compression of the caudal cervical vertebrae are associated with fatal postoperative complications, including vertebral body fracture, spinal cord edema, and implant failure.[13,19,23]

Postoperatively, horses are maintained on stall rest for 3 weeks and fed from a hay net to minimize motion at the surgery site. The duration of convalescence and rehabilitation after ventral stabilization is approximately 6 to 12 months. An individualized exercise program, determined by the projected use of the horse and the animal's neurologic status, should be designed to promote muscular strength. Extended exercise at slow speed, including ponying and lunging on inclines, is recommended during rehabilitation. A neurologic examination should be performed to determine the horse's ability to return to athletic function after surgery. It is unlikely that significant improvement in neurologic status will occur beyond the 1-year postoperative period.[19,23]

References

1. Berg LC, Nielsen JV, Thoefner MB, et al. Ultrasonography of the equine cervical region: a descriptive study in eight horses. Equine Vet J 2003;35:647–655.
2. Donawick WJ, Mayhew IG, Galligan DT, et al. Results of a low-protein low-energy diet and confinement on young horses with wobbles. Proceedings of the American Association of Equine Practitioners 1993;39:125–127.
3. Grisel RG, Grant BD, Rantanen NW. Arthrocentesis of the equine cervical facets. Amer Assoc Equine Pract 1996;42:197–198.
4. Hahn CN, Handel I, Green SL, et al. Assessment of the utility of using intra- and intervertebral minimum sagittal diameter ratios in the diagnosis of cervical vertebral malformation in horses. Vet Radiol Ultrasound 2008;49:1–6.
5. Hudson NPH, Mayhew IG. Radiographic and myelographic assessment of the equine cervical vertebral column and spinal cord. Eq Vet Educ 2005;17:43–48.
6. Kronfeld D. Dietary aspects of developmental orthopedic disease. Vet Clin North Am (Equine Pract) 1990;6:451–465.
7. Levine JM, Adam E, Mackay RJ, et al. Confirmed and presumptive cervical vertebral compressive myelopathy in older horses: A retrospective study (1992–2004). J Vet Intern Med 2007;21:812–819.
8. Levine JM, Ngheim PP, Levine GJ. Associations of sex, breed, and age with cervical vertebral compressive myelopathy in horses: 811 cases (1974–2007). J Am Vet Med Assoc 2008;233:1453–1458.
9. Matoon JS, Drost WT, Grguric MR, et al. Technique for equine cervical articular process joint injection. Vet Radiol Ultrasound 2004;45:238–240.
10. Mayhew IG, Donawick WJ, Green SL, et al. Diagnosis and prediction of cervical vertebral malformation in Thoroughbred foals based on semiquantitative radiographic indicators. Equine Vet J 1993;25:435–440.
11. Neuwirth L. Equine myelography. Compend Cont Educ Pract Vet 1992;14:72–79.
12. Nielsen JV, Berg LC, Thoefnert MB, et al. Accuracy of ultrasound-guided intra-articular injection of the cervical facet joints in horses: A cadaveric study. Equine Vet J 2003;35:657–661.
13. Nixon A, Stashak T, Ingram J. Dorsal laminectomy in the horse. III. Results in horses with cervical vertebral malformation. Vet Surg 1983;12:184–188.
14. Papageorges M, Gavin PR, Sande RD, et al. Radiographic and myelographic examination of the cervical vertebral column in 306 ataxic horses. Vet Radiol 1987;28:53–59.
15. Ricardi G, Dyson SJ. Forelimb lameness associated with radiographic abnormalities of the cervical vertebrae. Equine Vet J 1993;25:422–426.
16. Rose PL, Abutarbush SM, Duckett W. Standing myelography in the horse using a nonionic contrast agent. Vet Radiol Ultrasound 2007;48:535–538.
17. Rush Moore BR, Reed SM, Biller DS, et al. Assessment of vertebral canal diameter and bony malformations of the cervical part of the spine in horses with cervical stenotic myelopathy. Am J Vet Res 1994;55:5–13.
18. Rush Moore B, Holbrook TC, Stefanacci JD, et al. Contrast-enhanced computed tomography in six horses with cervical stenotic myelopathy. Equine Vet J 1992;24:197–202.
19. Rush Moore B, Reed SM, Robertson JT. Surgical treatment of cervical stenotic myelopathy in horses: 73 cases (1983–1992). J Am Vet Med Assoc 1993;203:108–112.
20. Stewart R, Reed S, Weisbrode S. The frequency and severity of osteochondrosis in cervical stenotic myelopathy in horses, Am J Vet Res 1991;52:873–879.
21. Van Biervliet J, Mayhew IG, de Lahunta A. Cervical vertebral compressive myelopathy: Diagnosis. Clin Tech Eq Pract 2006;5:54–59.
22. Van Biervliet J, Scrivani PV, Divers TJ, et al. Evaluation of decision criteria for detection of spinal cord compression based on cervical myelography in horses: 38 cases (1981–2001). Equine Vet. J. 2004;36:14–20.
23. Walmsley JP. Surgical treatment of cervical spinal cord compression in horses: A European experience. Eq Vet Educ 2005;2:49–53.

Foot Care and Farriery

BASIC FOOT CARE

Stephen E. O'Grady

INTRODUCTION

The equine foot is unique in that it is a biological entity (hoof structures) that follows the laws of physics (biomechanics). Biomechanics is the study of the mechanics of a biological structure, and it is essential that the veterinarian or farrier have a working knowledge of the foot's biomechanics to implement appropriate farriery.[10,15,27] Proper farriery promotes a healthy, functional foot, provides biomechanical efficiency, and prevents lameness.[17]

The structures of the hoof complex comprise the hoof capsule, sole, frog, digital cushion, ungual cartilages, and deep digital flexor tendon (DDFT). The equine foot has numerous functions: supporting the weight of the horse, dissipating the energy of impact as the foot strikes the ground, protecting the structures contained within the hoof capsule, and traction.

The veterinary and farrier literature often describes the "normal" foot. However, the concept of normal may be misleading because it does not consider genetics, breed, foot conformation, environmental influences, and the athletic pursuits of the individual horse. Thus, the terms good, ideal, or functional foot may be more appropriate, because they describe a foot that comprises:

1. A thick hoof wall
2. Adequate sole depth
3. Solid heel base
4. Growth rings below the coronet are of equal size at the toe and heel.
5. Acceptable foot conformation

See Figure 12.1.

Trimming and shoeing affects not only the external hoof capsule, but also the internal structures of the foot.

Adams and Stashak's Lameness in Horses, 6e, edited by Gary M. Baxter
© 2011 Blackwell Publishing, Ltd.

Often trimming and shoeing methods are based on theoretical assumptions and esthetic decisions derived from empiric experience rather than consistent guidelines that can be applied on an individual basis. Farriery assumes the dominant role in maintaining the health of the foot and preserving the integrity of its structures.[17]

The hoof care provided by the farrier depends on that individual's knowledge, training, experience, and skill level. Because the equine veterinarian is responsible for the overall soundness of the horse, a working knowledge of farriery is essential. A thorough knowledge of traditional horseshoeing enables the veterinarian to interact with the farrier at the farrier's level, which ultimately enhances the professional relationship and promotes quality hoof care.[4,12,17] This chapter focuses on basic, fundamental farriery: evaluation of the foot, foot trimming and preparation, shoeing principles, and farriery for common hoof disorders.

For clarity in this discussion, the hoof is defined as the distal end of the second phalanx, the hoof capsule, and structures within the hoof capsule. The digit refers to the limb distal to the metacarpo/metatarsophalangeal (fetlock) joint.

EVALUATION OF THE FOOT

Before any type of foot care or farriery is initiated, the hoof and digit should be visually evaluated, and the observations recorded mentally or as a written record. This evaluation should take place with the horse in the static position on a firm, flat surface and in motion in a straight line, again on a flat firm surface.

Static Observation

With the horse standing still and viewed from the lateral side, the hoof-pastern axis (HPA) should form a straight line. The dorsal hoof wall should be parallel to the dorsal surface of the pastern. In the ideal foot, the

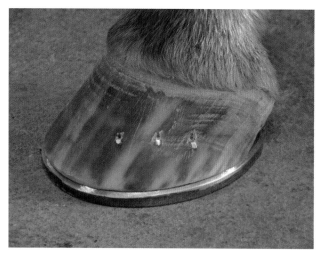

Figure 12.1. A shod foot that demonstrates what is considered good or ideal foot conformation.

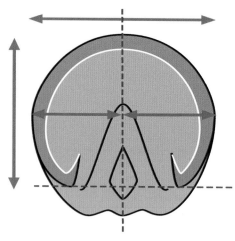

Figure 12.2. Schematic drawing showing ideal proportions for the solar surface of the foot.

angle of the hoof wall at the heel should approximate the angle at the toe of the dorsal hoof wall. However, this approximation of the toe and heel angle is generally not an accurate assessment because during movement, the heels of the hoof wall expand or move outward against the shoe—and to a lesser extent against the ground—when the animal is barefoot. This causes the hoof wall at the heels to wear relative to the hoof wall at the toe. Depending on the conformation of the foot and the amount of hoof mass present, this abrasive wear generally causes the hoof angle at the heel to be less than the angle at the toe. The angle of the foot appears to have taken on less importance recently since the hoof angles do not take into consideration the conformation of the horse's individual limbs.

It is generally thought that the foot is trimmed and/or shod appropriately and the hoof angle is correct when the dorsal hoof wall and the dorsal surface of the pastern are parallel.[1] The terms low hoof angle and high hoof angle describe a nonlinear relationship between the dorsal hoof wall and the dorsal pastern region (HPA). An imaginary line that bisects the third metacarpus (MC3) should intersect the ground at the most palmar aspect of the weight-bearing surface of the heels of the hoof capsule. Furthermore, an imaginary line extending from between the dorsal and palmar borders of the middle phalanx (palpated just above the coronet) to the ground should bisect the hoof capsule at approximately the widest part of the foot. The coronet should have an even, gentle slope from the toe to the heel.

Viewed from the dorsal aspect, a line bisecting the third metacarpus should bisect the phalanges and hoof so that the hoof is approximately symmetrical, including the mass of the hoof on either side of the line and the heights and angles of the walls. The phalanges are often offset to the lateral side as they enter the hoof capsule, which leads to disproportionate weight-bearing. A line drawn between 2 comparable points on the coronet should be parallel to the ground, and a vertical line bisecting the third metacarpal bone should be perpendicular to a line drawn across the coronet or the ground surface of the foot (Figure 2.55 in Chapter 2).

Viewing the hoof from the palmar aspect can help to note the height of the heels, whether there is a disparity between the heel height or heel conformation when compared to the contralateral limb, and whether there is a disparity in the heel bulb height when measured from the ground surface of the hoof to the hairline at the heel bulb on an individual foot. The difference in heel bulb length appears to arise from disproportionate weight-bearing and should be considered when trimming and shoeing the foot.

Viewed from the ground surface of the foot, the width and length of the hoof capsule of the forefoot should be approximately equal, although the hoof capsule may be slightly wider than it is long.[17] Stated another way, if a line is drawn across the widest part of the foot, a line from the widest part of the foot to the heels and a line from the widest part of the foot to the toe should approximate each other (Figure 12.2). The weight-bearing surface of the heels should extend to or coincide with the base of the frog. These 2 reference points can be used to evaluate both the shod or unshod foot and help determine whether previous farriery was appropriate.

Break-over is the phase of the stride between the heel lifting off the ground and the toe lifting off the ground. The point of break-over is best assessed from the ground surface and should be located in the center of the toe. However, the ideal point of break-over is widely disputed. In a traditionally trimmed and shod horse, break-over is positioned where the margin of the dorsal hoof wall intersects the ground. In a biomechanical sense, there are many situations in which it may be beneficial to position the break-over more palmarly.

The relationship between the longitudinal axis of the frog and the underlying distal phalanx is more constant than the longitudinal axis of the frog to the ground surface of the hoof. Ideally, the medial and lateral aspects of the ground surface of the foot should be symmetrical on either side of the central axis of the frog.[17] Another important reference point is the dimensions of the frog; the width of the frog should be 67% of the frog length.[28] The sole of the foot should be concave and possess sufficient depth such that it does not deform when pressure is applied.

Dynamic Observation

The key to observing the horse in motion is defining the placement of the foot as it strikes the ground. The strike pattern should be viewed from the side, and ideally the horse should either land slightly heel first or flat, with the toe and heel contacting the ground simultaneously. Toe-first landing is considered abnormal, and it may be an attempt by the horse to avoid landing on its heels if they are painful. Viewing the horse in motion from the front or from the rear allows the examiner to assess the mediolateral orientation of the heels as they strike the ground. Ideally, both heels should contact the ground simultaneously, but often horses with a narrow chest and a rotational limb deformity impact the ground on the lateral hoof wall and then load the medial side. This type of strike pattern results in the medial heel being displaced proximally, and this type of hoof capsule distortion is called a sheared heel.

Hoof Balance

Veterinarians and farriers often use the term hoof balance to describe the theoretically "ideal" shape or conformation of a foot, the position of the hoof relative to the limb above, and how the foot should be trimmed—yet hoof balance lacks an intrinsic definition.[10] The term has been further subdivided to describe various methods for achieving balance, including geometric, dynamic, 3-dimensional, and recently, natural balance. In practice, no single method of balance will achieve optimum foot conformation for every horse. For example, a problem may arise with the exclusive use of either geometric or dynamic balance to address both dorsal palmar/plantar and mediolateral trimming. If the landing pattern or limb conformation deviates from normal, one method of achieving hoof balance may produce a foot with a different shape from another or if the conformation of the limb causes the foot to assume a disproportionate load when landing, trimming the foot to land flat may be detrimental.[10,17]

"Hoof balance" is often used to communicate aspects of therapy to the farrier. A more effective option is to use a set of biomechanical principles or landmarks as guidelines with a universal meaning that can be applied to every horse, allowing the foot to be evaluated, trimmed, and/or shod in a consistent, reproducible manner (Table 12.1).

These guidelines standardize the basic approach to farriery by both veterinarians and farriers. Furthermore, they do not interfere with nor contradict the traditional concepts of static, geometric, or natural balance. The guidelines also can be used to modify existing hoof conformation, and improve hoof capsule distortions and landing patterns of the foot.

The guidelines or landmarks described in this chapter are applicable to both the fore- and hindfeet but for simplicity, only the forefeet are considered. In the section on foot preparation (trimming), the connotation of balance is replaced with anatomical landmarks along with dorsopalmar/plantar and lateromedial orientation.

Removing the Shoe

Removing the shoe may appear elementary, but it is extremely important that veterinarians master the technique to avoid damaging the hoof capsule during removal. Shoes are removed during lameness examinations to check the solar surface of the foot that is covered by the width of the shoe and during prepurchase examinations to evaluate the entire perimeter of the sole-wall junction (white line) for abnormalities. Shoes also should be removed for radiographs; otherwise, they prevent some of the structures from being imaged.

The first step in removing the shoe is to raise the clinch—the small square section of the nail that exits in the outer hoof wall and is bent over to secure the shoe—on the outer hoof wall. A clinch that is not straightened prior to pulling the shoe may damage the hoof wall as the shoe is removed. The clinch can be raised using a clinch-cutter, a small, chisel type tool (Figure 12.3). The clinch-cutter is placed under the clinch and a nylon hammer, which is quiet and prevents shock, is used to tap the clinch-cutter and straighten the bent clinch. An alternative method is to file the clinches off with a hoof rasp.

Shoe pullers (Figure 12.4) are then placed between the shoe and the hoof, starting at the heel and being levered forward, alternating from side to side toward the toe. The shoe is either removed in its entirety, or the it can be tapped back in place, exposing the nails above the surface of the shoe just in front of where the shoe was levered. The nails are then removed individually and the levering process repeated until all nails are removed. Another method is to use a creased nail puller

Table 12.1. Hoof parameters to use as guidelines to evaluate and trim the foot.

1. Hoof-pastern axis
2. The center of articulation
3. Heels of the hoof capsule extending to the base of the frog

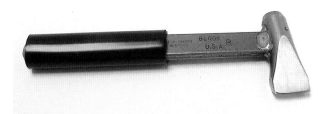

Figure 12.3. Clinch-cutter. (Courtesy of FPD Farrier Products Distribution, Shelbyville, KY 40066.)

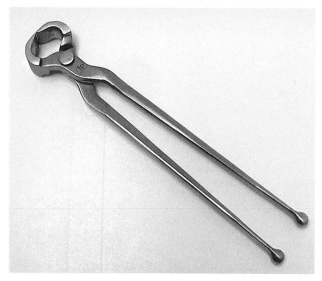

Figure 12.4. Shoe pullers. Note the knobs on the ends of the handles, which distinguish this tool from nippers (compare to nippers in Figure 12.15). (Courtesy of FPD Farrier Products Distribution, Shelbyville, KY 40066.)

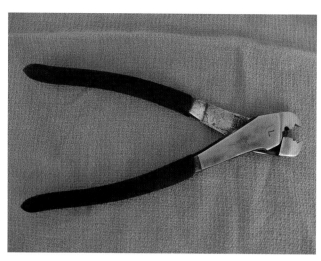

Figure 12.5. Creased nail pullers. Note the short handles, which can be readily used by veterinarians. (Courtesy of FPD Farrier Products Distribution, Shelbyville, KY 40066.)

(Figure 12.5) to grasp the nail head and remove each nail from within the crease or fuller of the horseshoe. The creased nail puller should always be used when removing therapeutic shoes to minimize trauma to an already compromised foot. If a horse loses a shoe or if the shoes must be removed and a farrier is not available, a layer of deformable impression material (Equilox International, Inc. Pine Island, MN) can be placed on the solar surface of the foot and attached by wrapping the foot with 2 or 3 inch elastic tape. This provides comfort and prevents damage to the hoof wall until the farrier replaces the shoe.

PRINCIPLES OF TRIMMING AND SHOEING

Stephen E. O'Grady

The author thanks Derek Poupard, CJF, for contributing to this section.

GUIDELINES FOR TRIMMING

The Importance of Hoof Conformation

Foot conformation (shape) defines the structures and is important because of its relationship to the foot's biomechanical function. Any changes made to the bottom of the horse's foot through farriery affect the angulation of the hoof, the hoof-pastern axis, and the alignment of the hoof capsule under the center of rotation.[6] Hoof conformation embraces the shape and function of the foot in relation to the ground, as well as the skeletal structures of the lower limb both at rest and in motion.[1,2,6] Each foot's conformation should be strong and protective and should maximize biomechanical efficiency. When this ideal conformation is theoretically achieved, it has been termed hoof balance. At present, there is no universal method to assess appropriate foot conformation or balance, nor is there a uniform method that implements guidelines when trimming the equine foot.

The Palmar Foot

The soft tissue structures that comprise and form the palmar/plantar section of the foot are often the limiting factor when trying to achieve and maintain good hoof conformation or shape.[18] These structures primarily include the frog, digital cushion, and ungual cartilages (Figure 12.6). The conformation of the palmar/plantar section of the foot is contingent on the accumulated mass provided by these structures. Unfortunately, attaining sufficient mass for good conformation is not always possible because the structures are influenced by genetics (certain breeds such as Thoroughbreds often have decreased mass), improper development or maturity, continuous repetitive overload when the structures are immature (especially common in young horses in training), and inappropriate farrier practices. Farriers generally need to address the heel area (trimming, manipulating, or supporting) to achieve the desired hoof-pastern axis, center of articulation, and hoof capsule extension to the base of the frog.

The Hoof-pastern Axis

The hoof-pastern axis (HPA) should be the first guideline considered when trimming the foot. With the horse standing still, the metacarpus/metatarsus should be perpendicular to the ground and when viewed from the lateral side, the HPA should form a straight line. When the HPA is parallel, a linear line passes through the middle of the phalanges (proximal, middle, and distal) from the metacarpophalangeal joint to the

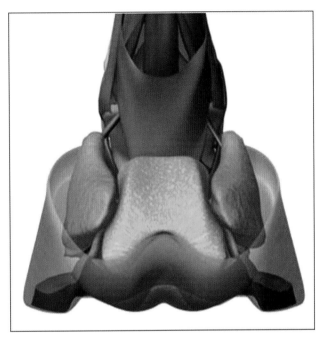

Figure 12.6. Foot model illustrating the structures in the palmar foot responsible for palmar foot conformation. Gray = ungual cartilages, pink = digital cushion, brown = frog. (Courtesy of Dr. Andrew Parks.)

ground. The straight alignment of the phalanges places the dorsopalmar orientation of the distal phalanx within the hoof capsule such that the solar surface of the distal phalanx assumes a similar alignment relative to the ground surface of the hoof capsule/ground. Ideally, the palmar angle of the distal phalanx is 3° to 5° greater than the dorsal angle of the distal phalanx; this allows the distal phalanx to descend in a distopalmar direction during weight bearing and use the physiology in the palmar/plantar section of the foot (Figure 12.7).[11]

The palmar angle of the distal phalanx generally depends on the conformation of the palmar/plantar section of the foot. The dorsopalmar/plantar orientation of the distal phalanx within the hoof capsule helps prevent disproportionate load concentration on the solar surface of the hoof capsule and changes in the position of the ground reaction force (GRF).[17,25,27] Changes in the GRF in a dorsal direction, such as the broken forward-hoof-pastern axis, or in a palmar direction, such as in the broken back-hoof-pastern axis, suggest disproportionate weight-bearing on the solar surface of the hoof capsule when the foot is loaded. Additional detrimental effects of either a broken

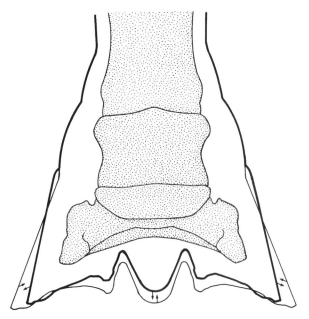

Figure 12.7. During weight-bearing, the frog and sole are forced downward, causing expansion of the hoof wall. The reverse occurs when the foot is unweighted.

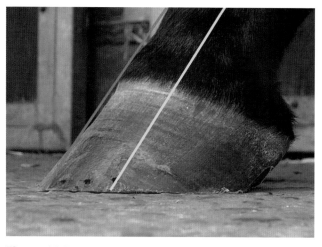

Figure 12.8. Hoof-pastern axis. Note that the dorsal surface of the pastern and the dorsal surface of the hoof wall form a straight line (red line). The yellow line depicts the corresponding digital alignment.

back- or broken-forward-hoof pastern axis have been well documented.[3,9,27]

The changes in hoof-pastern axis are always associated with 2 common hoof capsule distortions: low or underrun heels or upright or clubfeet. A broken back hoof-pastern axis is often caused by excessive toe length combined with a low heel or underrun heel. The low heel is generally combined with a lack of soft tissue mass in the palmar/plantar section of the foot. This decreases the ability of the foot to dissipate the energy of impact during landing and the forces acquired during landing are accepted by the laminar interface and the bone. The broken back-hoof-pastern axis also places the distal interphalangeal (DIP) and proximal interphalangeal (PIP) joints in dorsiflexion, promotes load bearing in the heel area of the foot, and increases the stresses in the DDFT.

In a broken forward-hoof-pastern axis, the heels grow long, which will bypass the soft tissue structures in the palmar/plantar section of the foot, causing the energy of impact generated during landing to be transferred directly through the laminar interface to bone. The DIP and PIP joints are placed in flexion and load bearing on the dorsal margin of the distal phalanx is promoted.

Until recently, the veterinary and farrier literature recommended that the normal hoof angle be 48° to 55° degrees for the forefeet and 52° to 60° degrees for the hindfeet. These recommendations have been shown to be erroneous, because they do not take into consideration the conformation of the horse's individual limb. Therefore, the foot is trimmed appropriately, and the hoof angle is correct for the individual horse when the dorsal hoof wall and the dorsal surface of the pastern region are aligned in parallel planes (Figure 12.8).[1,2,17] A parallel hoof-pastern-axis is easy to access

visually and can be confirmed radiographically when necessary.

The Center of Articulation

The second guideline or landmark for trimming the foot is the center of articulation. A vertical line drawn on a lateral radiograph from the center of the lateral condyle of the distal middle phalanx to the ground should bisect the bearing surface approximately in the middle of the foot (Figure 12.9A).[4,6,9,16–18] This line demarcates the theoretical center of articulation of the DIP joint and should coincide with a line drawn across the solar surface of the foot through the middle one-third of the frog or the widest part of the foot.

The widest part of the foot (center of articulation) forms a landmark on the solar surface of the foot that is repeatable, can be used as a reference point when trimming, and can also be used in the evaluation of foot conformation and the existing farriery that has been performed on the horse (Figure 12.9B). The widest part of the foot is also what farriers refer to as "Ducketts" bridge (Duckett D., Ambler, PA, personal communication, 2008)

The widest part of the foot is the one point on the solar surface of the foot that remains relatively constant regardless of the shape or length of the ground surface that is dorsal or palmar to this point. In a biomechanical sense, because the widest part of the foot is approximately under the center of rotation or biomechanical pivot point, there are moments created on either side of the center of rotation (Figure 12.10). Therefore, when considering biomechanical efficiency, the distance and force on either side of the line drawn through the widest part of the foot should approximate each other (equilibrium) when the horse is standing at rest. Following the trim, the ground surface of the ideal foot should be as wide as it is long and the ground surface of the hoof capsule at the heels should not project dorsal to the base of the frog.[10,17,25]

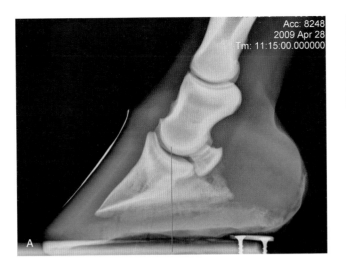

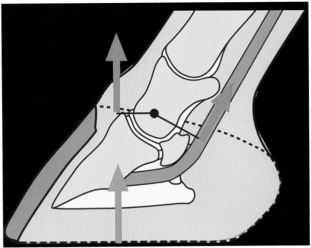

Figure 12.10. Schematic drawing illustrating both an extending force (dorsal red arrows) and a flexing force (palmar red arrow) on either side of the center of articulation.

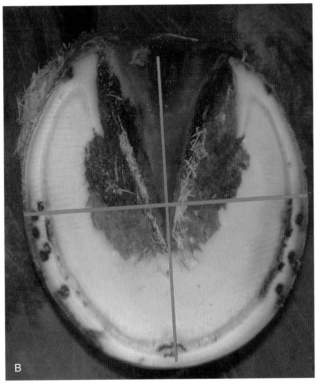

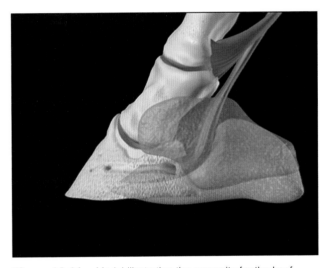

Figure 12.11. Model illustrating the necessity for the hoof capsule to approximate the frog to enclose the structures in the palmar foot. (Courtesy of Dr. Andrew Parks.)

Figure 12.9. A. Lateral radiograph demonstrating the center of articulation that should approximately bisect the weight-bearing surface of the foot (red line). B. Solar surface of the foot showing the middle or widest part of the foot, which should approximate the center of articulation. Note that the foot is basically as wide as it is long.

Heels of the Hoof Capsule Extending to the Base of the Frog

The third guideline is the heels of the hoof capsule extending to the base of the frog. Located within the hoof capsule dorsally are osseous structures that accept load through the lamellae interface and soft tissue structures palmarly/plantarly that are thought to absorb concussion during load bearing and dissipate the energy of impact.

Within the hoof capsule, the distal phalanx occupies approximately two-thirds of the space, and the soft tissue structures occupy one-third. For effective physiologic functioning of the foot, the osseous and soft tissue structures must be located on the same plane within the hoof capsule and complement each other (Figure 12.11). The hoof wall at the heels of the hoof capsule should extend to or approximate the base of the frog.

Appropriate or consistent trimming of the palmar/plantar section of the foot has always presented problems for the clinician, for a variety of reasons. Variations in hoof conformation, farrier training, empiric considerations, and owner pressure often dictate how the heels are trimmed. If the heels are left too long or are allowed to migrate dorsally toward the center of the foot, the function of the soft tissue structures is assumed by the laminar interface and the bones of the digit. Often there is limited soft tissue mass in the palmar foot, or the hoof wall at the heels cannot be trimmed to the base of the frog, which means that the branch of the shoe or some other form of farriery is used to extend the ground surface of the hoof capsule to the base of the frog. Farrier methods for the palmar section of the foot are discussed later in the chapter.

TRIMMING THE FOOT

The hoof care performed by the farrier is perhaps the most important routine procedure for maintaining and promoting the health of the equine foot. Farriery is a difficult occupation, and in order to provide the best service, the farrier should be provided with the best possible working conditions. It is important to spray the horse with an insecticide during the summer. There should be shade in warm weather and protection from cold weather in the winter. The area must be well lit and have an adequately sized space with a hard surface. Often the horse's owner or trainer must hold the horse to keep it quiet while being shod. If physical restraint is necessary, it should always be performed by the client rather than the farrier. When tranquilization or sedation is required, it is always best to have a veterinarian administer the medication.

The basic trim is the most significant aspect of proper farriery. The farrier uses landmarks—the hoof-pastern axis, center of articulation, and heels of the hoof capsule extending to the base of the frog—to carefully evaluate each foot. Sometimes good-quality radiographs are used to locate or confirm the guidelines and provide additional parameters for farriery.

The first observation should be of the hoof-pastern axis in the standing horse, as described above. To confirm that the hoof-pastern axis is parallel, the horse should stand squarely on all 4 feet with the third metacarpal bone positioned vertically to the ground, on a hard, level surface, and be viewed from the side. If the hoof-pastern axis is not straight and broken forward or backward, the initial trimming can correct the condition. The center of rotation also can be located and marked on the outer surface of the hoof capsule if necessary. A very practical technique is to palpate the dorsal and palmar border of the middle phalanx just above the coronet. Half the distance between the borders of the middle phalanx is determined, and from this point, a vertical line is dropped from the coronet to the ground (Figure 12.12). This line appears to have a good correlation with the widest part of the foot on the solar surface.

A leather apron should always be worn when trimming or shoeing the horse to protect the operator's legs. Trimming begins with picking up the foot and evaluating the structures on its solar surface. Before placing the foot between the farrier's legs, the ground surface of the foot is sighted by placing a hand on the dorsal distal surface of MC3 and allowing the distal limb (digit) to hang freely. The farrier's line of vision should be over the hoof to assess the lateral to medial orientation of the solar surface relative to the ground (Figure 12.13). If either the lateral or medial side of the hoof is excessively high or low relative to the opposing side, this can

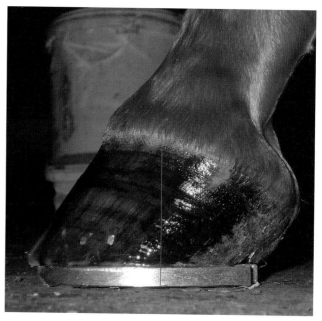

Figure 12.12. The vertical red line, as shown, usually approximates the center of rotation and the middle of the foot.

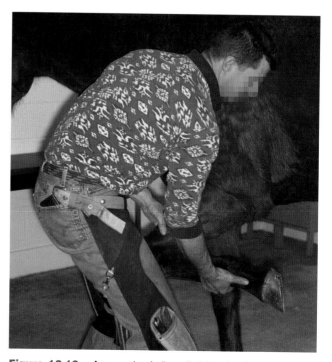

Figure 12.13. An examiner's line of vision should be placed over the hoof, which is permitted to hang in a relaxed position. This permits accurate assessment of mediolateral balance and inspection of the bottom of the foot.

be addressed during the trim. It is equally important to evaluate the height of the heel bulbs (measured from the hoof wall at the heel to the hairline) and note any marked disparity between them. A notable difference in height (greater than 5 mm) denotes a sheared heel hoof conformation and should be addressed during the trim.[28]

The size and position of the frog should be noted on the ground surface of the foot. The width of the frog

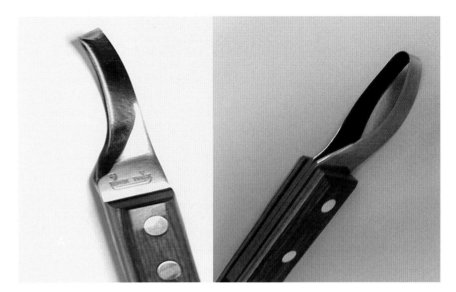

Figure 12.14. Offset hoof knife (left) and a loop hoof knife (right). (Courtesy of FPD Farrier Products Distribution, Shelbyville, KY 40066.)

should be 67% of its length and the surface of the frog should be on the same plane as the lateral and medial hoof wall at the heels of the hoof capsule.[17] The author believes that if the surface of the frog protrudes below the level of the hoof capsule at the heels or is recessed between the heels of the hoof capsule, this should be noted and corrected, if possible, during the trim. If the frog protrudes below the hoof capsule, as is most often seen in horses with low or underrun heels, the frog can be trimmed lightly to remove any excess horn and then the horse can be placed on a hard surface for 12 to 24 hours without shoes. This allows some compression of the frog and allows the heels of the hoof capsule to migrate distally, placing all of the structures on the same plane. If the frog is recessed between the heels, an attempt should be made to lower the heels of the hoof capsule to the point where all structures located on the ground surface of the palmar foot are on the same plane. The length of the frog far exceeding the width is a clear indication that there has been a chronic problem in which the proper physiology in the palmar foot has not been used. In this case the frog is usually accompanied by narrow heels and bars that show curvature instead of being straight; this is called contracted heels.

Next, a line is imagined or drawn (with a magic marker or felt tipped pen) across what is judged to be the widest part of the foot. This point can be measured with a ruler if desired. As described above, this line approximates the center of articulation (Figure 12.9) and can be used to determine the dorsal and palmar proportions of the foot.

Before beginning the trim, the ground surface of the foot is aggressively cleaned with a wire brush. The author removes no horny material from the solar surface of the foot other than any loose or exfoliating horn that is present over the frog or sole. In most cases, all horn material that remains after the foot is cleaned with a wire brush is left intact.

Excess length of the hoof wall at the toe and quarters of the hoof is determined by paring the sole/wall junction (white line) with an appropriate hoof knife (Figure 12.14) and then the excess horn is removed using hoof nippers (Figure 12.15), being careful to leave the adja-

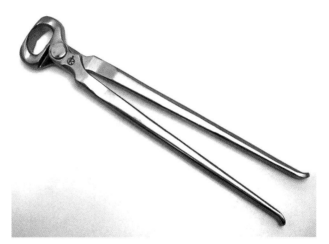

Figure 12.15. Hoof nippers. Note the flared ends to the handles that help distinguish these from shoe pullers (compare to Figure 12.4). (Courtesy of FPD Farrier Products Distribution, Shelbyville, KY 40066.)

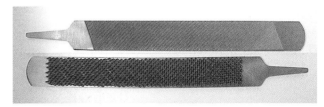

Figure 12.16. Hoof rasp. Note the coarse side of the rasp (bottom) that is used to remove hoof wall, and the smooth side (top) that is used to level the foot. (Courtesy of FPD Farrier Products Distribution, Shelbyville, KY 40066.)

cent sole for protection. The author removes the excess hoof wall length beginning just dorsal to the heels at the quarters with the nippers placed in a tapered position to start the cut and then moving in sequential increments to the opposite quarter. Using a hoof rasp (Figure 12.16), the heels of the hoof capsule are trimmed

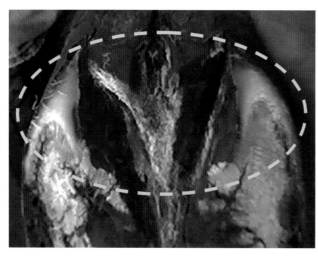

Figure 12.17. Heels of the hoof capsule trimmed to the base of the frog. Note that the hoof wall at the heels and the frog are on the same plane (yellow circle).

level with or blended into the toe and quarters, creating a level surface.

Other than when using the rasp at the toe, the author prefers to use the rasp in a side-to-side motion rather than in a forward motion. This allows better control and prevents uneven areas of the foot from being created. Particular attention is paid to extending the heels of the hoof capsule to the base of the frog when possible, with the intention of creating a solid heel base. If there is insufficient hoof wall for the end of the heel to reach the base of the frog, or if the heels are damaged, this distance can be lengthened by extending the branches of the shoe or by some other farriery method. The key to trimming the heels is to complete the trim at the heels with the hoof wall and the frog on the same plane if possible (Figure 12.17). The medial or lateral hoof wall can be trimmed cautiously relative to the other when changes to the lateral medial orientation of the foot are necessary, such as in the case of sheared heel conformation.

An imaginary line drawn from the initial line across the widest part of the foot to the base of the frog should approximate another line drawn from the widest part of the foot to the hoof wall at the toe. When making this final assessment, the distance from the middle of the foot to the toe is generally greater than the distance to the base of the frog. When this occurs, the foot can be placed on a foot stand and the outer perimeter of the dorsal hoof wall at the toe reduced with a rasp. This places the center of articulation in the middle of the foot or in the middle of the shoe when shod. The foot is further shaped by removing flares from the outer surface of the hoof capsule to concentrate weight-bearing on the hoof wall under the limb. A shoe can then be applied to complement the trim and protect the trim and change the biomechanics of the foot when necessary.

TRIMMING THE BAREFOOT HORSE

Recently, it has become popular to maintain horses in the barefoot or natural state. The author favors horses being maintained without shoes when possible. On the other hand, the author believes that horses can be shod in a physiologic manner such that minimal damage to the hoof capsule will occur. Factors to consider when making this decision include:

- Protection when hoof wear exceeds growth
- Traction, especially for athletic activities in performance horses
- Therapeutic shoes or devices to treat lameness or diseases of the hoof, or to address limb conformation

Any one or a combination of the above factors may dictate the necessity for shoes. The decision also depends on the intended use of the horse, the owners' expectations, and the hoof care the horse receives, especially during the transition period. Much of the horse industry is involved in competitive athletic disciplines and the question arises, "Can this horse compete and perform at a given standard without shoes?"

Wear vs. hoof wall growth takes into consideration the genetics and breed of the horse, structure and conformation of the hoof, working surface, and most importantly, the horse's intended use, all of which influence wear of the feet. The structure of the foot is usually the determining factor.

Maintaining the horse barefoot is best accomplished when—or potentially when—the hoof wall is thick and solid, there is good sole depth, and there are soft tissue structures in the palmar/plantar section of the foot that are of sufficient mass. Breeding practices have influenced the structure of the feet, and unfortunately, this has not always been for the better. Quarter horses have been bred for fashion, whereas Thoroughbreds have been bred for speed, and the result is often poor-quality feet. Usually, and especially in Thoroughbreds, the foot is prevented from growing and maturing into a so-called good or functional foot.[17]

Hoof development, particularly during the first 3 years, depends on stimulation from regular exercise and turn-out. Yearlings are often shod for sales. The majority of horse's feet remain healthy until the time they are broken and enter training, usually as 2-year-olds. As training begins, the hoof capsule and its related structures are still immature, the animal is confined to a stall or small paddock with exercise severely limited, a rider is placed on its back which leads to additional weight-bearing on the feet, and the horse begins to work. Training may lead to abnormal stresses being placed on an underdeveloped foot along with excessive wear. Next, the horse shows discomfort and shoes are then placed on the feet for protection. The first thing that happens when shoes are applied is that the solar surface of the foot loses contact with the ground. Next, how the foot is being trimmed and the application of shoes by the farrier must be considered.

The combination of the above factors can and often does change the structures of the foot forever, or the factors can lead to a weak foot that is hard to maintain without shoes. This observation can be proven by taking a digital photo of a horse's foot at the start of training and then taking another photo 6 months to a year later and comparing the difference. Shoes traditionally are placed on young horses too early, and often unnecessarily if just a few modifications were made in the training program to allow the feet to continue to develop.

The anticipated exercise program also is a key factor. Many horses fare well without shoes, as long as they are not asked to perform. Whereas light riding of barefoot horses may be feasible, competition may not be possible. Finally, the surface upon which the horse is kept and exercised influences the wear on the feet. A hard or abrasive surface, such as sand, is not as forgiving as a soft, deformable footing.

The need for traction on variable ground conditions can also dictate the choice of barefoot vs. shod. Shoes act as a traction device in addition to providing more cup to the foot. Shoes, and various traction devices that are added to shoes, allow horses to hold their footing, prevent slippage, and improve overall performance in competitions such as eventing, jumping, steeplechase racing, and polo. Equestrian sports that take place during the winter, such as fox hunting, are aided by traction devices because of the diverse weather and footing conditions. Traction devices protect the horse and give the horse and rider confidence while performing. Often overlooked is the fact that they also protect the rider, whether trail riding or competing. Borium or studs provide additional safety from slippage and allow a horse to be ridden, pull a carriage up and down hills, or to pull a sleigh on snow and ice.

Sliding plates used in reining horses may be considered anti-traction devices because they decrease the friction between the ground and the hoof.

Therapeutic shoeing generally is a component of or sometimes even the entire treatment for lameness confirmed to the foot. Lameness results from repetitive stresses or overload placed on a given structure(s) of the hoof capsule or within the hoof, leading to damage. Shoes can be used to change the forces/stresses on a given structure and unload damaged areas of the foot. They are used for realignment of the distal phalanx in laminitis, provide continuity of the hoof capsule after resection in white line disease (WLD), stabilize hoof cracks and distal phalanx fractures, and provide protection following a puncture wound or foot surgery. Angular or flexural deformities in young horses may be treated or aided by various types of shoes.

A transition period to allow the foot to adapt is generally needed when changing from shod to barefoot.[19] The hoof wall must toughen and the sole must become thicker to compensate for not wearing shoes. Horses are much easier to maintain in a barefoot manner if they have never had shoes. Another factor in the transition period is the length of time that the horse has worn shoes; this affects the length of time needed for the horse to develop the necessary sole protection once the shoes come off.

Often, the foot structures have inadequate mass or are irreversibly damaged and thus incapable of adaptation.

The horse should be taken out of work if a decision is made to remove the shoes. The author recommends a 30- to 90-day transition period during which time the structures of the horse's feet are allowed to toughen and adapt to going without shoes. At this point hoof care changes from trimming the foot to shaping the foot. The only tools necessary are a wire brush and a rasp.

Nothing is removed from the bottom of the foot. Using a rasp, the heels are moved back to the base of the frog (when possible) such that the heels of the hoof wall and the frog are on the same plane, and the hoof wall is not lowered but rather rasped on an angle (instead of a flat plane) to create a rounded edge. The angle of the hoof wall is created with the rasp placed at a 45° angle, starting on the outer side of the sole wall junction (white line). This manner of rasping creates a sharp edge that is then smoothed with a rasp, resulting in the rounded perimeter. Flares, or excess toe, are removed from the outer hoof wall (shaping). The shaping is finished by slightly beveling the toe on the ground surface of the foot from the toe quarters forward to promote sole growth and to toughen the sole wall junction. This bevel should not be created if firm pressure (using thumb pressure or hoof testers) on the sole causes the sole to deform.

The length of the adaptation phase often can be predicted according to the initial structure of the horse's foot, and should be modified as necessary. When there is minimal sole depth (as evidenced by hoof testers applied to the sole), the horse should be confined or placed in a small area of soft footing and walked daily on a firm surface until the structures of the foot begin to change and adapt. Placing the horse in a protective boot will protect the foot but may not provide the necessary stimulation for adaptation. At no time should the horse show marked discomfort, because this defeats the purpose. If the horse's sole has not become firmer and noticeable growth of sole does not appear on the inner border of the sole wall junction after 30 days, then it may be worthwhile to reconsider this method of hoof care in the best interest of the horse.

THE HORSESHOE

The basic configuration of a horseshoe is a curved bar made from a variety of materials that is rectangular in cross section and shaped to conform to the contour of the ground surface of the hoof wall. The shoe should be wide enough to cover the ground surface of the hoof wall, the sole wall junction (white line), and the adjacent sole. The shoe has 4 surfaces: the foot and ground surfaces and the inner and outer perimeter or margins. The parts of the shoe are named after the corresponding section of the hoof: toe, quarter, and heel. Each shoe has 2 branches, medial and lateral, that extend from the center of the toe to the medial and lateral heels, respectively. The width of the shoe is often referred to as the web. The shoe is punched or machine stamped with nail holes, 3 or 4 in each branch, 2 to 3 of which are generally used in each branch.

Materials and Size

Horseshoes may be made from steel, aluminum, titanium, synthetic polymers, or various composites; the construction material dictates the shoes' weight and durability. Most horseshoes are made of steel due to their durability, cost, and workability. However, aluminum is used frequently because of its lighter weight and ease of shaping for some farriers. Recently, shoes made from various synthetic polymers and composites have been recommended for specialty uses, but they have not replaced the traditional materials.

Shoes may be hand forged from steel or aluminum bar stock or manufactured. Handmade shoes offer few advantages over the manufactured shoes that are available today. It is more important that the farrier be skilled at forging, so he/she can modify manufactured shoes and hand forge a shoe from bar stock when necessary. Heating the shoe makes altering the shape much easier and it has advantages when fitting the shoe, such as seating clips (when used) and detecting uneven sections on the ground surface of the foot.

Bar stock is usually rectangular in cross section and available in sizes from 0.6 to 1.2 cm thick and 1.2 to 3.1 cm wide. The most common size is 0.8 to 1.9 cm. Concave bar stock has a crease stamped in the bar stock and is tapered from the crease toward the inner margin on the ground surface. A shoe made from this type of bar stock is thought to increase traction on all terrains and possess a self-cleaning action. It is frequently used in Europe but has not become as popular in the United States. Pre-made concave shoes can also be purchased.

Manufactured shoes, also referred to as keg shoes, are catalogued using numerical sizes. Although the sizes are usually consistent within and between a manufacturer's product lines, there is no universal standard for sizing keg horseshoes. Manufactured shoes may be generically shaped to the general shape of a horse's foot or specifically designed for a fore- or hindfoot. The dimensions of the stock of both manufactured and hand-forged shoes affect the weight and stiffness of the shoe, coverage of the ground surface of the foot, height to which the shoe elevates the foot off the ground, and rate at which the shoe wears.

Shoe weight influences the biomechanics of movement. The heavier the shoe, the more energy is expended accelerating and decelerating the limb at the beginning and end of each stride. Therefore the lightest possible shoe should be used that is compatible with protecting the wall and adjacent sole, and providing the stiffness and wear required. Shoes made from concave stock are lighter than those made from regular bar stock. The width and thickness of the shoe usually is uniform around the circumference of the shoe so that the biomechanical influences of shoe weight and the stresses imposed are generally balanced about the axis of the limb. Although the width or web of a shoe is related to the thickness of the hoof wall, and at least in part the size of the foot, it is common to increase the width of the web of the shoe to provide increased protection to the margins of the sole (Figure 12.18). The thickness of the shoe is related to the rate at which it is expected to wear and to a lesser extent the rigidity needed to prevent the shoe from losing shape. The height that the shoe raises the foot off the ground also is influenced by the thickness of the shoe, but this is usually a secondary consideration.

Several common modifications are made to the ground surface of the shoe by forging, and some modifications can be made with an electrical grinder. Softening the 90° angles at the junction of the shoe's ground surface and outer margin by beveling or rounding, called safing, increases the ease of break-over. A shoe with a rounded outside perimeter is thought to

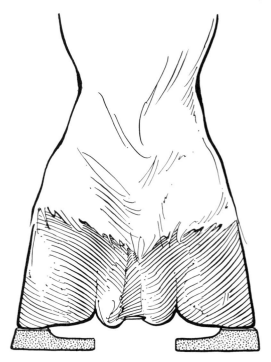

Figure 12.18. A wide-web shoe with a concave solar surface protects the sole without applying pressure to it.

improve the ease of break-over in any direction. A similar modification used by the author is achieved by using a half-round shoe, which is made from half-round bar stock that resembles a semi-circle in cross-section (Figure 12.19). Half-round shoes can be purchased, but the semi-circle does not have the same curvature as a shoe made from bar stock.

The toes of flat shoes frequently are rolled or beveled only at the toe to improve the ease of break-over. For enhancement of break-over, the author uses a grinder and starts the roll at the inner margin of the ground surface of the horseshoe and creates a tapered roll from this point to the outer margin. This decreases the thickness of the outer margin of the shoe by half the thickness of the material (Figure 12.20).

A similar effect can be achieved by rockering the toe, which is accomplished by bending the full thickness of the toe area of the shoe proximally. When rockering the toe of a horseshoe it is important to leave sufficient hoof wall mass at the toe to accommodate the rocker created in the horseshoe with the end result being an intimate fit between the shoe and the toe area of the foot. This intimate relation is created by burning the rocker in to the toe or by using a hoof rasp to create the bevel in the toe of the hoof to accept the rocker in the shoe. Less commonly, a flat shoe may be asymmetrically beveled or rounded to improve the ease of break-over toward a given side of the shoe to encourage a horse to break-over toward that side and direct or accommodate the flight of the foot. Rounding the outer margin of the medial branch of a shoe on the ground surface of the shoe with a hammer or grinder is called boxing. See Table 12.2 for a list of commonly used farrier terms.

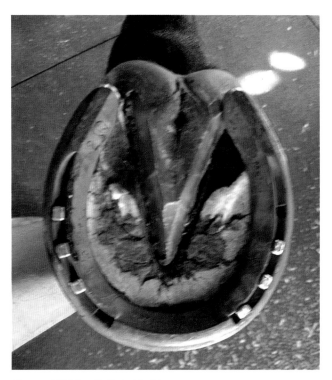

Figure 12.19. Half-round shoe.

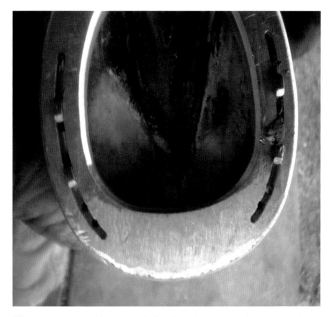

Figure 12.20. Using a grinder, break-over can be created in any shoe beginning at the inner margin of the shoe.

There is little traction between the flat surface of a steel or aluminum shoe and the ground. Grooves are created in the ground surface of the shoe, called fullering or creasing, to increase traction. A similar modification in racing or training plates is termed swedging. The fullering in the horseshoe becomes compacted with dirt; the friction between the dirt in the fullering and the dirt on the ground is greater than steel on dirt, thus aiding in traction. In addition, the nail heads are embedded within the crease with 1 to 2 mm of the nail head protruding above the crease, which also aids traction and helps to keep the nails tight.

The full circumference of the shoe may be fullered as in the concave shoe, or it may be limited to the branches of the shoe and less frequently just the toe. Fullering a single branch of the shoe enhances traction on one side and delays break-over on that side of the foot. When the branches of the shoe are fullered, the nail holes are centered in the groove, which conforms with the inside and outside of the nail heads. A classic example of a shoe that uses 2 of these modifications is a half round, half-swedge shoe worn on the hindfeet by harness horses. The inner branch is half round in cross-sectional profile and the lateral branch of the shoe is swedged. Thus, the medial branch, enhanced by the half round, breaks over rapidly, whereas the break-over of the lateral branch is delayed by the swedge.

The only common modification to the solar surface of the shoe is beveling of the inner half of the web toward the inside with a hammer or a grinder, called seating out or concaving. Horses with flat, thin soles benefit from a seated-out or concave shoe to decrease pressure on the sole adjacent to the wall. Safing decreases the likelihood of the shoe being stepped on by another foot and pulled off. Boxing the heels allows the farrier to fit the shoes with more expansion (width) at the heels without a ledge being present, which can easily be stepped on by another foot.

Clips are triangular-shaped projections that extend proximally from the periphery of the shoe (Figure 12.21). Clips are preformed on manufactured shoes or they may be forged in the shoe at the time of fitting. When a shoe is fitted, the outer surface of the clip is congruent with the surface of the hoof wall. Movement between the shoe and the hoof capsule is reduced, which decreases the shear stress on the hoof nails. A single clip placed in the center of the toe or side clips placed at the toe quarters can be used on fore shoes, while side clips placed at the toe quarters or quarters are generally used on the hind shoes. Clips may be positioned elsewhere around the periphery of the shoe when additional stability of the hoof capsule is necessary.

Extensions

An extension on a horseshoe is any projection of the shoe that extends outward beyond the perimeter of the foot in the horizontal plane. Extensions may be placed anywhere around the circumference of the foot. They may be forged into a shoe or welded onto the outside margin. An extension such as a wide lateral heel branch in a hind shoe is available as a manufactured shoe. A similar effect is obtained by using an oversized shoe fitted either forward or backward or by setting one branch of the shoe wide.

Every extension has the potential to cause the shoe to act as a lever. This lever action may be static, when the animal is not moving and the is foot bearing weight, or dynamic, particularly during the landing and break-over phases of the stride. When force is exerted on the extension by the ground, the forces are increased in the adjacent wall and decreased in the opposite wall as the point of action of the GRF shifts. In addition to

TABLE 12.2. Basic farriery terms.

Term	Definition or explanation
Forging	The act of changing the shape of a piece of steel by heating it in a forge and hammering it on an anvil.
Bar shoe	A horseshoe that is joined from 1 side to the other, commonly in the heel region. Common types are the straight-bar, egg-bar, heart-bar, patton-bar, and Z-bar.
Patton-bar Shoe	A shoe forged with marked heel elevation to allow the weight to be taken off the soft tissue structures in the back of the foot.
Square toe	A modification of a horseshoe in which the toe area is made flat to influence the break-over of the foot and decrease the amount of shoe and toe in the dorsal part of the foot. The square toe is generally limited to the hindfeet in most shoeing disciplines.
Rolled toe	A modification in which a bevel is created in the toe of the shoe to enhance break-over. Does not involve the plane on the bottom of the horse's hoof.
Rocker toe	A modification to the toe of a shoe in which a portion of the web at the toe of the shoe is bent toward the foot to enhance break-over. Involves the plane on the bottom of the horse's hoof.
Fullering	Through forging, a crease is cut into the web of a shoe with a handled chisel called a fuller or creaser. The crease is used for traction and the placement of nails. Also referred to as creasing.
Swedging	The act of hammering a piece of hot bar stock through a die that creates a swedge in the steel. The swedge created by the die is a V- shaped crease with a ridge on either side.
Boxing	Forging, grinding, or rasping a bevel on the hoof surface of the shoe where it extends beyond the perimeter of the foot.
Safing	Forging, grinding, or rasping a bevel on the ground surface of the shoe.
Clip	A small projection of metal on the outside perimeter of the shoe that extends up the hoof wall and takes the shearing strain off of the horseshoe nails.
Trailer	Extends the lateral heel of a hind shoe beyond the perimeter of the foot at the heel at an angle axial to the midline of the foot. Has a directional influence on the landing pattern and break-over of that foot. Not performed on the medial side or the front shoes for safety reasons.
Seating-out	Refers to forging, grinding, or rasping away the thickness on the inside, hoof surface of a horseshoe. Often done to avoid sole pressure or relieve sole pressure in flat and bruised hooves.
Floating	A section of the foot that has been trimmed such that there is no contact between the hoof wall and the shoe. A bar shoe is generally necessary for this procedure to be effective.
Jamming	Refers to any area around the circumference of the coronary band that has been displaced proximally relative to the remainder of the coronary band. Proximal displacement of the coronary band may be a more appropriate term.
Web	The width of the bar stock used to make a horseshoe or the width of the horseshoe.
Wide web	Refers to a width of stock that is larger than the normal factory-made shoe.
Expansion	The portion of the shoe that extends beyond the perimeter of the foot, generally from the widest point of the foot palmarly or plantarly. Shoes that have a lot of expansion are considered to be "fit full."
Stud	Small insert added to a shoe for traction or wear-ability. Studs are generally driven into a shoe or screwed into holes that are tapped in the shoe. Studs are available in many shapes, styles, and materials
Half round	Bar stock or manufactured shoes that have a cross section such as one-half of a circle. The flat portion of the stock goes against the hoof, while the rounded portion makes the ground surface.
Pour-ins	In farriery, this refers to the act of pouring a deformable material into the cavity in the solar surface of the foot between the branches of the shoe. Pour-ins can used to provide protection and have replaced pads in many therapeutic applications.

(Courtesy of Chris Gregory, CJF, FWCF)

1192

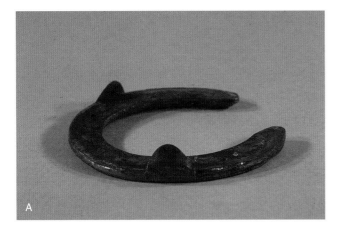

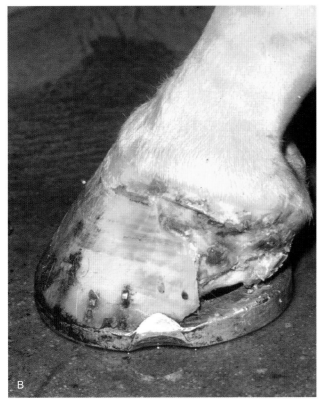

Figure 12.21. A steel shoe with quarter clips (A) and a clipped aluminum shoe used to stabilize the hoof wall after removal of a hoof avulsion (B).

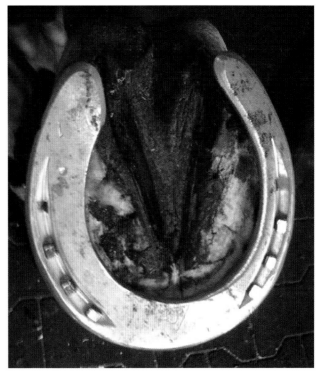

Figure 12.22. Shoe with one branch wider than the other, showing the flotation effect on one side of the foot.

acting as levers, extensions increase the surface area available for ground contact, which decreases the amount of shoe that descends into soft footing at that point in the circumference of the foot. The term floating, or flotation, refers to the web width of a section of the shoe that limits the amount of this part of the shoe that descends into soft footing (Figure 12.22).

Lateral or medial extensions may be used to force the opposite wall of the hoof capsule to the ground or support the wall adjacent to the extension. In doing so, the lever decreases the compression in the opposite wall and increases the compression in the side of the hoof on which the extension is being used. Heel extensions frequently are used on one side of the foot or bi-axially

(Figure 12.23). When used in performance horses, extensions are continuations of the heel of the shoe and are called trailers.

Trailers are used almost exclusively on the lateral branch of hind shoes. Egg-bar shoes that extend palmar/plantar to the heels of the hoof capsule act as heel extensions. They are most commonly used on the front feet but can also be used on the hindfeet when necessary. Force applied on the butt of an egg bar shoe decreases the moment about the DIP joint and the tension in the DDFT. Therefore, horses convalescing from a DDFT injury may benefit from heel extensions used in conjunction with some type of heel elevation. The egg-bar shoe acts as a palmar extension and when the horse is on a soft surface it reduces the sinking of the heels into the surface at the beginning of the stride and acts as a heel wedge during the support phase of the stride.[5] On the other hand, egg-bar shoes can be fitted too long and the extension beyond the heels acts as a lever, causing excess pressure on the heels of the hoof capsule. Heel wedges are known to decrease the force on the navicular bone.[5] The consequence of this benefit is that it is often used on horses with damaged heels and the heels are then placed under greater compressive stress. Heel extensions alter the way the foot strikes the ground. If, as happens frequently, the heels are closer to the ground at impact, the extension or butt of the egg-bar contacts the ground first. A lateral trailer, either in line with or diverging up to 45° from the mid-sagittal plane of the foot, forces the foot to pivot toward the side of the trailer as the foot lands. The toe of the foot is directed laterally after impact and break-over is redirected.

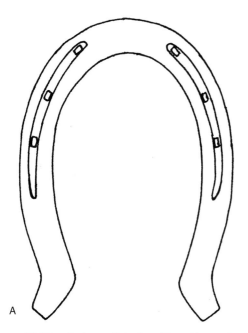

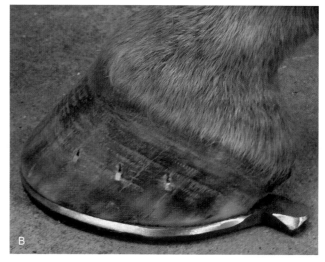

Figure 12.23. A shoe with trailers (A) and its application on the right hindfoot of a horse (B). The trailer should be as long as the width of the horse shoe.

Bar Shoes

A bar is the part of a shoe that extends from one branch of a shoe toward the other, forming a closed unit. In a complete bar shoe, one branch extends to the other. In a partial bar shoe, the bar extends part of the way across the shoe. Most bars extend from one heel to the other to form a closed shoe. A bar may extend from one quarter to the other, or even diagonally across the shoe. Several patterns of complete bar shoes are commonly used, including the straight bar, egg-bar, heart-bar, heart-bar–egg-bar (or full-support shoe), and Z-bar shoe (Figure 12.24).

Indications for a bar shoe include increased stability to the hoof capsule, increased ground surface area, local protection, recruitment of additional weight-bearing area of the foot, and ability to unload a section of the foot. Some type of bar shoe is frequently used, often in conjunction with other shoeing methods, to increase stability within the hoof capsule or distal phalanx. Bars that extend palmar/plantar to the normal position of the heel of the shoe act as a palmar/plantar extension. Bars that are set under the ground surface of the foot can be adjusted to protect that part of the foot from ground contact, apply pressure to that part of the foot, unload that part of the foot, or recruit that part of the foot for weight-bearing. A straight-bar shoe may decrease pressure on the palmar/plantar third of the frog and protect the underlying navicular bone. The heart-bar shoe is used to recruit or increase the role of the frog in weight-bearing, thus using the frog to create a weight-sharing relationship with the hoof wall and laminar interface. Heart-bar shoes also may be used to support the palmar/plantar aspect of the foot to reduce the stress in the adjacent wall and permit unloading of one or both heels.

A partial bar shoe extends part of the way across the ground surface of the foot, most commonly from one

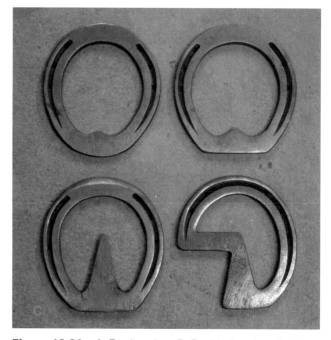

Figure 12.24. A. Egg-bar shoe. B. Straight-bar shoe. C. Heart-bar shoe. D. Z-bar shoe. (Courtesy of Jeff Ridley, CJF.)

heel onto the frog, which increases or reduces weight-bearing on a single heel. Farriers refer to this type of shoe as a half-bar or G-bar shoe. The bar of a Z-bar shoe is shaped with 2 90° bends that are incorporated into a three-quarter shoe, so that one leg of the Z is attached to the heel of one branch and the other is attached to the quarter of the opposite branch. It is very important that when the Z-bar shoe is fabricated, a frog plate is used to recruit the frog to share the load.

Traction Devices

Various devices can be added to the ground surface of a shoe to increase traction. Traction devices also can influence the speed and direction of landing and break-over. Calks are projections of almost any size and shape—although most are round, square, or rectangular—on the ground surface of a shoe (Figure 12.25). Blocks, stickers, and studs, made of steel or steel with a tungsten carbide core, are all different types of traction devices or calks. Toe grabs on racing plates are essentially curved, elongated calks. Borium, tungsten carbide particles in a brass matrix, is brazed onto the surface of a shoe with an acetylene torch to create a roughened surface to prevent slippage as well as wear of the shoe. Horseshoe nails with tungsten on the heads can be used to attach the shoe and simultaneously apply traction. These nails are helpful in cold areas with ice and snow.

Some calks are permanent, whereas others are temporary and can be removed. Permanent calks are forged into the heel of the shoe, molded into the shoe at the time of manufacture, or welded or brazed onto the shoe at the time of fitting. Drive-in calks are semi-permanent (can be changed if necessary) and are driven into a pre-drilled hole in the shoe. Temporary calks, called screw-in calks or studs, are screwed into drilled holes that have been tapped so they can be inserted and removed as needed. Plastic inserts or cotton can be used to plug the hole when not in use. The size and shape of the studs may be changed with the various athletic pursuits or ground conditions. Calks may be positioned at any point around the circumference of the shoe. The choice of whether to use calks, which type to use, and where to position them is usually is based on the trainer's and farrier's preference. Bilateral heel calks typically are used on jumpers and event horses. Racehorse plates may be equipped with toe grabs, with or without 1 or 2 heel calks (blocks or stickers). Draft animals usually have shoes with biaxial heel calks and less frequently a large toe calk.

Any traction device placed on the surface of the shoe inevitably alters the mechanics of the foot by altering the way it contacts the ground. The harder the ground surface or the taller the calk, the greater the effect. Calks concentrate stress in the wall immediately proximal to the calk. Therefore, the lowest, broadest calk compatible with adequate traction is recommended. A single calk at either the heel or toe alters mediolateral and dorsopalmar orientation. A single heel calk acts in much the same way as an extension or trailer, causing the foot to turn toward the side with the calk as the foot lands. Symmetrical placement of 2 pairs of calks, 1 pair on either side of the toe and 1 pair at the heels, encourages the foot to break-over in the center of the toe.

PLACEMENT AND APPLICATION OF THE SHOE

When a shoe is placed on the ground surface of a horse's foot, the horse is no longer standing on its foot; rather, it is standing on a shoe. Therefore, it is logical to place a shoe with biological congruency such that it is an extension of the trimmed foot. For example, most horses have a natural wear pattern on the toe of the front shoe; therefore, the shoe should incorporate some form of break-over enhancement to simulate the animal's natural wear pattern. If the shoe is considered an extension of the properly trimmed foot, it should be accurately fitted to the outline of the properly prepared hoof wall with the shoe placed central to the widest part of the foot (Figure 12.26). The shoe should be constructed from the lightest and simplest material that provides traction, protection, and adequate support to the foot for the work being performed.

The ground surface of the foot and the solar surface of the shoe must be flat and level to provide a tight fit between the surfaces. The shoe is fitted so that its outer margin closely follows the perimeter of the hoof wall from the toe to the last nail hole in the shoe. From the last nail hole to the end of the branch, the shoe should extend 0.0625 cm to 0.125 cm beyond the wall; or this distance can be varied according to the conformation of the foot. This protrusion of the shoe beyond the hoof wall is termed expansion.

The shoe should be placed (or the nail holes punched such that they allow the nails to be placed) in the white line. Nail hole location is important to prevent interference with the movement of the palmar/plantar foot—the last nail hole in the branch of the shoe should be located at or forward of the widest part of the foot. The abaxial end of the branch at the heel should be rounded to provide sufficient space between the frog and branches of the shoe to pass a hoof pick. The solar surface of the shoe can be concaved toward the inner margin to prevent sole pressure. The fitted shoe should lie central to the widest part of the foot with similar approximate distances from this point to break-over and from this

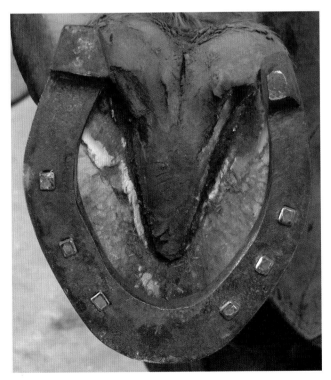

Figure 12.25. A roadster shoe with a lateral heel calk and a medial wedge to improve traction. (Courtesy of Jeff Ridley, CJF.)

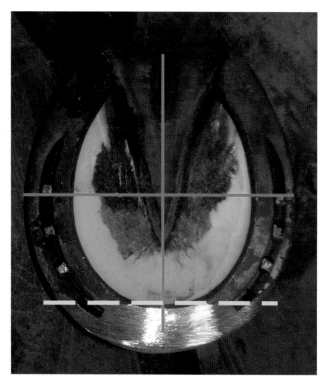

Figure 12.26. The shoe is fitted such that the widest part of the foot is located in the middle of the shoe (red lines). Note the break-over created in the shoe (dotted yellow line).

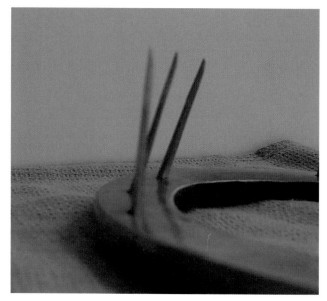

Figure 12.27. Nail pitch. Note the slope of the first 2 nails and the decreased pitch of the heel nail.

point to the base of the frog. If the heels of the hoof capsule are damaged or do not correlate with the base of the frog, the branch of the shoe can be used to increase the ground surface of the foot by extending the branch to the frog. If the shape of the solar surface of the foot is not ideal, the shoe should be fitted to provide even distribution of weight and, when possible, the shoe should be placed to accentuate the ideal shape.

Preparing the nail holes and driving the nails is often an overlooked part of farriery. If the hoof capsule is thought of as a cone, the necessity of driving the nails at the same angle becomes apparent. In this regard, hand-forged shoes provide an advantage of being able to angle the nail holes when the shoe is punched; this is called nail pitch (Figure 12.27). The nail holes in manufactured or machine shoes are stamped in bulk, so the opening on the solar surface of the shoe is closer to the outer margin of the shoe and the nail hole is not angled. When a nail is placed through a nail hole, the shank of the nail exits straight rather than being angled to the slope of the hoof capsule. This prevents the nail from gaining solid purchase and height within the hoof wall. Low nailing is usually a precursor to cracks and fissures in the hoof wall. This should and can be easily corrected by re-punching the nail hole at an angle and by back punching the nail hole on the solar surface of the shoe.

Back punching is accomplished by using a pritchel placed on an angle adjacent to the inner side of the nail hole and directed toward the outer side of the shoe. The pritchel is used to create a small notch by removing a

tiny piece of steel or aluminum material from the opening. This allows a nail inserted in the re-punched hole to immediately assume an appropriate angle.

The nail head must also have a tight fit within the nail hole. There should be no movement of the nail shank when the nail head is tapped down in the nail hole because movement will cause the shoe to loosen shortly after it is applied. If movement occurs, either a different nail with a different style of nail head should be used or the nail hole should be altered to accommodate the desired style of nail. The fewest number of nails and the smallest size of nail that will hold the shoe securely in place during the shoeing interval should be used to attach the horseshoe.

The horseshoe nail is unique in that there is a bevel next to the point that forms a short, single-sided wedge with the slanting side directed from within to without. On the same side of the bevel there is a pattern or trademark located on the head of the nail that can be seen and felt. To be driven into the foot properly, the bevel and roughened side of the nail head must face toward the inside or mid-sagittal section of the foot. Another way to remember this is that the frog must be able to see the pattern on the head of the nail. If the nail is placed with the bevel to the outside, the nail will not exit the hoof wall and may enter the sensitive structures of the foot.

Before nailing the shoe, the author removes a thin slice of sole adjacent to the white line from quarter to quarter to discourage sole pressure. Two or 3 nails are driven into each branch of the shoe without excessive pounding, paying strict attention to the sinking and sound of the nail as it is driven through the hoof wall. Nails should be driven in the direction in which it is desired that they pass through the hoof wall and exit approximately 2 cm above the junction of the shoe and the hoof or approximately one-third of the distance from the ground surface of the hoof and the coronary

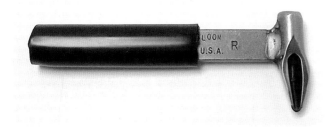

Figure 12.28. Hoof gouge. (Courtesy of FPD Farrier Products Distribution, Shelbyville, KY 40066.)

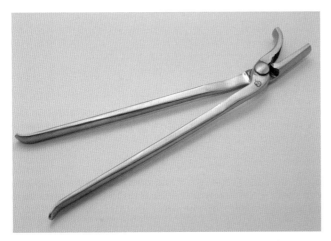

Figure 12.29. Clinching tongs. (Courtesy of FPD Farrier Products Distribution, Shelbyville, KY 40066.)

band. The ends of the nails that exit the hoof wall should be immediately wrung off or bent over against the hoof wall to prevent injury to the horse or farrier if the horse pulls its foot away. After the desired numbers of nails are placed in the shoe, the nails can be drawn up by placing a clinching block on the bent edge of the nail and striking the head of the nail with a hammer. The author does not perform this step because it often draws the shoe too tight against the sole wall junction, which can cause discomfort in a horse with a thin sole or hoof wall.

Finishing the foot is generally accomplished with the horse's foot placed on a foot stand. On the outer surface of the hoof wall, the bent ends or points of the nails should be cut with nail cutters so that approximately 3 to 4 mm of the nail protrudes, which will form the clinch. A rasp or a hoof gouge is used to clean or remove the disrupted horn from under the nail where it emerges from the hoof (Figure 12.28). Using clinching tongs, the end of the nail or clinch is pulled down firmly against the hoof wall (Figure 12.29). A clinch is sufficiently long when it equals the width of the nail at the bend. The holding power of the clinch is in the bend rather than the length of the clinch itself. Finally, the hoof wall and clinches are smoothed with a rasp and the entire area is sanded with a commercial sanding block to remove any rasp or file marks. This gives the finished hoof a natural appearance, especially if hoof dressings are applied.

NON-NAIL ALTERNATIVES IN FARRIERY

The use of various adhesives to attach shoes has become popular. The glue-on shoe can be attached to the hoof with an adhesive either by tabs or cuffs that are attached to the circumference of the shoe and extend proximally. The cuffs are made of semi-rigid plastic or synthetic cloth. Alternatively, the adhesive may be directly interposed between an aluminum shoe and the ground surface of the wall and immediately adjacent to the sole.[20] Recently, a mold has been introduced that allows a horseshoe to be formed from a composite that is applied to the ground surface of the foot.

Attaching a shoe with adhesives offers several advantages over nailing, such as when nailing is too painful, when there is insufficient wall for nailing the shoe, and as a therapeutic option. Depending on the specific application, adhesive attachment permits greater expansion of the foot. However, there are disadvantages as well. Glue-on shoes are more expensive and time consuming, and the application of adhesives to the side of the wall decreases the quality of the underlying wall over time. There is a also perception that glued-on shoes do not stay on as well as nailed-on shoes, but this impression is in part the result of poor case selection or poor application. Glue-on shoes should be considered a transient device to produce hoof mass or to treat a hoof disease or defect before reverting to traditional shoes or barefoot.

Glue-on shoeing has been used extensively since the introduction of the acrylics (polymethylmethacrylate) (Equilox International Inc., Pine Island, MN) and urethanes (Vettec Hoof Care Products, Oxnard, CA). These composites consist of a resin and a catalyst that polymerize in a matter of minutes when mixed together, forming a bond between the hoof wall and the shoe. Heat is generated in this process because it is an exothermic reaction. Once the composite has cured, it has a flexible consistency very similar to the outer hoof wall of the foot.

Indications for Glue-on Shoes

Glue-on shoes can be used for damaged hoof walls, hoof walls with poor horn consistency (especially during the summer months), or hoof walls that are thin and benefit from not using nails to attach the shoe. Occasionally, a horse will have its feet trimmed too short while being shod and become sore. In this case glue-on shoes lift the sole off the ground without placing nails in a short foot with minimal hoof wall. Soundness can be restored almost immediately.

In horses with chronic laminitis, realignment of the distal phalanx within the hoof capsule can be readily achieved with glue-on technology. Glue-on shoes permit alignment of the bottom of the distal phalanx with the ground. In white line disease, the accepted treatment is resection of the affected hoof wall along with thorough debridement. Often the farrier is left with inadequate hoof wall to attach a shoe with nails; in this case glue-on shoes provide a means to attach the shoe while leaving the resected area open for observation and daily treatment. Long-toe, underrun heel foot conformation often leads to a persistent low-grade lameness and has always

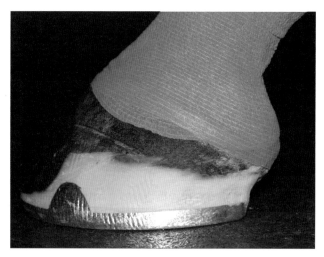

Figure 12.30. Direct method to apply a glue-on shoe in which the shoe is attached with a composite to the ground surface of the foot.

presented a challenge for veterinarians and farriers to manage. In this case, composite can be used to extend the heel further palmarly and when combined with the appropriate shoe, the extended or created heel is placed in a better functional position under the limb. Furthermore, the composite that is placed between the shoe and the foot prevents the abrasive movement of the heel of the foot against the shoe. This lack of movement prevents further wear, actually allowing re-growth of the hoof wall and bars at the heel. The composite between the foot and the shoe does not inhibit normal heel expansion and there have been no indications of contracted heels following their use.

Methods of Glue-on Farriery

There are 3 accepted methods to glue on a shoe. In the direct method, an aluminum shoe is attached with an adhesive (Equilox International, Inc., Pine Island, MN) to the ground surface of the foot (Figure 12.30). An aluminum horseshoe is preshaped to the hoof and the hoof-bearing surface of the shoe is roughened with a grinding disk to increase cohesion. A 2-part acrylic combined with fiberglass strands is used to bond the prepared shoe to the hoof wall. Meticulous attention

to preparation of the hoof is essential because the heat from the exothermic reaction may lead to an abscess and the outer hoof wall may degenerate with continued use.

The second method is the indirect method. Here, a patented aluminum, rubber-soled horseshoe is attached with a fabric cuff (Sound Horse Technologies, Unionville, PA). The appropriate size shoe is selected, the cuff is trimmed as necessary, and a composite is applied to the outer wall to bond to the cuff. Good sole depth can be attained with this shoe as the fabric cuff becomes the hoof wall, the urethane rim pad provides an interface to decrease concussion, and there is no sole pressure. However, the constrictive nature of the cuff encompassing the hoof wall must be questioned. Another indirectly applied shoe is an aluminum shoe encased in plastic with attached tabs around the circumference of the horseshoe; the shoe is glued to the hoof wall with cyanoacrylate adhesive (Equilox International, Inc., Pine Island, MN).

The third method is a new *in situ* shoe mold. Here a silicon mold is used to apply a horseshoe directly on to the surface of the hoof (QuixShoe, Dubai, United Arab Emirates). A 2-part urethane (Vettec Hoof Care Products, Oxnard, CA) is injected into the horseshoe-shaped cavity in the mold that is placed on the bearing surface of the hoof. Once the injected composite is set, the mold is removed and the cast horseshoe is attached to the hoof. Because the product originates as a liquid form and the molds are generic to standard-shaped feet of similar sizes, the shoe can be custom made for the individual hoof. Making a new mold for a specific foot or shoe can be time consuming and this technique has not been tested extensively under different conditions.

Glue-on shoes can be expensive and time consuming to apply. Success depends on proper hoof wall preparation, shoe fit, and composite application. Glue-on shoes should not be used to replace the necessary farrier skills that are used to resolve difficult foot cases, nor should glue-on technology be used to replace the basic fundamentals of proper horseshoeing.

All composites cure with an exothermic reaction; therefore, caution should be exercised when repeatedly applying these products to a thin or compromised hoof wall because the long-term effects on the hoof wall have not been determined. Nevertheless, glue-on shoe technology offers another option to attach horseshoes to the ground surface of the equine hoof when a non-nailing, nontraumatic alternative is indicated.

FARRIERY FOR COMMON HOOF PROBLEMS

Stephen E. O'Grady

CONDITIONS OF THE FOOT THAT RESPOND TO FARRIERY

The biomechanics of therapeutic shoeing and its scientific application have been described by Dr. Parks in chapter 8. In this section the basic principles of farriery will be applied to abnormal hoof conformation or hoof distortion and common hoof problems encountered in equine practice. The three types of hoof conformation that will be considered are the long toe, under-run heel, the club foot and the horse with sheared heels.

Long-toe, Low-heel Foot Conformation

A long toe/low or underrun heel conformation is defined as the angle of the heels being considerably less than the angle of the dorsal hoof wall. When this difference in angles is considerable, it is characterized by a broken back-hoof-pastern axis—the angle of the dorsal hoof wall is lower than the angle of the dorsal pastern. It is often the result of leaving the heels too long when trimming, which allows them to grow forward and lose their angle. This type of foot configuration is so common in equine practice, especially in Thoroughbred horses, that it is thought to be normal. In one study of foot-related lameness, it was found in 77% of the horses[8] and in another study of normal performance horses this condition was found in 52% of the horses.[14]

A low hoof angle results in dorsiflexion of the DIP joint, concentrates weight-bearing on the palmar section of the foot, and increases strain on the DDFT. This excess load, in turn, may cause increased stresses on the navicular apparatus and the soft tissue structures associated with the palmar foot. Excessive toe length is thought to delay the speed of break-over. This abnormal hoof conformation may contribute to palmar foot pain, chronic heel bruising, coffin joint synovitis, quarter and heel cracks, and interference problems. There is also experimental evidence that a low hoof angle compromises circulation in the heel area of the foot.[7]

The terms long-toe, low-heel (LT-LH) and long-toe, underrun heels are often use interchangeably; however, it may be helpful to distinguish between the two. In the case of a low heel, the angle of the heel is markedly lower than the angle of the dorsal hoof wall; however, the structure of the heel is relatively good in that the buttress, angle of the sole, tubular horn, and bars are intact, forming a base. In the underrun heel, the structure of the heels is compromised such that the hoof wall at the heels is thin, separated, and rolled under in an axial direction, the angle of the sole is missing, the bars are destroyed, and the heel-ground contact does not reach the base of the frog.

As low or underrun heels progress, this condition can be readily observed both visually and radiographically; the point at which the angle that the hoof capsule or

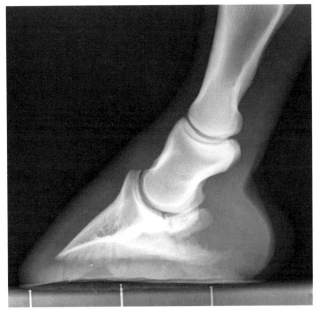

Figure 12.31. Lateral radiograph revealing a negative palmar angle to the distal phalanx. Note the lack of mass under the palmar process of the distal phalanx.

the distal phalanx forms with the ground is lower palmarly/plantarly than it is dorsally. A common error in routine farriery is not continually moving the ground surface of the hoof wall at the heels or the branch of the shoe to or toward the base of the frog. A negative palmar angle, as noted radiographically, means that the soft tissue structures (frog, digital cushion) are underdeveloped or have decreased in mass, usually due to damage, or they have prolapsed palmarly (Figure 12.31).[18] This type of hoof conformation alters the mechanics of the foot as the compromised heels lose the ability to accept weight and dissipate the energy of impact.

The treatment of low or underrun heels is difficult, and often the conformation of the heels can only be maintained rather than improved. The traditional treatment for underrun heels is to use an egg bar shoe, often accompanied by some form of heel elevation to raise the angle of the heels and correct the broken back-hoof-pastern axis that is associated with this condition. Traditionally, these shoes have been fit back to the bulbs of the heels with the idea that the increased ground surface of the shoe supports the palmar section of the foot and the egg bar supports the heels, thus correcting the problem. It is questionable whether support can be applied to compromised structures (heels) that no longer have the ability to accept weight. The egg bar shoe moves the GRF palmarly but in doing so acts as a moment arm or lever on the heels, creating excessive pressure. The egg-bar shoe places the bulk of the weight-bearing on the soft structures of the palmar foot with limited mass, which prevents further hoof wall growth at the coronet.

Farriery for this condition should be directed at using all of the structures in the palmar foot to share the load and elevate the heels as necessary. Various techniques have been successful, depending on the amount and integrity of the structures present. Foot preparation begins by visualizing the 2 basic landmarks on the ground surface of the foot: the widest part of the foot and the base of the frog. The palmar section of the foot is trimmed appropriately using the widest part of the foot as a starting point, and the heels are trimmed to healthy horn making sure that all of the structures of the heel and the frog are on the same plane. The toe is shortened accordingly, again using the widest part of the foot as a guideline. With LT-LH conformation, the frog is often situated lower than or below the level of the hoof wall at the heels. When a prolapsed frog is present, the shoe should be removed, excess horn trimmed from the frog, and the horse stood on a hard surface such as a rubber stall mat for 24 hours. An alternative to this is to fabricate a frog pad from a full wedge pad to place focal pressure on the frog, tape it on the foot, and stand the horse on a hard surface. This creates a level, flat surface in the palmar foot with all structures on the same plane. Following the trim, the heels are assessed with regard to the structural integrity and the structural mass present.

The trim is complemented by a shoe that attempts to place the load over the entire palmar foot, not just on the hoof capsule at the heels (load sharing concept), and provides the heel elevation to correct the hoof-pastern axis. If the structures of the heel are intact and the hoof wall angle simply needs to be raised, an open aluminum wedge shoe or an open steel or aluminum flat shoe with a bar wedge can be used to achieve the desired heel angle. If the heels are damaged or compromised, a load-sharing effect can be accomplished by using a straight-bar shoe or a properly fitted heart-bar shoe with a pad or degree pad placed between the shoe and the foot. The author is reluctant to use a heart-bar show if the frog and digital cushion lack sufficient mass. An open steel or aluminum shoe with a heel plate welded between the branches of the shoe or a plastic bar wedge placed between the shoe and the foot can also be used. Holes are drilled in the heel plate or bar wedge and some form of silastic material placed underneath the plate or wedge to create a deformable interface to spread the weight-bearing function over all the structures in the palmar foot. Impression material is placed on the ground surface of the palmar foot, starting in the middle of the frog and extending palmarly as far as desired. The shoe and pad or plate are placed on the foot and the heel of the shoe is pressed into the impression material. Two nails are placed in the toe of the shoe and the foot is held off the ground until the impression material cures (Figure 12.32). Glue-on technology, especially the application in which the shoe is formed from a composite using a mold, is helpful but should not be applied long-term because damage to the hoof wall is thought to occur from the heat generated by the composite.

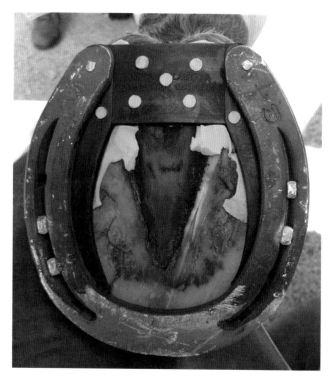

Figure 12.32. Impression material is placed in the palmar section of the foot and a pad is used to distribute the load.

Farriery for low heel conformation often is based on trial and error and combinations of various methods, and always depends on assessing the structures present, the footing, and the athletic pursuit of the horse. Any form of heel elevation should be accompanied by enhancing break-over. Moving break-over palmarly/plantarly can be accomplished in a variety of ways such as rolling or rockering the toe of the shoe or creating a rolled toe in the shoe using a hand grinder where the break-over begins at the toe quarters. Moving break-over palmarly/plantarly decreases the moment applied to the DIP joint and appears to decrease the maximum tension in the DDFT which occurs toward the end of the stance phase at the beginning of break-over.

Club Foot

A club foot is an upright conformation of the foot associated with a flexural deformity of the DIP joint. It is characterized by a broken forward-hoof-pastern axis which is a reflection of a hoof capsule where the angle of the dorsal hoof wall is higher than the angle of the dorsal pastern. This broken forward-hoof-pastern axis, or flexural deformity, is created by some degree of shortening of the musculotendinous unit (DDFT and associated muscle bellies), causing the DIP joint to be drawn into a flexed position.

Flexural deformities have been reported as a cause of decreased athletic performance and chronic low-grade lameness in the mature horse.[29] One reason is that with a shortening of the musculotendinous unit, there is a disparity of hoof wall growth with more growth at the heel than at the toe. The frog generally recedes due to excess hoof wall growth at the heels such that the energy of impact is assumed by the hoof wall, bypassing the soft tissue structures and transferring the load directly onto the bones of the digit through the laminar interface. Hoof abnormalities associated with club foot conformation are thin flat soles, poor hoof wall consistency, toe cracks, hoof wall separations, and white line disease. A high hoof angle leads to coffin joint flexion, promotes toe-first landing, and increases pressure in the dorsal section of the foot. Poor performance and injuries associated with a high hoof angle are thought to include DIP joint inflammation due to abnormal loading of the joint, sole bruising, and increased strain on the suspensory ligaments of the navicular bone.

High hoof angles with no or mild phalangeal misalignment can generally be improved by gradually lowering the heels in a tapered fashion from the apex of the frog to the heels (Figure 12.33). This increases the ground surface of the foot and attempts to re-establish weight-bearing on the entire solar surface of the foot. Break-over is moved palmarly at the same time to compensate for any increased tension in the DDFT created by lowering the heels.

Farriery for a high hoof angle with concurrent phalangeal misalignment is a greater challenge. Flexural deformities are usually diagnosed and treated while the horse is immature. However, mild flexural deformities are often ignored or treated improperly in foals. When these animals enter training, mild flexural deformities can be exacerbated by the type and the amount of exercise, ground surface, inappropriate farrier care such as improper or infrequent shoeing, or some type of underlying pathology. The object of farriery is to load the heels, compensate for the shortening of the DDFT, and improve the hoof-pastern axis when possible. Therefore, farriery is directed at lowering the heels, but the amount to remove can be hard to determine. In mild to moderate club feet, the amount of heel to be removed can be estimated by placing the thick end of a 2° or 3° pad under the toe of the foot and allowing the horse to stand on it. If the horse does not resent the tension placed on the DDFT, the thickness of the degree pad can be removed in a tapered fashion starting at the widest part

of the foot. The toe is shortened by backing up the dorsal hoof wall with a rasp. The trimmed foot is fitted with a shoe that has the break-over forged or ground into the shoe starting just dorsal to the apex of the frog and tapering toward the toe to further decrease the stresses on the DDFT.

With more advanced cases of club feet, the heels should still be lowered to load the heels and unload the toe, but heel elevation must be added to compensate for the shortening of the tendon unit. This can be determined after the trim by placing the trimmed foot palmar to the opposing limb to observe for space between the heels of the foot and the ground. The author uses a wedge shoe or places a wedge pad or a bar wedge between the heels of the foot and the shoe to compensate for the shortening of the tendon unit. This method allows the heels to be weight-bearing but at the same time decreases the stresses in the tendon unit. Break-over is applied as described above.

Severe flexural deformities can be treated by performing an inferior check ligament desmotomy combined with the appropriate farriery. See Chapter 11 for further information regarding this procedure.

Sheared Heels

Sheared heels are hoof capsule distortion resulting from displacement of one heel bulb proximally relative to the adjacent heel bulb (Figure 12.34).[28] This disparity between the lateral and medial heel bulb is generally 0.5 cm or more. When the weight of the horse is not distributed uniformly over the entire hoof during the landing phase of the stride, one focal area of the foot, usually a heel or heel and accompanying quarter, receives a disproportionate amount of the total load

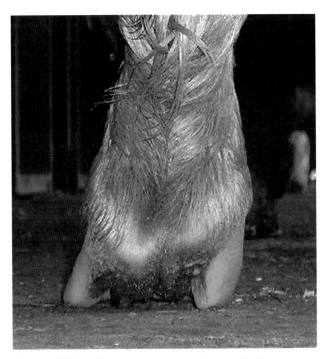

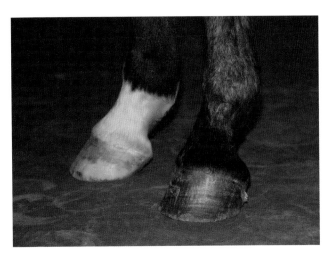

Figure 12.33. This young Warmblood has a mild club foot on the left forelimb that does not have phalangeal malalignment. Note the mismatched front feet.

Figure 12.34. Dorsopalmar view of a horse with sheared heels. Note the disparity between the length of the 2 heels and the deformation of the structures of the medial side of the foot.

during impact. The resultant force leads to a remodeling of the affected heel bulb. Although a number of sound horses have this type of hoof capsule distortion, the author believes that this type of hoof conformation can be a source of palmar foot pain in and of itself. The continual disproportionate loading and increased compressive stresses on one heel predisposes the foot to hoof capsule distortion, subsolar bruising, corns, quarter and heel cracks, fracture of the bar, deep fissures within the base of the frog, and thrush in narrow frogs. This type of foot conformation is readily observed by picking up the foot and noting the relative distances measured from the heel of the hoof capsule to the hairline at the bulbs of the heels between the lateral and medial heel.

The etiology of this condition is not completely understood. Inappropriate lateral medial orientation (balance) of the foot or a landing pattern in which the foot does not land flat has always been associated with improper trimming. However, there appears to be a correlation between limb conformations in which the limb has a rotational deformity (laterally) that changes the flight pattern of the limb and ultimately the manner in which the foot lands.[21] Furthermore, there appears to be a correlation between an offset distal phalanx and sheared heels. Commonly the distal phalanx is offset laterally within the hoof capsule rather than directly under the proximal and middle phalanges, placing additional load on the medial side of the foot with the ensuing forces causing the medial heel to displace. The unequal distribution of vertical forces on a given side of the foot over time appears to result in biological remodeling rather than the heel being pushed proximally, i.e., the heel is "growing out of shape rather than being pushed out of shape."[22]

The position of the coronary band is related to the balance between hoof wall growth at the coronary band and the rate of migration of the hoof wall distally. Furthermore, the rate of migration of the hoof wall is a balance between an active process occurring in the lamellae to cause them to move distally and the force on the wall from the ground reaction force. This appears to be the mechanism in horses with sheared heels/quarters. Displacement of the soft tissue due to mechanical stress also plays a role. To substantiate this statement, the author reviewed 50 dorsopalmar radiographs on horses with at least 1 heel bulb that was displaced proximally 0.5 cm or greater. In each case, the solar surface of the distal phalanx was horizontal (parallel) with the ground, indicating the disparity in heel height did not originate from the hoof wall located beneath the distal phalanx in the heel.

Farriery practices have always advocated trimming the horse with sheared heels so the ground surface of the foot is lower on the opposite side from the one that is being displaced proximally. Intuitively, if the heel is longer on the displaced side (measured ground surface to hairline), it is reasonable to lower the affected side. This in fact changes the landing pattern of the horse when observed in motion following this type of trim. Therefore, the author advocates trimming the heel and quarter lower on the side of the foot with the displaced heel bulb, unloading this section of the foot, and fitting a symmetrical straight-bar shoe. A wide-web steel or aluminum straight-bar shoe is fitted as symmetrically as possible underneath the long axis of the limb using the apex of the frog as a central marker.[22] The bar shoe effectively increases the surface area of the foot, provides more expansion (ground surface) on the displaced side that will have a straighter wall, and decreases the vertical movement of the heel bulbs. Before applying the shoe, the hoof wall under the affected heel and quarter that can be safely removed is trimmed away in a tapered fashion. This creates a space between the heel and the shoe that unloads the heel and quarter and allows the displaced heel to descend distally and settle into a more normal configuration (Figure 12.35). This type of selective trimming combined with a straight-bar shoe effectively decreases the disproportionate forces on the

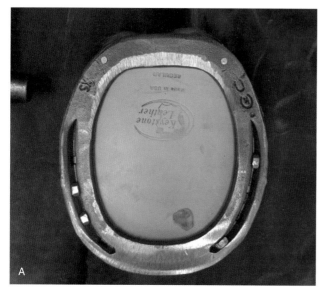 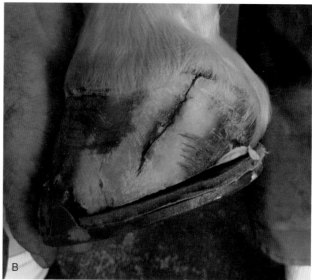

Figure 12.35. Straight bar shoe (A) with the medial heel unloaded (B). Note the quarter crack, which is often present with a sheared heel (B).

foot and allows the foot to assume a more acceptable conformation.

Note that in reviewing the common forms of abnormal hoof conformation, the guidelines or landmarks for trimming the foot can be applied to each of these situations and then used to initiate their correction.

RADIOGRAPHY AND FARRIERY

Radiography is both a diagnostic tool and an aid for assessing all structures of the foot. A radiograph is certainly not necessary for the majority of routine trimming and shoeing, but can be helpful when evaluating abnormal hoof conformation. Considerable information can be obtained from the image of the overall shape and mass of the hoof capsule, the soft tissue structures, and the position of the distal phalanx within the hoof capsule. Lack of performance or many subtle lameness conditions that are localized to the foot are caused by hoof capsule distortions, poor foot conformation, improper landing patterns, and soft tissue damage that result in inappropriate biomechanical stresses being placed on the navicular complex and the DIP joint.

Lateral to medial and dorsopalmar 0° views of the foot can be used as a precise guide to implement basic or therapeutic trimming and shoeing (Figure 12.36). From the lateral medial view, the hoof pastern axis, center of articulation, sole depth, palmar angle of the distal phalanx, break-over, and placement of the shoe can be assessed. When the solar plane of the distal phalanx shows a negative palmar angle, the need for heel elevation and the amount to apply, as well as whether the structures of the heel will accept it, can be determined. The dorsopalmar view allows the clinician to evaluate the lateral medial orientation of the distal phalanx within the hoof capsule, the position of the distal phalanx relative to the ground, and the effect of the position of the distal phalanx on the joint spaces of the digit. The need to assess the position of the hoof capsule relative to the long axis of the digit is often overlooked.

Hoof Wall Defects

Hoof wall defects constitute structural damage to the hoof capsule and can range from superficial to full thickness. The defect can be vertical occurring parallel to the horn tubules or horizontal occurring perpendicular to the horn tubules of the hoof wall. Defects or cracks can be classified according to their location in the hoof capsule, such as toe cracks, quarter cracks, and heel cracks.

A horizontal hoof wall crack originates at the coronet as a disruption of the coronary corium and moves distally as the hoof wall grows. The disruption of the coronary corium is caused by a rupture at this site, resulting from an abscess or infection or as a result of trauma to a section of the coronet. Once the coronet is healed, horizontal cracks do not generally enlarge and they grow out uneventfully. Quarter cracks are the most common hoof wall defect encountered and often cause foot lameness and/or decreased athletic performance in race and sport horses. A true quarter crack is full thickness, originates at the coronary band, and extends into the dermis of the hoof, leading to instability, inflammation, and/or infection. Quarter cracks often bleed as a result of the invasion into the dermis. Causes of quarter cracks may include trauma to the coronary band, preexisting damage to the corium from infection, abnormal hoof conformation, especially a sheared heel, short shoes, or an abnormal landing pattern when the foot strikes the ground. Any one of these causes may place continuous excessive stress or pressure on a focal area of the foot. Quarter cracks may result when these stresses exceed the hoof capsule's ability to deform. Various techniques for stabilizing and repairing quarter

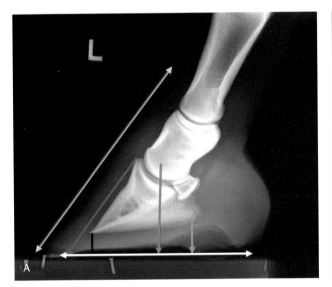 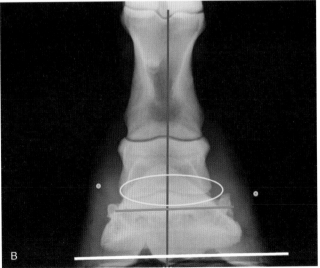

Figure 12.36. A. Lateral radiograph that illustrates hoof-pastern axis (yellow), center of articulation (red), sole depth (black) and palmar angle of distal phalanx (green), break-over (blue), and the placement of the shoe (white).

B. DP radiograph that illustrates the axial alignment of the digit (dark blue), position of the foramina in the distal phalanx relative to the ground (red), alignment of the joint space (yellow), and position of the coronary band at the heel bulbs (light blue).

cracks have been described; however, in the author's opinion, the most important aspect is to determine and correct the cause of the crack.

Farriery

The author prefers, when possible, to take the animal out of hard work and apply the necessary farriery to change the forces on the section of the foot with the defect, rather than repair the crack initially. If the appropriate farriery is applied, there will be substantial solid hoof wall growth at the next reset in 4 to 5 weeks, indicating the appropriate shoeing and trimming. Obviously, this approach is not an option in performance horses that must continue to compete.

Any abnormal hoof conformation should be evaluated and corrected. Short shoes leave insufficient ground surface under the heels and put the weight-bearing surface in front of the vertical axis of the limb. In such instances, a vertical line drawn from the origin of the quarter crack invariably coincides with the end of the shoe. The landing phase of the stride is of utmost importance. Many horses contact the ground asymmetrically, landing first on one side of the hoof and then impacting with the opposite side. This strike pattern is generally related to limb conformation and results in the sheared heel foot conformation. It is extremely rare to see a horse with a full-thickness quarter crack that is not accompanied by a sheared heel.[23] The foot is trimmed and the affected side below the crack is unloaded in the same manner as described for a sheared heel. Any horse with a full-thickness quarter crack should be placed in a bar shoe if possible. Various configurations of bar shoes such as a straight-bar, heart-bar or Z-bar shoe can be used. All of these shoes effectively increase the ground surface of the foot, provide palmar/plantar support, and decrease the independent vertical movement at the bulbs of the heels. No nails should be placed palmar/plantar to the defect in the foot.

The Repair

If the horse must continue in work, a repair should be performed along with the appropriate farriery. The objective is to stabilize the crack and promote healing. If a full-thickness crack is present, placing a composite over the defect generally does not provide stability and an implant should be placed and then covered with a composite. Infection at the origin of the quarter crack is characterized by marked lameness, pain on palpation, and a swollen, discolored coronary band above the defect. Occasionally, exudate can be expressed when digital pressure is applied to the coronet. If infection is present, the crack should be opened and bandaged with a suitable disinfectant agent for at least 48 hours before the repair.

A very easy and consistent repair technique will be described:[23] All loose undermined horn should be removed from the crack because it lacks mechanical strength. Two sets of paired 3/64-inch holes 0.25 inch apart are then drilled across from each other on either side of the crack, beginning at least 3/8 inch from the margin of the crack and ending within the depths of the trough. Stainless steel (21-gauge) wire is bent in a

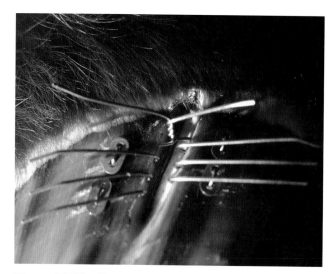

Figure 12.37. Placement of wires for a quarter crack repair.

hairpin shape 2.5 inches long and a small steel tab is placed on each wire unit (Tenderhoof Solutions, Morpeth, Ontario). One wire unit is passed through the holes from palmar to dorsal and another wire unit is passed through the opposing holes in a dorsal to palmar direction into the depth of the crack. Additional sets of wire units can be used according to the length of the defect or until the desired stabilization is achieved. The ends of all of the opposing wires are joined together and twisted until resistance is felt (Figure 12.37). The excess wire in front of the twist is cut off within the defect. The implant is then covered with an acrylic composite combined with fiberglass strands to form a patch.

Full-thickness toe cracks occur in the dorsal hoof wall extending from the coronet distally but rarely reaching the ground surface. The defect is movable; it opens when load is removed from the foot and closes when load is applied. The defect is usually associated with excessive length of the dorsal hoof wall with concavity, which can be noted with either a long toe or club foot conformation. Farriery is directed toward correcting hoof conformation if possible, decreasing the length of the toe, and shifting the weight-bearing palmarly in an attempt to unload the toe.

Unloading the toe can be accomplished by beginning the trim at the apex of the frog and trimming palmarly in a tapered manner. This creates 2 planes on the ground surface of the foot so when a shoe is placed on the foot, there will be a space between the hoof and the shoe at the toe. Farriers refer to this as floating the toe. Excess length of toe is removed from the dorsal surface of the hoof wall. Moving the break-over palmarly also helps decrease stresses in the dorsal hoof wall. The trim and application of the shoe in a manner that unloads the toe is often sufficient to stop the movement and promote healing. If further stabilization is needed, a metal or brass band can be fabricated and attached to the dorsal hoof wall with screws (Figure 12.38). The band should match the contour of the coronet and be placed at equal distances on either side of the defect. The band should be attached to the dorsal hoof wall with the foot in the

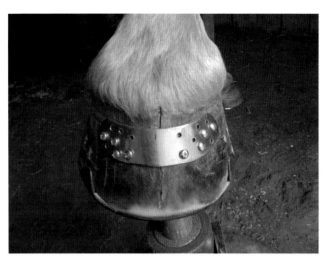

Figure 12.38. Brass band attached to dorsal hoof wall to stabilize a dorsal hoof wall defect. Note that the contour of the band matches the coronet.

unloaded position with the crack open to allow the horn papilla at the origin of the defect to produce new horn.

Heel cracks are generally associated with poor palmar foot conformation that lack mass such as low or underrun heels. This type of foot does not have sufficient ground surface under the heels to accept weight. This type of crack, although not as common as a toe or quarter crack, can recur and be difficult to treat. Some type of bar shoe is used to increase the ground surface in the palmar foot and unload the affected heel when possible. The horn in this section of the foot is generally too thin to accept an implant; therefore, the hoof wall palmar or plantar to the defect can be removed or the heel can be rebuilt using an appropriate composite.

White Line Disease

White line disease (WLD) is a keratolytic process on the solar surface of the hoof that is characterized by a progressive separation of the inner zone of the hoof wall.[24,26] The separation occurs in the nonpigmented horn at the junction between the stratum medium and stratum internum. A separation in the hoof wall is considered to be a delaminating process potentially brought on from mechanical stress, environmental conditions affecting the inner hoof wall attachment, and possibly some toxicity such as selenium.[27] The separation, which can originate at the toe, the quarter, and/or the heel, appears to be invaded by opportunistic bacteria/fungi leading to infection, which then progresses to varying heights and configurations proximally toward the coronet. This disease process always occurs secondary to a hoof wall separation.

Etiology

WLD can affect a horse of any age, sex, or breed. One or multiple hoofs may be involved and the affected hooves can be barefoot or shod. One or multiple horses on the same farm may be affected. The problem occurs worldwide. Multiple causes of white line disease have

been proposed, but none have been proven. These include excessive moisture and dryness that initiate and perpetuate separations and allow pathogens to invade, poor hygiene, and infectious organisms (bacteria, fungi, or a combination). The fact that WLD can be resolved with debridement alone further detracts from infection as a primary cause. Mechanical stress placed on the hoof wall that lead to a separation appear to be the logical cause. These include excessive toe length and various hoof capsule distortions such as long-toe, underrun heel, clubfoot, or sheared heels.

Clinical Signs and Diagnosis

White line disease presents no threat to the soundness of an animal until damage is sufficient to allow mechanical loss of the attachment between the external laminae and the inner hoof wall, resulting in displacement of the distal phalanx in a distal direction (rotation and/or sinking). In the early stages of WLD, the only noticeable change on the solar surface of the foot is a small powdery area located just abaxial to the hoof wall/sole junction. This area may remain localized or it may progress to involve a larger area of the hoof wall. As the separation becomes more extensive and extends into a quarter, a concavity (dish) can be seen forming along one side of the hoof and a bulge is present on the opposite side directly above the affected area at the coronary band. This occurs due to the loss of epidermal lamellae on the side with the separation. There may be slow hoof wall growth, poor consistency of hoof wall, and a hollow sound noted when the outer hoof wall is tapped with a hammer.[24] Often the disease goes undetected until the horse begins to show discomfort.

Radiology can be very informative and should be considered necessary. Good quality radiographs show the extent of the hoof wall separation and whether rotation of distal phalanx within the hoof capsule has occurred. They allow the clinician to differentiate between white line disease and laminitis. The radiographs can also be used as a guide when trimming and shoeing the horse.

Farriery

Correction of any hoof capsule distortion that may have contributed to the hoof wall separation is essential. Treatment for white line disease is directed toward protecting and unloading the damaged section of the foot with therapeutic farriery combined with resection of the hoof capsule overlying the affected area. Resection disrupts the continuity and weight-bearing strength of the hoof wall; therefore, some type of shoe is applied for protection, to stabilize the hoof wall, and move the weight-bearing to a nonaffected section of the foot. If the separated area of the foot is determined to be extensive, it is important to plan the method of support and the design of the shoe prior to the outer hoof wall being resected. Complete hoof wall resection (removal of outer hoof wall to expose diseased area) and debridement of all tracts and fissures in the affected area is necessary. The debridement should be continued proximally and marginally until there is a solid attachment between the hoof wall and external lamellae (Figure

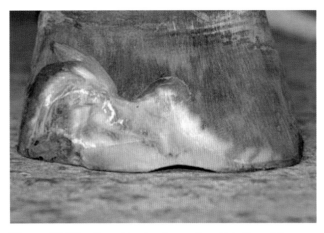

Figure 12.39. Dorsal hoof wall resection. Note the solid margins around the periphery of the resection.

12.39). The veterinarian or farrier should not reach blood during debridement.

Treatment with topical medications following hoof wall resection has been described and remains controversial.[16,24] None of the topical preparations have any proven efficacy. Disinfectants and astringents such as methiolate or 2% iodine may be helpful as a dye marker to outline the remaining tracts and aid in subsequent debridement. After thorough hoof wall resection, the affected area is left to grow out with debridement at frequent intervals. A wire brush is used daily to keep the resected area clean. The clinician should explore and debride any remaining tracts at 2-week intervals. When all tracts are resolved and grown out, a thorough examination is indicated at re-shoeing intervals every 4 to 5 weeks.

The type of shoe used and the method of attachment depend on the extent of the damaged hoof wall. Because the toe is involved in most cases of WLD, it is helpful to move the break-over in a palmar/plantar direction. The ground surface of the foot is trimmed from the apex of the frog palmarly/plantarly, thus creating 2 planes on the bottom of the foot. The shoe is fitted so break-over is placed just dorsal to the distal phalanx in an attempt to unload the dorsal hoof wall and remove the lever arm at the toe. This also stops the pinching effect that often occurs at the junction of normal hoof wall and the resection.

If the resection is extensive and/or if rotation of the distal phalanx is present, some type of bar shoe or a wooden shoe is used to stabilize the foot. An alternative method is to use a bar shoe or open shoe combined with some type of silastic material (Equilox International, Inc., Pine Island, MN). Attaching glue-on shoes to the ground surface of the foot is another useful method for shoeing the horse with WLD.[20] Acrylic repair following the resection is not recommended and should only be considered after all tracts are resolved.[24] The composite hides and/or fosters the organisms under the repair and the composite may weaken the surrounding normal hoof wall. Commitment from the owner to continue the treatment schedule for WLD as the hoof wall grows down is essential for success.

Canker

Equine canker is described as an infectious process that results in the development of a chronic hypertrophy of the horn-producing tissues.[13] It generally originates in the frog and may remain focal, but has the capacity to become diffuse and invade the adjacent sole, bars, and hoof wall. Canker can occur in one or multiple feet. The disease is commonly seen in draft breeds but can affect any breed or sex. The etiology remains elusive, but wet environmental or moist, unhygienic conditions have traditionally been thought to act as a stimulus; however, canker is commonly seen in horses that are well cared for and horses who receive regular hoof care.

Clinical Signs and Diagnosis

Canker generally originates in the frog and can be mistaken for thrush in the early stages. Thrush is limited to the lateral and medial sulci or the base of the frog if a fissure is present, whereas canker invades the horn of the frog anywhere throughout its structure. There is a proliferation of tissue with canker vs. a loss of tissue with thrush. In the early stages canker may present as a focal area of granulation tissue in the frog that bleeds easily when abraded. Canker is characterized by numerous, small, finger-like papillae of soft off-white material that resembles a cauliflower-like appearance.[15] The condition is frequently but not always accompanied by a foul odor and is covered with a caseous white exudate that resembles cottage cheese.

A presumptive diagnosis of canker is based on the gross appearance of the affected horny tissue along with a fetid odor; however, a definitive diagnosis may be confirmed with a biopsy. Histologically, the lesion is read as a chronic, hypertrophic, moist, pododermatitis of the frog.

Treatment and Prognosis

Canker always carries a guarded prognosis but recently a consistently successful treatment has been described.[13] Treatment consists of thorough, careful debridement of the affected tissue followed by a regimen of topical therapy applied daily and continued until the disease is resolved. The horse's foot is trimmed appropriately, removing all loose exfoliating sole as well as any excess toe or heel. The use of a tourniquet is essential. Debridement must be thorough and wide rather than aggressive and deep, which often removes the dermal tissue under the lesion that is necessary for cornification. Gauze sponges soaked in a solution of 10% benzyl peroxide in acetone (Franck's Pharmacy, Ocala, FL) and sprinkled with metronidazole powder are applied to the debrided area. The foot is then bandaged with a dry bandage. The affected area is cleaned daily with surgical scrub, rinsed with saline, dried with a paper towel, and the topical medication reapplied. It is crucial to keep the animal in a dry environment. Bandages are recommended until the affected area cornifies and then a shoe with a treatment plate can be used. A commitment is necessary from the owners, because aftercare takes several weeks, depending on the stage of the disease, until the affected tissue becomes cornified.

Fractures of the Distal Phalanx

Fracture of the distal phalanx is not an uncommon injury in equine practice. Although this fracture is quite common in racehorses, it can occur in any breed. Causes include racing on hard track, kicking an unyielding object, landing on blunt objects while exercising, and penetration of the hoof with a foreign body. The involvement of the DIP joint influences the outcome of the case and future soundness. Fractures that involve the articular surface usually account for increased lameness, a longer convalescence, and a poorer prognosis for a return to full athletic ability. On the other hand, nonarticular wing fractures carry a much better prognosis. See Chapter 5 for further information on distal phalanx fractures.

Affected horses show a moderate to severe supporting limb lameness that is acute in onset. Trotting on a hard surface generally accentuates the lameness. Increased digital pulse, sensitivity to hoof testers over the sole, and swelling around the coronary band are noted. With time, the sensitivity of the hoof testers becomes localized to the area of the fracture. Clinical signs are similar to those displayed by horses with a subsolar abscess or a severe sole bruise. Once the clinical examination has isolated a foot-related problem and no abscess is isolated, high-quality radiographs will often confirm a fracture. Nuclear scintigraphy often reveals the fracture in the acute stage before it becomes apparent on radiography. It is the author's opinion that digital nerve anesthesia should not be used prior to radiographs in acute lameness situations, even if clinical signs are minimal, because full weight-bearing on the foot may cause the fracture line to increase in length, become comminuted, or cause nonarticular fractures to become articular.

Farriery

The distal phalanx can be stabilized within the hoof capsule using 1 of 2 methods: a bar shoe with a continuous rim or contiguous clips or a foot cast. A straight-bar shoe with a continuous rim attached to the perimeter of the shoe, encasing the basal border of the hoof wall, prevents or limits expansion of the hoof wall, decreases the independent movement of the heels, and stabilizes the distal phalanx. The solar surface of the foot is packed with silastic material before applying the continuous rim shoe for a number of reasons. First, when any form of restrictive shoe is applied to the outer hoof wall, the foot tends to contract, especially at the heels, over a short period of time. Solar/frog support in any form appears to lessen this process quite markedly. Second, the distal phalanx descends in a distal palmar/plantar direction when weight is placed on the foot with no form of counter pressure below. Also, if the fracture is articular with the larger fragment being displaced ventrally, this added support may increase the stabilization in this direction. The full rim shoe is relatively easy to construct and has advantages over the bar shoe with side clips, which are placed randomly and apply limited focal pressure to the outer hoof wall.

The second method is to apply a foot cast. Foot casts are simple to apply and effectively stabilize the distal border of the hoof capsule. In preparation for casting, the hoof capsule should be clean and trimmed if needed. A piece of casting felt is cut to size, approximately 2 inches (5 cm) wide and long enough to extend approximately 1 to 1.5 inches dorsally from the heels both medially and dorsally, to cover the heel bulbs. The felt is positioned to cover the skin approximately 1 to 1.25 inches proximal to the heel bulbs, and may be held in place with white tape as the cast is applied. A roll of 2- or 3-inch fiberglass casting tape is then wound around the perimeter of the ground surface of the foot. Care must be taken to ensure that it does not contact the coronary band at the point at which the tape crosses over it just dorsal to the heel bulbs; either the coronary band must be protected by the casting felt or the tape cut away at the point of crossover. If needed, the concavity of the sole and the sulci may be filled with silicone putty to distribute the load of weight-bearing across the solar surface of the foot, and an acrylic may be applied to the ground surface of the cast to prevent the cast from wearing through.

Foot casts should be changed approximately every 3 weeks or as needed. The prolonged application of foot casts will cause some contraction of the foot and pressure sores on the skin immediately proximal to the heel bulbs.

Marginal fractures (type VI) occur at any site along the solar margin of the distal phalanx and are commonly secondary to another condition such as chronic sole bruising, pedal osteitis, chronic laminitis, or osteomyelitis, which may all represent a type of avascular necrosis. In general, these solar margin fractures are not of primary concern themselves, but rather an indication of another underlying condition. These horses respond to shoeing with a wide-web bar shoe that is well concaved (using a grinder or skilled forging) on the inner solar surface of the shoe.

MISCELLANEOUS CONDITIONS OF THE FOOT

Sole Bruising

Foot bruising and foot infections are 2 common causes of acute onset of severe foot lameness. Feet that lack sufficient sole depth to afford adequate protection are susceptible to bruising (Figure 12.40). Sole depth for a good foot should be greater than 15 mm and the sole should not deform when digital pressure or hoof testers are applied. Bruising can occur when the ground surface of the foot strikes a hard object or excessive trauma from working on a hard surface. It causes diffuse hemorrhage or hematoma formation in the dermal tissue above the horny sole. Clinical signs can range from mild to severe lameness, marked digital pulse, and marked response to hoof testers. Hoof tester response generally is diffuse rather than isolated to a small focal area. The diagnosis is made by ruling out the other common differentials, including laminitis, abscesses, puncture wounds, and distal phalanx fractures. The old adage of finding signs of bruising such as red discoloration in the sole of a lame horse at the time of examination or during farriery is not accurate, because these may result from previous hemorrhage in

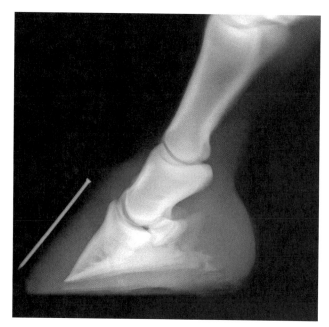

Figure 12.40. Lateral radiograph of a horse with thin soles that are prone to sole bruising.

the solar corium that has permeated into the horny sole over time.

The bruising resolves with stall confinement on deep sawdust bedding and a 3- to 5-day course of nonsteroidal anti-inflammatory drugs followed by a period of controlled exercise. The most important part of treatment is a farriery plan to improve sole depth. Farriery options include leaving the sole intact during trimming, evaluating the length of the toe when placing the shoe, modifying break-over, and adding some mild heel elevation. Placing a leather or plastic pad between the ground surface of the foot and the shoe protects the thin sole and provides comfort, but generally does not improve the structures of the foot.

Sole pressure often leads to sole bruising, and this type of bruising is usually noted shortly after the horse is trimmed or shod. In this case the hoof wall is trimmed shorter than the adjacent sole so that when a shoe is placed on the foot and clinched or when the horse stands on a hard surface, excess pressure is placed on the sole. Treatment for sole pressure is to concave the inner foot surface of the shoe to relieve the pressure on the sole or in the case of the horse without shoes, apply a shoe with the inner foot surface of the shoe concaved or deep seated to raise the solar surface of the foot off the ground.

The last form of bruising is the so-called corn, which is focal hemorrhage that occurs in the sole at the heels between the hoof wall and the bar (seat of the corn). The hemorrhage results from trauma, originates from the dermal lamellae, and appears as a small, focal, red discoloration in the seat of the corn. It may be present in one or both heels. There may be a marked hoof tester response and the source of pain can be confirmed using unilateral local anesthesia. Confusing the diagnosis are abscess, hoof wall separation, and fracture of the bars. The pressure is taken off the heel by unloading the heel with some form of bar shoe.

Hoof Abscesses

Hoof abscess, a localized accumulation of purulent exudate located between the germinal and keratinized layers of the epithelium, most commonly subsolar or submural, is probably the most common cause of acute lameness. Entry is either through a break or fissure in the sole-wall junction (white line), a misplaced nail, or a puncture wound somewhere in the solar surface of the foot. Organisms also may gain entry into the foot by way of a full-thickness hoof wall defect or crack.

Most horses with a foot abscess show an acute onset of lameness. The degree of lameness varies from being subtle in the early stages to nonweight-bearing. The digital pulse is usually bounding and with careful observation, unless the abscess is in the middle of the toe, the intensity of the digital pulse is much stronger on the side of the foot where the abscess is located. If the abscess is long-standing, there may be soft tissue swelling in the pastern or above the fetlock on the side of the limb corresponding to the side of the foot where the abscess is located. The site of pain can be localized to a small focal area through the careful use of hoof testers.

Treatment

The most important aspect of treating a subsolar/submural abscess is establishing drainage. The opening should be sufficient to allow drainage but not so extensive as to create further damage. When pain is localized with hoof testers, a small tract or fissure will commonly be found in the sole wall junction (white line). The wound or point of entry may not always be visible, because some areas of the foot such as the white line are somewhat elastic and wounds in this area tend to close. In this case, a suitable poultice should be applied to the foot daily in an attempt to soften the affected area and eventually a tract will become obvious.

The offending tract or fissure located within the sole wall junction is followed within the white line using a thin, small loop knife, hoof or bone curette, or other suitable probe (Figure 12.41). Just a small opening is

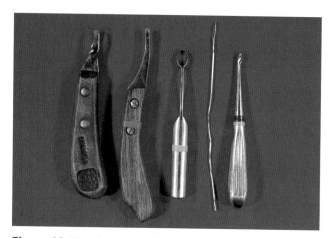

Figure 12.41. Small loop knives, hoof curettes, malleable probes, and bone curettes can be helpful to explore the foot in horses with suspected abscesses. (Courtesy of Dr. Gary Baxter.)

necessary to obtain proper drainage. Under no circumstances should a subsolar or submural abscess be approached through the sole. The application of a medicated poultice (3M Animal Care Products, St. Paul, MN) that has been soaked in hot water is applied to the foot for the first 24 to 48 hours. The author prefers the sheet version of this poultice rather than the poultice pad because the whole foot, including the coronet, should be enveloped in the poultice. Another method to encourage drainage is to apply a soak bandage. In this method, layers of practical cotton are crisscrossed to form a heavy bandage to envelope the foot. Magnesium sulfate (Epson salts) is placed in the inner foot surface of the bandage and the bandage is attached to the foot. The bandage is saturated with hot water and saturated periodically over the next 24 to 48 hours. Using either of these methods eliminates the need for continued foot soaking.

The horse should show marked improvement within 12 to 24 hours. Following the poultice or foot soak bandage, the hoof is kept bandaged with an appropriate antiseptic until all drainage has ceased and the wound is dry. The opening is filled with medicated hoof putty (Keratex Medicated Hoof Putty, Brookville, MD) and the shoe is replaced when the horse is sound. Often an abscess tract is identified but drainage cannot be established at the sole wall junction. A small vertical channel can be created adjacent to the abscess tract in the outer hoof wall using a small pair of half round nippers. Drainage can usually be established using a small probe in a horizontal plane.

Puncture Wound in the Sole

Another common cause of perceived subsolar abscesses is penetration of any region of the horny sole by a sharp object. This is not actually an abscess but rather a diffuse infection caused by the solar corium being inoculated with organisms from the penetrating object. Pain is immediate and usually followed by infection within 3 days. Using the hoof testers for guidance, the site of the puncture wound is easily identified. Drainage is the treatment of choice and the wound is opened carefully in a conical configuration using a small, thin loop knife.[11] The conical shape prevents the wound from closing prematurely and prevents dermal tissue from prolapsing and becoming trapped in the wound. The foot is bandaged with an appropriate antiseptic and use of systemic antibiotics is at the discretion of the clinician. When the wound has cornified, a shoe with a pad between the foot and the shoe is applied. Puncture wounds into the soft tissue structures of the foot are discussed further in Chapter 5.

Nail Abscess

Another form of abscess results from a horseshoe nail driven deep to the stratum corneum into dermal tissue. Dermal tissue can be inoculated by bacteria from a misplaced nail in 2 ways. First, the nail can be driven directly into the laminar corium. When the nail enters dermal tissue, the horse shows discomfort as the nail is driven into the foot and there is hemorrhage present where the nail exits the outer hoof wall. Blood observed at the exit of the offending nail alerts the farrier of the misplaced nail. The blood also acts as a physiologic rinse to dilute or eliminate bacterial contamination. Removal of the nail and application of an appropriate antiseptic usually prevent infection.

The second scenario that occurs frequently is when the farrier is driving a nail; the horse shows pain, indicating the nail is invading sensitive tissue. The farrier then generally removes the nail, places it in another spot or direction, and again drives it into the foot. The original nail (even if removed) may inoculate the dermis with organisms and contribute to an abscess. If the nail has entered the foot inside the sole–wall junction (white line), the owner should be alerted by the farrier to potential problems. To avert an abscess, the horse may be placed on a broad-spectrum antibiotic for 3 to 5 days as a prophylactic measure.

Finally, there is a "close nail," in which the nail is placed such that it lies against the border of the dermal corium just inside the hoof wall. Pressure against the corium—the movement of the horse combined with the organisms introduced with the nail—leads to an abscess as described above. There is usually a lag period of 7 to 14 days or even longer before clinical symptoms or lameness are observed. Treatment again revolves around removing the nail and establishing drainage.

References

1. Bach O, Butler D, White K, et al. Hoof balance and lameness: Improper toe length, hoof angle, and mediolateral balance. Compend Contin Educ Pract Vet 1995;17(10):1275–1282.
2. Bach O, White K, Butler D, et al. Hoof balance and lameness: Foot bruising and limb contact. Compend Contin Educ Pract Vet 1995;17(12):1505–1506.
3. Bach O, White K, Butler D. Factors involved in balancing equine hooves. J Am Vet Med Assoc 1991;198:180–9.
4. Butler KD. The prevention of lameness by physiologically-sound horseshoeing. Proceedings Am Assoc Equine Pract 1985;31: 465–475.
5. Chateau C, Deguerce C, Denoix JM. Effects of egg-bar shoes on the 3-dimensional kinematics of the distal forelimb in horses walking on a sand track. Equine Vet J Suppl. 2006;36:377.
6. Colles C. Interpreting radiographs 1. The foot. Equine Vet J 1983;15:297–303.
7. Colles C. Concepts of blood flow in the etiology and treatment of navicular disease. Proceedings Am Assoc Equine Pract 1983;29:265–270.
8. Curtis S. Farriery—Foal to race horse. R and W Publications, Newmarket, 1999, pp 1–11.
9. Dabareiner RM, Carter GK. Diagnosis, treatment and farriery for horses with chronic heel pain. Vet Clin North Am Equine Pract. 2003;19:2:417–428.
10. Denoix J-M. Functional anatomy of the equine interphalangeal joints. Proceedings Am Assoc Equine Pract 1999;41:174–177.
11. Fitzgerald BW, Honnas CM. Management of wounds in the foot. In Current Therapy in Equine Medicine, 6th ed. Robinson NE, ed. WB Saunders, Philadelphia, 2008, pp 535–540.
12. Hickman J, Humphrey M. Hickman's Farriery, 2nd ed. J.A. Allen, London, 1988, pp 136–175.
13. Honnas CM, O'Brien TR, Linford RL. Distal phalanx fractures in horses: A survey of 274 horses with radiographic assessment of healing in 36 horses. Vet Radiology 1988;29:98–107.
14. Kobluk C, Robinson R, Gordon B, et al. The effect of conformation and shoeing: A cohort study of 95 Thoroughbred racehorses. Proceedings Am Assoc Equine Pract 1989;35:259–274.
15. Leach DH, Da AI. A review of research on equine locomotion and biomechanics. Equine Vet J 1983;15:2:93–102.
16. Moyer W. Hoof wall defects: Chronic hoof wall separations and hoof wall cracks. Vet Clin North Am Equine Pract. 2003;19: 2:463–477.

17. O'Grady SE, Poupard DE. Proper physiologic horseshoeing. Vet Clin North Am Equine Pract. 2003;19:2:333–344.

18. O'Grady SE. Strategies for shoeing the horse with palmar foot pain. Proceedings Am Assoc Equine Pract 2006;52:209–214.

19. O'Grady SE. Basic farriery for the performance horse. Vet Clin North Am Equine Pract. 2008;24:1:203–218.

20. O'Grady SE, Watson E. How to glue on therapeutic shoes. Proceedings Am Assoc Equine Pract 1999;45:115–119.

21. O'Grady SE. Shoeing management of sheared heels. In Current Therapy in Equine Medicine, 5th ed. Robinson NE, ed. WB Saunders, Philadelphia, 2002, pp 528–532.

22. O'Grady SE. How to manage sheared heels. Proceedings Am Assoc Equine Pract 2005;451–456.

23. O'Grady SE. Quarter crack repair—An overview. Equine Vet Educ 2001;3:280–282.

24. O'Grady SE. White line disease—an update. Equine Vet Educ. 2002;3:66–72.

25. Parks AH. Form and function of the equine digit. Vet Clin North Am Equine Pract. 2003;19:2:285–296.

26. Pleasant RS, O'Grady SE. White line disease. In Current Therapy in Equine Medicine, 6th ed. Robinson NE, ed. WB Saunders, Philadelphia, 2008, pp 528–532.

27. Rooney JR. The Lame Horse, 2nd ed. Russell Meerdink Company, Wisconsin, 1998, pp 21–28.

28. Turner TA. The use of hoof measurements for the objective assessment of hoof balance. Proceedings Am Assoc Equine Pract 1992;38:389–395.

29. Turner TA, Stork C. Hoof abnormalities and their relation to lameness. Proceedings Am Assoc Equine Pract 1988;293–297.

NATURAL BALANCE TRIMMING AND SHOEING

Gene Ovnicek

INTRODUCTION

The term "natural balance" has been used for both labeling commercial products and describing an established protocol for trimming and shoeing horses. Natural Balance® Shoes have been developed and marketed by Equine Digit Support System, Inc. (EDSS) since the mid 1990s as a treatment and performance product. Additionally, EDSS has developed other complementary treatment and performance products with the Natural Balance name. The Natural Balance products are simply tools for farriers that are consistent and manufactured with specific design features to produce a given result.

Natural balance hoof care protocols, on the other hand, are hoof evaluation and preparation guidelines that farriers can use to treat hoof distortions which can lead to lameness or performance issues. The natural balance guidelines complement most good, conventional hoof care practices. The basic goal of the natural balance trimming and shoeing protocols is to establish equilibrium in and around the distal interphalangeal (DIP) joint by recognizing and eliminating hoof distortions that cause undue leverage and strain on the DIP joint and the hoof itself.

The structures that are used to evaluate distortions, balance the foot, and determine the quality of foot function include the frog, bars, exfoliated sole, and hoof wall. Other considerations that are employed when evaluating distortions and foot function are how the foot engages the ground (e.g., toe-first, flat, or heel-first), effort or leverage incurred at the time of breakover, and the use or discipline of the horse. For example, horses that are asked to turn sharp corners or circles at high speed may require a different amount or type of leverage reduction built into the shoe than those that only travel in a straight line. Moreover, horses that live and work in a consistent terrain may maintain better foot function and health if they are left barefoot rather than shod.

Many factors influence the decisions that farriers make in terms of how the foot is prepared and what shoeing application is used, if any. Natural balance hoof care protocols are designed to help farriers make those decisions using simple guidelines that are directed by the individual horse and each individual foot.

DISTORTIONS OF THE HOOF

Most of the original information behind natural balance was gleaned from the study and observation of feral horses and how they maintained their feet in their own natural environment.[1] Although there is much that we can take from the self maintained feet of horses living in the wild, there are environmental and use con-

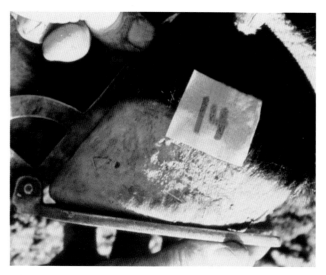

Figure 12.42. Lateral view of a feral horse's foot that lives in a dry, abrasive environment. Notice the rounded outer hoof wall in the front half of the foot.

siderations that must be factored in when applying that information to domestic horses.

In the wild, hoof wall wear depends upon the terrain. For example, in a very hard, dry, and abrasive terrain, the ground does not yield to the hoof wall. Rather, the outer hoof wall yields to the ground and becomes worn all the way around the foot to the level of the sole (Figure 12.42). In soft, sandy terrain, the ground yields to the hoof wall, so hoof wall wear occurs differently and more slowly. In this case, the wall is allowed to grow beyond the level of the sole. The further the wall grows beyond the level of the sole, the more susceptible it becomes to bending and breaking. Without the strength and support of the sole, the wall becomes vulnerable and eventually bends and breaks off systematically until it is again down to the level of the sole. Therefore, self maintenance does occur in a softer environment; it is just a longer and less kind process.

Horses that live in both a soft and wet environment have an even more difficult time with self maintenance. The hoof wall is less brittle due to the moisture, so breakage does not occur until the leverage becomes great. In these conditions, bacterial tracts or abscesses may be the vehicles that Mother Nature uses to initiate the maintenance process. In other words, a curled, badly distorted heel and bar can develop a bacterial tract that works its way to the sole corium and eventually causes a heel abscess. If the heel abscess is severe enough, it can eliminate the entire heel, thereby eliminating the distortion. It is not kind or aesthetically pleasing but effective for carrying out the necessary maintenance.

In addition to terrain factors, horses in the wild do not routinely turn circles repeatedly or at high speeds. They tend to travel at low to moderate speeds and in straight lines for the most part, yet the outer edge of their wall is rolled from one quarter, around the toe to the other quarter (Figure 12.42). Even with these conditions and activities, self maintained horses have reduced some leverage from a medial and lateral perspective. In the domestic equine world, we not only add the weight of a rider and tack, but we also ask horses to turn in repetitive circles at high speeds. With that, we see many soft tissue strains and injuries on the medial and lateral aspects of the distal joints.

Perhaps it is not possible to use the self-maintained horse as a model for the domestic equine. Maybe the parameters established in feral horse's feet still place too much stress and leverage on the distal joints of the domestic horse. Perhaps we need to relieve even more strain and leverage in domestic horses based on the increased loads and demands that they incur.

Most of the current natural balance guidelines and protocols have been adapted more specifically to the domestic equine through further anecdotal and field research and observations over the last 10 years. Practical applications by a large number of farriers in both treating lameness and improving performance over the last decade have helped to fine tune these methods of balancing feet as well. Through a better understanding of healthy foot function and anatomy, the natural balance guidelines have become a more widely used approach to trimming and shoeing domestic horses.

One difference between self-maintained feral horses and our domestic horses is the fact that domestic horses do not typically have the terrain, space, or activity to maintain their own feet, and are therefore susceptible to hoof distortions. Hoof distortions are generally the result of hoof structures (primarily hoof wall) that grow beyond the level of the sole in a direction that reduces support to the foot, or cause increased leverage to the foot. For example, a heel that grows beyond the level of the functional sole and forward becomes unstable and unable to support the weight and force of the horse as the foot engages and loads into the ground. A toe that grows much beyond the level of the sole can become a flare, which further increases the leverage at the time of break-over. A frog that fails to make contact with the ground because the heels have been allowed to grow beyond the level of the sole and has become narrow and atrophied from lack of use fails to absorb concussion and dissipate energy at the time of ground contact and load.

It is apparent that hoof distortions have a direct influence on function, support, and strain on the internal components of the foot and distal limb.[5,6] When a foot is subjected to increased strain on the soft tissue in and around the distal limb, lameness and pathology are likely to follow. Therefore, it is the job of the veterinarian and farrier to recognize these common hoof distortions and eliminate them at the time of trimming or shoeing to improve or eliminate lameness. Moreover, if these distortions can be dealt with early, or even prevented, then the prevention of lameness in horses can become a more realistic goal.

NATURAL BALANCE HOOF CARE GUIDELINES

A general understanding of the term functional sole plane is needed before discussing the detailed protocol. References have been made previously to the amount of wall that grows or extends beyond the level of the functional or live sole. The functional sole plane is established by scraping or paring the chalky or flaky appearing sole out of the foot until the smooth, waxy appearing surface is revealed. It is important that when exfoliating the sole, it is approached slowly and methodically so that the functional sole is not invaded or penetrated. If you go too far into the functional sole material, you will not only invade possible sensitive sole, but it also compromises the structures that will be used to balance the hoof wall and distal phalanx to the ground. The live, functional sole has been found (with few exceptions) to be an equal thickness beneath the medial and lateral aspect of the distal phalanx.[4] Therefore, if the goal is to balance the distal phalanx medially to laterally parallel to the ground surface, it is a very reliable guide.

NATURAL BALANCE EVALUATION, EXFOLIATION, AND MAPPING PROTOCOL

Recognizing Hoof Distortions

The first step in the natural balance hoof mapping protocol is to visually recognize hoof distortions in the heels, bars, frog, and toe (Figure 12.43). Heels that are curled, rolled over, crushed, or end dorsal to the widest part of the frog are distorted. Typically, the further dorsal the heels end to the back of the frog, the more distorted and less functional they have become. Similarly, the more curled, laid over, and fractured the bars are, the more distorted and less functional they are. The bars typically terminate into the frog commissures near the widest part of the foot. If the heels are allowed to grow forward, the bars must curve and bend, because the termination point of the bar cannot be moved forward, at least not at the corium level. Like hoof wall and sole material, bars can become overgrown. The overgrowth at the surface can grow forward of the widest part of the foot, and in some cases, such as laminitis, can grow completely around the frog apex. However, actual bar termination maintains its position near the widest part of the foot.

A frog that has become atrophied, narrow, and the central sulcus closed up is often lacking in function and has become distorted. At the same time, if the frog apex has become narrow and pointed, it is likely stretched and distorted as well. Furthermore, if the wall is allowed to grow much beyond the level of the sole, it will start to bend, flare, and become stretched forward. A thickened outer dorsal wall, inner wall, and white zone of the foot indicate that the extra leverage is stretching the components. It may be necessary to look closely at the dorsal wall to see a slight deviation below the coronary band, within the proximal 1 inch of the dorsal hoof wall. As a rule, noticeable flares start about half way down the hoof wall.

Identifying distortions and evaluating the degree of distortion in all aspects of the foot helps determine the

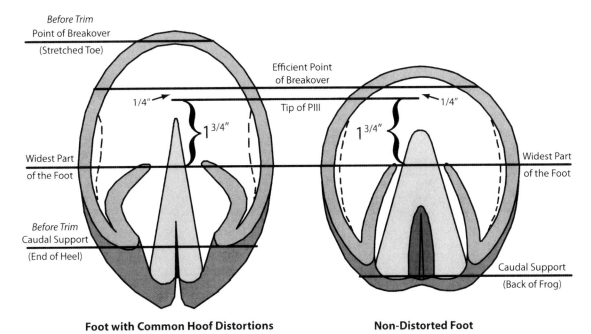

Foot with Common Hoof Distortions   **Non-Distorted Foot**

Figure 12.43. Drawings of 2 solar views. The solar view on the left is a foot with common hoof distortions. The solar view on the right is a non-distorted foot. Lines are drawn on the pictures to illustrate the point of break-over and where it should be on each foot, as well as the widest part of the foot (WPOTF) and caudal most aspect of support (either heels of the foot or back of the frog, depending on which structure contacts the ground first and primarily).

overall health of the foot. Having guidelines to overcome the distortions help detour lameness and improve performance.

Exfoliating the Foot

When leaving horses barefoot, the amount of exfoliating sole material to remove varies from one environment to another. To assess how much sole exists, first exfoliate and uncover the true frog apex where it blends in with the sole. This provides an idea as to how much nonfunctional sole exists. As a general rule, very little exfoliating in the toe region is tolerated by horses that live in hot, dry climates. Slightly more exfoliation can be done in soft, sod environments where horses get moderate amounts of moisture. In very wet or swampy environments, most feet need very little exfoliation, and most of the time simply wire brushing the bottom of the foot handles most of the exfoliation needs.

Usually where horses are left barefoot, it is a good idea to be conservative when exfoliating the sole. However, it is fairly safe to exfoliate the sole from the widest part of the foot back, so it is important to find the waxy appearing, functional sole in this region on each side of the foot. This will be the guide for establishing medial/lateral (M/L) balance later.

When applying shoes to horses, it is important to be more specific about removing the majority of exfoliating sole materials to get a clear picture of the functional sole plane. Nevertheless, starting in the back half of the foot is always recommended because it is a relatively safe zone in which to work. Once a clear picture of the functional sole is established in the back half of the foot,

move forward and exfoliate the sole in the toe region. Be extremely specific and careful when exfoliating the sole in the toe quarter (pillar) region of the foot. This is the primary guide when trimming the wall to balance the distal phalanx medially and laterally.

Mapping the Foot

The goal of mapping the foot is to gain an appreciation for the location of the distal phalanx and DIP joint within the hoof capsule. As part of their assessment to balance the foot, farriers have always tried to locate or picture the position of the distal phalanx within the hoof capsule, but have had largely varying results when using the hoof capsule itself as a guide. The hoof wall can become distorted and easily lose its relationship to the distal phalanx. However, more static references on the bottom of the foot help establish where the distal phalanx and DIP joint are relative to the hoof capsule.

Once the foot is exfoliated, a primary goal is to locate the widest part of the foot (WPOTF); there are 3 methods for locating this position.

1. Measure back approximately 1 inch from the true, exfoliated frog apex (on a medium size foot #00 to #2), and make a mark (Figure 12.44A).
2. Follow the bars to their termination point into the frog commissures. There is usually a slight bump or swell in the commissures to indicate this location. Make marks at these termination points (Figure 12.44B).

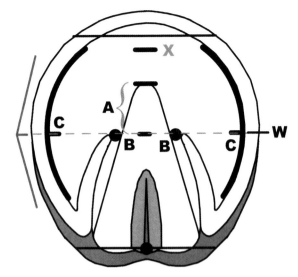

Figure 12.44. Drawings of the solar view of a foot that has the lines and marks used to locate (map) the widest part of the foot, which is generally the center of articulation. A. Measurement back from the true frog apex. B. The termination point of the bars into the frog commissures. C. The actual widest part of the sole. W. The widest part of the foot using the best 2 out of 3 marks. X. The tip of the distal phalanx as determined by a given distance forward of the WPOTF.

3. Scribe a line at the sole/wall junction in the quarters of the foot on each side. The peak or apex of this arc that has been drawn should be the widest part of the sole. Make a mark at the apex on each side of the foot (Figure 12.44C).

If all 3 locations line up, then draw a line connecting all of the marks that have been made (Figure 12.44W). If only 2 of the 3 locations line up, use those 2 and disregard the third set of marks.

Radiograph studies have shown that from the marked WPOTF, the dorsal tip of the distal phalanx is a consistent and predictable distance ahead of this mark.[2] On foot size #1 (5-inch-wide foot), measure 1.75 inches ahead of the WPOTF and make a mark. This is approximately the tip of the distal phalanx (Figure 12.44X). For foot sizes smaller and larger, the distance measured forward varies by no more than 1/8 inch/foot size. For example, a #00 foot is approximately 1.5 inches, while a number #2 foot is approximately 1.875 inches. These distances are accurate to within ± 1/8 inch.

As a standard starting point for the location of the point of break-over, measure forward 1/4 inch from the tip of the distal phalanx mark (Figure 12.43). In general, this position for the point of break-over (not the front of the shoe) seems to be effective for relieving excess strain and leverage on the DIP joint and excess tension on the deep digital flexor tendon at the time of break-over.[3]

Once the WPOTF and the point of break-over is established, the before-trimming and after-trimming ratios can be evaluated to compare how the foot has been and will be balanced around the WPOTF (Figure 12.43). The WPOTF is generally below the center of articulation (± 1/4 inch), depending on the angle of the distal phalanx.[4] If the distance from the WPOTF to the "before trim" heels is shorter than the distance from the WPOTF to the "before trim" point of break-over, then there are most likely hoof capsule distortions that can negatively affect the performance and soundness of the horse (Figure 12.43). Changing the ground surface ratios around the WPOTF or center of the foot so that there is equal or slightly more mass behind the WPOTF has been shown to improve the function of the foot and soundness of the horse.

NATURAL BALANCE BAREFOOT TRIMMING

The following natural balance hoof trimming procedure is used only on horses that will be left barefoot. The hoof preparation protocol for horses that are to be shod are slightly different and will be covered later.

Once the foot is exfoliated and mapped, it is time to trim the hoof wall to eliminate any distortions and achieve D/P and M/L balance. Begin by trimming the back two-thirds of the foot. Start just behind the toe quarter (pillar) region and follow the contour of the exfoliated sole, staying about 1/8 inch to 1/4 inch above the line of the sole (Figure 12.45). Next, trim the wall around the toe. Again, start behind the pillar and cut from one toe quarter around the toe to the other toe quarter. Stay at least 1/8 inch above the level of the sole all the way around the toe.

Once the rough cut has been made with nippers, a rasp is used to file the heels down to a flat landing that joins with a portion of the bar to form a solid base. The finished heel should be at or slightly lower than the ground surface of the frog, and should end close to the back of the frog. Both the medial and lateral heel should have a similar curvature and end at the same position relative to the back of the frog, and at the same height above the level of the functional sole plane. If the frog is atrophied, do not rasp the heel down so low that the functional sole plane in the heel region is invaded. With more use, the frog will eventually fill out and become a larger presence in the back of the foot.

With the heel prepared, a rasp is used to flatten the wall in the toe quarters so there is approximately 1/16 inch of gap between the sole and the ground surface of the wall. Make sure the gap is the same on both the medial and lateral sides. Once the toe is balanced with respect to the sole, bevel (or roll) the wall at a 10° to 15° angle from the break-over line forward (Figure 12.45). It is OK to touch some of the sole ahead of this point, because it is not sensitive. The objective is to produce a slight pivot point at the point of break-over that was marked earlier.

After the break-over roll is produced, a flattened area of wall about 3/4 inch to 1 inch in length should be left in the toe quarter region on each side of the foot. Behind that flattened area, relieve the wall in the quarters slightly to avoid flaring and chipping (Figure 12.45).

The final step in the barefoot trim is to dress the outer hoof wall to eliminate flares and produce a uniform wall thickness all the way around the foot (Figure 12.45). To eliminate sharp edges and avoid chipping, angle the rasp at a 45° angle to the wall and chamfer the distal border of the wall all the way around the foot.

Foot with Distortions - Before Trimming

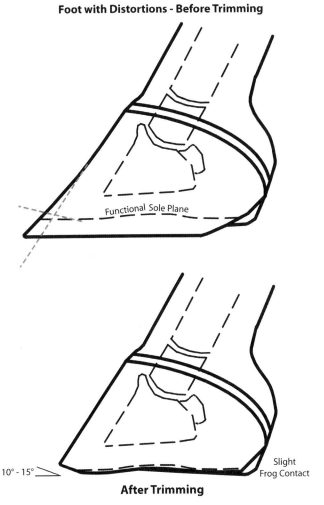

Functional Sole Plane

10° - 15°

Slight Frog Contact

After Trimming

Figure 12.45. Drawings of 2 lateral views. The top illustration is a foot with common distortions before trimming. The dashed line near the bottom of that foot is the functional or live sole contour used as a trimming guideline. The lighter, shorter dashed lines indicate how the flare is removed and how the toe is to be rolled (beveled). The bottom foot is an illustration of a natural balance barefoot trimmed foot. The wall has been prepared close to the level of the sole, the frog is in slight contact with the ground, and the toe has been rolled at a 10° to 15° angle to reduce leverage on the internal structures.

NATURAL BALANCE SHOEING

The following procedure is used for preparing feet that will have shoes applied to them.

Once the foot has been properly exfoliated and mapped as outlined previously, it is ready to be trimmed (Figure 12.46). Begin with nippers and trim the wall in the back half of the foot first. Unlike trimming for barefoot, the exact contour of the sole is not followed through the quarters. Instead, start with the nipper blades just behind the toe quarters and trim toward the heel leaving a gap of approximately 1/4 inch above the sole in the quarter region. Do the same on each side of the foot.

With the initial heel trim finished, start in the toe quarter region just behind the previous cut and trim the

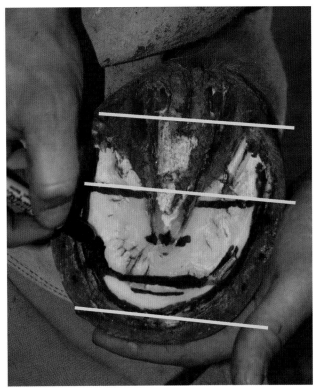

Figure 12.46. Sole view of a foot that has been exfoliated and mapped and is ready to be trimmed for shoes. Yellow lines have been drawn at the end of the heels, widest part of the foot, and at the "before trim" point of break-over.

wall from toe quarter to toe quarter. Make sure to leave at least 1/8 inch of wall above the level of the sole all the way around.

Once the rough-in trim is complete, use a rasp to file the heels so they are about 1/8 inch above the level of the functional sole in that region. Both the medial and lateral heel should have a similar curvature and have the same gap from the sole to the wall. The heels should also end evenly near the back of the frog. In cases of severely underrun and contracted heels, it may be necessary to rasp the heels down to the level of the sole to produce a good supportive landing and encourage better heel conformation. However, this should not need to be done every time the horse is shod. Once the heel growth becomes stronger and at a better angle, this more aggressive heel trimming should be stopped.

Once the heels are prepared exactly where desired, it is time to move to the toe. File the wall in the toe region so that there is a gap of approximately 1/16 inch from the exfoliated sole to the ground surface of the wall in the toe quarter region on each side. Although some horses are OK if rasped to the wall level with the sole, for safety measures it is recommended to leave a bit of wall above the sole. Either way, the gap should be exactly the same on both the medial and lateral sides, because this determines the balance of the distal phalanx to the ground once the shoe is applied.

When the heels and toe have been accurately prepared, proceed to rasping the wall in the quarters so

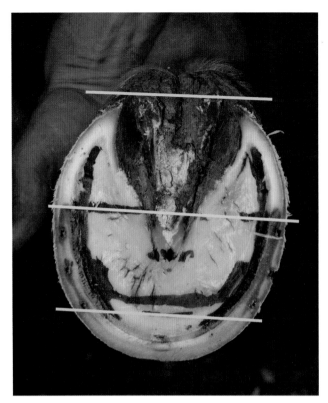

Figure 12.47. Solar view of a foot that has been exfoliated, mapped, and trimmed, and is ready for a shoe to be applied. Lines have been drawn at the end of the heels, widest part of the foot, and the position that the point of break-over of the shoe will be placed.

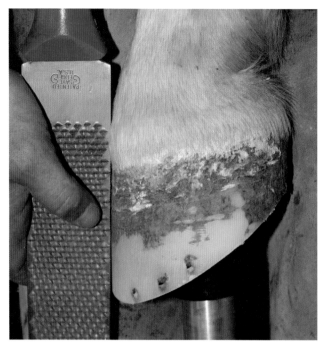

Figure 12.48. Lateral view of a foot in which the dorsal hoof wall has been groomed to a flat plane from the coronary band to the ground surface. All noticeable flares have been removed and uniform wall thickness has been achieved (as seen in Figure 12.47).

that the finished surface is perfectly flat to accept the flat shoe (Figure 12.47).

The final step before applying the shoe is to dress or groom all flares on the outer hoof wall to obtain a uniform wall thickness all the way around the foot (Figures 12.47 and 12.48). By dressing the wall prior to fitting the shoe, the chances of fitting the shoe to hoof capsule distortions are minimized.

Shoe fitting and design is an important part of dealing with lameness issues and improving performance. Basic shoe design for Natural Balance® applications should fit the following criteria:

1. Fairly symmetrical foot surface mass around the widest part of the shoe—the length of foot surface of the shoe should be the same ahead of and behind the widest part of the shoe.
2. Some leverage reduction considerations should be built into the toe of the shoe (i.e., rolled toe). In most lameness and performance situations, the roll should continue around the toe quarters for medial and lateral leverage considerations (Figure 12.49).
3. Wear plates in the toe of the shoe should be avoided so that the point of break-over is allowed to wear back into the shoe as the foot grows longer.

Shoe fitting is extremely important, so good forging skills are always necessary. When sizing the shoe, the heels of the shoe must extend to the back of the frog and the point of break-over of the shoe should align closely with the break-over line marked on the foot. The foot surface of the shoe should be divided equally around the widest part of the foot (Figures 12.49 and 12.50) The toe quarters of the shoe should fit to the groomed toe quarters of the foot, and the widest part of the shoe must align with the widest part of the foot.

When shaping the heels, they should have a gradual bend that follows the contour of the hoof, with the shoe becoming slightly wider than the heels as they progress from the widest part back. The finished heel of the shoe should be around 1/8 inch wider than the heel at the buttress.

The general shape of the shoe should be round on the foot surface with a slight boldness to the toe. However, the toe quarters of the shoe should maintain a width that is basically the same as the heels, meaning the toe quarters and heels should form a box (Figure 12.49).

Nailing on shoes and finishing the foot is basically the same as in any good conventional shoeing job. A quality nailing pattern with 3 or possibly 4 nails/side is generally required. Once the nails are clinched, grooming the wall is minimal, because the flares have been dressed prior to fitting the shoe. If there is any amount of toe that sticks out over the front of the shoe, simply position the rasp at a 30° angle and undercut the toe slightly (Figure 12.50). The angle of the undercut should be similar to the angle of the roll in the shoe. The amount of toe that extends ahead of the shoe depends on the amount of hoof capsule distortion that exists. Normally within 3 or 4 shoeing periods, the amount of toe over the front of the shoe will be minimal, as the

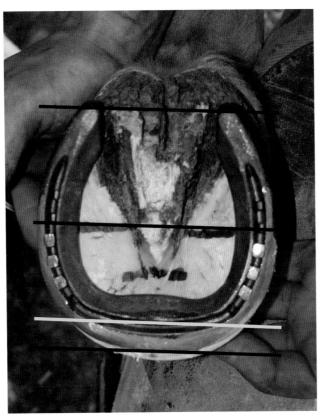

Figure 12.49. Solar view of a foot that has a Natural Balance® shoe applied to it. Black lines have been drawn at the back of the heels, the widest part of the foot, and the front of the shoe to illustrate that the foot surface of the shoe is divided up 50/50 around the widest part of the foot. The yellow line indicates the point of break-over of the shoe.

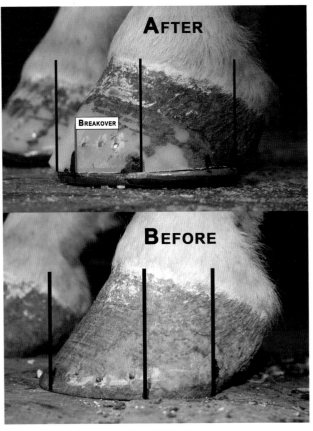

Figure 12.50. Lateral view of the same foot. Before trimming (bottom) and after trimming and shoeing (top) using Natural Balance guidelines. The black lines on the top image have been drawn at the front of the shoe, widest part of the foot, and back of the heels. The blue line is at the point of break-over of the shoe. The black lines on the bottom picture are at the "before trim" point of break-over, widest part of the foot, and the "before trim" back of the heels. The top picture illustrates better balance after trimming and shoeing around the widest part of the foot, which is generally the center of articulation of the DIP joint.

wall regains a better parallel relationship with the dorsal surface of the distal phalanx.

References

1. Ovnicek ED, Erfle J, Peters D. Wild horse hoof patterns offer a formula for preventing and treating lameness. Proceedings Am Assoc Eq Pract 1995;41:258–60.
2. Ovnicek ED. Widest Part of the Foot. Research paper presented at 6th Annual International Hoof Care Summit, 2009; February and at the 2010 British Equine Veterinary Association conference.
3. Page BT. Break-over of the hoof and its effects on structures and forces within the foot. *J Eq Vet Sci* 2002;22:258–264.
4. Savoldi M. Uniform Sole Thickness. www.americanfarriers.org. 2003;January-February.
5. Van Heel M. Shoeing today's equine athlete. The Farrier's Journal, 2006; No. 120.
6. Van Heel M, van Weeren PR, Back W. Shoeing sound Warmblood horses with a rolled-toe optimizes hoof-unrollment and lowers peak loading during break-over. *Equine Vet J* 2006;38:258–6.

INDEX

Adams and Stashak's Lameness in Horses, 6e, edited by
Gary M. Baxter
© 2011 Blackwell Publishing, Ltd.